FUNDAMENTAL NEUROSCIENCE

SECOND EDITION

FUNDAMENTAL NEUROSCIENCE

SECOND EDITION

Edited by

LARRY R. SQUIRE
VA Medical Center and University of California, San Diego
La Jolla, California

FLOYD E. BLOOM
The Scripps Research Institute
La Jolla, California

SUSAN K. McCONNELL
Stanford University
Stanford, California

JAMES L. ROBERTS
University of Texas Health Science Center
San Antonio, Texas

NICHOLAS C. SPITZER
VA Medical Center and University of California, San Diego
La Jolla, California

MICHAEL J. ZIGMOND
University of Pittsburgh
Pittsburgh, Pennsylvania

Illustrations by
Robert S. Woolley

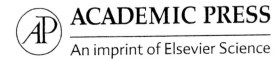

ACADEMIC PRESS
An imprint of Elsevier Science

Amsterdam   Boston   London   New York   Oxford   Paris
San Diego   San Francisco   Singapore   Sydney   Tokyo

Cover photo credit: Climbing Fiber-to Purkinje Cell Pathway. Varicose branches of a single climbing fiber (labeled blue with antiserum to lectin) cling to the proximal dendritic domain of an individual Purkinje cell arbor (labeled brown with antiserum to calbindin). Courtesy of Rossi, F., Borsello, T., Vaudano, E., and Strata, P. Neuroscience 53:759-778, 1993.

This book is printed on acid-free paper. ⊗

Academic Press
An imprint of Elsevier Science.
525 B Street, Suite 1900, San Diego, California 92101-4495, USA
http://www.academicpress.com

Academic Press
84 Theobald's Road, London WC1X 8RR, UK
http://www.academicpress.com

Library of Congress Catalog Card Number: 20022002109941

International Standard Book Number: 0-12-660303-0 (book)
International Standard Book Number: 0-12-660304-9 (CD-ROM)

PRINTED IN CHINA
02   03   04   05   06   07   RDC   9   8   7   6   5   4   3   2   1

Short Contents

VII
BEHAVIORAL AND COGNITIVE NEUROSCIENCE

Full Contents

I
NEUROSCIENCE

1. Fundamentals of Neuroscience
FLOYD E. BLOOM

2. The Architecture of Nervous Systems
LARRY W. SWANSON

II
CELLULAR AND MOLECULAR NEUROSCIENCE

3. Cellular Components of Nervous Tissue
PATRICK R. HOF, BRUCE D. TRAPP, JEAN DE VELLIS,
LUZ CLAUDIO, AND DAVID R. COLMAN

4. Subcellular Organization of the Nervous System: Organelles and Their Functions
SCOTT BRADY, DAVID R. COLMAN, AND PETER BROPHY

20. Synapse Elimination
RACHEL O. L. WONG AND JEFFREY W. LICHTMAN

21. Early Experience and Critical Periods
ERIC I. KNUDSEN

IV
SENSORY SYSTEMS

22. Fundamentals of Sensory Systems
STEWART H. HENDRY, STEVEN S. HSIAO, AND
M. CHRISTIAN BROWN

23. Sensory Transduction
PETER R. MacLEISH, GORDON M. SHEPHERD,
SUE C. KINNAMON, AND JOSEPH SANTOS-SACCHI

24. Chemical Senses: Taste and Olfaction
DAVID V. SMITH AND GORDON M. SHEPHERD

25. The Somatosensory System
STEWART H. HENDRY AND STEVEN S. HSIAO

26. Audition
M. CHRISTIAN BROWN

VII
BEHAVIORAL AND COGNITIVE NEUROSCIENCE

Preface to the First Edition

To our students, from whom we learn much.

Fundamental Neuroscience began with an ambitious set of objectives. We wished to produce a textbook that would: (1) introduce graduate students coming from diverse backgrounds to the full range of neuroscience, from molecular biology to clinical science; (2) assist instructors in offering an in-depth course in neuroscience to advanced undergraduates; (3) permit a research-oriented approach to neuroscience for medical students and others preparing for a professional career in the health sciences; and (4) provide a current resource for all who wish to familiarize themselves with this rapidly changing area. We also wished to contribute to the educational process in another way—by providing direct financial support.

This book reviews most of the major issues in neuroscience and some of the minor ones as well. We have included a large number of illustrations, almost all of them newly drawn. In addition, we have described many experiments to illustrate how information is gathered and conclusions are drawn and have included boxes that provide greater details and clinical correlations. Although we have focused on vertebrate neurobiology, particularly that of mammals, we have included examples from studies of invertebrates when that information was thought particularly useful to our objectives. And we have added a number of ethics cases for your consideration to emphasize our belief that good science and responsible conduct are inseparable.

To accomplish all this, the senior editors identified a group of section editors with experience both as researchers and as educators. These individuals were then asked to draft a table of contents for their sections and to find appropriate authors. Finally, the authors were asked to take part in an experiment—to try to produce a textbook that had the wisdom of a collection of individual reviews written by experts in their field and the cohesiveness of a single-authored volume. This required that the authors be willing to write material that would then be modified by others, often many others. We researchers don't like having our words—let alone our ideas—modified by anyone. And yet we assembled the team, and here, almost exactly six years after we began, our experiment has been completed.

The authors whom you will see listed under the titles of individual chapters and at the end of boxes are those people who accepted responsibility for preparing the initial drafts of material used in the textbook. In most cases they are listed in alphabetical order, although in some instances one individual played a substantially greater role than others and is listed first for that reason. There are instances in which the final chapter is very similar to that initially provided by the authors. In other cases a great deal of editing occurred. There are even chapters containing material taken from other chapters as well as chapters that were synthesized from several individual contributions. All this was done in an effort to provide you with the best possible textbook.

The Association of Neuroscience Departments and Programs (ANDP) was central to our efforts. The Council of the ANDP encouraged us to take on the task, and members of the ANDP provided critical input to the organization of the textbook. In particular, we thank the many individuals who commented on specific components of our project at various stages and thereby helped us to serve students and course instructors. These individuals include Yalchin Abdulaev, John Ashe, Jim Blankenship, John Bruno, Richard Burry, Dennis Choi, Avis Cohen, Gregory Cole, Ian Creese, Kathleen Dunlap, Gary Fiskum, Karen Gale, Glenn Hatton, John Hildebrand, John Kauer, James King, Kenneth Kratz, Richard Levine, Eve Marder, Alex Martin, Lorne Mendell, Ranney Mize, Sally Moody, Elisabeth Murray, Randolph

Nudo, David Potter, Dale Purves, George Rebec, Nicholas Spitzer, Glenn Stanley, and Paula Tallal. One-third of the royalties generated by sales of this textbook will be contributed to the ANDP to support their educational projects.

A number of other neuroscientists also participated in the formulation of this project. Anthony Movshon played a major role in organizing the section on sensory systems and recruiting its authors. Dennis O'Leary was instrumental in formulating the section on development. In addition, Darcy Kelley, Tom Reese, Patricia Goldman-Rakic, Tom Carew, Paula Tallal, Karl Herrup, Joseph LeDoux, Nick Spitzer, Richard Thompson, and Stephen Waxman participated in early discussions concerning the book.

Many others should be acknowledged, as well. Perhaps chief among them is Bob Woolley, our illustrator. For two years this project was a central component of Bob's life as he struggled to convert authors' sketches into final products, sought their input, handled their feedback, and met our deadlines. We hope that the results of his efforts, and those of Patrick Hof, who collaborated on many of the illustrations, will enrich your reading of this textbook and, through the use of visual aids that we can provide, enrich the classroom experience as well.

Craig Panner, acquisitions editor, provided day-to-day (and year-to-year) coordination of the entire endeavor, working well beyond the call of professional duty to keep together the thousand pieces. Susan Giegel, working at the University of Pittsburgh, oversaw many aspects of the project, arranged conference calls and meetings, read and wrote memos, answered queries, and provided pleasant and effective encouragement to meet deadlines. Cindy MacDonald, editorial manager, orchestrated a team of developmental editors and moderated discussions with often fiercely independent authors to provide a consistent text. These outstanding editors, who challenged the authors to clarify and simplify and then clarify again, were Matt Lee, Arkady Mak, Philippa Solomon, Lee Young, and Patty Zimmerman. Jacqueline Garrett, desk editor, scheduled the final production of the book and then "made it happen." Debby Bicher provided the interface between the illustrators and the typesetters. Cathy Reynolds designed the book, inside and out. Suzanne Rogers developed the marketing designs that inspired the cover, while Karen Steele and Charlotte Brabants orchestrated the marketing and promotions. Jasna Markovac provided essential advice in the early stages of the project and continued encouragement throughout. Erika Conner provided assistance at the outset of this project, and Karen Dempsey provided key administrative help all along the way.

Finally, there is Graham Lees. It was Graham, neuroscientist by training, editor by profession, who provided the most essential ingredient for this project form the very beginning—faith. Graham did more than encourage us from the sidelines, he was an active participant, suggesting editors and authors, commissioning paragraphs and boxes, critiquing content and style—even approving expensive modifications (e.g., multicolor figures) when he felt it would help the students, and all the while sending out a cheery newsletter, *FuNews*. There would be no textbook without Graham.

We hope we have achieved our initial goal—a textbook that will be of value to virtually anyone interested in neuroscience. We invite all of you to join us in the adventure of studying the nervous system. Indeed, we hope you will be active participants in that adventure. Earlier in this preface we stated that our experiment had been completed. Of course, that is not entirely true. As you read this we are already beginning to prepare the next edition. And we hope that you will participate in the process by sending comments to us at FN@acad.com. You also are invited to stay in touch with us through our web site (www.academicpress.com/fun). Here we will post material to supplement the textbook, including study questions, updates, and corrections.

A story is told that Charles Darwin once received a letter from a student who was just beginning his studies as a naturalist. The student is said to have asked what advice Mr. Darwin might offer to someone just starting this career. Darwin wrote back, "Try to discover one new fact." This book contains many facts, along with unifying ideas and principles that reflect our current knowledge of the nervous system. But it is also true that there is still much, much more to understand and that in some cases we do not yet even know what the questions are. We hope—we believe—that from among those of you who use this book will come the next generation of neuroscientists, individuals who will take up Darwin's challenge to discover things about the brain that no one knew before. It is to you that we dedicate *Fundamental Neuroscience*.

The Senior Editors
La Jolla, California

Preface to the Second Edition

In this second edition of *Fundamental Neuroscience*, we have tried to improve on the first edition and to produce a volume that effectively introduces students to the full range of contemporary neuroscience. Neuroscience is a large field founded on the premise that all of behavior and all of mental life have their origin in the structure and function of the nervous system. Today, the need for a single-volume introduction to neuroscience is greater than ever. Toward the end of the 20th century, the study of the brain became a central part of biological and psychological science. The maturation of neuroscience has meant that individuals from diverse backgrounds—molecular biologists, computer scientists, and psychologists—are interested in learning about the structure and function of the brain, about how the brain works. In addition, new techniques and tools have become available to study the brain with ever-increasing precision and detail. In the last 10 years, new genetic methods have been introduced to study the molecular biology of cells, neural systems, behavior, and neuroimaging techniques such as functional magnetic resonance imaging have been developed that permit study of the living human brain while it is engaged in cognition.

This second edition attempts to capture the promise and excitement of this fast-moving discipline. The new edition is shorter than that the first one but covers the same comprehensive range of topics. The first section of the volume begins with a new opening chapter that provides an overview of the discipline. A second chapter presents fundamental information about the architecture and anatomy of nervous systems. The remainder of the volume (sections II–VIII) presents the major topics of neuroscience. The second section (Cellular and Molecular Neuroscience) considers the cellular and subcellular organization of neurons, the physiology of nerve cells, and how signaling occurs between neurons. The third section (Nervous System Development) includes discussions of neurogenesis, migration, process outgrowth, and synapse formation. The fourth and fifth sections (Sensory Systems and Motor Systems) describe the neural organization of each sensory modality and the organization of the brain pathways and systems important for locomotion, voluntary action, and eye movements. The sixth section (Regulatory Systems) describes the variety of hypothalamic and extrahypothalamic systems that support motivation, reward, and internal regulation, including cardiovascular function, respiration, food and water intake, neuroendocrine function, circadian rhythms, and sleep and dreaming. The final section (Behavioral and Cognitive Neuroscience) describes the neural foundations of the so-called higher mental functions, including perception, attention, memory, language, and executive function. Each volume is accompanied by a CD of illustrations to increase the flexibility with which the material can be used.

Authors listed at the end of the chapters and boxes prepared drafts of their material, which were then edited by the senior editors. As in the first edition, the art program was under the excellent direction of Bob Woolley. We gratefully acknowledge the authors of the first edition for their valuable contributions, many of which served as the basis for chapters and boxes in the new edition. At Academic Press/Elsevier Science, the project was coordinated by Jasna Markovac (vice president and editorial director), and we are grateful to her for her vision, leadership, and advice throughout the project. In addition, Graham Lees helped produce the boxes, and Johannes Menzel and Lori Asbury very capably coordinated the production of the book.

The senior editors of *Fundamental Neuroscience*, all working neuroscientists, hope that users of this book, especially the students who will become the next generation of neuroscientists, find the subject matter of neuroscience as interesting and exciting as we do.

The Editors

Acknowledgments

The editors of the Second Edition would like to acknowledge the contributions of the section editors for the first edition: Thomas D. Albright, John H. Byrne, David R. Colman, Robert Y. Moore, Michael I. Posner, Edward M. Stricker, Larry W. Swanson, W. Thomas Thach, Leslie G. Ungerleider.

The editors and authors of the Second Edition also acknowledge those who contributed to chapters in the First Edition. Portions of this earlier material formed the basis for the revised chapters of the new edition, as indicated here.

Chapter 1.   Beth A Fischer and Story C. Landis
Chapter 2.   Thomas Lufkin and David R. Colman
Chapter 8.   Robert S. Zucker, Dimitri M. Kullman, and Mark Bennett
Chapter 10.   Steven E. Hyman
Chapter 15.   Nathaniel Heintz
Chapter 17.   Jonathan A. Raper
Chapter 18.   Susan M. Culican
Chapter 25.   Mary C. Bushnell
Chapter 28.   W. Thomas Thach
Chapter 32.   Amy J. Bastian and W. Thomas Thach
Chapter 36.   Alan F. Sved
Chapter 40.   Huda Akil, Serge Campeau, William E. Cullinan, Ronald M. Lechan, Roberto Toni, Stanley J. Watson, Robert Y. Moore, Lawrence A. Frohman, Judy Cameron, Phyllis M. Wise, and Michael J. Baum
Chapter 46.   Marilyn S. Albert, Adele D. Diamond, Roslyn Holly Fitch, Helen J. Neville, and Paula A. Tallal

Chapter 47.   Martha J. Farah and Glynn Humphreys
Chapter 49.   Gary S. Aston-Jones, Robert Desimone, Jonathan Driver, Steven J. Luck, and Michael I. Posner
Chapter 50.   John M. Beggs, Thomas H. Brown, Terry J. Crow, Kevin S. LaBar, Joseph E. LeDoux, and Richard F. Thompson
Chapter 51.   Lawrence F. Cahill, Mark A. Gluck, Michael E. Hasselmo, Frank C. Keil, Alex J. Martin, James L. McGaugh, Jaap Murre, Catherine Myers, Michael Petrides, Benno Roozendaal, Daniel L. Schacter, Daniel J. Simons, W. Carter Smith, and Cedric L. Williams
Chapter 52.   Thomas Carr and Randi Martin
Chapter 53.   Stanislas Dehaene and Manfred Spitzer

SECTION I

NEUROSCIENCE

CHAPTER

1

Fundamentals of Neuroscience

A BRIEF HISTORY OF NEUROSCIENCE

The name for the field of knowledge described in this book is *neuroscience*, the multidisciplinary bodies of science that analyze the nervous system to understand the biological basis for behavior. Modern studies of the nervous system have been ongoing since the middle of the 19th century. Neuroanatomists studied the brain's shape, its cellular structure, and its circuitry; neurochemists studied the brain's chemical composition, its lipids and proteins; neurophysiologists studied the brain's bioelectric properties; and psychologists and neuropsychologists investigated the organization and neural substrates of behavior and cognition.

The term neuroscience was introduced as an interdisciplinary term in the mid-1960s, signaling the beginning of an era in which each of these disciplines would work together cooperatively, sharing a common language, common concepts, and a common goal—to understand the structure and function of the normal and abnormal brain. Neuroscience today spans a wide range of research endeavors from the molecular biology of nerve cells (i.e, the genes necessary for provision of the proteins needed for nervous system function) to the biological basis of normal and disordered behavior, emotion, and cognition (i.e., the mental properties by which individuals interact with each other and with their environments).

Neuroscience is currently one of the most rapidly growing areas of science. Indeed, the brain is sometimes referred to as the last frontier of biology. In 1971, 1100 scientists convened at the first annual meeting of the Society for Neuroscience. In 2001, 23,009 scientists participated at the society's 31st annual meeting at which more than 14,000 research presentations were made.

THE TERMINOLOGY OF NERVOUS SYSTEMS IS HIERARCHICAL, DISTRIBUTED, DESCRIPTIVE, AND HISTORICALLY BASED

Beginning students of neuroscience could justifiably find themselves confused. Nervous systems of many organisms have their cell assemblies and macroscopically visible components named by multiple overlapping and often synonymous terms. With a necessarily gracious view to the past, this confusing terminology could be viewed as the intellectual cost of focused discourse with predecessors in the enterprise. The nervous systems of invertebrate organisms are often designated for their spatially directed collections of neurons responsible for local control of operations, such as the thoracic or abdominal ganglia, which receive sensations and direct motoric responses for specific body segments, all under the general control of a cepahalic ganglion whose role includes sensing the external environment.

In vertebrates, the components of the nervous system were named for both their appearance and their location. As noted by Swanson, and expanded upon in Chapter 2 of this volume, the names of the major parts of the brain were based on creative interpretations of early dissectors of the brain, attributing names to brain segments based on their appearance in the freshly dissected state: hippocampus (shaped like the sea horse) or amygdala (shaped like the almond), cerebrum (the main brain), and cerebellum (a small brain).

NEURONS AND GLIA ARE CELLULAR BUILDING BLOCKS OF THE NERVOUS SYSTEM

This book lays out our current understanding in each of the important domains that together define the full scope of modern neuroscience. The structure and function of the brain and spinal cord are most appropriately understood from the perspective of their highly specialized cells: the *neurons*, the interconnected, highly differentiated, bioelectrically driven, cellular units of the nervous system, and their more numerous support cells, the *glia*. Given the importance of these cellular building blocks in all that follows, a brief overview of their properties may be helpful

Neurons are Heterogeneously Shaped, Highly Active Secretory Cells

Neurons are classified in many different ways, according to function (sensory, motor, or interneuron), location (cortical, spinal, etc.), identity of the transmitter they synthesize and release (glutamatergic, cholinergic, etc.), and shape (pyramidal, granule, mitral, etc.). Microscopic analysis focuses on their general shape and, in particular, the number of extensions from the cell body. Most neurons have one *axon* to transmit signals to interconnected target neurons. Other processes, termed *dendrites*, extend from the nerve cell body (also termed the perikaryon—the cytoplasm surrounding the nucleus of the neuron) to receive synaptic contacts from other neurons; dendrites may branch in extremely complex patterns. Neurons exhibit the cytological characteristics of highly active secretory cells with large nuclei; large amounts of smooth and rough endoplasmic reticulum; and frequent clusters of specialized smooth endoplasmic reticulum (Golgi apparatus), in which secretory products of the cell are packaged into membrane-bound organelles for transport out of the cell body proper to the axon or dendrites. Neurons and their cellular extensions are rich in microtubules— elongated tubules approximately 24 nm in diameter. Microtubules support the elongated axons and dendrites and assist in the reciprocal transport of essential macromolecules and organelles between the cell body and the distant axon or dendrites.

Neurons Communicate Chemically through Specialized Contact Zones

The sites of interneuronal communication in the central nervous system (CNS) are termed *synapses* in the CNS and "junctions" in somatic motor and autonomic nervous systems. Paramembranous deposits of specific proteins essential for transmitter release, response, and catabolism characterize synapses and junctions morphologically. These specialized sites are presumed to be the active zone for transmitter release and response. Paramembranous proteins constitute a specialized junctional adherence zone, termed the synaptolemma. Like peripheral "junctions", central synapses are also denoted by accumulations of tiny (500 to 1500 Å) organelles, termed synaptic vesicles. The proteins of these vesicles have been shown to have specific roles in transmitter storage, vesicle docking onto presynaptic membranes, voltage- and Ca^{2+}-dependent secretion, and recycling and restorage of released transmitter.

Synaptic Relationships Fall into Several Structural Categories

Synaptic arrangements in the CNS fall into a wide variety of morphological and functional forms that are specific for the neurons involved. The most common arrangement, typical of hierarchical pathways, is either the axodendritic or the axosomatic synapse in which the axons of the cell of origin make their functional contact with the dendrites or cell body of the target. A second category of synaptic arrangement is more rare forms of functional contact between adjacent cell bodies (somasomatic) and overlapping dendrites (dendrodendritic). Within the spinal cord and some other fields of neuropil (relatively acellular areas of synaptic connections), serial axoaxonic synapses are relatively frequent. Here, the axon of an interneuron ends on the terminal of a long-distance neuron as that terminal contacts a dendrite or on the segment of the axon that is immediately distal to the soma, termed the initial segment, where action potentials arise. Many presynaptic axons contain local collections of typical synaptic vesicles with no opposed specialized synaptolemma. These are termed boutons en passant. The release of a transmitter may not always occur at such sites.

Synaptic Relationships Also Belong to Diverse Functional Categories

As with their structural representations, the qualities of synaptic transmission can also be functionally categorized in terms of the nature of the neurotransmitter that provides the signaling; the nature of the receptor molecule on the postsynaptic neuron, gland, or muscle; and the mechanisms by which the postsynaptic cell transduces the neurotransmitter signal into transmembrane changes. So-called "fast" or "classical" neurotransmission is the functional variety seen at the vast majority of synaptic and junc-tional sites, with a rapid onset and a rapid ending, generally employing excitatory amino acids (glutamate or aspartate) or inhibitory amino acids (γ-aminobutyrate, *GABA*, or glycine) as the transmitter. The effects of those signals are largely attributable to changes in postsynaptic membrane permeability to specific cations or anions and the resulting deploriza-tion or hyperpolarization, respectively. Other neurotransmitters, such as the monoamines (dopamine, norepinephrine, serotonin) and many neuropeptides, produce changes in excitability that are much more enduring. Here the receptors activate metabolic processes within the postsynaptic cells—frequently to add or remove phosphate groups from key intracellular proteins; multiple complex forms of enduring postsynaptic metabolic actions are under investigation. The brain's richness of signaling possibilities comes from the interplay on common postsynaptic neurons of these multiple chemical signals.

THE OPERATIVE PROCESSES OF NERVOUS SYSTEMS ARE ALSO HIERARCHICAL

As research progressed, it became clear that neuronal functions could best be fitted into nervous system function by considering their operations at four fundamental hierarchical levels: molecular, cellular, systems, and behavioral. These levels rest on the fundamental principle that neurons communicate chemically, by the activity-dependent secretion of *neurotransmitters*, at specialized points of contact named *synapses*.

At the *molecular level* of operations, the emphasis is on the interaction of molecules—typically proteins that regulate the transcription of genes and their posttrans-lational processing and proteins that mediate the intracellular processes of transmitter synthesis, storage, and release. Proteins also mediate the intracellular consequences of intercellular synaptic signaling. Such transductive mechanisms include the neurotransmitters' receptors, as well as the auxiliary molecules that allow these receptors to influence the short-term biology of responsive neurons (through regulation of ion

channels) and their longer-term regulation (through alterations in gene expression). The recent completion of the initial draft analyses of the human genome can be viewed as an extensive inventory of these molecular elements, more than half of which are thought to be either highly enriched in the brain or even exclusively expressed there (see later).

At the *cellular level* of neuroscience, the emphasis is on interactions between neurons through their synaptic transactions and between neurons and glia. Much current cellular level research focuses on the biochemical systems within specific cells that mediate such phenomena as pacemakers for the generation of circadian rhythms or that can account for activity-dependent adaptation. Research at the cellular level strives to determine which specific neurons and which of their most proximate synaptic connections may mediate a behavior or the behavioral effects of a given experimental perturbation.

At the *systems level*, emphasis is on the spatially distributed sensors and effectors that integrate the body's response to environmental challenges. There are sensory systems, which include specialized senses for hearing, seeing, feeling, tasting, and balancing the body. Similarly, there are motor systems for trunk, limb, and fine finger motions and internal regulatory systems for visceral regulation (e.g., control of body temperature, cardiovascular function, appetite, salt and water balance). These systems operate through relatively sequential linkages, and interruption of any link can destroy the function of the system.

Systems level research also includes research into cellular systems that innervate the widely distributed neuronal elements of the sensory, motor, or visceral systems, such as the pontine neurons with highly branched axons that innervate diencephalic, cortical, and spinal neurons. Among the best studied of these divergent systems are the monoaminergic neurons, which have been linked to the regulation of many behavioral outputs of the brain, ranging from feeding, drinking, thermoregulation, and sexual behavior. Monoaminergic neurons have also been linked to such higher functions as pleasure, reinforcement, attention, motivation, memory, and learning. Dysfunctions of these systems have been hypothesized as the basis for some psychiatric and neurological diseases, supported by evidence that medications aimed at presumed monoamine regulation provide useful therapy.

At the behavioral level of neuroscience research, emphasis is on the interactions between individuals and their collective environment. Research at the behavioral level centers on the integrative phenomena that link populations of neurons (often operationally or empirically defined) into extended specialized circuits, ensembles, or more pervasively distributed "systems" that integrate the physiological expression of a learned, reflexive, or spontaneously generated behavioral response. Behavioral research also includes the operations of higher mental activity, such as memory, learning, speech, abstract reasoning, and consciousness. Conceptually, "animal models" of human psychiatric diseases are based on the assumption that scientists can appropriately infer from observations of behavior and physiology (heart rate, respiration, locomotion, etc.) that the states experienced by animals are equivalent to the emotional states experienced by humans expressing these same sorts of physiological changes.

Some Principles of Brain Organization and Function

The central nervous system is most commonly divided into major structural units, consisting of the major physical subdivisions of the brain. Thus, mammalian neuroscientists divide the central nervous system into the brain and spinal cord and further divide the brain into regions readily seen by the simplest of dissections. Based on research that has demonstrated that these large spatial elements derive from independent structures in the developing brain, these subdivisions are well accepted. Mammalian brain is thusly divided into hindbrain, midbrain, and forebrain, each of which has multiple highly specialized regions within it. In deference to the major differences in body structure, invertebrate nervous systems are most often organized by body segment (cephalic, thoracic, abdominal) and by anterior–posterior placement.

Neurons within the vertebrate CNS operate either within layered structures (such as the olfactory bulb, cerebral cortex, hippocampal formation, and cerebellum or in clustered groupings (the defined collections of central neurons, which aggregate into "nuclei" in the central nervous system and into "ganglia" in the peripheral nervous system, and in invertebrate nervous systems). The specific connections between neurons within or across the macrodivisions of the brain are essen-tial to the brain's functions. It is through their pat-terns of neuronal circuitry that individual neurons form functional ensembles to regulate the flow of information within and between the regions of the brain.

CELLULAR ORGANIZATION OF THE BRAIN

Present understanding of the cellular organization of the CNS can be viewed simplistically according to three main patterns of neuronal connectivity (see Shepherd, 1997).

Three Basic Patterns of Neuronal Circuitry Exist

Long hierarchical neuronal connections typically are found in the primary sensory and motor pathways. Here the transmission of information is highly sequential, and interconnected neurons are related to each other in a hierarchical fashion. Primary receptors (in the retina, inner ear, olfactory epithelium, tongue, or skin) transmit first to primary relay cells, then to secondary relay cells, and finally to the primary sensory fields of the cerebral cortex. For motor output systems, the reverse sequence exists with impulses descending hierarchically from the motor cortex to the spinal motoneuron. It is at the level of the motor and sensory systems that beginning scholars of the nervous system will begin to appreciate the complexities of neuronal circuitry by which widely separated neurons communicate selectively. This hierarchical scheme of organization provides for a precise flow of information, but such organization suffers the disadvantage that destruction of any link incapacitates the entire system.

Local circuit neurons establish their connections mainly within their immediate vicinity. Such local circuit neurons frequently are small and may have relatively few processes. Interneurons expand or constrain the flow of information within their small spatial domain and may do so without generating action potentials, given their short axons.

Single source divergent circuitry is utilized by certain neuronal systems of the hypothalamus, pons, and medulla. From their clustered anatomical location, these neurons extend multiple branched and divergent connections to many target cells, almost all of which lie outside the brain region in which the neurons are located. Neurons with divergent circuitry could be considered more as interregional interneurons rather than as sequential elements within any known hierarchical system. For example, neurons of the locus coeruleus project from the pons to the cerebellum, spinal cord, hypothalamus, and several cortical zones to modulate synaptic operations within those regions.

Glia are Supportive Cells to Neurons

Neurons are not the only cells in the CNS. According to most estimates, neurons are outnumbered, perhaps by an order of magnitude, by the various nonneuronal supportive cellular elements (see Cherniak, 1990). Nonneuronal cells include macroglia, microglia, cells of the brain's blood vessels, cells of the choroid plexus that secrete the cerebrospinal fluid, and *meninges*, sheets of connective tissue that cover the surface of the brain and comprise the cerebrospinal fluid-containing envelope.

Macroglia are the most abundant supportive cells; some are categorized as astrocytes (nonneuronal cells interposed between the vasculature and the neurons, often surrounding individual compartments of synaptic complexes). Astrocytes play a variety of metabolic support roles, including furnishing energy intermediates and providing for the supplementary removal of excessive extracellular neurotransmitter secretions. A second prominent category of macroglia is myelin-producing cells, the oligodendroglia. Myelin, made up of multiple layers of their compacted membranes, insulates segments of long axons bioelectrically and accelerates action potential conduction velocity. Microglia are relatively uncharacterized supportive cells believed to be of mesodermal origin and related to the macrophage/monocyte lineage. Some microglia reside quiescently within the brain. During periods of intracerebral inflammation (e.g., infection, certain degenerative diseases, or traumatic injury), circulating macrophages and other white blood cells are recruited into the brain by endothelial signals to remove necrotic tissue and to try to defend against the infection.

The Blood–Brain Barrier Protects against Inappropriate Signals

The blood–brain barrier is an important permeability barrier to selected molecules between the bloodstream and the CNS. Evidence of a barrier is provided by the greatly diminished rate of access of most lipophobic chemicals from plasma to the brain unless there are specific energy-dependent transporter systems. Diffusional barriers retard the movement of substances from brain to blood as well as from blood to brain. The brain clears metabolites of transmitters into the cerebrospinal fluid by excretion through the acid transport system of the choroid plexus. This barrier is much less prominent in the hypothalamus and in several small, specialized organs (termed *circumventricular organs*) lining the third and fourth ventricles of the brain: the median eminence, area postrema, pineal gland, subfornical organ, and subcommissural organ. No such barrier occurs between the circulation and the peripheral nervous system (e.g., sensory and autonomic nerves and ganglia).

The Central Nervous System Can Initiate Limited Responses to Damage

Because neurons of the CNS are terminally differentiated cells, they do not undergo proliferative responses to damage, although evidence suggests the possibility of neural stem cell proliferation as a natural means for selected neuronal replacement in some restricted regions of the nervous system (see Gage, 2000). As a result, neurons have evolved other adaptive mechanisms to provide for the maintenance of function following injury. These adaptive mechanisms endow the brain with considerable capacity for structural and functional modification well into adulthood and may represent some of the same molecular mechanisms employed in memory and learning (see Squire and Kandel, 1999).

ORGANIZATION OF THIS TEXT

With these overview principles in place, which are detailed more extensively in Section II, we can resume our preview of this book. Another major domain of our field is nervous system development (Section III). How does a simple epithelium differentiate into specialized collections of cells and ultimately into distinct brain structures? How do neurons grow processes that find appropriate targets some distance away? How do nascent neuronal activity and embryonic experience shape activity?

Sensory systems and motor systems (Sections IV and V) encompass how the nervous system receives information from the external world and how movements and actions are produced, e.g., eye movements and limb movements. These questions range from the molecular level (how are odorants, photons, and sounds transduced into patterned neural activity?) to the systems and behavioral level (which brain structures control eye movements and what are the computations required by each structure?).

An evolutionarily old function of the nervous system is to regulate respiration, heart rate, sleep and waking cycles, food and water intake, and hormones. In this area of regulatory systems (Section VI), we explore how organisms remain in balance with their environment, ensuring that they obtain the energy resources needed to survive and reproduce. At the level of cells and molecules, the study of regulatory systems concerns the receptors and signaling pathways by which particular hormones or neurotransmitters prepare the organism to sleep, to cope with acute stress, or to seek food. At the level of brain systems, we ask such questions as what occurs in brain circuitry to produce thirst or to create a self-destructive problem such as drug abuse?

In recent years, the disciplines of psychology and biology have increasingly found common ground, and this convergence of psychology and biology defines the modern topics of behavioral and cognitive neuroscience (Section VII). These topics concern the so-called higher mental functions: perception, attention, language, memory, thinking, and the ability to navigate in space. Work on these problems has traditionally drawn on the techniques of neuroanatomy, neurophysiology, neuropharmacology, and behavioral analysis. More recently, behavioral and cognitive neuroscience has benefited from several new approaches: the use of computers to perform detailed formal analyses of how brain systems operate and how cognition is organized; noninvasive neuroimaging techniques, such as positron emission tomography and functional magnetic resonance imaging, to obtain pictures of the living human brain in action; and molecular biological methods, such as single gene knockouts in mice, which can relate genes to brain systems and to behavior.

THIS BOOK IS INTENDED FOR A BROAD RANGE OF SCHOLARS OF THE NEUROSCIENCES

This textbook is for anyone interested in neuroscience. In preparing it we have focused primarily on graduate students just entering the field, understanding that some of you will have majored in biology, some in psychology, some in mathematics or engineering, and even some like me, in German literature. It is hoped that through the text, the explanatory boxes, and, in some cases, the supplementary readings, you will find the book to be both understandable and enlightening. In many cases, advanced undergraduate students will find this book useful as well.

Medical students may find that they need additional clinical correlations that are not provided here. However, it is hoped that most medical scholars will at least be able to use our textbook in conjunction with more clinically oriented material. Finally, to those who have completed their formal education, it is hoped that this text can provide you with some useful information and challenging perspectives, whether you are active neuroscientists wishing to learn about areas of the field other than your own or individuals who wish to enter neuroscience from a different area of inquiry. We invite all of you to join us in the adventure of studying the nervous system.

CLINICAL ISSUES IN THE NEUROSCIENCES

Many fields of clinical medicine are directly concerned with the brain. The branches of medicine tied most closely to neuroscience are neurology (the study of the diseases of the brain), neurosurgery (the study of the surgical treatment of neurological disease), and psychiatry (the study of behavioral, emotional, and mental diseases). Other fields of medicine also make important contributions, including radiology (the use of radiation for such purposes as imaging the brain—initially with X rays and, more recently with positron emitters and magnetic waves) and pathology (the study of pathological tissue). To make connections to the many facets of medicine that are relevant to neuroscience, this book includes discussion of a number of clinical conditions in the context of basic knowledge in neuroscience.

THE SPIRIT OF EXPLORATION CONTINUES

As we begin the 21st century, the Hubble space telescope is providing us with information about as yet uncharted regions of the universe and the promise that we may learn something about the origin of the cosmos. This same spirit of adventure is also being directed to the most complex structure that exists in the universe—the human brain. The complexity of the human brain is enormous, describable only in astronomical terms. For example, the number of neurons in the human brain (about 10^{12} or 1000 billion) is approximately equal to the number of stars in our Milky Way galaxy. Whereas the possibility of understanding such a complex device is certainly daunting, it is nevertheless true that an enormous amount has already been learned. The promise and excitement of research on the nervous system have captured the attention of thousands of students and working scientists. What is at stake is not only the possibility of discovering how the brain works. It is estimated that diseases of the brain, including both neurological and psychiatric illnesses, affect as many as 50 million individuals annually in the United States alone, at an estimated societal cost of 40 billion dollars in clinical care and lost productivity. The prevention, treatment, and cure of these diseases will ultimately be founded in neuroscience research. Moreover, many of the issues currently challenging societies globally— instability within the family, illiteracy, poverty, and violence— could be illuminated by a better understanding of the brain.

THE GENOMIC INVENTORY IS A GIANT STEP FORWARD

The single largest event possibly in the history of biomedical research was publicly proclaimed in June 2000 and was presented in published form in February 2001: the initial "draft" inventory of the human genome. By using advanced versions of the powerful methods of molecular biology, several large scientific teams have been able to take apart all of an individual's human DNA in very refined ways, amplify the amounts of the pieces, determine the order of the nucleic acid bases in each of the fragments, and then put those fragments back together again across the 23 pairs of human chromosomes.

Having determined the sequences of the nucleic acids, it was possible to train computers to read the sequence information and spot the specific signals that identify the beginning and ending of sequences likely to encode proteins. Furthermore, the computer systems could then sort those proteins by similarity of sequences (motifs) within their amino acid building blocks. After sorting, the computers could next assign the genes and gene products to families of similar proteins whose functions had already been established. In this way, scientists were rapidly able to predict approximately how many proteins could be encoded by the human genome (all of the genes a human has).

Scientifically, this state of information is termed a "draft" because it is based on a very dense, but not yet complete, sample of the whole genome, and what has been determined still contains a very large number of interruptions and gaps. Some of the smaller genes, whose beginning and ending are most certain, could be thought of as parts in a reassembled Greek urn, held in place by bits of blank clay until further excavation is done. However, having even this draft has provided some important realities.

Similar routines allowed these scholars to determine how many of those were like genes we have already recognized in the smaller genomes of other organisms mapped out previously [yeast, worm (*C. aenorhabditis elegans*), and fruitfly (*Drosophila melangaster*)] and how many other gene forms may not have been encountered previously. Based on current estimates, it would appear that despite the very large number of nucleotides in the human and other mammalian genomes, about 30 times the length of the worms and more like 15 times the fruitfly, mammals may have only twice as many genes—perhaps 30–40,000. Compared to other completed genomes, the human genome has greatly increased its representation of genes related to nervous system function, tissue–specific developmental mechanisms, and immune function and blood coagulation. Importantly for diseases of the nervous system that are characterized by the premature death of neurons, there appears to have been a major expansion in the numbers of genes related to initiating the process of intentional cell death or apoptosis.

Two major future vistas can then be imagined. To create organisms as complex as humans from relatively so few genes probably means that the richness of the required proteins is based on their modifications, either during transcription of the gene or after translation of the intermediate messenger RNA into the protein. Second, while compiling this draft inventory represents a stunning technical achievement, there remains the enormously daunting task of determining, for example, where in the brain's circuits specific genes are normally expressed and how that expression pattern may be altered by the demands of illness or an unfriendly environment. That task, at present, is one for which there are as yet no tools equivalently as powerful as those used to acquire the flood of sequence data with which we are now faced. This stage has been referred to as the end of "naïve reductionism."

In order to benefit from the enormously rich potential mother lode of genetic information, we must next determine where these genes are expressed, what functions they can control, and what sorts of controls other gene products can exert over them. In the nervous system, where cell–cell interaction is the main operating system in relating molecular events to functional behavioral events, discovering the still murky properties of activity-dependent gene expression will require enormous investment.

NEUROSCIENCE TODAY: A COMMUNAL ENDEAVOR

As scientists, we draw from the work of those who came before us, using other scientists' work as a foundation for our own. We build on and extend previous observations and, it is hoped, contribute something to those who will come after us. The information presented in this book is the culmination of hundreds of years of research. To help acquaint you with some of this work, we have described many of the key experiments of neuroscience in the text or in boxes distributed throughout the book. We have also listed some of the classic papers of neuroscience and related fields at the end of each chapter and invite you to read some of them for yourselves.

The pursuit of science has not always been a communal endeavor. Initially, research was conducted in relative isolation. The scientific "community" that existed at the time consisted of intellectuals who shared the same general interests, terminology, and paradigms. For the most part, scientists were reluctant to collaborate or share their ideas broadly, because an adequate system for establishing priority for discoveries did not exist. However, with the emergence of scientific journals in 1665, scientists began disseminating their results and ideas more broadly because the publication record could be used as proof of priority. Science then began to progress much more rapidly, as each layer of new information provided a higher foundation on which new studies could be built.

Gradually, an interactive community of scientists evolved, providing many of the benefits that contemporary scientists enjoy: Working as part of a community allows for greater specialization and efficiency of effort. This not only allows scientists to study a topic in greater depth but also enables teams of researchers to attack problems from multidisciplinary perspectives. The rapid feedback and support provided by the community help scientists refine their ideas and maintain their motivation. It is this interdependence across space and time that gives science much of its power.

With interdependence, however, comes vulnerability. In science, as in most communities, codes of acceptable conduct have evolved in an attempt to protect the rights of individuals while maximizing the benefits they receive. Some of these guidelines are concerned with the manner in which research is conducted, and other guidelines refer to the conduct of scientists and their interactions within the scientific community. Let us begin by examining how new knowledge is created.

THE CREATION OF KNOWLEDGE

Over the years, a generally accepted procedure for conducting research has evolved. This process involves examining the existing literature, identifying an important question, and formulating a research plan. Often, new experimental pathways are launched when one scientist reads with skepticism the observations and interpretations of another and decides to test their validity. Sometimes the plan is purely "descriptive," e.g., determining the structure of a protein or the distribution of a neurotransmitter in brain. Descriptive initial research is essential to the subsequent inductive phase of experimentation, the movement from observations to theory, seasoned with wisdom and curiosity. Descriptive experiments are valuable both because of the questions that they attempt to answer and because of the questions that their results allow us to ask. Information obtained from descriptive experiments provides a base of knowledge on which a scientist may draw to develop hypotheses about cause and effect in the phenomenon under investigation. For example, once we identify the distribution of a particular transmitter within the brain or the course of a pathway of connections through descriptive work, we may then be able to develop a theory about what function that transmitter or pathway serves.

Once a hypothesis has been developed, the researcher then has the task of designing and performing experiments that are likely to disprove that hypothesis if it is incorrect. This is referred to as the deductive phase of experimentation, the movement from theory to observation. Through this paradigm the neuroscientist seeks to narrow down the vast range of alternative explanations for a given phenomenon. Only after attempting to disprove the hypothesis as thoroughly as possible may scientists be adequately assured that their hypothesis is a plausible explanation for the phenomenon under investigation.

A key point in this argument is that data may only lend support to a hypothesis rather than provide absolute proof of its validity. In part, this is because the constraints of time, money, and technology only allow a scientist to test a particular hypothesis under a limited set of conditions. Variability and random chance may also contribute to the experimental results. Consequently, at the end of an experiment, scientists generally only report that there is a statistical probability that the effect measured was due to intervention rather than to chance or variability.

Given that one can never prove a hypothesis, how do "facts" arise? At the conclusion of their experiments the researchers' first task is to report their findings to the scientific community. The dissemination of research findings often begins with an informal presentation at a laboratory or departmental meeting, eventually followed by presentation at a scientific meeting that permits the rapid exchange of information more broadly. One or more research articles published in peer-reviewed journals ultimately follow the verbal communications. Such publications are not simply a means to allow the authors to advance as professionals (although they are important in that respect as well). Publication is an essential component of the advancement of science. As we have already stated, science depends on sharing information, replicating and thereby validating experiments, and then moving forward to solve the next problem. Indeed, a scientific experiment, no matter how spectacular the results, is not completed until the results are published.

RESPONSIBLE CONDUCT

Although individuals or small groups may perform experiments, new knowledge is ultimately the product of the larger community. Inherent in such a system is the need to be able to trust the work of other scientists—to trust their integrity in conducting and reporting research. Thus, it is not surprising that much emphasis is placed on the responsible conduct of research.

Research ethics encompasses a broad spectrum of behaviors. Where one draws the line between sloppy science and unethical conduct is a source of much debate within the scientific community. Some acts are considered to be so egregious that despite personal differences in defining what constitutes ethical behavior, the community generally agrees that these behaviors do not. These unambiguously improper activities consist of *fabrication, falsification,* and *plagiarism*: Fabrication refers to making up data, falsification is defined as altering data, and plagiarism consists of using another person's ideas, words, or data without attribution. Each of these acts significantly harms the scientific community.

Fabrication and falsification in a research paper taint the published literature by undermining its integrity. Not only is the information contained in such papers misleading in itself, but other scientists may unwittingly use that information as the foundation for new research. If, when reported, these subsequent studies cite the previous, fraudulent publication, the literature is further corrupted. Thus, through a domino-like effect one paper may have a broad negative impact on the scientific literature. Moreover, when fraud is discovered, a retraction of the paper provides only a limited solution, as there is no guarantee that individuals who read the original article will see the retraction. Given the impact that just one fraudulent paper may have, it is not surprising that the integrity of published literature is a primary ethical concern for scientists.

Plagiarism is also a major ethical infraction. Scientific publications provide a mechanism for establishing priority for a discovery. As such, they form the currency by which scientists earn academic positions, gain research grants to support their research, attract students, and receive promotions. Plagiarism denies the original author of credit for his or her work. This hurts everyone: The creative scientist is robbed of credit, the scientific community is hurt by the disincentive to share ideas and research results, and the individual who has plagiarized—like the person who has fabricated or falsified data—may well find his or her career ruined.

In addition to the serious improprieties just described, which are in fact extremely rare, a variety of much more frequently committed "misdemeanors" in the conduct of research can also affect the scientific community. Like fabrication, falsification, and plagiarism, some of these actions are considered to be unethical because they violate a fundamental value, such as honesty. For example, most active scientists believe that honorary authorship—listing as an author someone who did not make an intellectual contribution to the work—is unethical because it misrepresents the origin of the research. In contrast, other unethical behaviors violate standards that the scientific community has adopted. For example, while it is generally understood that material submitted to a peer-reviewed journal as part of a research manuscript has never been published previously and is not under consideration by another journal, instances of retraction for dual publications can be found on occasion.

Scientific Misconduct Has Been Formally Defined by US Governmental Agencies

The serious misdeeds of fabrication, falsification, and plagiarism are generally recognized throughout the scientific community. These were broadly recognized by federal regulations in 1999 as a uniform standard of scientific misconduct by all agencies funding research. What constitutes a misdemeanor is less clear, however, because variations in the definitions of accepted practices are common. There are several sources of this variation. Because responsible conduct is based in part on conventions adopted by a field, it follows that there are differences among disciplines with regard to what is considered to be appropriate behavior. For example, students in neuroscience usually coauthor papers with their advisor, who typically works closely with them on their research. In contrast, students in the humanities often publish papers on their own even if their advisor has made a substantial intellectual contribution to the work reported. Within a discipline, the definition of acceptable practices may also vary from country to country. Because of animal use regulations, neuroscientists in the United Kingdom do relatively little experimental work with animals on the important topic of stress, whereas in the United States this topic is seen as an appropriate area of study so long as guidelines are followed to ensure that discomfort to the animals is minimized.

The definition of responsible conduct may change over time. For example, some protocols that were once performed on human and animal subjects may no longer be considered ethical. Indeed, ethics evolve alongside knowledge. We may not currently be able to know all of the risks involved in a procedure, but as new risks are identified (or previously identified risks refuted), we must be willing to reconsider the facts and adjust our policies as necessary. In sum, what is considered to be ethical behavior may not always be obvious, and therefore we must actively examine what is expected of us as scientists.

Having determined what is acceptable practice, we then must be vigilant. Each day neuroscientists are faced with a number of decisions having ethical implications, most of them at the level of misdemeanors: Should a data point be excluded because the apparatus might have malfunctioned? Have all the appropriate references been cited and are all the authors appropriate? Might the graphic representation of data mislead the viewer? Are research funds being used efficiently? Although individually these decisions may not significantly affect the practice of science, cumulatively they can exert a great effect.

Ethical Conduct among Scientists Is Critical to the Scientific Process

In addition to being concerned about the integrity of the published literature, we must be concerned with our public image. Despite concerns over the level of federal funding for research, neuroscientists are among the privileged few who have much of their work funded by taxpayer dollars. Highly publicized scandals damage the public image of our profession and hurt all of us who are dependent on continued public support for our work. They also reduce the public credibility of science and thereby lessen the impact that we can expect our findings to have. Thus, for our own good and that of our colleagues, the

scientific community, and the public at large, we must strive to act with integrity.

Behaving Responsibly Is Integral to Doing Good Science

Research and research ethics are inseparable. In that spirit, hypothetical dilemmas provide useful exercises in helping new scholars raise their sensitivity to the pitfalls than can befall a naïve investigator and the short cuts in execution and logical interpretation that may have made their way into the literature of neuroscience. Readers are encouraged to (1) think about these and other ethical issues as you explore neuroscience and (2) discuss your views with fellow students and faculty.

For example, imagine a young faculty member concerned about an upcoming evaluation for tenure, well aware that despite much effort on a difficult and challenging problem, her publication record is well below the standards of her institution. In her desk is a partially drafted manuscript of her initial successful experiments, as yet unreplicated. With more data in a strong paper, she believes her results could be seen as groundbreaking. However, any delays in publishing could jeopardize her suitability for tenure. A tempting thought occurs to her: suppose she were to submit a version of her manuscript that contains the means from the data she has collected but represents the data as being based on a larger number of replications than have yet been performed. Given her past experience that her manuscript will almost certainly require revision before it is accepted for publication, she reasons she will in the interim have plenty of time to do the replications and insert the corrected data. How would you advise her?

When such situations arise in real life, scientists can be faced with the need to choose between conflicting needs or obligations. In such situations, there is no magic formula for arriving at a resolution. However, ethicists have developed tools to assist us in analyzing such conflicts. One method for systematically examining the key components of an ethical dilemma has been outlined by Bebeau and colleagues (1995). The method consists of seeking answers to the questions of what conflicting rights or obligations form the basis of the dilemma, who will be affected by the decision, what are the possible actions to be taken, and what are the moral obligations of the decision maker.

Such an approach is particularly useful in working though a novel dilemma, e.g., one involving ethical issues arising from new technologies. The ethics of human cloning is one such situation. Only a few years ago the idea of cloning humans was the stuff of science fiction, and researchers did not need to give much thought to its ethical dimensions. Now we are faced with very real concerns over the use of such technologies.

SUMMARY

You are about to embark on a tour of fundamental neuroscience. Enjoy the descriptions of the current state of knowledge, read the summaries of some of the classic experiments on which that information is based, and consult the references that the authors have drawn on to prepare their chapters. Think also about the ethical dimensions of the science you are studying—your success as a professional and the future of our field depend on it.

References

Bebeau, M. J., Pimple, K. D., Muskavitch, K. M. T., and Smith, D. H. (1995). "Moral Reasoning in Scientific Research: Cases for Teaching and Assessment." The Poynter Center, Indiana University, Bloomington, IN.

Boorstin, D. J. (1983). "The Discoverers." Random House, New York.

Cherniak, C. (1990). The bounded brain: Toward quantitative neuroanatomy. *J. Cog. Neurosci.* **2**, 58–68.

Committee on the Conduct of Science (1995)."On Being a Scientist," 2nd Ed. National Academy Press, National Academy of Sciences, Washington, DC.

Cowan, W. M, and Kandel, E. R. (2001), Prospects for neurology and psychiatry. *JAMA* **285**, 594–600.

Day, R. A. (1994). "How to Write and Publish a Scientific Paper," 4th Ed. Oryx Press, Phoenix, AZ.

Kuhn, T. S. (1996). "The Structure of Scientific Revolutions," 3rd Ed. Univ. of Chicago Press, Chicago.

Popper, K. R. (1969). "Conjectures and Refutations: The Growth of Scientific Knowledge," 3rd Ed. Routledge and K. Paul, London.

Shepherd, G. M. (1997) "The Synaptic Organization of the Brain." Oxford Uni. Press, New York.

Squire, L., and Kandel, E. R. (1999). "Memory: From Mind to Molecules." W. H. Freeman, New York.

Swanson, L. (2000). What is the brain? *Trends Neurosci*, **23**, 519– 527.

Floyd E. Bloom

CHAPTER

2

The Architecture of Nervous Systems

These days the brain is often loosely compared to the CPU of a computer. The brain is a very special type of computer, however. It is a biological computer that has evolved over the course of hundreds of millions of years, and it is critical to appreciate that the brain really has no obvious correspondence at all with the computers you are familiar with on your desktop. The brain is a unique organ that thinks and feels, keeps the body alive and healthy, and enables reproduction of the species, which is its most important role from the grand perspective of evolution. From a strictly egocentric point of view, however, the brain is most precious to us simply because it is the organ of consciousness—as captured by René Descarte's famous 17th century aphorism: "I think therefore I am."

In any organ, or any machine for that matter, structure and function are two sides of the same coin—they are inextricably intertwined—with structure providing obvious physical constraints on function. Just compare the same tune played on a piano and on a flute. Nevertheless, as science has become more and more specialized, there has been a strong tendency to analyze the structure, function, and chemistry of the nervous system from somewhat different perspectives. The structural organization or architecture of the brain is the main theme of this chapter. What are the basic parts of the brain, and how are they related to one another physically? What are its basic design features, what are its major functional systems, and what are the organizing principles of its circuitry?

The brain is far and away the most complex object that we know of—there are roughly 100 billion neurons and 100 trillion interneuronal connections in the human brain. Traditionally, biologists have had great success in understanding complex problems by following two lines of research: embryology and evo-

lution. The reason that these two approaches are so powerful is obvious—they tend to proceed from a relatively simple state (which is more easily understood) to a much more complex state. They both explain the current or mature state historically, starting from the beginning. One remarkable conclusion that emerges from what they have taught us so far is that nerve cells in all animals—from jellyfish to humans—are basically the same in terms of cell biology; what changes most during embryogenesis and evolution is the *arrangement* of nerve cells into functional circuits—the architecture of the brain. The ultimate goal of neuroscience, of course, is to understand the structure and function of the human brain, but remarkable progress has been made by studying "lower" animals and early embryos. The other equally remarkable conclusion that emerges is that all vertebrates, from fish to humans, share a common fundamental plan of the brain, with the same basic parts and the same basic functional systems.

GENERAL PRINCIPLES FROM AN EVOLUTIONARY PERSPECTIVE

How does a nervous system add to or enhance the behavioral repertoire of an animal? From an evolutionary perspective, the answer is clear: a nervous system increases the chances that an individual animal will survive and reproduce, thereby increasing the chances for survival of the species as a whole. This chapter begins by examining some of the features of nervous systems that contribute to an increased likelihood of survival by focusing on nervous system organization in animals with relatively simple structures and behaviors. The simplest nervous system known in nature is the nerve net of the lowly invertebrate, hydra. What are its fundamental building blocks or units, and what is their basic organization?

The Nerve Net is the Simplest Type of Nervous System

In his influential book, "The Elementary Nervous System," G. H. Parker (1919) presented the broad outlines of a reasonable scenario for early nervous system evolution in the Darwinian sense. An updated version of his synthesis would begin with the first multicellular animals that evolved over half a billion years ago. They were probably similar to modern-day sponges, which are seemingly amorphous animals that spend most of their immobile lives attached to a rock or some other object submerged under water. The ingestive, defensive, and reproductive behaviors displayed by these animals are very simple and occur with no hint of a nervous system. Instead, their behavior is mediated by a set of primitive smooth muscle cells (myocytes) that by contracting control the flow of water through pores in the animal's body. These specialized cells are called *independent effectors* because their contraction is evoked by stimuli such as stretch or environmental chemicals that act directly on the membrane of the cell itself.

The first great phylum of animals to display a nervous system was the Cnidaria, which includes jellyfish, corals, anemones, and the very simple hydra. Whereas sponges are nonmotile, hydra locomote a little by somersaulting, and they feed with primitive tentacles (Fig. 2.1). These behaviors are coordinated and mediated by a nervous system, a network made up of specialized units or cells called *nerve cells* or *neurons* (Box 2.1).

Sensory Neurons

The body wall of hydra is constructed in a relatively simple way: there is an outer layer called *ecto-*

derm that faces and contacts the environment; an inner layer called *endoderm* that lines an internal body cavity and promotes food digestion and waste elimination; and a vague middle or *meso* layer in between. Neurons seem to have differentiated from the ectoderm. Perhaps the first to evolve were the *sensory neurons*. One end or pole of these spindle-shaped or bipolar cells facing the environment became specialized to detect stimuli much weaker than those detected by independent effectors, and the opposite pole became specialized to transmit information about these stimuli to a **group** of independent effectors (Fig. 2.3). The addition of sensory neurons provides at least four major selective advantages in evolution. First, there is greatly **increased sensitivity** to environmental stimuli. For example, weaker, more distant stimuli might now be detected. Second, it has been found that effector cell responses are typically **faster** after sensory neuron stimulation than after direct stimulation. Third, there are **stronger** behavioral responses because individual sensory neurons can innervate groups of effector cells. Fourth, sensory neurons with **different modalities** (classes of effective stimuli) can be distributed to **different regions of the body**. For example, chemoreceptors for food-related objects might be localized to the ends of tentacles.

The bipolar shape of sensory neurons is fundamentally important. The prototypical example of a theory about the organization of neural circuits was documented most thoroughly by Santiago Ramón y Cajal in his classical monograph, the "bible" of neuroanatomy, "The Histology of the Nervous System in Man and Vertebrates" (1911–1913). According to the theory of **functional polarity**, information normally flows in one direction through a nerve cell and thus through neural circuits—from the *dendrites* and *cell body* (soma, or perikaryon—the region surrounding the nucleus), which are the receptive or input parts of the neuron, to a single *axon*, which is the effector or output part. In other words, most neurons have two classes of process: one or more dendrites detecting inputs, and a single

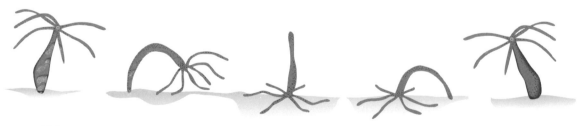

FIGURE 2.1 Locomotor behavior in hydra resembles a series of somersaults. The sequence of actions in one somersault is shown here, beginning at the left. The tiny black dot in the region between the tentacles in the figure at the far right is the mouth of the animal. Feeding behavior involves guiding particles of food into the mouth through coordinated movements of the tentacles.

BOX 2.1

THE NEURON DOCTRINE

The cell theory, which states that all organisms are composed of individual cells, was developed around the middle of the 19th century by Mattias Schleiden and Theodor Schwann. However, this unitary vision of the cellular nature of life was not immediately applied to the nervous system, as most biologists at the time believed in the cytoplasmic continuity of cells in the nervous system. Later in the century the most prominent advocate of this *reticularist* view was Camillo Golgi, who proposed that axons entering the spinal cord actually fuse with other axons (Fig. 2.2A). The reticularist view was challenged most thoroughly by Santiago Ramón y Cajal, a founder of contemporary neuroscience and without doubt the greatest observer of neuronal architecture. In beautifully written and carefully reasoned deductive arguments, Cajal presented us with what is now known as the *neuron doctrine*. This great concept in essence states that the cell theory applies to the nervous system: each neuron is an individual entity, the basic unit of neural circuitry (Fig. 2.2B). The acrimonious debate between reticularists and proponents of the neuron doctrine raged for decades. Over the years, the validity of the neuron doctrine has been supported by a wealth of accumulated data. Nevertheless, the reticularist view is not entirely incorrect because some neurons do act syncytially via specialized intercellular junctions, a feature that is more prominent during embryogenesis.

In 1897, Charles Sherrington postulated that neurons establish functional contact with each other and with other cell types via a theoretical structure he called the synapse (Greek *synaptein*, to fasten together). It was not until 50 years later that the structural existence of synapses was demonstrated by electron microscopy. In the electron micrograph shown in Fig. 2.2C, two axon terminals (At1 and At2) form synaptic junctions (s1 and s2) with a dendrite (Den). On the presynaptic (axonal) side of the junctions, synaptic vesicles that hold chemical neurotransmitters cluster near the presynaptic plasma membrane. The postsynaptic membrane, which is a specialization of the dendritic plasma membrane, has a prominent thickening that contains structural proteins, neurotransmitter receptors, intracellular signal transduction molecules, and cytoskeletal components. In the intercellular space that separates pre- and postsynaptic plasma membranes, an electron-dense "fuzz" is observed; its molecular constituents probably are involved in adhesion between the membranes.

The synaptic complex is built around an *adhesive* junction, and in this and other respects the complex is quite similar to the desmosome and the adherens junctions of epithelia (see Fannon and Colman, 1996). In fact, similarities in ultrastructure between the adherens junction and the synaptic complex of central nervous tissue were noted even in early electron microscopic studies (see Peters *et al.*, 1991).

Larry W. Swanson

References

Fennon, A., and Colman, D. R. (1996). A model for central synaptic junctional complex formation based on the differential adhesive specificities of the cadhesions. *Neuron*, **17**, 423–434.

Peters, A., Palay, S. L., and Webster, H. deF. (1991). "The Fine Structure of the Nervous System: Neurons and Their Supporting Cells," 3rd Ed. Oxford Univ. Press, New York.

axon conducting an output that can influence multiple cells by way of branching or *collateralization*. At least in early stages of development, sensory neurons in all animals have this fundamental bipolar shape. Over the course of evolution they have become specialized to detect a remarkable variety of stimuli from light, temperature, and a wide range of chemicals and ions, to vibration and other mechanical deformations.

Motor Neurons

A second stage of differentiation or complexity in the nervous system of hydra was the addition of neurons between sensory and effector. They are defined as motor neurons (*motoneurons*) because they directly innervate effector cells (typically muscle cells or gland cells), which in turn receive their inputs from sensory neurons (Fig. 2.2B). Conceptually, this provides a **two-layered nervous system**: the first or top layer consisting of sensory neurons and the second or bottom layer consisting of motor neurons. As a starting point, the connections of this prototypical network are such that sensory neurons project (send axon collaterals) to multiple motoneurons, and similarly each motoneuron projects to a set of effector cells, with the latter ensemble being defined as a **motor unit**. During an animal's normal behavior there is a unidirectional or polarized flow of information from one cell type, sensory neurons, to another cell type, motoneurons, to a third

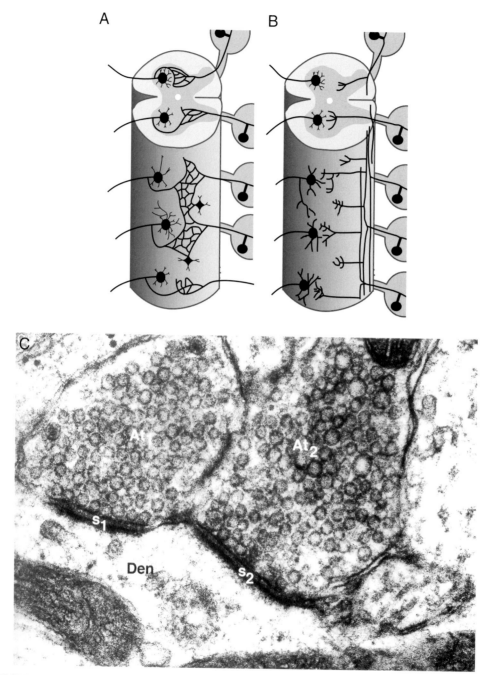

FIGURE 2.2 The nervous system is a reticulum versus the neuron doctrine. (A) Proponents of the reticularist's view of the nervous system believed that neurons are physically connected to one another, forming an uninterrupted network. (B) The neuron doctrine, in contrast, considers each neuron an individual entity that communicates with target cells across an appropriate intercellular gap. Adapted from Cajal (1911–1913). (C) The intercellular gap just referred to was found with the electron microscope in the 1950s to be a cleft that is typically about 20 nm wide. Synaptic junctions are shown here.

cell type, effector cells. This is the basic definition of a simple *reflex*, as defined by Charles Sherrington in his cornerstone of systems neuroscience, "The Integrative Action of the Nervous System" (1906).

In the hypothetical scenario we are discussing (Fig. 2.3), an environmental stimulus is detected by the dendrite of a sensory neuron and is then transmitted by its axon to the dendrites of a group of motoneurons. Then, the axon of each motoneuron in turn innervates a group of effector cells. This is the functional polarity theory applied to a simple two-neuron, sensory-motor network that mediates reflex behavior.

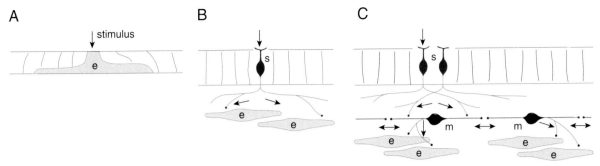

FIGURE 2.3 Activation of effector cells in simple animals. (A) Sponges lack a nervous system; stimuli act directly on effector cells (e), which are thus called independent effectors. (B) In cnidarians, bipolar sensory neurons (s) differentiate in the ectoderm (outer body wall layer). The outer process of the sensory neuron detects stimuli and is thus a dendrite. The inner process of some sensory neurons transmits information directly to effector cells and is thus an axon. Because this type of sensory neuron innervates effector cells directly, it is actually a sensorimotor neuron. (C) Most cnidarian sensory neurons send their axon to motor neurons (m), which in turn send an axon to effector cells. Motoneurons also have processes that interact with other motoneurons; in cnidarians, these processes typically conduct information in both directions (and are thus amacrine processes). Arrows show the direction of information flow.

In hydra, an additional feature of the two-layer nervous system has been observed: sensory neurons do not innervate each other whereas motoneurons do interact directly. In other words, motoneurons actually have two classes of projections: one to effector cells and another to other motoneurons. Structurally and functionally, these motoneurons also have two types of output processes. One is a typical axon that projects to the effector cells. However, the other is a process that contacts homologous processes from other motoneurons. Interestingly, many of these "horizontal" processes between cells of the motoneuron layer transmit information in either direction. Either motoneuron can transmit information to the other via these processes. Note that this is a violation of the functional polarity rule. Cajal (1911–1913) was well aware of this exception and called these processes *amacrine*. He noted that in fact neurons generate three functionally different types of process: dendrites that conduct toward the axon (and do not influence the neurons they contact; see Box 2.2), axons that conduct away from dendrites/soma (to influence cells that they contact), and **amacrine processes** that conduct in either direction.

The adaptive advantages of adding a second layer to the nervous system are obvious: they revolve mostly around increased capacity for response complexity and integration. To start with, consider a stimulus localized to one very specific part of the animal, perhaps even to one sensory neuron. The influence of this stimulus can radiate to distant parts of the animal because one sensory neuron innervates multiple motoneurons, those motoneurons innervate an even broader range of motoneurons, and each motoneuron innervates multiple effector cells. There can be a great deal of *divergence* between stimulus and the effector

cells producing a response, and the divergence pattern is a direct product of the architecture of any particular nervous system, i.e., how the neurons and their interconnections are arranged in the body. It is easy to imagine how this arrangement in hydra could be involved in coordinating all the tentacles to bring a morsel of food detected by just one of the tentacles to the mouth for entry into the central body cavity for digestion and absorption or how it could be involved in coordinating locomotion (Fig. 2.1).

A second fundamental consequence of this structural arrangement is *convergence* of information within the nervous system. Simply consider a particular motoneuron: it can receive inputs from more than one sensory neuron and from other motoneurons as well.

Nerve Nets

At first glance the nervous system of hydra is distributed fairly uniformly throughout the radially symmetrical body wall and tentacles (Fig. 2.4). Its essentially double-layer arrangement of distributed sensory neurons and motoneurons is called a *nerve net*. However, in certain regions of the body with specialized function, such as around the mouth or around the base of the tentacles, there may be a tendency for neurons to concentrate—a feature called *centralization* that will now be examined in more detail.

Flatworms are the Simplest Animals Exhibiting Centralization and Cephalization

Flatworms, with their bilateral symmetry, dorsal and ventral surfaces, and rostral and caudal ends, are distinctly more complex than cnidarians. The sensory receptors of a flatworm are more concentrated at the

BOX 2.2

CAJAL: ICONOCLAST TO ICON

Santiago Ramón y Cajal (1852–1934) is considered by many people to be the founder of modern neuroscience—a peer of Darwin and Pasteur in 19th-century biology. He was born in the tiny Spanish village of Petilla de Aragon on May 1, 1852, and as related in his delightful autobiography, he was somewhat mischievous as a child and was determined to become an artist, much to the consternation of his father, a respected local physician. However, he eventually entered the University of Zaragoza, and received a medical degree in 1873. As a professor of anatomy at Zaragoza, his interests were mostly in bacteriology (the 19th-century equivalent of molecular biology today in terms of an exciting biological frontier) until 1887, when he visited Madrid at age 35 and first saw through the microscope histological sections of brain tissue treated with the Golgi method, which had been introduced in 1873. Although very few workers had used this technique, Cajal saw immediately that it offered great hope in solving the most vexing problem of 19th-century neuroscience: how do nerve cells interact with each other? This realization galvanized and directed the rest of his scientific life, which was extremely productive in terms of originality, scope, and accuracy.

Shortly after Jacob Schleiden, Theodor Schwann, and Rudolf Virchow proposed the cell theory in the late 1830s, Joseph von Gerlach, Sr. and Otto Deiters suggested that nerve tissue was special in the sense that nerve cells are not independent units but instead form a continuous syncytium or reticular net (Fig. 2.2A). This concept was later refined by Camillo Golgi, who, based on the use of his silver chromate method, concluded that axons of nerve cells form a continuous reticular net, whereas dendrites do not anastomose but instead serve a nutritive role, much like the roots of a tree. Using the same technique, Cajal almost immediately arrived at the opposite conclusion, based first on his examination of the cerebellum and later of virtually all other parts of the nervous system. In short, he proposed that neurons interact by way of contact or contiguity rather than by continuity and are thus independent units, which was

finally proven when the electron microscope was used in the 1950s. This concept became known as the *neuron doctrine* (see Box 2.1).

Cajal's second major conceptual achievement was the theory of *functional polarity*, which stated that the dendrites and cell bodies of neurons receive information, whereas the single axon with its collaterals transmits information to the other cells. This theory allows one to predict the direction of information flow through neural circuits based on the morphology or shape of individual neurons forming them, and it was the cornerstone of Charles Sherrington's (1906) revolutionary physiological analysis of reflex organization in the mammal. Evidence that many dendrites transmit an action potential or graded potential in the retrograde direction would not violate the tenants of the functional polarity theory unless the potential led to altered membrane potentials in the associated presynaptic axon; if this were the case, the "dendrite" would be classed instead as an amacrine process (see text).

Around the close of the 19th century, Cajal made a remarkable series of discoveries at the cellular level. In addition to the two concepts just outlined, they include (1) the mode of axon termination in the adult CNS (1888), (2) the dendritic spine (1888), (3) the first diagrams of reflex pathways based on the neuron doctrine and functional polarity (1890), (4) the axonal growth cone (1890), (5) the chemotactic theory of synapse specificity (1892), and (6) the hypothesis that learning could be based on the selective strengthening of synapses (1895).

In one of the great ironies in the history of neuroscience, Cajal and Golgi shared the Nobel Prize for Medicine in 1906, although they had used the same technique to elaborate fundamentally different views on nervous system organization! The meeting in Stockholm may not have diminished the great personal friction between them. In 1931, Cajal wrote: "What a cruel irony of fate to pair like Siamese twins united by the shoulders, scientific adversaries of such contrasting characters."

Larry W. Swanson

rostral (head) end, where they encounter the oncoming environment as they locomote by swimming, or crawl along the substrate. Some, like planarians, are active predators (Fig. 2.5). These changes in body plan and behavior are accompanied by equally important changes in nervous system organization.

The cell bodies of many flatworm neurons are aggregated into clusters called *ganglia*, which are connected by longitudinal and transverse bundles of axons known as *nerve cords* (Fig. 2.5). This condensation of neural elements is called centralization and allows communication between neurons to be faster

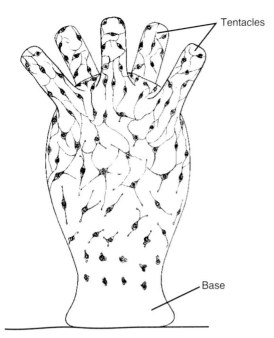

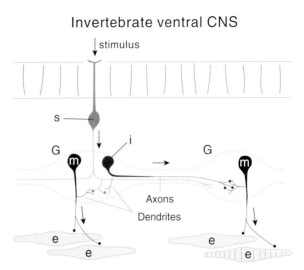

Invertebrate ventral CNS

FIGURE 2.6 There are usually two kinds of neuron in invertebrate ganglia (G): motor neurons (m) and interneurons (i), both of which are typically unipolar, with dendrites arising from a single axon. In a typical invertebrate ganglion, neuronal somata are arranged around the outside and synapses occur in the central region, called the neuropil. Sensory neurons (s) usually innervate motoneurons and interneurons but not effectors (e). Arrows show the usual direction of information flow.

FIGURE 2.4 The nerve net of the hydra, a simple cnidarian, is spread diffusely throughout the body wall of the animal. This drawing shows maturation of the nerve net in a hydra bud, starting near the base and finishing near the tentacles. Refer to McConnell (1932).

and therefore more efficient because cellular material is conserved and conduction times are reduced. The largest and most complex ganglia, the cephalic ganglia, are located rostrally where they receive infor-

mation from specialized sensory receptors. These ganglia constitute the simplest form of a brain. The concentration of neurons and sensory receptors at the rostral end is termed *cephalization*. Centralization and cephalization are two fundamental organizational trends in nervous system evolution.

Flatworms are the simplest animals to have a clearly distinct third type of neuron, the *interneuron*, which is interpolated between sensory and motor neurons (Fig. 2.6). Some interneurons might have only amacrine processes conducting impulses in either direction. Cajal referred to this special class as *amacrine neurons* (or, more precisely, as amacrine interneurons). However, most interneurons have a recognizable axon and dendrites and so presumably transmit information down the axon in only one direction. They are *typical neurons* that conform to the functional polarity rule.

One very important consequence of adding interneurons to the nervous system is simply to increase convergence and divergence of information processing, and thus ultimately increase the capacity for response complexity. However, there are at least two other critical functions that interneurons can serve. They can act as excitatory or inhibitory "**switches**" in chains of neurons, and they can act as *pacemakers* if they generate intrinsic rhythmical changes in activity.

By this definition, the vast majority of neurons in the vertebrate brain are interneurons. Thus it is useful from the beginning to recognize two classes of interneuron: local and projection. *Local interneurons*

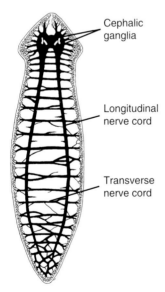

FIGURE 2.5 The nervous system of the planarian, a flatworm, includes longitudinal and transverse nerve cords associated with centralization and two fused cephalic ganglia in the rostral end associated with cephalization. Centralization and cephalization are probably related to the flatworm's bilateral symmetry and ability to swim forward rapidly. Refer to Lentz (1968). Reproduced with permission from Yale University Press.

have an axon that does nothing more than interact with other neurons in the immediate vicinity, and they are often called *local circuit neurons*. By way of distinction, *projection interneurons* send an axon to a distant, functionally distinct site, although it may also generate local collaterals; when confined entirely to the central nervous system (CNS) they are often referred to simply as *projection neurons*. In any event, all neurons throughout the animal kingdom may be classified broadly as sensory neurons, interneurons, or motoneurons.

The omnidirectional flow of information that is typical of cnidarian nerve nets is unusual in the rest of the animal kingdom. The vast majority of neurons in other animals are functionally polarized, with information flowing from the dendrites and soma to the axon. In invertebrates, however, most motoneurons and interneurons are unipolar: a single process, the axon, arises from the soma. Dendrites branch *from* the axons in the center of the ganglion—within the *neuropil*—where most synapses are made (Fig. 2.6). This arrangement of axon and dendrites is different from that found in vertebrates, where neurons are generally multipolar, with several dendrites, plus an axon extending from the soma or one of the dendrites (sometimes even from a secondary dendrite).

Certain features of simple nervous systems are preserved throughout evolution. For example, the part of the nervous system in the wall of the human gut (the enteric nervous system) has many features of a highly refined nerve net, and a "layer" of interneurons with amacrine processes is found in the human retina (see Fig. 2.17) and olfactory bulb.

The Nervous System of Annelids and Arthropods Is Segmented and Ventrally Located

Annelid worms and arthropods have even more complex body plans and behaviors than do flatworms, in part because of *segmentation*. Body segments, or metameres, are repeated serially along the rostrocaudal axis of the body. The segments presumably share a common underlying genetic program, although their terminal differentiation (adult structure) may vary. Because the same basic pattern is repeated in each segment, much of the genetic material from lower organisms is conserved even as a much more elaborate nervous system is produced. Annelids and all more complex invertebrates share another feature, a *ventral nerve cord*, consisting of a bilateral pair of ganglia (or a single fused ganglion) in each segment and longitudinal links to ganglia in adjacent segments via axon bundles (Fig. 2.7). Nerves also extend from each ganglion to the sensory structures and muscles in the same segment.

Basic Elements of the Vertebrate Nervous System are Present in the Lancelet

Vertebrates are a subphylum of the Chordates and they are the most complex representatives of the animal kingdom in terms of both structure and function. All vertebrates share a common basic body plan in which common organ systems are placed in a relatively strict anatomical relationship with each other (Box 2.3 and Fig. 2.8). Like other chordates, vertebrates possess two very important features during at least part of their life: a *notochord*, a stiff, cartilaginous rod that extends dorsally along the length of the body; and a more *dorsal nerve cord* that is hollow. In most vertebrates the body stiffening and protective functions of the notochord are taken over by the vertebral column and the bony skull, and the notochord is reduced to a series of cartilaginous cushions between or within the vertebrae. The vertebrate nerve cord is tremendously expanded, thickened, and folded to form the brain and spinal cord (the central nervous system).

The fundamental elements of the vertebrate nervous system are visible in the lancelet (amphioxus), a simple, nonvertebrate chordate (subphylum, Cephalochordata). The lancelet is a slender, fish-like filter-feeder that lives half buried in the sand in

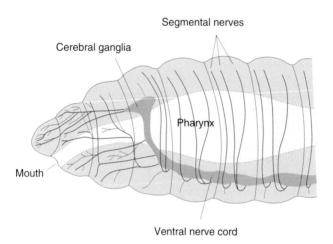

FIGURE 2.7 Organization of the nervous system in the rostral end of an annelid worm. A ventral nerve cord that contains more or less distinct ganglia connects with a fused pair of cerebral ganglia, which lie dorsal to the pharynx. Note the nerves arising from the ventral nerve cord and cerebral ganglia. Refer to Brusca and Brusca (1990).

BOX 2.3

ANATOMICAL RELATIONSHIPS IN THE VERTEBRATE BODY

To describe the physical relationships between structures in the nervous system and the rest of the vertebrate body, it is best to use terms that accurately and unambiguously describe the position of a given structure in three dimensions. The major axis of the body is the *rostrocaudal axis*, which extends along the length of the animal from the *rostrum* (beak) to the *cauda* (tail) (Fig. 2.8), as well as the length of the embryonic neural plate and neural tube (see Figs. 2.10 and 2.12). A second axis, the orthogonal *dorsoventral axis*, is vertical and runs from the *dorsum* (back) to the *ventrum* (belly). Finally, the third perpendicular axis, the *mediolateral axis*, is horizontal and runs from the midline (medial) to the lateral margin of the animal (lateral). Unfortunately, the rostrocaudal axis undergoes complex bending during embryogenesis, and the bending pattern is unique to each species. It would be ideal if the three cardinal axes were used in a topologically accurate way, say with reference to the body as it might appear with a "straightened out" rostrocaudal axis. In practice, however, this is rarely the

case, which leads to a certain degree of ambiguity, as is obvious when looking at the fish, frog, cat, and human bodies shown in Fig. 2.8.

The problem is especially difficult in human anatomy where use of an idiosyncratic terminology has a long, ingrained tradition. The basic principles are much easier to illustrate than to describe in writing (see Fig. 2.8), but one major source of confusion in the human brain is related to the fact that the rostrocaudal axis makes a 90° bend in the midbrain region (unlike in rodents and carnivores, for example, where the axis is relatively straight). The other source of confusion is simply the different names that are used. For example, in human anatomy the spinal cord has anterior and posterior horns, and posterior root ganglia, whereas in other mammals they are usually referred to as ventral and dorsal horns, and dorsal root ganglia. The merits of a uniformly applied nomenclature based on comparative structural principles seem obvious.

Larry W. Swanson

shallow, tropical marine waters (Fig. 2.9). Its dorsal nerve cord runs the length of the animal and sends out segmental nerves that innervate the muscles and organs. The body is stiffened by a dorsal notochord. Lancelets swim by alternately contracting segmental muscles, the *myotomes*, on the left and right sides of the body. Without the notochord these contractions would shorten the animal but would not produce forward propulsive force.

Although the typical brain regions found in vertebrates are not apparent in the rostral end of the lancelet nerve cord, specific genes specifying the head that are expressed very early in vertebrate embryogenesis are also expressed in the rostral part of the lancelet body. Thus, certain components of the molecular program specifying head development in modern vertebrates were present very early in chordate evolution (Holland and Holland, 1999).

Summary

Most of the basic cellular features of nervous system organization, including convergence and divergence of sensory and motor information, are found in the cnidarian nerve net. In the more complex

bilaterally symmetrical invertebrates, neurons and axons are aggregated in ganglia and nerve cords (centralization), and there is a higher concentration of neurons and sensory structures in the rostral end of the body (cephalization). Invertebrates with a segmented body plan have a ventral nerve cord that includes a bilateral pair of ganglia (or a single fused ganglion) in each segment. Basic features of vertebrate nervous system organization are found in the lancelet, a primitive chordate related to vertebrates.

DEVELOPMENT OF THE VERTEBRATE NERVOUS SYSTEM

One triumph of 19th century biology was the demonstration that early stages of embryogenesis are fundamentally the same in all vertebrates. The CNS, along with the heart, is one of the first organ systems to differentiate in the embryo, and the basic parts of the CNS that appear early in development are also common to all vertebrates. The names and arrangement of these parts are the starting point for regional or topographic neuroanatomical nomenclature (Swanson, 2000a).

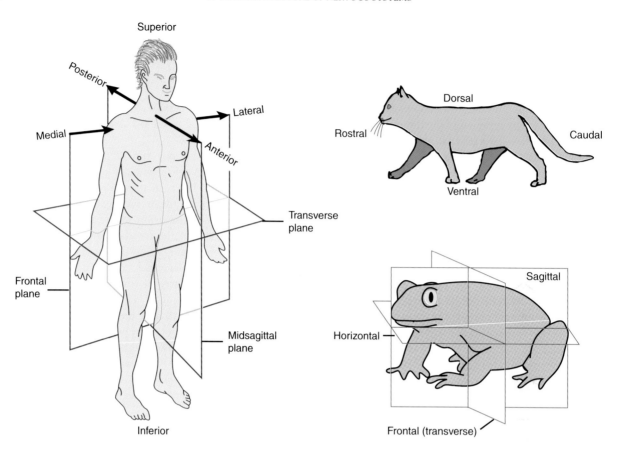

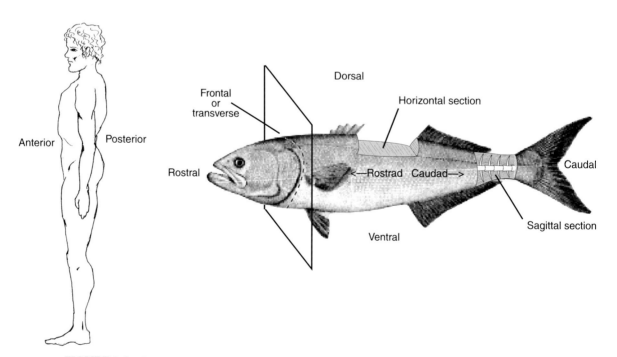

FIGURE 2.8 Orientation of the vertebrate body. Orientation planes for fish, quadrupeds, and bipeds are depicted. Associated with the three cardinal planes (rostrocaudal, dorsoventral, and mediolateral) are three orthogonal planes: horizontal, sagittal, and transverse (or frontal). For a further explanation, see Williams (1995).

A

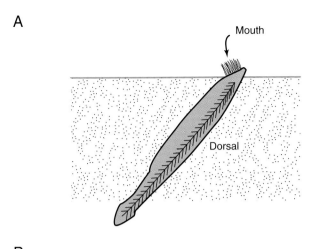

Mouth

Dorsal

B

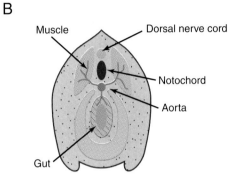

Muscle   Dorsal nerve cord

Notochord

Aorta

Gut

FIGURE 2.9 The lancelet (amphioxus) is a prototypic vertebrate. (A) Lateral view of the animal in its native environment under the ocean floor, with its mouth protruding above the sand. (B) A cross section of the lancelet showing the relationship among the dorsal nerve cord, the notochord, and the gut. Adapted from Cartmill *et al.* (1987).

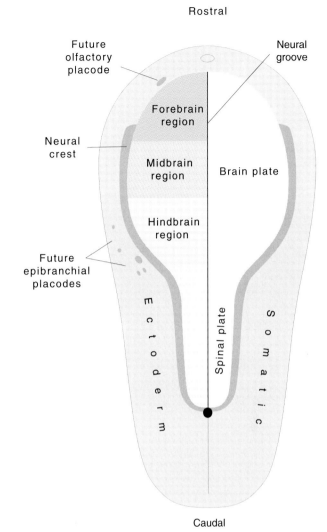

Rostral

Future olfactory placode

Neural groove

Forebrain region

Neural crest

Midbrain region

Brain plate

Hindbrain region

Future epibranchial placodes

Ectoderm

Spinal plate

Somatic

Caudal

FIGURE 2.10 The neural plate is a spoon-shaped region of ectoderm (neural ectoderm) that forms the CNS. Ectoderm that lies outside the neural plate is called somatic ectoderm. The neural plate is polarized (the rostral end is wider than the caudal end), bilaterally symmetrical (divided by the midline neural groove), and regionalized (the rostral half forms the brain, and the caudal half forms the spinal cord). The neural crest lies along the junction between somatic and neural ectoderm, and a series of placodes develops as "islands" within the somatic ectoderm. The neural crest and placodes generate neurons of the PNS. The approximate location of future major brain divisions in the neural plate is shown in color on the left. The same color scheme is used in Figs. 2.11 and 2.12. Refer to Swanson (1992).

Topographic Organization of the Nervous System Begins in the Neural Plate Stage

During embryogenesis the CNS develops as a hollow cylinder from a topologically flat sheet of cells, the *neural plate*, in a process called *neurulation*. The cellular and molecular mechanisms underlying neurulation are discussed in Chapter 14. What follows here is simply a description of the overall structural changes that occur during this transformation.

The neural plate is a spoon-shaped region in the one-cell-thick ectodermal layer of the trilaminar embryonic disc (Fig. 2.10). The wide end of the neural plate lies rostrally and becomes the brain, whereas the narrow end lies caudally and becomes the spinal cord; they are the two major divisions of the CNS. A *neural groove* runs down the middle of the neural plate, dividing it into right and left halves. Thus, the neural plate displays three cardinal features of morphogenesis: *polarity, bilateral symmetry*, and *regionalization*. The neural plate differentiates in a rostral to caudal direction, so that the brain plate is the first to show signs of

regionalization. These signs include the appearance of *optic vesicles*, which evaginate near the rostral end of the neural plate (in the presumptive hypothalamus); a midline *infundibulum*, which evaginates just caudal to the optic vesicles near the rostral end of the notochord; and the *otic rhombomere* (presumptive rhombomere 4), a swelling near the center of what will become the brain stem (Fig. 2.11, left).

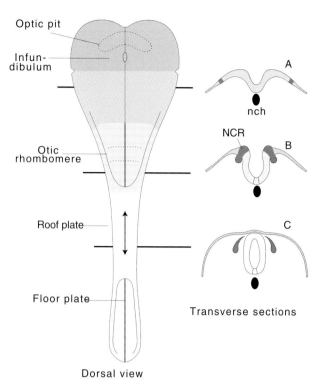

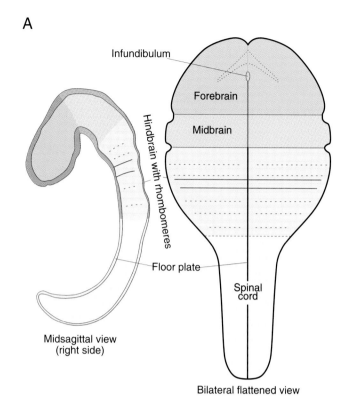

FIGURE 2.11 Optic pits, infundibulum, and otic rhombomere (dorsal view on left) are the earliest clear structural differentiations of the neural plate. The neural tube is formed by invagination of the neural ectoderm (transverse sections A and B), followed by fusion of the lateral edges of the neural plate (roughly in the cervical region in humans), and proceeds both rostrally and caudally (double arrow in roof plate). Note how the neural crest (NCR) pinches off in the process. Also note the position of the notochord (nch) just ventral to the neural groove. Refer to Swanson (1992).

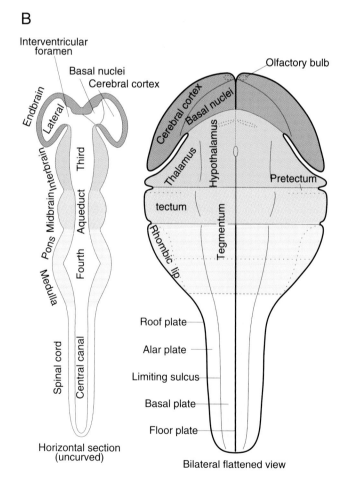

FIGURE 2.12 Formation and subdivision of the neural tube. (A) The brain region of the early neural tube develops three swellings: forebrain, midbrain, and hindbrain vesicles. The hindbrain vesicle develops a series of transverse swellings called rhombomeres. (B) As neurulation continues, the forebrain vesicle differentiates into right and left endbrain (cerebral hemisphere) vesicles and a medial interbrain vesicle; the hindbrain vesicle differentiates vaguely into pontine and medullary regions. The endbrain vesicle further divides into the cerebral cortex (including the olfactory bulb) and cerebral nuclei (basal ganglia); the interbrain vesicle divides into the thalamus and hypothalamus; the midbrain vesicle divides into the tectum and tegmentum; and the hindbrain divides into the rhombic lip, alar plate, and basal plate (tegmentum). Controversy exists about whether the pretectal region (sometimes called the synencephalon) is part of the interbrain or midbrain. At this stage of development, the major components of the adult ventricular system can be seen in the lumen of the neural tube. Refer to Swanson (1992) and Alvarez-Bolado and Swanson (1996).

At the junction between the neural plate and the rest of the ectoderm (which forms the epidermal layer of skin on the outside of the adult body) lies a narrow strip of tissue called the *neural crest* (Fig. 2.10). Extending around the spinal portion and approximately the caudal two-thirds of the brain portion of the neural plate, the neural crest is a distinctively vertebrate feature. It generates a variety of adult structures, including most neurons of the peripheral nervous system (PNS).

In summary, at the neural plate stage of vertebrate development the central and peripheral divisions of the nervous system are represented by the neural plate and neural crest, respectively. The two major divisions of the CNS—the brain and spinal cord—are also clear in the neural plate. At this stage the CNS is topologically quite simple: a bilaterally symmetrical, flat sheet that is one cell thick.

Further Regionalization Occurs in the Neural Tube Stage

As neurulation progresses, the two halves of the neural plate, now called *neural folds*, extend dorsally, away from the endoderm and midline mesoderm, so that the plate becomes V or U shaped (Fig. 2.11, right). Eventually the dorsal tips of the folds fuse to form a tube with two open ends. Even later, the ends of the tube, called *neuropores*, also fuse to produce a completely closed *neural tube* whose wall, the *neuroepithelium*, is still only one cell thick.

Marcello Malpighi, the great 17th century biologist who also discovered the capillary network between arteries and veins postulated by William Harvey in 1628, recognized that the early neural tube in the chick embryo displays three rostrocaudally arranged swellings now called the primary brain vesicles. They include the *forebrain* (prosencephalic) vesicle, which contains the optic stalks (vesicles) and infundibulum, the *midbrain* (mesencephalic) vesicle, and the *hindbrain* (rhombencephalic) vesicle, which contains the otic rhombomere (Fig. 2.12A). These vesicles are the fundamental structural or regional divisions of the brain. The most characteristic feature of the hindbrain vesicle is the appearance and rather swift disappearance of a series of transverse swellings called rhombomeres, which develop in association with the pharyngeal pouches and are discussed more fully in Chapter 14. As embryogenesis continues, the forebrain vesicle divides into the *endbrain* (telencephalic) and *interbrain* (diencephalic) vesicles, whereas the hindbrain vesicle differentiates somewhat into a rostral pontine (metencephalic) region and a caudal medullary (myelencephalic) region

(Fig. 2.12B). These divisions transform the "three primary vesicle stage" into the "five secondary vesicle stage."

The center of the neural tube remains in the adult as the *ventricular system* of the CNS (Fig. 2.12B, left). The shape of the ventricular system is determined by differentiation of the five secondary brain vesicles and the spinal cord. The left and right endbrain vesicles each contain a *lateral ventricle*, which is connected by an *interventricular foramen* to the third ventricle in the center of the interbrain vesicle. The *third ventricle* leads into the cerebral aqueduct in the midbrain vesicle, and the *aqueduct* in turn leads into the fourth ventricle in the hindbrain. Finally, the *fourth ventricle* becomes the *central canal* of the spinal cord. In older embryos and adults, the ventricular system contains *cerebrospinal fluid* (CSF), much of which is elaborated by specialized, highly vascular regions of *choroid plexus* in the roof of the lateral, third, and caudal fourth ventricles (see later).

Migrating Neurons Form the Mantle Layer

Through the five secondary vesicle stage, cells in the neural tube proliferate mitotically, but the neural tube remains one cell thick, a *pseudostratified epithelium*. Shortly thereafter, however, many of these cells begin to differentiate into neurons, which migrate away from the proliferation zone near the ventricles to form a new, more superficial zone, the *mantle layer* (see Chapter 15). In some regions of the CNS, neurons of the mantle layer become segregated into laminae that lie parallel to the surface of the CNS. In other regions, the neurons cluster in nuclei, relatively uniform collections of neurons (usually of several different types) that are structurally distinct from surrounding regions.

Mantle layer formation leads to further differentiation of the CNS (Figs. 2.12B). In the forebrain, the endbrain vesicle divides into the cerebral cortex (including the olfactory bulbs) dorsally and the cerebral nuclei (basal ganglia) ventrally, whereas the interbrain vesicle divides into the thalamus dorsally and the hypothalamus ventrally. The midbrain vesicle produces the laminated tectum dorsally and the nuclear tegmentum ventrally.

In the hindbrain and spinal cord, mantle layer formation results in clear regionalization because motoneurons are generated first and their site of differentiation is ventral in the neural tube (corresponding to medial in the neural plate). The early development of motoneurons correlates with the observation that gross, relatively uncoordinated motor behavior in the embryo begins well before

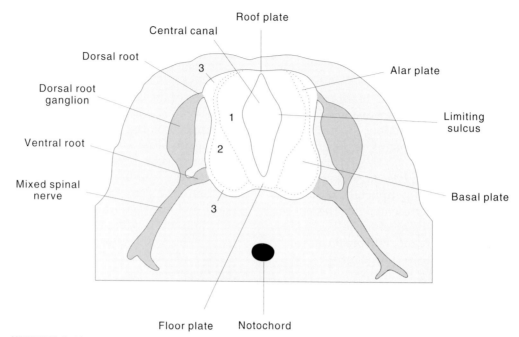

FIGURE 2.13   The early spinal cord and hindbrain are divided into dorsal (alar) and ventral (basal) plates by the limiting sulcus. This morphology reflects early ventral differentiation of the mantle layer (2), which is accompanied by an early ventral thinning of the neuroepithelial or ventricular layer of the neural tube (it remains as the ependymal lining of the adult ventricular system). The mantle layer develops into adult gray matter. This schematic drawing, which was traced from a transverse section of the spinal cord, also shows dorsal (sensory) and ventral (motor) roots of the spinal cord; dorsal root ganglia, which contain the somata of sensory neurons derived from the neural crest; and mixed (sensory and motor) spinal nerves distal to the ganglia. The peripheral area (3) is called the marginal zone and develops into the spinal cord white matter or funiculi, which contain ascending and descending fiber tracts.

sensory reflex pathways are established, implying that this behavior is generated endogenously, i.e., within the CNS itself (Hamburger, 1973).

The formation of a ventral mantle layer containing motoneurons is accompanied by the transient appearance of a longitudinal groove on the inner surface of the neural tube, the *limiting sulcus* (sulcus limitans). The great 19th century Swiss embryologist Wilhelm His pointed out that the limiting sulcus divides much of the neural tube on each side into a dorsal or *alar plate* and a ventral or *basal plate*, with sensory and motor functions, respectively (Fig. 2.13). His's observation complemented the earlier fundamental discovery by François Magendie and Charles Bell that sensory and motor fibers associated with the spinal cord are completely segregated within the spinal roots: sensory fibers enter through the dorsal roots and motor fibers leave through the ventral roots. It is now clear that the alar and basal plates are not purely sensory and motor because each contains interneurons. Nevertheless, it is helpful to think of the hindbrain and spinal cord as consisting of three longitudinal zones: sensory, integrative (reticular), and motor. Regionalization of the midbrain and forebrain does not fit as neatly into this scheme and is still relatively poorly understood.

The most dorsal region of the hindbrain alar plate forms a unique structure, the *rhombic lip*. In the pons, the rhombic lip generates the granule cells of the cerebellum, whereas more caudally in the hindbrain, the lip produces cell groups such as the precerebellar and vestibulocochlear nuclei. Cerebellar granule cells and neurons of the precerebellar nuclei are interesting because they migrate to their final destinations by traveling parallel to the surface of the neural tube rather than radially, like most CNS neurons (see Chapter 15).

This differentiation continues until the adult configuration of the CNS is achieved (Fig. 2.14). The most obvious late-developing structures are the cerebral hemispheres (endbrain) and the cerebellum.

Summary

The vertebrate CNS develops from a sheet of cells called the neural plate, which soon invaginates to form the neural tube. The rostral end of the tube then forms a series of swellings, or vesicles, that constitute the major regional parts of the brain. The caudal end of the tube forms the spinal cord. Most neurons of the PNS differentiate from the neural crest, which forms a narrow strip along the edge of the neural plate.

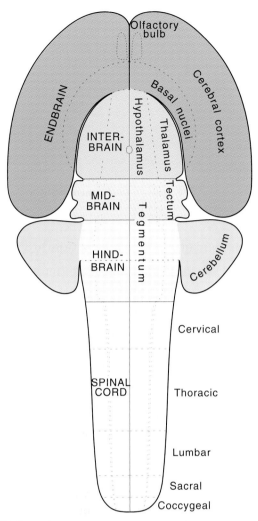

FIGURE 2.14 Major divisions of the adult CNS are derived from the regionalization of the neural plate and neural tube illustrated in Figs. 2.10–2.12. Modified from Swanson (1992).

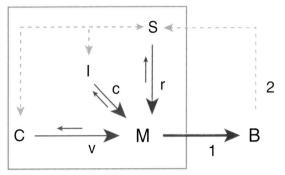

FIGURE 2.15 A model of the basic wiring diagram of the nervous system. This schematic view of how information flows through the nervous system (inside the box) postulates that behavior (B) is determined by the motor system (M), which is influenced by three classes of neural input: sensory (S), intrinsic behavioral state (I), and cognitive (C). Sensory inputs lead directly to reflex responses (r), cognitive inputs produce voluntary responses (v), and intrinsic inputs act as control signals (c) to regulate behavioral state. Motor system outputs (1) produce behaviors whose consequences are monitored by sensory feedback (2). Sensory feedback may be used by the cognitive system for perception and by the intrinsic system to generate affect (e.g., positive and negative reinforcement/pleasure and pain). The cognitive, sensory, and intrinsic systems are all interconnected, hence the arrowheads at the end of each dashed line within the box (nervous system). Refer to Swanson (2000c).

IDENTITY AND ORGANIZATION OF FUNCTIONAL SYSTEMS

How does the nervous system function from a systems rather than a cellular point of view? One way to approach this question is to analyze how the nervous system's basic functional subsystems are organized structurally. This approach should ultimately provide the fundamental circuit diagram for information processing in the nervous system. It seems prudent to begin this analysis without any biases or assumptions that may have been introduced by the strictly topographic or regional considerations dealt with in the preceding section.

One model of basic information processing in the nervous system is shown in Fig. 2.15. This model is a synthesis of basic neurobiological concepts pioneered by Cajal and Sherrington and basic cybernetic concepts pioneered by Norbert Wiener (1948) and John von Neumann (1958). In its simplest form, the model assumes that behavior is determined by the motor output of the CNS and that motor output is a function of three inputs: sensory (reflexive), cognitive (voluntary), and intrinsic behavioral state. The relative importance of these inputs in controlling motor output (behavior) varies from species to species and from individual to individual. Note that behavior elicits sensory feedback, which helps determine future motor activity and thus behavior. Each of the circuit's main components are now considered in more detail, bearing in mind that it is beyond the scope of this chapter to place all known parts of the CNS within this framework.

Motor Systems are Organized Hierarchically

There are three different types of motor system: skeletal, autonomic, and neuroendocrine. The first controls skeletal muscles responsible for voluntary behavior; the second controls smooth muscle and cardiac muscle, as well as many secretory glands; and the third controls hormone secretion from the pituitary gland. Because the skeletal motor system is the best understood of the three, it will serve as a prototype for considering the basic organizing principles of

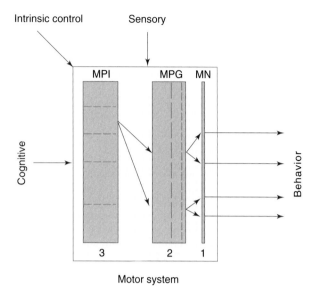

FIGURE 2.16 Hierarchical organization of the skeletal motor system. At the simplest level (1), pools of motoneurons (MN) innervate individual muscles that generate individual components of behavior. At the next higher level (2), interconnected pools of interneurons, referred to as motor pattern generators (MPG), innervate specific sets of motoneuron pools. At the highest level (3), additional interconnected pools of interneurons, referred to as motor pattern initiators (MPI), innervate specific sets of MPGs. MPIs can produce complex, stereotyped behaviors when they are activated (or inhibited) by specific patterns of sensory, intrinsic, and cognitive inputs. Note that MPGs and MPIs may themselves be organized hierarchically as indicated by the dashed lines and that sensory, intrinsic, and cognitive inputs may go directly to any level of the motor system. Refer to Swanson (2000c).

motor systems, which are presumably similar for all three.

The skeletal motor system is arranged hierarchically as diagrammed in Fig. 2.16. The lowest level in the hierarchy consists of α motoneurons, and their axons synapse directly on skeletal muscle fibers. The cell bodies of α motoneurons that innervate specific muscles are arranged within pools in the spinal cord and within nuclei in the brain stem. The next higher level consists of motor pattern generators (MPGs), circuits of interneurons that innervate unique sets of motoneuron pools or nuclei. The highest level is composed of motor pattern initiators (MPIs), which "recognize" or alter their output in response to specific input patterns and project to unique sets of MPGs. Ethologists refer to MPIs as "innate releasing mechanisms." One reason the organization of central neural circuitry is so complex is that each of the three types of input (sensory, intrinsic, cognitive) may go directly to each of the three general levels in the motor system hierarchy.

A hierarchical organization also exists within MPGs and MPIs themselves. At a conceptual level,

this organization is particularly easy to understand for the MPGs subserving locomotion. In the spinal cord, simple MPGs for locomotion coordinate the reciprocal innervation of antagonistic muscle pairs across individual joints, more complex MPGs coordinate the activity of simpler MPGs for all the joints in a given limb, and still more complex MPGs coordinate the activity of MPGs controlling all four limbs. Carrying the analysis to the next higher level, there is a separate hierarchy of MPIs in the brain for locomotion, which is activated by specific patterns of input and projects to the locomotor pattern generator network in the spinal cord.

Multiple Sensory Systems Function in Parallel

A set of sensory systems provides information to the CNS from various classes of receptors, and all of these systems can function at the same time. Cajal noted that pathways carrying unimodal sensory information generally branch in such a way that part of the information goes directly to the motor system and part goes to the cerebral cortex for sensation and perception. Information going directly to the motor system is typically reflexive in nature, whereas information going to the cerebral cortex has the potential to reach the level of consciousness and play an important role in cognition.

The various types of sensory systems are dealt with in Section IV, so only a few of their general features are mentioned here. First, the CNS receives a wide range of information about the external environment as well as the internal state of the body itself. Thus, sensory receptors can be found near the surface of the body (e.g., touch receptors and olfactory receptors), deep within the body (e.g., stretch receptors in the aorta), and even within the brain itself (e.g., osmoreceptors in the hypothalamus). Second, each of the three types of motor system receives a broad range of sensory inputs. Third, the range of sensory modalities is remarkably similar (although not identical) across vertebrate classes, and information relating to specific modalities enters the CNS through homologous cranial and spinal nerves in all vertebrates. Fourth, the number of synapses between a sensory receptor and the cerebral cortex may vary in different systems. For example, there is one synapse in the olfactory pathway and at least four in the visual pathway.

The Cognitive System Produces Anticipatory Behavior

There seems little doubt that the cerebral cortex—along with its cerebral nuclei or basal ganglia—is the most important part of the cognitive system, if not the only part, and that the cerebral cortex is responsible for planning, initiating, and evaluating the consequences of voluntary behavior (Section VII). The fundamental nature of voluntary behavior is obviously a difficult problem to address, but one useful approach is simply to compare it with reflexive behavior. Interestingly, many and perhaps all behaviors mediated by skeletal muscle can be initiated either reflexively or voluntarily, as Descartes pointed out long ago. What seems to distinguish reflexive and voluntary behavior most clearly is that the former is a stereotyped response to a defined stimulus, whereas the latter is anticipatory and impossible to predict with anywhere near the same degree of certainty.

Intrinsic Systems are Important in Controlling Behavioral State

The CNS generates a great deal of intrinsic activity (patterns of action potentials)—it is most definitely not simply a passive system waiting to respond to sensory input. In general, all parts of the CNS have a basal level of activity that can be either increased or decreased. In many cases, it is still not known whether particular neuronal cell types generate intrinsic activity patterns. It is clear, however, that motoneurons and related MPGs do generate intrinsic activity; the embryonic spinal cord produces motor output before sensory circuits develop, as noted earlier. Thus, in addition to the three extrinsic types of input to the motor system illustrated in Fig. 2.15, intrinsic activity within the motor system itself can produce behavior that is neither reflexive nor voluntary.

Certain regions of the CNS generate intrinsic activity patterns that are rhythmic. From a behavioral perspective, the most important rhythmic pattern is the sleep–wake cycle, which is entrained to the light–dark cycle by an endogenous circadian clock, the hypothalamic suprachiasmatic nucleus (Chapters 41 and 42). The sleep–wake cycle is profoundly significant because during sleep the body is maintained entirely by ongoing intrinsic and reflexive systems that control such behaviors as respiration and the sustained contraction of sphincters. In contrast, voluntary mechanisms come into play during periods of wakefulness, although reflexive and intrinsic mechanisms are vitally important then as well.

The control of behavioral state is thus a fundamental intrinsic property of the brain. One other aspect of behavioral state, arousal, is especially important during wakefulness. Arousal level is correlated in a general way with the motivational state—the level of

drive—of an animal (Chapter 43). The neural system mediating drive or motivation has not been elucidated, but it almost certainly involves the hypothalamus. However, the attainment of specific goal objects (foraging behavior) in motivated behavior involves the cognitive system. Therefore, arousal and drive may be controlled by subcortical systems, whereas the actual direction of behavior is mainly determined cortically.

One of the great mysteries of neuroscience is how systems elaborating pleasure and pain are organized at the level of specific neural systems. Many regard pleasure and pain as the conscious expression of positive and negative reinforcement, which determine whether a particular voluntary behavior is likely to be repeated or avoided in the future. In this context, reinforcement depends on sensory feedback related to the consequences of a particular behavior, and one suggestion is that the sensations of pleasure and pain, like those associated with drive, are elaborated subcortically within intrinsic control systems. According to this view, thinking or cognition is a product of the cerebral cortex, whereas feeling or affect is produced subcortically. However, it is also possible that all aspects of consciousness (both thinking and feeling) are strictly a product of neural activity within the cerebral cortex (see Chapters 25 and 43).

Pharmacological Systems and Genetic Networks: How are they Related to Functional Systems?

The incorporation of specific neurotransmitter systems into models of CNS function has become increasingly frequent since the mid-1970s. Two examples are the cholinergic and noradrenergic systems, defined as the total sets of neurons in the CNS that release acetylcholine or noradrenalin, respectively, as a neurotransmitter (Chapter 7). In general, these systems are not correlated in a straightforward way with traditional functional systems or with topographic subdivisions of the CNS. That is, they are not typically restricted to one functional system or to one major division of the brain, although there may be some exceptions. Thus, neurotransmitter systems are not functional systems in the traditional sense. However, they are conceptually important in helping define the circuits or functional systems that are influenced by the direct action of particular drugs. For example, the administration of a centrally acting agonist of acetylcholine receptors will influence synapses in a variety of traditional functional systems, and the set of these **functional systems** could be defined as a **pharmacological system** with a specific set of behavioral as well as other responses. If a drug is targeted for therapeutic reasons to a specific neural system (e.g., if a cholinergic agonist is targeted for the cerebral cortical cholinergic system in Alzheimer's disease (see Chapter 46), it will also act on other functional systems with appropriate cholinergic receptors (e.g., cholinergic receptors in the thalamus). Responses in these other systems produce "side effects," which may be good or bad.

Extending this line of thought further, the distribution of any gene product can also be used to define a chemical, molecular, or **gene expression system** in the brain, although the heuristic value of this approach is usually greater at cellular and molecular levels than at a functional systems level. For example, one could define a system in terms of all CNS neurons that express the calbindin or μ-opioid receptor gene, and it might be possible to prevent expression of the corresponding gene in a knockout mouse. This procedure may produce an obvious phenotype, but in most instances it can be assumed that the gene is normally expressed in multiple functional systems and will have complex (even if subtle) physiological and behavioral effects.

It is also important to remember that a genetic program is responsible for constructing the basic (macro) circuitry of the brain during embryogenesis. Determining the correspondence between gene expression networks and neural networks may be the ultimate achievement of systems neuroscience.

Summary

There does not appear to be a simple relationship between the topographic or the regional organization of the CNS and its functional organization. Thus, it is a mistake to assume *a priori* that information is processed in the CNS in a simple hierarchical way, with the spinal cord at the lowest level and the cerebral cortex at the highest level. An alternative view is that the CNS displays a network rather than a hierarchical mode of organization—where the motor system is driven by sensory, cognitive, and intrinsic behavioral state inputs, and future motor activity is determined in part by sensory feedback related to the consequences of the initial behavior.

Two major features complicate this simple network model. First, the motor system itself clearly displays aspects of hierarchical organization; the sensory system transmits a wide range of modalities in parallel, and this sensory information may reach each level in the motor hierarchy directly. Second, sensory information also reaches the intrinsic and cognitive systems. In fact, all three input systems are interconnected bidirectionally. Clearly, the basic plan of neural circuit architecture must be understood on its own terms, not through simple preconceived ideas or unfounded analogies with computers, telephone switchboards, or irrigation systems. How the traditional functional organization of the CNS is related to pharmacological systems and genetic networks remains to be determined.

SOME BASIC STRUCTURAL FEATURES OF THE NERVOUS SYSTEM

This section presents an overview of methods that structural neuroscientists have used to achieve the current, admittedly rather incomplete, understanding of nervous system architectural principles, as well as an introduction to some of the major nervous system components themselves. However, long experience has taught that nothing approaches actual dissection for gaining an appreciation of overall brain structure.

A Brief History of Structural Neuroscience Methods

Although the gross anatomical structure of the human brain was observed by early Greek physicians and philosophers, the astounding complexity of its circuitry was not really appreciated until the microscope was used effectively to identify individual tracts (axon bundles) and neuronal areas (recognizable aggregates of neuronal cell bodies). This occurred in the second half of the 19th century as neurohistologists applied reagents and reactions developed by the textile and photographic industries to thin sections of CNS tissue (Swanson, 2000b).

In retrospect, perhaps the single most enduring contribution of 19th century neurohistology was the silver impregnation method of Camillo Golgi, described in 1873. For the first time it was possible to see the full morphology of individual neurons (Fig. 2.17; Boxes 2.1 and 2.2)—their full dendritic tree, the shape of the cell body, the axon with all of its collateral branches, and the points of presumed functional contact with other cells, which Sherrington was to name the synapse in 1897. The Golgi method involves placing fresh brain tissue alternately in solutions of potassium dichromate and silver nitrate over a period of weeks, months, or even years. Mysteriously—the chemistry of the reaction is still elusive—only 1% or so of the neurons are filled (seemingly at random) with a dense precipitate. The precipitate reveals the entire architecture of each metal-impregnated cell, from the tiniest dendritic branches

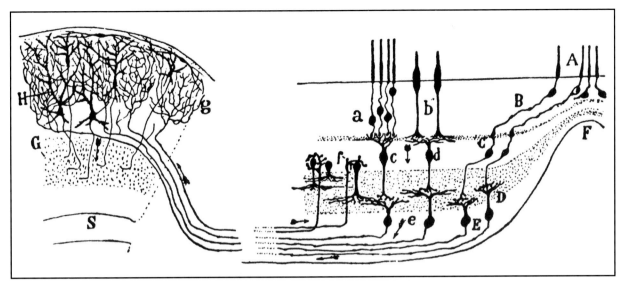

FIGURE 2.17 This drawing of neural architecture was prepared by Cajal (1911–1913) and is based on the Golgi method. It shows the organization of certain cell types in the retina (on the right) and the projection from the retina to the optic tectum (superior colliculus, on the left). Application of the neuron doctrine and theory of functional polarity (Boxes 2.1 and 2.2) to essentially the entire vertebrate nervous system by Cajal and many other workers about a century ago led to the "classical" way neuronal cell types have been defined in structural terms ever since, a view that is illustrated beautifully here. Note that three major cell types tend to fall into specific layers in the retina: photoreceptors of several subtypes (a, b, A, B), bipolar cells of several subtypes (c, d), and ganglion cells of several subtypes (e, D, E). The cardinal feature of a specific cell type is the distribution of its axon—what the cell does in terms of its output. Photoreceptors detect light and their axon innervates bipolar cells; the latter in turn innervate ganglion cells, and finally the latter send a projection axon through the optic nerve to the superior colliculus. Photoreceptors are classical sensory neurons (Fig. 2.3), bipolar neurons are local circuit neurons, and ganglion cells are projection neurons. Also note a second class of local circuit neuron in the retina, the amacrine cell (f). Cajal pointed out that neuronal cell bodies in the retina are arranged in three layers (outer nuclear for photoreceptors, inner nuclear for local circuit neurons, and ganglion cell layer), with synaptic neuropil zones in between (the outer and inner plexiform layers, shown as gray). Cajal also illustrated a clear gradient in retinal structural organization—due in this specific case to the presence of a foveal region (F) with much higher visual acuity because of many structural features, some of which are obvious in the drawing. The power of Cajal's theory of functional polarity is evident here: he drew arrows to indicate the presumed normal direction of information flow through the circuit based on the arrangement of axons and dendrites of individual cell types in the circuit.

and spines to the swollen tips of axons, against a light yellow background of unstained tissue. Thus, the Golgi method reveals more by staining less. Today, selective labeling of individual neurons can also be achieved by injecting a dye or other marker into a living neuron with a micropipette, which can be used simultaneously to study the electrical activity of the neuron.

Unfortunately, the Golgi method provided very little information about the longer connections within the CNS: axonal projections between nonadjacent cell groups. This was approached in the second half of the 19th century with methods that selectively stained fibers that are degenerating because of pathological or experimental lesions. These degeneration methods evolved from studies by Augustus Waller, who showed in 1850 that transection of a nerve eventually causes degeneration of the distal segment of the nerve (Wallerian, anterograde degeneration). This led Waller to propose that the cell body is the "trophic center" of

the nerve cell and that the axon is dependent upon it for survival. About 30 years later Bernard von Gudden showed that this degeneration may be accompanied under certain conditions by pathological changes in the somata of neurons whose axons are in the nerve. This degeneration suggested the retrograde transport of "trophic factors" from axon to cell body. The first selective degeneration method for central pathways was developed in 1885 by Marchi and Algeri. It revealed degenerating myelin sheaths around severed axons as black particles on a light background, effectively isolating the degenerating sheaths from healthy ones in a tissue section. After producing discrete brain lesions in experimental animals and waiting a few weeks for fiber degeneration to occur, anatomists could, in principle, use this method to reveal the course of nerve tracts that arise in specific regions of the brain. The method was quite limited, however, because it did not stain unmyelinated or thinly myelinated axons, or the (unmyelinated) terminal fields of myelinated axons. There were also many "false positive" results due to transection of fibers merely passing through the lesion site (interrupting fibers-of-passage).

In the middle of the 20th century, selective silver impregnation and degeneration methods were combined by Walle J.H. Nauta and others in techniques to reveal degenerating unmyelinated axons and their terminal fields. Essentially the entire CNS was remapped at much finer resolution with these methods, although they still suffered from the fiber-of-passage problem ("false positive" results) and were not nearly as sensitive as the next generation of techniques, which were developed around 1970. Instead of relying on pathological changes due to lesion or nerve section, the next (current) generation relied on (1) physiological mechanisms in healthy neurons and (2) the histochemical detection of antibodies and complementary strands of nucleic acids. The physiological mechanism taken advantage of was fast intraaxonal transport of markers in both anterograde and retrograde directions.

The first successful anterograde tract tracer method was based on the injection of radiolabeled amino acids. They are taken up and incorporated into proteins only in the cell body (and to a lesser extent in dendrites) and then shipped anterogradely throughout the axon and all of its collaterals. Autoradiographs of tissue sections through the brain reveal the site of injection and the three-dimensional pattern of axonal transport from labeled neurons confined to the injection site. This method proved even more sensitive than experimental degeneration and did not involve fibers-of-passage (which do not have protein synthetic machinery), but did not show the morphology of labeled axons—only hazy patterns of silver grains in autoradiograms. In 1984, Gerfen and Sawchenko introduced the use of a plant lectin (PHAL) as an anterograde tracer that is not taken up by fibers-of-passage. It is extremely sensitive, at least in small animals, and because it is detected immunohistochemically, it shows the morphology of labeled axons with the clarity of a Golgi impregnation. It is in effect an experimental Golgi method for tracing longer pathways in the nervous system. Since then several other very useful anterograde tracers have been introduced.

A variety of tracers are also taken up by axon terminals (and usually by axons themselves) and are transported retrogradely through the axon to cells of origin. These invaluable methods reveal the distribution of all neurons in the nervous system that contribute to a terminal field (or nerve, or fiber tract) that is injected with the tracer. When more than one differentiable tracer is used in the same animal, patterns of multiple simultaneous labeling can be used to iden-

tify neuron populations that send collateral projections to more than one terminal field.

Beginning around 1970, immunohistochemical methods were also developed for localizing within tissue sections the precise cellular distribution of any molecule (antigen) that can be the target of a specific antibody. The approach was quickly applied to characterize the distribution of neurons that synthesize specific neurotransmitters or their synthetic enzymes, but now the method is used for a broad range of molecules from ATP to neurotransmitter receptor subunits. This approach was extended about 15 years later to the histochemical localization of nucleic acid sequences, especially mRNAs. Thus, using *in situ* hybridization, the distribution of cells that express one or another mRNA can be mapped in great detail.

Today, it is common to combine axonal transport methods with histochemical techniques for localizing antigens and nucleic acid sequences. Thus, the spatial distribution of neural circuits may be determined experimentally, and this information may be complemented with information about the identity and amount of specific molecules within specific components (neuronal cell types) of the circuitry.

Last, but certainly not least, it is important to note that beginning in the 1950s the electron microscope opened a whole world of ultrastructure that was previously only guessed at. It provided the first glimpses of synapses (the cleft is only about 20 nm wide, far below the resolution of the light microscope), myelin sheath organization, and many cellular organelles. It also allowed biologists to examine in detail the biosynthetic apparatus that resides within each cell.

These methods have provided a far more detailed picture of CNS connectivity patterns or circuit organization than ever before in many species of animals. As a result, comparative neuroanatomy has flourished and forms a solid structural foundation on which contemporary physiological and behavioral studies are based.

The Peripheral Nervous System is Divided into Sensorimotor, Autonomic, and Enteric Divisions

Early in embryogenesis, the cells that make up the neural crest bud off laterally from the neural tube and begin to migrate through the embryo. The neural crest ultimately generates major parts of the head and jaw, as well as almost all of the neurons of the PNS (some cranial nerve sensory neurons derive from placodes or islands of somatic ectoderm; Fig. 2.10). Thus, migrating neural crest cells lay down most of the peripheral ganglia and their derivatives, the

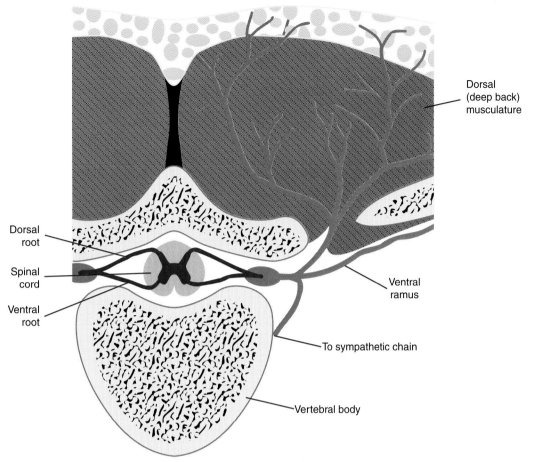

FIGURE 2.18 A cross section of the midthoracic region of the adult human illustrating the appearance of the spinal cord *in situ* with dorsal and ventral roots coalescing to form the mixed spinal nerve. This nerve sends fibers (axons) dorsally to the postural (deep) muscles of the back through dorsal rami and also generates ventral rami that innervate the muscles and skin of the thoracic cage. The mixed spinal nerve also sends fibers to the sympathetic chain, which is part of the sympathetic division of the autonomic nervous system.

interconnections between them, and the neurons of the enteric nervous system in the wall of the digestive tract. Other neural crest cells penetrate the adrenal gland and develop into its medulla, which secretes neuroactive hormones, including adrenalin.

Functionally, and to some extent structurally, the PNS may be divided into a sensory ganglion component with accompanying nerves, the motor part of the autonomic nervous system (ANS), and the enteric nervous system. The first component, which includes sensory or dorsal root ganglia and all peripheral nerves, is really defined by gross anatomical considerations rather than principles of circuit organization (Fig. 2.18). The sensory part consists of dorsal root ganglia sensory neurons with one process (embryologically and phylogenetically the axon) entering the brain through the dorsal roots and the other process (embryologically and phylogenetically the dendrite)

coursing through a peripheral nerve(s) to various sites throughout the body. However, the peripheral nerves also contain the axons of skeletal motoneurons whose cell bodies are found in the spinal cord and brain stem; near the spinal cord the initial part of the axon courses through a ventral root. Thus, most peripheral nerves carry *afferent* (sensory) information toward the CNS and *efferent* (motor) information toward the body. Sensory neurons carry afferent information about stimuli detected in the skin, skeletal muscles, tendons, joints, blood vessels, and deep viscera. The autonomic and enteric nervous systems consist of a network of efferent pathways, ganglia, and nerve nets that control peristaltic movements of the gut, a wide range of glandular secretions, dilation and contraction of blood vessels, and many other functions of the deep organs. The output of the autonomic and enteric nervous systems is modulated by both somatic and visceral afferents. Thus, a typical peripheral nerve

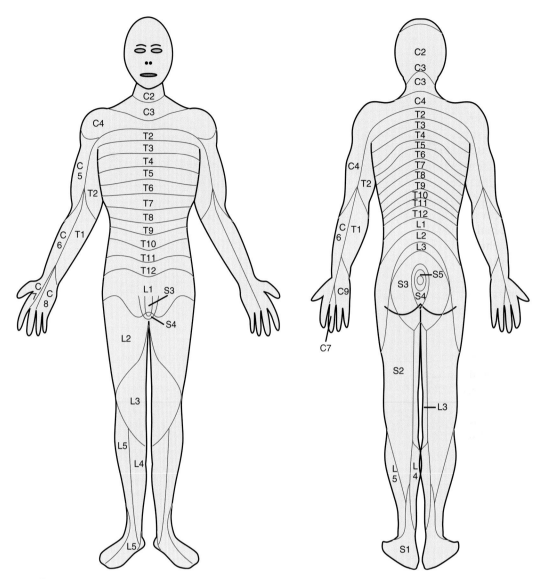

FIGURE 2.19   A dermatome map of the human body. The spinal cord level that selectively innervates each dermatome is indicated. Note twisting of dermatomes in the lower limb, which arises from rotation of that limb as it develops to accommodate bipedal locomotion.

carries a mixture of afferents and efferents that innervate the body wall and the deep organs.

Somatic afferents are distributed near the body surface in a manner that reflects the segmental origins of the body wall itself. Each spinal nerve innervates a relatively narrow mediolateral band of skin called a *dermatome* (Fig. 2.19), although it is important bear in mind that in fact adjacent nerves innervate overlapping territories (otherwise interruption of a nerve would lead to complete loss of sensation in a band of skin, which is not the case). The segmental pattern of dermatomes is best seen in the torso, where very little differential growth of the body wall occurs. In contrast, dermatomes in the upper and lower limbs are

distorted because they form before the limbs grow out in the embryo. In humans, the lower limbs also rotate after they are formed, causing the dermatomes to rotate as well.

Peripheral nerves often ramify and join with nerves from other segments to form *plexi* (singular: plexus; literally, a "braid"). Plexi serve as crossroads and distribution centers for peripheral nerves, allowing axons to reorganize themselves into complex nerve bundles that innervate body structures. Brachial and lumbosacral plexi at the base of the upper and lower limbs, respectively, are the largest examples of these perplexing structures. The ANS also has a bewildering variety of plexi in which nerves converge and redistribute axons to their target organs.

The Two Divisions of the ANS Generally Exert Opposing Actions

The ANS consists of two anatomically and functionally distinct systems: the *sympathetic* and *parasympathetic* divisions (Chapter 35). The pathways of the sympathetic division originate with neurons whose somata lie in the thoracic and upper lumbar levels of the spinal cord. In the parasympathetic division, the neurons of origin are in the brain stem and sacral levels of the spinal cord. Therefore, the sympathetic and parasympathetic divisions are sometimes called the thoracolumbar and craniosacral divisions, respectively. Anatomically, the two divisions are constructed quite differently, and their anatomy reveals much about the differences in their function.

The two divisions function in a kind of "push–pull" relationship with each other. It is never the case that one is completely on or off. Instead, there are degrees of sympathetic and parasympathetic "tone." During sleep, certain involuntary functions such as digestion are accelerated. The glands that take part in digestion are activated parasympathetically, and the sympathetic tone is correspondingly decreased. However, as noted by Walter B. Cannon three-quarters of a century ago, during the characteristic "fight or flight" reaction in defensive behavior, sympathetic tone is enhanced markedly and parasympathetic tone is reduced sharply.

Sympathetic outflow is vastly amplified and coordinated through a series of sympathetic ganglia and the adrenal medulla. As a consequence of this arrangement, sympathetic function occurs more or less synchronously throughout the body. In contrast, the parasympathetic system is relatively finely tuned. For example, digestion requires the coordinated stimulation of glandular secretion through the gastrointestinal tract, from the stomach and the small intestine to the large bowel. This coordination is accomplished partly through local increases in parasympathetic tone.

The Spinal Cord Generates a Series of Dorsal and Ventral Roots

The human spinal cord, roughly as thick as an adult's little finger, is surrounded and protected by the vertebral column (Fig. 2.18), which forms during early embryogenesis from sclerotome cells. They initially enclose the neural tube, but later clefts form at regularly spaced intervals that eventually separate adjacent vertebrae. In cross section, the spinal cord can be seen to contain two basic types of nervous tissue: *gray matter* and *white matter*. Gray matter occurs in a "butterfly" configuration surrounding the central canal (spinal part of the ventricular system) and is composed primarily of neuronal cell bodies and neuropil. White matter surrounds gray matter in the spinal cord and consists mostly of axons collected into poorly differentiated, mostly overlapping fiber bundles. Many of the axons are surrounded by a myelin sheath, a uniquely vertebrate feature that allows very rapid conduction of nerve impulses (see Chapter 6). The paracrystalline arrangement of lipids and proteins in myelin, together with the unusually high lipid/protein ratio of myelin, gives white matter its pale appearance.

The adult spinal cord presents a segmented appearance because of the bilateral pairs of dorsal and ventral roots attached at regular intervals along its length. The pairs of dorsal and ventral roots have been grouped into five sets: cervical (in the neck above the rib cage), thoracic (associated with the rib cage), lumbar (in the abdominal region), sacral (near the pelvis), and coccygeal (associated with the tail vertebrae). Although noted earlier, it is worth emphasizing that dorsal roots transmit sensory, afferent information to the spinal cord, whereas ventral roots transmit motor, efferent information from the cord. Dorsal and ventral roots unite a short distance from the spinal cord (just past the dorsal root ganglion) to form mixed (sensory and motor) spinal nerves, which then pass through the vertebral column via the interventricular foramina. In humans, there are usually 31 pairs of spinal nerves (8 cervical, 12 thoracic, 5 lumbar, 5 sacral, and 1 coccygeal), which are named according to the intervertebral foramen through which they pass (Fig. 2.20A).

In the early fetus the spinal cord extends the full length of the vertebral column, but as development proceeds, the vertebral column outgrows the spinal cord. At birth, the spinal cord ends at the level of the third lumbar vertebra, and by adulthood it reaches only to the first lumbar vertebra. This differential growth does not, however, affect the correct distribution of spinal nerves through the intervertebral foramina. As a result, spinal nerves from caudal segments of the cord travel long distances inside the vertebral canal (Fig. 2.20B). Their parallel arrangement caudal to the termination of the spinal cord gives them the appearance of a horse tail and is the basis for their name, *cauda equina*. It is at the level of the cauda equina where a sample of CSF may be removed for analysis by aspiration through a lumbar puncture. This "spinal tap" is done at or below the level of the second lumbar vertebra to avoid the risk of injuring the spinal cord.

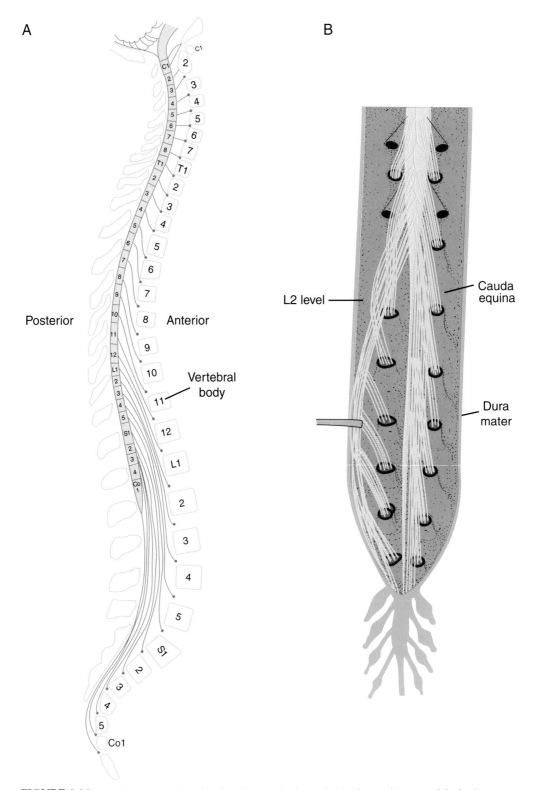

FIGURE 2.20   The human spinal cord within the spinal column. (A) Midsagittal section of the back region. The spinal cord is considerably shorter than the vertebral column (made up of vertebral bodies, or simply verte-brae) that encases it. The spinal cord extends only to level L1–L2, but the nerve rootlets emanating from each segment continue down to the appropriate vertebral column exit point. (B) The cauda equina ("horse tail") is formed from the collected nerve roots. The cauda equina exits the vertebral canal through the dura mater, which surrounds the spinal column.

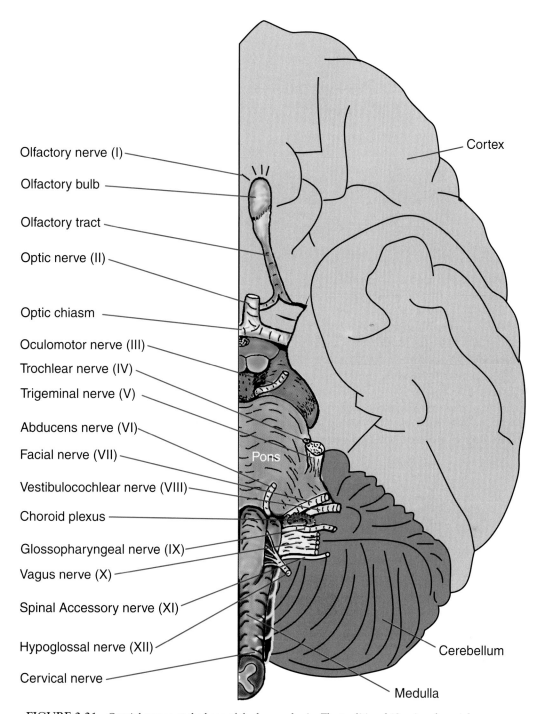

Olfactory nerve (I)

Olfactory bulb

Olfactory tract

Optic nerve (II)

Optic chiasm

Oculomotor nerve (III)

Trochlear nerve (IV)

Trigeminal nerve (V)

Abducens nerve (VI)

Facial nerve (VII)

Vestibulocochlear nerve (VIII)

Choroid plexus

Glossopharyngeal nerve (IX)

Vagus nerve (X)

Spinal Accessory nerve (XI)

Hypoglossal nerve (XII)

Cervical nerve

Cortex

Pons

Cerebellum

Medulla

FIGURE 2.21 Cranial nerves at the base of the human brain. The traditional 12 pairs of cranial nerves are seen as they exit from the brain. "Cervical nerve" refers to the ventral root of the first spinal nerve—the first of 31 pairs of spinal nerves discussed in the text.

Cranial Nerves Transmit Sensory and Motor Information between Brain and Periphery

Based on gross dissections of the human brain stem, Samuel Thomas von Soemmerring in 1778 recognized a sequence of 12 pairs of cranial nerves (Fig. 2.21), and this classification scheme has become traditional for vertebrates in general, although it is problematic in terms of completeness (e.g., not including the terminal nerve, associated with the nasal cavity) and nonconformance with contemporary fate maps of cranial nerve nucleus development (e.g., motoneurons for nerve VII are generated rostral to those for nerve VI). Be that as it may, cranial nerves are much more heterogeneous than spinal nerves, and indeed it is probably safe to say that no two pairs of cranial nerves have the same composition of functionally defined fiber types.

In humans, seven cranial nerves transmit information about the so-called special senses associated with the head: olfaction (I, the olfactory nerve), vision (II, the optic nerve), hearing and balance (VIII, the vestibuloacoustic nerve), and taste (V, VII, IX, and X; parts of the trigeminal, facial, glossopharyngeal, and vagus nerves, respectively). Nerves III (oculomotor), IV (trochlear), and VI (abducens) primarily control eye movements, although the third nerve is also involved in the parasympathetically mediated pupillary light reflex and accommodation of the lens. Major parts of the fifth nerve carry sensory axons from the face (a rostral extension of the spinal somatic sensory system) and motor axons that innervate the muscles used for mastication (chewing). The seventh nerve controls the muscles of facial expression and also innervates the salivary and lacrimal glands—its role in the expression of human emotion is obvious. The ninth nerve innervates the pharynx and mediates the swallowing reflex. The vagus nerve ("the wanderer") has an exception-

ally complex and widespread innervation pattern, including the muscles of the larynx used in speech, and the parasympathetic innervation of most viscera in the thorax and abdomen. Of particular note, vagal stimulation slows the heart by increasing parasympathetic tone. The XIth nerve (spinal accessory) innervates the trapezius muscle, a trapezoid-shaped muscle that sits high on the back and helps steady the shoulder blade (scapula). Finally, the XIIth nerve (hypoglossal) innervates muscles of tongue.

Cerebral Hemispheres are Divided into Cortex and Nuclei

The most extraordinary growth of the mammalian brain occurs in the endbrain or cerebral hemispheres (Fig. 2.22), which consist of both cortex and deep nuclei (or basal ganglia). Qualitatively they develop more or less as mirror images of one another and are divided down the dorsal midline by the deep interhemispheric (longitudinal) fissure. However, there are asymmetries, e.g., in humans the speech centers are lateralized (Chapter 52), and the patterns of gyri and sulci are different on the two sides (and different in each individual). The size of the hemispheres is restricted by the capacity of the bony skull or cranium within which the brain grows. As the hemispheres

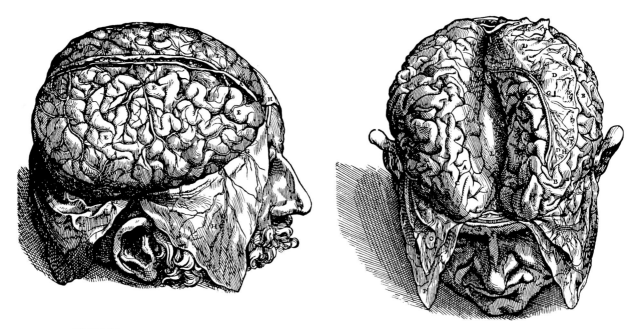

FIGURE 2.22   The surface structure of the human cerebral cortex, which is thrown into folds (gyri) separated by depressions (sulci). In the figure on the right, the two hemispheres have been pulled apart at the interhemispheric or longitudinal fissure to reveal the corpus callosum that interconnects the two cerebral hemispheres. This is from perhaps the most important book in the history of medicine, the "Fabric of the Human Body," published in 1543 by Andreas Vesalius.

grow during embryogenesis they develop folds (*gyri*) separated by invaginations (*sulci* and, when deeper, *fissures*). This folding allows the cortex of the hemispheres to have a greater surface area. The extent and pattern of folding vary stereotypically between species, although like any trait there are quantitative differences between individuals of a particular species. Two major grooves, the central sulcus and the lateral (Sylvian) fissure, are used as anatomical landmarks in human cerebral hemispheres. The central sulcus extends more or less vertically along the lateral surface of the hemisphere where it approaches the horizontally oriented lateral fissure. Together they divide arbitrarily the external surface of the cerebral cortex into four lobes— *frontal*, *parietal*, *occipital*, and *temporal*—named after the corresponding cranial bones that lie over them. In addition, the *insular lobe* is folded completely inside the hemisphere (actually about two-thirds of the folded cortical surface lies buried and unexposed to the outer surface of the hemisphere), and the *limbic lobe* forms the medial border of the hemisphere along the interhemispheric fissure.

These lobes are only crude guides to the functional organization of the cerebral hemisphere. Over the course of the last century and a half, progressively better analysis has divided the cortical mantle into a mosaic of on the order of 50 to 100 areas with more or less distinct structural and functional characteristics. Perhaps the most famous and enduring maps of **cortical regionalization** were generated by Korbinian Brodmann in the first decade of the 20th century (Fig. 2.23), although refinements and alternative interpretations abound. Nevertheless, regionalization maps of the cerebral cortex are fundamentally important guides for understanding CNS architecture. Just as one example, virtually the entire thalamus projects topographically on the cortical mantle, which in turn projects topographically on the cerebral nuclei (basal ganglia). In one way or another, information from every sensory modality reaches the cerebral cortex, and it in turn sends inputs to virtually all parts of the motor system.

Most areas of each cerebral hemisphere modulate activity on the opposite or contralateral side of the

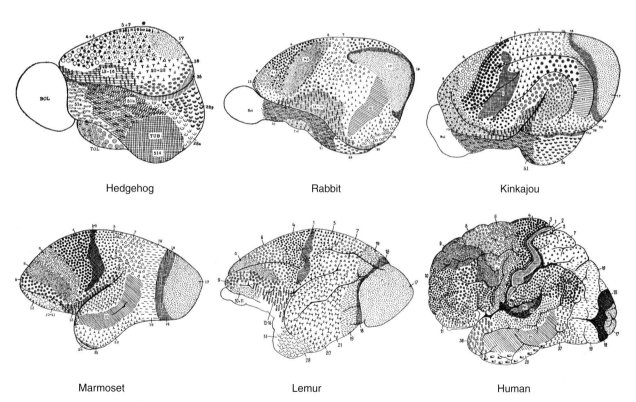

Hedgehog   Rabbit   Kinkajou

Marmoset   Lemur   Human

FIGURE 2.23 Regionalization of the mammalian cerebral cortex according to the work of Korbinian Brodmann (1909). His parceling of the cortex was based on regional differences in how neuronal cell bodies tend to be arranged in layers, an approach referred to as cytoarchitectonics. This figure illustrates his findings in six species, with different regions, or "areas" as he called them, indicated with different symbols and numbers. He distinguished 47 areas in the human cerebral cortex and showed that generally similar patterns apply to all nine of the mammalian species he studied.

body by way of descending pathways that eventually decussate (cross the midline) to reach parts of the motor system in the opposite side of the CNS. Furthermore, bundles of axons called *commissures* connect areas in the cerebral cortex of one hemisphere with the same or related areas in the opposite hemisphere, and different areas within the same hemisphere are interconnected by way of so-called **association pathways**. Commissural and association pathways allow comparison and integration of information between cortical areas within the same hemisphere, as well as between the two hemispheres.

Communication between the hemispheres is completely eliminated by commissurotomy, the surgical division of all the cerebral commissures. This procedure is sometimes performed as a treatment for severe cases of epilepsy to prevent epileptic activity that originates in one hemisphere from spreading to the other hemisphere, thus affecting both sides of the

body. Incredibly, commissurotomy patients function extremely well under most conditions, and behavioral studies of such patients have yielded some remarkable information about cerebral cortical organization. Axon bundles (tracts or pathways) that connect very dissimilar structures on the two sides of the CNS are usually referred to as *decussations* (in contrast to commissures, as discussed earlier).

The Nervous System is Protected by Membranous Coverings

The brain and spinal cord are completely surrounded by three connective tissue membranes: *pia mater*, *arachnoid mater*, and *dura mater*. Collectively, they are known as *meninges*. The pia ("faithful") is a very thin, vascular membrane. As its name suggests, the pia adheres closely to the surface of the CNS, even in regions where there are substantial invaginations,

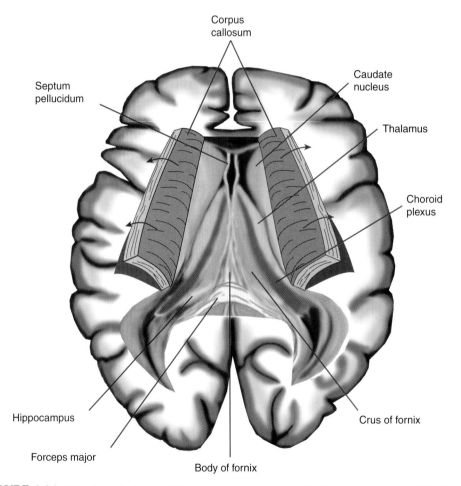

FIGURE 2.24 The choroid plexus of the ventricular system. In this horizontal section of the human brain, the ventricular system, normally filled with cerebrospinal fluid (CSF), is opened and the choroid plexus, which produces the CSF, is visible in the lateral ventricles (in red).

such as the surface of the cerebral and cerebellar cortex. Exterior to the pia is the arachnoid ("spidery"), which has a tenuous, web-like structure, but is histologically similar to the pia. The dura ("hard" or "strong") is a thick, inelastic covering that is closely apposed to the inner surface of the skull and vertebral canal. Membranes covering the CNS are continuous with similar coverings of the PNS, where the terminology is different.

In certain regions of the CNS neural tissue is absent but meninges persist. In these regions, ependymal cells of the ventricular system (the monolayer vestige of the embryonic neuroepithelium that ends up lining the adult ventricular system) fuse with the pia and arachnoid layers to form structures known as the *choriod plexus* (Fig. 2.24). The choroid plexus contains abundant blood vessels and serves as a component of the blood–brain barrier (the blood–CSF barrier). It produces CSF, which fills the ventricles of the brain and central canal of the spinal cord. CSF passes out of the interior of the brain through paired foramina (holes) in the fourth ventricle under the cerebellum and through a single foramen in the roof plate of the medulla. All of these openings lead to the subarachnoid space, which lies between the pia and arachnoid and is also filled with CSF.

The Brain is a Well-Vascularized Structure

The human brain consumes a full 20% of the body's oxygen supply at rest, even though it usually only weighs just over a kilogram. Therefore, the brain must continuously receive a voluminous blood supply, on the order of a liter per minute. Blood reaches the brain through two arterial roots: *vertebral* and *internal carotid* arteries. These arteries anastomose at the circle of Willis, located at the base of the brain (essentially surrounding the base of the hypothalamus, and stalk of the pituitary gland; Fig. 2.25). The importance of this anastomosis cannot be overemphasized because after this point there is a marked reduction in the extent of anastomoses between brain arteries. As a result, blockage or rupture of even a small artery or arteriole can rapidly deprive a brain region of oxygen, producing the condition known as a *stroke*.

After entering the skull through the foramen magnum along with the spinal cord, the paired vertebral arteries fuse into a single *basilar artery*, giving off the cerebellar arteries and the posterior cerebral arteries, which supply caudal regions of the cerebral hemispheres. The internal carotid arteries divide to form the anterior and middle cerebral arteries; the former

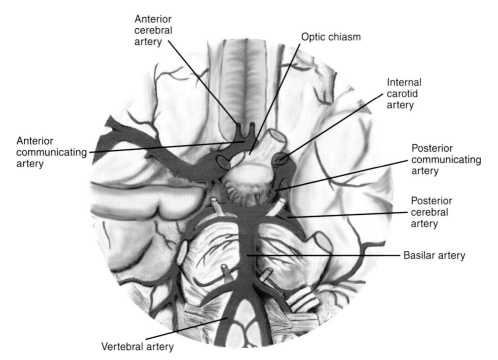

FIGURE 2.25 The circle of Willis (circulosis arteriosis or arterial circle) is located at the base of the brain. The circle consists of several arteries, which anastomose with each other, forming an alternative circulatory pathway when one of the arteries is compromised for whatever reason.

supplies the medial surface of each cerebral hemisphere, where it presses against the other hemisphere in the region of the limbic lobe, whereas the latter supplies the rest of the hemispheres (including the speech and somatic motor areas). By and large, the major arteries course along the cerebral surface before abruptly diving into the brain and dividing into arterioles and capillaries.

Numerous large *venous sinuses* collect blood from the capillary beds in the brain and return it to the heart, mostly via internal jugular veins. The major venous sinuses lie within the dura mater, whose inelasticity essentially holds the sinuses open. Blood flow through the sinuses is not very rapid, nor is it under great pressure. The presence of thin-walled venous sinuses surrounded by the tough and immovable dura sets the stage for serious injury to the sinuses when the head is subjected to physical trauma. Perhaps the best-known example is the traumatic injury to the great cerebral vein in the midline that can occur when a boxer is struck in the head. The impact of the blow causes the brain to recoil in its CSF cushion, exerting a shearing force against the dura, which remains attached to the skull. This force effectively ruptures the great cerebral vein, leading to serious hemorrhage of venous blood into the subdural space (between dura and arachnoid).

Summary

This chapter has considered some approaches to the problem of understanding the fundamental structure and wiring diagram of the nervous system—the basic plan or architecture. One approach is to examine a series of increasingly complex animals from an evolutionary perspective to gain insight into basic organizing principles. Such an examination reveals tendencies toward centralization, cephalization, bilateral symmetry, and regionalization of the nervous system. It also suggests that basic cellular (and molecular) mechanisms of neuronal function have changed little since the appearance of the simplest nervous systems in jellyfish and other cnidarians.

Another approach is to follow the development of the vertebrate nervous system from embryo to adult. At early stages of development, the CNS of all vertebrates has the same basic structure. A polarized, bilaterally symmetrical, regionalized neural plate of ectodermal origin invaginates to form a neural tube. The neural tube has three swellings in its rostral half—the forebrain, midbrain, and hindbrain vesicles—and the caudal half forms the primitive spinal cord. These four basic divisions of the CNS go on to subdivide repeatedly until all of the laminated and nuclear cell groups of the adult CNS are formed. A topographic or regional description of the CNS emerges from such a developmental approach.

How the functional systems or circuitry of the CNS is arranged into a unified whole is an unsolved problem. In the model discussed in this chapter, behavior is equated with motor output, which is driven by sensory, intrinsic behavioral state, and cognitive inputs, as well as by endogenous neuronal activity within the motor system itself. Future behavior is determined in part by sensory feedback related to the consequences of the original behavior. In the present state of knowledge, the relationship between functional systems and the regional architecture of the CNS is not obvious. The correspondence between functional neural systems and gene expression networks is even more obscure, although promising results are beginning to emerge in the developing spinal cord and brain stem cranial nerve nuclei.

References

Alvarez-Bolado, G., and Swanson, L. W. (1996). "Developmental Brain Maps: Structure of the Embryonic Rat Brain." Elsevier, Amsterdam.

Brodmann, K. (1909). "Vergleichende Lokalisationslehre der Grosshirnrinde in ihren Prinzipien dargestellt auf Grund des Zellenbaues." Barth, Leipzig. Translated as "Brodmann's 'Localisation in the Cerebral Cortex'" by L. J. Garey. Gordon-Smith, London, 1994.

Brusca, R. C., and Brusca, G. J. (1990). "Invertebrates." Sinauer, Sunderland.

Cajal, S. Ramón y (1911–1913). "Histologie du système nerveux de l'homme et des vertébrés," in 2 vols., Maloine, Paris. Translated as "Histology of the Nervous System of Man and Vertebrates" by N. Swanson and L. W. Swanson. Oxford Univ. Press, New York, 1995.

Cartmill, M., Hylander, W. L., and Shafland, J. (1987). "Human Structure." Harvard Univ. Press, Cambridge.

Hamburger, V. (1973). Anatomical and physiological basis of embryonic motility in birds and mammals. In "Studies on the Development of Behavior and the Nervous System" (G. Gottlieb, ed.), Vol. 1, p. 51076. Academic Press, New York.

Holland, L. Z., and Holland, N.D. (1999). Chordate origins of the vertebrate central nervous system. *Curr. Opin. Neurobiol.* **9**, 596–602.

Lentz, T. L. (1968). "Primitive Nervous Systems." Yale Univ. Press, New Haven.

McConnell, C. H. (1932) Development of the ectodermal nerve net in the buds of *Hydra. Quart. J. Micr. Sci.* **75**, 495–509.

Parker, G. H. (1919). "The Elementary Nervous System." Lippincott, Philadelphia.

Sherrington, C. S. (1906). "The Integrative Action of the Nervous System." Scribner's, New York. [Reprinted, Yale University Press, New Haven, 1947]

Swanson, L. W. (1992). "Brain Maps: Structure of the Rat Brain." Elsevier, Amsterdam.

Swanson, L. W. (2000a). What is the brain? *Trends Neurosci.* **23**, 519–527.

Swanson, L. W. (2000b) A history of neuroanatomical mapping. *In* "Brain Mapping: The Applications" (A. W. Toga and J. C. Mazziotta, eds.), pp. 77–109. Academic Press, San Diego.

Swanson, L. W. (2000c). Cerebral hemisphere regulation of motivated behavior. *Brain Res.* **886**, 113–164.

Von Neumann, J. (1958). "The Computer and the Brain." Yale Univ. Press, New Haven.

Wiener, N. (1948). "Cybernetics, or Control and Communication in the Animal and Machine." Wiley, New York.

Williams, P. L. (ed.) (1995). "Gray's Anatomy," 38th (British) ed. Churchill Livingstone, New York.

Suggested Readings

Bergquist, H., and Källén, B. (1954). Notes on the early histogenesis and morphogenesis of the central nervous system in vertebrates. *J. Comp. Neurol.* **100**, 627–659.

Björklund, A., and Hökfelt, T. (1983-present). "Handbook of Chemical Neuroanatomy." Elsevier, Amsterdam.

Descartes, R. (1972). "Treatise on Man." French text with translation by T. S. Steele. Harvard Univ. Press, Cambridge.

Herrick, C. J. (1948), "The Brain of the Tiger Salamander." University of Chicago Press, Chicago.

Kingsbury, B. F. (1922). The fundamental plan of the vertebrate brain. *J. Comp. Neurol.* **34**, 461–491.

Lorenz, K. (1978). "Behind the Mirror." Harcourt Brace Jovanovich, Orlando.

Nieuwenhuys, R., Voogd, J., and van Huijzen, C. (1988). "The Human Central Nervous System: A Synopsis and Atlas," 3rd Ed. Springer-Verlag, Berlin.

Russell, E. S. (1916). "Form and Function: A Contribution to the History of Animal Morphology." John Murray, London.

Tinbergen, N. (1951). "The Study of Instinct." Oxford Univ. Press, London.

Larry W. Swanson

CELLULAR AND MOLECULAR NEUROSCIENCE

3

Cellular Components of Nervous Tissue

Several types of cellular elements are integrated to yield normally functioning brain tissue. The neuron is the communicating cell, and a wide variety of neuronal subtypes are connected to one another via complex circuitries usually involving multiple synaptic connections. Neuronal physiology is supported and maintained by neuroglial cells, which have highly diverse and incompletely understood functions. These include myelination, secretion of trophic factors, maintenance of the extracellular milieu, and scavenging of molecular and cellular debris from it. Neuroglial cells also participate in the formation and maintenance of the blood–brain barrier, a multicomponent structure that is interposed between the circulatory system and the brain substance and that serves as the molecular gateway to the brain parenchyma.

THE NEURON

Neurons are highly polarized cells, meaning that they develop, in the course of maturation, distinct subcellular domains that subserve different functions. Morphologically, in a typical neuron, three major regions can be defined: (1) the cell body, or perikaryon, which contains the nucleus and the major cytoplasmic organelles; (2) a variable number of dendrites, which emanate from the perikaryon and ramify over a certain volume of gray matter and which differ in size and shape, depending on the neuronal type; and (3) a single axon, which extends, in most cases, much farther from the cell body than the dendritic arbor (Fig. 3.1). Dendrites may be spiny (as in pyramidal cells) or nonspiny (as in most interneurons), whereas the axon is generally smooth and emits

a variable number of branches (collaterals). In vertebrates, many axons are surrounded by an insulating myelin sheath, which facilitates rapid impulse conduction. The axon terminal region, where contacts with other cells are made, displays a wide range of morphological specializations, depending on its target area in the central or peripheral nervous system. Classically, two major morphological types of contacts, or *synapses*, may be recognized by electron microscopy: asymmetric synapses, responsible for the transmission of excitatory inputs, and symmetric or inhibitory synapses.

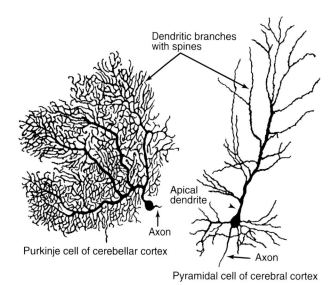

FIGURE 3.1 Typical morphology of projection neurons. (Left) A Purkinje cell of the cerebellar cortex and (right) a pyramidal neuron of the neocortex. These neurons are highly polarized. Each has an extensively branched, spiny apical dendrite, shorter basal dendrites, and a single axon emerging from the basal pole of the cell.

The cell body and dendrites are the two major domains of the cell that receive inputs, and dendrites play a critically important role in providing a massive receptive area on the neuronal surface. In addition, there is a characteristic shape for each dendritic arbor, which is used to classify neurons into morphological types. Both the structure of the dendritic arbor and the distribution of axonal terminal ramifications confer a high level of subcellular specificity in the localization of particular synaptic contacts on a given neuron. The three-dimensional distribution of dendritic arborization is also important with respect to the type of information transferred to the neuron. A neuron with a dendritic tree restricted to a particular cortical layer may receive a very limited pool of afferents, whereas the widely expanded dendritic arborizations of a large pyramidal neuron will receive highly diversified inputs within the different cortical layers in which segments of the dendritic tree are present (Fig. 3.2) (Mountcastle, 1978). The structure of the dendritic tree is maintained by surface interactions between adhesion molecules and, intracellularly, by an array of cytoskeletal elements (microtubules, neurofilaments, and associated proteins), which also take part in the movement of organelles within the dendritic cytoplasm.

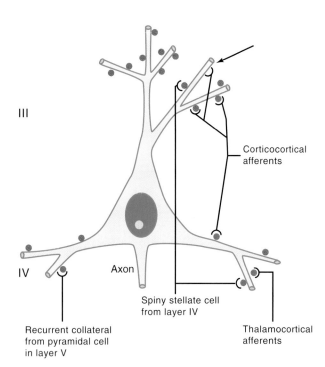

FIGURE 3.2 Schematic representation of four major excitatory inputs to pyramidal neurons. A pyramidal neuron in layer III is shown as an example. Note the preferential distribution of synaptic contacts on spines. Spines are labeled in red. Arrow shows a contact directly on the dendritic shaft.

An important specialization of the dendritic arbor of certain neurons is the presence of large numbers of dendritic spines, which are membrane-limited organelles that project from the surface of dendrites. They are abundant in large pyramidal neurons and are much sparser on the dendrites of interneurons. Spines are more numerous on the apical shafts of pyramidal neurons than on basal dendrites. As many as 30,000 to 40,000 spines are present on the largest pyramidal neurons. Spines constitute the region of the dendritic arborization that receives most of the excitatory input. Each spine generally contains one asymmetric synapse; thus, the approximate density of excitatory input on a neuron can be inferred from an estimate of its number of spines. The cytoplasm within the spines is characterized by the presence of polyribosomes and a variety of filaments, including actin and α- and β-tubulin, as well as a spine apparatus comprising cisternae, membrane vesicles, and stacks of dense lamellar material (see Box 3.1).

The perikaryon contains the nucleus and a variety of cytoplasmic organelles. Stacks of rough endoplasmic reticulum are conspicuous in large neurons and, when interposed with arrays of free polyribosomes are referred to as Nissl substance. Another feature of the perikaryal cytoplasm is the presence of a rich cytoskeleton composed primarily of neurofilaments and microtubules, discussed in detail in Chapter 4. These cytoskeletal elements are dispersed in "bundles" that extend into the axon and dendrites. Whereas dendrites and the cell body can be characterized as domains of the neuron that receive afferents, the axon, at the other pole of the neuron, is responsible for transmitting neural information. This information may be primary, in the case of a sensory receptor, or processed information that has already been modified through a series of integrative steps. The morphology of the axon and its course through the nervous system are correlated with the type of information processed by the particular neuron and by its connectivity patterns with other neurons. The axon leaves the cell body from a small swelling called the axon hillock. This structure is particularly apparent in large pyramidal neurons; in other cell types, the axon sometimes emerges from one of the main dendrites. At the axon hillock, microtubules are packed into bundles that enter the axon as parallel fascicles. The axon hillock is the part of the neuron from which the action potential is generated. The axon is generally unmyelinated in local circuit neurons (such as inhibitory interneurons), but it is myelinated in neurons that furnish connections between different parts of the nervous system. Axons usually have higher

BOX 3.1

SPINES

Spines are protrusions on the dendritic shafts of neurons and are the site of a large number of axonal contacts. Use of the silver impregnation techniques of Golgi or of the methylene blue used by Ehrlich in the late 19th century led to the discovery of spiny appendages on dendrites of a variety of neurons. The best known are those on pyramidal neurons and Purkinje cells, although spines occur on neuron types at all levels of the central nervous system. In 1896, Berkley observed that terminal boutons were closely apposed on spines and suggested that spines may be involved in conducting impulses from neuron to neuron. In 1904, Santiago Ramón y Cajal suggested that spines could collect the electrical charge resulting from neuronal activity. He also noted that spines substantially increase the receptive surface of the dendritic arbor, which may represent an important factor in receiving the contacts made by the axonal terminals of other neurons. It has been calculated that the approximately 4000 spines of a pyramidal neuron account for more than 40% of its total surface area (Peters *et al.*, 1991).

More recent analyses of spine electrical properties have demonstrated that spines are dynamic structures that can regulate many neurochemical events related to synaptic transmission and modulate synaptic efficacy. Spines are also known to undergo pathologic alterations and have a reduced density in a number of experimental manipulations (such as deprivation of a sensory input) and in many developmental, neurologic, and psychiatric conditions (such as dementing illnesses, chronic alcoholism, schizophrenia, trisomy 21). Morphologically, spines are characterized by a narrow portion emanating from the dendritic shaft, the neck, and an ovoid bulb or head. Spines have an average length of 2 μm despite considerable variability in morphology. At the ultrastructural level (Fig. 3.3), spines are characterized by the presence of asymmetric synapses and a few vesicles and contain fine and quite indistinct filaments. These filaments most likely consist of actin and α- and β-tubulins. Microtubules and neurofilaments present in dendritic shafts do not penetrate the spines. Mitochondria and free ribosomes are infrequent, although many spines contain polyribosomes in their head and neck. Interestingly, most polyribosomes in dendrites are located at the bases of spines, where they are associated with endoplasmic reticulum, indicating that spines possess the machinery necessary for the local synthesis of proteins.

Another classic feature of the spine is the presence of confluent tubular cisterns in the spine head that represent an extension of the dendritic smooth endoplasmic reticulum. Those cisterns are referred to as the spine apparatus. The function of the spine apparatus is not fully understood but may be related to the storage of calcium ions during synaptic transmission.

Patrick R. Hof, Bruce D. Trapp, Jean de Vellis, Luz Claudio, and David R. Colman

Reference

Peters, A., Polay, S. L., and Welston, H. deF. (1991). "The Fine Structure of the Nervous System: Neurons and Their Supporting Cells," 3rd Ed. Oxford Univ. Press, New York.

numbers of neurofilaments than dendrites, although this distinction can be difficult to make in small elements that contain fewer neurofilaments. In addition, the axon may be extremely ramified, as in certain local circuit neurons; it may give out a large number of recurrent collaterals, as in neurons connecting different cortical regions; or it may be relatively straight in the case of projections to subcortical centers, as in cortical motor neurons that send their very long axons to the ventral horn of the spinal cord. At the interface of axon terminals with target cells are the synapses, which represent specialized zones of contact consisting of a presynaptic (axonal) element, a narrow synaptic cleft, and a postsynaptic element on a dendrite or perikaryon. The fine structure of synapses is discussed later. In the next section, we turn our attention to the principal morphologic features of several neuronal types from the cerebral cortex, subcortical structures, and periphery as typical examples of the cellular diversity in the nervous system.

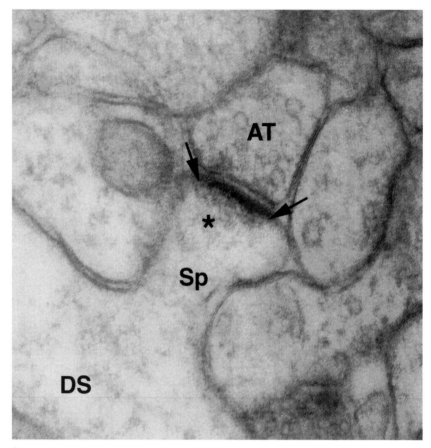

FIGURE 3.3   Ultrastructure of a single dendritic spine (Sp). Note the narrow neck emanating from the main dendritic shaft (DS) and the spine head containing filamentous material, cisterns of the spine apparatus, and the postsynaptic density of an asymmetric synapse (arrows). AT, axon terminal.

Pyramidal Cells Are the Main Excitatory Neurons in the Cerebral Cortex

All of the cortical output is mediated through pyramidal neurons, and the intrinsic activity of the neocortex can be viewed simply as a means of finely tuning their output. A pyramidal cell is a highly polarized neuron, with a major orientation axis perpendicular (or orthogonal) to the pial surface of the cerebral cortex. In cross section, the cell body is roughly triangular (Fig. 3.2), although a large variety of morphologic types exist with elongate, horizontal, or vertical fusiform, or inverted perikaryal shapes. A pyramidal neuron typically has a large number of dendrites that emanate from the apex and form the base of the cell body. The span of the dendritic tree depends on the laminar localization of the cell body, but it may, as in giant pyramidal neurons, spread over several millimeters. The cell body and dendritic arborization may be restricted to a few layers or, in some cases, may span the entire cortical thickness, (Jones, 1984).

In most cases, the axon of a large pyramidal cell extends from the base of the perikaryon and courses toward the subcortical white matter, giving off several collateral branches that are directed to cortical domains generally located within the vicinity of the cell of origin (as explained later). Typically, a pyramidal cell has a large nucleus, a cytoplasmic rim that contains, particularly in large pyramidal cells, a collection of granular material chiefly composed of lipofuscin. The deposition of lipofuscin increases with age and is considered a benign change. Although all pyramidal cells possess these general features, they can also be subdivided into numerous classes based on their morphology, laminar location, and connectivity (Fig. 3.4) (Jones, 1975). For instance, small pyramidal neurons in layers II and III of the neocortex have restricted dendritic trees and form vast arrays of axonal collaterals with neighboring cortical domains, whereas medium-to-large pyramidal cells in deep layer III and layer V have much more extensive dendritic trees and furnish long corticocortical connec-

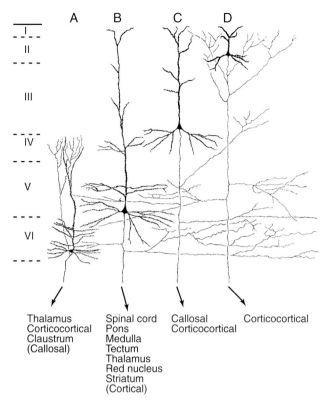

Thalamus
Corticocortical
Claustrum
(Callosal)

Spinal cord
Pons
Medulla
Tectum
Thalamus
Red nucleus
Striatum
(Cortical)

Callosal
Corticocortical

Corticocortical

FIGURE 3.4 Morphology and distribution of neocortical pyramidal neurons. Note the variability in cell size and dendritic arborization, as well as the presence of axon collaterals, depending on the laminar localization (I–VI) of the neuron. Also, different types of pyramidal neurons with a precise laminar distribution project to different regions of the brain. Adapted from Jones (1984).

tions. Layer V also contains very large pyramidal neurons arranged in clusters or as isolated, somewhat regularly spaced elements. These neurons project to subcortical centers such as the basal ganglia, brain stem, and spinal cord. Finally, layer VI pyramidal cells exhibit a greater morphologic variability than pyramidal cells in other layers and are involved in certain corticocortical as well as corticothalamic projections.

The excitatory inputs to pyramidal neurons can be divided into intrinsic afferents, such as recurrent collaterals from other pyramidal cells and excitatory interneurons, and extrinsic afferents of thalamic and cortical origin. Neurotransmitters in these excitatory inputs are thought to be glutamate and possibly aspartate. Although this division may appear relatively simplistic, the complexity and heterogeneity of excitatory transmission in the neocortex may not be derived from the presynaptic side, but rather from the postsynaptic side of the synapse. In other words, at the molecular level, a variety of glutamate receptor subunit combinations may confer different functional

capacities on a given glutamatergic synapse (see Chapter 9).

Pyramidal cells not only furnish the major excitatory output of the neocortex, but also act as a major intrinsic excitatory input through axonal collaterals. The collaterals of the main axonal branch that exits from the cortex are referred to as recurrent collaterals because they ascend back to superficial layers; thus, the collateral branches of a pyramidal cell synapse in layers superficial to their origin, although a deep or local system of branches is also present (see Fig. 3.4). Although many of these branches ascend in a radial, vertical pattern of arborization, there is a separate set of projections that travel horizontally over long distances (in some instances as much as 7–8 mm). One of the major functions of the vertically oriented component of the recurrent collaterals may be to interconnect layers III and V, the two major output layers of the neocortex. In layer III pyramidal cells, 95% of the synaptic targets of recurrent cells are other pyramidal cells. This is true of both vertical and distant horizontal recurrent projections. In addition, the majority of these synapses are on dendritic spines and, to some degree, on dendritic shafts. It is possible that there are regional and laminar specificities to these synaptic arrangements, although such fine patterns are not yet fully elucidated. These recurrent projections function to set up local excitatory patterns and coordinate multineuronal assemblies into an excitatory output.

Spiny Stellate Cells Are Excitatory Interneurons

The other major excitatory input to pyramidal cells of cortical origin is provided by the interneuron class referred to as spiny stellate cells, small multipolar neurons with local dendritic and axonal arborizations. These neurons resemble pyramidal cells in that they are the only other cortical neurons with large numbers of dendritic spines, but they differ from pyramidal neurons in that they lack an apical dendrite. Although the dendritic arbor of these neurons tends to be local, it can vary from a primarily radial orientation to one that is more horizontal. The relatively restricted dendritic arbor of these neurons is presumably a manifestation of the fact that they are high-resolution neurons that gather afferents to a very restricted region of the cortex. Dendrites rarely leave the layer in which the cell body resides. The spiny stellate cell also resembles the pyramidal cell in that it provides asymmetric synapses that are presumed to be excitatory, and, like pyramidal cells, these neurons are thought to use either glutamate or aspartate as their neurotransmitter.

Spiny stellate cells exhibit extensive regional and laminar specificities in their distribution. Spiny stellate cells are found in highest concentration in layers IVC and IVA of the primary visual cortex, where they constitute the predominant neuronal type. They are also found in high numbers in layer IV of other primary sensory areas. However, several cortical regions have relatively few of these neurons, and even in areas in which these neurons are well represented, they are vastly outnumbered by aspiny interneurons (Peters and Jones, 1984).

The axons of spiny stellate neurons are primarily intrinsic in their targets and radial in orientation and appear to play an important role in forming links among layer IV, the major thalamorecipient layer, and layers III, V, and VI, the major projection layers (Fig. 3.5). In some respects, the axonal arbor of spiny stellate cells mirrors the vertical plexuses of recurrent collaterals; however, they are more restricted than recurrent collaterals. Given its axonal distribution, the spiny stellate neuron appears to function as a high-fidelity translator of thalamic inputs, maintaining

strict topographic organization and setting up initial vertical links of information transfer within sensory areas. Presumably, both pyramidal cells and aspiny nonpyramidal cells receive these radially limited inputs of the spiny stellate neuron, suggesting that this interneuron plays a key role in setting up the excitatory component of a functional cortical domain (Peters and Jone, 1984).

Basket, Chandelier, and Double Bouquet Cells Are Inhibitory Interneurons

A large variety of inhibitory interneuron types are present in the cerebral cortex and in subcortical structures. These neurons contain the inhibitory neurotransmitter γ-aminobutyric acid (GABA) and exert strong local inhibitory effects. Three major subtypes of cortical interneurons are discussed in this section as examples. In all three cases, dendritic and axonal arborizations offer important clues to their role in the regulation of pyramidal cell function. In addition, for several GABAergic interneurons, a subtype of a given morphologic class can be defined further by a particular set of neurochemical characteristics. Although the following examples are taken from neurons prevalent in the neocortex and hippocampus of primates, inhibitory interneurons are present throughout the cerebral gray matter and exhibit a rich variety of morphologies, depending on the brain region, as well as on the species studied.

Basket Cells

This class of GABAergic interneuron takes its name from the fact that its axonal endings form a basket of terminals surrounding a pyramidal cell soma (see Fig. 3.6) (Somogyi et al., 1983). Basket cells can be divided into large and small cells. This cell class provides most of the inhibitory GABAergic synapses to the somas and proximal dendrites of pyramidal cells, although basket cells also synapse on the shaft of the apical dendrite. One basket cell may contact numerous pyramidal cells, and, in turn, several basket cells can contribute to the pericellular basket of one pyramidal cell. The basket cells have relatively large somas and multipolar morphology, with dendrites extending in all directions for several hundred micrometers such that the vertically oriented dendrites cross several layers. The axonal pattern is the defining characteristic of this cell. The axon arises vertically, bifurcates quickly, and travels long distances (1–2 mm), forming multiple pericellular arrays as it spreads horizontally. Basket cells predominate in layers III and V in the neocortex and preferentially innervate the pyramidal cells within these layers,

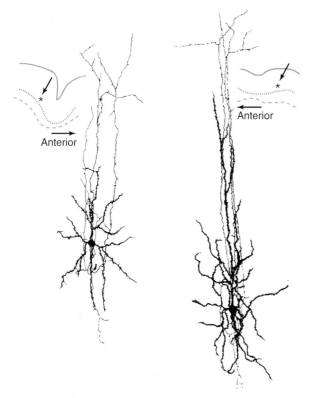

FIGURE 3.5 Drawing of Golgi-impregnated spiny stellate neurons in layer IV of the primary somatosensory cortex. Insets show the cortical localization of each neuron. The coarse branches represent the dendrites and fine branches represent the axonal plexus. Note that the axon is organized vertically. Adapted from Jones (1975).

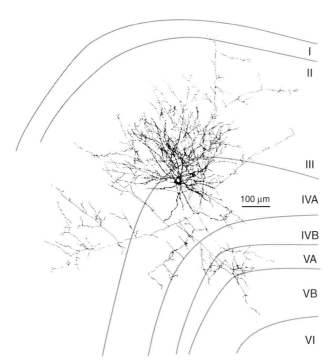

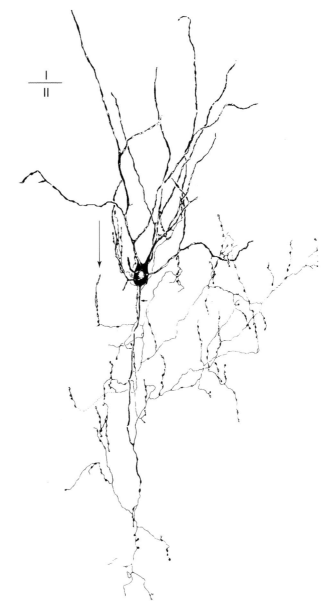

FIGURE 3.6 Drawing of a Golgi-impregnated basket cell from layer IVA of the primary visual cortex. Note the widely ramified dendritic tree and the wide horizontal spread of the axon that makes contact with many local neuronal perikarya. Cortical layers are indicated by Roman numerals. Adapted from Somogyi *et al.* (1983).

although they do not synapse exclusively on pyramidal cells. They are also numerous amid pyramidal neurons in the hippocampus. Thus, the basket cell is the primary source of horizontally directed inhibitory inputs to the soma, proximal dendrites, and apical shaft of a pyramidal neuron. Interestingly, these cells are also characterized by certain biochemical features in that the majority of them contain the calcium-binding protein parvalbumin, and cholecystokinin appears to be the most likely neuropeptide in large basket cells.

Chandelier Cells

The chandelier cell generally has a bitufted or multipolar dendritic tree, but the dendritic tree of this neuron is quite variable (Fig. 3.7) (Freund *et al.*, 1983). The defining characteristic of this cell class is the very striking appearance of its axonal endings. In Golgi or immunohistochemical preparations, axon terminals appear as vertically oriented "cartridges," each consisting of a series of axonal boutons, or swellings, linked together by thin connecting pieces. These axonal specializations look like old-style chandeliers, which explains why this cell type is so named. The most salient characteristic of the chandelier cell is the extraordinary specificity of its synaptic target. These

FIGURE 3.7 Drawing of an axoaxonic chandelier neuron from layer II of the primary visual cortex. The dendritic spread of this neuron is quite limited. Note the typical axon terminal specializations (arrow). Adapted from Freund *et al.* (1983).

neurons synapse exclusively on the axon initial segment of pyramidal cells. This characteristic is responsible for their alternate name, axoaxonic cells. Most of the chandelier cells are located in layer III, and their primary target appears to be layer III pyramidal cells, although they also synapse to a lesser extent on pyramidal cells in deep layers. One pyramidal cell may receive inputs from multiple chandelier cells, and one chandelier cell may innervate more than one pyramidal cell. Because of the high density of chandelier cell axon endings in layer III,

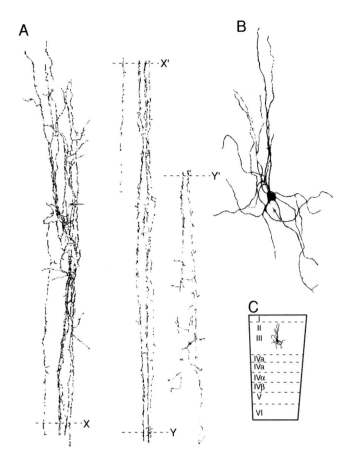

FIGURE 3.8 Drawing of a double bouquet cell in layer III of the primary visual cortex. The axonal tree (A) has been broken into three segments contiguous at X–X' and Y–Y' in order to display its entire radial extent. The arrow in B corresponds to the arrow in A. This neuron has very long radial axonal extensions, but very limited horizontal spread. Its location is shown in the inset C. Adapted from Somogyi and Cowey (1981).

this particular neuron may be highly involved in controlling corticocortical circuits. In addition, because the strength of the synaptic input is correlated directly with its proximity to the axon initial segment, there can be no more powerful inhibitory input to a pyramidal cell than that of the chandelier cell. Presumably, this interneuron is in a position that enables it to completely shut down the firing of a pyramidal cell (Freund *et al.*, 1983; DeFelipe *et al.*, 1989).

Double Bouquet Cells

The cell bodies of double bouquet cells are most prevalent in layers II and III, as well as being present in layer V of the neocortex. These interneurons are characterized by a vertical bitufted dendritic tree and a tight bundle of vertically oriented varicose axon collaterals that traverse layers II through V (Fig. 3.8)

(Somogyi and Cowey, 1981) and are therefore entirely different from those of chandelier and basket cells.

Of the inhibitory interneurons, the double bouquet cell serves as perhaps the best example of the emerging concept of cell typology in which connectivity, location, morphology, and neurochemical phenotype are all features the considered in "typing" a given cell. It is clear that neurochemical phenotype subdivides the double bouquet cell into multiple classes. For example, a GABA–calbindin–somatostatin double bouquet cell appears to be localized primarily in layers II and III and has 40% of its synapses on spines and the remaining synapses primarily on the distal shafts of pyramidal and nonpyramidal cells. Large numbers of this particular subtype of double bouquet cell are present in association cortices, with fewer in primary sensory cortices. Its regional, laminar, and synaptic organization suggests that it plays a crucial role in the regulation of pyramidal cells that furnish corticocortical projections. A different subclass of double bouquet cell contains calbindin and tachykinins as peptide neuromodulators. This subclass appears to have similar synaptic targets but is present primarily in layer V and thus presumably regulates the activity of a different group of pyramidal cells.

Other Interneuron Subtypes

Several other subtypes of interneurons can be distinguished on the basis of their morphology and neurochemical characteristics. A particularly interesting neuron is the poorly understood "clutch cell," which is driven primarily by thalamocortical inputs and, in turn, targets the spiny stellate cell of layer IV. Thus, this inhibitory interneuron is in essence situated so that it can regulate the firing rate of the spiny stellate cell in a fashion similar to how the three GABAergic neurons (basket, chandelier, and double bouquet) regulate the firing rate of pyramidal cells. Another important interneuron type is the bipolar neuron, which is characterized by elongated apical and basal dendrites and a locally ramifying axonal plexus, presumably making contacts with the apical dendrites of neighboring pyramidal cells. This cell is highly prevalent in the neocortex of rodents and has a modulatory role in the integration of cortical activity with noradrenergic projections from the brain stem. In the rat brain, some of these bipolar neurons may also contain the calcium-binding protein calretinin, but their homologue, if any, in the primate cortex remains to be determined.

Noncortical Neurons Have Distinct Morphological Characteristics

This section, reviews characteristics of four neuronal types found in subcortical structures: the medium-sized spiny cells of the basal ganglia, the dopaminergic neurons of the pars compacta of the substantia nigra, the Purkinje cell of the cerebellum, and the α motor neuron of the ventral horn of the spinal cord. The rationale for choosing these particular neurons as representative is that each plays a determinant role in the pathogenetic mechanisms of severe neurologic disorders that affect humans. Thus, degeneration of medium-sized spiny neurons is a central feature of Huntington disease; the death of dopaminergic neurons is the neuropathologic signature of Parkinson disease; the loss of Purkinje cells is seen in familial cerebellar cortical degeneration; and the degeneration of spinal cord motor neurons is the hallmark of lower motor neuron disease, a form of amyotrophic lateral sclerosis.

Medium-Sized Spiny Cells

These neurons are unique to the striatum, a part of the basal ganglia that comprises the caudate nucleus and putamen (see Chapter 31), where they are present in large numbers (as many as 10^8 in humans). Medium-sized spiny cells are scattered throughout the caudate nucleus and putamen and are recognized by their relatively large size, compared with other cel-

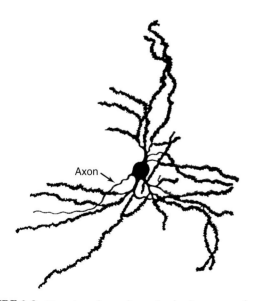

Axon

FIGURE 3.9 Drawing of a medium-sized spiny neuron from the striatum. Note the highly ramified dendritic arborization radiating in all directions and the very high density of spines. Adapted from Carpenter and Sutin (1983).

lular elements of the basal ganglia, and by the fact that they are generally isolated neurons. These neurons differ from all others in the striatum in that they have a highly ramified dendritic arborization radiating in all directions and densely covered with spines (Fig. 3.9) (Carpenter and Sutin, 1983). Medium-sized spiny neurons are central to the function of the basal ganglia because they furnish a major output from the caudate nucleus and putamen and receive a highly diverse input from, among other sources, the cerebral cortex, thalamus, and certain dopaminergic neurons of the substantia nigra. They have long axons that leave the basal ganglia and also form a large array of recurrent collaterals that innervate neighboring medium-sized spiny cells. These neurons are neurochemically quite heterogeneous, contain GABA, and may contain several neuropeptides such as enkephalin, dynorphin, substance P, and the calcium-binding protein calbindin. In Huntington disease, a neurodegenerative disorder of the striatum characterized by involuntary movements and progressive dementia, an early and dramatic loss of medium-sized spiny cells occurs. Interestingly, medium-sized spiny neurons that contain somatostatin appear to be relatively resistant to the degenerative process.

Dopaminergic Neurons of the Substantia Nigra

The substantia nigra is characterized by a rich diversity of neuronal types that exhibit differential distributions among the various functional compartments. Of these neurons, the most conspicuous are the large dopaminergic neurons that reside mostly within the pars compacta of the substantia nigra and in the ventral tegmental area. A distinctive feature of these cells is the presence of a pigment, neuromelanin, in compact granules in the cytoplasm. These neurons are medium-sized to large, fusiform, and frequently elongated; they have several large radiating dendrites. The axon emerges from the cell body or from one of the dendrites and projects to large expanses of cerebral cortex and to the basal ganglia. These neurons contain the catecholamine-synthesizing enzyme tyrosine hydroxylase, as well as the monoamine dopamine as their neurotransmitter; some of them colocalize calbindin and calretinin. These neurons are affected severely and selectively in Parkinson disease—a movement disorder different from Huntington disease and characterized by resting tremor and rigidity—and their specific loss is the neuropathologic hallmark of this disorder.

Purkinje Cells

The structure of the cerebellar cortex, in contrast with that of the cerebral cortex, is basically identical all over; it is composed of three layers that contain very distinct neuronal types. One of these layers contains Purkinje cells, which are the most salient cellular elements of the cerebellar cortex. They are arranged in a single row throughout the entire cerebellar cortex between the molecular (outer) layer and the granular (inner) layer. They are the largest cerebellar neurons and have a round perikaryon with a highly branched dendritic tree shaped like a candelabrum and extending into the molecular layer where they are contacted by incoming systems of afferent, parallel fibers from granule neurons as well as other afferents from the brain stem (see Chapter 31). The apical dendrites of Purkinje cells have an enormous number of spines (more than 80,000 per cell). A particular feature of the dendritic tree of the Purkinje cell is that it is distributed in one plane, perpendicular to the longitudinal axes of the cerebellar folds, and each dendritic arbor determines a separate domain of cerebellar cortex (Fig. 3.1). The axons of Purkinje neurons course through the cerebellar white matter and contact deep cerebellar nuclei or vestibular nuclei. They also furnish recurrent collaterals, mostly within the granular layer. Humans have approximately 15 million Purkinje cells. These neurons contain the inhibitory neurotransmitter GABA and the calcium-binding protein calbindin. A severe disorder combining ataxic gait and impair-ment of fine hand movements, accompanied by dysarthria and tremor, has been documented in some families and is related directly to Purkinje cell degeneration.

Spinal Motor Neurons

Motor cells of the ventral horns of the spinal cord, also called α motor neurons, have their cell bodies within the spinal cord and send their axons outside the central nervous system to innervate the muscles. Different types of motor neurons are distinguished by their targets. The alpha motor neurons innervate skeletal muscles, but smaller motor neurons (the γ motor neurons, forming about 30% of the motor neurons) innervate the spindle organs of the muscles (see Chapter 28). The α motor neurons are some of the largest neurons in the entire central nervous system (CNS) and are characterized by a multipolar perikaryon and a very rich cytoplasm that renders them very conspicuous on histological preparations. They have a large number of spiny dendrites that arborize locally within the ventral horn. The α motor neuron axon leaves the central nervous system through the ventral root of the peripheral nerves. The cell bodies are arranged in a nonrandom fashion in the ventral horn so that they are grouped in functional vertical columns that span a certain number of spinal segments. This disposition corresponds to a somatotopic representation of the muscle groups of the limbs and axial musculature (Brodal, 1981). Spinal motor neurons use acetylcholine as their neurotransmitter. Large motor neurons are severely affected in lower motor neuron disease (a form of amyotrophic lateral sclerosis), a neurodegenerative disorder characterized by progressive muscular weakness that affects, at first, one or two limbs and that can be initially asymmetric. As the disease progresses, it becomes symmetric and affects more and more of the body musculature, which shows signs of wasting as a result of denervation. Neuropathologically, a massive loss of ventral horn motor neurons occurs, and the remaining motor neurons appear shrunken and pyknotic.

Retinal Photoreceptors and Cochlear Hair Cells Are Examples of Specialized Sensory Receptors

Retinal photoreceptors and cochlear hair cells are modified neuroepithelial cells that are specialized in the initial transduction of visual and acoustic stimuli, respectively. Comparable specialized neuronal types exist for other sensory modalities; i.e. that is, olfactory, gustatory, and vestibular inputs. In contrast, somatosensory inputs are transmitted by peripheral nerve cells whose endings are associated with a variety of sensory structures in the peripheral tissues. Receptor neurons are extremely polarized cells, with one uniquely diversified end that is responsible for the reception of the sensory stimulus. This morphology is particularly well demonstrated in retinal photoreceptors. Photoreceptor cells are of two types, the rod and the cone, which are specialized for scotopic (light/dark) and color vision, respectively (see Chapter 27). The rods are slender cells, with an elongated cylindrical outer portion, whereas the cones are smaller elements, with shorter, conical outer portions (Fig. 3.10) (Krebs and Krebs, 1991). Each cell type consists of an outer and an inner segment. The inner segments of both rods and cones contain the metabolic machinery necessary for protein and lipid synthesis and oxidative metabolism. In rods, the outer segment is composed of a very large number of parallel lamellae stacked perpendicularly to the main axis of the cylinder. These lamellae are closed, flattened membranous discs that appear in thin-section electron microscopy as pairs of parallel membranes. In cones, these lamellar stacks are less numerous. These structures are responsible for the mechanisms of phototransduction and contain several visual pigments, located inside the membranous discs, that are necessary for the absorption of light. Cochlear (and vestibular) hair cells are also highly polarized and present striking apical differentiation specialized in the detection of

endolymphatic movements in the inner ear. In the cochlea, receptor hair cells that detect stimuli produced by sound are short, goblet-like cells embedded in supporting cells (the phalangeal cells of Deiters). Their apical domain contains a U-shaped row of stereocilia (hairs) that are in contact with the tectorial membrane of the organ of Corti. Vibrations of this membrane, generated by sound waves in the endolymph, displace the hairs and initiate transduction of the acoustic stimulus (see Chapter 26). The other pole of the hair cell contains the nucleus and a dense population of mitochondria and receives synaptic contacts from afferent and efferent fibers from the cochlear nerve, which spreads around the lower third of the receptor cell (Fig. 3.11) (Hudspeth, 1983).

Enteric Motor Neurons Form an Independent Neural Plexus in the Gut Wall

The enteric nervous system constitutes a part of the autonomic nervous system that innervates the gastrointestinal tract, as do the sympathetic and parasympathetic systems. Although all three systems take part in the regulation of intestinal function, the enteric system is by far the most important and has the unique feature that it can function relatively independent of the control of higher centers. The enteric system consists of an extremely rich plexus of nerve fibers and neurons disseminated among all of the layers that form the wall of the intestinal tract (Fig. 3.12). It contains nerve cells arranged in ganglia interconnected by complex bundles of fibers that extend from the lower third of the esophagus to the internal anal sphincter. In humans, this system contains about 107 to 108 neurons.

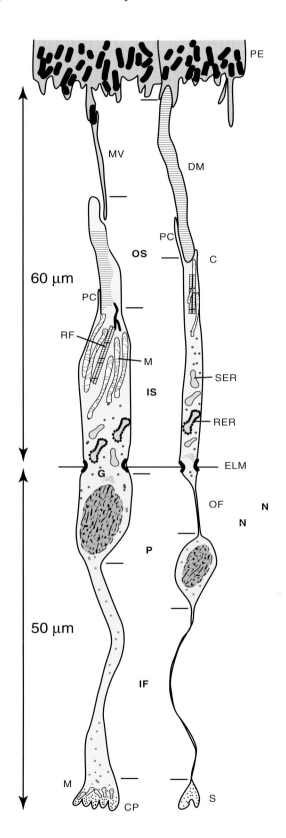

FIGURE 3.10 Drawing of a cone (left) and a rod (right) from monkey retina. Note the difference in shape and size of these cells. They are composed of an outer segment (OS), an inner segment (IS), a perikaryon (P), and an inner fiber (IF). The outer segment is connected to the inner segment by a thin connecting cilium (C). The outer fiber (OF) is thin and well visible in rods, whereas the perikaryon of both cell types has a comparable appearance. In cones, the inner fiber is thicker and ends as a large cone pedicle, whereas in rods, the inner fiber is rather thin and terminates in a unique spherule. Cone pedicles (CP) and rod spherules (S) are specialized synaptic endings where photoreceptors make contact with specific subtypes of retinal relay neurons. DM, membranous discs (lamellae); ELM, external limiting membrane; G, Golgi apparatus; M, mitochondria, MV, microvilli of pigment epithelium; N, nucleus; PC, calycoid process; PE, pigment epithelium; RER, SER, rough and smooth endoplasmic reticulum; RF, rootlet fibers. Adapted from Krebs and Krebs (1991).

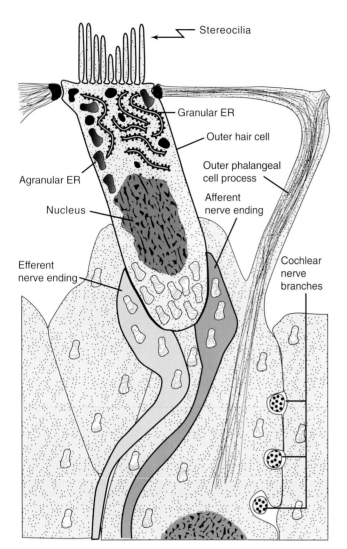

FIGURE 3.11   Schematic drawing of an electron micrograph of an outer hair cell and its relationships to supporting (outer phalangeal) cell and cochlear nerve endings. Note the apical domain containing stereocilia. The other pole of the hair cell contains the nucleus and a dense population of mitochondria and receives synaptic contacts from the cochlear nerve, which spread around the lower third of the receptor cell.

The principal enteric plexus is located between circular and longitudinal layers of the muscularis and is known as the myenteric plexus of Auerbach. It is composed of ganglia, each containing from 3 to 50 neurons linked by unmyelinated fibers and forming a continuous network. The cells in this plexus are of two main morphological types. One is a large multipolar neuron with short dendrites in direct contact with similar nearby cells and a long axon that contacts different cell types in neighboring ganglia. These cells are thought to be association interneurons. The other cell type, considered an enteric motor

neuron, is by far more dominant and demonstrates more variable morphology. These cells make extensive contacts with neurons of either type within the same ganglia or with distant cells. Other ganglia are found within the submucosal plexus of Meissner. Their relatively large multipolar neurons form a network interconnecting the outer nerve bundles with the submucosal tissue.

The neurochemistry of the enteric system is extremely complex and still poorly understood. A large number of classical neurotransmitters, such as acetylcholine, GABA, and noradrenaline, have been identified in enteric nerve fibers and ganglionic neurons. In addition, enteric neurons in both myenteric and submucosal plexuses contain a variety of neuropeptides. Neurons in the submucosal plexus are enriched in somatostatin, substance P, and vasoactive intestinal peptide but do not seem to contain Leu-enkephalin, which is observed in myenteric nerve cells. It is not clear, however, whether these neuropeptides are the principal transmitters of subclasses of enteric neurons or are colocalized compounds that act as local neuromodulators.

Summary

The neuron is one of the more highly specialized cell types and is the critical cellular element in

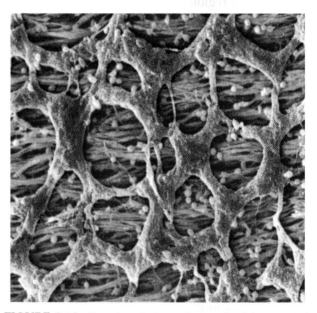

FIGURE 3.12   Scanning electron micrograph of the myenteric plexus in the intestine. Note dense axonal bundles and synaptic boutons (pseudo-colored green) and the network of large multipolar neurons with relatively short extensions contacting neighboring cells (pseudo-colored red).

the brain. All neurological processes are dependent on complex cell–cell interactions between single neurons and/or groups of related neurons. Neurons can be described according to their size, shape, neurochemical characteristics, location, and connectivity.

The size, shape, and neurochemistry of the neuron are important determinants of that particular functional role of the neuron in the brain. In this respect, there are three general classes of neurons: the inhibitory GABAergic interneurons that make local contacts, the local excitatory spiny stellate cells in the cerebral cortex, and the excitatory glutamatergic efferent neurons, exemplified by cortical pyramidal neurons. Within these general classes, the structural variation of neurons is systematic, and careful analyses of the anatomic features of neurons have led to various categorizations and to the development of the concept of cell type. The grouping of neurons into descriptive cell types (such as chandelier, double bouquet, or bipolar cells) allows the analysis of populations of neurons and the linking of specified cellular characteristics with certain functional roles. The relevant characteristics may include morphology, location, connectivity, and biochemistry.

Also, neurons form circuits, and these circuits constitute the structural basis for brain function. Macrocircuits involve a population of neurons projecting from one brain region to a distant region, and microcircuits reflect the local cell–cell interactions within a brain region. The detailed analysis of these macro- and microcircuits is an essential step in understanding the neuronal basis of a given cortical function in the healthy and the diseased brain. Thus, these cellular characteristics allow us to appreciate the special structural and biochemical qualities of that neuron in relation to its neighbors and to place it in the context of a specific neuronal subset, circuit, or function.

NEUROGLIA

The term neuroglia, or "nerve glue," was coined in 1859 by Rudolph Virchow, who conceived of the neuroglia as an inactive "connective tissue" holding neurons together in the central nervous system. The metallic staining techniques developed by Ramón y Cajal and del Rio-Hortega allowed these two great pioneers to distinguish, in addition to the ependyma lining the ventricles and central canal, three types of supporting cells in the CNS: oligodendrocytes, astrocytes, and microglia. In the peripheral nervous system

(PNS), the Schwann cell is the major neuroglial component.

Oligodendrocytes and Schwann Cells Synthesize Myelin

The more complex the brain, the more interconnections must be formed and maintained. As shown in depth later, there is a practical limit to how fast an individual bare axon can conduct an action potential. Thus, neurons and their associated processes cannot communicate with each other extremely rapidly through the action potential without some help. Organisms have developed two kinds of solutions for enhancing rapid communication between neurons and their effector organs. In invertebrates, the diameters of individual axons that must conduct rapidly are enlarged. In vertebrates, the myelin sheath (Fig. 3.13) has evolved to permit rapid nerve conduction.

Axon enlargement accelerates the rate of conduction of the action potential greatly, which increases with axonal diameter. The net effect, therefore, is that small axons conduct at a much slower rate than larger ones. The largest axon in the invertebrate kingdom is the squid giant axon, which is about the thickness of a mechanical pencil lead. It conducts the action potential extremely rapidly, and the axon itself mediates an escape reflex, which must be rapid if the animal is to survive. An obvious trade-off in a nervous system with 10 billion neurons, as in the human brain, is that all axons cannot be as thick as pencil lead, or each human head would be very large indeed.

Thus, along the invertebrate evolutionary line, there is a natural, insurmountable limit—a constraint imposed by axonal size—to increasing the processing capacity of the nervous system beyond a certain point. Vertebrates, however, devised a way to get around this problem through evolution of the myelin sheath, allowing the tremendous evolutionary advantage of increased rapidity of conduction of the nerve impulse along axons with fairly minute diameters. As we know, neurons interact in complex ways with the other cell types that exist within the nervous system. Virtually all axons, for example, are wrapped or ensheathed by cells that subserve what is vaguely termed a "supportive" or "trophic" function. This is true in invertebrate as well as vertebrate nervous systems. Along the vertebrate lineage, however, certain ensheathing cells have become highly specialized to generate vast quantities of plasma membrane that is compacted to form the myelin sheath, which supports rapid nerve conduction.

Not all axons in central or peripheral nervous systems are myelinated, and one of the puzzles is to

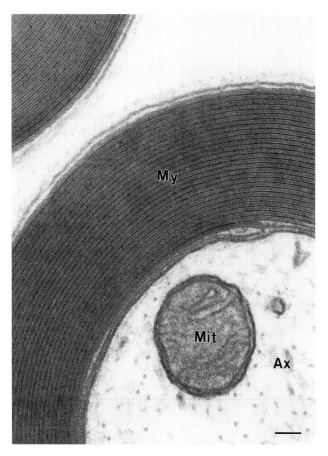

FIGURE 3.13 An electron micrograph of a transverse section through part of a myelinated axon from the sciatic nerve of a rat. The tightly compacted multilayer myelin sheath (My) surrounds and insulates the axon (Ax). Mit, mitochondria. Scale bar: 75 nm.

not have to be regenerated continually along the axonal segment that is covered by the myelin membrane sheath. This leaping of the action potential from node to node allows axons with fairly small diameters to conduct extremely rapidly (Ritchie, 1984). The jumping of the action potential from node to node along a given axon is called saltatory conduction.

The evolution of a system in which a single oligodendrocyte cell body is responsible for the construction and maintenance of several myelin sheaths (Fig. 3.14) and the removal of the cytoplasm between each turn of the myelin lamellae so that only the thinnest layer of plasma membrane is left have resulted in saving a huge amount of intracranial space. Brain volume is thus reserved for further expansion of neuronal populations.

Conservation of space in the peripheral nervous system does not seem to have presented such a pressing problem. Myelin in the PNS is generated by Schwann cells (Fig. 3.15), each of which wraps only a single axonal segment. The biochemical composition of the myelin derived in the CNS and the composition of that derived in the PNS differ somewhat, although there are common proteins found in each nervous system subdivision. Myelin has a high lipid-to-protein ratio, and the lipids are specialized. The myelin sheath has become an excellent model system for studying the generation or formation of specialized plasma membrane and membrane adhesionbecause each layer of the multilayered myelin sheath must adhere to the adjacent layers. This adhesion is largely accomplished by protein–protein interactions, which have been best studied in the PNS.

The major integral membrane protein of peripheral nerve myelin is protein zero (P0), a member of a very large family of proteins termed the immunoglobulin gene superfamily. These proteins have in common recognition or adhesion functions or both and, although the primary amino acid sequences differ among the members of this family, all members are related to one another by certain common structural motifs. Members of the immunoglobulin (Ig) gene superfamily have one or more Ig-like domains that contain cysteines placed about 100 amino acids or so apart. These cysteines are linked to one another by disulfide bridges. Most of these Ig domains are displayed on the extracellular surfaces of cells, where they can act as ligands or receptors. Protein zero is relatively simple in primary structure, consisting of a single Ig-like domain, a transmembrane segment, and a highly charged (basic) cytoplasmic domain. This protein makes up about 80% of the protein complement of peripheral nerve myelin. Interactions between the extracellular domains of P0 molecules

determine why some are selected for myelination and others remain unmyelinated. It is believed that early in the nervous system development of an organism, signals relayed between the axon and the myelinating cell determine whether the "myelination program" is triggered in that cell. These signals have not yet been identified.

In the central nervous system, the myelin sheath (Fig. 3.14) is elaborated by oligodendrocytes, nonneuronal glial cells that, during brain development, send out a few cytoplasmic processes that engage adjacent axons, some of which go on to become myelinated (Bunge, 1968). Myelin itself consists of a single sheet of oligodendrocyte plasma membrane, which is wrapped tightly around an axonal segment. Each myelinated segment of an axon is termed an internode because, at the end of each segment, there is a bare portion of the axon, the node of Ranvier, that is flanked by another internode. Physiologically, myelin has insulating properties such that the action potential can "leap" from node to node and therefore does

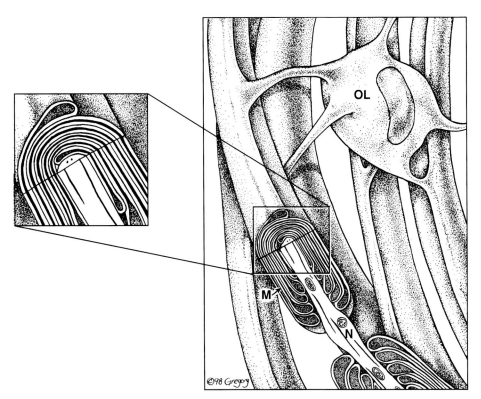

FIGURE 3.14 An oligodendrocyte (OL) in the central nervous system is depicted myelinating several axon segments. A cutaway view of the myelin sheath is shown (M). Note that the internode of myelin terminates in paranodal loops that flank the node of Ranvier (N). (Inset) An enlargement of compact myelin with alternating dark and light electron-dense lines that represent intracellular (major dense lines) and extracellular (intraperiod line) plasma membrane appositions, respectively.

expressed on one layer of the myelin sheath with those of the apposing layer yield a characteristic regular periodicity that can be seen by thin-section electron microscopy (Fig. 3.13). This zone, called the intraperiod line, represents the extracellular apposition of the myelin bilayer as it wraps around itself. On the other side of the bilayer, the cytoplasmic side, the highly charged P0 cytoplasmic domain probably functions to neutralize the negative charges on the polar head groups of the phospholipids that make up the plasma membrane itself, allowing the membranes of the myelin sheath to come into close apposition with one another. In electron microscopy, this cytoplasmic apposition is a bit darker than the intraperiod line and is termed the major dense line. In peripheral nerves, although other molecules are present in small quantities in compact myelin and may have important functions, compaction (i.e., the close apposition of membrane surfaces without intevening cytoplasm) is accomplished solely by P0–P0 interactions at both extracellular and intracellular (cytoplasmic) surfaces.

Protein zero is a "perfect" plasma-membrane compactor, allowing the close apposition of adjacent bilayers such that the space between them effectively prevents the passage of anything but small ions and water along the compacted bilayer surfaces. It is in effect a "streamlined" Ig superfamily molecule that probably arose *de novo* with development of the myelin sheath. Curiously, P0 is not present in all myelin sheaths in the central nervous system of every species—an evolutionary paradox that has attracted much attention. In fish, P0 is present in both central and peripheral nervous systems, where it performs its compaction function, as the major integral membrane protein. However, in terrestrial vertebrates (reptiles, birds, and mammals), P0 is limited to the PNS and so is not found in the central nervous system. Instead, the compaction function is probably subserved by totally unrelated molecules, the DM-20 protein and its insertion isoform, the myelin proteolipid protein (PLP). These two proteins are generated from the same gene and are identical to each other with the exception that the proteolipid protein has, in addition, a positively charged segment exposed on the cytoplasmic aspect of the bilayer. Both PLP and DM20 are extremely hydrophobic and traverse the bilayer four times, and so have hydrophilic segments exposed on both cytoplasmic and extracellular surfaces of the

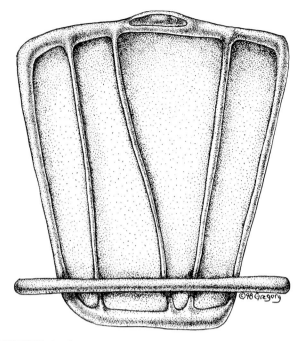

FIGURE 3.15   An "unrolled" Schwann cell in the PNS is illustrated in relation to the single axon segment that it myelinates. The broad stippled region is compact myelin surrounded by cytoplasmic channels that remain open even after compact myelin has formed, allowing an exchange of materials among the myelin sheath, the Schwann cell cytoplasm, and perhaps the axon as well.

bilayer. In this respect, the topology of these molecules is very similar to that of connexins and other polypeptides that are known to function in channel or pore formation.

A large number of naturally occurring neurological mutations can affect the proteins specific to the myelin sheath. These mutations have been named according to the phenotype that is produced: the shiverer mouse, the shaking pup, the rumpshaker mouse, the jimpy mouse, the myelin-deficient rat, the quaking mouse, and so forth. Many of these mutations have been well characterized, and their analyses have allowed us to begin to understand at a molecular level what the proteins affected by each mutation actually do in the formation and maintenance of the myelin sheath (see Box 3.2).

The first neurologic mutation that was studied in this respect was the shiverer mouse, in which the gene that encodes a major set of peripheral membrane proteins, the myelin basic proteins (MBPs), is functionally deleted. Normally, these proteins serve to seal the cytoplasmic aspects of the myelin bilayer, possibly by charge neutralization similar in function to the cytoplasmic tail of P0. When gene expression of these proteins is completely compromised, as in the shiverer, the cytoplasmic aspects fail to appose and do not

fuse, and a mouse that exhibits tremors and convulsions ("shivers") as it walks is produced. This is a naturally occurring mutation and was the first neurological mutation whose effects were cured by gene transfer. This was accomplished by the introduction of an intact MBP gene into the shiverer genome. The shiverer mutation is autosomal recessive, but even a single allele of the gene (i.e., the heterozygote MBP+/MBP–) produces sufficient myelin to phenotypically at least "cure" the shiverer of its overtly abnormal shivering behavior. These heterozygotes myelinate to somewhat less extent than normal, but the fact that the shiverer phenotype is eliminated in the heterozygote even though the number of myelin sheaths around each axon is reduced indicates that there is a built-in safety factor in the normal situation.

Astrocytes Play Important Roles in CNS Homeostasis

As the name suggests, astrocytes are star-shaped, process-bearing cells distributed throughout the central nervous system. They constitute from 20 to 50% of the volume of most brain areas. Astrocytes come in many shapes and forms. The two main forms, protoplasmic and fibrous astrocytes, predominate in gray and white matter, respectively (Fig. 3.16). Embryonically, astrocytes develop from radial glial cells, which transversely compartmentalize the neural tube. Radial glial cells serve as scaffolding for the migration of neurons and play a critical role in defining the cytoarchitecture of the CNS (Fig. 3.17). As the CNS matures, radial glia retract their processes and serve as progenitors of astrocytes. However, some specialized astrocytes of a radial nature are still found in the adult cerebellum and the retina and are known as Bergmann glial cells and Müller cells, respectively.

Astrocytes "fence in" neurons and oligodendrocytes. Astrocytes achieve this isolation of the brain parenchyma by extending long processes projecting to the pia mater and the ependyma to form the glia limitans, by covering the surface of capillaries, and by making a cuff around the nodes of Ranvier. They also ensheath synapses and dendrites and project processes to cell somas (Fig. 3.18). Astrocytes are connected to each other by gap junctions, forming a syncytium that allows ions and small molecules to diffuse across the brain parenchyma. Astrocytes have in common unique cytological and immunological properties that make them easy to identify, including their star shape, the glial end feet on capillaries, and a unique population of large bundles of intermediate filaments. These filaments are composed of an

BOX 3.2

INHERITED PERIPHERAL NEUROPATHIES

The peripheral myelin protein-22 (PMP22) is a very hydrophobic glycoprotein and is highly expressed in compact PNS myelin. It has been mapped to the previously defined Tr locus on mouse chromosome 11. Comparison of marker genes on mouse chromosome 11 and human chromosome 17 revealed that PMP22 was also a candidate gene for the most common form of autosomal-dominant demyelinating hereditary peripheral neuropathy in humans, Charcot–Marie–Tooth disease type 1A (CMT1A). Indeed, the entire PMP22 gene is contained within a 1.5-Mb intrachromosomal duplication on chromosome 17p11.2, a genetic abnormality that had been linked to CMT1A by human molecular genetics. Consistent with these results, PMP22 is overexpressed in CMT1A patients who carry the characteristic duplication. The crucial role of PMP22 in the etiology of CMT1A was confirmed by generating transgenic mice and rats with increased PMP22 gene dosage, which resulted in severe PNS myelin deficits.

CMT is one of the more frequent hereditary diseases of the nervous system, with an overall prevalence of approximately 1 in 4000, and CMT1A duplication accounts for around 70% of all cases. Why is this chromosomal abnormality so common? Detailed analysis of the CMT1A locus suggests that the duplication is due to crossing over involving repetitive sequences that flank the monomeric region. If correct, such a mechanism should also generate an allele carrying the reciprocal deletion of the same region. Indeed, the expected deletion is associated with the relatively mild recurrent neuropathy hereditary neuropathy with liability to pressure palsy (HNPP). Thus, overexpression and underexpression of the myelin protein PMP22 are associated with myelin deficiencies in distinct human diseases. Although one might speculate from these data that correct stochiometry of myelin protein expression is crucial for a myelinating Schwann cell, the exact disease mechanism remains to be clarified. Interestingly, the finding that a myelin protein was responsible for CMT1A led to the discovery that two other components of PNS myelin are mutated in rare forms of CMT1. The adhesion protein P0, which is largely responsible for PNS myelin compaction, is affected in CMT1B, and an X-linked form of CMT (CMTX) has been linked to mutations in the gap junction protein connexin-32. In contrast to PMP22 and P0, connexin-32 is located in uncompacted lamellae of PNS myelin, where it is thought to facilitate the exchange of small molecules via reflexive gap junctions between adaxonal and abaxonal aspects of myelinating Schwann cells.

Finally, there is a striking correlation between the role of PMP22 in the PNS and that of PLP/DM20 in the CNS with respect to biology and involvement in disease; both genes can be affected by various genetic mechanisms, including gene duplication and gene deletion. However, despite our vast knowledge derived from human molecular genetics, the molecular functions of both proteins are largely unknown. Given the findings that PMP22 and PLP/DM20 are members of extended gene families and may be involved in the control of cell proliferation and cell death, these proteins may have broader functions than simply being stabilizing building blocks of compact myelin.

In summary, the combination of basic and clinical sciences has led to substantial progress in our current understanding of common hereditary neuropathies. Using clinical, genetic, and cell biology approaches in concert, we will continue to learn more about disease mechanisms involved in neuropathies to the benefit of the clinic as much as to our understanding of myelin biology.

Ueli Suter

astroglial-specific protein commonly referred to as glial fibrillary acidic protein (GFAP). S-100, a calcium-binding protein, and glutamine synthetase are also astrocyte markers. Ultrastructurally, gap junctions (connexins), desmosomes, glycogen granules, and membrane orthogonal arrays are distinct features used by morphologists to identify astrocytic cellular processes in the complex cytoarchitecture of the nervous system.

For a long time, astrocytes were thought to physically form the blood–brain barrier (considered later in this chapter), which prevents the entry of cells and diffusion of molecules into the CNS. In fact, astrocytes are indeed the blood–brain barrier in lower species. However, in higher species, astrocytes are responsible for inducing and maintaining the tight junctions in endothelial cells that effectively form the barrier. Astrocytes also take part in angiogenesis, which may

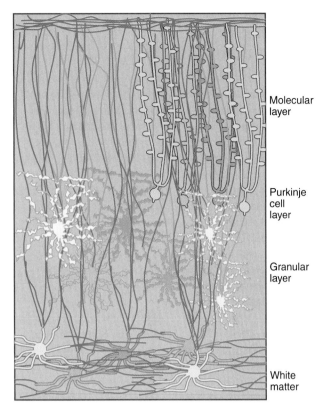

FIGURE 3.16 The arrangement of astrocytes in human cerebellar cortex. Bergmann glial cells are in red, protoplasmic astrocytes are in green, and fibrous astrocytes are in blue.

be important in the development and repair of the CNS. However, their role in this important process is still poorly understood.

Astrocytes Have a Wide Range of Functions

There is strong evidence for the role of radial glia and astrocytes in the migration and guidance of neurons in early development. Astrocytes are a major source of extracellular matrix proteins and adhesion molecules in the CNS; examples are nerve cell–nerve cell adhesion molecule (N-CAM), laminin, fibronectin, cytotactin, and the J-1 family members janusin and tenascin. These molecules participate not only in the migration of neurons, but also in the formation of neuronal aggregates, so-called nuclei, as well as networks.

Astrocytes produce, *in vivo* and *in vitro*, a very large number of growth factors. These factors act singly or in combination to selectively regulate the morphology, proliferation, differentiation, or survival, or all four, of distinct neuronal subpopulations. Most of the growth factors also act in a specific manner on the development and functions of astrocytes and oligodendrocytes. The production of growth factors and cytokines by astrocytes and their responsiveness to these factors is a major mechanism underlying the developmental function and regenerative capacity of

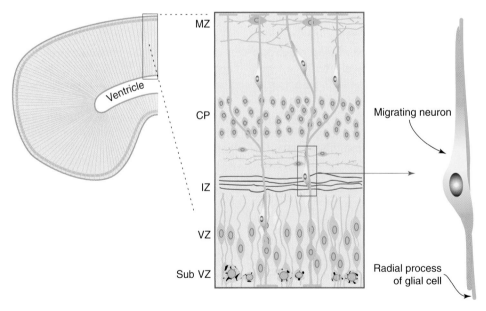

FIGURE 3.17 Radial glia perform support and guidance functions for migrating neurons. In early development, radial glia span the thickness of the expanding brain parenchyma. (Inset) Defined layers of the neural tube from the ventricular to the outer surface: VZ, ventricular zone; IZ, intermediate zone; CP, cortical plate; MZ, marginal zone. The radial process of the glial cell is indicated in blue, and a single attached migrating neuron is depicted at the right.

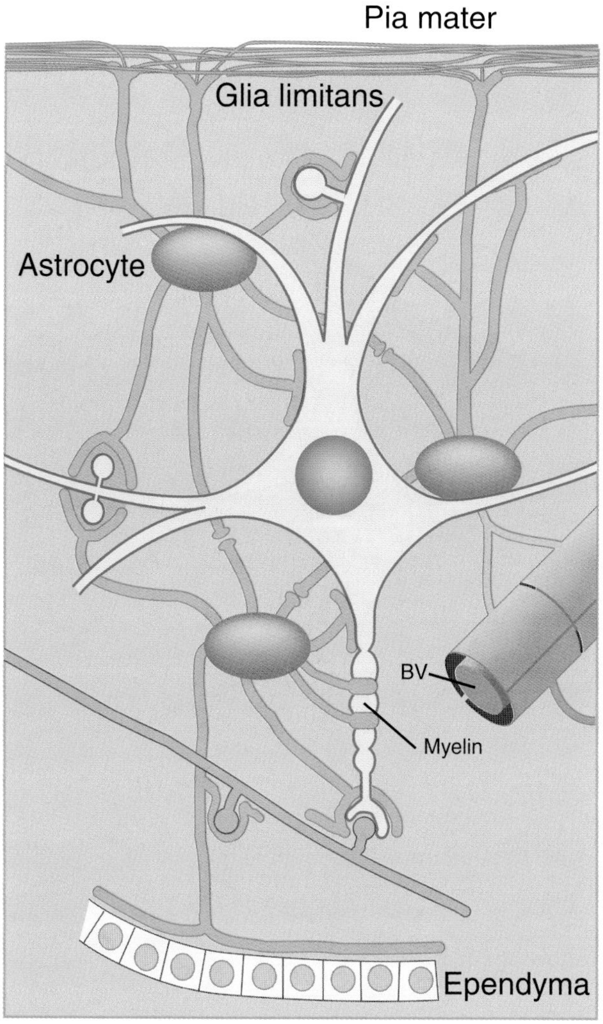

Pia mater

Glia limitans

Astrocyte

BV

Myelin

Ependyma

FIGURE 3.18 Astrocytes (in orange) are depicted *in situ* in schematic relationship with other cell types with which they are known to interact. Astrocytes send processes that surround neurons and synapses, blood vessels, and the region of the node of Ranvier and extend to the ependyma, as well as to the pia mater, where they form the glial limitans.

the CNS. During neurotransmission, neurotransmitters and ions are released at high concentration in the synaptic cleft. The rapid removal of these substances is important so that they do not interfere with future synaptic activity. The presence of astrocyte processes around synapses positions them well to regulate neurotransmitter uptake and inactivation (Kettenman and Ransom, 1995). These possibilities are consistent with the presence in astrocytes of transport systems for many neurotransmitters. For instance, glutamate reuptake is performed mostly by astrocytes, which convert glutamate into glutamine and then release it into the extracellular space. Glutamine is taken up by neurons, which use it to generate glutamate and γ-

aminobutyric acid, potent excitatory and inhibitory neurotransmitters, respectively (Fig. 3.19). Astrocytes contain ion channels for K^+, Na^+, Cl^-, HCO_3, and Ca^{2+}, as well as displaying a wide range of neurotransmitter receptors. K+ ions released from neurons during neurotransmission are soaked up by astrocytes and moved away from the area through astrocyte gap junctions. This is known as "spatial buffering." Astrocytes play a major role in detoxification of the CNS by sequestering metals and a variety of neuroactive substances of endogenous and xenobiotic origin.

In response to stimuli, intracellular calcium waves are generated in astrocytes. Propagation of the Ca^{2+} wave can be visually observed as it moves across the cell soma and from astrocyte to astrocyte. The generation of Ca^{2+} waves from cell to cell is thought to be mediated by second messengers, diffusing through gap junctions (see Chapter 11). Because they develop postnatally in rodents, gap junctions may not play an important role in development. In the adult brain, gap junctions are present in all astrocytes. Some gap junctions have also been detected between astrocytes and neurons. Thus, they may participate, along with astroglial neurotransmitter receptors, in the coupling of astrocyte and neuron physiology.

In a variety of CNS disorders–neurotoxicity, viral infections, neurodegenerative disorders, HIV, AIDS, dementia, multiple sclerosis, inflammation, and trauma–astrocytes react by becoming hypertrophic and, in a few cases, hyperplastic. A rapid and huge upregulation of GFAP expression and filament formation is associated with astrogliosis. The formation of reactive astrocytes can spread very far from the site of origin. For instance, a localized trauma can recruit astrocytes from as far as the contralateral side, suggesting the existence of soluble factors in the mediation process. Tumor necrosis factor (TNF) and ciliary neurotrophic factors (CNTF) have been identified as key factors in astrogliosis.

Microglia are Mediators of Immune Responses in Nervous Tissue

The brain has traditionally been considered an "immunologically privileged site," mainly because the blood–brain barrier (see later) normally restricts the access of immune cells from the blood. However, it is now known that immunological reactions do take place in the central nervous system, particularly during cerebral inflammation. Microglial cells have been termed the tissue macrophages of the CNS, and they function as the resident representatives of the

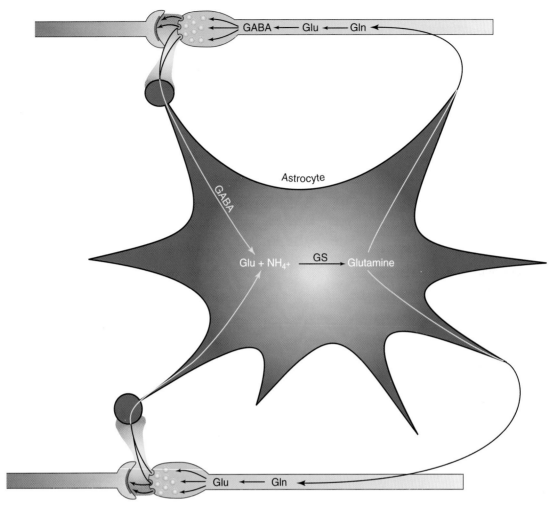

FIGURE 3.19 The glutamate–glutamine cycle is an example of a complex mechanism that involves an active coupling of neurotransmitter metabolism between neurons and astrocytes. The systems of exchange of glutamine, glutamate, GABA, and ammonia between neurons and astrocytes are highly integrated. The postulated detoxification of ammonia and the inactivation of glutamate and GABA by astrocytes are consistent with the exclusive localization of glutamine synthetase in the astroglial compartment.

immune system in the brain. These cells are perhaps the least understood of the CNS cells. Although the function of microglia in the normal adult CNS remains to be clarified, a rapidly expanding literature describes microglia as major players in CNS development and in the pathogenesis of CNS disease. The notion that the CNS is an immune-privileged organ is no longer valid. A hallmark of microglia cells is their ability to become reactive and to respond to pathological challenges in a variety of ways.

The first description of microglia cells can be traced to Franz Nissl (1899), who used the term "rod cell" to describe a population of glial cells that reacted to brain pathology. He postulated that rod-cell function was similar to that of leukocytes in other organs. Cajal

described microglia as part of his "third element" of the CNS—cells that he considered to be of mesodermal origin and distinct from neurons and astrocytes (Ramón y Cajal, 1913).

Del Rio-Hortega (1932) divided Cajal's third element into oligodendrocytes and microglia, two cell types with different morphology, function, and origin. He used silver impregnation methods to visualize the ramified appearance of microglia in the adult brain, and he concluded that ramified microglia could transform into cells that were migratory, ameboid, and phagocytic. A fundamental question raised by Del Rio-Hortega's studies was the origin of microglial cells. Although he provided evidence that microglia originated from cells that migrate into the brain from the pial surface, he also raised the possibility that microglia originate from blood "mononuclears." Controversy over the lineage of microglia still exists today.

Microglia Have Diverse Functions in Developing and Mature Nervous Tissue

Four different sources of microglia have been proposed (Dolman, 1991): (1) bone marrow-derived monocytes, (2) mesodermal pial elements, (3) neural epidermal cells, and (4) capillary-associated pericytes. On the basis of current knowledge, it appears that most ramified microglia cells are derived from bone marrow-derived monocytes, which enter the brain parenchyma during early stages of brain development. These cells help phagocytose degenerating cells that undergo programmed cell death as part of normal development. They retain the ability to divide and have the immunophenotypic properties of monocytes and macrophages. In addition to their role in remodeling the CNS during early development, microglia may secrete cytokines or growth factors that are important in fiber tract development, gliogenesis, and angiogenesis. After the early stages of development, ameboid microglia cells transform into the ramified microglia cells that persist throughout adulthood (Altman, 1994).

Little is known about microglial function in the normal adult vertebrate CNS. Microglia constitute a formidable percentage (5–20%) of the total cells in the mouse brain. Microglia are found in all regions of the brain, and there are more in gray than in white matter. The phylogenetically newer regions of the CNS (cerebral cortex, hippocampus) have more microglia than older regions (brain stem, cerebellum). Species variations have also been noted, as human white matter has three times more microglia than rodent white matter.

Microglia usually have small rod-shaped somas from which numerous processes extend in a rather symmetrical fashion. Processes from different microglia rarely overlap or touch, and specialized contacts between microglia and other cells have not been described in the normal brain. Although each microglial cell occupies its own territory, microglia collectively form a network that covers much of the CNS parenchyma. Because of the numerous processes, microglia present extensive surface membrane to the CNS environment. Regional variation in the number and shape of microglia in the adult brain suggests that local environmental cues can affect microglial distribution and morphology. On the basis of these morphological observations, it is likely that

microglia play a role in tissue homeostasis. The nature of this homeostasis remains to be elucidated. It is clear, however, that microglia can respond quickly and dramatically to alterations in the CNS microenvironment.

Microglia Become Activated in Pathological States

"Reactive" microglia can be distinguished from resting microglia by two criteria: (1) change in morphology and (2) upregulation of monocyte–macrophage molecules (Fig. 3.20). Although the two phenomena generally occur together, reactive responses of microglia can be diverse and restricted to subpopulations of cells within a microenvironment. Microglia not only respond to pathological conditions involving immune activation, but also become activated in neurodegenerative conditions that are not considered immune mediated. This latter response is indicative of the phagocytic role of microglia. Microglia change their morphology and antigen expression in response to almost any form of CNS injury.

Summary

Neuroglia are a set of cell types that together subserve supportive and trophic roles critical for the normal functioning of nervous tissue. Certain glial cells e.g., the myelinating cells, have clearly shaped nervous system evolution and development in that they evolved to facilitate rapid conduction of the action potential along small-caliber axons. The coordinated integrative functions of the vertebrate brain therefore depend on a normal complement of myelinated axons. Astrocytes and microglial cells also have major and extremely important functions in development and in tissue injury, but these roles are not as well understood as yet. In pathological states of all kinds (autoimmune, toxic insult, trauma), these cells react to contain and limit tissue damage. They also contribute in a major way to repair mechanisms.

CEREBRAL VASCULATURE

Blood vessels form an extremely rich network in the central nervous system, particularly in the cerebral cortex and subcortical gray masses, whereas the white matter is less densely vascularized (Fig. 3.21) (Duvernoy et al., 1981). The vascular bed is supplied by perforating arteries that arise from a relatively

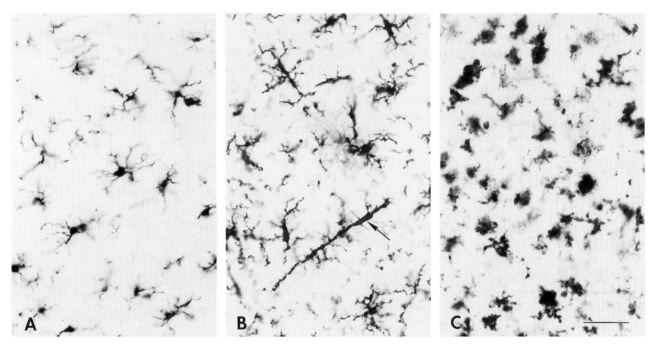

FIGURE 3.20 Activation of microglial cells in a tissue section from human brain. Resting microglia in normal brain (A). Activated microglia in diseased cerebral cortex (B) have thicker processes and larger cell bodies. In regions of frank pathology (C) microglia transform into phagocytic macrophages, which can also develop from circulating monocytes that enter the brain. Arrow in B indicates rod cell. Sections stained with antibody to ferritin. Scale bar = 40 μm.

small number of large, peripheral arterial trunks. The main trunks give off smaller cerebral arteries whose branches penetrate the subarachnoidal space, where they divide into many subbranches before penetrating the brain tissue. Within the cerebral gray matter, these penetrating arteries divide into a large number of small arterioles that eventually form an extremely rich, highly anastomotic capillary bed. At the other end of the capillary network are veinules, draining into larger cerebral veins, which are the tributaries of large venous sinuses responsible for returning blood to the general circulation. The brain vascular system has no end arteries, and there is a relatively free circulation throughout the central nervous system. There are, however, distinct regional patterns of microvessel distribution in the brain. These patterns are particularly clear in certain subcortical structures that constitute discrete vascular territories and in the cerebral cortex, where regional and laminar patterns are striking. For example, layer IV of the primary visual cortex possesses an extremely rich capillary network in comparison with other layers and adjacent regions (Fig. 3.21). Interestingly, most of the inputs from the visual thalamus terminate in this particular layer. Whether similar functional correlations may be derived from comparable vascular patterns in other brain regions remains to be determined. Nonetheless,

capillary densities are higher in regions containing large numbers of neurons and where synaptic density is high. Penetrating arteries and draining veins have well-defined, tree-shaped branching patterns. With regard to cortical vessels, some arteries divide in the upper cortical layers, whereas others penetrate to the lower layers before dividing. The branches of penetrating arteries define local vascular fields of approximately similar size and shape around the vessel of origin, which cover the entire cortical mantle in a continuous network.

Pathologic factors that affect the patency of brain microvessels may result in the development of an ischemic injury localized to a variable amount of tissue, depending on the size and location of the affected arteries. For instance, progressive occlusion of a large arterial trunk, as seen in stroke, induces an ischemic injury that may eventually lead to necrosis of the brain tissue. The size of the resulting infarction is determined in part by the worsening of the blood circulation through the cerebral microvessels. In fact, occlusion of a large arterial trunk results in rapid swelling of the capillary endothelium and surrounding astrocytes, which may reduce the capillary lumen to about one-third of its normal diameter, preventing red blood cell circulation and oxygen delivery to the tissue. The severity of these changes subsequently

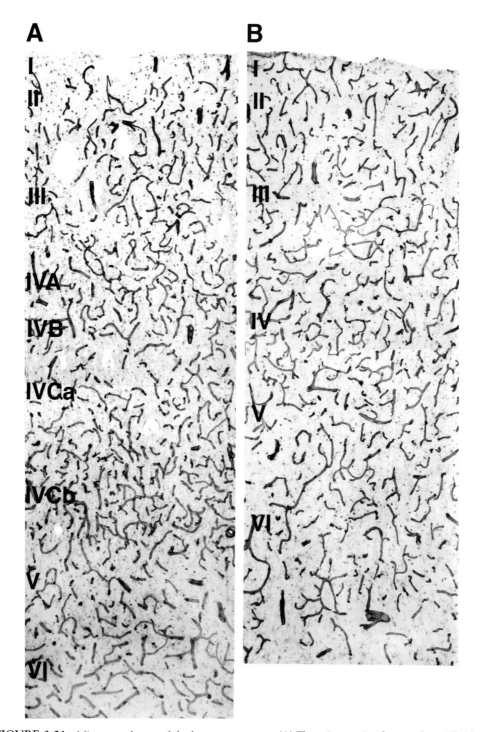

FIGURE 3.21 Microvasculature of the human neocortex. (A) The primary visual cortex (area 17). Note the presence of segments of deep penetrating arteries that have a larger diameter than the microvessels and run from the pial surface to the deep cortical layers, as well as the high density of microvessels in the middle layer (layers IVCA and IVCb). (B) The prefrontal cortex (area 9). Cortical layers are indicated by Roman numerals. Microvessels are stained using an antibody against heparan sulfate proteoglycan core protein, a component of the extracellular matrix.

determines the time course of neuronal necrosis, as well as the possible recovery of the surrounding tissue and the neurological outcome of the patient. In addition, the presence of multiple microinfarcts caused by occlusive lesions of small cerebral arterioles may lead to a progressively dementing illness, referred to as vascular dementia, affecting elderly humans.

The Blood–Brain Barrier Maintains Intracerebral Milieu

Capillaries of the central nervous system form a protective barrier that restricts the exchange of solutes between blood and brain. This distinct function of brain capillaries is called the blood–brain barrier (Figs. 3.22 and 3.23) (Bradbury, 1979). Capillaries of the retina have similar properties and are termed the blood–retina barrier. It is thought that the blood–brain and blood–retina barriers function to maintain a constant intracerebral milieu, critical for neuronal function. This function is important because of the nature of intercellular communication in the CNS, which includes chemical signals across intercellular spaces. Without a blood–brain barrier, circulating factors in the blood, such as certain hormones, which can also act as neurotransmitters, would interfere with synaptic communication. When the blood–brain barrier is disrupted, edema fluid accumulates in the brain,

leading to neurological impairments. Increased permeability of the blood– brain barrier plays a central role in many neuropathological conditions, including multiple sclerosis, AIDS, and childhood lead poisoning, and may also play a role in Alzheimer disease. (Box 3.3). The blood–brain barrier is composed of three cellular components—endothelial cells, pericytes, and astrocytes—and one noncellular component—the basement membrane. These components interact with each other to produce a highly selective and dynamic barrier system.

In general, the cerebral capillaries are comparable to those seen in other tissues (Peters *et al.*, 1991). The capillary wall is composed of an endothelial cell surrounded by a very thin (about 30 nm) basal lamina, similar to that seen in capillaries in peripheral tissues. End feet of perivascular astrocytes are apposed against this continuous basal lamina. Around the capillary lies a virtual perivascular space occupied by another cell type, the pericyte, which surrounds the capillary walls. The endothelial cell forms a thin monolayer around the capillary lumen, and a single endothelial cell can completely surround the lumen of the capillary (Fig. 3.23). The cytoplasm is rich in actin

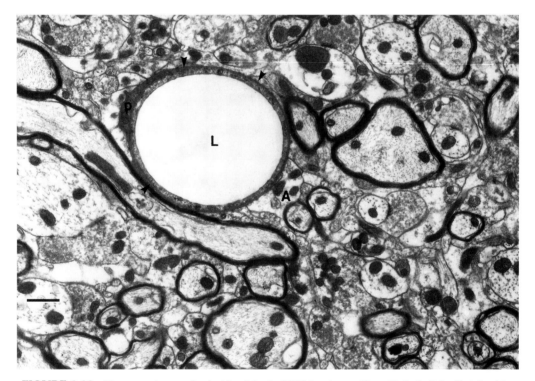

FIGURE 3.22 Electron micrograph of a blood–brain (BBB) barrier capillary. Endothelial cells joined by tight junctions form continuous capillaries with no fenestrations and restrict the passage of solutes between blood and brain. Pericytes (P) are present within the basement membrane (arrowheads) of these capillaries, serve to control vascular tone, and can also be phagocytic in the brain. Astrocyte foot processes (A) surround the basement membrane and are responsible for the induction of BBB properties on endothelial cells. L, lumen of the capillary. Bar: 2 μm.

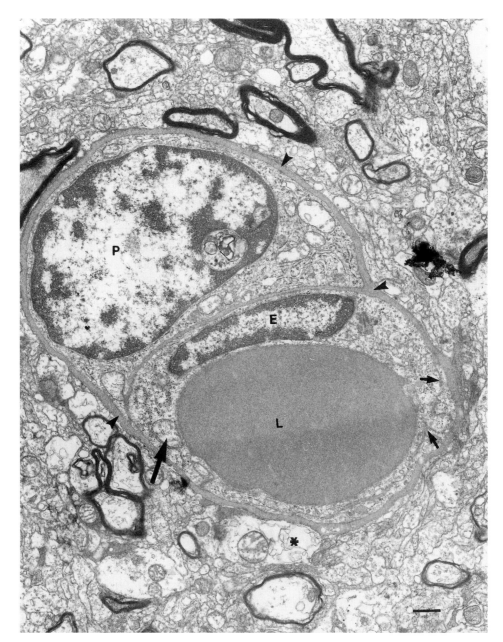

FIGURE 3.23 Human cerebral capillary obtained at biopsy. Blood–brain barrier (BBB) capillaries are characterized by the paucity of transcytotic vesicles in endothelial cells (E), a high mitochondrial content (large arrow), and the formation of tight junctions (small arrows) between endothelial cells that restrict the transport of solutes through the interendothelial space. The capillary endothelium is encased within a basement membrane (arrowheads), which also houses pericytes (P). Outside the basement membrane are astrocyte foot processes (asterisk), which may be responsible for the induction of BBB characteristics on the endothelial cells. L, lumen of the capillary. Bar: 1 μm. From Claudio *et al.* (1995).

filaments and contains an extensive Golgi apparatus and high numbers of mitochondria.

A fundamental difference between brain endothelial cells and those of the systemic circulation is the presence in brain of interendothelial tight junctions, also known as zonula occludens. In the systemic circulation, the interendothelial space serves as a diffusion pathway that offers little resistance to most blood solutes entering the surrounding tissues. In contrast, blood–brain barrier tight junctions effectively restrict the intercellular route of solute transfer. The blood–brain barrier interendothelial junctions are not static

BOX 3.3

HIV-ASSOCIATED DEMENTIA COMPLEX

Infection with the human immunodeficiency virus (HIV) begins with an acute flu-like syndrome that is followed by a chronic, subclinical infection. Years to decades later, CD4 T lymphocytes are depleted and the patient develops acquired immune deficiency syndrome (AIDS). Approximately a quarter of AIDS patients develop a neurodegenerative disorder termed HIV-associated dementia complex (HIVD). The clinical syndrome HIVD is notable for cognitive, motor, and behavioral abnormalities that suggest a preponderance of subcortical damage. Early neurological symptoms appear to be reversible; however, a progressive neurological deficit becomes fixed later.

Autopsy studies have shown an unusual encephalitis associated with HIVD. Abundant activated macrophages are distributed throughout deep gray and white matter structures and less so in neocortical gray matter. HIV itself was found at high levels in the CNS of demented patients and associated with the peculiar neuropathology. However, the abundance of HIV in these lesions remains controversial.

There are two groups of theories regarding the pathogenesis of neuronal damage in HIVD. The first group builds on the possibility that HIV proteins are neurotoxic. In support of this possibility, retroviral envelope proteins in general are known to be cytotoxic, and HIV envelope proteins in particular have been shown to be neurotoxic. A variety of direct and indirect mechanisms have been suggested to mediate this neurotoxicity. More recently the HIV transcription factor tat has been suggested to act through a novel receptor mechanism to mediate neuroglial dysfunction. In some of the model systems of HIV neurotoxicity, macrophages and/or astrocytes form critical intermediaries in propagating the neurotoxicity. The second group of theories suggests that neuronal degeneration results from the release of a wide variety of macrophage factors. Studies of CSF and brain tissues of AIDS cases have demonstrated a wide variety of such factors. The emerging consensus of these studies is that there is a variable presence of lymphokines and a more consistent presence of monokines and chemokines in the CNS of AIDS subjects. Thus, it is possible that these factors trigger neuronal degeneration.

Pharmacological control of systemic HIV replication slows the progression of AIDS and has increased patient survival dramatically. Unfortunately, even with optimal therapy, immunosuppression eventually develops and patients succumb to AIDS. How the pharmacological manipulation of systemic HIV infection will impact the CNS infection is not clear. However, at the present time, even with highly active antiretroviral therapy, immunosuppression eventually develops and HIVD continues to appear in approximately one-quarter of infected individuals.

Clayton A. Wiley

Suggested Readings

Budka, H. (1991). Neuropathology of human immunodeficiency virus infection. *Brain Pathol.* **1**, 163–175.
Sanders, V. J., Wiley, C. A., and Hamilton, R. L. (2001). The mechanisms of neuronal damage in retroviral infections of the nervous system. *Curr. Top. Microbiol. Immunol.* **253**, 179–201.

seals; rather they are a series of active gates that can allow certain small molecules to penetrate. One such molecule is the lithium ion, used in the control of manic depression.

Another characteristic of endothelial cells of the brain is their low transcytotic activity. This is illustrated by the paucity of transcytotic vesicles in the cytoplasm compared with endothelial cells of the systemic circulation. The frequency of transcytotic vesicles tends to increase with increasing permeability of an endothelium. Brain endothelium, therefore, is by this index not very permeable. It is of interest that certain regions of the brain, such as the area postrema and periventricular organs, lack a blood–brain barrier.

In these regions, the perivascular space is in direct contact with the nervous tissue, and endothelial cells are fenestrated and show many pinocytotic vesicles. In these brain regions, neurons are known to secrete hormones and other factors that require rapid and uninhibited access to the systemic circulation.

Because of the high metabolic requirements of the brain, blood–brain barrier endothelial cells must have transport mechanisms for the specific nutrients needed for proper brain function. One such mechanism is glucose transporter isoform 1 (GLUT-1), which is expressed asymmetrically on the surface of blood–brain barrier endothelial cells. In Alzheimer disease, the expression of GLUT-1 on brain endothelial cells is reduced. This reduction may be due to a lower metabolic requirement of the brain after extensive neuronal loss. Other specific transport mechanisms on the cerebral endothelium include the large neutral amino acid carrier-mediated system that transports, among other amino acids, L-3,4-dihydroxyphenylalanine (L-dopa), used as a therapeutic agent in Parkinson disease. Also on the surface of blood–brain barrier endothelial cells are transferrin receptors that allow the transport of iron into specific areas of the brain. The amount of iron that is transported into the various areas of the brain appears to depend on the concentration of transferrin receptors on the surface of endothelial cells of that region. Thus, the transport of specific nutrients into the brain is regulated during physiological and pathological conditions by blood–brain barrier transport proteins distributed according to the regional and metabolic requirements of brain tissue.

Basement Membrane, Pericytes, and Astrocytes Are Also Blood–Brain Barrier Components

Basement membranes are not true membranes but are extracellular matrices with a width varying from 20 to 300 nm, composed mainly of collagens, glycoproteins, laminin, proteoglycans, and other proteins. In the cerebral microvasculature, the basement membrane surrounds the endothelium and the adjacent pericytes. The nature of the basement membrane surrounding the blood vessels varies with the type of vasculature and during pathological conditions. The composition and structure of the basement membrane affect the permeability of the vessel. For example, *in vitro* studies of endothelial monolayers in which the underlying matrix was composed primarily of collagen type I restricted the passage of albumin, suggesting a role for the basement membrane in blood–brain barrier permeability. Replacement of collagen type I with fibronectin resulted in an increased permeability to albumin. This finding correlates with the lack of fibronectin around blood–brain barrier vessels.

Pericytes (Fig. 3.22) are present within the basement membrane of all vessels in the body, including the nervous system. The functions of pericytes include the secretion of basement membrane components, the regulation of revascularization and repair, and the regulation of vascular tone in capillaries. In the central nervous system, pericytes may act as part of the vascular barrier by increased phagocytosis after blood–brain barrier injury.

The processes of astrocytes form a sheath around blood–brain barrier microvessels. These processes are termed astrocyte foot processes or end feet and assist in inducing the blood–brain barrier properties of brain endothelia.

Disruption of the Blood–Brain Barrier Causes Edema

In general, disruption of the blood–brain barrier causes perivascular or vasogenic edema, which is the accumulation of fluids from the blood around the blood vessels of the brain. This is one of the main features of multiple sclerosis. In multiple sclerosis, inflammatory cells, primarily T cells and macrophages, invade the brain by migrating through the blood–brain barrier and attack cerebral elements as if these elements were foreign antigens. It has been observed by many investigators that the degree of edema accumulation causes the neurological symptoms experienced by people suffering from multiple sclerosis.

Studying the regulation of blood–brain barrier permeability is important for several reasons. Therapeutic treatments for neurological disease need to be able to cross the barrier. Attempts to design drug delivery systems that take therapeutic drugs directly into the brain have been made by using chemically engineered carrier molecules that take advantage of receptors such as that for transferrin, which normally transports iron into the brain. Development of an *in vitro* test system of the blood–brain barrier is of importance in the creation of new neurotropic drugs that are targeted to the brain. This could be especially useful in the treatment of neurodegenerative diseases and the AIDS dementia complex (Box 3.4).

Summary

The hallmark of the brain vasculature is the blood–brain barrier, a multicomponent gateway between brain tissue and other organ systems. We can consider the blood–brain barrier the gateway to the brain because it restricts access to macromolecules present in the blood. It also serves as the interface between the immune and the nervous systems, acting as the "meeting site" for communication between the two.

References

Altman, J. (1994). Microglia emerge from the fog. *Trends Neurosci.* **17**, 47–49.

Bradbury, M. W. B. (1979). "The Concept of a Blood-Brain Barrier," pp. 381–407. Wiley, Chichester.

Brodal, A. (1981). "Neurological Anatomy in Relation to Clinical Medicine," 3rd Ed. Oxford Univ. Press, New York.

Bunge, R. P. (1968). Glial cells and the central myelin sheath. *Physiol. Rev.* **48**, 197–251.

BOX 3.4

VIRAL VECTORS AND GENE THERAPY

It is somewhat ironic that infectious agents can be used as therapeutic gene delivery systems. Novel genes intended to correct an inherent genetic flaw can be introduced into weakened forms of viruses, "**viral vectors**," and used in gene therapy. In *ex vivo* gene therapy, cells are removed from an individual, grown in tissue culture, and modified with a viral vector. The cells are then introduced by injection back into the host individual. In *in vivo* gene therapy, viral vectors are injected directly into specific sites in the brain of the host, enter local neurons or glial cells, and then selectively destroy or transform them.

Viruses naturally shuttle their own genetic material into host cells for replication by the hosts' genetic apparatus. Viral proteins often cause toxicity or death of the host cell. The immune system responds with a strong inflammatory response that can also cause profound local tissue damage. Viral vectors have been designed to capitalize on the high efficiency of transfer of genetic material while attempting to limit the toxicity caused by viral replication.

The viruses available to neurobiology each afford advantages and disadvantages. Retroviruses, with only an RNA genome, must be converted into a complementary DNA (cDNA) copy by the viral enzyme reverse transcriptase. This process requires a sufficient pool of DNA precursors present only in actively dividing cells and, thus, retroviruses have been used to direct genes into dividing cells during development and into brain tumors. A third application has been to introduce genes into dividing cells in tissue culture prior to transplantation in animal models of neurological disorders such as Parkinson and Alzheimer diseases. Although clinical trials with retroviruses were promising, the slow rate of division of most brain tumor cells favors the use of other vectors, which infect nondividing cells, such as the non-replicating form of human immunodeficiency virus (HIV). This retrovirus, a lentivirus, can be used to efficiently and safely transfer genes into mammalian brain neurons *in vivo* without the expression of HIV proteins. Recombinant HSV vectors with deletions in certain DNA synthetic enzymes (such as thymidine kinase or ribonucleotide reductase) have also been used as potential treatments for brain tumors. These genes are only necessary to promote DNA synthesis in nondividing cells, but they are dispensable in actively dividing cells. These vectors replicate in and destroy dividing tumor cells (which contain adequate DNA precursors) while sparing normal, nondividing brain cells. This approach has shown promise in preclinical studies in rodent and primate brain tumors.

Adenoviruses (AD) and herpesviruses (HSV), which contain DNA genomes, are potentially more useful agents for gene transfer into either neurons or glial cells of the adult brain because they do not require cell division for the efficient uptake and expression of their genetic material. Two general classes of vectors have been created on the basis of these viruses: *recombinant vectors* and *defective vectors*. Recombinant vectors contain deletions of one or more genes that promote viral replication or cause cellular toxicity, and the gene of interest is inserted into the mutated viral chromosome. Defective vectors contain a gene of interest attached to recognition signals that permit replication and packaging of the DNA into a viral coat. No viral genes are present, and the necessary viral proteins are provided either by a "helper" virus or by a cell line that constitu-

Carpenter, M. B., and Sutin, J. (1983). "Human Neuroanatomy." Williams & Wilkins, Baltimore, MD.

van Domburg, P. H. M. F., and ten Donkelaar, H. J. (1991). The human substantia nigra and ventral tegmental area. *Adv. Anat. Embryol. Cell Biol.* **121**, 1–132.

Claudio, L., Raine, C. S., and Brosnan, C. F. (1995). Evidence of persistent blood-brain barrier abnormalities in chronic-progressive multiple sclerosis. *Acta Neuropathol.* **90**, 228–238.

del Ro-Hortega, P. (1932). Microglia. *In* "Cytology and Cellular Pathology of the Nervous System" (W. Penfield, ed.), Vol. 2, pp. 481–534. Harper (Hoeber), New York.

DeFelipe, J., Hendry, S. H. C., and Jones, E. G. (1989). Visualization of chandelier cell axons by parvalbumin immunoreactivity in monkey cerebral cortex. *Proc. Natl. Acad. Sci. USA* **86**, 2093–2097.

Dolman, C. L. (1991). Microglia. *In* "Textbook of Neuropathology" (R. L. Davis and D. M. Robertson, eds.), pp. 141–163. Williams & Wilkins, Baltimore, MD.

Duvernoy, H. M., Delon, S., and Vannson, J. L. (1981). Cortical blood vessels of the human brain. *Brain Res. Bull.* **7**, 519–579.

Freund, T. F., Martin, K. A. C., Smith, A. D., and Somogyi, P. (1983). Glutamate decarboxylase-immunoreactive terminals of Golgi-impregnated axoaxonic cells and of presumed basket cells in synaptic contact with pyramidal neurons of the cat's visual cortex. *J. Comp. Neurol.* **221**, 263–278.

Hudspeth, A. J. (1983). Transduction and tuning by vertebrate hair cells. *Trends Neurosci.* **6**, 366–369.

Jones, E. G. (1984). Laminar distribution of cortical efferent cells. *In* "Cellular Components of the Cerebral Cortex" (A. Peters and E. G. Jones, eds.), Vol. 1, pp. 521–553. Plenum, New York.

BOX 3.4 (cont'd)

tively expresses such genes. The packaged vector is incapable of replication, and no viral proteins are ever expressed in target cells. The major advantage of this class of vectors is that all elements responsible for viral toxicity have been eliminated. However, these vehicles are technically very difficult to synthesize and the potentially toxic "helper" virus must be eliminated completely.

Recombinant vectors developed from AD and HSV are as yet the most common vehicles used for gene transfer in neurobiology. AD recombinants are simpler to construct, and deletion of multiple genes is easier compared with HSV, largely due to factors related to the smaller size and fewer number of genes present in the AD genome. A variety of recombinant herpesviruses have been used as transneuronal tracers for the neuroanatomical analysis of brain circuits. For example, weakened strains of herpesviruses can be microinjected into a specific peripheral site (e.g., visceral organ or muscle) or the brain itself, and after several days, an infection spreads in a hierarchial manner within the chain of neurons that regulate this target. The wave of infection can be detected in first-, second-, and often third-order neurons of a neural network by histochemical methods. In addition, this technology has used to study the physiology of neurons as well.

Defective HSV and adeno-associated virus (AAV) vectors are the major types of defective DNA viral vectors in use. Defective HSV vectors contain an HSV origin of DNA replication and packaging signal, but the vector contains no viral genes. HSV proteins are provided by a helper virus or through a potentially safer, multiple plasmid system. An advantage of this system is that many copies of the viral gene are packaged into a single viral particle, thereby amplifying expression of the gene of interest.

AAV is a parvovirus that requires coinfection of a cell by adenovirus (or herpesvirus) to efficiently replicate and package new AAV virions. The AAV vector is transfected with a second plasmid containing all AAV genes without the replication and packaging sequences. Disadvantages of this system include its small size (only 5 kb of foreign DNA can be packaged) and the technical difficulty in producing large amounts of high-titer virus stocks.

Both AAV and defective HSV systems have been used for a variety of basic and clinical neuroscience applications, including *in vivo* promoter analysis, study of genes influencing neuronal regeneration, and gene therapy in animal models of Parkinson and Alzheimer diseases, epilepsy, and stroke.

Viral vectors offer unique molecular tools with which to alter CNS diseases, as well as to study basic cellular functions of both neurons and glial cells. Amelioriation of certain human diseases may be achieved by carefully tailoring the type of genetic message and packaging system used.

Michael G. Kaplitt and Arthur D. Loewy

Suggested Readings

Kaplitt, M. G., and Loewy, A. D. (1995). Viral Vectors: Tools for the Study and Genetic Manipulation of the Nervous System. Academic Press, San Diego.

Loewy, A. D. (1998). Viruses as transneuronal tracers for defining neural circuits. *Neurosci. Biobehav. Rev.* **22**, 679–684.

Irnaten, M., Neff, R. A., Wang, J., Loewy, A. D., Mettenleiter, T. C., and Mendelowitz, D. (2001). Activity of cardiorespiratory networks revealed by transsynaptic virus expressing GFP. *J. Neurophysiol.* **85**, 435–438.

Jones, E. G. (1975). Varieties and distribution of non-pyramidal cells in the somatic sensory cortex of the squirrel monkey. *J. Comp. Neurol.* **160**, 205–267.

Kettenman, H., and Ransom, B. R., eds. (1995). "Neuroglia." Oxford Univer. Press, Oxford.

Krebs, W., and Krebs, I. (1991). "Primate Retina and Choroid: Atlas of Fine Structure in Man and Monkey." Springer-Verlag, New York.

Mountcastle, V. B. (1978). An organizing principle for cerebral function: The unit module and the distributed system. *In* "The Mindful Brain: Cortical Organization and the Group-Selective Theory of Higher Brain Function" (V. B. Mountcastle and G. Eddman, eds.), pp. 7–50. MIT Press, Cambridge, MA.

Nissl, F. (1899). Üeber einige Beziehungen zwischen Nervenzellenerkränkungen und gliö sen Erscheinungen bei verschiedenen Psychosen. *Arch. Psychol.* **32**, 1–21.

Peters, A., and Jones, E. G., eds. (1984). "Cellular Components of the Cerebral Cortex," Vol. 1. Plenum, New York.

Peters, A., Palay, S. L., and Webster, H. de F. (1991). "The Fine Structure of the Nervous System: Neurons and Their Supporting Cells," 3rd ed. Oxford Univer. Press, New York.

Ramón y Cajal, S. (1913). Contribucion al conocimiento de la neuroglia del cerebro humano. *Trab. Lab. Invest. Biol.* **11**, 255–315.

Ritchie, J. M. (1984). Physiological basis of conduction in myelinated nerve fibers. *In* "Myelin" (P. Morell, ed.), pp. 117–146. Plenum, New York.

Somogyi, P., and Cowey, A. (1981). Combined Golgi and electron microscopic study on the synapses formed by double bouquet cells in the visual cortex of the cat and monkey. *J. Comp. Neurol.* **195**, 547–566.

Somogyi, P., Kisvárday, Z. F., Martin, K. A. C., and Whitteridge, D. (1983). Synaptic connections of morphologically identified and physiologically characterized bastret cells in the striate cortex of cat. *Neuroscience* **10**, 261–294.

Suggested Readings

Brightman, M. W., and Reese, T. S. (1969). Junctions between intimately apposed cell membranes in the vertebrate brain. *J. Cell Biol.* **40**, 648–677.

Broadwell, R. D., and Salcman, M. (1981). Expanding the definition of the BBB to protein. *Proc. Natl. Acad. Sci. USA* **78**, 7820–7824.

Fernandez-Moran, H. (1950). EM observations on the structure of the myelinated nerve sheath. *Exp. Cell Res.* **1**, 143–162.

Gehrmann, J., Matsumoto, Y., and Kreutzberg, G. W. (1995). Microglia: Intrinsic immuneffector cell of the brain. *Brain Res. Rev.* **20**, 269–287.

Kimbelberg, H., and Norenberg, M. D. (1989). Astrocytes. *Sci. Am.* **26**, 66–76.

Kirschner, D. A., Ganser, A. L., and Caspar, D. W. (1984). Diffraction studies of molecular organization and membrane interactions in myelin. *In* "Myelin" (P. Morell, ed.), pp. 51–96. Plenum, New York.

Lum, H., and Malik, A. B. (1994). Regulation of vascular endothelial barrier function. *Am. J. Physiol.* **267**, L223–L241.

Rosenbluth, J. (1980). Central myelin in the mouse mutant shiverer. *J. Comp. Neurol.* **194**, 639–728.

Rosenbluth, J. (1980). Peripheral myelin in the mouse mutant shiverer. *J. Comp. Neurol.* **194**, 729–753.

Patrick R. Hof, Bruce D. Trapp, Jean de Vellis,
Luz Claudio, and David R. Colman

4

Subcellular Organization of the Nervous System: Organelles and Their Functions

Cells have many features in common, but each cell type also possesses a functional architecture related to its unique physiology. In fact, cells may become so specialized in fulfilling a particular function that virtually all cellular components may be devoted to it. For example, the machinery inside mammalian erythrocytes is completely dedicated to the delivery of oxygen to the tissues and the removal of carbon dioxide. Toward this end, this cell has evolved a specialized plasma membrane, an underlying cytoskeletal matrix that molds the cell into a biconcave disk, and a cytoplasm rich in hemoglobin. Modification of the cell machinery extends even to the discarding of structures such as the nucleus and the protein synthetic apparatus, which are not needed after the red blood cell matures. In many respects, the terminally differentiated, highly specialized cells of the nervous system exhibit comparable commitment—the extensive development of subcellular components reflects the roles that each plays.

The neuron serves as the cellular correlate of information processing and, in aggregate, all neurons act together to integrate responses of the entire organism to the external world. It is therefore not surprising that the specializations found in neurons are more diverse and complex than those found in any other cell type. Single neurons commonly interact in specific ways with hundreds of other cells—other neurons, astrocytes, oligodendrocytes, immune cells, muscle, and glandular cells. This chapter defines the major functional domains of the neuron, describes the subcellular elements that compose the building blocks of these domains, and examines the processes that create and maintain neuronal functional architecture.

AXONS AND DENDRITES: UNIQUE STRUCTURAL COMPONENTS OF NEURONS

Neurons and glial cells are remarkable for their size and complexity, but they do share many features with other eukaryotic cells (Peters *et al.*, 1991) As discussed in Chapter 3, the perikaryon, or cell body, contains a nucleus and its associated protein synthetic machinery. Most neuronal nuclei are large and typically contain a preponderance of euchromatin. This is consistent with the need to create and maintain a large cellular volume. Because protein synthesis must be kept at a high level just to maintain the neuronal extensions, transcription levels in neurons are generally high. In turn, the wide variety of different polypeptide constituents associated with cellular domains in a neuron requires that a large number of different genes be transcribed constantly.

When specific mRNAs have been synthesized and processed, they move from the nucleus into a subcellular region that can be termed the translational cytoplasm (Lasek and Brady, 1982) comprising cytoplasmic ("free") and membrane-associated polysomes, the intermediate compartment of the smooth endoplasmic reticulum, and the Golgi complex. The constituents of translational cytoplasm are thus associated with the synthesis and processing of proteins. Neurons in particular have relatively large amounts of translational cytoplasm to accommodate a high level of protein synthesis. This protein synthetic machinery is arranged in discrete intracellular "granules" termed Nissl substance (Box 4.1) after the histologist who first discovered these structures in the 19th century. The Nissl substance is actually a

BOX 4.1

THE NISSL SUBSTANCE

"It is interesting that Nissl recognized the composite nature of the substance named for him, although he could not have resolved either of its components ..."

The preceding quote and the following discussion of the Nissl substance appeared in Sanford, *et al.* (1955):

As imaged in the electron microscope, the crowded cytoplasm of the neuron contrasts sharply with the relatively open cytoplasm of many other cell types. As this compact appearance stems largely from the extensive meshwork of Nissl substance, the neuron resembles, even at the electron microscope level, certain protein-secreting glandular cells, such as those of the pancreatic acini and the salivary glands.

Like the basophilic substance or ergastoplasm of glandular cells, the Nissl substance is a composite material constructed of endoplasmic reticulum and fine granules, both of which have been revealed by electron microscopy. The first component of the Nissl substance appears to be part of the general endoplasmic reticulum of the neuron. The reticulum extends throughout the entire cytoplasm, but is considerably more condensed within the area of the Nissl bodies than in the rest of the cell. These condensations not only determine the size and shape of each Nissl body, but also constitute a membranous framework upon which the other components are arranged. In many types of neurons, meshes of the endoplasmic reticulum are distributed at random in three dimensions but in all neurons, and especially in the large motor neurons, the endoplasmic reticulum may display a distinctly orderly arrangement within the Nissl bodies. This orientation consists of a layering of reticular sheets, at more or less regular intervals. Each sheet is a reticulum developed predominantly in two dimensions and comprising tubules, strings of vesicles, and numerous large and flat cisternae. Even in such highly ordered forms as the Nissl bodies of motor neurons, the continuity of the reticulum persists, as indicated by frequent branches and anastomoses between layers.

The second component of the Nissl substance is represented by small granules disposed in patterned arrays either in close contact with the outer membranes of the endoplasmic reticulum or scattered in the intervening matrix. This matrix may be considered as a third component of the Nissl substance. It is evident, therefore, that although Nissl bodies are differentiated parts of the cytoplasm, they are continuous with it by virtue of the continuity of the endoplasmic reticulum and the matrix. No interface or membrane separates them from the rest of the cytoplasm. In this respect, as well as in general architecture, they are comparable to the ergastoplasm of glandular cells. The only differences lie in (a) a different intracellular distribution, (b) a lesser degree of preferred orientation of the endoplasmic reticulum, and (c) an apparently greater concentration of fine granules within the areas of Nissl bodies.

We now recognize that the electron-dense "granules" are ribosomes, arranged in cytoplasmic "free" polysomal rosettes, or attached to the surface of the endoplasmic reticulum membrane. The lumen of the ER compartment (arrow) contains a "fuzz" that probably is formed by the numerous nascent chains being inserted cotranslationally into the ER lumen, some resident proteins that take part in the translation process, and certain structural components of the ER membrane.

Scott Brady, David R. Colman, and Peter Brophy

Reference

Sanford, L., Palay, M. D., and Palade, G. E. (1955). The fine structure of neurons. *J. Biophys. Biochem. Cytol.* **88**, 69–88.

combination of stacks of rough endoplasmic reticulum (RER), interposed with rosettes of free polysomes (Box 4.1 and Fig. 4.1). This arrangement is unique to neurons, and its functional significance is unknown. Most, but by no means all, proteins used throughout the neuron are synthesized in the perikaryon. During or after synthesis and processing, proteins are packaged into membrane-limited organelles, incorporated into cytoskeletal elements, or remain as soluble constituents of the cytoplasm. After proteins have been packaged appropriately, they are transported to their sites of function.

With a few exceptions, vertebrate neurons have two discrete functional domains or compartments, the axonal and the somatodendritic compartments, each of which encompasses a number of sub- or microdomains (Fig. 4.2). The axon is perhaps the most familiar functional domain of a neuron and is classi-

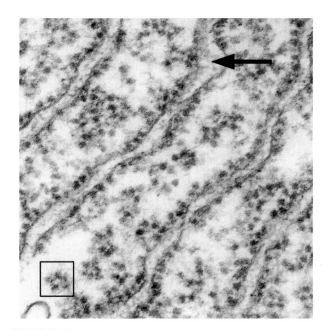

FIGURE 4.1 The "Nissl body" in neurons is an array of cytoplasmic-free polysomal rosettes (boxed) interspersed between rows of rough endoplasmic reticulum (RER) studded with membrane-bound ribosomes. Nascent polypeptide chains emerging from the ribosomal tunnel on the RER are inserted into the lumen (arrow), where they may be processed before transport out of the RER. The relationship between the polypeptide products of these "free" and "bound" polysome populations in the Nissl body, an arrangement that is unique to neurons, is unknown.

cally defined as the cellular process by which a neuron makes contact with a target cell to transmit information, providing a conducting structure for transmitting the action potential to a synapse, a specialized subdomain for transmission of a signal from neuron to target cell (neuron, muscle, etc.), most often by release of appropriate neurotransmitters. Consequently, most axons end in a presynaptic terminal, although a single axon may have many (hundreds or even thousands in some cases) presynaptic specializations known as en passant synapses along its length. Characteristics of presynaptic terminals are presented in greater detail later.

The axon is the first neuronal process to differentiate during development. A typical neuron has only a single axon that proceeds some distance from the cell body before branching extensively. Usually the longest process of a neuron, axons come in many sizes. In a human adult, axons range in length from a few micrometers for small interneurons to a meter or more for large motor neurons, and they may be even longer in large animals (such as giraffes, elephants, and whales). In mammals and other vertebrates, the longest axons generally extend approximately half the body length.

Axonal diameters also are quite variable, ranging from 0.1 to 20 µm for large myelinated fibers in vertebrates. Invertebrate axons grow to even larger diameters, with the giant axons of some squid species achieving diameters in the millimeter range. Invertebrate axons reach such large diameters because they lack the myelinating glia that speed conduction of the action potential. As a result, axonal caliber must be large to sustain the high rate of conduction needed for the reflexes that permit escape from predators and capture of prey. Although axonal caliber is closely regulated in both myelinated and nonmyelinated fibers, this parameter is critical for those organisms that are unable to produce myelin.

The region of the neuronal cell body where the axon originates has several specialized features. This domain, called the axon hillock, is distinguished most readily by a deficiency of Nissl substance. Therefore, protein synthesis cannot take place to any appreciable degree in this region. Cytoplasm in the vicinity of the axon hillock may have a few polysomes but is dominated by the cytoskeletal and membranous organelles that are being delivered to the axon. Microtubules and neurofilaments begin to align roughly parallel to each other, helping to organize membrane-limited organelles destined for the axon. The hillock is a region where materials either are committed to the axon (cytoskeletal elements, synaptic vesicle precursors, mitochondria, etc.) or are excluded from the axon (RER and free polysomes, dendritic microtubule-associated proteins). The molecular basis for this sorting is not understood. Cytoplasm in the axon hillock does not appear to contain a physical "sizing" barrier (like a filter) because large organelles such as mitochondria enter the axon readily, whereas only a small number of essentially excluded structures such as polysomes are occasionally seen only in the initial segment of the axon and not in the axon proper. An exception to this general rule is during development when local protein synthesis does take place at the axon terminus or growth cone. In the mature neuron, the physiological significance of this barrier must be considerable because axonal structures are found to accumulate in this region in many neuropathologies, including those due to degenerative diseases (such as amyotrophic lateral sclerosis) and to exposure to neurotoxic compounds (such as acrylamide).

The initial segment of the axon is the region of the axon adjacent to the axon hillock. Microtubules generally form characteristic fascicles, or bundles, in the initial segment of the axon. These fascicles are not seen elsewhere. The initial segment and, to some extent, the axon hillock also have a distinctive specialized plasma membrane. Initially, the plasmalemma

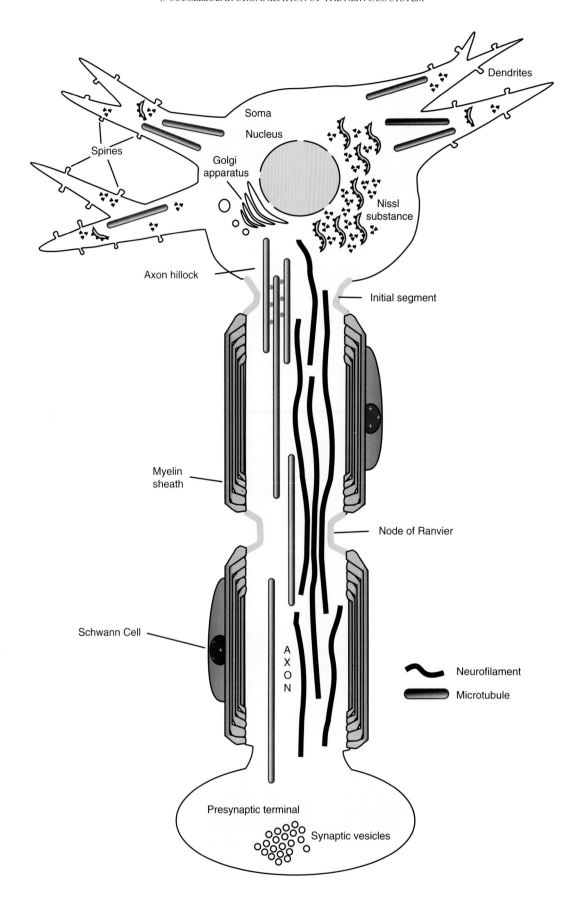

was thought to have a thick electron-dense coating actually attached to the inner surface of the membrane, but this dense undercoating is in reality separated by 5–10 nm from the plasma membrane inner surface and has a complex ultrastructure. Neither the composition nor the function of this undercoating is known. Curiously, the undercoating is present in the same regions of the initial segment as the distinctive fasciculation of microtubules, although the relationship is not understood. The plasma membrane is specialized in the initial segment and axon hillock in that it contains voltage-sensitive ion channels in large numbers, and most action potentials originate in this domain.

Ultimately, axonal structure is geared toward the efficient conduction of action potentials at a rate appropriate to the function of that neuron. This can be seen from both the ultrastructure and the composition of axons. Axons are roughly cylindrical in cross section with little or no taper. As discussed later, this diameter is maintained by regulation of the cytoskeleton. Even at branch points, daughter axons are comparable in diameter to the parent axon. This constant caliber helps ensure a consistent rate of conduction. Similarly, the organization of membrane components is regulated to this end. Voltage-gated ion channels are distributed to maximize conduction. Sodium channels are distributed more or less uniformly in small nonmyelinated axons, but are concentrated at high density in the regularly spaced unmyelinated gaps, known as nodes of Ranvier. An axon so organized will conduct an action potential or train of spikes long distances with high fidelity at a defined speed. These characteristics are essential for maintaining the precise timing and coordination seen in neuronal circuits.

Most vertebrate neurons have multiple dendrites arising from their perikarya. Unlike axons, dendrites branch continuously and taper extensively with a reduction in caliber in daughter processes at each branching. In addition, the surface of dendrites is covered with small protrusions, or spines, which are postsynaptic specializations. Although the surface area of a dendritic arbor may be quite extensive, dendrites in general remain in the relative vicinity of the perikaryon. A dendritic arbor may be contacted by the axons of many different and distant neurons or innervated by a single axon making multiple synaptic contacts.

The base of a dendrite is continuous with the cytoplasm of the cell body. In contrast to the axon, Nissl substance extends into dendrites, and certain proteins are synthesized predominantly in dendrites. There is evidence for the selective placement of some mRNAs in dendrites as well (Steward, 1995). For example, whereas RER and polysomes extend well into the dendrites, the mRNAs that are transported and translated in dendrites are a subset of the total neuronal mRNA, deficient in some mRNA species (such as neurofilament mRNAs) and enriched in mRNAs with dendritic functions (such as microtubule-associated protein, MAP2, mRNAs). Also, certain proteins appear to be targeted, postsynthesis, to the dendritic compartment as well.

The shapes and complexity of dendritic arborizations may be remarkably plastic. Dendrites appear relatively late in development and initially have only limited numbers of branches and spines. As development and maturation of the nervous system proceed, the size and number of branches increase. The number of spines increases dramatically, and their distribution may change. This remodeling of synaptic connectivity may continue into adulthood, and environmental effects can alter this pattern significantly. Eventually, in the aging brain, there is a reduction in complexity and size of dendritic arbors, with fewer spines and thinner dendritic shafts. These changes correlate with changes in neuronal function during development and aging.

As defined by classical physiology, axons are structural correlates for neuronal output, and dendrites constitute the domain for receiving information. A neuron without an axon or one without dendrites might therefore seem paradoxical, but such neurons do exist. Certain amacrine and horizontal cells in the vertebrate retina have no identifiable axons, although they do have dendritic processes that are morphologically distinct from axons. Such processes may have both pre- and postsynaptic specializations or may have gap junctions that act as direct electrical connections between two cells. Similarly, the pseudounipolar sensory neurons of dorsal root ganglia (DRG) have no dendrites. In their mature form, these DRG sensory neurons give rise to a single axon that extends a few hundred micrometers before branching. One long branch extends to the periphery, where it may form a sensory nerve ending in muscle spindles or skin. Large DRG peripheral branches are myelinated and

◀ FIGURE 4.2 Basic elements of neuronal subcellular organization. The neuron consists of a soma, or cell body, in which the nucleus, multiple cytoplasm-filled processes termed dendrites, and the (usually single) axon are placed. The neuron is highly extended in space; a neuron with a cell body of the size shown here could easily maintain an axon several miles in length! The unique shape of each neuron is the result of a cooperative interplay between plasma membrane components (the lipid matrix and associated proteins) and cytoskeletal elements. Most large neurons in vertebrates are myelinated by oligodendrocytes in the CNS and by Schwann cells in the PNS. The compact wraps of myelin encasing the axon distal to the initial segment permit the rapid conduction of the action potential by a process termed "saltatory conduction" (see Chapter 3).

TABLE 4.1 Functional and Morphological Hallmarks of Axons and Dendrites[a]

Axons	Dendrites
With rare exceptions, each neuron has a single axon	Most neurons have multiple dendrites arising from their cell bodies
Axons appear first during neuronal differentiation	Dendrites begin to differentiate only after the axon has formed
Axon initial segments are distinguished by a specialized plasma membrane containing a high density of ion channels and distinctive cytoskeletal organization	Dendrites are continuous with the perikaryal cytoplasm, and the transition point cannot be distinguished readily
Axons typically are cylindrical in form with a round or elliptical cross section	Dendrites usually have a significant taper and small spinous processes that give them an irregular cross section
Large axons are myelinated in vertebrates, and the thickness of the myelin sheath is proportional to the axonal caliber	Dendrites are not myelinated, although a few wraps of myelin may occur rarely
Axon caliber is a function of neurofilament and microtubule numbers with neurofilaments predominating in large axons	The dendritic cytoskeleton may appear less organized, and microtubules dominate even in large dendrites
Microtubules in axons have a uniform polarity with plus ends distal from the cell body	Microtubules in proximal dendrites have mixed polarity, with both plus and minus ends oriented distal to the cell body
Axonal microtubules are enriched in tau protein with a characteristic phosphorylation pattern	Dendritic microtubules may contain some tau protein, but MAP2 is not present in axonal compartments and is highly enriched in dendrites
Ribosomes are excluded from mature axons, although a few may be detectable in initial segments	Both rough endoplasmic reticulum and cytoplasmic polysomes are present in dendrites, with specific mRNAs being enriched in dendrites
Axonal branches tend to be distal from the cell body	Dendrites begin to branch extensively near the perikaryon and form extensive arbors in the vicinity of the perikaryon
Axonal branches form obtuse angles and have diameters similar to the parent stem	Dendritic branches form acute angles and are smaller than the parent stem
Most axons have presynaptic specializations that may be *en passant* or at the ends of axonal branches	Dendrites are rich in postsynaptic specializations, particularly on the spinous processes that project from the dendritic shaft
Action potentials are usually generated at the axon hillock and conducted away from the cell body	Some dendrites can generate action potentials, but more commonly they modulate the electrical state of the perikaryon and initial segment
Traditionally, axons are specialized for conduction and synaptic transmission, i.e., neuronal output	Dendritic architecture is most suitable for integrating synaptic responses from a variety of inputs, i.e., neuronal input

[a] Neurons typically have two classes of cytoplasmic extensions that may be distinguished using electrophysiological, morphological, and biochemical criteria. Although some neuronal processes may lack one or more of these features, enough parameters can generally be defined to allow unambiguous identification.

have the morphological characteristics of an axon, but they contain neither pre- nor postsynaptic specializations. The other branch extends into the central nervous system, where it forms synaptic contacts. In DRG neurons, the action potential is generated at distal sensory nerve endings and is then transmitted along the peripheral branch to the central branch and the appropriate central nervous system (CNS) targets, bypassing the cell body. The functional and morphological hallmarks of axons and dendrites are listed in Table 4.1.

Summary

Neurons are polarized cells that are specialized for membrane and protein synthesis, as well as for conduction of the nerve impulse. In general, neurons have a cell body, a dendritic arborization that is usually located near the cell body, and an extended axon that may branch considerably before terminating to form synapses with other neurons.

PROTEIN SYNTHESIS IN NERVOUS TISSUE

Both neurons and glial cells have strikingly extended morphologies. This cytoarchitecture is ideal for a tissue whose functions depend on multiple intercellular contacts locally and at great distances. Protein and lipid components are synthesized and assembled into the membranes of these cell extensions through pathways of membrane biogenesis that have been elucidated primarily in other cell types, including the yeast *Saccharomyces cerevisiae*. However, some adaptations of these general mechanisms have been necessary, due to the specific requirements of cells in the nervous system. Neurons, for example, have devised mechanisms for ensuring that the specific components of the axonal and dendritic plasma membranes are selectively delivered (targeted) to each plasma membrane subdomain.

The distribution to specific loci of organelles, receptors, and ion channels is critical to normal neuronal function. In turn, these loci must be "matched" appropriately to the local microenvironment and specific cell–cell interactions. Similarly, in myelinating glial cells during the narrow developmental window when the myelin sheath is being formed, these cells synthesize vast sheets of insulating plasma membrane at an unbelievably high rate. To understand how the plasma membrane of neurons and glia might be modeled to fit individual functional requirements, it is necessary to review the progress that has been made so far in our understanding of how membrane components and organelles are generated in eukaryotic cells.

There are two major categories of membrane proteins: integral and peripheral. Integral membrane proteins, which include the receptors for neurotransmitters (e.g., the acetylcholine receptor subunits) and polypeptide growth factors (e.g., the dimeric insulin receptor), have segments that are either embedded in the lipid bilayer or bound covalently to molecules that insert into the membrane, such as those proteins linked to glycosyl phosphatidylinositol at their C termini (e.g., Thy-1). A protein with a single membrane-embedded segment and an N terminus exposed at the extracellular surface is said to be of type I, whereas type II proteins retain their N termini on the cytoplasmic side of the plasma membrane. Peripheral membrane proteins are localized on the cytoplasmic surface of the membrane and do not cross any membrane during their biogenesis. They interact with the membrane either by means of their associations with membrane lipids or the cytoplasmic tails of integral proteins or by means of their affinity for other peripheral proteins (e.g., platelet-derived growth factor receptor-Grb2-Sos-Ras complex). In some cases, they may bind directly to the polar head groups of the lipid bilayer (e.g., myelin basic protein).

Integral Membrane and Secretory Polypeptides Are Synthesized *de Novo* in the Rough Endoplasmic Reticulum

The subcellular destinations of integral and peripheral membrane proteins are determined by their sites of synthesis. In the secretory pathway, integral membrane proteins and secretory proteins, are synthesized in the rough endoplasmic reticulum, whereas the

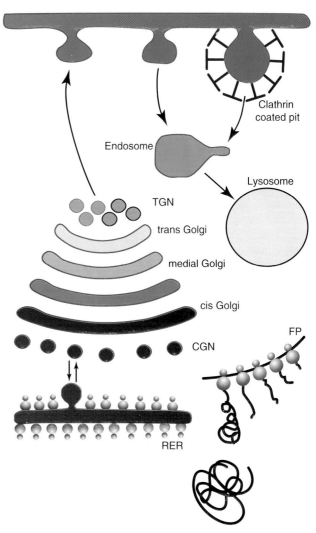

FIGURE 4.3 The secretory pathway. Transport and sorting of proteins in the secretory pathway occur as they pass through the Golgi complex before reaching the plasma membrane. Sorting occurs in the *cis*-Golgi network (CGN), also known as the intermediate compartment, and in the *trans*-Golgi network (TGN). Proteins exit from the Golgi complex at the TGN. The default pathway is the direct route to the plasma membrane. Proteins bound for regulated secretion or for transport to endosomes and from there to lysosomes are diverted from the default path by means of specific signals. In endocytosis, one population of vesicles is surrounded by a clathrin cage and is destined for late endosomes. Another population appears to be coated in a lace-like structure whose composition is yet to be defined.

mRNAs encoding peripheral proteins are translated on cytoplasmic "free" polysomes, which are not membrane associated but which may interact with cytoskeletal structures.

The pathway by which secretory proteins are synthesized and exported was first postulated through the elegant ultrastructural studies on the pancreas by George Palade and colleagues (Palade, 1975). Pancreatic acinar cells were an excellent choice for this work because they are extremely active in secretion, as revealed by the abundance of their RER network, a property they share with neurons. Nissl deduced, in the 19th century, that pancreatic cells and neurons would be found to have common secretory properties because of similarities in the distribution of the Nissl substance (Fig. 4.3).

Pulse–chase autoradiography has revealed that newly synthesized secretory proteins move from the RER to the Golgi apparatus, where the proteins are packaged into secretory granules and transported to the plasma membrane from which they are released by exocytosis. Pulse–chase studies in neurons reveal a similar sequence of events for proteins transported into the axon. Unraveling of the detailed molecular mechanisms of the pathway began with the successful reconstitution of secretory protein biosynthesis *in vitro* and the direct demonstration that, very early during synthesis, secretory proteins are translocated into the lumen of RER vesicles, prepared by cell fractionation, termed microsomes. A key observation here was that the fate of the protein was sealed as a result of encapsulation in the lumen of the RER at the site of synthesis. This cotranslational insertion model provided a logical framework for understanding the synthesis of integral membrane proteins with a transmembrane orientation.

The process by which integral membrane proteins are synthesized closely follows the secretory pathway, except that integral proteins are of course not released from the cell, but instead remain within cellular membranes. Synthesis of integral proteins begins with synthesis of the nascent chain on a polysome that is not yet bound to the RER membrane (Fig. 4.4). Emergence of the N terminus of the nascent protein from the protein-synthesizing machinery allows a ribonucleoprotein, a signal recognition particle (SRP), to bind to an emergent hydrophobic signal sequence and prevent further translation (Walther and Johnson 1994). Translation arrest is relieved when SRP docks with its cognate receptor in the RER and dissociates from the signal sequence in a process that requires GTP. Synthesis of transmembrane proteins on RER is an extremely energy-efficient process. The passage of a fully formed and folded protein through a membrane is, thermody-

namically, formidably expensive; it is infinitely "cheaper" for cells to thread amino acids, in tandem, through a membrane during initial protein synthesis.

Protein synthesis then resumes, and the emerging polypeptide chain is translocated into the RER membrane through a conceptualized "aqueous pore" termed the translocon. Several proteins have been identified in cross-linking experiments as possible components of the translocon, including translocating chain-associating membrane protein (TRAM) and translocon-associated protein a (TRAP), which is a component of the mammalian homologue of the yeast sec 61 complex. Many others are strikingly similar to proteins that were originally discovered in yeast, revealing the common conserved nature of this process in organisms as diverse as yeasts and humans.

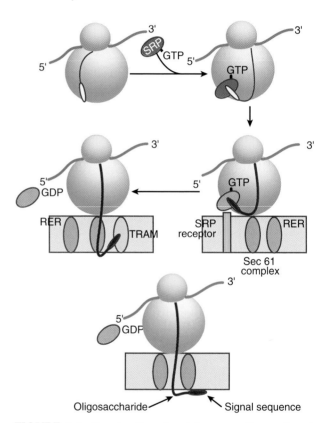

FIGURE 4.4 Translocation of proteins across the rough endoplasmic reticulum (RER). Integral membrane and secretory protein synthesis begins with partial synthesis on a free polysome not yet bound to the RER. The N terminus of the nascent protein emerges and allows a ribonucleoprotein, signal recognition particle (SRP), to bind to the hydrophobic signal sequence and prevent further translation. Translation arrest is relieved once the SRP docks with its receptor at the RER and dissociates from the signal sequence in a process that requires GTP. Once protein synthesis resumes, translocation occurs through an aqueous pore termed the translocon, which includes translocating chain-associating membrane protein (TRAM) and translocon-associated protein (TRAP). The signal sequence is removed by a signal peptidase located in the lumen of the RER.

A few polypeptides deviate from the common pathway for secretion. For example, certain peptide growth factors, such as basic fibroblast growth factor and ciliary neurotrophic factor, are synthesized without signal peptide sequences but are potent biological modulators of cell survival and differentiation. These growth factors appear to be released under certain conditions, although the mechanisms for such release are still controversial. One possibility is that release of these factors may be associated primarily with cellular injury.

Two cotranslational modifications are commonly associated with the emergence of the polypeptide on the luminal face of the RER. First, an N-terminal hydrophobic signal sequence that is used for insertion into the RER is usually removed by a signal peptidase. Second, oligosaccharides rich in mannose sugars are transferred from a lipid carrier, dolichol phosphate, to the side chains of asparagine residues (Kornfield and Kornfield, 1985). The asparagines must be in the sequence N X T (or S), and they are linked to mannose sugars by two molecules of *N*-acetylglucosamine. Although the prevention of glycosylation of some proteins causes their aggregation and accumulation in the RER and Golgi apparatus, for most glycoproteins, the significance of glycosylation is not apparent. Neither is it a universal feature of integral membrane proteins: some proteins, such as the proteolipid proteins of CNS myelin, neither lose their signal sequence nor become glycosylated. One clear case of a proved function for a carbohydrate moiety is the targeting of proteins to lysosomes in the *trans*-Golgi by means of the mannose 6-phosphate receptor. Intercellular adhesion molecules, such as selectins, which affect the sticking of lymphocytes to blood vessel walls, appear to interact with lectin-like proteins through their oligosaccharide chains. Similarly, the sialic acid side chains of the neural cell adhesion molecule (NCAM) are essential for modulation of cell–cell adhesion mediated by NCAMs. Thus, for the vast majority of polypeptides destined for release from the cell (secretory polypeptides), an N-terminal "signal sequence" first mediates the passage of the protein into the RER and is cleaved immediately from the polypeptide by a signal peptidase residing on the luminal side of the RER. For proteins destined to remain as permanent residents of cellular membranes (and these form a particularly important and diverse category of plasma membrane proteins in neurons and myelinating glial cells), however, many variations on this basic theme have been found. Simply stated:

1. Signal sequences for membrane insertions need not be only N-terminal; those that lie within a polypeptide sequence are not cleaved.

2. A second type of signal, a "halt" or "stop" transfer signal, functions to arrest translocation through the membrane bilayer. The halt transfer signal is also hydrophobic and is usually flanked by positive charges. This arrangement effectively stabilizes a polypeptide segment in the RER membrane bilayer.

3. The sequential display in tandem of insertion and halt transfer signals in a polypeptide as it is being synthesized ultimately determines its disposition with respect to the phospholipid bilayer, and thus its final topology in its target membrane. By synthesizing transmembrane polypeptides in this way, virtually any topology may be generated.

Newly Synthesized Polypeptides Exit from the RER and Are Moved through the Golgi Apparatus

When the newly synthesized protein has established its correct transmembrane orientation in the RER, it is incorporated into vesicles and must pass through the Golgi complex before reaching the plasma membrane (Fig. 4.3). For membrane proteins, the Golgi serves two major functions: (1) it sorts and targets proteins and, (2) it performs further posttranslational modifications, particularly on the oligosaccharide chains that were added in the RER. Sorting takes place in the *cis*-Golgi network (CGN), also known as the intermediate compartment, and in the *trans*-Golgi network (TGN), whereas sculpting of oligosaccharides is primarily the responsibility of the *cis*-, *medial*-, and *trans*-Golgi stacks. The TGN is a tubulovesicular network wherein proteins are targeted to the plasma membrane or to organelles.

In addition to the processing of carbohydrates in the Golgi, posttranslational modifications can take place in other subcellular compartments. Some protein glycosylations are modified further post-Golgi in components of the smooth endoplasmic reticulum or transport vesicles, as described later in this section. Finally, some neuropeptides (vasopressin, enkephalins, etc.) are synthesized as sequence domains in large precursor proteins that must be cleaved in transit by specific proteases to form the biologically active form.

The CGN serves an important sorting function for proteins entering the Golgi from the RER. Because most proteins that move from the RER through the secretory pathway do so by default, any resident endoplasmic reticulum proteins must be restrained from exiting or returned promptly to the RER from the CGN should they escape. Although no retention signal has been demonstrated for the endoplasmic reticulum, two retrieval signals have been identified:

a Lys-Asp-Glu-Leu or KDEL sequence in type I proteins and the Arg-Arg or RR motif in the first five amino acids of proteins with a type II orientation in the membrane. The KDEL tetrapeptide binds to a receptor called Erd 2 in the CGN, and the receptor–ligand complex is returned to the RER. There may also be a receptor for the N arginine dipeptide; alternatively, this sequence may interact with other components of the retrograde transport machinery, such as microtubules.

Movement of proteins between Golgi stacks proceeds by means of vesicular budding and fusion (Rothman, 1994). Through the use of a cell-free assay

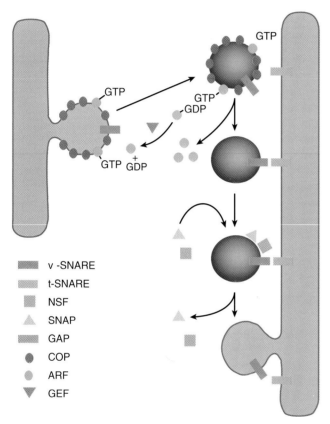

v -SNARE
t-SNARE
NSF
SNAP
GAP
COP
ARF
GEF

FIGURE 4.5 General mechanisms of vesicle targeting and docking in the ER and Golgi. The assembly of coat proteins (COPs) around budding vesicles is driven by ADP-ribosylation factors (ARFs) in a GTP-dependent fashion. Dissociation of the coat is triggered when hydrolysis of the GTP bound to ARF is stimulated by a GTPase-activating protein (GAP) in the Golgi membrane. The cycle of coat assembly and disassembly can continue when the replacement of GDP on ARF by GTP is catalyzed by a guanine-nucleotide exchange factor (GEF). Fusion of vesicles with their target membrane in the Golgi is regulated by a series of proteins, N-ethylmaleimide-sensitive factor (NSF), soluble NSF attachment proteins (SNAPs), and SNAP receptors (SNAREs), which together assist the vesicle in docking with its target membrane. SNAREs on the vesicle (v-SNAREs) are believed to associate with corresponding t-SNAREs on the target membrane.

containing Golgi-derived vesicles, the essential mechanisms for budding and fusion have been shown to require coat proteins (COPs) in a manner that is analogous to the role of clathrin in endocytosis. Currently, two main types of COP complex, COPI and COPII, have been distinguished. Although both have been shown to coat vesicles that bud from the endoplasmic reticulum, they may have different roles in membrane trafficking. Coat proteins provide the external framework into which a region of a flattened Golgi cisternae can bud and vesiculate. A complex of these COPs forms the coatomer (coat protomer) together with a p200 protein, AP-1 adaptins, and a family of GTP-binding proteins called ADP-ribosylation factors (ARFs), originally named for their role in the action of cholera toxin. Immunolocalization of one of the coatamer proteins, β-COP, predominantly to the CGN and cis-Golgi indicates that these proteins may also take part in vesicle transport into the Golgi (Fig. 4.5). The function of ARF is to drive the assembly of the coatamer and therefore vesicle budding in a GTP-dependent fashion. Dissociation of the coat is triggered when hydrolysis of the GTP bound to ARF is stimulated by a GTPase-activating protein (GAP) in the Golgi membrane. The cycle of coat assembly and disassembly can continue when the replacement of GDP on ARF by GTP is catalyzed by a guanine-nucleotide exchange factor (GEF). The importance of this GDP–GTP exchange to normal vesicular traffic is illustrated dramatically by the effects of brefeldin A, a fungal metabolite that specifically inhibits GTP exchange and disperses the Golgi complex by preventing the return of Golgi components from the intermediate compartment.

Fusion of vesicles with their target membrane in the Golgi apparatus is believed to be regulated by a series of proteins, N-ethylmaleimide-sensitive factor (NSF), soluble NSF attachment proteins (SNAPs), and SNAP receptors (SNAREs), which together assist the vesicle in docking with its target membrane. In addition, Rabs, a family of membrane-bound GTPases, act in concert with their own GAPs, GEFs, and a cytosolic protein that dissociates Rab–GDP from membranes after fusion called guanine-nucleotide dissociation inhibitor. Rabs are believed to regulate the action of SNAREs, the proteins directly engaged in membrane–membrane contact prior to fusion. The tight control necessary for this process and the importance of ensuring that vesicle fusion takes place only at the appropriate target membrane may explain why eukaryotic cells contain so many Rabs, some of which are known to specifically take part in the internalization of endocytic vesicles at the plasma membrane (Fig. 4.3).

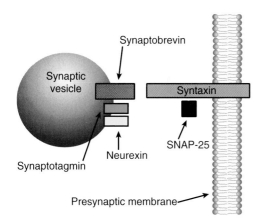

FIGURE 4.6 Mechanisms of vesicle targeting and docking in the synaptic terminal. The synaptic counterpart of v-SNARE is synaptobrevin (also known as vesicle-associated membrane protein), and syntaxin corresponds to t-SNARE. SNAP-25 is an accessory protein that binds to syntaxin. Synaptotagmin is believed to be the Ca^{2+}-sensitive regulatory protein in the complex that binds to syntaxin. Neurexins appear to have a role in conferring Ca^{2+} sensitivity to these interactions.

Exocytosis of the neurotransmitter at the synapse must occur in an even more finely regulated manner than endocytosis. The proteins first identified in vesicular fusion events in the secretory pathway (namely NSF, SNAPs, and SNAREs or closely related homologues) appear to play a part in the fusion of synaptic vesicles with the active zones of the presynaptic neuronal membrane (Fig. 4.6).

The synaptic counterpart of v-SNARE is synaptobrevin [also known as vesicle-associated membrane protein (VAMP)], and syntaxin corresponds to t-SNARE. SNAP-25 is an accessory protein that binds to syntaxin. In the constitutive pathway, such as between the RER and Golgi apparatus, assembly of the complex at the target membrane promotes fusion. However, at the presynaptic membrane, Ca^{2+} influx is required to stimulate membrane fusion at the presynaptic membrane. Synaptotagmin is believed to be the Ca^{2+}-sensitive regulatory protein in the complex that binds syntaxin. Neurexins appear to have a role in regulation as well, because, in addition to interacting with synaptotagmin, they are the targets of black widow spider venom (α)-latrotoxin, which deregulates the Ca^{2+}-dependent exocytosis of the neurotransmitter.

The comparison between secretion in slow-releasing cells, such as the pancreatic (β)-cell, and neurotransmitter release at the neuromuscular junction is much like the comparison between a hand-held pocket calculator for balancing a checkbook and a state-of-the-art desktop computer. Two differences stand out. First, the speed of neurotransmitter release is much greater both in release from a single vesicle and in total release in response to a specific signal. Releasing the contents of a single synaptic vesicle at a mouse neuromuscular junction takes from 1 to 2 ms, and the response to an action potential involving the release of many synaptic vesicles is over in approximately 5 ms. In contrast, releasing the insulin in a single secretory granule by a pancreatic (β)-cell takes from 1 to 5 s, and the full release response may take from 1 to 5 min. A 103- to 105-fold difference in rate is an extraordinary range, making neurotransmitter release one of the fastest biological events routinely encountered, but this speed is critical for a properly functioning nervous system.

A second major difference between slow secretion and fast secretion is seen in the recycling of vesicles. In the pancreas, secretory vesicles carrying insulin are used only once, and so new secretory vesicles must be assembled *de novo* and released from the TGN to meet future requirements. In the neuron, the problem is that the synapse may be at a distance of 1 m or more from the protein synthetic machinery of the perikaryon, and so newly assembled vesicles even traveling at rapid axonal transport rates (see later) may take more than a day to arrive. Now, the number of synaptic vesicles released in 15 min of constant stimulation at a single frog neuromuscular junction has been calculated to be on the order of 105 vesicles, but a single terminal may have only a few hundred vesicles at any one time. These measurements would make no sense if synaptic vesicles had to be replaced constantly through new synthesis in the perikaryon, as is the case with insulin-carrying vesicles. The reason that these numbers are possible is that synaptic vesicles are taken up locally by endocytosis, refilled with neurotransmitter, and reutilized at a rate fast enough to keep up with normal physiological stimulation levels. This takes place within the presynaptic terminal, and evidence shows that these recycled synaptic vesicles are used preferentially (Heuser and Reese, 1973). Such recycling does not require protein synthesis because the classical neurotransmitters are small molecules, such as acetylcholine, or amino acids, such as glutamate, that can be synthesized or obtained locally. Significantly, neurons have fast and slow secretory pathways operating in parallel in the presynaptic terminal (Sudhof, 1995). Synapses that release classical neurotransmitters (acetylcholine, glutamate, etc.) with these fast kinetics also contain dense core granules containing neuropeptides (calcitonin gene-related peptide, substance P, etc.) that are comparable to the secretory granules of the pancreatic (β)-cell. These are used only once because neuropeptides are produced from large polypeptide precursors that must be made by protein synthesis in the cell body. The release of neuropeptides is relatively slow; as is the case in endocrine release, neuropeptides serve primarily as modulators of synaptic function. The small clear synaptic vesicles containing the classic neurotransmitters can in fact be depleted pharmacologically from the presynaptic terminal, while the dense core granules remain. These observations indicate that even though fast and slow secretory mechanisms have many similarities and may even have common components, in neurons they can operate independent of one another.

Proteins Exit the Golgi Complex at the *trans*-Golgi Network

Most of the N-linked oligosaccharide chains acquired at the RER are remodeled in the Golgi cisternae, and while the proteins are in transit, another type of glycosyl linkage to serine or threonine residues through *N*-acetylgalactosamine can also be made. Modification of existing sugar chains by a series of glycosidases and the addition of further sugars by glycosyl transferases occur from the *cis* to the *trans* stacks. Some of these enzymes have been localized to particular cisternae. For example, the enzymes (β)-1,4-galactosyltransferase and (α)-2,6-sialyltransferase are concentrated in the *trans*-Golgi. How they are retained there is a matter of some debate. One idea is that these proteins are anchored by oligomerization. Another view is that the progressively rising concentration of cholesterol in membranes more distal to the ER in the secretory pathway increases membrane thickness, which in turn anchors certain proteins and causes an arrest in their flow along the default route.

The default or constitutive pathway seems to be the direct route to the plasma membrane taken by vesicles that bud from the TGN (Fig. 4.3). This is how, in general, integral plasma membrane proteins reach the cell surface. Proteins bound for regulated secretion or for transport to endosomes and from there to lysosomes are diverted from the default path by means of specific signals. It has been assumed that the sorting of proteins for their eventual destination takes place at the TGN itself. However, recent analyses of the three-dimensional structure of the TGN have provoked a revision of this view. These studies have shown that the TGN is tubular, with two major types of vesicles that bud from distinct populations of tubules. The implication is that sorting may already have occurred in the *trans*-Golgi prior to the proteins' arrival at the TGN. One population of vesicles consists of those surrounded by the familiar clathrin cage, which are destined for late endosomes. The other population appears to be coated in a lace-like structure, which may prove to be made from the elusive coat protein required for vesicular transport to the plasma membrane. The β-COP protein and related coatomer proteins active in more proximal regions of the secretory pathway are absent from the TGN.

Endocytosis and Membrane Cycling Occurs in the *trans*-Golgi Network

Two types of membrane invagination occur at the surface of mammalian cells and are clearly distinguishable by electron microscopy. The first type is a caveola, which has a thread-like structure on its surface made of the protein caveolin. Caveolae mediate the uptake of small molecules such as vitamin folic acid by a process called potocytosis. They may also have a role in concentrating proteins linked to the plasma membrane by the glycosylphosphatidylinositol anchor. Demonstration of the targeting of protein tyrosine kinases to caveolae by the tripeptide signal MGC (Met-Gly-Cys) also suggests that caveolae may function in signal transduction cascades.

The other type of endocytic vesicle at the cell surface is that coated with the distinctive meshwork of clathrin triskelions. The triskelion comprises three copies of a clathrin heavy chain and three copies of a clathrin light chain (Pley and Parham, 1993). The ease with which these triskelions can assemble into a cage structure demonstrates how they promote the budding of a vesicle from a membrane invagination. Clathrin binds selectively to regions of the cytoplasmic surface of membranes that are selected by adaptins. The AP-2 complex, which is primarily active at the plasma membrane, consists of 100-kDa α and β subunits and two subunits of 50 and 17 kDa each. AP-1 complexes localize to the TGN and have γ and β subunits of 100 kDa together with smaller polypeptides of 46 and 19 kDa. Adaptins bind to the cytoplasmic tails of membrane proteins, thus recruiting clathrin for budding at these sites.

A further component of the endocytic complex at the plasma membrane is GTPase dynamin, which seems to be required for the normal budding of coated vesicles during endocytosis. Dynamins are a family of 100-kDa GTPases found in both neuronal and nonneuronal cells and may interact with the AP-2 component of a clathrin-coated pit (deCamilli *et al.*, 1995). Dynamin I is found primarily in neurons, whereas dynamin II has a widespread distribution. Oligomers of dynamin form a ring at the neck of a budding clathrin-coated vesicle, and GTP hydrolysis appears to be necessary for the coated vesicle to pinch off from the plasma membrane. The existence of a specific neuronal form of dynamin may be a manifestation of the unusually rapid rate of synaptic vesicle recycling.

The primary function of clathrin-coated vesicles at the plasma membrane is to deliver membrane proteins together with any ligands bound to them to the early endosomal apparatus. The other major site of action of clathrin is in vesicles that bud from the TGN carrying lysosomal enzymes en route to late endosomes. Early endosomes have a tubulovesicular morphology. Receptors that will be recycled back to the plasma membrane partition into the tubules; those endocytosed proteins destined for lysosomes concentrate in the vesicular regions. Recycling seems to be the default pathway, whereas proteins must be actively targeted to lysosomes. However, the precise signals for this are unknown.

Regulation of membrane cycling in the endosomal compartment is likely to include the Rab family of small GTP-binding proteins. Indeed, each stage of the endocytic pathway may have its own Rab protein to ensure efficient targeting of the vesicle to the appropriate membrane. Rab6 is believed to have a role in transport from the TGN to endosomes, whereas Rab9 may regulate vesicular flow in the reverse direction. In neurons, Rab5a has a role in regulating the fusion of endocytic vesicles and early endosomes and appears to function in endocytosis from both somatodendritic domains and the axon. The association of the protein with synaptic vesicles in nerve terminals, attached presumably by means of its isoprenoid tail, also suggests that early endosomal compartments may have a role in the packaging and recycling of synaptic vesicles.

Lysosome Is the Target Organelle in Several Inherited Diseases That Affect the Nervous System

Lysosomes were first isolated and characterized as a distinct organelle fraction bounded by a single membrane and separable from mitochondria by differential and sucrose gradient centrifugation. Because of their high content of acid hydrolases, the classic view is that lysosomes are organelles of terminal degradation. Indeed, the latency of hydrolase activity before membrane permeabilization by agents such as nonionic detergents has been used biochemically as a measure of the purity and intactness of lysosomal

preparations. However, in addition to their well-established function in lipid and protein breakdown, tubulovesicular lysosomes may overlap in sorting functions with early endosomes, particularly during antigen processing in macrophages.

Inherited deficiencies in lipid metabolism in the lysosome often have particularly devastating consequences on the nervous system because of the abundance of the lipid-rich membrane myelin. Metachromatic leukodystrophy is an autosomal recessive disease caused by a deficiency in arylsulfatase A activity, which is also responsible for degrading the myelin lipid cerebroside sulfate (sulfatide). Oligodendrocytes accumulate sulfatide in metachromatic granules, causing severe disruption of myelination. Peripheral nerve myelination is also affected, as are other organs that normally contain much lower amounts of sulfatide, such as the kidney, the liver, and the endocrine system. Krabbe disease, or globoid cell leukodystrophy, is also a dysmyelinating disease in which there is an almost complete lack of oligodendrocytes and therefore myelin, caused by a deficiency in the β-galactosidase responsible for hydrolyzing galactocerebroside to ceramide and galactose. Galactocerebroside is particularly abundant in myelin, constituting about 25% of myelin lipid. Mice that lack galactocerebroside have the ability to assemble multilamellar myelin; however, this myelin does not support adequate nerve conduction, neither is it stable. Unlike metachromatic leukodystrophy, Krabbe disease is limited to the CNS and peripheral nervous system (PNS). However, why a buildup of galactocerebroside should prove particularly toxic to oligodendrocytes is not entirely clear. One hypothesis is that a metabolite of galactocerebroside, galactosphingosine (psychosine), is the primary culprit. Because there is an authentic mouse model for Krabbe disease, twitcher, gene therapy provides some hope of correcting the disease.

How are proteins destined to operate in lysosomes targeted to these organelles? Soluble lysosomal hydrolase enzymes acquire a phosphorylated mannose on their oligosaccharide chains by a two-step process in the Golgi apparatus. This mannose 6-phosphate label is recognized by specific mannose 6-phosphate receptors, which carry the proteins to late endosomes. In contrast, lysosomal membrane proteins are targeted by means of cytoplasmic tail signals that contain either leucine or tyrosine of type LJ or type YXXJ or NXXY, where J is any hydrophobic amino acid. The LJ signal seems to be essential for efficient delivery directly to endosomes, whereas the second type of signal seems to be more important in the recovery of proteins destined for lysosomes from the plasma membrane. The majority of lysosomal membrane proteins have the YXXJ but do not have the LJ signal. The implication of these observations is that many of the lysosomal membrane proteins make their way to lysosomes from the TGN endosomes through the plasma membrane.

What are the receptors for the type LJ or the type YXXJ or NXXY motifs at the TGN? Because transport from the TGN to the endosomes occurs in clathrin-coated vesicles, the proteins that link such vesicles to membranes, the adaptins, may play a role. The weight of the evidence suggests that AP-1 recognizes the LJ sequence, whereas AP-2 identifies the YXXJ and NXXY motifs. Once the ligands are bound, these adaptins would direct transport of their respective ligands to the endosomes from the TGN or through the plasma membrane, respectively.

At present, it is not clear how proteins in the late endosome, such as mannose 6-phosphate receptors, that cycle back to the Golgi are sorted from those whose ultimate destination is a lysosome.

How Are Peripheral Membrane Proteins Targeted to their Appropriate Destinations?

Peripheral membrane proteins are synthesized in the same type of free polysome in which the bulk of the cytosolic proteins are made. However, the cell must ensure that these membrane proteins are sent to the plasma membrane rather than allowed to attach in a haphazard way to other intracellular organelles. The fact that a complex machinery has evolved to ensure the correct delivery of integral membrane proteins suggests that some equivalent targeting mechanism must exist for proteins that attach to the cytoplasmic surface of the plasma membrane. Such proteins are translated on "free" polysomes, but these polysomes are associated with cytoskeletal structures and are not distributed uniformly throughout the cell body. In a number of cases, mRNAs that encode soluble cytosolic proteins are concentrated in discrete regions of the cell, resulting in a local accumulation of the translated protein close to the site of action. For some peripheral membrane proteins, this is the plasma membrane.

Evidence that this mechanism might operate in peripheral membrane protein synthesis came from studies showing biochemically and by *in situ* hybridization that mRNAs encoding the myelin basic proteins are concentrated in the myelinating processes that extend from the cell body of oligodendrocytes (Colman *et al.*, 1982). Myelin basic protein may be a special case because of its very strong positive charge and consequent propensity for binding promiscu-

ously to the negatively charged polar head groups of membrane lipids. Nevertheless, the fact that actin mRNAs are localized to the leading edge of cultured myocytes and mRNA for the microtubule-associated protein MAP2b is concentrated in the dendrites of neurons suggest that targeting by local synthesis is more common than originally thought. This mechanism is probably less important for peripheral membrane proteins that associate with the cytoplasmic surface of the plasma membrane by means of strong specific associations with proteins already located at the membrane because such proteins would act as specific receptors. Because only selected cytoplasmic mRNAs are localized to the periphery, the process is specific. However, no mRNAs are localized exclusively to the periphery, and a significant fraction are typically localized proximal to the nucleus in a region rich with the translational and protein-processing machinery of the cell (the Nissl substance or translational cytoplasm).

Special Mechanisms Are Used to Target Proteins to Mitochondria and Peroxisomes

The inner membrane of the mitochondrion is the site of oxidative phosphorylation in which the step-by-step transfer of electrons from oxygen intermediary metabolites to molecular oxidation is coupled to proton transport and ATP synthesis. Thus, this organelle has an essential role in providing the large amount of ATP required for the electrical activity of neurons. The fact that, in a resting adult, about 40% of the total energy consumption is required for ion pumping in the CNS accounts for the exquisite sensitivity of the brain to damage from oxygen deprivation. The sensitivity of neurons to interruptions in the provision of ATP by the mitochondrion is also seen in cases of uremia, where a buildup of ammonium ions depletes the Krebs cycle of α-oxoglutaric acid by converting it into glutamate.

Although the mitochondrion has its own circular DNA that encodes some proteins, most mitochondrial proteins are synthesized in the nucleocytoplasmic system. This poses the problem of how these proteins once made in the cytoplasm gain entry into the mitochondrion. Furthermore, because the mitochondrion has an inner and an outer membrane, some proteins must cross two membranes to gain access to the inner matrix. This group of proteins includes the enzymes of the Krebs cycle and the fatty acid β-oxidation pathway.

Unlike proteins inserted into the RER, mitochondrial proteins can be imported either posttranslationally or cotranslationally with the use of a cleavable amphipathic helical signal sequence usually at the N terminus. At the RER, the signal sequence of a nascent polypeptide chain can be translocated across the membrane because the polypeptide remains small and unfolded due to the arrest of translation caused by a signal-recognition particle. However, mitochondrial proteins are typically synthesized on cytoplasmic or free polysomes and must be folded at least partially to prevent degradation. For posttranslational import, mitochondria rely on a group of molecular chaperones to prevent complete folding of the polypeptides. These hsp70 and hsp60 proteins were originally identified because they are upregulated during heat shock. Their role in binding to proteins and maintaining them in specific conformations helps explain why these proteins have an important function in protecting proteins against the stress of elevated temperatures as well as facilitating the proper folding of newly synthesized polypeptides. In yeast, a second protein, Ydj1p, whose bacterial homologue DnaJ regulates chaperone function has been identified. Ydj1p possesses an isoprenoid tail linked to its C-terminal amino acid, which may serve to anchor the protein to the outer membrane. The third factor that has been implicated is the mitochondrial stimulation factor, which is a heterodimer possessing an ATP-dependent protein "unfoldase" activity. This factor may be more important in cotranslational import where polysomes are known to be associated with the mitochondrial outer membrane.

Most of our current understanding of protein translocation from the mitochondrial outer membrane inward has come from studies on either the fungus *Neurospora crassa* or the yeast *S. cerevisiae*. In both yeast and higher eukaryotes, the partially folded polypeptide targeted for the mitochondrion may be stabilized by a cytoplasmic chaperone that is a member of the hsp70 family, but this interaction is not required for import. However, several proteins in the outer membrane form an essential complex that acts as a receptor and pore for protein translocation. This complex can in turn interact with an inner membrane complex at specialized contact sites that minimize the distance across the two membranes, thereby facilitating the movement of proteins to the inner matrix. Although both pores can function independently, they contact and cooperate when there is a transmembrane potential across the inner membrane. This accounts for early observations showing that importation of subunits of the F1-ATPase, an inner membrane protein, required an active electron transport chain but did not need ATP synthesis. The mitochondrial import sequence extends through the pore into the

inner matrix, where a second member of the hsp70 family binds and facilitates movement into the inner matrix. After proteins have crossed into the inner matrix, they must dissociate from hsp70 in order to fold properly, a process that requires another kind of molecular chaperone, hsp60.

Peroxisomes are so named because they contain oxidases that generate H_2O_2 and the enzyme catalase, which is responsible for detoxifying it. In addition, these organelles contain many other enzymes that take part in lipid, purine, and amino acid metabolism. Peroxisomes are of interest because of the number of inherited diseases associated with defects either in certain enzymes or indeed in the assembly of the organelle itself (Moser, 1987). Some of these diseases manifest as particularly damaging to the nervous system and include adrenoleukodystrophy (accumulation of very long chain fatty acids due to insufficient lignoceryl-CoA ligase activity caused by inefficient import of the protein) and Refsum disease (buildup of phytanic acid due to defective α-oxidation), both of which cause demyelination.

Like many mitochondrial proteins, peroxisomal proteins are imported posttranslationally. Although cytosolic factors are implicated in peroxisomal biogenesis, no peroxisomal chaperones analogous to the hsp70 family have yet been shown to function in protein import. Therefore, unfolding and refolding are assumed not to play a role in the accumulation of proteins inside the peroxisome. Among these cytosolic proteins is presumed to be the receptor for the tripeptide C-terminal import signal SKL (Ser-Lys-Leu) known as peroxisomal targeting signal 1 (PTS1). In addition to C-terminal PTS1, some peroxisomal proteins have a cleavable N-terminal sequence called PTS2, which signals their import. A quite distinct translocation machinery appears to operate for PTS1 and PTS2 proteins. Two possible receptor proteins in the peroxisomal membrane, one of which is the adrenoleukodystrophy protein (ALDP), have been identified. ALDP is a member of a larger family known as ABC ATP-dependent membrane transporters.

A characteristic feature of peroxisomal biogenesis is that it is stimulated by drugs whose detoxification requires peroxisomal activity. It is possible that mature peroxisomes are recruited from a pool of precursor organelles, and there is some evidence for the existence of such a population in rat liver. Although the mature organelle appears to be spherical, electron microscopic evidence suggests a peroxisomal reticulum at which synthesis and protein import may take place. Mature peroxisomes might then arise from this reticulum by a process of budding.

Cytoplasmic Proteins Are Also Compartmentalized

Membrane-bound organelles are the most familiar form of compartmentation in cells, but cytoplasmic regions of the cell containing metabolic compartments exist as well. Regions of the neuronal or glial cytoplasm may have highly specialized polypeptide compositions that are important for function. For example, the neuronal phosphoprotein synapsin is highly enriched in presynaptic terminals, where it participates in the localization and targeting of synaptic vesicles. Similarly, calmodulin and the glycolytic enzyme aldolase have been localized in muscle cells to the region of the I band, where they are thought to facilitate coupling of ATP production to contractility.

As mentioned earlier, cytoplasmic proteins are synthesized on cytoplasmic polysomes, termed "free" polysomes to reflect an absence of underlying ER membrane, even though they may be restricted to specific domains of the cell cytoplasm. This restriction is particularly obvious in the neuronal perikaryon, where both cytoplasmic polysomes and membrane-associated polysomes are concentrated in areas near the nucleus and Golgi complex. In addition, cytoplasmic polysomes containing specific mRNAs may be localized to certain regions of the cell, such as the proximal dendrite (those encoding the microtubule-associated protein MAP-2) and the processes of oligodendrocytes (those encoding myelin basic protein). In contrast, the protein synthetic machinery of the polysome appears to be effectively excluded from the mature axon. Therefore, cytoplasmic polysomes are representative of cytoplasmic compartmentation for proteins and nucleic acids.

In most cases, localized cytoplasmic proteins interact with cytoskeletal structures in the cytoplasm (see next section), but macromolecular complexes that form in order to make a cellular process more efficient or free from error have been described. Evidence exists that glycolytic enzymes of neurons and muscle cells may be organized in a labile complex that facilitates energy metabolism, but the existence of such complexes remains controversial.

Perhaps the best characterized cytoplasmic macromolecular complex is the proteasome, which is a large protein complex (2×10^6 Da, sedimenting as a 20S particle) that contains several distinct enzymatic activities, including catalytic sites for both ubiquitin-dependent and ubiquitin-independent proteolysis (Hochstrasser, 1995). Ubiquitin is a small, highly conserved polypeptide that is added covalently to cytoplasmic proteins targeted for degradation. The catalytic core of the proteasome is a barrel-shaped structure formed by four heptameric stacked rings, but additional proteins (about 16 polypeptides) may interact with the 20S core to form a larger 26S particle. Because proteasomes constitute the primary cytoplasmic pathway for protein degradation (i.e., nonlysosomal pathways), they serve a number of important physiological functions, including regulation of cell proliferation and processing of antigens for presentation. In the nervous system, however, proteasomes are likely to be most important for homeostasis, allowing turnover of cytoplasmic polypeptides at specific sites so that the elaborate cellular extensions of neurons and glia may be maintained.

Cytoplasmic proteins may also be compartmentalized effectively by posttranslational modification. Two types of modification may be particularly important for this kind of compartmentalization. Local activation of kinases can lead to the phosphorylation of proteins in specific domains of the neuron. For example, the reversible phosphorylation of synapsin in the presynaptic terminal appears to be responsible for the targeting of synaptic vesicles to the terminal and for the mobilization of vesicles during prolonged stimulation. An impressive variety of cytoplasmic protein kinases that may be selectively activated to modify serines or threonines presented in distinctive consensus sequences have been described. Distinct from these serine or threonine kinases, a number of other kinases that specifically modify tyrosines can be found in the brain. In some cases, the tyrosine kinase is linked directly to a membrane-spanning receptor and phosphorylates cytoplasmic proteins in the vicinity of the receptor after activation. Completing the cycle of phosphorylation and dephosphorylation are a number of phosphatases with varying specificities. The properties and physiological roles for kinases and phosphatases are discussed in greater detail later.

A second common posttranslational modification of cytoplasmic proteins is the addition of carbohydrate moieties. Whereas modification of membrane-associated proteins in the Golgi complex proceeds by the addition of complex carbohydrates through N linkages on selected asparagines, glycosylated cytoplasmic proteins have simpler carbohydrates added through O linkages to serine or threonine hydroxyls. This modification was first recognized as a feature of many nuclear proteins and components of the nuclear membrane, but subsequent studies showed that a number of cytoplasmic proteins also have O-linked carbohydrates. Unlike phosphorylation, relatively little is known about the functional significance of cytoplasmic glycosylation. Remarkably, however, serines and threonines subject to O-linked glycosylation would also be good sites for phosphorylation by various kinases as well. This congruence raises the possibility that glycosylation and phosphorylation of some cytoplasmic proteins may serve complementary functions.

Summary

Membrane biogenesis and protein synthesis in neurons and glial cells are accomplished by the same mechanisms that have been worked out in great detail in other cell types. Integral membrane proteins are synthesized in the rough endoplasmic reticulum, and peripheral membrane proteins are products of cytoplasmic-free ribosomes that are found in the cell sap. For transmembrane proteins and secretory polypeptides, synthesis in the RER is followed by transport to the Golgi apparatus, where membranes and proteins are sorted and targeted for delivery to precise intracellular locations. It is likely that the neuron and glial cell have evolved additional highly specialized mechanisms for membrane and protein sorting and targeting because these cells are so greatly extended in space, although these additional mechanisms have yet to be fully described. The basic features of the process of secretion, which includes neurotransmitter delivery to presynaptic terminals, are beginning to be understood as well. The key features of this process are apparently common to all cells, including yeast, although the neuron has developed certain specializations and modifications of the secretory pathway that reflect its unique properties as an excitable cell.

CYTOSKELETONS OF NEURONS AND GLIAL CELLS

The cytoskeleton of eukaryotic cells is an aggregate structure formed by three classes of cytoplasmic structural proteins: microtubules (tubulins), microfilaments (actins), and intermediate filaments (Fig. 4.7). Each of these elements exists concurrently and independently in overlapping cellular domains. Most cell types contain one or more examples of each class of cytoskeletal structure, but there are exceptions. For example, mature mammalian erythrocytes contain neither microtubules nor intermediate filaments, but they do have elaborate and highly specialized actin cytoskeletons. Among cells of the nervous system, the oligodendrocyte is unusual in that it contains no cytoplasmic intermediate filaments. Typically, each cell type in the nervous system has a unique complement of cytoskeletal proteins that are important for the differentiated function of that cell type.

Although the three classes of cytoskeletal elements interact with each other and with other cellular structures, all three are dynamic structures rather than passive structural elements. Their aggregate properties form the basis of cell morphologies and plasticity in the nervous tissue. In many cases, biochemical specialization in the cytoskeleton is characteristic of a particular cell type, function, and developmental stage. Each type of cytoskeletal element has unique functions that are essential for a working nervous system.

Microtubules Are an Important Determinant of Cell Architecture

Microtubules (Fig. 4.7) are nearly ubiquitous components of the cytoskeleton in eukaryotes (Hyams and Lloyd, 1994). They play key roles in intracellular transport, are a primary determinant of cell morphology, are the structural correlate of the mitotic spindle, and form the functional core of cilia and flagella. Microtubules are very abundant in the nervous system, and tubulin subunits of microtubules may

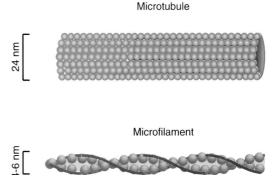

FIGURE 4.7 Two major classes of cytoskeletal structures found in all cellular components of the nervous system are microtubules and microfilaments. These structures constitute the substrates for the various motor proteins of cells. In electron micrographs, microtubules appear as hollow tubes with walls formed by 12–14 protofilaments. Each protofilament consists of a series of α- and β-tubulin dimers organized in a polar fashion, giving the microtubule a plus (fast growing) end and a minus (slow growing) end. In axons, microtubules have their plus ends distal from the cell body, whereas dendritic microtubules may have either polarity. Microtubules are approximately 24 nm in diameter and may be more than 100 μm in length. Various polypeptides called microtubule-associated proteins (MAPs) are typically associated with the surface of the microtubule. These MAPs may help regulate assembly and organization of the microtubules. In contrast, actin microfilaments form from two twisted strands of actin subunits that form filaments only 4–6 nm in diameter. The length of microfilaments is quite variable, but most neuronal filaments are short, in the range of 200–500 nm. Many different proteins have been shown to interact with microfilaments in cells, including cross-linking, bundling, severing, and capping proteins (see Table 4.3).

constitute more than 10% of total brain protein. As a result, many fundamental properties of microtubules have been defined by using microtubule protein prepared from brain extracts. At the same time, the microtubule cytoskeleton of the neuron has a variety of biochemical specializations that meet the unique demands imposed by the size and shape of the neuron.

Of the various functions defined for microtubules, intracellular transport and the generation of cellular morphology are the most important roles played by microtubules in cells of the nervous system. In part, this comes from their ability to organize cytoplasmic polarity. Microtubules *in vitro* are dynamic, polar structures with plus and minus ends that correspond to the fast- and slow-growing ends, respectively. In contrast, both stable and labile microtubules can be identified *in vivo*, where they help define both microscopic and macroscopic aspects of intracellular organization in cells. Microtubule organization, stability, and composition in nervous tissue are all highly regulated in the nervous system.

By electron microscopy, microtubules appear as hollow tubes 25 nm in diameter and in axons can be up to hundreds of micrometers in length. High-resolution electron micrographs also reveal that the walls of microtubules typically comprise 13 protofilaments formed by a linear arrangement of globular subunits, although microtubules with 12 to 14 protofilaments exist in some tissues and organisms. Globular subunits in the walls of a microtubule are heterodimers of α- and β-tubulin, whereas a variety of microtubule-associated proteins bind to the surface of microtubules.

Neuronal microtubules are remarkable for their genetic and biochemical diversity. Multiple genes exist for both α- and β-tubulins. These genes are expressed differentially according to cell type and developmental stage. Some of these genetic isotypes are expressed ubiquitously, whereas others are only turned on at specific times in development, in specific cell types, or both. Most tubulin genes are expressed in nervous tissue, and some appear to be enriched or specific to neurons. When specific isotypes are prepared in a pure form, they show variability in assembly kinetics and ability to bind ligands. However, when more than one isotype is expressed in a single cell, such as a neuron, they coassemble into microtubules with mixed composition.

A variety of posttranslational modifications of tubulins have been described, the most common of which are tyrosination–detyrosination, acetylation–deacetylation, and phosphorylation. The first two of these pathways are associated intimately with the assembly of microtubules, but relatively little is known about physiological functions for any of these modified tubulins. Most α-tubulin isotypes are synthesized with a Glu-Tyr dipeptide at the C terminus (Tyr-tubulin), but the tyrosine can be removed by a specific tubulin carboxypeptidase after assembly into a microtubule, leaving a terminal glutamate (Glu-tubulin). When microtubules containing detyrosinated α-tubulins are disassembled, the liberated α-tubulins are retyrosinated rapidly by a specific tubulin tyrosine ligase. The result is that microtubules that have been assembled for an extended period of time will tend to be rich in Glu-tubulin. The tyrosination state of α-tubulin does not affect its assembly–disassembly kinetics *in vitro*, but evidence suggests that detyrosination may affect the interaction of microtubules with other cellular structures. In parallel with detyrosination, α-tubulins are also substrates for a specific acetylation reaction. Acetylation of tubulin was initially described for flagellar tubulins, but subsequent work demonstrated that this modification was widespread in neurons and many other cell types. Because the acetylase acts preferentially on α-tubulin assembled into microtubules, long-lived or stable microtubules tend to be rich in acetylated α-tubulin. However, the distribution of microtubules rich in acetylated tubulin may not be identical with that of Glu-tubulin. Acetylated α-tubulin is also deacetylated rapidly upon disassembly of microtubules, although acetylation does not alter the stability of microtubules *in vitro*.

In contrast with these modifications, tubulin phosphorylation involves a β-tubulin and appears to be restricted to an isotype expressed preferentially in neurons and neuron-like cells. A variety of kinases have been shown to phosphorylate tubulin *in vitro*, but the endogenous kinase has not been identified. The effect of phosphorylation on assembly is unknown, but phosphorylation is upregulated during neurite outgrowth. As with α-tubulin modifications, the physiological role of phosphorylation on neuronal β-tubulin has yet to be determined. A variety of additional posttranslational modifications have been reported, but their significance and distribution in the nervous system are not well documented.

The biochemical diversity of microtubules is increased through the association of different MAPs with different populations of microtubules (Table 4.2). The significance of microtubule diversity is not completely understood, but it may include functional differences as well as variations in assembly and stability. In particular, MAP composition may be used to define specific neuronal domains. For example, one type of MAP, MAP-2, appears to be restricted to den-

TABLE 4.2 Major Microtubule Proteins and Microtubule Motors in Mammalian Brain

	Location and function
Tubulins	
α- and β-tubulins	Neurons, glia, and nonneuronal cells except mature mammalian erythrocytes. Multigene family with some genes expressed preferentially in brain, whereas others are ubiquitous. Primary structural polypeptides of microtubules
γ-Tubulin	Present in all microtubule-containing cells, but restricted to region of microtubule-organizing center. Needed for nucleation of microtubules
Microtubule-associated proteins (MAPs)	
MAP-1a/1b	Widely expressed in neurons and glia, including both axons and dendrites. Forms are developmentally regulated phosphoproteins.
MAP-2a/2b MAP-2c	Dendrite-specific MAPs. The smaller MAP-2c is, regulated developmentally, becoming restricted to spines in adults, whereas 2a and 2b are major phosphoproteins in adult brain
LMW tau HMW tau	Tau proteins are enriched in axons and have a distinctive phosphorylation pattern in the axon, but may be found in other compartments. A single gene with multiple forms due to alternative splicing. The HMW tau is found in adult peripheral axons
Motor proteins	
Kinesin Neuron-specific kinesin	Present in all microtubule-containing cells. Associated with membrane-bound organelles and serves to move them along microtubules in fast axonal transport. The neuron-specific form is the product of a specific gene expressed in nervous tissue
Kinesin-related proteins	A diverse set of motor proteins with a kinesin-related motor domain and varied tails. Some are regulated developmentally and some are restricted to dividing cells, where they act as mitotic motors.
Axonemal dynein Cytoplasmic dynein (MAP-1c)	A set of minus-end-directed microtubule motors. Axonemal forms are associated with cilia and flagella. In nervous tissue, these may be associated with the ependyma. Cytoplasmic forms may be involved in the transport of either organelles or cytoskeletal elements

dritic regions of the neuron, whereas another class of MAPs, tau proteins, are modified differentially in axons. A recently identified isoform of MAP-2 is similar to MAP-2c but includes an additional repeat within the microtubule-binding site; hence it is known as 4-repeat MAP-2c, or MAP-2d.57. Oligodendrocyte progenitors transiently express this novel isoform of MAP-2c in their cell bodies but not in their processes, suggesting that MAP-2d might have a role separate from its known capacity to bundle microtubules (Vouyiouklis and Brophy, 1995).

MAPs in nervous tissue fall into two heterogeneous groups: tau proteins and high molecular weight MAPs. Tau proteins have been the subject of intense interest because posttranslationally modified tau proteins are the primary polypeptide constituents of neurofibrillary tangles from the brains of Alzheimer patients. Tau proteins appear to be neuronal MAPs, although reports of tau immunoreactivity outside neurons have appeared. Tau proteins bind to microtubules during assembly–disassembly cycles with a constant stoichiometry and can promote microtubule assembly and stabilization. Tau exists in a number of molecular weight isoforms that vary with region of the nervous system and developmental stage. For

example, tau proteins in the adult CNS are typically from 60 to 75 kDa, whereas PNS axons contain a higher molecular mass tau of approximately 100 kDa. The different isoforms of tau protein are generated from a single mRNA by alternative splicing, and additional heterogeneity is produced by phosphorylation.

In contrast with tau MAPs, high molecular weight MAPs are a diverse group of largely unrelated proteins found in a variety of tissues, although some are brain specific. All have apparent molecular mass of 1300 kDa and form side arms protruding from the walls of microtubules. Many of them may participate in microtubule assembly and cytoskeletal organization. Traditionally, the high molecular weight MAPs comprise five polypeptides: MAPs 1a, 1b, 1c, 2a, and 2b. MAP-2 proteins are closely related and are located primarily in dendrites. In contrast, the three polypeptides known as MAP-1 are unique polypeptides with little sequence homology. MAP-1c is a cytoplasmic form of dynein (see the section on molecular motors later in this chapter). MAPs 1a and 1b are widespread and appear to be regulated developmentally. MAPs 1a, 1b, and 2 are all thought to play important roles in stabilizing and organizing the microtubule cytoskeleton.

In most cell types, cytoplasmic microtubules appear to be relatively dynamic structures, although stable microtubules or microtubule segments are found in all cells. In nonneuronal cells such as astrocytes and other glial cells, microtubules are typically anchored in centrosomal regions that serve as microtubule-organizing centers. As a result, their cytoplasmic microtubules are oriented so that plus ends are distal to the cell center. The biochemistry of microtubule-organizing centers is not fully understood, but they contain a novel tubulin subunit, γ-tubulin, which is thought to function as a nucleating site for microtubules. In contrast, dendritic and axonal microtubules of neurons are not continuous with the microtubule-organizing center, so alternate mechanisms must exist for stabilization and organization of these microtubules. The situation is complicated further by the fact that dendritic and axonal microtubules differ in both composition and organization. Studies show that both axonal and dendritic microtubules are nucleated at the microtubule-organizing center but are subsequently released for delivery to the appropriate compartment. Surprisingly, axonal and dendritic compartments are not equivalent. There are two striking differences. First, MAPs of dendritic and axonal microtubules are different in both identity and phosphorylation state. Second, microtubule orientation in axons is similar to that seen in other cell types with the plus end distal, but microtubules in dendrites may exhibit both polarities. Perhaps due to these differences, dendritic microtubules are less likely to be aligned with one another and appear less regular in their spacing.

Stabilization of axonal and dendritic microtubules is essential because of the volume of cytoplasm and distance from sites of protein synthesis for tubulin. Because microtubules play critical roles in both dendritic and axonal function, mechanisms to ensure their proper extent and organization must exist. A common side effect of one class of antineoplastic drugs, the vinca alkaloids, underscores the importance of microtubule stability in axons. Vincristine and other vinca alkaloids act by destabilizing spindle microtubules, but dosage must be monitored carefully to prevent the development of peripheral neuropathies due to loss of axonal microtubules.

Axonal microtubules contain a particularly stable subset of microtubule segments that are resistant to depolymerization by antimitotic drugs, cold, and calcium. The stable microtubule segments are biochemically distinct and may constitute more than half of the axonal tubulin. Stable domains in microtubules may serve to regulate the axonal cytoskeleton by nucleating and organizing microtubules as well as stabilizing them. The biochemical basis of microtubule stability is not completely understood but probably includes posttranslational modification of the tubulin, the presence of stabilizing proteins, or both. There are indications that levels of cold-insoluble tubulin correlate with axonal plasticity. In contrast, relatively little is known about the regulation of dendritic microtubules, but local synthesis of MAP-2 in dendrites may play a role in regulating their stability.

Microfilaments and the Actin-Based Cytoskeleton Are Involved in Intracellular Transport and Cell Movement

The actin cytoskeleton is universally present in eukaryotes, although actin microfilaments are most familiar as the thin filaments of skeletal muscle. Microfilaments (Table 4.3) play a critical role in contractility for both muscle and nonmuscle cells. Actin and its contractile partner myosin are particularly abundant in nervous tissue relative to other nonmuscle tissues. In fact, one of the earliest descriptions of nonmuscle actin and myosin was in brain (Berl et al., 1973). In neurons, actin microfilaments are most abundant in presynaptic terminals, dendritic spines, growth cones, and the subplasmalemmal cortex. Although concentrated in these regions, microfilaments are also present throughout the cytoplasm of both neurons and glia in the form of short filaments from 4 to 6 nm in diameter and from 400 to 800 nm in length.

As with tubulin, multiple actin genes exist in both vertebrates and invertebrates. Four α-actin human genes have been cloned. Each of these α-actin genes is expressed specifically in a different muscle cell type (skeletal, cardiac, vascular smooth, and enteric smooth muscle). In addition to α-actins, two nonmuscle actin genes (β- and γ-actin) are present in humans. β-Actin and γ-actin genes are expressed ubiquitously, and both are abundant in nervous tissue. The functional significance of these different genetic isotypes is not clear because the actins are highly conserved proteins. Across the range of known actin sequences, the amino acids are identical at approximately two of three positions. Even the positions of introns within different actin genes are highly conserved across many species and genes. Despite this high degree of conservation, differences in the distribution of specific isotypes within a single neuron have been reported. For example, β-actin may be enriched in growth cones. The prominent actin bundles seen in fibroblasts and some other nonneuronal cells in culture are not

TABLE 4.3   Selected Proteins of the Microfilament
Cytoskeleton in Brain

Actins
   α-Actin (smooth muscle)
   β-actin and γ-actin (neuronal and nonneuronal cells)

Actin monomer-binding proteins
   Profilin
   Thymosin β4 and β10

Capping proteins
   Ezrin/radixin/moesin
   Schwannomin/merlin

Gelsolin family
   Gelsolin
   Villin
   Scinderin

Cross-linking and bundling proteins
   Spectrin (fodrin)
   Dystrophin, utrophin, and related proteins
   α-Actinin

Tropomyosin

Proteins with nonmicrofilament functions
   MAP-2
   Tau

Myosins
   Iβ
   II
   V
   VI
   VII

characteristic of neurons, and most neuronal actin microfilaments are less than 1 μm in length.

Many microfilament-associated proteins have been described in nervous tissue (myosin, tropomyosin, spectrin, α-actinin, etc.), but less is known about their distribution and normal function in neurons and glia. Myosins and myosin-associated proteins are considered later in the section on molecular motors, but several categories of actin-binding proteins can be defined (Table 4.3). Monomer actin-binding proteins such as profilin and thymosin β4 or β10 are abundant in the developing brain and are thought to help regulate the amount of actin assembled into microfilaments by sequestering actin monomers. These monomers can be mobilized rapidly in response to appropriate signals. For example, phosphatidylinositol 4,5-bisphosphate causes the actin–profilin complex to dissociate, freeing the monomer for microfilament assembly. Such regulation may play a key role in growth cone motility, where actin assembly is an important mechanism for filopodial extension.

Several proteins that can cap actin microfilaments, serving to anchor them to other structures or to regulate microfilament length, have been identified. The ezrin–radixin–moesin gene family encodes barbed-end capping proteins that are concentrated at sites where the microfilaments meet the plasma membrane, suggesting a role in anchoring microfilaments or linking them to extracellular components through membrane proteins. A mutation in a member of this family expressed in Schwann cells, merlin or schwannomin, is thought to be responsible for the human disease neurofibromatosis type 2. Development of numerous tumors with a Schwann cell lineage in neurofibromatosis type 2 suggests that this microfilament-binding protein acts normally as a tumor suppressor.

Whereas some membrane proteins can interact directly with actin microfilaments of the membrane cytoskeleton, others interact with the actin cytoskeleton through intermediaries such as spectrin. Proteins such as spectrin (fodrin), α-actinin, and dystrophins cross-link, or bundle, microfilaments, giving rise to higher order complexes. Spectrin is enriched in the cortical membrane cytoskeleton and is thought to have a role in the localization of integral membrane proteins such as ion channels and receptors. Dystrophin is the best known member of a family of related proteins that all appear to be essential for the clustering of receptors in muscle and nervous tissue. A mutation in dystrophin is responsible for Duchenne muscular dystrophy. Positioning of integral membrane proteins on the cell surface is likely to be an essential function of the actin-rich membrane cytoskeleton, acting in concert with a new class of proteins that contain the protein-binding module, the PDZ domain.

Members of the gelsolin family have multiple activities. They can not only cap the barbed end of a microfilament, but also sever microfilaments and nucleate microfilament assembly under some circumstances. These severing-capping proteins may be essential for reorganizing the actin cytoskeleton. Because gelsolin severing activity is Ca^{2+} activated, it may provide a mechanism for altering the membrane cytoskeleton in response to Ca^{2+} transients. Other second messengers, such as phosphatidylinositol 4,5-bisphosphate, may also serve as regulators of gelsolin function, suggesting an interplay between different classes of actin-binding proteins such as gelsolin and profilin. Oligodendrocytes are the only neural cells in the CNS that express significant amounts of the actin-binding and microfilament-severing protein gelsolin (Tanaka and Sobue, 1994).

Proteins with other functions may also interact directly with actin or actin microfilaments. For example, the enzyme DNase I binds actin tightly, inhibiting both DNase activity and actin assembly.

The physiological function of this interaction is unclear, but it has proved a useful tool for probing actin structure and function. Some membrane proteins, such as the epidermal growth factor receptor, bind actin microfilaments directly, which may be important in anchoring these membrane components at a particular location on the cell surface. Other cytoskeletal structures may have specific interactions. Both MAP-2 and tau microtubule-associated proteins have been shown to interact with actin microfilament *in vitro* and have the potential to mediate interactions between microtubules and microfilaments. Finally, the synaptic vesicle-associated phosphoprotein, synapsin I, has a phosphorylation-sensitive interaction with microfilaments that appears to be important for the targeting and storage of synaptic vesicles in the presynaptic terminal (de Camilli *et al.*, 1990). Many of these interactions have been defined by *in vitro*-binding studies, and their physiological significance is not always clearly established. However, there is little doubt that interactions occur between the actin cytoskeleton and a variety of other cellular structures.

The presence of actin as a major component of both pre- and postsynaptic specializations, as well as in the growth cone, gives the actin cytoskeleton special significance in the nervous system. The enrichment of microfilaments and associated proteins in the membrane cytoskeleton means that they are the cytoskeletal components most subject and most responsive to changes in the local external environment of the neuron.

Microfilaments also play a critical role in positioning the various receptors and ion channels at specific locations on the neuronal surface. Although many studies have emphasized enrichment of the microfilament cytoskeleton at the plasma membrane, microfilaments are also abundant in the deep cytoplasm. In many respects, the microfilaments may be best regarded as a uniquely plastic component of the neuronal cytoskeleton that plays a critical role in local trafficking of both cytoskeletal and membrane components.

Intermediate Filaments Are Prominent Constituents of Nervous Tissue

Intermediate filaments of the nervous system appear as solid, rope-like fibrils from 8 to 12 nm in diameter that may be many micrometers long (Lee and Cleveland, 1996). Intermediate filament proteins constitute a superfamily of five classes, which have distinctive patterns of expression specific to cell type and developmental stage (Table 4.4).

Type I and type II intermediate filament proteins are keratins, which are hallmarks of epithelial cells.

TABLE 4.4 Intermediate Filament Proteins of the Nervous System

Class and name	Cell type
Types I and II	
Acidic and basic keratins	Epithelial and endothelial cells
Type III	
Glial fibrillary acidic protein	Astrocytes and nonmyelinating Schwann cells
Vimentin	Neuroblasts, glioblasts, fibroblasts, etc.
Desmin	Smooth muscle
Peripherin	A subset of peripheral and central neurons
Type IV	
NF triplet (NFH, NFM, NFL)	Most neurons, expressed at highest level in large myelinated fibers
α-Internexin	Developing neurons, parallel fibers of cerebellum
Nestin	Early neuroectodermal cells. The most divergent member of this class; some have classified it as a sixth type
Type V	
Nuclear lamins	Nuclear membranes

Keratins are not associated with nervous tissue and will not be considered further here. In contrast, all nucleated cells contain type V intermediate filament proteins, the nuclear lamins. Lamins are encoded by the most evolutionarily divergent of the intermediate filament genes, with a distinctive pattern of introns and exons, as well as having a different polypeptide domain structure. Intermediate filaments in the nervous system are all produced by either type III or type IV intermediate filament proteins.

Type III intermediate filaments are a diverse family that includes, among others, vimentin (characteristic of fibroblasts and many embryonic tissues such as embryonic neurons) and glial fibrillary acidic protein (GFAP, a marker for astrocytes and Schwann cells). Type III intermediate filament subunits typically have a molecular mass between 45 and 60 kDa and consist of a conserved rod domain and relatively small gene-specific amino- and carboxy-terminal sequences. As a result, intermediate filaments formed from type III subunits form smooth filaments without side arms. Type III polypeptides can form homopolymers but may also coassemble with other type III intermediate filament subunits.

A recently described type III intermediate filament protein, peripherin, is unique to neurons and may be coexpressed with neurofilament triplet proteins. Peripherin has a characteristic expression during development and regeneration in specific neuronal populations. It has been shown to coassemble with neurofilament triplet proteins both *in vitro* and *in vivo*, where presumably it can substitute for the low molecular weight neurofilament (NFL). However, whether coassembly is generally the case is not known. Physiological roles for neuron-specific type III intermediate filament polypeptides are uncertain. Unlike type IV intermediate filaments, intermediate filaments made from type III subunits tend to disassemble more readily under physiological conditions. Thus, the presence of type III intermediate filament subunit proteins may produce more dynamic structures, which could be important during development or regeneration.

Although other type III intermediate filament proteins are found in the nervous system, they are generally restricted to glia or to neurons at early stages of differentiation. Vimentin is abundant in a wide variety of cells during early development, including both glioblasts and neuroblasts. Some Schwann cells and astrocytes contain vimentin. Curiously, mature oligodendrocytes do not appear to have any intermediate filaments; an exception to the general rule that most metazoan cells contain all three classes of cytoskeletal structures. Oligodendrocyte precursors do, however, express vimentin and may express GFAP transiently.

In neurons, intermediate filaments typically have side arms that limit packing density, whereas glial intermediate filaments lack side arms and may be very tightly packed. Neuronal intermediate filaments have an unusual degree of metabolic stability, which makes them well suited to the role of stabilizing and maintaining neuronal morphology. The existence of neurofilaments was established for many years before much was known about their biochemistry or function. Neurofilaments could be seen in early electron micrographs, and many traditional histological procedures visualize neurons as a result of a specific interaction of metals with neurofilaments. Recent work on the biochemistry and molecular genetics of intermediate filaments has illuminated many aspects of their function in the nervous system.

The primary type of intermediate filament in neurons is formed from three subunits, the neurofilament triplet, each encoded by a separate gene. Neurofilament triplet proteins are from type IV intermediate filament genes, which are generally expressed only in neurons and have a characteristic domain structure that can be recognized in both primary sequence and gene structure. The polypeptides were initially identified from axonal transport studies. Apparent molecular mass for the neurofilament subunits vary widely across species, but mammalian forms typically range from 180 to 200 kDa for the high molecular weight subunit (NFH), from 130 to 170 kDa for the medium subunit (NFM), and from 60 to 70 kDa for the NFL. Interestingly, Schwann cells in damaged peripheral nerves also transiently express NFM and NFL. Neurofilament subunits are phosphorylated in axons, with NFM and NFH having unusually high levels of phosphorylation. In some species, NFH has 50 or more repeats of a consensus phosphorylation site at its carboxy terminus, and levels of NFH phosphorylation indicate that most of these sites are phosphorylated *in vivo*. This high level of phosphorylation in neurofilament subunit tail domains is a distinctive characteristic of neurofilaments.

A second motif characteristic of neurofilaments is the presence of a glutamate-rich region in the tail adjacent to the core rod domain. This glutamate region has particular significance for neuroscientists because it appears to be the basis for the reaction of the classic neurofibrillary silver stains for neurons. These stains were first introduced in the late 19th century and have been used extensively by neurohistologists and neuroanatomists from Ramon y Cajal's time to the present day. However, the molecular basis of these neurofibrillary stains was not known until 1968, when F. O. Schmitt showed that neurofibrils were formed by 10-nm-diameter neurofilaments. Remarkably, the ability of isolated neurofilament subunits to react with silver histological stains is retained even after separation in gel electrophoresis for neurofilaments from organisms as diverse as humans, squid, and the marine fanworm, *Myxicola*. Conservation of the glutamate-rich domain suggests both an important functional role for this motif and the early divergence of neurofilaments from the other intermediate filament families.

Neurofilaments formed from neurofilament triplet proteins play a critical role in determining axonal caliber. As mentioned earlier, neurofilaments have characteristic side arms, unique among intermediate filaments; these side arms are formed by NFM and NFH carboxy-terminal regions. Although all three neurofilament subunits contribute to the neurofilament central core, the side arms are formed only by the NFM and NFH subunits. Phosphorylation of NFH and NFM side arms alters charge density on the neurofilament surface, repelling adjacent neurofilaments with a similar charge. The high density of surface charge due to phosphate groups on neurofilaments makes it difficult to imagine a stable interaction between neurofilaments and other structures of like charge. Although many reports refer to cross bridges between neurofilaments, direct studies of interactions between neurofilaments provide little evidence of stable cross-links between neurofilaments or between neurofilaments and other cytoskeletal structures. However, dynamic interactions between neurofilaments and cellular structures or proteins may be critical for many aspects of neurofilament function and metabolism.

Alteration in expression levels for neurofilament subunits or mutations in neurofilament genes can lead to specific neuropathologies. Overexpression of genes encoding normal NFH or expression of some mutant NFL genes in transgenic mouse models leads to the accumulation of neurofilaments in the cell body and proximal axon of spinal motor neurons. These accumulations are similar to those seen in amyotrophic lateral sclerosis and related motor neuron diseases, leading to the hypothesis that the disruption of normal neurofilament function is a common intermediate in the pathogenesis of motor neuron disease. Similarly, an early indicator of neuropathies caused by neurotoxins such as acrylamide and hexanedione is the accumulation of neurofilaments in either proximal or distal regions of the axon. Disruption of neurofilament organization is a hallmark of pathology for many degenerative diseases of the nervous system, particularly those affecting large myelinated axons such as those of spinal motor neurons. Although pathology can be produced by altering neurofilament organization, the question of whether neurofilament defects are a primary event in pathogenesis or a manifestation of an underlying metabolic pathology remains controversial in most cases.

Another member of the type IV intermediate filament family, α-internexin, has also been identified. Like neurofilament triplet proteins, α-internexin is expressed only in neurons. Unlike the triplet proteins, α-internexin is expressed preferentially early in development of the nervous system and then disappears from most neurons during maturation. Intermediate filaments containing α-internexin do persist in portions of the adult nervous system, such as the branched axons of granule cells in the cerebellar cortex. Evidence show that α-internexin can coassemble with members of the neurofilament triplet, but it also forms homopolymeric filaments. The primary sequence of α-internexin has features in common with both NFL and NFM that are thought to form the basis for assembly properties distinct from those of other type IV intermediate filaments.

The final type of intermediate protein present in the nervous system is nestin, which is expressed transiently during early development. Nestin is also expressed in Schwann cells and in the progenitors of oligodendrocytes, which appear late in the development of the embryonic nervous system. Remarkably, nestin appears to be expressed almost exclusively in ectodermal cells after commitment to the neuroglial lineage, but prior to terminal differentiation. At 1250 kDa, nestin is the largest intermediate filament subunit and is the most divergent in sequence with several distinctive features, leading some to classify nestin as a sixth type of intermediate filament protein, whereas others group it with type IV intermediate filaments. Relatively little is known about the assembly properties of nestin *in vivo* or the physiological function of nestin intermediate filaments in neuroectodermal cells.

How Do the Various Cytoskeletal Systems Interact?

Each class of cytoskeletal structures may be found without the others in some cellular domains, but all three classes—microtubules, microfilaments, and intermediate filaments—coexist in many domains. As a result, they inevitably interact. This is not to say that individual cytoskeletal elements are necessarily cross-linked to one another. As mentioned earlier, microtubules and neurofilaments have highly phosphorylated side arms that project from their surfaces. The high density of negative charge on the surface tends to repel structures with a like charge such as other microtubules and neurofilaments. This does not mean that microtubules and neurofilaments do not interact with each other, but it does suggest that such interactions may be transient.

One location containing longer microfilaments and more elaborate organization is the growth cone, which contains bundles of microfilaments in the filopodia, as well as a more dispersed actin network. Neurofilaments are largely excluded from the growth cone, typically extending no further than the neck of the growth cone. In contrast, microtubules and microfilaments play complementary roles in the growth cone itself. Microfilaments are critical in sprouting but appear less critical for elongation, at least over short distances. Disruption of microtubules in the distal neurite does not affect sprouting but does inhibit neurite elongation.

Summary

The intracellular framework that gives shape to the neuron and glial cell is the cytoskeleton, a complicated set of filaments and tubules and their associated proteins. These organelles are responsible as well for intracellular movement of materials and, during development, for cell migration and plasma membrane extension within nervous tissue.

MOLECULAR MOTORS IN THE NERVOUS SYSTEM

Until 1985, our knowledge of molecular motors in vertebrate cells of any type was restricted to myosins and flagellar dyneins. Myosins had been identified in nervous tissue, but their functions were uncertain. Because the preponderance of evidence indicated that fast axonal transport was microtubule based, there was considerable interest in dyneins in cell cytoplasm. Despite a number of studies, no evidence for a functional cytoplasmic dynein emerged. Worse yet, the characteristic properties of fast organelle movements appeared inconsistent with both myosins and dyneins. Over the past decade, however, we have developed a good but still incomplete understanding of how these motors may work inside cells (Brady, 1991, Brady and Sperry, 1995).

Myosins and dyneins can be distinguished pharmacologically by their differential susceptibility to inhibitors of ATPase activity, but the spectrum of inhibitors active against fast axonal transport fails to match the properties of either myosin or dynein. The most striking difference between inhibitor effects on axonal transport and on myosin or dynein motors was seen in the effect of a nonhydrolyzable analog of ATP. Adenylyl-imidodiphosphate (AMP-PNP) is a weak competitive inhibitor of both myosin and dynein, requiring a 10- to 100-fold excess of analog. In contrast, within minutes of AMP-PNP perfusion into isolated axoplasm, both anterograde and retrograde axonal transport stop. Inhibition by AMP-PNP occurs even in the presence of stoichiometric concentrations of ATP. Organelles moving in both directions freeze in place and remain attached to microtubules. AMP-PNP weakens the interaction of myosin with microfilaments and of dynein with microtubules, but stabilizes the binding of membrane-bound organelles to microtubules. Thus, the effects of AMP-PNP indicate that movement of membrane-bound organelles in fast axonal transport must require another type of motor, distinct from myosins and dyneins.

The effects of AMP-PNP both demonstrated the existence of a new type of mechanochemical ATPase and provided a basis for identifying its constituent polypeptides. Binding of ATPase to microtubules should be increased by AMP-PNP and decreased by ATP. Polypeptides meeting this criterion were soon identified. The new ATPase was named kinesin, based initially on an ability to move microtubules across glass coverslips as first described in axoplasmic extracts. Studies soon established that kinesin was a microtubule-activated ATPase with minimal basal activity. This combination of ATPase activity and

motility *in vitro* confirmed that kinesin was a new class of microtubule-based motor (Brady and Sperry, 1995; Bloom and Endow, 1995).

Kinesin has now been identified in a variety of organisms and tissues, leading to an extensive characterization of many biochemical, pharmacological, immunochemical, and molecular properties. Electron microscopic and biophysical analyses reveal kinesin as a long, rod-shaped protein, approximately 80 nm in length. Neuronal kinesin is a heterotetramer with two heavy chains (molecular mass 115–130 kDa) and two light chains (62–70 kDa). Localization of antibodies specific for kinesin subunits by high-resolution

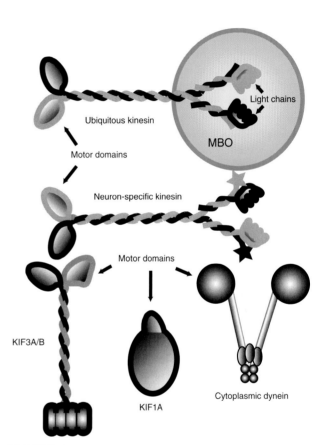

FIGURE 4.8 Examples of microtubule motor proteins in the mammalian nervous system. The first microtubule motor identified in nervous tissue was the ubiquitous form of kinesin, but subsequent studies showed that a neuron-specific form of kinesin was found in mammalian brain. Motor domains are well conserved by tail domains and appear to be specialized for interaction with various targets, such as different membrane-bound organelles. After the sequence of the kinesin heavy chain was established, the presence of additional genes that contained sequences homologous to the motor domain of kinesin was soon recognized. The molecular organization of these various motor proteins is quite diverse, including monomers (KIF1A), trimers (KIF3A/3B), and tetramers (ubiquitous and neuron-specific kinesins). Many kinesin-related proteins have been implicated in the processes of cell division, but a number can also be found in postmitotic cells such as neurons.

electron microscopy of bovine brain kinesin indicates that the two heavy chains are arranged in parallel, forming the heads and much of the shaft, whereas light chains are localized to the fan-shaped tail region (Fig. 4.8).

A variety of approaches have demonstrated that the ATP-binding and microtubule-binding domains of kinesin are in the head regions of the heavy chains, whereas the light chains in the tail region of kinesin appear to bind to membranes. When *in vitro* motility assays are employed for analysis of brain kinesins, movements are directed toward the plus ends of microtubules. Because axonal microtubules are oriented with their plus ends distal from the cell body, this movement would be appropriate for a motor that moves organelles in the anterograde direction.

Neuronal kinesin appears associated with a variety of membrane-bound organelles, including synaptic vesicles, mitochondria, coated vesicles, and lysosomes. The interaction of kinesin and other molecular motors with membrane surfaces is not well understood. In the case of kinesin, the interaction is thought to involve the light chains of kinesin along with the carboxy termini of the heavy chains.

Kinesins have now been shown to be a family of related proteins with a highly conserved domain that includes ATP- and microtubule-binding domains. Many of these kinesin-related polypeptides appear associated with cell division, and kinesin-related proteins in vertebrate tissues are not well characterized. However, multiple members of the kinesin superfamily are expressed in both adult and developing brains. This proliferation of motor proteins has dramatically altered the questions being asked about motor function in the brain. The discovery that ncd, a kinesin-related protein from Drosophila, can move structures toward the minus end of microtubules increases the number of potential functions that kinesin family members might serve in nervous tissue still further, perhaps including a role in retrograde transport. Further study is needed to establish specific functions for each member of the kinesin superfamily expressed in neurons or glial cells.

As an indirect result of the discovery of kinesin, one of the high molecular weight microtubule-associated proteins of brain, MAP-1c, was found to be the long sought cytoplasmic form of dynein. Both MAP-1c dynein and kinesin can be isolated from bovine brain by incubation of microtubules with nucleotide-free soluble extracts. Both are bound to microtubules under these conditions and released by ATP. MAP-1c dynein moved microtubules *in vitro* with a polarity opposite that seen with kinesin and was identified as a two-headed cytoplasmic dynein using both struc-

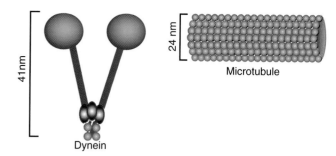

FIGURE 4.9 Biochemical studies on kinesin in brain led to the description of a cytoplasmic form of dynein that was distinct from axonemal dyneins. Cytoplasmic dynein may interact with membrane-bound organelles and cytoskeletal structures. Genetic methods have established that there may be as many as 30 kinesin-related proteins and 15 dynein heavy chains in a single organism. The diversity of microtubule-based motors is consistent with the extent of the microtubule cytoskeleton in the nervous system.

tural and biochemical criteria. Concurrently, a similar protein was identified in nematodes.

MAP-1c dyneins form a 40-nm-long complex of molecular mass 1.6×10^6 Da, which includes two heavy chains and a number of light chains (Figs. 4.8 and 4.9). Less information is available about the distribution and properties of MAP-1c dyneins than about kinesin. Immunocytochemical studies in nonneuronal cells showed immunoreactivity on mitotic spindles. In addition, a punctate pattern of immunoreactivity also present in interphase cells was thought to be due to dynein bound to membrane-bound organelles. Dyneins are widely thought to be the motor for fast retrograde axonal transport but are also a candidate for a motor in slow axonal transport.

Myosins from muscle were the first molecular motors identified, but in recent years interest in nonmuscle myosins has increased (Hammer, 1994; Hasson and Mooseker, 1995). Nonmuscle myosins may be categorized as belonging to one of eight classes, but only a subset has been clearly demonstrated in the nervous system. Nonmuscle myosins in this subset share considerable homology in their motor domains but diverge widely in other domains.

The most familiar of the myosins are the myosin II proteins (Fig. 4.10), which are found in the thick filaments of smooth and skeletal muscle but are also present in nonmuscle cells. Two heavy chains of myosin II form a dimer that may interact with other myosin II dimers to form bipolar filaments. Under tissue culture conditions, many cells contain bundles of actin microfilaments, known as stress fibers, that exhibit a characteristic distribution of myosin II into distinct patterns that may be sarcomeric equivalents, but stress fibers are not apparent in neurons and other cells of the nervous system *in situ*. However, bipolar

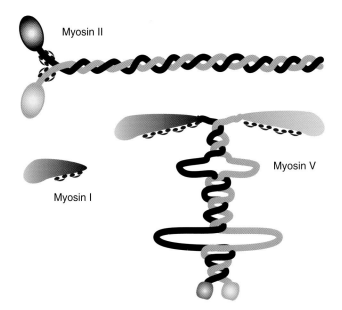

Myosin II

Myosin V

Myosin I

FIGURE 4.10 Examples of myosin motor proteins found in the mammalian nervous system. Myosin heavy chains contain the motor domain, whereas light chains serve to regulate motor function. Myosin II was the first molecular motor characterized biochemically from skeletal muscle and brain. Biochemical and genetic approaches have now defined > 11 classes of myosin, many of which can be found in brain. Myosin II is a classic two-headed myosin that forms thick filaments in nonmuscle cells. Myosin I motors have single motor domains, but may interact with actin microfilaments or membranes. Myosin V motors were initially identified as a mouse mutation that affected coat color and produced seizures. Myosin V has multiple binding sites for calmodulin that act as light chains. Mutations in other classes of myosin have been linked to deafness. Other myosins, including myosins I, II, and V, have been detected in growth cones as well as in mature neurons. The specific roles of these various myosins in the nervous system remain to be established.

thick filaments assembled from myosin II dimers can be isolated from nervous tissues. Many of the cellular contractile events described in nonneuronal cells, such as the contractile ring in mitosis, are thought to include myosin II. Although brain myosin II was one of the first nonmuscle myosins to be described, relatively little is known about the function of myosin II in neurons. Myosin II has been localized in the neurites of neurons in primary culture.

Myosin I proteins have a single, smaller heavy chain that does not form filaments but possesses a homologous actin-activated ATPase domain. One exciting aspect of myosin I is its ability to interact directly with membrane surfaces, which may generate movements of plasma membrane components or intracellular organelles. Myosin I has been purified from neural and neuroendocrine tissues. At least three genes in this family have been found in mammals, and multiple forms are present in brain. An interest-

ing aspect of myosin IB is its expression in the stereocilia of hair cells in the cochlea and vestibular system, where it may play a role in mechanotransduction. Both myosin I and myosin II molecules have been proposed to have a role in the motility of lamelipodia at the leading edge of growth cones, but they are also expressed at substantial levels in adult nervous tissue in which growth cones are rare.

The mouse mutation dilute, which affects coat color, was shown to result from a mutation in a gene that encodes a novel myosin heavy chain distinct from both myosins I and II. Similar myosin molecules have been identified in other cell types and organisms and are classified as myosin V. The change in coat color seen in the dilute mouse is due to an inability of skin dendritic pigment cells to deliver the pigment to developing hairs. There are complex neurological deficits in dilute mutants, including seizures that eventually lead to death in severely altered alleles of the dilute mutation. Myosin V was also discovered independently in extracts from chicken and mammalian brain. The specific cellular localization and function of myosin V in the nervous system remain unclear, although it has been reported in growth cones. However, neurons in dilute mice without one allele of myosin V clearly develop axons and make connections. The seizures do not begin until early adulthood.

Representatives from two more classes of myosin have been identified in nervous tissue. Genes for a myosin VI and a myosin VIIA have been identified in brain as well as in other tissues. Both have been implicated in forms of congenital deafness. Myosin VI appears to be the gene responsible for Snell's Waltzer deafness, and myosin VIIA has been identified as the gene responsible for a human disease involving both deafness and blindness, Usher syndrome type 1B. Both of these myosins are expressed in mechanosensory hair cells of the cochlea and vestibular apparatus, and they exhibit a different localization from each other and from myosin IB.

The diversity of brain myosins and their distinctive localization suggests that the various myosins may have narrowly defined functions. However, relatively little is known about specific neuronal functions for myosins despite intensive study of myosins in the nervous system. The axonal transport of myosin II-like proteins has been described, but little further progress has been made on the functions of myosin II in the mature nervous system. Even less is known about myosin I in the nervous system. However, myosins likely play roles in growth cone motility, synaptic plasticity, and even neurotransmitter release. There are few instances in our knowledge of neuronal function in which we fully understand the role played by specific molecular motors, but members of all three classes are abundant in nervous tissue. This proliferation of different motor molecules and their isoforms suggests that some physiological activities may require multiple classes of motor molecules.

Summary

The concept is now firmly in place that neurons and glial cells, like other cells, contain certain molecular motors responsible for moving discrete populations of molecules, particles, and organelles through intracellular compartments.

BUILDING AND MAINTAINING NERVOUS SYSTEM CELLS

The functional architecture of neurons comprises many specializations in cytoskeletal and membranous components. Each of these specializations is dynamic, constantly changing, and being renewed at a rate determined by the local environment and cellular metabolism. The processes of axonal transport represent a key to understanding neuronal dynamics and provide a basis for exploring neuronal development, regeneration, and neuropathology. Recent advances are important sources of insight into the molecular mechanisms underlying axonal transport, although many questions remain.

Slow Axonal Transport Moves Soluble Components and Cytoskeletal Structures

Slow axonal transport has two major components, both representing the movement of cytoplasmic constituents (Fig. 4.11). The cytoplasmic and cytoskeletal elements of the axon in axonal transport move at rates at least two orders of magnitude more slowly than fast transport. Slow component a is composed largely of cytoskeletal proteins, neurofilaments, and microtubule protein. Slow component b is a complex and heterogeneous rate component, including hundreds of distinct polypeptides ranging from cytoskeletal proteins such as actin (and tubulin in some nerves) to soluble enzymes of intermediary metabolism (such as glycolytic enzymes). Many characteristics of axonal transport have been described, and these characteristics provide the foundation for our understanding of mechanisms.

Neurofilaments and microtubules move as discrete cytological structures (Brady, 1992). Studies on the

transport of neurofilament protein indicate that little degradation or metabolism occurs until neurofilaments reach nerve terminals, where they are degraded rapidly. Comparable results have been obtained in studies labeling microtubule protein by radioactivity or fluorescence. Under favorable conditions, movement of individual microtubules can be detected in neurites or growth cones. Both radiolabeling studies and direct observations of individual microtubules indicate that all microtubules and neurofilaments move down the axon, but the motor protein involved is uncertain. Differential metabolism appears to be a key to the targeting of cytoplasmic and cytoskeletal proteins. Proteins with slow degradative rates accumulate and reach higher steady-state concentrations. Alteration of degradation rates changes the steady-state concentration of a protein. The concentration of actin in presynaptic terminals is explained by a slower turnover in terminals relative to neurofilament proteins and tubulin, and inhibition of calpain causes neurofilament rings to appear in presynaptic terminals. Differential turnover may be accomplished by specific proteases or posttranslational modifications that affect the susceptibility to degradation.

The coherent movement of neurofilaments and microtubule proteins provides strong evidence for the "structural hypothesis." For example, pulse-labeling experiments show that radiolabeled neurofilament proteins move as a bell-shaped wave with little or no trailing of neurofilament protein. This fits with the observed stability of neurofilaments under physiological conditions, which suggests that any soluble pool of neurofilament subunits is negligible. Similarly, the

FIGURE 4.11   Slow axonal transport represents the delivery of ▶ cytoskeletal and cytoplasmic constituents to the periphery. Cytoplasmic proteins are synthesized on free polysomes and organized for transport as cytoskeletal elements or macromolecular complexes (1). Microtubules are formed by nucleation at the microtubule-organizing center near the centriolar complex (2) and then released for migration into the axon or dendrites. The molecular mechanisms are not as well understood as those for fast axonal transport, but slow transport appears to be unidirectional with no retrograde component. Studies suggest that motors like cytoplasmic dynein may interact with the axonal membrane cytoskeleton to move the microtubules with their plus ends leading (3). Neurofilaments may not be able to move on their own, but may hitchhike on microtubules (4). Other cytoplasmic proteins may do the same or may be moved by other motors. Once cytoplasmic structures reach their destinations, they are degraded by local proteases (5) at a rate that allows either growth (in the case of growth cones) or maintenance of steady-state levels. The different composition and organization of the cytoplasmic elements in dendrites suggest that different pathways may be involved in the delivery of cytoskeletal and cytoplasmic materials to the dendrite (6). In addition, some mRNAs are transported into the dendrites, but not into axons.

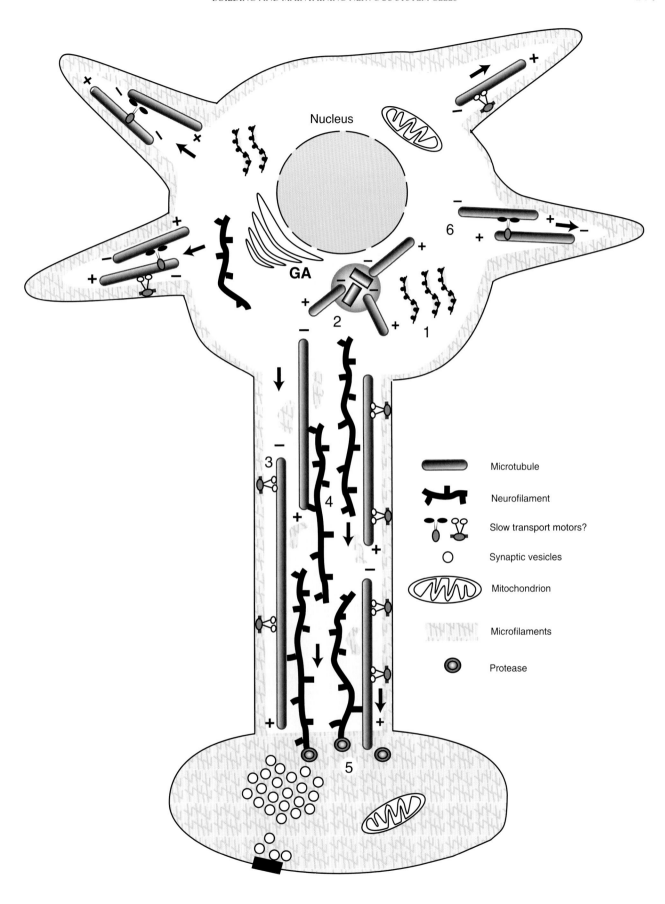

Nucleus

GA

Microtubule

Neurofilament

Slow transport motors?

Synaptic vesicles

Mitochondrion

Microfilaments

Protease

coherent transport of tubulin and MAPs makes sense only if microtubules are moved because MAPs do not interact with unpolymerized tubulin.

A striking demonstration of microtubule movement can be seen with fluorescent analogs of tubulin (Tanaka and Kirschner, 1991; Reinsch *et al.*, 1991). Tubulin labeled with caged fluorescein can be injected into one cell of a fertilized Xenopus oocyte at the two-cell stage. Such tubulins are fluorescent only after photoactivation. The injected oocyte is then allowed to develop into an embryo. The injected tubulin equilibrates with endogenous tubulin and is incorporated into the microtubules of all cells derived from the original injected cell. Because protein synthesis is minimal in early cell divisions of embryonic development, the labeled tubulin is reused by daughter cells until diluted out by newly synthesized tubulin. When early embryonic neurons are cultured, the caged fluorescent tubulin may be photoactivated and visualized.

When local segments of an axon are photoactivated, patches of fluorescent tubulin can be seen to move down the growing neurite. The fluorescent patches remain discrete during movements in the anterograde direction at slow transport rates. Observations of full microtubules can also be made in embryonic Xenopus neurons by using rhodamine-labeled tubulin. In favorable areas of axons and growth cones, individual fluorescent microtubules can be visualized. Such microtubules can be seen to move down axons and into growth cones. The forces are sufficient to bend these microtubules in conjunction with growth cone movements. When studies of axonal transport using radiolabels are combined with direct observations of individual microtubules by video microscopy, there is little doubt that microtubules and neurofilaments can and do move in the axon as intact, individual cytoskeletal elements.

Fast Axonal Transport Is the Means by Which Membrane Vesicles and their Contents Are Rapidly Moved Long Distances within a Neuron

Early biochemical and morphological studies established that the material moving in fast axonal transport was associated with membrane-bound organelles (Fig. 4.12) (Lasek and Brady, 1982; Lasek, 1967). A variety of materials could be shown to move in fast transport. In anterograde transport, materials being moved include membrane-associated enzyme activities, neurotransmitters, and neuropeptides. Many of the materials moving down the axon in anterograde transport are returned in retrograde

transport (Lasek, 1967; LaVail and LaVail, 1972), in some cases after modification in the terminal. In addition, a number of exogenous materials taken up in the distal regions of the axon are moved back to the cell body by retrograde transport (Fig. 4.12). Exogenous materials in retrograde transport include neurotrophic factors, such as nerve growth factor, and viral particles invading the nervous system. The uptake of neurotrophic factors may play a critical role in the process of regeneration.

Electron microscopic analysis of materials accumulated at a ligation or crush demonstrated that organelles moving in the anterograde direction were morphologically distinct from those moving in the retrograde direction (Smith, 1980; Tsukita and Ishikawa, 1980). Consistent with the ultrastructural differences, radiolabel and immunocytochemical studies indicate that there are both quantitative and qualitative differences between anterograde and retrograde moving material. Differences between anterograde and retrograde transport indicate that some processing or repackaging events must occur as part of turnaround in axonal transport. Turnaround pro-

FIGURE 4.12 Fast axonal transport represents the transport of ▶ membrane-associated materials, having both anterograde and retrograde components. For anterograde transport, most polypeptides are synthesized on membrane-bound polysomes, also known as rough endoplasmic reticulum (1), and then transferred to the Golgi apparatus for processing and packaging into specific classes of membrane-bound organelles (2). Proteins following this pathway include both integral membrane proteins and secretory polypeptides in the lumen of vesicles. Cytoplasmic peripheral membrane proteins such as kinesins are synthesized on the cytoplasmic or free polysomes. Once vesicles have been assembled and the appropriate motors associate with them, they are moved down the axon at a rate of 100–400 mm per day (3). Different membrane structures are delivered to different compartments and may be regulated independently. For example, dense core vesicles and synaptic vesicles are both targeted for the presynaptic terminal (4), but the release of vesicle contents involves distinct pathways. After vesicles merge with the plasma membrane, their protein constituents are taken up by coated pits and vesicles via the receptor-mediated endocytic pathway and delivered to a sorting compartment (5). After proper sorting into appropriate compartments, membrane proteins are either committed to retrograde axonal transport or recycled (6). Retrograde moving organelles are morphologically and biochemically distinct from anterograde vesicles. These larger vesicles have an average velocity about half that of anterograde transport. The retrograde pathway is an important mechanism for the delivery of neurotrophic factors to the cell body. Material delivered by retrograde transport typically fuses with cell body compartments to form mature lysosomes (7), where most constituents are recycled. However, neurotrophic factors and neurotrophic viruses can act at the level of the cell body. Although evidence shows that vesicle transport also occurs into dendrites (8), less is known about this pocess. Dendritic vesicle transport is complicated by the fact that dendritic microtubules may have mixed polarity.

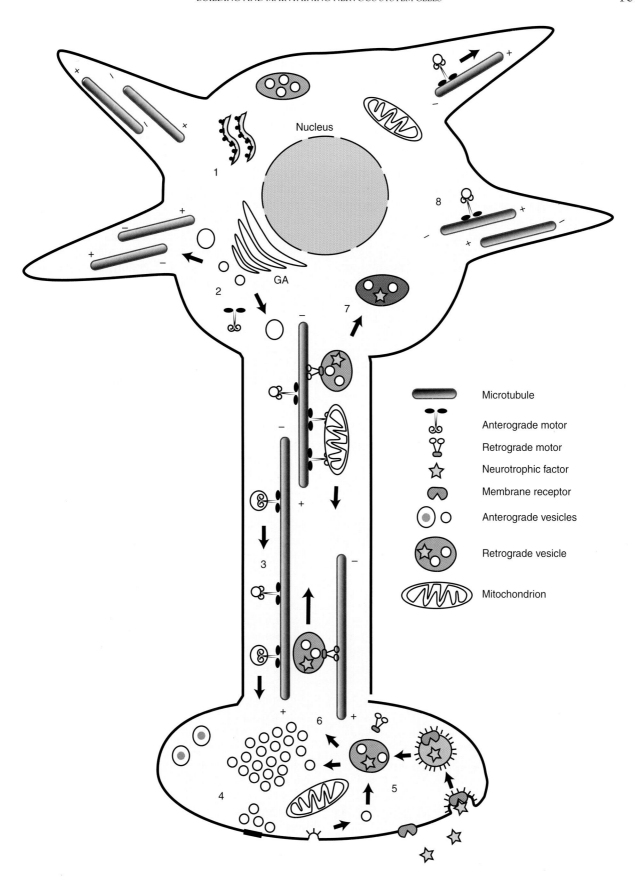

cessing appears to require a proteolytic event because certain protease inhibitors inhibit turnaround without affecting anterograde and retrograde transport.

Biochemical and morphological approaches resulted in considerable progress toward a description of the materials being transported in fast axonal transport but were not suitable for identifying the molecular motors used in translocation. A different technology that permitted direct observation of organelle movements and precise control of experimental conditions was required. Such experiments became possible with the advent of video microscopic techniques (Brady, 1991).

An early use of video-enhanced contrast (VEC) microscopy was to characterize the bidirectional movement of membrane-bound organelles in giant axons from the squid *Loligo pealeii*. Years before, studies had shown that axoplasm could be extruded from the giant axon as an intact cylinder. Properties of the isolated axoplasm had been characterized in some detail, making VEC microscopic analysis of axoplasm a natural choice. Remarkably, fast axonal transport continued unabated in isolated axoplasm for hours. Isolated axoplasm from the giant axon has no plasma membrane or other permeability barriers but can be readily maintained in an active state. Combining VEC microscopy with isolated axoplasm permitted rigorous dissection of the mechanisms for fast axonal transport with the use of biochemical and pharmacological approaches. A number of insights into axonal transport mechanisms have resulted from these studies. Most importantly, studies in isolated axoplasm have led to the identification of several families of molecular motors that may take part in axonal transport.

How Is Axonal Transport Regulated?

The diversity of polypeptides in each axonal transport rate component and the coherent movement of proteins having many different molecular weights produce a conundrum. How can so many different polypeptides move down the axon as a group? In theory, one could propose that each protein has a motor of its own. In that case, each rate component might represent movements due to a specific class of motors or to variable affinities for a smaller number of motors. However, the relatively small numbers of motor molecules and the logistical difficulties associated with such a model effectively preclude this possibility.

The structural hypothesis mentioned earlier was formulated in response to the observation that rate components of axonal transport move as discrete waves, each with a characteristic rate and a distinctive composition (Figs. 4.11 and 4.12). The hypothesis is deceptively simple: Axonal transport represents the movement of discrete cytological structures (Brady, 1992). Proteins in axonal transport do not move as individual polypeptides. Instead, they move as part of a cytological structure or in association with a cytological structure. The only assumption made is that a limited number of elements can interact directly with transport motors so transported material must be packaged appropriately to be moved. The different rate components result from packaging of transported material into different cytologically identifiable structures. In other words, membrane-associated proteins move as membrane-bound organelles (vesicles, mitochondria, etc.), whereas tubulin and MAPs move as microtubules, and neurofilaments move as neurofilaments.

The structural hypothesis does not require movement of a cross-linked microtubule–neurofilament complex in the form of a solid axoplasmic column. Evidence for existence of a cross-linked complex of microtubules and neurofilaments is not compelling in any case. Instead, the hypothesis specifically predicts that individual microtubules and neurofilaments move rather than tubulin dimers or neurofilament monomers. No assumptions are made about higher-order interactions between cytoskeletal structures or membranous structures. Indeed, one variant of the structural hypothesis proposes that cytoskeletal proteins move in the form of small oligomers rather than polymers, although there is no evidence for the presence of such oligomers *in vivo*. For example, to the limits of detection, neurofilaments exist only as the polymer under *in vivo* conditions. Similarly, tubulin interchanges between dimer and polymer with no known oligomeric intermediate. Because a number of experiments indicate that microtubules and neurofilaments can move *in vivo* as intact polymers, there is no compelling reason to postulate additional oligomeric forms.

Because synthesis of proteins takes place at some distance from many functional domains of a neuron, transport to distal regions of the neuron is necessary, but not sufficient, for proper function. Specific materials must also be delivered to their proper site of utilization and should not be left in inappropriate locations. For example, because a synaptic vesicle has no known function in axons or the cell body, it must be delivered to a presynaptic terminal along with other components necessary for regulated neurotransmitter release. The traditional picture places the presynaptic terminal at the end of an axonal process. Such images imply that a synaptic vesicle need only

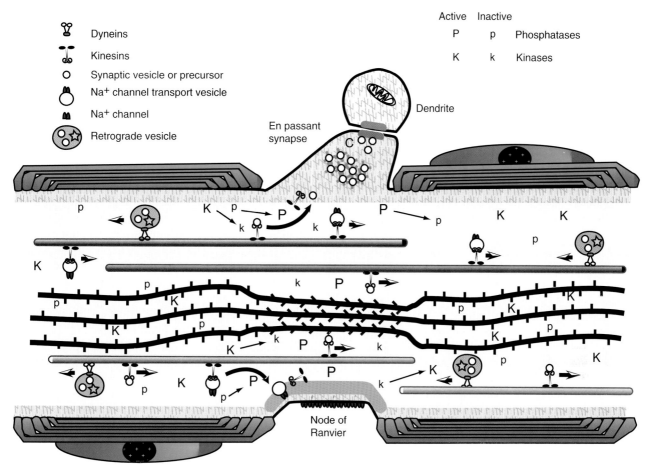

FIGURE 4.13 Axonal dynamics in a myelinated axon from the peripheral nervous system (PNS). Axons are in a constant flux with many concurrent dynamic processes. This diagram illustrates a few of the many dynamic events occurring at a node of Ranvier in a myelinated axon from the PNS. Axonal transport moves cytoskeletal structures, cytoplasmic proteins, and membrane-bound organelles from the cell body toward the periphery (from right to left). At the same time, other vesicles return to the cell body by retrograde transport (retrograde vesicle). Membrane-bound organelles are moved along microtubules by motor proteins such as the kinesins and cytoplasmic dyneins. Each class of organelles must be directed to the correct functional domain of the neuron. Synaptic vesicles must be delivered to a presynaptic terminal to maintain synaptic transmission. In contrast, organelles containing sodium channels must be targeted specifically to nodes of Ranvier for saltatory conduction to occur. Cytoskeletal transport is illustrated by microtubules (rods in the upper half of the axon) and neurofilaments (bundle of rope-like rods in the lower half of the axon) representing the cytoskeleton. They move in the anterograde direction as discrete elements and are degraded in the distal regions. Microtubules and neurofilaments interact with each other transiently during transport, but their distribution in axonal cross sections suggests that they are not stably cross-linked. In axonal segments without compact myelin, such as the node of Ranvier or following focal demyelination, a net dephosphorylation of neurofilament side arms allows the neurofilaments to pack more densely. Myelination is thought to alter the balance between kinase (K indicates an active kinase; k is an inactive kinase) and phosphatase (P indicates an active phophatase; p is an inactive phosphatase) activity in the axon. Most kinases and phosphatases have multiple substrates, suggesting a mechanism for targeting vesicle proteins to specific axonal domains. Local changes in the phosphoryation of axonal proteins may alter the binding properties of proteins. The action of synapsin I in squid axoplasm suggests that dephosphorylated synapsin cross-links synaptic vesicles to microfilaments. When a synaptic vesicle encounters the dephosphorylated synapsin and actin-rich matrix of a presynaptic terminal, the vesicle is trapped at the terminal by inhibition of further axonal transport, effectively targeting the synaptic vesicle to a presynaptic terminal. Similarly, a sodium channel-binding protein may be present at nodes of Ranvier in a high-affinity state (i.e., dephosphorylated). Transport vesicles for nodal sodium channels (Na channel vesicle) would be captured upon encountering this domain, effectively targeting sodium channels to the nodal membrane. Interactions between cells could in this manner establish the functional architecture of the neuron.

BOX 4.2

BATTEN DISEASE

One of the most common hereditary neurodegenerative disorders of children is Batten disease, also known by the rather imposing name of neuronal ceroid lipofuscinosis. The disease was long considered a model for accelerated aging in the nervous system because the hallmark of the disease is the accumulation of abnormal yellowish-brown autofluorescent pigments (ceroid) that resemble pigments that accrue with age (lipofuscin).

The molecular basis for Batten disease has been discovered only recently. The underlying problem seems to lie in the abnormal degradation of proteins in the lysosome. The lysosome is an acidic "recycling" compartment that contains over 74 hydrolytic enzymes, and deficiences in about 40 of these enzymes have been described in humans. Many of these disorders affect the central nervous system profoundly. Batten disease is caused by autosomal recessive mutations in one of at least eight genes (designated CLN1 through CLN8) and is characterized clinically by visual failure, loss of previously attained developmental milestones, and seizures. The diagnosis is considered when an infant or child has symptoms and signs indicating gray matter disease. When tests for other metabolic disorders are unremarkable, a tissue biopsy reveals characteristic cellular inclusion bodies that strongly suggest the diagnosis.

There are three major forms of Batten disease, each with a distinctive age of onset and electron microscopic appearance of the storage material. The most severe is the infantile form (Santavuori–Haltia disease), which begins before age 2 with microcephaly, cognitive and motor decline, and seizures. The characteristic inclusion body in this form of Batten disease is the granular osmiophilic deposit (or GROD). The late-infantile form (Jansky–Bielschowsky disease) occurs at age 2–4 with seizures as the predominant symptom. The residual bodies have a curvilinear appearance in this disease. Classical juvenile-onset Batten disease (Batten–Spielmeyer–Vogt disease) begins at ages 5 to 9 with visual failure. Children with juvenile Batten disease are often diagnosed as having a retinal form of blindness, such as retinitis pigmentosum, and enter schools for the blind, but later develop problems in their school work and have behavioral problems. At that point, the neurodegenerative nature of the underlying disease is suspected. A tissue biopsy showing the characteristic

"fingerprint" inclusions or a genetic test for Batten disease confirms the sad diagnosis.

Identification of the genes underlying the major forms of Batten disease has been extremely important in providing a better understanding of the disease. The infantile form of Batten disease is caused by deficiency in a lysosomal enzyme, palmitoyl-protein thioesterase. The enzyme removes the fatty acid palmitate from lipid-modified proteins. Many proteins are palmitoylated, particularly on cysteine residues, and the fatty acid serves to make the protein more hydrophobic, promoting membrane attachment or protein–protein interactions. The deficiency of the enzyme causes fatty acylated peptides to accumulate in the lysosome and form indigestible residual bodies, eventually leading to neuronal loss by apoptosis. The late-infantile form is caused by lack of another enzyme, tripeptidyl aminopeptidase, whose function is to clip off three amino acids from the amino termini of proteins undergoing degradation in the lysosome. In this form of the disorder (also in juvenile-onset disease), a major mitochondrial protein (subunit c of mitochondrial ATP synthase) accumulates. This very hydrophobic mitochondrial protein probably represents one of the most abundant substrates for the aminopeptidase. The juvenile-onset form is caused by autosomal recessive mutations in a lysosomal membrane protein (CLN3 protein, or battenin) whose function is unknown.

No proven treatment exists for any form of Batten disease. Approaches to these disorders include substrate deprivation using small molecule inhibitors, enzyme replacement therapy (for those forms caused by deficiencies in soluble lysosomal enzymes), and gene therapy. Mouse models exist for most forms of Batten disease and will facilitate the development of treatments for these disorders.

Sandra L. Hofmann

References/Suggested Readings

Hofmann, S.L., and Peltonen, L. (2001). The neuronal ceroid lipofuscinoses. *In* "The Metabolic and Molecular Bases of Inherited Disease" (C. R. Scriver, A. L. Beaudet, W. S. Sly, B. Childs, and B. Vogelstein, eds.), 8th Ed. McGraw-Hill, New York.

Wisniewski, K. E., and Zhong, N. (2001). Batten disease: Diagnosis, treatment and research, *Adv. Genet.* **45**, 225–236.

move along the axonal microtubules until it reaches microtubule ends in the presynaptic terminal. However, many CNS synapses are not at the end of an axon. Numerous terminals are located sequentially along a single axon, making en passant contacts with multiple target cells along the way. Targeting of synaptic vesicles then becomes a more complex problem and targeting ion channels or neurotransmitter receptors to nodes of Ranvier or other appropriate sites on the neuronal surface is equally challenging.

Although the specific details of this targeting are not well understood, a simple model for the targeting of synaptic vesicles serves to illustrate how such targeting may occur (Fig. 4.13). Synapsin I is a cytoplasmic protein enriched in presynaptic terminals that can bind reversibly to both actin microfilaments and synaptic vesicles. Both binding activities are regulated by the phosphorylation of synapsin, and this phosphorylation is known to be increased during stimulation. If nonphosphorylated synapsin were present at the border between the axon and the presynaptic terminal, then a fraction of the synaptic vesicles (or their precursors) traveling down the axon in fast axonal transport would be bound and cross-linked to the actin cytoskeleton that is enriched in the presynaptic terminal. These bound synaptic vesicles would become part of the reserve pool in the terminal at some distance from active zones. As the terminal was stimulated, local calmodulin-activated kinases would phosphorylate synapsin and allow these reserve synaptic vesicles to be mobilized. Consistent with this model, dephosphorylated synapsin has been shown to inhibit fast axonal transport when introduced directly into the axoplasm at concentrations comparable to those seen in the presynaptic terminal.

Although such a model is speculative at present, it does satisfy several criteria that any mechanism for targeting to specific neuronal subdomains must address. Specifically, the mechanism must be local because distances to the cell body can be quite large. There must be some means to connect the targeting signal to an external microenvironment, such as an appropriate target cell. Finally, there must be a way of distinguishing subdomains so that synaptic vesicles are not delivered to nodes of Ranvier and voltage-gated sodium channels are not all targeted to the presynaptic terminal. The careful segregation of different organelles and polypeptides to different regions within a neuron suggests that highly efficient targeting mechanisms do exist.

Summary

A well-studied feature of the neuron is the phenomenon of axonal transport, which has been described in both anterograde and retrograde directions. The axonal transport system is responsible for the delivery of materials from the cell body to distant parts of the neuron, for membrane retrieval and circulation, and for uptake of materials from presynaptic terminals and dendrites and their delivery to the cell soma. The precise molecular mechanisms by which anterograde and retrograde transport can be targeted within an individual dendrite and/or axon are not understood at present.

Neurons and glial cells may have unusually large cell volumes enclosed within extensive plasma membrane surfaces. Nature has evolved a number of "universal" mechanisms in other systems and adapted them for the special needs of nervous tissue cells. The synthesis and delivery of components, and in particular proteins, to cytoplasmic organelles and cell surface subdomains engage general and evolutionarily conserved molecular mechanisms and pathways that are employed in single-cell yeasts as well as in cells in complex nervous tissue.

Once synthesized and sorted, most intracellular organelles (vesicles destined for axonal or dendritic domains, mitochondria, cytoskeletal components) must be distributed, and targeted, to precise intracellular locations. Because they are so extended in space, neurons and glial cells have adapted and developed to a high degree common mechanisms that operate to distribute components within all cells. In the neuron, movement of materials within the axon has been the central focus of most studies. The phenomenon of axoplasmic flow or transport is now in some measure understood at the molecular level.

References

Berl, S., Puszkin, S., and Nicklas, W. J. K. (1973). Actomyosin-like protein in brain. *Science* **179**, 441–446.

Brady, S. T. (1991). Molecular motors in the nervous system. *Neuron* **7**, 521–533.

Brady, S. T. (1992). Axonal dynamics and regeneration. *In* "Neuroregeneration" (A. Gorio, ed.), pp. 7–36. Raven Press, New York.

Brady, S. T., and Sperry, A. O. (1995). Biochemical and functional diversity of microtubule motors in the nervous system. *Curr. Opin. Neurobiol.* **5**, 551–558.

Bloom, G. S., and Endow, S. A. (1995). Motor proteins 1: Kinesins. *Protein Profile* **2**, 1109–1171.

Colman, D. R., Kreibich, G., Frey, A. B., and Sabatini, D. D. (1982). Synthesis and incorporation of myelin polypeptides into CNS myelin. *J. Cell Biol.* **95**, 598–608.

de Camilli, P., Benfenati, F., Valtorta, F., and Greengard, P. (1990). The synapsins. *Annu. Rev. Cell Biol.* **6**, 433–460.

de Camilli, P., Takei, K., and McPherson, P. S. (1995). The function of dynamin in endocytosis. *Curr. Opin. Neurobiol.* **5**, 559–565.

Hammer, J. A. (1994). The structure and function of unconventional myosins: A review. *J. Muscle Res. Cell Motil.* **15**, 1–10.

Hasson, T., and Mooseker, M. S. (1995). Molecular motors, membrane movements and physiology—emerging roles for myosins. *Curr. Opin. Cell Biol.* **7**, 587–594.

Heuser, J. E., and Reese, T. S. (1973). Evidence for recycling of synaptic vesicle membrane during transmitter release at the frog neuromuscular junction. *J. Cell Biol.* **57**, 315–344.

Hochstrasser, M. (1995). Ubiquitin, proteasomes, and the regulation of intracellular protein degradation. *Curr. Opin. Cell Biol.* **7**, 215–223.

Hyams, J. S., and Lloyd, C. W. (1994). Microtubules. *In* "Modern Cell Biology" (J. B. Harford, ed.), p. 439. Wiley-Liss, New York.

Kornfeld, R., and Kornfeld, S. (1985). Assembly of asparagine-linked oligosaccharides. *Annu. Rev. Biochem.* **54**, 631–664.

Lasek, R. J. (1967). Bidirectional transport of radioactively labeled axoplasmic components. *Nature (Lond.)* **216**, 1212–1214.

Lasek, R. J., and Brady, S. T. (1982). The axon: A prototype for studying expressional cytoplasm. *In* "Organization of the Cytoplasm, pp. 113–124. Cold Spring Harbor Laboratory Press, Cold Spring Harbor, NY.

LaVail, J. H., and LaVail, M. M. (1972). Retrograde axonal transport in the central nervous system. *Science.* **176**, 1416–1417.

Lee, M. K., and Cleveland, D. W. (1996). Neuronal intermediate filaments. *Annu. Rev. Neurosci.* **19**, 187–217.

Moser, H. W. (1987). New approaches in peroxisomal disorders. *Dev. Neurosci.* **9**, 1.

Palade, G. E. (1975). Intracellular aspects of the process of protein synthesis. *Science.* **189**, 347–358.

Peters, A., Palay, S. L., and Webster, H. D. (1991). The Fine Structure of the Nervous System: Nervous and Their Supporting Cells, 3rd Ed. Oxford Univ. Press, New York.

Pley, U., and Parham, P. (1993). Clathrin: Its role in receptor-mediated vesicular transport and specialized functions in neurons. *Crit. Rev. Biochem. Mol. Biol.* **28**, 431–464.

Reinsch, S. S., Mitchison, T. J., and Kirschner, M. (1991). Microtubule polymer assembly and transport during axonal elongation. *J. Cell Biol.* **115**, 365–380.

Rothman, J. E. (1994). Mechanism of intracellular protein transport. *Nature (Lond.)* **372**, 55–63.

Smith, R. S. (1980). The short term accumulation of axonally transported organelles in the region of localized lesions of single myelinated axons. *J. Neurocytol.* **9**, 39–65.

Steward, O. (1995). Targeting of mRNAs to subsynaptic microdomains in dendrites. *Curr. Opin. Neurobiol.* **5**, 55–61.

Sudhof, T. C. (1995). The synaptic vesicle cycle—a cascade of protein–protein interactions. *Nature (Lond.)* **375**, 645–653.

Tanaka, E. M., and Kirschner, M. (1991). Microtubule behavior in the growth cones of living neurons during axon elongation. *J. Cell Biol.* **115**, 345-364.

Tanaka, J., and Sobue, K. (1994). Localization and characterization of gelsolin in nervous tissues: Gelsolin is specifically enriched in myelin-forming cells. *J. Neurosci.* **14**, 1038–1052.

Tsukita, S., and H. Ishikawa. (1980). The movement of membranous organelles in axons. Electron microscopic identification of anterogradely and retrogradely transported organelles. *J. Cell Biol.* **84**, 513–530.

Vouyiouklis, D. A., and Brophy, P. J. (1995). Microtubule-associated proteins in developing oligodendrocytes: Transient expression of a MAP2c isoform in oligodendrocyte precursors. *J. Neurosci. Res.* **42**, 803–817.

Walter, P., and Johnson, A. E. (1994). Signal sequence recognition and protein targeting to the endoplasmic-reticulum membrane. *Annu. Rev. Cell Biol.* **10**, 87–119.

*Scott Brady, David R. Colman,
and Peter Brophy*

5

Electrotonic Properties of Axons and Dendrites

Neurons characteristically have elaborate dendritic trees arising from their cell bodies and single axons with their own terminal branching patterns (see Chapters 3 and 4). With this structural apparatus, neurons carry out five basic functions (Fig. 5.1):

1. Generate intrinsic activity (at any given site in the neuron through voltage-dependent membrane properties and internal second-messenger mechanisms).
2. Receive synaptic inputs (mostly in dendrites, to some extent in cell bodies, and in some cases in axon terminals).
3. Integrate signals (combine synaptic responses with intrinsic membrane activity).
4. Encode output patterns (in graded potentials or action potentials).
5. Distribute synaptic outputs (from axon terminals and, in some cases, from cell bodies and dendrites).

In addition to synaptic inputs and outputs, neurons may receive and send nonsynaptic signals in the form of electric fields, volume conduction of neurotransmitters and gases, and release of hormones into the bloodstream.

TOWARD A THEORY OF NEURONAL INFORMATION PROCESSING

A **fundamental goal of neuroscience** is to develop quantitative descriptions of these functional operations and their coordination within the neuron that enable it to function as an integrated **information-**

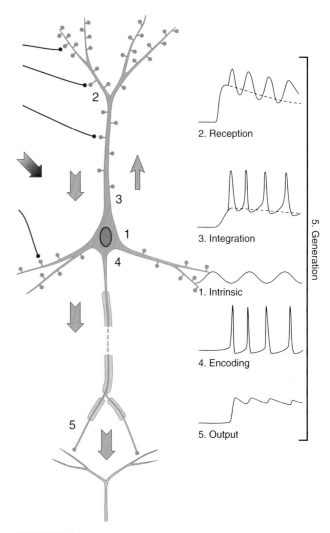

FIGURE 5.1 Nerve cells have four main regions and five main functions. Electrotonic potential spread is fundamental for coordinating the regions and their functions.

115

processing unit. This is the necessary basis for testing experiment-driven hypotheses that can lead to **realistic empirical computational models** of neurons, neural systems, and networks and their roles in information processing and behavior.

Toward these ends, the first task is to understand how activity spreads within and between different parts of the neuron. To do this for the single axon is difficult enough; for the branching dendrites it becomes extremely challenging. It is no exaggeration to say that the task of understanding how intrinsic activity, synaptic potentials, and active potentials spread through and are integrated within the complex geometry of dendritic trees is one of the last frontiers of molecular and cellular neuroscience.

This chapter begins with the passive properties of the membrane that underlie spread of most types of neuronal activity. Chapter 12 considers the active membrane properties that contribute to more complex types of information processing, particularly the types that take place in dendrites. Together, the two chapters provide an integrated theoretical framework for understanding the neuron as a complex information processing unit. Both draw on other chapters for the specific properties—membrane receptor (Chapter 9), internal receptors (Chapter 10), synaptically gated membrane channels (Chapter 9), intrinsic voltage-gated channels (Chapter 6), and second-messenger systems (Chapter 10)—that mediate the operations of the neuron.

BASIC TOOLS: CABLE THEORY AND COMPARTMENTAL MODELS

Slow spread of neuronal activity is by ionic or chemical diffusion or active transport. Our main interest in this chapter is in rapid spread by electric current. What are the factors that determine this spread? The most basic are *electrotonic properties*.

The origins of the study of electrotonic properties are summarized in Box 5.1, which highlights the interesting fact that our understanding of electrotonus arose from a merging of the study of current spread in nerve cells and muscle with the development of cable theory for transmission through electrical cables on the ocean floor. The electrotonic properties of neurons are therefore often referred to as *cable properties*. As indicated in Box 5.1, electrotonic theory was first applied mathematically to the nervous system in the late 19th century for spread of electric current through nerve fibers. By the 1930s and 1940s, it was applied to simple invertebrate (crab and squid) axons—the first steps toward the development of the Hodgkin–Huxley equations (Chapter 6) for the action potential in the axon.

Mathematically, the analytical approach is impractical for the complexity of dendritic systems, but the development of computational compartmental methods for dendritic trees by Rall (1964, 1967, 1977), and Rall and Shepherd, (1968), beginning in the 1960s,

---

BOX 5.1

ORIGINS OF ELECTROTONUS

The mathematical treatment of axonal electrotonus began in the 1870s with the work of Hermann, supported by Weber's mathematical analysis of the external field in the surrounding volume conductor. Hermann recognized the mathematical analogy of this problem with the problems in heat conduction, but the analogy with Kelvin's treatment of the submarine telegraph cable in the 1850s was first recognized by Hoorweg in 1898. This cable analogy was developed independently by Cremer and by Hermann early in the 20th century and has been widely used since that time. These mathematical analogies are important because of the extensive literature devoted to both general mathematical methods and special solutions applicable to problems of this kind (Carslaw and Jaeger, 1959). Important papers on the steady-state distributions of axonal electrotonus are

those of Rushton and of Cole and Hodgkin published in the 1920s and 1930s. The two most useful mathematical presentations of axonal electrotonus (including consideration of transients) are those provided by Hodgkin and Rushton and by Davis and Lorente de No in the 1940s [detailed references can be found in Rall (1958)].

Wilfrid Rall

References

Carslaw, H. S., and Jaeger, J. C. (1959). "Conduction of Heat in Solids." Oxford Univ. Press, London.
Rall, W. (1958). Dendritic cement distribution and whole neuron properties. Nav. Med. Res. Inst. Res. Rep. NM 0105.01.02, 479–525.

opened the way to *compartmental models*. Together with the analytical methods of cable theory, these models have provided a sound basis for a theory of dendritic function (Segev *et al.*, 1995, Jack *et al.*, 1975). Combined with mathematical models for the generation of synaptic potentials and action potentials, they provide the basis for a complete theoretical description of neuronal activity.

A variety of software packages now makes it possible for even a beginning student to explore functional properties and construct realistic neuron models (Bower and Beeman, 1995; Shepherd and Brayton, 1979; Hines, 1984; Ziv *et al.*, 1994). We therefore present modern electrotonic theory within the context of constructing these compartmental models. Exploration of these models will aid the student greatly in understanding the complexities that are present in even the simplest types of passive spread of current in axons and dendrites.

SPREAD OF STEADY-STATE SIGNALS

Modern Electrotonic Theory Depends on Simplifying Assumptions

The successful application of cable theory to nerve cells requires that it be based as closely as possible on the structural and functional properties of neuronal processes. The problem confronting the neuroscientist is that most of these processes are quite complicated. As discussed in Chapters 3 and 4, a segment of axon or dendrite may be filled with various organelles, bounded by a plasma membrane with its own complex structure and irregular outline and surrounded by myriad neighboring processes (see Fig. 5.2A).

Constructing a model of the spread of electric current through such a segment therefore requires some carefully chosen simplifying assumptions, which allow the construction of an *equivalent circuit* of the electrical properties of such a segment. These are summarized in Box 5.2. Students should work their way through this series of simple equations; for the mathematically disinclined, a grasp of the principles is important. The main message of Box 5.2 is that even the simplest representation of the passive spread of electrotonic potential during a steady-state input to a neuron requires a number of assumptions. Understanding them is essential for describing electrotonic spread under the different conditions that the nervous system presents. It is important for the student to gain at least an intuitive feel for the way that the complexity of the neuron is reduced by these assumptions

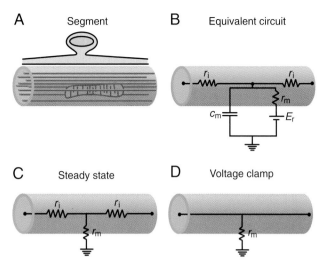

FIGURE 5.2 Construction of a compartmental model of the passive electrical properties of a nerve cell process begins with (A) identification of a segment of the process and its organelles followed by (B) abstraction of an equivalent electrical circuit based on the membrane capacitance (c_m), membrane resistance (r_m), resting membrane potential (E_r), and internal resistance (r_i); (C) abstraction of the circuit for steady-state electrotonus, in which c_m and E_r can be ignored. (D)The space clamp used in voltage-clamp analysis reduces the equivalent circuit even further to only the membrane resistance (r_m), usually depicted as membrane conductances (g) for different ions. In a compartmental modeling program, the equivalent circuit parameters are scaled to the size of each segment.

in order to extract principles that give insight into function.

Electrotonic Spread Depends on the Characteristic Length

In order to describe the passive spread of electrotonic potential, we use the assumptions in Box 5.2 to represent a segment of a process as an internal resistance r_i connected both to the r_i of the next segment and through the membrane resistance r_m to ground (see Fig. 5.2B). Let us first consider the spread of electrotonic potential under steady-state conditions (Fig. 5.2C). In standard cable theory, this is described by

$$V = \frac{I_m}{r_i} \cdot \frac{d^2V}{dx^2}. \tag{5.1}$$

This equation states that if there is a steady-state current input at point $x = 0$, the electrotonic potential (V) spreading along the cable is proportional to the second derivative of the potential (d^2V) with respect to distance and the ratio of the membrane resistance (r_m) to the internal resistance (r_i) over that distance. The steady-state solution of this equation for a cable of infinite extension for positive values of x gives

$$V = V_0 e^{-x/\lambda}, \tag{5.2}$$

BOX 5.2

BASIC ASSUMPTIONS UNDERLYING CABLE THEORY

1. Segments are cylinders. A segment is assumed to be a cylinder with constant radius.

This is the simplest assumption; however, compartmental simulations can readily incorporate different geometrical shapes with differing radii if needed (Fig. 5.2B).

2. The electrotonic potential is due to a change in the membrane potential. At any instant of time, the "resting" membrane potential (E_r) at any point on the neuron can be changed by several means: injection of current into the cell, extracellular currents that cross the membrane, and changes in membrane conductance (caused by a driving force different from that responsible for the membrane potential). Electric current then begins to spread between that point and the rest of the neuron, in accord with

$$V = V_m - E_r,$$

where V is the electrotonic potential and V_m is the changed membrane potential.

Modern neurobiologists recognize that the membrane potential is rarely at rest. In practice, "resting" potential means the membrane potential at any given instant of time other than during an action potential or rapid synaptic potential.

3. Electrotonic current is ohmic. Passive electrotonic current flow is usually assumed to be ohmic, i.e., in accord with the simple linear equation

$$E = IR,$$

where E is the potential, I is the current, and R is the resistance.

This relation is largely inferred from macroscopic measurements of the conductance of solutions having the composition of the intracellular medium, but is rarely measured directly for a given nerve process. Also largely untested is the likelihood that at the smallest dimensions (0.1 μm diameter or less), the processes and their internal organelles may acquire submicroscopic electrochemical properties that deviate significantly from macroscopic fluid conductance values; compartmental models permit the incorporation of estimates of these properties.

4. In the steady state, membrane capacitance is ignored. The simplest case of electrotonic spread occurs from the point on the membrane of a steady-state change (e.g., due to injected current, a change in synaptic conductance, or a change in voltage-gated conductance) so that time-varying properties (transient charging or discharging of the membrane) due to the membrane capacitance can be ignored (Fig. 5.2C).

5. The resting membrane potential can usually be ignored. In the simplest case, we consider the spread of electrotonic potential (V) relative to a uniform resting potential (E_r) so that the value of the resting potential can be ignored. Where the resting membrane potential may vary spatially, V must be defined for each segment as

$$V_m = E_r.$$

6. Electrotonic current divides between internal and membrane resistances. In the steady state, at any point on a process, current divides into two local resistance paths: further within the process through an internal (axial) resistance (r_i) or across the membrane through a membrane resistance (r_m) (see Fig. 5.2C).

7. Axial current is inversely proportional to diameter. Within the volume of the process, current is assumed to be distributed equally (in other words, the resistance across the process, in the Y and Z axes, is essentially zero). Because resistances in parallel sum to decrease the overall resistance, axial current (I) is inversely proportional to the cross-sectional area ($I \propto \frac{1}{A} \propto \frac{1}{\pi r^2}$); thus, a thicker process has a lower overall axial resistance than a thinner process. Because the axial resistance (r_i) is assumed to be uniform throughout the process, the total cross-sectional axial resistance of a segment is represented by a single resistance,

$$r_i = R_i / A,$$

where r_i is the internal resistance per unit length of cylinder (in ohms per centimeter of axial length), R_i is the specific internal resistance (in ohms centimeter, or ohm cm), and A ($= \pi r^2$) is the cross-sectional area.

The internal structure of a process may contain membranous or filamentous organelles that can raise the effective internal resistance or provide high-conductance submicroscopic pathways that can lower it. In voltage-clamp experiments, the space clamp eliminates current through r_i, so that the only current remaining is through r_m, thereby permitting isolation and analysis of different ionic membrane conductances, as in the original experiments of Hodgkin and Huxley (Fig. 5.2D; see also Chapter 6).

8. Membrane current is inversely proportional to membrane surface area. For a unit length of cylinder, the membrane current (i_m) and the membrane resistance (r_m) are assumed to be uniform over the entire surface. Thus, by the same rule of the summing of parallel resistances, the membrane current is inversely proportional to the

---

BOX 5.2   (cont'd)

membrane area of the segment so that a thicker process has a lower overall membrane resistance. Thus,

$$r_m = R_m/c,$$

where r_m is the membrane resistance for unit length of cylinder (in ohm cm of axial length), R_m is the specific membrane resistance (in ohm cm), and c ($= 2\pi r$) is the circumference. For a segment, the entire membrane resistance is regarded as concentrated at one point; i.e., there is no axial current flow within a segment but only between segments (see Fig. 5.2C).

Membrane current passes through ion channels in the membrane. The density and types of these channels vary in different processes and indeed may vary locally in different segments and branches. These differences are incorporated readily into compartmental representations of the processes.

9. The external medium along the process is assumed to have zero resistivity. In contrast with the internal axial resistivity (r_i), which is relatively high because of the small dimensions of most nerve processes, the external medium has a relatively low resistivity for current because of its relatively large volume. For this reason, the resistivity of the paths either along a process or to ground is generally regarded as negligible, and the potential outside the membrane is assumed to be everywhere equivalent to ground (see Fig. 5.2C). This greatly simplifies the equations that describe the spread of electrotonic potentials inside and along the membrane.

Compartmental models can simulate any arbitrary distribution of properties, including significant values for extracellular resistance where relevant. Particular cases in which external resistivity may be large, such as the special membrane caps around synapses on the cell body or axon hillock of a neuron, can be addressed by suitable representation in the simulations. However, for most simulations, the assumption of negligible external resistance is a useful simplifying first approximation.

10. Driving forces on membrane conductances are assumed to be constant. It is usually assumed that ion concentrations across the membrane are constant during activity.

Changes in ion concentrations with activity may occur, particularly in constricted extracellular or intracellular compartments; these changes may cause deviations from the assumptions of constant driving forces for the membrane currents, as well as the assumption of uniform E_r. For example, accumulations of extracellular K^+ may change local E_r (Pongracz et al., 1992), and intracellular accumulations of ions within the tiny volumes of spine heads may change the driving force on synaptic currents (Qian and Sejnowski, 1989). These special properties are easily included in most compartmental models.

11. Cables have different boundary conditions. In classical electrotonic theory, a cable such as one used for long-distance telecommunication is very long and can be considered of infinite length (one customarily assumes a semi-infinite cable with $V = 0$ at $x = 0$ and only positive values of length x). This assumption carries over to the application of cable theory to long axons, but most dendrites are relatively short. This imposes boundary conditions on the solutions of the cable equations, which have very important effects on electrotonic spread.

In highly branched dendritic trees, boundary conditions are difficult to deal with analytically but are readily represented in compartmental models.

Gordon M. Shepherd

References

Pongracz, F., Poolos, N. P., Kocsis, J. D., and Shepherd, G. M. (1992). A model of NMDA receptor-mediated activity in dendrites of hippocampal CA1 pyramidal neurons. *J. Neurophysiol.* **68**(6), 2248–2259.

Qian, N., and Sejnowski, T. J. (1989). An electro-diffusion model for computing membrane potentials and ionic concentration in branching dendrites, spines and axons. *Biol. Cybernet.* **62**, 1–15.

---

where λ is defined as the square root of r_m/r_i (in centimeters) and V_0 is the value of V at $x = 0$.

Inspection of this equation shows that when $x = \lambda$, the ratio of V to V_0 is $e - 1 = 1/e = 0.37$. Thus, λ is a critical parameter defining the length over which the electrotonic potential spreading along an infinite cable, with given values for internal and membrane resistance, decays (is attenuated) to a value of 0.37 of the value at the site of the input. It is accordingly

referred to as the *characteristic length* (space constant, length constant) of the cable. The higher the value of the specific membrane resistance (R_m), the higher the value of r_m for that segment, the larger the value for λ, and the greater the spread (the less the attenuation) of electrotonic potential through that segment (Fig. 5.3). Specific membrane resistance (R_m) is thus an important variable in determining the spread of activity in a neuron. Most of the passive electrotonic current may be carried by K⁺ "leak" channels, which are open at "rest" and are largely responsible for holding the cell at its resting potential. However, as mentioned earlier, many cells or regions within a cell are seldom at "rest" but are constantly active, in which case electrotonic current is carried by a variety of open channels. Thus, the effective Rm can vary from values of less than 1000Ω cm² to more than $100,000\Omega$ cm² in different neurons and in different parts of a neuron. Note that λ varies with the square root of R_m, so a 100-fold difference in R_m translates into only a 10-fold difference in λ.

Conversely, the higher the value of the specific internal resistance (R_i), the higher the value of r_i for that segment, the smaller the value of λ, and the less the spread of electrotonic potential through that segment (see Fig. 5.3). Traditionally, the value of R_i has been believed to be in the range of approximately $50–100\Omega$ cm based on muscle cells and the squid

axon. In mammalian neurons, estimates now tend toward a value of 200Ω cm. This limited range may suggest that R_i is less important than R_m in controlling passive current spread in a neuron. The square-root relation further reduces the sensitivity of l to R_i. However, as noted in assumption 7 in Box 5.2, the membranous and filamentous organelles in the cytoplasm may alter the effective R_i. The presence of these organelles in very thin processes, such as distal dendritic branches, spine stems, and axon preterminals, may thus have potentially significant effects on the spread of electrotonic current through them. Furthermore, the relative significance of R_i and R_m depends greatly on the length of a given process, as will be seen shortly.

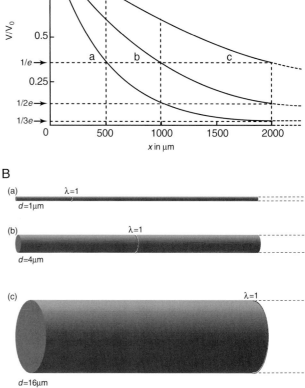

FIGURE 5.4 The space constant governing the spread of electrotonic potential through a nerve cell process also depends on the square root of the diameter of the process. (A) Potential profiles for processes with three different diameters but fixed values of R_i and R_m. (B) The three axon profiles in A. Note that to double λ, the diameter must be quadrupled.

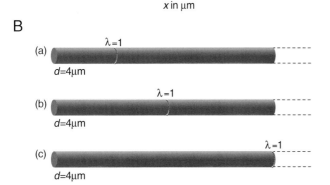

FIGURE 5.3 The space constant governing the spread of electrotonic potential through a nerve cell process depends on the square root of the ratio between the specific membrane resistance (R_m) and the specific internal resistance (R_i). (A) Potential profiles for processes with three different values of λ. (B) Dotted lines represent the location of l on each of the three processes.

Electrotonic Spread Depends on the Diameter of a Process

The space constant (λ) depends not only on the internal and membrane resistance, but also on the diameter of a process (Fig. 5.4). Thus, from the relations between r_m and R_m, and r_i and R_i, discussed in the preceding section,

$$\lambda = \sqrt{\frac{I_m}{r_i}} = \sqrt{\frac{R_m}{R_i} \cdot \frac{d}{4}}. \qquad (5.3)$$

Neuronal processes vary widely in diameter. In the mammalian nervous system, the thinnest processes are the distal branches of dendrites, the necks of some dendritic spines, and the cilia of some sensory cells; these processes may have diameters of only 0.1 μm or less (the thinnest processes in the nervous system are approximately 0.02 μm). In contrast, the thickest processes in the mammal are the largest myelinated axons and the largest dendritic trunks, which may have diameters as large as 20 to 25 μm. This means that the range of diameters is approximately three orders of magnitude (1000-fold). Note, again, that the relation to λ is the square root; thus, over a 10-fold difference in diameter, the difference in λ is only about 3-fold (Fig. 5.4).

Electrotonic Properties Must Be Assessed in Relation to the Lengths of Neuronal Processes

Application of classical cable theory to neuronal processes assumes that the processes are infinitely long (assumption 11 in Box 5.2). However, because neuronal processes have finite lengths, the length of a given process must be compared with λ to assess the extent to which λ accurately describes the actual electrotonic spread in that process. One of the largest processes in any nervous system, the squid giant axon, has a diameter of approximately 1 mm. R_m for this axon has been estimated as 600Ω cm^2 (a very low value compared to most values of R_m in mammals), and R_i as vapproximately 80Ω cm, the value of Ringer solution (note that the very large diameter is counterbalanced by the very low R_m). Putting these values into Eq. (5.3) gives a λ of approximately 5.5 mm. The real length of the giant axon is several centimeters; to relate real length to characteristic length, we define *electrotonic length* (L) as

$$L = x/\lambda \qquad (5.4)$$

Thus, if $x = 30$ mm, then $L = 30$ mm/4.5 mm = 7; i.e., the real length of the giant axon is seven λ. The electrotonic potential decays to only a small percentage of the original value by only three characteristic lengths (see Fig. 5.4), so for this case the assumption of an infinite length is justified. A reason often given for why the nervous system needs action potentials is that they overcome the severe attenuation of passively spreading potentials that occurs over the considerable lengths required for transmission of signals by axons.

In contrast to axons, dendritic branches have lengths that are usually much shorter than three characteristic lengths. In dendrites, therefore, the branching patterns come to dominate the extent of potential spread. We discuss the methods for dealing with these branching patterns later in this chapter.

The relative importance of R_i and R_m in controlling current spread depends on the length of a segment relative to its characteristic length λ. Consider, for example, a neuronal process (large axon or dendrite) 10 μm in diameter, with $R_i = 100\Omega$ cm and $R_m = 10,000\Omega$ cm^2. By the preceding definitions, the longitudinal resistance r_i per unit length (1 cm) would equal 130 MΩ, whereas the membrane resistance r_m would be only 3 MΩ. Thus, the relatively low specific internal resistance has a relatively large effect over the unit distance (cm) because of the small diameter of the nerve process. Such a process would have a characteristic length of 1500 μm, where, by definition [see Eq. (5.4)], $r_m = r_i$, and the current would be equally divided between the two. At shorter distances, more current tends to flow through r_i as the membrane area is reduced (and r_m thereby increases); this becomes an important factor in shaping current flow through small dendritic branches and dendritic spines (as will be seen shortly and in Chapter 12).

Summary

Passive spread of electrical potential along the cell membrane underlies all types of electrical signaling in the neuron. It is thus the foundation for understanding how the diverse functions of the neuron are coordinated within the neuron so that the neuron can generate, receive, integrate, encode, and send signals in interacting with its neighboring neurons and glial cells.

Electrotonic spread shares properties with electrical transmission through electrical cables; the study of cable transmission has put these properties on a sound quantitative basis. The theoretical basis for extension of cable theory to complex dendritic trees has been developed in parallel with compartmental modeling methods for simulating dendritic signal processing.

Cable theory depends on a number of reasonable simplifying assumptions about the geometry of neuronal processes and current flow within them. Steady-state electrotonus in dendrites depends, to begin with, on passive resistance of the membrane and of the internal cytoplasm and on the diameter and length of a nerve process.

SPREAD OF TRANSIENT SIGNALS

Electrotonic Spread of Transient Signals Depends on Membrane Capacitance

Until now, we have considered only the passive spread of steady-state inputs. However, the essence of many neural signals is that they change rapidly. In mammals, fast action potentials characteristically last from 1 to 5 ms, and fast synaptic potentials last from 5 to 30 ms. How do the electrotonic properties affect spread of these rapid signals?

Rapid signal spread depends not only on all of the factors discussed thus far, but also on the membrane capacitance (c_m), which is due to the lipid moiety of the plasma membrane. Classically, the value of the specific membrane capacitance (C_m) has been considered to be 1 mF cm^{-2}. However, a value of 0.6– 0.75 mF cm^{-2} is now preferred for the lipid moiety itself, with the remainder being due to gating charges on membrane proteins (Jack et al., 1975).

The simplest case demonstrating the effect of membrane capacitance on transient signals is that of a single segment or a cell body with no processes (a very unrealistic assumption, but a simple starting point). In the equivalent electrical circuit for a neural process, the membrane capacitance is placed in parallel with ohmic components of the membrane conductance and the driving potentials for ion flows through those conductances (see Fig. 5.2B). Again neglecting the resting membrane potential, we take as an example the injection of a current step into a soma; in this case, the time course of the current spread to ground is described by the sum of the capacitative and resistive current (plus the input current, I_{pulse}):

$$C \frac{dV_m}{dt} + \frac{V_m}{R} = I_{pulse}. \qquad (5.5)$$

Rearranging,

$$RC \frac{dV_m}{dt} + V_m = I_{pulse} \cdot R, \qquad (5.6)$$

where $RC = \tau$ (τ is the time constant of the membrane).

The solution of this equation for the response to a step change in current (I) is

$$V_m(T) = I_{pulse} R(1 - e^{-T}). \qquad (5.7)$$

When the pulse is terminated, the decay of the initial potential (V_0) to rest is given by

$$V_m(T) = V_0 e^{-T}. \qquad (5.8)$$

These "on" and "off" transients are shown in Fig. 5.5. The significance of τ is shown in the diagram; it is the time required for the voltage change across the membrane to reach $1/e = 0.37$ of its final value. This time constant of the membrane defines the transient voltage response of a patch of membrane to a current step in terms of the electrotonic properties of the patch, analogous to the way that the length constant defines the spread of voltage change over distance in terms of the electrotonic properties of a segment.

A Two-Compartment Model Defines the Basic Properties of Signal Spread

These spatial and temporal cable properties can be combined in a two-compartment model (Shepherd and Koch, 1998) that can be applied to the generation and spread of any arbitrary transient signal (Fig. 5.6).

In the simplest case, current is injected into one of the compartments. For a positive current pulse, the positive charge injected into compartment A attempts to flow outward across the membrane, partially

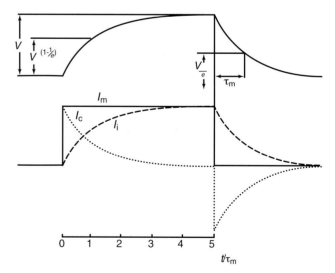

FIGURE 5.5 The equivalent circuit of a single isolated compartment responds to an injected current step by charging and discharging along a time course determined by the time constant, τ. In actuality, because nerve cell segments are parts of longer processes (axonal or dendritic) or larger branching trees, the actual time courses of charging or discharging are modified. V steady-state voltage; I_m, injected current applied to membrane; I_c, current through the capacitance; I_i, current through the ionic leak conductance; τ_m, membrane time constant. From Jack et al. (1975).

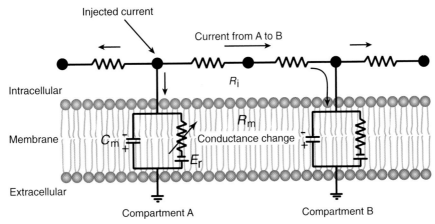

Injected current

Current from A to B

Intracellular

R_i

Membrane

C_m

R_m
Conductance change

E_r

Extracellular

Compartment A

Compartment B

FIGURE 5.6 The equivalent circuit of two neighboring compartments or segments (A and B) of an axon or dendrite shows the pathways for current spread in response to an input (injected current or increase in membrane conductance) at segment A.

opposing the negative charge on the inside of the lipid membrane (the charge responsible for the negative resting potential), thereby depolarizing the membrane capacitance (C_m) at that site. At the same time, the charge begins to flow as current across the membrane through the resistance of the ionic membrane channels (R_m) that are open at that site. The proportion of charge divided between C_m and R_m determines the rate of charge of the membrane, i.e., the membrane time constant, τ. However, charge also starts to flow through the internal resistance (R_i) into compartment B, where the same events take place. The charging (and discharging) transient in compartment A departs from the time constant of a single isolated compartment, being faster because of the impedance load (e.g., current sink) of the rest of the cable (represented by compartment B). Thus, the time constant of the system no longer describes the charging transient in the system because of the conductance load of one compartment on another (this is analogous to the way that the conductance load makes the electrotonic potential more attenuated than the space constant). The system is entirely passive and invariant; the response to a second current pulse sums linearly with that of the first.

This case is a useful starting point because an experimenter often uses electrical currents as stimuli in analyzing nerve function. However, a neuron normally generates current spread by means of a localized conductance change across the membrane. Consider such a change in the example of compartment A in Fig. 5.6. Assume a change in the ionic conductance for Na^+, as in the initiation of an action potential or an excitatory postsynaptic potential, producing an inward positive current in compartment A.

The charge transferred to the interior surface of the membrane attempts to follow the same paths followed by the injected current just described by opposing the negativity inside the membrane capacitance, crossing the membrane through the open membrane channels to ground, and spreading through the internal resistance to the next compartment, where the charge flows are similar.

Thus, the two cases start with different means of transferring positive charge within the cell, but from that point the current paths and the associated spread of the electrotonic potential are similar. The electrotonic current that spreads between the two segments is referred to as the *local current*. Note again that the charging transient in compartment A is faster than the time constant of the resting membrane; this difference is due both to the conductance load of compartment B and to the fact that the imposed conductance increase in compartment A reduces the time constant of compartment A (by reducing effective R_m). This illustrates a critical point first emphasized by Wilfrid Rall (1964): changes in membrane conductance alter the system so that it is no longer a linear system, even though it is a passive system. Thus, passive electrotonic spread is not so simple as most people think! Nonlinear summation of synaptic responses is further discussed later in this chapter.

Summary

In addition to the properties underlying steady-state electrotonus, passive spread of *transient* potentials depends on the membrane capacitance. Initiation of electrotonic spread by intracellular injection of a transient electrical current pulse produces an electrotonic potential that spreads by passive local currents from point to point. It is more attenuated in amplitude than the steady-state case as it spreads along an axon or dendrite due to the low-pass filtering action of the membrane capacitance. Simultaneous current pulses at that site or other sites produce potentials that add linearly because the passive properties are invariant. However, transient conductance changes, as in synaptic responses, generate electrotonic potentials that do not sum linearly because of the nonlinear interactions of the conductances.

ELECTROTONIC PROPERTIES UNDERLYING PROPAGATION IN AXONS

Impulses Propagate in Unmyelinated Axons by Means of Local Electrotonic Currents

Let us apply our knowledge of electrotonic current properties to propagation of an action potential in an unmyelinated axon, i.e., one that is not surrounded by myelin or other membranes that restrict the spread of extracellular current. Details on the ionic mechanisms of the nerve impulse can be found in Chapter 6. The local current spreading through the internal resistance to the neighboring compartment enables the action potential to propagate along the membrane of the axon. The rate of propagation is determined by both the passive cable properties and the kinetics of the action potential mechanism.

Each of the cable properties is relevant in specific ways. For brief signals such as the action potential, C_m is critical in controlling the rate of change of the membrane potential. For long processes such as axons, R_i increasingly opposes electrotonic current flow as the value of r_i increases beyond the characteristic length, whereas the effect of r_m decreases, due to the increased membrane area for parallel current paths (see earlier). This effect is greater in thinner axons, which have shorter characteristic lengths. Finally, R_m is a parameter that can vary widely. Thus, each of these parameters must be assessed in order to understand the exquisite effects of passive variables on the rates of impulse propagation in axons.

A high value of R_m, for example, forces current further along the membrane, increasing the characteristic length and consequently the spread of electrotonic potential, as we have seen; however, at the same time, it increases the membrane time constant, thus slowing the response of a neighboring compartment to a rapid change. Increasing the diameter of the axon lowers the effective internal resistance of a compart-

ment, thereby also increasing the characteristic length, but without a concomitant effect on the time constant. Thus, changing the diameter is a direct way of affecting the rate of impulse propagation through changes in passive electrotonic properties. The conduction rate of any given axon depends on the particular combination of these properties (Rushton, 1951, Ritchie, 1995). For example, in the squid giant axon, the very large diameter (as large as 1 mm) promotes rapid impulse propagation; the very low value of R_m (600 gV cm) lowers the time constant (promoting rapid current spread) but also decreases the length constant (limiting the spatial extent of current spread).

The effects of these passive properties on impulse velocity also depend on other factors. For example, on the basis of the cable equations, we can show that the conduction velocity should be related to the square root of the diameter (Rushton, 1951). However, the density of Na$^+$ channels in fibers of different diameters is not constant; thus, the binding of saxitoxin molecules, for example, to Na$^+$ channels varies greatly with diameter, from almost 300 μm^{-2} in the squid axon to only 35 μm^{-2} in the garfish olfactory nerve (Ritchie, 1995). Thus, both active and passive properties must be assessed in order to understand a particular functional property.

Myelinated Axons Have Membrane Wrappings and Booster Sites for Faster Conduction

The evolution of larger brains to control larger bodies and more complex behavior required communication over longer distances within the brain and body. This requirement placed a premium on the ability of axons to conduct impulses as rapidly as possible. As noted in the preceding section, a direct way of increasing the rate of conduction is by increasing the diameter, but larger diameters mean fewer axons within a given space, and complex behavior must be mediated by many axons. Another way of increasing the rate of conduction is to make the kinetics of the impulse mechanism faster; i.e., make the rate of increase in Na$^+$ conductance with increasing membrane depolarization faster. The Hodgkin–Huxley equations (Chapter 6) for the action potential in mammalian nerves in fact have this faster rate.

As we have seen, the rapid spread of local currents is promoted by an increase in R_m but is opposed by an associated increase in the time constant. What is needed is an increase in R_m with a concomitant decrease in C_m. This is brought about by putting more resistances in series with the membrane resistance (because resistances in series add) while putting more capacitances in series with the membrane capacitance (capacitances in series add as the reciprocals, much like resistances in parallel, as noted earlier). The way the nervous system does this is through a special satellite cell called a Schwann cell, a type of glial cell. As described in Chapters 3 and 4, Schwann cells wrap many layers of their plasma membranes around an axon. The membranes contain special constituents and together are called myelin. Myelinated nerves contain the fastest conducting axons in the nervous system. A general empirical finding known as the Hursh factor (Hursh, 1939) states that the rate of propagation of an impulse along a myelinated axon in meters per second is six times the diameter of the axon in micrometers. Thus, the largest axons in the mammalian nervous system are approximately 20 μm in diameter, and their conduction rate is approximately 120 m s^{-1}, whereas the thin myelinated axons of about 1 μm in diameter have conduction rates of approximately 5 to 10 m s^{-1}.

As discussed in Chapter 4 , myelinated axons are not myelinated along their entire length; at regular intervals (approximately 1 mm in peripheral nerves), the myelin covering is interrupted by a node of Ranvier. The node has a complex structure. The density of voltage-sensitive Na$^+$ channels at the node is high (10,000 μm^{-2}), whereas it is very low (20 μm^{-2}) in the internodal membrane. This difference in density means that the impulse is actively generated only at the node; the impulse jumps, so to speak, from node to node, and the process is therefore called *saltatory conduction*. A myelinated axon therefore resembles a passive cable with active booster stations.

In rapidly conducting axons the impulse may extend over considerable lengths; e.g., in a 20-μm-diameter axon conducting at 120 ms^{-1}, at any instant of time an impulse of 1-ms duration extends over a 120-mm length of axon, which includes more than 100 nodes of Ranvier. It is therefore more appropriate to conceive that the impulse is generated simultaneously by many nodes, with their summed local currents spreading to the next adjacent nodes to activate them.

The specific membrane resistance (R_m) at the node is estimated to be only 50Ω cm^2, due to a large number of open ionic channels at rest. This value of R_m reduces the time constant of the nodal membrane to approximately 50 ms, which enables the nodal membrane to charge and discharge quickly, aiding rapid impulse generation greatly. For axons of equal cross-sectional area, myelination is estimated to increase the impulse conduction rate 100-fold.

In all axons, a critical relation exists between the amount of local current spreading down an adjacent axon and the threshold for opening Na$^+$ channels in the membrane of the adjacent axon so that propaga-tion of the impulse can continue. This introduces the notion of a safety factor, i.e., the amount by which the electrotonic potential exceeds the threshold for acti-vating the impulse. The safety factor must protect against a wide range of operating conditions, includ-ing adaptation (during high-frequency firing), fatigue, injury, infection, degeneration, and aging.

Normally, an excess of local current ensures an adequate margin of safety against these factors. In the squid axon, the safety factor ranges from 4 to 5. In myelinated axons, an exquisite matching between internodal electrotonic properties and nodal active properties ensures that the electrotonic potential reaching a node has an adequate amplitude and the node has sufficient Na$^+$ channels to generate an action potential that will spread to the next node. The safety factors for myelinated axons range from 5 to 10. Thus, the interaction of passive and active properties under-lies the safety factors for impulse propagation in axons. Similar considerations apply to the ortho-dromic spread of signals in dendritic branches and the backpropagation of action potentials from the axon hillock into the soma and dendrites.

Theoretically, the conduction velocity, space con-stant, and impulse wavelength of myelinated fibers scale linearly with fiber diameter (Rushton, 1951; Ritchie, 1995), as indeed is indicated in the aforemen-tioned Hursh factor. This difference between myeli-nated and unmyelinated fibers in their dependence on diameter is thus related to the scaling of the internodal length. At approximately 1 μm in diameter, the Hursh factor breaks down; at less than 1 μm in diameter, there is an advantage, all other factors being equal, for an axon to be unmyelinated. However, myelinated axons are found down to a diameter of only 0.2 μm, which has been correlated with shorter internodal dis-tances (Waxman and Bennett, 1972). Thus, conduction velocity in myelinated nerve depends on a complex interplay between passive and active properties.

Summary: Passive Spread and Active Propagation

A frequent source of confusion in describing nerve activity is the use of the terms *spread* and *propagation*. Rall has used these terms to make the distinction between electrotonus and action potential conduction. Thus, electrotonic potentials are said to *spread*, where-as action potentials (impulses) are said to propagate. These and related terms are discussed further in Chapter 12.

Impulses propagate continuously through unmyeli-nated fibers because the local currents spread directly to neighboring sites on the membrane. The rate of propagation is directly determined by the electrotonic properties of the fiber. In myelinated axons, the impulse propagates discontinuously from node to node. The electrotonic properties of both the nodal and internodal regions determine not only the rate of impulse propagation, but also the safety factor for impulse transmission.

ELECTROTONIC SPREAD IN DENDRITES

Dendrites are the main neuronal compartment for the reception of synaptic inputs. The spread of synaptic responses through the dendritic tree depends critically on the electrotonic properties of the dendrites. Because dendrites are branching structures, understanding the rules governing dendritic electrotonus and the resulting integration of synaptic responses in dendrites is much more difficult than understanding the rules of simple spread in a single axon.

Dendritic Electrotonic Spread Depends on Boundary Conditions of Dendritic Termination and Branching

As noted earlier, compared with axons, dendrites are relatively short, and their length becomes an important factor in assessing their electrotonic properties. Consider, in the mammalian nervous system, a moderately thin dendrite of 1 μm (three orders of magnitude smaller than the squid axon) that has a typical R_m of 60,000Ω cm^{-2} (two orders of magnitude larger than that of the squid axon) and an R_i of 240Ω cm (three times the squid value). Inserting these values into the equation for characteristic length [Eq. (5.3)] gives a λ of approximately 790 μm. This illustrates that λ tends to be relatively long in comparison with the actual lengths of the dendrites; in other words, because of the relatively high membrane resistance, the electrotonic spread of potentials is relatively effective within a dendritic branching tree.

This essential property underlies the integration of signals in dendrites. The effective spread immediately leads to a second property. The assumption of infinite length no longer holds; dendritic branches are bounded by their terminations, on the one hand, and the nature of their branching, on the other. These are termed *boundary conditions*. The spread of electrotonic potentials is therefore exquisitely sensitive to the boundary conditions of the dendrites.

This problem is approached most easily by considering two extreme types of termination of a dendritic branch. First, consider that at $x = a$ the branch ends in a sealed end with infinite resistance. In this case, the axial component of the current can spread no further and must therefore seek the only path to ground, which is across the membrane of the cylinder. This current is added to the current already crossing the membrane; in the equation for Ohm's law ($E = IR$), I is increased, giving a larger E. The membrane will thus be more depolarized up to the terminal point a; in fact, near point a, axial current is negligible and almost all the current is across the membrane, which amounts to a virtual space clamp near point a (Fig. 5.7). If at point a the infinite resistance is replaced by the more realistic assumption of an end that is sealed with surface membrane, only a small amount of current crosses this membrane and attenuation of electrotonic potential is only slightly greater. Infinite resistance is therefore a useful approximation for assessing the effects of a sealed end on electrotonic spread in a terminal dendritic branch.

At the other extreme, consider that at point a a small dendritic branch opens out into a very large

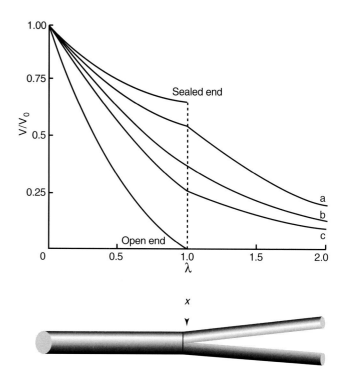

FIGURE 5.7 The spread of electrotonic potential through a short nerve cell process such as a dendritic branch is governed by the space constant and by the size of the branches; the latter imposes a boundary condition at the branch point. Curves a–c represent a range of realistic assumptions about the sizes of the branches relative to the size of the stem, together with the limiting conditions of an open circuit (corresponding to an infinite conductance load) and a closed circuit (corresponding to a sealed tip).

conductance. Examples are, in the extreme, a hole in the membrane; less extreme are a very small dendritic branch on a large soma and a small twig or spine on a large dendritic branch. Recall that large processes sum their resistances in parallel, which gives low current density and small voltage changes. Therefore, a current spreading through the high resistance of a small branch into a large branch encounters a very low resistance. For steady-state current spread, this situation is referred to as a large conductance load; for a transient current, we refer to it as a low impedance (which includes the effect of the membrane capacitance). This introduces the key principle of *impedance matching* between interacting compartments, an important principle generally in biological systems. In our example, an impedance mismatch exists between the high impedance thin branch and the lower impedance thick branch. This mismatch reduces any voltage change due to the current and, in the extreme, effectively clamps the membrane to the resting potential (E_r) at that point. The electrotonic potential is thus attenuated through the branch much more rapidly than would be predicted by the characteristic length (see Fig. 5.7). This does not invalidate l as a measure of electrotonic properties; rather, it means that, as with the time constant, each cable property must be assessed within the context of the size and branching of the dendrites.

All the different types of branching found in neuronal dendrites lie between these two extremes with a corresponding range of boundary conditions at $x = a$. Consider a segment of dendrite that divides into two branches at $x = a$. We can appreciate intuitively that the amount of spread of electrotonic potential into the two branches will be governed by the factors just considered. One possibility is that the two branches have very small diameters, so their input impedance is higher than that of the segment; in this case, the situation will tend toward the sealed-end case (Fig. 5.7, top trace). In contrast, the segment may give rise to two very fat branches, so the situation will tend toward the large conductance load case (Fig. 5.7, bottom trace).

For many cases of dendritic branching, the input impedance of the branches is between the two extremes (see Fig. 5.7, traces a–c), providing for a reasonable degree of impedance matching between the stem branch and its two daughter branches. This situation thus approximates the infinite cylinder case, in which by definition the input impedance at one site matches that at its neighboring site along the cylinder. The general rules for impedance matching at branch points were worked out by Rall (1959, 1964, 1967), who showed that the input conductance of a dendritic

segment varies with the diameter raised to the 3/2 power. There is electrotonic continuity at a branch point equivalent to the infinitely extended cylinder if the diameter of the segment raised to the 3/2 power equals the sum of the diameters raised to the 3/2 power of all the daughter branches. An idealized branching pattern that satisfies this rule is shown in Fig. 5.8. When the branching tree reduces to a single chain of compartments, as in this case, it is called an "equivalent cylinder." When the branching pattern departs from the d 3/2 rule, the compartment chain is referred to as an "equivalent dendrite" (Rall and Shepherd, 1968).

Dendritic Synaptic Potentials Are Delayed and Attenuated by Electrotonic Spread

We are now in a position to assess the effects of cable properties on the time course of the spread of synaptic potentials through dendritic branches and trees. Consider in Fig. 5.8 the case of recording from a soma while delivering a brief excitatory synaptic conductance change to different locations in the dendritic tree. The response to the nearest site is a rapidly rising synaptic potential that peaks near the end of the conductance change and then decays rapidly toward baseline. When the input is delivered to the middle of the chain of compartments, the response in the soma begins only after a delay, rises more slowly, reaches a much lower peak (which is reached after the end of the conductance change in the soma), and decays slowly toward baseline. For input to the terminal compartment, the voltage delay at the soma is so long that the response has scarcely started by the end of the conductance change in the distal dendrite; the response rises slowly to a delayed (several milliseconds) and prolonged plateau that subsides very slowly (see Fig. 5.8).

Although the synaptic potentials thus decrease in amplitude as they spread, the rate of electrotonic spread can be calculated in terms of the half-amplitude at any point. If distance is expressed in units of λ and time in units of τ, then for spread through a semi-infinite cable, we have the simple equation (Jack *et al.*, 1975)

$$\text{Velocity} = 2 \frac{\lambda}{\tau}. \qquad (5.9)$$

Thus, if we ignore boundary effects, for the 10-mm process mentioned earlier in which $\lambda = 1500$ and $\tau = 10$ ms, the velocity of spread would be 0.3 ms^{-1}, or 300 mms^{-1}. It can be seen that electrotonic spread can be relatively fast over short distances within a dendritic tree but is very slow in comparison with impulse transmission for an axon of this diameter

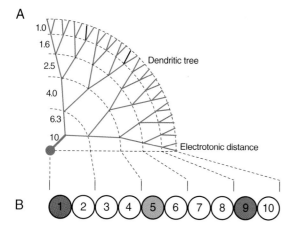

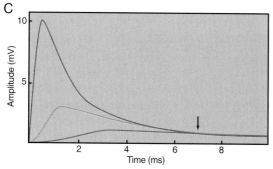

FIGURE 5.8   The spread of electrotonic potentials is accompanied by a delay and an attenuation of amplitude. (A) Dendritic diameters (left) satisfy the *3/2d* rule so that the tree can be portrayed by an equivalent cylinder. An excitatory postsynaptic potential (EPSP) is generated in compartment 1, 5, or 9 (B) while recordings are made from compartment 1. (C) Short latency, large amplitude, and rapid transient response in compartment 1 at the site of input, as well as the later, smaller, and slower responses recorded in compartment 1 for the same input to compartments 5 and 9. Despite the initial differences in time course, the responses converge at the arrow to decay together. Based on Rall (1967).

(60 ms^{-1}). Thus, both the severe decrement and the slow velocity make passive spread by itself ineffective for transmission over long distances.

These general rules of delay and attenuation govern the passive spread of all transient potentials in dendritic branches and trees. As a rule of thumb, spread within one space constant (see the decrement between compartments 1 and 5 in Fig. 5.8) mediates relatively effective linkage for rapid signal integration, whereas spread over one or two space constants (see the decrement between compartments 1 and 9 in Fig. 5.8) is limited to slower background modulation. In real dendrites, these limitations are often overcome through boosting the signals at intermediate sites by voltage-gated properties (see Chapter 12).

The spread of electrotonic potential from a point of input involves the *equalization of charge* on the membrane throughout the system. After cessation of the input, a time is reached when charge has become equalized and the entire system is equipotential; from this time on, the remaining electrotonic potential decays equally at every point in the system. This time is indicated by the vertical arrow in Fig. 5.8C. Before this time, the decaying transients are governed by equalizing time constants, indicating electrotonic spread, which can be identified by "peeling" on semilogarithmic plots of the potentials (Rall, 1977). After this time, the decay of electrotonic potential is governed solely by the membrane time constant, τ. In experimental recordings of synaptic potentials, the overall electrotonic length of the dendritic system, considered as an "equivalent cylinder" or "equivalent dendrite" (see earlier discussion), can be estimated from measurements of the membrane time constant and the equalizing time constants. The electrotonic lengths of the dendritic trees of many neuron types lie between 0.3 and 1.5.

What is the spread of the postsynaptic potential throughout the system when a synaptic input is delivered to a single terminal dendritic branch (Fig. 5.9) (Rall and Rinzel, 1973, Rinzel and Rall, 1974). Let us begin by considering a steady-state potential. Two main factors are involved. First, in the terminal branch, both the effective membrane resistance and the internal resistance are very large; hence, the branch has a very high input resistance, which produces a very large voltage change for any given synaptic conductance change. Balanced against this high input resistance is a second factor: the small branch has a very large conductance load on it because of the rest of the dendritic tree. As a result, there is a steep decrement in the electrotonic potential spreading from the branch through the tree to the cell body (see Fig. 5.9A). For comparison, a direct input to the soma produces only a small potential change there because of the relatively very low input resistance at that site.

For a transient synaptic input, a third factor—membrane capacitance—must be taken into account. The small surface area of a terminal branch has little capacitance, according to our earlier calculations, so the amplitude of a transient response differs little from a steady-state response in the branch. However, in spreading out from a small process (such as a distal dendritic twig or spine), the transient synaptic potential is attenuated by the impedance mismatch between the process and the rest of the dendritic tree. Spread of the transient through the dendritic tree is attenuated further by the need to charge the capacitance of the dendritic membrane and is slowed by the time taken for the charging. The amount of slowing is

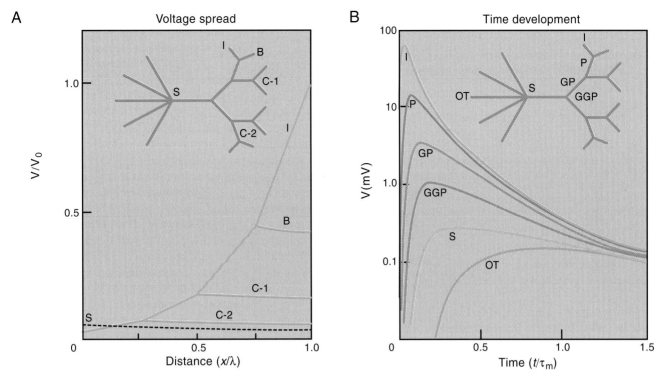

FIGURE 5.9 Electrotonic spread from a single small dendritic branch. (A) For steady-state input (*I*), the electrotonic potential (*V*), relative to the initial potential (*V*$_0$) at the site of input, spreads from the distal branch through the dendritic tree, with a large decrement into the parent branch (due to the large conductance load) but a small decrement into neighboring branches B, C–1, and C–2 (due to the small conductance loads). The resulting potential in the soma (*S*) is much reduced, as is the response to the same input delivered directly to the soma (because of the low input resistance at the soma and the large conductance load of the dendritic tree). The dashed line indicates the response when the same amount of current is injected into the soma. (B) For transient input (*I*) to a distal branch, transient electrotonic potentials decrease sharply in amplitude and are delayed and slower as they spread toward the soma through the parent (P), grandparent (GP), and great-grandparent (GGP) branches, eventually reaching the soma (S) and output trunk (OT). Modified from Segev (1995) based on Rall and Rinzel (1973, 1974).

so precise that the relative distance of a synapse in the dendritic tree from the soma can be calculated from experimental measurements in the soma of the time to peak of the recorded synaptic potential (Rall, 1977; Johnston and Wu, 1995). For these reasons, the peak of a synaptic potential transient spreading from distal dendrites toward the soma may be severely attenuated, severalfold more than for the case of steady-state attenuation. This is often referred to as the *filtering effect* of the cable properties. However, the integrated response (the area under the transient voltage) is approximately equivalent to the steady-state amplitude, indicating that there is only a small loss of total charge (see Fig. 5.9B).

DYNAMIC PROPERTIES OF PASSIVE ELECTROTONIC STRUCTURE

Electrotonic Structure of the Neuron Changes Dynamically

These considerations show that, compared with the anatomical structure of a dendritic system, which is relatively fixed over short periods of time, electrotonic properties have complex, shifting, effects on signal integration. The effects depend on multiple factors, including the directions of signal spread, inhomogeneities in passive properties, rates of signal transfer, and interactions between synaptic or active conduc-

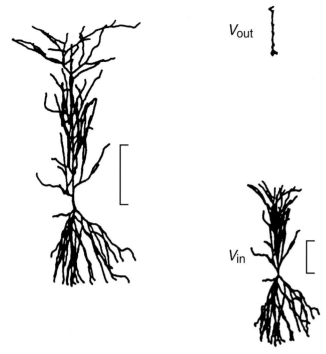

FIGURE 5.10 The electrotonic structure of a neuron varies with the direction of spread of signals. (Left) Stained CA1 pyramidal neuron. (Right) Electrotonic transform of the stained morphology for the case of a voltage spreading toward the cell body (bottom, V_{in}) and away from the cell body (top, V_{out}). Calibration, 1 electrotonic length. See text. From Carnevale *et al.* (1997).

tances, to name a few. The effects can be illustrated in a graphic fashion for the entire soma–dendritic system by taking a stained neuron and replacing it with a representation based on its electrotonic properties. This is termed a *morpho-electrotonic transform* (MET) or *neuromorphic transform.*

The method is illustrated in Fig. 5.10 for a CA1 hippocampal pyramidal cell. The problem is to compare the spread of a signal from the soma to the dendrites (voltage out, V_{out}) with spread from the dendrites to the soma (voltage in, V_{in}). On the left is the stained neuron, giving rise to a long apical dendrite with many branches and shorter basal dendrites and their branches. In the right lower diagram is an electrotonic representation of the neuron for signals spreading from the distal dendrites toward the soma. There is severe decrement from each distal branch (cf. Fig. 5.9) so that apical and basal dendritic trees have electrotonic lengths of approximately 3 and 2, respectively. By comparison, in the right upper diagram is an electrotonic representation of this neuron for a signal spreading from the soma to the dendrites. The basal dendrites have shrunk to almost nothing, indicating that they are nearly isopotential. This is because they are relatively short compared with their electrotonic lengths and because the sealed-end boundary condition greatly reduces the decrement of electrotonic potential through them (cf. Fig. 5.7). The apical

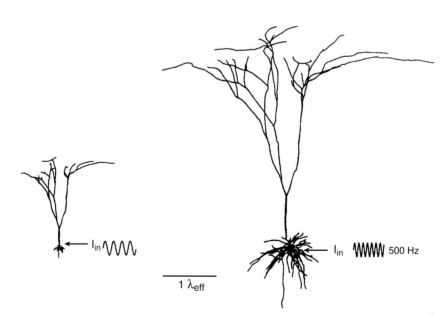

FIGURE 5.11 The electrotonic structure of a neuron varies with the rapidity of signals. (Left) Electrotonic transform of a pyramidal neuron in response to a sinusoidal current of 100 Hz injected into the soma (i.e., this is an example of V_{out}). (Right) Electrotonic transform of same cell in response to 500 Hz. Calibration, 1 electrotonic length. See text. From Zador *et al.* (1995).

dendrite has shrunk to an electrotonic length of approximately 1. Thus, distal synaptic responses decay considerably in spreading all the way to the soma, which active properties help to overcome, as we shall see in Chapter 12. However, signals at the soma "see" a relatively compact dendritic tree.

The analysis in Fig. 5.10 applies to spread of steady-state or very slowly changing signals. What about spread of rapid signals? We have seen that membrane capacitance makes the dendrites act as a low-pass filter, further reducing rapid signals. The electrotonic transforms can include this effect, as shown in Fig. 5.11. On the left, the electrotonic representation of a pyramidal neuron is shown for a slow (100 Hz) current injected in the soma. The form is similar to that of the cell in Fig. 5.10, with tiny, virtually isopotential basal dendrites and a longer apical dendritic tree of electrotonic length of approximately 1.5. By comparison, a rapid (500 Hz) signal is severely attenuated in spreading into the dendrites, as shown by the basal dendrites with L of approximately 1 and the apical dendritic tree electrotonic lengths of 4–5. Thus, a somatic action potential could backpropagate into the basal dendrites rather effectively, but would

require active properties to invade very far into the apical dendrites. There is direct evidence for these properties underlying backpropagating action potentials in apical dendrites (Chapter 12).

The electrotonic structure of a neuron is not necessarily fixed, but may vary under synaptic control. An example is shown in Fig. 5.12 for the case of a medium spiny cell in the basal ganglia. During low levels of resting excitatory synaptic input, the electrotonic transform of this cell type is relatively large (left) because of the action of a specific K+ current (known as I_h) in the dendrites that holds them relatively hyperpolarized (see arrow at –90 mV). When synaptic excitation increases, the K+ current is deactivated, reducing the membrane conductance and thereby increasing the input resistance of the cell; the dendritic tree becomes more compact electrotonically (middle) so that synaptic inputs are more effective in activating the cell. As the cell responds to the synaptic excitation, the resulting depolarization activates other K+ currents, which expand the electrotonic structure again (right). This example illustrates how cable properties and voltage-gated properties interact to control the integrative actions of the neuron.

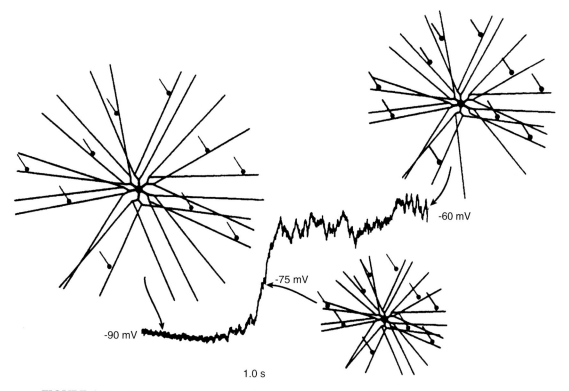

FIGURE 5.12   The electrotonic structure of a neuron can vary with shifts in the resting membrane potential. In this medium spiny cell, the electrotonic transform varies with the resting membrane potential, which in turn reflects the combination of resting voltage-gated K+ currents and excitatory synaptic currents. See text. From Wilson (1998).

Synaptic Conductances in Dendrites Tend to Interact Nonlinearly

Dynamic interactions also occur between synaptic conductances. It is often assumed that synaptic responses sum linearly, but we have already noted that this is not generally true. In an electrical cable, responses to simultaneous current inputs sum linearly (they show "superposition") because the cable properties remain invariant at all times (see Fig. 5.6). However, as noted in that case, synaptic responses in real neurons generate current by means of changes in the membrane conductance at the synapse. In addition to generating current, the change in synaptic conductance alters the overall membrane resistance of that segment and with it the input resistance, thereby changing the electrotonic properties of the whole system. As pointed out by Rall (1964), excitatory and inhibitory conductance changes involve "a change in a conductance which is an element of the system; the

system itself is perturbed; the value of a constant coefficient in the linear differential equation is changed; hence the simple superposition rules do not hold."

This effect is easily illustrated by the two-compartment model of Fig. 5.6. Consider a synaptic input to compartment A, which decreases the membrane resistance of that compartment. Now consider a simultaneous synaptic input to compartment B, which has the same effect on the membrane resistance of that compartment. The internal current flowing between the two compartments encounters a much lower impedance and hence has much less effect on the membrane potential than would have been the case for current injection. The integration of these two responses therefore gives a smaller summed potential than the summation of the two responses taken individually. This effect is referred to as *occlusion*. In essence, each compartment partially short circuits the other through a larger conductance load, thus reducing the combined response.

These properties mean that, as noted earlier, synaptic integration in dendrites in general is not linear even for purely passive electrotonic properties. The further apart the synaptic sites, the fewer the interactions between the conductances, and the more linear the summation becomes (see Fig. 5.13). These nonlinear properties of passive dendrites, combined with the nonlinear properties of voltage-gated channels at local sites on the membrane, contribute to the complexity of signal processing that takes place in dendrites, as will be discussed in Chapter 12.

Significance of Active Conductances in Dendrites Depends on Their Relation to Cable Properties

In electrophysiological recordings from the cell body, dendritic synaptic responses often appear small and slow (cf. Fig. 5.8). However, at their sites of origin in the dendrites, the responses tend to have a large amplitude (because of the high input resistances of the thin distal dendrites) and a rapid time course (because of the small membrane capacitance) (cf. Fig. 5.9). These properties have important implications for the signal processing that takes place in dendrites. In particular, the fact that distal dendrites contain sites of voltage-gated channels means that local integration, local boosting, and local threshold operations can take place. These most distal responses need spread no further than to neighboring local active sites to be boosted by these sites; thus, a rapid integrative sequence of these actions ultimately produces significant effects on signal integration at the

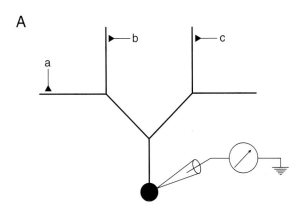

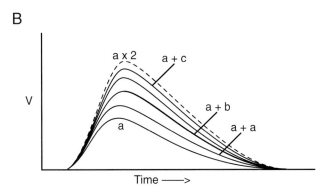

FIGURE 5.13 Schematic diagram of a dendritic tree to illustrate graded effects of nonlinear interactions between synaptic conductances. (A) Three sites of synaptic input (a–c) are shown, with a recording site in the soma. (B) The voltage response (*V*) is shown for the response to a single input at a, the theoretical linear summation for two inputs at a (a × 2), and the gradual reduction in summation from c to a due to increasing shunting between the conductances. See text. From Shepherd and Koch (1990).

cell body. These properties will be considered further in Chapter 12.

In addition to their role in local signal processing, the cable properties of the neuron are also important for (1) controlling the spread of synaptic potentials from the dendrites through the soma to the site of action potential initiation in the axon hillock initial segment and (2) backpropagation of an action potential into the soma–dendritic compartments, where it can activate dendritic outputs and interact with the active properties involved in signal processing. These properties are discussed further in Chapter 12.

Dendritic Spines Form Electrotonic and Biochemical Compartments

The rules governing electrotonic interactions within a dendritic tree also apply at the level of the smallest process of a nerve cell, called a spine. This may vary from a bump on a dendritic branch to a twig to a lollipop-shaped process several micrometers long (Fig. 5.14). A dendritic spine usually receives a single excitatory synapse; an axonal initial segment spine characteristically receives an inhibitory synapse.

Dendritic spines receive most of the excitatory inputs to pyramidal neurons in the cerebral cortex and to Purkinje cells in the cerebellum, as well as to a variety of other neuron types, so an understanding of

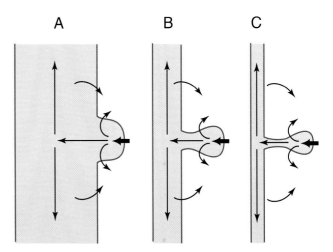

FIGURE 5.14 Diagrams illustrating different types of spines and current flows generated by a synaptic input. (A) Stubby spine arising from a thick process. (B) Moderately elongated spine from a medium diameter branch. (C) Spine with a long stem originating from a thin branch. Parallel considerations apply to diffusion between the spine head and dendritic branch. Modified from Shepherd (1974).

their properties is critical for understanding brain function (Shepherd, 1996; Zandor and Koch, 1994; Harris and Kater, 1994; Yuste and Tank, 1996). As with the whole dendritic tree, one begins with their electrotonic properties. Given the rules we have built

---

BOX 5.3

SOME BASIC ELECTROTONIC PROPERTIES OF DENDRITIC SPINES

a. High input resistance. The smaller the size and the narrower the stem, the higher the input resistance; this gives a large amplitude synaptic potential for a given synaptic conductance. Such a large depolarizing EPSP can have powerful effects on the local environment within the spine.

b. Low total membrane capacitance. The small size also means a small total membrane capacitance, implying that synaptic (and any active) potentials may be rapid; this means that spines on dendrites can potentially be involved in rapid information transmission.

c. Increases in total dendritic membrane capacitance. Although the membrane capacitance of an individual spine is small, the combined spine population increases the total capaciticance of its parent dendrite. This increases the filtering effect of the dendrite on transmission of signals through it.

d. Decrement of potentials spreading from the spine. There is an impedance mismatch between the spine head and its parent dendrite; this means that potentials spreading from the spine to the dendrite will suffer considerable decrement unless there are active properties of the dendrite or of neighboring spines to boost the signal.

e. Ease of potential spread into the spine. The other side of the impedance mismatch is that membrane potential changes within the dendrite spread into the spine with little decrement; thus, the spine tends to follow the potential of its dendrite, except for the transient large-amplitude responses to its own synaptic input. This means that a spine can serve as a *coincidence detector* for nearby synaptic responses or for an action potential backpropagating into the dendritic tree.

Gordon M. Shepherd

earlier in this chapter, by simple inspection of spine morphology as shown in Fig. 5.14, we can postulate several distinctive features that may have important functional implications (see Box 5.3).

In addition to its electrotonic properties, the spine may have interesting biochemical properties. The same cable equations that govern electrotonic properties also have their counterparts in describing the diffusion of substances (as well as the flow of heat). Thus, as already noted, accumulations of only small numbers of ions are needed within the tiny volumes of spine heads to change the driving force on an ion species or to affect significant changes in the concentrations of subsequent second messengers. This interest is intensifying, as the ability to image ion fluxes, such as for Ca^{2+}, and to measure other molecular properties of individual spines increases with new technology such as two-photon microscopy (reviewed in Matus and Shepherd, 2000). The interpretation of those results for the integrative properties of the neuron will require considerations in the biochemical domain that parallel those discussed in the electrotonic domain. The range of properties and possible functions of spines are discussed further in Chapter 12.

Summary

In addition to being dependent on membrane properties, the spread of electrotonic potentials in branching dendritic trees is dependent on the boundary conditions set by the modes of branching and termination within the tree. In general, other parts of the dendritic tree constitute a conductance load on activity at a given site; the spread of activity from that site is determined by the impedance match or mismatch between that site and the neighboring sites. Rules governing these impedance relations have been worked out relative to the case in which the sum of the daughter branch diameters raised to the 3/2 power is equal to that of the parent branch, in which case the system of branches is an "equivalent cylinder," resembling a single continuous cable. This provides a starting point in analyzing synaptic integration, which can be adapted for different types of branching patterns in terms of "equivalent dendrites."

Synchronous synaptic potentials in several branches spread relatively effectively through most dendritic trees. Responses in individual branches may be relatively isolated because of the decrement of passive spread and require local active boosting for effective communication with the rest of the tree. Passive spread can be characterized in terms of several measures, including characteristic length of the equivalent cylin-

der. There is scaling within individual branches, such that electrotonic in finer branches spread is relatively effective over their shorter lengths. Integration of synaptic potentials in passive dendrites is fundamentally nonlinear because of interactions between the synaptic conductances. The rules for electrotonic spread in dendrites are the basis for understanding the contributions of active properties of dendrites (see Chapter 12).

RELATING PASSIVE TO ACTIVE POTENTIALS

We can now begin to gain insight into the relation between passive and active potentials in a neuron. We consider a model, the olfactory mitral cell, in which we apply the principles of this chapter and look forward to the principles underlying active properties in Chapter 12.

A basic problem is to understand the factors that decide where the action potential will be initiated with different levels of excitatory or inhibitory inputs. The possible sites are anywhere from the axon through the soma to the most distal dendrites. The mitral cell is advantageous for this analysis (1) because all the excitatory synaptic input is through olfactory nerve terminals that make their synapses on the distal dendritic tuft and (2) because the primary dendrite that connects the tuft to the cell body is an unbranched cylinder. Applying depolarizing current to distal dendrite or soma, the experimental findings were counterintuitive: with weak distal inputs the action potential initiation site is far away, in the axon, but with increasing excitation it shifts to the distal dendrite, as illustrated in Fig. 5.15A (Chen et al., 1997). How can the weak response spread so far passively, and why does not it excite the active dendrites along the way?

FIGURE 5.15 Interactions of passive and active potentials in ▶ the olfactory mitral cell. (A) Insets show diagrams of a mitral cell with recording sites at soma and distal dendrite. Curves show fitting of experimental and computed responses to weak and strong depolarizing currents injected into the distal primary dendrite. Note the nearly exact superposition of experimental (solid lines) and computed (dashed lines) responses. (B) Longitudinal distribution of membrane potential changes during responses to weak distal dendritic excitation. (C) Same to strong distal dendritic excitation. Blue lines, predominantly passively generated potentials; red lines, predominantly actively generated potentials. d, dendrite; s, soma; c, passive charging; o, onset of action potential; sp, spike peak; r, recovery. See text. Adapted from Shen et al. 1999.

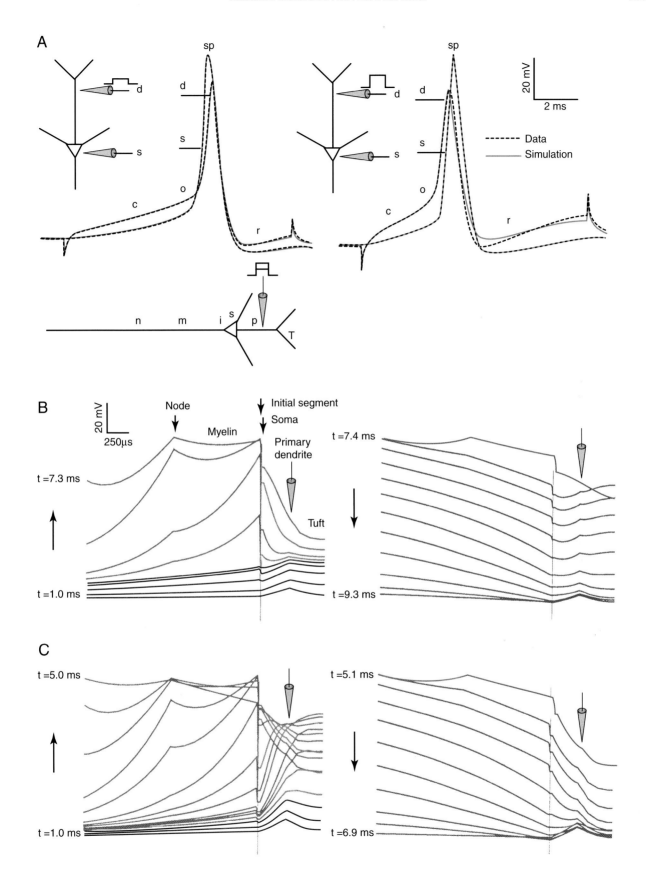

This is much too complex a problem to solve in your head or with "back of the envelope" calculations. The only effective method is a computational simulation. A compartmental model of the mitral cell was therefore constructed, with Na^+ and K^+ conductances scaled to the structure of the mitral cell. Fitting of computed with experimental responses was carried out under stringent constraints, with minimization of eight simultaneous simulations (distal and soma recording sites, distal and soma sites of excitatory current input; strong and weak levels of excitation) (Shen *et al.*, 1999).

We will analyze the active properties in Chapter 12; here we focus on fitting the passive properties. Two steps were essential. First, each experimental recording began with a period of passive charging of the mitral cell membrane (c in Fig. 5.15A). Figure 5.15A shows that the model gave a very accurate simulation, even when the charging was long lasting (left, weak stimulation). This was a critical fit for giving the correct latency of action potential initiation. Second, the longitudinal spread of passive current between the axon and the distal dendrite was calculated. This showed that with weak distal excitation (Fig. 5.15B), the electrotonic current spread with a shallow gradient from the site of injection along the dendrite to the axon (bottom traces); the action potential arose first in the axon because of the much higher density of Na^+ channels there compared with the dendrite. However, with strong distal excitation *(C)*, the direct depolarization of the less excitable distal dendrite led the weaker electrotonic depolarization of the more excitable axon, and dendritic action potential initiation occurred first. This can be explored online at senselab.med.yale.edu/modeldb.

The computational simulations thus show precisely how the interactions of passive and active potentials control the sites of action potential initiation in the neuron. This is a model for the complex integrative properties of the neuron, which is explored further in Chapter 12.

References

Bower, J., and Beeman, D. (eds.) (1995). "The Book of Genesis." Springer-Verlag (Telos), New York.

Carnevale, N. T., Tsai, K. Y., Claiborne, B. J., and Brown, T. H. (1997). Comparative electrotonic analysis of 3 classes of rat hippocampal neurons. *J. Neurophysiol.*

Chen, W. R., Midtgaard, J., and Shepherd, G. M. (1997). Forward and backward propagation of dendritic impulses and their synaptic control in mitral cells. *Science* 278, 463–467.

Harris, K. M., and Kater, S. B. (1994). Dendritic spines, Cellular specializations imparting both stability and flexibility to synaptic function. *Annu. Rev. Neurosci.* 17, 341–371.

Hines, M. (1984). Efficient computation of branched nerve equations. *Int. J. Bio-Med. Comput.* 15, 69–76.

Hursh, J. B. (1939). Conduction velocity and diameter of nerve fibers. *Am. J. Physiol.* 127, 131–139.

Jack, J. J. B., Noble, D., and Tsien, R. W. (1975). "Electrical Current Flow in Excitable Cells." Oxford Univ. Press (Clarendon), London.

Johnston, D., and Wu, S. M. S. (1995). "Foundations of Cellular Neurophysiology." MIT Press, Cambridge.

Matus, A., and Shepherd, G.M. (2000). The millenium of the dendrite? *Neuron.*

Rall, W. (1959). Branching dendritic trees and motoneuron membrane resistivity. *Exp. Neurol.* 1, 491–527.

Rall, W. (1964). Theoretical significance of dendritic trees for neuronal input-output relations. *In* "Neural Theory and Modelling" (R. F. Reiss, ed.), pp. 73–97. Stanford Univ. Press, Stanford, CA.

Rall, W. (1967). Distinguishing theoretical synaptic potentials computed for different soma-dendritic distributions of synaptic input. *J. Neurophysiol.* 30, 1138–1168.

Rall, W. (1977). Core conductor theory and cable properties of neurons. *In* "The Nervous System, Cellular Biology of Neurons" (E. R. Kandel, ed.), Vol. 1; pp. 39–97. Am. Physiol. Soc., Bethesda, MD.

Rall, W., and Rinzel, J. (1973). Branch input resistance and steady attenuation for input to one branch of a dendritic neuron model. *Biophys. J.* 13, 648–688.

Rall, W., and Shepherd, G. M. (1968). Theoretical reconstruction of field potentials and dendrodendritic synaptic interactions in olfactory bulb. *J. Neurophysiol.* 3(6), 884–915.

Rinzel, J., and Rall, W. (1974). Transient response in a dendritic neuron model for current injected at one branch. *Biophys. J.* 14, 759–790.

Ritchie, J. M. (1995). Physiology of axons. *In* "The Axon, Structure, Function, and Pathophysiology" (S. G. Waxman, J. D. Kocsis, and P. K. Stys, eds.), pp. 68–69. Oxford Univ. Press, New York.

Rushton, W. A. H. (1951). A theory of the effects of fibre size in medullated nerve. *J. Physiol. (Lond.)* 115, 101–122.

Segev, I. (1995). Cable and compartmental models of dendritic trees. *In* "The Book of Genesis" (J. M. Bower and D. Beeman, eds.), pp. 53–82. Springer-Verlag (Telos), New York.

Segev, I., Rinzel, J., and Shepherd, G. M. (eds.) (1995). "The Theoretical Foundation of Dendritic Function." MIT Press, Cambridge, MA.

Shen, G., Chen, W. R., Midtgaard, J., Shepherd, G. M. and Hines, M. L. (1999) Computational analysis of action potential initiation in mitral cell soma and dendrites based on dual patch recordings. *J. Neurophysiol.* 82, 3006–3020.

Shepherd, G. M. (1974). "The Synaptic Organization of the Brain." Oxford Univ. Press, New York.

Shepherd, G. M. (1996). The dendritic spine, A multifunctional integrative unit. *J. Neurophysiol.* 75, 2197–2210.

Shepherd, G. M., and Brayton, R. K. (1979). Computer simulation of a dendrodendritic synaptic circuit for self- and lateral-inhibition in the olfactory bulb. *Brain Res.* 175, 377–382.

Shepherd, G. M., and Koch, C. (1990). Dendritic electrotonus and synaptic integration. *In* "The Synaptic Organization of the Brain" (G. M. Shepherd, ed.), 3rd Ed., pp. 439–574. Oxford Univ. Press, New York.

Waxman, S. G., and Bennett, M. V. L. (1972). Relative conduction velocities of small myelinated and nonmyelinated fibres in the central nervous system. Nature, New Biol. 238, 217.

Wilson, C. J. (1998). Basal ganglia. *In* "The Synaptic Organization of the Brain" (G. M. Shepherd, ed.), 4th Ed., pp. 329–376. Oxford Univ. Press, New York.

Yuste, R., and Tank, D. (1996). Dendritic integration in mammalian neurons, a century after Cajal. *Neuron.* **13**, 23–43.

Zador, A., and Koch, C. (1994). Linearized models of calcium dynamics, Formal equivalence to the cable equation. *J. Neurosci.* **14**, 4705–4715.

Zador, A. M., Agmon-Snir, H., and Segev, I. (1995). The morpho-electrotonic transform, A graphical approach to dendritic function. *J. Neurosci.* **15**, 1169–1682.

Ziv, I., Baxter, D. A., and Byrne, J. H. (1994). Simulator for neural networks and action potentials, Description and application. *J. Neurophysiol.* **71**, 294–308.

Gordon M. Shepherd

6

Membrane Potential and Action Potential

The communication of information between neurons and between neurons and muscles or peripheral organs requires that signals travel over considerable distances. A number of notable scientists have contemplated the nature of this communication through the ages. In second century A.D., the great Greek physician Claudius Galen proposed that "humors" flowed from the brain to the muscles along hollow nerves. A true electrophysiological understanding of nerve and muscle, however, depended on the discovery and understanding of electricity itself. The precise nature of nerve and muscle action became clearer with the advent of new experimental techniques by a number of European scientists, including Luigi Galvini, Emil Du Bois-Reymond, Carlo Matteucci, and Hermann von Helmholtz, to name a few (Brazier, 1988). Through the application of electrical stimulation to nerves and muscles, these early electrophysiologists demonstrated that the conduction of commands from the brain to the muscle for the generation of movement was mediated by the flow of electricity along nerve fibers.

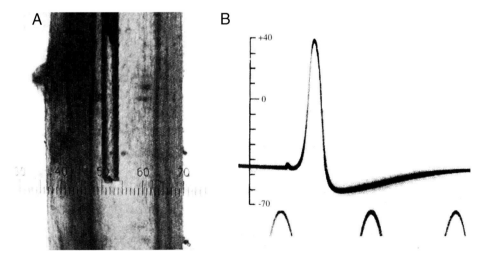

FIGURE 6.1 Intracellular recording of the membrane potential and action potential generation in the squid giant axon. (A) A glass micropipette, about 100 μm in diameter, was filled with seawater and lowered into the giant axon of the squid after it had been dissected free. The axon is about 1 mm in diameter and is transilluminated from behind. (B) One action potential recorded between the inside and the outside of the axon. Peaks of a sine wave at the bottom provided a scale for timing, with 2 ms between peaks. From Hodgkin and Huxley (1939).

With the advancement of electrophysiological techniques, electrical activity recorded from nerves revealed that the conduction of information along the axon was mediated by the active generation of an electrical potential, called the action potential. But what precisely was the nature of these action potentials? To know this in detail required not only a preparation from which to obtain intracellular recordings but also one that could survive *in vitro*. The squid giant axon provided precisely such a preparation. Many invertebrates contain

unusually large axons for the generation of escape reflexes; large axons conduct more quickly than small ones and so the response time for escape is reduced (see Chapter 5). The squid possesses an axon approximately 0.5 mm in diameter, large enough to be impaled by even a course micropipette (Fig. 6.1). By inserting a glass micropipette filled with a salt solution into the squid giant axon, Alan Hodgkin and Andrew Huxley demonstrated in 1939 that axons at rest are electrically polarized, exhibiting a resting membrane potential of approximately –60 mV inside versus outside. In the generation of an action potential, the polarization of the membrane is removed (referred to as depolarization) and exhibits a rapid swing toward, and even past, 0 mV (Fig. 6.1). This depolarization is followed by a rapid swing in the membrane potential to more negative values, a process referred to as hyperpolarization. The membrane potential following an action potential typically becomes even more negative than the original value of approximately –60 mV. This period of increased polarization is referred to as the afterhyperpolarization or the undershoot.

The development of electrophysiological techniques to the point that intracellular recordings could be obtained from the small cells of the mammalian nervous system revealed that action potentials in these neurons are generated through mechanisms similar to that of the squid giant axon.

It is now known that action potential generation in nearly all types of neurons and muscle cells is accomplished through mechanisms similar to those first detailed in the squid giant axon by Hodgkin and Huxley. This chapter considers the cellular mechanisms by which neurons and axons generate a resting membrane potential and how this membrane potential is briefly disrupted for the purpose of propagation of an electrical signal, the action potential.

MEMBRANE POTENTIAL

Membrane Potential Is Generated by the Differential Distribution of Ions

Through the operation of ionic pumps and special ionic buffering mechanisms, neurons actively maintain precise internal concentrations of several important ions, including Na^+, K^+, Cl^-, and Ca^{2+}. The mechanisms by which they do so are illustrated in Figs. 6.2 and 6.3. The intracellular and extracellular concentrations of Na^+, K^+, Cl^-, and Ca^{2+} differ markedly (see Fig. 6.2); K^+ is actively concentrated inside the cell, and Na^+, Cl^-, and Ca^{2+} are actively extruded to the extracellular space. However, this does not mean that the cell

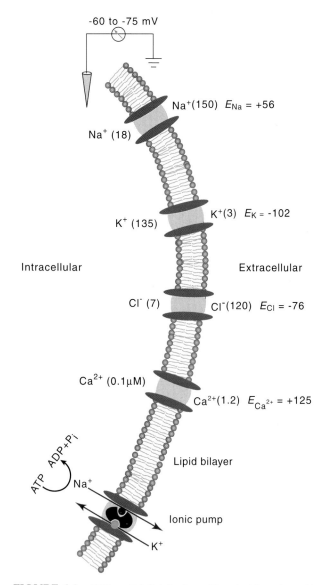

FIGURE 6.2 Differential distribution of ions inside and outside plasma membrane of neurons and neuronal processes, showing ionic channels for Na^+, K^+, Cl^-, and Ca^{2+}, as well as an electrogenic Na^+–K^+ ionic pump (also known as Na^+, K^+-ATPase). Concentrations (in millimoles except that for intracellular Ca^{2+}) of the ions are given in parentheses; their equilibrium potentials (*E*) for a typical mammalian neuron are indicated.

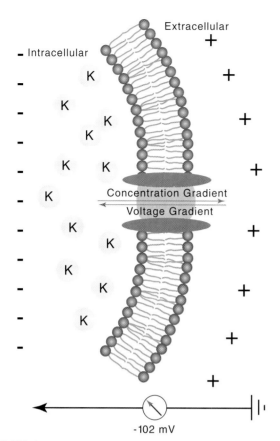

FIGURE 6.3 The equilibrium potential is influenced by the concentration gradient and the voltage difference across the membrane. Neurons actively concentrate K⁺ inside the cell. These K⁺ ions tend to flow down their concentration gradient from inside to outside the cell. However, the negative membrane potential inside the cell provides an attraction for K⁺ ions to enter or remain within the cell. These two factors balance one another at the equilibrium potential, which in a typical mammalian neuron is –102 mV for K⁺.

is filled only with positive charge; anions (denoted A⁻) to which the plasma membrane is impermeant are also present inside the cell and almost balance the high concentration of K⁺. The osmolarity inside the cell is approximately equal to that outside the cell.

Electrical and Thermodynamic Forces Determine the Passive Distribution of Ions

Ions tend to move down their concentration gradients through specialized ionic pores, known as ionic channels, in the plasma membrane. Through simple laws of thermodynamics, the high concentration of K⁺ inside glial cells, neurons, and axons results in a tendency for K⁺ ions to diffuse down their concentration gradient and leave the cell or cell process (see Fig. 6.3). However, the movement of ions across the membrane also results in a redistribution of electrical charge. As K⁺ ions move down their concentration

gradient, the intracellular voltage becomes more negative, and this increased negativity results in an electrical attraction between the negative potential inside the cell and the positively charged, K⁺ ions, thus offsetting the outward flow of these ions. The membrane is selectively permeable, i.e., it is impermeable to the large anions inside the cell, which cannot follow the potassium ions across the membrane. At some membrane potential, the "force" of the electrostatic attraction between the negative membrane potential inside the cell and the positively charged K⁺ ions will exactly balance the thermal "forces" by which K⁺ ions tend to flow down their concentration gradient (see Fig. 6.3). In this circumstance, it is equally likely that a K⁺ ion exits the cell by movement down the concentration gradient as it is that a K⁺ ion enters the cell due to the attraction between the negative membrane potential and the positive charge of this ion. At this membrane potential, there is no net flow of K⁺, and these ions are said to be in equilibrium. The membrane potential at which this occurs is known as the equilibrium potential. (See Box 6.1 for calculation of the equilibrium potential.)

To illustrate, let us consider the passive distribution of K⁺ ions in the squid giant axon as studied by Hodgkin and Huxley. The K⁺ concentration $[K^+]$ inside the squid giant axon is about 400 mM, whereas the $[K^+]$ outside the axon is about 20 mM. Because $[K^+]_i$ is greater than $[K^+]_o$, potassium ions will tend to flow down their concentration gradient, taking positive charge with them. The equilibrium potential (at which the tendency for K⁺ ions to flow down their concentration gradient will be exactly offset by the attraction for K⁺ ions to enter the cell because of the negative charge inside the cell) at a room temperature of 20°C can be calculated by the Nernst equation as such:

$$E_K = 58.2 \log_{10}(20/400) = -76 \text{ mV}.$$

Therefore, at a membrane potential of –76 mV, K⁺ ions have an equal tendency to flow either into or out of the axon. The concentrations of K⁺ in mammalian neurons and glial cells differ considerably from that in the squid giant axon. By substituting 3.1 mM for $[K^+]_o$ and 140 mM for $[K^+]_i$ in the Nernst equation, with T = 37°C, we obtain

$$E_K = 61.5 \log_{10}(3.1/140) = -102 \text{ mV}.$$

Movements of Ions Can Cause either Hyperpolarization or Depolarization

In mammalian cells, at membrane potentials positive to –102 mV, K⁺ ions tend to flow out of the cell.

BOX 6.1

NERNST EQUATION

The equilibrium potential is determined by (1) the concentration of the ion inside and outside the cell, (2) the temperature of the solution, (3) the valence of the ion, and (4) the amount of work required to separate a given quantity of charge. The equation that describes the equilibrium potential was formulated by a German physical chemist named Walter Nernst in 1888:

$$E_{ion} = RT/zF \cdot \ln\big([ion]_o/[ion]_i\big)$$

Here, E_{ion} is the membrane potential at which the ionic species is at equilibrium, R is the gas constant [8.315 J per Kelvin per mole (J K^{-1} mol^{-1})], T is the temperature in Kelvins ($T_{Kelvin} = 273.16 + T_{Celcius}$), F is Faraday's

constant [96,485 coulombs per mole (C mol^{-1})], z is the valence of the ion, and $[ion]_o$ and $[ion]_i$ are the concentrations of the ion outside and inside the cell, respectively. For a monovalent, positively charged ion (cation) at room temperature (20°C), substituting the appropriate numbers and converting natural log (ln) into log base 10 (log$_{10}$) result in

$$E_{ion} = 58.2 \log_{10}\big([ion]_o/[ion]_i\big);$$

at a body temperature of 37°C, the Nernst equation is

$$E_{ion} = 61.5 \log_{10}\big([ion]_o/[ion]_i\big).$$

David A. McCormick

Increasing the ability of K$^+$ ions to flow across the membrane, i.e., increasing the conductance of the membrane to K$^+$ (gK) causes the membrane potential to become more negative, or hyperpolarized, due to the exiting of positively charged ions from inside the cell (Fig. 6.4).

At membrane potentials negative to –102 mV, K$^+$ ions tend to flow into the cell; increasing the membrane conductance to K$^+$ causes the membrane potential to become more positive, or depolarized, due to the flow of positive charge into the cell. The membrane potential at which the net current "flips" direction is referred to as the reversal potential. If the channels conduct only one type of ion (e.g., K$^+$ ions), then the reversal potential and the Nernst equilibrium potential for that ion coincide (see Fig. 6.4A). Increasing the membrane conductance to K$^+$ ions while the membrane potential is at the equilibrium potential for K$^+$ (E_K) does not change the membrane potential because no net driving force causes K$^+$ ions to either exit or enter the cell. However, this increase in membrane conductance to K$^+$ decreases the ability of other species of ions to change the membrane potential because any deviation of the potential from E_K increases the drive for K$^+$ ions to either exit or enter the cell, thereby drawing the membrane potential back toward E_K (see Fig. 6.4B).

The exiting and entering of the cell by K$^+$ ions during generation of the membrane potential give rise to a curious problem. When K$^+$ ions leave the cell to generate a membrane potential, the concentration of K$^+$ changes both inside and outside the cell. Why does this change in concentration not alter the equilibrium

potential, thus changing the tendency for K$^+$ ions to flow down their concentration gradient? The reason is that the number of K$^+$ ions required to leave the cell to achieve the equilibrium potential is quite small. For example, if a cell were at 0 mV and the membrane suddenly became permeable to K$^+$ ions, only about 10^{-12} mol of K$^+$ ions per square centimeter of membrane would move from inside to outside the cell in bringing the membrane potential to the equilibrium potential for K$^+$. In a spherical cell of 25 μm diameter, this would amount to an average decrease in intracellular K$^+$ of only about 4 μM (e.g., from 140 to 139.996 mM). However, there are instances when significant changes in the concentrations of K$^+$ may occur, particularly during the generation of pronounced activity, such as that related to an epileptic seizure. During the occurrence of a tonic–clonic generalized (grand mal) seizure, large numbers of neurons discharge throughout the cerebral cortex in a synchronized manner. This synchronous discharge of large numbers of neurons significantly increases the extracellular K$^+$ concentration, by as much as a couple of millimoles, resulting in a commensurate positive shift in the equilibrium potential for K$^+$. This shift in the equilibrium potential can increase the excitability of affected neurons and neuronal processes and thus promote the spread of the seizure activity. Fortunately, the extracellular concentration of K$^+$ is tightly regulated and is kept at normal levels through uptake by glial cells, as well as by diffusion through the fluid of the extracellular space.

As is true for K$^+$ ions, each of the membrane-permeable species of ions possesses an equilibrium

A

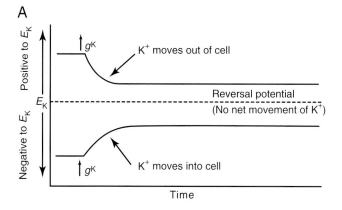

B

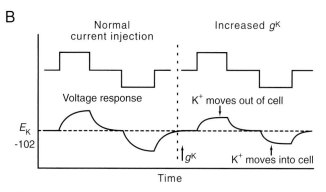

FIGURE 6.4 Increases in K⁺ conductance can result in hyperpolarization, depolarization, or no change in membrane potential. (A) Opening K⁺ channels increases the conductance of the membrane to K⁺, denoted gK. *If the membrane potential is positive to the equilibrium potential (also known as the reversal potential) for K⁺, then increasing gK will cause some K⁺ ions to leave the cell, and the cell will become hyperpolarized. If the membrane potential is negative to E_K when gK is increased, then K⁺ ions will enter the cell, therefore making the inside more positive (more depolarized). If the membrane potential is exactly E_K when gK is increased, then there will be no net movement of K⁺ ions. (B) Opening K⁺ channels when the membrane potential is at E_K does not change the membrane potential; however, it reduces the ability of other ionic currents to move the membrane potential away from E_K. For example, a comparison of the ability of the injection of two pulses of current, one depolarizing and one hyperpolarizing, to change the membrane potential before and after opening K⁺ channels reveals that increases in gK decrease the responses of the cell noticeably.

potential that depends on the concentration of that ion inside and outside the cell. Thus, equilibrium potentials may vary between different cell types, such as those found in animals adapted to live in salt water versus mammalian neurons. In mammalian neurons, the equilibrium potential is approximately 56 mV for Na⁺, approximately –76 mV for Cl⁻, and about 125 mV for Ca²⁺ (see and Fig. 6.2). Thus, increasing the membrane conductance to Na⁺ (gNa) through the opening of Na⁺ channels depolarizes the membrane potential toward 56 mV; increasing the membrane conductance to Cl⁻ brings the membrane potential closer to

–76 mV; and finally increasing the membrane conductance to Ca²⁺ depolarizes the cell toward 125 mV.

Na⁺, K⁺, and Cl⁻ Contribute to the Determination of the Resting Membrane Potential

If a membrane is permeable to only one ion and no electrogenic ionic pumps are operating (see next section), then the membrane potential is necessarily at the equilibrium potential for that ion. At rest, the plasma membrane of most cell types is not at the equilibrium potential for K⁺ ions, indicating that the membrane is also permeable to other types of ions. For example, the resting membrane of the squid giant axon is permeable to Cl⁻ and Na⁺, as well as K⁺, due to the presence of ionic channels that not only allow these ions to pass but also are open at the resting membrane potential. Because the membrane is permeable to K⁺, Cl⁻, and Na⁺, the resting potential of the squid giant axon is not equal to E_K, E_{Na}, or E_{Cl}, but is somewhere in between these three. A membrane permeable to more than one ion has a steady-state membrane potential whose value is between those of the equilibrium potentials for each of the permeant ions (Box 6.2).

Different Types of Neurons Have Different Resting Potentials

Intracellular recordings from neurons in the mammalian central nervous system (CNS) reveal that different types of neurons exhibit different resting membrane potentials. Indeed, some types of neurons do not even exhibit a true "resting" membrane potential; they spontaneously and continuously generate action potentials even in the total lack of synaptic input. In the visual system, intracellular recordings have shown that photoreceptor cells of the retina—the rods and cones—have a membrane potential of approximately –40 mV at rest and are hyperpolarized when activated by light. Cells in the dorsal lateral geniculate nucleus, which receive axonal input from the retina and project to the visual cortex, have a resting membrane potential of approximately –70 mV during sleep and –55 mV during waking, whereas pyramidal neurons of the visual cortex have a resting membrane potential of about –75 mV. Presumably, the resting membrane potentials of different cell types in the central and peripheral nervous system are highly regulated and are functionally important. For example, the depolarized membrane potential of photoreceptors presumably allows the membrane potential to move in both negative and positive directions

BOX 6.2

GOLDMAN–HODGKIN–KATZ EQUATION

An equation developed by Goldman and later used by Alan Hodgkin and Bernard Katz describes the steady-state membrane potential for a given set of ionic concentrations inside and outside the cell and the relative permeabilities of the membrane to each of those ions:

$$V_m = \frac{RT}{F} \cdot \ln\left[\frac{(p_K[K^+]_o + p_{Na}[Na^+]_o + p_{Cl}[Cl^-]_i)}{(p_K[K^+]_i + p_{Na}[Na^+]_i + p_{Cl}[Cl^-]_o)}\right].$$

The relative contribution of each ion is determined by its concentration differences across the membrane and the relative permeability (p_K, p_{Na}, p_{Cl}) of the membrane to each type of ion. If a membrane is permeable to only one ion, then the Goldman–Hodgkin–Katz equation reduces to the Nernst equation. In the squid giant axon, at resting membrane potential, the permeability ratios are

$$p_K : p_{Na} : p_{Cl} = 1.00 : 0.04 : 0.45.$$

The membrane of the squid giant axon, at rest, is most permeable to K^+ ions, less so to Cl^-, and least permeable to Na^+. (Chloride appears to contribute considerably less to the determination of the resting potential of mammalian neurons.) These results indicate that the resting membrane potential is determined by the resting permeability of the membrane to K^+, Na^+, and Cl^-. In theory, this resting membrane potential may be anywhere between E_K (e.g., –76 mV) and E_{Na} (55 mV). For the three ions at 20°C, the equation is

$$V_m = \frac{58.2 \log_{10}\{(1 \cdot 20 + 0.04 \cdot 440 + 0.45 \cdot 40)}{(1 \cdot 400 + 0.04 \cdot 50 + 0.45 \cdot 560)\}}$$

$$= -62 \text{ mV}.$$

This suggests that the squid giant axon should have a resting membrane potential of –62 mV. In fact, the resting membrane potential may be a few millivolts hyperpolarized to this value through the operation of the electrogenic Na^+–K^+ pump.

David A. McCormick

in response to changes in light intensity. The hyperpolarized membrane potential of thalamic neurons during sleep (–70 mV) dramatically decreases the flow of information from the sensory periphery to the cerebral cortex, presumably to allow the cortex to be relatively undisturbed during sleep, and the 20-mV membrane potential between the resting potential and the action potential threshold in cortical pyramidal cells may permit the subthreshold computation and integration of multiple neuronal inputs in single neurons (see Chapters 5 and 12).

Ionic Pumps Actively Maintain Ionic Gradients

Because the resting membrane potential of a neuron is not at the equilibrium potential for any particular ion, ions constantly flow down their concentration gradients. This flux becomes considerably larger with the generation of electrical and synaptic potentials because ionic channels are opened by these events. Although the absolute number of ions traversing the plasma membrane during each action potential or synaptic potential may be small in individual cells, the collective influence of a large neural network of cells, such as in the brain, and the presence of ion fluxes even at rest can substantially change the distribution of ions inside and outside neurons. Cells have solved this problem with the use of active transport of ions against their concentration gradients. The proteins that actively transport ions are referred to as ionic pumps, of which the Na^+-K^+ pump is perhaps the most thoroughly understood (Lauger, 1991). The Na^+–K^+ pump is stimulated by increases in the intracellular concentration of Na^+ and moves Na^+ out of the cell while moving K^+ into it, achieving this task through the hydrolysis of ATP (see Fig. 6.2). Three Na^+ ions are extruded for every two K^+ ions transported into the cell. Because of the unequal transport of ions, the operation of this pump generates a hyperpolarizing electrical potential and is said to be electrogenic. The Na^+–K^+ pump typically results in the membrane potential of the cell being a few millivolts more negative than it would be otherwise.

The Na^+–K^+ pump consists of two subunits, α and β, arranged in a tetramer $(\alpha\beta)_2$. The α subunit has a molecular mass of about 100 kDa and six hydrophobic regions capable of forming transmembrane helices. The β subunit is smaller (about 38 kDa) and has only one hydrophobic membrane-spanning region. The Na^+–K^+ pump is believed to operate through conformational changes that alternatively expose a Na^+-binding site to the interior of the cell (followed by the release of Na^+) and a K^+ binding site

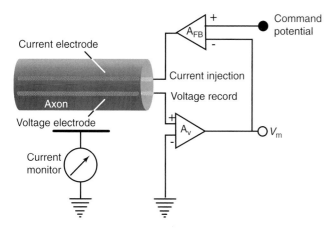

FIGURE 6.5 The voltage-clamp technique keeps the voltage across the membrane constant so that the amplitude and time course of ionic currents can be measured. In the two-electrode voltage-clamp technique, one electrode measures the voltage across the membrane while the other injects current into the cell to keep the voltage constant. The experimenter sets a voltage to which the axon or neuron is to be stepped (the command potential). Current is then injected into the cell in proportion to the difference between the present membrane potential and the command potential. This feedback cycle occurs continuously, thereby clamping the membrane potential to the command potential. By measuring the amount of current injected, the experimenter can determine the amplitude and time course of the ionic currents flowing across the membrane.

to the extracellular fluid (see Fig. 6.2). Such a conformation change may be due to the phosphorylation and dephosphorylation of the protein.

The membranes of neurons and glia contain multiple types of ionic pumps, used to maintain the proper distribution of each ionic species important for cellular signaling. Many of these pumps are operated by the Na^+ gradient across the cell, whereas others operate through a mechanism similar to that of the Na^+–K^+ pump (i.e., the hydrolysis of ATP). For example, the calcium concentration inside neurons is kept to very low levels (typically 50–100 nM) through the operation of both types of ionic pumps, as well as special intracellular Ca^{2+} buffering mechanisms. Ca^{2+} is extruded from neurons through both a Ca^{2+}, Mg^{2+}-ATPase and a Na^+–Ca^{2+} exchanger. The Na^+–Ca^{2+} exchanger is driven by the Na^+ gradient across the membrane and extrudes one Ca^{2+} ion for each Na^+ ion allowed to enter the cell.

The Cl^- concentration in neurons is actively maintained at a low level through operation of a chloride-bicarbonate exchanger, which brings in one ion of Na^+ and one ion of HCO_3^- for each ion of Cl^- extruded. Intracellular pH can also markedly affect neuronal excitability and is therefore tightly regulated, in part by a Na^+–H^+ exchanger that extrudes one proton for each Na^+ allowed to enter the cell.

Summary

The membrane potential is generated by the unequal distribution of ions, particularly K^+, Na^+, and Cl^-, across the plasma membrane. This unequal distribution of ions is maintained by ionic pumps and exchangers. K^+ ions are concentrated inside the neuron and tend to flow down their concentration gradient, leading to a hyperpolarization of the cell. At the equilibrium potential, the tendency of K^+ ions to flow out of the cell will be exactly offset by the tendency of K^+ ions to enter the cell due to the attraction of the negative potential inside the cell. The resting membrane is also permeable to Na^+ and Cl^- and therefore the resting membrane potential is approximately –75 to –40 mV, in other words, substantially positive to E_K.

ACTION POTENTIAL

An Increase in Na^+ and K^+ Conductance Generates Action Potentials

Hodgkin and Huxley not only recorded the action potential with an intracellular microelectrode (see Fig. 6.1), but also went on to perform a remarkable series of experiments that explained qualitatively and quantitatively the ionic mechanisms by which the action potential is generated (Hodgkin and Huxley, 1952a, b). As mentioned earlier, these investigators found that during the action potential, the membrane potential of the cell rapidly overshoots 0 mV and approaches the equilibrium potential for Na^+. After generation of the action potential, the membrane potential repolarizes and becomes more negative than before, generating an afterhyperpolarization. These changes in membrane potential during generation of the action potential were associated with a large increase in conductance of the plasma membrane, but to what does the membrane become conductive in order to generate the action potential? The prevailing hypothesis was that there was a nonselective increase in conductance causing the negative resting potential to increase toward 0 mV. Since publication of the experiments of E. Overton in 1902, the action potential had been known to depend on the presence of extracellular Na^+. Reducing the concentration of Na^+ in the artificial seawater bathing the axon resulted in a marked reduction in the amplitude of the action potential. On the basis of these and other data, Hodgkin and Katz proposed that the action potential is generated through a rapid increase in the conductance of the membrane to Na^+ ions. A quantitative

BOX 6.3

VOLTAGE-CLAMP TECHNIQUE

In the voltage-clamp technique, two independent electrodes are inserted into the squid giant axon: one for recording the voltage difference across the membrane and the other for intracellularly injecting the current (Fig. 6.5). These electrodes are then connected to a feedback circuit that compares the measured voltage across the membrane with the voltage desired by the experimenter. If these two values differ, then current is injected into the axon to compensate for this difference. This continuous feedback cycle, in which the voltage is measured and current is injected, effectively "clamps" the membrane at a particular voltage. If ionic channels were to open, then the resultant flow of ions into or out of the axon would be compensated for by the injection of positive or negative current into the axon through the current-injection electrode. The current injected through this electrode is necessarily equal to the current flowing through the ionic channels. It is this injected current that is measured by the experimenter. The benefits of the voltage-clamp technique are twofold. First, the current injected into the axon to keep the membrane potential "clamped" is necessarily equal to the current flowing through the ionic channels in the membrane, thereby giving a direct measurement of this current. Second, ionic currents are both voltage and time dependent; they become active at certain membrane potentials and do so at a particular rate. Keeping the voltage constant in the voltage clamp allows these two variables to be separated; the voltage dependence and the kinetics of the ionic currents flowing through the plasma membrane can be measured directly.

David A. McCormick

proof of this theory was lacking, however, because ionic currents could not be observed directly. Development of the voltage-clamp technique by Kenneth Cole at the Marine Biological Laboratory in Massachusetts resolved this problem and allowed quantitative measurement of the Na^+ and K^+ currents underlying the action potential (Cole, 1949; Box 6.3).

Hodgkin and Huxley (1952) used the voltage-clamp technique to investigate the mechanisms of generation of the action potential in the squid giant axon. Axons and neurons have a threshold for the initialization of an action potential of about –45 to –55 mV. Increasing the voltage from –60 to 0 mV produces a large, but transient, flow of positive charge into the cell (known as inward current). This transient inward current is followed by a sustained flow of positive charge out of the cell (the outward current). By voltage clamping the cell and substituting different ions inside or outside the axon or both, Hodgkin, Huxley, and colleagues demonstrated that the transient inward current is carried by Na^+ ions flowing into the cell and the sustained outward current is mediated by a sustained flux of K^+ ions moving out of the cell (Fig. 6.6) (Hodgkin and Huxley, 1952a, b; Hille, 1977).

Na^+ and K^+ currents (I_{Na} and I_K, respectively) can be blocked, allowing each current to be examined in isolation (see Fig. 6.6B). Tetrodotoxin (TTX), a powerful poison found in the puffer fish *Spheroides rubripes*, selectively blocks voltage-dependent Na^+ currents (the puffer fish remains a delicacy in Japan and must be prepared with the utmost care by the chef). Using TTX, one can selectively isolate I_K and examine its voltage dependence and time course (see Fig. 6.6B).

Another compound, tetraethylammonium (TEA), is a useful pharmacological tool for selectively blocking I_K (see Fig. 6.6B). The use of TEA to examine the voltage dependence and time course of the Na^+ current underlying action-potential generation (see Fig. 6.6B) reveals some fundamental differences between Na^+ and K^+ currents. First, the inward Na^+ current activates, or "turns on," much more rapidly than the K^+ current (giving rise to the name "delayed rectifier" for this K^+ current). Second, the Na^+ current is transient; it inactivates, even if the membrane potential is maintained at 0 mV (see Fig. 6.6A). In contrast, the outward K^+ current, once activated, remains "on" as long as the membrane potential is clamped to positive levels; i.e., the K^+ current does not inactivate, it is sustained. Remarkably, from one experiment, we see that the Na^+ current both activates and inactivates rapidly, whereas the K^+ current only activates slowly. These fundamental properties of the underlying Na^+ and K^+ channels allow the generation of action potentials.

Hodgkin and Huxley proposed that K^+ channels possess a voltage-sensitive "gate" that opens by depolarization and closes by the subsequent repolarization of the membrane potential. This process of "turning on" and "turning off" the K^+ current came to be known as activation and deactivation. The Na^+ current also exhibits voltage-dependent activation and deactivation (see Fig. 6.6), but the Na^+ channels also become inactive despite maintained depolarization. Thus, the Na^+

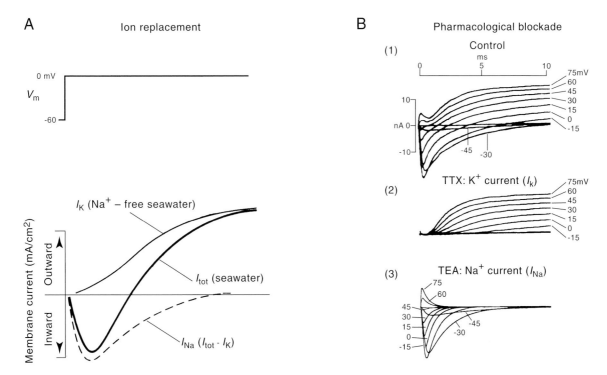

FIGURE 6.6 Voltage-clamp analysis reveals ionic currents underlying action potential generation. (A) Increasing the potential from –60 to 0 mV across the membrane of the squid giant axon activates an inward current followed by an outward current. If the Na^+ in seawater is replaced by choline (which does not pass through Na^+ channels), then increasing the membrane potential from –60 to 0 mV results in only the outward current, which corresponds to I_K. Subtracting I_K from the recording in normal seawater illustrates the amplitude–time course of the inward Na^+ current, I_{Na}. Note that I_K activates more slowly than I_{Na} and that I_{Na} inactivates with time. From Hodgkin and Huxley (1952) (B) These two ionic currents can also be isolated from one another through the use of pharmacological blockers. (1) Increasing the membrane potential from –45 to 75 mV in 15–mV steps reveals the amplitude–time course of inward Na^+ and outward K^+ currents. (2) After the block of I_{Na} with the poison tetrodotoxin (TTX), increasing the membrane potential to positive levels activates I_K only. (3) After the block of I_K with tetraethylammonium (TEA), increasing the membrane potential to positive levels activates I_{Na} only. From Hille (1977).

current not only activates and deactivates, but also exhibits a separate process known as inactivation, whereby the channels become blocked even though they are activated. Removal of this inactivation is achieved by removal of depolarization and is a process known as deinactivation. Thus, Na^+ channels possess two voltage–sensitive processes: activation–deactivation and inactivation-deinactivation. The kinetics of these two properties of Na^+ channels are different: inactivation takes place at a slower rate than activation.

The functional consequence of the two mechanisms is that Na^+ ions are allowed to flow across the membrane only when the current is activated but not inactivated. Accordingly, Na^+ ions do not flow at resting membrane potentials because the activation gate is closed (even though the inactivation gate is not). Upon depolarization, the activation gate opens, allowing Na^+ ions to flow into the cell. However, this depolarization also results in closure (at a slower rate) of the inactivation gate, which then blocks the flow of Na^+ ions. Upon

repolarization of the membrane potential, the activation gate once again closes and the inactivation gate once again opens, preparing the axon for generation of the next action potential (Fig. 6.7). Depolarization allows ionic current to flow by virtue of activation of the channel. The rush of Na^+ ions into the cell further depolarizes the membrane potential and more Na^+ channels become activated, forming a positive feedback loop that rapidly (within 100 ms or so) brings the membrane potential toward E_{Na}. However, the depolarization associated with generation of the action potential also inactivates Na^+ channels, and, as a larger and larger percentage of Na^+ channels become inactivated, the rush of Na^+ into the cell diminishes. This inactivation of Na^+ channels and the activation of K^+ channels result in the repolarization of the action potential. This repolarization deactivates the Na^+ channels. Then, the inactivation of the channel is slowly removed, and the channels are ready, once again, for the generation of another action potential (see Fig. 6.7).

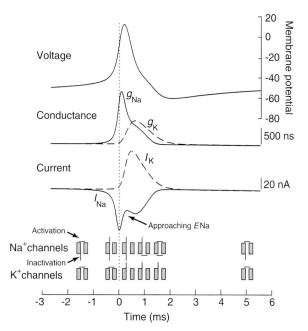

FIGURE 6.7 Generation of the action potential is associated with an increase in membrane Na^+ conductance and Na^+ current followed by an increase in K^+ conductance and K^+ current. Before action potential generation, Na^+ channels are neither activated nor inactivated (illustrated at the bottom of the figure). Activation of Na^+ channels allows Na^+ ions to enter the cell, depolarizing the membrane potential. This depolarization also activates K^+ channels. After activation and depolarization, the inactivation particle on the Na^+ channels closes and the membrane potential repolarizes. The persistence of the activation of K^+ channels (and other membrane properties) generates an afterhyperpolarization. During this period, the inactivation particle of the Na^+ channel is removed and the K^+ channels close.

By measuring the voltage sensitivity and kinetics of these two processes, activation–deactivation and inactivation–deinactivation of the Na^+ current, as well as the activation–deactivation of the delayed rectifier K^+ current, Hodgkin and Huxley generated a series of mathematical equations that quantitatively described the generation of the action potential (calculation of the propagation of a single action potential required an entire week of cranking a mechanical calculator). According to these early experimental and computational neuroscientists, the action potential is generated as follows. Depolarization of the membrane potential increases the probability of Na^+ channels being in the activated, but not yet inactivated, state. At a particular membrane potential, the resulting inflow of Na^+ ions tips the balance of the net ionic current from outward to inward (remember that depolarization will also increase K^+ and Cl^- currents by moving the membrane potential away from E_K and

E_{Cl}). At this membrane potential, known as the action potential threshold (typically about –55 mV), the movement of Na^+ ions into the cell depolarizes the axon and opens more Na^+ channels, causing yet more depolarization of the membrane; repetition of this process yields a rapid, positive feedback loop that brings the axon close to E_{Na}. However, even as more and more Na^+ channels are becoming activated, some of these channels are also inactivating and therefore no longer conducting Na^+ ions. In addition, the delayed rectifier K^+ channels are also opening, due to the depolarization of the membrane potential, and allowing positive charge to exit the cell. At some point, close to the peak of the action potential, the inward movement of Na^+ ions into the cell is exactly offset by the outward movement of K^+ ions out of the cell. After this point, the outward movement of K^+ ions dominates, and the membrane potential is repolarized, corresponding to the fall of the action potential. The persistence of the K^+ current for a few milliseconds following the action potential generates the afterhyperpolarization. During this afterhyperpolarization, which is lengthened by the membrane time constant, inactivation of the Na^+ channels is removed, preparing the axon for generation of the next action potential (see Fig. 6.7). The occurrence of an action potential is not associated with substantial changes in the intracellular or extracellular concentrations of Na^+ or K^+, as shown earlier for the generation of the resting membrane potential. For example, generation of a single action potential in a 25-μm-diameter hypothetical spherical cell should increase the intracellular concentration of Na^+ by only approximately 6 μM (from about 18 to 18.006 mM). Thus, the action potential is an electrical event generated by a change in the distribution of charge across the membrane and not by a marked change in the intracellular or extracellular concentration of Na^+ or K^+.

Refractory Periods Prevent "Reverberation"

The ability of depolarization to activate an action potential varies as a function of the time since the last generation of an action potential, due to the inactivation of Na^+ channels and the activation of K^+ channels. Immediately after the generation of an action potential, another action potential usually cannot be generated regardless of the amount of current injected into the axon. This period corresponds to the absolute refractory period and is largely mediated by the inactivation of Na^+ channels. The relative refractory period occurs during the action potential afterhyperpolarization and follows the absolute refractory period. The relative refractory period is characterized by a requirement for the increased injection of ionic current into the cell to generate another action potential and results from persistence of the outward K^+ current. The practical implication of refractory periods is that action potentials are not allowed to "reverberate" between the soma and the axon terminals.

The Speed of Action Potential Propagation Is Affected by Myelination

Axons may be either myelinated or unmyelinated. Invertebrate axons or small vertebrate axons are typically unmyelinated, whereas larger vertebrate axons are often myelinated. As described in Chapter 4, sensory and motor axons of the peripheral nervous system are myelinated by specialized cells (Schwann cells) that form a spiral wrapping of multiple layers of myelin around the axon (Fig. 6.8). Several Schwann cells wrap around an axon along its length; between the ends of successive Schwann cells are small gaps (nodes of Ranvier). In the central nervous system, a single oligodendrocyte, a special type of glial cell, typically ensheaths several axonal processes.

In unmyelinated axons, the Na^+ and K^+ channels taking part in action potential generation are distributed along the axon, and the action potential propagates along the length of the axon through local depolarization of each neighboring patch of membrane, causing that patch of membrane to also generate an action potential (see Fig. 6.8). In myelinated axons, however the Na^+ channels are concentrated at the nodes of Ranvier. The generation of an action potential at each node results in depolarization of the next node and subsequently generation of an action potential with an internode delay of only about 20 μs (see Chapter 5), referred to as saltatory conduction (from the Latin saltare, "to leap"). Growing evidence indicates that, between the nodes of Ranvier and underneath the myelin covering, K^+ channels may play a role in determining the resting membrane potential and repolarization of the action potential. A cause of some neurological disorders, such as multiple sclerosis and Guillain–Barre syndrome, is the

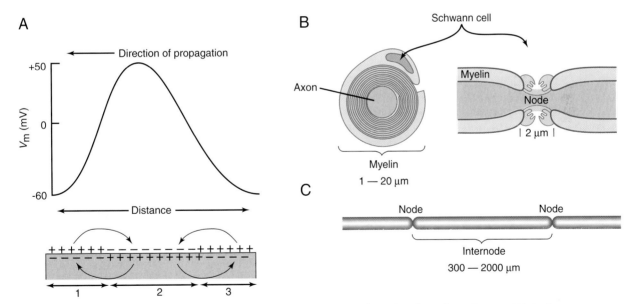

FIGURE 6.8   Propagation of the action potential in unmyelinated and myelinated axons. (A) Action potentials propagate in unmyelinated axons through the depolarization of adjacent regions of membrane. In the illustrated axon, region 2 is undergoing depolarization during the generation of the action potential, whereas region 3 has already generated the action potential and is now hyperpolarized. The action potential will propagate further by depolarizing region 1. (B) Vertebrate myelinated axons have a specialized Schwann cell that wraps around them in many spiral turns. The axon is exposed to the external medium at the nodes of Ranvier (Node). (C) Action potentials in myelinated fibers are regenerated at the nodes of Ranvier, where there is a high density of Na^+ channels. Action potentials are induced at each node through the depolarizing influence of the generation of an action potential at an adjacent node, thereby increasing conduction velocity.

demyelination of axons, resulting in a block of conduction of the action potentials.

Ion Channels Are Membrane-Spanning Proteins with Water-Filled Pores

The generation of ionic currents useful for the propagation of action potentials requires the movement of significant numbers of ions across the membrane in a relatively short time. The rate of ionic flow during the generation of an action potential is far too high to be achieved by an active transport mechanism and results instead from the opening of ion channels. Although the existence of ionic channels in the membrane has been postulated for decades, their properties and structure have only recently become known in detail. The powerful combination of electrophysiological and molecular techniques has enhanced our knowledge of the structure–function relations of ionic channels greatly (Box 6.4).

Various neural toxins were particularly useful in the initial isolation of ionic channels. For example, three subunits (α, $\beta1$, $\beta2$) of the voltage-dependent Na^+ channel were isolated with the use of a derivative of a scorpion toxin. The α subunit of the Na^+ channel is a large glycoprotein with a molecular mass of 270 kDa, whereas the $\beta1$ and $\beta2$ subunits are smaller polypeptides of molecular masses 39 and 37 kDa, respectively (Fig. 6.9). The α subunit, of which there are at least nine different isoforms, is the building block of the water-filled pore of the ionic channel, whereas the β subunits have some other role, such as in the regulation or structure of the native channel (Catterall, 2000a).

The α subunit of the Na^+ channel contains four internal repetitions (see Fig. 6.9B). Hydrophobicity analysis of these four components reveals that each contains six hydrophobic domains that may span the membrane as an α-helix. Of these six membrane–spanning components, the fourth (S4) has been pro-

---

BOX 6.4

ION CHANNELS AND DISEASE

Cells cannot survive without functional ion channels. It is therefore not surprising that an ever-increasing number of diseases have been found to be associated with defective ion channel function. There are a number of different mechanisms by which this may occur.

1. Mutations in the coding region of ion channel genes may lead to gain or loss of channel function, either of which may have deleterious consequences. For example, mutations producing enhanced activity of the epithelial Na^+ channel are responsible for Liddle's syndrome, an inherited form of hypertension, whereas other mutations in the same protein that cause reduced channel activity give rise to hypotension. The most common inherited disease in Caucasians is also an ion channel mutation. This disease is cystic fibrosis (CF), which results from mutations in the epithelial chloride channel, known as CFTR. The most common mutation, deletion of a phenylalanine at position 508, results in defective processing of the protein and prevents it from reaching the surface membrane. CFTR regulates chloride fluxes across epithelial cell membranes, and this loss of CFTR activity leads to reduced fluid secretion in the lung, resulting in potentially fatal lung infections.

2. Mutations in the promoter region of the gene may cause under- or overexpression of a given ion channel.

3. Other diseases result from defective regulation of channel activity by cellular constituents or extracellular ligands. This defective regulation may be caused by mutations in the genes encoding the regulatory molecules themselves or defects in the pathways leading to their production. Some forms of maturity-onset diabetes of the young (MODY) may be attributed to such a mechanism. ATP-sensitive potassium (K-ATP) channels play a key role in the glucose-induced insulin secretion from pancreatic β cells, and their defective regulation is responsible for one form of MODY.

4. Autoantibodies to channel proteins may cause disease by downregulating channel function—often by causing internalization of the channel protein itself. Well-known examples are myasthenia gravis, which results from antibodies to skeletal muscle acetylcholine channels, and Lambert–Eaton myasthenic syndrome, in which patients produce antibodies against presynaptic Ca^{2+} channels.

5. Finally, a number of ion channels are secreted by cells as toxic agents. They insert into the membrane of the target cell and form large nonselective pores, leading to cell lysis and death. The hemolytic toxin produced by the bacterium *Staphylococcus aureus* and the toxin secreted by the protozoan *Entamoeba histolytica*, which causes amebic dysentery, are examples.

BOX 6.4 *(cont'd)*

Natural mutations in ion channels have been invaluable for studying the relationship between channel structure and function. In many cases, genetic analysis of a disease has led to the cloning of the relevant ion channel. The first K$^+$ channel to be identified (Shaker), for example, came from the cloning of the gene that caused Drosophila to shake when exposed to ether. Likewise, the gene encoding the primary subunit of a cardiac potassium channel (KCNQ1) was identified by positional cloning in families carrying mutations that caused a cardiac disorder known as long QT syndrome (see later). Conversely, the large number of studies on the relationship between Na$^+$ channel structure and function has greatly assisted our understanding of how mutations in Na$^+$ channels produce their clinical phenotypes.

Many diseases are genetically heterogeneous, and the same clinical phenotype may be caused by mutations in different genes. Long QT syndrome is a relatively rare inherited cardiac disorder that causes abrupt loss of consciousness, seizures, and sudden death from ventricular arrhythmia in young people. Mutations in five different genes, two types of cardiac muscle K$^+$ channels (HERG, KCNQ1, KCNE1, KCNE2) and the cardiac muscle sodium channel (SCN1A), give rise to long QT syndrome. The disorder is characterized by a long QT interval in the electrocardiogram, which reflects the delayed repolarization of the cardiac action potential. As might therefore be expected, mutations in the cardiac Na$^+$ channel gene that cause long QT syndrome enhance the Na$^+$ current (by reducing Na$^+$ channel inactivation), whereas those in potassium channel genes cause loss of function and reduce the K$^+$ current.

Mutations in many different types of ion channels have been shown to cause human diseases. In addition to the examples listed earlier, mutations in water channels cause nephrogenic diabetes insipidus; mutations in gap junction channels cause Charcot–Marie–Tooth disease (a form of peripheral neuropathy) and hereditary deafness; mutations in the skeletal muscle Na$^+$ channel cause a range of disorders known as periodic paralyses; mutations in intracellular Ca^{2+}-release channels cause malignant hyperthermia (a disease in which inhalation anesthetics trigger a potentially fatal rise in body temperature); and mutations in neuronal voltage-gated Ca^{2+} channels cause migraine and episodic ataxia. The list increases daily. As is the case with all single gene disorders, the frequency of these diseases in the general population is very low. However, the insight they have provided into the relationship between ion channel structure and function, and into the physiological role of the different ion channels, has been invaluable. As William Harvey said in 1657 "nor is there any better way to advance the proper practice of medicine than to give our minds to the discovery of the usual form of nature, by careful investigation of the rarer forms of disease."

Frances M. Ashcroft

posed to be critical to the voltage sensitivity of the Na$^+$ channels. Voltage-sensitive gating of Na$^+$ channels is accomplished by the redistribution of ionic charge ("gating charge") in the channel. Positive charges in the S4 region may act as voltage sensors such that an increase in the positivity of the inside of the cell results in a conformational change of the ionic channel. In support of this hypothesis, site-directed mutagenesis of the S4 region of the Na$^+$ channel to reduce the positive charge of this portion of the pore also reduces the voltage sensitivity of activation of the ionic channel.

The mechanisms of inactivation of ionic channels have been analyzed with a combination of molecular and electrophysiological techniques. The most convincing hypothesis is that inactivation is achieved by a block of the inner mouth of the aqueous pore. Ionic channels are inactivated without detectable movement of ionic current through the membrane; thus inactivation is probably not directly gated by changes in the membrane potential alone. Rather, inactivation is triggered or facilitated as a secondary consequence of activation. Site-directed mutagenesis or the use of antibodies has shown that the part of the molecule between regions III and IV may be allowed to move to block the cytoplasmic side of the ionic pore after the conformational change associated with activation.

Neurons of the Central Nervous System Exhibit a Wide Variety of Electrophysiological Properties

The first intracellular recordings of action potentials in mammalian neurons by Sir John Eccles and colleagues revealed a remarkable similarity to those of the squid giant axon and gave rise to the assumption that the electrophysiology of neurons in the CNS was really rather simple: when synaptic potentials

A

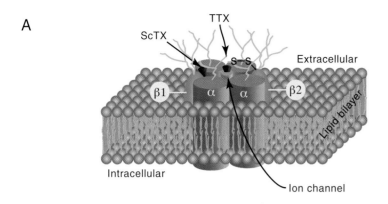

B

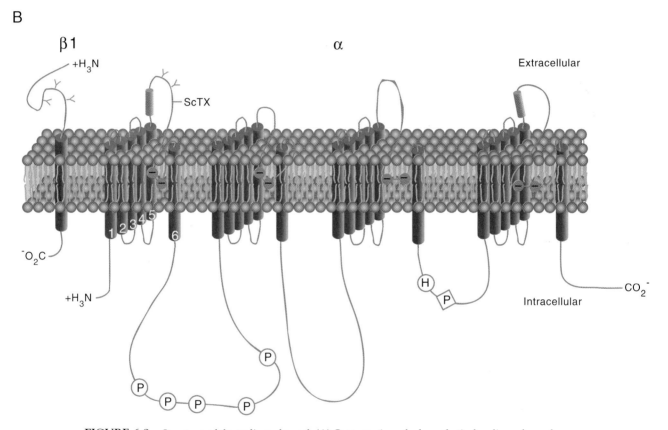

FIGURE 6.9   Structure of the sodium channel. (A) Cross section of a hypothetical sodium channel consisting of a single transmembrane α subunit in association with a $\beta1$ subunit and a $\beta2$ subunit. The α subunit has receptor sites for α-scorpion toxins (ScTX) and tetrodotoxin (TTX). (B) Primary structures of α and $\beta1$ subunits of sodium channel illustrated as transmembrane-folding diagrams. Cylinders represent probable transmembrane α-helices.

brought the membrane potential positive to action potential threshold, action potentials were produced through an increase in Na^+ conductance followed by an increase in K^+ conductance, as in the squid giant axon. The assumption, therefore, was that the complicated patterns of activity generated by the brain during the resting, sleeping, or active states were brought about as an interaction of the very large numbers of neurons present in the mammalian CNS. However, intracellular recordings of invertebrate neurons revealed that different cell types exhibit a wide variety of different electrophysiological behaviors, indicating that neurons may be significantly more complicated than the squid giant axon. Elucidation of the basic electrophysiology and synaptic physiology of different types of neurons and neuronal

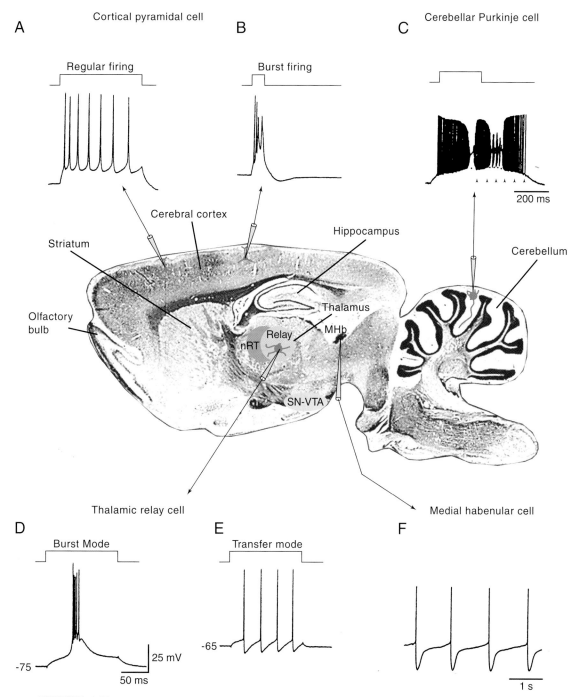

FIGURE 6.10 Neurons in the mammalian brain exhibit widely varying electrophysiological properties. (A) Intracellular injection of a depolarizing current pulse in a cortical pyramidal cell results in a train of action potentials that slow down in frequency. This pattern of activity is known as "regular firing." (B) Some cortical cells generated bursts of three or more action potentials, even when depolarized only for a short period of time. (C) Cerebellar Purkinje cells generate high-frequency trains of action potentials in their cell bodies that are disrupted by the generation of Ca^{2+} spikes in their dendrites. These cells can also generate "plateau potentials" from the persistent activation of Na^+ conductances (arrowheads). Thalamic relay cells may generate action potentials either as bursts (D) or as tonic trains of action potentials (E) due to the presence of a large low-threshold Ca^{2+} current. (F) Medial habenular cells generate action potentials at a steady and slow rate in a "pacemaker" fashion.

pathways within the mammalian CNS was facilitated by the *in vitro* slice technique, in which thin (~0.5 mm) slices of brain can be maintained for several hours. Intracellular recordings from identified cells revealed that neurons of the mammalian nervous system, such as those of invertebrate networks, can generate complex patterns of action potentials entirely through intrinsic ionic mechanisms and without synaptic interaction with other cell types. For example, Rodolfo Llinás and colleagues discovered that Purkinje cells of the cerebellum can generate high-frequency trains (>200 Hz) of Na$^+$- and K$^+$-mediated action potentials interrupted by Ca^{2+} spikes in the dendrites, whereas a major afferent to these neurons, the inferior olivary cell, can generate rhythmic sequences of broad action potentials only at low frequencies (<15 Hz) through an interaction between various Ca^{2+}, Na$^+$, and K$^+$ conductances (Fig. 6.10). These *in vitro* recordings confirmed a major finding obtained with earlier intracellular recordings *in vivo*: each morphologically distinct class of neuron in the brain exhibits distinct electrophysiological features. Just as cortical pyramidal cells are morphologically distinct from cerebellar Purkinje cells, which are distinct from thalamic relay cells, the electrophysiological properties of each of these different cell types are also markedly distinct (Llinás, 1988).

Although no uniform classification scheme has been formulated in which all the different types of neurons of the brain can be classified, a few characteristic patterns of activity seem to recur. The first general class of action potential generation is characterized by those cells that generate trains of action potentials one spike at a time. The more prolonged the depolarization of these cells, the more prolonged their discharge. The more intensely these cells are depolarized, the higher the frequency of action potential generation. This type of relatively linear behavior is typical for brain stem and spinal cord motor neurons functioning in muscle contraction. A modification of this basic pattern of "regular firing" is characterized by the generation of trains of action potentials that exhibit a marked tendency to slow down in frequency with time, a process known as spike frequency adaptation. Examples of cells that discharge in this manner are cortical and hippocampal pyramidal cells.

In addition to these regular firing cells, many neurons in the central nervous system exhibit the intrinsic propensity to generate rhythmic bursts of action potentials (see Fig. 6.10). Examples of such neurons are thalamic relay neurons, inferior olivary neurons, and some types of cortical and hippocampal pyramidal cells. In these cells, clusters of action potentials can occur together when the membrane is brought above the firing threshold. These clusters of action potentials are typically generated through the activation of specialized Ca^{2+} currents that, through their slower kinetics, allow the membrane potential to be depolarized for a sufficient period to result in the generation of a burst of regular, Na$^+$- and K$^+$-dependent action potentials (discussed in the next section).

Yet another general category of neurons in the brain comprises cells that generate relatively short duration (<1 ms) action potentials and can discharge at relatively high frequencies (>300 Hz). Such electrophysiological properties are often found in neurons that release the inhibitory amino acid γ-aminobutyric acid (see Fig. 6.10) and some types of interneurons in the cerebral cortex, thalamus, and hippocampus. Finally, the last general category of neurons consists of those that spontaneously generate action potentials at relatively slow frequencies (e.g., 1–10 Hz). This type of electrophysiological behavior is often associated with neurons that release neuromodulatory transmitters, such as acetylcholine, norepinephrine, serotonin, and histamine. Neurons that release these neuromodulatory substances often innervate wide regions of the brain and appear to set the "state" of the different neural networks of the CNS in a manner similar to the modulation of the different organs of the body by the sympathetic and parasympathetic nervous systems.

Each of these unique intrinsic patterns of activity in the nervous system is due to the presence of a distinct mixture and distribution of different ionic currents in the cells. As in classical studies of the squid

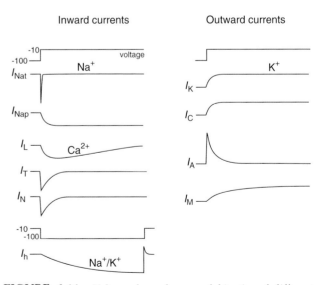

FIGURE 6.11 Voltage dependence and kinetics of different ionic currents in the mammalian brain. Depolarization of the membrane potential from −100 to −10 mV results in the activation of currents entering or leaving neurons.

giant axon, these different ionic currents have been characterized, at least in part, with voltage-clamp and pharmacological techniques, and the basic electrophysiological properties have been replicated with computational simulations (see Figs. 6.7 and 6.12).

Neurons Have Multiple Active Conductances

The search for the electrophysiological basis of the varying intrinsic properties of different types of neurons of vertebrates and invertebrates revealed a wide variety of ionic currents. Each type of ionic current is characterized by several features: (1) the type of ions conducted by the underlying ionic channels (e.g., Na^+, K^+, Ca^{2+}, Cl^-, or mixed cations), (2) their voltage and time dependence, and (3) their sensitivity to second messengers. In vertebrate neurons, two distinct Na^+ currents have been identified and six distinct Ca^{2+} currents and more than seven distinct K^+ currents are known (Fig. 6.11). This is a minimal number, as these currents are formed from a much greater pool of channel subunits. The following sections briefly review these classes of ionic currents and their ionic channels, relating them to the different patterns of behavior mentioned earlier for neurons in the mammalian CNS.

Na⁺ Currents are Both Transient and Persistent

Depolarization of many different types of vertebrate neurons results not only in the activation of the rapidly activating and inactivating Na^+ current (I_{Nat}) underlying action potential generation, but also in the rapid activation of a Na^+ current that does not inactivate and is therefore known as the "persistent" Na^+ current (I_{Nap}). The threshold for activation of the persistent Na^+ current is typically about -65 mV, i.e., below the threshold for the generation of action potentials. This property gives this current the interesting ability to enhance or facilitate the response of the neuron to depolarizing, yet subthreshold, inputs. For example, synaptic events that depolarize the cell will activate I_{Nap}, resulting in an extra influx of positive charge and therefore a larger depolarization than otherwise would occur. Likewise, hyperpolarizations may result in deactivation of I_{Nap}, again resulting in larger hyperpolarizations than would otherwise occur. In this manner, the persistent Na^+ current may play an important regulatory function in the control of the functional responsiveness of the neuron to synaptic inputs and may contribute to the dynamic coupling of the dendrites to the soma.

Persistent activation of I_{Nap} may also contribute to another electrophysiological feature of neurons: the generation of plateau potentials. A plateau potential refers to the ability of many different types of neurons to generate, through intrinsic ionic mechanisms, a prolonged (from tens of milliseconds to seconds) depolarization and action potential discharge in response to a short-lasting depolarization (see Fig. 6.10C). One can wonder whether such plateau potentials contribute to persistent firing in neurons during the performance of visual memory tasks, as has been found in some types of neurons in the frontal neocortex and superior colliculus of behaving primates.

K⁺ Currents Vary in Their Voltage Sensitivity and Kinetics

Potassium currents that contribute to the electrophysiological properties of neurons are numerous and exhibit a wide range of voltage-dependent and kinetic properties (reviewed in Chandy and Gutman, 1995). Perhaps the simplest K^+ current is that characterized by Hodgkin and Huxley: this K^+ current, I_K, activates rapidly on depolarization and does not inactivate (see Fig. 6.11). Other K^+ currents activate with depolarization but also inactivate with time. For example, the rapid activation and inactivation of I_A give this current a transient appearance (see Fig. 6.11), and I_A is believed to be important in controlling the rate of action potential generation, particularly at low frequencies (Fig. 6.12). Like the Na^+ channel, I_A channels are inactivated by the plugging of the inner mouth of the pore through movement of an inactivation particle.

Another broad class of K^+ channels consists of those that are sensitive to changes in the intracellular concentration of Ca^{2+}. These K^+ currents are collectively referred to as I_{KCa} (see Fig. 6.11). Still other K^+ channels are not only activated by voltage, but are also modulated by the activation of various modulatory neurotransmitter receptors (e.g., I_M; see Fig. 6.11). Between these classic examples of K^+ currents are a variety of other types that have not been fully characterized, including K^+ currents that vary from one another in their voltage sensitivity, kinetics, and response to various second messengers.

Molecular biological studies of voltage-sensitive K^+ channels, first done in Drosophila and later in mammals, have revealed the presence of a large number of genes that generate K^+ channels. They consist of four distinct subfamilies: Kv1, Kv2, Kv3, and Kv4 (reviewed in Chandy and Gutman, 1991). These genes generate a wide variety of different K^+ channels, not only due to the large number of genes

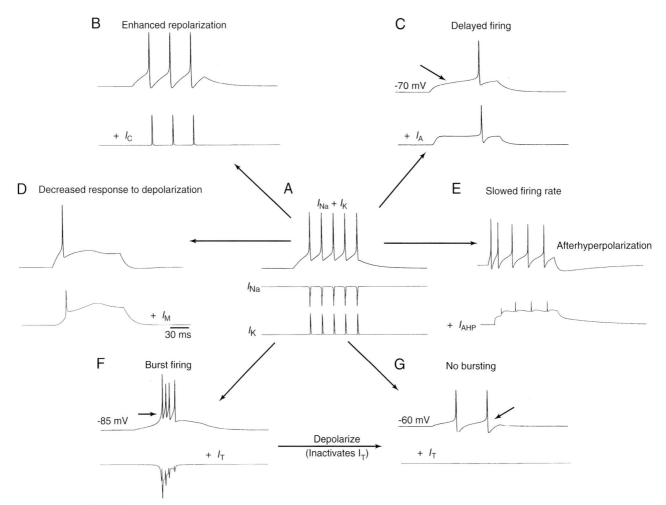

FIGURE 6.12   Simulation of the effects of the addition of various ionic currents to the pattern of activity generated by neurons in the mammalian CNS. (A) The repetitive impulse response of the classical Hodgkin–Huxley model (voltage recordings above, current traces below). With only I_{Na} and I_K, the neuron generates a train of five action potentials in response to depolarization. Addition of I_C (B) enhances action potential repolarization. Addition of I_A (C) delays the onset of action potential generation. Addition of I_M (D) decreases the ability of the cell to generate a train of action potentials. Addition of I_{AHP} (E) slows the firing rate and generates a slow afterhyperpolarization. Finally, addition of the transient Ca^{2+} current I_T results in two states of action potential firing: (F) burst firing at –85 mV and (G) tonic firing at –60 mV. From Huguenard and McCormick (1994).

involved, but also due to alternative RNA splicing, gene duplication, and other posttranslational mechanisms. Functional expression of different K^+ channels reveals remarkable variation in the rate of inactivation, such that some are rapidly inactivating (A current like), whereas others inactivate more slowly and, finally, some K^+ channels do not inactivate, such as I_K. One of the largest subfamilies of K^+ channels are those that give rise to the resting membrane potential, so-called "leak channels." Interestingly, these channels appear to be opened by gaseous anesthetics, indicating that hyperpolarization of central neurons is a major component of general anesthesia. It is now clear that each type of neuron in the nervous system contains a unique set of functional voltage-sensitive

K^+ channels, selected, modified, and placed in particular spatial locations in the cell in a manner that facilitates the unique role of that cell type in neuronal processing.

An additional current that also regulates the responsiveness of neurons to depolarizing inputs is the voltage-sensitive K^+ current known as the M current (Figs. 6.11 and 6.12D). By investigating the ionic mechanisms by which the release of acetylcholine from preganglionic neurons in the brain results in prolonged changes in the excitability of neurons of the sympathetic ganglia, Brown and Adams (1980) discovered a unique K^+ current that slowly (over tens of milliseconds) turns on with depolarization of the neuron (see Fig. 6.12D). The slow activation of this K+ current results in a decrease in the responsiveness of the cell to depolarization, and therefore regulates how the cell responds to excitation. This K+ current, like I_{AHP}, is reduced by the activation of a wide variety of receptors, including muscarinic receptors, for which it is named. Reduction of I_M results in a marked increase in responsiveness of the affected cell to depolarizing inputs and again may contribute to the mechanisms by which neuromodulatory systems control the state of activity in cortical and hippocampal networks (reviewed in McCormick, 1992).

Ca²⁺ Currents Control Electrophysiological Properties and Ca²⁺-Dependent Second-Messenger Systems

Ionic channels that conduct Ca²⁺ are present in all neurons. These channels are special in that they serve two important functions. First, Ca²⁺ channels are present throughout the different parts of the neuron (dendrites, soma, synaptic terminals) and contribute greatly to the electrophysiological properties of these processes. Second, Ca²⁺ channels are unique in that Ca²⁺ is an important second messenger in neurons, and entry of Ca²⁺ into the cell can affect numerous physiological functions, including neurotransmitter release, synaptic plasticity, neurite outgrowth during development, and even gene expression. On the bases of their voltage sensitivity, their kinetics of activation and inactivation, and their ability to be blocked by various pharmacological agents, Ca²⁺ currents can be separated into at least six separate categories, three of which are I_T ("transient"), I_L ("long lasting"), and I_N ("neither"), illustrated in Fig. 6.11A. A fourth, I_P, is found in Purkinje cells of the cerebellum, as well as in many different cell types of the CNS. These Ca²⁺ channels are formed from at least 10 different α subunits as well as a variety of β and γ subunits, indicating that there an even greater number of Ca²⁺ currents are yet to be characterized.

Neurons Possess Multiple Subtypes of High-Threshold Ca²⁺ Currents

High voltage-activated Ca²⁺ channels are activated at membrane potentials positive to approximately –40 mV and include the currents I_L, I_N, and I_P. L-type calcium currents exhibit a high threshold for activation (about –10 mV) and give rise to rather persistent, or long-lasting, ionic currents (see Fig. 6.11A). Dihydropyridines, Ca²⁺ channel antagonists, are clinically useful for their effects on the heart and vascular smooth muscle (e.g., for the treatment of arrhythmias,

angina, and migraine headaches) and selectively block L-type Ca²⁺ channels. In contrast with I_L, I_N is not blocked by dihydropyridines: it is blocked selectively by a toxin found in Pacific cone shells (ω-conotoxin-GVIA). N-type Ca²⁺ channels have a threshold for activation of about –20 mV, inactivate with maintained depolarization, and are modulated by a variety of neurotransmitters. In some cell types, I_N has a role in the Ca²⁺-dependent release of neurotransmitters at presynaptic terminals. The P-type calcium channel is distinct from N and L types in that it is not blocked by either dihydropyridines or ω-conotoxin-GVIA but is blocked by a toxin (ω-agatoxin-IVA) present in the venom of the Funnel web spider. This type of calcium channel activates at relatively high thresholds and does not inactivate. Prevalent in Purkinje cells, as well as other cell types, as mentioned earlier, the P-type Ca²⁺ channel participates in the generation of dendritic Ca²⁺ spikes, which can strongly modulate the firing pattern of the neuron in which it resides (see Fig. 6.10C; Llinás, 1988).

Collectively, high threshold-activated Ca²⁺ channels contribute to the generation of action potentials in mammalian neurons. The activation of Ca²⁺ currents adds somewhat to the depolarizing part of the action potential, but, more importantly, these channels allow Ca²⁺ to enter the cell, which has the secondary consequence of activation of various Ca²⁺-activated K+ currents and protein kinases (see Chapter 10). As mentioned earlier, activation of these K+ currents modifies the pattern of action potentials generated in the cell (see Figs. 6.10 and 6.12).

High-threshold Ca²⁺ channels are similar to the Na+ channel in that they are composed of a central α1 subunit that forms the aqueous pore and several regulatory or auxiliary subunits. As in the Na+ channel, the primary structure of the α1 subunit of the Ca²⁺ channel consists of four homologous domains (I–IV), each containing six regions (S1–S6) that may generate transmembrane α-helices. Genes for at least 10 different Ca²⁺ channel α subunits have been cloned and are separated into three subfamilies (Cav1, Cav2, and Cav3). The properties of the products of these genes indicate that I_L is likely to correspond to the Cav1 subfamily, whereas I_N corresponds to Cav2.2 and I_T is formed from the Cav3 subfamily (see Catterall, 2000b).

Low-Threshold Ca²⁺ Currents Generate Bursts of Action Potentials

Low-threshold Ca²⁺ currents (see Fig. 6.11A) often take part in the generation of rhythmic bursts of action potentials (see Figs. 6.10 and 6.12). The low-threshold Ca^{2+} current is characterized by a threshold for activation of about −65 mV, which is below the threshold for generation of typical Na^+-K^+-dependent action potentials (−55 mV). This current inactivates with maintained depolarization. Because of these properties, the role of low-threshold Ca^{2+} currents differs markedly from that of the high-threshold Ca^{2+} currents. Through activation and inactivation of the low-threshold Ca^{2+} current, neurons can generate slow (about 100 ms) Ca^{2+} spikes, which can result, due to their prolonged duration, in generation of a high-frequency "burst" of short-duration Na^+-K^+ action potentials (see Fig. 6.10 and Box 6.5).

In the mammalian brain, this pattern is especially well exemplified by the activity of thalamic relay neurons; in the visual system, these neurons receive direct input from the retina and transmit this information to the visual cortex. During periods of slow wave sleep, the membrane potential of these relay neurons is relatively hyperpolarized, resulting in the removal

---

BOX 6.5

JELLYFISH–WHAT A NERVE!

An insight into how whole animal behavior depends on the properties and distribution of ion channels within nerves axons comes from research on the jellyfish *Aglantha digitale*. Feeding and locomotion in *Aglantha* are determined by activity in 14 simple nerve circuits. The jellyfish can swim slowly when feeding or quickly if escaping from predators just through contractions of a single muscle sheet coupled to this simply organized nervous system.

The reason *Aglantha* can do so much with so little is that its motor axons can develop two entirely different propagating action potentials (Mackie and Meech, 1985). Each "giant" motor nerve axon not only has voltage-dependent sodium channels and three types of potassium channel, but also crucial T-type calcium channels. These T-type channels contribute to a truncated calcium spike that propagates along the motor axon without gaining amplitude or decrementing in the way that electrotonic potentials do. The motor axon makes direct synaptic contact with the muscle epithelium that makes up the bell of the jellyfish and so the propagating calcium spike induces weak contractions responsible for propulsion during the regular slow swimming the animal performs when feeding.

Aglantha lives in the colder waters of the world at a depth of about 100 m. Studied in their natural habitat by Claudia Mills and George Mackie, they are seen to avoid predators by generating an all-together stronger form of swimming. In the laboratory, this "escape" swimming can be reproduced by stimulating vibration-sensitive receptors at the base of the bell of the animal. The stronger synaptic depolarization that this stimulus induces in each of the eight giant motor axons drives its membrane potential beyond the peak of the calcium spike and induces a full-sized sodium action potential. Because the sodium spike propagates more rapidly than the slow swim calcium spike, there is a coordinated contraction of the body wall that drives the animal forward.

Sodium and calcium spikes like those seen in *Aglantha* have been recorded from a variety of sites in the mammalian CNS (Llinás, 1998). However, unlike in *Aglantha*, the peak of the calcium spike usually exceeds the threshold of the sodium spike and the two impulses fuse to form a single complex signal. Patch-clamp analysis of *Aglantha* axons has revealed a family of potassium channels that are responsible for setting thresholds and repolarizing each of the two different impulses. Each potassium channel has an identical unitary conductance and appears to be organized in a mosaic fashion over the suface of the axon. Sodium and T-type calcium channels are clustered together into well-defined "hot spots". The significance of the clustering is not known, but inserted channels would age together and, if retained in clusters, could be eliminated together.

Robert W. Meech

References

Llinás, R. R. (1988). The intrinsic electrophysiological properties of mammalian neurons: Insights into central nervous system function. *Science* 242, 1654–1664.

Mackie, G. O., and Meech, R. W. (1985). Seperate sodium and calcium spikes in the same axon. *Nature* **313**, 791–793.

of inactivation (deinactivation) of the low-threshold Ca^{2+} current. This deinactivation allows these cells to spontaneously generate low-threshold Ca^{2+} spikes and bursts of from two to five action potentials (Fig. 6.13). The large number of thalamic relay cells bursting during sleep in part gives rise to the spontaneous synchronized activity that early investigators were so surprised to find during recordings from the brains of sleeping animals. It has even proved possible to maintain one of the sleep-related brain rhythms (spindle waves) intact in slices of thalamic tissue maintained *in vitro*, due the generation of this rhythm by the interaction of a local network of thalamic cells and their electrophysiological properties.

The transition to waking or the period of sleep when dreams are prevalent (rapid eye movement sleep) is associated with a maintained depolarization of thalamic relay cells to membrane potentials ranging from about –60 to –55 mV. The low-threshold Ca^{2+} current is inactivated and therefore the burst discharges are abolished. In this way, the properties of a single ionic current (I_T) help explain in part the remarkable changes in brain activity taking place in the transition from sleep to waking (Fig. 6.13).

Hyperpolarization-Activated Ionic Currents Are Involved in Rhythmic Activity

In most types of neurons, hyperpolarization negative to approximately –60 mV activates an ionic current, known as I_h, that conducts both Na^+ and K^+ ions (see Fig. 6.11). This current typically has very slow kinetics, turning on with a time constant on the order of tens of milliseconds to seconds. Because the channels underlying this current allow the passage of both Na^+ and K^+ ions, the reversal potential of I_h is typically about –35 mV—between E_{Na} and E_K. Because this current is activated by hyperpolarization below approximately –60 mV, it is typically dominated by the inward movement of Na^+ ions and is therefore depolarizing. For what purpose could neurons use a depolarizing current that activates when the cell is hyperpolarized? A clue comes from cardiac cells in which this current, known as I_f for "funny," is

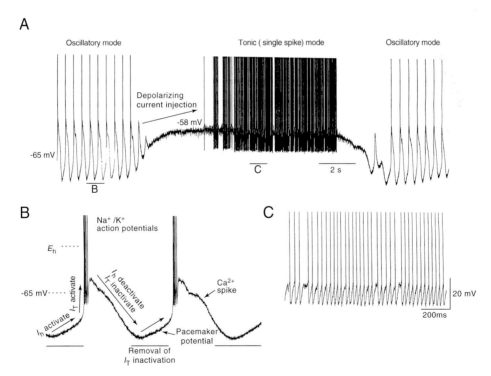

FIGURE 6.13   Two different patterns of activity generated in the same neuron, depending on membrane potential. (A) The thalamic neuron spontaneously generates rhythmic bursts of action potentials due to the interaction of the Ca^{2+} current I_T and the inward "pacemaker" current I_h. Depolarization of the neuron changes the firing mode from rhythmic burst firing to tonic action potential generation in which spikes are generated one at a time. Removal of this depolarization reinstates rhythmic burst firing. This transition from rhythmic burst firing to tonic activity is similar to that which occurs in the transition from sleep to waking. (B) Expansion of detail of rhythmic burst firing. (C) Expansion of detail of tonic firing. From McCormick and Pape (1990).

important for determining heart rate. Activation of I_f results in a slow depolarization of the membrane potential between adjacent cardiac action potentials. The more that I_f is activated, the faster the membrane depolarizes between beats and therefore the sooner the threshold for the next action potential is reached and the next beat is generated. In this manner, the amplitude, or sensitivity to voltage, of I_f can modify the heart rate. Interestingly, the sensitivity of I_f to voltage is adjusted by the release of noradrenaline and acetylcholine; the activation of adrenoceptors by noradrenaline increases I_f and therefore increases the heart rate, whereas the activation of muscarinic receptors decreases I_f, thereby decreasing the heart rate (see DiFrancesco, 1993). This continual adjustment of I_f results from a "push–pull" arrangement between β-adrenergic and muscarinic cholinergic receptors and is mediated by the adjustment of intracellular levels of cyclic AMP. Indeed, the recent cloning of H channels reveals that their structure is similar to that of cyclic nucleotide-gated channels.

Could I_h play a role in neurons similar to that of I_f in the heart? Possibly. Synchronized rhythmic oscillations in the membrane potential of large numbers of neurons, in some respects similar to those of the heart, are characteristic of the mammalian brain. Oscillations of this type are particularly prevalent in thalamic relay neurons during some periods of sleep, as mentioned earlier. Intracellular recordings from these thalamic neurons reveal that they often generate rhythmic "bursts" of action potentials mediated by the activation of a slow spike that is generated through the activation of the low-threshold, or transient, Ca^{2+} current, I_T (see Fig. 6.13). Between the occurrence of each low-threshold Ca^{2+} spike is a slowly depolarizing membrane potential generated by activation of the mixed Na^+-K^+ current I_h, as with I_f in the heart. The amplitude, or voltage sensitivity, of I_h adjusts the rate at which the thalamic cells oscillate, and, as with the heart, this sensitivity is adjusted by the release of modulatory neurotransmitters. In a sense, the thalamic neurons are "beating" in a manner similar to that of the heart.

Summary

An action potential is generated by the rapid influx of Na^+ ions followed by a slightly slower efflux of K^+ ions. Although the generation of an action potential does not disrupt the concentration gradients of these ions across the membrane, the movement of charge is sufficient to generate a large and brief deviation in the membrane potential. Propagation of the action potential along the axon allows communication of the output of the cell to its synapses. Neurons possess many different types of ionic channels in their membranes, allowing complex patterns of action potentials to be generated and complex synaptic computations to occur within single neurons.

References

Brazier, M. A. B. (1988). "A History of Neurophysiology in the 19th Century." Raven Press, New York.

Brown, D. A., and Adams, P. R. (1980). Muscarinic suppression of a novel voltage sensitive K^+ current in a vertebrate neurone. Nature (London) 283, 673–676.

Carbonne, E., and Lux, H. D. (1984). A low voltage-activated, fully inactivating Ca channel in vertebrate sensory neurones. Nature (London) 310, 501–502.

Catterall, W.A. (2000a) From ionic currents to molecular mechanisms, The structure and function of voltage-gated sodium currents. Neuron 26, 13–25.

Catterall, W.A. (2000b). Structure and regulation of voltage-gated Ca^{2+} channels. Annu. Rev. Cell Dev. Biol. 16, 521–555.

Chandy, K. G., and Gutman, G. A. (1995). Voltage-gated potassium channel genes. In "Ligand- and Voltage-Gated Channels" (A. North, ed.), pp. 1–72. CRC Press, Boca Raton, FL.

Cole, K. S. (1949). Dynamic electrical characteristics of the squid axon membrane. Arch. Sci. Physiol. 3, 253–258.

DiFrancesco, D. (1993). Pacemaker mechanisms in cardiac tissue. Annu. Rev. Physiol. 55, 455–472.

Hille, B. (1977). Ionic basis of resting potentials and action potentials. In "Handbook of Physiology" (E. R. Kandel, ed.), Sect. 1, Vol. 1, pp. 99–136. Am. Physiol. Soc., Bethesda, MD.

Hodgkin, A. L. (1976). Chance and design in electrophysiology, An informal account of certain experiments on nerve carried out between 1934 and 1952. J. Physiol. (Lond.) 263, 1–21.

Hodgkin, A. L., and Huxley, A. F. (1939). Action potentials recorded from inside a nerve fiber. Nature (Lond.) 144, 710–711.

Hodgkin, A. L., and Huxley, A. F. (1952). Currents carried by sodium and potassium ions through the membrane of the giant axon of Loligo. J. Physiol. (Lond.) 116, 449–472.

Hodgkin, A. L., and Huxley, A. F. (1952). A quantitative description of membrane current and its application to conduction and excitation in nerve. J. Physiol. (Lond.) 117, 500–544.

Lauger, P. (1991)."Electrogenic Ion Pumps." Sinauer, Sunderland, MA.

Llinás, R. R. (1988). The intrinsic electrophysiological properties of mammalian neurons: Insights into central nervous system function. Science 242, 1654–1664.

Ludwig, A., Zong, X., Jeglitsch, M., Hofmann, F., and Biel, M. (1998). A family of hyperpolarization-activated mammalian cation channels. Nature 393, 587–591.

McCormick, D. A. (1992). Neurotransmitter actions in the thalamus and cerebral cortex and their role in neuromodulation of thalamocortical activity. Prog. Neurobiol. 39, 337–388.

McCormick, D. A., and Pape, H.-C. (1990). Properties of a hyperpolarization-activated cation current and its role in rhythmic oscillation in thalamic relay neurones. J. Physiol. (Lond.) 431, 291–318.

Nicoll, R. A. (1988). The coupling of neurotransmitter receptors to ion channels in the brain. Science 241; 545–551.

Nowycky, M. C., Fox, A. P., and Tsien, R. W. (1985). Three types of neuronal calcium channel with different calcium agonist sensitivity. Nature (Lond.) 316, 440–443.

Reithmeier, R. A. F. (1994). Mammalian exchangers and cotransporters. Curr. Opin. Cell Biol. 6, 583–594.

Suggested Readings

Hille, B. (2001) "Ionic Channels of Excitable Membranes," 3rd Ed. Sinauer, Sunderland, MA.

Hodgkin, A. L. (1992). "Chance and Design." Cambridge Univ. Press, Cambridge.

Huguenard, J., and McCormick, D. A. (1994). "Electrophysiology of the Neuron." Oxford Univ. Press, New York.

Johnston, D., and Wu, S. M-S. (1995). "Foundations of Cellular Neurophysiology." MIT press.

Koch, C. (1999). "Biophysics of Computation." Oxford Univ. Press, New York.

David A. McCormick

7

Neurotransmitters

Neuroscience a century ago was a tumultuous period marked by claim and counterclaim, confusion, and recrimination—not unlike politics today, or for that matter science. The reason was the revolt against the idea that the brain is one continuous network (a syncytium), with each cell in physical contact. The pioneering studies of Santiago Ramon y Cajal revealed a very different picture, in which the units of the brain (neurons) were independent structures (see Shepherd, 1991). Although final confirmation of this view awaited electron microscopic verification, a general acceptance of neurons as the independent building blocks of the nervous system emerged. This brought about a new debate: what is the mode of communication between neurons? The answer has not been static, but has evolved continuously. This chapter discusses briefly several means through which cells communicate with each other and then discusses in considerable detail one such mechanism: chemical synaptic transmission.

Neurons vary widely in function but share certain structural characteristics. They have a cell body (soma) from which processes emerge; the processes (axons and dendrites) represent polarized compartments of the cell. Axons can be short or long and can be local or project to distant areas. In contrast, dendrites are local. The general concept arose that axons transmit information, which is conveyed to dendrites or soma of follower cells. The critical gap between the transmitting element of the neurons (axon) and the recipient zone of the follower cell (e.g., the dendrite) is the area across which the transmission of information occurs. This area was termed the "synapse" by Charles Sherrington (see Shepherd, 1991) and defined pre- and postsynaptic cells. This general conceptual

framework remains in place today, although there are many exceptions, including dendrites that release neuroactive substances and axons that receive inputs from other neurons. One other characteristic proposed by Sherrington that is central to the concept of chemical communication between neurons is that synaptic transmission does not follow all-or-none rules, but is graded in strength and flexible.

SEVERAL MODES OF NEURONAL COMMUNICATION EXIST

A debate on whether neuronal communication was chemical or electrical raged for the first half of the 20th century, even though some evidence was marshaled in support of the chemical argument midway through the 19th century. In 1849, Claude Bernard noted that curare, which is an active constituent of a poison applied to arrows in South America, blocked nerve-to-muscle neurotransmission. This effect was subsequently shown to be due to the binding of curare to postsynaptic receptors for the neurotransmitter acetylcholine (ACh), thus blocking neuromuscular transmission. Half a century later Thomas Elliott observed that epinephrine resulted in the contraction of smooth muscle that had been deprived of its neural innervation, suggesting that muscle contraction depended on the action of chemical molecules liberated from nerves. In a seminal series of studies using the isolated frog heart, Otto Loewi provided firm evidence of chemical neurotransmission by showing that ACh was released upon nerve stimulation and activated a target muscle.

It is now clear that the major means of interneuronal communication is chemical in nature, but neurons also use some other processes for intercellular communication. These include electrical synaptic transmission, ephaptic interactions, and autocrine, paracrine, and long-range signaling, to which molecules produced by both neural and non-neural cells contribute. The nonsynaptic mode of intercellular communication with the longest range (distance) is humoral signaling. For example, some hormones made outside of the brain can enter the central nervous system (CNS) to exert effects on neurons expressing appropriate receptors for the hormones. These hormone actions may occur over the short term (such as changes in neuronal activity) or, more often, over a longer time frame (e.g., long-lasting changes in gene expression).

Molecules produced by neurons can also be used in intercellular communication that does not require synaptic specializations. Factors that are secreted by neurons or diffuse passively from the cells in which they are generated include classical neurotransmitters, neuropeptides, and neurosteroids, as well as the gases nitric oxide and carbon monoxide. These factors may act through autocrine mechanisms (activating receptors on the same cell that releases them) or paracrine pathways to nearby cells. The gases nitric oxide and carbon monoxide and the endogenous cannabinoid anandamide act as retrograde signaling molecules, providing chemically coded information to a presynaptic neuron from the next cell in "line." Soluble factors can act on high- or low-affinity receptors at local or distant sites. The role of such molecules is thought to be primarily in modulating neural activity, although they may also provide guidance cues for neurons that are growing toward their final targets in the brain and for the establishment and maintenance of synaptic connections (see Chapter 20).

CHEMICAL TRANSMISSION

Chemically mediated transmission is the major mode of neuronal communication. The acceptance of chemical neurotransmission as the dominant mode of information flow between neurons led to the establishment of specific criteria for a compound to be accepted as a neurotransmitter. These "classical" criteria for transmitters have resulted in a relatively small number of compounds being recognized as "classical" transmitters. Over the past generation it has become apparent that there are a large number of chemical messengers that broadly qualify as intercellular transmitters, although these compounds often do not meet (and may serve as exceptions) the classical criteria.

Several Criteria Have Been Established for a Neurotransmitter

Neurotransmitters are endogenous substances that are released from neurons, act on receptor sites that are typically present on membranes of postsynaptic cells, and produce a functional change in the properties of the target cell. Over the years there has been general agreement that several criteria should be met before a substance is designated a neurotransmitter.

1. A neurotransmitter must be synthesized by and released from neurons. This means that the presynaptic neuron should contain a transmitter and the appropriate enzymes need to synthesize that neurotransmitter. Synthesis in the *axon terminal* is not an absolute requirement. For example, peptide transmitters are synthesized in the *cell body* and transported to distant sites, where they are released .

2. The substance should be released from nerve terminals in a chemically or pharmacologically identifiable form. Thus, one should be able to isolate the transmitter and characterize its structure using biochemical or other techniques.

3. A neurotransmitter should reproduce at the postsynaptic cell the specific events (such as changes in membrane properties) that are seen after stimulation of the presynaptic neuron.

FIGURE 7.1　The multiple modes of intercellular signaling. (A) Substances (purple) produced outside the nervous system (1) or by cells within the CNS (2, 3) can affect neuronal activity, acting through (1) humoral, (2) paracrine, and (3) autocrine mechanisms. (B) Ephaptic transmission. Two apposed cell membranes showing regions of low (1, green label indicating channels) and high (2, sawtooths, representing tight junctions) resistances. The equivalent electrical circuit is shown below. Communication between these cells is permitted through membrane areas of low resistance (1). The presence of tight junctions (2) between apposed cells favors an increase of current density by preventing current flow into the bulk extracellular space. Charges accumulate in the narrow intercellular space and affect capacitance and resistive components of the cell membranes. (C) Electrical synapses. Gap junction channels provide low-resistance pathways between adjacent cells, allowing direct communication between the cytoplasm of both cells. In contrast with the ephaptic mode of transmission, current flows directly from cell to cell and not through the extracellular space. The electrical equivalent circuit is shown below, differing from that of the ephapse in B primarily in the absence of a resistance to ground. (D) Chemical synapses. Neurotransmitters released from the presynaptic terminal (on the left) diffuse across the cleft to bind to postsynaptic receptors, where they interact with specific receptors to produce currents that excite or inhibit the cell.

4. The effects of a putative neurotransmitter should be blocked by competitive antagonists of the transmitter in a dose-dependent manner. In addition, treatments that inhibit synthesis of the transmitter candidate should block the effects of presynaptic stimulation.

5. There should be active mechanisms to terminate the action of the putative neurotransmitter. Such mechanisms can include reuptake of the substance into the presynaptic neuron or glial cells through specific transporter molecules, or enzymatic inactivation.

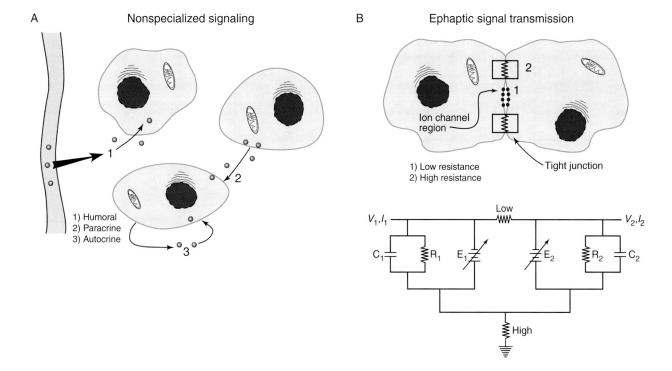

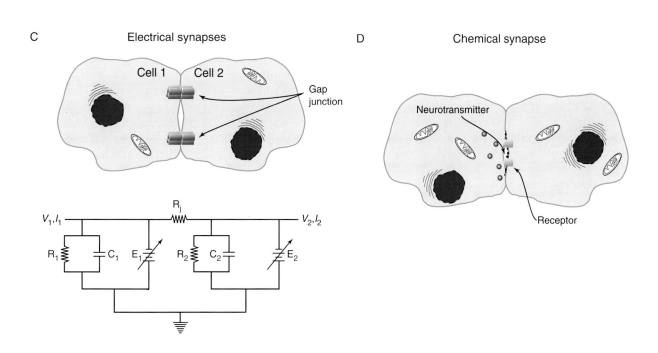

The Process of Chemical Neurotransmission Can Be Divided into Five Steps

Synaptic transmission consists of a number of steps. The general mechanisms of chemical synaptic transmission are depicted in Fig 7.1.

1. *Synthesis of the neurotransmitter in the pre-synaptic neuron.* In order for the transmitter to be synthesized, precursors should be present in the appropriate places within neurons. Enzymes taking part in the conversion of the precursor(s) into the transmitter should be present in an active form and localized to the appropriate compartment in the neuron, and any necessary cofactors for enzyme activity should be present. Drugs affecting the synthesis of neurotransmitters have long been of value in medicine. An example is α-methyl-*p*-tyrosine, a drug used to treat an adrenal gland tumor that causes very high blood pressure by releasing massive amounts of norepinephrine (NE). α-Methyl-*p*-tyrosine blocks the synthesis of NE, thereby lowering blood pressure.

2. *Storage of the neurotransmitter and/or its precursor in the presynaptic nerve terminal.* Classical and peptide transmitters are stored in synaptic vesicles, where they are sequestered and protected from enzymatic degradation, and are ready for quick release. In the case of so-called classical neurotransmitters (acetylcholine, biogenic amines, and amino acids), the synaptic vesicles are small (~50 nm in diameter), whereas neuropeptide transmitters are found in large dense-core vesicles (~100 nm in diameter) and are typically released in response to repetitive stimulation or burst firing of neurons. Because most neurotransmitters are synthesized in the cytosol of neurons, there must be some mechanism through which the transmitter gains entry into the vesicle. This mechanism is the vesicular transporter protein.

3. *Release of the neurotransmitter into the synaptic cleft.* The vesicle in which the transmitter is stored fuses with the cell membrane and releases the transmitter. Neurons use two pathways to secrete proteins. The release of most neurotransmitters occurs by a regulated pathway that is controlled by extracellular signals. The neurotransmitter release process is discussed more fully in the next chapter (Chapter 8). A second (constitutive) pathway is not triggered by extracellular stimulation and is used to secrete membrane components, viral proteins, and extracellular matrix molecules; some unconventional transmitters (e.g., growth factors) may be synthesized and released by the constitutive and regulated pathways.

4. *Binding and recognition of the neurotransmitter by target receptors.* Neurotransmitters that are released interact with receptors located on the target (postsynaptic) cell. These receptors fall into two broad classes. The first are membrane proteins called metabotropic receptors, which are coupled to intracellular G proteins as effectors (see Chapter 9). Ionotropic receptors form channels through which ions such as Na^+ and Ca^{2+} flow. Receptors can be found on neurons that are postsynaptic to the cell releasing the transmitter or on presynaptic neurons, where they respond to the transmitter released from the same cell. Such autoreceptors regulate transmitter release, synthesis, or impulse flow and can be thought of as homeostatic feedback mechanisms.

5. *Termination of the action of the released transmitter.* If a cell lacks the means to terminate the actions of neurotransmitters, it will suffer the consequences. For example, the sustained activation of postsynaptic targets can result in tetanus (in muscles) or seizures (in the brain). Neurotransmitter actions may be terminated actively or passively. Among the active mechanisms are reuptake of the neurotransmitter through specific transporter proteins on the presynaptic neuron and enzymatic degradation to an inactive substance. In some cases, glial cells can accumulate released transmitters. Diffusion away from the synaptic region is a passive mechanism that halts the continued activity of a transmitter.

These five steps form a logical scaffold for understanding chemical neurotransmission. There are, however, differences across the various transmitters, and our knowledge of the different transmitters varies widely. One class of neurotransmitters, the catecholamines, has been studied extensively. We discuss in detail catecholamine neurotransmitters to illustrate the various steps of chemical neurotransmission and then examine the particulars of chemical neurotransmission for other classical neurotransmitters. We also discuss differences between classical and other (nonclassical) neurotransmitters or chemical messengers, including peptide transmitters and unconventional transmitters such as nitric oxide and growth factors.

CLASSICAL NEUROTRANSMITTERS

The term classical is used to differentiate acetylcholine, the biogenic amines, and the amino acid transmitters from other transmitters. Although the designation is somewhat arbitrary, several criteria can be used to distinguish the two groups of transmitters. For example, storage vesicles for classical transmitters are smaller. In addition, classical transmitters are subject to active reuptake by the presynaptic cell and thus can be viewed as homoeostatically conserved; in contrast, there is no energy-dependent, high-affinity reuptake process for nonclassical transmitters. Finally, most classical transmitters are synthesized in the nerve terminal by enzymatic action; peptides, however, are synthesized in the soma from a precursor protein and are then transported to the nerve terminal. The remainder of this chapter deals with the biochemistry of several different transmitter groups, discussing their synthesis, storage, and release. Chapter 8, we will discusses in much more detail a specific issue—transmitter release. Finally, Chapter 9 discusses in some depth the receptors on which various transmitters act.

Catecholamine Neurotransmitters

Catecholamines are organic compounds that contain a catechol nucleus (a benzene ring with two adjacent hydroxyl substitutions) and an amine group. In practice the term is usually used to describe the three transmitters: dopamine (DA), NE, and epinephrine (Epi). These three neurotransmitters are formed by successive enzymatic steps requiring distinct enzymes (see Fig 7.2 and 7.3). The localization of specific synthesizing enzymes in different cells results in distinct

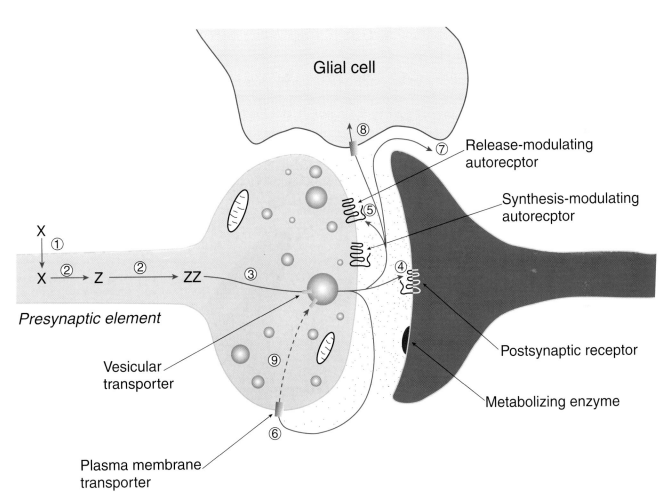

FIGURE 7.2 Schematic representation of the life cycle of a classical neurotransmitter. After accumulation of a precursor amino acid into the neuron (1), the amino acid precursor is metabolized sequentially (2) to yield the mature transmitter. The transmitter is then accumulated into vesicles by the vesicular transporter (3), where it is poised for release and protected from degradation. Once released, the transmitter can interact with postsynaptic receptors (4) or autoreceptors (5) that regulate transmitter release, synthesis, or firing rate. Transmitter actions are terminated by means of a high-affinity membrane transporter (6) that is usually associated with the neuron that released the transmitter. Alternatively, tranmitter actions may be terminated by diffusion from the active sites (7) or accumulation into glia through a membrane transporter (8). When the transmitter is taken up by the neuron, it is subject to metabolic inactivation (9).

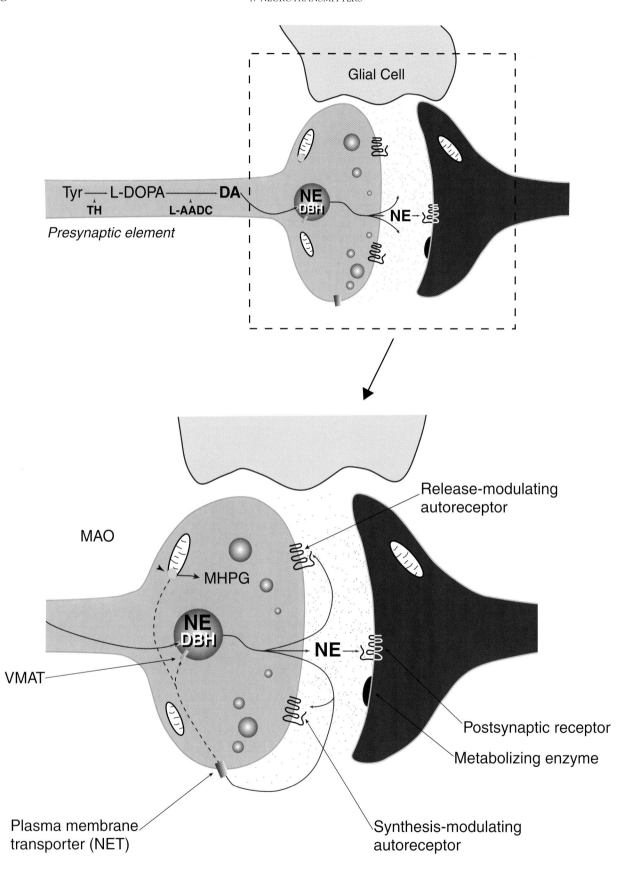

DA-, NE-, and Epi-containing neurons in the brain. Catecholamines also have transmitter roles in the peripheral nervous system and certain hormonal functions.

In the peripheral nervous system, DA has significant biological activity in the kidney but is mainly present as a NE precursor. NE is the transmitter of the sympathetic nervous system in mammals, whereas Epi is the sympathetic transmitter in frogs. Despite this species difference, biochemical aspects of neurotransmission are remarkably constant across different vertebrate species and even invertebrates.

Biosynthesis of Catecholamines

The amino acids phenylalanine and tyrosine are precursors for catecholamines. Both amino acids are present in the plasma and brain in high concentrations. In mammals, tyrosine can be formed from dietary phenylalanine by the enzyme phenylalanine hydroxylase, found in large amounts in the liver. Insufficient amounts of phenylalanine hydroxylase result in phenylketonuria (see Box 7.1).

Catecholamine synthesis is usually considered to begin with tyrosine, which represents a branch point for many important biosynthetic processes in animal tissues. The enzyme tyrosine hydroxylase (TH) converts the amino acid L-tyrosine into 3,4-dihydroxyphenylalanine (DOPA). The purification of TH and other enzymes in the catecholamine biosynthetic pathway allowed detailed analyses of these enzymes and aided in the development of useful inhibitors of the enzymes. The development of antibodies against the purified enzymes led to immunohistochemical mapping of the location of neurons in which the enzymes are found.

The hydroxylation of L-tyrosine by TH results in the formation of the DA precursor *DOPA*, which is

metabolized quickly to DA by L-aromatic amino acid decarboxylase (AADC; see Cooper *et al.*, 1996). This step occurs so rapidly that it is very difficult to measure DOPA in the brain without first inhibiting AADC. In neurons that use DA as the transmitter, the decarboxylation of DOPA to DA is the final step in transmitter synthesis. However, in neurons using NE (also known as noradrenaline) or epinephrine (adrenaline) as transmitters, the enzyme dopamine β-hydroxylase (DBH) is present; this enzyme oxidizes DA to yield NE. Finally, in still other neurons in which Epi serves as the transmitter, a third enzyme (phenylethanolamine *N*-methyltransferase, PNMT) converts NE into Epi. Thus, an adrenergic cell that uses Epi as its transmitter contains four enzymes (TH, AADC, DBH, and PNMT), whereas NE neurons contain only three enzymes (lacking PNMT) and DA cells only two (TH and AADC). A summary of catecholamine synthesis is shown in Fig. 7.4.

Tyrosine Hydroxylase

In human beings, a single TH gene is alternatively spliced to yield four TH mRNAs and four distinct TH protein isoforms. However, in most primates, only two TH isoforms are present, and the rat possesses but a single form of TH. It has been speculated that different TH forms in human beings are associated with differences in activity of the enzyme, but conclusive data addressing this point are lacking.

The function of TH and other enzymes is determined by two factors: changes in enzyme activity (the rate at which the enzyme converts precursor into its product) and changes in the amount of enzyme protein. The primary determinant of TH activity is phosphorylation of the enzyme (Fig. 7.4), which can occur at four different serine sites. Another means of regulating enzyme activity is through end product inhibition: catecholamines can inhibit the activity of TH by competing for a required cofactor (tetrahydrobiopterine, BH4) for the enzyme (Cooper *et al.*, 1996).

Increased neuronal demand for catecholamines can be met by synthesizing new TH protein or increasing TH activity. The degree to which increases in catecholamine synthesis depend on *de novo* synthesis of new enzyme protein or changes in activity differs across brain regions. For example, in brain stem NE neurons, increases in TH gene expression and synthesis of the enzyme are readily seen under conditions requiring more catecholamine synthesis, whereas phosphorylation is more important in midbrain DA neurons.

The synthesis of catecholamines starts with the entry of tyrosine (or phenylalanine) into the brain.

FIGURE 7.3 Characteristics of a norepinephrine (NE)-containing catecholamine neuron. Tyrosine (Tyr) is accumulated by the neuron and is then metabolized sequentially by tyrosine hydroxylase (TH) and L-aromatic amino acid decarboxylase (L-AADC) to dopamine (DA). The DA is then taken up through the vesicular monoamine transporter into vesicles. In DA neurons, this is the final step. However, in this NE-containing cell, DA is metabolized to NE by dopamine-b-hydroxylase (DBH), which is found in the vesicle. Once NE is released, it can interact with postsynaptic noradrenergic receptors or presynaptic noradrenergic autoreceptors. The accumulation of NE by the high-affinity membrane NE transporter (NET) terminates the actions of NE. Once taken back up by the neuron, NE can be metabolized to inactive compounds (DHPG) by degradative enzymes such as monoamine oxidase (MAO) or taken back up by the vesicle.

BOX 7.1

PKU AND METABOLISM

Phenylketonuria (PKU) is a genetic disease caused by mutations in the enzyme phenylalanine hydroxylase (PAH) that result in the loss of the enzyme's ability to hydroxylate phenylalanine (Phe) to tyrosine, from which catecholamine transmitters are synthesized. If PAH levels are low or absent (as in PKU), blood levels of Phe are massively elevated. A tiny fraction of the increased Phe is converted to phenylpyruvic acid, which is excreted in the urine; hence, the name of the disease.

Elevated Phe levels in PKU spare the body, but spoil—indeed, devastate—the developing brain. Severe mental retardation ensues unless steps are taken to limit dietary Phe intake. PKU patients also have a somewhat higher incidence of seizures. The mechanism by which elevated Phe levels damage the developing brain is unknown, but may involve competition with the brain uptake of other essential amino acids.

Phenylalanine hydroxylase functions *in vivo* as part of a complex multicomponent system consisting of two other enzymes (a reductase and dehydratase) and a nonprotein coenzyme (tetrahydrobiopterin or BH4). There are (rare) variant forms of PKU caused by lack of one of the other components of the hydroxylating system; these forms are much more severe.

PKU is inherited as an autosomal recessive trait. The vast majority of PKU babies are conceived when both parents are heterozygotes, each one harboring one normal gene and one PKU gene. Thus, on average, one-fourth of children born to such parents are PKU, one-fourth are normal, and half are heterozygotes. The incidence of heterozygosity for PKU is about 1 in 55. If one can dare say that there is anything fortunate about this dreadful disease, it is that it is rare. The frequency, however, varies widely among different ethnic groups, ranging from 1/200,000 in Japan to 1/5000 in Ireland. One auspicious feature of the disease is that the affected infants are essentially normal at birth. This raised the hope that there might be a way to prevent the intellectual deterioration of PKU. This hope was realized 50 years ago with the introduction of a low (not a no!) Phe diet, which has proven to be largely if not totally effective in preventing brain damage and permits normal IQ if the diet is started shortly after birth. However, the low Phe diet is a heavy burden for both patients and their families. Although it was once hoped that the diet could be stopped after 6 or 7 years, it now appears that a longer period is beneficial. Since the sine qua non of successful dietary treatment of PKU is to start the diet as soon as possible after birth, its success was closely tied to the development of an inexpensive and rapid test for PKU. The Guthrie test, which was introduced in 1961, gives a semiquantitative measure of Phe levels in a drop of blood and is widely used for the screening of newborns.

PKU is noteworthy in that the brain is the only organ that is damaged by mutations in an enzyme that is found only in the liver in humans. This provides a valuable lesson: metabolically, no organ in the body is an island unto itself.

Seymour Kaufman

This process is an energy-dependent one in which tyrosine competes with large neutral amino acids as a substrate for the transporter. Because brain tyrosine levels are high enough to saturate TH, catecholamine synthesis cannot be increased by tyrosine administration under normal conditions. Exceptions to this rule are catecholamine synthesis in cells that are very active, such as DA neurons that innervate the prefrontal cortex, and under certain pathological conditions. Because TH is saturated by tyrosine, tyrosine hydroxylation is the rate-limiting step in catecholamine synthesis under basal conditions. However, under conditions of neuronal activation, the enzyme responsible for NE synthesis (DBH) becomes rate limiting, and thus tyrosine availability regulates catecholamine synthesis under certain conditions.

TH is a mixed function oxidase with moderate substrate specificity, hydroxylating phenylalanine as well as tyrosine. The actions of TH require a biopterin cofactor and iron (Fe^{2+}). BH4 is an essential cofactor for TH and some other enzymes, including the tryptophan hydroxylase, the enzyme that synthesizes the indolamine serotonin (5-hydroxyptryptamine, 5-HT), which is discussed in the next section. Because BH4 is not present in saturat-

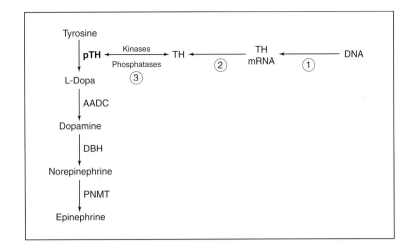

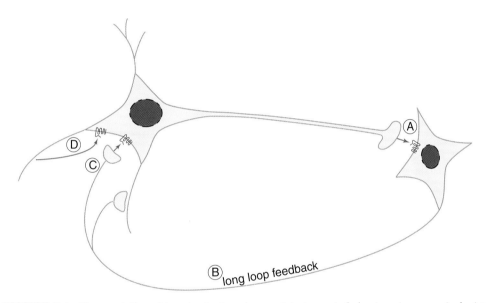

FIGURE 7.4   The regulation of tyrosine hydroxylase protein in a catecholaminergic neuron is depicted schematically. Ways in which the synthesis of catecholamines can be regulated. (1) There may be a change in TH gene expression. (2) Catecholamine synthesis can be regulated by changes in translation of the TH transcript, either enhancing translation or alternatively stabilizing the transcript. (3) TH activity is regulated by the actions of specific kinases on four serine residues of the enzyme (leading to phosphorylated pTH). (Bottom) How both long loop feedback projections (B) and local regulation by relase of catecholamines from dendritic processes (D) can regulate the activity of catecholaminergic neurons. Target neurons that receive a catecholaminergic neuron input (A) can regulate activity of the catecholamine neuron by projecting back (long-loop feedback) onto the catecholamine cell (B); the long-loop feedback axons may terminate onto either dendrites or soma of the catecholamine neuron (C). Local feedback by catecholamines released from dendrites (D) are also critically involved in regulating the activity of catecholamine neurons.

ing concentrations under basal conditions, the BH4 cofactor is crucial for the regulation of TH activity. Intracellular levels of BH4 are determined by its synthesizing enzyme, GTP cyclohydrolase. Mutations in the gene encoding GTP cyclohydrolase result in a movement disorder called DOPA responsive dystonia.

L-Aromatic Amino Acid Decarboxylase

The hydroxylation of tyrosine by TH generates DOPA, which is then decarboxylated to dopamine (DA) by L-aromatic amino acid decarboxylase (AADC; also sometimes referred to as DOPA decarboxylase). AADC has low substrate specificity and decarboxylates tryptophan as well as tyrosine. Because this enzyme is present in both catecholamine and 5-HT neurons, it plays an important role in the synthesis of both groups of transmitters. In dopaminergic neurons, AADC is the final enzyme of the synthetic pathway.

DA does not cross the blood–brain barrier, but its precursor DOPA enters the brain readily. AADC acts so quickly that DOPA is converted into DA almost instantaneously. It appears that AADC is regulated mainly by the induction of new protein rather than changes in activity. DOPA has achieved fame as a means of treating Parkinson's disease, which is due to loss of DA in the striatum (see Chapter 34). Although DOPA enters the brain readily, decarboxylating enzymes in the liver and capillary endothelial cells degrade DOPA rapidly in the periphery. DOPA is therefore administered in combination with a peripheral decarboxylase inhibitor that does not enter the brain; this inhibitor protects DOPA from being metabolized before it enters the brain, and thereby sharply increases central DA concentrations. Although DOPA is used extensively in Parkinson's disease, chronic treatment with DOPA may decrease the activity of endogenous AADC. This is an illustration of the rule that drugs have both side and therapeutic effects, and can even exert countertherapeutic effects.

Dopamine β-Hydroxylase

Noradrenergic and adrenergic neurons contain the enzyme dopamine-β-hydroxylase (DBH), an oxidase that converts DA into NE. In noradrenergic neurons, this is the final step in catecholamine synthesis. Humans have two different DBH mRNAs that are generated from a single gene. DBH mRNAs in the brain are restricted to NE and Epi neurons.

DBH does not have a high degree of substrate specificity and *in vitro* it oxidizes almost any phenylethylamine to its corresponding phenylethanolamine. For example, in addition to forming NE from DA, DBH converts tyramine into octopamine. Interestingly, receptors that have a high affinity for the trace amines tyramine and octopamine have just been discovered. Many of the structurally similar metabolites that arise from the actions of DBH on substrates other than DA can act as false neurotransmitters for NE.

Phenylethanolamine N-Methyltransferase

Phenylethanolamine *N*-methyltransferase (PNMT) is present at high levels in the adrenal medulla, where it methylates NE to form Epi, the major adrenal catecholamine. A single PNMT gene is found in the adrenal gland and in certain brain stem neurons. The actions of PNMT require *S*-adenosylmethionine as the methyl donor for the methylation of NE; PNMT has modest substrate specificity and will transfer methyl groups to the nitrogen on a variety of b-hydroxylated amines. The regulation of PNMT activity in the brain has not been studied extensively; in the adrenal gland, glucocorticoids and nerve growth factor regulate PNMT.

Storage of Catecholamines and Their Enzymes

Vesicular Storage

Catecholamines are found in vesicles, which are specialized subcellular organelles. Vesicular storage of transmitters serves as a depot until the molecule is released by appropriate physiological stimuli (see Chapter 8). The vesicles are concentrated in the presynaptic terminal, near the synapse, where they are ready for fusion with the cellular membrane and exocytosis. Catecholamine storage in vesicles offers protection from metabolic inactivation by intraneuronal enzymes or attack by toxins that have gained entry into the neuron.

The NE-synthesizing enzyme DBH differs from the other enzymes in catecholamine synthesis by being localized to the vesicle rather than the cytosol. This means that only *after* DA is accumulated into the vesicles by the vesicular monoamine transporter (VMAT) is it metabolized to NE. The vesicular storage of DBH has one other interesting consequence: DBH is actually released from cells when its product (NE) is released.

Vesicular Monoamine Transporters

The ability of vesicles to take up DA or other catecholamines depends on the VMAT (Weihe and Eiden, 2000). The VMAT is distinct from the neuronal membrane transporter (see later) in terms of substrate affinity and localization. Two VMAT genes have been cloned: VMAT1 is found in adrenal cells that synthesize and release monoamines and VMAT2 is found in the brain in catecholamine and 5-HT neurons. VMAT2 is not highly specific and transports catecholamines, indoleamines, and histamine into vesicles. Both VMATs are Mg^{2+} dependent and are inhibited by reserpine, a drug that disrupts the vesicular storage of monoamines.

Reserpine has been used for centuries in India as a folk medicine to treat high blood pressure and psychoses. The discovery that reserpine depletes vesicular stores of monoamines was critical to our understanding of how reserpine alleviates psychotic symptoms and also shed light on the mechanisms through which certain toxins can cause a Parkinson's disease-like syndrome. The use of reserpine to treat hypertension and psychoses was reported in international journals in the early 1930s, but these therapeutic actions were not widely appreciated in Western medicine until a generation later. At that time, Brodie and co-workers discovered that reserpine depleted brain 5-HT. The contemporaneous discovery that the hallucinogen LSD is structurally similar to 5-HT led to the proposal that the antipsychotic actions of reserpine were due to its ability to deplete brain 5-HT stores. However, it was soon realized that reserpine depletes *both* 5-HT and catecholamines in the brain; thus, the antipsychotic effects of reserpine might be due to 5-HT or catecholamine depletion, or both.

To determine which transmitters were more important, Arvid Carlsson and colleagues administered catecholamine and 5-HT precursors to reserpine-treated rats in order to replenish monoamine levels; they then examined locomotor activity, which is severely depressed by reserpine treatment. Motor function was restored by the DA precursor DOPA but not by the 5-HT precursor 5-hydroxytryptophan. This work led to the characterization of DA as a neurotransmitter, and DOPA treatment of reserpinized animals was shown to increase brain DA concentrations. This suggested that the primary mechanism through which reserpine exerts antipsychotic effects is through its ability to disrupt DA transmission and contributed to the hypothesis that the dysfunction of central DA systems underlies schizophrenia. Interestingly, recent studies suggest that drugs that are antagonists at both DA and 5-HT receptors may be therapeutically superior to pure DA antagonists in the treatment of schizophrenia.

Vesicles store transmitters for subsequent release. Data have suggested that vesicular storage determines the quantal release of transmitters (see Chapter 8). For example, transfecting VMAT2 into DA neurons results in overexpression of the vesicular transporter in small synaptic vesicles and increases in both quantal size and frequency of release.

VMATs have significant homology with a group of bacterial antibiotic drug resistance transporters, suggesting a role of VMAT in detoxification. This is indeed the case: VMAT allows the vesicles to sequester toxins, thereby reducing toxicity. This is best exemplified by studies in heterozygous mice bearing one copy of VMAT2. In these mice, the parkinsonian toxin MPTP (see Chapter 31) causes a greater loss of DA neurons, as there is less VMAT to sequester the toxin in vesicles and MPTP can disrupt mitochondrial function more freely.

Release of Catecholamines

Catecholamine release typically occurs by the same Ca^{2+}-dependent exocytotic process used by other transmitters (see Chapter 8), but can also occur through at least two other mechanisms. First, catecholamines can be released by a reversal of the catecholamine transporters DAT and NET. This occurs in response to certain drugs (such as amphetamine) and has been reported to occur following the application of excitatory amino acids as well. Second, DA (and perhaps other catecholamines) can be released from dendrites through a process that does not appear to involve Ca^{2+}.

Regulation of Catecholamine Synthesis and Release by Autoreceptors

Enzymes that control the synthesis of catecholamines can be regulated at both the transcriptional level and by posttranslational modifications that alter enzymatic activity. In addition, DA and NE *synthesis* can be regulated by the interaction of released catecholamine with specific DA or NE "autoreceptors" located on the nerve terminal. Similarly, the *release* of catecholamines is regulated by autoreceptors, as is the *firing rate* of catecholaminergic neurons.

DA autoreceptors are perhaps the best characterized of the catecholamine autoreceptors. Autoreceptors exist on most parts of the neuron and are defined functionally by the events that they regulate. Synthesis-, release-, and impulse-modulating DA autoreceptors have been described (see Cooper *et al.*, 1996). All three types of DA autoreceptors belong to the D2 family of DA receptors, which includes three different receptors (D_2, D_3, and D_4). It is clear that D_2 autoreceptors exist, but considerable controversy surrounds the presence of D_3 autoreceptors; there do not appear to be D_4 autoreceptors. Because there are three functionally different DA autoreceptors, the same receptor protein may serve different autoreceptor roles through distinct transduction mechanisms.

The autoreceptor functions as a feedback mechanism. Thus, DA that is released from a neuron stimulates an autoreceptor to inhibit further transmitter release. *Release-modulating autoreceptors* are not only found on DA neurons; in fact, they are a common regulatory feature on neurons that use classical transmitters. Because intracellular DA levels regulate tyrosine hydroxylase activity by interfering with the binding of BH4 to TH, changes in the release of DA may also alter transmitter synthesis. Separate *synthesis-modulating autoreceptors* also directly regulate DA synthesis: DA release decreases DA synthesis whereas DA antagonists increase synthesis. Interestingly, synthesis-modulating autoreceptors are not found on all DA neurons: some midbrain and hypothalamic DA neurons lack synthesis-modulating autoreceptors. Because release-modulating autoreceptors may regulate synthesis indirectly, the presence of synthesis-modulating autoreceptors may not be necessary in certain neurons. Finally, *impulse-modulating autoreceptors* found on the soma and dendrites of DA neurons regulate the firing rate of these cells. As noted earlier, because the release of DA can alter synthesis of the transmitter, it follows that impulse-modulating autoreceptors also change DA synthesis. Thus, all three types of DA autoreceptors may ultimately regulate synthesis. The interdependence of regulatory processes governing DA cells is characteristic of monoaminergic neurons.

Autoreceptors also regulate NE release. There are two NE autoreceptors, one of which (an *α* receptor) inhibits NE release while a second (a *β* receptor) actually facilitates release. Synthesis-modulating NE autoreceptors that directly regulate NE *synthesis* have not been reported, and little is known about the autoreceptor regulation of Epi release in the brain.

Inactivation of Catecholamine Neurotransmission

Continuous stimulation of neuronal receptors is not a physiological condition. Neuronal activity is not continuous, but fluctuates as neurons fire more rapidly or slowly. Continuous transmitter stimulation would fail to convey accurate information to the follower cell about the dynamic activity of the presynaptic neuron. Moreover, continuous stimulation of certain receptors is pathological and damages postsynaptic cells. One such example involves receptors for the excitatory transmitter glutamate (Glu), which are discussed in a later section of this chapter.

There are several different mechanisms for terminating the actions of a catecholamine. The simplest is diffusion away from the receptor followed by dilution in extracellular fluid to subthreshold concentrations. In addition, there are active modes of halting transmitter action, including catecholamine uptake by membrane-associated transporter proteins and enzymatic inactivation.

Enzymatic Inactivation of Catecholamines

Enzymatic inactivation was originally thought to be the major means of terminating catecholamine actions in the CNS. It is now thought to play a secondary role, although it remains the major mechanism of terminat-

ing catecholamine effects in the bloodstream. Two enzymes contribute to catecholamine catabolism: monoamine oxidase (MAO) and catechol-*0*-methyltransferase (COMT). The two enzymes can act independently or can act on the products generated by the other enzyme, leading to catecholamine metabolites that are deaminated, *O*-methylated, or both. COMT is a relatively nonspecific enzyme that transfers methyl groups from the donor *S*-adenosylmethionine (SAM) to the *m*-hydroxy group of catechols. COMT is found in both peripheral tissues and central nervous system and is the major means of inactivating catecholamines that are released from the adrenal gland.

Two forms of MAO have been identified. MAO_A has high affinities for NE and 5-HT and is selectively inhibited by certain drugs such as clorgyline. In contrast, MAO_B has a higher affinity for *o*-phenylethylamines and is selectively inhibited by different compounds such as deprenyl. Both MAO isoforms are associated with the outer mitochondrial membrane. MAOs oxidatively deaminate catecholamines and their *o*-methylated derivatives to form inactive and unstable aldehyde derivatives, which can be further degraded by other enzymes. This process can be clinically important: drugs that target the enzymatic inactivation of catecholamines have been central to the treatment of several neuropsychiatric disorders (see Box 7.2).

Neuronal Catecholamine Transporters

The reuptake of a transmitter released by a neuron is the major mode of inactivation of the released transmitter in the brain. Accumulation of the transmitter also allows intracellular enzymes that degrade the transmitter to act, thus bolstering the actions of extracellular enzymes.

Several characteristics define the high-affinity neuronal reuptake of transmitters (Clark and Amara, 1993). The process is energy dependent and saturable, depends on Na^+ cotransport, and requires extracellular Cl^-. Because reuptake depends on coupling to the Na^+ gradient across the neuronal membrane, toxins that inhibit Na^+, K^+-ATPase inhibit reuptake. Under certain conditions, the coupling of transporter function to Na^+ flow may cause local changes in membrane Na^+ gradients and thereby paradoxically extrude ("release") the transmitter.

Membrane catecholamine transporters are not Mg^{2+} dependent and are not inhibited by reserpine. These characteristics distinguish the neuronal and vesicular membrane transporters (see earlier discussion). Catecholamine transporters are localized to neurons. Although there appears to be a reuptake process that can accumulate catecholamines into glia,

BOX 7.2

MAO AND COMT INHIBITORS IN THE TREATMENT OF NEUROPSYCHIATRIC DISORDERS

One hypothesis of the pathophysiology of depression posits a decrease in noradrenergic levels in the brain. MAO_A inhibitors, such as tranylcypromine, effectively increase NE levels (as well as DA and 5-HT concentrations) and were once a mainstay in the treatment of depression. However, the use of MAO inhibitors in depression has been largely supplanted by the introduction of drugs that increase extracellular NE levels by blocking the NE transporter (tricyclic antidepressants) and other agents that increase 5-HT or DA levels by blocking SERT or DAT (such as Prozac and Welbutrin). The treatment of depression with MAO_A inhibitors, although still useful for certain patients who do not respond to other antidepressants, is marred by a large number of side effects. Among the most serious is hypertensive crisis. Patients treated with MAO_A inhibitors cannot metabolize tyramine efficiently, which is present in large amounts in certain foods, such as aged cheeses and red wines. Because tyramine releases catecholamines peripherally, small amounts of tyramine increase blood pressure significantly and may lead to a high risk for stroke.

Deprenyl, a specific inhibitor of MAO_B, has been used as an initial treatment for Parkinson's disease (PD; see Chapter 31). The use of deprenyl in the treatment of PD and the rationale for its use were based on data from studies of a neurotoxin, 1-methyl-4-phenyl-1,2,3,6-tetrahydropyridine (MPTP). MPTP results in the degeneration of midbrain DA neurons and a parkinsonian syndrome. MPTP-induced parkinsonism was first noted in a group of opiate addicts. In an attempt to synthesize a designer drug, the structurally related MPTP was inadvertently produced; addicts who injected this drug developed a severe parkinsonian syndrome. Subsequent animal studies showed that MPTP itself is not toxic, but that its active metabolite, MPP^+, is highly toxic. The for-

mation of MPP^+ from MPTP is catalyzed by MAO_B, and treatment with MAO inhibitiors such as deprenyl can prevent MPTP toxicity. The realization that MPTP administration rather faithfully reproduces the cardinal signs and symptoms of PD reawakened interest in environmental toxins as a cause of PD. The MPTP saga also led to the idea that deprenyl treatment might slow the progression of PD by preventing metabolism of an environmental compound to an active toxin such as MPP^+. Although clinical studies were initially interpreted to suggest that there was a slowing of clinical progression of Parkinson's disease in response to deprenyl, later studies showed that deprenyl increases DA levels slightly and thus gives some symptomatic relief.

Catechol O-methyl transferase, which together with MAO degrades catecholamines, also plays a role in the treatment of PD. Two COMT, inhibitors are used to prevent the enzymatic inactivation of DOPA. By inhibiting COMT, these drugs prolong the therapeutic action of DOPA and may smooth out fluctuations in the therapeutic response to DOPA.

Changes in catecholamine function have also been the object of intense scrutiny in schizophrenia, with recent attention focusing on possible changes in dopamine. One allelic variant of the COMT gene results in a much reduced activity of the enzyme. Data have examined COMT alleles for full vs low COMT activity in normal subjects and schizophrenics. Individuals bearing the allele that confers lower COMT activity display improved performance on cognitive tasks that involve DA actions in the prefrontal cortex; the performance of schizophrenic persons on these tasks is impaired. It has therefore been proposed that high COMT activity may confer an increased risk to schizophrenia.

Ariel Y. Deutch and Robert H. Roth

---

the process does have a high affinity for the amines and its functional significance is unknown.

Two distinct mammalian catecholamine transporter proteins—DA (DAT) and NE (NET) transporters—have been cloned and characterized pharmacologically. The two are closely related members of a class of transporter proteins (including 5-HT and amino acid transmitter transporters) with 12 transmembrane domains. Neither transporter is specific, with each

accumulating both DA and NE. In fact, NET has a higher affinity for DA than for NE. An epinephrine transporter has been identified in the frog but not in mammals.

The regional distribution of DAT and NET largely follows the expected localization to DA and NE neurons, respectively. However, DAT does not appear to be expressed in all DA cells. Certain hypothalamic cells that release DA into the blood system of the pituitary lack detectable DAT mRNA and protein. Because DA released from these neurons is carried away in the blood, the existence of a transporter protein on these DA cells would be superfluous.

Immunohistochemical studies of the subcellular localization of DAT led to an unexpected finding. DAT is typically expressed *outside* of the synapse instead of at the synaptic junction. This suggests that the transporter may be used to inactivate (accumulate) DA that has escaped from the synaptic cleft, and thus suggests that diffusion is the initial process by which DA is removed from the synapse. The extrasynaptic localization is also consistent with studies indicating that perisynaptic concentrations of DA are ≥ 1.0 mM, a value roughly comparable to the affinity of the cloned DAT for DA. The extrasynaptic localization of the catecholamine transporters and the fact that receptors for DA and other transmitters are also found extrasynaptically suggest that extrasynaptic ("paracrine" or volume) neurotransmission may be of considerable importance for catecholamine signaling.

Mice with targeting mutations of the DAT have been particularly useful in clarifying the function of transporters. Transgenic mice that lack constitutive expression of DAT have a remarkably wide array of deficits in DA function, ranging from increased extracellular DA levels and delayed clearance of released DA to a striking decrease in tissue concentrations of DA in the face of increased DA synthesis (Gainetdinov *et al.*, 1998). There is also a complete loss of autoreceptor-mediated tone, including deficits in release-, synthesis-, and impulse-modulating autoreceptor function. These deficits in DAT knockout mice have been suggested to reflect a disinhibition of tyrosine hydroxylase due to a lack of intraneuronal DA (which provides feedback inhibition of the enzyme), and hence a marked increased in the synthesis and release of DA.

Cocaine exerts its effects by increasing extracellular catecholamine and 5-HT levels. Psychostimulants such as cocaine and amphetamine increase catecholamine levels by blocking transporters. In particular, cocaine shows a very high affinity for DAT; amphetamine is a less potent inhibitor but also induces release (via transporter reversal) of catecholamines. Studies in DAT knockout mice have surprisingly revealed that these mice will still self-administer cocaine. However, mice with double knockouts of both the DAT and the 5-HT transporter (often abbreviated as SERT, for serotonin transporter) fail to self-administer cocaine, suggesting that both transmitters are critical for the effects of cocaine.

NET is the molecular target of tricyclic antidepressant drugs. These agents potently inhibit NE reuptake, with much weaker effects on DA and 5-HT transporters. Mice with targeted null mutations of NET act like antidepressant-treated mice. Drugs that inhibit NET selectively without significantly altering 5-HT or DA uptake have just entered into clinical use.

Serotonin

One hundred and fifty years ago scientists became aware of a substance in the blood that induces powerful contractions of smooth muscle organs. More than a century passed until Page and collaborators succeeded in isolating the compound (which they advanced as a possible cause of high blood pressure) from platelets. At the same time, Italian researchers were studying a substance found in high concentrations in intestinal mucosa that caused contractions of the intestinal smooth muscle. The material isolated from platelets was called "serotonin," and the substance isolated from the intestinal tract was named "enteramine." Purification of the two substances revealed them to be the identical substance, which we will abbreviate as 5-HT for its chemical name, 5-hydroxytryptamine. For example, when 5-HT that was prepared synthetically was compared with the purified compound isolated from platelets, it was found to have all of the biological features of the natural substance.

5-HT is found in neurons and in several types of peripheral cells. In fact, the brain accounts for only about 1% of body stores of 5-HT. Although the purification and identification of 5-HT were based on studies of peripheral processes, much of the impetus for 5-HT research has been the involvement of 5-HT in psychiatric disorders. The finding that the chemical structure of 5-HT is similar to that of LSD led to theories that associated abnormalities in 5-HT function to schizophrenia and depression.

FIGURE 7.5 Example of a serotonergic neuron. Tryptophan ▶ (Trp) in the neuron is metabolized sequentially by tryptophan hydroxylase (TrypOHase) and L-AADC to yield serotonin (5-HT). 5-HT is accumulated by the vesicular monoamine transporter. When released, 5-HT can interact with both postsynaptic receptors and presynaptic autoreceptors. 5-HT is taken up by the high-affinity 5-HT transporter (SERT), and once inside the neuron it can be reaccumulated by vesicular transporter or inactivated metabolically by MAO and other enzymes.

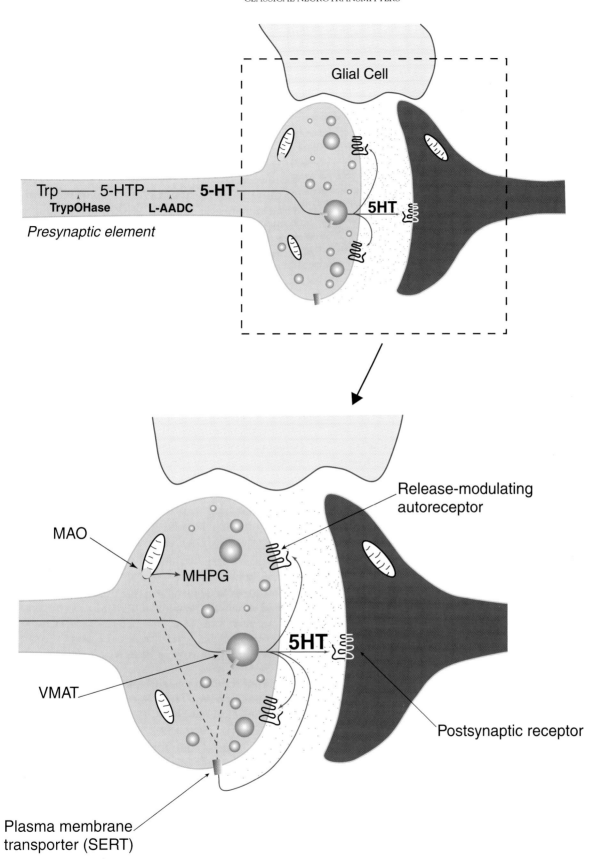

Synthesis of 5-HT

The basic process of 5-HT biosynthesis is very similar to that of catecholamine transmitters: a peripheral amino acid (tryptophan) gains entry into the brain and is metabolized in serotonergic neurons via a series of enzymatic steps that culminate in the synthesis of 5-HT. Once tryptophan enters the serotonergic neuron, it is hydroxylated by tryptophan hydroxylase, the rate-limiting step in 5-HT synthesis (see Fig. 7.5), giving rise to the 5-HT precursor 5-hydroxytryptophan (5-HTP), which is then decarboxylated by L-aromatic amino acid decarboxylase. Thus, only two critical enzymes (tryptophan hydroxylase and AADC) are involved in the synthesis of 5-HT (Cooper et al., 1996; Frazer and Hensler, 1994).

5-HT is the final product of this synthetic pathway in almost all neurons. The exception is in the pineal gland, where 5-HT is metabolized to the hormone melatonin. Although 5-HT is not metabolized to other transmitters in most of the brain, steps in tryptophan metabolism result in the formation of several potent non-transmitter molecules.

Tryptophan Hydroxylase

The rate-limiting step in 5-HT synthesis is tryptophan hydroxylation. This step is similar in many ways to that mediated by TH in the case of catecholamine biosynthesis. However, the availability of the 5-HT precursor tryptophan, an amino acid, is very important in regulating 5-HT synthesis; in sharp contrast, catecholamine synthesis under normal conditions is not regulated by precursor availability. Because 5-HT cannot cross the blood–brain barrier, brain cells must synthesize the amine. Tryptophan is present in high levels in plasma, and changes in dietary tryptophan can substantially alter brain levels of 5-HT. An active uptake process facilitates the entry of tryptophan into the brain. However, other large neutral aromatic amino acids compete for this transporter, and brain levels of tryptophan are therefore determined by plasma concentrations of competing neutral amino acids as well as tryptophan itself.

It appears that increases in intracellular 5-HT levels do not significantly decrease further 5-HT synthesis in vivo; in contrast, transmitter synthesis in catecholamine cells is influenced by end product inhibition. In both 5-HT and catecholamine synthesis, activation of the key synthetic enzyme occurs by phosphorylation. The need for long-term increases in 5-HT availability is met by the induction of new tryptophan hydroxylase protein.

L-Aromatic Amino Acid Decarboxylase

L-Aromatic amino acid decarboxylase metabolizes 5-HTP to 5-HT. This is the same enzyme that was already discussed in the context of catecholamine biosynthesis. In both catecholamine and 5-HT cells, the precursor (DOPA in DA neurons and 5-HTP in 5-HT neurons) is almost instantaneously converted (into DA and 5-HT) by AADC. Because AADC is not saturated with 5-HTP under basal conditions, it is possible to increase the content of 5-HT in brain not only by increasing dietary tryptophan, but also by administering 5-HTP, which enters the brain readily.

Alternative Tryptophan Metabolic Pathways

Although 5-HT is typically the final transmitter product of tryptophan synthesis, 5-HT in the brain and periphery can be metabolized further to yield important active products. In the pineal gland, 5-HT is metabolized through two enzymatic steps to form 5-methoxy-N-acetyltryptamine (melatonin), a hormone that is thought to play an important role in both sexual behavior and sleep. In peripheral tissues, most tryptophan is not metabolized to 5-HT but is instead metabolized by the kynurenine pathway. Data indicate that this kynurenine shunt is also present in the brain and leads to the accumulation of several interesting active substances. The two major tryptophan metabolites generated by the kynurenine shunt are quinolinic and kynurenic acids. Quinolinic acid is a potent agonist at N-methyl-D-aspartate (NMDA) Glu receptors, which are discussed in Chapter 9. Quinolinic acid causes cell loss and convulsions; in contrast, kynurenine is an antagonist at NMDA receptors. These compounds are the focus of considerable clinical interest.

Storage and Release of 5-HT

5-HT is stored in vesicles and is released by an exocytotic mechanism. The vesicular amine transporter that accumulates 5-HT is the same as that in catecholamine neurons (VMAT2). Because catecholamines and 5-HT share a common vesicular transporter, it is not surprising that reserpine, which depletes vesicular stores of catecholamines, also depletes 5-HT from serotonergic neurons.

As in catecholamine neurons, functionally dissociable somatodendritic and terminal autoreceptors regulate the release and firing rate of 5-HT neurons. The responsible receptor, designated 5-HT$_{1A}$, is one of about 15 different 5-HT receptors!

Inactivation of Released 5-HT

Like the catecholamines, 5-HT that is released into the synapse is inactivated primarily by reuptake through SERT. This transporter belongs to the same family of 12 transmembrane domain transporters as the catecholamine transporters and shares many characteristics with other transporter family members. SERT is an important clinical target for therapeutic drugs. For example, antidepressant drugs such as fluoxetine (Prozac) are selective 5-HT reuptake inhibitors. Because antidepressant drugs increase 5-HT or NE levels by either blocking SERT or NET or disrupting enzymatic inactivation of these monoamines, the dominant theories of the pathogenesis of depression posit critical modulatory roles for NE and 5-HT. Cocaine, which blocks both SERT and DAT, has been used in the past as an antidepressant.

The enzymatic degradation of 5-HT is catalyzed by monoamine oxidase (MAO). The product of this reaction, 5-hydroxyindole acid aldehyde, can be oxidized further to 5-hydroxy-indole acetic acid, which is the primary metabolite of 5-HT. MAO inhibitors increase 5-HT levels and have been used as antidepressants (see Box 7.2).

γ-Aminobutyric Acid: The Major Inhibitory Neurotransmitter

A number of amino acids fulfill most of the criteria for consideration as neurotransmitters. The best studied of these are γ-aminobutyric acid (GABA), the major inhibitory transmitter in brain, and glutamate (Glu), which is the major excitatory transmitter in brain (Paul, 1995). Although certain aspects of the synthesis of amino acid transmitters are less well understood than for catecholamines, many of the principles outlined in the discussion of catecholamines apply to amino acid transmitters.

A major difference between catecholamine and amino acid transmitters is that the latter are derived from glucose metabolism. This dual role for amino acid transmitters means that mechanisms must exist to segregate the transmitter and general metabolic pools of the amino acid transmitters (see Delorcy and Olsen, 1994). A second difference between amino acid and catecholamine transmitters is that the former are taken up readily by glia as well as neurons.

GABA was discovered in 1950 by Eugene Roberts, whose subsequent studies revealed that GABA has a neurotransmitter role. GABA is ubiquitous in the CNS, as might be expected for a transmitter derived from the metabolism of glucose. Although the transmitter GABA is widespread, it nonetheless has a distinct distribution in different types of cells in the brain.

GABA Biosynthesis

Several aspects of the synthesis of GABA differ from that of the monoamines (see Fig. 7.6). Most of these differences relate to precursors of GABA being part of cellular intermediary metabolism rather than dedicated solely to a neurotransmitter synthetic pool.

The GABA Shunt and GABA Transaminase

GABA is ultimately derived from glucose metabolism. α-Ketoglutarate formed by the Krebs (tricarboxylic acid) cycle is transaminated to the amino acid glutamate by the enzyme GABA-oxoglutarate transaminase (GABA-T). In those cells in which GABA is used as a transmitter, the presence of the enzyme glutamic acid decarboxylase (GAD) permits the formation of GABA from Glu derived from α-ketoglutarate (Paul, 1995).

One unusual feature of GABA synthesis is that intraneuronal GABA is inactivated by the actions of GABA-T, which appears to be associated with mitochondria (Fig. 7.6). Thus, GABA-T is both a key synthetic enzyme and a degradative enzyme! GABA-T metabolizes GABA to succinic semialdehyde, but only if α-ketoglutarate is present to receive the amino group that is removed from GABA. This unusual GABA shunt serves to maintain supplies of GABA.

Glutamic Acid Decarboxylase

As with other classical transmitters, the biosynthesis of GABA requires a critical biosynthetic enzyme, glutamic acid decarboxylase. This enzyme is found exclusively in neurons in which GABA is a neurotransmitter. Two isoforms of GAD are encoded by two genes (Erlander and Tobin, 1991). These two isoforms, designated GAD65 and GAD67 in accord with their molecular weights, exhibit somewhat different intracellular distributions, suggesting that the two isoforms may be regulated in different ways. This appears to be the case. GAD65 and GAD67 differ significantly in their affinity for the pyridoxal cofactor: GAD65 shows a relatively high affinity for the cofactor, whereas the larger GAD isoform does not. The affinity of GAD65 for cofactor results in the ability of GAD65 to be regulated efficiently by increasing enzymatic activity. In contrast, increased demand for GAD67 usually involves the synthesis of a new enzyme.

A major question concerning amino acid transmitters is how the transmitter pools are kept distinct from the general metabolic pools in which the amino acids serve. GAD is required for the synthesis of the

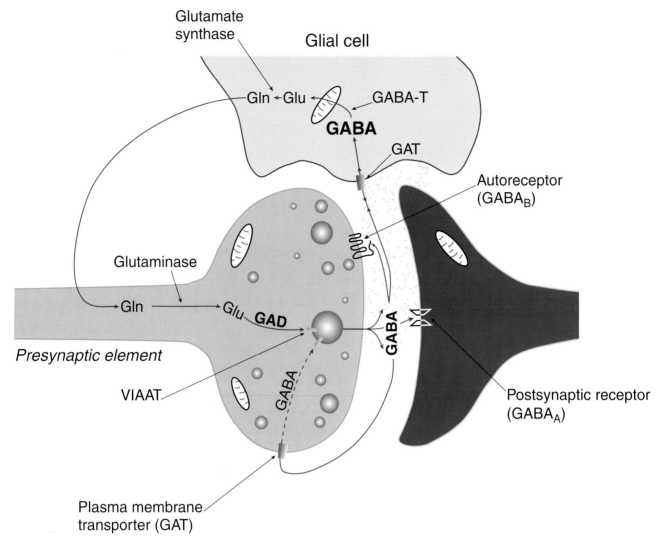

FIGURE 7.6 Schematic depiction of the life cycle of a GABAergic neuron. α-Ketoglutarate formed in the Krebs cycle is transaminated to glutamate (Glu) by GABA transaminase (GABA-T). The transmitter GABA is formed from the Glu by glutamic acid decarboxylase (GAD). GABA that is released is taken by high-affinity GABA transporters (GAT) present on neurons and glia.

transmitter GABA, and the presence of GAD is a marker of GABAergic neurons. GAD is a cytosolic enzyme, but GABA-T, which converts α-ketoglutarate into the GAD substrate glutamate, is present in mitochondria. Thus, the metabolic pool is present in mitochondria, and Glu destined for the transmitter pool must be exported from mitochondria to the cytosol. This process is poorly understood.

Glu is not only a precursor to the formation of GABA, but is also the major excitatory neurotransmitter (see later). GAD is usually not present in neurons in which Glu is a transmitter, and thus glutamatergic neurons do not use GABA as a transmitter. Why GABA

neurons fail to use the precursor Glu as a transmitter may involve two different biosynthetic enzymes for the transmitter and metabolic pools of Glu and different vesicular transporters for Glu and GABA. A neuronal enzyme that is localized to vesicles has been proposed to be responsible for the synthesis of the transmitter pool of Glu. Because GABA hyperpolarizes cells rapidly, wheares Glu depolarizes neurons rapidly, it is not surprising that the two amino acid transmitter pools are not generally colocalized. However, in some brain regions, isolated neurons are seen in which GABA and Glu have been reported. The functional significance of such an arrangement is not clear.

Storage and Release of GABA

Vesicular Inhibitory Amino Acid Transporter

A vesicular GABA transporter has been identified. This transporter was cloned on the basis of homology to a related protein (unc-47) in the worm *Caenorhabditis elegans*. The strategy of moving from invertebrate to mammalian species has proven a very useful approach in identifying a variety of mammalian transmitter-related genes. The vesicular GABA transporter has 10 transmembrane domains, and thus differs from the vesicular monoamine transporters. The vesicular GABA transporter shares with the VMATs, however, a lack of substrate specificity, and will transport the inhibitory transmitter glycine as well as GABA. Consistent with this pharmacology, the vesicular GABA transporter has been found in glycine- as well as GABA-containing neurons. Accordingly, the protein is more accurately called the vesicular inhibitory amino acid transporter. Some rare GABA cells may lack the transporter, raising the specter of a related transporter or some unique functional attribute of these cells.

Regulation of GABA Release by Autoreceptors

The major postsynaptic GABA receptor is the GABA$_A$ receptor, which contains the chloride ion channel (see Chapter 9). Pharmacological studies indicate that the autoreceptor-mediated regulation of GABA neurons takes place predominantly through GABA$_B$ receptors located on GABAergic nerve terminals. Anatomical studies have revealed that both GABA$_B$ and GABA$_A$ receptors are present on postsynaptic non-GABAergic neurons. It is possible that these postsynaptic GABA$_B$ sites respond to GABA released from a neuron that is presynaptic to another GABA neuron. However, an anatomical arrangement of one GABA neuron terminating on another GABA cell would have the same functional consequence as an autoreceptor (decreasing subsequent transmitter release).

Inactivation of Released GABA

The ability of glia cells to accumulate GABA and Glu distinguishes amino acid from classical transmitters. This dual glial–neuronal reuptake process may have arisen because amino acids play dual roles as both transmitters and metabolic intermediaries.

GABA Transporter Proteins

Reuptake is the primary mode of inactivation of the transmitter GABA. At least three specific GABA transporter (GAT) proteins are expressed in the CNS,

providing a diverse means of regulating GABA neurons. In addition, a betaine transporter that accumulates GABA has been cloned. Early studies defined two types of GABA transporters as neuronal or glial, based on pharmacological criteria. However, the cloning of GABA transporters and subsequent anatomical studies revealed that one of the GATs found in brain (defined as a glial transporter on pharmacological grounds) is present in both neurons and glia.

The presence of multiple neuronal transporters for the same transmitter is seen in amino acid but not catecholamine or indoleamine neurons (which express a single membrane-associated transporter protein with relatively poor substrate specificity). The reason for multiple GABA transporters is not clear. GATs are expressed in both GABAergic and non-GABAergic cells (presumably cells that receive a GABA innervation). It is possible that different transporters are targeted differently in the cell, with one found in dendrites and another in axons, with somewhat different functional roles. Another possibility is that GATs may be cotransporters for other amino acids; transporters for β-alanine and taurine have not been cloned, but these amino acids are accumulated by GATs. Finally, it is possible that one or more of these transporters often works in the outward direction, serving to "release" GABA.

Enzymatic Inactivation of GABA

GABA transaminase (GABA-T) is both a synthetic and a degradative enzyme, with both enzymatic functions conserving the transmitter pool of GABA. GABA-T is found in non-GABAergic and GABA-containing neurons and in a number of peripheral tissues. Electron microscopic studies suggest that GABA-T is associated with mitochondria. However, pharmacological studies of different subcellular fractions suggest that the activity of GABA-T observed in synaptosomes that contain mitochondria is less than that seen in synaptosomal membrane fractions that lack mitochondria. Thus, GABA may be metabolized either extraneuronally or in postsynaptic neurons.

Glutamate and Aspartate: Excitatory Amino Acid Transmitters

Excitatory amino acid transmitters account for most of the fast synaptic transmission that occurs in the mammalian brain. Glu and aspartate are the major excitatory amino acid neurotransmitters, and several related amino acids, such as *N*-acetylaspartylglutamate, are also thought to have neurotransmitter roles. Excitatory amino acids, like the inhibitory amino acid GABA, participate in both intermediary metabolism and neuronal communication. The intertwining of the roles of amino acids as transmitters and key players in cellular metabolism has made it difficult for investigators to demonstrate that these compounds fulfill all of the criteria for neurotransmitter status. Nonetheless, it is now accepted that glutamate and aspartate are excitatory neurotransmitters.

Biosynthesis of Glutamate

Neither Glu nor aspartate crosses the blood–brain barrier. Brain levels of these transmitters are derived only by local synthesis from glucose. Two processes lead to Glu synthesis in the nerve terminal. As discussed earlier, Glu is formed from glucose through the Krebs cycle and transamination of α-ketoglutarate. In addition, Glu can be formed directly from glutamine (see Fig. 7.7). Because glutamine is synthesized in glial cells, both neurons and glia are impor-

tant in determining the transmitter pool of glutamate. Glutamine is exported from glia and is transported into nerve terminals before being converted into Glu by a glutaminase enzyme (Dingledine and McBain, 1994). A mitochondrial phosphate-activated glutaminase (PAG) has been advanced as the specific form of glutaminase that gives rise to the transmitter pool of Glu. However, PAG is also found in high concentrations in tissues such as the liver. The process by which Glu is exported from the mitochondrion to allow vesicular glutamate storage is not understood.

Storage and Release of Glutamate

Vesicular Glutamate Transporter

Glutamate is released from synaptic vesicles by a calcium-dependent process. Although the vesicular

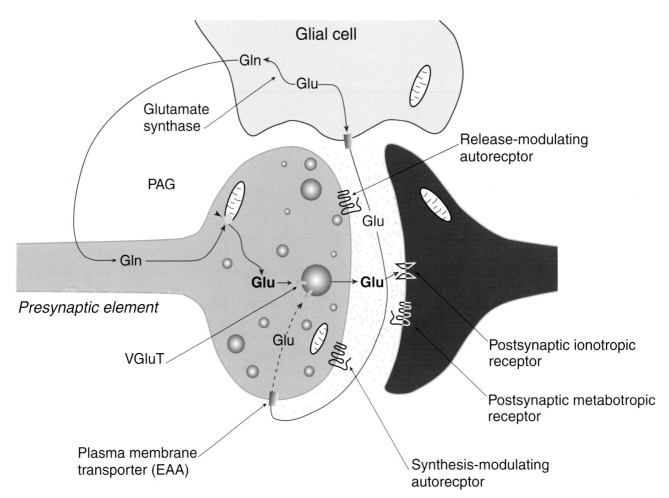

FIGURE 7.7 Depiction of an excitatory amino acid (glutamate) synapse. Glutamate, synthesized via metabolic pathways, is concentrated through a vesicular transporter into secretory granules. After release from the presynaptic terminal, glutamate can interact with postsynaptic and/or release-modulating receptors. Glutamate is then cleared from the synaptic region by high-affinity plasma membrane transporters or by recycling through adjacent glia.

storage of glutamate has been known for quite some time, the vesicular Glu transporter has been cloned only recently. This is related in part to the fact that the vesicular Glu transporter is not related to other transmitter transporters, although it has significant sequence homology with a worm protein implicated in glutamatergic transmission. The vesicular Glu transporter is the same protein that was suggested previously to mediate the sodium-dependent transport of inorganic phosphate. It is found predominantly in axon terminals.

Regulation of Glutamate Release

Glutamate release is regulated by an autoreceptor. Three broad classes of postsynaptic excitatory amino acid receptors that form ion channels (see Chapter 9). However, the autoreceptor that regulates Glu release is a metabotropic rather than ionotropic receptor. Eight different receptors (and various splice variants) that comprise three classes of metabotropic Glu receptors have been identified. The release-modulating autoreceptor is a member of one class (group II) of metabotropic receptors that is coupled negatively to adenylyl cyclase. Both members of the group II family (the mGluR2 and mGluR3 receptors) are found on presynaptic glutamatergic axon terminals, and a large number of studies have revealed that class II receptors function as release-modulating Glu receptors. Electrophysiological studies have also suggested an impulse-modulating Glu autoreceptor, suggested to be either an mGluRl or an mGluR5 site. The eight different metabotropic Glu receptors subserve an extremely broad array of functions and appear to be critically involved in regulating not only Glu function, but also the activity (including release) of a several other transmitters, ranging from classical transmitters such as DA to peptide transmitters such as substance P (see Cartmell and Schoepp, 2000).

Inactivation of Glutamate

Glu inactivation occurs predominantly by reuptake through plasma membrane transporters. In contrast to GABA and other classical transmitters, there does not appear to be a significant role for the enzymatic inactivation of Glu. The extent to which diffusion regulates synaptic and extracellular levels of Glu is not clear.

Five Glu transporters have been cloned, with some localized to glia and others to neurons. Electron microscopic studies suggest that Glu transporters are expressed heavily in astrocytes but expressed weakly in neurons. Glu transporters accumulate L-Glu and D- and L-aspartate. The affinities of the different Glu transporters are similar for Glu itself but differ for other amino acids. The transporters have distinct brain distributions, and even the glial transporters exhibit regional and intracellular differences in expression (Chaudhry *et al.*, 1996), underscoring the heterogeneity of glia as well as neurons.

The presence of certain Glu transporters on glial cells is consistent with the intricate interplay of glial and neuronal elements. Because Glu released from neurons is accumulated by glia and is then metabolized to glutamine, there is an ultimate recycling of the released amino acid. The fate of Glu accumulated by the neuronal Glu transporter is unclear. It has not been established if Glu released from a given neuron is taken up by a Glu transporter on that particular neuron or, alternatively, by Glu transporters on other neurons or glia.

Acetylcholine

The fundamental concepts of chemical synaptic transmission are based on early studies of acetylcholine, which was first proposed to be a transmitter over a century ago. A key reason for ACh playing such a prominent role in guiding early studies of neurotransmitters is the relative ease with which ACh can be studied. Acetylcholine is the transmitter at the neuromuscular junction of mammals. The ability to expose and maintain isolated preparations of the neuromuscular junction permitted electrophysiological and biochemical studies of synaptic transmission. Electrophysiological studies revealed fast excitatory responses of muscle fibers to the stimulation of nerves innervating the muscle. The presence of miniature end plate potentials (mEPPs) in muscle fiber was noted, and in the early 1950s, Fatt and Katz demonstrated that these mEPPs resulted from the slow "leakage" of ACh, with each mEPP representing the release of transmitter in one vesicle (termed a quantum). Overt depolarization generated an increase in the number of quanta released over a given period of time (see Chapter 8).

Over the past half century many of the rules that govern ACh neurotransmission have been shown to be general principles that apply to other transmitters. For example, the concept of the quantal nature of neurotransmission is central to current ideas of transmitter release. Although the discovery of different neurotransmitters has expanded our knowledge, studies of ACh continue to provide a foundation for modern concepts of chemical neurotransmission.

Acetylcholine Synthesis

The synthesis of ACh is among the simplest of any transmitter, having but a single step: the acetyl group from acetyl-coenzyme A is transferred to choline by

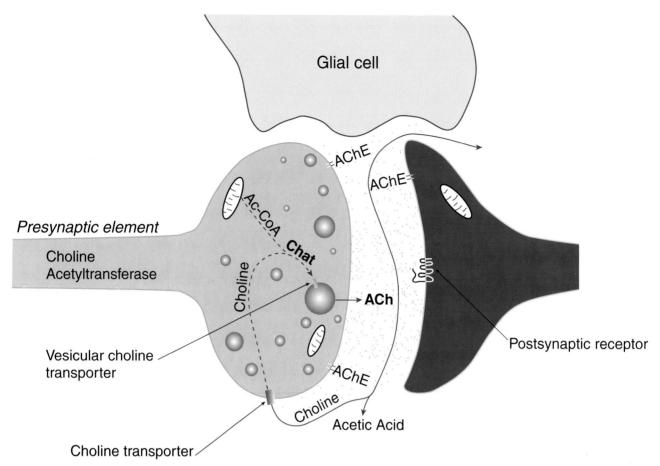

FIGURE 7.8   Acetylcholine (ACh) synthesis, release, and termination of action are shown. A choline transporter accumulates choline. The enzyme choline acetyltransferase (ChAT) acetylates the choline using acetyl-CoA (Ac-CoA) to form the transmitter ACh, which is accumulated into vesicles by the vesicular transporter. The released ACh may interact with postsynaptic muscarinic or nicotinic cholinergic receptors or can be taken up into the neuron by a choline transporter. Acetylcholine can be degraded after release by the enzyme acetylcholine esterase (AChE).

the enzyme choline acetyltransferase (ChAT). There are correspondingly few requirements for ACh synthesis: the presence of the substrate choline, the donor acetyl-coenzyme A, and ChAT (see Fig. 7.8).

The acetyl-CoA that serves as the donor is derived from pyruvate generated by glucose metabolism. This obligatory dependence on a metabolic intermediary is similar to the situation present in GABA synthesis, where the immediate precursor Glu is formed from α-ketoglutarate. Acetyl-CoA is localized to mitochondria. Because the synthetic enzyme ChAT is cytoplasmic, acetyl-CoA must exit the mitochondria to gain access to ChAT.

Choline Acetyltransferase

Choline acetyltransferase is the definitive marker for cholinergic neurons. Multiple mRNAs encode ChAT, resulting from the differential use of three pro-

moters and alternative splicing of the 5′ noncoding region of the gene. In the rat, the different transcripts encode the same protein, but in human give rise to multiple forms of the enzyme, including both active and inactive (truncated) forms. The functional significance of the different transcripts under normal and disease conditions is a topic of considerable interest.

Although ChAT is the sole enzyme involved in the synthesis of ACh, it is not the rate-limiting step in ACh synthesis. The full enzymatic activity of ChAT is not expressed *in vivo*: ChAT activity, when measured *in vitro*, is much greater than would be expected on the basis of ACh synthesis *in vivo*. The reason for this discrepancy has been suggested to be related to the requirement that acetyl-CoA be transported from the mitochondria to the cytoplasm, a process that may be rate limiting. Alternatively, intracellular choline concentrations may determine the rate of ACh synthesis. This latter idea has led to the use of choline precursors in attempts to enhance ACh synthesis in Alzheimer disease, in which there is a marked decrease of cortical ACh levels. Attempts have been made to treat Alzheimer disease with lecithin, a choline precursor; unfortunately, lecithin does not diminish dementia, but does cause bad breath.

Acetylcholine Storage and Release

Vesicular Cholinergic Transporter

ACh is synthesized by ChAT and is taken up into storage vesicles by the vesicular cholinergic transporter (VAChT). This transporter is distinct from the membrane transporter that accumulates choline. The VAChT is expressed in cholinergic neurons throughout the brain.

The cloning of human VAChT revealed that the gene was localized to chromosome 10, near the ChAT gene for ChAT. It was then demonstrated that the entire VAChT coding region is contained in the first intron of the ChAT gene. This suggested that both genes are coordinately regulated, a suspicion that was subsequently confirmed.

Cholinergic Autoreceptor Function

Cholinergic release-modulating autoreceptors have been identified in peripheral tissues and in the brain.

This receptor is a muscarinic cholinergic receptor, rather than the nicotinic receptor found at the neuromuscular junction (see Chapter 9). It appears that the brain ACh release-modulating autoreceptor is an M2 receptor, one of five muscarinic cholinergic receptors. There is scant evidence for a synthesis-modulating cholinergic autoreceptor.

Inactivation of Acetylcholine

Acetylcholinesterase

The primary mode of inactivation of ACh appears to be enzymatic, which is simply the hydrolysis of ACh to choline. Two groups of cholinesterases have been defined on the basis of substrate specificity: acetylcholinesterases (AChEs) and butyrylcholinesterases (Taylor and Brown, 1994). The former are relatively specific for ACh and are found in high concentration in the brain, whereas butyrylcholinesterases (which also efficiently hydrolyze choline esters) are enriched in the liver and are present in lower levels in the brain (see Box 7.3).

Several AChE species are encoded by a single gene that is alternatively spliced, with tissue-specific expression of different transcripts. One of the multiple mRNAs encoding AChE represents the primary form of the enzyme expressed in brain and muscle. AChE is present in high concentrations in cholinergic neurons. However, AChE is also present in moderately high

---

BOX 7.3

ACETYLCHOLINESTERASE INHIBITORS, NERVE GASES, AND PHARMACOTHERAPY

The enzymatic inactivation of acetylcholine (ACh) has been fertile ground for the development of a large number of pharmaceutical agents. Anticholinesterases such as sarin are potent neurotoxins and have been used as nerve gases since World War I. Other anticholinesterases include organophosphates (such as parathion), which are widely used insecticides. Anticholinesterases, whether the target is a human or a tomato hornworm, function in the same way: instead of the released ACh leading to discrete single depolarizations of muscle fibers, the accumulation of acetylcholine at the neuromuscular junction leads to muscle fibrillation and ultimately depolarization inactivation of the muscle, i.e., the muscle is so excited it stops!

Anticholinesterases have some less aggressive uses as well. Competitive neuromuscular blocking agents such as succinylcholine are used as an adjunct to anesthetics during surgery to increase muscle relaxation; conversely, anticholinergics can be used to reverse the muscle paralysis caused by succinylcholine. Anticholinesterases are the mainstay of the treatment of myasthenia gravis, a disorder of the neuromuscular junction that is usually marked by the presence of antinicotinic receptor antibodies. Attempts have also been made to treat Alzheimer's disease, in which there is a sharp decrease in cortical ACh, by administering an anticholinesterase to inhibit the breakdown of ACh. Unfortunately, this approach has not proven very effective.

Ariel Y. Deutch and Robert H. Roth

concentrations in some noncholinergic neurons that receive cholinergic inputs (i.e., that are cholinoceptive). This observation is consistent with the fact that AChE is a secreted enzyme that is associated with the cell membrane. Thus, ACh hydrolysis takes place extracellularly, and the choline generated is conserved by the high-affinity reuptake process.

In addition to its role in inactivating acetylcholine, AChE has been proposed to be a chemical messenger in the CNS (Greenfield, 1991). AChE release from central neurons is calcium dependent and cerebellar release is elicited by the electrical stimulation of cerebellar afferents. Electrophysiological studies have revealed that AChE elicits changes in the threshold for Ca^{2+} spikes, and local application of AChE enhances the responses of cerebellar neurons to Glu and aspartate, transmitters present in the axons innervating the cerebellum.

High-Affinity Choline Transporter

A low-affinity reuptake process for choline is widely distributed in the body, and choline is present in the blood in high concentration. Both low and high affinity choline uptake processes are present in brain. Cholinergic neurons in the brain express a sodium-dependent transporter that is saturated at plasma levels of choline, consistent with high affinity choline uptake.

In contrast to other plasma membrane transmitter transporters, the choline transporter is not involved directly in termination of the action of release transmitter. Because ACh is hydrolyzed by AChE, enzymatic inactivation is the major means of terminating cholinergic transmission. In the absence of direct evidence that choline binds with high affinity to cholinergic receptor, it appears that the function of the choline transporter is conservation of transmitter stores.

Summary of Classical Transmitters

Classical neurotransmitters are small molecules that are derived from either amino acids or intermediary metabolism. They are usually synthesized by the sequential actions of key enzymes, in the general vicinity of where they are to be released. Release is elicited by depolarization and is calcium dependent. Once released, the transmitter is inactivated by a specific reuptake mechanism, by enzymatic means, or both mechanisms.

Criteria for transmitter status are based in large part on experiments conducted in peripheral sites such as the neuromuscular junction. The relatively high concentrations of classical transmitters made measurement of transmitter release a key criterion, but one that would prove difficult to meet for those transmitters discovered since the 1970s. Nevertheless, the increasing sensitivity of analytical techniques, coupled with the ingenuity of neuroscientists, led to the uncovering of a large number of peptides, growth factors, and even gases that functioned as transmitters. The next section explores the similarities and differences of the classical transmitters with these new kids on the block. These differences have often illuminated unknown fundamental processes of neurons and expanded our concept of information flow between neurons.

NONCLASSICAL NEUROTRANSMITTERS

There are many more peptide transmitters than classical transmitters. Although there are clear differences between classical and peptide transmitters and "unconventional" transmitters, the different classes of transmitters have much in common. For example, both classical and peptide transmitters are often remarkably well conserved across species; many of the peptide transmitters or closely related peptides were initially isolated from amphibian species. In addition, both classical and peptide transmitters are synthesized in neurons, where they are stored in vesicles and released in a Ca^{2+}-dependent manner. However, the biosynthetic mechanisms and the modes of inactivation of peptide and classical transmitters are quite different. We will first consider the question of the significance of multiple neurotransmitters, then turn to the general principles of peptide transmitter biosynthesis and inactivation, which are illustrated by examining the details of the life cycle of neurotensin, and finally discuss unconventional transmitters.

Why Do Neurons Have So Many Transmitters?

About a dozen classical transmitters and dozens of neuropeptides function as transmitters. If the role of transmitters is to serve as a chemical bridge that conveys information between two spatially distinct cells, why have so many chemical messengers? Several different factors, ranging from the intracellular localization of transmitters to the different firing rates and patterns of neurons, probably contribute to the need for multiple transmitters.

Afferent Convergence on a Common Neuron

Perhaps the simplest explanation for multiple transmitters is that many afferent nerve terminals synapse onto a single neuron. A neuron must be able to distinguish between the multiple inputs that bring information to it. This need can be met in part by segregating the place on the neuron at which an input terminates: the soma, axon, or dendrite. However, because many afferents terminate in close proximity, another means of distinguishing inputs and their information is necessary: chemical coding of the inputs. Information conveyed by distinct transmitters is then distinguished by the different receptors present on the targeted neuron.

Colocalization of Neurotransmitters

Over the past generation it has become clear that a single neuron can use more than one neurotransmitter. The idea that a neuron is limited to one transmitter can be traced to Henry Dale or more accurately, to an informal restatement of what is termed Dale's principle. In the 1940s, Dale posited that a metabolic process that takes place in the cell body can reach or influence events in all the processes of the neuron. Sir John Eccles restated Dale's view to suggest that a neuron releases the same transmitter at all its processes. Illustrating the dangers of the scientific equivalent of sound bites, this principle was soon misinterpreted to indicate that only a single transmitter can be present in a given neuron.

We now know that this is not the case and that neurons can contain and use two or more transmitters. For example, a neuron can use both a classical transmitter (such as DA) and a peptide transmitter (such as neurotensin). It now appears that few, if any, neurons contain only one transmitter, and in many cases three or more transmitters are found in a single neuron.

The presence of multiple transmitters in a single neuron may indicate that different transmitters are used by a neuron to signal different functional states to its target cell. For example, the firing rates of the neurons that terminate on a postsynaptic cell differ considerably, and it may be useful to encode fast firing by one transmitter and slower firing by a transmitter in the cell. The firing *pattern* of neurons is also a means of conveying information. For example, a neuron may discharge (fire) at a rate of five times every second. This frequency can reflect a neuron discharging every 200 ms or, alternatively, a cell that fires a burst of five discharges during an initial 200-ms period followed by 800 ms of silence. Peptide transmitters are often released at higher firing rates and particularly under burst-firing patterns.

In many ways, the different synthetic steps in peptides and classical transmitters may lead to differen-

tial release. Classical transmitters can be replaced rapidly because their synthesis occurs in nerve terminals. In contrast, peptide transmitters must be synthesized in the cell body and transported to the terminal. Thus, it is useful to conserve peptide transmitters for situations of high demand because they would otherwise be depleted rapidly.

Transmitter Release from Different Processes

The restatement of Dale's principle by Eccles held that a transmitter is found in all processes of a neuron. However, in invertebrate species, it has been demonstrated that a transmitter can be localized to different parts of a neuron. It is clear that many proteins in mammalian neurons are distributed in a highly specialized manner in neurons. Although differential targeting of transmitters in mammalian neurons remains to be demonstrated conclusively, if a transmitter were restricted to a particular part of a neuron, it follows that the neuron would need multiple transmitters to account for different release sites. Receptors are very specific in their locations on neurons, and certain receptors that respond to excitatory amino acid transmitters are recruited to hot spots on neurons by the activity patterns of presynaptic inputs.

Synaptic Specializations versus Nonjunctional Appositions between Neurons

In addition to the diversity in transmitters that may result from transmitters being targeted to different intraneuronal sites, anatomical relations between one cell and its follower may contribute to the need for different transmitters. We typically think of synaptic specializations (see Chapter 3) as the morphological substrate of communication between two neurons. However, there may also be nonsynaptic communication between two neurons. These could occur across distances that are larger than conventional synaptic arrangements. In such a situation the requirements for transmitter action would differ from those discussed previously because the distance traversed by the transmitter molecule would be farther than at a synaptic apposition. Thus, transmitters that lack an efficient reuptake system, such as peptide transmitters, might be favored at nonsynaptic sites. Because a single neuron can form both synaptic and nonsynaptic specializations, a single neuron may require more than one neurotransmitter.

Fast versus Slow Responses of Target Neurons to Neurotransmitters

Different firing rates or patterns may be accompanied by changes in the type or relative amounts of a transmitter being released from a neuron. Postsynaptic responses to transmitters occur over different time scales. For example, stimulation of receptors that form ion channels leads to very rapid changes, but metabotrophic receptors that respond to catecholamines and peptide transmitters and are coupled to intracellular events through specific transduction molecules such as G proteins have slower response characteristics. The difference in temporal response characteristics is useful because it allows the receptive neuron to respond differently to a stimulus, depending on the antecedent activity in the cell. A transmitter can change the response characteristics of a particular cell to subsequent stimuli on the order of seconds or even minutes, and thus short-term changes can occur independent of changes in gene expression.

PEPTIDE TRANSMITTERS

Synthesis and Storage of Peptide Transmitters

Classical transmitters are typically synthesized in the process, such as the axon, from which they are released; peptide transmitters are usually not. In most cases, genes encoding peptide transmitters give rise to a prohormone, which is incorporated into secretory

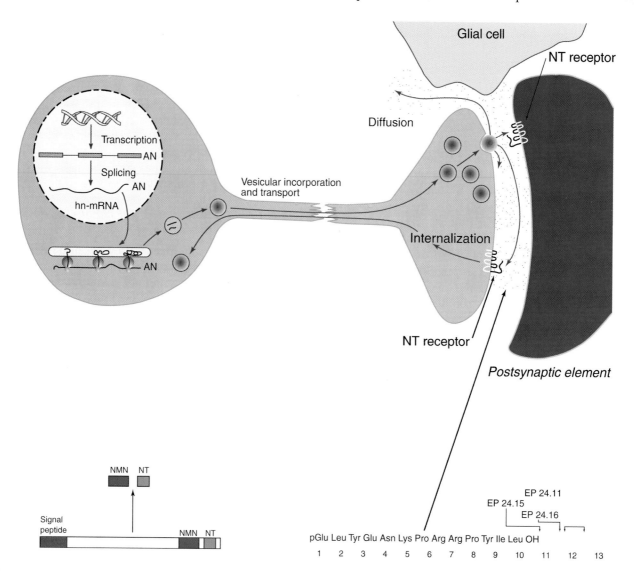

FIGURE 7.9 Schematic illustration of the synthesis, release, and termination of action of the peptide transmitter neurotensin (NT). The illustrative panels of the bottom show processing of NT from the prohormone (left) and enzymatic inactivation of NT (right).

granules after transcription; it is then acted on by peptidases to form the peptide transmitter (see Fig. 7.9). This process typically occurs in the cell body, and the peptide-containing vesicles are then transported to the axon. A few small peptide transmitters, such as carnosine (β-alanyl-L-histidine), can be synthesized enzymatically.

In neurons that use classical transmitters, the neuron meets demands for increased amounts of transmitter by increasing local synthesis of the transmitter. However, increasing the amount of a peptide transmitter requires an increase in gene expression to yield a prohormone and the subsequent delivery of peptide-containing granules to the terminal by axonal transport, which takes hours or even days. Thus, classical transmitters can respond to increased demand rapidly, but peptide transmitters cannot. This difference in biosynthetic strategies contributed to the initial difficulties in localizing the sources of peptide-containing inputs to certain brain regions. Because peptides are transported from the soma immediately after translation from mRNA and processing of the prohormone, the cell body regions and proximal processes of these neurons typically contain very low concentrations of the peptide transmitters.

The storage of peptides and classical transmitters also differs. Classical neurotransmitters are generally stored in small (approximately 50 nm) synaptic vesicles. In contrast, neuropeptide transmitters are stored in large (approximately 100 nm) dense-core vesicles. Because peptide transmitters are typically released at a high neuronal firing frequency or in a burst-firing pattern, it is reasonable to assume that there are different mechanisms for the exocytosis and subsequent release of peptide and classical transmitter vesicles. Although the release of peptide transmitters, like that of classical transmitters, is calcium dependent, data suggest that distinct but related molecular mechanisms subserve the release of small and large dense-core vesicles.

Inactivation of Peptide Transmitters

The different strategies employed for the synthesis of peptide and classical transmitters are paralleled by differences in inactivation of the released transmitter. Classical transmitters have high-affinity reuptake processes to remove the transmitter from the extracellular space. In contrast, peptide transmitters are inactivated enzymatically or by diffusion, but lack a high-affinity active reuptake process. The enzymatic inactivation of peptide transmitters also differs from that of classical transmitters. Because peptide transmitters are short chains of amino acids, the inactivating enzymes show specificity for certain types of dipeptides but are not specific to any single peptide. For example, a metalloendopeptidase that inactivates enkephalins, small pentapeptide opioid-like transmitters, is frequently called enkephalinase but is also critically involved in the inactivation of several other neuropeptides.

One final difference in the inactivation of peptide and classical transmitters is the product. Once classical transmitters are catabolized, the resultant metabolites are inactive at the transmitter receptor. However, certain peptide fragments derived from the enzymatic "inactivation" of peptide transmitters are biologically active. An example is angiotensin, in which the angiotensin I is metabolized to yield angiotensin II and III, each successively more active than the parent angiotensin I. It is therefore sometimes difficult to distinguish between synthetic processing and inactivation. The peptide that is stored in vesicles and then released is therefore considered the transmitter, although the actions of certain peptidases may lead to other biologically active fragments.

Approaches to the Study of Neuropeptide Synthesis, Release, and Inactivation

The aspects of peptide transmitter biosynthesis and inactivation that differ from those observed with classical transmitters have resulted in different methods being emphasized in the study of the two types of transmitters.

Anatomical approaches are used extensively to define those neurons in which peptides function as neurotransmitters. Using antibodies that recognize peptide transmitter prohormones can be used to identify neurons in which peptide transmitters are synthesized. Similarly, antibodies against the peptides themselves can be used to localize the transmitter to cell bodies, particularly when axonal transport has been blocked and thus prevents export of the peptide to the nerve terminals. *In situ* hybridization histochemistry has been used more recently; cRNA or cDNA probes or oligonucleotides complementary to a defined sequence of a peptide mRNA bind to the mRNA and thus identify those cells in which the peptide is found.

Biochemical studies of peptide synthesis and inactivation also emphasize different approaches from those undertaken in the study of classical transmitters. The synthesis of peptide transmitters has been studied extensively by following the rapid incorporation of radiolabeled amino acids into peptides in so-called pulse–chase experiments. More recent studies have emphasized molecular approaches because the prohormone from which the peptide will be cleaved is transcribed directly from mRNA.

The release of peptides has been studied in slices of brain, as has release of classical transmitters. However, *in vivo* studies of release of peptides were not possible until relatively recently. The measurement of metabolites as an index of transmitter release, which has been used extensively for monoamine neurons, is not applicable to peptidergic neurons for two reasons. The peptide fragments derived from the parent peptide may be similar to those of other peptides, thus confounding identification of the source. Moreover, larger peptide fragments are often degraded further to smaller peptide fragments.

In vivo microdialysis has proven useful for measuring extracellular concentrations of neuropeptides, particularly small peptides. Because the released peptide diffuses quickly across the dialysis membrane, whereas the peptidases are generally too large to do so, one can obtain measurable levels of peptides in the dialysate, provided that very sensitize and specific analytical methods are used. Because dialysis does not offer good temporal or spatial resolution, a related method has been to insert electrodes coated with antibodies into a specific area of the brain for a short period of time. Upon removal the probes are exposed to a radiolabeled peptide, which binds to receptors that are not already occupied by peptide.

Neurotensin Is a Peptide Neurotransmitter

Neurotensin (NT) is a peptide that is widely expressed in the central nervous system and in certain peripheral tissues, such as the small intestine. A related peptide, neuromedin N, is transcribed from the gene that encodes NT in mammals (see Fig. 7.8); a related peptide (LANT-6) is found in birds. Mammalian peptide transmitters are often structurally similar to peptides present in nonmammalian organisms; many peptide transmitters were originally identified in extracts of the skin of certain toads. An example is the neurotensin-like octapeptide xenopsin.

Neurotensin Synthesis

A 170 amino acid prohormone precursor of NT is encoded by a single gene that is transcribed to yield two mRNAs. The smaller transcript is the major form in the intestine; the two mRNA species are equally abundant in most brain areas. The precursor contains one copy each of NT and NMN. The molar ratios of NT/NMN differ across different tissues, suggesting different enzymatic processing of the prohormone or, alternatively, the generation of different transcripts.

Because NT and NMN are contained in the same exon of the NT-NMN gene, differences in relative abundance of the two are due to differential processing of the precursor.

NT and most peptide transmitters are stored in large dense-core vesicles. The characteristics of NT and NMN release are similar to those seen for classical transmitters. Thus, depolarization evokes the Ca^{2+}-dependent release of both NT and NMN (Kitabgi *et al.*, 1992). The impulse-dependent release of NT varies as a function of frequency and pattern of impulses. Higher frequencies of firing elicit greater NT release. The release of NT is enhanced in response to burst firing of neurons (Bean and Roth, 1992).

Inactivation of Neurotensin

There is no reuptake process by membrane transporters for peptides; instead, peptides are inactivated by enzymatic actions or diffusion. NT is inactivated by a group of enzymes called metalloendopeptidases. Three of these endopeptidases (known with great flair as 24.11, 24.15, and 24.16) degrade NT (Kitabgi *et al.*, 1992). Endopeptidase 24.11 (also known as enkephalinase for its well-characterized actions on the enkephalin peptide transmitters) cleaves NT at two specific sites to yield a decapeptide, and endopeptidase 24.16 acts at the same two sites (see Fig. 7.8); the other endopeptidase acts at a different set of amino acid residues. Because these enzymes act at dipeptides that are found in many peptides and proteins, and two of the three act at the same site, it is obvious that enzymes that inactivate peptides are not very specific.

Although there are no known membrane transporters for peptide transmitters, peptides can be accumulated by neurons. This occurs by internalization of the peptide bound to its receptor. G protein-coupled receptors undergo internalization via an endocytotic mechanism, where they are either recycled to the membrane after various steps or shipped to lysosomes for degradation (Tsao *et al.*, 2001). Receptor-bound peptides can also be internalized through this process and once inside the cell dissociate from the receptor.

The internalization of NT in midbrain DA neurons that project to the striatum, a forebrain site, has been relatively well described. What is quite unusual in this case is that NT accumulated by axon terminals in the striatum is retrogradely transported back to the cell bodies of origin in the midbrain. The functional significance of this is unclear. NT may serve as a growth factor that regulates targeted ingrowth and survival of NT-containing afferents to the striatum. Another intriguing possibility is that the peptide may function over a relatively extended period to alter gene expression in the cell that accumulates the peptide.

Coexistence of Neurotensin and Classical Transmitters

Colocalization of transmitters in mammalian neurons appears to be the norm rather than exception. For example, NT it is colocalized with DA in certain hypothalamic and midbrain neurons of the rat. The colocalization of NT and DA has provided a useful system in which to explore the interrelationships between two colocalized transmitters. In the prefrontal cortex of the rat, NT is found only in DA axons. Neurotensin release in the prefrontal cortex is increased when neuronal firing is increased or when DA neurons enter into a burst-like firing pattern (Bean and Roth, 1992). In addition, the release-modulating dopaminergic autoreceptor on DA axons appears to be closely associated with NT release. Autoreceptor-selective doses of DA agonists (which decrease DA release) enhance NT release from colocalized DA–NT axons; conversely, antagonists at the DA autoreceptor decrease NT release but enhance DA release. Thus, the release of NT and DA are regulated reciprocally by actions at a DA autoreceptor.

Summary of Peptide Transmitters

Peptide transmitters differ from classical transmitters by being synthesized in the soma rather than axon terminal. The active transmitter thus must be transported in vesicles to the nerve terminal. This suggests that transmitter release must be regulated carefully so that depletion of an important intercellular communication molecule does not occur. The termination of peptide transmitter actions differs from that of classical transmitters, being achieved mainly by enzymatic means and diffusion, and there is much less specificity in the inactivation of peptide transmitters. These differences between peptide and classical transmitters were originally viewed as inconsistent with a transmitter role of the peptides, and the common acceptance of peptides as transmitters met with considerable resistance. However, once this battle was won, the gate was opened for the consideration of radically different molecules as transmitters.

UNCONVENTIONAL TRANSMITTERS

Criteria used to define neurotransmitters were formulated early in the modern neuroscience era and were arrived at on the basis of studies of acetylcholine in peripheral sites, such as the neuromuscular junction and superior cervical ganglion. In the century since ACh was advanced as a transmitter compound, remarkable technical advances have allowed us to measure substances in the brain that are present in minute quantities or are very unstable. This has forced us to consider the possibility that substances that do not meet the established requirements for neurotransmitters may indeed be transmitters. This possibility obviously requires changing the definition of a transmitter. One simple approach would be to designate a neurotransmitter any compound that permits information flow from one neuron to another. This definition circumvents the matter of glial contribution to the ionic milieu of the neuron, which certainly imparts information concerning the function of the glia (and parenthetically points to the increasing awareness of the active roles that glia play in the CNS). However, such a definition is very similar to that of a hormone and lacks awareness of the temporal characteristics of transmitter action and the distance of the target cell from the transmitter release site. Finally, this definition does not accommodate unconventional roles for transmitters, such as the regulation of neuronal development or intracellular trafficking of proteins. Because of these considerations, we will now discuss what we have elected to call "unconventional" transmitters.

Nitric Oxide and Carbon Monoxide Are Unconventional Transmitters

Nitrates have been extensively used in the treatment of angina pectoris, characterized by chest pain due to insufficient blood delivery to the heart muscle. Nitrates dilate cardiac blood vessels, thereby increasing blood flow and relieving angina pain. However, the mechanisms by which nitroglycerine and similar nitrates elicit vasodilatation were not known until recently. In 1980, an endothelial-derived relaxing factor contained in the cells lining blood vessels was shown to dilate blood vessels potently and rapidly. This factor was soon shown to be the gas nitric oxide (NO). In addition, Glu, acting at NMDA receptors, was observed to release a factor that caused vasodilatation in brain. It soon became apparent that the endothelial-derived relaxing factor and the Glu-induced factor that caused cerebrovascular vasodilatation were the same compound and that NO was present in neurons as well as vasculature. These data, coupled with the identification of neuronal and vascular isoforms of the synthetic enzyme that makes NO [nitric oxide synthase (NOS)], led to the proposal that NO may serve as a molecule taking part in inter-

BOX 7.4

GOING FOR GASES AS NEUROTRANSMITTER

One of the most rewarding experiences for a scientist is to find that long-held prejudices are altogether wrong and that a new, correct insight reveals a novel scientific principle. In the late 1950s, only acetylcholine and the biogenic amines were known to be neurotransmitters. The next decade saw amino acids acknowledged as neurotransmitters. The discovery of enkephalins and endorphins in the mid-1970s reinforced gradually accumulating evidence that peptides are transmitters, and now we find that there are over 100 different bioactive brain peptides.

In the 1970s and early 1980s, nitric oxide (NO) was found to mediate the ability of macrophages to kill tumor cells and bacteria and to regulate blood vessel relaxation. A short report suggested that NO can be formed in brain tissue. Progress in the NO field at that time was slow because assaying NO synthase (NOS), the enzyme that oxidizes the amino acid arginine to NO, was quite tedious, based on the accumulation of nitrite formed from the NO. A much simpler approach was to monitor the conversion of [^{3}H]arginine into [^{3}H]citrulline, which is formed simultaneously with NO; this assay could process 100 or more samples in an hour. Research on blood vessels revealed that NO acts by stimulating cyclic GMP formation. In the brain, the excitatory neurotransmitter glutamate was known to augment cyclic GMP levels. Glutamate, acting through

its NMDA receptor, triples NO synthase activity in a matter of seconds, and arginine derivatives that inhibit NOS activity block the elevation of cyclic GMP. This finding causally linked the actions of so prominent a neurotransmitter as glutamate to NO.

To determine if NO was a neurotransmitter, it was necessary to ascertain whether NOS was localized in neurons. The most straightforward approach would be to generate an antibody to use in anatomical studies. However, purifying NOS protein to generate an antibody proved very difficult because the enzyme lost its activity in attempts to purify it. The addition of calmodulin was found to stabilize the enzyme. Because calmodulin is a calcium-binding protein, this finding immediately explained how NO formation can be triggered rapidly by synaptic activation through glutamate. When glutamate activates its NMDA receptor, Ca^{2+} rushes into the cell, binds to calmodulin, and activates NOS.

The ability of purified NOS led to antibodies being developed and NOS being localized by immunohistochemistry. The neuronal form of NOS (nNOS) is present in only about 1% of the neurons in the brain. However, these cells give rise to processes that ramify so extensively that probably every neuron in the brain is exposed to NO. The purified NOS protein also allowed an amino acid sequence to be obtained and the gene for the enzyme cloned. The

---

cellular communication, including neurotransmission (see Box 7.4 and Fig. 7.10).

Nitric oxide is a well-known air pollutant and thus, at the very least, an unconventional candidate for a neurotransmitter. The idea that an unstable toxic gas could serve as a transmitter led to several incredulous questions concerning the nature of neurotransmission, the most obvious being how can a gas be stored for release in an impulse-dependent manner? The answer is simple: it is not stored. If one accepts the argument that NO is a transmitter, the classical definition of a neurotransmitter becomes blurred or untenable, depending on one's perspective. Many theories can accommodate one exception. However, NO is not the only gaseous neurotransmitter; carbon monoxide and hydrogen sulfide play similar transmitter-like roles (Baranano et al., 2001).

The list of exceptions posed by NO to the dogma of traditional neurotransmitters is rather long. For example, NO is not stored in cells, is not released in

an exocytotic manner, lacks an active process that terminates its action, does not interact with specific membrane receptors on target cells, and regulates the function of axon terminals presynaptic to the neuron in which NO is synthesized. It is therefore not difficult to understand the skepticism that first met the hypothesis that NO is a neurotransmitter or to have some sympathy for those who expressed the view that NO is not a transmitter but an alien event, benign or otherwise, intent on making neuroscientists question their most cherished beliefs. The reader is referred to Box 7.4 for a discussion of NO and CO as neuronal signaling molecules.

Growth Factors as Unconventional Transmitters

The section on nitric oxide presented several striking differences between conventional and unconventional transmitters. Another class of unconventional

BOX 7.4 *(cont'd)*

structure of NOS revealed that it is regulated by many more factors than virtually any other enzyme in biology, including at least five oxidative–reductive cofactors, four phosphorylating enzymes, and three binding proteins. This makes sense because of the unique properties of NO as a gaseous neurotransmitter. Most neurotransmitters are stored in vesicles with large storage pools so that only a small amount of the transmitter is released with each nerve impulse. In contrast, every time a neuron wishes to release a molecule of NO, it must activate NOS—hence, a requirement for exquisitely subtle regulation of the enzyme.

Neurotransmitters come in chemical classes such as biogenic amines, amino acids, and peptides. Might there be at least one other gaseous neurotransmitter? Carbon monoxide (CO) is normally formed in the body by the enzyme heme oxigenase, which is primarily responsible for degrading heme in aging red blood cells. It cleaves the heme ring to form biliverdin, which is reduced rapidly to bilirubin, the pigment that accounts for jaundice in patients with a degradation of red blood cells. When the enzyme cleaves the heme ring, CO is released as a single carbon fragment.

The biosynthetic enzyme for a transmitter should be localized to selected neuronal populations. Heme oxigenise-2, the neuronal form of the enzyme, was shown to be localized to discrete neuronal populations through-out the brain. To seek a neurotransmitter function, the peripheral nervous system (in which synaptic transmission is characterized more readily than in the brain) was used. The myenteric plexus of nerves regulates intestinal peristalsis. A previously unidentified neurotransmitter of myenteric plexus neurons accounts for the relaxation phase of peristalsis. nNOS had already been localized to neurons of the myenteric plexus, and some functional evidence showed that NO might be a neurotransmitter of this pathway. Heme oxigenise-2 was found to be localized to the same myenteric plexus neurons as NOS. Mice with targeted deletions of the genes for nNOS or heme oxigenise-2 were used to elucidate function. In both types of gene knockout mice, intestinal relaxation evoked by neuronal depolarization was reduced about 50%, implying that NO and CO each contribute half of the relaxation. This finding, along with other evidence, established transmitter functions for both NO and CO and suggested that they are functioning as cotransmitters, although exactly how they interact remains a mystery. Such a cotransmitter role reminds us of the fact that most neurons in the brain contain at least two and sometimes more neurotransmitters. Thus, in addition to overturning a number of dogmas about neurotransmission, NO and CO may help resolve the riddle of cotransmission. (See also Fig. 7.10 in text.)

Solomon H. Snyder

transmitters, the growth factors, has certain features in common with the transmitter gases but differs in other ways. These molecules are discussed in detail in Chapters 18 and 19. However, we will discuss them in the context of serving as signaling molecules.

Growth factors are a group of proteins that regulate the survival, differentiation, and growth of various cell types, including neurons. Both neurotrophic factors and NO are capable of influencing presynaptic cells. NO diffuses out of cells and alters transmitter release from presynaptic axons, whereas neurotrophic factors provide support for developing axons that are growing into an area in which the target cells express growth factors. There are several different classes of growth factors, each class with multiple growth factors. Because our knowledge of the basic cellular biology of any single growth factor is incomplete, we will draw on examples from different growth factors to illustrate general characteristics of the life cycle of these transmitters.

Synthesis of Growth Factors

Early studies of growth factors typically examined crude extracts of tissue or biological fluids on some bioassay of cell survival, followed by purification and isolation of a growth factor from the crude extracts. Today the identification of growth factors often emphasizes cloning of cDNAs on the basis of sequence homology; the cloned genes are then expressed in various cell lines and tested in different bioassays.

Molecular approaches have often provided interesting and unexpected information on the synthesis of growth factors. For example, some growth factors are translated from multiple mRNAs. Brain derived neurotrophic factor (BDNF) is a growth factor that is distributied heterogeneously in the brain and has several functions, some classically associated with growth factors and others more transmitter-like. The BDNF gene has five different exons that encode the mature BDNF protein. Each of four 5' exons has a

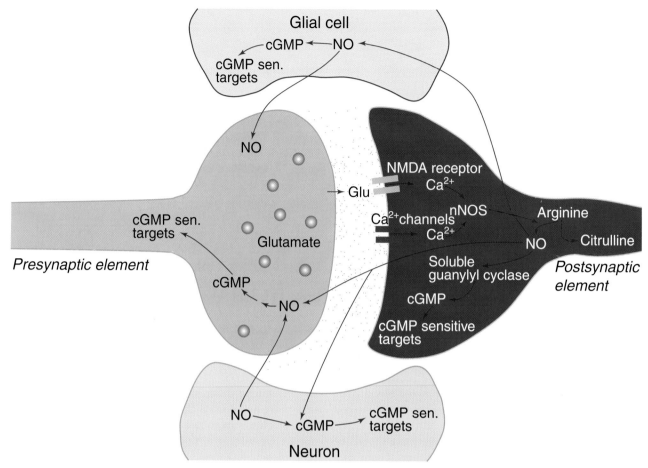

FIGURE 7.10 Schematic representation of a nitric oxide (NO)-containing neuron. NO is formed from arginine by the actions of different nitric oxide synthases (NOS). NO diffuses freely across cell membranes and can thereby influence both presynaptic neurons (such as the glutamatergic presynaptic neuron in the figure) or other cells that are not apposed directly to the NOS-containing neuron; these other cells can be neurons or glia.

separate promoter, and alternative use of these promoters and differential splicing gives rise to eight different BDNF mRNAs! Despite the complexity of the molecular "synthesis" of BDNF, there is only one mature BDNF protein; it has been speculated that various BDNF transcripts may produce BDNF protein under different conditions or give rise to different amounts of protein.

Our current knowledge of the posttranslational processing of most growth factors is limited. In the case of nerve growth factor (NGF), the mature protein is cleaved from a prohormone, similar to the synthesis of peptide transmitters. NGF prohormone processing is unique, however, in that NGF has three subunits, one of which is an enzyme that is thought to cleave the prohormone to yield the mature protein. The identity and specificity of the enzymes responsible for processing of most grown factors are only now being determined.

Storage and Release of Growth Factors

Neurons secrete proteins by two distinct processes. The constitutive pathway for secretion is not triggered by extracellular stimulation and is used to secrete membrane components, viral proteins, and extracellular matrix molecules. In contrast, the release of conventional neurotransmitters is controlled by extracellular signals and uses the so-called regulated pathway. For example, a peptide protein precursor contains an N-terminal signal sequence that allows the protein to be targeted to the endoplasmic reticulum and then to the Golgi network and ultimately be packaged into vesicles. Some growth factors lack a signal sequence, including BNDF and the related neurotrophin-3 (NT-3). Nonetheless, BDNF is often stored in vesicles and released through the regulated pathway. NT-3 is normally committed to the constitutive pathway but can be diverted to the regulated pathway, as happens in cells that are transfected with both BDNF and NT-3 (Farhadi *et al.*, 2000). It now appears that BDNF and NGF under basal conditions are constitutively released from the soma and proximal dendrites, but that depolarization leads to regulated release, which is seen in distal axons as well as in dendrites (Kohara *et al.*, 2001). This activity-dependent release does not appear to depend on extracellular Ca^{2+} but instead on intracellular Ca^{2+} stores. This is quite different from conventional transmitters, which are not released in the absence of extracellular Ca^{2+}. Thus, the release of at least certain growth factors differs from that of conventional transmitters by occurring through both constitutive and regulated pathways and by not being dependent on extracellular Ca^{2+}.

Functional Significance of Growth Factors as Neurotransmitters

Growth factors support the development, differentiation, and maintenance of neurons (see Chapter 20). The survival of neurons and targeted axonal ingrowth of the processes of neurons to their final targets requires certain factors elaborated by the target region. However, it is not clear if release of the growth factor in this context is a chemical signal that conveys information to neurons, provides critical sustenance, or both.

What information supports the contention that growth factors may be unconventional transmitters, even under the broad definition that we have used? First, growth factors are stored and released from neurons via regulated as well as constitutive pathways. Some data are consistent with the speculation that BDNF is stored in vesicles. The synthesis and release of growth factors are also under transynaptic control. For example, NGF and BDNF expression is controlled by neuronal activity, with Glu and ACh increasing expression and GABA decreasing expression of these neurotrophic factors. Moreover, the induction of BDNF by various treatments is regionally, spatially, and temporally distinct. All these characteristics suggest that the synthesis and release of these growth factors are regulated by neuronal activity, and thus growth factors both receive information and convey information across cells. Receptors for growth factors are expressed in neurons, and neurotrophic factor-induced activation of such receptors regulates certain key intracellular signaling pathways. For example, BDNF stimulates phosphoinositide turnover in neurons and thus shares with NO the ability to regulate a key intracellular transduction mechanism.

Summary

Molecules such as gases and growth factors almost seem to be designed as challenges to the criteria for classical transmitters. They may be synthesized by the constitutive as well as the regulated pathway, are not necessarily stored, do not obligatorily depend on calcium and fusion of vesicles with the membrane for release, and make a mockery of the designation of neurons as pre- and postsynaptic because their influence can be on one or even two or more neurons away.

SYNAPTIC TRANSMISSION IN PERSPECTIVE

Several of the key proteins involved in regulating chemical neurotransmission in mammals have been identified on the basis of homologies to proteins found in invertebrates such as the worm *C. elegans* and the fly *Drosophila melanogaster*. It now appears that some of the molecules used as neurotransmitters are even found in plants, as are their receptors! As nervous systems have become elaborated evolutionarily, many transmitter-related proteins have maintained roles that are not directly related to transmitter function or, alternatively, are involved in less discrete and more spatially elaborate signaling.

An example is acetylcholine, the synthesis of which depends on the cytosolic enzyme choline acetyltransferase. ChAT mRNA is also found in the testes, leading to the appearance of ACh in spermatazoa. There is even one form of ChAT that is targeted to the nucleus of cells. ChAT mRNA has also been reported to be present in lymphocytes, as have certain muscarinic cholinergic receptors. Also found in these white blood cells are AChE mRNAs, and both acetylcholinesterase and butyrylcholinesterase enzyme activity has been reported decreased in Alzheimer's disease. Still another example is the presence of AChE in bone marrow cells and peripheral blood cells in certain leukemias; recent data indicate that inhibition of AChE gene expression in bone marrow suppresses apoptosis, or programmed cell death (see Chapters 19 and 20).

We have discussed chemically coded synaptic transmission. However, one cannot discuss the biochemistry and pharmacology of synaptic transmission without referring to and appreciating critical information about the structure (anatomy) and function (physiology and behavior) of neurons. Neuroscience is multidisciplinary, requiring an understanding of different aspects of cellular function to come to grips with the basic principles of synaptic communication.

Our concepts of synaptic transmission are in flux, requiring frequent reevaluation and revision. This can be seen most clearly in the evolving definition of a neurotransmitter. Classical transmitters are but one part of the family of transmitters, with other relatives being peptides, gases, and growth factors. The somewhat bewildering number of transmitters becomes still more confusing when one considers that multiple transmitters are found in single neurons. Some transmitters are stored, whereas others are synthesized quickly in response to key stimuli. Use of the terms "conventional" and "unconventional" in discussing transmitters is indicative of our current unease with the expanding definition of transmitters. This dynamic state of affairs is seen in all areas of neuroscience and helps make neuroscience such an exciting discipline.

References

Baranano, D. E., Ferris, C. D., and Snyder, S. H. (2001). Atypical neural messengers. *Trends Neurosci.* **24**, 99–106.

Bean, A. J., and Roth, R. H. (1992). Dopamine-neurotensin interactions in mesocortical neurons, Evidence from microdialysis studies. *Ann. N.Y. Acad. Sci.* **668**, 43–53.

Cartmell, J., and Schoepp, D. D. (2000). Regulation of neurotransmitter release by metabotropic glutamate receptors. *J. Neurochem.* **75**, 889–907.

Chaudhry, F. A., Lehre, K. P., van Lookeren Campagne, M., Otterson, O. P., Danbolt, N. C., and Storm-Mathisen, J. (1996). Glutamate transporters in glial plasma membranes, Highly differentiated localizations revealed by quantitative ultrastructural immunocytochemistry. *Neuron* **15**, 711–720.

Cooper, J. R., Bloom, F. E., and Roth, R. H. (1996). "The Biochemical Basis of Neuropharmacology," 7th Ed. Oxford Univ. Press, New York.

Farhadi, H. F., Mowla, S. J., Petrecca, K., Morris, S. J., Seidah, N. G., and Murphy, R. A. (2000). Neurotrophin-3 sorts to the constitutive secretory pathway of hippocampal neurons and is diverted to the regulated secretory pathway by coexpression with brain-derived neurotrophic factor. *J. Neurosci.* **20**(11), 4059–4068.

DeLorcy, T. N., and Olsen, R. W. (1994). GABA and glycine. *In* "Basic Neurochemistry" (G. J. Siegel, B. W. Agranoff, R. W. Albers, and P. B. Molinoff, eds.), 5th Ed., pp. 389–400. Raven Press, New York.

Dingeldine, R., and McBain, C. J. (1994). Excitatory amino acid transmitters. *In* "Basic Neurochemistry" (G. J. Siegel, B. W. Agranoff, R. W. Albers, and P. B. Molinoff, eds.), 5th Ed., pp. 367–388. Raven Press, New York.

Erlander, M. G., and Tobin, A. J. (1991). The structural and functional heterogeneity of glutamic acid decarboxylase, A review. *Neurochem. Res.* **16**, 215–226.

Frazer, A., and Hensler, J. G. (1994). Serotonin. *In* "Basic Neurochemistry" (G. J. Siegel, B. W. Agranoff, R. W. Albers, and P. B. Molinoff, eds.), 5th Ed., pp. 283–309. Raven Press, New York.

Gainetdinov, R. R., Jones, S. R., Fumagalli, F., Wightman, R. M., and Caron, M. G. (1998). Re-evaluation of the role of the dopamine transporter in dopamine system homeostasis. *Brain Res. Rev.* **26**, 148–153.

Greenfield, S. A. (1991). A non-cholinergic role of AChE in the substantia nigra, From neuronal secretion to the generation of movement. *Mol. Cell. Neurobiol.* **11**, 55–77.

Kitabgi, P., De Nadal, F., Rovere, C., and Bidard, J.-N. (1992). Biosynthesis, maturation, release, and degradation of neurotensin and neuromedin N. *Ann. N.Y. Acad. Sci.* **668**, 30–42.

Kohara, K., Kitamura, A., Morishima, M., and Tsumoto, T. (2001). Activity-dependent transfer of brain-derived neurotrophic factor to postsynaptic neurons. *Science* **291**, 2419–2423.

Paul, S. P. (1995). GABA and glycine. *In* "Neuropyschopharmacology: The Fourth Generation of Progress" (F. E. Bloom and D. J. Kupfer, eds.), pp. 87–94. Raven Press, New York.

Poo, M. M. (2001). Neurotrophins as synaptic modulators. *Nature Rev. Neurosci.* **2**, 24–32.

Shepherd, G. M. (1991). "Foundations of the Neuron Doctrine." Oxford Univ. Press, New York.

Taylor, P., and Brown, J. H. (1994). Acetylcholine. *In* "Basic Neurochemistry" (G. J. Siegel, B. W. Agranoff, R. W. Albers, and P. B. Molinoff, Eds.), 5th Ed. Raven Press, New York.

Tsao, P., Cao, T., and von Zastrow, M. (2001). Role of endocytosis in mediating downregulation of G-protein-coupled receptors. *Trends Pharmacol. Sci.* **22**, 91–6.

Weihe, E., Eiden, L. E. (2000). Chemical neuroanatomy of the vesicular amine transporters. *FASEB J.* **14**, 2435–2449.

Xu, F., Gainetdinov, R. R., Wetsel, W. C., Jones, S. R., Bohn, L. M., Miller, G. W., Wang, Y. M., and Caron, M. G. (2000). Mice lacking the norepinephrine transporter are supersensitive to psychostimulants. *Nature Neurosci.* **3**, 465–471.

Ariel Y. Deutch and Robert H. Roth

Release of Neurotransmitters

The synapse is the primary place at which information is transmitted from neuron to neuron or from neuron to peripheral target, be it a gland or a muscle. Most synapses rely on a chemical intermediary, or transmitter, secreted in response to an action potential in the presynaptic cell in order to influence the activity of the postsynaptic cell. In chemical transmission, a single action potential in a small presynaptic terminal can generate a large *postsynaptic potential* (PSP) (as large as tens of millivolts). This is accomplished by the release of thousands to hundreds of thousands of molecules of transmitter that can bind to postsynaptic receptor molecules and open (or close) thousands of ion channels in about 1 ms. The effect can be either excitatory or inhibitory, depending on the ions that permeate the channels operated by the receptor. The resulting responses are either *excitatory postsynaptic potentials* (EPSPs) or *inhibitory postsynaptic potentials* (IPSPs), depending on whether they drive the cell toward a point above or below its firing threshold, as discussed in Chapter 11.

Why are most synapses chemical? The simpler alternative might appear to be the electrical synapse (see Chapter 11) in which the electrical signal from one cell can cross directly into the next through the electrically conducting pathway of the gap junction. Even when pre- and postsynaptic elements are coupled in this manner, however, a presynaptic spike of 100 mV would likely cause only a 1-mV change in the postsynaptic cell because relatively little charge can flow through these junctions to charge the large membrane capacitance of the postsynaptic cell. More efficient electrical transfer requires that the presynaptic terminal be as large as or larger than the postsynaptic

element and therefore only a few presynaptic cells could converge on a given postsynaptic cell. Such synapses would further limit the computational capacity of the brain because they could only induce excitation, not inhibition, in response to a presynaptic action potential. Chemical synapses are characterized by great flexibility. Different afferents can have different effects, with different strengths and time courses, on each other as well as on postsynaptic cells. These differences depend on the identity of the transmitter(s) released and the receptors present (see Chapters 7 and 9). Chemical synapses are often modified by prior activity in the presynaptic neuron. Chemical synapses are also particularly subject to the modulation of presynaptic ion channels by substances released by the postsynaptic or neighboring neurons. This flexibility is essential for the complex processing of information that neural circuits must accomplish, and it provides an important locus for modifying neural circuits in adaptive processes such as learning (Chapters 50 and 51).

TRANSMITTER RELEASE IS QUANTAL

In order to secrete thousands of transmitter molecules rapidly and simultaneously, nerve terminals, like other secretory cells, package the transmitter into membrane-enclosed organelles. When one of these *synaptic vesicles* fuses with the plasma membrane, the contents of the vesicle (approximately 5000 molecules) can diffuse into the extracellular space and encounter receptors on the postsynaptic cell within hundreds of microseconds. The transport rates of known membrane carriers are far slower. A consequence of releasing transmitter by the fusion of vesicles with the plasma membrane (called *exocytosis*) is that synaptic transmission is *quantal*— responses are built from signals with a discrete amplitude corresponding to a single vesicle. In the absence of presynaptic electrical activity, transmitter is released spontaneously as individual quanta. Each packet generates a small postsynaptic signal—either a *miniature excitatory* or a *miniature inhibitory postsynaptic potential* (MEPSP or MIPSP, respectively, or just "mini")—that can be detected by microelectrode recording (Katz, 1969) . An action potential accelerates tremendously, but very briefly, the rate of secretion of quanta and synchronizes them to evoke a PSP. At a synapse between two neurons, this might represent the release of 1 to 10 vesicles. At the vertebrate neuromuscular junction, a remarkably large and specialized synapse, hundreds of vesicles, can be released, and the response is, to a first approximation, the sum of the individual quanta. Evidence that the biophysical phenomenon of quanta corresponds to the release of transmitter by synaptic vesicles is summarized in Box 8.1.

The anatomical specializations of the synapse and the properties of the presynaptic ion channels and postsynaptic receptors unite to achieve fast, quantal transmission (Figs. 8.1 and 8.2). The chief anatomical feature of the terminal is the profusion of synaptic vesicles, typically 50 nm in diameter, that cluster near the synapse and dock at specialized sites called *active zones* along the presynaptic membrane (Fig. 8.1). The vesicles may differ in their appearance depending on the transmitter they enclose: thus glutamate and acetylcholine are stored in small clear vesicles, whereas peptide neurotransmitters occupy large dense-cored vesicles. Athough it may appear as indistinct fuzz on electron micrographs, the active zone is likely to be a highly structured specialization of the membrane and cytoskeleton (Figure 8.1 and see discussion later). Action potentials release transmitter by depolarizing the presynaptic membrane and opening Ca^{2+} channels that are in the active zone. The local intense rise in Ca^{2+} concentration triggers the exocytosis of docked vesicles with the plasma membrane (Figs. 8.1B and 8.1C) and the release of their contents into the narrow *synaptic cleft* (about 100 nm wide) separating the presynaptic terminal from high concentrations of postsynaptic receptors. At neuromuscular junctions, one of the best studied synapses, transmitter from one vesicle diffuses across the synaptic cleft in 2 ms and

---

BOX 8.1

EVIDENCE THAT A QUANTUM IS A VESICLE

Transmitter is released from vesicles:

1. All chemically transmitting synaptic terminals contain presynaptic vesicles.

2. Synaptic vesicles concentrate and store transmitter.

3. Rapid freezing of neuromuscular junctions during stimulation shows vesicle exocytosis occurring at the moment of transmitter release.

4. Intravesicular proteins appear on the external terminal surface after secretion.

5. Pharmacologically retarding the filling of vesicles generates a class of small MEPSPs that probably represent partially filled vesicles; drugs that enhance vesicle loading increase MEPSP size. In contrast, quantal size can be independent of the cytoplasmic acetylcholine concentration.

6. Synaptic vesicles formed by endocytosis load with extracellular electron-dense and fluorescent dyes (horseradish peroxidase and FM1-43, respectively) after nerve stimulation; the dye is released by subsequent stimulation.

7. Clostridial toxins that interfere with the synaptic vesicle-plasma membrane interaction block neurosecretion.

One quantum is one vesicle:

1. The number of acetylcholine molecules in isolated vesicles corresponds to the number of molecules released in a quantum.

2. When release is enhanced and the collapse of vesicle fusion images is prolonged by treatment with the potassium channel blocker 4-aminopyridine to broaden action potentials, the number of vesicle fusions observed corresponds to the number of quanta released by an action potential. Under these special circumstances, several vesicles are released at each active zone (Fig. 8.1C).

3. The number of vesicles present in nerve terminals corresponds to the total store of releasable quanta under conditions where endocytosis is blocked.

but rather to the concentration in a *microdomain* in the immediate vicinity of the Ca^{2+} channels (Fig. 8.3). In these microdomains, very high concentrations of Ca^{2+} are reached very quickly and drop rapidly to near-resting levels within microseconds of the closing of the channels. Presently, there are no Ca^{2+} dyes that are sufficiently local, sensitive, and fast that one can measure the concentration changes in these microdomains directly. Instead, our understanding of these signals comes from diffusion modeling, from modifying the buffering capacity of the cytosol, and from using indirect indicators of the local Ca^{2+} concentration, such as the gating of Ca^{2+}-activated K^+ channels or transmitter release itself (Roberts, 1994; Schneggenburger and Neher, 2000).

In the brief period for which the Ca^{2+} channels are open, the cytosol that lies within 100 nm of the mouth of each channel is flooded with Ca^{2+}, and the local Ca^{2+} concentration is likely to reach 100 µM or higher, the closer to the channel; the higher the concentration (Figs. 8.3A and 8.3B). The further from the channel, the more dilute the Ca^{2+} becomes and the greater the chance that it has been bound up by the high Ca^{2+}-buffering capacity of the cytosol. After the channels close, diffusion and buffering bring the Ca^{2+} concentration of the microdomains to near resting levels within a few milliseconds: the concentration gradient that existed around the mouth of the channel completely dissipates, and only the small net rise of total Ca^{2+} in the terminal remains (Fig. 8.3C). This signal, some-

times called residual Ca^{2+}, is what is detected by fluorescent indicator dyes. The effect may be compared to dumping a bucket of water into a swimming pool—a dramatic rise in water level occurs at one spot but it is very transient and gives rise to just a small net rise in the level of the entire pool. This view of excitation–secretion coupling is born out by anatomical studies. At neuromuscular junctions that are fast frozen during the act of secretion, vesicle fusion images are seen in freeze-fracture planes of the presynaptic membrane about 50 nm from intramembranous particles thought to be Ca^{2+} channels (see Fig. 8.1C).

The Active Zone Has Many Ca^{2+} Channels

When individual Ca^{2+} channels are labeled with biotinylated ω-conotoxin tagged with colloidal gold particles, more than 100 channels per active zone are seen. Any vesicle docked at such an active zone is likely to be surrounded by as many as 10 Ca^{2+} channels within a 50-nm distance. Even though not all these channels will open during each action potential, more than one channel is likely to open, and therefore Ca^{2+} entering through several nearby channels can influence a vesicle. At the squid giant synapse, more than 50 channels open in each ~0.6 µm² active zone, whereas 10 channels open within the more compact active zones of frog saccular hair cells (Yamada and Zucker 1992; Roberts, 1994). The Ca^{2+} microdomains of these channels overlap at single vesicles and cooperate in triggering secretion of a vesicle (Fig. 8.3). Ca^{2+} channels have been divided into several classes based on their biophysical and pharmacological properties. N and P/Q types of Ca^{2+} channels appear to be the most prevalent at CNS synapses, although R types are also reported and L types are seen at certain frog synapses. These channels can coexist at a single active zone and a single vesicle may be influenced by the influx through both N and P channels.

The Exocytosis Trigger Must Have Fast, Low-Affinity, Cooperative Ca^{2+} Binding

The sensor that detects the Ca^{2+} so as to trigger release must also have special properties to achieve fast and transient exocytosis. Estimates have now been made in several synapses and cell types, including retinal bipolar cells, crayfish neuromuscular junctions, hair cells, and the Calyx of Held that seem to converge on a value in the 10–100 µM range. This affinity is suited to the relatively high concentrations of Ca^{2+} in the microdomains near channels. The on rate must be particularly fast. This is confirmed by the

FIGURE 8.3 Microdomains with high Ca^{2+} concentrations form in the cytosol near open Ca^{2+} channels and trigger the exocytosis of synaptic vesicles. (A) In this adaptation of a model of Ca^{2+} dynamics in the terminal, a set of Ca^{2+} channels is spaced along the x axis, as if in a cross section of a terminal. The channels have opened and, while they are open, the cytosolic Ca^{2+} concentration (y axis) is spatially inhomogeneous. Near the mouth of the channel, the influx of Ca^{2+} drives the local concentration to as high as 800 µM, but within just 50 nm of the channel, the concentration drops off to 100 µM. Channels are spaced irregularly but are often sufficiently close to one another that their clouds of Ca^{2+} can overlap and sum. (B) In the active zone (gray), an action potential has opened a fraction of the Ca^{2+} channels, and microdomains of high cytosolic Ca^{2+} (pink) arise around these open channels as Ca^{2+} flows into the cell. In the rest of the cytoplasm, the Ca^{2+} concentration is at resting levels (0.10 µM), but within these microdomains, particularly near the channel mouth, Ca^{2+} concentrations are much higher, as in A. Synaptic vesicles docked and primed at the active zone may come under the influence of one or more of these microdomains and thereby be triggered to fuse with the membrane. (C) A few milliseconds after the action potential, the channels have closed and the microdomains have dispersed. The overall Ca^{2+} concentration in the terminal is now slightly higher (0.11 µM) than before the action potential. If no other action potentials occur, the cell will pump the extra Ca^{2+} out across the plasma membrane and restore the initial condition after several 100 ms.

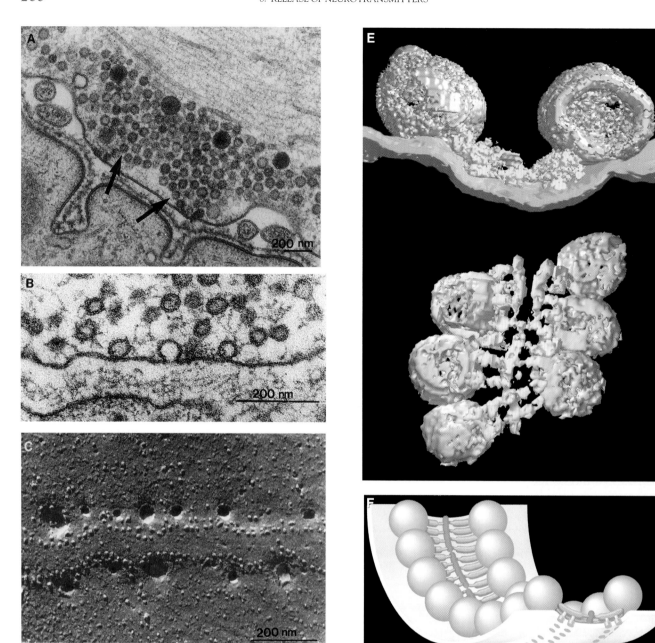

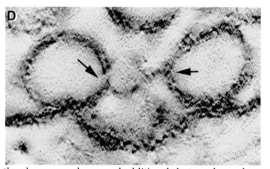

FIGURE 8.1 Ultrastructural images of exocytosis and active zones. (A–C) Synapses from frog sartorius neuromuscular junctions were quick-frozen milliseconds after stimulation in conditions that enhance transmission. (A) A thin section showing vesicles clustered in the active zone, some docked at the membrane (arrows). (B) Shortly (5 ms) after stimulation, vesicles were seen to fuse with the plasma membrane. (C) After freezing, presynaptic membranes were freeze-fractured and a platinum replica was made of the external face of the cytoplasmic membrane leaflet. Vesicles fuse about 50 nm from rows of intramembranous particles thought to include Ca²⁺ channels. (D–F) The fine structure of the active zone at a frog neuromuscular junction as seen with electron tomography. (D) In a cross-sectional image from tomographic data, two vesicles are docked at the plasma membrane and additional electron-dense elements are seen. When these structures are traced and reconstructed through the volume of the EM section (E), proteins of the active zone (gold) appear to form a regular structure adjacent to the membrane that connects the synaptic vesicles (silver) and plasma membrane (white). Viewed from the cytoplasmic side (E, lower image), proteins are seen to extend from the vesicles and connect in the center. (F) Schematic rendering of an active zone based on tomographic analysis. An ordered structure aligns the vesicles and connects them to the plasma membrane and to one another. Parts A and B from Heuser (1977); part C from Heuser *et al.* (1979). Part B reproduced from the *Journal of Cell Biology* **88**, 564–580 (1981). (D–F) After Harlow *et al.* (2001).

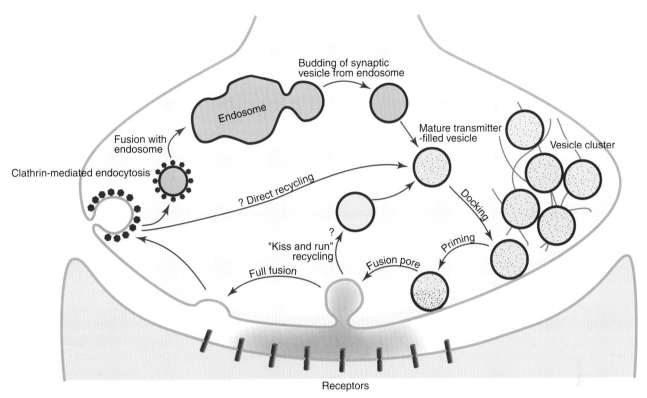

FIGURE 8.2 The life cycle of synaptic vesicles. Transmitter-filled vesicles can be observed in clusters in the vicinity of the active zone. Some vesicles are recruited to sites within the active zone in a process called docking. These vesicles are subsequently primed for release. The rise in cytosolic Ca^{2+} that occurs during an action potential triggers the opening of a fusion pore between some of the primed, docked vesicles and the plasma membrane. Transmitter exits through this fusion pore. Three pathways are proposed by which the now empty vesicle can be recovered and returned to the releasable pool: (1) by a direct reclosing of the fusion pore and reformation of the vesicle, often called "kiss and run", (2) by complete fusion (i.e., the flattening of the vesicle onto the membrane surface) followed by clathrin-mediated endocytosis, removal of the clathrin coat, and return of the vesicle to the releasable pool; and (3) by complete fusion and recycling as in the second pathway, but the endocytosed vesicle fuses first with an endosome and mature vesicles are subsequently formed by budding from the endosome. After or during this recycling process, the vesicle must be refilled with transmitter.

reaches a concentration of about 1 mM at the postsynaptic receptors. A large number of these receptors (up to 2000) will bind transmitter rapidly, and if a receptor binds two molecules of transmitter simultaneously, the receptor will open a postsynaptic ion channel (see Chapter 9). Each channel has a 25 pS conductance and remains open for about 1.5 ms, admitting a net inflow of 35,000 positive ions. Thus, a single vesicle can cause 70 million ions to cross the membrane and give rise to a mini of a few millivolts. The neuromuscular junction is also specialized for efficiency. A single action potential in a motor neuron can release 300 quanta within about 1.5 ms along a junction that contains about 1000 active zones. The resulting postsynaptic depolarization, which begins after a synaptic delay of about 0.5 ms and reaches a peak of tens of millivolts, is typically sufficient to generate an action potential in the muscle fiber.

The anatomy and physiology are somewhat different at fast central synapses. Postsynaptic cells make contact with presynaptic axon swellings that are called *varicosities* when they occur along fine axons and are called *boutons* when they are located at the tips of axons. The postsynaptic cell can be contacted on the cell body, but often the synapse is made onto a fine dendritic branch or tiny spine with a length of a few micrometers (Fig. 8.5). These fine processes can have a very high input resistance and can be capable of generating active propagating responses. A typical varicosity or bouton contains one to four active zones. At any single active zone, an action potential may release zero, one, or perhaps two vesicles. However, with multiple active zones between two cells, the action of each zone will be additive in determining the response of the postsynaptic cell. At a representative excitatory glutamatergic synapse, each action potential releases from

5 to 10 quanta. Each quantum that is released elevates transmitter concentration in the cleft to about 1 mM, as at the neuromuscular junction, but because there are fewer receptors clustered beneath these synapses, each quantum activates only 30 or so ion channels as compared with the 1000–2000 channels activated at the neuromuscular junction. At excitatory synapses, the release of a quantum may be sufficient to generate EPSPs of 1 mV or less in amplitude, clearly subthreshold for generating action potentials. However, central neurons often receive thousands of inputs, each of which has a "vote" on how the cell should respond. A comparison of these excitatory synapses at small neurons and the vertebrate neuromuscular junction at the much larger skeletal muscle fiber illustrates two important points: (1) the fundamental quantal nature of the chemical synapse is universal and (2) the different physiological requirements of particular synapses, such as synapses onto small or large cells, can be met by differences in any of several parameters, including the number of receptors activated per quantum, the number of active zones connecting two cells, the probability of a given active zone releasing a vesicle, and the conductance of the postsynaptic receptor channel. In describing synaptic transmission, two parameters are particularly important. *Quantal size* or quantal amplitude describes the unitary response to release of a single quantum (vesicle), whereas *quantal content* refers to the average number of quanta released by a single impulse. These parameters are discussed further later.

EXCITATION–SECRETION COUPLING

The action potential is an electrical event—a change in the voltage gradient across the plasma membrane. How is this electrical change converted to the fusion of synaptic vesicles and the release of neurotransmitter? The classical studies of Bernard Katz and colleagues (Katz, 1969) established that this coupling is achieved by the use of Ca^{2+} as an intracellular messenger. Ca^{2+} inside the cell is normally buffered to very low levels (~100 nM), and both concentration and electrical gradients provide a strong driving force for Ca^{2+} entry. Thus, when a voltage-dependent Ca^{2+} channel opens in response to the depolarization of the membrane during an action potential, there is the potential for the intracellular Ca^{2+} concentration to increase a thousandfold. In this manner, the electrical signal is converted to a dramatic chemical signal, and Ca^{2+} sensors in the fusion machinery can trigger vesicle fusion. The mechanism

of fusion itself is discussed later, but first the nature of the Ca^{2+} signal and the evidence for its centrality must be understood.

It has been known for over 100 years that Ca^{2+} must be present in the extracellular saline for transmission to occur. Subsequently (Katz, 1969), it was shown that Ca^{2+} need only be present at the moment of invasion of the nerve terminal by the action potential. If the timing or amount of Ca^{2+} entry is altered, transmission is similarly altered. Thus, if a very large depolarization occurs in the nerve terminal, the influx of Ca^{2+} is inhibited by the electrical gradient, despite the opening of the channels. When the cell repolarizes, a large Ca^{2+} influx occurs. In experimental conditions, release can be delayed in this fashion until after the depolarization. Similarly, divalent cations that block Ca^{2+} channels, such as Co^{2+} and Mn^{2+}, block transmission. Elevating intracellular Ca^{2+}, e.g., by using an ionophore that lets Ca^{2+} ions flow across the membrane, causes transmitter release. However, because this results in a steady change in the Ca^{2+} concentration rather than a pulse, this release appears as an acceleration of the spontaneous release of quanta rather than as a synchronous postsynaptic response. It has also become possible to fill a terminal with a caged form of the Ca^{2+} ion, i.e., with Ca^{2+} ions bound up within a chemical carrier. A flash of light can rearrange this carrier, uncaging the Ca^{2+}, and thereby cause an abrupt increase in cytosolic Ca^{2+} and a sudden increase in secretion as well Finally, loading the terminal with Ca^{2+} chelators to prevent increases in cytosolic Ca^{2+} can prevent release.

Vesicles Are Released by Calcium Microdomains

The opening of Ca^{2+} channels during a single action potential allows in enough Ca^{2+} to raise the concentration in the bouton from approximately 100 to 110 nM. How can a mere 10% change in the concentration cause an enormous shift in the activity of the fusion machinery? Ca^{2+}-sensitive enzymes, for comparison, do not alter their rates a thousandfold in response to 10% changes in Ca^{2+}. Furthermore, because Ca^{2+} pumps and exchangers on the plasma membrane work relatively slowly, this small rise in Ca^{2+}, which can be detected with fluorescent Ca^{2+} indicator dyes, persists for hundreds of milliseconds after the action potential. Why does the relatively long-lasting change in Ca^{2+} in the bouton drive transmitter secretion that only occurs for a millisecond or so after the action potential? The answer to both of these questions lies in the fact that the release mechanism is *not* responding to the general concentration of Ca^{2+} in the bouton,

A

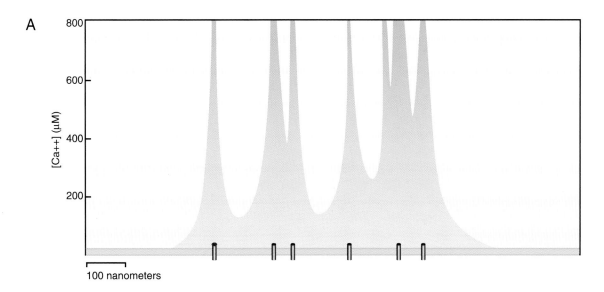

100 nanometers

B

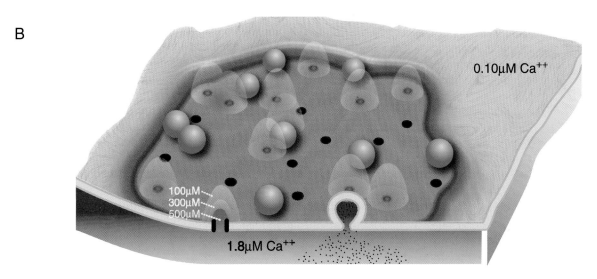

0.10μM Ca⁺⁺

100μM
300μM
500μM

1.8μM Ca⁺⁺

C

0.11μM Ca⁺⁺

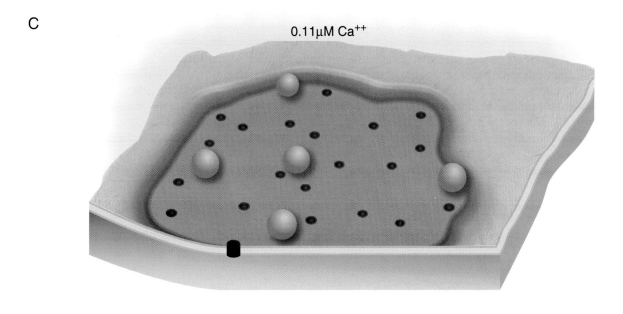

finding that presynaptic injection of relatively slow Ca^{2+} buffers such as ethylene glycol bis(β-aminoethyl ether)-N,N'-tetraacetic acid (EGTA) have almost no effect on transmitter release to single action potentials. Only millimolar concentrations of fast Ca^{2+} buffers such as 1,2-bis(2-aminophenoxy)ethane-$N,N,$ N',N'-tetraacetic acid (BAPTA), with on rates of about 5×10^8 M^{-1} s^{-1}, can capture Ca^{2+} ions before they bind to the secretory trigger, indicating that the on-rate of Ca^{2+} binding to this trigger is similarly fast. At a rate of 5×10^8 M^{-1} s^{-1}, 100 μM Ca^{2+} reaches equilibrium with its target in about 50 μs. The off rate of Ca^{2+} dissociation from these sites must also be fast, at least 10^3 s^{-1}, to account for the rapid termination of transmitter release (0.25 ms time constant) after Ca^{2+} channels close and Ca^{2+} microdomains collapse.

Importantly, the relationship of Ca^{2+} influx or cytosolic Ca^{2+} in microdomains to the amount of release is not linear at most synapses. By plotting this relationship on a log–log plot, a Hill coefficient can be determined, and values as high as 3 or 4 are commonly obtained. This value implies a high cooperativity in the action of Ca^{2+} inside the terminal, perhaps because multiple Ca^{2+} -binding sites must be occupied in order to trigger release efficiently (Schneggenburger and Neher, 2000) . The interesting physiological consequence of this steep relationship is that small modulations of Ca^{2+} channels that increase or decrease Ca^{2+} influx can have a large effect on the strength of a synapse. For example, at a synapse from a parallel fiber onto a Purkinje cell in the cerebellum, when the activation of modulatory presynaptic GABA receptors inhibits Ca^{2+} channels sufficiently to reduce Ca^{2+} influx by 25%, the amplitude of transmission decreases by 70%.

Summary

Chemical synapses permit one neuron to rapidly and effectively excite or inhibit the activity of another cell. A diversity of transmitters and receptors allows varied postsynaptic responses. The packaging of transmitter into vesicles and its release in quanta enable a single action potential to secrete hundreds of thousands of molecules of transmitter almost instantaneously onto another cell. Ca^{2+} acts as an intracellular messenger tying the electrical signal of presynaptic depolarization to neurosecretion. At fast synapses, Ca^{2+} enters through clusters of channels near docked synaptic vesicles in active zones. This Ca^{2+} acts at extremely short distances (tens of nanometers) in remarkably little time (200 μs) and at very high local concentrations (~100 μM), in calcium microdomains, by binding cooperatively to a low-affinity receptor

with fast kinetics to trigger exocytosis. When Ca^{2+} channels close, these microdomains of high Ca^{2+} return to near resting concentrations quickly and the evoked response is terminated. Speed, efficiency, and flexibility are the hallmarks of this process.

MOLECULAR MECHANISMS OF THE NERVE TERMINAL

To release neurotransmitter in response to an action potential, a synaptic vesicle must fuse with the plasma membrane of the nerve terminal with great rapidity and fidelity, and thus the synapse requires an effective and well-regulated molecular machine. This machine must include the means to load the vesicle with transmitter, to dock the vesicle near the membrane so that it can fuse with a short latency, to define a release site on the plasma membrane, to restrict fusion to the active zone rather than other points on the surface of the terminal or axon, and to cause the release itself. Additionally, a reserve of synaptic vesicles must be held near the active zone (e.g., Fig. 8.5) and those vesicles must be recruited to the plasma membrane as needed. The number of vesicles that are ready and waiting to fuse must be strictly determined, and the protein and lipid components of the vesicle must be recycled to form a new vesicle after fusion has occurred. For each of these processes, a molecular understanding remains incomplete, but a decade of rapid scientific progress in this field has resulted in considerable headway.

Most Neurons Require A Cycle of Membrane Trafficking

Active neurons are in constant need of transmitter-filled vesicles ready to release their contents. A bouton in the CNS, for example, may contain a store of 200 vesicles, but if it releases even one of these with each action potential and if the cell is firing at an unexceptional rate such as 5 Hz, the store of vesicles would be consumed within less than a minute. Transport of newly synthesized vesicles from the cell body would be far too slow to support such a demand and the axonal traffic needed to supply an entire arbor of nerve terminals would be staggering.

In short, active neurons need an efficient mechanism to recycle and reload vesicles within the terminal. The exception is peptidergic neurons because peptides must be synthesized in the endoplasmic reticulum (ER) and then sent down the axon. Not surprisingly, therefore, vesicles with peptide transmitters are

BOX 8.2

HISTOLOGICAL TRACERS CAN BE USED TO FOLLOW VESICLE RECYCLING

Much of our understanding of the life history of synaptic vesicles (Fig. 8.2) comes from studies using electron-dense or fluorescent markers of intracellular regions that have been in contact with the extracellular space. Horseradish peroxidase (HRP) is an enzyme that catalyzes the oxidation of diaminobenzidine, forming an electron-dense product that can be identified easily in the electron microscope; FM1-43 is an amphipathic styryl dye that becomes highly fluorescent on partitioning into cell membranes. When frog muscles were soaked in HRP and the motor neurons were stimulated for 1 min, the enzyme appeared in coated vesicles in nerve terminals in regions outside active zones. After more prolonged stimulation, most of the HRP collected in endosomal cisternae due to the fusion of endocytotic vesicles with these organelles. When the HRP was washed out and the neurons were rested for an hour before fixation, HRP appeared in small clear synaptic vesicles in active zones. When rested neurons were stimulated again before fixation, this time in the absence of HRP, the filled vesicles gradually disappeared due to their release by exocytosis (Heuser and Reese, 1973). In this manner, the route from coated vesicle to endosome to releasable synaptic vesicle was established. FM1–43 can be similarly taken up into living motor nerve terminals and its accumulation or release can be monitored with the use of confocal fluorescence microscopy. High-frequency stimulation for just 15s in FM1–43 was marked by uptake of dye into nerve terminals. More prolonged stimulation followed by a period of rest without the dye in the bath resulted in the persistent staining of synaptic vesicles in active zones. Subsequent stimulation at 10 Hz gradually destained the terminals in minutes; destaining required the presence of Ca^{2+} in the medium and represented exocytosis of stained vesicles. After about 1 min, the rate of destaining decreased as the vesicle pool began to be diluted with unstained vesicles newly recovered by endocytosis (Betz and Bewick, 1993). Exposing dissociated hippocampal neurons to FM1-43 at various times after stimulation showed that endocytosis proceeded for about 1 min after exocytosis. Cells loaded with dye and then restimulated began to destain about 30 s after endocytosis, which is a measure of the time needed for the recycling of recovered vesicles into the pool of releasable vesicles. Changes in fluorescence corresponding to the release or uptake of a single vesicle have been reported. These experiments provide a dynamic view of the life cycle of synaptic vesicles.

References

Betz, W. J., and Bewick, G. S. (1993). Optical monitoring of transmitter release and synaptic vesicle recycling at the frog neuromuscular jucntion. *J. Physiol.* **460**, 287–309.

Heuser, J. E., and Reese, T. S. (1973). Evidence for recycling of synaptic vesicle membrane during transmitter release at the frog neuromuscular junction. *J. Cell. Biol.* **57**(2), 315–344.

released at very low rates. For most neurotransmitters, however, the exocytosis of a synaptic vesicle is followed rapidly by its endocytosis (see later and Box 8.2) and within approximately 30 s the vesicle is again available for release. This pathway is sometimes referred to as the exo-endocytic cycle (Fig. 8.2). This chapter is concerned primarily with the movement of synaptic vesicle proteins and membranes through this cycle.

The transmitter content of the vesicle has its own cycle of synthesis, loading into vesicles, secretion, clearance from the cleft, and, in many cases, reuse; these pathways are discussed in Chapter 7. The exo-endocytic cycle, however, is central to understanding synaptic transmission. If we start with a transmitter-filled vesicle in the cytosol, we can outline its progression through this cycle (Fig. 8.2). The vesicle will eventually be mobilized from the reserve pool in the cytosol to the readily releasable pool by translocating to the active zone and becoming "docked" at the plasma membrane. Biochemical priming steps may occur at this point that will enable the vesicle to fuse within microseconds once the Ca^{2+} signal is given. Exocytosis may involve a complete merging of the vesicle membrane with the plasma membrane or it may involve only a transient connection of the two. In the latter case, the vesicle, having emptied its contents, may return directly to the vesicle pool and be refilled with transmitter. If fusion is complete, however, the vesicle needs to be reformed with a clathrin cage and pinched off the plasma membrane. In some cases, these endocytosed vesicles seem to fuse with endosomes or large membranous sacs called cisternae, and mature synaptic vesicles then bud from this compartment. In other cases, the mature vesicle may be formed directly from the plasma membrane.

Histological tracers have provided both anatomical and physiological means to follow this cycle (Box 8.2). A defect in any single step in the cycle will halt transmitter release. Moreover, each step in this cycle represents a potential control point for modulating the efficacy of the synapse. Modulation of the strength or fidelity of synaptic signaling, commonly known as synaptic plasticity (see Chapter 50), plays an important role both in the development of synaptic connections (see Chapters 18, 19, 20, and 21) and in the functioning of the mature nervous system. Indeed, regulation by Ca^{2+} and other second messenger systems is known to affect the docking, fusing, and recycling of vesicles at some synapses and is also likely to regulate the balance between reserve stores and those vesicles actively engaged in the exo-endocytic cycle. Understanding the mechanisms of this modulation is an important goal and will certainly require the detailed understanding of the fundamental machinery itself. The question has been approached through the combined use of biochemical, genetic, and biophysical techniques.

Transmitter Release Is Rapid

As discussed earlier in this chapter, the delay between the arrival of an action potential at a terminal and the secretion of the transmitter can be less than 200 μs. This places some severe constraints on the fusion mechanism. Vesicles must already be present at the release sites, as there is no time to mobilize them from a distance. A catalytic cascade during fusion, such as that involved in phototransduction or in excitation–contraction coupling in smooth muscle, would also be far too slow for excitation–secretion coupling at the nerve terminal. Indeed, even a single bimolecular catalytic step might be too slow for such short latencies. Models therefore favor the idea that a fusion-ready complex of the vesicle and plasma membrane is preassembled at release sites and that Ca^{2+} binding need only trigger a simple conformation change in this complex to open a pathway for the transmitter to exit the vesicle.

Because the volume of the synaptic vesicle is small, the diffusion of transmitter from the vesicle proceeds almost instantaneously as soon as a pore has opened up between the vesicle lumen and the extracellular space. This structure is referred to as the fusion pore, but its biochemical nature is unknown. Thus, the time-critical steps come between the influx of Ca^{2+}

and the formation of the fusion pore, and these steps establish the latency between arrival of the action potential and transmitter diffusion into the cleft. Any further step, such as the complete merging of the vesicle and plasma membrane, if it occurs at all, can occur on a slower time course, after the transmitter has left the vesicle. The tethering of the vesicle at the release site (often called docking) and any biochemical events that need to occur in order for the vesicle to reach the fusion-ready state (often called priming) can also be slower. Docking and priming a vesicle cannot be *too* slow, however; a central nervous system (CNS) synapse is estimated to have 2 to 20 vesicles in this fusion-ready state; therefore, if a synapse is to respond faithfully to a sustained train of action potentials, it must be able to replace the fusion-ready vesicles with a time course of seconds. The rate at which this occurs may determine some of the dynamic properties of the synapse.

The short latency of transmission would seem to preclude the involvement of ATP hydrolysis at the fusion step because such a reaction would be too slow. This is born out by numerous physiological studies in which exocytosis persists after Mg^{2+}-ATP has been dialyzed from the cell and in which all the Mg^{2+} has been chelated. (Lack of Mg^{2+} would render any residual ATP inert to most enzymes.) Thus, if energy is needed to fuse the membranes, it must be stored in the fusion-ready state of the vesicle–membrane complex and released upon addition of Ca^{2+}.

Transmitter Release Is A General Cell Biological Question

Exocytosis and endocytosis are not unique to neurons; these processes go on in every eukaryotic cell. Moreover, exocytosis itself is only one representative of a general class of membrane-trafficking steps in which one membrane-bound compartment must fuse with another. Other examples would include the fusion of recycling vesicles with endosomes, transport from the ER to the Golgi, or transport from endosomal compartments to lysosomes. In each case, the same biophysical problem must be overcome, and the mechanisms for all these membrane fusion steps appear to have much in common.

For a vesicle to fuse with the plasma membrane, or any other target, there is a large energy barrier to surmount. To bring the lipid bilayers within a few nanometers of one another so that they can fuse, the hydration shell around the polar lipid head groups must be disrupted. Simply to split open each membrane so that the bilayer of one could be connected to the bilayer of the other would require exposing the hydrophobic core of each membrane to the aqueous milieu of the cytoplasm and this barrier is sufficiently great that it does not occur under normal conditions. Thus, a specialized mechanism is required to bring the membranes close together and then drive fusion.

At present, it appears that all the membrane-trafficking steps within the cell use a similar set of proteins to accomplish this task (Fig. 8.7). As discussed later, homologues of proteins found at the synapse and known to be essential for exocytosis have also been shown to function in ER to Golgi transport in mammalian cells, in endosomal fusion, and in exocytosis in yeast. Indeed, it appears that representatives of this core set of proteins are present on every trafficking vesicle or target membrane and are required for every fusion step. This discovery, which grew from the conjunction of independent studies of different model systems (Bennett and Scheller, 1993), has led to the exciting hypothesis that all intracellular membrane fusions will be united by a single and universal mechanism. To the extent that this proves true, it will be a great boon to cell biology: experiments in one model system, e.g., the highly developed genetic analysis of membrane fusion in yeast, can be absorbed into neuroscience. Similarly, the abundance of synaptic vesicles for biochemical analysis and the unparalleled precision of electrophysiological assays of single vesicle fusions can deepen the understanding of other cellular events. Will these disparate membrane fusion events be truly identical in their mechanisms? The jury is still out. Most likely, however, different membrane fusions will present variations on a common theme; the fundamental processes will be adapted to the specific requirements of each physiological step.

Perhaps an instructive analogy may be drawn with muscle contraction: actin and myosin offer a fundamentally conserved mechanism for producing force and movement, and every muscle contains isoforms of actin, heavy and light myosin chains, troponins, and tropomyosins. However, skeletal muscle and smooth muscle differ enormously in the details of how Ca^{2+} interacts with these proteins and regulates their activity. Regulation via troponins or via myosin light chain kinase, differences in the intrinsic ATPase rates of the myosins, and other critical features have adapted these related sets of proteins to their particular purpose in the individual type of muscle. Similarly, the need for extremely tight control of fusion in the nerve terminal—for rapid rates of fusion with very short latencies to occur in brief bursts at precise points on the plasma membrane—may cause some profound differences in how the synaptic isoforms of these proteins function compared to the isoforms involved in general cellular traffic.

Synaptic Proteins Have Been Identified from Purified Vesicles

Synaptic vesicles are abundant in nervous tissue and, due to their unique physical properties (uniform small diameter and low buoyant density), they can be purified to homogeneity by simple subcellular fractionation techniques. As a result, at a biochemical level, synaptic vesicles are among the most thoroughly characterized organelles. One of the first sources for the purification of synaptic vesicles was the electric organ of marine elasmobranchs. This structure, a specialized adaptation of the neuromuscular junction, is highly enriched in synaptic vesicles. It has also proven simple to isolate synaptic vesicles from mammalian brain. The protein compositions of synaptic vesicles from these sources are remarkably similar, demonstrating the evolutionary conservation of synaptic vesicle function. This similarity also points to the fact that many of the proteins present on the synaptic vesicle membrane perform general functions that are not restricted to a single class of transmitter.

Our knowledge of many of the important proteins in vesicle fusion commenced with the purification and characterization of synaptic vesicles. These vesicles contained a discrete set of abundant proteins, and individual proteins could be isolated and subsequently cloned. The major constituents of the synaptic vesicle are shown in Fig. 8.4. For some of these proteins, there are well-established functions, but for others, the functions remain uncertain (Table 8.1). The proton transporter, for example, is an ATPase that acidifies the lumen of the vesicle. The resulting proton gradient provides the energy by which transmitter is moved into the vesicle. This task is carried out by another vesicular protein, a vesicular transporter that allows protons to move down their electrochemical gradient and out of the vesicle in exchange for transmitter that moves into the lumen. Several vesicular transporters are known, all structurally related, and by their substrate selectivity they help specialize a terminal for release of the appropriate transmitter (see later). Two other large proteins with multiple transmembrane domains are abundant in vesicles: synaptic vesicle protein 2 (SV2) and synaptophysin. The functional significance of these proteins remains elusive despite extensive biochemical and genetic characterization. Other vesicular proteins are discussed later in this chapter.

Transmitter release depends on more than just vesicular proteins, however; proteins of the plasma membrane and cytoplasm are also important. In many cases, the identification of these additional components or an appreciation of their importance to the

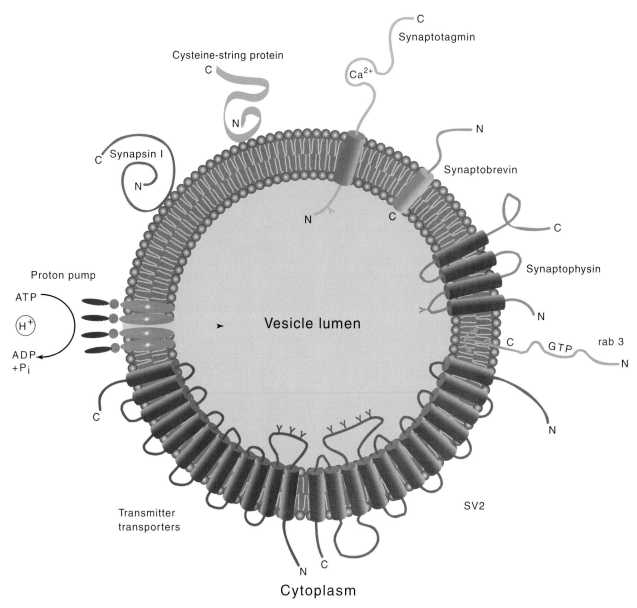

FIGURE 8.4   Schematic representation of the structure and topology of major synaptic vesicle membrane proteins (see also Table 8.1).

synapse derived from investigations of vesicular proteins. Two examples will serve to illustrate this point.

The first example begins with synaptotagmin, an integral membrane protein of the synaptic vesicle that was purified from synaptic vesicles and cloned. The portion of synaptotagmin that extends into the cytoplasm (the majority of the protein, see Fig. 8.4) was subsequently used for affinity column chromatography. In this manner, a protein called syntaxin was identified as a synaptotagmin-binding protein. This protein resides in the plasma membrane and is now appreciated as one of the critical players in vesicle fusion (see later). More recently, yeast two-hybrid

screens have been conducted and used to identify proteins that bind to syntaxin. One such protein, syntaphilin, may serve as a regulator or modulator of syntaxin function. Thus, subsequent to the isolation of an abundant vesicular protein, biochemical assays have led to a fuller picture.

A second and similar example (Gonzalez and Scheller, 1999) began with the realization that an abundant small GTP-binding protein, rab3, was present on the vesicle surface. This protein, discussed further later, may regulate vesicle availability or docking to release sites. Subsequently, rabphilin was identified on the basis of its affinity for the GTP-

TABLE 8.1 Function of Synaptic Vesicle Proteins

Protein	Function
Proton pump	Generation of electrochemical gradient of protons
Vesicular transmitter transporter	Transmitter uptake into vesicle
VAMP/synaptobrevin	Component of SNARE complex; acts in a late, essential step in vesicle fusion
Synaptotagmin	Ca^{2+} binding; possible trigger for fusion and component of vesicle docking at release sites via interactions with SNARE complex and lipid; promotes clathrin-mediated endocytosis by binding AP-2 complex
Rab3	Possible role in regulating vesicle targeting and availability
Synapsin	Likely to tether vesicle to actin cytoskeleton
Cysteine string protein	Promotes reliable coupling of action potential to exocytosis
SV2	Unknown
Synaptophysin	Unknown

bound form of rab3. Rabphilin lacks a transmembrane domain but is recruited to the surface of the synaptic vesicle by binding to rab3. Rabphilin may have a role in modulating transmission, particularly in mossy fiber terminals of the hippocampus. Still later, many additional rab3-binding proteins were identified, including RIM, a component of the active zone. Rab3 can exist in either GTP- or GDP-bound states, and additional factors that regulate these states were also identified: a GDP dissociation inhibitor (GDI), a GDP/GTP exchange protein (GEP), and a GTPase activating protein (GAP). Thus, from the identification of a synaptic vesicle protein, an array of additional factors has come to light, all of which are likely to figure in the exo-endocytic cycle.

Genetic Screens Have Led to the Identification of Synaptic Proteins

Genetic screens have provided an independent method for identifying the machinery of transmitter release. One of the most fertile screens was carried out not in the nervous system per se, but rather in yeast. Because membrane trafficking in yeast is closely parallel to vesicle fusion at the terminal, mutations that alter the secretion of enzymes from yeast can be a springboard for the identification of synaptic proteins.

In the early 1980s, a series of such screens was carried out, and a collection of over 50 mutants was obtained. Many of these were shown to accumulate in post-

TABLE 8.2 Additional Proteins Implicated in Transmitter Release

Protein	Function
Syntaxin	SNARE protein present on plasma membrane (and on synaptic vesicles to a lesser extent); forms core complex with SNAP-25 and VAMP/synaptobrevin; essential for late step in fusion
SNAP-25	SNARE protein present on plasma membrane (and on synaptic vesicles to a lesser extent); forms core complex with syntaxin and VAMP/synaptobrevin; essential for late step in fusion
Nsec-1/munc-18	Syntaxin-binding protein required for all membrane traffic to the cell surface; likely bound to syntaxin when syntaxin is not in a SNARE complex
Synaphin/complexin	Syntaxin-binding protein; may oligomerize core complexes
Syntaphilin	Binds syntaxin; prevents formation of SNARE complex (?)
Snapin	Binds SNAP-25; associated with synaptic vesicles; unknown function
NSF	ATPase that can disassemble SNARE complex; likely to disrupt complexes after exocytosis
α-SNAP	Cofactor for NSF in SNARE complex disassembly
unc-13/munc-13	Active zone protein; vesicle priming for release; modulation of transmission by diacyl glycerol
Rabphilin	C2 domain protein; Ca^{2+}-binding protein; binds rab3 and associates with synaptic vesicle; modulation of transmission (?)
DOC2	C2 domain protein; Ca^{2+}-binding protein; binds Munc-18; unknown function
RIM1 and related proteins	Active zone proteins; bind rab3; modulation of transmission (?)
Piccolo	Likely scaffolding protein to tether vesicles near active zone
Bassoon	Likely scaffolding protein to tether vesicles near active zone
Exocyst (sec6/8 complex)	Marks plasma membrane sites of vesicle fusion in yeast; synaptic role uncertain

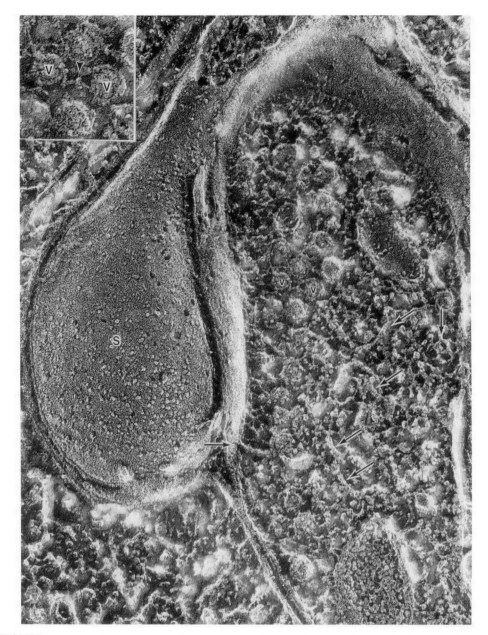

FIGURE 8.5 Structure of a synapse between a parallel fiber and a Purkinje cell spine in the cerebellum. The sample was frozen rapidly and then freeze fractured, shallow etched, and rotary shadowed to reveal the details of the synaptic architecture. From Landis *et al.* (1988). Copyright by Cell Press.

Golgi vesicles in the cytoplasm and thus appeared to block a late stage of transport, such as the targeting or fusion of these vesicles at the plasma membrane. Screens for suppressors and enhancers of these secretion mutations uncovered further components.

Subsequently, excellent *in vitro* assays have been established in which to study the fusion of vesicles derived from yeast with their target organelles. Among the secretion mutants and their interacting genes were homologues of some of the proteins dis-

cussed earlier: sec4 encodes a small GTP-binding protein like rab3 and Sso1 and Sso2 encode plasma membrane proteins that are homologues of syntaxin. The sec1 gene encodes a soluble protein with a very high affinity for Sso1, and the mammalian homologue of this protein, n-sec1, is bound tightly to syntaxin in nerve terminals and has an essential function in transmission. Yeast is not the only organism in which a genetic screen uncovered an important protein for the synapse: the unc-13 mutation of *Caenorhabditis elegans*, e.g., identified a component of the active zone mem-

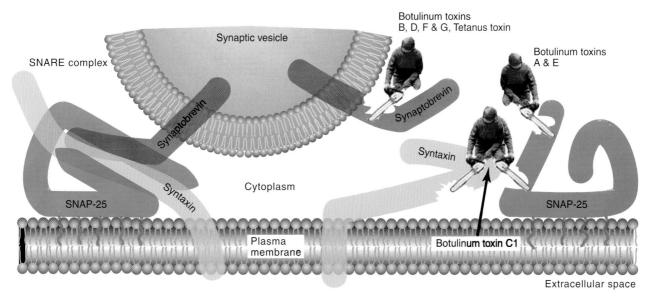

FIGURE 8.6 SNARE proteins and the action of clostridial neurotoxins. The SNARE complex shown at the left brings the vesicle and plasma membranes into close proximity and likely represents one of the last steps in vesicle fusion. Vesicular VAMP, also called synaptobrevin, binds with syntaxin and SNAP-25 that are anchored to the plasma membrane. Tetanus toxin and the botulinum toxins, proteases that cleave specific SNARE proteins as shown, can block transmitter release.

brane that is important in priming vesicles for fusion and in modulation of the synapse.

Genetics has further contributed to our understanding of synaptic proteins by allowing tests of the significance of an identified protein for synaptic transmission. Such studies have been carried out in *C. elegans, Drosophila*, and mice and can reveal either an absolute requirement for the protein (as in the case of syntaxin mutants in *Drosophila*) or relatively subtle effects (as in the case of rab3 mutations in mice).

From biochemical purifications, *in vitro* assays, genetic screens, and fortuitous discoveries, an ever-growing list of nerve terminal proteins has been assembled (Tables 8.1 and 8.2). The manner in which these proteins coordinate the release of transmitter, as well as all the other cell biological functions of the exo-endocytic cycle, remains uncertain, but a consensus has emerged in recent years that puts one set of proteins at the core of the vesicle fusion.

SNAREs and the Core Complex Are Key to Membrane Fusions

Three synaptic proteins, vesicle-associated membrane protein (VAMP)/synaptobrevin, syntaxin, and the synaptosomal associated protein of 25 kDa (SNAP-25), are capable of forming an exceptionally tight complex with one another that is generally referred to as either the *core complex* or the SNAP

receptor (SNARE) *complex* (Sollner *et al.*, 1993; Sutton *et al.*, 1998) . The interaction of these three proteins is essential for synaptic transmission and is likely to lie very close to or indeed at the final fusion step of exocytosis (Figs. 8.6 and 8.7). What are these proteins?

VAMP (also called synaptobrevin) was among the first synaptic vesicle proteins to be cloned. It is anchored to the synaptic vesicle by a single transmembrane domain and has a cytoplasmic domain that contributes a coiled-coil strand to the core complex. Syntaxin has a very similar structure but is located primarily in the plasma membrane (although some is present on vesicles as well). SNAP-25 is also a protein primarily of the plasma membrane but, unlike the others, lacks a transmembrane domain and is instead anchored in its central region by acylations. SNAP-25 contributes two strands to the SNARE coiled coil.

The interactions of these proteins can be envisioned as closely juxtaposing the two membranes meant to fuse. The proteins of this complex are archetypes of a class of membrane-trafficking protein collectively called **SNAREs**. Vesicle-associated proteins, such as VAMP, are referred to as **v-SNAREs** and those of the target membrane, such as SNAP-25 and syntaxin, are referred to as **t-SNAREs**.

A SNARE complex is found at each membrane-trafficking step within a eukaryotic cell (Fig. 8.7). Through a combination of SNARE proteins on the

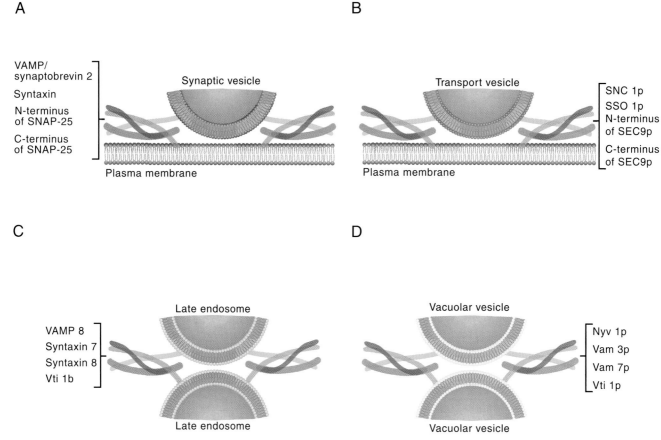

FIGURE 8.7 Neurotransmitter release shares a core mechanism with many membrane fusion events within eukaryotic cells. The fusion of synaptic vesicles (A) is driven by a particular complex of four coiled-coil domains contributed by three different proteins. Exocytosis in yeast (B), the fusion of late endosomes in mammalian cells (C), and the fusion of vacuolar vesicles in yeast (D) exemplify the closely related four-stranded coiled-coil complexes required to drive fusion in other membrane-trafficking steps.

opposing membranes, a four-stranded coiled coil is formed. Alongside the example of the synapse in Fig. 8.7A, three analogous cases are shown from exocytosis in yeast (Fig. 8.7B), the fusion of late endosomes with one another (Fig. 8.7C), and the fusion of vesicles that form the yeast vacuole (Fig. 8.7D).

Abundant genetic and biochemical data argue for an essential role of SNAREs, and the combination of yeast genetics, *in vitro* assays, biochemical analyses, and synaptic physiology has had a synergistic effect in advancing the field. For example, the discovery that secretory mutations in yeast were homologues of synaptic SNAREs provided some of the first functional data on these proteins (Bennett and Scheller, 1993), whereas data from synapses first placed the proteins on vesicles and the plasma membrane. In addition, the crystal structure was solved first for synaptic proteins (Sutton *et al.*, 1998). Because transmembrane domains and of course the membranes themselves, were absent from the crystallized samples, it was not possible to

conclude from the structure alone that SNAREs form a bridge between the membranes rather than forming complexes within the same membrane. Instead, an *in vitro* assay with purified yeast vesicles established this point.

Some of the strongest evidence for an essential role of SNAREs at the synapse has come from the study of a potent set of eight neurotoxins produced by clostridial bacteria. These toxins (tetanus toxin and the family of related botulinum toxins) have long been known to block the release of neurotransmitter from the terminal. The discovery that they do so by proteolytically cleaving individual members of the SNARE complex provided neurobiologists with a set of tools with which to probe SNARE function (Fig. 8.6).

Each of the toxins comprises a heavy and a light chain that are linked by disulfide bonds. The heavy chain binds the toxin to surface receptors on neurons, thereby enabling the toxin to be endocytosed. Once inside the cell, the disulfide bond is reduced and the free light chain enters the cytoplasm of the cell. This light chain is the active portion of the toxin and is a member of the Zn^{2+}-dependent family of proteases. The catalytic nature of the toxin accounts for its astonishing potency; a few tetanus toxin light chains, for example, at a synapse can suffice to proteolyse all the VAMP/synaptobrevin, thereby shutting down transmitter release. The toxins are highly specific, recognizing unique sequences within an individual SNARE protein, as summarized in Fig. 8.6. VAMP/synaptobrevin can be cleaved not only by tetanus toxin but by the botulinum toxins of types B, D, F, and G, and each toxin cleaves at a different peptide bond within the structure. SNAP-25 is cleaved by botulinum toxins A and E, but again at different sites from one another. Botulinum toxin C1 cleaves both syntaxin and, less efficiently, SNAP-25.

What precisely is the function of SNARE proteins in promoting transmitter release? How does the assembly of this complex relate to membrane fusion? Studies with botulinum toxins, yeast mutants, mutants of *Drosophila* and *C. elegans*, and permeabilized mammalian cells all place SNAREs late in the process. Synapses that lack an individual SNARE, e.g., synapses whose VAMP has been mutated or cleaved by toxin, have the expected population of synaptic vesicles, and these vesicles accumulate at active zones in the expected manner. Indeed, as judged by electron microscopy, there may even be an excess of docked vesicles in close proximity to the plasma membrane at the active zone. Yet these synapses are incapable of secreting transmitter. Thus, SNAREs appear to be essential for a step that comes after the docking of the vesicle at the release site, but before the fusion pore opens and transmitter can diffuse into the cleft. The details of how the complex functions, however, are less certain.

One attractive model is that the energy released by the formation of this very high-affinity complex is used to drive together the two membranes. A loose complex of the SNARES would form and then "zipper up" and pull the membranes together. This may correspond to the actual fusion of the membranes or, alternatively, to a priming step that requires a subsequent rearrangement of the lipids in order to open the pore that will connect the vesicle lumen to the extracellular space. Evidence from the fusion of yeast vacuolar vesicles implicates a distinct downstream step, regulated by Ca^{2+}/calmodulin and involving subunits of the proton pump, but whether this is true of neurons as well remains unknown. Vesicles consisting of only lipid bilayers and SNAREs can fuse *in vitro*, suggesting that no other proteins will be essential for the fusion step.

One additional function may reside with SNARE proteins: identification of an appropriate target membrane. Within a cell, there are myriad membrane compartments with which a transport vesicle can fuse: how then is specificity achieved? The great diversity of SNAREs (Fig. 8.7) may account for some of this specificity because not all combinations of vesicle-associated and target-associated SNAREs (v- and t-SNAREs) will form functional complexes. This potential mechanism, however, is likely to be only a part of the story. Particularly in the nerve terminal, it appears that synaptic vesicles can find the active zone even in the absence of the relevant SNAREs, e.g., when a SNARE has been cleaved by a clostridial toxin or in a mutant lacking a SNARE. In addition, the t-SNAREs syntaxin and SNAP-25 can be present along the entire axon and thus are inadequate to explain the selective release of transmitter at synapses and active zones.

NSF—An ATPase for Membrane Trafficking

At some point as vesicles move through their exo-endocytic cycle, energy must be added to the system. *N*-Ethylmaleimide sensitive factor (NSF), an ATPase involved in membrane trafficking, is one likely source. NSF was first identified as a required cytosolic factor in an *in vitro* trafficking assay (Block *et al.*, 1988). The importance of NSF was confirmed when it was found to correspond to the yeast sec18 gene, an essential gene for secretion. NSF hexamers bind a cofactor called α-SNAP (soluble NSF attachment protein), or sec17, and this complex in turn can bind to the SNARE complex. When Mg-ATP is hydrolyzed, the SNARE complex is disrupted into its component proteins (Sollner *et al.*, 1993) . Originally it was speculated that this disassembly of the complex might correspond to fusion—that the action of NSF might catalytically rearrange the SNAREs so that the membranes were brought together. As discussed earlier, however, a late role for ATP is unlikely in transmitter release, and SNAREs can stimulate fusion *in vitro* without NSF present. More recent models put NSF action well before or after the fusion step. If SNARE complexes form between VAMP, syntaxin, and SNAP-25 all in the same membrane, these futile complexes can be split apart by NSF so that productive complexes bridging the membrane compartments can be formed. After fusion, the tight SNARE complex needs to be disrupted so that the VAMP can be recycled to synaptic vesicles while the other SNAREs remain on the plasma membrane. If, indeed, the energy of forming a tight SNARE complex is part of the energy that drives fusion, NSF, by restoring the SNAREs to their dissociated, high-energy state, will be an important part of the energetics of membrane fusion.

Docking and Priming Vesicles Prepares Them for Fusion

As discussed earlier and outlined in Fig. 8.2, many preparatory and regulatory steps may precede the action of SNAREs and the membrane fusion step at which SNAREs appear to act. These preparatory steps must tether the vesicle at an appropriate release site in the active zone and hold the vesicle in a fusion-ready state. These mechanisms remain among the most obscure of the processes involved in exocytosis, but there is a growing list of proteins that may participate. One example is the protein n-sec1 (also called munc18), the neuronal homologue of the product of the yeast sec1 gene. This protein binds to syntaxin with a very high affinity and, when so bound, prevents syntaxin from binding to SNAP-25 or VAMP. Mutations of this protein prevent trafficking in both yeast and higher organisms. It appears likely that n-sec1 serves two functions: it may promote membrane fusion by priming syntaxin so that, once it has dissociated, it can participate correctly in fusion, but it may also be a negative regulator, keeping syntaxin inert until an appropriate vesicle or signal displaces n-sec1 and allows a SNARE complex to form.

Rab3 is another protein for which a priming or regulatory role is often invoked at the synapse. This small GTP-binding protein, mentioned earlier, is the homologue of the yeast sec4 gene product. In yeast, and at other membrane-trafficking steps within mammalian cells, rab proteins have essential roles. They appear to help a vesicle to recognize its appropriate target and begin the process of SNARE complex formation. At the synapse, however, the significance of rab3 is still uncertain. Although it is clearly associated with synaptic vesicles, genetic disruption of rab3 has a surprisingly slight phenotype and causes only subtle alterations in synaptic properties. Whether this is due to additional, redundant rab proteins or whether the rab family has been relegated to a more minor role at the synapse remains to be determined.

Because synaptic vesicles dock and fuse specifically at the active zone, this region of the nerve terminal membrane must have unique properties that promote docking and priming. The special nature of this domain is easily discernible in electron micrographs: an area of electron-dense material can be observed opposite the postsynaptic density (Fig. 8.1). In some synapses, such as photoreceptors, hair cells, and many insect synapses, the structures are more elaborate and include ribbons, dense bodies, and T bars that extend into the cytoplasm and appear to have a special relationship with the nearby pool of vesicles.

Advances in electron microscopy have allowed a more detailed look at the association of vesicles and plasma membrane at the active zone (Harlow et al., 2001). At the neuromuscular junction of the frog (Fig. 8.1), the electron-dense material adjacent to the presynaptic plasma membrane is actually a highly ordered structure—a lattice of proteins that connect the vesicles to a cytoskeleton, to one another, and to the plasma membrane. The molecules that correspond to these structures are not yet known. A few proteins, however, are known to be concentrated in the active zone or in the cloud of vesicles near the active zone. These proteins, piccolo, bassoon, RIM1, and unc-13, may be a part of the machinery that defines the active zone as the appropriate target for synaptic vesicle fusion.

In addition to the specializations of the active zone, additional machinery must be present to preserve a dense cluster of synaptic vesicles extending approximately 200 nm back from the active zone (Fig. 8.1). The vesicles in this domain are not likely to be releasable within microseconds of the arrival of an action potential but are instead likely to represent a reserve pool from which vesicles can be mobilized to release sites on the plasma membrane. The equilibrium between this pool and vesicles actually at the membrane may be an important determinant of the number of vesicles released per impulse, but remains poorly understood.

One protein likely to play a role in the maintenance of the reserve pool is synapsin, a family of peripheral membrane proteins on synaptic vesicles. Synapsins can also bind actin filaments and thus may provide a linker that tethers the vesicles in the cluster to the synaptic cytoskeleton. Disruption of this link can cause the vesicle cluster to be diminished and reduce the number of vesicles in the releasable pool of the terminal. Synapsin has attracted considerable interest because it is the substrate for phosphorylation by both cAMP and Ca^{2+}-dependent protein kinases. These phosphorylations may influence the availability of reserve vesicles for recruitment to release sites.

Ca^{2+}-Binding Proteins Are Candidates for Coupling the Action Potential to Exocytosis

The most striking difference between synaptic transmission and traffic between other cellular compartments is the rapid triggering of fusion by action potentials. As discussed previously, the opening of Ca^{2+} channels and the focal rise of intracellular Ca^{2+} activate the fusion machinery. How does the terminal sense the rise in Ca^{2+}? What is the Ca^{2+} trigger and how does it open the fusion pore? Is it a single Ca^{2+}-binding protein or do several components respond to the altered Ca^{2+} concentration? Does Ca^{2+} remove a brake that normally prevents a docked, primed vesicle from fusing or does Ca^{2+} induce a conformational change that is actively required to promote fusion? How does the steep, exponential relationship of release to intracellular Ca^{2+} arise? These questions are an active area of investigation and debate.

Some clues may come from other systems: Ca^{2+}-dependent membrane fusion is not unique to the synapse. Ca^{2+} can trigger both exocrine and endocrine secretion. Furthermore, Ca^{2+} released from intracellular stores now appears to be essential in trafficking steps in yeast that previously had been viewed as constitutive and unregulated. In yeast vacuolar fusion, for example, calmodulin senses a local increase in Ca^{2+} and triggers fusion. Calmodulin, however, has not been the leading candidate for the synaptic trigger. The affinity of calmodulin for Ca^{2+} has generally been thought to be too high to explain the relatively high levels of Ca^{2+} (at least 10 μM) that are needed to evoke transmitter release. However, the apparent affinity of calmodulin for Ca^{2+} is very dependent on the proteins to which calmodulin binds, and the four Ca^{2+}-binding sites of free calmodulin probably have an average affinity of about 10 μM. Evidence for an involvement of calmodulin in synaptic transmission continues to arise, suggesting that yeast vacuolar traffic and synaptic transmission may not be as divergent as one might think. At present, however, a modulatory role for calmodulin is favored over a requirement in the final triggering step at the synapse.

The leading candidate for being the synaptic Ca^{2+} sensor is synaptotagmin, an integral membrane protein of the synaptic vesicle (Fig. 8.4). Synaptotagmin has a large cytoplasmic portion that comprises two Ca^{2+}-binding C2 domains, called C2A and C2B. These domains can also interact with the SNARE complex proteins and with phospholipids in a Ca^{2+}-dependent manner. It has been hypothesized that one or more of these interactions is the molecular correlate of the triggering event for fusion. Consistent with this hypothesis, mutations that remove synaptotagmin profoundly reduce synaptic transmission in flies, worms, and mice, while having little effect on or enhancing the rate of spontaneous release of transmitter. Whether this reduction in evoked release is due specifically to the loss of the Ca^{2+} trigger, however, is harder to demonstrate. Synaptotagmin is likely to be involved in endocytosis and potentially in vesicle docking as well, which has complicated the analysis.

These processes, as mentioned earlier, are also likely to be regulated by Ca^{2+}, and the Ca^{2+}-binding sites on synaptotagmin may be relevant for this regulation as well.

Transmitter Must Be Packaged into the Vesicle

A central requirement of quantal synaptic transmission is the synchronous release of thousands of molecules of transmitter from the presynaptic nerve terminal. This requirement is partly met by the capacity of synaptic vesicles to accumulate and store high concentrations of transmitter. In cholinergic neurons, for example, the concentration of acetylcholine within the synaptic vesicle can reach 0.6 M, more than 1000-fold greater than that in the cytoplasm. Two synaptic vesicle proteins mediate the uptake of transmitter: the vacuolar proton pump and a family of transmitter transporters. The vacuolar proton pump is a multisubunit ATPase that catalyzes the translocation of protons from the cytoplasm into the lumen of a variety of intracellular organelles, including synaptic vesicles. The resulting transmembrane electrochemical proton gradient is utilized as the energy source for the active uptake of transmitter by transmitter transporters.

Transmitter uptake has been characterized in isolated synaptic vesicle preparations in which at least four types of distinct transporters have been identified: one for acetylcholine, another for catecholamines and serotonin, a third for the excitatory amino acid glutamate, and the fourth for the inhibitory amino acids GABA and glycine. At least one gene for each of these classes of transmitter transporter has now been cloned. As expected, these distinct transporters are expressed differentially by neurons. The type of transporter in a cell dictates the type of transmitter stored in the synaptic vesicles of a particular neuron, and when investigators drive the expression of a glutamate transporter, e.g., in a GABA-releasing neuron, they can trick the cell into now releasing glutamate.

Vesicular transporters are integral membrane proteins with 12 membrane-spanning domains that display sequence similarity with bacterial drug resistance transporters. Synaptic vesicle transporters are clearly distinct from the plasma membrane transmitter transporters that remove transmitter from the synaptic cleft and thereby contribute to the termination of synaptic signaling (see Fig. 8.2). The distinguishing characteristics include their transport topology, energy source, pharmacology, and structure. The sequestration of transmitter into vesicles, in addition to its obviously essential role for transmitter exocytosis, has some further benefits to the cell. Sequestration can prevent high cytosolic concentrations of the transmitter from inhibiting the biosynthetic enzymes for transmitter synthesis and can protect the transmitter from catabolic enzymes. In addition, in some cell types, sequestration may protect the cell from damage caused by the oxidation of labile transmitters, particularly dopamine.

In contrast to small chemical transmitters, proteinaceous signaling molecules, including neuropeptides and hormones, are typically stored in granules that are larger and have a higher electron density than synaptic vesicles. The contents of these granules are not recycled at the release sites; as a result, their replenishment requires new protein synthesis followed by packaging into secretory vesicles in the cell body. Because of the slow kinetics of their release, the slow responsiveness of their postsynaptic receptors, and their inability to be recycled locally, proteinaceous signaling molecules typically mediate regulatory functions.

Endocytosis Recovers Synaptic Vesicle Components

After exocytosis, the components of the synaptic vesicle membrane must be recovered from the presynaptic plasma membrane, as discussed previously. Vesicle recycling could theoretically be accomplished by either of two mechanisms (Fig. 8.2). The first is simply a reversal of the fusion process. In this case, a fusion pore opens to allow transmitter release and then closes rapidly to reform a vesicle. Often nicknamed "kiss and run," it has the theoretical advantage that it would allow all the vesicular components to remain together on a single vesicle that would be available immediately for reloading with transmitter. The mechanism is potentially quick and energetically efficient. This mechanism is employed in some nonneuronal cells, but its relevance for the synapse is an unresolved issue.

The predominant pathway for synaptic vesicle recycling is more likely to be a second mechanism, endocytosis. Endocytosis of synaptic vesicle components, like receptor-mediated endocytosis in other cell types, is mediated by vesicles coated with the protein clathrin. Accessory proteins select the cargo incorporated into these vesicles as they assemble. One class of accessory protein known as AP-2 displays a high affinity for synaptotagmin, which may be important, therefore, in recruiting the clathrin coat to the vesicle. The final pinching off of clathrin-coated vesicle requires the protein dynamin, which can form a ring-like collar around the neck of an endocytosing vesicle. A crucial role for dynamin in synaptic vesicle recy-

cling is demonstrated most clearly in a temperature-sensitive *Drosophila* mutant known as *shibire*. The *shibire* gene encodes the *Drosophila* homologue of dynamin. At the nonpermissive temperature, shibire mutant flies become paralyzed rapidly due to a nearly complete depletion of synaptic vesicles from their nerve terminals. When the components of the synaptic vesicle membrane are recovered in clathrin-coated vesicles, recycling is completed by vesicle uncoating and, perhaps, passage through an endosomal compartment in the nerve terminal (see Fig. 8.2).

Summary

The life of the synaptic vesicle involves much more than just the Ca^{2+}-dependent fusion of a vesicle with the plasma membrane. It is a cyclical progression that must include endocytosis, transmitter loading, docking, and priming steps as well. In many regards, this cell biological process shares mechanistic similarities with membrane trafficking in other parts of the cell and with simpler organisms such as yeast. Interaction of vesicular and plasma membrane proteins of the SNARE complex—VAMP/synaptobrevin, syntaxin, and SNAP-25—is an essential late step in fusion. Many other proteins have been identified that are likely to precede the action of the SNAREs, regulate the SNAREs, and recycle them. Components of the synaptic vesicle membrane, the presynaptic plasma membrane, and the cytoplasm all contribute to the regulation of synaptic vesicle function. Together, these proteins build on the fundamental core apparatus to create an astonishingly accurate, fast, and reliable means of delivering transmitter to the synaptic cleft.

QUANTAL ANALYSIS: PROBING SYNAPTIC PHYSIOLOGY

A quantitative description of the signal passing across a synapse can be a source of insight into the biophysics of transmission and its regulation. As discussed earlier, the response to an action potential in the presynaptic cell reflects the release of discrete packets of transmitter, called quanta, that are a direct consequence of the vesicular release of transmitter. A given synapse, however, will not secrete exactly the same number of vesicles in response to each stimulus. Instead, the probabilistic nature of the presynaptic apparatus typically causes the amount released to fluctuate from trial to trial in a quantal manner; i.e., the postsynaptic response adopts preferred levels, which arise from the summation of various numbers of vesicle fusions (Katz, 1969). Thus, although a particular synapse may release an average of two vesicles per action potential, it may release one vesicle in response to one stimulation and three vesicles in response to the next. To the third stimulus, the synapse may fail to release any transmitter at all. From a full description of the properties of the synapse, the size of the individual quantum response can be estimated, as well as the average number of quanta released for a given presynaptic action potential. This approach, called quantal analysis, is also a source of insight into the probabilistic processes underlying transmitter release from the presynaptic terminal and into the mechanisms by which transmission can be modified by physiological, pharmacological, and pathological phenomena.

A Standard Model of Quantal Transmission Can Describe Many Synapses

The quantal nature of transmission was first demonstrated in the early 1950s by Bernard Katz and colleagues, who studied the frog neuromuscular junction. By recording from a muscle fiber immediately under a branch of the motor axon, they measured the postsynaptic potential both at rest and in response to stimulation of the axon. Spontaneous signals that were approximately 1/100 of the signal evoked by stimulating the presynaptic axon were observed to occur at random intervals. At any one site, these spontaneous minis were of roughly constant amplitude, with a coefficient of variation of 30%. As discussed previously, a neuromuscular junction normally releases hundreds of quanta per impulse, but when extracellular Ca^{2+} was lowered to reduce transmitter

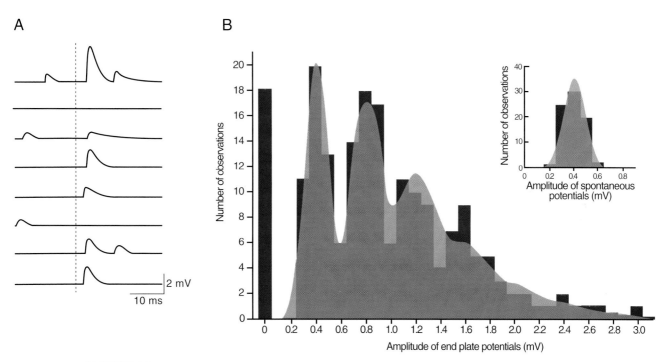

FIGURE 8.8   Quantal transmission at the neuromuscular junction. (A) Intracellular recordings from a rat muscle fiber in response to repeated presynaptic stimulation of the motor axon. Low extracellular [Ca^{2+}] and high [Mg^{2+}] restricted Ca^{2+} entry and so kept transmission to a very low level. The stimulus was given at the time marked by the dotted line. The size of the postsynaptic response fluctuated from trial to trial, with some trials giving failures of transmission. Spontaneous minis occurring in the background (e.g., those events that occur before the dotted line) had approximately the same amplitude as the smallest evoked responses, implying that they arose from the release of single quanta of acetylcholine. From Liley (1956), (B) Peak amplitudes of 200 evoked responses [end plate potentials (EPPs)] from a similar experiment, plotted as an amplitude histogram. Eighteen trials resulted in failures of transmission (indicated by the bar at 0 mV), and the rest gave EPPs whose amplitude tended to cluster at integral multiples of 0.4 mV. This coincides with the mean amplitude of the spontaneous minis, whose amplitude distribution is shown in the insert together with a Gaussian fit. Shading through the EPP histogram is a fit obtained by assuming a Poisson model of quantal release. Roman numerals indicate the number of quanta corresponding to each component in the distribution. From Boyd and Martin, (1956).

release to very low levels, the evoked response fluctuated from trial to trial between preferred amplitudes, which coincided with integral multiples of the mini amplitude (Fig. 8.8).

We now understand this to arise from the fact that minis are the fusion of a single vesicle and that evoked responses can represent one or more of these same vesicles. Before the vesicle hypothesis was established, however, Katz and colleagues inferred that the mini is the quantal building block, variable numbers of which are released to make up the evoked signal. The relative numbers of trials resulting in 0, 1, 2, ... quanta were well described by a Poisson distribution—a statistical distribution that arises in many instances where a random process operates, implying that the process governing quantal release may also depend on a simple underlying mechanism.

On the basis of this evidence, Katz and colleagues proposed the following model of transmission, which has gained wide acceptance and will be referred to as the standard Katz model.

- Arrival of an action potential at the presynaptic terminal briefly raises the probability of release of quanta of transmitter (i.e., the fusion of synaptic vesicles).
- Several quanta (synaptic vesicles) are available to be released, and every quantum gives roughly the same electrical signal in the postsynaptic cell. This is the quantal size or amplitude, Q, which sums linearly with all other quanta released.
- The average number of quanta released, m, is given by the product of n, the number of available quanta, and p, the average release probability: $m = np$. The average response to a stimulus is the product of the quantal size and the average number of quanta per stimulus, Qm or Qnp.
- The relative probability of observing 0, 1, 2, ..., n quanta released is then given by a binomial distribution, with parameters n and p.
- Under conditions of depressed transmission, p is low and the system approximates a Poisson process. This is the limiting case of the binomial distribution where p tends to 0 and n is very large and the distribution is determined by the unique parameter m.

The value of Q has a clear underlying basis: the efficacy of an individual synaptic vesicle fusion in altering the conductance of the postsynaptic membrane. The binomial parameters, n and p, however, are formalisms whose underlying meanings are harder to pin down. n may correspond to the number of vesicles in a primed, fusion-ready state at the active zone or to discrete release sites competent for release,

or even to the number of active zones. Correspondingly, p may represent the probability of fusion of any individual vesicle or the probability of fusion at a given release site or active zone. For some mechanisms, therefore, it is difficult to say whether n or p is altered. For example, if additional vesicles are recruited to release sites, that change may be manifest as a change in n because there are more releaseable quanta or as a change in p because the probability of fusion at a given release site has increased because it is more likely to be charged with a vesicle.

These quantal parameters remain a useful description of the synapse, however, despite their obscurity on a mechanistic level. For example, it is often useful to classify synapses as having a high or low probability of release (p) to explain their behavior during trains of stimuli (see later). In a synapse with few releasable vesicles and a high p, a train is predicted to deplete the releasable pool rapidly and the strength of transmission declines, a phenomenon known as synaptic depression. Another synapse might have the same average quantal content, but accomplish this with a large releasable pool and a low probability of fusion for any individual vesicle in the pool. Such a synapse would be less prone to depression and indeed both types of synapse are encountered.

A major impetus for the accurate measurement of quantal parameters is that it may help determine the locus of modulatory effects on synaptic transmission, or the site of action of a drug. A blocker of postsynaptic receptors, for example, will not alter the mini frequency or the number of quanta released, but will decrease the amplitudes of both spontaneous minis and the quantal components of evoked responses. A change in the loading of transmitter into a vesicle could cause a similar change. In contrast, a synaptic modulator that decreased Ca^{2+} channel opening or a blocker of those channels would decrease the probability of presynaptic release and be recognized as a decrease in quantal content, m. Many modulators of presynaptic transmission cause a parallel change in quantal content and in the frequency of spontaneous minis. This sort of analysis has been instrumental in understanding synaptic plasticity and in determining whether a given alteration occurs at the presynaptic terminal or the postsynaptic membrane.

The Standard Katz Model Does Not Always Apply

Incorrectly applying the Katz model and quantal analysis to synapses at which its assumptions do not hold has been a frequent source of error. Although a superb description of transmission at the neuromuscular junction, it is not uniformly applicable to central nervous system synapses, and the technical difficulties of isolating and accurately sampling the physiology of an individual synapse in the CNS can make the determination of quantal parameters exceptionally difficult. Here we discuss five issues with which the standard Katz model is unable to deal adequately.

Quantal Uniformity

In order for the quantal amplitude to be constant at different release sites, a uniform population of vesicles must be available to be released, as well as receptors with identical properties opposite each release site. Although true at the neuromuscular junction, this may not uniformly be the case in CNS synapses. Vesicles may be charged with different amounts of transmitter and different active zones may face very different populations of receptors. Moreover, it is possible that at some synapses vesicle fusion does not release the entire transmitter content of the vesicle. Whereas the amplitudes of minis form a relatively tight distribution at the frog neuromuscular junction, they are often highly variant and do not have a normal distribution at many CNS synapses, particularly when multiple synapses with different properties connect two cells. When there is high variability in the underlying quantal sizes, the evoked responses are not likely to form perfectly clean peaks of 0, 1, 2… quanta (as in Fig. 8.8), but rather tend to blur into one another. Also, when the population of quantal events is highly variable, accurately detecting the true quantal size can be difficult: the smallest events are often lost in the noise. Furthermore, when scores of neurons converge on the cell from which the recording is made, it is typically not possible to determine what synapse is contributing any given spontaneous event. For these reasons, analysis of quantal transmission in the CNS must be done with great care.

Uniform and Independent Release Probabilities

For the Katz model to apply, the release sites must be identical, with a uniform probability of exocytosis. If this condition were not satisfied, evoked signals would still cluster at integral multiples of the quantal amplitude, but the relative proportion of trials resulting in 0, 1, …, n quanta would no longer be described by a simple binomial (or Poisson) distribution. Release sites at many synapses are unlikely to be uniform. For example, when different vesicles at a synapse see different isoforms of Ca^{2+} channels in different phosphorylation states of those channels with different probabilities of opening, and when the fusion machinery itself may be in different regulatory states, this assumption of uniformity is a poor approximation of reality. Another violation of the independence of release sites may arise at some CNS synapses where it has been hypothesized that the fusion of a single vesicle at an active zone temporarily inhibits the fusion of others.

Postsynaptic Distortion of Signals and Receptor Saturation or Variability

Postsynaptic currents or potentials arising from different release sites must sum linearly, i.e., the response to two vesicles fusing should be twice the response to a single vesicle. Under experimental conditions, however, the opening and closing of voltage-dependent ion channels in the postsynaptic membrane can distort summation. Another source of nonlinear summation arises at some CNS synapses where receptor number is low and a single quantum is sufficient to activate the majority of the receptors and give a near-maximal response. Indeed, a major difference between some vertebrate CNS synapses and the neuromuscular junction is that the quantal amplitude is often determined not by the vesicle contents, but by the number of available receptors. At some excitatory synapses, the glutamate content of a quantum appears to be sufficient to bind most available postsynaptic receptors. The trial-to-trial variability of the quantal amplitude at an individual site is therefore determined principally by receptor and channel properties. In the mammalian CNS, relatively few channels (fewer than 100) open, compared with 1000–2000 at the neuromuscular junction. In the extreme case of a developing synapse, the variation from impulse to impulse might depend as much on whether one, two, or three receptors were activated per vesicle fusion as whether one, two, or three vesicles fused.

Silent Synapses

In the standard Katz model, the postsynaptic membrane is a constant array of receptors, and the variability of responses derives solely from the alteration in the number of quanta released at the active zone. In this scheme, when a synapse is observed to increase its frequency of minis and increase the amplitude of the evoked response without a change in the quantal size, it must be due to an increased probability of release. In recent years, increasing evidence has mounted that this, too, may not hold at certain CNS synapses. At particular glutamate synapses, for example, some active zones may be secreting transmitter without producing a physiological response because no receptors (in particular AMPA receptors, see Chapter 9) are present in the postsynaptic membrane. These so-called "silent synapses" can spring to life when a set of receptors is inserted into the postsynaptic membrane in a concerted fashion. Because more active zones are now contributing to the detected physiological response, mini frequency will be higher and evoked release increased, although the quantal size will not have changed. Thus, many of the requirements for the standard Katz model cannot realistically be expected to hold in all cases and the evidence that these simple probabilistic models are correct is far from compelling. However, the fact that evoked synaptic signals are often found clustered at integral multiples of an underlying unit strongly argues that evoked responses do indeed arise from the summation of individual quanta. Despite the technical difficulties and theoretical caveats, the analysis of mini frequency, quantal size, quantal content, and synaptic probability has been the foundation of our description of synaptic transmission and the source of great insight into synaptic modulation.

It has been possible to augment this understanding with independent methods, including the ability to observe vesicle fusion by optical means that will quantitatively describe presynaptic activity without depending on the postsynaptic membrane to report the event (see Box 8.2). Another method of indirectly estimating release probability at glutamatergic synapses makes use of a blocker of NMDA receptors, MK-801, that will only act in the open state. From the rate of blockade during a train of stimuli, the probability of the channel having been opened by a given impulse can be inferred.

Summary

Quantal analysis has improved our understanding of biophysical and pharmacological mechanisms of transmission greatly by describing normal transmission and by offering a tool to distinguish and characterize presynaptic and postsynaptic actions of drugs or endogenous agents that modify the strength of a synapse. Numerical methods can be used to estimate the probability of transmitter release and the size of the postsynaptic effect of an individual quantum of neurotransmitter. Although these methods must be applied with caution, they yield a unique insight into the mechanisms of synaptic plasticity, both at the neuromuscular junction and in the central nervous system.

SHORT-TERM SYNAPTIC PLASTICITY

Chemical synapses are not static transmitters of information. Their effectiveness waxes and wanes, depending on the frequency of stimulation and the

history of prior activity. Because information processing in the nervous system in not conducted by individual action potentials at widely spaced intervals, this plasticity is of the utmost importance to the function of the synapse within its physiological circuit. At most synapses, repetitive high-frequency stimulation (called a *tetanus*) is initially dominated by a growth in successive PSP amplitudes, called synaptic *facilitation* (Fig. 8.9). This process builds to a steady state within about 1 s and decays equally rapidly when stimulation stops. Decay is measured by single test stimuli given at various intervals after a conditioning train. Facilitation does not require a train to be observed; at many synapses it can be seen after a single action potential. Thus, when two stimuli are given with very close spacing, the second one can be as much as twice the amplitude of the first. This is called *paired-pulse facilitation* (Fig. 8.9). At most synapses, a slower phase of increase in efficacy, which has a characteristic time constant of several seconds and is called *augmentation*, succeeds facilitation. Finally, with prolonged stimulation, some synapses display a third phase of growth in PSP amplitude that lasts minutes and is called *potentiation*.

Often, a phase of decreasing transmission, called synaptic *depression*, is superimposed on these processes (Fig. 8.9). Synaptic depression leads to a dip in transmission during repetitive stimulation, which often tends to overlap and obscure the augmentation and potentiation phases. At some synapses, it is manifest after only a single action potential and gives rise to *paired-pulse depression*. When stimulation ceases, recovery from the various processes occurs in the same order as their development during the tetanus, with facilitation decaying first, then depression and augmentation, and finally potentiation. Thus, potentiation is often visible in isolation only long after a tetanus and is thus called *posttetanic potentiation* (PTP).

FIGURE 8.9 Short-term synaptic plasticity. (A) An idealized synapse in which facilitation predominates. Two stimuli (paired pulses) are given to the presynaptic nerve in each line and postsynaptic voltage responses are shown. Closely spaced stimuli (top line) facilitate strongly but as the interval between stimuli increases, the degree of facilitation diminishes. The fifth line illustrates how facilitation can accumulate during a train of stimuli. (B) An idealized synapse in which synaptic depression predominates. (C) At most synapses, both depression and facilitation occur and, depending on the nature of the individual synapse and the time course of facilitation, depression, augmentation, and potentiation, any of these phenomena may predominate at a given moment. Thus, in a realistic pattern of activity, with unevenly spaced action potentials arriving at a terminal, the strength of transmission can depend greatly on the previous history of the synapse.

A   Facilitation

B   Depression

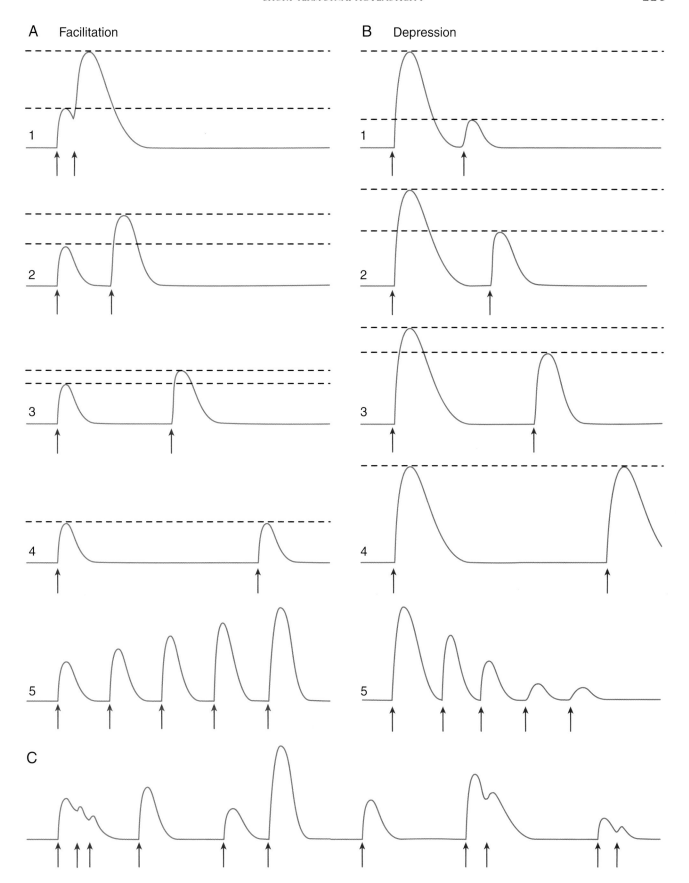

Additional forms of use-dependent plasticity, called long-term potentiation and long-term depression (LTP and LTD), have received considerable attention as likely correlates of some forms of learning and are discussed elsewhere (Chapter 50). Most frequently, at synapses in which a quantal analysis has been done, all these forms of synaptic plasticity (except some forms of cortical LTP) are due to changes in the number of quanta released by action potentials.

The propensity to facilitation or depression can be quite different at different types of synapse and thus contributes to the diversity of synaptic communication and the flexibility of information processing by synapses. At a given synapse, the frequency and

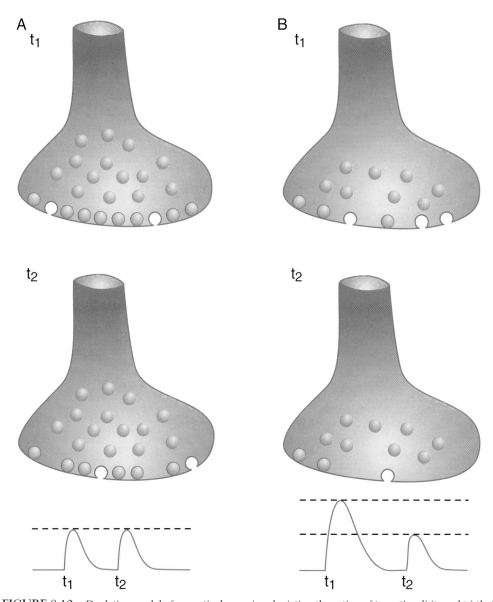

FIGURE 8.10   Depletion model of synaptic depression depicting the action of two stimuli (t_1 and t_2) that arrive so closely spaced that no vesicles have been recruited to the releasable pool to replace those that fused in response to the first stimulus. (A) A synapse in which the releasable pool (n) is large and the probability of fusion for a given vesicle (p) is low shows little or no depression. Because only a small fraction of the docked, releasable vesicles fused in response to the first stimulus, the second response is comparable in amplitude. (B) A synapse in which the releasable pool (n) is small but the probability of fusion (p) is high is likely to be strongly depressing. Vesicles released by the first impulse deplete half the fusion-competent pool, leaving n at t_2 equal to half its value at t_1. If p has not changed at t_2, the second stimulus will release half as many quanta.

duration of a train can alter whether facilitation or depression is most in evidence. In a physiologically realistic setting of irregularly spaced stimuli, all of these phenomena may be simultaneously at play and one or another may predominate for any given response, depending on the preceding history of stimulation. Thus, responses in the postsynaptic cell will be anything but a constant response to each action potential in the train.

Synaptic Depression May Arise from Depletion of Readily Releasable Vesicles, Autoinhibition, or Receptor Desensitization

The rate at which synaptic depression develops usually depends on stimulation frequency, whereas recovery from depression proceeds with a single time constant of seconds to minutes in different preparations. At many synapses, depression is relieved when transmission is reduced by lowering Ca^{2+} or raising Mg^{2+} in the medium. When little or no release occurs, there is little depression of the subsequent response. These characteristics are consistent with depression being due to the depletion of a readily releasable store of docked or nearly docked vesicles and recovery being due to their replenishment from a nearby supply (Fig. 8.10) (Zucker, 1989). The parameters of such a depletion model can be estimated from the rate of recovery from depression, which gives the rate of refilling the releasable store, and the fractional drop in PSPs given at short intervals, which gives the fraction of the releasable store liberated by each action potential.

As mentioned previously, synapses with a high probability of release from a relatively small pool of vesicles will be the most prone to this form of depression. Recovery from this form of depression appears to be influenced by cytosolic Ca^{2+} as well, consistent with a hypothetical ability of elevated Ca^{2+} in the cytosol to enhance the recruitment of reserve vesicles to release sites. Alternative models are tenable in which a release site is temporarily inactivated by the fusion of a vesicle.

Vesicle depletion cannot account for all forms of synaptic depression. At some synapses, depression is due to an inhibitory action of released transmitter on presynaptic receptors called autoreceptors. For example, in rat hippocampal cortex, the depression of GABA responses is blocked by antagonists of presynaptic GABAB receptors. Presumably, GABA acts to hyperpolarize nerve terminals and block transmitter release. At other synapses, desensitization of postsynaptic receptors contributes heavily to the observed depression.

Facilitation, Augmentation, and Potentiation Are Due to Effects of Residual Ca^{2+}

With few exceptions, all the phases of increased short-term plasticity are Ca^{2+} dependent in the sense that little or no facilitation, augmentation, or potentiation is generated by stimulation in Ca^{2+}-free medium. Originally, these phases of increased transmission were thought to be due to the effect of residual Ca^{2+} remaining in active zones after presynaptic activity and summating with Ca^{2+} influx during subsequent action potentials to generate slightly higher peaks of Ca^{2+} (Katz and Miledi, 1968; Zucker, 1989). Due to the highly nonlinear dependence of transmitter release on Ca^{2+}, a small residual amount could activate a substantial increase in phasic transmitter release during an action potential, while having only a small effect on mini frequency itself. However, as this relationship was examined more closely and with Ca^{2+} indicators to actually measure the residual intracellular Ca^{2+}, this hypothesis became unlikely. These findings led to the proposal that Ca^{2+} acts to increase transmission at one or more targets distinct from the sites triggering exocytosis, in addition to summating with peak Ca^{2+} transients to drive fusion. Unlike the triggering site, the facilitation site for Ca^{2+} binding should be a high-affinity site that can be influenced by the relatively low levels of residual Ca^{2+}. Other second messenger systems and kinases may also be involved.

Potentiation lasts for a long period after a strong tetanus because residual Ca^{2+} is present for the duration of PTP, presumably due to overloading of the processes responsible for removing excess Ca^{2+} from neurons. These processes include Ca^{2+} extrusion pumps, such as plasma membrane ATPase and Na^+-Ca^{2+} exchange, and Ca^{2+} uptake into organelles such as endoplasmic reticulum and mitochondria.

Summary

Short-term synaptic plasticity allows synaptic strength to be modulated as a function of prior activity and can cause large changes in responses during physiologically relevant patterns of stimulation. Synapses may show a decline in transmission (depression) or an increase in synaptic efficacy with time constants ranging from seconds (facilitation and augmentation) to minutes (potentiation or PTP) to hours (LTP); many synapses show a mixture of several of these phases. Synaptic depression may be due to depletion of a readily releasable supply of vesicles, to the inhibitory action of transmitter on presynaptic autoreceptors, or to the desensitization of postsynaptic receptors. Depression makes synapses selectively responsive to brief stimuli or to changes in level of activity. Frequency-dependent increases in synaptic efficacy are due to the effects of residual presynaptic Ca^{2+} acting to modulate the release process, probably through a high-affinity binding site. These frequency-dependent increases in synaptic efficacy allow synapses to distinguish significant signals from noise and to respond to selected patterns of activity.

References

Bennett, M. K., and Scheller, R. H. (1993). The molecular machinery for secretion is conserved from yeast to neurons. *Proc. Natl. Acad. Sci. USA* **90**(7), 2559–2563.

Block, M. R., Glick, B. S., Wilcox, C. A., Wieland, F. T., and Rothman, J. E. (1988). Purification of an N-ethylmaleimide-sensitive protein catalyzing vesicular transport. *Proc. Natl. Acad. Sci. USA* **85**(21), 7852–7856.

Boyd, I. A., and Martin, A. R. (1956). Spontaneous subthreshold activity at mammalian neuromuscular junctions. *J. Physiol. (Lond.)* **132**, 74–91.

Davies, C. H., Davies, S. N., and Collingridge, G. L. (1990). Paired-pulse depression of monosynaptic GABA-mediated inhibitory postsynaptic responses in rat hippocampus. *J. Physiol.* **424**, 513–531.

Gonzalez, L., and Scheller, R. H. (1999). Regulation of membrane trafficking: Structural insights from a Rab/effector complex. *Cell* **96**(6), 755–758.

Harlow, M. L., Ress, D., Stoschek, A., Marshall, R. M., and McMahan, U. J. (2001). The architecture of active zone material at the frog's neuromuscular junction. *Nature* **409**(6819), 479–484.

Heuser, J. E. (1977). Synaptic vesicle exocytosis revealed in quick-frozen frog neuromuscular junctions treated with 4-aminopyridine and given a single electrical shock. *Soc. Neurosci. Symp.* **2**, 215–239.

Heuser, J. E., Reese, T. S., Dennis, M. J., Jan, Y., Jan, L., and Evans, L. (1979). Synaptic vesicle exocytosis captured by quick freezing and correlated with quantal transmitter release. *J. Cell Biol.* **81**(2), 275–300.

Katz, B. (1969). The Release of Neural Transmitter Substances. Thomas, Springfield, IL.

Katz, B., and Miledi, R. (1968). The role of calcium in neuromuscular facilitation. *J. Physiol.* **195**(2), 481–492.

Landis, D. M., Hall, A. K., Weinstein, L. A., and Reese, T. S. (1988). The organization of cytoplasm at the presynaptic active zone of a central nervous system synapse. *Neuron* **1**(3), 201–209.

Liley, A. W. (1956). The quantal components of the mammalian end-plate potential. *J. Physiol.* **133**, 560–573.

Roberts, W. M. (1994). Localization of calcium signals by a mobile calcium buffer in frog saccular hair cells. *J. Neurosci.* **14**(5 Pt 2), 3246–3262.

Schneggenburger, R., and Neher, E. (2000). Intracellular calcium dependence of transmitter release rates at a fast central synapse. *Nature* **406**(6798); 889–893.

Sollner, T., Bennett, M. K., Whiteheart, S. W., Scheller, R. H., and Rothman, J. E. (1993a). A protein assembly-disassembly pathway in vitro that may correspond to sequential steps of synaptic vesicle docking, activation, and fusion. *Cell* **75**(3); 409–418.

Sollner, T., Whiteheart, S. W., Brunner, M., Erdjument-Bromage, H., Geromanos, S., Tempst, P., and Rothman, J. E. (1993b). SNAP receptor implicated in vesicle targeting and fusion. *Nature* **362**(6418); 318–324.

Sutton, R. B., Fasshauer, Jahn, R., and Brunger, A. T. (1998). Crystal structure of a SNARE complex involved in synaptic exocytosis at 2.4 A resolution. *Nature* **395**(6700); 347–353.

Yamada, W. M., and Zucker, R. S. (1992). Time course of transmitter release calculated from simulation of a calcium diffusion model. *Biophys J* **61**(3); 671–682.

Zucker, R. S. (1989) Short-term synaptic plasticity. *Annu. Rev. Neurosci.* **12**; 13–31.

Suggested Readings

Chen, Y. A., and Scheller, R. H. (2001). SNARE-mediated membrane fusion. *Nature Rev. Mol. Cell Biol.* **2**(2); 98–106.

De Camilli, P., Takei, K., and McPherson, P. S. (1995). The function of dynamin in endocytosis. *Curr. Opin. Neurobiol.* **5**(5); 559–565.

Dittman, J. S., and Regehr, W. G. (1998). Calcium dependence and recovery kinetics of presynaptic depression at the climbing fiber to Purkinje cell synapse. *J. Neurosci.* **18**(16); 6147–6162.

Liao, D., Hessler, N. A., and Malinow, R. (1995). Activation of postsynaptically silent synapses during pairing-induced LTP in CA1 region of hippocampal slice. *Nature* **375**(6530); 400–404.

Novick, P., Field, C., and Schekman, R. (1980). Identification of 23 complementation groups required for post-translational events in the yeast secretory pathway. *Cell* **21**(1); 205–215.

Peters, C., Bayer, M. J., Buhler, S., Andersen, J. S., Mann, M., and Mayer, A. (2001). Trans-complex formation by proteolipid channels in the terminal phase of membrane fusion. *Nature* **409**(6820); 581–588.

Rothman, J. E., and Warren, G. (1994). Implications of the SNARE hypothesis for intracellular membrane topology and dynamics. *Curr. Biol.* **4**(3); 220–233.

Ryan, T. A., Li, L., Chin, L. S., Greengard, P., and Smith, S. J. (1996). Synaptic vesicle recycling in synapsin I knock-out mice. *J. Cell Biol.* **134**(5); 1219–1227.

Ryan, T. A., Reuter, H., Wendland, B., Schweizer, F. E., Tsien, R. W., and Smith, S. J. (1993). The kinetics of synaptic vesicle recycling measured at single presynaptic boutons. *Neuron* **11**(4); 713–724.

Schiavo, G., Rossetto, O., Tonello, F., and Montecucco, C. (1995). Intracellular targets and metalloprotease activity of tetanus and botulism neurotoxins. *Curr. Top. Microbiol. Immunol.* **195**; 257–274.

Thomas L. Schwarz

9

Neurotransmitter Receptors

Chemical synaptic transmission plays a fundamental role in neuron-to-neuron and neuron-to-muscle communication. The type of receptors present in the plasma membrane determines in large part the nature of a neuron or muscle cell's response to a neurotransmitter. These receptors can either mediate the direct opening of an ion channel (ionotropic receptors) or alter the concentration of intracellular metabolites (metabotropic receptor). The sign of a given response can be inhibitory or excitatory, and the response magnitude is determined by receptor number, the "state" of the receptors, and the amount of transmitter released. Finally, the temporal and spatial summation of information conveyed by the activation of multiple receptors determines whether that neuron will fire an action potential or the muscle will contract. As one can see, there is remarkable flexibility and diversity in molding the response to neurotransmitter by constructing a synapse with the desired receptor types.

Two broad classifications exist for receptors. An *ionotropic receptor* is a relatively large, multisubunit complex typically composed of four or five individual proteins that combine to form an ion channel through the membrane (Fig. 9.1A). In the absence of neurotransmitter, these ion channels exist in a closed state and are largely impermeable to ions. Neurotransmitter binding induces rapid conformational changes that open the channel, permitting ions to flow down their electrochemical gradients. Changes in membrane current resulting from ligand binding to ionotropic receptors are generally measured on a millisecond time scale. The ion flow ceases when transmitter dissociates from the receptor or when the

receptor becomes desensitized, a process discussed in more detail later in this chapter.

In contrast, a *metabotropic receptor* is composed of a single polypeptide (Fig. 9.1B) and exerts its effects not through the direct opening an ion channel, but through binding to and activating GTP-binding proteins (often referred to as G-proteins). Transmitters that activate metabotropic receptors typically produce responses of slower onset and longer duration (from tenths of seconds to potentially hours) due to the series of enzymatic steps necessary to produce a response. The metabotropic receptors have more recently been named G-protein-coupled receptors, or GPCRs for short, to more accurately capture their properties; the latter nomenclature is adopted in this chapter.

We consider the structure of the ionotropic receptor family first and then turn to a description of the structure of the GPCRs. In each section, information is presented to establish a general structural model of each receptor type. These models are then used to guide the description of other related ionotropic or GPCRs. The order in which receptor types are presented is based predominantly on structural relatedness and should not be interpreted as representing their relative importance in the function of the nervous system.

IONOTROPIC RECEPTORS

All ionotropic receptors are membrane-bound protein complexes that form an ion-permeable pore in the membrane. By comparing the amino acid sequence

225

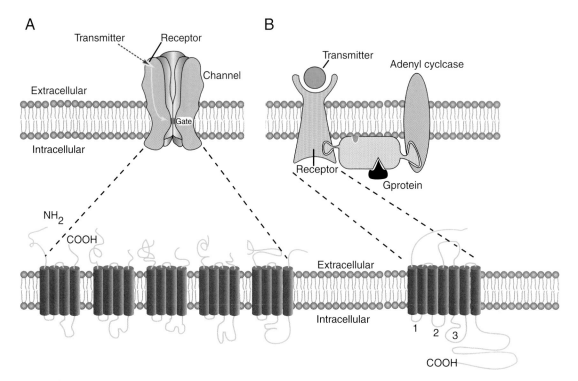

FIGURE 9.1   Structural comparison of ionotropic and metabotropic receptors. (A) *Ionotropic receptors* bind transmitter, and this binding translates directly into the opening of the ion channel through a series of conformational changes. Ionotropic receptors are composed of multiple subunits. The five subunits that together form the functional nAChR are shown. Note that each of the nAChR subunits wraps back and forth through the membrane four times and that the mature receptor is composed of five subunits. (B) *Metabotropic receptors* bind transmitter and, through a series of conformational changes, bind to G-proteins and activate them. G-proteins then activate enzymes such as adenylate cyclase to produce cAMP. Through the activation of cAMP-dependent protein kinase, ion channels become phosphorylated, which affects their gating properties. Metabotropic receptors are single subunits. They contain seven transmembrane-spanning segments, with the cytoplasmic loops formed between the segments providing the points of interactions for coupling to G-proteins. Adapted from Kandel (1991).

of cloned ionotropic receptors, one can deduce that they are similar in overall structure, although two independent ancestral genes have given rise to two distinct families. One family includes one of the receptors for acetylcholine (ACh), the nicotinic ACh receptor (nAChR), a receptor for γ-aminobutyric acid (GABA), the GABA_A receptor, the glycine receptor, and one subclass of serotonin (5-HT) receptors, the 5HT3 receptor. The other family comprises the many types of ionotropic glutamate receptors (Hollmann and Heinemann, 1994).

Our understanding of ionotropic receptor structure and function has expanded enormously since the mid-1970s. Molecular approaches have provided elegant and extensive descriptions of gene families encoding different receptors, and systems for expressing cloned cDNAs have permitted detailed structure–function analysis of each receptor subtype. The expression of subunits independently and together has clarified the role that specific combinations of subunits play in deter-

mining the responses mediated by ionotropic receptor families. With the addition of biophysical and X-ray structural analysis, events associated with the opening of at least one ionotropic receptor, the nAChR, are available at nearly atomic resolution (Unwin, 1995).

nAChR Is a Model for the Structure of Ionotropic Receptors

The nAChR is so named because the plant alkaloid nicotine can bind to the ACh-binding site and activate the receptor. Nicotine is therefore called an *agonist* of ACh because it binds to the receptor and opens it. In contrast, *antagonists* are molecules that bind to the receptor and inhibit its function. Agonists and antagonists are powerful tools that permit characterization of the structure and function of individual receptor subtypes.

We know more about the structure of the nAChR than about any other ionotropic receptor, primarily

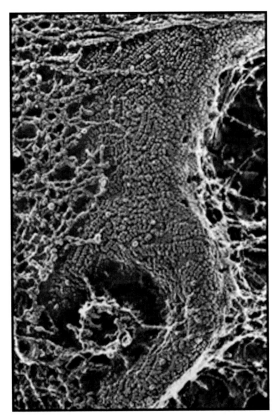

FIGURE 9.2   Panoramic view of the postsynaptic membrane of an electrocyte in the *Torpedo* electric organ, revealed by "deep-etch" electron microscopy. To the left, a lace-like basal lamina lies above the membrane, obscuring it from view. Near the bottom center, the basal lamina assumes a ring-like appearance as it dips down into a dark postsynaptic invagination. In the center of the field, the basal lamina has been fractured away to reveal the true external surface of the postsynaptic membrane. Clusters and linear arrays of 8- to 9-nm protrusions can be clearly seen. These represent AChR oligomers. To the right, the postsynaptic membrane has been freeze-fractured away, thus revealing an underlying meshwork of cytoplasmic filaments that supports the postsynaptic membrane and its receptors. ×175,000. Original courtesy of J. Heuser.

nAChR Is a Heteromeric Protein Complex with a Distinct Architecture

The structure of nAChR is typical of ionotropic receptors. The nAChR purified as described from *Torpedo* is composed of five subunits (see Fig. 9.1) and has a native molecular mass of approximately 290 kDa. The subunits are designated α, β, γ, and δ, and each receptor complex contains two copies of the α subunit. The subunits are homologous membrane-bound proteins that assemble in the bilayer to form a ring enclosing a central pore. Pioneering electron microscopic analyses by Nigel Unwin have provided the best image of the structural appearance of the nAChR receptor (Fig. 9.3). In fact, nAChR is the only membrane-bound neurotransmitter receptor for which high-resolution structural information is available. The extracellular domain of each subunit together forms a funnel-shaped opening that extends approximately 100 Å outward from the outer leaflet of the plasma membrane. The funnel at the outer portion of the receptor has an inside diameter of 20–25 Å. The funnel shape is thought to concentrate and force ions and transmitter to interact with amino acids in the limited space of the pore without producing a major barrier to diffusion. This funnel narrows near the center of the lipid bilayer to form the domain of the receptor that determines the opened or closed state of the ion pore. The intracellular domain of the receptor forms short exits for ions traveling into the cell and an entrance for ions traveling out of the cell. The intracellular domain also establishes the association of the receptor with other intracellular proteins that determine the subcellular localization of the nAChR. The arrangement of the subunits in the receptor is somewhat debatable. However, most data support a model whereby the β subunit lies between the two α subunits (Unwin, 1995).

Each nAChR Subunit Has Multiple Membrane-Spanning Segments

The primary structure of each nAChR subunit was obtained by the efforts of Shosaka Numa and colleagues. The deduced amino acid sequence from cloned mRNAs indicates that nAChR subunits range in size from 40 to 65 kDa. A general domain structure for each subunit was derived from primary sequence data and toxin and antibody-binding studies. Each subunit consists of four transmembrane (TM)-spanning segments referred to as TM1–TM4 (Fig. 9.4). Each segment is composed mainly of hydrophobic amino acids that stabilize the domain within the hydrophobic environment of the lipid membrane. The

because electric organs of certain species of fish, such as the *Torpedo* ray, contain nearly crystalline arrays of this molecule (Fig. 9.2). The electric organ is a specialized form of skeletal muscle that has the potential to generate large voltages (as much as 500 V in some cases) from the simultaneous opening of arrays of ion channels activated through the binding of ACh. Purification of nAChRs was aided significantly by utilization of a toxin from snake venom called α-bungarotoxin. Affinity columns constructed with α-bungarotoxin bind to the nAChR with high affinity and specificity, providing a means of purifying nearly homogeneous nAChRs in a single chromatographic step.

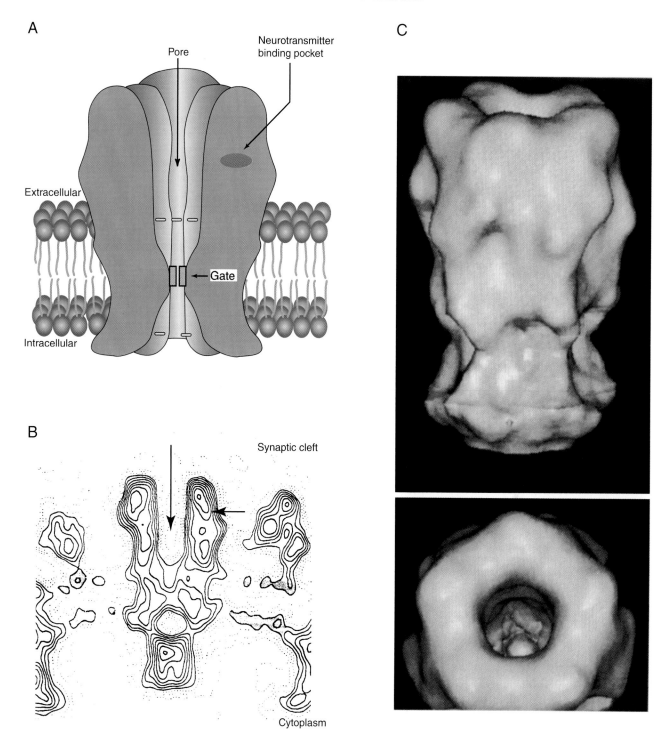

FIGURE 9.3 (A) Vertical section diagramming the structure of the nAChR as it is believed to exist in the membrane. Note that the funnel-shaped structure narrows to a small central point referred to as the gate. Strategically placed rings of negatively charged amino acids on both sides of the gate form part of the selectivity filter for positively charged ions. The approximate position of the neurotransmitter-binding site is shown in relation to the gate and the plasma membrane. (B) Protein density map derived from reconstructions of the nAChR imaged by cryo-electron microscopy. The vertical arrow indicates the direction of ion flow from outside to inside within the funnel-shaped part of the receptor. The horizontal arrow indicates the predicted position of the neurotransmitter-binding site that resides approximately 30 Å above the bilayer. The additional protein density attached to the bottom of the receptor is suggested to be a protein that anchors the nAChR to synapses. (C) Three-dimensional computer rendering of the nAChR. (Top) Side view of the nAChR similar to that in A. The darker shaded area near the bottom of the receptor delineates the approximate location where the receptor contacts the lipid bilayer. (Bottom) A view looking down into the funnel-shaped opening of the receptor. Note that the funnel narrows forming the gate. Original figure adapted from Unwin (1993).

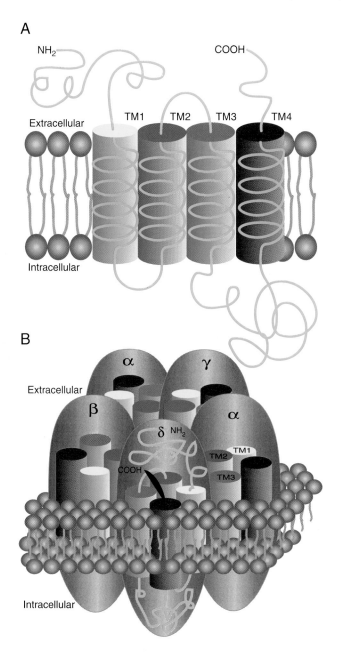

A

NH₂   COOH

Extracellular

TM1   TM2   TM3   TM4

Intracellular

B

α   γ

Extracellular

β

α

δ NH₂

COOH

TM2   TM1

TM3

Intracellular

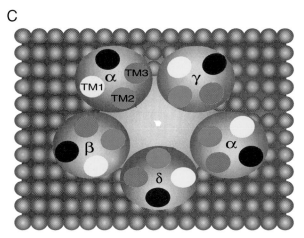

C

α   TM3

TM1

TM2

γ

β

α

δ

four transmembrane domains are arranged in an antiparallel fashion, wrapping back and forth through the membrane. The N terminus of each subunit extends into the extracellular space, as does the loop connecting TM2 and TM3, as well as the C terminus. Amino acids linking TM1 and TM2 and those linking TM3 and TM4 form short loops that extend into the cytoplasm.

Structure of the Channel Pore Determines Ion Selectivity and Current Flow

In the model shown in Fig. 9.4C, each subunit of the nAChR can be seen to contribute one cylindrical component (representing a membrane-spanning segment) that presents itself to a central cavity that forms the ion channel through the center of the complex. The membrane-spanning segments that line the pore are the five TM2 regions, one contributed by each subunit. The amino acids that compose the TM2 segment are arranged in such a way that three rings of negatively charged amino acids are oriented toward the central pore of the channel (Fig. 9.5). These rings of negative charge appear to provide much of the selectivity filter of the channel, ensuring that only cations can pass through the pore. Anions are largely excluded due to charge repulsion (Imoto *et al.*, 1988). The nAChR is permeable to most cations, such as Na^+, K^+, and Ca^{2+}, although monovalent cations are preferred. This mechanism for selectivity is poor in relation to the selectivity described for the family of voltage-gated ion channels (e.g., voltage-gated Ca^{2+} channels; see Chapter 8). The restricted physical dimensions of the pore—9–10 Å in the open state—contribute greatly to the selectivity for particular ions (Unwin, 1995). A coarse filtering that also influences selectivity appears to be a shielding effect produced by other negatively charged amino acids surrounding the outer channel region of the receptor.

Ions do not directly enter or exit through the central pore of the cytoplasmic end of the nAChR.

FIGURE 9.4 (A) Diagram highlighting the orientation of membrane-spanning segments of one subunit of the nAChR. The amino and carboxy termini extend in the extracellular space. The four membrane-spanning segments are designated TM1–TM4. Each forms an α helix as it traverses the membrane. (B) Side view of the five subunits in their approximate positions within the receptor complex. There are two α subunits present in each nAChR. (C) Top view of all five subunits highlighting the relative positions of their membrane-spanning segments, TM1–TM4, and the position of TM2 that lines the channel pore. Adapted from Kandel, (1991).

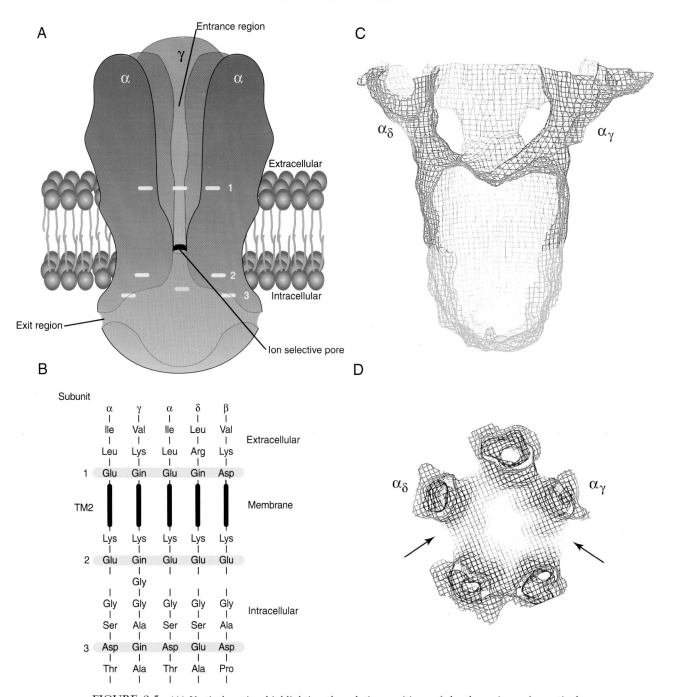

FIGURE 9.5 (A) Vertical section highlighting the relative positions of the three rings of negatively charged amino acids that help form the cation selectivity of the nAChR. Regions where ions exit or enter from the intracellular side of the receptor are disposed laterally at the base of the receptor. (B) Amino acid sequence of each of the TM2 membrane-spanning segments of the five nAChR subunits. Numbers 1–3 correspond to the positions of the amino acids taking part in the formation for the three rings of negatively charged amino acids that determine the cation selectivity of the pore. Aspartate (Asp) and glutamate (Glu) are negatively charge amino acids. (C) Wire frame portrayal of the protein density distribution of the intracellular portion of the nAChR. The front portion of the receptor was cut away to reveal the inverted cone-shaped cavity of the intracellular domain. The green wire frame represents protein density contributed by the anchoring protein rapsyn. (D) Wire frame portrayal of the protein density distribution of the intracellular domain of the nAChR looking downward from within the receptor. Arrows indicate major gaps in the lateral walls of the receptor where ions enter and exit. Adapted from Miyazawa (1999).

A

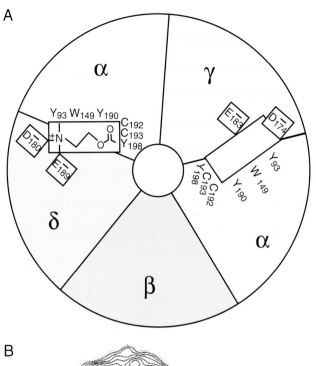

B

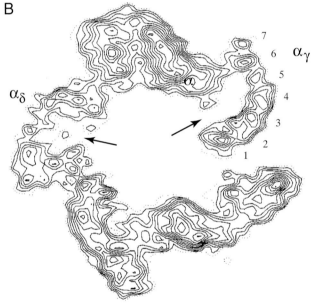

C

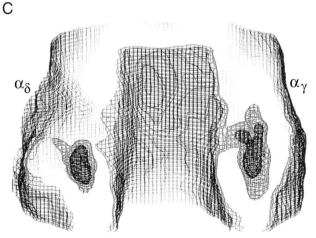

Two narrow openings are present on the lateral aspects of the cytoplasmic portion of the receptor through which ions must travel to exit or gain access to the central pore (Fig. 9.5) (Miyazawa *et al.*, 1999). α-Helical rods extending down from each subunit form an inverted pentagonal cone to produce these openings. While too large (8 × 15 Å) to be a significant barrier to ion flow, these lateral pores could serve as an additional filtering step for the passage of certain ions. Collectively, these physical characteristics of the pore—together with the electrochemical gradient across the plasma membrane—determine the possibility of ionic movements. Thus, when the pore of the nAChR opens, anions remain restricted from movement across the membrane while positively charged cations move down their respective electrochemical gradients, resulting in an influx of Na^+ and Ca^{2+} and an efflux of K^+.

There are Two Binding Sites for ACh on nAChR

Each receptor complex has two ACh-binding sites that reside in the extracellular domain and lie approximately 30 Å from the outer leaflet of the membrane (see Fig. 9.3). The ACh-binding site is formed for the most part by six amino acids in α subunits; however, amino acids in both γ and δ subunits also contribute to binding (Fig. 9.6A). Mutations introduced at these critical amino acids in the α subunit significantly attenuate ligand binding. The two binding sites are

FIGURE 9.6 (A) Diagram of the relative positions of amino acids that form the Ach-binding site in the nAChR. The view is from above the receptor looking down into the pore. Each subunit is represented by a wedge. At the left, Ach is shown bound to its site at the interface between α and δ subunits. The length of the binding site is shown slightly contracted relative to the site (between α and γ subunits) without bound Ach. Critical amino acids for transmitter binding are indicated. Residues shown in boxes are amino acids predicted to make contact with the positively charged part of the Ach molecule. Note that many of the residues important for ACh binding are contributed by the α subunit. Cys residues at positions 192 and 193 form a disulfide bond essential for stabilizing the ACh-binding pocket. Adapted from Karlin (1993). (B) A top-down view of the protein density map of nAChR sliced through the area where the ACh-binding areas reside. Note that ACh molecules must gain access to their binding sites through channels whose openings are on the inside of the funnel-shaped portion of the receptor. (C) A lateral view of a wire frame portrayal of nAChR at the level of Ach-binding sites. A portion of the receptor was cut away to highlight the fact that cavities where Ach bind must be accessed from the pore of the receptor through short channels. Adapted from Miyazawa (1999).

not equivalent because of the asymmetry of the receptor due to the different neighboring subunits (either γ or δ) adjacent to the two α subunits. Significant cooperativity also exists within the receptor molecule, and so binding of the first molecule of ACh enhances binding of the second. A higher resolution structure of the nAChR (Miyazawa *et al.*, 1999) has revealed that access to ACh-binding sites appears to be through small channels that open into the interior mouth of the pore (Figs. 9.6B and 9.6C). Thus, ACh molecules must enter the pore and traverse these channels to gain access to their binding sites. Attractive forces similar to those that bring positively charged ions into the pore may also attract positively charged ACh molecules into the channels that lead to ACh-binding sites. Two adjacent Cys residues (Cys-192 and Cys-193) in each α subunit form a disulfide bond that also appears to contribute to the stability of the ACh-binding pocket (Fig. 9.6A). These Cys residues are highly conserved in most ionotropic receptors and must form an essential bond for stabilizing high-affinity neurotransmitter binding. α-Bungarotoxin binds to the α subunit in close proximity to the two adjacent Cys residues.

Opening of nAChR Occurs through Concerted Conformational Changes Induced by ACh Binding

When nAChR binds two molecules of ACh, the channel opens almost instantaneously (time constants for opening are approximately 20 μs), thus permitting the passage of ions. A model developed from electron micrographic reconstructions of the nicotine-bound form of nAChR indicates that the closed-to-open transition is associated with a rotation of the TM2 segments (Fig. 9.7; Unwin, 1995). The TM2 segments are helical and exhibit a kink in their structure that forces a Leu residue from each segment into a tight ring that effectively blocks the flow of ions through the central pore of the receptor. When the TM2 segments rotate because of ACh binding, the kinks also rotate, relaxing the constriction formed by the Leu ring, and ions can then permeate through the pore. The rotation also orients a series of Ser and Thr residues (amino acids with a polar character) into the central area of the pore, which facilitates the permeation of water-solvated cations. As the resolution of the structure increases, refinements in this model are likely to be

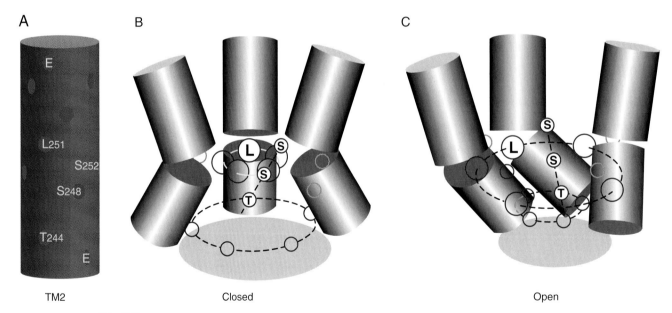

FIGURE 9.7 (A) Relative positions of amino acids in the TM2 segment of one of the nAChR α subunits modeled as an α helix. Glutamate residues (E) that form parts of the negatively charged rings for ion selectivity are shown at the top and bottom of the helix. (B) Arrangement of three of the TM2 segments of the nAChR modeled with the receptor in the closed (ACh-free) configuration. In the closed configuration, leucine (L) residues form a right ring in the center of the pore that blocks ion permeation. (C) Arrangement of the three TM2 segments after ACh binds to the receptor. In the open configuration, construction formed by the ring of leucine (L) residues opens as the helices twist about their axes. Note that polar serine (S) and threonine (T) residues align when ACh binds, which apparently helps the water-solvated ions travel though the pore. Adapted from Unwin (1995).

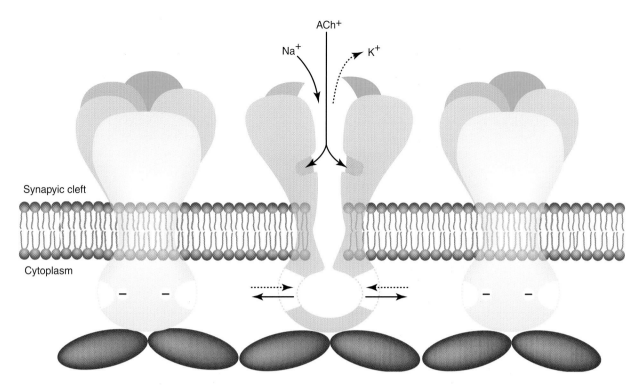

FIGURE 9.8 Summary figure highlighting structural features of nAChR. The ACh-free form of the receptor remains closed to ion flow. ACh gains access to its binding site by entering the outer portion of the central pore of the nAChR that produces a relaxation of the central pore and an expansion of the holes in the lateral walls of the intracellular portion of the receptor. The protein rapsyn, represented by the gray ovals, anchors nAChR to synapses by interacting with the intracellular domain. Adapted from Miyazawa (1999).

forthcoming. However the architecture of nAChR is well established and provides a structural framework to which all other ionotropic receptors can be compared.

Main features of the nAChR transition from a closed to open state are summarized in Fig 9.8. ACh gains access to its binding sites by entering the central pore of the receptor where it then enters small channels that provide access to the binding sites. Once both binding sites are occupied, the receptor opens rapidly to permit ion flow. The twisting of TM2 segments induced by ACh binding gates open the ion pore. In addition to negatively charged rings spaced within the central channel, charge screening also occurs in the lateral openings of the cytoplasmic domain of the receptor (Fig. 9.8). The ion selectivity of nAChR for positively charged ions (Na$^+$ and K$^+$ mainly) comes from the charge screening at these different levels and the physical constriction of the gate of the pore.

The Muscle Form of nAChR Is Very Similar to nAChR from *Torpedo*

nAChRs at the neuromuscular junction are a concentrated collection of homogeneous receptors having a structure similar to that of the *Torpedo* electric organ. This similarity is not surprising because the electric organ is a specialized form of muscle tissue. The adult form of the muscle receptor has the pentameric structure $\alpha_2\beta\epsilon\delta$. An embryonic form of the receptor has an analogous structure, except that the ϵ subunit is replaced by a unique γ subunit. The embryonic and adult subunits of both mouse and bovine muscle receptors have been cloned and expressed in heterologous systems, such as the *Xenopus laevis* oocyte (Box 9.1), and the receptors differ in both channel kinetics and channel conductance. These differences in channel properties appear to be necessary for the proper function of the nAChRs as they undergo the transition from developing to mature neuromuscular junction synapses.

BOX 9.1

THE *XENOPUS* OOCYTE

The *Xenopus* oocyte has been used extensively to study the properties of cDNAs encoding receptor subunits and their mutated forms. In addition, the oocyte has been used to study how combinations of different subunits interact to produce receptors with different properties. The large size and efficient translational machinery of *Xenopus* oocytes make them ideal for electrophysiological analyses of cDNAs encoding prospective receptors and channels. For example, mRNAs produced by an *in vitro* transcription of cDNAs encoding each of the individual nAChR subunits were introduced into oocytes by microinjection (panel A). Several days later, oocytes were voltage clamped to study the properties of the expressed channels (panel B). When ACh was applied through a separate pipette, a significant inward current was detected in the oocyte (panel C, trace 1). The response was specifically blocked by addition of an antagonist, tubocurarine (panel C, trace 2), and the block was reversed by a 15-min wash (panel C, trace 3). Details of this study indicate that all four of the nAChR subunits (α, β, γ, and δ) were required for ACh to produce an electrophysiological response. More recently, the patch-clamp technique has also been applied to oocyte expression of receptors to analyze the behavior of single channels. Adapted from Mishina *et al.* (1984).

M. Neal Waxham

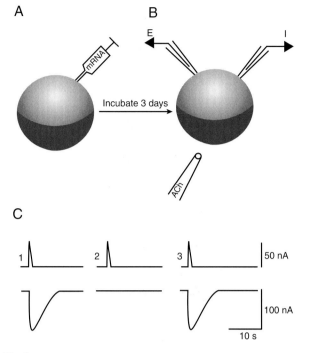

Reference

Mishina, M., Kurosaki, T., Tobimatsu, T., Morimoto, Y., Noda, M., Yamamoto, T., Terao, M., Lindstrom, J., Takahashi, T., Kuno, M., and Numa, S. (1984). Expression of functional acetylcholine receptor from cloned cDNAs. *Nature (Lond.)* **307**, 604–608.

nAChR Matures as a Typical Membrane-Bound Protein and Has Well-Ordered Assembly

The pathway of nAChR assembly in muscle is a tightly regulated process. For example, the five subunits of nAChR have the potential to assemble randomly into 208 different combinations. Nevertheless, in vertebrate muscle, only one of these configurations ($\alpha_2\beta\epsilon\delta$) is typically found in mature tissue, indicating a very high degree of coordinated assembly and, ultimately, little structural variability. The well-ordered assembly of specific intermediates is essential for this coordinated process, and the intermediates formed appear to start with a dimer between α and either ϵ

(γ in mature muscle) or δ. The heterodimers then bind to β and to each other to form the final receptor. An alternative pathway in which α, β, and γ first form a trimer has also been proposed. All of this assembly takes place within the endoplasmic reticulum. During intracellular maturation, each subunit is glycosylated, and, if glycosylation is inhibited, the production of mature nAChRs decreases. Two highly conserved disulfide bonds in the N-terminal extracellular domain are essential for efficient assembly of the mature receptor. The first is between two adjacent Cys residues (Cys-192 and Cys-193) and, as noted, resides very close to the ACh-binding site on the receptor (see Fig. 9.6A). The second bond is between two Cys residues 15 amino acids apart, forming a loop in the extracellular domain.

Phosphorylation Is a Common Posttranslational Modification of Receptors

Many ionotropic receptors, such as nAChR, are phosphorylated, although the functional significance of the phosphorylation is not always evident. nAChR is phosphorylated by at least three protein kinases. cAMP-dependent protein kinase (PKA) phosphorylates the γ and δ subunits, Ca^{2+}/phospholipid-dependent protein kinase (PKC) phosphorylates the δ subunit, and an unidentified tyrosine kinase phosphorylates the β, γ, and δ subunits. The phosphorylation sites are all found in the intracellular loop between TM3 and TM4 membrane-spanning segments. Phosphorylation by these three protein kinases appears to increase the rapid phase of desensitization of the receptor. Desensitization of receptors is a common observation, and this process limits the amount of ion flux through a receptor by producing transitions into a closed state (one that does not permit ion flow) in the continued presence of neurotransmitter. For the nAChR, the rate of desensitization has a time constant of approximately 50–100 ms. This rate appears to be too slow to have much significance in shaping the synaptic response at the neuromuscular junction, where the response typically lasts from 5 to 10 ms. This slow desensitization is not true of the brain forms of nAChR and is discussed further later.

Structures of Other Ionotropic Receptors Are Variations of the nAChR Structure

On the basis of similarity of structure, clear evolutionary relationships exist for the family of ionotropic receptors. Figure 9.9 shows an evolutionary tree for the family of ionotropic receptors related to nAChR. An early major subdivision separates those receptors permeable to anions from those permeable to cations. The former group includes GABA$_A$ and glycine receptors, whereas the latter group includes 5-HT3 and ACh receptors. One can begin to appreciate that structural similarities can predict a degree of functional similarity. Each of these receptor types is described in the next section.

Neuronal nAChRs Contain Two Types of Subunits

Neuronal nAChRs are similar, yet distinct in structure to the *Torpedo* isoform of the receptor (Figs. 9.9 and 9.10). For example, neuronal nAChR is composed of only two types of subunits, α and β, which combine to produce the functional receptor, and the majority of these receptors do not bind to α-bungarotoxin. At least nine different α subtypes ($\alpha1$ being the muscle α subunit) have been identified, and some are species specific ($\alpha8$ is found only in chicken and $\alpha9$ is found only in rat). Four different β subtypes ($\beta1$ being the muscle β subunit) have been identified. The neuronal β subunits are not closely related to the muscle $\beta1$ subunit and are sometimes referred to simply as non-α subunits. One structural feature that distinguishes neuronal α subunits from β subunits is the presence of particular Cys residues in the extracellular domain of the α subunit. Two of these Cys residues are adjacent to one another and form a disulfide bond. β subunits do not have these adjacent Cys residues. Because these Cys residues are critical for ACh binding, α subunits of neuronal AChRs, like muscle α subunits, contain the main contact points for ACh binding (Fig. 9.10). All of the α and β genes encode proteins with four transmembrane-spanning segments (TM1–TM4). Although the physical structure of this receptor family has not been well characterized, it appears that each functional receptor is a pentameric assembly.

Structural Diversity of Neuronal nAChRs Produces Channels with Unique Properties

Neuronal nAChRs have diverse functions and are the receptors presumed to be responsible for the psychophysical effects of nicotine addiction. One major function of nAChRs in the brain is to modulate excitatory synaptic transmission through a presynaptic action. The diversity in function of nAChRs can be related to the heterogeneous structure contributed by the thousands of possible combinations between the different α and β subunits. Control mechanisms for receptor assembly in neurons do not appear to be as stringent as those of the nAChR in *Torpedo* and muscle. Functional neuronal nAChRs can be assembled from a single subunit (e.g., $\alpha7$, $\alpha8$, or $\alpha9$), and a single type of α subunit can also be assembled with multiple types of β subunits (e.g., $\alpha3$ with $\beta2$ or $\beta4$ or both) and vice versa (Fig. 9.10). These additional possibilities produce a staggering array of potential receptor molecules, each with distinct properties, including differences in single channel kinetics and rates of desensitization. This type of diversity is not unique to neuronal nAChRs. For most receptor classes studied in detail, diversity is the rule and not the exception. It is intriguing to speculate that subunit composition may also play roles in targeting the receptors to different intracellular locations.

Neuronal nAChRs exhibit a range of single-channel conductances between 5 and 50 pS, depending on the tissue or the specific subunits expressed. Most, but

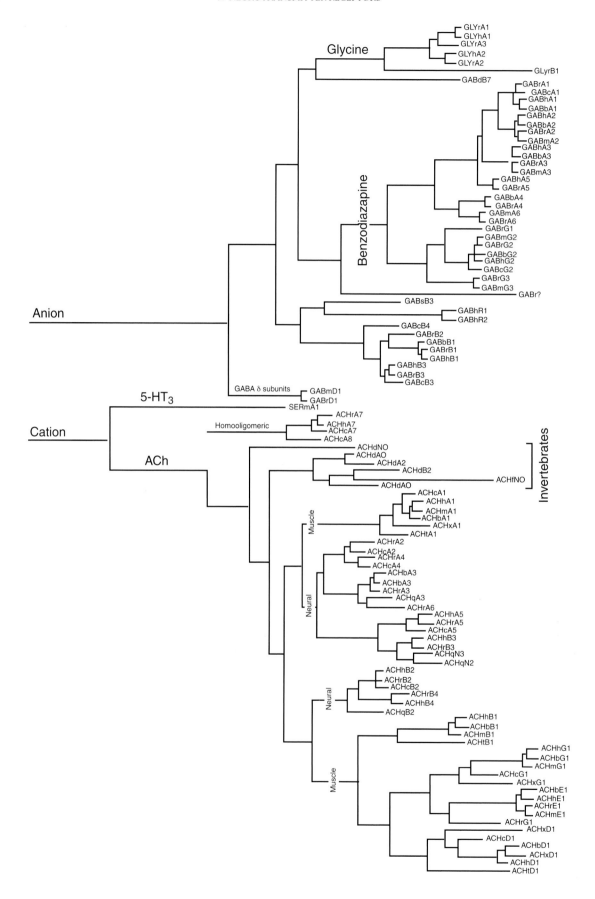

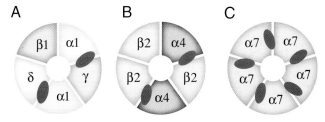

FIGURE 9.10 Diagrams of top-down views of AChR from muscle (A), one of the neuronal AChRs composed of $\alpha 2$ and $\beta 4$ subunits (B), and the homoligomeric form of the neuronal AChR produced by the assembly of $\alpha 7$ subunits (C). Purple ovals represent the Ach-binding sites on each receptor complex. ACh receptors from brain are diverse in both structure and properties due to the variety of different receptor complexes produced from subunit mixing.

not all, of these receptors are blocked by neuronal bungarotoxin, a snake venom distinct from α-bungarotoxin. All of the neuronal nAChRs are cation-permeable channels that, in addition to permitting the influx of Na^+ and the efflux of K^+, permit an influx of Ca^{2+}. The Ca^{2+} permeability for neuronal nAChR is greater than that for the muscle nAChR and is variable among the different neuronal receptor subtypes. Indeed, some receptors have very high Ca^{2+}/Na^+ permeability ratios; e.g., $\alpha 7$ nAChRs exhibit a Ca^{2+}/Na^+ permeability ratio of nearly 20, whereas other neuronal isoforms exhibit Ca^{2+}/Na^+ permeability ratios of about 1.0–1.5. The Ca^{2+} permeability of the $\alpha 7$ nAChR can be eliminated by the mutation of a single amino acid residue in TM2 (Glu-237 for Ala) without significantly affecting other aspects of the receptor. This key Glu residue presumably lies within the pore of the receptor and enhances the passage of Ca^{2+} ions through an interaction with its negatively charged side chain. Activation of $\alpha 7$ receptors through the binding of ACh could therefore produce a significant increase in the level of intracellular Ca^{2+} without the opening of voltage-gated Ca^{2+} channels. Subunits $\alpha 7$, $\alpha 8$, and $\alpha 9$ are also the α-bungarotoxin-binding subtypes of neuronal nAChRs.

FIGURE 9.9 Evolutionary relationships of the family of cloned ionotropic receptor subunits. The nomenclature used to describe each receptor subunit is RRRsS#, where RRR represent the type of receptor, s the organism, S the subunit type, and # the subunit number. Type of receptor (RRR): ACh, acetylcholine; GAB, GABA; GLY, glycine; and SER, serotonin. Organism (s): b, bovine; c, chicken; d, *Drosophila*; f, filaria; g, goldfish; h, human; l, locust; m, mouse; n, nematode; r, rat; s, snail; t, *Torpedo*; and x, *Xenopus*. Subunit type (S): A, α; B, β; G, γ; D, δ; E, ϵ; R, rho; N, non-α; and ?, undetermined. Adpated from Ortells and Lunt (1995).

Neuronal nAChRs Desensitize Rapidly

For the nAChR from muscle, desensitization is minor and probably is not of physiological significance in determining the shape of the synaptic response at the neuromuscular junction. However, for some neuronal nAChRs, desensitization likely plays a major role in determining the effects of the actions of ACh. Receptors composed of $\alpha 7$, $\alpha 8$, and certain α/β combinations exhibit desensitization time constants of between 100 and 500 ms, whereas others exhibit desensitization constants between 2 and 20 s. Given the diverse functions of neuronal nAChRs, the variable rates of desensitization likely play important roles whereby this inherent property of the receptor shapes the physiological response generated from binding ACh.

One Serotonin Receptor Subtype, 5-HT3, Is Ionotropic and Is a Close Relative of nAChR

5-HT is historically thought of as a metabotropic transmitter that binds to and activates only GPCRs (described in more detail later). The 5-HT3 subclass is an exception forming an ionotropic receptor activated by binding 5-HT. The 5-HT3 receptor is permeable to Na^+ and K^+ ions and is similar in many ways to nAChR in that both desensitize rapidly and are blocked by tubocurarine. From expression studies of the cloned cDNA, it appears that the 5-HT3 receptor is a homomeric complex composed of five copies of the same subunit. The deduced amino acid sequence of the cDNA indicates that the protein is 487 amino acids long (56 kDa) and has a structure most analogous to the $\alpha 7$ subtype of neuronal nAChRs (see Fig. 9.9), which also forms a homooligomeric receptor.

The 5-HT3 receptor is mostly impermeable to divalent cations. For example, Ca^{2+} is largely excluded from permeation and in fact effectively blocks current flow through the pore, even though the predicted pore size of the channel (7.6 Å) is approximately the same as that for the nAChR (8.4 Å). Apparently, other physical or electrochemical barriers limit the capacity of divalent ions to permeate the 5-HT3 pore. Dose–response studies indicate that at least two ligand-binding sites must be occupied for the channel to open; however, the binding of agonist and/or opening of the channel appears to be approximately 10 times slower than for most other ligand-gated ion channels. The functional significance or physical explanation of this slow opening is not known. The native 5-HT3 receptor also exhibits desensitization (time constant 1–5 s), although the reported desensitization rate varies widely, depending on the methodology used for analysis and the source of receptor. Interestingly, this desensitization can be significantly slowed or enhanced by single amino acid substitutions at a Leu residue in the TM2 segment of the subunit.

5-HT3 receptors are distributed sparsely on primary sensory nerve endings in the periphery and are distributed widely at low concentrations in the mammalian CNS. The 5-HT3 receptor is clinically significant because antagonists of 5-HT3 receptors have important applications as antiemetics, anxiolytics, and antipsychotics.

GABA$_A$ Receptors Are Related in Structure to nAChRs, but Exhibit an Inhibitory Function

Synaptic inhibition in the mammalian brain is mediated principally by GABA receptors. The most widespread ionotropic receptor activated by GABA is designated GABA$_A$. The subunits composing the GABA$_A$ receptor have sequence homology with the nAChR subunit family, and the two families have presumably diverged from a common ancestral gene. In fact, the general structure of the two receptors appears to be quite similar. The GABA$_A$ receptor is composed of multiple subunits, probably forming a heteropentameric complex of approximately 275 kDa. Five different types of subunits are associated with GABA$_A$ receptors and are designated α, β, γ, δ, and ϵ. An additional subunit, ρ, is found predominantly in the retina, whereas the other subunits are distributed widely in the brain. Each subunit group also has different subtypes; e.g., six different α, four β, four γ, and two ρ subunits have been identified. The predicted amino acid sequences indicate that each of these subunits has a molecular mass ranging between 48 and 64 kDa. Like neuronal nAChR, these subunits mix in a heterogeneous fashion to produce a wide array of GABA$_A$ receptors with different pharmacological and electrophysiological properties. The predominant GABA$_A$ receptor in brain and spinal cord is $\alpha1$, $\beta2$, and $\gamma2$ with a likely stoichiometry of two $\alpha1$s, two $\beta2$s, and one $\gamma2$. Expression of subunit cDNAs in oocytes indicates that the α subunit is essential for producing a functional channel. The α subunit also appears to contain the high-affinity binding site for GABA.

The ion channel associated with the GABA$_A$ receptor is selective for anions (in particular, Cl$^-$), and the selectivity is provided by strategically placed positively charged amino acids near the ends of the ion channel. When GABA binds to and activates this receptor, Cl$^-$ flows into the cell, producing a hyperpolarization by moving the membrane potential away

from the threshold for firing an action potential. The neuronal GABA$_A$ receptor exhibits multiple conductance levels, with the predominant conductance being 27–30 pS. Measurements and modeling of single-channel kinetics suggest that two sequential binding sites exist for anions within the pore.

The GABA$_A$ Receptor Binds Several Compounds That Affect Its Properties

The GABA$_A$ receptor is an allosteric protein, its properties are modulated by the binding of a number of compounds. Two well-studied examples are barbiturates and benzodiazepines, both of which bind to the GABA$_A$ receptor and potentiate GABA binding. The net result is that in the presence of barbiturates, benzodiazepines, or both, the same concentration of GABA will cause increased inhibition. Benzodiazepine binding is conferred on the receptor by the γ subunit, but the presence of α and β subunits is necessary for the qualitative and quantitative aspects of benzodiazepine binding. The benzodiazepine-binding site appears to lie along the interface between α and γ subunits and only certain subtypes are sensitive to benzodiazepines. Benzodiazepine binding to GABA$_A$ receptors requires $\alpha1$, 2, or 5 and $\gamma2$ or 3; other subunit combinations are insensitive to benzodiazepines.

Picrotoxin, a potent convulsant compound, appears to bind within the channel pore of the GABA$_A$ receptor and prevent ion flow. Single-channel experiments indicate that picrotoxin either slowly blocks an open channel or prevents the GABA receptor from undergoing a transition into a long-duration open state. Apparently, barbiturates produce similar changes in channel properties, but they potentiate rather than inhibit GABA$_A$ receptor function. Bicuculline, another potent convulsant, appears to inhibit GABA$_A$ receptor channel activity by decreasing the binding of GABA to the receptor. Steroid metabolites of progesterone, corticosterone, and testosterone also appear to have potentiating effects on GABA currents that are similar in many ways to the action of barbiturates; however, the binding sites for these steroids and the barbiturates are distinct. Finally, penicillin directly inhibits GABA receptor function, apparently by binding within the pore and thus is designated an open channel blocker.

The physiological effects of compounds such as picrotoxin, bicuculline, and penicillin are striking. Each of these compounds at a sufficiently high concentration can produce widespread and sustained seizure activity. Conversely, many, but not all, of the sedative properties associated with barbiturates and benzodiazepines can be attributed to their ability to augment inhibition in the brain through enhancing the inhibitory potency of GABA.

Interestingly, ρ-subunit-containing GABA receptors, found in abundance in the retina, are pharmacologically unique. They are resistant to the inhibitory action of bicuculline, although they remain sensitive to blockage by picrotoxin. In addition, these retinal receptors are not sensitive to modulation by barbiturates or benzodiazepines. Thus, ρ-containing receptors are distinct from $GABA_A$ receptors and are similar to receptors earlier designated $GABA_C$.

Several studies indicate that phosphorylation of the $GABA_A$ receptor likely modifies its functions; however, whether the receptor itself is phosphorylated *in vivo* or whether phosphorylation increases or decreases the current flowing through the channel remains debated. $GABA_A$ receptors are modulated by protein kinase A, protein kinase C, Ca^{2+}–calmodulin-dependent protein kinase, and an undefined protein kinase.

Glycine Receptor Structure Is Closely Related to $GABA_A$ Receptor Structure

Glycine receptors are the major inhibitory receptors in the spinal cord and the brain stem. Glycine receptors are similar to $GABA_A$ receptors in that both are ion channels selectively permeable to the anion Cl^- (see Fig. 9.9). The structure of the glycine receptor is indicative of this similarity in properties. The native complex is approximately 250 kDa and is composed of two main subunits: α (48 kDa) and β (58 kDa). The receptor appears to be pentameric, most likely composed of three α and two β subunits. Apparently, three molecules of glycine must bind to the receptor to open it to ion flow, suggesting that the α subunit may contain the glycine-binding site. The glycine receptor has an open channel conductance of approximately 35–50 pS, similar to that of the $GABA_A$ receptor. Strychnine is a potent antagonist of the glycine.

Four distinct α subunits and one β subunit of the glycine receptor have been cloned. Each exhibits the typical predicted four transmembrane segments and are approximately 50% identical with one another at the amino acid level. Expression of a single a subunit in oocytes is sufficient to produce functional glycine receptors, indicating that the α subunit is the pore-forming unit of the native receptor. β subunits play exclusively modulatory roles, affecting, for example, sensitivity to the inhibitory actions of picrotoxin. They are widespread in the brain, and their distribution does not specifically colocalize with glycine receptor α subunit mRNA. β subunits may serve other functions independent of their association with glycine receptor.

Certain Purinergic Receptors Are Also Ionotropic

Purinergic chemical transmission is distributed throughout the body and is considered in greater detail in a later section on GPCRs. Purinergic receptors bind to ATP (or other nucleotide analogs) or its breakdown product adenosine. ATP is released from certain synaptic terminals in a quantal manner and is often packaged within synaptic vesicles containing another neurotransmitter, the best described being ACh and catecholamines.

Although not included in our listing of ionotropic receptors (Fig. 9.9), two subtypes of ATP-binding purinergic receptors (P2x and P2z) have been discovered to be ionotropic receptors, but data on their functions and properties are sparse. P2x receptors appear to mediate a fast depolarizing response in neurons and muscle cells to ATP by the direct opening of a nonselective cation channel. cDNAs encoding the P2x receptor indicate that its structure comprises only two transmembrane domains, with some homology in its pore-forming region with K^+ channels. The P2z receptor is also a ligand-gated channel that permits permeation of either anions or cations and even molecules as large as 900 Da.

Glutamate Receptors Are Derived from a Different Ancestral Gene and Are Structurally Distinct from Other Ionotropic Receptors

Glutamate receptors are widespread in the nervous system where they are responsible for mediating the vast majority of excitatory synaptic transmission in the brain and spinal cord. Early studies suggested that the glutamate receptor family is composed of several distinct subtypes. In the 1970s, Jeffrey Watkins and colleagues advanced this field significantly by developing agonists that could pharmacologically distinguish between different glutamate receptor subtypes. Four of these agonists—N-methyl-D-aspartate (NMDA), amino-3-hydroxy-5-methylisoxazoleproprionic acid (AMPA), kainate, and quisqualate—are distinct in the type of receptors to which they bind and have been used extensively to characterize the glutamate receptor family (Watkins *et al.*, 1990; Hollmann and Heinemann, 1994). A convenient distinction for describing ionotropic glutamate receptors has been to classify them as either NMDA or non-NMDA subtypes, depending on whether they bind the agonist NMDA. Non-NMDA receptors also bind the agonist kainite or AMPA. Both NMDA and non-NMDA receptors are ionotropic. Quisqualate is unique within this group in having the capacity to activate both

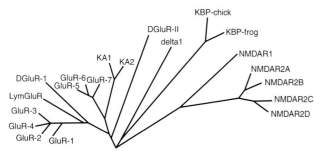

FIGURE 9.11 Evolutionary relationships of the ionotropic glutamate receptor family. Adapted from Hollmann and Heinemann (1994).

ionotropic and GPCR glutamate receptor subtypes (Hollmann and Heinemann, 1994). A family tree highlighting the evolutionary relationship of the glutamate receptors is shown in Fig. 9.11.

Non-NMDA Receptors Are a Diverse Family

In 1989, the isolation of a cDNA that produced a functional glutamate-activated channel when expressed in *Xenopus* oocytes was reported (Hollmann *et al.*, 1989). The initial glutamate receptor was termed GluR-K1, and the cDNA encoded a protein with an estimated molecular mass of 99.8 kDa. Not long after this original report, several groups (Boulter *et al.*, 1990; Keinanen *et al.*, 1990; Nakanishi *et al.*, 1990) independently reported the isolation of families of glutamate receptor subunits, termed either GluR1-GluR4 or GluRA-GluRD. Each GluR subunit consists of approximately 900 amino acids and has four predicted membrane-spanning segments (TM1–TM4); however, there is an important distinction in the TM2 domain making the GluRs distinct from the nAChR family. The native form of GluR subunits appears to be a tetrameric complex with an approximate molecular mass of 600 kDa. Thus, the size of the glutamate receptor is almost twice that of the nAChR, mostly because of the large extracellular domain where glutamate binds to the receptor.

Unique Properties of Non-NMDA Receptors Are Determined by Assembly of Different Subunits

When cDNAs encoding these receptors were expressed in either oocytes or HeK-293 cells, application of the non-NMDA receptor agonist AMPA produced substantial inward currents. In these same experiments, the agonist kainate was demonstrated to

produce larger currents, mainly because of rapid and significant desensitization of the receptor when AMPA was used as the agonist. A striking observation from these expression studies was that when the GluR2 subunit alone was expressed in the oocytes, little current was obtained when the preparation was exposed to agonist, unlike the large currents found when either GluR1 or GluR3 was expressed (Verdoorn *et al.*, 1991; Nakanishi *et al.*, 1990). GluR2 subunits by themselves appear to form poorly conducting receptors. However, when GluR2 is expressed with either GluR1 or GluR3, the behavior of the heteromeric receptor is distinctly different.

Examination of I/V plots indicates that when GluR1 and GluR3 are expressed alone or together, they produce channels with strong inward rectification. Coexpression of GluR2 with either GluR1 or GluR3 produces a channel with little rectification and a near linear I/V plot. Further analyses indicated that GluR1 and GluR3, either independently or when coexpressed, exhibited channels permeable to Ca^{2+} (Hollmann and Heinemann, 1994). In contrast, any combination of receptor that included the GluR2 subunit produced channels impermeable to Ca^{2+}. Earlier single-channel analyses of glutamate receptors expressed in embryonic hippocampal neurons indicated that two distinct receptors are present: one relatively impermeable to Ca^{2+}, exhibiting a linear I/V plot, and another significantly permeable to Ca^{2+}, exhibiting a rectifying I/V plot. Clearly, the properties of glutamate receptors can be quite different and can initiate unique intracellular responses, depending on the subunit composition expressed in a particular neuron. In a series of elegant studies, the replacement of a single amino acid (Arg for Gln) in TM2 of the GluR2 subunit (see Fig. 9.12B for identification of this amino acid) was shown to switch its behavior from a non-Ca^{2+}-permeable to a Ca^{2+}-permeable channel (Burnashev *et al.*, 1992). Apparently, an Arg at this position blocks Ca^{2+} from traversing the pore formed in the center of the GluR channel.

Functional Diversity in GluRs Is Produced by mRNA Splicing and RNA Editing

Analysis of mRNAs encoding GluR subunits indicated that each could be expressed in one of two splice variants, termed flip and flop. These flip and flop modules are small segments (38 amino acids) just preceding the TM4 domain in all four GluR subunits. The receptor channel expressed from these splice variants has distinct properties, depending on which of the two modules is present. Specifically, flop-containing receptors desensitize more during glutamate application. Therefore, GluRs with flop modules express smaller steady-state currents than GluRs with flip modules. Both flip- and flop-containing GluRs are widely expressed in the brain with a few exceptions. One unique cell type appears to be pyramidal CA3 cells in the rat hippocampus, where the GluRs are deficient in flop modules. In neighboring CA1 pyramidal cells and dentate granule cells, flop-containing GluRs appear to dominate. The significance of these splice variations for information processing in the brain is not known, but the physiological prediction would be that CA3 neurons exhibit larger steady-state glutamate-activated currents due to decreased desensitization from the absence of flop modules.

Typically, one believes that there is absolute fidelity in the process of transcribing DNA into mRNA and then into protein; i.e., that nucleotides present in the DNA are accurate predictors of the ultimate amino acid sequence of the protein. However, a novel mechanism in the neuronal nucleus was discovered that edits mRNAs post transcriptionally, and at least three of the four GluR subunits are subjected to this process (Sommer *et al.*, 1991). In fact, one of the sites edited is the critical Arg residue regulating Ca^{2+} permeability in the GluR2 subunit. At another edited site, Gly replaces Arg-764 in the GluR2 subunit, and this editing also takes place in GluR3 and GluR4. The Arg-to-Gly conversion at amino acid 764 produces receptors that exhibit significantly faster rates of recovery from the desensitized state. The extent to which other receptors or other protein molecules undergo this form of editing is an area rich for investigation. At a minimum, this editing mechanism produces dramatic differences in the function of GluRs.

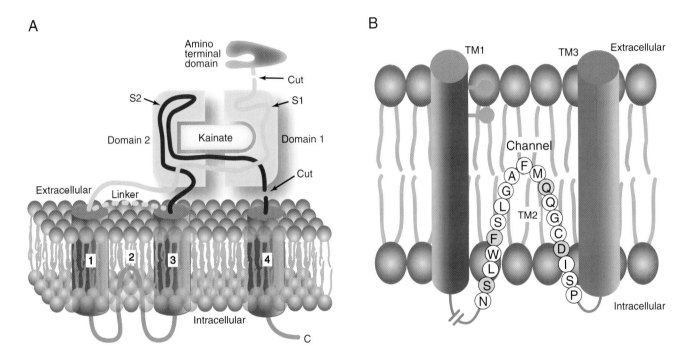

FIGURE 9.12 (A) Model of one of the subunits of the ionotropic glutamate receptor. Ionotropic glutamate receptors have four membrane-associated segments; however, unlike nAChR, only three of them completely traverse the lipid bilayer. TM2 forms a loop and reexits into the cytoplasm. Thus, the large N-terminal region extends into the extracellular space, whereas the C terminus extends into the cytoplasm. Two domains in the extracellular segments associate with each other to form the binding site for transmitter, in this example kainate, a naturally occurring agonist of glutamate. (B) Enlarged area of the predicted structure and amino acid sequence of the TM2 region of the glutamate receptor, GluR3. TM1 and TM3 are drawn as cylinders in the membrane flanking TM2. The residue that determines Ca^{2+} permeability of the non-NMDA receptor is the glutamine residue (Q) highlighted in gray. In NMDA receptors, an asparagine residue at this same position is the proposed site of interaction with Mg^{2+} ions that produce the voltage-dependent channel block. Serine (S) and phenylalanine (F), also shaded in gray, are highly conserved in the non-NMDA receptor family. The aspartate (D) residue is also conserved and is thought to form part of the internal cation-binding site. The break in the loop between TM1 and TM2 indicates a domain that varies in length among ionotropic glutamate receptors. Adapted from Wo and Oswald (1995).

Glutamate Receptors Do Not Conform to the Typical Four Transmembrane-Spanning Segment Structures Described for nAChR

Although the field of glutamate receptors is advancing at a rapid pace, we have little structural data on the native molecule or on the topology of any single GluR subunit as it exists in the membrane. The receptor has a large extracellular domain that serves as the binding site for glutamate (Fig. 9.12A). Through some sophisticated genetic engineering, it was possible to obtain a crystal structure of the glutamate-binding site for the GluR in the presence of the agonist kainite. Intricate interactions between the extracellular loops of the GluR subunits form the kainate binding sites (Fig. 9.12A).

Superficially, the remainder of the receptor was originally thought to resemble the nAChR in having four transmembrane segments that wrap back and forth through the membrane in an antiparallel fashion. However, that model has now been proven incorrect by a number of elegant molecular and biochemical studies. The most recent information indicates that the TM2 segment does not traverse the membrane completely (Fig. 9.12). Instead, it forms a kink within the membrane and enters back into the cytoplasm, similar in some ways to the pore-forming domain (P segment) of voltage-activated K^+ channels. An enlargement of this P segment (Fig. 9.12B) highlights the amino acids conserved in all the GluRs and further identifies the critical Gln residues responsible for Ca^{2+} permeability of the receptor. It also appears that glutamate receptors do not conform to the five subunit structure of the nAChR. Both biochemical (Armstrong and Gouaux, 2000) and electrophysiological (Rosenmund et al., 1998) evidence indicates that functional glutamate receptors are composed of four, not five subunits. Thus, it appears that glutamate receptors are a rather highly divergent form of the nAChR receptor family. In fact, their structure conforms more closely to the family of K^+ channels in that both appear tetrameric and both have a unique P segment that forms the selectivity filter.

Other Non-NMDA GluRs Have Poorly Characterized Functions

Three other members, GluR5–7, now form a second non-NMDA receptor subfamily, whose contribution to producing functionally distinct receptors is less well understood. Their overall structure is similar to that of GluR1–4, and they exhibit about 40% sequence homology; however, their agonist-binding profile and their electrophysiological properties are distinct. They are expressed at lower levels in the brain than the GluR1–4 family (Hollmann and Heinemann, 1994).

Two members of the glutamate receptor family, KA-1 and KA-2, are the high-affinity kainate-binding receptors found in brain. Clearly distinct from the glutamate receptors discussed so far, KA-1 and KA-2 are more similar to the GluR5–7 subfamily than to the GluR1–4 subfamily. Neither KA-1 nor KA-2 produces a functional channel when expressed in cells or oocytes, even though high-affinity kainate-binding sites were detected. KA-1 does not appear to form functional receptors or channels with any of the other GluR subunits, and its physiological relevance remains obscure. It is expressed at high concentrations in only two cell types, hippocampal CA3 and dentate granule cells. KA-2 exhibits interesting properties when combined with other GluR subunits. For example, coexpression of GluR6 and KA-2 produces functional receptors that respond to AMPA, although neither subunit itself responds to this agonist. This information indicates that agonist-binding sites are at least partly formed at the interfaces between subunits.

Although other kainate-binding proteins and glutamate receptors have been described, their functions and biological significance are not currently understood. These receptors include two kainate-binding proteins, one from chicken and the other from frog, several invertebrate glutamate receptors, and two "orphan" receptors termed $\alpha 1$ and $\delta 2$ (Hollmann and Heinemann, 1994).

NMDA Receptors Are a Family of Ligand-Gated Ion Channels That Are Also Voltage Dependent

NMDA receptors appear to be at least partly responsible for aspects of development, learning and memory, and neuronal damage due to brain injury. The particular significance of this receptor to neuronal function comes from two of its unique properties. First, the receptor exhibits associativity. For the channel to be open, the receptor must bind glutamate and the membrane must be depolarized. This behavior is due to a Mg^{2+}-dependent block of the receptor at normal membrane resting potentials. Second, the receptor permits a significant influx of Ca^{2+}, and increases in intracellular Ca^{2+} activate a variety of processes that alter the properties of the neuron. Excess Ca^{2+} is also toxic to neurons, and the hyperactivation of NMDA receptors is thought to contribute to a variety of neurodegenerative disorders.

Many pharmacological compounds produce their effects through interactions with the NMDA receptor. For example, certain hallucinogenic compounds, such as phencyclidine (PCP) and dizocilpine (MK-801), are effective blockers of the ion channel associated with the NMDA receptor (Fig. 9.13). These potent antagonists require the receptor channel to be open to gain access to their binding sites and are therefore referred to as open-channel blockers. They also become trapped when the channel closes and are therefore difficult to wash out of the channel of the NMDA receptor. Antagonists for the glutamate-binding site have also been developed, and some of the most well known are AP-5 and AP-7. These and other antagonists specific for the glutamate-binding site also produce hallucinogenic effects in both animal models and humans. NMDA remains a specific agonist for this receptor; however, it is about one order of magnitude less potent than L-Glutamate for receptor activation. L-Glutamate is the predominant neurotransmitter that activates the NMDA receptor; however, L-aspartate can also activate the receptor, as can an endogenous dipeptide in the brain, N-acetylaspartylglutamate (Hollmann and Heinemann, 1994).

NMDA Receptor Subunits Show Similarity to Non-NMDA Receptor Subunits

The primary structure of the NMDA receptor was revealed in 1990 when the first cDNA encoding a subunit of the NMDA receptor was isolated (Moriyoshi et al., 1991). The first cloned subunit was aptly named NMDAR1, and the deduced amino acid sequence indicated a protein of approximately 97 kDa, similar to other members of the GluR family. Four potential transmembrane domains were identified, and the current assumption is that four individual subunits compose the macromolecular NMDA receptor complex. However, recall that the transmembrane organization of GluR subunits indicates that TM2 does not fully transverse the membrane. It seems likely that the NMDA receptor subunits will also follow this recent modification of the model. The TM2 segment of each subunit clearly lines the pore of the NMDA receptor channel, as does the TM2 segment of the GluR subunits. In fact, a single Asn residue, analogous to that in the GluR2 subunit, regulates the Ca^{2+} permeability of the NMDA receptor. Mutation of this Asn residue reduces Ca^{2+} permeability markedly.

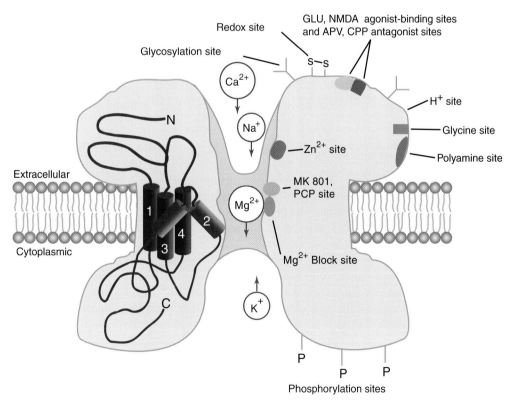

FIGURE 9.13   Diagram of a NMDA receptor highlighting binding sites for numerous agonists, antagonists, and other regulatory molecules. The location of these sites is a crude approximation for the purpose of discussion. Adapted from Hollmann and Heinemann (1994).

Three of the best-characterized facets of the NMDA receptor were found when the NMDAR1 subunit was initially expressed by itself in oocytes, although currents were relatively small. These characteristics are (1) a Mg^{2+}-dependent, voltage-sensitive ion channel block, (2) a glycine requirement for effective channel opening, and (3) Ca^{2+} permeability (Moriyoshi et al., 1991). As described later, other NMDAR subunits contribute to assembly of the receptors thought to exist in the nervous system.

Functional Diversity of NMDA Receptors Occurs through RNA Splicing

At least eight splice variants have now been identified for the NMDAR1 subunit and these variants produce differences, ranging from subtle to significant, in the properties of the expressed receptor (Hollmann and Heinemann, 1994). For example, NMDAR1 receptors lacking a particular N-terminal insert due to alternative splicing exhibit enhanced blockade by protons and exhibit responses that are potentiated by Zn^{2+} in micromolar concentrations. Zn^{2+} has classically been described as an NMDA receptor antagonist that significantly blocks its activation. Clearly, the particular splice variant incorporated into the receptor complex affects the types of physiological response generated. Spermine, a polyamine found in neurons and in the extracellular space, also slightly increases the amplitude of NMDA responses, and this modulatory effect also appears to be associated with a particular splice variant. The physiologic role of spermine in regulating NMDA receptors remains unclear.

Multiple NMDA Receptor Subunit Genes Also Contribute to Functional Diversity

Four other members of the NMDA receptor family have been cloned (NMDAR2A–2D), and their deduced primary structures are highly related. These four NMDA receptor subunits do not form channels when expressed singly or in combination unless they are coexpressed with NMDAR1. Apparently, NMDAR1 serves an essential function for the formation of a functional pore by which activation of NMDA receptors permits the flow of ions. NMDA receptors 2A–2D play important roles in modulating the receptor activity when mixed as heteromeric forms with NMDAR1. Coexpression of NMDAR1 with any of the other subunits produces much larger currents (from 5- to 60-fold greater) than when NMDAR1 is expressed in isolation, and NMDA receptors expressed in neurons are likely to be heterooligomers of NMDAR1 and

NMDAR2 subunits. The C-terminal domains of NMDAR2A–2D are quite large relative to the NMDAR1 C-terminus and appear to play roles in altering channel properties and in affecting the subcellular localization of the receptors. All of the NMDAR subunits have an Asn residue at the critical point in the TM2 domain essential for producing Ca^{2+} permeability. This Asn residue also appears to form at least part of the binding site for Mg^{2+}, which suggests that the sites for Mg^{2+} binding and Ca^{2+} permeation overlap.

The distribution of NMDAR2 subunits is generally more restricted than the homogeneous distribution of NMDAR1, with the exception of NMDAR2A, which is expressed throughout the nervous system. NMDAR2C is mostly restricted to cerebellar granule cells, whereas 2B and 2D exhibit broader distributions. As noted, the large size of the C terminus of the NMDAR2 subunit suggests a potential role in association with other proteins, possibly to target or restrict specific NMDA receptor types to areas of the neuron. Mechanisms related to receptor targeting are now becoming understood and will clearly play major roles in determining the efficacy of synaptic transmission.

NMDA Receptors Exhibit Complex Channel Properties

The biophysical properties of the NMDA receptor are complex. Single-channel conductance has a main level of 50 pS; however, subconductances are evident, and different subunit combinations produce channels with distinct single-channel properties. A binding site for the Ca^{2+}-binding protein calmodulin has also been identified on the NMDAR1 subunit. Binding of Ca^{2+}–calmodulin to NMDA receptors produces a fourfold decrease in open-channel probability. Ca^{2+} influx through the NMDA receptor could induce calmodulin binding and lead to an immediate short-term feedback inhibition, decreasing ion flow through the receptor.

Summary

A general model for ionotropic receptors has emerged mainly from analyses of nAChR. Ionotropic receptors are large membrane-bound complexes generally composed of five subunits. The subunits each have four transmembrane domains, and the amino acids in TM2 form the lining of the pore. Transmitter binding induces rapid conformational changes that are translated into an increase in the diameter of the pore, permitting ion influx. Cation or anion selectivity is obtained through the coordination of specific negatively or positively charged amino acids at strategic locations in the receptor pore. How well the details of structural information obtained for the nAChR will generalize to other ionotropic receptors awaits structural analyses of these other members. However, it is already clear that this model does not adequately describe the orientation of the transmembrane domains or the subunit number of the glutamate receptor family. The TM2 domain of glutamate receptors forms a hairpin instead of traversing the membrane completely, causing the remainder of the receptor to adopt a different architecture than that described for the nAChR family. It also appears that glutamate receptors are composed of four, not five, subunits. These differences are perhaps not surprising given that the nAChR family and the glutamate receptor family appear to have arisen from two different ancestral genes.

G-PROTEIN COUPLED RECEPTORS

The number of members in the G-protein coupled receptor family is enormous, with over already 1000 identified. Historically, the term *metabotropic* was used to describe the fact that intracellular metabolites are produced when these receptors bind ligand. However, there are now clearly documented cases where the activation of "metabotropic" receptors does not produce alterations in metabolites but instead produce their effects by interacting with G-proteins that alter the behavior of ion channels. Thus, these receptors are now referred to as G-protein-coupled receptors (GPCRs).

When a GPCR is activated, it couples to a G-protein initiating the exchange of GDP for GTP, activating the G-protein. Activated G-proteins then couple to many downstream effectors and most alter the activity of other intracellular enzymes or ion channels. Many of the G-protein target enzymes produce diffusible second messengers (metabolites) that stimulate further downstream biochemical processes, including the activation of protein kinases (see Chapter 12). Time is required for each of these coupling events, and the effects of GPCR activation are typically slower in onset than those observed following the activation of ionotropic receptors. Because there is a lifetime associated with each intermediate, the effects produced by GPCR activation are also typically longer in duration than those produced by the activation of ionotropic receptors. Most small neurotransmitters, such as ACh, glutamate, 5-HT, and

GABA, can bind to and activate both ionotropic and GPCRs. Thus, each of these transmitters can induce both fast responses (milliseconds), such as typical excitatory or inhibitory postsynaptic potentials, and slow-onset and longer duration responses (from tenths of seconds to, potentially, hours). Other transmitters, like neuropeptides, produce their effects largely by binding only to GPCRs. These effects across multiple time domains provide the nervous system with a rich source for temporal information processing that is subject to constant modification. Currently, the GPCR family can be divided into three subfamilies on the basis of their structures: (1) the rhodopsin-adrenergic receptor subfamily, (2) the secretin-vasoactive intestinal peptide receptor subfamily, and (3) the metabotropic glutamate receptor subfamily.

GPCR Structure Conforms to a General Model

A GPCR consists of a single polypeptide with a generally conserved structure. The receptor contains seven membrane-spanning helical segments that wrap back and forth through the membrane (Fig. 9.14). G-protein-coupled receptors are homologous to rhodopsin from both mammalian and bacterial sources, and detailed structural information on rhodopsin has been used to provide a framework for developing a general model for GPCR structures. Aside from rhodopsin, two of the best structurally characterized GPCRs are the β-adrenergic receptor (βAR) and the muscarinic acetylcholine receptor (mAChR), and biochemical analyses to date support the use of rhodopsin as a structural framework for the family of GPCRs.

The most conserved feature of GPCRs is the seven membrane-spanning segments; however, other generalities can be made about their structure. The N terminus of the receptor extends into the extracellular space, whereas the C terminus resides within the cytoplasm (Fig. 9.14). Each of the seven transmembrane domains between N and C termini consists of approximately 24 mostly hydrophobic amino acids. These seven domains associate together to form an oblong ring within the plasma membrane (Fig. 9.14B). Between each transmembrane domain is a loop of amino acids of various sizes. The loops connecting TM1 and TM2, TM3 and TM4, and TM5 and TM6 are intracellular and are labeled i1, i2, and i3, respectively, whereas those between TM2 and TM3, TM4 and TM5, and TM6 and TM7 are extracellular and are labeled e1, e2, and e3, respectively (see Fig. 9.14A for examples).

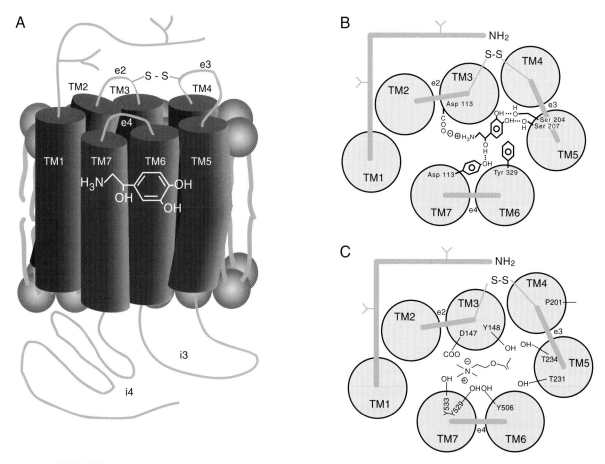

FIGURE 9.14 (A) Diagram showing the approximate position of the catecholamine-binding site in βAR. The transmitter-binding site is formed by amino acids whose side chains extend into the center of the ring produced by the seven transmembrane domains (TM1–TM7). Note that the binding site exists at a position that places it within the plane of the lipid bilayer. (B) A view looking down on a model of the βAR receptor identifying residues important for ligand binding. The seven transmembrane domains are represented as gray circles labeled TM1 though TM7. Amino acids composing the extracellular domains are represented as green bars labeled e1 through e4. The disulfide bond (-S-S-) that links e2 to e3 is also shown. Each of the specific residues indicated makes stabilizing contact with the transmitter. (C) A view looking down on a model of the mAChR identifying residues important for ligand binding. Stabilizing contacts, mainly through hydroxyl groups (–OH), are made with the transmitter on four of the seven transmembrane domains. The chemical nature of the transmitter (i.e., epinephrine versus Ach) determines the type of amino acids necessary to produce stable interactions in the receptor-binding site (compare B and C). Adapted from Strosberg, (1990).

The Neurotransmitter-Binding Site Is Buried in the Core of the Receptor

The neurotransmitter-binding site for many GPCRs (excluding the metabotropic glutamate, GABA_B and neuropeptide receptors) resides within a pocket formed in the center of the seven membrane-spanning segments (Fig. 9.14A). In the βAR, this pocket resides at least 10.9 Å into the hydrophobic core of the receptor, placing the ligand-binding site within the plasma membrane lipid bilayer (Kobilka, 1992). Strategically positioned charged and polar residues in the mem-

brane-spanning segments point inward into a central pocket that forms the binding site for the ligand. For example, Asn residues in the second and third segments, two Ser residues in the fifth segment, and a Phe residue in the sixth segment provide major contact points in the βAR-binding site for the transmitter (Fig. 9.14B; Kobilka, 1992). Replacing the Asp in TM3 with a Glu reduced transmitter binding by more than 100-fold, and replacement with a less conserved amino acid, such as Ser, reduces binding by more than 10,000-fold. Two Ser residues in TM5 are also essential for efficient transmitter binding and

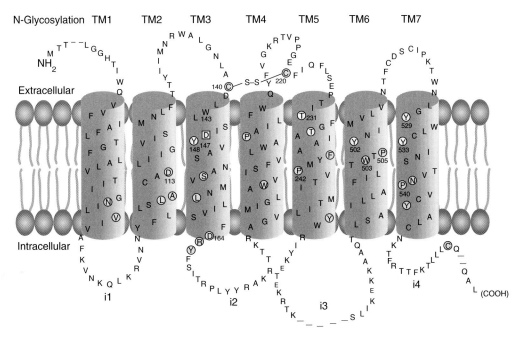

FIGURE 9.15 Amino acid sequence and predicted domain topology of the M3 isoform of mAChR. Transmembrane domains are TM1–TM7. The NH₂ terminus of the protein is at the left and extends into the extracellular space. The COOH terminus is intracellular and is at the right; i1 to i4 are the four intracellular domains. The conserved disulfide bond (-S-S-) connects extracellular loop 2 to 3. Dashes in the amino acid sequence represent inserts of various lengths that are not shown. Conserved amino acids for all members of the G-protein-coupled receptor family of receptors are marked in purple. Amino acids taking part in ACh binding to the receptor are highlighted in yellow. Note that all amino acids associated with ligand binding lie in approximately the same horizontal plane across the receptor.

receptor activation, as is an Asp residue in TM2 and a Phe residue in TM6. In total, the two Asp, the two Ser, and the Phe residues are highly conserved in all receptors that bind catecholamines. Variations in the amino acids at these five positions appear to provide the specificity between binding of different transmitters to the individual GPCRs.

The neurotransmitter-binding site of mAChRs, like that of the β2AR, has been investigated in great detail (Fig. 9.14C). The Asp residue in TM3 is also critical for ACh binding to mAChRs. Mutagenesis studies indicate important roles for Tyr and Thr residues in TM3, TM5, TM6, and TM7 in contributing to the ligand-binding site for ACh. Interestingly, many of these mutations do not affect antagonist binding, indicating that distinct sets of amino acids participate in binding agonists and antagonists. When the transmembrane domains are examined from a side view (Fig. 9.15), all of the key amino acids implicated in agonist binding lie at about the same level within the core of the receptor structure, buried approximately 10–15 Å from the surface of the plasma membrane (Fig. 9.15, yellow boxed amino acids). An additional amino acid identified as essential for agonist binding of the

mAChR is a Pro residue in TM4. This residue is also highly conserved among GPCRs, and structural predictions suggest that it affects ligand binding not by interacting with agonist directly but by stabilizing a conformation essential for high-affinity binding. Structural predictions also place this Pro residue in the same plane as the Asp, Tyr, and Thr residues that form the ligand-binding site of the mAChR (Fig. 9.15).

Transmitter Binding Causes a Conformational Change in the Receptor and Activation of G-Proteins

Proposed models for GPCR activation assume that the receptor can isomerize spontaneously between inactive and active states (Premont et al., 1995). Only the active state interacts with G-proteins in a productive fashion. This isomerization is analogous to the spontaneous isomerization proposed for ion channels as they oscillate between open and closed states. At equilibrium, in the absence of agonist, the inactive state of GPCRs is favored, and little G-protein activation occurs. Agonist binding stabilizes the active conformation and shifts the equilibrium toward the active form, and G-protein activation ensues. Conversely, receptor antagonists block G-protein activation through two proposed mechanisms: (1) negative antagonism in which antagonists bind to the inactive state of the receptor, thus favoring an equilibrium to the inactive form; and (2) neutral antagonism in which antagonists bind to both the active and inactive forms, thus stabilizing both and preventing a complete transition into the active form. This kinetic model indicates that agonist binding is not necessary for the receptor to undergo transition into the active state; instead, it stabilizes the activated state of the receptor. This proposed model is supported by observations of both spontaneously arising and engineered mutants of βAR and αAR receptors. Specific amino acid replacements produced receptors that exhibit constitutive activity in the absence of agonists (Premont et al., 1995). The amino acid changes apparently stabilize the active conformation of the molecule in a state more similar to the agonist-bound form of the receptor, leading to productive interactions with G proteins in the agonist-free state.

The Third Intracellular Loop Forms a Major Determinant for G-Protein Coupling

Extensive studies using site-directed mutagenesis and the production of chimeric molecules have revealed the domains and amino acids essential for G-protein coupling to GPCRs. Receptor domains within the second (i2) and third (i3) intracellular loops (Fig. 9.15) appear largely responsible for determining the specificity and efficiency of coupling for adrenergic and muscarinic cholinergic receptors and are the likely sites for G-protein coupling of the entire GPCR family. In particular, the 12 amino acids of the N-terminal region of the third intracellular loop significantly affect the specificity of G-protein coupling. Other regions in the C terminus of the third intracellular loop and the N-terminal region of the C-terminal tail appear to be more important for determining the efficiency of G-protein coupling than for determining its specificity (Kobilka, 1992). The third intracellular loop varies enormously in size among the different G-protein-coupled receptors, ranging from 29 amino acids in the substance P receptor to 242 amino acids in the mAChR (Strader et al., 1994). The intracellular loop connecting TM5 and TM6 is the main point of receptor coupling to G-proteins, and ligand binding to amino acids in TM5 and TM6 may be responsible for triggering the G-protein–receptor interaction by transmitting a conformational change to the third intracellular loop.

Specific Amino Acids Are Involved in Transducing Transmitter Binding into G-Protein Coupling

Residues associated with transmitting the conformational change induced by ligand binding to the activation of G-proteins have been investigated with the use of mAChRs. These studies revealed that an Asp residue in TM2 is important for the receptor activation of G-proteins, and altering the Asp by site-directed mutagenesis has a major negative effect on G-protein–receptor activation. A Thr residue in TM5 and a Tyr residue in TM6 are also essential. Because these residues are connected by i3, they are assumed to play fundamental roles in transmitting the conformational change induced by ligand binding to the area of i3 essential for G-protein coupling and activation. When mutated, a Pro residue on TM7 produces a major impairment in the ability of the TM3 segment to induce the activation of phospholipase C through a G-protein and presumably is another key element in propagating the conformational changes necessary for efficient coupling to G-proteins. As informative as mutagenesis studies can be, a true molecular understanding of the conformational changes induced by agonist binding will likely require a structural approach similar to that applied by Nigel Unwin to nAChR.

As mentioned earlier, GPCRs are single polypeptides; however, they are clearly separable into distinct functional domains. For example, β2AR can be physically split, with the use of molecular techniques, into two fragments: one fragment containing TM1–TM5 and the other containing TM6 and TM7. In isolation, neither of these fragments can produce a functional receptor; however, when coexpressed in the same cell, functional β2ARs that can bind ligand and activate G-proteins are produced. This remarkable experiment indicates that physical contiguity in the primary sequence is not essential for producing functional β2ARs and also emphasizes the contribution of domains in the separate fragments (TM1–TM5 and TM6 and TM7) to both ligand binding and G-protein coupling. Like β2AR, m2 and m3 members of the mAChR family can form functional receptors even if split into two separate domains. A fragment containing the first five transmembrane domains forms a functional receptor when expressed with a fragment containing TM6 and TM7 (Fig. 9.16).

GPCRs Also Exist as Homo- or Heterooligomers

The observation that GPCRs can be physically split through genetic engineering and produced functional channels when recombined provided the first hint that full-length GPCRs might also oligomerize with each other into functional molecules. A test of this hypothesis was accomplished by making chimeric receptors composed of the transmembrane domains 1–5 of the α2-AR and the transmembrane domains 6 and 7 of the m3 muscarinic receptors and vice versa (Fig. 9.16B). When either of these chimeric molecules was expressed in isolation, neither formed a functional receptor. However, when coexpressed, receptors were formed that bind both muscarinic and adrenergic ligands and ligand binding led to functional activation of downstream effectors. Through domain swapping, the ligand-binding sites for both receptor ligands were reconstituted by oligomerization of the two chimeric receptors into one bifunc-

tional chimeric dimer (Fig. 9.16B). Oligomerization of GPCRs is also supported by cross-linking and immunoprecipitation experiments and with experiments examining the direct biophysical association of the receptors in living cells (Overton and Blumer, 2000). While some debate remains, evidence now seems overwhelming that oligomerization of GPCRs is adding a new layer of complexity and diversity to the study of these receptors. The functional impacts of GPRR oligomerization are just beginning to be appreciated. Important functional consequences could relate to alterations in (1) ligand binding, (2) efficiency and specificity of coupling to downstream effectors, (3) subcellular localization, and (4) receptor desensitization. The evolving and apparently widespread nature of direct receptor–receptor interactions leads

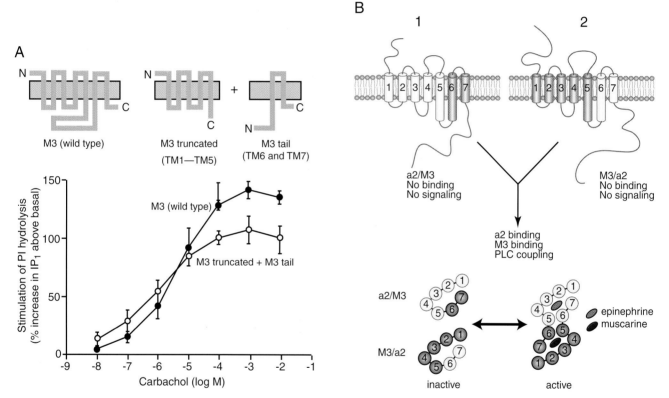

FIGURE 9.16 Oligomerization of GPCRs. (A) The mAChR can be split into two physically separated domains that, when added back together, retain the ability to bind transmitter and activate G-proteins. (Upper left) Model of the full-length mAChR. (Upper right) Two engineered pieces of the receptor. The graph indicates that when coexpressed in the same cells, the two fragments can produce a functional mAChR that responds to the agonist carbachol producing activation of G-protein and subsequent activation of an enzyme that hydrolyzes phosphatidylinositol (PI). (B) Some GPCRs can function as dimers. In this example, chimeric receptors were produced between α2AR (α2) and mAChR (M3) by swapping certain transmembrane domains through genetic engineering. When α2/M3 or M3/α2 is expressed separately, they are not active. However, if both chimeric molecules are expressed in the same cells, they form receptors that can be activated by either epinephrine or muscarine. Adapted from Salahpour et al., (2000). (Bottom) A top-down view of how this domain swapping might occur when two molecules dimerize to produce receptors that can respond to both transmitters. Adapted from Lee et al., (2000). Inhibition of cell surface expression by mutant receptors demonstrates that D2 dopamine receptors exist as oligomers in the cell. Mol. Pharmacol. 58: 120–128.

one to believe that our current understanding of neurotransmitter receptors and their biological impact will be undergoing continual modifications for many years to come.

G-Protein Coupling Increases Affinity of the Receptor for Neurotransmitter

The affinity of a GPCR for agonist increases when the receptor is coupled to the G-protein. This positive feedback effectively increases the lifetime of the agonist-bound form of the receptor by decreasing the dissociation rate of the agonist. An excellent demonstration of this effect comes from studies using engineered βAR receptors that are constitutively active in their ability to couple to G-proteins. These mutant receptors show a significantly increased affinity for agonists. When the G-protein dissociates, the agonist-binding affinity of the receptor returns to its original state. Changes induced by ligand binding apparently stabilize the receptor in a conformation with both higher affinity for ligand and higher affinity for coupling to G-proteins.

Specificity and Potency of G-Protein Activation Are Determined by Several Factors

GPCRs associate with G-proteins to transduce ligand binding into intracellular effects. This coupling step can lead to diverse responses, depending on the type of G-protein and the type of effector enzyme present. Ligand binding to a single subtype of GPCR can activate multiple G-protein-coupled pathways. For example, activated α2ARs have been shown to couple to as many as four different G-proteins in the same cell (Strader *et al.*, 1994). Some of the specificity for G-protein activation can be determined by the specific conformations assumed by the receptor, and a single receptor can assume multiple conformations. For example, α2ARs can isomerize into at least two states. One state interacts with a G-protein that couples to phospholipase C, and a second state interacts with G-proteins that couple to both phospholipase C and phospholipase A_2. Thus, a single GPCR can produce a diversity of responses, making it difficult to assign specific biological effects to individual receptor subtypes in all settings.

Activated GPCRs are free to couple to many G-protein molecules, permitting a significant amplification of the initial transmitter-binding event. This catalytic mechanism is referred to as "collision coupling," whereby a transient association between the activated receptor and the G-protein is sufficient to produce the exchange of GDP for GTP, activating the G-protein. For example, because adenylate cyclase appears to be tightly coupled to the G-protein, the rate-limiting step in the production of cAMP is the number of successful collisions between the receptor and the G-protein. A constant GTPase activity hydrolyzes GTP, bringing the G-protein and therefore the adenylate cyclase back to the basal state. Transmitter concentration clearly plays a role in the number of activated receptors present at any given time, and GPCRs exhibit saturable dose–response curves. The apparent maximal rate is achieved when all of the G-protein–cyclase complexes have become activated or, more accurately, when the rate of formation is maximal with respect to the rate of GTP hydrolysis. A less intuitive consequence of these models is that receptor number can significantly affect the concentration of transmitter that produces a half-maximal response of cAMP accumulation. Thus, the larger the receptor number, the greater the probability that a productive collision will occur between an agonist-bound receptor and the G-protein. Experimental evidence for this prediction was obtained for the βAR receptor expressed at various levels in eukaryotic cells. Increasing concentrations of βAR produced a decrease in the concentration of agonist required to produce half-maximal production of cAMP. Apparently, the cell can adjust the magnitude of its response by adjusting the number of receptors available for transmitter interaction. Additionally, the important process of receptor desensitization can also regulate the number of receptors capable of productive G-protein interactions.

Receptor Desensitization Is a Built-in Mechanism for Decreasing the Cellular Response to Transmitter

Desensitization is a very important process whereby cells can decrease their sensitivity to a particular stimulus to prevent saturation of the system. Desensitization involves a complex series of events (Kobilka, 1992). For GPCRs, desensitization is defined as an increase in the concentration of agonist required to produce half-maximal stimulation of, for example, adenylate cyclase. In practical terms, desensitization of receptors produces less response for a constant amount of transmitter.

There are two known mechanisms for desensitization. One mechanism is a decrease in response brought about by the covalent modifications produced by receptor phosphorylation and is quite rapid (seconds to minutes). The other mechanism is the physical removal of receptors from the plasma membrane (likely through a mechanism of receptor-mediated endocytosis) and tends to require greater periods of time (minutes to hours). The latter process can be either reversible (sequestration) or irreversible (down-regulation).

The Rapid Phase of GPCR Desensitization Is Mediated by Receptor Phosphorylation

Desensitization of the βAR appears to involve at least three protein kinases: PKA, PKC, and β-adrenergic receptor kinase [βARK; also referred to as a G-protein receptor kinase (GRK)]. Phosphorylation of ARs by PKA does not require that the agonist be bound to the receptor and appears to be a general mechanism by which the cell can reduce the effectiveness of all receptors, independent of whether they are in the agonist-bound or unbound state (Fig. 9.17). This process is also referred to as heterologous desensitization because the receptor does not require bound-agonist (for simplicity PKA is shown phosphorylating only the agonist-bound form of the receptor in Fig 9.17). PKA and PKC phosphorylate sites on the third intracellular loop and possibly the C-terminal cytoplasmic domain. Phosphorylation of these sites interferes with the ability of the receptor to couple to G-proteins, thus producing the desensitization (Fig. 9.17). Whether the same sites on the βAR are phosphorylated by both PKA and PKC is controversial. Some researchers conclude that the effects of phosphorylation by either kinase on decreasing coupling of the receptor to G-proteins are similar, suggesting that the sites phosphorylated are similar. Others find that the effects are additive. Although the details of the role played by each of these kinases are ambiguous, phosphorylation by either enzyme desensitizes the receptor.

GRKs can also phosphorylate GPCRs and lead to receptor desensitization. Six members of the GRK family of kinases have been identified: rhodopsin kinase (GRK1), βARK (GRK2), and GRK3 through GRK6 (Premont *et al.*, 1995). GRK2 (originally called β-AR receptor kinase or βARK) is a Ser- and Thr-specific protein kinase initially identified by its capacity to phosphorylate βAR. GRK2 phosphorylates only the agonist-bound form of the receptor, usually when agonist concentrations reach the micromolar level, as typically found in the synaptic cleft. This process is referred to as homologous desensitization because the regulation is specific for those receptor molecules that are in the agonist-bound state. Phosphorylation of βAR by GRK2 does not interfere substantially with coupling to G-proteins. Instead, an additional protein, arrestin, binds the GRK2-phosphorylated form of the receptor, thus blocking receptor–G-protein coupling (Fig. 9.17). This process is analogous to the desensitization of the light-sensitive receptor molecule rhodopsin produced by GRK1 phosphorylation and the binding of arrestin. Phosphorylation sites on βAR for GRK2 reside on the C-terminal cytoplasmic domain and are distinct from those phosphorylated by PKA.

The cycle of homologous desensitization starts with the activation of a GPCR, which induces activation of G-proteins and dissociation of the $\beta\gamma$ subunit complex from α subunits. At least one role for the $\beta\gamma$ complex appears to be to bind to GRKs, which leads to their recruitment to the membrane in the area of the locally activated G-protein–receptor complex. The recruited GRK is then activated, leading to phosphorylation of the agonist-bound receptor and subsequent binding of arrestin. Arrestin binds to the same domains on the receptor necessary for coupling to G-proteins, thus terminating the actions of the activated receptor (Fig. 9.17). The ensuing process of sequestration follows GPCR phosphorylation and arrestin binding.

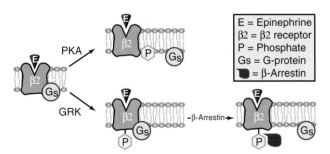

FIGURE 9.17 Different modes of desensitization of GPCRs. This diagram indicates that the epinephrine (E)-bound form of β2AR normally couples to the G-protein, G_s. PKA can phosphorylate the receptor, leading to an inhibition of binding to G_s. The G-protein receptor kinase (GRK) can also phosphorylate the receptor; however, this phosphorylation does not interfere directly with binding to G_s. GRK phosphorylation is needed for the binding of another protein, β-arrestin, which by its association with the receptor, prevents G_s from binding. Adapted from Kobilka (1992).

Desensitization Can Also Be Produced by Loss of Receptors from the Cell Surface

Desensitization of GPCRs is also produced by removal of the receptor from the cell surface. This process can be either reversible (sequestration, or internalization) or irreversible (downregulation). Sequestration is the term used to describe the rapid (within minutes) but reversible endocytosis of receptors from the cell surface after agonist application (Fig. 9.18). Neither G-protein coupling nor receptor phosphorylation appears to be absolutely essential for this process, but phosphorylation by GRKs clearly

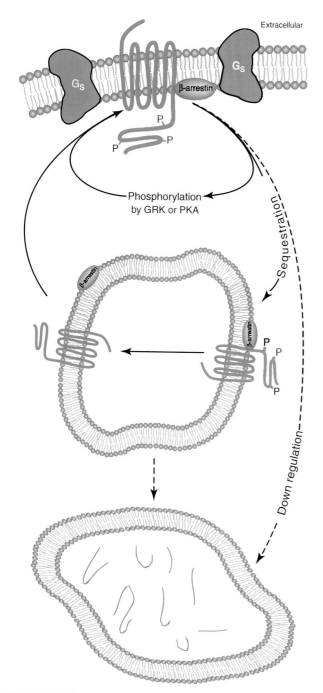

FIGURE 9.18 Additional intracellular pathways associated with desensitization of GPCRs. GPCRs are phosphorylated (noted with P) on their intracellular domains by PKA, GRK, and other protein kinases. The phosphorylated form of the receptor can be removed from the cell surface by a process called sequestration with the help of the adapter protein β-arrestin; thus fewer binding sites remain on the cell surface for transmitter interactions. In intracellular compartments, the receptor can be dephosphorylated and returned to the plasma membrane in its basal state. Alternatively, phosphorylated receptors can be degraded (downregulated) by targeting to a lysosomal organelle. Degradation requires replenishment of the receptor pool through new protein synthesis. Adapted from Kobilka (1992).

enhances the rate of sequestration. The binding of arrestins to the phosphorylated receptor also enhances sequestration (Ferguson *et al.*, 1996). Thus, arrestin binding appears to promote not only rapid desensitization by disrupting the receptor–G-protein interaction, but also receptor sequestration. Because the receptor can be uncoupled functionally from the G-protein through the rapid phosphorylation-dependent phase of desensitization, the physiological roles of sequestration remain an open issue, although decreasing the number of receptor molecules on the cell surface would contribute to the overall process of desensitization to agonist. Receptor cycling through intracellular organelles is a trafficking mechanism that leads to an enhanced rate of dephosphorylation of the phosphorylated receptor, returning it to the cell surface in its basal state (Fig. 9.18).

Downregulation occurs more slowly than sequestration and is irreversible (Fig. 9.18). The early phase (within 4 h) may involve both a PKA-dependent and a PKA-independent process. This early phase of downregulation is apparently due to receptor degradation after endocytotic removal from the plasma membrane. The later phases (>14 h) of downregulation appear to be further mediated by a reduction in receptor biosynthesis through a decrease in the stability of the receptor mRNA and a decreased transcription rate.

Other Posttranslational Modifications Are Required for Efficient Metabotropic Receptor Function

Like many proteins expressed on the cell surface, GPCRs are glycosylated, and the N-terminal extracellular domain is the site of carbohydrate attachment. Relatively little is known about the effect of glycosylation on the function of GPCRs. Glycosylation does not appear to be essential to the production of a functional ligand-binding pocket (Strader *et al.*, 1994), although prevention of glycosylation may decrease membrane insertion and alter intracellular trafficking of the β2AR.

Another important structural feature of most GPCRs is the disulfide bond formed between two Cys residues present on the extracellular loops (e2 and e3; Figs. 9.14 and 9.15). Apparently, the disulfide bond stabilizes a restricted conformation of the mature receptor by covalently linking the two extracellular domains, and this conformation favors ligand binding. Disruption of this disulfide bond significantly decreases agonist binding (Kobilka, 1992).

A third Cys residue, in the C-terminal domain of GPCRs (Fig. 9.15, pink circled C in i4), appears to serve as a point for covalent attachment of a fatty acid (often palmitate). Presumably, fatty acid attachment stabilizes an interaction between the C-terminal domain of a GPCR and the membrane. The full consequences of this posttranslational modification are not understood because replacing the normally palmitoylated Cys with an amino acid that cannot be acylated appears to have little effect on receptor binding; however, G-protein coupling may not be as efficient.

GPCRs Can Physically Associate with Ionotropic Receptors

There is now good evidence that metabotropic and ionotropic receptors can interact directly with each other (Liu et al., 2000). GABA$_A$ receptors (ionotropic) were shown to couple to DA (D5) receptors (metabotropic) through the second intracellular loop of the γ subunit of the GABA$_A$ receptor and the C-terminal domain of the D5, but not the D1, receptor. DA binding to D5 receptors produced downregulation of GABA$_A$ currents, and pharmacologically blocking the GABA$_A$ receptor produced decreases in cAMP production when cells were stimulated with DA. It further appeared that ligand binding to both receptors was necessary for their stable interaction. Whether this form of receptor regulation is unique to this pair of partners or is a widespread phenomenon remains an open question ripe for further investigation.

GPCRs All Exhibit Similar Structures

The family of GPCRs exhibits structural similarities that permit the construction of "trees" describing the degree to which they are related evolutionarily (Fig. 9.19). Some remarkable relations become evident in such an analysis. For example, the D1 and D5 subtypes of DA receptors are related more closely to the α2AR than to the D2, D3, and D4 DA receptors. The similarities and differences among GPCR families are highlighted in the remainder of this chapter.

Muscarinic ACh Receptors

Muscarine is a naturally occurring plant alkaloid that binds to muscarinic subtypes of the AChRs and activates them. mAChRs play a dominant role in mediating the actions of ACh in the brain, indirectly producing both excitation and inhibition through binding to a family of unique receptor subtypes. mAChRs are found both presynaptically and postsynaptically and, ultimately, their main neuronal effects appear to be mediated through alterations in the properties of ion channels. Presynaptic mAChRs

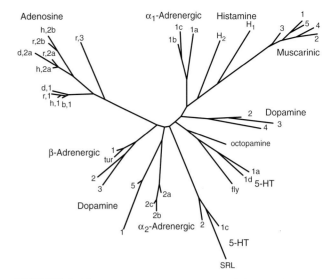

FIGURE 9.19 Evolutionary relationship of the metabotropic receptor family. To assemble this tree, sequence homologies in the transmembrane domains were compared for each receptor. Distance determines the degree of relatedness. r, rat; d, dog; h, human; tur, turkey; SRL, a putative serotonin receptor; and 5-HT, 5-hydroxytryptamine (serotonin). Adapted from Linden (1994). Original tree construction was by William Pearson and Kevin Lynch, University of Virginia.

take part in important feedback loops that regulate ACh release. ACh released from the presynaptic terminal can bind to mAChRs on the same nerve ending, thus activating enzymatic processes that modulate subsequent neurotransmitter release. This modulation is typically an inhibition; however, activation of m5 AChR produces an enhancement in subsequent release. These *autoreceptors* are an important regulatory mechanism for the short-term (milliseconds to seconds) modulation of neurotransmitter release (see Chapter 7).

The family of mAChRs now includes five members (m1–m5), ranging from 55 to 70 kDa, and each of the five subtypes exhibits the typical architecture of seven transmembrane domains. Much of the diversity in this family of receptors resides in the third intracellular loop (i3) responsible for the specificity of coupling to G-proteins. The m1, m3, and m5 mAChRs couple predominantly to G-proteins that activate the enzyme phospholipase C. m2 and m4 receptors couple to G-proteins that inhibit adenylate cyclase, as well as to G-proteins that regulate K$^+$ and Ca^{2+} channels directly. As is the case for other GPCRs, the domain near the N terminus of i3 is important for the specificity of G-protein coupling. This domain is conserved in m1, m3, and m5 AChRs, but is unique in m2 and m4. Several other important residues have also been identified for G-protein coupling. A particular

Asp residue near the N-terminus of the second intracellular loop (i2) is important for G-protein coupling, as are residues residing in the C-terminal region of the i3 loop.

Major mAChRs found in the brain are m1, m3, and m4, and each is distributed diffusely. The m2 subtype is the heart isoform and is not highly expressed in other organs. Genes for m4 and m5 lack introns, whereas those encoding m1, m2, and m3 contain introns, although little is known concerning alternatively spliced products of these receptors. Atropine is the most widely utilized antagonist for mAChR and binds to most subtypes, as does N-methylscopolamine. The antagonist pirenzipine appears to be relatively specific for the m1 mAChR, and other antagonists, such as AF-DX116 and hexahydrosiladifenidol, appear to be more selective for m2 and m3 subtypes.

Adrenergic Receptors

The catecholamines epinephrine (adrenaline) and norepinephrine (noradrenaline) produce their effects by binding to and activating adrenergic receptors. Interestingly, epinephrine and norepinephrine can both bind to the same adrenergic receptor. Adrenergic receptors are currently separated into three families: $\alpha1$, $\alpha2$, and β. Each of the $\alpha1$ and $\alpha2$ families is further subdivided into three subclasses. Similarly, the β family also contains three subclasses ($\beta1$, $\beta2$, and $\beta3$). The main adrenergic receptors in the brain are the $\alpha2$ and $\beta1$ subtypes. $\alpha2$ARs have diverse roles, but the function that is best characterized (in both central and peripheral nervous tissue) is their role as autoreceptors. Different AR subtypes bind to G-proteins that can alter the activity of phospholipase C, Ca^{2+} channels, and, probably the best studied, adenylate cyclase. For example, activation of $\alpha2$ARs produces inhibition of adenylate cyclase, whereas all βARs activate the cyclase.

Only a few agonists or antagonists cleanly distinguish the AR subtypes. One of them, isoproterenol, is an agonist that appears to be highly specific for βARs. Propranolol is the best-known antagonist for β receptors, and phentolamine is a good antagonist for α receptors but binds weakly at β receptors. The genomic organization of the different AR subtypes is unusual. Like many G-protein-coupled GPCRs, $\beta1$ and $\beta2$ARs are encoded by genes lacking introns. $\beta3$ARs, which apparently have a role in lipolysis and are poorly characterized, are encoded by an intron-containing gene, as are αARs, providing an opportunity for alternative splicing as a means of introducing functional heterogeneity into the receptor.

Dopamine Receptors

Some 80% of the DA in the brain is localized to the corpus striatum, which receives major input from the substantia nigra and takes part in coordinating motor movements. DA is also found diffusely throughout the cortex, where its specific functions remain largely undefined. However, many neuroleptic drugs appear to exert their effects by blocking DA binding, and imbalances in the dopaminergic system have long been associated with neuropsychiatric disorders.

DA receptors are found both pre- and postsynaptically, and their structure is homologous to that of the receptors for other catecholamines (Civelli et al., 1993). Five subtypes of DA receptors can be grouped into two main classes: D1-like and D2-like receptors. D1-like receptors include D1 and D5, whereas D2-like receptors include D2, D3, and D4 (see Fig. 9.19). The main distinction between these two classes is that D1-like receptors activate adenylate cyclase through interactions with G_s, whereas D2-like receptors inhibit adenylate cyclase and other effector molecules by interacting with G_i/G_o. D1-like receptors are also slightly larger in molecular mass than D2-like receptors. An additional point of interest, as noted earlier, is that D5 receptors selectively associate with $GABA_A$ receptors, impacting their function and vice versa (Liu et al., 2000). The deduced amino acid sequence for the entire family ranges from 387 amino acids (D4) to 477 amino acids (D5). Main structural differences between D1-like and D2-like receptors are that the intracellular loop between the sixth and the seventh transmembrane segments is larger in D2-like receptors and D2-like receptors have smaller C-terminal intracellular segments. Two isoforms of the D2 receptor have been isolated that are called D2 long and D2 short; alternative splicing generates these isoforms. D2 long contains a 29 amino acid insert in the large intracellular loop between TM5 and TM6. Functional or anatomical differences have yet been fully resolved for the short and long forms of D2.

D1-like receptors, like βARs, are transcribed from intronless genes. Conversely, all D2-like receptors contain introns, thus providing for possibilities of alternatively spliced products. Posttranslational modifications include glycosylation at one or more sites, disulfide bonding of the two Cys residues in e2 and e3, and acylation of the Cys residue in the C-terminal tail (analogous to the β2AR). The DA-binding site includes two Ser residues in TM5 and an Asp residue in TM3, analogous to the βAR.

Because of the presumed role of DA in neuropsychiatric disorders, enormous effort has been put into developing pharmacological tools for manipulating this system. DA receptors bind bromocriptine, lisuride, clozapine, melperone, fluperlapine, and haloperidol. Because these drugs do not show great specificity for receptor subtypes, their usefulness for dissecting effects specifically related to binding to one or another DA receptor subtype is limited. However, their role in the treatment of human neuropsychiatric disorders is enormous (see Chapter 44).

Purinergic Receptors

Purinergic receptors bind to ATP or other nucleotide analogs and to its breakdown product adenosine. While ATP is a common constituent found within synaptic vesicles, adenosine is not and is therefore not considered a "classic" neurotransmitter. However, the multitude of receptors that bind and are activated by adenosine indicates that this molecule has important modulatory effects on the nervous system. Situations of high metabolic activity that consume ATP and situations of insufficient ATP-regenerating capacity can lead to the accumulation of adenosine. Because adenosine is permeable to membranes and can diffuse into and out of cells, a feedback loop is established in which adenosine can serve as a local diffusible signal that communicates the metabolic status of the neuron to surrounding cells and vice versa (Linden, 1994).

The original nomenclature describing purinergic receptors defined adenosine as binding to P1 receptors and ATP as binding to P2 receptors. Families of both P1 and P2 receptors have since been described, and adenosine receptors are now identified as A-type purinergic receptors, consisting of A1, A2a, A2b, and A3. ATP receptors are designated as P type and consist of P2x, P2y, P2z, P2t, and P2u. Recall that P2x and P2z subtypes are ionotropic receptors (see earlier discussion).

A-type receptors exhibit the classic arrangement of seven transmembrane-spanning segments but are typically shorter than most GPCRs, ranging in size between 35 and 46 kDa. The ligand-binding site of A-type receptors is unique in that the ligand, adenosine, has no inherent charged moieties at physiological pH. A-type receptors appear to utilize His residues as their points of contact with adenosine, and, in particular, a His residue in TM7 is essential because its mutation eliminates agonist binding. Other His residues in TM6 and TM7 are conserved in all A-type receptors and may serve as other points of contact with agonists. Work with chimeric A-type receptors has further substantiated the importance of residues in TM5, TM6, and TM7 for ligand binding. A1 receptors are highly expressed in the brain, and their activation downregulates adenylate cyclase and increases

phospholipase C activity. The A2a and A2b receptors are not as highly expressed in nervous tissue and are associated with the stimulation of adenylate cyclase and phospholipase C, respectively. The A3 subtype exhibits a unique pharmacological profile in that binding of xanthine derivatives, which blocks the action of adenosine competitively, is absent. Very low levels of the A3 receptor are found in brain and peripheral nervous tissue. The A3 receptor appears to be coupled to the activation of phospholipase C.

The human A1 receptor has a unique mode of receptor expression (Olah and Stiles, 1995). Introns in the 5'-untranslated sequence of the mRNA, spliced in a tissue-specific manner, are capable of affecting the translational efficiency of the mRNA. Two extra start codons upstream from the start codon that initiates translation of the A1 receptor exert a negative effect on translation. Mutating these two extra start codons can relieve the translational repression. This process is an effective way of controlling the level of receptor expression and may serve as a more general model for translational regulation for other mRNAs.

The P-type receptors, P2y, P2t, and P2u, are typical G-protein-linked GPCRs, mostly localized to the periphery. However, direct effects of ATP have been detected in neurons, and often the response is biphasic; an early excitatory effect followed, with its breakdown to adenosine, by a secondary inhibitory effect. Interestingly, P-type receptors exhibit a higher degree of homology to peptide-binding receptors than they do to A-type purinergic receptors. As in A-type receptors, P-type receptors have a His residue in the third transmembrane domain; however, other sites for ligand binding have not been specifically identified.

Serotonin Receptors

Cell bodies containing serotonin (5-HT) are found in the raphe nucleus in the brain stem and in nerve endings distributed diffusely throughout the brain. 5-HT has been implicated in sleep, modulation of circadian rhythms, eating, and arousal. 5-HT also has hormone-like effects when released in the bloodstream, regulating smooth muscle contraction and affecting platelet-aggregating and immune systems.

5-HT receptors are classified into four subtypes, 5-HT1 to 5-HT4, with a further subdivision of 5-HT1 subtypes. Recall that the 5-HT3 receptor is ionotropic (see earlier discussion). The other 5-HT receptors exhibit the typical seven transmembrane-spanning segments and all couple to G-proteins to exert their effects. For example, 5-HT1a, 1b, 1d, and 4 either activate or inhibit adenylate cyclase. 5-HT1c and 5-HT2 receptors preferentially stimulate activation of phospholipase C to produce increased intracellular levels of diacylglycerol and inositol 1,4,5-trisphosphate.

5-HT receptors can also be grossly distributed into two groups on the basis of their gene structures. Both 5-HT1c and 5-HT2 are derived from genes that contain multiple introns. In contrast, similar to the βAR family, 5-HT1 is coded by a gene lacking introns. Interestingly, 5-HT1a is more closely related ancestrally to the βAR family than it is to other membranes of the 5-HT receptor family and was originally isolated by utilizing cDNA for the β2AR as a molecular probe. This observation helps explain some pharmacological data suggesting that both 5-HT1a and 5-HT1b can bind certain adrenergic antagonists.

Glutamate GPCRs

GPCRs that bind glutamate [metabotropic glutamate receptors (mGluRs)] are similar in general structure in having seven transmembrane-spanning segments to other GPCRs; however, they are divergent enough to be considered to have originated from a separate evolutionary-derived receptor family (Hollmann and Heinemann, 1994; Nakanishi, 1994). In fact, sequence homology between the mGluR family and other GPCRs is minimal except for the GABA$_B$ receptor. The mGluR family is heterogeneous in size, ranging from 854 to 1179 amino acids. Both the N-terminal and the C-terminal domains are unusually large for G-protein-coupled receptors. One great difference in the structures of mGluRs is that the binding site for glutamate resides in the large N-terminal extracellular domain and is homologous to a bacterial amino acid-binding protein (Armstrong and Gouaux, 2000). In most of the other families of GPCRs, the ligand-binding pocket is formed by transmembrane segments partly buried in the membrane. Additionally, mGluRs exist as functional dimers in the membrane in contrast to the single subunit forms of most GPCRs (Liu et al., 2000). These significant structural distinctions support the idea that mGluRs evolved separately from other GPCRs. The third intracellular loop, thought to be the major determinant responsible for G-protein coupling, of mGluRs is relatively small, whereas the C-terminal domain is quite large. The coupling between mGluRs and their respective G-proteins may be through unique determinants that exist in the large C-terminal domain.

Currently, eight different mGluRs can be subdivided into three groups on the basis of sequence homologies and their capacity to couple to specific enzyme systems. Both mGluR1 and mGluR5 activate a G-protein coupled to phospholipase C. mGluR1 activation can also lead to the production of cAMP and of arachidonic acid by coupling to G-proteins that activate adenylate cyclase and phospholipase A$_2$. mGluR5 seems more specific, activating predominantly the G-protein-activated phospholipase C.

The other six mGluR subtypes are distinct from one another in favoring either trans-1-aminocyclopentane-1,3-dicarboxylate (mGluR2, 3, and 8) or 1-2-amino-4-phosphonobutyrate (mGluR4, 6, and 7) as agonists for activation. mGluR2 and mGluR4 can be further distinguished pharmacologically by using the agonist 2-(carboxycyclopropyl)glycine, which is more potent at activating mGluR2 receptors. Less is known about the mechanisms by which these receptors produce intracellular responses; however, one effect is to inhibit the production of cAMP by activating an inhibitory G-protein.

mGluRs are widespread in the nervous system and are found both pre- and postsynaptically. Presynaptically, they serve as autoreceptors and appear to participate in the inhibition of neurotransmitter release. Their postsynaptic roles appear to be quite varied and depend on the specific G-protein to which they are coupled. mGluR1 activation has been implicated in long-term synaptic plasticity at many sites in the brain, including long-term potentiation in the hippocampus and long-term depression in the cerebellum (see Chapter 55).

GABA$_B$ Receptor

GABA$_B$ receptors are found throughout the nervous system, where they are sometimes colocalized with ionotropic GABA$_A$ receptors. GABA$_B$ receptors are present both pre- and postsynaptically. Presynaptically, they appear to mediate inhibition of neurotransmitter release through an autoreceptor-like mechanism by activating K$^+$ conductances and diminishing Ca^{2+} conductances. In addition, GABA$_B$ receptors may affect K$^+$ channels through a direct physical coupling to the K$^+$ channel, not mediated through a G-protein intermediate. Postsynaptically, GABA$_B$ receptor activation produces a characteristic slow hyperpolarization (termed the slow inhibitory postsynaptic potential) through the activation of a K$^+$ conductance. This effect appears to be through a pertussis toxin-sensitive G-protein that inhibits adenylate cyclase.

Cloning of the GABA$_B$ receptor (GABA$_B$R1) revealed that it has high sequence homology to the family of glutamate GPCRs, but shows little similarity to other G-protein-coupled receptors. The large N-terminal extracellular domain of the GABA$_B$ receptor is the presumed site of GABA binding. With the exception of this large extracellular domain, the GABA$_B$ receptor structure is typical of the GPCR family, exhibiting seven transmembrane domains. The initial cloning of the GABA$_B$ receptor was made possible by the development of the high-affinity, high-specificity antagonist CGP64213. This antagonist is several orders of magnitude more potent at inhibiting GABA$_B$ receptor function than the more widely known antagonist saclofen. Baclofen, an analog of saclofen, remains the best agonist for activating GABA$_B$ receptors.

Functional GABA$_B$ receptors appear to exist primarily as dimers in the membrane. Expression of the cloned GABA$_B$R1 isoform does not produce significant functional receptors. However, when coexpressed with the GABA$_B$R2 isoform, receptors that are indistinguishable functionally and pharmacologically from those in brain were produced. In addition, GABA$_B$ dimers exist in neuronal membranes, and all data point to the conclusion that GABA$_B$ receptors dimerize and that the dimer is the functionally important form of the receptor. As noted earlier (Fig. 9.17B), GPCRs can interact with themselves and other receptors. It is well to keep in mind that these types of direct receptor interactions may be more widespread than currently appreciated.

Peptide Receptors

Neuropeptide receptors form an immense family. Because of their diversity, they cannot be covered in detail in this chapter. Despite this diversity, however, none of the receptors that bind peptides appears to be coupled directly to the opening of ion channels. Neuropeptide receptors exert their effects either through the typical pathway of activation of G-proteins or through a more recently described pathway related to activation of an associated tyrosine kinase activity.

The peptide-binding domain of neuropeptide receptors includes residues in both the large N-terminal extracellular domain and the transmembrane domain. These additional stabilizing contacts presumably provide the receptors with their remarkably high affinity for neuropeptides (in the nanomolar concentration range). For example, residues in the first and second extracellular domains, as well as those in at least four of the transmembrane domains of the NK1 neurokinin receptor, interact with substance P to form stabilizing contacts. Many small molecule antagonists are known to inhibit activation of the NK1 receptor, and these antagonists bind to some, but not all, of the same amino acids in the transmembrane segments as substance P. The possible mechanisms for inhibition of the peptide receptors range from complete structural overlap between agonist and antagonist binding to complete allosteric exclusion. Knowledge of the

activated structure of the neuropeptide receptors provides remarkable opportunities for future drug design.

Summary

GPCRs are single polypeptides composed of seven transmembrane-spanning segments. In general, the binding site for neurotransmitter is located within the core of the circular structure formed by these segments. Transmitter binding produces conformational changes in the receptor that expose parts of the i3 region, among others, for binding to G-proteins. G-protein binding increases the affinity of the receptor for transmitter. Desensitization is common among GPCRs and leads to a decreased response of the receptor to neurotransmitter by several distinct mechanisms. mGluRs are structurally distinct from other GPCRs; mGluRs have large N-terminal extracellular domains that form the binding site for glutamate. Otherwise, the basic structure of mGluRs appears to be similar to that of the rest of the GPCR family.

References

Armstrong, N., and Gouaux, E. (2000). Mechanisms for activation and antagonism of an AMPA-sensitive glutamate receptor: Crystal structures of the GluR2 ligand binding core. *Neuron* **28**, 165–181.

Boulter, J., Hollmann, M., O'Shea-Greenfield, A., Hartley, M., Deneris, E., Maron, C., and Heinemann, S. (1990). Molecular cloning and functional expression of glutamate receptor subunit genes. *Science* **249**, 1033–1037.

Civelli, O., Bunzow, J. R., and Grandy, D. K. (1993). Molecular diversity of the dopamine receptors. *Annu. Rev. Pharmacol. Toxicol.* **33**, 281–307.

Ferguson, S. S. G., Downey, W. E., Colapietro, A.-M., Barak, L. S., Menard, L., and Caron, M. G. (1996). Role of arrestin in mediating agonist-promoted G-protein coupled receptor internalization. *Science* **271**, 363–366.

Hollmann, M., and Heinemann, S. (1994). Cloned glutamate receptors. *Annu. Rev. Neurosci.* **17**, 31–108.

Hollmann, M., O'Shea-Greenfield, A., Rogers, S. W., and Heinemann, S. (1989). Cloning by functional expression of a member of the glutamate receptor family. *Nature (Lond.)* **342**, 643–648.

Imoto, K., Busch, C., Sakmann, B., Mishina, M., Konno, T., Nakai, J., Bujo, H., Mori, Y., Fukuda, K., and Numa, S. (1988). Rings of negatively charged amino acids determine the acetylcholine receptor channel conductance. *Nature (Lond.)* **335**, 645–648.

Kandel, E. R., Schwartz, J. H., and Jessell, T. M. (1991). "Principles of Neurol Science," 3rd Ed. Elsevier, New York.

Karlin, A. (1993). Structure of nicotinic acetylcholine receptors. *Curr. Opin. Neurobio.* **3**, 299–309.

Keinanen, K., Wisden, W., Sommer, B., Werner, P., Herb, A., Verdoorn, T. A., Sakmann, B., and Seeburg, P. H. (1990). A family of AMPA-selective glutamate receptors. *Science* **249**, 556–560.

Kobilka, B. (1992). Adrenergic receptors as models for G-protein-coupled receptors. *Annu. Rev. Neurosci.* **15**, 87–114.

Lee, S. P., O'Dowd, B. F., Ng., G. Y. K., Varghese, G., Akil, H., Mansour, A., Nguyen, T., and George, S. R. (2000). Inhibition of cell surface expression by mutant receptors demonstrates that D2 dopamine receptors exist as oligomers in the cell. *Mol. Pharmacol.* **58**, 120–128.

Linden, J. (1994). *In* "Basic Neurochemistry" (G. J. Siegel, B. W. Agranoff, R. W. Albers, and P. B. Molinoff, eds.), pp. 401–416. Raven Press, New York.

Liu, F., Wan, Q., Pristupa, Z.B., Yu, X.–M., Want, Y.T., and Niznik, H.B. (2000). Direct protein-protein coupling enables cross-talk between dopamine D5 and γ-aminobutyric acid A receptors. *Nature* **403**, 274–278.

Miyazawa, A., Fujiyoshi, Y., Stowell, M., and Unwin, N. (1999). Nicotinic acetylcholine receptor at 4.6A resolution: Transverse tunnels in the channel wall. *J. Mol. Biol.* **288**, 765–786.

Moriyoshi, K., Masu, M., Ishii, T., Shigemoto, R., Mizuno, N., and Nakanishi, S. (1991). Molecular cloning and characterization of the rat NMDA receptor. *Nature (Lond.)* **354**, 31–37.

Nakanishi, S. (1994). Metabotropic glutamate receptors: Synaptic transmission, modulation, and plasticity. *Neuron* **13**, 1031–1037.

Nakanishi, N., Shneider, N. A., and Axel, R. (1990). A family of glutamate receptor genes: Evidence for the formation of heteromultimeric receptors with distinct channel properties. *Neuron* **5**, 569–581.

Olah, M. E., and Stiles, G. L. (1995). Adenosine receptor subtypes: Characterization and therapeutic regulation. *Annu. Rev. Pharmacol. Toxicol.* **35**, 581–606.

Ortells, M. O., and Lunt, G. G. (1995). Evolutionary history of the ligand-gated ion channel superfamily of the reseptors. *Trends Neurosci.* **18**, 122.

Overton, M.C., and Blumer, K.J. (2000) G-protein-coupled receptors function as oligomers in vivo. *Curr. Bio.* **10**, 341–344.

Premont, R. T., Inglese, J., and Lefkowitz, R. J. (1995). Protein kinases that phosphorylate activated G-protein-coupled receptors. *FASEB J.* **9**, 175–182.

Rosenmund, C., Stern-Bach, Y., and Stevens, C.F. (1998). The tetrameric structure of a glutamate receptor channel. *Science* **280**, 1596–1599.

Salahpour, A., Angers, S., and Bouvier, M. (2000). Functional significance of oligomerization of G-protein-coupled receptors. *Trends Endocrinol. Metab.* **11**, 163–168.

Sommer, B., Kohler, M., Sprengel, R., and Seeburg, P. H. (1991). RNA editing in brain controls a determinant of ion flow in glutamate-gated channels. *Cell (Cambridge, Mass.)* **67**, 11–19.

Strader, C. D., Fong, T. M., Tota, M. R., Underwood, D., and Dixon, R. A. (1994). Structure and function of G-protein-coupled receptors. *Annu. Rev. Biochem.* **63**, 101–132.

Strosberg, A. D. (1990). Biotechnology of β-adrenergic reseptors. *Mol. Neurobiol.* **4**, 211–250.

Unwin, N. (1993). Neurotransmitter action: Opening of ligand-gated ion channel. *Cell* **7**, 31–41.

Unwin, N. (1995). Acetylcholine receptor channel imaged in the open state. *Nature (Lond.)* **373**, 37–43.

Watkins, J. C., Krogsgaard-Larsen, P., and Honore, T. (1990). Structure activity relationships in the development of excitatory amino acid receptor agonists and competitive antagonists. *Trends Pharmacol. Sci.* **11**, 25–33.

Wo, Z. G., and Oswald, R. E. (1995), Unraveling the modulor design of glutamate-gated ion channels. *Trends Neurosci.* **18**, 161–168.

M. Neal Waxham

10

Intracellular Signaling

Almost all aspects of neuronal function, from its maturation during development, to its growth and survival, cytoskeletal organization, gene expression, neurotransmission, and use-dependent modulation, are dependent on intracellular signaling initiated at the cell surface. The response of a neuron to neurotransmitters, growth factors, and other signaling molecules is determined by its complement of receptors, pathways available for transducing signals into the neuron and transmitting these signals to its intracellular compartments, and the enzymes, ion channels, and cytoskeletal proteins that ultimately mediate the effects of the neurotransmitters in the cytoplasm or nucleus. Molecules involved in signal transmission and transduction are highly represented in mammalian and invertebrate genomes. Individual neuronal responses are further determined by the concentration and localization of signal transduction components and are modified by the prior history of neuronal activity. Several primary classes of signaling systems, operating at different time courses, provide great flexibility for intercellular communication. One class comprises ligand-gated ion channels, such as the nicotinic receptor considered in Chapter 9. This class of signaling system provides fast transmission that is activated and deactivated within 10 ms. It forms the underlying "hard wiring" of the nervous system that makes rapid multisynaptic computations possible. A second class consists of receptor tyrosine kinases, which typically respond to growth factors and to trophic factors and produce major changes in the growth, differentiation, or survival of neurons (Chapter 19). A third class utilizes G-protein-linked signals and constitutes the largest number of receptors. This signaling system

requires several steps for transduction and transmission of the signal, thus slowing the response from 100–300 ms to many minutes. The relatively slow speed is offset, however, by a richness in the diversity of its modulation and its inherent capacity for amplification and plasticity. The initial steps in this signaling system typically generate a second messenger inside the cell, and this second messenger then activates a number of proteins, including protein kinases that modify cellular processes. Signal transduction also modulates the level of transcription of genes, which determine the differentiated and functional state of cells.

SIGNALING THROUGH G-PROTEIN-LINKED RECEPTORS

Signal transduction through G-protein-linked receptors requires three membrane-bound components: (1) a cell surface receptor that determines to which signal the cell can respond; (2) a G protein on the intracellular side of the membrane that is stimulated by the activated receptor; and (3) either an effector enzyme that changes the level of a second messenger or an effector channel that changes ionic fluxes in the cell in response to the activated G protein. The human genome encodes for more than 600 receptors for catecholamines, odorants, neuropeptides, and light that couple to one or more of the 27 identified G proteins. These, in turn, regulate one or more of more than two dozen different effector channels and enzymes. The key feature of this information flow is the ability of G proteins to detect the presence of activated receptors and to amplify the signal by altering the activity of appropriate effector enzymes and channels.

G proteins are GTP-binding proteins that couple the activation of seven-helix receptors by neurotransmitters at the cell surface to changes in the activity of effector enzymes and effector channels. A common effector enzyme is adenylate cyclase, which synthesizes cyclic AMP—an intracellular surrogate for the neurotransmitter, the first messenger. Phospholipase C (PLC), another effector enzyme, generates diacylglycerol (DAG) and inositol 1, 4, 5-trisphosphate (IP_3), the latter of which releases intracellular stores of Ca^{2+}. Information from an activated receptor flows to the second messengers that typically activate protein kinases, which modify a host of cellular functions. Cyclic AMP, Ca^{2+}, and DAG have in common the ability to activate protein kinases with broad substrate specificities. They phosphorylate key intracellular proteins, ion channels, enzymes, and transcription factors taking part in diverse cellular biological processes. The activities of protein kinases and phosphatases are in balance, constituting a highly regulated process, as revealed by the phosphorylation state of these targets of the signal transduction process. In addition to regulating protein kinases, second messengers such as cAMP, cGMP, Ca^{2+}, and arachidonic acid can directly gate, or modulate, ion channels. G proteins can also couple directly to ion channels without the interception of second messengers or protein kinases. In these diverse ways, a neuro-

transmitter outside the cell can modulate essentially every aspect of cell physiology and encode the history of cell stimuli in the form of altered activity and expression of its cellular constituents. An overview of G-protein signaling to protein kinases is presented in Fig. 10.1.

G-Protein Signaling Operates on Common Principles

The many types of G proteins and the many types of effector enzymes have certain features in common (Hille, 1992). First, each receptor can couple to one or only a few G proteins, thus specifying the stimulus response. Second, second messengers are typically synthesized in one or two steps from a precursor (e.g., ATP) that is readily available in those cells at high concentration but is itself inactive as a signaling molecule. G proteins can also stimulate enzymes that eliminate second messengers. Third, the initial signal can be amplified greatly: each receptor can activate many G-protein molecules; each adenylate cyclase can synthesize many cAMP molecules; and each protein kinase can phosphorylate many copies of each of its substrates. Fourth, the process is slower in onset and persists longer than ligand-gated ion channel signaling. A fifth feature of G-protein signaling is the ability to orchestrate a variety of effects through the same second messenger. For example, the cyclic AMP-dependent protein kinase (PKA), stimulated by serotonin activity on sensory neurons, phosphorylates and inhibits a K^+ channel. This inhibition results in a prolonged action potential and a greater influx of Ca^{2+} with each stimulation of the sensory neuron and in a sensitization of the gill response regulated by this circuit. On a slower time course, cAMP and PKA can also modify carbohydrate metabolism to keep up with activity and the transcription of genes and translation of proteins that ultimately modify the number of synaptic contacts made by the sensory neuron after prolonged periods of activity or inactivity. A nervous system with information flow by fast transmission alone would be capable of stereotyped or reflex responses. Modulation of this transmission and changes in other cellular functions by G-protein-linked systems and by receptor-tyrosine kinase-linked systems enables an orchestrated response. The large diversity of signaling molecules and their intracellular targets offer nearly unlimited flexibility of response over a broad time scale and with high amplification. This signaling is a key feature of neuronal plasticity, regulating every step of the way from neurotransmitter receptors and ion channels, signal transduction pathways, neurotransmitter synthesis, and release to

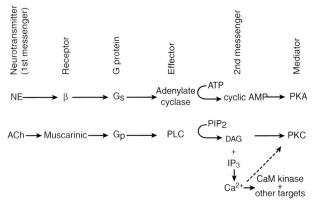

FIGURE 10.1 Overview of G-protein signaling to protein kinases. Norepinephrine (NE) and acetylcholine (ACh) can stimulate certain receptors that couple through distinct G proteins to different effectors, which results in increased synthesis of second messengers and activation of protein kinases (PKA and PKC). PLC, phospholipase C; PIP2, phosphatidylinositol bisphosphate; DAG, diacylglycerol; CaM, Ca^{2+}–calmodulin dependent; IP_3, inositol 1, 4, 5-triphosphate.

the expression of genes in the nucleus that underlie synaptic changes linked to learning and memory.

Receptors Catalyze the Conversion of G Proteins into the Active GTP-Bound State

G proteins undergo a molecular switch between two interconvertible states that are used to "turn on" or "turn off" downstream signaling. G proteins taking part in signal transduction utilize a regulatory motif that is seen in other GTPases engaged in protein synthesis and in intracellular vesicular traffic. G proteins are switched on by stimulated receptors, and they switch themselves off after a time delay. Whether a G protein is turned on or off depends on the guanine nucleotide to which it is bound. G proteins are inactive when GDP is bound and are active when GTP is bound. The sole function of seven-helix receptors in activating G proteins is to catalyze an exchange of GTP for GDP. This is a temporary switch because G proteins are designed with a GTPase activity that hydrolyzes the bound GTP and converts the G protein back into the GDP-bound, or inactive, state. Thus, a G protein must continuously sample the state of activation of the receptor, and it transmits downstream information only while the neuron is exposed to neurotransmitter. A fast GTPase means that the signal transduction pathway is very responsive to the presence of neurotransmitter outside, whereas a slow GTPase provides greater amplification but is less responsive to the elimination of the neurotransmitter. A cell cannot produce distinct responses to each stimulus presented at high frequency when the participating G protein has a slow GTPase. The benefit of a slow GTPase is that it allows amplification of the signal by permitting a given receptor to activate many G proteins and allows G proteins to produce changes in many effector enzymes for each G-protein cycle. The GTPase activity of G proteins serves both as a timer and as an amplifier (Fig. 10.2).

The G-Protein Cycle

G proteins are trimeric structures composed of two functional units: (1) an α subunit (39–52 kDa) that catalyzes GTPase activity and (2) a $\beta\gamma$ dimer (35 and 8 kDa, respectively) that interacts tightly with the α subunit when bound to GDP (Stryer and Bourne, 1986; Neer, 1995). The role of the three subunits in the G-protein cycle is depicted in Fig. 10.3. In the basal state, GDP is bound tightly to the α subunit, which is associated with the $\beta\gamma$ pair to form an inactive G protein. In addition to blocking interaction of the α subunit with its effector, the $\beta\gamma$ pair increases the affinity of the a subunit for activated receptors. Binding of the neurotransmitter to the receptor produces a conformational change that positions previously buried residues that promote increased affinity of the receptors for the inactive G protein. A given receptor can interact with only one or a limited number of G proteins, and the α subunit produces most of this specificity. Coupling with the activated receptor reduces the affinity of the α subunit for GDP, facilitating its dissociation and thus leaving the nucleotide-binding site empty. Either GDP or GTP can bind the vacant site; however, because the level of GTP in the cell is much greater than the level of GDP, the dissociation of GDP is usually followed by the binding of GTP. Thus, the receptor effectively catalyzes an exchange of GTP for GDP. Binding of

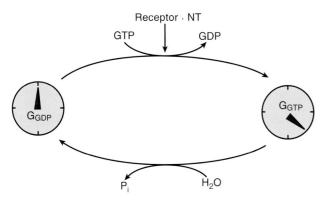

FIGURE 10.2 GTPase activity of G proteins serves as a timer and amplifier. Receptors activated by neurotransmitters (NT) initiate the GTPase timing mechanism of G proteins by displacement of GDP by GTP. Neurotransmitters thus convert GGOP ("turned-off state") to GGTP (time-limited "turned-on" state).

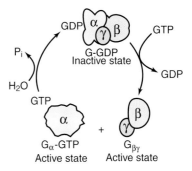

FIGURE 10.3 Interconversion, catalyzed by excited receptors, of G-protein subunits between inactive and active states. Displacement of GDP with GTP dissociates the inactive heterotrimeric G protein, generating α-GTP and $\beta\gamma$, both of which can interact with their respective effectors and activate them. The system converts into the inactive state after GTP has been hydrolyzed and the subunits have reassociated. From Stryer (1995). Used with permission of W. H. Freeman and Company.

TABLE 10.1   Functions of α Subunits of G Proteins[a]

Class	Member	Modifying toxin	Some functions
α_s	α_s, α_{olf}	Cholera	Stimulate adenylate cyclase, regulate Ca^{2+} channels
α_i	α_{i-1}, α_{i-2}, α_{i-3}, α_o, α_z	Pertussis	Inhibit adenylate cyclase, regulate K^+ and Ca^{2+} channels
α_t	α_{gust}, α_{t-1}, α_t^{-2}	Cholera and pertussis	Activate cGMP phosphodiesterase
α_q	α_q, α_{11}, α_{14}, α_{15}, α_{16}	—	Activate PLC
α_{12}	α_{12}, α_{13}	—	Regulate Na^+/K^+ exchange

[a]Summarized from Neer (1995).

GTP has two consequences: (1) it dissociates the G protein into α-GTP and $\beta\gamma$ and (2) the α-GTP subunit has a reduced affinity for the stimulated receptor, leading to dissociation of the complex.

GTP–GDP exchange is inherently very slow because the amount of activation energy required to open the nucleotide-binding site is large. This slow exchange ensures that very little of the G protein is in the on state under basal conditions. The stimulated receptor does not provide the energy for the cycle, but it lowers the amount of free energy for the dissociation from the nucleotide-binding site and accelerates the exchange reaction greatly. When the stimulated receptor increases GTP–GDP exchange, the GTPase reaction becomes the rate-limiting step of the cycle and α-GTP accumulates. The level of G protein in the on state can increase from being 1% to being more than 50% of all G protein. The direction of the cycle is determined by the GTPase reaction, which uses the energy of GTP to make the reaction irreversible and to maintain a low level of α-GTP in the basal state (Stryer and Bourne, 1986).

Information Flow Thru G-Protein Subunits

One of the more tense and public debates in signal transduction has been the question whether the a subunit alone conveys information that specifies which effector is activated or whether the $\beta\gamma$ pair has a role. One of the contestants even paid for a vanity license plate proclaiming "α not β." The α subunit was thought to be responsible for specifying which effector enzyme was activated by a G protein, with $\beta\gamma$ playing a nonspecific role in keeping the α subunit inactive while presenting it to receptors for activation. This notion was eventually changed because of the finding that $\beta\gamma$ can directly activate certain K^+ channels. The historic association of G-protein function with α has persisted for the purpose of nomenclature, with G_s and α_s referring to the G protein and its corresponding α subunit, which stimulates adenylate cyclase. These names have been retained even though it is now apparent that α and $\beta\gamma$ subunits can both

modify effector enzymes and channels and that a given α subunit may combine with a number of $\beta\gamma$ pairs. The α subunits may act either independently or in concert with $\beta\gamma$ (Clapham and Neer, 1993). Furthermore, β and γ subunits in a $\beta\gamma$ pair can combine in many different ways. The terms G_i, G_p, and G_o were used for G-protein activities that inhibited adenylate cyclase, stimulated phospholipase, or were presumed to have other effects, respectively. At this stage, cloning and genomic sequencing has outpaced functional studies; the human genome encodes 27 distinct genes for α subunits, along with five βs and 13 γs. Known functions of the different subunits are summarized in Tables 10.1 and 10.2. Because the protein composition of most G proteins is not known, a cell may contain $\alpha_i\beta_2\gamma_3$ and $\alpha_i\beta_1\gamma_4$, each having different properties. The inherent affinities of $\beta\gamma$ pairs for a particular α and spatial segregation of G proteins probably limit the number of combinations of subunits greatly. (see Box 10.1).

Effector Enzymes, Channels, and Transporters Decode Receptor-Mediated Cell Stimulation in the Cell Interior

The function of the trimeric G proteins is to decode information about the concentration of neurotransmitters bound to appropriate receptors on the cell

TABLE 10.2   Effector Functions of β/γ Dimers of G Proteins

Inhibition of adenylate cyclase
Stimulation of adenylate cyclase types II and IV (with α)

Stimulation of phospholipase Cβ
Stimulation of K^+ channel
Stimulation of Ca^{2+} channel

Stimulation of phospholipase A_2
Stimulation of phosphatidylinositol-3-kinase

BOX 10.1

WHY ARE G-PROTEIN-REGULATED SYSTEMS SO COMPLEX?

Transmembrane signaling systems all contain two fundamental elements: one that recognizes an extracellular signal (a receptor) and another that generates an intracellular signal. These elements can be incorporated easily into a single molecule, e.g., in receptor tyrosine kinases and guanylyl cyclases. Why then are G-protein-regulated systems so complex, minimally containing five gene products in the basic module (receptor, heterotrimeric G protein, and effector)? The design of these systems permits both integration and branching at its two interfaces—between receptor and G protein and between G protein and effector. Each component of the system can thus be regulated independently—transcriptionally, posttranslationally, or by interactions with other regulatory proteins. Furthermore, hundreds of genes encode receptors for hormones and neurotransmitters, dozens of genes encode G protein subunits (α, β, and γ), and dozens more genes encode G-protein-regulated effectors. Each cell in an organism thus has the opportunity to sample the genome and construct a highly customized and sophisticated switchboard in its plasma membrane, permitting the organism to make an extraordinary variety of responses to complex situations. The choices that each cell makes include much more than just the components of the basic modules, extending as well to regulators of G-protein-mediated pathways such as receptor kinases and GTPase-activating proteins. The identity and concentrations of the components of the switchboard can also be sculpted within minutes or hours to permit adaptation to developmental needs or environmental stresses.

The classical stress response of mammals to the hormone epinephrine provides an elegant example of the power of modular signal transduction systems. A single hormone is utilized to initiate responses of opposite polarity in very similar cells. Thus, vascular smooth muscle in skin contracts to minimize bleeding (if there is a wound) and to maintain blood pressure, whereas vascular smooth muscle in skeletal muscle relaxes to provide increased blood flow during heightened physical activity. Smooth muscle in the intestine relaxes, whereas cardiac muscle is powerfully stimulated. In addition, hepatocytes hydrolyze glycogen to glucose, adipocytes hydrolyze triglycerides and release free fatty acids for fuel, and certain endocrine and exocrine secretions are stimulated or inhibited. Several distinct receptors for epinephrine are selectively expressed in various cell types to achieve this beneficial orchestration of stimulatory and inhibitory events. These receptors vary in their capacities to interact with G proteins from three different subfamilies (G_s, G_i, and G_q) and thus to activate or inhibit several effects to achieve the desired responses. Each cell's choices of particular receptors, G proteins, and effectors permit additional choices of regulators of each of these components to adjust the magnitude and/or the kinetics of the response.

The past two decades of research in this area have witnessed identification and characterization of the molecular players involved in G-protein-mediated signaling and appreciation of the basic mechanisms that underlie the protein–protein interactions that drive these systems. Current research is expanding this basic core of knowledge—on the one hand, toward greater understanding of how the individual modules contribute to the integrated networks of intact cells and, on the other, toward elucidation of the physical and structural bases of these complex cellular reactions. We can begin to construct a movie of G-protein-mediated signaling at atomic resolution, and many of its most important frames are shown in Fig. 10.4 (see next page).

Alfred G. Gilman and Stephen R. Sprang

surface and convert this information into a change in the activity of enzymes and channels that mediate the effects of the neurotransmitter. The effector can be an enzyme that synthesizes or degrades a diffusible second messenger or it can be an ion channel. The number of identified effectors of G-protein signaling has increased markedly in the past few years and now also includes membrane-transport proteins.

Response Specificity in G-Protein Signaling

The modular design of G-protein signaling may appear to be incapable of providing specificity. Receptors can stimulate one or more G proteins, G proteins can couple to one or more effector enzymes or channels, and the resulting second messengers will affect many cellular processes. Signals originating from activated receptors can either converge or diverge,

BOX 10.1 (cont'd)

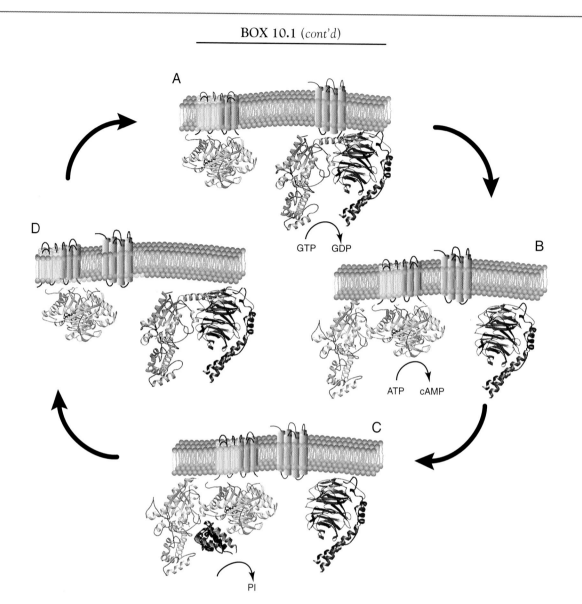

FIGURE 10.4 (A) G proteins are held in an inactive state because of very high affinity binding of GDP to their a subunits. When activated by agonist, membrane-bound seven helical receptors (Fig. 10.4 right, glowing magenta) interact with heterotrimeric G proteins (a, amber; b, teal; g, burgundy) and stimulate dissociation of GDP. This permits GTP to bind to and activate a, which then dissociates from the high-affinity dimer of b and g subunits. (B) Both activated (GTP-bound) a (lime) and bg are capable of interacting with downstream effectors. Figure 10.4 shows the interaction of GTP-a$_S$ with adenylate cyclase (catalytic domains are mustard and ash). Adenylate cyclase then catalyzes the synthesis of the second messenger cyclic AMP (cAMP) from ATP. (C) Signaling is terminated when a hydrolyzes its bound GTP to GDP. In some signaling systems, GTP hydrolysis is stimulated by GTPase-activating proteins or GAPs (cranberry) that bind to a and stablize the transition state for GTP hydrolysis. (D) Hydrolysis of GTP permits GDP-a to dissociate from its effector and associate again with bg. The heterotrimeric G protein is then ready for another signaling cycle if an activated receptor is present. This figure is based on the original work of Mark Wall and John Tesmer.

depending on the receptor and on the complement of G proteins and effectors in a given neuron (Fig. 10.5).

How can a neurotransmitter produce a specific response if G-protein coupling has the potential for

such a diversity of effectors? A given neuron has only a subset of receptors, G proteins, and effectors, thereby limiting possible signaling pathways. Transducin, for example, is confined to the visual system, where

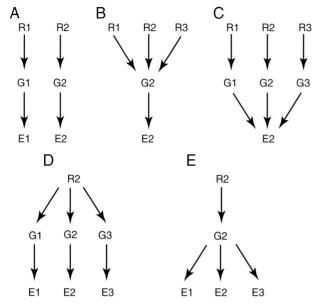

FIGURE 10.5 Signals can converge or diverge on the basis of interactions between receptors (R) and G proteins (G) and between G proteins and effectors (E). The complement of receptors, G proteins, and effectors in a given neuron determines the degree of integration of signals, as well as whether cell stimulation will produce a focused response to a neurotransmitter or a coordination of divergent responses. Adapted from Ross (1989).

the predominant effector is the cGMP phosphodiesterase and not adenylate cyclase. A number of other factors combine to increase signal specificity.

Specificity and choice   Receptors and G proteins have higher intrinsic affinities and efficacies for modulating the activity of the "correct" G protein(s) and effector(s), respectively. Some coupling obtained when high concentrations of these components are generated by overexpression in cell lines or in reconstitution experiments with purified proteins does not occur at concentrations found *in vivo*.

Spatial compartmentalization   Second-messenger systems can be compartmentalized, thus adding specificity and localized control of signaling. The same receptor may regulate a Ca^{2+} channel through one G protein at a nerve terminal and regulate PLCβ at a distal dendrite through another G protein. Although addition of the neurotransmitter in culture would produce both effects, synaptic inputs would be able to elicit specific effects at nerve terminals or at dendrites.

GTPase activity   The degree of amplification by the G protein (based on GTPase) and by the effector (based on its specific activity or conductance) can

determine which of the possible pathways is more prominent. Furthermore, some effectors appear to act as GTPase-activating proteins (GAPs), which modify the intrinsic GTPase activity of the G protein. Such an effector terminates signaling faster when stimulated by one G protein relative to another and fine-tunes the flow of information through the various forks of the signaling system. The signaling strength (i.e., the speed and efficiency) of any branch of the pathway can be modulated. Inherent affinities, level of expression of the various components, compartmentation, GTPase rates, and GAP activity combine to produce either a well-focused response by a single pathway or a richer and more diffuse response through several pathways.

Fine-Tuning of cAMP by Adenylate Cyclases

The level of cAMP is highly regulated due to a balance between synthesis by adenylate cyclases and degradation by cAMP phosphodiesterases (PDEs). Each of these enzymes can be regulated and manipulated independently. Adenylate cyclase was the first G-protein effector to be identified, and now a group of related adenylate cyclases are known to be regulated differentially by both α and $\beta\gamma$ subunits (Taussig and Gilman, 1995). G proteins can both activate and inhibit adenylate cyclases either synergistically or antagonistically.

Adenylate cyclases are large proteins of approximately 120 kDa. All the known classes of adenylate cyclase consist of a tandem repeat of the same structural motif—a short cytoplasmic region followed by six putative transmembrane segments and then a highly conserved catalytic domain of approximately 35 kDa on the cytoplasmic side. Catalytic domains resemble each other as well as the catalytic domain of guanylate cyclase. It is therefore likely that these two domains interact with G_s, bind ATP, and catalyze its conversion into cyclic AMP. Some isoforms are activated by calmodulin and have one calmodulin-binding domain in the link between the first catalytic domain and the second set of transmembrane sequences.

Differential regulation of adenylate cyclase isoforms

The most common and familiar pathway for modulating adenylate cyclase is activation through α_s. As more isoforms were cloned and studied, however, it became clear that, although all were activated by α_s, they differed in the degree and type of regulation by other G proteins. The activity of adenylate cyclase corresponds to input from receptors that are stimulatory or inhibitory and whose concurrent action can be additive or synergistic. Mammals have at least nine adenylate cyclase isoforms, designated I–IX (not including alternative splicing), that differ in their regulatory properties and tissue distribution. Many isoforms are found throughout the body, but type I is largely restricted to nerve cells and type III to the olfactory bulb. Additional isoforms, such as type II, are also prominent in the brain. Types V and VI may be the predominant forms of adenylate cyclase in peripheral tissues.

All adenylate cyclase isoforms are stimulated by G_s through its α_s subunit. Known isoforms can be divided minimally into at least three groups on the basis of additional regulatory properties (Fig. 10.6). Group A (types I, III, and VIII) possesses a calmodulin-binding domain and is activated by Ca^{2+}–calmodulin. Group B (types II and IV) is weakly responsive to direct interaction with α_s or $\beta\gamma$ but is highly activated when both are present. As described later, this synergistic effect enables this cyclase to function as a coincidence detector. Group C is typified by types V and VI (and IX), which differ from group A cyclases in their inhibitory regulation.

Inhibition of adenylate cyclases   Adenylate cyclases are also subject to several forms of inhibitory control. First, activation of all adenylate cyclases can be antagonized to some extent by $\beta\gamma$ released from abundant G proteins, such as G_i, G_o, and G_z, which complex with α_s-GTP and shift the equilibrium toward an inactive trimer by mass action. Second, either α or $\beta\gamma$ subunits derived from G_i, G_o, or G_z can directly inhibit group A cyclases, and the α subunit from G_i or G_z can inhibit group C cyclases. Many G proteins can generate $\beta\gamma$ subunits capable of directly inhibiting group A and activating group B adenylate cyclases. However, not all G proteins are sufficiently abundant to produce enough $\beta\gamma$ to bring about these effects. The level of $\beta\gamma$ required for these actions is higher than the level needed for α subunits to produce their effects. The level of G_s in particular is low; thus, α_s derived from G_s is sufficient to activate adenylate cyclases, but the $\beta\gamma$ derived from it is insufficient to directly inhibit or activate adenylate cyclases. Therefore, the sources of $\beta\gamma$ for modulation of type I and II adenylate cyclases are likely the abundant G proteins, such as G_i and G_o. This explains the apparent paradox that receptors that couple to G_s produce effects only through α_s, whereas receptors that couple to G_i produce effects through both α_i and $\beta\gamma$ even though they can share the same $\beta\gamma$.

Receptors coupling to adenylate cyclase   Dozens of neurotransmitters and neuropeptides work through cyclic AMP as a second messenger and do so by the activation of either G_s to stimulate adenylate cyclase or G_i or G_o to inhibit adenylate cyclase. Among the neurotransmitters that increase cyclic AMP are the amines norepinephrine, epinephrine, dopamine, serotonin, and histamine and the neuropeptides vasointestinal peptide (VIP) and somatostatin. In the olfactory system, a special form of G-protein α subunit, termed α_{olf}, serves the same function as α_s. Odorants are detected by several hundred seven-helix receptors that activate G_{olf}, which in turn activates the type III adenylate cyclase in the neuroepithelium. Many of the same neurotransmitters activate distinct receptors that couple to G_i or G_o. They include acetylcholine, dopamine, serotonin, norepinephrine, and opiate peptides.

Adenylate cyclases as coincidence detectors   The properties of adenylate cyclases described in Fig. 10.6 suggest an integrative capacity for adenylate cyclase. Type I and type II adenylate cyclases appear to be specifically designed to detect concurrent stimulation of neurons by two or more neurotransmitters (Bourne and Nicoll, 1993).

Type I adenylate cyclase is stimulated by neurotransmitters that couple to G_s and by neurotransmitters that elevate intracellular Ca^{2+}. This adenylate cyclase can convert the depolarization of neurons into an increase in cAMP. Cells possess many mechanisms for increasing intracellular Ca^{2+}, including voltage-gated Ca^{2+} channels that allow Ca^{2+} influx in response to depolarization and a G_q-coupled pathway. This class of adenylate cyclase has been implicated in several associative forms of learning, a role that may be related to its ability to link cAMP-based and Ca^{2+}-based signals.

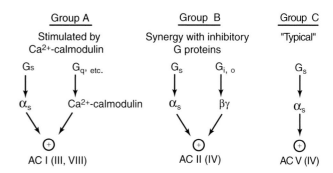

FIGURE 10.6   Isoforms of adenylate cyclase (AC). All isoforms are stimulated by α_s but differ in the degree of interaction with Ca^{2+}–calmodulin and with $\beta\gamma$ derived from inhibitory G proteins. Not shown is the ability of excess $\beta\gamma$ to complex with α_s and inhibit group A and group C adenylate cyclases. Adapted from Taussig and Gilman (1995).

Stimulation of type II adenylate cyclase by α_s is conditional on the presence of $\beta\gamma$ derived from a G protein other than G_s, thus enabling the cyclase to serve as a coincidence detector. As indicated earlier, $\beta\gamma$ derived from G_s is not sufficient to produce synergistic activation of this enzyme. Thus, activation of a second receptor, presumably coupled to the abundant G_i and G_o, is needed to provide the $\beta\gamma$. In tissues lacking the type II adenylate cyclase, neurotransmitters can couple to G_i and inhibit the other adenylate cyclases. In tissues, such as cortex and hippocampus, that contain the type II adenylate cyclase, the same neurotransmitters can couple to G_i and potentiate increases in cyclic AMP resulting from concurrent stimulation by neurotransmitters coupled to G_s.

Sources of Second Messengers: Phospholipids

Two phospholipids, phosphatidylinositol 4,5-bisphosphate (PIP_2) and phosphatidylcholine (PC), are primary precursors for a G-protein-based second-messenger system. Three second messengers, diacylglycerol, arachidonic acid and its metabolites, and elevated Ca^{2+}, are ultimately produced. A single step converts inert phospholipid precursors into lipid messengers. The elevation of Ca^{2+} levels is accomplished by the regulated entry of Ca^{2+} from a concentrated pool sequestered in the endoplasmic reticulum or from outside the cell into the lumen of the cytosol or nucleus, where its concentration is low. DAG action is mediated by protein kinase C (PKC) (Tanaka and Nishizuka, 1994). Ca^{2+} has many cellular targets but mediates most of its effects through calmodulin, a Ca^{2+}-binding protein that activates many enzymes after it binds Ca^{2+}. One class of calmodulin-dependent enzymes is a family of protein kinases that enable Ca^{2+} signals to modulate a large number of cellular process by phosphorylation (Braun and Schulman, 1995).

Generation of DAG and IP₃ from Gq and Gi coupled to PLCβ

Generation of DAG and IP₃ from G_q and G_i coupled to PLCβ The phosphatidylinositide-signaling pathway is just as prominent in neuronal signaling as the cyclic AMP pathway and is similar to it in overall design. Stimulation of a large number of neurotransmitters and hormones [including acetylcholine (M1, M3), serotonin ($5HT_2$, $5HT_{1C}$), norepinephrine (α_{1A}, α_{1B}), glutamate (metabotropic), neurotensin, neuropeptide Y, and substance P] is coupled to the activation of a phosphatidylinositide-specific PLC. Turnover of phosphatidylinositol—its degradation followed by resynthesis in response to a large variety of neurotransmitters and hormones—has been a curiosity for decades. Only recently has it become clear that in addition to their function as membrane phospho-

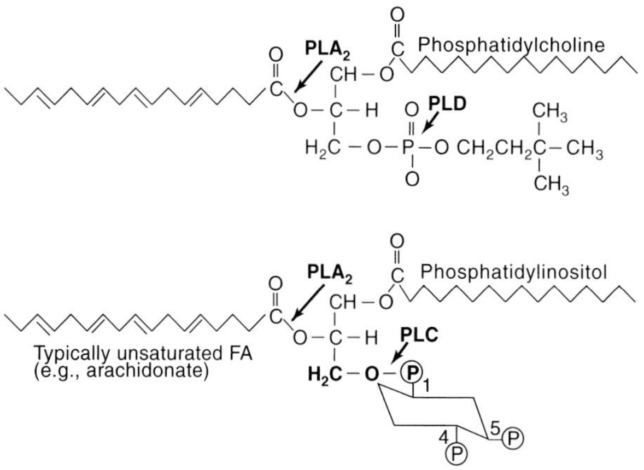

FIGURE 10.7 Structures of phosphatidylinositol and phosphatidylcholine. The sites of hydrolytic cleavage by PLC, PLD, and PLA2 are indicated by arrows. FA, fatty acid.

lipids, phosphoinositides are precursors for second messengers.

Phosphatidylinositol (PI) is composed of a diacylglycerol backbone with *myo*-inositol attached to the *sn*-3 hydroxyl by a phosphodiester bond (Fig. 10.7). The six positions of the inositol are not equivalent: the 1 position is attached by a phosphate to the DAG moiety. PI is phosphorylated by PI kinases at the 4 position and then at the 5 position to form PIP_2. In response to the appropriate G-protein coupling, PLC hydrolyzes the bond between the *sn*-3 hydroxyl of the DAG backbone and the phosphoinositol to produce DAG, a hydrophobic molecule, and IP_3, which is water soluble (Fig. 10.8). Three classes of PLC that hydrolyze PIP_2 with some selectivity have been cloned and characterized. Two dozen genes encode the three classes designated PLCβ, PLCγ, and PLCδ—soluble enzymes that have in common a catalytic domain structure but differ in their regulatory properties. G proteins couple to several variants of PLCβ. PLCγ is regulated by growth factor tyrosine kinases. In contrast, PLCδ in brain is primarily glial, and its mode of regulation is not well understood, although it may be activated by arachidonic acid.

PLCβ is coupled to neurotransmitters by G_i and G_q. At least two G proteins were suspected because PLC stimulation was fully inhibited by pertussis toxin in some systems and only partially inhibited in others. The pertussis toxin-sensitive pathway is mediated by G_i. However, the $\beta\gamma$ rather than the α subunit of G_i is responsible. The pertussis toxin-insensitive pathway is mediated by a number of isoforms referred to as G_q and α_q. G_q couples to PLCβ through its α subunit. There are several PLCβ isoforms, and they show distinct regulation by G proteins. One isoform is most sensitive to α_q, another is more sensitive to $\beta\gamma$ (e.g.,

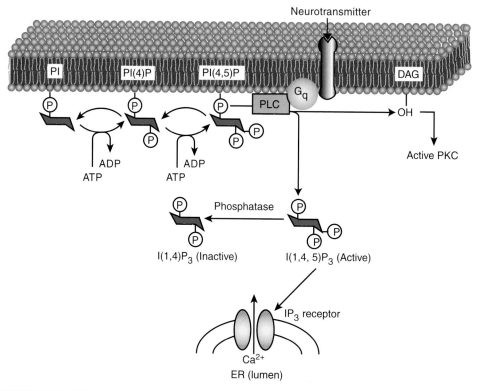

FIGURE 10.8   Schematic pathway of IP_3 and DAG synthesis and action. Stimulation of receptors coupled to G_q activates PLCβ, which leads to the release of DAG and IP_3. DAG activates PKC, whereas IP_3 stimulates the IP_3 receptor in the endoplasmic reticulum (ER), leading to mobilization of intracellular Ca^{2+} stores. Adapted from Berridge (1993).

from G_i), and a third shows little activation by either G protein.

DAG derived from activation of phospholipase D

The time course of DAG production after cell stimulation suggests a complex process. DAG is initially derived from PIP_2 as a direct consequence of G-protein coupling to PLCβ. This DAG activates PKC, and its action is terminated quickly by conversion into phosphatidic acid and recycling into phospholipids. However, a second phase of DAG synthesis often follows, and this phase produces a level of DAG far in excess of that available from PIP_2. This second phase can last many minutes and may include the hydrolysis of a major cellular phospholipid, phosphatidylcholine, by a phospholipase D (PLD) activity. PLD cleaves phosphatidylcholine at the phosphodiester bond to produce phosphatidic acid and choline. Dephosphorylation of phosphatidic acid produces DAG. The PLD pathway may be used by some mitogens and growth factors and likely contains a variety of activation schemes that may include G proteins. Stimulation of the cell generates a transient cleavage of IP_3 and DAG

from PIP_2 and a transient rise in Ca^{2+} due to IP_3-mediated release of intracellular stores. This produces the early activation of PKC. Activation is sustained in the cell in which PLD is stimulated, leading to the second phase of DAG, from phosphatidylcholine. If PLA_2 is activated, arachidonic acid is released from PIP_2 and phosphatidylcholine.

Regulation of PLCγ by receptor tyrosine kinases DAG and IP_3 is also produced when certain receptor tyrosine kinases are activated. This G-protein-independent pathway utilizes PLCγ rather than PLCβ. Stimulation of receptor tyrosine kinases such as epidermal growth factor (EGF) leads to their autophosphorylation on tyrosine residues and activation. Specific phosphotyrosine moieties on the receptor then recruit effector enzymes, such as PLCγ, that possess Src homology 2 (SH2) domains. These structural elements specifically recognize certain protein sequences with phosphotyrosine and lead to the translocation of effectors such as PLCγ to the receptor at the membrane. After binding to the receptor, PLCγ is activated by phosphorylation on tyrosine and hydrolyzes PIP_2 to DAG and IP_3.

Additional lipid messengers PLA$_2$ cleaves the fatty acid at the *sn*-2 position of the DAG backbone (Fig. 10.7). The fatty acid composition of phospholipids is quite heterogeneous; PIP$_2$ is largely composed of stearic acid at the *sn*-1 position and arachidonic acid at the *sn*-2 position. Thus, arachidonic acid is released in response to PLA$_2$ hydrolysis of PIP$_2$. This fatty acid is a 20-carbon *cis*-unsaturated fatty acid with four double bonds. PLA$_2$ can be activated by $\beta\gamma$ and α subunits of G proteins, but the identity of the endogenous G proteins that mediate this activation is not known. A cytosolic PLA$_2$ has been cloned and shown to be activated by mitogen-activated protein (MAP) kinases in response to growth factor signaling. Phosphorylation leads to its translocation to the membrane, where it can act on membrane phospholipids. Arachidonic acid has biological activity of its own in addition to serving as a precursor for prostaglandins and leukotrienes. Arachidonic acid and other *cis*-unsaturated fatty acids can modulate K$^+$ channels, PLCγ, and some forms of PKC. Other lipids may also generate signaling molecules.

A subfamily of lipid kinases that are specific for addition of a phosphate moiety on the 3 position, phosphoinositide 3-kinases (PI-3 kinases), also play a regulatory role. Depending on their preferred lipid substrate, they can produce PI-3-P, PI-3,4-P$_2$, PI-3,5-P$_2$, and PI-3,4,5-P$_3$. A number of signals, including growth factors, activate PI-3 kinases to generate these lipid messengers. In turn, these lipids then bind directly to a number of proteins and enzymes to modify vesicular traffic, protein kinases involved in survival and cell death. There is also evidence that another lipid, sphingomyelin, is a precursor for intracellular signals as well.

IP$_3$, a potent second messenger that produces its effects by mobilizing intracellular Ca^{2+} The main function of IP$_3$ is to stimulate the release of Ca^{2+} from intracellular stores. The concentration of cytosolic-free Ca^{2+} is approximately 100 nM in unstimulated neurons, whereas its concentration in the extracellular space is 1.5–2.0 mM. This provides a tremendous driving force for movement down its concentration gradient; its reversal potential is more than 100 mV. Ca^{2+} is the most common second messenger in neurons, yet it can be neurotoxic. Neurons have therefore developed several mechanisms for maintaining a low interstimulus level of free Ca^{2+}. A Ca^{2+}–ATPase and a Na$^+$–Ca^{2+} exchanger in the plasma membrane catalyze the active transport of Ca^{2+} to the extracellular space, and a different Ca^{2+}–ATPase in the ER membrane sequesters Ca^{2+} in the ER network. Much of the Ca^{2+} in the ER is complexed with low-affinity-binding proteins that enable the ER to concentrate Ca^{2+} yet enable Ca^{2+} to readily flow down its concentration gradient into the cell lumen upon opening of Ca^{2+} channels in the ER. The ER is the major IP$_3$-sensitive Ca^{2+} store in cells (Fig. 10.8).

The IP$_3$ receptor is a macromolecular complex that functions as an IP$_3$ sensor and a Ca^{2+} release channel. It has a broad tissue distribution but is highly concentrated in the cerebellum. Purification and cloning of the IP$_3$ receptor show it to be a 313-kDa membrane glycoprotein with a single IP$_3$-binding site at its N-terminal, facing the cytoplasm. The functional channel is composed of four such subunits. The C-terminal half of the molecule contains eight putative transmembrane domains; four such sets of transmembrane segments combine to form a relatively nonselective channel or pore. Ca^{2+} release by IP$_3$ is highly cooperative, with a Hill coefficient of 2.7. Thus, a small change in IP$_3$ has a large effect on Ca^{2+} release from the ER. The IP$_3$ receptor has low activity at either high or low levels of cytoplasmic Ca^{2+}, with peak release requiring 200–300 nM Ca^{2+}, a property that may be used in the generation of some Ca^{2+} waves. The mouse mutants *pcd* and *nervous* have deficient levels of the IP$_3$ receptor and exhibit defective Ca^{2+} signaling, and a genetic knockout of the IP$_3$ receptor leads to motor and other deficits.

The structure of the IP$_3$ receptor is quite similar to that found earlier for the ryanodine receptor, which serves as a Ca^{2+}-sensitive Ca^{2+} channel in muscle and brain. The ryanodine receptor is a tetramer composed of 560-kDa subunits. In muscle, it is activated by voltage changes that are detected by the dihydropyridine receptor and conveyed to the ryanodine receptor by direct protein–protein interaction. In other cells, the ryanodine receptor is gated by Ca^{2+} or by cyclic ADP-ribose. Localizations of the IP$_3$ and the ryanodine receptors in the brain are distinct, suggesting that they subserve different aspects of Ca^{2+} signaling. For example, the IP$_3$ receptor is more enriched in cerebellar Purkinje cells and hippocampal CA1 neurons, whereas the ryanodine receptor is more enriched in the dentate gyrus and CA3 neurons in hippocampus. Electron microscopy reveals that IP$_3$ receptors in the hippocampus are often on dendritic shafts and cell bodies, whereas ryanodine receptors are in axons and in dendritic spines and the nearby shaft.

Termination of the IP$_3$ signal IP$_3$ is a transient signal terminated by dephosphorylation to inositol. Inactivation is initiated either by dephosphorylation to inositol 1,4-bisphosphate (Fig. 10.9) or by an initial phosphorylation to a tetrakisphosphate form that is

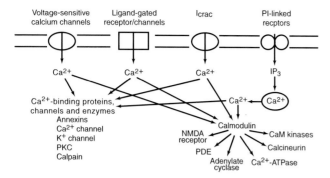

FIGURE 10.9 Multiple sources of Ca^{2+} converge on calmodulin and other Ca^{2+}-binding proteins. Cellular levels of Ca^{2+} can rise either by influx (e.g., through voltage-sensitive channels or ligand-gated channels) or by redistribution from intracellular stores triggered by IP$_3$. Calcium modulates dozens of cellular processes by the action of the Ca^{2+}–calmodulin complex on many enzymes, and calcium has some direct effects on enzymes such as PKC and calpain. CaM kinase, Ca^{2+}–calmodulin-dependent kinase.

dephosphorylated by a different pathway. Both pathways have in common an enzyme that cleaves the phosphate on the 1 position. Complete dephosphorylation yields inositol, which is recycled in the biosynthetic pathway. Recycling is important because most tissues do not contain *de novo* biosynthetic pathways for making inositol. Thus, phosphatases not only terminate the signal, but also serve as a salvage step that may be particularly important when cells are actively undergoing PI turnover. It is intriguing that the simple salt Li$^+$ selectively inhibits the salvage of inositol by inhibiting the enzyme that dephosphorylates the 1 position and is common to the two pathways. This simple salt is the drug used to treat manic-depressive disorders. At therapeutic doses of Li$^+$, the reduced salvage of inositol in cells with high phosphoinositide signaling may lead to a depletion of PIP$_2$ and a selective inhibition of this signaling pathway in active cells.

Calcium Ion

Calcium has a dual role as a carrier of electrical current and as a second messenger. Its effects are more diverse than those of other second messengers such as cyclic AMP and DAG because its actions are mediated by a much larger array of proteins, including protein kinases (Carafoli and Klee, 1999). Furthermore, many signaling pathways directly or indirectly increase cytosolic Ca^{2+} concentration from 100 nM to 0.5–1.0 mM. The source of elevated Ca^{2+} can be either the ER or the extracellular space (Fig. 10.9). As indicated earlier, mobilization of ER Ca^{2+} is mediated by IP$_3$ derived from PLCβ activation through G proteins and from PLCγ activation by receptor tyrosine

kinases acting on the IP$_3$ receptor. In addition, Ca^{2+} can activate its own mobilization through the ryanodine receptor on the ER. Mechanisms for Ca^{2+} influx from outside the cell include several voltage-sensitive Ca^{2+} channels and ligand-gated cation channels that are permeable to Ca^{2+} [e.g., nicotinic receptor and *N*-methyl-d-aspartate (NMDA) receptor]. In the Drosophila visual system and in nonexcitable mammalian cells, depletion of Ca^{2+} from the cytosol and ER initiates an unknown signal that stimulates a low-conductance influx current called I_{CRAC} (Ca^{2+} release-activated current) across the plasma membrane. In mammalian cells, a unique channel protein responsible for the current provides a slow but prolonged rise in intracellular Ca^{2+} that not only serves as a second messenger but also replenishes ER stores. Ca^{2+} is sequestered efficiently in the ER and is extruded out of the cell, which can lower Ca^{2+} to baseline levels rapidly.

Dynamics of Ca^{2+} signaling revealed by fluorescent Ca^{2+} indicators We know a great deal about the spatial and temporal regulation of Ca^{2+} signals because of the development of fluorescent Ca^{2+} indicators. A variety of fluorescent compounds related to the Ca^{2+} chelator ethylene glycol bis (β-aminoethyl ether)-N,N'-tetraacetic acid selectively bind Ca^{2+} at various concentration ranges and change their fluorescent properties upon binding Ca^{2+}. They have dissociation constants in the physiological range of Ca^{2+} and provide a rapid and fairly accurate measurement of ionized Ca^{2+}. Digital fluorescence imaging can be used to detect Ca^{2+} in subcellular compartments such as dendrites and spines, the nucleus, and the cytosol and has demonstrated localized changes in free Ca^{2+}. Some cells also undergo oscillations in free Ca^{2+} with a frequency that is increased by an increased concentration of hormone. Stimulation of cultured astrocytes with glutamate generates Ca^{2+} oscillations, which propagate as a wave that spreads across a multicellular network and may coordinate some actions of glia.

Lack of uniformity in Ca^{2+} levels The concentration of Ca^{2+} entering the cytosol through voltage-sensitive Ca^{2+} channels in the plasma membrane or through the IP$_3$ receptor in the ER is extremely high because of the large concentration gradient across these membranes. Relatively low-affinity Ca^{2+}-dependent processes can produce effects of Ca^{2+} near the membrane, such as synaptic release and modulation of Ca^{2+} channels. However, by the time Ca^{2+} diffuses a few membrane diameters away, it is buffered rapidly by many Ca^{2+}-binding proteins, and its concentration drops from

100 to 1 μM or less. The diffusion of Ca^{2+} is slowed greatly in biological fluid because of the high concentration of binding proteins (0.2–0.3 mM). Ca^{2+} diffuses a distance of 0.1–0.5 μm, and diffusion lasts approximately 30 ms before Ca^{2+} is bound. Ca^{2+} is therefore a second messenger that acts locally, a feature that makes Ca^{2+} subdomains possible where Ca^{2+} signaling is segregated spatially. In contrast, IP_3 is a global intermediate with an effective range that can span a typical soma before being terminated by dephosphorylation.

Calmodulin-Mediated Effects of Ca^{2+}

Ca^{2+} acts as a second messenger to modulate the activity of many mediators. The predominant mediator of Ca^{2+} action is calmodulin. This abundant and ubiquitous 17-kDa calcium binding is highly conserved across phyla. Ca^{2+} binds to calmodulin in the physiological range and converts it into an activator. Calmodulin has no intrinsic enzymatic activity. It serves a central regulatory role by modulating the activity of various cellular targets (Cohen and Klee, 1988). Binding of Ca^{2+} to calmodulin produces a conformational change that greatly increases its affinity for a number of target enzymes. Ca^{2+}–calmodulin binds and activates more than 20 eukaryotic enzymes, including cyclic nucleotide PDEs, adenylate cyclase, nitric oxide synthase, Ca^{2+}-ATPase, calcineurin (a phophoprotein phosphatase), and several protein kinases (Fig. 10.9). This activation of calmodulin allows neurotransmitters that change Ca^{2+} to affect dozens of cellular proteins, presumably in an orchestrated fashion. Ca^{2+} also affects proteins and enzymes independently of calmodulin, including calcium-binding proteins and enzymes such as calpain and PKC. Ion channels (K channels and IP_3 receptors or channels) are modulated directly by Ca^{2+} (Fig. 10.9). First discovered as a protein factor necessary for Ca^{2+}-dependent activation of a cyclic nucleotide PDE, the substance was renamed calmodulin (Ca^{2+} response modulator) when it was subsequently found to modulate many enzymes in addition to PDE.

Calmodulin interacts with its targets in several ways. The "conventional" interaction with enzyme targets requires a stimulated rise in Ca^{2+} so that the four Ca^{2+}-binding sites on calmodulin become occupied and it can bind. At basal Ca^{2+}, however, much of calmodulin may be bound to a diverse group of proteins such as GAP-43 (neuromodulin), neurogranin, and unconventional myosins. Interactions with these targets are not well understood and may serve to localize calmodulin near other targets or to "buffer" calmodulin so that the level of free calmodulin is kept very low and is less likely to activate the conventional

targets at basal Ca^{2+}. A third group of enzymes, which includes the inducible form of nitric oxide synthase, bind calmodulin in a manner that makes it sensitive to basal Ca^{2+}, and the enzymes are therefore active at basal Ca^{2+}.

Regulation of guanylate cyclase by nitric oxide

An important target of Ca^{2+}–calmodulin is the enzyme nitric oxide synthase (NOS) (see Chapter 8). This enzyme synthesizes one of the simplest known messengers, the gas NO (Baranano et al., 2001). Nitric oxide was first recognized as a signaling molecule that mediates the action of acetylcholine on smooth muscle relaxation. An intercellular signal was necessary to explain how the stimulation of endothelial cells by acetylcholine could produce a relaxation in tone of the underlying smooth muscle cells that surround the vessels. A labile substance operationally termed endothelium-derived relaxing factor (EDRF) was detected and has since been shown to be NO. Acetylcholine stimulates the PI signaling pathway in the endothelium to increase intracellular Ca^{2+}, which activates NOS so that more NO is made. NO then diffuses radially from the endothelial cells across two cell membranes to the smooth muscle cell, where it activates guanylate cyclase to make cyclic GMP. This in turn activates a cyclic GMP-dependent protein kinase that phosphorylates proteins, leading to a relaxation of muscle. In 1998, Robert F. Furchgott, Louis J. Ignarro, and Ferid Murad received the Nobel Prize for their discoveries concerning nitric oxide as a signaling molecule and therapeutic mediator in the cardiovascular system.

Let us now turn to the details of the NO pathway. We will see that other pathways can activate NOS, mediate the actions of NO, stimulate guanylate cyclases, and mediate the actions of cyclic GMP.

Nitric oxide is derived from L-arginine in a reaction catalyzed by NOS, a complex enzyme that has one equivalent each of flavin adenine dinucleotide (FAD), flavin mononucleotide (FMN), tetrahydrobiopterin, and heme (iron protoporphyrin IX) per monomer. NOS converts L-arginine and O_2 into NO and L-citrulline in a five-electron oxidation reaction that requires nicotinamide adenine dinucleotide phosphate (NADPH) as a cofactor. NOS likely produces the neutral-free radical NO as the active agent. As we have already seen in the generation of second messengers, stimulation of a single step converts a common inert precursor (in this case, L-arginine) into a powerful intercellular and intracellular signal (NO). Although NO is stable in oxygen-free water, it is labile and lasts only a few seconds in biological fluids because of its inactivation by superoxides and its complex formation with heme-containing proteins such as oxyhemoglobin. Thus, no specialized processes are needed to inactivate this particular signaling molecule.

As a gas, NO is soluble in both aqueous and lipid media and can diffuse readily from its site of synthesis across the cytosol or cell membrane and affect targets in the same cell or in nearby neurons, glia, and vasculature (Baranano et al., 2001). Neuronal communication by synaptic vesicles is unidirectional, from presynaptic to postsynaptic neuron. NO provides the capability for a retrograde message and thus reverses the usual flow of information, i.e., information can travel from a postsynaptic site of synthesis to a presynaptic site of modulation. When synaptic activity stimulates NO production at a spine, NO signals are unlikely to be restricted to that synapse alone, the consequences of which are important for models of long-term potentiation that propose NO as a messenger.

NO produces a variety of effects, including relaxation of smooth muscle (as mentioned earlier) of the peripheral vasculature and perhaps control of cerebral blood flow, relaxation of smooth muscle of the gut in peristalsis, and killing of foreign cells by macrophages. It was first recognized as a neuronal messenger that couples glutamate receptor stimulation to increases in cyclic GMP. Analogs of L-arginine, such as nitroarginine and monomethyl arginine, block NOS unless there is an excess of L-arginine. Such inhibitors of NO synthase have been used to implicate NO in long-term potentiation and long-term depression in the hippocampus and cerebellum, respectively.

Three classes of NO synthase have been characterized. Two of them are constitutively expressed and activated by Ca^{2+}–calmodulin formed when intracellular Ca^{2+} is elevated. The constitutive forms are designated neuronal or endothelial on the basis of their original source, although they overlap in this tissue distribution. The third class of NOS is an inducible form; its level is increased markedly by transcription and protein synthesis in response to cell stimulation, and it is prominent in macrophages stimulated by cytokines. After translation, the inducible form is active at basal Ca^{2+} levels because it has a tightly bound calmodulin in a conformation that enhances its Ca^{2+} sensitivity greatly. Because NOS is a major flavin-containing enzyme, it possesses NADPH diaphorase activity. It reduces nitroblue tetrazolium to formazan, a reaction that can be used as a cytochemical stain for NOS because much of the diaphorase staining in the brain is due to this enzyme. This family of enzymes displays distinct regional distributions in the brain, suggesting some regional

specificity in the use of NO as a signaling molecule in the brain. The constitutive neuronal isoform is concentrated in cerebellar granule cells and likely provides the NO that activates guanylate cyclase in nearby Purkinje cells during the induction of long-term depression in the cerebellum (see Chapter 32).

The action of NO is often mediated by guanylate cyclase and cyclic GMP. However, a number of physiological and pathological effects of NO are independent of cyclic GMP. NO stimulates ADP-ribosylation of a number of proteins in the brain and other tissues. The nature of ADP-ribosyltransferases and their effects is not known. Another effect of NO is stimulation of release of neurotransmitters, apparently in a Ca^{2+}-independent fashion.

Activation of guanylate cyclases Two types of guanylate cyclase, a soluble one regulated by NO and a membrane-bound enzyme regulated directly by neuropeptides, synthesize cyclic GMP from GTP in a reaction similar to the synthesis of cyclic AMP from ATP. The soluble enzyme is a heterodimer, with catalytic sites resembling those of adenylate cyclase and a heme group. NO activates the soluble enzyme by binding to the iron atom of the heme moiety. This is the basic mechanism for the regulation of soluble guanylate cyclases. Stimulation of guanylate cyclase is the major, but not only, effect of NO in the brain and other tissues. A number of therapeutic muscle relaxants, such as nitroglycerin and nitroprusside, are NO donors that produce their effects by stimulating cyclic GMP synthesis.

Membrane-bound guanylate cyclases are transmembrane proteins with a binding site for neuroendocrine peptides on the extracellular side of the plasma membrane and a catalytic domain on the cytosolic side. Several isoforms of membrane-bound guanylate cyclase, each with a binding site for a distinct neuropeptide, such as atrial natriuretic peptide and brain natriuritic peptide, have been characterized. In the periphery, these peptides regulate sodium excretion and blood pressure; in the brain, their functions are less clear.

Cyclic GMP Phosphodiesterase, an Effector Enzyme in Vertebrate Vision

The versatility of G-protein signaling is illustrated in vertebrate phototransduction, in which a specialized G protein called transducin (G_t) is activated by light rather than by a hormone or neurotransmitter. Transducin stimulates cyclic GMP phosphodiesterase, an effector enzyme that hydrolyzes cyclic GMP and ultimately turns off the dark current (see Chapter 27). Nature has evolved an elegant mechanism for using photons of light to modify a hormone-like molecule, retinal, that activates a seven-helix receptor called rhodopsin. This receptor has a built-in prehormone that is converted into the active form by light. Light photoisomerizes the inactive 11-*cis*-retinal to the active all-*trans*-retinal, which functions as a neurotransmitter to activate its receptor. Activated rhodopsin triggers the GTP–GDP exchange of transducin, leading to dissociation of its α_t and $\beta\gamma$ subunits. The active species in transducin is the α subunit. It activates a soluble cyclic GMP phosphodiesterase by binding to and displacing an inhibitory subunit of the enzyme. In the dark, retinal rods contain high levels of cyclic GMP, which maintains a cyclic GMP-gated channel permeable to Na^+ and Ca^{2+} in the open state and thus provides a depolarizing dark current. As the levels of cyclic GMP drop, the channel closes to hyperpolarize the cell.

Rods can detect a single photon of light because the signal-to-noise ratio of the system is very low due to a very low spontaneous conversion of the 11-*cis*- into the all-*trans*-retinal. Furthermore, the amplification factor is quite high; one rhodopsin molecule stimulated by a single photon can activate 500 transducins. Transducin remains in the "on" state long enough to activate 500 PDEs. PDE is designed for speed and can hydrolyze 105 cyclic GMP molecules in the second before it is deactivated by GTP hydrolysis and dissociation from transducin. Cyclic GMP in rods regulates a cyclic GMP-gated cation channel, leading to additional amplification of the signal.

Modulation of Ion Channels by G Protein

Each neuron has a set of ion channels that it uses to integrate incoming signals, propagate action potentials, and introduce Ca^{2+} into terminals specialized for the release of neurotransmitters. Because the repertoire of ion channels gives neurons their individual response signatures, it is not surprising that several types of mechanisms regulate these channels. Second messengers derived from G protein and other pathways activate protein kinases that phosphorylate ion channels. In addition, certain ion channels are effector proteins that are directly modulated by G proteins.

The first ion channel demonstrated to undergo regulation by G proteins was the cardiac K^+ channel that mediates slowing of the heart by acetylcholine released from the vagus nerve. When this I_{KACh} channel is examined in a membrane patch delimited by the seal of a cell-attached electrode, the addition of acetylcholine within the electrode increases the frequency of channel opening dramatically, whereas the addition of acetylcholine to the cell surface outside the seal does not. Although acetylcholine stimulates mus-

carinic M2 receptors when added either inside or outside the seal, the receptors outside do not have access to the channels being recorded in the sealed patch because this signaling pathway does not include diffusible second messengers that can affect the channel. The process is therefore described as membrane delimited, which is explained most simply by a direct interaction between the G protein and the channel. Subsequent studies have shown that the pathway is pertussis toxin sensitive and that purified G_i activated by GTPγS added to the underside of the patch will activate the channel.

Whether the active component of G_i is the α or the $\beta\gamma$ subunit was controversial. Dogmas do not die easily and, for many years, $\beta\gamma$ was not considered a direct activator or inhibitor of effector enzymes and channels. The I_{KACh} channel appears to be composed of heteromultimers of two types of subunits that can be activated by either α_i or $\beta\gamma$. The α_i subunit is more potent in regulating the channel, but the membrane contains enough $\beta\gamma$ to enable $\beta\gamma$ to activate the channel as well. Different combinations of channel subunits may be activated preferentially by α_i and by $\beta\gamma$ subunits.

Of the ion channels other than the K^+ channel, evidence is most compelling for the stimulation or inhibition of Ca^{2+} channel subtypes by G proteins. The central role played by Ca^{2+} in muscle contraction, in synaptic release, and in gene expression makes the modulation of Ca^{2+} influx a common target for regulation by neurotransmitters. In the heart, where L-type Ca^{2+} channels are critical for the regulation of contractile strength, the Ca^{2+} current is enhanced by α_s formed by β-adrenergic stimulation of G_s. In contrast, N-type Ca^{2+} channels, which modulate synaptic release in nerve terminals, are often inhibited by muscarinic and α-adrenergic agents and by opiates acting at receptors coupled to G_i and G_o. In sympathetic ganglia, norepinephrine reduces synaptic release by inhibiting Ca^{2+} influx through the N channel. The G protein couples to the channel in a membrane-delimited process that shifts the temporal distribution of gating modes, favoring the time spent in a low-open probability mode, thereby effectively lowering the open time of the channel.

Inhibition of L-type Ca^{2+} currents can exhibit strict G-protein specificity for both α and $\beta\gamma$ subunits. In GH3 cells, a pituitary cell line, antisense oligonucleotides that eliminate expression of α_{o1} and α_{o2} blocks the inhibitory effect of muscarinic agents (at M4 receptors) and of somatostatin, respectively. Microinjection of antisense oligonucleotides to β_1 and β_3 blocked inhibition by somatostatin and muscarinic agents, respectively. Finally, the γ subunit subtype was also critical. Thus, γ_3 was required for coupling to the somatostatin receptor, whereas γ_4 coupled to muscarinic receptors. Thus, in the same cell, somatostatin couples to Ca^{2+} channels through $\alpha_{o2}\,\beta_1\,\gamma_3$, whereas the muscarinic receptor couples to $\alpha_{o1}\,\beta_3\,\gamma_4$. $\beta\gamma$ subunits may affect the channels directly, perhaps in synergy with the α subunit or as a requirement for the appropriate presentation of the α subunits to the correct receptor.

G-Protein Signaling Gives Special Advantages in Neural Transmission

The G-protein-based signaling system provides several advantages over fast transmission (Hille, 1992; Neer, 1995). These advantages include amplification of the signal, modulation of cell function over a broad temporal range, diffusion of the signal to a large cellular volume, cross talk, and coordination of diverse cell functions.

Amplification

Several thousandfold amplification can be initiated by a single neurotransmitter–receptor complex that activates numerous G proteins, each of which activates many effector enzymes and channels. Each enzyme can generate many second-messenger molecules, and each channel allows the flux of many ions. As shown in the next section, second messengers often activate protein kinases that phosphorylate many substrates before deactivation.

Temporal Range

The sacrifice in speed relative to signaling by ligand-gated ion channels is compensated by a broad range of signaling that facilitates integration of signals by the G-protein system. Transmission through membrane-delimited coupling of ion channels to G proteins is relatively fast, with only some sacrifice in speed. Signaling that includes second messengers is much slower. It can be as fast as 100–300 ms, as in olfactory signaling in which cAMP and IP_3 take part, or it can take from seconds to minutes.

Spatial Range

A slower time frame means that cellular processes that are quite distant from the receptor can be modulated. Diffusion of second messengers such as IP_3, Ca^{2+}, and DAG can extend neurotransmission through the cell body and to the nucleus to alter gene expression.

Cross Talk

Both the signal transduction machinery and the ultimate mediators of their responses, such as the protein kinases, are capable of cross talk. This is seen in coincident detection of signals from two receptors converging on type I and type II adenylate cyclase.

Coordinated Modulation

Neurotransmitters acting through G proteins can elicit a coordinated response of the cell that can modulate synaptic release, resynthesis of neurotransmitter, membrane excitability, the cytoskeleton, metabolism, and gene expression.

Summary

A major class of signaling utilizing G-protein-linked signals affords the nervous system a rich diversity of modulation, amplification, and plasticity. Signals are mediated through second messengers activating proteins that modify cellular processes and gene transcription. A key feature is the ability of G proteins to detect the presence of activated receptors and to amplify the signal through effector enzymes and channels. Phosphorylation of key intracellular proteins, ion channels, and enzymes activates diverse, highly regulated cellular processes. The specificity of response is ensured through receptors reacting only with a limited number of G proteins. The response of the system is determined by the speed of activation of GTPase. The function of G-protein subunits is now being elucidated. In addition to the speed of response, the spatial compartmentalization of the system enables specificity and localized control of signaling. Phospholipids and phosphoinositols provide substrates for second-messenger signaling for G proteins. Stimulation of release of intracellular calcium is often the mediator of the signal. Calcium itself has a dual role as a carrier of electrical current and as a second messenger. Calmodulin is a key regulator that provides complexity and enhances specificity of the signaling system. Sensitivity of the system is imparted by an extremely robust amplification system, as seen in the visual system, which can detect single photons of light.

MODULATION OF NEURONAL FUNCTION BY PROTEIN KINASES AND PHOSPHATASES

Protein phosphorylation and dephosphorylation are key processes that regulate cellular function. They play a fundamental role in mediating signal transduction initiated by neurotransmitters, neuropeptides, growth factors, hormones, and other signaling molecules. The primary determinants of morphology and function of a cell are the protein constituents expressed in that cell. However, the functional state of many of these proteins is modified by phosphorylation–dephosphorylation, the most ubiquitous posttranslational modification in eukaryotes. About 4% of mammalian genes probably encode a kinase or phosphatase, and a fifth of all proteins may serve as targets for kinases and phosphatases. Phosphorylation can rapidly modify the function of enzymes, structural and regulatory proteins, receptors, and ion channels taking part in diverse processes, without a need to change the level of their expression. Phosphorylation and dephosphorylation can also produce long-term alterations in cellular properties by modulating transcription and translation and changing the complement of proteins expressed by cells.

Protein kinases catalyze the transfer of the terminal, or γ, phosphate of ATP to the hydroxyl moieties of Ser, Thr, or Tyr residues at specific sites on target proteins. Most protein kinases are either Ser/Thr kinases or Tyr kinases, with only a few designed to phosphorylate both categories of acceptor amino acids. Protein phosphatases catalyze the hydrolysis of the phosphoryl groups from phosphoserine–phosphothreonine, phosphotyrosine, or both types of phosphorylated amino acids on phosphoproteins.

Protein phosphatases reverse the effects of protein kinases, and protein kinases reverse the effect of protein phosphatases (Fig. 10.10). This statement may seem odd only because signal transduction schemes typically depict unidirectional and not bidirectional regulation; i.e. a stimulus activates a kinase that phos-

phorylates a substrate protein, and basal phosphatase activity dephosphorylates the substrate protein after kinase activity subsides. In fact, regulation of the phosphorylation state of proteins is bidirectional, and the phosphorylation state of proteins *in vivo* ranges widely, from minimal to almost fully phosphorylated, even in the absence of cell stimulation (Rosenmund *et al.*, 1994, Greengard *et al.*, 1998). The phosphorylation state can be altered dynamically either upward or downward from the steady state, depending on the inputs of the cell and its complement of kinases and phosphatases. Although phosphatases clearly serve to reverse a stimulated phosphorylation, our lack of understanding of phosphatase regulation is largely to blame for our viewing phosphatases in this limited role.

The activity of protein kinases and protein phosphatases is typically regulated either by a second messenger (e.g., cAMP or Ca^{2+}) or by an extracellular ligand (e.g., nerve growth factor). In general, second-messenger-regulated kinases modify Ser and Thr, whereas receptor-linked kinases modify Tyr. Among the thousands of protein kinases and protein phosphatases in neurons, a relatively small number serve as master regulators to orchestrate neuronal function. The cAMP-dependent protein kinase is a prototype for the known regulated Ser/Thr kinases; they are similar in overall structure and regulatory design. PKA is emphasized here because the experimental strategies currently being used in the study of kinases have come from the investigation of PKA-mediated processes. As its name implies, cyclic AMP-dependent protein kinase carries out the posttranslational modification of numerous protein targets in response to signal transduction processes that act through G proteins and alter the level of cAMP in cells. PKA is the predominant mediator for signaling through cAMP, the only other being a cAMP-liganded ion channel in olfaction. In a similar fashion, the related cGMP-dependent protein kinase (PKG) mediates most of the actions of cGMP. Ca^{2+}–calmodulin-dependent protein kinase II and several other kinases mediate many of the actions of stimuli that elevate intracellular Ca^{2+}. Finally, the PI signaling system increases both DAG and Ca^{2+}, which activate any of a family of protein kinases collectively called protein kinase C. Each of these kinases has a broad substrate specificity and is therefore able to phosphorylate diverse substrates throughout the cell. The activities of protein kinases and phosphatases are balanced, as revealed by the phosphorylation state of these targets of the signal transduction process. Here, again, although there are thousands of protein phosphatases, a relatively small number exemplified by protein

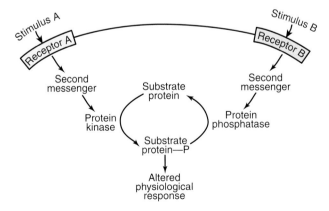

FIGURE 10.10 Regulation by protein kinases and protein phosphatases. Enzymes and other proteins serve as substrates for protein kinases and phosphoprotein phosphatases, which modify their activity and control them in a dynamic fashion. Multiple signals can be integrated at this level of protein modification. Adapted from Greengard *et al.* (1996).

phosphatase 1 (PP-1), protein phosphatase 2A (PP-2A), and protein phosphatase 2B (PP-2B, or calcineurin) are responsible for most of the dephosphorylation at Ser and Thr residues on phosphoproteins that are under the regulation of the aforementioned kinases. The Nobel Prize for Physiology and Medicine was awarded to Edwin G. Krebs and Edmund H. Fischer in 1992 for their pioneering work on the regulation of cell function by protein kinases and phosphatases.

Certain Principles Are Common in Protein Phosphorylation and Dephosphorylation

Protein kinases and protein phosphatases are described either as multifunctional if they have a broad specificity and therefore modify many protein targets or as dedicated if they have a very narrow substrate specificity and may modify only a single protein target. The Ser/Thr kinases and phosphatases described here are multifunctional, giving them the ability to coordinate the regulation of many cellular processes in response to cell stimulation, but how is response specificity achieved with kinases and phosphatases that are designed to recognize many substrates? These enzymes are by no means promiscuous; their substrates conform either to a consensus sequence along the primary protein sequence (for the kinases) or to general features of the three-dimensional structure of the phosphoprotein (for the phosphatases). Furthermore, spatial positioning of kinases and their substrates in the cell either increases or decreases the likelihood of phosphorylation–dephosphorylation of a given substrate.

The amplification of signal transduction described earlier is continued during transmission of the signal by protein kinases and protein phosphatases. In some cases, the kinases are themselves subject to activation by phosphorylation in a cascade in which one activated kinase phosphorylates and activates a second, and so on, to provide amplification and a switch-like response termed ultrasensitivity.

Kinases and phosphatases integrate cellular stimuli and encode the stimuli as the steady-state level of phosphorylation of a large complement of proteins in the cell (Hunter, 1995). Phosphorylation and dephosphorylation are reversible processes, and the net activity of the two processes determines the phosphorylation state of each substrate. The phosphorylation state depends on the degree of activation or inactivation of the protein kinase or protein phosphatase, the affinity of the protein target for these enzymes, and the concentration and access of the kinase, phosphatase, and target protein. Some proteins are largely phosphorylated in the basal state and are primarily subject to the regulation of phosphatases. Distinct signal transduction pathways can converge on the same or different target substrates. In some cases, these substrates can be phosphorylated by several kinases at distinct sites.

Phosphorylation produces specific changes in the function of a target protein, but these changes are completely dependent on the site of phosphorylation and the nature of the target protein. Phosphorylation may increase or decrease the catalytic activity of an enzyme or its affinity for its substrate or cofactor. It can modify interactions between the phosphoprotein and other proteins, DNA, phospholipids, or other cellular constituents and thereby alter the function of the phosphoprotein in gene expression, synaptic vesicle recycling, and membrane transport. Phosphorylation can regulate desensitization of receptors, their coupling to other signaling molecules, or their localization at synaptic sites. Any of several characteristics of ion channels can be altered by phosphorylation, including voltage dependence, probability of being opened, open and close time kinetics, and conductance. The number of possible effects is almost limitless and enables the fine-tuning of numerous cellular processes over broad time scales, from milliseconds to hours. Kinases and phosphatases do this fine-tuning by regulating the presence of a highly charged and bulky phosphoryl moiety on Ser, Thr, or Tyr at a precise location on the substrate protein. The phosphate may introduce a steric constraint at the surface of the protein in interactions with other cellular constituents, or the negative charge of the phosphoryl moiety may elicit a conformational change because of attractive or repulsive ionic interactions between the phosphorylated segment and other charged amino acids on the protein.

Finally, each of the three kinases described here is capable of functioning as a cognitive kinase, i.e., a kinase capable of a molecular memory. Although each is activated by its respective second messenger, it can undergo additional modification that reduces its requirement for the second messenger. This molecular memory potentiates the activity of these kinases and may enable them to participate in aspects of neuronal plasticity.

cAMP-Dependent Protein Kinase Was the First Well-Characterized Kinase

Neurotransmitters that stimulate the synthesis of cAMP exert their intracellular effects primarily by activating PKA. The functions (and substrates) regulated by PKA include gene expression [cAMP response element-binding protein (CREB)], catecholamine synthesis (tyrosine hydroxylase), carbohydrate metabolism (phosphorylase kinase), cell morphology [microtubule-associated protein 2 (MAP-2)], postsynaptic sensitivity (AMPA receptor), and membrane conductance (K channel). Paul Greengard and Eric Kandel received the Nobel Prize for Medicine in 2000 (along with Arvid Carlsson) for their discoveries concerning signal transduction via PKA and phosphoprotein phosphatases in the nervous system. PKA is a tetrameric protein composed of two types of subunits: (1) a dimer of regulatory (R) subunits (either two RI subunits for type I PKA or two RII subunits for type II PKA) and (2) two catalytic subunits (C subunit). Two or more isoforms of the RI, RII, and C subunits have distinct tissue and developmental patterns of expression but appear to function similarly. The C subunits are 40-kDa proteins that contain the binding sites for protein substrates and ATP. The R subunits are 49- to 51-kDa proteins that contain two cAMP-binding sites. In addition, the R subunit dimer contains a region that interacts with cellular anchoring proteins that serve to localize PKA appropriately within the cell.

The binding of second messengers by PKA and the other second-messenger-regulated kinases relieves an inhibitory constraint and thus activates the enzymes (Fig. 10.11). The C subunit has intrinsic protein kinase activity that remains inhibited as long as the C subunit is complexed with the R subunits in the tetrameric holoenzyme. As each R subunit binds two molecules of cAMP, its affinity for the C subunit is reduced greatly, and the C subunit dissociates as a free active kinase. Cyclic AMP therefore activates the C subunit by relieving it of its inhibitory R subunits. The steady-state level of cAMP determines the frac-

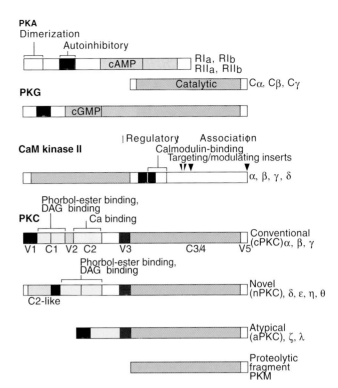

FIGURE 10.12 Domain structure of protein kinases. Protein kinases are encoded by proteins with recognizable structural sequences that encode specialized functional domains. Each of the kinases [PKA, PKG, CaM (Ca²⁺-calmodulin-dependent) kinase II, and PKC] has homologous catalytic domains that are kept inactive by the presence of an autoinhibitory segment (blue lines). Regulatory domains contain sites for binding second messengers such as cAMP, cGMP, Ca²⁺-calmodulin, DAG, and Ca²⁺-phosphatidylserine. Alternative splicing creates additional diversity.

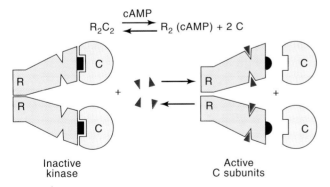

FIGURE 10.11 Activation of PKA by cyclic AMP. An autoinhibitory segment (blue) of the regulatory subunit (R) dimer interacts with the substrate-binding domain of the catalytic (C) subunits of PKA, blocking access of substrates to their binding site. Binding of four molecules of cyclic AMP reduces the affinity of R for C, resulting in dissociation of constitutively active C subunits.

tion of PKA that is in the dissociated or active form. In this way PKA decodes cAMP signals into the phosphorylation of proteins and the resultant change in various cellular processes.

PKA is a member of a large family of protein kinases that have in common a significant degree of homology in their catalytic domains and are likely derived from an ancestral gene (Fig. 10.12). This homology extends to the three-dimensional crystal structure based on X-ray crystallography of PKA and a few other kinases. The catalytic domain comprises approximately 280 amino acids that may be in a subunit distinct from the regulatory domain, as in PKA, or in the same subunit, as in PKC and Ca²⁺-calmodulin-dependent (CaM) kinases. The crystal structure of the C subunit complexed to a segment of protein kinase inhibitor (PKI), a selective high-affinity inhibitor of PKA, reveals that the C subunit is composed of two lobes. A small N-terminal lobe contains a highly conserved region that binds Mg²⁺-ATP in a cleft between the two lobes. A larger C-terminal lobe contains the protein–substrate recognition sites and the appropriate amino acids for catalyzing transfer of the phosphoryl moiety from ATP to the polypeptide chain of the substrate. Inhibition by PKI is diagnostic of PKA involvement; PKI contains an autoinhibitory sequence resembling PKA substrates and is positioned in the catalytic site like a substrate, thus blocking access for substrates.

How can protein kinases have a common structural homology yet exhibit phosphorylation target specificity? Although the C-terminal lobes of all kinases may utilize a similar scaffold for their peptide-binding and catalytic sites, distinct amino acids are positioned on this scaffold to produce specificity in peptide binding. Dedicated protein kinases, such as myosin light chain kinase (MLCK), which phosphorylates only certain myosin light chains, have numerous sites of contact between the catalytic domain and the phosphorylation site on the substrate and therefore have high specificity. In contrast, PKA has a smaller number of contact sites, thus enabling a much larger yet specific set of substrates to bind. Some substrates have been found to contain a distinct docking site for the kinase that regulates them that may serve to further increase the selectivity of phosphorylation.

PKA phosphorylates Ser or Thr at specific sites in dozens of proteins. The sequences of amino acids at the phosphorylation sites are not identical, but a consensus sequence can be deduced from a comparison of these sequences. PKA phosphorylates at sites with the consensus sequence Arg-Arg-X-Ser/Thr-Y, in which X can be one of many different amino acids and Y is a hydrophobic amino acid. Each kinase has a characteristic consensus sequence that forms the basis for distinct substrate specificities (Table 10.3). These consensus sequences are often used to identify putative sites of phosphorylation on newly cloned proteins, although many substrates are phosphorylated

at "anomalous" sites, thus reducing the reliability of these predictions. Secondary and tertiary structures probably have a role in substrate recognition, and the finding of anomalous phosphorylation sites may simply be due to our lack of knowledge of exactly how substrates are recognized. The consensus sites of PKA, CaM kinase II, and PKC all include a basic residue on the substrate, and these kinases do share some target substrates.

A regulatory theme common to PKA, CaM kinase II, and PKC is that their second messengers activate them by displacing an autoinhibitory domain from the active site [i.e., they relieve an inhibitory constraint rather than stabilizing a conformation of the kinase that has higher activity (Kemp et al., 1994)]. Some of the contacts between C and R subunits PKA resemble those between the C subunit with its protein substrates. The R subunit blocks access of substrates by positioning a pseudosubstrate or autoinhibitory domain in the catalytic site. This segment of R resembles a substrate and binds to C as would a substrate or PKI. Binding of cAMP to the R subunit near this autoinhibitory domain must disrupt its binding to the C subunit, thus leading to dissociation of an active C subunit. CaM kinase II and PKC likewise have autoinhibitory segments that are near the second-messenger-binding sites and may be activated similarly (see Figure 10.12).

Functional differences between type I and type II PKA (which have C subunits in common but have different R subunits) may arise from differential targeting in cells and from differences in regulation by autophosphorylation. RII, but not RI, is autophosphorylated by its C subunit when it is in the holoenzyme form. This potentiates cAMP action by reducing the rate of reassociation of RII and C after a stimulus. Only anchoring proteins for RII have been characterized thus far.

Multifunctional CaM Kinase II Decodes Diverse Signals That Elevate Intracellular Ca²⁺

Most of the effects of Ca^{2+} in neurons and other cell types are mediated by calmodulin, and many of the effects of Ca^{2+}–calmodulin are mediated by protein phosphorylation–dephosphorylation. In contrast with the cAMP system, both dedicated and multifunctional kinases are found in the Ca^{2+}-signaling system (Schulman and Braun, 1999). Two kinases, MLCK and phosphorylase kinase, are each dedicated to the phosphorylation of a single substrate—myosin light chains and phosphorylase, respectively. The Ca^{2+}-signaling system also contains a family of Ca^{2+}–calmodulin-

TABLE 10.3   Consensus Phosphorylation Sites of Some Protein Kinases[a]

Protein kinase	Consensus phosphorylation site[b]
PKA	R-R/K-X-S*/T*
PKG	R/K$_{2-3}$-X-S*/T*
cPKC	(R/K$_{1-3}$-X$_{2-0}$)-S*/T*-(X$_{2-0}$-R/K$_{1-3}$)
CaM kinase II	R-X-X-S*/T*
MLCK (smooth muscle)	(K/R$_2$-X)-X$_{1-2}$-K/R$_3$-X$_{2-3}$-R-X$_2$-S*-N-V-F

[a]Adapted from Kennelly and Krebs (1991).
[b]R, Arg; K, Lys; S*, phospho-Ser; T*, phospho-Thr; X, polar amino acid; N, Asp; V, Val; F, Phe.

dependent protein kinases with broad substrate specificity, including CaM kinases I, II, and IV; of these, CaM kinase II is the best characterized. CaM kinase II phosphorylates tyrosine hydroxylase, MAP-2, synapsin I, calcium channels, Ca^{2+}–ATPase, transcription factors, and glutamate receptors and thereby regulates synthesis of catecholamines, cytoskeletal function, synaptic release in response to high-frequency stimuli, calcium currents, calcium homeostasis, gene expression, and synaptic plasticity, respectively. The enzyme is activated by Ca^{2+} regardless of whether it is elevated by influx through Ca^{2+} channels or ligand-gated Ca^{2+} channels or is released from intracellular stores following stimulation of the PI-signaling pathway. This kinase is found in every tissue but is particularly enriched in neurons, where it may account for as much as 2% of all hippocampal protein. This level is 50 times as high as the level of the kinase in other tissues; thus, CaM kinase II likely serves some special functions in such brain regions. It is found in the cytosol, in the nucleus, in association with cytoskeletal elements, and in postsynaptic thickening termed the postsynaptic density found in asymmetric synapses. It is a large multimeric enzyme, consisting of 12 subunits derived from four homologous genes (α, β, γ, and δ) that encode different isoforms of the kinase that range from 54 to 65 kDa per subunit. Multimers and heteromultimers of α- and β-CaM kinase II isoforms are found predominantly in brain, whereas γ- and δ-CaM kinases are found throughout the body, including the brain.

The domain structure of CaM kinase II isoforms is shown in Fig. 10.12. Unlike those of PKA, the catalytic, regulatory, and targeting domains are all contained within a single polypeptide. The N-terminal half of each isoform contains the catalytic domain that is highly homologous to the catalytic subunit of PKA and other Ser/Thr kinases. The middle region constitutes the regulatory domain, which contains an autoinhibitory domain with an overlapping calmodulin-binding sequence. The C-terminal end contains an association domain that allows 12 subunits (two rings of six catalytic domains each) to assemble into a multimer, as well as targeting sequences that direct the kinase to distinct intracellular sites.

Regulation of the kinase by autophosphorylation is a critical feature of CaM kinase II. The basic three-dimensional conformation of the catalytic domain is likely to be similar to the structures determined for PKA and CaM kinase I. The kinase is inactive in the basal state because an autoinhibitory segment is positioned in the catalytic site, sterically blocking access to its substrates. Peptides corresponding to this region are useful inhibitors for functional studies and inhibit the kinase by competing for binding of both ATP and protein substrates. Elevation of Ca^{2+} generates a Ca^{2+}–calmodulin complex that wraps around the calmodulin-binding domain of the kinase, which overlaps with part of the autoinhibitory domain. Thus, binding of Ca^{2+}–calmodulin displaces the autoinhibitory domain from the catalytic site and thus activates the kinase by enabling ATP and protein substrates to bind. Displacement of this domain also exposes a binding site for anchoring proteins that the activated kinase can bind to, perhaps positioning it for more selective phosphorylation. The site occupied by one particular amino acid in the autoinhibitory domain of all isoforms of this kinase, Thr-286 (in α-CaM kinase II), must be crucial in allowing the autoinhibitory domain to keep the active site shut before activation. If the kinase is activated, it can autophosphorylate this particular Thr residue. Phosphorylation disables the autoinhibitory segment by preventing it from reblocking the active site after calmodulin dissociates and thereby locks the kinase in a partially active state that is independent, or autonomous, of Ca^{2+}–calmodulin.

An additional dramatic effect of autophosphorylation is that it enhances the affinity of the bound calmodulin by 400-fold, which it achieves by reducing the rate of dissociation of calmodulin from the kinase after Ca^{2+} levels are reduced below threshold. In essence, autophosphorylation traps bound calmodulin for several seconds and keeps the kinase active for a while after Ca^{2+} levels decline to baseline. The consequence of calmodulin trapping and disruption of the autoinhibitory domain is to prolong the active state of the kinase, a potentiation that led to its description as a cognitive kinase.

CaM kinase II responds to a large number of neurotransmitter receptors subserved by various signal transduction systems *in situ*, and stimulation of these pathways increases the autonomous activity of the enzyme. The level of autonomous activity (8–15% in brain) may reflect the integration of multiple cellular inputs, and autonomous activity may be adjusted either upward or downward.

CaM kinase II is targeted to distinct cellular compartments. Differences between the four genes encoding CaM kinase II and between the two or more isoforms that are encoded by each gene by apparent alternative splicing reside primarily in a variable region at the start of the association domain (see Fig. 10.12). In some isoforms, this region contains an additional sequence of 11 amino acids that targets those isoforms to the nucleus. One unusual isoform termed αKAP has a short hydrophobic segment in place of the catalytic domain and serves to target catalytically competent subunits that coasseble with it to membranes. The major neuronal isoform, α-CaM kinase II, is largely cytosolic but is also found attached to postsynaptic densities and to synaptic vesicles and may therefore have several targeting sequences. Targeting to the NMDA type glutamate receptor occurs only after calmodulin activates the kinase and exposes a binding site.

Protein Kinase C Is the Principal Target of the PI Signaling System

Protein kinase C is a collective name for members of a relatively diverse family of protein kinases most closely associated with the PI-signaling system. PKC is a multifunctional Ser/Thr kinase capable of modulating many cellular processes, including exocytosis and endocytosis of neurotransmitter vesicles, neuronal plasticity, gene expression, regulation of cell growth and cell cycle, ion channels, and receptors. A major breakthrough in understanding of the PI-signaling pathway was the realization that DAG and Ca^{2+}, two products of this pathway, function as second messengers to activate PKC. The role of DAG in PI signaling was unclear until its link to PKC was established. Many PKC isoforms also require an acidic phospholipid such as phosphatidylserine for appropriate activation. The kinase is also of interest because it is the target of a class of tumor promoters called phorbol esters. They activate PKC by simulating the action of DAG, bypassing the normal receptor-based pathway, and somehow stimulating cell growth inappropriately.

We now understand that the PKC family of kinases is diverse in structure and regulatory properties. Unlike PKA, PKC is a monomeric enzyme (78–90 kDa) with catalytic, regulatory, and targeting domains all on one polypeptide. Each isoform has a regulatory domain, with several subdomains, in its N-terminal half and a catalytic domain at the C-terminal (see Fig. 10.12). Only the first PKC isoforms to be characterized, now termed the conventional isoforms (or cPKC), have all of the domains. The domains are referred to as (1) V1, which contains the auto-inhibitory or pseudosubstrate sequence present in all isoforms; (2) C1, a cysteine-rich domain that binds DAG and phorbol esters; (3) C2, a region necessary for Ca^{2+} sensitivity and for binding to phosphatidylserine and to anchoring proteins; (4) V3, a protease-sensitive hinge; (5) C3/4, the catalytic domain; and (6) V5, which may also mediate anchoring. Subsequent cloning revealed a larger and more diverse group of isoforms than that of cPKC (Fig. 10.12). One class of isoforms, termed novel PKCs (nPKC), lacks a true C2 domain and is therefore not Ca^{2+} sensitive. Another class is considered atypical (aPKC) because it lacks C2

and the first of two cysteine-rich domains that are necessary for DAG (or phorbol ester) sensitivity. This class is neither Ca^{2+} nor DAG sensitive.

Activation of PKC is best understood for the conventional isoforms. Generation of DAG resulting from stimulation of the PI-signaling pathway increases the affinity of cPKC isoforms for Ca^{2+} and phosphatidylserine. Although triglyceride lipases also generate DAG, the sn-1,2-diacylglycerol isomer is derived only from PI turnover, and it is the only isomer effective in activating PKC. Cell stimulation results in the translocation of cPKC from a variety of sites to the membrane or cytoskeletal elements where it interacts with PS–Ca^{2+}–DAG at the membrane. Binding of the second messengers to the regulatory domain disrupts the nearby autoinhibitory domain, leading to a reversible activation of PKC by deinhibition, as is found for PKA and CaM kinase II.

Translocation is not restricted to the plasma membrane. Some PKC isoforms translocate to intracellular sites enriched with certain anchoring proteins for the activated form of PKC, termed receptors for activated C kinase (RACK). Distinct PKC isoforms can translocate to the cytoskeleton, membrane, perinuclear area, and nucleus, probably by binding of the C2 and/or the V1 and V5 domains to distinct anchoring proteins. In the inactive state, a segment of PKC may occupy this RACK-binding domain, thus preventing translocation until the activation of PKC exposes this domain. Activation may therefore consist of both displacement of the autoinhibitory segment to unblock the catalytic site and displacement of an "auto-anchoring" site to unblock the RACK-binding site. Whether DAG is synthesized only in the plasma membrane and the PKC–PS–DAG complex subsequently diffuses to distant RACKs or whether some DAG is generated intracellularly is not known. The early phase of DAG derived from PI is followed by a longer phase in which DAG derived from PC is more prominent. After termination of the signal, DAG is recycled into phospholipids, and PKC is redistributed to its initial sites.

Prolonged activation of PKC can be produced by the addition of phorbol esters, which simulate activation by DAG but remain in the cell until they are washed out. In a matter of hours to days, such persistent activation by phorbol esters leads to a degradation of PKC. Either PKC may be more susceptible to proteolysis when activated or some of the compartments to which it translocates have a higher level of protease activity. This phenomenon is sometimes used experimentally to produce a PKC-depleted cell (at least for phorbol ester-binding isoforms) and thereafter to test for a loss of putative PKC functions.

Spatial Localization Regulates Protein Kinases and Phosphatases

Protein kinases and protein phosphatases are often positioned spatially near their substrates or they translocate to their substrates upon activation to improve speed and specificity in response to neurotransmitter stimulation. PKA is targeted to intracellular sites on the cytoskeleton, membrane, and Golgi through interactions between the RII subunit and specific anchoring proteins. MAP-2 is an anchoring protein for RII, which concentrates PKA near its substrate (including MAP-2) in dendrites. Anchoring proteins with no previously known function are referred to as A kinase anchoring proteins (AKAPs). One such anchor, AKAP79, is an anchor for PKA, for PKC, and for calcineurin, the Ca^{2+}–calmodulin-dependent phosphatase (Klauck et al., 1996). The three signaling molecules bind to different sites on this anchoring protein. Better coordination of the phosphorylation–dephosphorylation of the same or different substrates may be achieved by placing calcineurin, PKC, and PKA in the same compartment through AKAPs. Another example of a signaling complex is the protein termed yotiao, which binds to the NMDA type glutamate receptor and serves as an anchor for both PKA and a phosphatase (PP-1).

The use of anchoring proteins has several consequences. First, it enhances the rate of phosphorylation when kinases or phosphatases are placed near some substrates. Specificity is enhanced when these enzymes are concentrated near proteins that are to be substrates and away from other proteins that are not to be substrates in a given cell. Second, it increases the signal-to-noise ratio for substrates that are not near anchoring proteins because phosphorylation–dephosphorylation would be reduced in the basal state. For example, PKA is anchored on the Golgi away from the nucleus in the basal state. Brief stimuli lead to the transient dissociation of C subunits and provide for the localized regulation of nearby substrates but little phosphorylation of nuclear proteins. Prolonged stimuli enable some C subunits to diffuse passively through nuclear pores and into nuclei, where they can participate in the regulation of gene expression. Termination of the nuclear action of C subunits is aided by PKI, which binds and inhibits the C subunit in the nucleus and hastens its export out of the nucleus, where it can reassociate with R subunits. A high signal-to-noise ratio can be achieved with PKC by translocation toward substrates only after activation. Interaction with anchoring proteins should increase the rate and specificity of phosphorylation and may also prolong the active state of PKC by stabi-

lizing it. Third, anchoring enables significant basal phosphorylation of substrates near anchoring proteins. Basal phosphorylation would be high if PKA were highly concentrated by an anchoring protein near high-affinity substrates. For example, if an anchoring protein concentrates PKA 50-fold relative to the rest of the cell, then the local concentration of free C subunits will be high at basal cAMP even though the percentage of dissociated C subunits is low. Such an arrangement provides for novel ways of blocking the pathway through disruption of anchoring. When a peptide similar to the site at which RII binds to the AKAP is introduced into a neuron, it disrupts the ability of an AKAP to concentrate PKA near the AMPA receptor and leads to decreased modulation of the AMPA receptor in the basal state (Rosenmund et al., 1994).

PKA, CaM Kinase II, and PKC Are Cognitive Kinases

The ability of three major Ser/Thr kinases (PKA, CaM kinase II, and PKC) in brain to initiate or maintain synaptic changes that underlie learning and memory may require that they themselves undergo some form of persistent change in activity. As mentioned earlier, they have been described as cognitive kinases because they are capable of sustaining their activated states after their second messengers return to basal level and because their target substrates modulate synaptic plasticity.

cAMP-Dependent Protein Kinase

A role for PKA as a cognitive kinase can be seen in long-term facilitation of the gill-withdrawal reflex in Aplysia and in long-term potentiation in the rodent hippocampus. In the gill-withdrawal reflex, stimulation of the tail facilitates the withdrawal of the gill and siphon in response to a light touch. A shock to the tail stimulates the release of serotonin from tail sensory neurons onto motor neurons that control gill withdrawal, which increases cAMP and PKA activity in the motor neurons. Repetitive stimulation of the tail produces a sensitization, based on prolonged PKA activity, that can last for several days. Sensitization is an elementary form of learning in which a response to one stimulus is facilitated by another stimulus. This pathway is a crude approximation of what happens when Aplysia finds itself in turbulent waters. Where is the molecular memory of tail stimulation retained? In motor neuron cultures, a single exposure to serotonin or cAMP produces short-term facilitation and a short-term increase in the phosphorylation of more than a

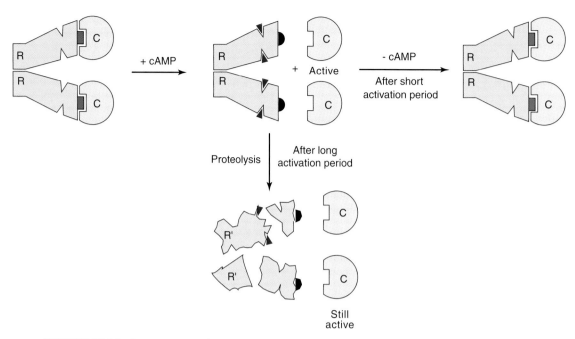

FIGURE 10.13   Long-term stimulation can convert PKA into a constitutively active enzyme. Dissociation of PKA R and C subunits is reversible with short-term elevation of cyclic AMP. More prolonged activation results in loss of R subunits to proteolysis, resulting in an insufficient amount of R subunits to associate with and inhibit all C subunits after the cAMP stimulus terminates.

dozen PKA substrates in these cells. However, repeated or prolonged exposure to these agents leads to long-term facilitation and an enhanced state of phosphorylation of the same set of proteins. This phenomenon is due to a PKA that is persistently active despite the fact that cAMP is no longer elevated (Chain *et al.*, 1999). A possible scheme for this phenomenon is shown in Fig. 10.13. The RII subunit is autophosphorylated on its autoinhibitory segment by the C subunit in the holoenzyme. Phospho-RII and C subunits dissociate upon elevation of cAMP and reassociate when cAMP levels subside. However, the reassociation rate is reduced greatly by the presence of phosphate on the RII subunit, thus prolonging the phosphorylation of various target proteins by the C subunit. Furthermore, RII subunits are more susceptible than C subunits to proteolytic degradation in their dissociated state. Thus, prolonged or repetitive stimulation leads to a preferential decrease in the inhibitory RII subunits and thus a slight excess of C subunits that remain persistently active because of insufficient RII subunits. The various targets of PKA can then be phosphorylated by this active C subunit long after cAMP levels return to basal or prestimulus levels. Prolonged activation of PKA enables the C subunit to enter the nucleus and induce gene expression, and one of these genes facilitates further proteolysis of RII.

Although short-term facilitation does not require transcription of new genes or protein synthesis, the long-term effects on phosphorylation and on facilitation do require transcription of new genes and protein synthesis. In this interesting process, a molecular memory of appropriate stimulation by serotonin is encoded by a persistence of PKA activity that is regenerative.

PKA may also function as a cognitive kinase in hippocampal long-term potentiation. This phenomenon is seen most clearly in the short- and long-term phases of long-term potentiation in CA3 neurons stimulated by means of the mossy fiber pathway, one of several sites of long-term potentiation in the hippocampus. Induction of both the early and the late phase of long-term potentiation at this site requires PKA. The persistent phase of long-term potentiation requires both RNA synthesis and new protein synthesis, with the likelihood of PKA-mediated increases in gene expression. Although the induction of long-term potentiation requires a rise in Ca^{2+}, rather than of cAMP, one of the Ca^{2+}-stimulated adenylate cyclases appears to convert some of the Ca^{2+} signal into a rise in cAMP. Mutant mice lacking one such cyclase isoform show a marked reduction in Ca^{2+}-sensitive cyclase and cAMP accumulation, a reduced long-term potentiation in hippocampal slices, and a weaker spatial memory in behavioral tests.

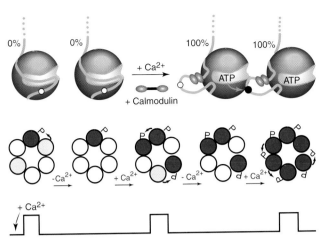

FIGURE 10.14 Frequency-dependent activation of CaM kinase II. Autophosphorylation occurs when both neighboring subunits in a holoenzyme are bound to calmodulin. At a high frequency of stimulation (rapid Ca^{2+} spikes), the interspike interval is too short to allow significant dephosphorylation or dissociation of calmodulin, thereby increasing the probability of autophosphorylation with each successive spike. In a simplified CaM kinase with only six subunits, calmodulin-bound subunits are shown in pink and autophosphorylated subunits with trapped calmodulin are shown in red. Adapted from Hanson and Schulman (1992).

Ca^{2+}–Calmodulin-Dependent Protein Kinase

CaM kinase II has features of a cognitive kinase because it has a molecular memory of its activation that is based on autophosphorylation and it phosphorylates proteins that modulate synaptic plasticity (Lisman *et al.*, 2002). The biochemical properties of CaM kinase II suggest mechanisms by which appropriate stimulus frequencies can generate an autonomous enzyme (Fig. 10.14). The critical site of phosphorylation is in the autoinhibitory segment within the ring of catalytic-regulatory domains in the holoenzyme. Each subunit can bind and be activated by calmodulin independently but requires neighboring subunits for autophosphorylation. Autophosphorylation takes place within each holoenzyme but requires the phosphorylation of one subunit by a proximate neighbor. Furthermore, calmodulin must be bound to the subunit that is to be phosphorylated, apparently to displace the autoinhibitory domain and expose the phosphorylation site to the active subunit. Individual stimuli may be too brief and available calmodulin may be limited so a single stimulus may lead to binding and activation of only a few subunits per holoenzyme. Thus, each stimulus achieves only submaximal activation of the kinase. When two neighboring subunits are bound concurrently to calmodulin during a stimulus, autophosphorylation is achieved. Autophosphorylation leads to potentiation

because the phosphorylated subunit traps its bound calmodulin for several seconds and thus remains active, longer than the Ca^{2+} signal. Even after calmodulin dissociates, the autophorylated subunit remains partially active until dephosphorylated. At low stimulus frequency, the time between stimuli is sufficient for calmodulin to dissociate and the kinase to be dephosphorylated, and the same submaximal activation will occur with each stimulus. However, at higher frequencies, some subunits will remain autophosphorylated and bound to calmodulin so successive stimuli will result in more calmodulin bound per holoenzyme, which will make autophosphorylation and subsequent calmodulin trapping more probable. The enzyme is therefore able to decode the frequency of cellular stimulation; low-frequency stimulation leads to submaximal activation of the kinase at each stimulus, whereas higher frequencies exceed a threshold beyond which stimulation leads to the recruitment of additional calmodulin and a higher level of activation and autonomy with each spike.

CaM kinase phosphorylates a number of substrates that affect synaptic strength. For example, phosphorylation of synapsin I, a synaptic vesicle protein, by CaM kinase II reduces the attachment of synaptic vesicles to actin at nerve terminals. Phosphorylation of synapsin I by CaM kinase II enables synaptic release to be maintained at high stimulus frequencies, perhaps by facilitating movement of vesicles toward release sites. Inhibition of CaM kinase II in hippocampal slices or just elimination of its autophosphorylation by an α-CaM kinase II mouse knockin in which the critical Thr was replaced by Ala blocks the induction of long-term potentiation. Although the kinase has normal activity *in vitro*, it shows no frequency-dependent activation and its activity cannot be prolonged without autophosphorylation. These mice are deficient in learning spatial navigational cues, one of the functions of the rodent hippocampus. The basis for its role is uncertain but may be the phosphorylation of AMPA receptors and their recruitment to the membrane, leading to a greater postsynaptic response (Lisman *et al.*, 2002). The enzyme can therefore be described appropriately as a cognitive kinase with regard to its own molecular memory as well as its functional role in mediating aspects of synaptic plasticity.

Protein Kinase C

PKC can also be converted into a form that is independent, or autonomous, of its second messenger and can be described as a cognitive kinase. Before Ca^{2+} and DAG were known to have roles in the reversible activation of PKC, PKC was identified as an inactive precursor that was activated *in vitro* by Ca^{2+}-dependent proteolysis to a constitutively active fragment termed protein kinase M (PKM). Physiological activation of PKC may also convert it into a PKM-like species. Standard protocols lead to transient activation of both Ca^{2+}-dependent and Ca^{2+}-independent forms of PKC. However, during the persistent phase of long-term potentiation, some of the PKC remains active but is autonomous of Ca^{2+} and DAG. The activity appears to be a PKM or other modified form of an atypical PKC. PKC has also been implicated in long-term potentiation, and its substrates include NMDA and AMPA receptors.

Protein Tyrosine Kinases Take Part in Cell Growth and Differentiation

Protein kinases that phosphorylate tyrosine residues on key proteins participate in numerous cellular process and are usually associated with the regulation of cell growth and differentiation. Signal transduction by protein tyrosine kinases often includes a cascade of kinases phosphorylating other kinases, eventually activating Ser/Thr kinases, which carry out the intended modification of a cellular process. There are two classes of protein tyrosine kinases. The first is a family of receptor tyrosine kinases that are activated by the binding of extracellular growth factors such as nerve growth factor, epidermal growth factor, insulin, and platelet-derived growth factor. The second family

of protein tyrosine kinases, such as c-Src, are soluble kinases that also participate in the regulation of cell growth, as well as in neuronal plasticity, but are activated by extracellular ligands indirectly.

Why have two sets of amino acids been chosen as targets for phosphorylation? First, the consequences of leaky, or "promiscuous," phosphorylation by a protein Ser/Thr kinase of an unintended target may affect metabolic activity or synaptic function but do not typically initiate irreversible and global functions such as cell growth and differentiation. The consequence of such inappropriate stimulation is seen in the effect of a variety of oncogenes that utilize altered forms of receptor tyrosine kinases or intermediates in their cascades to subvert normal cell growth. The cellular concentrations of protein Ser/Thr kinases and their targets are much higher than those of protein tyrosine kinases and their substrates. Inadvertent phosphorylation of targets that play critical roles in cell growth is less likely if these targets are regulated at tyrosine residues, which are not well recognized by the numerous protein Ser/Thr kinases. Second, introduction of a phosphotyrosine structure into a protein has a greater regulatory potential than introduction of a phosphoserine or phosphothreonine. The three phosphorylated amino acids have in common an ability to produce conformational changes due to the extra charge or bulk of the phosphate. For example, in the activation of receptor tyrosine kinases, autophosphorylation displaces an inhibitory domain. In addition, however, the phosphotyrosine and nearby

TABLE 10.4 Categories of Protein Phosphatases[a]

Phosphatase	Characteristic	Other inhibitors
PP-1	Sensitive to phospho-inhibitor-1, phospho-DARPP-32, and inhibitor-2; has targeting subunits	Weakly sensitive to okadaic acid
PP-4	Nuclear	Highly sensitive to okadaic acid
PP-5	Nuclear	Mildly sensitive to okadaic acid
PP-2A	Regulatory subunits Does not require divalent cation	Highly sensitive to okadaic acid
PP-2B (calcineurin)	Ca^{2+}/calmodulin-dependent CnB regulatory subunit	FK506, cyclosporin
PP-2C	Requires Mg^{2+}	EDTA
Receptor PTPs[b]	Plasma membrane	Vanadate, tyrphosphtin, erbstatin
Nonreceptor PTPs	Various cellular compartments	Vanadate, tyrphosphtin
Dual specificity PTPs	Nuclear (e.g., cdc25A/B/C and VH family)	Vanadate

[a]From Hunter (1995).

[b]Protein phosphotyrosine phosphatases.

amino acid sequences can be recognized by various signal transduction effectors, such as PLCγ, that contain structural domains that bind to the tyrosine-phosphorylated kinase. The receptor tyrosine kinase thus becomes a platform for concentrating various signaling molecules at specific phosphotyrosine sites in its sequence. These signaling molecules are either activated directly by binding or activated after having been phosphorylated by the receptor tyrosine kinase. It is easier to bind with the necessary strict specificity to segments of protein around phosphotyrosines because of the aromatic side chain in tyrosine, which may be an additional reason for use of Tyr as phosphotransferase targets.

Protein Phosphatases Undo What Kinases Create

Protein phosphatases in neuronal signaling are categorized as either phosphoserine–phosphothreonine phosphatases (PSPs) or phosphotyrosine phosphatases (PTPs) (Hunter, 1995; Price and Mumby, 1999). The enzymes catalyze the hydrolysis of the ester bond of the phosphorylated amino acids to release inorganic phosphate and the unphosphorylated protein. Phosphatases control all of the cellular processes of protein kinases, including neurotransmission, neuronal excitability, gene expression, protein synthesis, neuronal plasticity, and cell growth. A limited number of multifunctional PSPs account for most of such phosphatase activity in cells (Hunter, 1995). They are categorized into six groups (1, 4, 5, 2A, 2B, and 2C) on the basis of their substrates, inhibitors, and divalent cation requirements (Table 10.4). An additional historical distinction is that phosphatase 1 (PP-1) preferentially dephosphorylates the β subunit of phosphorylase kinase, whereas protein phosphatase 2A preferentially dephosphorylates its a subunit. Of these PSPs, only protein phosphatase 2B (PP-2B, or calcineurin) responds directly to a second messenger; it responds to increases in cellular Ca^{2+}. PP-1, -4, -5, -2A, and calcineurin are structurally related and differ from PP-2C. Little is known about the basis of substrate specificity of these phosphatases; examination of the primary sequences of their dephosphorylation sites reveals no obvious consensus. The specificity of PP-1 and PP-2A is particularly broad, and each can remove phosphates that were transferred by any of the protein kinases discussed herein as well as many other kinases. Phosphotyrosine phosphatases constitute a distinct and larger class of phosphatases, including PTPs with dual specificity for both phosphotyrosines and phosphoserine–phosphothreonines. PTPs are

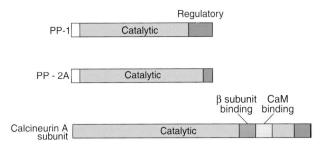

FIGURE 10.15 Domain structure of the catalytic subunits of some Ser/Thr phosphatases. The three major phosphoprotein phosphatases, PP-1, PP-2A, and calcineurin, have homologous catalytic domains but differ in their regulatory properties.

either soluble enzymes or membrane proteins with variable extra cellular domains that enable regulation by extracellular binding of either soluble or membrane-bound signals.

Structure and Regulation of PP-1 and Calcineurin

PP-1 and calcineurin are the best characterized phosphatases with regard to both structure and regulation. The domain structures of the catalytic subunits of PP-1 and calcineurin are depicted in Fig. 10.15. PP-1 is a protein of 35–38 kDa; most of the sequence forms the catalytic domain; its C-terminal is the site of regulatory phosphorylation. The catalytic domains of PP-1, PP-2A, and calcineurin are highly homologous (Price and Mumby, 1999).

Although PP-1 and PP-2A are usually prepared as free catalytic subunits, they are normally complexed in cells with specific anchoring or targeting subunits. For example, PP-1 is attached to glycogen particles in liver, myofibrils in muscle, and unidentified targeting subunits in brain. Phosphorylation of the PP-1 targeting subunit in liver releases the catalytic subunit and results in reduced dephosphorylation of substrates near the targeting subunit because diffusion reduces the local concentration of PP-1. Targeting of PP-1 also modulates its regulation by natural inhibitors. As PP-1 dissociates from targeting subunits, it becomes susceptible to inhibition by inhibitor-2.

Inhibition of PP-1 by two other inhibitors, inhibitor-1 and its homologue DARPP-32 (dopamine and cAMP-regulated phosphoprotein; M_r 32,000), is conditional on the phosphorylation state of these inhibitors. Inhibitor-1 has a broader distribution in brain than DARPP-32, which is largely found in the medium spiny neurons in the neostriatum and in their terminals in the globus pallidus and substantia nigra. Both proteins inhibit only after they are phosphorylated by PKA or PKG. PKA also increases the susceptibility of PP-1 to inhibition by stimulating its release from targeting subunits. Because the substrates for PKA and PP-1 overlap to a great extent, the rate and extent of phosphorylation of such substrates are enhanced by the ability of PKA to catalyze their phosphorylation while blocking their dephosphorylation. Inhibitor-1, DARPP-32, and inhibitor-2 are all selective for PP-1. Highly selective inhibitors capable of penetrating the cell membrane are available for these phosphatases. Okadaic acid, a natural product of marine dinoflagellates, is a tumor promoter but, unlike phorbol esters, it acts on PP-2A and PP-1 rather than on PKC. The steady-state level of phosphorylation of dozens of proteins is elevated when cells are treated by okadaic acid and its derivatives.

Protein phosphatase 1 The X-ray structure of the catalytic subunit of PP-1 bound to the toxin microcystin, a cyclic peptide inhibitor, reveals PP-1 to be a compact ellipsoid with hydrophobic and acidic surfaces forming a cleft for binding substrates. PP-1 is a metalloenzyme requiring two metals in the active site that likely take part in electrostatic interactions with the phosphate on substrates that aid in catalyzing the hydrolytic reaction. The phosphate would be positioned at the intersection of two grooves on the surface of the enzyme where binding to amino acid residues on the substrate would occur. Such binding would be blocked when phospho-inhibitor-1 or microcrystin LR binds to this surface. The same general structure of the catalytic domain is seen in calcineurin.

Calcineurin (PP-2B) Calcineurin is a Ca^{2+}–calmodulin-dependent phosphatase that is highly enriched in the brain. It is a heterodimer with a 60-kDa A subunit (CnA) that contains an N-terminal catalytic domain and a C-terminal regulatory domain that includes an autoinhibitory segment, a calmodulin-binding domain, and a binding site for the 19-kDa regulatory B subunit (CnB). CnB is a calmodulin-like Ca^{2+}-binding protein that binds to a hinge region of CnA. Regulation of calcineurin takes place in this region because it controls the access of phosphoproteins to the catalytic site. Some activation of calcineurin is attained by binding of Ca^{2+} to CnB. Stronger activation is obtained by the binding of Ca^{2+}–camodulin.

The substrate specificity of calcineurin does not appear to be as broad as that of PP-1, and that of calcineurin and CaM kinase II has little overlap. Thus, a rise in Ca^{2+} does not lead to a futile cycle of phosphorylation and dephosphorylation by these Ca^{2+}–calmodulin-dependent enzymes. However, their Ca^{2+}–calmodulin sensitivity is quite different, and

weak or low-frequency stimuli may selectively activate calcineurin, whereas strong or high-frequency stimuli activate CaM kinase II and calcineurin. This difference may play a role in the bidirectional control of synaptic strength by low- and high-frequency stimulation.

Additional regulation may be accorded by interaction of this hinge region with cyclophilin and FKBP, proteins that bind the immunosuppressive agents cyclosporin and FK506, respectively. The FK506-binding protein (FKBP) is highly abundant in the brain, and its distribution resembles that of calcineurin. Both FK506 and cyclosporin A are membrane permeant and are highly potent and selective inhibitors of calcineurin. They are referred to as immunophilins because their ability to block the essential role of calcineurin in lymphocyte activation makes them effective immunosuppressants. The X-ray structure of calcineurin complexed with FK506 reveals a ternary complex in which FK506 is bound at the interface between FKBP and the regulatory domain of CnA. Unlike calmodulin, CnB does not completely wrap around its target. CnB binds to one surface of an extended regulatory domain and FKBP–FK506 binds to the opposite surface. The FK506–FKBP complex is wedged between the regulatory domain and the catalytic site and likely inhibits calcineurin by making it difficult for phosphoproteins to have access to the catalytic site. It is unclear whether there is an endogenous FK506-like molecule that similarly functions to facilitate the interaction of calcineurin and FKBP.

Protein Kinases, Protein Phosphatases, and Their Substrates Are Integrated Networks

Cross talk between protein kinases and protein phosphatases is key to their ability to integrate inputs into neurons (Cohen, 1992). Such cross talk is exemplified by the interaction of cyclic AMP and Ca^{2+} signals through PKA and calcineurin, respectively. The medium spiny neurons in the neostriatum receive cortical inputs from glutamatergic neurons that are excitatory and nigral inputs by dopaminergic neurons that inhibit them. A possible signal transduction scheme for this regulation is shown in Fig. 10.16. The key to regulation is the bidirectional control of DARPP-32 phosphorylation (Greengard *et al.*, 1998) (see Box 10.2). Glutamate activates calcineurin by increasing intracellular Ca^{2+}, leading to the dephosphorylation and inactivation of phospho-DARPP-32. This releases inhibition of PP-1, which can then dephosphorylate a variety of substrates, including

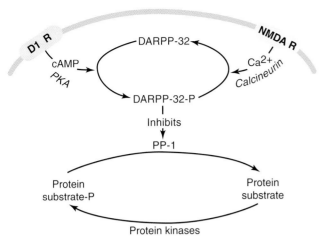

FIGURE 10.16   Cross talk between kinases and phosphatases. The state of phosphorylation of protein substrates is regulated dynamically by protein kinases and phosphatases. In the striatum, for example, dopamine stimulates PKA, which converts DARPP-32 into an effective inhibitor of PP-1. This increases the steady-state level of phosphorylation of a hypothetical substrate subject to phosphorylation by a variety of protein kinases. This action can be countered by NMDA receptor stimulation by another stimulus that increases intracellular Ca^{2+} and activates calcineurin. PP-1 is deinhibited and dephosphorylates the phosphorylated substrate when calcineurin deactives DARPP-32-P. Adapted from Greengard et al. (1996).

Na^+, K^+-ATPase, and lead to membrane depolarization. This is countered by dopamine, which stimulates cAMP formation and activation of PKA, which then converts DARPP-32 into its phosphorylated (i.e., PP-1 inhibitory) state. Although PKA and calcineurin are acting in an antagonistic manner, they are not doing it by phosphorylating and dephosphorylating the ATPase. By their actions upstream, at the level of DARPP-32, the regulation of numerous target enzymes (e.g., Ca^{2+} channels and Na^+ channels) in addition to the ATPase can be coordinated.

Studying Cellular Processes Controlled by Phosphorylation–Dephosphorylation Requires a Set of Criteria

Major goals of signal transduction research are to delineate pathways by which signals such as neurotransmitters transduce their signals, usually across the plasma membrane, and to determine how the transduced signal is transmitted to the ultimate cellular components that are to be modified by the extracellular signal. Many signaling components have yet to be discovered; in other circumstances, which of the known pathways are utilized by a given physiological stimulus is unclear. For the transmission of the signal,

the question is often "Which kinase(s) and which phosphatase(s) are responsible for the phosphorylation?" Cellular and biochemical assays can often identify the entire signaling pathway, from stimulation of receptor, to generation of a second-messenger activation of a kinase or phosphatase, change in the phosphorylation state of the substrate and an ultimate change in its functional state. Such investigations utilize a variety of pharmacological inhibitors or activators of the signaling molecules complemented by genetic approaches that utilize transfection of activated forms of the kinases or phosphatases in question, transgenic animals, and mice with individual signaling components knocked out.

Summary

The morphology of a cell is determined by protein constituents. Its function is regulated by the phosphorylation or dephosphorylation of the proteins. Phosphorylation modifies the function of regulatory proteins subsequent to their genetic expression. The activities of the protein kinases and protein phosphatases are typically regulated by second messengers and extracellular ligands. Kinases and phosphatases integrate and encode stimulation of a large group of cellular receptors. The number of possible effects is almost limitless and enables the tuning of cellular processes over a broad time scale. The kinases that regulate phosphorylation can exhibit conformational changes that potentiate the activity of the kinase. This may be one of the key elements in molecular memory and neuronal plasticity. Most of the effects of Ca^{2+} in cells are mediated by calmodulin, which in turn mediates changes in protein phosphorylation–dephosphorylation. The phosphoinositol signaling system is mediated through PKC, which modulates many cellular processes from exocytosis to gene expression. All three classes of enzymes discussed have been described as cognitive kinases because they are capable of sustaining their activated states after their second-messenger stimuli have returned to basal levels. PKA has been implicated in learning and memory in Aplysia and in hippocampus, where it is involved in long-term potentiation. Protein phosphatases play an equally important role in neuronal signaling by dephosphorylating proteins. Cross talk between protein kinases and protein phosphatases is key to their ability to integrate inputs into neurons. A major effort of signal transduction research is to delineate the pathways through which the neurotransmitters' signals across the plasma membrane are transmitted to the ultimate cellular components to be modified.

BOX 10.2

INTERACTIONS OF SIGNAL TRANSDUCTION PATHWAYS IN THE BRAIN

An understanding of the signal transduction mechanisms by which neurotransmitters produce their effects on their target neurons and of the mechanisms by which coordination of various signal transduction pathways is achieved represents a major area of research in cellular neurobiology. The dopaminoceptive medium-sized spiny neurons, located in the neostriatum, have been studied in great detail with regard to these mechanisms. Figure 10.17 illustrates a portion of what is now known about interactions of signaling mechanisms in these neurons. Activation by dopamine of D1 receptors increases cAMP, causing activation of PKA (cAMP-dependent protein kinase) and phosphorylation of DARPP-32 (dopamine + cAMP-regulated phosphoprotein; M_r, 32,000) on threonine-34. Conversely, glutamate, acting on NMDA receptors, increases $[Ca^{2+}]_i$, leading to the activation of PP2B (protein phosphatase 2B; calcineurin) and dephosphorylation of phosphothreonine-34-DARPP-32. VIP, NO (nitric oxide), and some other neurotransmitters increase the phosphorylation of DARPP-32 through a variety of signaling mechanisms. Dopamine (acting on D2 receptors), CCK, GABA, and some other neurotransmitters regulate the state of phosphorylation of DARPP-32 through a variety of other signaling mechanisms. CK1 (casein-kinase I) and CK2 (casein-kinase II) phosphorylate DARPP-32 on residues

other than threonine-34, causing it to undergo conformational changes. These changes result in phosphothreonine-34-DARPP-32 becoming a poorer substrate for PP2B (in the case of CKI) or a better substrate for PKA (in the case of CKII). Antipsychotic drugs such as haldol increase the state of phosphorylation of DARPP-32 on threonine-34 by blocking the dopamine-induced D2 receptor-mediated activation of PP2B.

The physiological consequences of phosphorylation of DARPP-32 on threonine-34 are profound. Thus, DARPP-32 in its threonine-34 phosphorylated, but not dephosphorylated, form acts as a potent inhibitor of PP-1 (protein phosphatase 1). PP-1 is a major serine–threonine protein phosphatase, which controls the state of phosphorylation of a variety of phosphoprotein substrates in the brain. These substrates include Na^+ channels, L-, N-, and P-type Ca^{2+} channels, the electrogenic ion pump Na^+, K^+-ATPase, the NR-1 subclass of glutamate receptors, and many more.

In summary, the DARPP-32/PP-1 cascade provides a mechanism by which a large number of neurotransmitters act in a complex, but coordinated, fashion to regulate the state of phosphorylation and activity of a variety of ion channels, ion pumps, and neurotransmitter receptors.

Paul Greengard

INTRACELLULAR SIGNALING AFFECTS NUCLEAR GENE EXPRESSION

The first part of this chapter describes how signaling systems regulate the function of cellular proteins already expressed; another critical level of control exerted by these systems is their ability to regulate the synthesis of cellular proteins by regulating the expression of specific genes. For all living cells, regulation of gene expression by intracellular signals is a fundamental mechanism of development, homeostasis, and adaptation to the environment. Protein phosphorylation and regulation of gene expression by intracellular signals are the most important mechanisms underlying the remarkable degree of plasticity exhibited by neurons. Alterations in gene expression underlie many forms of long-term changes in neural functioning, with a time course that ranges from hours to

many years. Indeed, as discussed earlier, evidence now suggests that formation of long-term memories in many neural systems requires changes in gene expression and new protein synthesis.

Interactions of Specific DNA Sequences with Regulatory Proteins Control Both Basal and Signal-Regulated Transcription

As a stable, linear polymer, the double helix of DNA is an ideal molecule for the storage of information; when transiently unwound, it can be readily replicated or serve as a template for the synthesis of other macromolecules: enzymes processing down its length can add a succession of nucleotides complementary to those in the template strand. However, its chemical simplicity and relatively rigid helical structure limit its functions in the cell to information storage and transfer. Information contained within

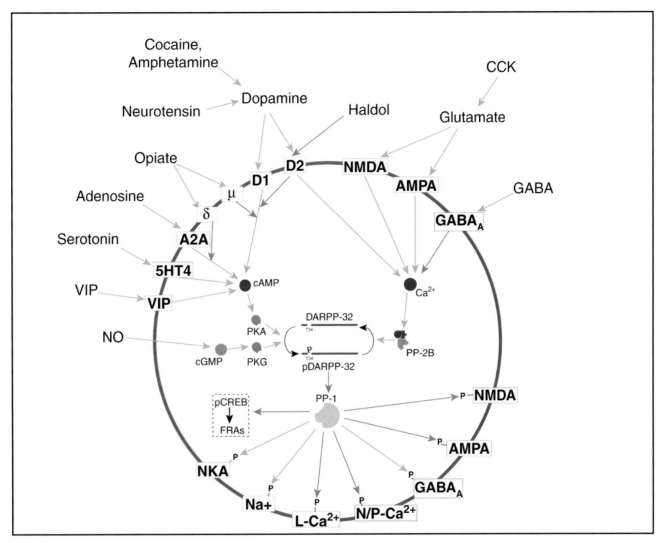

FIGURE 10.17 Signaling pathways in the neostriatum. Activation by dopamine of the D 1 subclass of dopamine receptors stimulates the phosphorylation of DARPP-32 at Thr-34. This is achieved through a pathway involving the activation of adenylyl cyclase, the formation of cAMP, and the activation of PKA. Activation by dopamine of the D2 subclass of dopamine receptors causes the dephosphorylation of DARPP-32 through two synergistic mechanisms: D2 receptor activation (i) prevents the D 1 receptor-induced increase in cyclic AMP formation and (ii) raises intracellular calcium, which activates a calcium-dependent protein phosphatase, namely PP2B, calcium/calmodulin-dependent protein phosphatase, or calcineurin. Activated PP-2B dephosphorylates DARPP-32 at Thr-34. Glutamate acts as both a fast-acting and a slow-acting neurotransmitter. Activation by glutamate of AMPA receptors causes a rapid response through the influx of sodium ions, depolarization of the membrane, and firing of an action potential Slow synaptic transmission, in respoAse to glutamate, results in part from activation of the AMPA and NMDA subclasses of glutamate the glutamate receptor, which increases intracellular calcium and the activity of PP2B, and causes the dephosphorylation of DARPP-32 on Thr-34. All other neurotransmitters that have been shown to act directly to alter the physiology of dopaminoceptive neurons also alter the phosphorylation state of DARPP-32 on Thr-34 through the indicated pathways. Neurotransmitters that act indirectly to affect the physiology of these dopaminoceptive neurons also regulate DARPP-32 phosphorylation; e.g., neurotensin, through stimulating the release of dopamine, increases DARPP-32 phosphorylation; conversely, cholecystokinin (CCK), by stimulating the release of glutamate, decreases DARPP-32 phosphorylation. Antischizophrenic drugs and drugs of abuse, all of which affect the physiology of these neurons, also regulate the state of phosphorylation of DARPP-32 on Thr-34. For example, the antischizophrenic drug haldol, which blocks the activation by dopamine of the D2 subclass of dopamine receptor, increases DARPP-32 phosphorylation. Agonists for the μ and δ subclasses of opiate receptors block Dl and A2A receptor-mediated increases in cAMP, respectively, and the resultant increases in DARPP-32 phosphorylation. Cocaine and amphetamine, through increasing extracellular dopamine levels, increase DARPP-32 phosphorylation. Marijuana, nicotine, alcohol, and LSD, all of which affect the physiology of the dopaminoceptive neurons, also regulate DARPP-32 phosphorylation. Finally, all drugs of abuse have greatly reduced biological effects in animals with targeted deletion of the DARPP-32 gene. 5HT4, 5 hydroxytryptophan (serotonin) receptor 4; NKA, Na+,K+/ATPase; VIP, vasoactive intestinal peptide; L- and N/P-Ca²⁺, L-type and N/P-type calcium channels. From Greengard (2001).

DNA must therefore be expressed through other molecules: RNA and proteins. The human genome contains approximately 40,000 genes that encode structural RNAs or protein-coding messenger RNAs (mRNAs). Within genes, a fundamental distinction can be made between DNA sequences that code for RNAs—and, in the case of protein-coding genes, mRNAs that will eventually be translated—and DNA sequences that exert control functions. Certain control sequences determine the beginnings and ends of segments of DNA that can be transcribed into RNA. Other closely linked DNA sequences determine whether a potentially transcribed segment is actually transcribed in a particular cell and, if so, under what circumstances. Regulated gene expression conferred by the nucleotide sequence of the DNA itself is called *cis* regulation because the control regions are linked physically on the DNA to regions that can potentially be transcribed. The *cis* regulatory sequences function by serving as high-affinity binding sites for regulatory proteins called transcription factors (or *trans*-acting factors because they may be encoded anywhere in the genome rather than on the same stretch of DNA that they regulate).

The transcription of specific genes into mRNA is carried out by a complex enzyme called RNA polymerase II. This process is often divided into three steps: initiation of RNA synthesis, RNA chain elongation, and chain termination. While biologically significant regulation may occur at any of these steps, it is at the step of transcription initiation that extracellular signals, such as neurotransmitters, hormones,

drugs, and growth factors, exert their most significant control over the processes that gate the flow of information out of the genome.

Transcription initiation requires two critical processes: (1) positioning of RNA polymerase II at the correct start site of the gene to be transcribed and (2) controlling the efficiency of initiations to produce the appropriate transcriptional rate for the circumstances of the cell (Tjian and Maniatis 1994). The *cis*-regulatory elements that set the transcription start sites of genes are called the basal promoter. Other *cis*-regulatory elements tether additional activator and repressor proteins to the DNA to regulate the overall transcriptional rate (Fig. 10.18).

The Basal Promoter

The promoters for RNA polymerase II transcribed genes contain a distinct basal promoter element on which a basal transcription complex is assembled. This complex is composed of a set of proteins, some of which recognize the specific DNA structural elements and some of which bind and position RNA polymerase II to the gene. The basal promoter of most of these genes is a sequence rich in the nucleotides adenine (A) and thymine (T) located between 25 and 30 bases upstream of the transcription start site. This sequence is called the TATA box. Certain RNA polymerase II transcribed promoters, most commonly those controlling "housekeeping genes," lack a TATA box; in such cases, other specialized guanosine–cytosine (GC)-rich nucleotide sequences stand in for the TATA box.

Sequence-Specific Transcription Factors

The basal transcription apparatus is not adequate to initiate more than low levels of transcription. To achieve significant levels of transcription, this multiprotein assembly requires help from transcriptional activators that recognize and bind *cis*-regulatory elements found elsewhere within the gene. Because they are tethered to DNA by specific *cis*-regulatory recognition sequences, such proteins have been described as sequence-specific transcription factors.

Functional *cis*-regulatory elements are generally found within several hundred base pairs of the start site of the gene to which they are linked, but they can occasionally be found many thousands of nucleotides away, upstream or downstream of the start site. They are generally composed of small "modular" DNA sequences, generally 7–12 in length and structured as a palindrome, each of which is a specific binding site for one or more transcription factors. Each gene has a particular combination of *cis*-regulatory elements, the nature, number, and spatial arrangement of which determine the gene's unique pattern of expression,

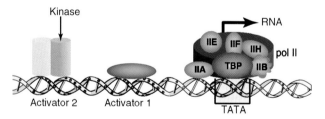

FIGURE 10.18 Schematic of a generalized RNA polymerase II promoter showing three separate *cis*-regulatory elements along a stretch of DNA. These elements are two hypothetical activator protein-binding sites and the TATA element. The TATA element is shown binding the TATA-binding protein (TBP). Multiple general transcription factors (IIA, IIB, etc.) and RNA polymerase II (pol II) associate with TBP. Each transcription factor comprises multiple individual proteins complexed together. This basal transcription apparatus recruits RNA polymerase II into the complex and also forms the substrate for interactions with the activator proteins binding to the activator elements shown. Activator 2 is shown to be a substrate for a protein kinase.

including the cell types in which it is expressed, the times during development in which it is expressed, and the level at which it is expressed in adults both basally and in response to physiological signals.

Sequence-specific transcription factors commonly comprise several physically distinct functional domains. In particular, such transcription factors frequently contain (1) a domain that recognizes and binds a specific nucleotide sequence (i.e., a *cis*-regulatory element), (2) a transcription activation domain that interacts with general transcription factors to form an active transcription complex, and (3) a multimerization domain that permits the formation of homo- and heteromultimers with other transcription factors (Tjian and Maniatis, 1994).

Many transcription factors are active only as dimers or higher order complexes. Multimerization domains are diverse and include so-called leucine zippers (which are described in the next section), Src homology SH2 domains, and certain a-helical motifs. Within active transcription-factor dimers, whether homodimers or heterodimers, both partners commonly contribute jointly to both the DNA-binding domain and the activation domain. Dimerization can be a mechanism of either positive or negative control of transcription. Overall, the ability of transcription factors to form heterodimers and other multimers increases the diversity of transcription-factor complexes that can form in cells and, as a result, increases the types of specific regulatory information that can be exerted on gene expression.

Sequence-specific transcriptional activator and repressor factors may produce an active transcription complex by contacting one or more proteins within the basal transcription complex. Frequently, however, they do not interact with the basal transcription apparatus directly but through the mediation of adapter proteins (Fig. 10.19). In either of these scenarios, transcription factors that bind at a distance from the basal promoter can interact with the basal transcription apparatus because the DNA forms loops that bring distant regions in contact with each other. In many cases, these adapter proteins are enzymes themselves with the ability to modify the structure of the proteins associated with the DNA. Remember, rather than being a linear duplex of DNA, in the nucleus the genome is wrapped in a complex stucture with DNA-binding proteins called histones. These histones "compact" the DNA, wrapping it into structures refered to as nucleosomes. Some of these adapter proteins, such as the CBP shown in Fig. 10.19, are histone acetyl transferases, which modify the histone structure, weakening the binding to DNA, thus enhancing the access of the transcription complex to the promoter and allowing transcription to occur more efficiently. Other adapter proteins are histone deacetylases, which remove acetate side chains from histone, tightening their grip on the DNA and inhibiting the transcription process. Finally, there are histone methyl transferases and demethylases that can have similar effects. The sum of all of these processes is to properly align the RNA polymerase II complex on the gene and then have it transcribed at a rate appropriate for the current state of the cell.

A Significant Consequence of Intracellular Signaling is the Regulation of Transcription

Intracellular signals play a major role in the regulation of gene expression. Many activator proteins can participate in the assembly of the mature transcription apparatus only after a signal-directed change in subcellular localization (e.g., from the cytoplasm to the nucleus) or a posttranslational modification, most commonly phosphorylation. Such alterations in location or conformation permit information obtained by the cell from its different signaling systems to regulate gene expression appropriate to the status of the cell.

All diploid cells within an organism, starting with the fertilized one-cell embryo, contain a complete copy of the organism's genome. Differential expression of this common genome is required for the formation of distinct cell types during development, of crucial importance in the differentiation of thousands

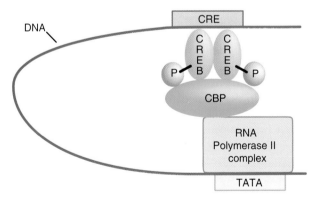

FIGURE 10.19 Looping of DNA permits activator (or repressor) proteins binding at a distance to interact with the basal transcription apparatus. The basal transcription apparatus is shown as a single box (pol II complex) bound at the TATA element. The activator protein (CREB) is shown as having been phosphorylated. On phosphorylation, many activators, such as CREB, are able to recruit adaptor proteins that mediate between the activator and the basal transcription apparatus. An adaptor protein that binds phosphorylated CREB is called a CREB-binding protein (CBP).

of distinct types of neurons found in the brain (see Chapter 3). The mechanisms by which these differentiated cells form are highly dependent on intercellular signaling. Much work in this area has been done in Drosophila and Xenopus, organisms in which viable embryos can be well studied in isolation.

In certain cases, restriction of the expression of a gene to specific cell types depends on the presence of critical transcription factors only in those cell types. For example, pituitary hormones—growth hormone and prolactin—are expressed only in pituitary lactotrophs and somatotrophs because their required activator transcription factor, Pit 1, is expressed only in those two cell types in the mature organism. In other cases, genes contain cis-regulatory elements that bind transcriptional repressor proteins; the presence of repressor proteins in a particular cell type blocks expression of those genes in that cell type.

The sequential expression, during development, of hierarchies of activator and repressor proteins depends initially on the asymmetric distribution of critical signaling molecules within the embryo, leading to differential gene expression within embryonic cells. As cells gain individual identities during development, cell–cell interactions mediated by contact or by the elaboration of intercellular autocrine, paracrine, or longer range signaling continue the process of specifying the complement of genes expressed in target cells. Genes that are silent during particular phases of development may become unavailable for subsequent activation because they become wrapped in inactive chromatin structures. The mechanisms by which a subset of genes is permanently silenced in some cells and rendered potentially active in others are not well understood.

Transcriptional Regulation by Intracellular Signals

As discussed earlier, all protein-encoding genes contain cis-regulatory elements that permit the genes to which they are linked to be activated or repressed by physiological signals. Intracellular signals can activate transcription factors through a variety of different general mechanisms, but each requires a translocation step by which the signal is transmitted through the cytoplasm to the nucleus. Some transcription factors are themselves translocated to the nucleus. For example, the transcription factor NF-κB is retained in the cytoplasm by its binding protein IκB; this interaction masks the NF-κB nuclear localization signal. Signal-regulated phosphorylation of IκB by protein kinase C and other protein kinases leads to dissociation of NF-κB, permitting it to enter the nucleus. Other transcription factors must be directly phosphorylated or dephosphorylated to bind DNA.

For example, in many cytokine-signaling pathways, plasma membrane receptor tyrosine phosphorylation of transcription factors known as signal transducers and activators of transcription (STATs) permits their multimerization, which in turn permits both nuclear translocation and construction of an effective DNA-binding site within the multimer. Yet other transcription factors are already bound to their cognate cis-regulatory elements within the nucleus under basal conditions and become able to activate transcription after phosphorylation. The transcription factor CREB, for example, is bound constitutively to cAMP response elements (CREs) found within many genes. The critical nuclear translocation step in CREB activation involves not the transcription factor itself, but the catalytic subunit of protein kinase A, which, upon entering the nucleus, can phosphorylate CREB. Phosphorylation of CREB converts it into its active state by permitting it to interact with the adapter protein CBP, which can then contact the basal transcription apparatus (see Fig. 10.19).

Role of cAMP and Ca^{2+} in the Activation Pathways of Transcription

As described earlier, the cAMP second-messenger pathway is among the best characterized intracellular signaling pathways; a major feature of signaling by this pathway is the regulation of a large number of genes. Cyclic AMP response elements, with the consensus nucleotide sequence of TGACGTCA, have been identified in many genes expressed in the nervous system.

The consensus CRE sequence illustrates a common feature of many transcription factor-binding sites; it is a palindrome. Examination of the sequence TGACGTCA readily reveals that the sequences on the two complementary strands, which run in opposite directions, are identical. Many cis-regulatory elements are perfect or approximate palindromes because many transcription factors bind DNA as dimers, in which each member of the dimer recognizes one of the "half-sites." CREB binds to CREs as a homodimer, with a higher affinity for perfectly palindromic than for asymmetric CREs.

When bound to a CRE, CREB activates transcription when it is phosphorylated on its Ser-133. It does so, as described earlier, because phosphorylated CREB, but not unphosphorylated CREB, can recruit the adapter protein, CBP, into the transcription complex. CBP, in turn, interacts with the basal transcription complex and modifies histones to enhance the efficiency of transcription.

The regulation of CREB activation by phosphorylation illustrates several general principles, including

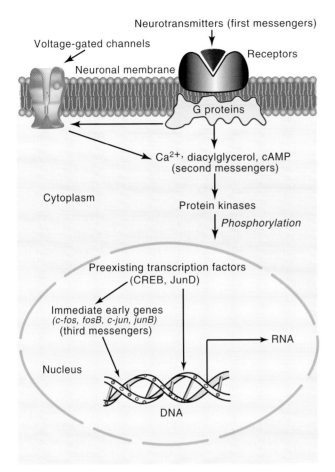

FIGURE 10.20 Signal transduction to the nucleus. In this schematic, activation of a neurotransmitter receptor activates cellular signals (G proteins and second-messenger systems). These signals, in turn, regulate the activation of protein kinases, which translocate to the nucleus. Within the nucleus, protein kinases can activate genes regulated by constitutively synthesized transcription factors. A subset of these genes encodes additional transcription factors (third messengers), which can then activate multiple downstream genes.

the requirement for nuclear translocation of protein kinases in cases where transcription factors are already found in the nucleus under basal conditions and the role of phosphorylation in regulating protein–protein interactions. An additional important principle illustrated by CREB is the convergence of signaling pathways. CREB is phosphorylated on Ser-133 by the free catalytic subunit of the cAMP-dependent protein kinase (Fig. 10.20). However, CREB Ser-133 can also be phosphorylated by Ca^{2+}–calmodulin-dependent protein kinase types II and IV and by RSK2, a kinase activated in growth factor pathways, including Ras and MAP kinase. When each individual signal is relatively weak, convergence may be a critical mechanism resulting in specificity of gene regulation, with some genes being activated only when

multiple pathways are stimulated. Some genes that contain CREs are known to be induced in more than an additive fashion by the interaction of cAMP and Ca^{2+}, but how convergent phosphorylation on the same serine might produce synergy is not yet clear. Synergy is understood more readily in cases in which a particular protein is modified at two different sites, causing interacting conformational changes. In addition to Ser-133, CREB contains sites for phosphorylation by a variety of protein kinases, including glycogen synthase kinase 3 (GSK3), but the biological effects of phosphorylating these additional serines are not fully understood. These additional phosphorylation events may fine-tune the regulation of CREB-mediated transcription.

CREB illustrates yet another important principle of transcriptional regulation: CREB is a member of a family of related proteins. Many transcription factors are members of families; this permits complex forms of positive and negative regulation. CREB is closely related to other proteins called activating transcription factors (ATFs) and CRE modulators (CREMs), which result from alternative splicing of a single CREM gene. All of these proteins bind CREs as dimers; many can dimerize with CREB itself. ATF-1 appears to be very similar to CREB in that it can be activated by both cAMP and Ca^{2+} pathways. Many of the other ATF proteins and CREM isoforms can activate transcription; however, certain CREMs may act to repress it. These CREM isoforms lack the glutamine-rich transcriptional activation domain of CREB-ATF family members that are activators of transcription. Thus CREB–CREM homodimers may bind DNA but fail to activate transcription. Like CREB, many of the ATF proteins are synthesized constitutively, but ATF 3 and certain CREM isoforms are inducible in response to environmental stimuli. The new synthesis of transcription factors is yet another mechanism of gene regulation.

The dimerization domain used by CREB–ATF proteins and several other families of transcription factors is called a leucine zipper. This domain was first identified in transcription factor C/EBP and is also utilized by the AP-1 family of transcription factors. The so-called leucine zipper actually forms a coiled-coil. The dimerization motif is an α helix in which every seventh residue is a leucine; based on the periodicity of α helices, the leucines line up along one face of the helix two turns apart. The aligned leucines of the two dimerization partners interact hydrophobically and stabilize the dimer. In CREB, C/EBP, and the AP-1 family of proteins, the leucine zipper is at the carboxy terminus of the protein. Just upstream of the leucine zipper is a region of highly basic amino acid residues that forms the DNA-binding domain.

Dimerization by means of the leucine zipper domain juxtaposes the adjacent basic regions of each of the partners; these juxtaposed basic regions undergo a conformational change when they bind DNA. The interaction of these proteins with DNA has been described as a "scissors grip." This combination of motifs is why this superfamily of proteins is referred to as basic leucine zipper proteins (bZIPs).

AP-1 Transcription Factors

Activator protein 1 (AP-1) is another family of bZIP transcription factors that play a central role in the regulation of neural gene expression by extracellular signals. The AP-1 family comprises multiple proteins that bind as heterodimers (and a few as homodimers) to the DNA sequence TGACTCA, the consensus AP-1 element that forms a palindrome flanking a central C or G. While the AP-1 sequence differs from the CRE sequence by only a single base, this one-base difference strongly biases protein binding away from the CREB family of proteins. AP-1 sequences confer responsiveness to the PKC pathway.

AP-1 proteins generally bind DNA as heterodimers composed of one member each of two different families of related bZIP proteins, the Fos family and the Jun family. Known members of the Fos family are c-Fos, Fra-1 (Fos-related antigen-1), Fra-2, and FosB; there is also evidence for posttranslationally modified forms of FosB. Known members of the Jun family are c-Jun, JunB, and JunD. Heterodimers form between proteins of the Fos family and proteins of the Jun family by means of the leucine zipper. Unlike Fos proteins, c-Jun and JunD, but not JunB, can form homodimers that bind to AP-1 sites, albeit with far lower affinity than Fos–Jun heterodimers. The potential complexity of transcriptional regulation is greater still because some AP-1 proteins can heterodimerize through the leucine zipper with members of the CREB–ATF family, e.g., ATF2 with c-Jun. AP-1 proteins can also form higher–order complexes with unrelated families of transcription factors. AP-1 proteins can complex with and thus apparently inhibit the transcriptional activity of steroid hormone receptors (discussed later).

Among the known Fos and Jun proteins, only JunD is expressed constitutively at high levels in many cell types. The other AP-1 proteins tend to be expressed at low or even undetectable levels under basal conditions, but, with stimulation, may be induced to high levels of expression. Thus, unlike genes that are regulated by constitutively expressed transcription factors such as CREB, genes that are regulated by c-Fos–c-Jun heterodimers require new transcription and translation of their required regulatory factors.

Cellular Immediate-Early Genes

Genes that are activated transcriptionally by synaptic activity, drugs, and growth factors have often been classified roughly into two groups. Genes, such as the c-fos gene itself, that are activated rapidly (within minutes), transiently, and without requiring new protein synthesis are often described as cellular immediate-early genes (IEGs). Genes that are induced or repressed more slowly (within hours) and are dependent on new protein synthesis have been described as late-response genes. The term IEG was initially applied to describe viral genes that are activated "immediately" upon infection of eukaryotic cells by utilization of preexisting host-cell transcription factors. Viral immediate-early genes generally encode transcription factors needed to activate viral "late" gene expression. This terminology has been extended to cellular (i.e., nonviral) genes with varying success. The terminology is problematic because many cellular genes are induced independent of protein synthesis, but with a time course intermediate between "classical" IEGs and late-response genes. In fact, some genes may be regulated with different time courses or requirements for protein synthesis in response to different intracellular signals. Moreover, many cellular genes regulated as IEGs encode proteins that are not transcription factors. Despite these caveats, the concept of IEG-encoded transcription factors in the nervous system is a useful heuristic. Because of their rapid induction from low basal levels in response to neuronal depolarization (the critical signal being Ca^{2+} entry) and second-messenger and growth factor pathways, several IEGs have been used as cellular markers of neural activation, permitting novel approaches to functional neuroanatomy (see Chapter 39, Box 39.4).

The protein products of those cellular IEGs that function as transcription factors bind to cis-regulatory elements contained within a subset of late-response genes to activate or repress them. As illustrated in Fig. 10.20, IEGs such as c-fos have therefore been termed third messengers in signal transduction cascades, with neurotransmitters designated as intercellular first messengers and small intracellular molecules, such as cAMP and Ca^{2+}, as second messengers. However, IEGs are not always a necessary step the in signal-regulated expression of genes having roles in the differentiated function of neurons. In fact, many such genes, including many genes encoding neuropeptides such as proenkephalin and prodynorphin and some genes encoding neurotrophic factors, are activated in response to neuronal depolarization or cAMP by phosphorylation of the constitutively expressed transcription factor CREB rather than by

IEG third messengers. In sum, neural genes that are regulated by extracellular signals are activated or repressed with varying time courses by reversible phosphorylation of constitutively synthesized transcription factors and by newly synthesized transcription factors, some of which are regulated as IEGs.

Activation of the c-fos Gene

The c-fos gene is activated rapidly by neurotransmitters or drugs that stimulate the cAMP pathway or Ca^{2+} elevation. Both pathways produce phosphorylation of transcription factor CREB. The c-fos gene contains three binding sites for CREB. The c-fos gene can also be induced by the Ras/MAP kinase pathway, which is activated by a number of growth factors. For example, neurotrophins, such as nerve growth factor (NGF), bind a family of receptor tyrosine kinases (Trks); NGF interacts with Trk A, which activates Ras. Ras then acts through a cascade of protein kinases including Raf and the cytoplasmic MAP kinase kinases (MAPKKs) MEK1/MEK2, which phosphorylate the MAP kinases ERK1/ERK2. These kinases translocate into the nucleus, where they can activate RSK2 to phosphorylate CREB, but they can also apparently directly phosphorylate other transcription factors such as the ternary complex factor Elk-1. Elk-1 binds along with the serum response factor (SRF) to the serum response element (SRE) within the c-fos gene and many other growth factor-inducible genes. Cross talk between neurotransmitter and growth factor-signaling pathways has been documented with increasing frequency and likely plays an important role in the precise tuning of neural plasticity to diverse environmental stimuli.

Regulation of c-Jun

Expression of most of the proteins of the Fos and Jun families that constitute transcription factor AP-1 and the binding of AP-1 proteins to DNA is regulated by extracellular signals. However, both Fos and Jun family members are phosphoproteins themselves, and AP-1-mediated transcription requires not only the new synthesis of AP-1 proteins, but also the phosphorylation of proteins within AP-1 complexes. Phosphorylation of c-Jun within its N-terminal activation domain has been shown to markedly enhance its ability to activate transcription without affecting its ability to form dimers or bind DNA. Other phosphorylation sites within c-Jun regulate its ability to bind DNA.

Phosphorylation and activation of c-Jun can result from the action of Jun N-terminal kinase (JNK). JNK is a member of the mitogen-activated protein kinase (MAPK) family of protein kinases whose mammalian members include ERKs, p38, and JNK. In addition to cellular stressors, the inflammatory cytokines interleukin-1β (IL-1β) and tumor necrosis factor α (TNFα) have been shown to activate both JNK and p38. JNK has also been shown to be activated by neurotransmitters, including glutamate. Thus, AP-1-mediated transcription within the nervous system requires multiple steps, beginning with the activation of genes encoding AP-1 proteins.

Cytokines as Inducers of Gene Expression in the Nervous System

With regard to function, the boundary between trophic, or growth, factors and cytokines in the nervous system has become increasingly arbitrary. However, cell-signaling mechanisms offer a useful means of distinction. Growth factors, such as neurotrophins (e.g., nerve growth factor, brain-derived neurotrophic factor, and neurotrophin 3), epidermal growth factor (EGF), and fibroblast growth factor (FGF), act through receptor protein tyrosine kinases, whereas cytokines, such as leukemia inhibitory factor (LIF), ciliary neurotrophic factor (CNTF), and interleukin-6 (IL-6), act through nonreceptor protein tyrosine kinases.

LIF, CNTF, and IL-6 subserve a wide array of overlapping functions inside and outside the nervous system, including hematopoietic and immunologic functions outside the nervous system and regulation of neuronal survival, differentiation, and, in certain circumstances, plasticity within the nervous system. These peptides have marked homologies of their tertiary structures rather than their primary sequences, which presumably permits them to interact with related receptor complexes that contain a common signal-transducing subunit, gp130. Receptors for these cytokines consist of a signal-transducing β component, which includes gp130 and, in some cases, additional subunits. As is typical of cytokine receptors, cytoplasmic tails of the signal-transducing β components of the IL-6, LIF, and CNTF receptors lack kinase domains. Rather, the cytoplasmic domains interact with nonreceptor protein tyrosine kinases (PTKs) of the Janus kinase (Jak) family, which include Jak1, Jak2, and Tyk2. Some cytokine receptors, such as the prolactin receptor, which interacts exclusively with Jak2, can interact only with a single Jak PTK. In contrast, IL-6, LIF, and CNTF receptors can interact with multiple Jak PTKs, including Jak1, Jak2, and Tyk2. Presumably, the dimerization of receptors on ligand binding permits Jak family PTKs to cross-phosphorylate each other.

Signal transduction to the nucleus includes tyrosine phosphorylation by the Jak PTKs of one or more

BOX 10.3

THE CELLULAR BASIS OF ALZHEIMER'S DISEASE

The brain of a patient with Alzheimer's disease (AD) contains three primary pathological features, two that are visible (senile plaques and neurofibrillar tangles) and one that is not (neuronal loss). The accumulation of plaques and tangles correlates with a decline in functional status and neuronal loss is an early and prominent event. Neuronal loss appears to involve degenerative pathways related to apoptosis.

Data in cell culture have shown that brain neurons are particularly vulnerable to degeneration by apoptosis. Further, the inducers that activate the program (e.g., β-amyloid, oxidative damage, low energy metabolism) correspond to conditions present in the AD brain. This suggests the possibility that apoptosis may be one of the mechanisms contributing to neuronal loss in this disease. Indeed, some neurons in vulnerable regions of the AD brain show evidence of DNA damage, nuclear apoptotic bodies, chromatin condensation, and the induction of select genes characteristic of apoptosis in cell culture and animal models. This suggests the existence of apoptosis in the AD brain, a hypothesis also consistent with evolving research in one of the regulatory functions of the presenilin genes. However, DNA damage is also present in the majority of neurons in vulnerable regions in early and mild cases. In most tissues, cells in fully activated apoptosis degenerate and are removed within hours to days and thus it seems all DNA damage is unlikely to signify terminal apoptosis. The presence of extensive DNA damage suggests an acceleration of damage, faulty repair process, loss of protective mechanisms, or an activation and arrest of aspects of the apoptotic program. DNA damage is unlikely to be an artifact of postmortem delay or agonal state.

The existence of protective mechanisms for neurons may also exist, as these cells are nondividing and essential. In this context, it is interesting that Bcl-2 is upregulated in most neurons with DNA damage. Further, at least one DNA repair enzyme is also unregulated. Thus, it appears as if neurons are in a struggle between degeneration and repair.

As research advances, it is critical to reduce the stimuli that cause the neuronal damage and to discover the key intervention points to assist neurons in the repair processes.

Carl W. Cotman

of the STAT proteins mentioned earlier. The first STAT family members were identified as proteins binding to interferon-regulated genes but have subsequently been found to take part in the activity of multiple cytokines. Upon phosphorylation, STAT proteins form dimers through the association of SH2 domains, an important type of protein interaction domain described earlier. Dimerization is thought to trigger translocation to the nucleus, where STATS bind their cognate cytokine response elements. Different STATs become activated by different cytokine receptors, not because of differential use of Jak PTKs, but because of specific coupling of certain STATs to certain receptors. Thus, for example, the IL-6 receptor preferentially activates STAT1 and STAT3; the CNTF receptor preferentially activates STAT3. The c-*fos* gene, for example, contains an element called the SIS-inducible element (SIE), which binds STAT proteins; thus, c-*fos* gene expression can also be induced by cytokines. Cytokine response elements have now been identified within many neural genes, including vasoactive intestinal polypeptide and several other neuropeptide genes.

Steroid Hormone Receptors

The differentiation of many cells types in the brain is established by exposure to steroids. For example, exposure to estrogen or testosterone during critical developmental periods results in the sexually dimorphic development of certain nuclei. Steroid hormones, including glucocorticoids, sex steroids, mineralocorticoids, retinoids, thyroid hormone, and vitamin D, are small lipid-soluble ligands that can diffuse across cell membranes. They act on their receptors within the cell cytoplasm in marked distinction to the other types of intercellular signals described herein. Another unique feature of steroid hormones is that their receptors are themselves transcription factors. Like other transcription factors described in this chapter, steroid hormone receptors are modular in nature. Each has a transcriptional-activation domain at its amino terminus, a DNA-binding domain, and a hormone-binding domain at its carboxy terminus. DNA-binding domains recognize specific palindromic DNA sequences, steroid hormone response elements, within the regulatory regions of specific genes.

After having been bound by hormone, activated steroid hormone receptors translocate into the nucleus, where they bind to their cognate response elements. Such binding then increases or decreases the rate at which these target genes are transcribed, depending on the precise nature and DNA sequence context of the element.

Summary

The formation of long-term memories requires changes in gene expression and new protein synthesis. Control sequences on DNA determine which segments of DNA can be transcribed into RNA. It is at transcription initiation that extracellular signals such as neurotransmitters, hormones, drugs, and growth factors exert their most significant control. The transcription itself is carried out by RNA polymerases. The transcription is modulated by transcription factors that recruit the polymerases to the DNA. For example, the critical nuclear translocation step in the activation of transcription factor CREB involves the catalytic subunit of PKA, which can phosphorylate CREB on entering the nucleus. In addition, increasing evidence indicates that at least some forms of long-term memory require new gene expression.

Genes that encode the transcription factors themselves may respond quickly or slowly. These genes have been coined third messengers in signal transduction cascades. Cross talk between neurotransmitter and growth factor-signaling pathways is likely to play an important role in the precise tuning of neuronal plasticity to diverse environmental stimuli.

The active, mature transcription complex is a remarkable architectural assembly of proteins assembled at the basal promoter—in most cases, at a sequence called the TATA box. In addition to RNA polymerase II, this complex includes a large number of associated general transcription factors, sequence-specific transcription factors, and intervening adapters. A wide variety of transcription factors bound to *cis*-regulatory elements elsewhere in the gene, but permitted to interact by the looping of DNA, join in the formation of the active transcription complex. This remarkable mechanism permits cells to exert exquisite control of the genes being transcribed in a variety of situations, e.g., to govern appropriate entry or exit from the cell cycle, to maintain appropriate cellular identity, and to respond appropriately to extracellular signals.

Transcription can be regulated by many different extracellular signals modulated by a large array of signaling pathways (many including reversible phosphorylation) and a complex array of transcription factors. Most of these factors are members of families and regulate transcription only as multimers. Given this complexity, the potential for very precise regulation is clear, but the mechanisms by which such precision is achieved are not fully understood. In this chapter, regulation has been illustrated by only a few of the families of transcription factors. Those chosen appear to play important roles in the nervous system and illustrate many of the basic principles of gene regulation.

References

Baranano, D. E., Ferris, C. D., and Snyder, S. H. (2001). Atypical neural messengers. *Trends Neurosci.* **24**, 99–106.

Berridge, M. J. (1993). Inositol trisphosphate and calcium signalling. *Nature* **361**, 315–325.

Bourne, H. R., and Nicoll, R. (1993). Molecular machines integrate coincident synaptic signals. *Cell* **72**, 65–75.

Braun, A. P., and Schulman, H. (1995). The multifunctional calcium/calmodulin-dependent protein kinase: From form to function. *Annu. Rev. Physiol.* **57**, 417–445.

Chain, D. G., Casadio, A., Schacher, S., Hegde, A. N., Valbrun, M., Yamamoto, N., Goldberg, A. L., Bartsch, D., Kandel, E. R., and Schwartz, J. H. (1999). Mechanisms for generating the autonomous cAMP-dependent protein kinase required for long-term facilitation in *Aplysia*. *Neuron* **22**, 147–156.

Clapham, D. E., and Neer, E. J. (1993). New roles for G-protein $\beta\gamma$-dimers in transmembrane signalling. *Nature* **365**, 403–406.

Cohen, P. (1992). Signal integration at the level of protein kinases, protein phosphatases and their substrates. *TIBS* **17**, 408–413.

Greengard, P. (2001). The neurobiology of slowsynaptic transmession. *Science* **294**, 1024–1030.

Greengard, P., Nairn, A. C., Girault, J.-A., Quimet, C. C., Snyder, G. L., Fisone, G., Allen, P. B., Fienberg, A., and Nishi, A. (1998). The DARPP-32/protein phosphatase-1 cascade: A model for signal integration. *Brain Res. Rev.* **26**, 274–284.

Hanson, P. I., and Schulman, H. (1992). Neuronal Ca^{2+}/calmodulin-dependent protein kinases. *Annu. Rev. Biochem.* **61**, 559–601.

Hille, B. (1992). G protein-coupled mechanisms and nervous signaling. *Neuron* **9**, 187–195.

Hunter, T. (1995). Protein kinases and phosphatases: The yin and yang of protein phosphorylation and signaling. *Cell* **80**, 225–236.

Kemp, B. E., Faux, M. C., Means, A. R., House, C., Tiganis, T., Hu, S.-H., and Mitchelhill, K. I. (1994). Structural aspects: Pseudo-substrate and substrate interactions. *In* "Protein Kinases" (J. R. Woodgett, ed.), pp. 30–67.

Kennelly, P. J., and Krebs, E. G. (1991). Consensus sequences as substrate specificity determinants for protein kinases and protein phosphatases. *J. Biol. Chem.* **266**, 15555–15558.

Klauck, T. M., Faux, M. C., Labudda, K., Langeberg, L. K., Jaken, S., and Scott, J. D. (1996). Coordination of three signaling enzymes by AKAP79, a mammalian scaffold protein. *Science* **271**, 1589–1592.

Lisman, J., Schulman, H., and Cline, H. (2002). The molecular basis of CaMKII function in synaptic plasticity and behavioural memory. *Nat. Rev. Neurosci.* **3**, 175–190.

Neer, E. J. (1995). Heterotrimeric G proteins: organizers of transmembrane signals. *Cell* **80**, 249–257.

Price, N. E., and Mumby, M. C. (1999). Brain protein serine/threonine phosphatases. *Curr. Opin. Neurobiol.* **9**, 336–342.

Rosenmund, C., Carr, D. W., Bergeson, S. E., Nilaver, G., Scott, J. D., and Westbrook, G. L. (1994). Anchoring of protein kinase A is required for modulation of AMPA/kainate receptors on hippocampal neurons. *Nature* **368**, 853–856.

Ross, E. M. (1989). Signal sorting and amplification through G protein-coupled receptors. *Neuron* **3**, 141–152.

Schulman, H., and Braun, A. (1999), Ca²⁺/calmodulin-dependent protein kinases. *In* "Calcium as a Cellular Regular" (E. Carafoli and C. Klee, eds.), pp. 311–343. Oxford Univ. Press, New York.

Stryer, L., and Bourne, H. R. (1986). G proteins: A family of signal transducers. *Annu. Rev. Cell Biol.* **2**, 391–419.

Tanaka, C., and Nishizuka, Y. (1994). The protein kinase C family for neuronal signaling. *Annu. Rev. Neurosci.* **17**, 551–567.

Taussig, R., and Gilman, A. G. (1995). Mammalian membrane-bound adenylyl cyclases. *J. Biol. Chem.* **270**, 1–4.

Tjian, R., and Maniatis, T. (1994). Transcription activation: A complex puzzle with few easy pieces. *Cell* **77**, 5–8.

Stryer, L. (1995). "Biochemistry," 4th Ed. Freeman, New York.

Suggested Readings

Carafoli, E., and Klee, C. (1999). "Calcium as a Cellular Regulator." Oxford Univ. Press, New York.

Cohen, P., and Klee, C. B. (1988). Calmodulin. *In* "Molecular Aspects of Cellular Regulation," Vol. 5. Elsevier, Amsterdam.

Greengard, P., Snyder, G., Fisone, G., and Aperia, A. (1996). Interactions of signal transduction pathways in the nervous system. *In* "Challenges and Perspectives in Neuroscience" (D. Ottoson, ed.), pp. 3–26. Pergamon, London.

Nairn, A. C., Hemmings, H. C., Jr., and Greengard, P. (1985). Protein kinases in the brain. *Annu. Rev. Biochem.* **54**, 931–976.

Howard Schulman and James L. Roberts

11

Postsynaptic Potentials and Synaptic Integration

The study of synaptic transmission in the central nervous system (CNS) provides an opportunity to learn more about the diversity and richness of mechanisms underlying this process and to learn how some of the fundamental signaling properties of the nervous system, such as action potentials and synaptic potentials, work together to process information and generate behavior.

Postsynaptic potentials (PSPs) in the CNS can be divided into two broad classes on the basis of mechanisms and, generally, duration of these potentials. One class is based on the direct binding of a transmitter molecule(s) with a receptor–channel complex; these receptors are ionotropic. The structure of these receptors is discussed in detail in Chapter 9. The resulting PSPs are generally short lasting and hence are sometimes called fast PSPs; they have also been referred to as "classical" because they were the first synaptic potentials to be recorded in the CNS (Eccles, 1964; Spencer, 1977) The duration of a typical fast PSP is about 20 ms.

The other class of PSPs is based on the indirect effect of a transmitter molecule(s) binding with a receptor. The receptors that produce these PSPs are metabotropic. As discussed in Chapter 9, the receptors activate G proteins that affect the channel either directly or through additional steps in which the level of a second messenger is altered. The responses mediated by metabotropic receptors can be long lasting and are therefore called slow PSPs. The mechanisms for fast PSPs mediated by ionotropic receptors are considered first.

IONOTROPIC RECEPTORS: MEDIATORS OF FAST EXCITATORY AND INHIBITORY SYNAPTIC POTENTIALS

The Stretch Reflex Is Useful to Examine the Properties and Functional Consequences of Ionotropic PSPs

The stretch reflex, one of the simpler behaviors mediated by the central nervous system, is a useful example with which to examine the properties and functional consequences of ionotropic PSPs. The tap of a neurologist's hammer to a ligament elicits a reflex extension of the leg, as illustrated in Fig. 11.1. The brief stretch of the ligament is transmitted to the extensor muscle and is detected by specific receptors in the muscle and ligament (Chapter 29). Action potentials initiated in the stretch receptors are propagated to the spinal cord by afferent fibers (Chapter 29). The receptors are specialized regions of sensory neurons with somata located in the dorsal root ganglia just outside the spinal column. Axons of the afferents enter the spinal cord and make excitatory synaptic connections with at least two types of postsynaptic neurons. First, a synaptic connection is made to the extensor motor neuron. As the result of its synaptic activation, the motor neuron fires action potentials that propagate out of the spinal cord and ultimately invade the terminal regions of the motor axon at neuromuscular junctions. There, acetylcholine (ACh) is released, nicotinic ACh receptors are activated, an end plate potential (EPP) is produced, an action

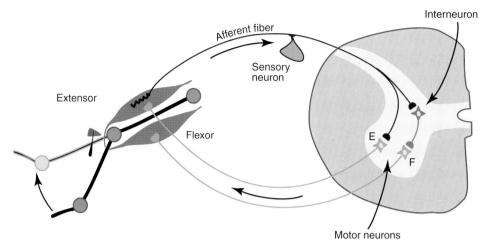

FIGURE 11.1 Features of the vertebrate stretch reflex. Stretch of an extensor muscle leads to the initiation of action potentials in the afferent terminals of specialized stretch receptors. The action potentials propagate to the spinal cord through afferent fibers (sensory neurons). The afferents make excitatory connections with extensor motor neurons (E). Action potentials initiated in the extensor motor neuron propagate to the periphery and lead to the activation and subsequent contraction of the extensor muscle. The afferent fibers also activate interneurons that inhibit the flexor motor neurons (F).

potential is initiated in the muscle cell, and the muscle cell is contracted, producing the reflex extension of the leg. Second, a synaptic connection is made to another group of neurons called interneurons (nerve cells interposed between one type of neuron and another). The particular interneurons activated by the afferents are inhibitory interneurons because activation of these interneurons leads to the release of a chemical transmitter substance that inhibits the flexion motor neuron. This inhibition tends to prevent an uncoordinated (improper) movement (i.e., flexion) from occurring. The reflex system illustrated in Fig. 11.1 is also known as the monosynaptic stretch reflex because this reflex is mediated by a single ("mono") excitatory synapse in the central nervous system. Spinal reflexes are described in greater detail in Chapter 29.

Figure 11.2 illustrates procedures that can be used to experimentally examine some of the components of synaptic transmission in the reflex pathway for the stretch reflex. Intracellular recordings are made from one of the sensory neurons, the extensor and flexor motor neurons, and an inhibitory interneuron. Normally, the sensory neuron is activated by stretch to the muscle, but this step can be bypassed by simply injecting a pulse of depolarizing current of sufficient magnitude into the sensory neuron to elicit an action potential. The action potential in the sensory neuron leads to a potential change in the motor neuron known as an excitatory postsynaptic potential (EPSP; Fig. 11.2).

Mechanisms responsible for fast EPSPs mediated by ionotropic receptors in the CNS are fairly well

known. Moreover, the ionic mechanisms for EPSPs in the CNS are essentially identical with the ionic mechanisms at the skeletal neuromuscular junction. Specifically, the transmitter substance released from the presynaptic terminal (Chapters 7 and 8) diffuses across the synaptic cleft, binds to specific receptor sites on the postsynaptic membrane (Chapter 9), and leads to a simultaneous increase in permeability to Na^+ and K^+, which makes the membrane potential move toward a value of about 0 mV. However, the processes of synaptic transmission at the sensory neuron–motor neuron synapse and the motor neuron–skeletal muscle synapse differ in two fundamental ways: (1) in the transmitter used and (2) in the amplitude of the PSP. The transmitter substance at the neuromuscular junction is ACh, whereas that released by the sensory neurons is an amino acid, probably glutamate. Indeed, glutamate is the most common transmitter that mediates excitatory actions in the CNS. The amplitude of the postsynaptic potential at the neuromuscular junction is about 50 mV; consequently, each PSP depolarizes the postsynaptic cell beyond threshold so there is a one-to-one relation between an action potential in the spinal motor neuron and an action potential in the skeletal muscle cell. Indeed, the EPP must depolarize the muscle cell by only about 30 mV to initiate an action potential, allowing a safety factor of about 20 mV. In contrast, the EPSP in a spinal motor neuron produced by an action potential in an afferent fiber has an amplitude of only about 1 mV. The mechanisms by which these small PSPs can trigger an action potential in the post-

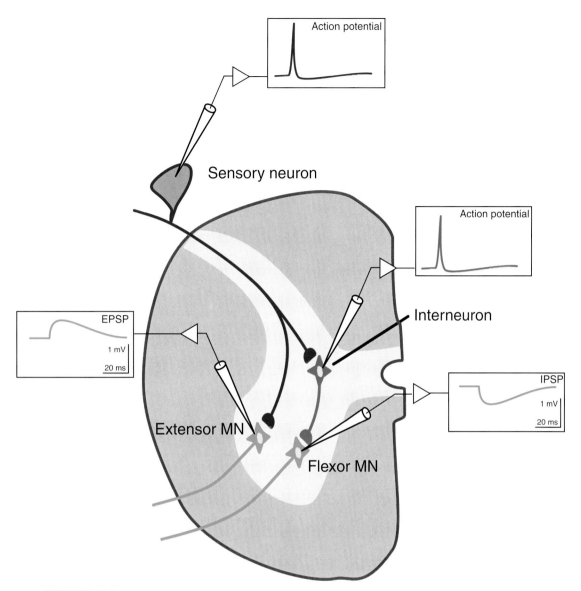

FIGURE 11.2 Excitatory (EPSP) and inhibitory (IPSP) postsynaptic potentials in spinal motor neurons. Idealized intracellular recordings from a sensory neuron, interneuron, and extensor and flexor motor neurons (MNs). An action potential in the sensory neuron produces a depolarizing response (an EPSP) in the extensor motor neuron. An action potential in the interneuron produces a hyperpolarizing response (an IPSP) in the flexor motor neuron.

synaptic neuron are discussed in a later section of this chapter and in Chapter 12.

Macroscopic Properties of PSPs are Determined by the Nature of Gating and Ion-Permeation Properties of Single Channels

Patch-Clamp Techniques

Patch-clamp techniques (Hamill, 1981), with which current flowing through single isolated receptors can be measured directly, can be sources of insight into

both the ionic mechanisms and the molecular properties of PSPs mediated by ionotropic receptors. This approach was pioneered by Erwin Neher and Bert Sakman in the 1970s and led to their being awarded the Nobel Prize in Physiology or Medicine in 1991.

Figure 11.3A illustrates an idealized experimental arrangement of an "outside-out" patch recording of a single ionotropic receptor. The patch pipette contains a solution with an ionic composition similar to that of the cytoplasm, whereas the solution exposed to the outer surface of the membrane has a composition similar to that of normal extracellular fluid. The electrical potential across the patch, and hence the transmembrane potential (V_m), is controlled by the patch-clamp amplifier. The extracellular (outside) fluid is considered "ground." Transmitter can be delivered by applying pressure to a miniature pipette filled with an agonist (in this case, ACh), and the current (I_m) flowing across the patch of membrane is measured by the patch-clamp amplifier (Fig. 11.3B).

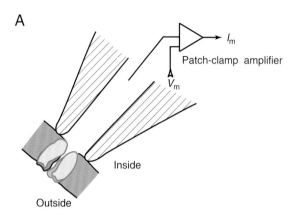

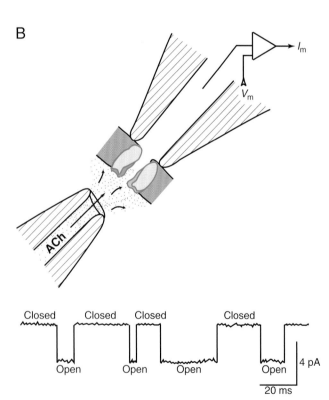

FIGURE 11.3 Single-channel recording of ionotropic receptors and their properties. (A) Experimental arrangement for studying properties of ionotropic receptors. (B) Idealized single-channel currents in response to application of ACh.

Pressure in the pipette that contains ACh can be continuous, allowing a constant stream of ACh to contact the membrane, or can be applied as a short pulse to allow a precisely timed and discrete amount of ACh to contact the membrane. The types of recordings obtained from such an experiment are illustrated in the traces in Fig. 11.3. In the absence of ACh, no current flows through the channel (Fig. 11.3A). When ACh is applied continuously, current flows across the membrane (through the channel), but remarkably, the current does not flow continuously; instead, small step-like changes in current are observed (Fig. 11.3B). These changes represent the probabilistic (random) opening and closing of the channel.

Channel Openings and Closings

As a result of the type of patch-recording techniques heretofore described, three general conclusions about the properties of ligand-gated channels can be drawn. First, ACh, as well as other transmitters that activate ionotropic receptors, causes the opening of individual ionic channels (for a channel to open, usually two molecules of transmitter must bind to the receptor). Second, when a ligand-gated channel opens, it does so in an all-or-none fashion. Increasing the concentration of transmitter in the ejection microelectrode does not increase the permeability (conductance) of the channel; it increases its probability (P) of being open. Third, the ionic current flowing through a single channel in its open state is extremely small (e.g., 10^{-12} A); as a result, current flowing through any single channel makes only a small contribution to the normal postsynaptic potential. Physiologically, when a larger region of the postsynaptic membrane, and thus more than one channel, is exposed to a released transmitter, the net conductance of the membrane increases due to the increased probability that a larger population of channels will be open at the same time. The normal PSP, measured with standard intracellular recording techniques (see, e.g., Fig. 11.2), is then proportional to the sum of the currents that flow through these many individual open channels. The properties of voltage-sensitive channels (see Chapter 6) are similar in that they, too, open in all-or-none fashion, and, as a result, the net effect on the cell is due to the summation of currents flowing through many individual open ion channels. The two types of channels differ, however, in that one is opened by a chemical agent, whereas the other is opened by changes in membrane potential.

Statistical Analysis of Channel Gating and Kinetics of the PSP

The experiment illustrated in Fig. 11.3B was performed with continuous exposure to ACh. Under

A

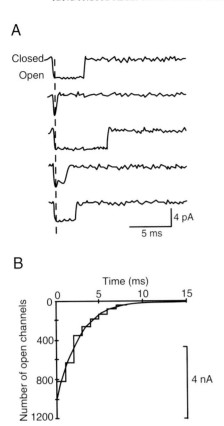

FIGURE 11.4 Determination of the shape of the postsynaptic response from single-channel currents. (A) Each trace represents the response of a single channel to a repetitively applied puff of transmitter. Traces are aligned with the beginning of the channel opening (dashed line). (B) The addition of 1000 of the individual responses. If a current equal to 4 pA were generated by the opening of a single channel, then a 4-nA current would be generated by 1000 channels opening at the same time. Data are fitted with an exponential function having a time constant equal to $1/\alpha$ (see text). Reprinted with permission from Sakmann (1992). American Association for the Advancement of Science, © 1992 The Nobel Foundation.

such conditions, the channels open and close repeatedly. When ACh is applied by a brief pressure pulse to more accurately mimic the transient release from the presynaptic terminal, the transmitter diffuses away before it can cause a second opening of the channel. A set of data similar to that shown in Fig. 11.4A would be obtained if an ensemble of these openings were collected and aligned with the start of each opening. Each individual trace represents the response to each successive "puff" of ACh. Note that, among the responses, the duration of the opening of the channel varies considerably—from very short (less than 1 ms) to more than 5 ms. Moreover, channel openings are independent events. The duration of any one channel opening does not have any relation to the duration of a previous opening. Figure 11.4B illustrates a plot that is obtained by adding 1000 of

these individual responses. Such an addition roughly simulates the conditions under which a transmitter released from a presynaptic terminal leads to the near simultaneous activation of many single channels in the postsynaptic membrane. (Note that the addition of 1000 channels would produce a synaptic current equal to about 4 nA.) This simulation is valid given the assumption that the statistical properties of a single channel over time are the same as the statistical properties of the ensemble at one instant of time (i.e., an ergotic process). The ensemble average can be fit with an exponential function with a decay time constant of 2.7 ms. An additional observation (discussed below) is that the value of the time constant is equal to the mean duration of the channel openings. The curve in Fig. 11.4B is an indication of the probability that a channel will remain open for various times, with a high probability for short times and a low probability for long times.

The ensemble average of single-channel currents (Fig. 11.4B) roughly accounts for the time course of the EPSP. However, note that the time course of the aggregate synaptic current can be somewhat faster than that of the excitatory postsynaptic potential in Fig. 11.2. This difference is due to charging of the membrane capacitance by a rapidly changing synaptic current. Because the single-channel currents were recorded with the membrane voltage clamped, the capacitive current [$I_c = C_m*(dV/dt)$] is zero. In contrast, for the recording of the postsynaptic potential in Fig. 11.2, the membrane was not voltage clamped, and therefore as the voltage changes (dV/dt), some of the synaptic current charges the membrane capacitance [see Eq. (7)].

Analytical expressions that describe the shape of the ensemble average of the open lifetimes and the mean open lifetime can be derived by considering that single-channel opening and closing is a stochastic process (Johnston and Wu, 1995; Sakmann, 1992). Relations are formalized to describe the likelihood (probability) of a channel being in a certain state. Consider the following two-state reaction scheme:

$$C \overset{\beta}{\underset{\alpha}{\Leftrightarrow}} O$$

In this scheme, α represents the rate constant for channel closing and β the rate constant for channel opening. The scheme can be simplified further if we consider a case in which the channel has been opened by the agonist and the agonist is removed instantaneously. A channel so opened (at time 0) will then close after a certain random time (Fig. 11.4). It can be shown that the mean open time = $1/\alpha$ (Johnston and Wu, 1995; Sakmann, 1992).

Gating Properties of Ligand-Gated Channels

Although statistical analysis can be a valuable source of insight into the statistical nature of the gating process and the molecular determinants of the macroscopic postsynaptic potential, the description in the preceding section is a simplification of the actual processes. Specifically, a more complete description must include the kinetics of receptor binding and unbinding and the determinants of the channel opening, as well as the fact that channels display rapid transitions between open and closed states during a single agonist receptor occupancy. Thus, the open states illustrated in Figs. 11.3B and 11.4A represent the period of a burst of extremely rapid openings and closings. If the bursts of rapid channel openings and closings are thought of, and behave functionally, as a single continuous channel closure, the formalism developed in the preceding section is a reasonable approximation for many ligand-gated channels. Nevertheless, a more complex reaction scheme is necessary to quantitatively explain available data. Such a scheme would include the following states,

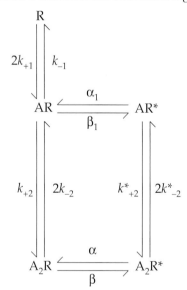

where R represents the receptor, A the agonist, and the α, β, and k values the forward and reverse rate constants for the various reactions. A_2R^* represents a channel opened as a result of the binding of two agonist molecules. The asterisk indicates an open channel. (Note that the lower part of the reaction scheme is equivalent to the one developed earlier, i.e.,

$$C \underset{\alpha}{\overset{\beta}{\Longleftrightarrow}} O$$

With the use of probability theory, equations describing transitions between the states can be determined. The approach is identical to that used in the simplified two-state scheme. However, the mathematics and analytical expressions are more complex because of the interactions among transitions and the multiple dimensionality of the variables. For some receptors, additional states must be represented. For example, as described in Chapter 9, some ligand-gated channels exhibit a process of desensitization in which continued exposure to a ligand results in channel closure.

Null (Reversal) Potential and Slope of I–V Relations

What ions are responsible for the synaptic current that produces the EPSP? Early studies of the ionic mechanisms underlying the EPSP at the skeletal neuromuscular junction yielded important information. Specifically, voltage-clamp and ion-substitution experiments indicated that the binding of transmitter to receptors on the postsynaptic membrane led to a simultaneous increase in Na^+ and K^+ permeability that depolarized the cell toward a value of about 0 mV (Fatt and Katz, 1951; Takeuchi and Takeuchi, 1960). These findings are applicable to the EPSP in a spinal motor neuron produced by an action potential in an afferent fiber and have been confirmed and extended at the single-channel level.

Figure 11.5 illustrates the type of experiment in which the analysis of single-channel currents can be a source of insight into the ionic mechanisms of EPSPs. A transmitter is delivered to the patch while the membrane potential is varied systematically (Fig. 11.5A). In the upper trace, the patch potential is –40 mV. The ejection of transmitter produces a sequence of channel openings and closings, the amplitudes of which are constant for each opening (i.e., about 4 pA). Now consider the case in which the transmitter is applied when the potential across the patch is –20 mV. The frequency of the responses, as well as the mean open lifetimes, is about the same as when the potential was at –40 mV, but now the amplitude of the single-channel currents is decreased uniformly. Even more interesting, when the patch is depolarized artificially to a value of about 0 mV, an identical puff of transmitter produces no current in the patch. If the patch potential is depolarized to a value of about 20 mV and the puff is delivered again, openings are again observed, but the flow of current through the channel is reversed in sign; a series of upward deflections indicate outward single-channel currents. In summary, there are downward deflections (inward currents) when the membrane potential is at –40 mV, no deflections (currents) when the membrane is at 0 mV,

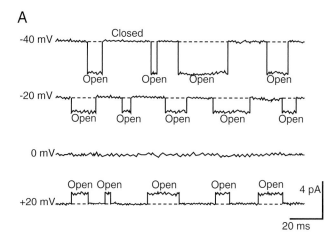

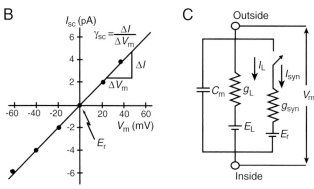

FIGURE 11.5 Voltage dependence of the current flowing through single channels. (A) Idealized recording of an ionotropic receptor in the continuous presence of agonist. (B) I–V relation of the channel in A. (C) Equivalent electrical circuit of a membrane containing that channel. γ_{SC}, single-channel conductance; I_L, leakage current; I_{SC}, single-channel current; g_L, leakage conductance; g_{syn}, macroscopic synaptic conductance; E_L, leakage battery; E_r, reversal potential.

and upward deflections (outward currents) when the membrane potential is moved to 20 mV.

The simple explanation for these results is that no matter what the membrane potential, the effect of the transmitter binding with receptors is to produce a permeability change that tends to move the membrane potential toward 0 mV. If the membrane potential is more negative than 0 mV, an inward current is recorded. If the membrane potential is more positive than 0 mV, an outward current is recorded. If the membrane potential is at 0 mV, there is no deflection because the membrane potential is already at 0 mV. At 0 mV, the channels are opening and closing as they always do in response to the agonist, but there is no net movement of ions through them. This 0–mV level is known as the synaptic null potential or reversal potential because it is the potential at which the sign of the synaptic current reverses. The fact that the experimentally determined reversal potential equals

the calculated value obtained by using the Goldman–Hodgkin–Katz (GHK) equation (Chapter 6) provides strong support for the theory that the EPSP is due to the opening of channels that have equal permeabilities to Na^+ and K^+. Ion-substitution experiments also confirm this theory. Thus, when the concentration of Na^+ or K^+ in the extracellular fluid is altered, the value of the reversal potential shifts in a way predicted by the GHK equation. (Some other cations, such as Ca^{2+}, also permeate these channels, but their permeability is low compared with that of Na^+ and K^+.)

Different families of ionotropic receptors have different reversal potentials because each has unique ion selectivity. In addition, it should now be clear that the sign of the synaptic action (excitatory or inhibitory) depends on the value of the reversal potential relative to the resting potential. If the reversal potential of an ionotropic receptor channel is more positive than the resting potential, opening of that channel will lead to depolarization (i.e., an EPSP). In contrast, if the reversal potential of an ionotropic receptor channel is more negative than the resting potential, opening of that channel will lead to hyperpolarization, i.e., an inhibitory postsynaptic potential (IPSP), which is the topic of a later section in this chapter.

Plotting the average peak value of single-channel currents (I_{sc}) versus the membrane potential (transpatch potential) at which they are recorded (Fig. 11.5B) can be a source of quantitative insight into the properties of the ionotropic receptor channel. Note that the current–voltage (I–V) relation is linear; it has a slope, the value of which is the single-channel conductance, and an intercept at 0 mV. This linear relation can be put in the form of Ohm's law ($I = G^*\Delta V$). Thus

$$I_{sc} = \gamma_{sc} * (V_m - E_r), \qquad (1)$$

where γ_{sc} is the single-channel conductance and E_r is the reversal potential (here, 0 mV).

Summation of Single-Channel Currents

We now know that the sign of a synaptic action can be predicted by knowledge of the relation between the resting potential (V_m) and the reversal potential (E_r), but how can the precise amplitude be determined? The answer to this question lies in understanding the relation between synaptic conductance and extra synaptic conductances. These interactions can be rather complex (see Chapter 12), but some initial understanding can be obtained by analyzing an electrical equivalent circuit for these two major conductance branches. We first need to move from a consideration of single-channel conductances and currents to that of macroscopic conductances and currents. The postsynaptic membrane contains thousands of any one type of ionotropic receptor, and each of these receptors could be activated by a transmitter released by a single action potential in a presynaptic neuron. Because conductances in parallel add, the total conductance change produced by their simultaneous activation would be

$$g_{syn} = \gamma_{sc} * P * N, \tag{2}$$

where γ_{sc}, as before, is the single-channel conductance, P is the probability of opening of a single channel (controlled by the ligand), and N is the total number of ligand-gated channels in the postsynaptic membrane. The macroscopic postsynaptic current produced by the transmitter released by a single presynaptic action potential can then be described by

$$I_{syn} = g_{syn} * (V_m - E_r). \tag{3}$$

Equation (3) can be represented physically by a voltage (V_m) measured across a circuit consisting of a resistor (g_{syn}) in series with a battery (E_r). An equivalent circuit of a membrane containing such a conductance is illustrated in Fig. 11.5C. Also included in this circuit is a membrane capacitance (C_m), a resistor representing the leakage conductance (g_L), and a battery (E_L) representing the leakage potential. (Voltage-dependent Na^+, Ca^{2+}, and K^+ channels that contribute to the generation of the action potential have been omitted for simplification.)

The simple circuit allows the simulation and further analysis of the genesis of the PSP. Closure of the switch simulates the opening of the channels by transmitter released from some presynaptic neuron [i.e., a change in P of Eq. (2) from 0 to 1]. When the switch is open (i.e., no agonist is present and the ligand-gated channels are closed), the membrane potential (V_m) is equal to the value of the leakage battery (E_L). Closure of the switch (i.e., the agonist opens the channels) tends to polarize the membrane potential toward the value of the battery (E_r) in series with the synaptic conductance. Although the effect of the channel openings is to depolarize the postsynaptic cell *toward* E_r (0 mV), this value is never achieved because ligand-gated receptors are only a small fraction of the ion channels in the membrane. Other channels (such as the leakage channels, which are not affected by the transmitters) tend to hold the membrane potential at E_L and prevent the membrane potential from reaching the 0–mV level. In terms of the equivalent electrical circuit (Fig. 11.5C), g_L is much greater than g_{syn}.

An analytical expression that can be a source of insight into the production of an EPSP by the engage-

ment of a synaptic conductance can be derived by examining the current flowing in each of the two conductance branches of the circuit in Fig. 11.5C. As shown previously [Eq. (3)], current flowing in the branch representing the synaptic conductance is equal to

$$I_{syn} = g_{syn} * (V_m - E_r).$$

Similarly, the current flowing through the leakage conductance is equal to

$$I_L = g_L * (V_m - E_L). \tag{4}$$

By conservation of current, the two currents must be equal and opposite. Therefore,

$$g_{syn} * (V_m - E_r) = -g_L * (V_m - E_L).$$

Rearranging and solving for V_m, we obtain

$$V_m = \frac{g_{syn} E_r + g_L E_L}{g_{syn} + g_L}. \tag{5}$$

Note that when the synaptic channels are closed (i.e., switch open), g_{syn} is 0 and

$$V_m = E_L.$$

Now consider the case of ligand-gated channels being opened by the release of transmitter from a presynaptic neuron (i.e., switch closed) and a neuron with $g_L = 10$ nS, $E_L = -60$ mV, $g_{syn} = 0.2$ nS, and $E_r = 0$ mV. Then

$$V_m = \frac{(0.2 \times 10^{-9} * 0) + (10 \times 10^{-9} * -60)}{10.2 \times 10^{-9}}$$

$$= -59 \text{ mV}$$

Thus, as a result of the closure of the switch, the membrane potential has changed from its initial value of −60 mV to a new value of −59 mV; i.e., an EPSP of 1 mV has been generated.

The preceding analysis ignored membrane capacitance (C_m), the charging of which makes the synaptic potential slower than the synaptic current. Thus, a more complete analytical description of the postsynaptic factors underlying the generation of a PSP must account for the fact that some of the synaptic current will flow into the capacitive branch of the circuit. Again, by conservation of current, the sum of the currents in the three branches must equal 0. Therefore,

$$0 = C_m \frac{dV_m}{dt} + I_L + I_{syn}, \tag{6}$$

$$0 = C_m \frac{dV_m}{dt} + g_L * (V_m - E_L) + g_{syn}(t) * (V_m - E_r), \tag{7}$$

where $C_m (dV_m/dt)$ is the capacitive current.

By solving for V_m and integrating the differential equation, we can determine the magnitude and time course of a PSP. An accurate description of the kinetics of the PSP requires that the simple switch closure (all-or-none engagement of the synaptic conductance) be replaced with an expression $[g_{syn}(t)]$ that describes the dynamics of the change in synaptic conductance with time.

Nonlinear I–V Relations of Some Ionotropic Receptors

For many PSPs mediated by ionotropic receptors, the current–voltage relation of the synaptic current is linear or approximately linear (Fig. 11.5B). Such ohmic relations are typical of nicotinic ACh channels and non-NMDA (N-methyl-D-aspartate) glutamate channels (as well as many receptors mediating IPSPs). The linear I–V relation is indicative of a channel whose conductance is not affected by the potential across the membrane. Such linearity should be contrasted with the steep voltage dependency of the conductance of channels underlying the initiation and repolarization of action potentials (Chapter 6).

NMDA glutamate channels are a class of ionotropic receptors that have nonlinear current–voltage relations. At negative potentials, the channel conductance is low even when glutamate is bound to the receptor. As the membrane is depolarized, conductance increases and current flowing through the channel increases, resulting in the I–V relation illustrated in Fig. 11.6A. This nonlinearity is represented by an arrow through the resistor representing this synaptic conductance in the equivalent circuit of Fig. 11.6B. The nonlinear I–V relation of the NMDA receptor can be explained by a voltage-dependent block of the channel by Mg^{2+} (Fig. 11.7). At normal values of the resting potential, the pore of the channel is blocked by Mg^{2+}. Thus, even when glutamate binds to the receptor (Fig. 11.7B), the blocked channel prevents ionic flow (and an EPSP). The block can be relieved by depolarization, which presumably displaces Mg^{2+} from the pore (Fig. 11.7B). When the pore is unblocked, cations (i.e., Na^+, K^+, and Ca^{2+}) can flow readily through the channel, and this flux is manifested in the linear part of the I–V relation (Fig. 11.6A). Non-NMDA channels (Fig. 11.7A) are not blocked by Mg^{2+} and have linear I–V relations (Fig. 11.5B).

Inhibitory Postsynaptic Potentials Decrease the Probability of Cell Firing

Some synaptic events decrease the probability of generating action potentials in the postsynaptic cell. Potentials associated with these actions are called inhibitory postsynaptic potentials. Consider the inhibitory interneuron illustrated in Fig. 11.2. Normally, this interneuron is activated by summating EPSPs from converging afferent fibers. These EPSPs summate in space and time such that the membrane potential of the interneuron reaches threshold and fires an action potential. This step can be bypassed by artificially depolarizing the interneuron to initiate an action potential. The consequences of that action potential from the point of view of the flexor motor neuron are illustrated in Fig. 11.2. The action potential in the interneuron produces a transient increase in the membrane potential of the motor neuron. This transient hyperpolarization (the IPSP) looks very much like the EPSP, but it is reversed in sign.

What are the ionic mechanisms for these fast IPSPs and what is the transmitter substance? Because the membrane potential of the flexor motor neuron is about –65 mV, one might expect an increase in the conductance to some ion (or ions) with an equilibrium potential (reversal potential) more negative than –65 mV. One possibility is K^+. Indeed, the K^+ equilibrium potential in spinal motor neurons is about –80 mV; thus, a transmitter substance that produced a selective increase in K^+ conductance would lead to an IPSP. The K^+-conductance increase would move the membrane potential from –65 mV toward the K^+ equilibrium potential of –80 mV. Although an increase in K^+ conductance mediates IPSPs at some inhibitory synapses (see later), it does not at the synapse between the inhibitory interneuron and the spinal motor neuron. At this particular synapse, the IPSP seems to be due to a selective increase in Cl^- conductance. The equilibrium potential for Cl^- in spinal motor neurons is about –70 mV. Thus, the transmitter substance released by the inhibitory neuron diffuses

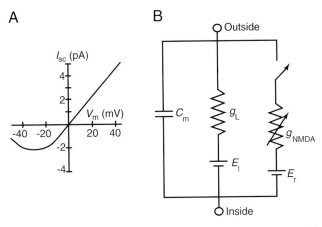

FIGURE 11.6 (A) I–V relation of the NMDA receptor. (B) Equivalent electrical circuit of a membrane containing NMDA receptors.

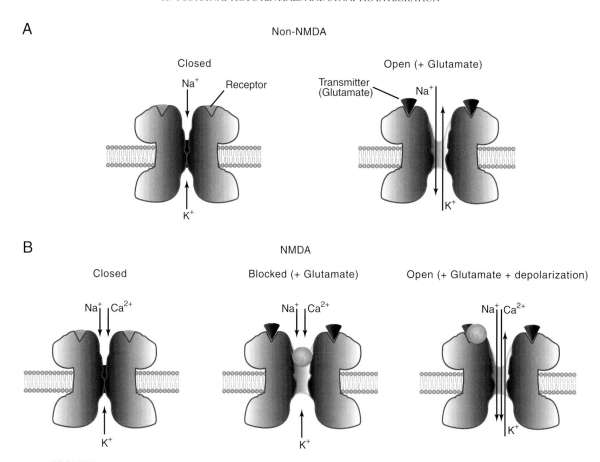

FIGURE 11.7 Features of non-NMDA and NMDA glutamate receptors. (A) Non-NMDA receptors: (left) in the absence of agonist, the channel is closed, and (right) glutamate binding leads to channel opening and an increase in Na^+ and K^+ permeability. (B) NMDA receptors: (left) in the absence of agonist, the channel is closed; (middle) the presence of agonist leads to a conformational change and channel opening, but no ionic flux occurs because the pore of the channel is blocked by Mg^{2+}; and (right) in the presence of depolarization, the Mg^{2+} block is removed and the agonist-induced opening of the channel leads to changes in ion flux (including Ca^{2+} influx into the cell).

across the cleft and interacts with receptor sites on the postsynaptic membrane. These receptors are normally closed, but when opened they become selectively permeable to Cl^-. As a result of the increase in Cl^- conductance, the membrane potential moves from a resting value of -65 mV toward the Cl^- equilibrium potential of -70 mV.

As in the sensory neuron–spinal motor neuron synapse, the transmitter substance released by the inhibitory interneuron in the spinal cord is an amino acid, but in this case the transmitter is glycine. The toxin strychnine is a potent antagonist of glycine receptors. Although glycine was originally thought to be localized to the spinal cord, it is also found in other regions of the nervous system. The most common transmitter associated with inhibitory actions in many areas of the brain is γ–aminobutyric acid (GABA; see Chapter 8).

GABA receptors are divided into three major classes: $GABA_A$, $GABA_B$, and $GABA_C$ (Bormann and

Fiegenspan, 1995; Billinton *et al.*, 2001; Bowery, 1993; Cherubini and Conti, 2001; Gage, 1992; Moss and Smart, 2001). As discussed in Chapter 9, $GABA_A$ receptors are ionotropic receptors, and, like glycine receptors, binding of transmitter leads to an increased conductance to Cl^-, which produces an IPSP. $GABA_A$ receptors are blocked by bicuculline and picrotoxin. A particularly striking aspect of $GABA_A$ receptors is their modulation by anxiolytic benzodiazepines. Figure 11.8 illustrates the response of a neuron to GABA before and after treatment with diazepam (Bormann, 1988). In the presence of diazepam, the response is potentiated greatly. In contrast to $GABA_A$ receptors that are pore-forming channels, $GABA_B$ receptors are G-protein coupled (see also Chapter 9). $GABA_B$ receptors can be coupled to a variety of different effector mechanisms in different neurons. These mechanisms include decreases in Ca^{2+} conductance, increases in K^+ conductance, and modulation of voltage-dependent A-type K^+ current. In hippocampal pyramidal neurons, the $GABA_B$-mediated IPSP is due an increased in K^+ conductance. Baclofen is a potent agonist of $GABA_B$ receptors, whereas phaclofen is a selective antagonist. $GABA_C$ receptors are pharmacologically distinct from $GABA_A$ and $GABA_B$ receptors and are found predominantly in the vertebrate retina. $GABA_C$ receptors, like $GABA_A$ receptors, are Cl^- selective pores.

Ionotropic receptors that lead to the generation of IPSPs and ionotropic receptors that lead to the generation of EPSPs have biophysical features in common. Indeed, analyses of the preceding section are generally applicable. A quantitative understanding of the effects of the opening of glycine or $GABA_A$ receptors can be obtained by using the electrical equivalent circuit of Fig. 11.5C and Eq. (5), with the values of g_{syn} and E_r appropriate for the respective ionotropic receptor. Interactions between excitatory and inhibitory conductances can be modeled by adding additional branches to the equivalent circuit (see Fig. 11.15D and Chapter 12).

Some PSPs Have More Than One Component

The transmitter released from a presynaptic terminal diffuses across the synaptic cleft, where it binds to ionotropic receptors. In many cases, the postsynaptic receptors are homogeneous. In other cases, the same transmitter activates more than one type of receptor. A major example of this type of heterogeneous postsynaptic action is the simultaneous activation by glutamate of NMDA and non-NMDA receptors on the same postsynaptic cell. Figure 11.9 illustrates such a dual-component glutamatergic EPSP in the CA1 region of the hippocampus. The cell is voltage clamped at various fixed holding potentials, and the macroscopic synaptic currents produced by activation of the presynaptic neurons are recorded. The experiment is performed in the presence and absence of the agent 2-amino-5-phosphonovalerate (APV), which is a specific blocker of NMDA receptors. When the cell is held at a potential of 20 or -40 mV, APV leads to a dramatic reduction of the late, but not the early, phase of the excitatory postsynaptic current (EPSC). In contrast, when the potential is held at -80 mV, the EPSC is unaffected by APV. These results indicate that PSP consists of two components: (1) an early non-NMDA component and (2) a late NMDA component. In addition, results indicate that conductance of the non-NMDA component is linear, whereas conductance of the NMDA component is nonlinear. The I–V relations of the early (peak) and late (at approximately 25 ms) components of the EPSC are plotted in Fig. 11.9 (Hestrin *et al.*, 1990). Note the similarity in form of

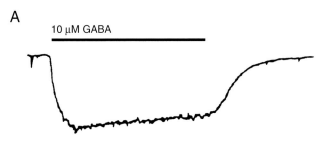

A

10 µM GABA

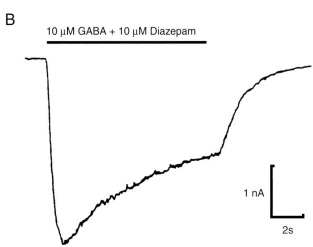

B

10 µM GABA + 10 µM Diazepam

1 nA

2s

FIGURE 11.8 Potentiation of GABA responses by benzodiazepine ligands. (A) Brief application (bar) of GABA leads to an inward Cl^- current in a voltage-clamped spinal neuron. (B) In the presence of diazepam, the response is enhanced significantly. From Bormann (1988).

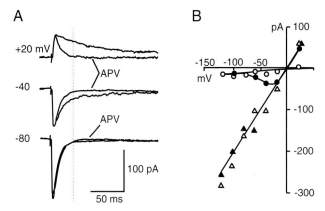

A

+20 mV

-40

APV

-80

APV

100 pA

50 ms

B

pA — 100

-150 -100 -50
mV

-100

-200

-300

FIGURE 11.9 Dual-component glutamatergic EPSP. (A) The excitatory postsynaptic current was recorded before and during the application of APV at the indicated membrane potentials. (B) Peak current–voltage relations are shown before (▲) and during (△) the application of APV. Current–voltage relations measured 25 ms after the peak of the EPSC [dotted line in (A)] before (•) and during (O) application of APV are also shown. Reprinted with permission from Hestrin *et al.* (1990).

these plots of macroscopic currents to the plots of single-channel currents in Figs. 11.5B and 11.6A.

Dual-component IPSPs are also observed in the CNS, but here the transmitter (GABA) that mediates the inhibitory actions may be released from different neurons that converge on a common postsynaptic neuron. Stimulation of afferent pathways to the hippocampus results in an IPSP in a pyramidal neuron, which has a fast initial inhibitory phase followed by a slower inhibitory phase (Fig. 11.10). Application of GABA$_A$ antagonists blocks the early inhibitory phase, whereas the GABA$_B$ receptor antagonist phaclofen blocks the late inhibitory phase (not shown). Early and late IPSPs can also be distinguished based on their ionic mechanisms. Hyperpolarizing the membrane potential to –78 mV nulls the early response, but at this value of membrane potential the late response is still hyperpolarizing (Figs. 11.10A and 11.10B). Hyperpolarizing the membrane potential to values more negative than –78 mV reverses the sign of the early response, but the slow response does not reverse until the membrane is made more negative than about –100 mV (Thalmann, 1988). The reversal

potentials are consistent with a fast Cl⁻-mediated IPSP, mediated by fast opening of GABA$_A$ receptors and a slower K⁺-mediated IPSP mediated by G-protein GABA$_B$ receptors.

Dual-component PSPs need not be strictly inhibitory or excitatory. For example, a presynaptic cholinergic neuron in the mollusk *Aplysia* produces a diphasic excitatory–inhibitory (E–I) response in its postsynaptic follower cell. The response can be simulated by local discrete application of ACh to the postsynaptic cell (Fig. 11.11) (Blankenship *et al.*, 1971). The ionic mechanisms underlying this synaptic action were investigated in ion-substitution experiments, which revealed that the dual response is due to an early Na⁺-dependent component followed by a slower Cl⁻-dependent component. Molecular mechanisms underlying such slow synaptic potentials are discussed next.

Summary

Synaptic potentials mediated by ionotropic receptors are the fundamental means by which information

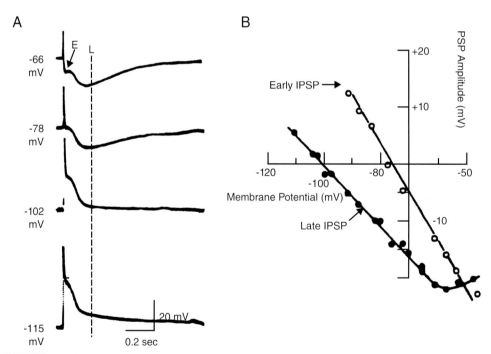

FIGURE 11.10 Dual-component IPSP. (A) Intracellular recordings from a pyramidal cell in the CA3 region of the rat hippocampus in response to activation of mossy fiber afferents. With the membrane potential of the cell at the resting potential, afferent stimulation produces an early (E) and late (L) IPSP. With increased hyperpolarizing produced by injecting constant current into the cell, the early component reverses first. At more negative levels of the membrane potential, the late component also reverses. This indicates that the ionic conductance underlying the two phases is distinct. (B) Plots of the change in amplitude of the early (measured at 25 ms) and the late (measured at 200 ms, dashed line in A) response as a function of membrane potential. Reversal potentials of the early and late components are consistent with a GABA$_A$-mediated chloride conductance and a GABA$_B$-mediated potassium conductance, respectively. From Thalmann (1988).

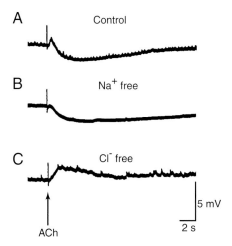

FIGURE 11.11 Dual-component cholinergic excitatory–inhibitory response. (A) Control in normal saline. Ejection of ACh produces a rapid depolarization followed by a slower hyperpolarization. (B) In Na$^+$-free saline, ACh produces a purely hyperpolarizing response, indicating that the depolarizing component in normal saline includes an increase in g_{Na}. (C) In Cl–free saline, ACh produces a purely depolarizing response, indicating that the hyperpolarizing component in normal saline includes an increase in g_{Cl}. Reprinted with permission from Blankenship *et al.* (1971).

is transmitted rapidly between neurons. Transmitters cause channels to open in an all-or-none fashion, and the currents through these individual channels summate to produce the macrosynaptic postsynaptic potential. The sign of the postsynaptic potential is determined by the relationship between the membrane potential of the postsynaptic neuron and the ion selectivity of the ionotropic receptor.

METABOTROPIC RECEPTORS: MEDIATORS OF SLOW SYNAPTIC POTENTIALS

A common feature of the types of synaptic actions heretofore described is the direct binding of the transmitter with the receptor–channel complex. An entirely separate class of synaptic actions has as its basis the indirect coupling of the receptor with the channel. So far, two types of coupling mechanisms have been identified: (1) coupling of the receptor and channel through an intermediate regulatory protein, such as a G-protein; and (2) coupling through a diffusible second-messenger system. Because coupling through a diffusible second-messenger system is the most common mechanism, it is the focus of this section.

A comparison of the features of direct, fast ionotropic-mediated and indirect, slow metabotropic-mediated synaptic potentials is shown in Fig. 11.12.

Slow synaptic potentials are not observed at every postsynaptic neuron, but Fig. 11.12A illustrates an idealized case in which a postsynaptic neuron receives two inputs, one of which produces a conventional fast EPSP and the other of which produces a slow EPSP. An action potential in neuron 1 leads to an EPSP in the postsynaptic cell with a duration of about 30 ms (Fig. 11.12B). This type of potential might be produced in a spinal motor neuron by an action potential in an afferent fiber. Neuron 2 also produces a postsynaptic potential (Fig. 11.12C), but its duration (note the calibration bar) is more than three orders of magnitude greater than that of the EPSP produced by neuron 1.

How can a change in the postsynaptic potential of a neuron persist for many minutes as a result of a single action potential in the presynaptic neuron? Possibilities include a prolonged presence of the transmitter

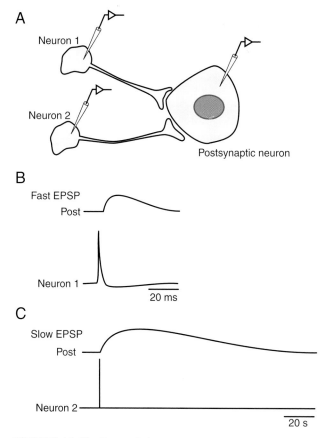

FIGURE 11.12 Fast and slow synaptic potentials. (A) Idealized experiment in which two neurons (1 and 2) make synaptic connections with a common postsynaptic follower cell (Post). (B) An action potential in neuron 1 leads to a conventional fast EPSP with a duration of about 30 ms. (C) An action potential in neuron 2 also produces an EPSP in the postsynaptic cell, but the duration of this slow EPSP is more than three orders of magnitude greater than that of the EPSP produced by neuron 1. Note the change in the calibration bar.

due to continuous release, to slow degradation, or to slow reuptake of the transmitter, but the mechanism here involves a transmitter-induced change in the metabolism of the postsynaptic cell. Figure 11.13 compares the general mechanisms for fast and slow synaptic potentials. Fast synaptic potentials are produced when a transmitter substance binds to a channel and produces a conformational change in the channel, causing it to become permeable to one or more ions (both Na^+ and K^+ in Fig. 11.13A). The increase in permeability leads to a depolarization associated with the EPSP. The duration of the synaptic event critically depends on the amount of time during which the transmitter substance remains bound to the receptors. Acetylcholine, glutamate, and glycine remain bound only for a very short period. These transmitters are removed by diffusion, enzymatic breakdown, or reuptake into the presynaptic cell. Therefore, the duration of the synaptic potential is directly related to the lifetimes of the opened channels, and these lifetimes are relatively short (see Fig. 11.4B).

One mechanism for a slow synaptic potential is shown in Fig. 11.13B. In contrast with the fast PSP for which the receptors are actually part of the ion channel complex, channels that produce slow synaptic potentials are not coupled directly to the transmitter receptors. Rather, the receptors are separated physically and exert their actions indirectly through changes in metabolism of specific second-messenger systems. Figure 11.13B illustrates one type of response in *Aplysia* for which the cAMP–protein kinase A (PKA) system is the mediator, but other slow PSPs use other second-messenger kinase systems (e.g., the protein kinase C system). In the cAMP-dependent slow synaptic responses in *Aplysia*, transmitter binding to membrane receptors activates G-proteins and stimulates an increase in the synthesis of cAMP. Cyclic AMP then leads to the activation of cAMP-dependent protein kinase (PKA), which phosphorylates a channel protein or protein associated with the channel (Siegelbaum *et al.*, 1982). A conformational change in the channel is produced, leading to a change in ionic conductance. Thus, in contrast with a direct conformational change produced by the binding of a transmitter to the receptor–channel complex, in this case, a conformational change is produced by protein phosphorylation. Indeed, phosphorylation-dependent channel regulation is a fairly general feature of slow PSPs. However, channel regulation by second messengers is not produced exclusively by phosphorylation. In one family of ion channels, the channels are gated or regulated directly by cyclic nucleotides. These cyclic nucleotide-gated channels require cAMP or cGMP to open but have other features in common with members of the superfamily of voltage-gated ion channels (Kaupp, 1995; Zimmermann, 1995).

Another interesting feature of slow synaptic responses is that they are sometimes associated with decreases rather than increases in membrane conductance. For example, the particular channel illustrated in Fig. 11.13B is selectively permeable to K^+ and is normally open. As a result of the activation of the second messenger, the channel closes and becomes less permeable to K^+. The resultant depolarization may seem paradoxical, but recall that the membrane potential is due to a balance between resting K^+ and Na^+ permeability. K^+ permeability tends to move the membrane potential toward the K^+ equilibrium potential (–80 mV), whereas Na^+ permeability tends to move the membrane potential toward the Na^+ equilibrium potential (55 mV). Normally, K^+ permeability predominates, and the resting membrane potential is close to, but not equal to, the K^+ equilibrium potential. If K^+ permeability is decreased because some of the channels close, the membrane potential will be biased toward the Na^+ equilibrium potential and the cell will depolarize.

At least one reason for the long duration of slow PSPs is that second-messenger systems are slow (from seconds to minutes). Take the cAMP cascade as an example. Cyclic AMP takes some time to be synthesized, but, more importantly, after synthesis, cAMP levels can remain elevated for a relatively long period (minutes). The duration of the elevation of cAMP depends on the actions of cAMP-phosphodiesterase, which breaks down cAMP. However, duration of an effect could outlast the duration of the change in the second messenger because of persistent phosphorylation of the substrate protein(s). Phosphate groups are removed from substrate proteins by protein phosphatases. Thus, the net duration of a response initiated by a metabotropic receptor depends on the actions of not only the synthetic and phosphorylation processes, but also the degradative and dephosphorylation processes.

Activation of a second messenger by a transmitter can have a localized effect on the membrane potential through phosphorylation of membrane channels near the site of a metabotropic receptor. The effects can be more widespread and even longer lasting than depicted in Fig. 11.13B. For example, second messengers and protein kinases can diffuse and affect more-distant membrane channels. Moreover, a long-term effect can be induced in the cell by altering gene expression. For example, protein kinase A can diffuse to the nucleus, where it can activate proteins that regulate gene expression. Detailed descriptions of

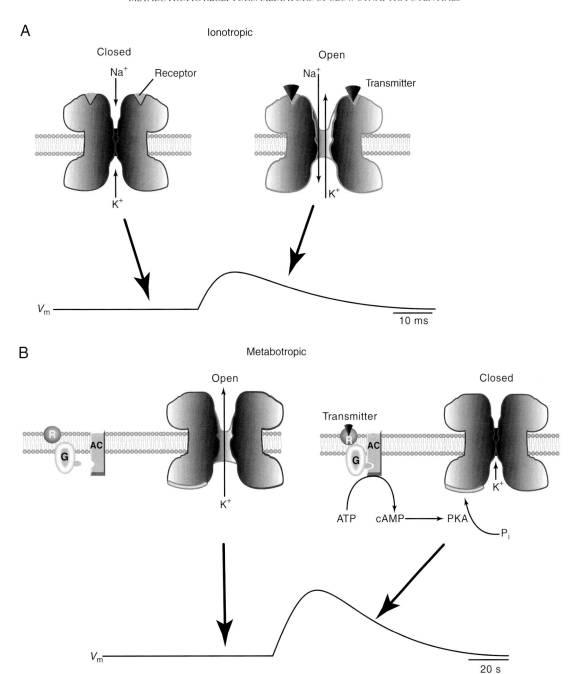

FIGURE 11.13 Ionotropic and metabotropic receptors and mechanisms of fast and slow EPSPs. (A, left) Fast EPSPs are produced by binding of the transmitter to specialized receptors that are directly associated with an ion channel (i.e., a ligand-gated channel). When the receptors are unbound, the channel is closed. (A, right) Binding of the transmitter to the receptor produces a conformational change in the channel protein such that the channel opens. In this example, the channel opening is associated with a selective increase in the permeability to Na^+ and K^+. The increase in permeability results in the EPSP shown in the trace. (B, left) Unlike fast EPSPs, which are due to the binding of a transmitter with a receptor–channel complex, slow EPSPs are due to the activation of receptors (metabotropic) that are not coupled directly to the channel. Rather, coupling takes place through the activation of one of several second-messenger cascades, in this example, the cAMP cascade. A channel that has a selective permeability to K^+ is normally open. (B, right) Binding of the transmitter to the receptor (R) leads to the activation of a G-protein (G) and adenylyl cyclase (AC). The synthesis of cAMP is increased, cAMP-dependent protein kinase (protein kinase A, PKA) is activated, and a channel protein is phosphorylated. The phosphorylation leads to closing of the channel and the subsequent depolarization associated with the slow EPSP shown in the trace. The response decays due to both the breakdown of cAMP by cAMP-dependent phosphodiesterase and the removal of phosphate from channel proteins by protein phosphatases (not shown).

second messengers and their actions are given in Chapter 10.

Summary

In contrast to the rapid responses mediated by ionotropic receptors, responses mediated by metabotropic receptors are generally relatively slow to develop and persistent. These properties arise because metabotropic responses can involve the activation of second-messenger systems. By producing slow changes in the resting potential, metabotropic receptors provide long-term modulation of the effectiveness of responses generated by ionotropic receptors. Moreover, these receptors, through the engagement of second-messenger systems, provide a vehicle by which a presynaptic cell cannot only alter the membrane potential, but also produce widespread changes in the biochemical state of a postsynaptic cell.

INTEGRATION OF SYNAPTIC POTENTIALS

The small amplitude of the EPSP in spinal motor neurons (and other cells in the CNS) poses an interesting question. Specifically, how can an EPSP with an amplitude of only 1 mV drive the membrane potential of the motor neuron (i.e., the postsynaptic neuron) to threshold and fire the spike in the motor neuron that is necessary to produce the contraction of the muscle? The answer to this question lies in the principles of temporal and spatial summation.

When the ligament is stretched (Fig. 11.1), many stretch receptors are activated. Indeed, the greater the stretch, the greater the probability of activating a larger number of the stretch receptors; this process is referred to as recruitment. However, recruitment is not the complete story. The principle of frequency coding in the

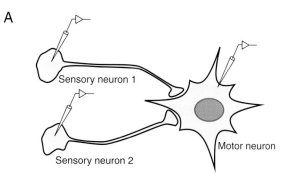

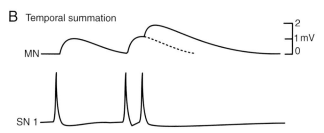

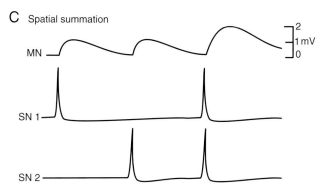

FIGURE 11.14 Temporal and spatial summation. (A) Intracellular recordings are made from two idealized sensory neurons (SN1 and SN2) and a motor neuron (MN). (B) Temporal summation. A single action potential in SN1 produces a 1-mV EPSP in the MN. Two action potentials in quick succession produce a dual-component EPSP, the amplitude of which is approximately 2 mV. (C) Spatial summation. Alternative firing of single action potentials in SN1 and SN2 produce 1-mV EPSPs in the MN. Simultaneous action potentials in SN1 and SN2 produce a summated EPSP, the amplitude of which is about 2 mV.

FIGURE 11.15 Modeling the integrative properties of a neuron. (A) Partial geometry of a neuron in the CNS revealing the cell body and pattern of dendritic branching. (B) The neuron modeled as a sphere connected to a series of cylinders, each of which represents the specific electrical properties of a dendritic segment. (C) Segments linked with resistors representing the intracellular resistance between segments, with each segment represented by the parallel combination of the membrane capacitance and the total membrane conductance. Reprinted with permission from Koch and Segev (1989). Copyright 1989 MIT Press. (D) Electrical circuit equivalent of the membrane of a segment of a neuron. The segment has a membrane potential V and a membrane capacitance C_m. Currents arise from three sources: (1) m voltage-dependent conductances ($g_{vd_1}-g_{vd_m}$), (2) n conductances due to electrical synapses ($g_{es_1}-g_{es_n}$), and (3) n times o time-dependent conductances due to chemical synapses with each of the n presynaptic neurons ($g_{cs_{1,1}}-g_{cs_{n,o}}$). E_{vd} and E_{cs} are constants and represent the values of the equilibrium potential for currents due to voltage-dependent conductances and chemical synapses, respectively. V_1-V_n represent the value of the membrane potential of the coupled cells. Reprinted with permission from Ziv et al. (1994).

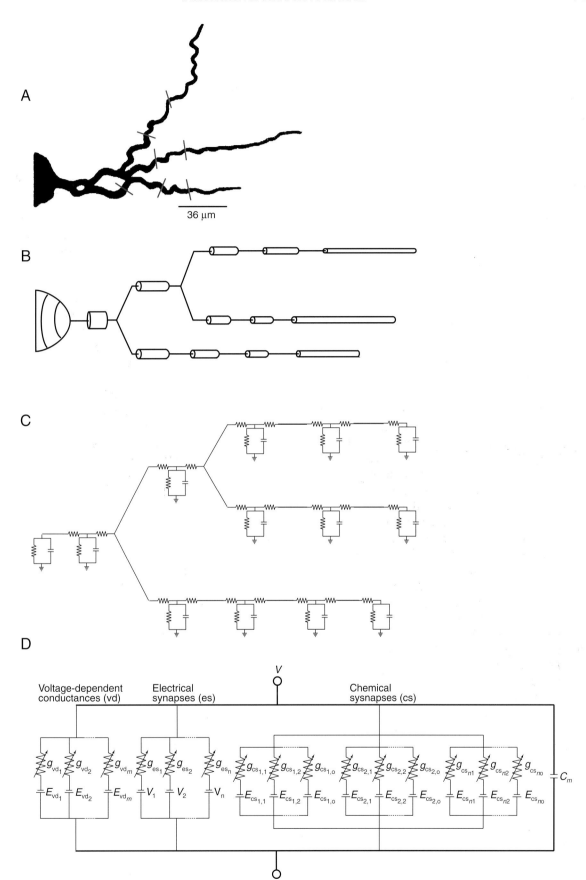

A

36 μm

B

C

D

Voltage-dependent   Electrical   Chemical
conductances (vd)   synapses (es)   sysnapses (cs)

nervous system specifies that the greater the intensity of a stimulus, the greater the number of action potentials per unit time (frequency) elicited in a sensory neuron. This principle applies to stretch receptors as well. Thus, the greater the stretch, the greater the number of action potentials elicited in the stretch receptor in a given interval and therefore the greater the number of EPSPs produced in the motor neuron from that train of action potentials in the sensory cell. Consequently, the effects of activating multiple stretch receptors add together (spatial summation), as do the effects of multiple EPSPs elicited by activation of a single stretch receptor (temporal summation). Both of these processes act in concert to depolarize the motor neuron sufficiently to elicit one or more action potentials, which then propagate to the periphery and produce the reflex.

Temporal Summation Allows Integration of Successive PSPs

Temporal summation can be illustrated by firing action potentials in a presynaptic neuron and monitoring the resultant EPSPs. For example, in Figs. 11.14A and 11.14B, a single action potential in sensory neuron 1 produces a 1-mV EPSP in the motor neuron. Two action potentials in quick succession produce two EPSPs, but note that the second EPSP occurs during the falling phase of the first, and the depolarization associated with the second EPSP adds to the depolarization produced by the first. Thus, two action potentials produce a summated potential that is about 2 mV in amplitude. Three action potentials in quick succession would produce a summated potential of about 3 mV. In principle, 30 action potentials in quick succession would produce a potential of about 30 mV and easily drive the cell to threshold. This summation is strictly a passive property of the cell. No special ionic conductance mechanisms are necessary. Specifically, the postsynaptic conductance change [g_{syn} in Eq. (3)] produced by the second of two successive action potentials adds to that produced by the first. In addition, the postsynaptic membrane has a capacitance and can store charge. Thus, the membrane temporarily stores the charge of the first EPSP, and the charge from the second EPSP is added to that of the first. However, the "time window" for this process of temporal summation very much depends on the duration of the postsynaptic potential, and temporal summation is possible only if the presynaptic action potentials (and hence postsynaptic potentials) are close in time to each other. The time frame depends on the duration of changes in the synaptic conductance and the time constant (Chapter 5). Temporal summation, however, is rarely observed to be linear as

in the preceding examples, even when the postsynaptic conductance change [g_{syn} in Eq. (3)] produced by the second of two successive action potentials is identical with that produced by the first (i.e., no presynaptic facilitation or depression) and the synaptic current is slightly less because the first PSP reduces the driving force (V_m–E_r) for the second. Interested readers should try some numerical examples.

Spatial Summation Allows Integration of PSPs from Different Parts of a Neuron

Spatial summation (Fig. 11.14C) requires a consideration of more than one input to a postsynaptic neuron. An action potential in sensory neuron 1 produces a 1-mV EPSP, just as it did in Fig. 11.14B. Similarly, an action potential in a second sensory neuron by itself also produces a 1-mV EPSP. Now, consider the consequences of action potentials elicited simultaneously in sensory neurons 1 and 2. The net EPSP is equal to the summation of the amplitudes of the individual EPSPs. Here, the EPSP from sensory neuron 1 is 1 mV, the EPSP from sensory neuron 2 is 1 mV, and the summated EPSP is approximately 2 mV (Fig. 11.14C). Thus, spatial summation is a mechanism by which synaptic potentials generated at different sites can summate. Spatial summation in nerve cells is influenced by the space constant—the ability of a potential change produced in one region of a cell to spread passively to other regions of a cell (see Chapter 5).

Summary

Whether a neuron fires in response to synaptic input depends, at least in part, on how many action potentials are produced in any one presynaptic excitatory pathway and on how many individual convergent excitatory input pathways are activated. The summation of EPSPs in time and space is only part of the process, however. The final behavior of the cell is also due to the summation of inhibitory synaptic inputs in time and space, as well as to the properties of the voltage-dependent currents (Fig. 11.15) in the soma and along the dendrites (Koch and Segev, 1989; Ziv et al., 1994). For example, voltage-dependent conductances such as A-type K+ conductance have a low threshold for activation and can thus oppose the effectiveness of an EPSP to trigger a spike. Low-threshold Na+ and Ca2+ channels can boost an EPSP. Finally, we need to consider that spatial distribution of the various voltage-dependent channels, ligand-gated receptors, and metabotropic receptors is not uniform. Thus, each segment of the neuronal membrane can perform selective integrative functions.

Clearly, this system has an enormous capacity for the local processing of information and for performing logical operations. The flow of information in dendrites and the local processing of neuronal signals are discussed in Chapter 12.

References

Billinton, A., Ige, A. O., Bolam, J. P., White, J. H., Marshall, F. H., and Emson, P.C. (2001). Advances in the molecular understanding of GABA$_B$ receptors. *Trends Neurosci.* **24**, 277–282.

Blankenship, J. E., Wachtel, H., and Kandel, E. R. (1971). Ionic mechanisms of excitatory, inhibitory and dual synaptic actions mediated by an identified interneuron in abdominal ganglion of *Aplysia. J. Neurophysiol.* **34**, 76–92.

Bormann, J. (1988). Electrophysiology of GABA$_A$ and GABA$_B$ receptor subtypes. *Trends Neurosci.* **11**, 112–116.

Bormann, J., and Feigenspan, A. (1995). GABA$_C$ receptors. *Trends Neurosci.* **18**, 515–519.

Bowery, N. G. (1993). GABA$_B$ receptor pharmacology. *Annu. Rev. Pharmacol. Toxicol.* **33**, 109–147.

Cherubini, E., and Conti, F. (2001). Generating diversity at GABAergic synapses. *Trends Neurosci.* **24**, 155–162.

Eccles, J. C. (1964). "The Physiology of Synapses." Springer-Verlag, New York.

Fatt, P., and Katz, B. (1951). An analysis of the end-plate potential recorded with an intra cellular electrode. *J. Physiol. (Lond.)* **115**, 320–370.

Gage, P. W. (2001). Activation and modulation of neuronal K$^+$ channels by GABA. *Trends Neurosci.* **15**, 46–51.

Hamill, O. P., Marty, A., Neher, E., Sakmann, B., and Sigworth, J. (1981). Improved patch-clamp techniques for high-resolution current recording from cells and cell-free membrane patches. *Pflüg Arch.* **391**, 85–100.

Hestrin, S., Nicoll, R. A., Perkel, D. J., and Sah, P. (1990). Analysis of excitatory synaptic action in pyramidal cells using whole-cell recording from rat hippocampal slices. *J. Physiol. (Lond.)* **422**, 203–225.

Johnston, D., and Wu, S. M.-S. (1995). "Foundations of Cellular Neurophysiology." MIT Press, Cambridge, MA.

Kaupp, U. B. (1995). Family of cyclic nucleotide gated ion channels. *Curr. Opin. Neurobiol.* **5**, 434–442.

Koch, C., and Segev, I. (1989). "Methods in Neuronal Modeling." MIT Press, Cambridge, MA.

Moss, S. J., and Smart, T. G. (2001). Constructing inhibitory synapses. *Nature Rev. Neurosci.* **2**, 240–250.

Sakmann, B. (1992). Elementary steps in synaptic transmission revealed by currents through single ion channels. *Science* **256**, 503–512.

Siegelbaum, S. A., Camardo, J. S., and Kandel, E. R. (1982). Serotonin and cyclic AMP close single K$^+$ channels in *Aplysia* sensory neurones. *Nature (Lond.)* **299**, 413–417.

Spencer, W. A. (1977). The physiology of supraspinal neurons in mammals. *In* "Handbook of Physiology" (E. R. Kandel, Ed.), Vol. 1, Part 2, Sect. 1, pp. 969–1022. American Physiological Society, Bethesda, MD.

Takeuchi, A., and Takeuchi, N. (1960). On the permeability of end-plate membrane during the action of transmitter. *J. Physiol. (Lond.)* **154**, 52–67.

Thalmann, R. H. (1988). Evidence that guanosine triphosphate (GTP)-binding proteins control a synaptic response in brain: Effect of pertussis toxin and GTPγS on the late inhibitory postsynaptic potential of hippocampal CA3 neurons. *J. Neurosci.* **8**, 4589–4602.

Zimmermann, A. L. (1995). Cyclic nucleotide gated channels. *Curr. Opin. Neurobiol.* **5**, 296–303.

Ziv, I., Baxter, D. A., and Byrne, J. H. (1994). Simulator for neural networks and action potentials: Description and application. *J. Neurophysiol.* **71**, 294–308.

Suggested Readings

Burke, R. E. and Rudomin, P. (1977). Spatial neurons and synapses. *In* "Handbook of Physiology" (E. R. Kandel, ed.), Sect. 1, Vol. 1, Part 2, pp. 877–944. American Physiological Society, Bethesda, MD.

Byrne, J. H., and Schultz, S. G. (1994). "An Introduction to Membrane Transport and Bioelectricity," 2nd Ed. Raven Press, New York.

Cowan, W. M., Sudhof, T. C., and Stevens, C. F., eds. (2001). "Synapses." Johns Hopkins Univ. Press.

Hille, B., ed. (2001). "Ion Channels of Excitable Membranes," 3rd Ed. Sinauer, Sunderland, MA.

Shepherd, G. M., ed. (2001). "The Synaptic Organization of the Brain," 4th Ed. Oxford Univ. Press, New York.

John H. Byrne

12

Information Processing in Complex Dendrites

One of the hallmarks of neurons is the variety of their dendrites. The branching patterns are dazzling and the range of size is astounding, from the large trees of cortical pyramidal neurons to the tiny size of a retinal bipolar cell, which would fit comfortably within the cell body of a pyramidal neuron (see Fig. 12.1)! The functions of these dendritic trees have drawn increasing interest in recent years(Segev *et al.*, 1995; Yuste and Tank, 1996; Wilson, 1998; Stuart *et al.*, 1999; Segev and London, 2000; Matus and Shepherd, 2000; Stern and Marx, 2000). The fundamental questions asked in this chapter are (1) what are the principles of information processing in complex dendritic trees and (2) how are they adapted for the specific operational tasks of a particular type of dendrite?

STRATEGIES FOR STUDYING COMPLEX DENDRITES

As we discussed in Chapter 5, the neuron processes information through five basic types of activity: intrinsic, reception, integration, encoding, and output. Understanding how these activities are integrated within the neuron starts with the rules of passive current spread. We now ask how active, voltage-gated channels are involved in *complex information processing*, particularly within branching dendritic trees.

Many of the principles were first worked out in the dendrites of neurons that lack axons or the ability to generate action potentials. There are many examples in invertebrate ganglia. In vertebrates, they include the retinal amacrine cell and the olfactory

granule cell. Studies of these neurons are covered in Shepherd (1991). In summary, a dendritic tree by itself is capable of performing many of the basic functions required for information processing, such as the generation of intrinsic activity, input-output functions for feature extraction, parallel processing, signal-to-noise enhancement, and oscillatory activity. These cells demonstrate that there is no one thing that dendrites do; they do whatever is required to process information within their particular neuron or neuronal circuit.

Information in dendrites can take many forms. There are actions of neuropeptides on membrane receptors and internal cytoplasmic or nuclear receptors; actions of second and third messengers within the neuron; movement of substances within the dendrites by diffusion or by active transport; and changes occurring during development. All of these types of cellular traffic and information flow in dendrites are coming under direct study (Stuart *et al.*, 1999; Matus and Shepherd, 2000). The student should review these subjects in earlier chapters. This chapter focuses on information processing involving electrical signaling mechanisms by synapses and voltage-gated channels and considers how this takes place in neurons with axons.

Among cells with axons, long axon (output) cells tend to be larger than short axon (local) cells and have therefore been more accessible to experimental analysis. Indeed, virtually everything known about the functional relations between dendrites and axons has been obtained from studies of long axon cells. Much of what we think we understand about those relations in short axon cells is only by inference.

319

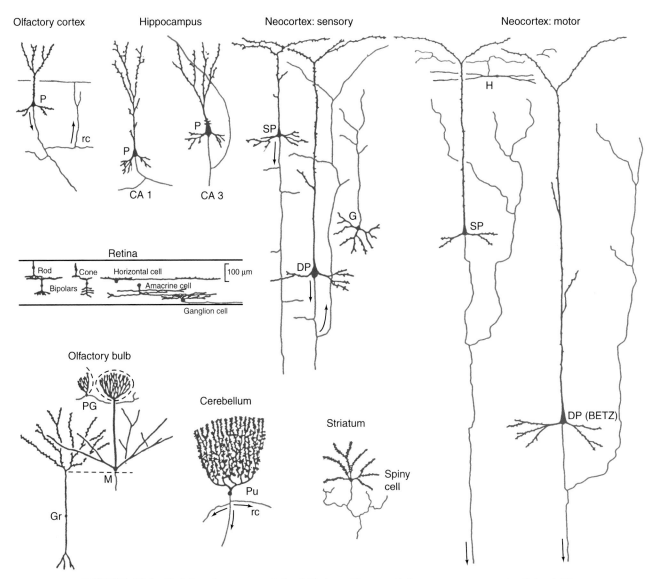

FIGURE 12.1 Varieties of neurons and dendritic trees. P, pyramidal neuron; rc, recurrent collateral; SP, small pyramidal neuron; DP, deep pyramidal neuron; G, granule cell; Gr, granule cell (olfactory); M, mitral cell; PG, periglomerular cell; Pn, Purkinje cell. Modified from Shepherd (1992).

As in the analysis of the passive properties of neurons, there are a number of sites on the web that support the computational analysis of complex neurons and their active dendrites; for orientation, consult senselab. med. yale. edu/move/db.

AN AXON PLACES CONSTRAINTS ON DENDRITIC PROCESSING

We immediately recognize that the presence of an axon places critical constraints on dendritic processing (Fig. 12.2).

The first principle is: **if a neuron has an axon, it has only one**. This near universal single axon rule is remarkable and still little understood. It results from developmental mechanisms that provide for differentiation of a single axon from among early undifferentiated processes; these mechanisms are especially being analyzed in neuronal cultures (Craig and Banker, 1994). The principle, which can be regarded virtually as a law for neurons, means that for dendritic integration to lead to output from the neuron to distant targets, all of the activity within the dendrites must eventually be funneled into the origin of the axon in the single axon hillock. Therefore, in these cells the flow of information in dendrites has an overall orientation, just as sur-

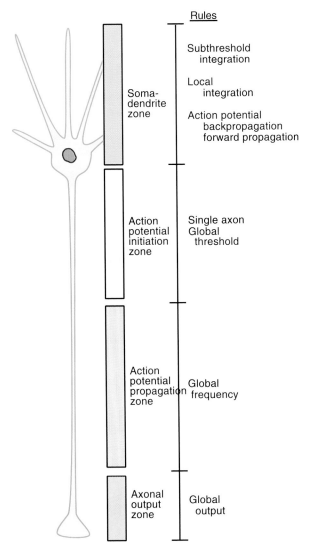

FIGURE 12.2 The presence of a single axon forces several organizational rules onto a neuron. See text for details.

mised by the classical neuroanatomists. We thus have a principle of **global output**.

> In order to transfer information between regions, the information distributed at different sites within a dendritic tree of an output neuron must be encoded. for global output at a single site at the origin of the axon.

A related principle, and virtually another universal rule, is that the main function of the axon in long axon cells is to support the generation of action potentials in the axon hillock-initial segment region. By definition, action potentials have thresholds for generation; thus, the principle of **frequency encoding of global output** in an axonal neuron is:

> The results of dendritic integration affect the output through the axon only by initiating or modulating action

potential generation in the axon hillock-initial segment. Global output from dendritic integration is therefore encoded in impulse frequency in a single axon.

A further consequence of the spatial separation of dendrites and axon is the presence of **subthreshold dendritic activity**:

> A considerable amount of subthreshold activity, including local active potentials, can affect the integrative states of the dendrites and their local outputs but not necessarily directly or immediately affect the global output of the neuron.

We turn now to the functional properties that allow dendritic trees to process information within these constraints.

DENDRODENDRITIC INTERACTIONS BETWEEN AXONAL CELLS

We first recognize that with axonal cells, as with anaxonal cells, output can be through the dendrites (see principle of subthreshold dendritic activity discussed earlier). This is against the common wisdom, which assumes that if a neuron has an axon, all the output goes through the axon. There are many examples in invertebrates.

Neurite–Neurite Synapses in Lobster Stomatogastric Ganglion

One of the first examples in invertebrates was in the stomatogastric ganglion of the lobster (Selverson *et al.*, 1976). Neurons were recorded intracellularly and stained with Procion yellow. Serial electron micrographic reconstructions showed the synaptic relations between stained varicosities in the processes and their neighbors (the processes are equivalent to dendrites, but are often referred to as neurites in theinvertebrate literature). In many cases, a varicosity could be seen to be not only presynaptic to a neighboring varicosity, but also postsynaptic to that same process. It was concluded that synaptic inputs and outputs are distributed over the entire neuritic arborization. Polarization was not from one part of the tree to another. "Bifunctional" varicosities appeared to act as local input–output units, similar to the manner in which granule cell spines appear to operate (see later). Similar organization has been found in other types of stomatogastric neurons (Fig. 12.3A).

Sets of these local input–output units, distributed throughout the neuritic tree, participate in the generation and coordination of oscillatory activity involved

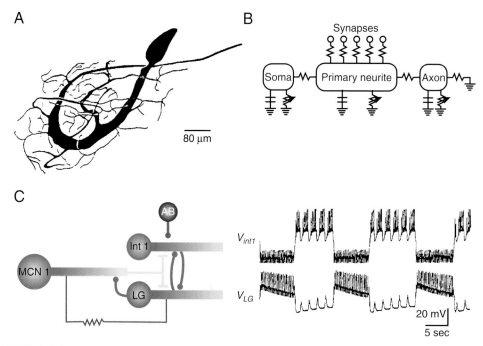

FIGURE 12.3   Local synaptic input–output sites are widely found within the neuropil of invertebrate ganglia. (A) Output neuron with many neurite branches in the gastric mill ganglion of the lobster, (B) compartmental representation of stomatogastric neuron, (C) model of rhythm generating circuit of the gastric mill of the lobster, involving neurite–neurite interactions. A and B from Golowasch and Marder (1992); C from Manor *et al.* (1999).

in controlling the rhythmic movements of the stomach. In a current model of this oscillatory circuit, these interactions are mutually inhibitory (Fig. 12.3B).

In summary, **a cell with an axon can have local outputs through its dendrites as well as its axon**, which may be involved in specific functions such as oscillatory circuits.

PASSIVE DENDRITIC TREES CAN PERFORM COMPLEX COMPUTATIONS

Another principle that carries over from axonless nonspiking cells is the ability of axonal cells to carry out complex computations in dendritic trees with mostly passive properties. This is exemplified by neurons that are motion detectors.

Motion detection is a fundamental operation carried out by the nervous systems of most species; it is essential for detecting prey and predator alike. In invertebrates, motion detection has been studied especially in the brain of the blowfly. In the lobula plate of the third optic neuropil are tangential cells (LPTCs) that respond to preferential direction (PD) of motion with increased depolarization due to sequential responses across their dendritic fields. This response has been modeled by Reichardt and colleagues by a

series of elementary motion detectors (EMDs) in the dendrites. A compartmental model (Single and Borst, 1998) reproduces the experimental results and theoretical predictions by showing how local modulations at each EMD are smoothed by integration in the dendritic tree to give a smoothed high-fidelity global output at the axon (see Fig. 12.4A). In the model, spatial integration is largely independent of specific electrotonic properties but depends critically on the geometry and orientation of the dendritic tree.

In vertebrates, motion detection is built into the visual pathway at various stages in different species, principally the retina, midbrain (optic tectum), and cerebral cortex. Studies in the optic tectum have revealed cells with splayed uniplanar dendritic trees and specialized distal appendages that appear highly homologous across reptiles, birds, and mammals (Fig. 12.4B) (Luksch *et al.*, 1998). These are presumed to mediate motion detection. Physiological studies are needed to test the hypothesis that these cells perform operations through their dendritic fields similar to those of LPTC cells in the insect. To the extent that this is borne out, it will support a principle of **motion detection through spatially distributed dendritic computations** that is conserved across vertebrates and invertebrates. This kind of directional selectivity of dendritic processing was predicted by Rall (1964) from his studies of dendritic electrotonus (see Chapter 5).

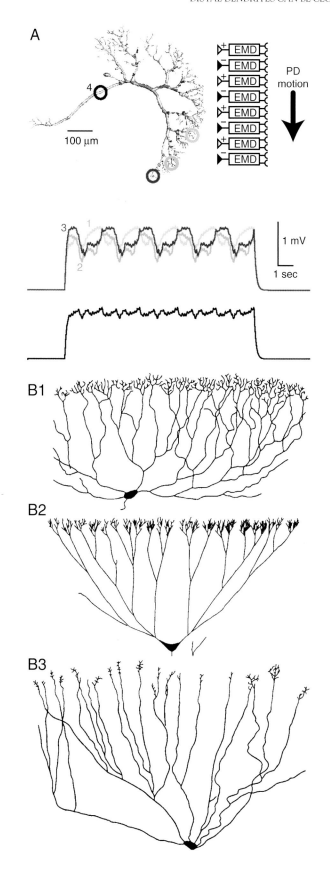

DISTAL DENDRITES CAN BE CLOSELY LINKED TO AXONAL OUTPUT

An obvious problem for a neuron with an axon is that the distal branches of dendritic trees are a long distance from the site of axon origin at or near the cell body. As mentioned earlier, the common perception is that these distal dendrites are too distant from the site of axonal origin and impulse generation to have more than a slow and weak background modulation of impulse output.

This perception is disproved by many kinds of neurons in which specific inputs are located preferentially on their distal dendrites. Such is true of the mitral and tufted cells in the olfactory bulb, where the input from the olfactory nerves ends on the most distal dendritic branches in the glomeruli; in rat mitral cells, this may be 400–500 μm or more from the cell body, in turtle, 600–700 μm. The same applies to their targets, the pyramidal neurons of the olfactory cortex, where the input terminates on the spines of the most distal dendrites in layer I. In many other neurons, a given type of input terminates over much or all of the dendritic tree; such is the case, for example, for climbing fiber and parallel fiber inputs to the cerebellar Purkinje cells. The relative significance of the more distal inputs in these cells is not so apparent. All of these examples are shown in Fig. 12.1.

How do distal dendrites effectively control axonal output? We consider several important properties.

Large Synaptic Conductances

Of key importance is the amplitude of the conductance generated by the synapse itself (Fig. 12.5A). In motor neurons, conductances of the most distal excitatory synapses may be many times the amplitude of proximal synapses (Redman and Walmsley, 1983). This would account for the fact that the peak unitary synaptic response recorded at the soma varies in time course according to synaptic location but has a constant amplitude of approximately 100 μV (Fig. 12.5A).

FIGURE 12.4 Dendritic systems as motion detectors. (A) A computational model of a motion detector neuron in the visual system of the fly, consisting of elementary motion detector (EMD) units in its dendritic tree activated by the preferential direction (PD) of motion. Local modulations of the individual EMDs are integrated in the dendritic tree to give smooth global output in the axon (Single and Borst, 1998). (B) Dendritic trees of neurons in the optic tectum of lizard (B1), chick (B2), and gray squirrel (B3). The architecture of the dendritic branching patterns and distal specialization for the reception of retinal inputs is highly homologous [references in Luksch *et al.* (1998)].

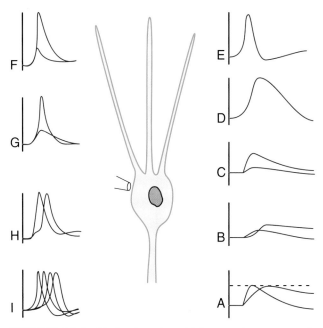

FIGURE 12.5 Mechanisms by which synaptic responses in distal dendrites can have an enhanced effect in controlling impulse output from the axon-hillock-initial segment region. Schematized neuron with patch recording from the soma. (A) Larger distal syaptic conductances (the response is slower because of the electrotonic delay in the intervening dendrites). (B) Higher membrane resistance (the response is slowed by the larger time constant). Voltage-gated channels may increase EPSP amplitude (C), give rise to slow action potentials (D), give rise to forward propagating full action potentials (E), set up fast prepotentials (F), or function as coincidence detectors (G), which give rise to "pseudosaltatory conduction" toward the soma through individual sites (H) or clusters (I). (see text).

Studies have provided evidence for a similar increase in synaptic conductance in the distal dendrites of cortical pyramidal neurons (Magee, 2000).

High Specific Membrane Resistance

A second key property is the specific membrane resistance (R_m) of the dendritic membrane. Traditionally, the argument was that if R_m is relatively low, the characteristic length of the dendrites will be relatively short, the electrotonic length will be correspondingly long, and synaptic potentials will therefore decrement sharply in spreading toward the axon hillock. However, as discussed in Chapter 5, intracellular recordings indicated that R_m is sufficiently high that the electrotonic lengths of most dendrites are in the range of 1–2 (Johnston and Wu, 1995), and patch recordings suggest much higher R_m values, indicating electrotonic lengths less than 1. Thus, a relatively high R_m seems adequate for close electrotonic linkage, at least in the steady state (Fig. 12.5B).

Low K Conductances

An important factor controlling effective membrane resistance is K conductances. Chapter 5 discussed how a K channel, I_h, can affect the summation of EPSPs in striatal spiny cells. There is increasing evidence for the control of dendritic input conductance by different types of K currents (Midtgaard *et al.*, 1993; Magee, 1999). When dendritic K conductances are turned off, R_m increases and dendritic coupling to the soma is enhanced. These conductances also control backpropagating action potentials, as discussed later.

Voltage-Gated Depolarizing Conductances

For transient responses, the electrotonic linkage becomes weaker because of the filtering effect of the capacitance of the membrane, and it is made worse by a higher R_m, which increases the membrane time constant, thereby slowing the spread of a passive potential (see Chapter 5). This disadvantage can be overcome by depolarizing voltage-gated conductances, Na, Ca, or both (Fig. 12.5C–I). Box 12.1 discusses the variety of mechanisms by which these voltage-gated conductances can operate.

Summary

These examples illustrate an important principle of **distal dendritic processing**:

Distal dendrites can mediate relatively rapid, specific information processing, even at the weakest levels of detection, in addition to slower modulation of overall neuronal activity. The spread of potentials to the site of global output from the axon is enhanced by multiple passive and active mechanisms.

DEPOLARIZING AND HYPERPOLARIZING DENDRITIC CONDUCTANCES INTERACT DYNAMICALLY

We see that depolarizing conductances increase the excitability of distal dendrites and the effectiveness of distal synapses, whereas K conductances reduce the excitability and control the temporal characteristics of the dendritic activity. This balance is thus crucial to the functions of dendrites. Figure 12.7 summarizes data showing how these conductances vary along the extents of the dendrites of mitral cells, hippocampal and neocortical pyramidal neurons, and Purkinje cells.

The significance of a particular density of channel needs to be judged in relation to the electrotonic prop-

BOX 12.1

VOLTAGE-GATED COMPUTATIONS IN DENDRITES

Active sites within branches or spines may act as *coincidence detectors* (Fig. 12.5G) of simultaneous synaptic responses. Through such mechanisms, simple logic gates are set up, which can perform the basic logic operations of AND, OR, and AND-NOT (Fig. 12.6). Other types of computation in dendrites include linearization of synaptic interactions and basic types of arithmetic processing: addition, subtraction, multiplication, and division (Koch 1999).

There may be a sequence of coincidence detection as an active response spreads from site to site through the branching tree. This means that the effectiveness of a distal EPSP may depend not on spreading all the way to the soma, but rather on spreading to the nearest site containing voltage-gated Na^+ or $Ca2^+$ channels, for coincidence detection and conduction to the next local site, and so on. Sequential spread of local active potentials from site to site provides for "pseudosaltatory conduction" through the dendritic tree (Fig. 12.5H). This may occur between individual sites or multiple sites forming clusters (Fig. 12.5I).

There is experimental and/or theoretical evidence for all of these mechanisms, some of which is considered later.

How does forward propagation of active responses in dendrites fit with the classical model of action potential initiation at the axonal initial segment? We will see that there are cells in which the initiation site actually shifts between the initial segment and the distal dendrite depending on the strengths and locations of synaptic excitation and inhibition. The site of action potential initiation thus can vary depending on the dynamic state of the neuron. It is also important to recognize that, because of the filtering effect of the dendritic cable properties, dendritic action potentials that spread to the soma may be indistinguishable at the soma from EPSPs (Fig. 12.6B; see Chapter 5). Thus, dendritic EPSPs that trigger the action potential at the initial segment, as in the classical model, may actually include significant contributions from active dendritic depolarization.

Gordon M. Shepherd

erties discussed in Chapter 5. For instance, a given conductance has more effect on membrane potential in smaller distal branches because of the higher input resistance (see Fig. 5.14). The significance of these conductance interactions for the firing properties of these different cell types is discussed later. Dendritic conductances can be crucial in setting the intrinsic excitability state of the neuron. In the motor neuron, for example, the neuron can alternate between bistable states dependent on the activation of dendritic metabotropic glutamate receptors (Svirskie *et al.*, 2001).

Summary

The combination of conductances at different levels of the dendritic tree involves a delicate balance between depolarizing and hyperpolarizing actions acting over different time periods. The combination of conductances at different levels of the dendritic tree is characteristic for different morphological types of neurons.

THE AXON HILLOCK-INITIAL SEGMENT ENCODES GLOBAL OUTPUT

In cells with long axons, activity in the dendrites eventually leads to activation and modulation of

action potential output in the axon. A key question is the precise site of origin of this action potential. This question was one of the first to be addressed in the rise of modern neuroscience; historical background is summarized in Box 12.2.

These studies established the classical model: the lowest threshold site for action potential generation is in the *axonal initial segment*.

Further testing had to await the development of methods for recording directly from dendrites in tissue slices. In CA1 hippocampal pyramidal neurons, weak synaptic potentials elicited action potentials near the cell body (Richardson *et al.*, 1987), but this site shifted to proximal dendrites with stronger synaptic excitation (Turner *et al.*, 1991). This confirmed the suggestion of Fuortes and colleagues that the site can shift under different stimulus conditions and was consistent with the stretch receptor, where larger receptor potentials shift the initiation site closer to the cell body.

Definitive analysis was achieved by Stuart and Sakmann (1994) using dual patch recordings from cortical pyramidal neurons under infrared differential contrast microscopy. As shown in Fig. 12.10, with depolarization of the distal dendrites by injected current or excitatory synaptic inputs, a large amplitude depolarization is produced in the dendrites, which spreads to the soma. Despite its lower amplitude, soma depolarization is the first to initiate the action potential.

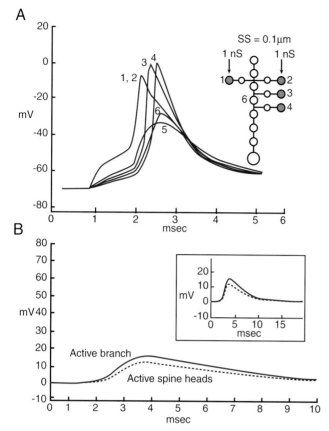

FIGURE 12.6 Logic operations are inherent in coincidence detection by active dendritic sites. The example is an AND operation performed by two dendritic spines with Hodkin–Huxley-type active kinetics, with intervening passive dendritic membrane. (A) Simultaneous synaptic input of 1 nS conductance to spines 1 and 2 gives rise to action potentials within both spines, which spread passively to activate action potentials in spines 3 and 4. Sequential coincidence detection by active spines can thus bring boosted synaptic responses close to the soma. From Shepherd and Brayton (1987). (B) Recording of boosted spine responses at the soma shows their similarity to the slow time course of classical EPSPs due to the electrotonic properties of the intervening dendritic membrane (see text). SS, spine stem diameter. From Shepherd *et al.* (1989).

Subsequent studies with triple patch electrodes have shown that the action potential actually arises first in the initial segment and first node (as shown in Chapter 5, Fig. 5.14). This approach has provided the breakthrough for subsequent analyses of dendritic properties and their coupling to the axon, as is discussed later.

RETROGRADE IMPULSE SPREAD INTO DENDRITES CAN HAVE SEVERAL FUNCTIONS

In addition to identifying the preferential site for action potential initiation in the axonal initial seg-

ment, the experiments of Stuart and Sackmann (1994) showed clearly that the action potential does not merely spread passively back into the dendrites but actively backpropagates. Note that we distinguish between passive "spread" and active "propagation" of the action potential.

What is the function of the backpropagating action potential? Experimental evidence shows that it can have a variety of functions.

Dendrodendritic Inhibition

A clear function for a backpropagating action potential was first suggested for the olfactory mitral cell, where mitral-to-granule dendrodendritic synapses are triggered by the action potential spreading from the soma into the secondary dendrites (Fig. 12.11). Because of the delay in activating the reciprocal inhibitory synapses from the granule cells, self-inhibition of the mitral cell occurs in the wake of the passing impulse; the two do not collide. The mechanism functions similarly with both active backpropagation and passive electrotonic spread into the dendrites, as tested in computer simulations (Rall and Shepherd, 1968). Functions of dendrodendritic inhibition include center-surround antagonism mediating the abstraction of molecular determinants underlying the discrimination of different odor molecules, storing of olfactory memories at the reciprocal synapses, and generation of oscillating activity in mitral and granule cell populations.

Boosting Synaptic Responses

In several types of pyramidal neurons, active dendritic properties appear to boost action potential invasion so that summation with EPSPs occurs that makes them effective in spreading to the soma.

Resetting Membrane Potential

A possible function is that the Na$^+$ and K$^+$ conductance increases associated with active propagation wipe out the existing membrane potential, resetting the membrane potential for new inputs.

Synaptic Plasticity

The action potential in the dendritic branches presumably depolarizes the spines (because of the favorable impedance matching, as discussed in Chapter 5), which means that the impulse depolarization would summate with the synaptic depolarization of the spines. This process would enable the spines to func-

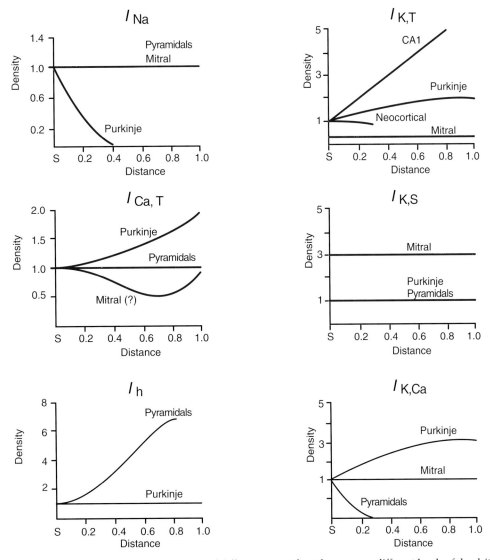

FIGURE 12.7 Graphs of the distribution of different types of conductances at different levels of dendritic trees in different types of neurons. S, soma. From Magee (1999).

tion as coincidence detectors and implement Hebb-like changes in synaptic plasticity. This postulate is being tested by electrophysiological recordings (Spruston *et al.*, 1995) and Ca²⁺ imaging (Yuste *et al.*, 1994). Activity-dependent changes of dendritic synaptic potency are not seen with passive retrograde depolarization but appear to require actively propagating retrograde impulses (Spruston *et al.*, 1995).

Frequency Dependence

Trains of action potentials generated at the soma–axon hillock can invade the dendrites to varying extents. Proximal dendrites appear to be invaded throughout a high-frequency burst, whereas distal dendrites appear to be invaded mainly by the early

action potentials (Regehr *et al.*, 1989; Callaway and Ross, 1995; Yuste *et al.*, 1994; Spruston *et al.*, 1995). Activation of Ca²⁺-activated K⁺ conductances by early impulses may effectively switch off the distal dendritic compartment.

Retrograde Actions at Synapses

The retrograde action potential may contribute to the activation of neurotransmitter release from the dendrites. Dynorphin released by synaptically stimulated dentate granule cells can affect the presynaptic terminals (Simmons *et al.*, 1995). In the cerebral cortex there is evidence that GABAergic interneuronal dendrites act back on axonal terminals of pyramidal cells and that glutamatergic pyramidal cell dendrites act

BOX 12.2

CLASSICAL STUDIES OF THE ACTION POTENTIAL INITIATION SITE

Fuortes and colleagues (1957) were the first to deduce that an EPSP spreads from the dendrites through the soma to initiate the action potential in the region of the axon hillock and the initial axon segment. They suggested that

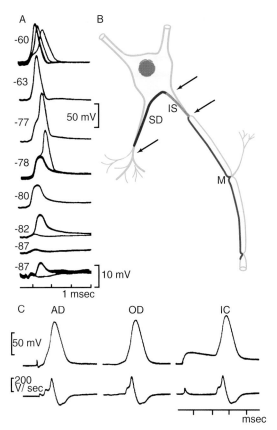

FIGURE 12.8   Classical evidence for the site of action potential initiation. Intracellular recordings were from the cell body of the motor neuron of an anesthetized cat. (A) Differential blockade of an antidromic impulse by adjusting the membrane potential by holding currents. Recordings reveal the sequence of impulse invasion in the myelinated axon (recordings at –87 mV, two amplifications), the initial segment of the axon (first component of the impulse beginning at –82 mV), and the soma–dendritic region (large component beginning at –78 mV). (B) Sites of the three regions of impulse generation (M, myelinated axon; IS, initial segment; SD, soma and dendrites); arrows show probable sites of impulse blockade in A. (C) Comparison of intracellular recordings of impulses generated antidromically (AD), synaptically (orthodromically, OD), and by direct current injection (IC). Lower traces indicate electrical differentiation of these recordings showing the separation of the impulse into the same two components and indicating that the sequence of impulse generation from the initial segment into the soma–dendritic region is the same in all cases. From Eccles (1957).

the action potential has two components: (1) an A component that is normally associated with the axon hillock and initial segment and (2) a B component that is normally associated with retrograde invasion of the cell body. Because the site of action potential initiation can shift under different membrane potentials, they preferred the noncommittal terms "A" and "B" for the two components as recorded from the cell body. In contrast, Eccles (1957) referred to the initial component as the initial-segment (IS) component and to the second component as the soma-dendritic (SD) component (Fig. 12.8).

Apart from the motor neuron, the best early model for intracellular analysis of neuronal mechanisms was the crayfish stretch receptor, described by Eyzaguirre and Kuffler (1955). Intracellular recordings from the cell body showed that stretch causes a depolarizing receptor potential equivalent to an EPSP, which spreads through the cell to initiate an action potential. It was first assumed that this action potential arose at or near the cell body. Edwards and Ottoson (1958), working in

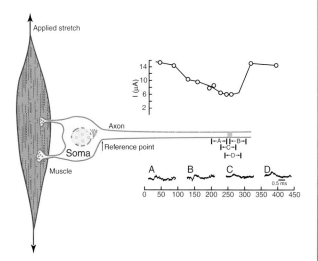

FIGURE 12.9   Classical demonstration of the site of impulse initiation in the stretch receptor cell of the crayfish. Moderate stretch of the receptor muscle generated a receptor potential that spread from the dendrites across the cell body into the axon. Paired electrodes recorded the longitudinal extracellular currents at positions A–D, showing the site of the trigger zone (green region). The excitability curve (shown at the top), obtained by passing current between the electrodes and finding the current (I) intensity needed to evoke an impulse response, also shows the trigger zone to be several hundred micrometers out on the axon. From Ringham (1971).

Kuffler's laboratory, tested this postulate by recording the local extracellular current in order to locate precisely the site of inward current associated with action potential initiation. Surprisingly, this site turned out to be far out on the axon, some 200 μm from the cell body (Fig. 12.9). This result showed that potentials generated in the distal dendrites can spread all the way through the dendrites and soma well out into the initial segment of the axon to initiate impulses. It further showed that the action potential recorded at the cell body is the backward spreading impulse from the initiation site. Edwards and Ottoson's study was important in establishing the basic model of impulse

initiation in the axonal initial segment.

Gordon M. Shepherd

References

Eccles, J. C. (1957). "The Physiology of Nerve Cells." Johns Hopkins Univ. Press, Baltimore.

Edwards, C., and Ottoson, D. (1958). The site of impulse initiation in a nerve cell of a crustacean sretch receptor. *J. Physiol. (Lond.)* **143**, 138–148.

Eyzaguirre, C., and Kuffler, S. W. (1955). Processes of excitation in the dendrites and in the soma of single isolated sensory nerve cells of the lobster and crayfish. *J. Gen. Physiol.* **39**, 87–119.

Fuortes, M. G. F., Frank, K., and Banker, M. C. (1957). Steps in the production of motor neuron spikes, *J. Gen. Physiol.* **40**, 735–752.

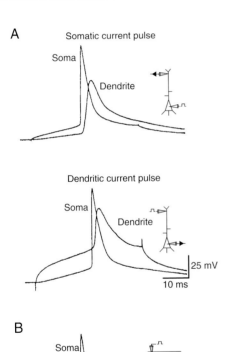

FIGURE 12.10   Direct demonstration of the impulse-initiation zone and backpropagation into dendrites using dual-patch recordings from soma and dendrites of a layer V pyramidal neuron in a slice preparation of the rat neocortex. (A) Depolarizing current injection in either the soma or the dendrite elicits an impulse first in the soma. (B) The same result is obtained with synaptic activation of layer I input to distal dendrites. Note the close similarity of these results to the earlier findings in the motor neuron (Fig. 12.8). From Stuart and Sakmann (1994).

back on axonal terminals of the interneurons (Fig. 12.12). The combined effects of the axonal and dendritic compartments of both neuronal types regulate the normally excitability of pyramidal neurons and may be a factor in the development of cortical hyperexcitability and epilepsy (Zilberter, 2000).

Conditional Axonal Output

Because of the long distance between distal dendrites and initial axonal segment, we may hypothesize that the coupling between the two is not automatic. Indeed, conditional coupling dependent on synaptic inputs and intrinsic activity states at intervening dendritic sites appears to be fundamental to the relation between local dendritic inputs and global axonal output (Spruston, 2000).

EXAMPLES OF HOW VOLTAGE-GATED CHANNELS TAKE PART IN DENDRITIC INTEGRATION

It is commonly believed that active dendrites are a modern concept, but in fact this idea is as old as Cajal. Box 12.3 gives a short history of this idea and the experimental evidence that has been obtained over the years.

Detailed analysis of active dendritic properties began with computational studies of olfactory mitral cells and experimental studies of cerebellar Purkinje cells. Since then, studies of active dendritic properties have proliferated, particularly since introduction of the patch recording method. Several types of neurons

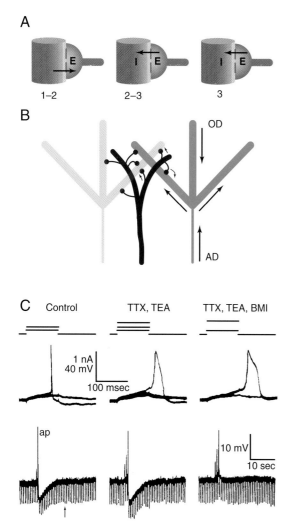

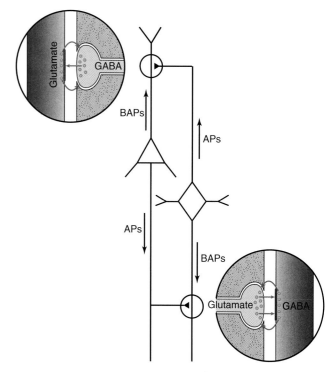

FIGURE 12.12 Pyramidal neurons and interneurons in the cerebral cortex interact through axo–dendritic and dendro–axonic contacts. APs, action potentials in axons; BAPs, backpropagating action potentials in dendrites. See text. Modified from Zilberter (2000).

FIGURE 12.11 Dendrodendritic interactions in the olfactory bulb. (A) Depolarization by an action potential in time period 1–2 activates excitatory output from the mitral cell dendrite, setting up an EPSP (E) in a granule cell spine. During time period 2–3, the granule spine EPSP activates a reciprocal inhibitory synapse, setting up an IPSP (I) in the mitral cell dendrite, which lasts into time period 3. (B) Either orthodromic (OD) or antidromic (AD) activation of the mitral cell sets up a backspreading/backpropagating impulse into the secondary dendrites, activating both feedback and lateral inhibition of the mitral cells through the dendrodendritic pathway. From Rall and Shepherd (1968). (C) Experimental demonstration of the dendrodendritic pathway. (Left) In an intracellular recording from a mitral cell in an isolated turtle olfactory bulb, injected depolarizing current elicits an action potential [fast trace and action potential (ap) in slow trace below] followed by a long-lasting hyperpolarizing IPSP; downward deflections are reduced during the IPSP, indicating an increase in membrane conductance during the IPSP. (Center) Depolarizing current elicits a lower amplitude and slower action potential when the preparation is bathed in TTX (which blocks the Na$^+$ component of the impulse) and TEA (which blocks K$^+$ conductances that would shunt the remaining Ca^{2+} component). The IPSP persists, activated by the Ca^{2+} action potential (bottom trace). (Right) Addition of bicuculline (BMI) to the bath blocks the IPSP (bottom trace), presumably by blocking the granule-to-mitral reciprocal synapse. Adapted from Jahr and Nicoll (1982).

have provided important models for the possible functional roles of active dendritic properties.

Purkinje Cells

The cerebellar Purkinje cell has the most elaborate dendritic tree in the nervous system, with more than 100,000 dendritic spines receiving synaptic inputs from parallel fibers and mossy fibers. The basic distribution of active properties in the Purkinje cell was indicated by the pioneering experiments of Llinas and Sugimori (1980) in tissue slices (Fig. 12.14). The action potential in the cell body and axon hillock is due mainly to fast Na$^+$ and delayed K$^+$ channels; there is also a Ca^{2+} component. The action potential correspondingly has a large amplitude in the cell body and decreases by electrotonic decay in the dendrites. In contrast, recordings in the dendrites are dominated by slower "spike" potentials that are Ca^{2+} dependent due to a P-type Ca^{2+} conductance (see Fig. 12.14). These spikes are generated from a plateau potential due to a persistent Na p current.

There are two distinct operating modes of the Purkinje cell in relation to its distinctive inputs. Climbing fibers mediate strong depolarizing EPSPs throughout most of the dendrites that appear to give

BOX 12.3

CLASSICAL STUDIES OF ACTIVE DENDRITIC PROPERTIES

The first intracellular recordings of active properties of dendrites were obtained in 1958 by Eccles and collaborators from motor neurons undergoing chromatolytic degeneration after amputation of their axons (Eccles *et al.*, 1958). Small spikes could be seen riding on EPSPs, which were thought to be due to impulse "booster" sites in the dendrites. Similar activity was seen in the first intracellular recordings from hippocampal pyramidal neurons (Spencer and Kandel, 1961). These "fast prepotentials" appeared to intervene between the EPSP in the dendrite and the impulse initiation in the soma–axon hillock region (Fig. 12.13). These active sites were suggested to be at branch points in the apical dendrite, where they would serve to boost EPSPs generated by more distal dendritic inputs. This boosting property has provided an important model for the possible significance of active dendritic properties. Active properties of dendrites were the subject of increasing study from the 1950s on, with extracellular (see Fatt, 1957; Anderson, 1960) and intracellular recordings. The use of dual-patch recordings finally enabled direct recordings from dendrites and comparisons with soma recordings, as discussed in the text.

Gordon M. Shepherd

References

Anderson, P. (1960). Interhippocampal impulses. II. Aprical dendritic activation of CA1 neurons. *Acta Physiol. Scand.* **48**, 178–208.

Eccles, J. C., Libet, B., and Young, R. R. (1958). The behaviour of chromatolysed motoneurons studied by intracellular recording. *J. Physiol.* (*Lond.*) **143**, 11–40

Fatt. P. (1957). Sequence of events in synaptic activation of a motoneurone. *J. Neurophysiol.* **20**, 61–80.

Spencer, W. A, and Kandel, E. R. (1961). Electrophysiology of hippocampal neurons. IV. Fast potentials. *J. Neurophysiol.* 272–285.

A

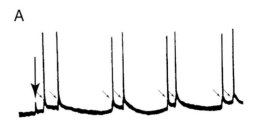

B

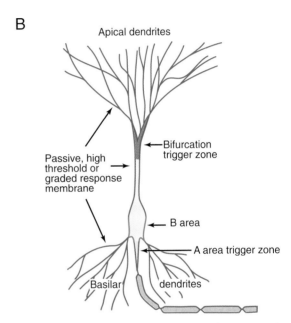

FIGURE 12.13 Early evidence of active dendritic properties in normal adult neurons. (A) Intracellular recordings from the soma of a hippocampal pyramidal neuron in an anesthetized cat; large spontaneous action potentials are preceded by a small "fast prepotential" (small arrows), which occasionally occurs in isolation (large arrow). (B) Conceptual schema of how a "trigger zone" at bifurcating dendritic branches could give rise to the fast prepotential and boost the distal dendritic response. From Spencer and Kandel (1961).

rise to synchronous Ca^{2+} dendritic action potentials throughout the dendritic tree, which then spread to the soma to elicit the bursting "complex spike" in the axon hillock. In contrast, parallel fibers are active in small groups, giving rise to smaller populations of individual EPSPs possibly targeted to particular dendritic regions (compartments). In this mode, *subthreshold amplification* through active dendritic proper-

ties may enhance the effect of a particular set of input fibers in controlling or modulating the frequency of Purkinje cell action potential output in the axon hillock. The Purkinje cell is subjected to *local inhibitory control* by stellate cell synapses targeted to specific dendritic compartments and to *global inhibitory control* of axonal output by basket cell synapses on the axonal initial segment.

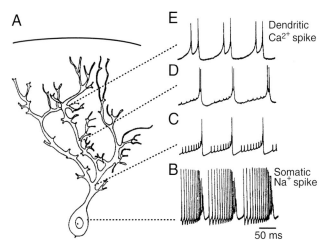

FIGURE 12.14 Classical demonstration of the difference between soma and dendritic action potentials. (A) Drawing of a Purkinje cell in the cerebellar slice. (B) Intracellular recordings from the soma showing fast Na$^+$ spikes. (C–E) Intracellular recordings from progressively more distant dendritic sites; fast soma spikes become small due to electrotonic decrement and are replaced by large-amplitude dendritic Ca^{2+} spikes. Spread of these spikes to the soma causes an inactivating burst that interrupts the soma discharge. Adapted from Llinas and Sugimori (1980).

Pyramidal Neurons

Active properties of the apical dendrite of hippocampal pyramidal neurons have been amply documented by patch recordings (Magee and Johnston, 1995). In contrast to the Purkinje cell, both fast Na$^+$ and Ca^{2+} conductances have been shown throughout the dendritic tree of the pyramidal neuron by electrophysiological and dye-imaging methods (see Fig. 12.7). Activation of low-threshold Na$^+$ channels is believed to play an important role in triggering the higher-threshold Ca^{2+} channels. Similar results have been obtained in studies of pyramidal neurons of the cerebral cortex.

The output pattern of a neuron depends on its dendritic properties and their interaction with the soma. This is exemplified by the generation of a burst response in a pyramidal neuron. EPSPs spread through the dendrite, activating fast Na$^+$ and then high-threshold (HT) Ca^{2+} channels that give a subthreshold boost to the EPSP. The enhanced EPSP spreads to the soma-axon hillock, triggering a Na$^+$ action potential. This propagates into the axon and also backpropagates into the dendrites, eliciting a slower all-or-nothing Ca^{2+} action potential. This large-amplitude, slow depolarization then spreads through the dendrites and back to the soma, triggering a train of action potentials that form a burst response.

This sequence of events is contained in a two-compartment model representing the soma and dendritic

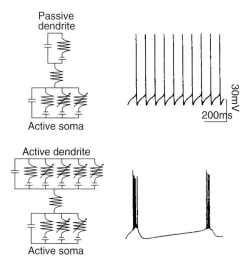

FIGURE 12.15 Generation of a burst response by interactions between soma and dendrites. From Pinsky and Rinzel (1994).

compartments (Fig. 12.15). The sequence emphasizes not only the importance of the interplay between the different types of channels, but also the critical role of the compartmentation of the neuron into dendritic and somatic compartments so that they can interact in controlling the intensity and time course of the impulse output.

Does the specific form of the input–output transformation depend on a specific distribution of active channels in the dendritic tree? Na$^+$ and Ca^{2+} channels are distributed widely in pyramidal neuron dendrites. In computational simulations, grouping channels in different distributions may have little effect on the input–output functions of a neuron (Mainen and Sejnowski, 1995). However, evidence shows that subthreshold amplification by voltage-gated channels may tend to occur in the more proximal dendrites of some neurons (Yuste and Denk, 1995). In addition, the dendritic trees of some neurons are clearly divided into different anatomical and functional subdivisions, as discussed in the next section.

Medium Spiny Cell

A third instructive example of the role of active dendritic properties is found in the medium spiny cell of the neostriatum (Figs. 12.16A and 12.16B). The passive electrotonic properties of this cell are described in Chapter 5 (Fig. 5.12). Inputs to a given neuron from the cortex are widely distributed, meaning that a given neuron must summate a significant number of synaptic inputs before generating an impulse response. The responsiveness of the cell is controlled by its cable properties; individual responses in the spines are filtered out by the large

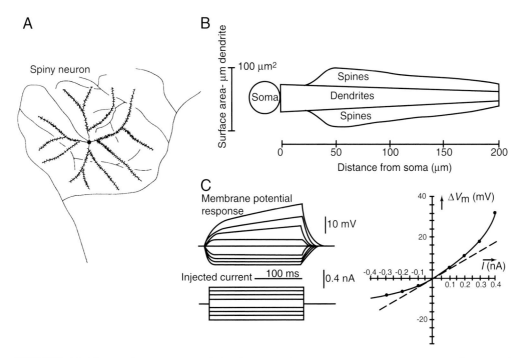

FIGURE 12.16 Dendritic spines and dendritic membrane properties interact to control neuronal excitability. (A) Diagram of a medium spiny neuron in the caudate nucleus; (B) plot of surface areas of different compartments showing a large increase in surface area due to spines; and (C) intracellular patch-clamp analysis of medium spiny neuron showing inward rectification of the membrane that controls the response of the dendrites to excitatory synaptic inputs (cf. Chapter 5, Fig. 5.12). From Wilson (1998).

capacitance of the many dendritic spines so that individual EPSPs recorded at the soma are small.

With synchronous specific inputs, larger summated EPSPs depolarize the dendritic membrane strongly. The dendritic membrane contains inwardly rectifying channels (I_h) (Fig. 12.16C), which reduce their conductance upon depolarization and thereby increase the effective

membrane resistance and shorten the electrotonic length of the dendritic tree. Large depolarization also activates HT Ca^{2+} channels, which contribute to large-amplitude, slow depolarizations. These combined effects change the neuron from a state in which it is insensitive to small noisy inputs into a state in which it gives a large response to a specific input and is maxi-

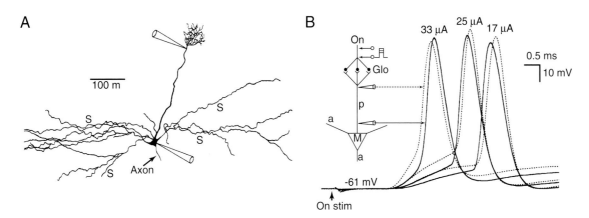

FIGURE 12.17 Shift of action potential initiation site between soma and distal dendrite. (A) A mitral cell in a slice preparation from the rat olfactory bulb stained with biocytin showing placement of dual patch recording electrodes, one on the soma and one at the distal end of the primary dendrite 300 mm from the soma near the distal dendritic tuft in the glomerulus. (B) In another cell, an electrode site near the soma is paired with a distal dendritic site. With weak shocks to the olfactory nerves (17 μA), the soma action potential arises first; as the shocks are strengthened to 33 μA, the action potential initiation shifts to the distal dendrite recording site. From Chen *et al*. (1997).

mally sensitive to additional inputs. Through this voltage-gated mechanism, a neuron can enhance the effectiveness of distal dendritic inputs, not by boosting inward Na^+ and K^+ currents, but by reducing outward shunting K^+ currents. This exemplifies the principle of dynamic control over dendritic properties mentioned earlier.

MULTIPLE IMPULSE INITIATION SITES ARE UNDER DYNAMIC CONTROL

Can the active properties of dendrites give rise to full dendritic action potentials that propagate toward the cell body and precede the action potential in the soma–axon hillock-initial segment region? Evidence for this began with extracellular recordings of a "population spike" that appears to propagate along the apical dendrites toward the cell body in hippocampal pyramidal cells (Anderson, 1960), supported by the recording of "fast prepotentials" (see earlier discussion) and by current source density calculations in cortical pyramidal neurons (Herreras, 1990). However, because of the indirect nature of this evidence, it is possible (Stuart., *et al.* 1997) that these active properties of distal dendrites can boost dendritic synaptic responses but may be too slow to lead to action potential initiation and forward propagation.

Evidence on this question has been obtained from the olfactory mitral cell, whose excitatory inputs are on its distal dendritic tuft (see Fig. 12.17A). At weak levels of electrical shocks to the olfactory nerves, the site of action potential initiation is at or near the soma, as in the classical model (17 μA in Fig. 12.17B). This shows that despite its long length, the primary dendrite is not an impediment to the transfer of an EPSP carrying specific sensory information from the distal dendrite to the soma and initial axonal segment. It adds another nail to the coffin of the common misconception that, in neurons with axons, specific excitatory inputs must be targeted near the axon hillock and that distal dendrites can mediate only slow background modulation of that site.

As the level of distal excitatory input is increased, dual-patch recordings show clearly that the action potential initiation site is not fixed; instead, the site shifts gradually from the soma to the distal dendrite (see 25 and 33 μA in Fig. 12.17B). Thus the site of impulse initiation is not fixed in the mitral cell, but varies with the intensity of distal excitatory input. The action potential is due to tetrodotoxin-sensitive Na channels distributed along the extent of the primary dendrite. The way that passive potential spread along the dendrite controls the site of action potential initiation in these experiments has been discussed in Chapter 5 (Fig. 5.15). The site can also be shifted to distal dendrites by synaptic inhibition applied to the soma through dendrodendritic synapses.

Summary

These are only a few examples of the range of operations carried out by complex dendrites. These dendritic operations are embedded in the circuits that control behavior. Many further examples could be mentioned; for instance, the way that motoneuron intrinsic properties are involved in the activation patterns of motor units controlling the limbs (Gorassini *et al.*, 1999). Thus, for each neuron, the dendritic tree constitutes an expanded unit essential to the circuits underlying behavior.

DENDRITIC SPINES ARE MULTIFUNCTIONAL MICROINTEGRATIVE UNITS

The very small size of dendritic spines has made it difficult to study them directly. However, examples have already been given of spines with complex information processing capacities, such as granule cell

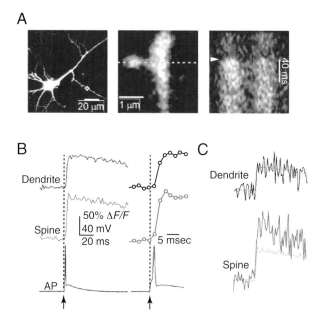

FIGURE 12.18 Calcium transients can be imaged in single dendritic spines in a rat hippocampal slice. (A) Fluo-4, a calcium-sensitive dye, injected into a neuron enables an individual spine to be imaged under two-photon microscopy. (B) An action potential (AP) induces an increase in Ca^{2+} in the dendrite and a larger increase in the spine (averaged responses). (C) Fluctuation analysis indicated that spines likely contain up to 20 voltage-sensitive Ca channels; single channel openings could be detected, which had a high (0.5) probability of opening following a single action potential. From Sabatini and Svoboda (2000).

spines in the olfactory bulb and spines of medium spiny neurons in the striatum. In cortical neurons, spines have been implicated in cognitive functions from observations of dramatic changes in spine morphology in relation to different types of mental retardation and different hormonal exposures. Activity-dependent changes in spine morphology could be a mechanism contributing to learning and memory (summarized in Harris and Krater, 1994; Shepherd, 1996; Yuste and Denk, 1995).

Computational models have been very useful in testing these hypotheses, as well as suggesting other possible functions, such as the dynamic changes of electrotonic structure in medium spiny cells of the basal ganglia (see earlier discussion). With the development of more powerful light microscopical methods, such as two-photon laser confocal microscopy, it has become possible to image Ca^{2+} fluxes in individual spines in relation to synaptic inputs and neuronal activity (Fig. 12.18). Evidence for active properties of dendrites

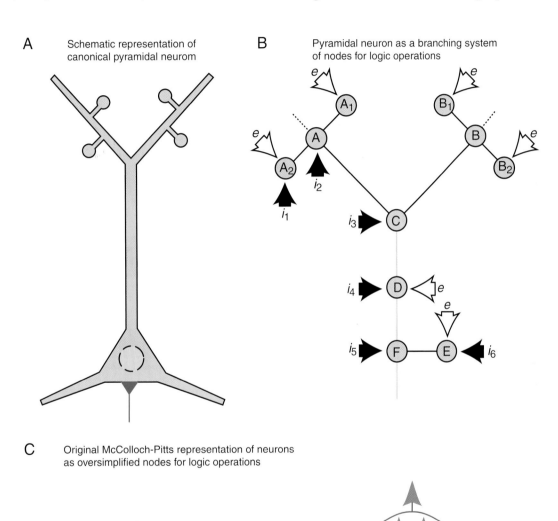

FIGURE 12.19 The dendritic tree as a complex system of computational nodes. (C) Contrast A and B with the concept of McCulloch and Pitts (1943) in which the dendritic tree is ignored and the entire neuron is reduced to a single computational node. *e*, excitatory synapse; *i*, inhibitory synapse. From Shepherd (1994).

has suggested that the spines may also have active properties. Thus, spines may be devices for nonlinear thresholding operations, either through voltage-gated ion channels (see Fig. 12.6) or through voltage-dependent synaptic properties such as N-methyl-D-aspartate (NMDA) receptors. However, spines may also function as compartments to isolate changes at the synapse, such as excess Ca^{2+}, that would be harmful to the rest of the neuron (Volfovsky et al., 1999).

The range of functions that have been hypothesized for spines is partly a reflection of how little direct evidence we have of specific properties of spines. It also indicates that the answer to the question "What is the function of the dendritic spine?" is unlikely to be only one function but rather a range of functions that is tuned in a given neuron to the specific operations of that neuron. The spine is increasingly regarded as a microcompartment that integrates a range of functions (Harris and Kater, 1994; Shepherd, 1996; Yuste and Denk, 1995). A spiny dendritic tree is thus covered with a large population of microintegrative units. As discussed previously, the effect of any given one of these units on the action potential output of the neuron should therefore not be assessed with regard only to the far-off cell body and axon hillock, but rather with regard first to its effect on its neighboring microintegrative units.

SUMMARY: THE DENDRITIC TREE AS A COMPLEX INFORMATION PROCESSING SYSTEM

Dendrites are the primary information processing substrate of the neuron. They allow the neuron wide flexibility in carrying out the operations needed for processing information in the spatial and temporal domains within nervous centers. The main constraints on these operations are the rules of passive electrotonic spread (Chapter 5), and the rules of nonlinear thresholding at multiple sites within the complex geometry of dendritic trees discussed in this chapter. Cells with and without axons and action potentials demonstrate many specific types of information processing that are possible in dendrites, such as motion detection, oscillatory activity, lateral inhibition, and network control of sensory processing and motor control. These types are possible for cells with axons, which in addition operate within constraints that govern local vs global outputs and sub vs suprathreshold activities.

Spines add a dimension of local computation to dendritic function that is especially relevant to mechanisms for learning and memory. Although spines seem to distance synaptic responses from directly affecting axonal output, many cells demonstrate that distal spine inputs carry specific information.

The key to understanding how all parts of the dendritic tree, including its distal branches and spines, can participate in mediating specific types of information processing is to recognize the tree as a complex system of active nodes. From this perspective, if a spine can affect its neighbor, and that spine its neighbor, a dendritic tree becomes a cascade of decision points, with multiple cascades operating over multiple overlapping time scales (see Fig. 12.19). Far from being a single node, as in the classical concept of McCulloch and Pitts (1943) and classical neural network models, the complex neuron is a system of nodes in itself, within which **the dendrites constitute a kind of neural microchip for complex computations**. The neuron as a single node, so feeble in its information processing capacities, is replaced by the neuron as a complex multinodal system. The range of operations of which this complex system is capable continues to expand (Poirazi and Mel, 2000). Exploring the information processing capacities of the brain at the level of real dendritic systems, by both experimental and theoretical methods, thus presents one of the most exciting challenges for neuroscientists in the future.

References

Anderson, P. (1960). Interhippocampal impulses. II. Apical dendritic activation of CA1 neurons. Acta Physiol. Scand. **48**, 178–208.

Callaway, J. C., and Ross, W. N. (1995). Frequency-dependent propagation of sodium action potentials in dendrites of hippocampal CA1 pyramidal neurons. J. Neurophysiol. **74**, 1395–1403.

Chen, W. R., Midtgaard, J., and Shepherd, G. M. (1997). Forward and backward propagation of dendritic impulses and their synaptic control in mitral cells. Science **278**, 463–467.

Craig, A. M., and Banker, G. (1994). Neuronal polarity. Annu. Rev. Neurosci. **17**, 267–310.

Golowasch, J., and Marder, E. (1992). Ionic currents of the lateral pyloric neuron of the stomatogastric ganglion of the crab. J. Neurophysiol. **67**, 2, 318–331.

Gorassini, M., Bennett, D. J., Kiehn, O., Eken, T., and Hultborn, H. (1999). Activation patterns of hindlimb motor units in the awak rat and their relation to motoneuron intrinsic properties. J. Neurophysiol. **82**, 709–717.

Harris, K. M., and Kater, S. B. (1994). Dendritic spines: Cellular specializations imparting both stability and flexibility to synaptic function. Annu. Rev. Neurosci. **17**, 341–371.

Herreras, O. (1990). Propagating dendritic action potential mediates synaptic transmission in CA1 pyramidal cells in situ. J. Neurophysiol. **64**, 1429–1441.

Jahr, C. E., and Nicoll, R. A. (1982). An intracellular analysis of dendrodendritic inhibition in the turtle in vitro olfactory bulb. J. Physiol. (Lond.) **326**, 213–234.

Johnston, D. A., and Wu, S. M.-S. (1995). "Foundations of Cellular Neurophysiology." MIT Press, Cambridge, MA.

Koch, C. (1999). "Biophysics of Computation: Information Processing in Single Neurons." Oxford Univ. Press, New York,

Llinas, R., and Sugimori, M. (1980). Electrophysiological properties of in vitro Purkinje cell dendrites in mammalian cerebellar slices. *J. Physiol. (Lond.)* **305**, 197–213.

Luksch, H., Cox, K., and Karten, H. J. (1998). Bottlebrush dendritic endings and large dendritic fields: motion-detecting neurons in the tectofugal pathway. *J. Comp. Neurol.* **396**, 399–414.

Magee, J. C. (1999). Voltage-gated ion channels in dendrites. *In* "Dendrites" (G. Stuart, N. Spruston, and M. Hausser, eds.), pp. 139–160. Oxford Univ. Press, New york.

Magee, J. C. (2000). Dendritic integration of excitatory synaptic input. *Nature Neurosci.* **1**, 181–190.

Magee, J. C., and Johnston, D. (1995). Characterization of single voltage-gated Na$^+$ and Ca^{2+} channels in apical dendrites of rat CA1 pyramidal neurons. *J. Physiol. (Lond.)* **487**, 67–90.

Mainen, Z. F., and Sejnowski, T. J.(1995). Influence of dendritic structure on firing pattern in model neocortical neurons. *Nature* **382**, 363–365.

Manor, Y., Nadim, F., Epstein, S., Ritt, J., Marder, E., and Kopell, N. (1999). Network oscillations generated by balancing graded asymmetric reciprocal inhibition in passive neurons. *J. Neurosci.* **19**,2765–2779.

Matus, A., and Shepherd, G. M. (2000). The millennium of the dendrite? *Neuron* **27**, 431–434.

McCulloch, W. S., and Pitts, W. H. (1943). A logical calculus of the ideas immanent in nervous activity. *Bull. Math. Biophys.* **5**, 115–133.

Midtgaard, J., Lasser-Ross, N., and Ross, W. N. (1993). Spatial distribution of Ca^{2+} influx in turtle Purkinje cell dendrites in vitro: Role of a transient outward current. *J. Neurophysiol.* **70**, 2455–2469.

Pinsky, P. F., and Rinzel, J. (1994). Intrinsic and network rhythmogenesis in a reduced Traub model for CA3 neurons. *J. Comput. Neurosci.* **1**,39–60.

Poirazi, P., and Mel, B. W. (2000). Impact of active dendrites and structural plasticity on the memory capacity of neural tissue.

Rall, W. (1964). Theoretical significance of dendritic trees for neuronal input-output relations. *In* "Neural Theory and Modelling" (R. F. Reiss, ed.), pp. 73–97. Stanford University Press.

Rall, W., and Shepherd, G. M. (1968). Theoretical reconstruction of field potentials and dendrodendritic synaptic interactions in olfactory bulb. *J. Neurophysiol.* **31**, 884–915.

Redman, S. J., and Walmsley, B. (1983). Amplitude fluctuations in synaptic potentials evoked in cat spinal motoneurons at identified group in synapses. *J. Physiol. (Lond.)* **343**, 135–145.

Regehr, W. G., Connor, J. A., and Tank, D. W. (1989). Optical imaging of calcium accumulation in hippocampal pyramidal cells during synaptic activation. *Nature (Lond.)* 533–536.

Richardson, T. L., Turner, R. W., and Miller, J. J. (1987). Action-potential discharge in hippocampal CA1 pyramidal neurons. *J. Neurophysiol.* **58**, 98–996.

Ringham, G. L. (1971). Origin of nerve impulse in slowly adapting stretch receptor of crayfish. *J. Neurophysiol.* **33**, 773–786.

Sabatini , B. L., and Svoboda, K. (2000). Analysis of calcium channels in single spines using optical fluctuation analysis. *Nature* **408**, 589–593.

Segev, I., and London, M. (2000). Untangling dendrites with quantitative models. *Science* **290**, 744–750.

Segev, I., Rinzel, J., and Shepherd, G. M. (eds.). (1995). "The Theoretical Foundation of Dendritic Function. Selected Papers of Wilfrid Rall." MIT Press, Cambridge.

Selverston, A. I., Russell, D. F., and Miller, J. P. (1976). The stomatogastric nervous system: Structure and function of a small neural network. *Prog. Neurobiol.* **37**, 215–289.

Shepherd, G. M., and Brayton, R. K. (1987). Logic operations are properties of computer-simulated interactions between excitable dendritic spines. *Neurosci.* **21**, 151–166.

Shepherd, G. M., Woolf, T. B., and Cernevals, N. T. (1989). Comparisons between active properties of distal dendritic branches and spines: implications for neuronal computations. *J. Cogn. Neurosci.* **1**, 273–286.

Shepherd, G. M. (1991). "Foundations of the Neuron Doctrine." Oxford Univ. Press, New York.

Shepherd, G. M. (1992). Canonical neurons and their computational organization. *In* "Single Neuron Computation" (T. McKenna, J. Davis, and S. F. Zornetzer, eds.), pp. 27–59. MIT Press, Cambridge.

Shepherd, G. M. (1994). "Neurobiology," (3rd Ed.). Oxford Univ. Press, New York.

Shepherd, G. M. (1996). The dendritic spine: A multifunctional integrative unit. *J. Neurophysiol.* **75**, 2197–2210.

Simmons, M. L., Terman, G. W., Gibbs, S. M., and Chavkin, C. (1995). L -type calcium channels mediate dynorphin neuropeptide release from dendrites but not axons of hippocampal granule cells. *Neuron* **14**, 1265–1272.

Single, S., and Borst, A. (1998). Dendritic integration and its role in computing image velocity. *Science* **281**, 1848–1850.

Spruston, N., Schiller, Y., Stuart, G., and Sakmann, B. (1995). Activity-dependent action potential invasion and calcium influx into hippocampal CA1 dendrites. *Science* **268**, 297–300.

Spruston, N. (2000). Distant synapses raise their voices. *Nature Neurosci.* **3**,849–851.

Stern, P., and Marx, J. (2000). Beautiful, complex and diverse specialists. *Science* **290**, 735.

Stuart, G., Spruston, N., and Hausser, M. (1999). "Dendrites." Oxford Univ. Press, New York.

Stuart, G., Spruston, N., Sakmann, B., and Hausser, M. (1997). Action potential initiation and backpropagation in neurons of the mammalian central nervous system. *Trends Neurosci.* **20**,125–131.

Stuart, G. J., and Sakmann, B. (1994). Active propagation of somatic action potentials into neocortical pyramidal cell dendrites. *Nature (Lond.)* **367**, 6–72.

Svirskie, G., Gutman, A., and Hounsgaard, J. (2001). Electrotonic structure of motoneurons in the spinal cord of the turtle: Inferences for the mechanisms of bistability. *J. Neurophysiol.* **85**, 391–399.

Turner, R. W., Meyers, E. R., Richardson, D. L., and Barker, J. L. (1991). The site for initiation of action potential discharge over the somatosensory axis of rat hippocampal CA1 pyramidal neurons. *J. Neurosci.* **11**, 2270–2280.

Volfovsky, N., Parnas, H., Segal M., and Korkotian, E. (1999). Geometry of dendritic spines affects calcium dynamics in hippocampal neurons: Theory and experiments. *J. Neurophysiol.* **82**, 450–462.

Wilson, C. (1998). Basal ganglia. *In* "The Synaptic Organization of the Brain" (G. Shepherd, ed.), 4th Ed., pp. 329–375. Oxford Univ. Press, New York.

Yuste, R., and Denk, W. (1995). Dendritic spines as basic functional units of neuronal integration in dendrites. *Nature (Lond.)* **375**, 682–684.

Yuste, R., Gutnick, M. J., Saar, D., Delaney, K. D., and Tank, D. W. (1994). Calcium accumulations in dendrites from neocortical neurons: An apical band and evidence for functional compartments. *Neuron* **13**, 23–43.

Yuste, R., and Tank, D. (1996). Dendritic integration in mammalian neurons, a century after Caj al. *Neuron* **13**, 23–43.

Zilberter, Y. (2000). Dendritic release of glutamate suppresses synaptic inhibition of pyramidal neurons in rat neocortex. *J. Physiol.* **528**, 489–496.

Gordon M. Shepherd

13

Brain Energy Metabolism

All the processes described in this textbook require energy. Ample clinical evidence indicates that the brain is exquisitely sensitive to perturbations of energy metabolism. This chapter covers the topics of energy delivery, production, and utilization by the brain. Careful consideration of the basic mechanisms of brain energy metabolism is an essential prerequisite to a full understanding of the physiology and pathophysiology of brain function. I review the features of brain energy metabolism at the global, regional, and cellular levels and, at the cellular level, extensively describe recent advances in the understanding of neuron–glial metabolic exchanges. A particular focus is the cellular and molecular mechanisms that tightly couple neuronal activity to energy consumption. This tight coupling is at the basis of functional brain-imaging techniques, such as positron emission tomography (PET) and functional magnetic resonance imaging.

ENERGY METABOLISM OF THE BRAIN AS A WHOLE ORGAN

Glucose is the Main Energy Substrate for the Brain

The human brain constitutes only 2% of the body weight, yet the energy-consuming processes that ensure proper brain function account for approximately 25% of total body glucose utilization. With a few exceptions that will be reviewed later, glucose is the obligatory energy substrate of the brain (Edvinsson et al., 2001). In any tissue, glucose can follow various metabolic pathways; in the brain, glucose is almost entirely oxidized to CO_2 and water through its sequen-

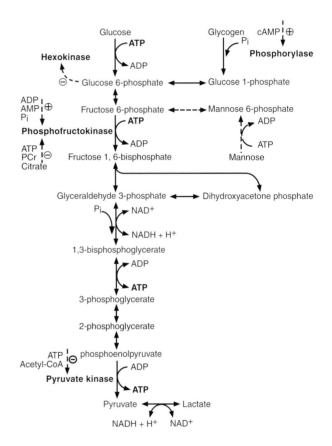

FIGURE 13.1 Glycolysis (Embden–Meyerhof pathway). Glucose phosphorylation is regulated by hexokinase, an enzyme inhibited by glucose 6-phosphate. Glucose must be phosphorylated to glucose 6-phosphate to enter glycolysis or to be stored as glycogen. Two other important steps in the regulation of glycolysis are catalyzed by phosphofructokinase and pyruvate kinase. Their activity is controlled by the levels of high-energy phosphates, as well as of citrate and acetyl-CoA. Pyruvate, through lactate dehydrogenase, is in dynamic equilibrium with lactate. This reaction is essential to regenerate NAD^+ residues necessary to sustain glycolysis downstream of glyceraldehyde 3-phosphate. PCr, phosphocreatine.

tial processing by glycolysis (Fig. 13.1), the tricarboxylic acid (TCA) cycle (Fig. 13.2), and the associated oxidative phosphorylation, which yield, on a molar basis, 38 ATP per glucose. Indeed, the oxygen consumption of the brain, which accounts for almost 20% of the oxygen consumption of the whole organism, is 160 mmol per 100 g of brain weight per minute and roughly corresponds to the value determined for CO_2 production. This O_2/CO_2 relation corresponds to what is known in metabolic physiology as a respiratory quotient of nearly 1 and demonstrates that carbohydrates, and glucose in particular, are the exclusive substrates for oxidative metabolism. This rather detailed information of whole brain energy metabolism was obtained using an experimental approach in which the concentration of a given substrate in the arterial blood entering the brain through the carotid artery is compared with that present in the venous blood draining the

brain through the jugular vein (Kety and Schmidt, 1948). If the substrate is utilized by the brain, the arteriovenous (A-V) difference is positive; in certain cases, the A-V difference may be negative, indicating that metabolic pathways resulting in the production of the substrate predominate. In addition, when the rate of cerebral blood flow (CBF) is known, the steady-state rate of utilization of the substrate can be determined per unit time and normalized per unit brain weight according to the following relation: CMR = CBF (A-V), where CMR is the cerebral metabolic rate of a given substrate. This approach was pioneered by Seymour Kety and C. F. Schmidt in the late 1940s and was further developed in the 1950s and 1960s. In normal adults, CBF is approximately 57 ml per 100 g of brain weight per minute, and the calculated glucose utilization by the brain is 31 mmol per 100 g of brain weight per minute, as determined with the A-V difference method (Kety and Schmidt, 1948). This value is slightly higher than that predicted from the rate of oxygen consumption of the brain. Thus, in an organ such as the brain with a respiratory quotient of 1, the stoichiometry would predict that 6 mmol of oxygen are needed to fully oxidize 1 mmol of the six-carbon molecule of glucose; given an oxygen consumption rate of 160 mmol per 100 g of brain weight per minute, the predicted glucose utilization would be 26 mmol per 100 g of brain weight per minute (160:6), yet the actual measured rate is 31 mmol. What then is the fate of the excess 4.4 mmol? First, glucose metabolism may proceed, to a very limited extent, only through glycolysis, resulting in the production of lactate without oxygen consumption (see Fig. 13.1); glucose can also be incorporated into glycogen (Fig. 13.1). Second, glucose is an essential constituent of macromolecules such as glycolipids and glycoproteins present in neural cells. Finally, glucose enters the metabolic pathways that result in the synthesis of three key neurotransmitters of the brain: glutamate, GABA, and acetylcholine (see Chapter 8).

Ketone Bodies Become Energy Substrates for the Brain in Particular Circumstances

In particular circumstances, substrates other than glucose can be utilized by the brain. For example, breast-fed neonates have the capacity to utilize the ketone bodies acetoacetate (AcAc) and D-3-hydroxybutyrate (3-HB), in addition to glucose, as energy substrates for the brain. This capacity is an interesting example of a developmentally regulated adaptive mechanism because maternal milk is highly enriched in lipids, resulting in a lipid-to-carbohydrate ratio much higher than that present in postweaning

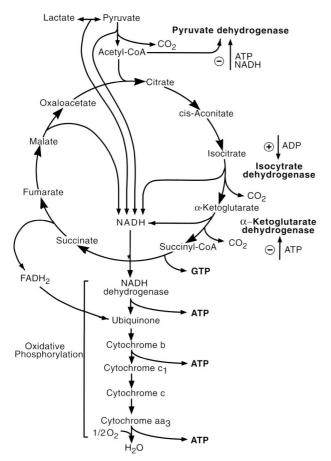

FIGURE 13.2 Tricarboxylic acid cycle (Krebs' cycle) and oxidative phosphorylation. Pyruvate entry into the cycle is controlled by pyruvate dehydrogenase activity that is inhibited by ATP and NADH. Two other regulatory steps in the cycle are controlled by isocitrate and α-ketoglutarate dehydrogenase, whose activity is controlled by the levels of high-energy phosphates.

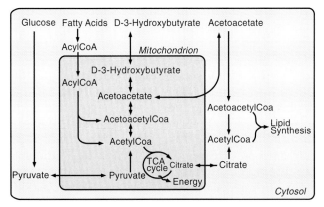

FIGURE 13.3 Relationship between lipid metabolism and the TCA cycle. Under particular dietary conditions, such as lactation in newborns or fasting in adults, the ketone bodies acetoacetate and D-3-hydroxybutyrate and circulating fatty acids can provide substrates to the TCA cycle after conversion into acetyl-CoA. Carbon atoms for lipid synthesis can be provided by glucose through citrate produced in the TCA cycle, a particularly relevant process for the developing brain.

nutrients. Indeed, lipids account for approximately 55% of the total calories contained in human milk, in contrast with 30–35% for a balanced postweaning diet. In addition to the ketone bodies AcAc and 3-HB, other products of lipid metabolism, relevant to brain metabolic processes, are free fatty acids. Acetoacetate, 3-HB, and free fatty acids can all be processed to acetyl-CoA, thus providing ATP through the TCA cycle (Fig. 13.3). We will see later that brain energy metabolism is highly compartmentalized, with certain metabolic pathways specifically localized in a given cell type. It is therefore not surprising that whereas ketone bodies can be oxidized by neurons, oligodendrocytes, and astrocytes, the β-oxidation of free fatty acids is localized exclusively in astrocytes. Another consideration regarding the lipid-rich diet provided during the suckling period relates to its contribution to the process of myelination. The question is whether the polar lipids and cholesterol that make up myelin are derived from dietary sources or are synthesized within the brain. Evidence shows that brain lipids can be synthesized from blood-borne precursors such as ketone bodies. In addition, when suckling rats are fed a diet low in ketones, carbon atoms for lipogenesis can also be provided by glucose. To summarize, ketone bodies and AcAc are energy substrates, as well as precursors for lipogenesis during the suckling period; however, the developing brain appears to be metabolically quite flexible because glucose, in addition to its energetic function, can be metabolized to generate substrates for lipid synthesis.

Starvation and diabetes are two situations in which the availability of glucose to tissues is inadequate and

in which plasma ketone bodies are elevated because of enhanced lipid catabolism. Under these conditions, the adaptive mechanisms described for breast-fed neonates become operative in the brain, allowing it to utilize AcAc or 3-HB as energy substrates (Owen *et al.*, 1967).

Mannose, Lactate, and Pyruvate Serve as Instructive Cases

A number of metabolic intermediates have been tested as alternative substrates to glucose for brain energy metabolism. Among the numerous molecules tested, mannose is the only one that can sustain normal brain function in the absence of glucose. Mannose crosses the blood–brain barrier readily and, in two enzymatic steps, is converted into fructose 6-phosphate, an intermediate of the glycolytic pathway (see Fig. 13.1). However, mannose is not normally present in the blood and therefore is not considered a physiological substrate for brain energy metabolism.

Lactate and pyruvate can be sources of insight into the intrinsic properties of isolated brain tissue versus those of the brain as an organ receiving substrates from the circulation. Lactate and pyruvate can sustain the synaptic activity of isolated brain samples, usually thin slices, maintained *in vitro* in a physiological medium lacking glucose (Schurr *et al.*, 1999). In vivo, until recently, it was thought that their permeability across the blood–brain barrier was limited, hence preventing circulating lactate or pyruvate to substitute for glucose to maintain brain function adequately. However, evidence from magnetic resonance spectroscopy (MRS) experiments indicates that the permeability of circulating lactate across the blood–brain barrier may actually be higher than previously thought; in addition, the presence of monocarboxylate transporters on intraparenchymal brain capillaries has been documented. Thus there is a need for the reappraisal of the use by the brain of monocarboxylates. In any case, as shown later, if formed within the brain parenchyma from glucose that has crossed the blood–brain barrier, lactate and pyruvate may in fact become the preferential energy substrates for activated neurons.

Summary

Glucose is the obligatory energy substrate for brain, and it is almost entirely oxidized to CO_2 and H_2O. This simple statement summarizes, with few exceptions, over four decades of careful studies of brain energy metabolism at organ and regional levels. Under ketogenic conditions, such as starvation and diabetes and during breast-feeding, ketone bodies may provide an energy source for the brain. Lactate and pyruvate, formed from glucose within the brain parenchyma, are adequate energy substrates as well.

COUPLING OF NEURONAL ACTIVITY, BLOOD FLOW, AND ENERGY METABOLISM

A striking characteristic of the brain is its high degree of structural and functional specialization. Thus, when we move an arm, motor areas and their related pathways are activated selectively (see Chapter 30); intuitively, one can predict that as "brain work" increases locally (e.g., in motor areas), the energy requirements of the activated regions will increase in a temporally and spatially coordinated manner. Because energy substrates are provided through the circulation, blood flow should increase in the modality-specific activated area. More than a century ago, the British neurophysiologist C. Sherrington showed, in experimental animals, increases in blood flow localized to the parietal cortex in response to sensory stimulation (Roy and Sherrington, 1890). He postulated that "the brain possesses intrinsic mechanisms by which its vascular supply can be varied locally in correspondence with local variations of functional activity." With remarkable insight, he also proposed that "chemical products of cerebral metabolism" produced in the course of neuronal activation could provide the mechanism to couple activity with increased blood flow.

Which Mechanisms Couple Neuronal Activity to Blood Flow?

Since Sherrington's seminal work, the search for the identification of chemical mediators that can couple neuronal activity with local increases in blood flow has been intense. These signals can be broadly grouped into two categories: (1) molecules or ions that transiently accumulate in the extracellular space after neuronal activity and (2) specific neurotransmitters that mediate the coupling in anticipation or at least in parallel with local activation (neurogenic mechanisms). The increases in extracellular K^+, adenosine, and lactate and the related changes in pH are all a consequence of increased neuronal activity, and all have been considered mediators of neurovascular coupling because of their vasoactive effects (Villringer and Dirnagl, 1995). However, the spatial

and temporal resolution achieved by these mediators may not be sufficient to entirely account for the activity-dependent coupling between neuronal activity and blood flow. Indeed, these vasoactive agents are formed with a certain delay (seconds) after the initiation of neuronal activity and can diffuse at considerable distance. In this respect, neurogenic mechanisms appear to be better fitted. Brain microvessels are richly innervated by neuronal fibers. These fibers may have an extrinsic origin (e.g., in the autonomic ganglia) or be part of neuronal circuits intrinsic to the brain, such as local interneurons or long projections that originate in the brainstem (e.g., those containing monoaminergic neurotransmitters) (see Chapter 8). In addition, functional receptors coupled to signal transduction pathways have been identified for several neurotransmitters on intraparenchymal microvessels. Neurotransmitters with potential roles in coupling neuronal activity with blood flow include the amines noradrenaline, serotonin, and acetylcholine and the peptides vasoactive intestinal peptide, neuropeptide Y (NPY), calcitonin gene-related peptide (CGRP), and substance P (SP). The neurogenic mode of neurovascular coupling implies that vasoactive neurotransmitters are released from perivascular fibers as excitatory afferent volleys activate a discrete and functionally defined brain volume.

A recent and very attractive addition to the list of potential mediators for coupling neuronal activity to blood flow is nitric oxide (NO). Indeed, NO is an ideal candidate; it is formed locally by neurons and glial cells under the action of a variety of neurotransmitters likely to be released by depolarized afferents to an activated brain area. Nitric oxide is a diffusible and potent vasodilator whose short half-life spatially and temporally restricts its domain of action. However, in several experimental models in which the activity of NO synthase, the enzyme responsible for NO synthesis, was inhibited, a certain degree of coupling was still observed, indicating that NO is probably only one of the regulators of local blood flow acting in synergy with others (Iadecola et al., 1994).

In summary, several products of activity-dependent neuronal and glial metabolism such as lactate, H+, adenosine, and K^+ have vasoactive effects and are therefore putative mediators of coupling, although the kinetics and spatial resolution of this mode do not account for all the observed phenomena. As attractive as it is, an exclusively neurogenic mode of coupling neuronal activity to blood flow is unlikely and, moreover, still awaits firm functional confirmation *in vivo*. Nitric oxide is undoubtedly a key element in coupling, particularly in view of the fact that glutamate, the principal excitatory neurotransmitter, triggers a receptor-mediated NO formation in neurons and glia; this is consistent with the view that whenever a functionally defined brain area is activated and glutamate is released by the depolarized afferents, NO may be formed, thus providing a direct mechanism contributing to the coupling between activity and local increases in blood flow.

Through the activity-linked increase in blood flow, more substrates—namely, glucose and oxygen—necessary to meet the additional energy demands are delivered to the activated area per unit time. The cellular and molecular mechanisms involved in oxygen consumption and glucose utilization are treated in a later section.

Blood Flow and Energy Metabolism Can Be Visualized in Humans

Modern functional brain-imaging techniques enable the *in vivo* monitoring of human blood flow and the two indices of energy metabolism: glucose utilization and oxygen consumption (Box 13.1). For instance, with the use of PET and appropriate positron-emitting isotopes such as ^{18}F and ^{15}O, basal rates, as well as activity-related changes in local blood

---

BOX 13.1

POSITRON EMISSION TOMOGRAPHY (PET) AND FUNCTIONAL MAGNETIC RESONANCE IMAGING (fMRI)

We have seen that neuronal activity is tightly coupled to blood flow and metabolism. With the advent of sophisticated imaging procedures such as PET and fMRI, it is now possible to detect the signals generated by the metabolic processes associated with neuronal activity, thus providing a unique opportunity to see the "brain at work." Indeed, local changes in blood flow, glucose utilization, and oxygen consumption can be monitored noninvasively under basal and activated conditions in human subjects. How is this possible?

For PET, a solution containing slightly radioactive molecules is injected into the circulation, and its sites of brain uptake can be visualized. The molecule is labeled radioactively with an unstable radionuclide possessing an excess number of protons; as a consequence of normal radioactive decay, the excess proton is converted into a neutron. In this process, a positron (a positively charged electron) is emitted and collides with an electron, releasing energy in the form of two photons with opposite trajectories. The photons are sensed by specialized detectors placed around the head; when two photons simultaneously reach two detectors positioned at 180° of each other, the origin of the positron–electron collision can be localized with a resolution of 5 to 10 mm. Commonly used positron-emitting radionuclides are oxygen-15 (^{15}O), carbon-11 (^{11}C), and fluorine-18 (^{18}F). Blood flow is monitored with ^{15}O-labeled water and glucose utilization with ^{18}F-2-deoxyglucose. Oxygen consumption is visualized directly with ^{15}O. With the use of sophisticated algorithms to process data, the localization of activity to specific brain areas during a given task (sensory, motor,

cognitive) can be achieved. Thus, the activity of neuronal ensembles, and of the associated glia, coupled to increased blood flow and glucose utilization results in a localized signal due to the augmented concentration of ^{15}O-labeled water (monitoring blood flow) and ^{18}F-2-deoxyglucose (assessing glucose utilization) in the activated area.

PET is one of the ways in which brain work can be visualized. An increasingly popular technique, fMRI relies on the magnetic signals detected in an activated brain region in relation to its degree of oxygenation. Depending on the degree to which it is saturated by oxygen, hemoglobin (by acting as a paramagnetic contrast agent) can alter the magnetic signal detected in a tissue exposed to the magnetic fields used for structural MRI. In other words, different MRI signals can be obtained depending on the oxyhemoglobin/deoxyhemoglobin ratio in a given brain area. Local activation of a brain area results in increased blood flow. Although the precise mechanisms are still being discussed, it is currently thought that this phenomenon, by leading to a localized enrichment in oxyhemoglobin, alters the oxyhemoglobin/deoxyhemoglobin ratio, providing the signal for fMRI. Functional MRI is a remarkably convenient and powerful technique: the signal acquisition time is extremely rapid (on the order of seconds) and the resolution equals that of PET (i.e., a few millimeters). In addition, fMRI is totally noninvasive and can thus be repeated frequently on the same subject, who can then serve as its own control.

Pierre J. Magistretti

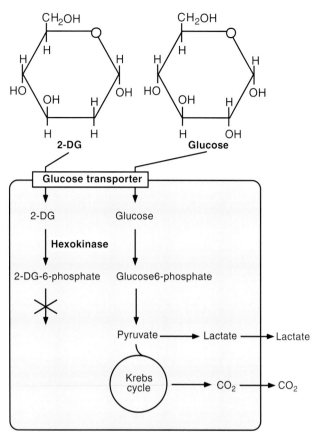

FIGURE 13.4 Structure and metabolism of glucose and 2-deoxyglucose (2-DG). 2-DG is transported into cells through glucose transporters and phosphorylated by hexokinase to glucose 6-phosphate without significant further processing or dephosphorylation back to glucose. Therefore, when labeled radioactively, 2-DG used in tracer concentrations is a valuable marker of glucose uptake and phosphorylation, which directly indicates glucose utilization.

flow or oxygen consumption, can be studied using ^{15}O-labeled water or ^{15}O, respectively (Frackowiak et al., 1980). Local rates of glucose utilization [also defined as local cerebral metabolic rates for glucose (LCMRglu)] can be determined with ^{18}F-labeled 2-deoxyglucose (2-DG) (Phelps et al., 1979). The use of 2-DG as a marker of LCMRglu was pioneered by Louis Sokoloff and associates at the National Institutes of Health, first in laboratory animals (Sokoloff, 1981). The method is based on the fact that 2-DG crosses the blood–brain barrier, is taken up by brain cells, and is phosphorylated by hexokinase with kinetics similar to that for glucose; however, unlike glucose 6-phosphate, 2-deoxyglucose 6-phosphate cannot be metabolized further and therefore accumulates intracellularly (Fig. 13.4).

For studies in laboratory animals, tracer amounts of radioactive 2-DG are injected intravenously; the animal is subjected to the behavioral paradigms of interest and sacrificed at the end of the experiment. Serial thin sections of the brain are prepared and processed for autoradiography. This autoradiographic method provides, after appropriate corrections, an accurate measurement of LCMRglu with a spatial resolution of approximately 50–100 mm. Using this method, researchers have determined LCMRglu in virtually all structurally and functionally defined brain structures in various physiological and pathological states, including sleep, seizures, and dehydration, and after a variety of pharmacological treatments (Sokoloff, 1981). Furthermore, glucose utilization increases in the pertinent brain areas during motor tasks or activation of pathways subserving specific modalities, such as visual, auditory, olfactory, or somatosensory stimulation (Sokoloff, 1981). For example, in mice, sustained stimulation of the whiskers results in marked increases in LCMRglu in discrete areas of the primary sensory cortex called the barrel fields, where each whisker is represented with an extreme degree of topographical specificity (see Chapter 26). Basal glucose utilization of the gray matter as determined by 2-DG autoradiography varies, depending on the brain structure, between 50 and 150 mmol per 100 g of wet weight per minute in the rat.

In humans, LCMRglu determined by PET with the use of ^{18}F-2-DG is approximately 50% lower than that in rodents, and physiological activation of specific modalities increases LCMRglu in discrete areas of the brain that can be visualized with a spatial resolution of a few millimeters. For example, visual stimulations presented to subjects as checkerboard patterns reversing at frequencies ranging from 2 to 10 Hz selectively increase LCMRglu in the primary visual cortex and a few connected cortical areas. With the use of this stimulation paradigm, the combined PET analysis of local cerebral blood flow (LCBF) and local oxygen consumption (LCMRO$_2$), in addition to LCMRglu, has revealed a unique and unexpected feature of human brain energy metabolism regulation. The canonical view was that the three metabolic parameters were tightly coupled, implying that, if, for example, CBF increased locally during physiological activation, LCMRglu and LCMRO$_2$ would increase in parallel. In what is now referred to as the phenomenon of "uncoupling," physiological stimulation of the visual system increases LCBF and LCMRglu (both by 30–40%) in the primary visual cortex without a commensurate increase in LCMRO$_2$ (which increases only 6%) (Fox et al., 1988), indicating that the additional glucose utilized during neuronal activation can be processed through glycolysis rather than through the tricarboxylic acid (TCA) cycle and oxidative phosphorylation. The phenomenon of uncoupling has been confirmed in other cortical areas, although its magnitude may differ depending on the modality, and may actually be absent in certain cases. A glance at the metabolic pathways reveals that if glucose does not enter the TCA cycle to be oxidized, then lactate will be produced (see Figs. 13.1 and 13.2). Lactate, like several other metabolically relevant molecules, can be determined with the technique of magnetic resonance imaging (MRI) spectroscopy for ^1H, which provides a means of unequivocally identifying in living tissues the presence of molecules that bear the naturally occurring isotope ^1H. Consistent with the prediction that if during activation glucose is predominantly processed glycolytically, then lactate should be produced locally in the activated region, a transient increase in the lactate signal is detected with ^1H MRI spectroscopy in the human primary visual cortex during appropriate visual stimulation. These observations support the view that to face the local increases in energy demands linked to neuronal activation, the brain transiently resorts to glycolysis followed by at least oxidative phosphorylation (Magistretti and Pellerin, 1999). This transient uncoupling may vary in amplitude depending on the modalities of activation and is likely to occur in different cellular compartments, i.e., astrocytes vs neurons (Frackowiak *et al.*, 2001).

Summary

Studies at the whole organ level, based on the A-V differences of metabolic substrates, have revealed a great deal about the global energy metabolism of the brain. They have indicated that, under normal conditions, glucose is virtually the sole energy substrate for the brain and that it is entirely oxidized. New techniques that allow imaging of the three fundamental parameters of brain energy metabolism—namely, blood flow, oxygen consumption, and glucose utilization—provide a more refined level of spatial resolution and demonstrate that brain energy metabolism is regionally heterogeneous and is coupled tightly to the functional activation of specific neuronal pathways (Magistretti *et al.*, 1999).

ENERGY-PRODUCING AND ENERGY-CONSUMING PROCESSES IN THE BRAIN

What are the cellular and molecular mechanisms that underlie the regulation of brain energy metabo-

lism revealed by the foregoing studies at global and regional levels? In particular, what are the metabolic events taking place in the cell types that make up the brain parenchyma? How is it possible to reconcile whole organ studies indicating complete oxidation of glucose with transient activation-induced glycolysis at the regional level? These and other related questions will be addressed here and in the next sections.

Glucose Metabolism Produces Energy

Before we move on to an analysis of the cell-specific mechanisms of brain energy metabolism, it seems appropriate to briefly review some basic aspects of the energy balance of the brain. Because glucose, in normal circumstances, is the main energy substrate of the brain, the overview will be restricted to its metabolic pathways. Glucose metabolism in the brain is similar to that in other tissues and includes three principal metabolic pathways: glycolysis, the tricarboxylic acid cycle, and the pentose phosphate pathway. Because of the global similarities with other tissues, these pathways are simply summarized in Figs. 13.1, 13.2, and 13.5, and only a few aspects specific to the nervous tissue will be discussed.

Glycolysis

Glycolysis (Embden–Meyerhof pathway) is the metabolism of glucose to pyruvate (see Fig. 13.1). It results in the net production of only two molecules of ATP per glucose molecule; indeed, four ATPs are formed in the processing of glucose to pyruvate, whereas two ATPs are consumed to phosphorylate glucose to glucose 6-phosphate and fructose 6-phosphate to fructose 1,6-bisphosphate, respectively (see Fig. 13.1). Under anaerobic conditions, pyruvate is converted into lactate, allowing the regeneration of nicotinamide adenine dinucleotide (NAD$^+$), which is essential to maintain a continued glycolytic flux. Indeed, if NAD$^+$ were not regenerated, glycolysis could not proceed beyond glyceraldehyde 3-phosphate (see Fig. 13.1). Another situation in which the end product of glycolysis is lactate rather than pyruvate is when oxygen consumption does not match glucose utilization, implying that the rate of pyruvate production through glycolysis exceeds pyruvate oxidation by the TCA cycle (see Fig. 13.2). This condition has been well described in skeletal muscle during intense exercise and appears to share similarities with the transient uncoupling observed between glucose utilization and oxygen consumption that has been described in the human cerebral cortex during activation with the use of PET (Fox *et al.*, 1988).

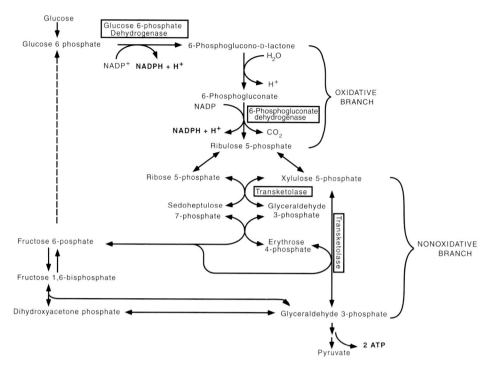

FIGURE 13.5 The pentose phosphate pathway. In the oxidative branch of the pentose phosphate pathway, two NADPH are generated per glucose 6-phosphate. The first rate-limiting reaction of the pathway is catalyzed by glucose-6-phosphate dehydrogenase; the second NADPH is generated through the oxidative decarboxylation of 6-phosphogluconate, a reaction catalyzed by glucose-6-phosphogluconate dehydrogenase. The nonoxidative branch of the pentose phosphate pathway provides a reversible link with glycolysis by regenerating the two glycolytic intermediates glyceraldehyde 3-phosphate and fructose 6-phosphate. This regeneration is achieved through three sequential reactions. In the first, catalyzed by transketolase, xylulose 5-phosphate and ribose 5-phosphate (which originate from ribulose 5-phosphate, the end product of the oxidative branch) yield glyceraldehyde 3-phosphate and sedoheptulose 7-phosphate. Under the action of transaldolase, these two intermediates yield fructose 6-phosphate and erythrose 4-phosphate. This latter intermediate combines with glyceraldehyde 3-phosphate, in a reaction catalyzed by transketolase, to yield fructose 6-phosphate and glyceraldehyde 3-phosphate. Thus, through the nonoxidative branch of the pentose phosphate pathway, two hexoses (fructose 6-phosphate) and one triose (glyceraldehyde 3-phosphate) of the glycolytic pathway are regenerated from three pentoses (ribulose 5-phosphate).

Tricarboxylic Acid Cycle

Under aerobic conditions, pyruvate is oxidatively decarboxylated to yield acetyl-CoA in a reaction catalyzed by the enzyme pyruvate dehydrogenase (PDH). Acetyl-coenzyme A condenses with oxaloacetate to produce citrate (see Fig. 13.2). This is the first step of the tricarboxylic acid cycle, in which three pairs of electrons are transferred from NAD^+ to NADH—and one pair from flavin adenine dinucleotide (FAD) to its reduced form ($FADH_2$)—through four oxidation–reduction steps (see Fig. 13.2). NADH and $FADH_2$ transfer their electrons to molecular O_2 through the mitochondrial electron transfer chain to produce ATP in the process of oxidative phosphorylation. Thus, under aerobic conditions (i.e., when glucose is fully oxidized through the TCA cycle to CO_2 and H_2O), NAD^+ is regenerated, and glycolysis

proceeds to pyruvate, not lactate. However, as soon as a mismatch, even a transient one, occurs between glucose utilization and oxygen consumption, lactate is produced. As discussed earlier, such a transient production of lactate appears to occur in the human brain during activation. Experiments performed in freely moving rats have also demonstrated a transient increase in lactate content in the extracellular space of discrete brain regions during physiological sensory stimulation. In these experiments, lactate was determined in the extracellular fluid collected by microdialysis.

Pentose Phosphate Pathway

Although glycolysis, the TCA cycle, and oxidative phosphorylation are coordinated pathways that produce ATP, using glucose as a fuel, ATP is not the only form of metabolic energy. Indeed, for several biosynthetic reactions in which the precursors are in a more oxidated state than the products, metabolic energy in the form of reducing power is needed in addition to ATP. This is the case for the reductive synthesis of free fatty acids from acetyl-CoA, which are components of myelin and of other structural elements of neural cells, such as the plasma membrane. In cells of the brain, as in other organs, the reducing power is provided by the reduced form of nicotinamide adenine dinucleotide phosphate (NADPH). The processing of glucose through the pentose phosphate pathway produces NADPH. The first reaction in the pentose phosphate pathway is the conversion of glucose 6-phosphate into ribulose 5-phosphate (Fig. 13.5). This dehydrogenation, in which two molecules of NADPH are generated per molecule of glucose 6-phosphate, is the rate-limiting step of the pentose phosphate pathway. The NADP/NADPH ratio is the single most

important factor regulating the entry of glucose 6-phosphate into the pentose phosphate pathway. Thus, if a high reducing power is needed, NADPH levels decrease and the pentose phosphate pathway is activated to generate new reducing equivalents. In addition to reductive biosynthesis, NADPH is needed for the scavenging of reactive oxygen species (ROS). The superoxide anion, hydrogen peroxide, and the hydroxy radical are three ROS, generated by the transfer of single electrons to molecular oxygen as by-products of certain physiological cellular processes. Examples of such processes are the electron transfer chain associated with oxidative phosphorylation and the activities of monoamine oxidase, tyrosine hydroxylase, nitric oxide synthase, and the eicosanoid-forming enzymes lipoxygenases and cyclooxygenases. Reactive oxygen species are highly damaging to cells because they can cause DNA disruption and mutations, as well as activation of enzymatic cascades, including proteases and lipases that can eventually lead to cell death.

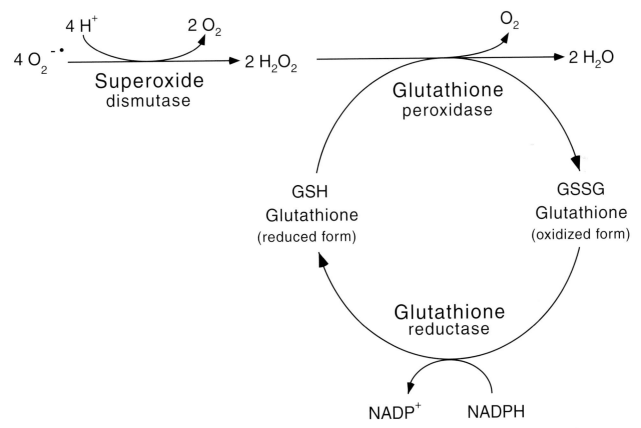

FIGURE 13.6 Enzymatic reactions for scavenging reactive oxygen species (ROS). The toxic superoxide anion (O2$^-$) formed by a variety of physiological reactions, including oxidative phosphorylation, is scavenged by superoxide dismutase, which converts the superoxide anion into hydrogen peroxide (H_2O_2) and molecular oxygen. Glutathione peroxidase converts the still toxic hydrogen peroxide into water; reduced glutathione (GSH) is required for this reaction, in which it is converted into its oxidized form (GSSG). GSH is regenerated through the action of glutathione reductase, a reaction requiring NADPH.

Scavenging of ROS is ensured by the sequential action of superoxide dismutase (SOD) and glutathione peroxidase (Fig. 13.6). Thus, two superoxide anions formed by the aforementioned cellular processes are converted by SOD into H_2O_2, still a ROS. Glutathione peroxidase converts H_2O_2 into H_2O and O_2 at the expense of reduced glutathione, which is regenerated by glutathione reductase in the presence of NADPH. In addition to the scavenging mechanisms for ROS, the pentose phosphate pathway is also tightly connected to glycolysis through two enzymes, transketolase and transaldolase, which recycle ribulose 5-phosphate to fructose 6-phosphate and glyceraldehyde 3-phosphate, two intermediates of glycolysis (see Fig. 13.5).

The Wernicke–Korsakoff Syndrome: A Neuropsychiatric Disorder Due to a Dysfunction of Energy Metabolism

A well-characterized neuropsychiatric disorder, the Wernicke–Korsakoff syndrome, is caused by transketolase hypoactivity. The Wernicke–Korsakoff syndrome is characterized by a severe impairment of memory and of other cognitive processes accompanied by balance and gait dysfunction and by paralysis of oculomotor muscles. The syndrome is due to a lack of thiamine (vitamin B_1) in the diet; it affects only susceptible persons who are also alcoholics or chronically undernourished. Thiamine pyrophosphate is a thiamine-containing cofactor essential for the activity of transketolase. In patients with the Wernicke–Korsakoff syndrome, thiamine pyrophosphate binds 10 times less avidly to transketolase compared with the enzyme of normal persons. This enzymatic dysfunction renders patients with the Wernicke–Korsakoff syndrome much more vulnerable to thiamine deficiency. This syndrome illustrates how an anomaly in a discrete metabolic pathway of energy metabolism may result in severe alterations in behavior and motor function.

Processes Linked to Neuronal Function Consume Energy

The main energy-consuming process of the brain is the maintenance of ionic gradients across the plasma membrane, a condition that is crucial for excitability. Maintenance of these gradients is achieved predominantly through the activity of ionic pumps fueled by ATP, particularly Na^+, K^+-ATPase, localized in neurons as well as in other cell types such as glia. Activity of these pumps accounts for approximately 50% of basal glucose oxidation in the nervous system (Erecinska, 1999). Very recently elegant theoretical calculations of the cost of synaptic transmission have

been provided by Attwell and Laughlin (2001). They estimated the energy budget of an average glutamatergic pyramidal neuron firing at 4 Hz, with the assumption that >80% of cortical neurons are pyramidal cells and that >90% of the synapses release glutamate. First, the cost of the recycling of released glutamate via reuptake and metabolism in astrocytes and the restoration of the post- synaptic ion gradient has been estimated. Glutamate recycling requires 2.67 ATP/glutamate molecule; since one vesicle contains 4 $\times 10^3$ molecules of glutamate, the cost of transmitter recycling is $\sim 1.1 \times 10^4$ ATP/vesicle. The restoration of postsynaptic ionic gradients disrupted by the activity of NMDA and non-NMDA receptors is $\sim 1.4 \times 10^5$ ATP/vesicle, giving a total of 1.51×10^5 ATP/vesicle. By estimating the total number of synapses formed by a single pyramidal neuron at 8×10^3 (Braitenberg and Schüz, 1998) and a firing rate of 4 Hz (implying a 1:4 chance that an active potential releases one vesicle), the figure of 3.2×10^8 ATP/action potential/neuron is obtained.

Contrary to previous estimates based on the measurement of heat production in peripheral *unmyelinated* nerves, the cost of action potential propagation is rather elevated. Thus by considering that an action potential actively depolarizes the cell body and axons by 100 mV and passively the dendrites by 50 mV, the calculation yields a value of 3.8×10^8 ATP/neuron. This calculation is based on the estimate of the minimal Na^+ influx required to depolarize the cell (Attwell and Laughlin, 2001). If calculations also include Ca^{2+}-mediated depolarization of dendrites, the cost is increased by 7%. Remember that these energetic costs are due to the activation of ATPases needed to restore ion gradients. Thus, the overall cost of synaptic transmission plus action potential propagation for a pyramidal neuron firing at 4 Hz would be 2.8×10^9 ATP/neuron/s. The basal energy consumption for maintenance of the resting potential based on the estimates of input resistance, reversal potential and membrane conductance yields values of 3.4×10^8 ATP/cell/s for neurons and 1×10^8 ATP/cell/s for glia, thus a combined consumption of 3.4×10^9 ATP/ cell/s assuming a 1:1 ratio between neurons and glia. On the basis of this calculation, one can conclude that $\sim 87\%$ of total energy consumed reflects the activity of glutamate-mediated neurotransmission and 13% reflects the energy requirements of resting potential maintenance (Fig. 13.7). This value is in remarkable agreement with estimates made *in vivo* using MRS. If the total energy consumption per neuron and the associated glia is compounded per gram of tissue per minute (the conventional form for expressing glucose utilisation), the figure obtained is 30 μM ATP/g/min, a value that is very close to that

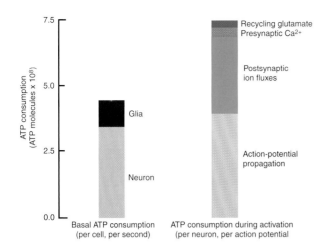

FIGURE 13.7 Energy budget for the rodent central cortex (Attwell and Laughlin, 2001). Relative rates of ATP consumption by resting neurons and glia (left). The relative cost of the various processes is associated with a firing rate of 4 Hz for a glutamatergic pyramidal neuron (modified from Frackowiak *et al.*, 2001).

determined *in vivo* for brain glucose utilization, i.e., 30–50 μM ATP/g/min (Clarke and Sokoloff, 1999).

In addition to the maintenance of ionic gradients that are disrupted during activity, other energy-consuming processes exist in neurons. Thus, the permanent synthesis of molecules needed for communications, such as neurotransmitters, or for general cellular purposes consumes energy. Axonal transport of molecules synthesized in the nucleus to their final destination along the axon or at the axon terminal is yet another process fueled by cellular energy metabolism.

Summary

Exactly as in other tissues, the metabolism of glucose, the main energy substrate of the brain, produces two forms of energy: ATP and NADPH. Glycolysis and the TCA cycle produce ATP, whereas energy in the form of reducing equivalents stored in the NADPH molecule is produced predominantly through the pentose phosphate pathway. Maintenance of the electrochemical gradients, particularly for Na^+ and K^+, needed for electrical signaling via the action potential and for chemical signaling through synaptic transmission is the main energy-consuming process of neural cells.

BRAIN ENERGY METABOLISM AT THE CELLULAR LEVEL

Glia and Vascular Endothelial Cells, in Addition to Neurons, Contribute to Brain Energy Metabolism

Neurons exist in a variety of sizes and shapes and express a large spectrum of firing properties (see Chapter 6). These differences are likely to imply specific energy demands; for example, large pyramidal cells in the primary motor cortex, which must maintain energy-consuming processes such as ion pumping over a large membrane surface or axonal transport along several centimeters, have considerably larger energy requirements than local interneurons. However, it is now clear that other cell types of the nervous system—glia and vascular endothelial cells—not only consume energy but also play a crucial role in the flux of energy substrates to neurons. Arguments for such an active role for nonneuronal cells—in particular, glia—are both quantitative and qualitative. Glial cells make up approximately half of the brain volume. A conservative figure is a 1:1 ratio between the number of astrocytes, one of the predominant glial cell types (see Chapter 3), and neurons. Higher ratios have been described, depending on the regions, developmental ages, or species. Indeed, the astrocyte-to-neuron ratio increases with the size of the brain and is thus high in humans. It is therefore clear that glucose reaching the brain parenchyma provides energy substrates to a variety of cell types, only some of which are neurons.

Even more compelling for the realization of the key role that astrocytes play in providing energy substrates to active neurons are the cytological relations that exist among brain capillaries, astrocytes, and neurons. These relations, which are illustrated in Fig. 13.8, are as follows. First, through specialized processes, called end feet, astrocytes surround brain capillaries (Kacem *et al.*, 1998). This implies that astrocytes form the first cellular barrier that glucose entering the brain parenchyma encounters and make them a likely site of prevalent glucose uptake and energy substrate distribution. More than a century ago, the Italian histologist Camillo Golgi and his pupil Luigi Sala sketched such a principle. A lucid formulation of it was presented by the British neuropathologist W. L. Andriezen in an article describing the features of the perivascular glia (Andriezen, 1893): "The development of a felted sheath of neuroglia fibers in the ground-substance immediately surrounding the blood vessels of the Brain seems therefore ... to allow the free passage of lymph and metabolic products which enter into the fluid and general metabolism of the nerve cells." In addition to perivascular end feet, astrocytes bear processes that ensheathe synaptic contacts. Astrocytes also express receptors and uptake sites with which neurotransmitters released during synaptic activity can interact (Chapter 8). These features endow astrocytes with an exquisite sensitivity to

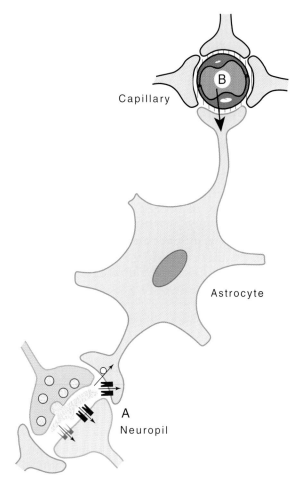

FIGURE 13.8 Schematic representation of cytological relations existing among intraparenchymal capillaries, astrocytes, and the neuropil. Astrocyte processes surround capillaries (end feet) and ensheathe synapses; in addition, receptors and uptake sites for neurotransmitters are present on astrocytes. These features make astrocytes ideally suited to sense synaptic activity (A) and to couple it with uptake and metabolism of energy substrates originating from the circulation (B).

detect increases in synaptic activity. In summary, because of the foregoing structural and functional characteristics, astrocytes are ideally suited to couple local changes in neuronal activity with coordinated adaptations in energy metabolism (see Fig. 13.8).

A Tightly Regulated Glucose Metabolism Occurs in All Cell Types of the Brain, Neuronal and Nonneuronal

Given the high degree of cellular heterogeneity of the brain, understanding the relative role played by each cell type in the flux of energy substrates has largely depended on the availability of purified preparations, such as primary cultures enriched in

neurons, astrocytes, or vascular endothelial cells. Such preparations have some drawbacks because they may not necessarily express all the properties of the cells *in situ*. In addition, one of the parameters of energy metabolism *in vivo*—namely, blood flow—cannot be examined in cultures. Despite these limitations, *in vitro* studies in primary cultures have proved very useful in identifying the cellular sites of glucose uptake and its subsequent metabolic fate, particularly, glycolysis and oxidative phosphorylation, thus providing illuminating correlations of two parameters of brain energy metabolism that are monitored *in vivo*: (1) glucose utilization and (2) oxygen consumption.

Glucose Transporters in the Brain

Glucose is a highly hydrophilic molecule that enters cells through a facilitated transport mediated by specific transporters. Eleven genes, encoding glucose transporter proteins, have been identified and cloned so far; these are designated GLUT1 to GLUT11. Glucose transporters belong to a family of rather homologous glycosylated membrane proteins with 12 transmembrane-spanning domains, and both amino and carboxyl terminals are exposed to the cytoplasmic surface of the membrane. In the brain, three transporters are expressed predominantly in a cell-specific manner, GLUT1, GLUT3, and GLUT5 (Maher *et al.*, 1994).

Two forms of GLUT1 with molecular masses of 55 and 45 kDa, respectively, are detected in the brain, depending on their degree of glycosylation. The 55-kDa form of GLUT1 is essentially localized in brain microvessels, choroid plexus, and ependymal cells. In microvessels, the distribution of GLUT1 is asymmetric, with a higher density on the ablumenal (parenchymal) side than on the vascular side. An intracellular pool of GLUT1 has also been identified in vascular endothelial cells. In the brain *in situ*, the 45-kDa form of GLUT1 is localized predominantly in astrocytes. Under culture conditions, all neural cells, including neurons and other glial cells, express GLUT1; however, this phenomenon appears to be due to the capacity of GLUT1 to be induced by cellular stress.

The glucose transporter specific to neurons is GLUT3. Its cellular distribution appears to predominate in the cell bodies rather than in the axon terminal compartment.

GLUT5 is localized to microglial cells, the resident macrophages of the brain, taking part in the immune and inflammatory responses of the nervous system. In peripheral tissues, particularly in the small intestine (from which it was cloned), GLUT5 functions as a transporter for fructose, whose concentrations are very low in the brain. In the nervous system, therefore, GLUT5 may have diverse transport functions.

Another glucose transporter, GLUT2, has been localized selectively in astrocytes of discrete brain areas, such as certain hypothalamic and brain stem nuclei, which participate in the regulation of feeding behavior and in the central control of insulin release. The insulin-sensitive glucose transporter GLUT4 has been localized in brain vascular endothelium.

It is clear that glucose uptake into the brain parenchyma is a highly specified process regulated in a cell-specific manner by glucose transporter subtypes. Figure 13.9 summarizes this process: Glucose enters the brain through 55-kDa GLUT1 transporters localized on endothelial cells of the blood–brain barrier. Uptake into astrocytes is mediated by 45-kDa GLUT1 transporters, whereas GLUT3 transporters mediate this process in neurons. GLUT2 transporters on astrocytes may "sense" glucose, a function of this glucose transporter subtype in pancreatic β cells. Finally, GLUT5 mediates the uptake of an unidentified substrate into microglial cells. Other glucose transporters

recently identified on neurons are GLUT×1 (or GLUT8) and GLUT9.

Cell-Specific Glucose Uptake and Metabolism

As we have seen, glucose utilization can be assessed with radioactively labeled 2-DG. To determine the cellular site of basal and activity-related glucose utilization, this technique has been applied to homogeneous cultures of astrocytes or neurons. For quantitative purposes and to allow comparisons with *in vivo* studies, these *in vitro* experiments, in which radioactive 2-DG is used as a tracer, must be conducted in a medium containing a concentration of glucose near that measured *in vivo* in the extracellular space of the brain, for which values ranging between 0.5 and 2.0 mM have been reported (Fellows *et al.*, 1992). The basal rate of glucose utilization is higher in astrocytes than in neurons, with values of about 20 and 6 nmol per milligram of protein per minute, respectively (Magistretti and Pellerin, 1999). These values are of the same order as those determined *in*

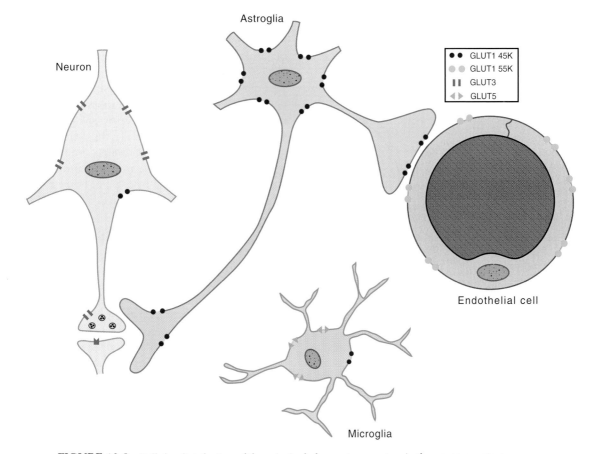

FIGURE 13.9 Cellular distribution of the principal glucose transporters in the nervous system.

vivo for cortical gray matter (10–20 nmol mg^{-1} min^{-1}) with the 2-DG autoradiographic technique. In view of this difference and of the quantitative preponderance of astrocytes compared with neurons in the gray matter, these data reveal a significant contribution by astrocytes to basal glucose utilization as determined by 2-DG autoradiography or PET *in vivo*.

The contribution of astrocytes to glucose utilization during activation is even more striking. *In vitro*, acti-

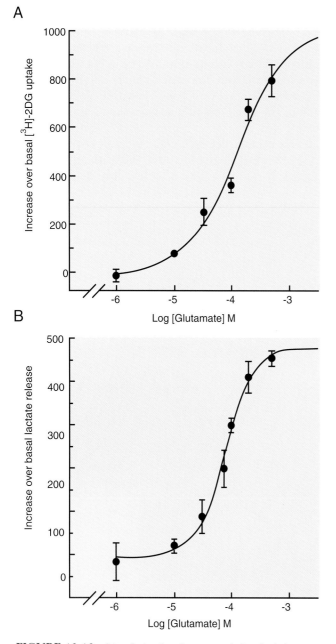

FIGURE 13.10 Stimulation by glutamate of glycolysis in astrocytes. Glutamate stimulates glucose uptake and phosphorylation (A) and lactate production (B) in astrocytes. This effect is concentration dependent with an EC$_{50}$ of ~60 mM.

vation can be mimicked by exposure of the cells to glutamate, the principal excitatory neurotransmitter (Chapter 8), because, during activation of a given cortical area, the concentration of glutamate in the extracellular space increases considerably due to its release from the axon terminals of activated pathways. As shown in Fig. 13.10A, L–glutamate stimulates 2-DG uptake and phosphorylation by astrocytes in a concentration-dependent manner, with an EC$_{50}$ of 60 to 80 mM (Pellerin and Magistretti, 1994; Takahashi *et al.*, 1995). Unlike other actions of glutamate, stimulation of glucose utilization in astrocytes is mediated not by specific glutamate receptors, but by glutamate transporters. Indeed, in addition to the maintenance of extracellular K$^+$ homeostasis, one of the well-established functions of astrocytes is to ensure the reuptake of certain neurotransmitters, particularly, that of glutamate at excitatory synapses (Danbolt, 2001). At least three glutamate transporter subtypes have been cloned in various species, including humans. The GLT-1 subtype is localized exclusively in astrocytes, whereas the EAAC1 subtype is exclusively neuronal; GLAST, the third subtype, is expressed both in glia and in neurons, with a predominant distribution in astrocytes. The density of GLT-1 and GLAST is particularly high on astrocytes that surround nerve terminals and dendritic spines, consistent with the prominent role of these transporters in the reuptake of synaptically released glutamate (Danbolt, 2001). The driving force for glutamate uptake through the specific transporters is the transmembrane Na$^+$ gradient; indeed, glutamate is cotransported with Na$^+$ in a ratio of one glutamate for every two or three Na$^+$ ions. The selective loss of GLT-1, the astrocyte-selective glutamate transporter, has been demonstrated in the motor cortex and spinal cord of patients who died of amyotrophic lateral sclerosis, a neurodegenerative disease affecting motor neurons.

Glutamate-Stimulated Uptake of Glucose by Astrocytes is a Source of Insight into the Cellular Bases of ^{18}F–2–DG PET *in Vivo*

The glutamate-stimulated uptake of glucose by astrocytes is a source of insight into the cellular bases of the activation-induced local increase in glucose utilization visualized with ^{18}F–2–DG PET *in vivo*. As we have seen, focal physiological activation of specific brain areas is accompanied by increases in glucose utilization; because glutamate is released from excitatory synapses when neuronal pathways subserving specific modalities are activated, the stimulation by glutamate of glucose utilization in astrocytes provides a direct mechanism for coupling neuronal activity to

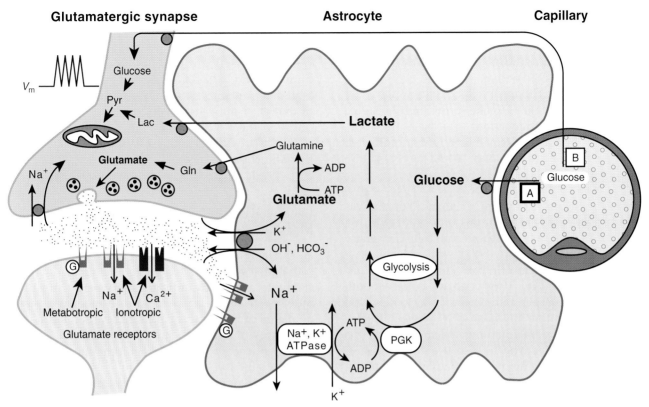

FIGURE 13.11 Schematic representation of the mechanism for glutamate-induced glycolysis in astrocytes during physiological activation. At glutamatergic synapses, presynaptically released glutamate depolarizes postsynaptic neurons by acting at specific receptor subtypes. The action of glutamate is terminated by an efficient glutamate uptake system located primarily in astrocytes. Glutamate is cotransported with Na$^+$, resulting in an increase in the intraastrocytic concentration of Na$^+$, leading to an activation of the astrocyte Na$^+$,K$^+$-ATPase. Activation of Na$^+$,K$^+$-ATPase stimulates glycolysis (i.e., glucose utilization and lactate production). The stoichiometry of this process is such that for one glutamate molecule taken up with three Na$^+$ ions, one glucose molecule enters astrocytes, two ATP molecules are produced through glycolysis, and two lactate molecules are released. Within the astrocyte, one ATP fuels one "turn of the pump," while the other provides the energy needed to convert glutamate to glutamine by glutamine synthase (see Fig. 13.13). Once released by astrocytes, lactate can be taken up by neurons and serve as an energy substrate. (For graphic clarity only lactate uptake into presynaptic terminals is indicated. However, this process could also take place at the postsynaptic neuron.) In accord with recent evidence, glutamate receptors are also shown on astrocytes. This model, which summarizes *in vitro* experimental evidence indicating glutamate-induced glycolysis, is taken to show cellular and molecular events occurring during activation of a given cortical area (arrow labeled A, activation). Direct glucose uptake into neurons under basal conditions is also shown (arrow labeled B, basal conditions). Pyr, pyruvate; Lac, lactate; Gln, glutamine; G, G protein. Modified from Pellerin and Magistretti (1994).

glucose utilization in the brain (Fig. 13.11). The intracellular molecular mechanism of this coupling requires Na$^+$, K$^+$-ATPase because ouabain completely inhibits the glutamate-evoked 2-DG uptake by astrocytes (Pellerin and Magistretti, 1994). The astrocytic Na$^+$, K$^+$-ATPase responds predominantly to increases in intracellular Na$^+$ (Na^+_i) for which it shows a K_m of about 10 mM (Erecinska, 1989). In astrocytes, the Na^+_i concentration ranges between 10 and 20 mM, and so Na$^+$, K$^+$-ATPase is set to be activated readily when Na^+_i rises concomitantly with glutamate uptake. These observations indicate that a major determinant of glucose utilization is the activity of Na$^+$, K$^+$-ATPase. In this context, we should note that, *in vivo*, the main

mechanism that accounts for activation-induced 2-DG uptake is the activity of Na$^+$, K$^+$-ATPase.

It is important here to briefly consider the relative participation of the neuronal and astrocytic Na$^+$, K$^+$-ATPases in glucose utilization. When glutamate is released from depolarized neuronal terminals, it is taken up predominantly into astrocytes. The stoichiometry of glutamate reuptake being one molecule of glutamate cotransported with three Na$^+$ ions, the increase in intracellular astrocytic Na$^+$ concentration associated with glutamate reuptake massively activates the pump. Thus, although the tonic activity of the Na$^+$, K$^+$-ATPase is needed to maintain the transmembrane neuronal and glial ionic gradients and accounts for basal glucose utilization, on a short-term temporal scale (from milliseconds to seconds), when glutamate is released from depolarized axon terminals of modality-specific afferents, the astrocytic Na^+, K^+-ATPase is briskly activated, due to the massive increase (by at least 10 mM) in intracellular Na^+ associated with glutamate reuptake, providing the signal for the activation-dependent glucose utilization. Increases of glutamate as small as 10 μM are sufficient to double the activity of Na^+, K^+-ATPase (Chattan et al., 2000).

How does activation of Na^+, K^+-ATPase cause increased glucose utilization? The mechanism was explained by pioneering studies on erythrocytes by Joseph Hoffmann and colleagues at Yale University (Proverbio and Hoffman, 1977), which have been confirmed in a number of other cell systems, including brain (Erecinska, 1989) and vascular smooth muscle. The increase in pump activity consumes ATP, which is a negative modulator of phosphofructo-kinase, the principal rate-limiting enzyme of glycolysis (see Fig. 13.1). Thus, when ATP concentration is low, phosphofructokinase activity is stimulated, resulting in increased glucose utilization. The activity of hexokinase, the enzyme responsible for glucose and 2-DG phosphorylation (see Fig. 13.4), is also increased under these conditions. This explains why the increase in glucose utilization, associated with the stimulation of Na^+,K^+-ATPase, can be monitored with 2-DG, which is not processed beyond the hexokinase step.

A compartmentalization of glucose uptake during activation has also been unequivocally found by Marco Tsacopoulos and colleagues in the honeybee drone retina (Tsacopoulos et al., 1988). In this highly organized, crystal-like nervous tissue preparation, photoreceptor cells form rosette-like structures that are surrounded by glial cells. In addition, mitochondria are exclusively present in the photoreceptor neurons. Light activation reveals an increase in radioactive 2-DG uptake in the glial cells surrounding the rosettes but not in the photoreceptor neurons. An increase in O_2 consumption is nevertheless measured in photoreceptor neurons. After activation of photoreceptors by light, glucose is probably taken up predominantly by glial cells, which then release a metabolic substrate to be oxidized by photoreceptor neurons.

In summary, as indicated in the operational model described in Fig. 13.11, upon activation of a particular brain area, glutamate released from excitatory terminals is taken up by a Na^+-dependent transporter located on astrocytes. The ensuing local increase in intracellular Na^+ concentration activates Na^+, K^+-ATPase, which in turn stimulates glucose uptake by astrocytes. This model delineates a simple mechanism for coupling synaptic activity to glucose utilization; in addition, it is consistent with the notion that the signals detected during physiological activation in humans with ^{18}F-2-DG PET and autoradiography in laboratory animals may predominantly reflect uptake of the tracer into astrocytes. This conclusion does not question the validity of the 2-DG-based techniques; rather, it provides a cellular and molecular basis for these functional brain-imaging techniques (Magistretti et al., 1999).

Lactate Released by Astrocytes May Be a Metabolic Substrate for Neurons

The fact that the increase in glucose uptake during activation can be ascribed predominantly, if not exclusively, to astrocytes indicates that energy substrates must be released by astrocytes to meet the energy demands of neurons. As indicated earlier, lactate and pyruvate are adequate substrates for brain tissue in vitro (Schurr et al., 1999). In fact, synaptic activity can be maintained in vitro in cerebral cortical slices with only lactate or pyruvate as a substrate (Schurr et al., 1999). Lactate is quantitatively the main metabolic intermediate released by cultured astrocytes at a rate of 15 to 30 nmol per milligram of protein per minute. Other quantitatively less important intermediates released by astrocytes are pyruvate (approximately 10 times less than lactate) and α-ketoglutarate, citrate, and malate, which are released in marginal amounts. For lactate (or pyruvate) to be a metabolic substrate for neurons, particularly during activation, two additional conditions must be fulfilled: (1) that indeed during activation lactate release by astrocytes increases and (2) lactate uptake by neurons must be demonstrated. Both mechanisms have been demonstrated. Mimicking activation in vitro by exposing cultured astrocytes to glutamate results in a marked release of lactate and, to a lesser degree, pyruvate (Pellerin and Magistretti, 1994) (see Fig. 13.10B). This glutamate-evoked lactate release shows the same pharmacology and time course as glutamate-evoked glucose utilization and indicates that glutamate stimulates the processing of glucose through glycolysis. In vivo ^{1}H MRI studies in humans that show a transient lactate peak in the primary visual cortex during physiological stimulation are consistent with the notion of activation-induced glycolysis. In addition, lactate levels in the rat somatosensory cortex transiently increase subsequent to forepaw stimulation. Finally, monocarboxylate transporters have been demonstrated on neurons and astrocytes in addition to capillaries (Pierre et al., 2000).

Thus, a metabolic compartmentation whereby glucose taken up by astrocytes and metabolized glycolytically to lactate is then released in the extracellular space to be utilized by neurons is consistent with biochemical and electrophysiological observations (Magistretti *et al.*, 1999; Tsacopoulos and Magistretti, 1996). This array of *in vitro* and *in vivo* experimental evidence is summarized in the model of cell-specific metabolic regulation illustrated in Fig. 13.11.

Studies of the well-compartmentalized honeybee drone retina and of isolated preparations of guinea pig retina containing photoreceptors attached to Mueller (glial) cells corroborate the existence of such metabolic fluxes between glia and neurons. In addition to the glial localization of glucose uptake during activation, glycolytic products have been shown to be released. In particular, during activation, glial cells in the honeybee drone retina release alanine produced from pyruvate by transamination; the released alanine is taken up by photoreceptor neurons and, after reconversion into pyruvate, can enter the TCA cycle to yield ATP through oxidative phosphorylation (see Fig. 13.2). In the guinea pig retina, lactate, formed glycolytically from glucose, is released by Mueller cells to fuel photoreceptor neurons.

Although plasma lactate is unlikely to be a substitute for glucose as a metabolic substrate for the brain, lactate formed within the brain parenchyma (e.g., through glutamate-activated glycolysis in astrocytes) can fulfill the energetic needs of neurons. Lactate, after conversion into pyruvate by a reaction catalyzed by lactate dehydrogenase (LDH), can provide, on a molar basis, 18 ATP through oxidative phosphorylation. Conversion of lactate into pyruvate does not require ATP, and, in this regard, lactate is energetically more favorable than the first obligatory step of glycolysis in which glucose is phosphorylated to glucose 6-phosphate at the expense of one molecule of ATP (see Fig. 13.1). Another metabolic fate for lactate has been shown *in vitro* and *in vivo* by MRS. Thus, once converted to pyruvate, lactate may enzymatically yield glutamate and hence be a substrate for the replenishment of the neuronal pool of glutamate. Because this reaction is not associated with oxygen consumption, part of the uncoupling between glucose utilization and oxygen consumption described in certain paradigms of activation may be explained by the processing of glucose-derived lactate into the glutamate neuronal pool.

Glycogen, the Storage Form of Glucose, Is Localized in Astrocytes

Glycogen is the single largest energy reserve of the brain (Magistretti *et al.*, 1993); it is mainly localized in astrocytes, although ependymal and choroid plexus cells, as well as certain large neurons in the brain stem, contain glycogen. When compared to the contents in liver and muscle, the glycogen content of the brain is exceedingly small, about 100 and 10 times inferior, respectively. Thus, the brain can hardly be considered a glycogen storage organ, and here the function of glycogen should be viewed as that of providing a metabolic buffer during physiological activity.

Glycogen Metabolism Is Coupled to Neuronal Activity

Glycogen turnover in the brain is extremely rapid, and glycogen levels are finely coordinated with synaptic activity (Magistretti *et al.*, 1993). For example, during general anesthesia, a condition in which synaptic activity is markedly attenuated, glycogen levels rise sharply. Interestingly, however, the glycogen content of cultures containing exclusively astrocytes is not increased by general anesthetics; this observation indicates that the *in vivo* action of general anesthetics on astrocyte glycogen is due to the inhibition of neuronal activity, stressing the existence of a tight coupling between synaptic activity and astrocyte glycogen. Accordingly, reactive astrocytes, which develop in areas where neuronal activity is decreased or absent as a consequence of injury, contain high amounts of glycogen.

In addition to glycogen, glucose is incorporated into other macromolecules such as proteins (glycoproteins) and lipids (glycolipids) at rates specific for the turnover of each macromolecule, which can span from a few minutes to a few days.

Certain Neurotransmitters Regulate Glycogen Metabolism in Astrocytes

Glycogen levels in astrocytes are tightly regulated by various neurotransmitters. Several monoamine neurotransmitters—namely, noradrenaline, serotonin, and histamine—are glycogenolytic in the brain, in addition to certain peptides, such as vasoactive intestinal peptide (VIP) and pituitary adenylate cyclase activating peptide (PACAP), and adenosine and ATP (Magistretti *et al.*, 1993). The effects of all these neurotransmitters are mediated by their cogent specific receptors coupled to second messenger pathways that are under the control of adenylate cyclase or phospholipase C. The initial rate of glycogenolysis activated by VIP and noradrenaline is between 5 and 10 nmol per milligram of protein per minute, a value that is remarkably close to glucose utilization of the gray matter, as determined by the 2-DG auto-radiographic method. This correlation indicates that glycosyl units mobilized in response to glycogenolytic neurotransmitters can provide quantitatively adequate substrates for the energy demands of the brain parenchyma. At present, whether the glycosyl units mobilized through glycogenolysis are used by astrocytes to meet their energy demands during activation or are metabolized to a substrate such as lactate, which is then released for the use of neurons, is not clear. It appears, however, that glucose is not released by astrocytes after glycogenolysis, supporting the view that the activity of glucose-6-phosphatase (see Fig. 13.1) in astrocytes is very low. *In vitro* evidence suggests that lactate may be the metabolic intermediate produced through glycogenolysis and exported from astrocytes.

These observations show that neuronal signals (e.g., certain neurotransmitters) can exert receptor-mediated metabolic effects on astrocytes in a manner similar to peripheral hormones on their target cells. However, the action of this type of neurotransmitter is temporally specified and spatially restricted to activated areas. Indeed, brain glycogenolysis visualized by autoradiography in laboratory animals has also been demonstrated *in vivo* after physiological activation of a modality-specific pathway (Swanson *et al.*, 1992). Repeated stimulation of whiskers resulted in a marked decrease in the density of glycogen-associated autoradiographic grains in the somatosensory cortex of rats (barrel fields), as well as in the relevant thalamic nuclei (Swanson *et al.*, 1992). These observations indicate that the physiological activation of specific neuronal circuits results in the mobilization of glial glycogen stores.

Summary

Under basal conditions, glucose uptake and metabolism occur in every brain cell type. Glucose uptake is mediated by specific transporters that are distributed in a cell-specific manner. Astrocytes play a critical role in the utilization of glucose coupled to excitatory synaptic transmission. The molecular mechanisms of this coupling are stoichiometrically directed: for each synaptically released glutamate molecule taken up with three Na^+ ions by an astrocyte, one glucose molecule enters the same astrocyte, two ATP molecules are produced through glycolysis, and two lactate molecules are released and consumed by neurons to yield 18 ATPs through oxidative phosphorylation. Neuronal signals, e.g., certain neurotransmitters, can exert receptor-mediated glycogenolysis in astrocytes in a manner similar to peripheral hormones

on their target cells. However, this type of effect by neurotransmitters is temporally specified and spatially restricted within activated areas, possibly to provide additional energy substrates in register with local increases in neuronal activity.

GLUTAMATE AND NITROGEN METABOLISM: A COORDINATED SHUTTLE BETWEEN ASTROCYTES AND NEURONS

As has been shown, synaptically released glutamate is removed rapidly from the extracellular space by a transporter-mediated reuptake system that is particularly efficient in astrocytes (Danbolt, 2001). This mechanism contributes in a crucial manner to the fidelity of glutamate-mediated neurotransmission. Indeed, glutamate levels in the extracellular space are low (<3 μM), allowing for optimal glutamate-mediated signaling after depolarization while preventing overactivation of glutamate receptors, which could eventually result in excitotoxic neuronal damage.

One may wonder how astrocytes dispose of the glutamate that they take up, because, unlike carbohydrates or lipids, amino acids cannot be stored. The predominant pathway in peripheral tissues for disposing of amino acids is the transfer of their α amino group to a corresponding α-keto acid; this reaction is catalyzed by aminotransferases (Fig. 13.12). In astrocytes, the α amino group of glutamate can be transferred to oxaloacetate to yield α-ketoglutarate (α-KG) and aspartate in a reaction catalyzed by aspartate

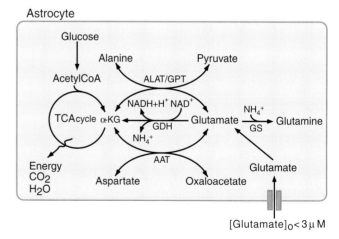

FIGURE 13.12 Metabolic fate of glutamate taken up by astrocytes. ALAT, alanine aminotransferase; GDH, glutamate dehydrogenase; GS, glutamine synthase; AAT, aspartate aminotransferase; GPT, glutamate dehydrogenase; α-KG, α-ketoglutarate.

amino transferase (AAT). The α-KG generated is an intermediate of the TCA cycle and is therefore oxidized further. Another transamination reaction catalyzed by alanine amino transferase (ALAT) transfers the α amino group of glutamate to pyruvate, resulting in the formation of alanine and α-KG.

Two other pathways exist in astrocytes to metabolize glutamate. First, glutamate can be converted directly into α-KG through an NAD-requiring oxidative deamination catalyzed by glutamate dehydrogenase (GDH) (see Fig. 13.12). Glutamate, by entering the TCA cycle indirectly (through AAT or ALAT) or directly (through GDH), is an energy substrate for astrocytes. Second, the quantitatively predominant metabolic pathway of glutamate in astrocytes is its amidation to glutamine, an ATP-requiring reaction in which an ammonium ion is fixed on glutamate (see Fig. 13.12) (Van den Berg and Garfinkel, 1971). This reaction is catalyzed by glutamine synthase (GS), an enzyme almost exclusively localized in astrocytes,

and provides an efficient means of disposing not only of glutamate but also of ammonium (Box 13.2). Glutamine is released by astrocytes and is taken up by neurons, where it is hydrolyzed back to glutamate by the phosphate-dependent mitochondrial enzyme glutaminase (Erecinska and Silver, 1990). This metabolic pathway, often referred to as the glutamate–glutamine shuttle, is a clear example of cooperation between astrocytes and neurons (Fig. 13.13). It allows the removal of potentially toxic excess glutamate from the extracellular space, while returning to the neuron a synaptically inert (glutamine does not affect neurotransmission) precursor with which to regenerate the neuronal pool of glutamate.

However, not all glutamate is regenerated through the glutamate–glutamine shuttle because some of the glutamate released by neurons enters at the α-KG level, the TCA cycle in astrocytes; therefore, *de novo* synthesis is required to maintain the neuronal glutamate pool. Glutamate can be synthesized through NADPH–

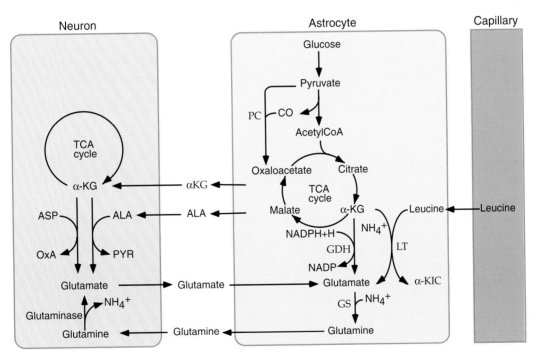

FIGURE 13.13 Metabolic intermediates are released by astrocytes to regenerate the glutamate neurotransmitter pool in neurons. Glutamine, formed from glutamate in a reaction catalyzed by glutamine synthase (GS), is released by astrocytes and taken up by neurons, which convert it into glutamate under the action of glutaminase. GS is an enzyme selectively localized in astrocytes. This metabolic cycle is referred to as the glutamate–glutamine shuttle. Other quantitatively less important sources of neuronal glutamate are lactate, alanine, and α-ketoglutarate (α-KG). In astrocytes, glutamate is synthesized *de novo* from α-KG in a reaction catalyzed by glutamate dehydrogenase (GDH). The carbon backbone of glutamate is exported by astrocytes after conversion into glutamine under the action of GS; the conversion of leucine into α-ketoisocaproate (α-KIC), catalyzed by leucine transaminase (LT), provides the amino group for the synthesis of glutamine from glutamate. Carbons "lost" from the TCA cycle as α-KG is converted into glutamate are replenished by oxaloacetate (OxA) formed from pyruvate in a reaction catalyzed by pyruvate carboxylase, another astrocyte-specific enzyme.

BOX 13.2

HEPATIC ENCEPHALOPATHY IS A DISORDER OF ASTROCYTE FUNCTION RESULTING IN A NEUROPSYCHIATRIC SYNDROME

Hepatic encephalopathy is observed in patients with severe liver failure. The disease can be in one of two forms: an acute form, called fulminant hepatic failure, and a chronic form, portosystemic encephalopathy. The neuropsychiatric symptoms of fulminant hepatic failure are delirium, coma, and seizures associated with acute toxic or viral hepatic failure. Patients having porto-systemic encephalopathy may present personality changes, episodic confusion, or stupor and, in the most severe cases, coma. The current view on the pathophysiology of hepatic encephalopathy is that, due to liver failure, "toxic" substances that affect brain function accumulate in the circulation.

One of the substances thought to be responsible for neuropsychiatric "toxicity" is ammonia. The neuropathological findings are rather striking: astrocytes are the brain cells that appear principally affected. In the acute form, astrocyte swelling is prominent and likely to be the cause of the observed acute brain edema. In portosystemic encephalopathy, astrocytes adopt morphological features characteristic of what is defined as an Alzheimer type II astrocyte: in these cells, the nucleus is pale and enlarged, chromatin is marginated, and a prominent nucleolus is often observed. Lipofuscin deposits may be present, and the amount of the astrocyte-specific protein glial fibrillary acidic protein (see Chapter 4) is decreased. Neurons appear structurally normal. All the foregoing histopathological changes have been reproduced *in vitro* by acutely or chronically applying ammonium chloride to primary astrocyte cultures. As mentioned earlier, detoxification of ammonium is an ATP-requiring, astrocyte-specific reaction catalyzed by glutamine synthase (see Fig. 13.12). It is therefore not surprising that excess ammonia perturbs energy metabolism; indeed, ammonia stimulates glycolysis whereas it inhibits TCA cycle activity. In addition, ammonia decreases the glycogen content of astrocytes markedly.

In summary, while the precise pathophysiological mechanisms of the neuropsychiatric syndrome in hepatic encephalopathy are still unknown, this clinical condition provides a striking illustration of the fundamental importance of neuron–astrocyte metabolic interactions because structural and functional alterations apparently restricted to astrocytes result in severe behavioral perturbations.

Pierre J. Magistretti

dependent reductive amination of α-KG catalyzed by GDH (note that here the cofactor is NADPH, whereas, for the opposite reaction also catalyzed by GDH, the oxidant is NAD; see Figs. 13.12 and 13.13) (Erecinska and Silver, 1990). For the synthesis of glutamate, glucose provides the carbon backbone as α-KG through the TCA cycle, whereas an exogenous source of nitrogen is necessary (see Fig. 13.13). Convincing evidence, obtained by using ^{15}N-labeled amino acids whose metabolic fate was determined by gas chromatography and mass spectrometry, indicates that plasma leucine provides the nitrogen required for net glutamate synthesis from α-KG. Thus, leucine taken up from the circulation at astrocytic end feet provides the amino group to α-KG in a reaction catalyzed by leucine transaminase (LT), resulting in the formation of glutamate and α-ketoisocaproate (α-KIC) (see Fig. 13.13). Because this reaction takes place in astrocytes, to replenish the neuronal glutamate pool, the astrocytes export glutamate as glutamine. As noted earlier, the neuronal glutamate pool could also be replenished by lactate released by astrocytes.

Finally, another potential pathway described by Arne Schousboe and colleagues exists for the *de novo* synthesis of glutamate in neurons from substrates provided by astrocytes. With the use of uniformly labeled ^{13}C compounds in combination with magnetic resonance spectroscopy, astrocytes have been shown to release significant amounts of alanine and α-KG. Both metabolic intermediates are taken up by neurons and can be converted into glutamate and pyruvate in a transamination reaction catalyzed by ALAT (see Fig. 13.12). In this case, as for the glutamate–glutamine shuttle (Fig. 13.13), astrocytes provide the substrate(s) necessary for glutamate synthesis in neurons.

Note that because α-KG is used for glutamate synthesis, metabolic intermediates downstream of α-KG must be available to maintain a sustained flux through the TCA cycle in astrocytes (see Fig. 13.13). This need is met by the activity of the enzyme pyruvate carboxylase (PC), which fixes CO_2 on pyruvate to generate oxaloacetate, which, by condensing with acetyl-CoA, maintains the flux through the TCA cycle. The carboxylation of pyruvate to oxaloacetate is referred to as an anaplerotic (Greek for "fill up") reaction. Interestingly, like glutamine synthase, PC is selectively localized in astrocytes. The fact that these two enzymes are localized in astrocytes in conjunction with the existence of a glutamate–glutamine shuttle stresses that astrocytes are essential for maintaining the neuronal glutamate pool used for neurotransmission (see Fig. 13.13).

As noted earlier, the metabolic intermediate α-KG lies at the branching point of glucose and glutamate metabolism (see Fig. 13.12). Any change in the activities of the enzymes that convert α-KG into glutamate or into succinyl-CoA, the next intermediate in the TCA cycle, may affect the efficacy of the TCA cycle or glutamate levels. Interestingly, a marked decrease in the activity of α-ketoglutarate dehydrogenase (α-KGDH), the enzyme catalyzing the conversion of α-KG into succinyl-CoA, was found in a very high proportion of postmortem brains from patients with Alzheimer disease; in addition, a similar decrease in α-KGDH activity has been demonstrated in the fibroblasts of patients affected by the familial form of Alzheimer disease.

Summary

A key function of astrocytes is to remove synaptically released glutamate. A large proportion of glutamate is transformed to glutamine through an energy- requiring process that also allows for the detoxification of ammonium. Glutamine released by astrocytes regenerates the neuronal glutamate pool. Some of the glutamate is also regenerated from lactate and through fixation of the amino group of leucine onto the TCA intermediate α-KG, providing another indication of the tight link existing between glutamate and nitrogen metabolism and of the crucial function that astrocytes play in maintaining the neuronal glutamate pool at levels that ensure the maintenance of synaptic transmission.

THE ASTROCYTE–NEURON METABOLIC UNIT

From a strictly energetic viewpoint, the brain can be seen as an almost exclusive glucose-processing machine producing H_2O and CO_2. However, the metabolism of glucose in the brain is specified temporally, spatially, and functionally. Thus, glucose metabolism increases with exquisite spatiotemporal precision in register with neuronal activity. The site of this increase is not the neuronal cell body; rather, it is the neuropil,

where presynaptic terminals, postsynaptic elements, and astrocytes ensheathing synaptic contacts are localized (Sokoloff, 1981). This cytological relation between astrocytes and neurons is also manifested by a functional metabolic partnership: in response to a neuronal signal (glutamate), astrocytes release a glucose-derived metabolic substrate for neurons (lactate). Glucose also provides the carbon backbone for regeneration of the neuronal pool of glutamate. This process results from a close astrocyte– neuron cooperation. Indeed, the selective localization of pyruvate carboxylase in astrocytes, indicating the need to replenish the TCA cycle with carbon backbones, strongly suggests that glucose-derived metabolic intermediates are used for glutamate (and other amino acid) synthesis. The newly synthesized glutamate is not provided as such by astrocytes to neurons; rather, it is converted into glutamine by-glutamine synthase, another enzyme localized selectively in astrocytes. Glutamate, taken up by astrocytes during synaptic activity, undergoes the same metabolic process, also being released as glutamine (the glutamate–glutamine shuttle).

Summary

In conclusion, the axon terminal of glutamatergic neurons, which are the main communication lines in the nervous system, and the astrocytic processes that surround them should be viewed as a metabolic unit in which the neuron furnishes the activation signal (glutamate) to the astrocyte and the astrocyte provides not only the precursors needed to maintain the neurotransmitter pool (glutamine and, in part, lactate

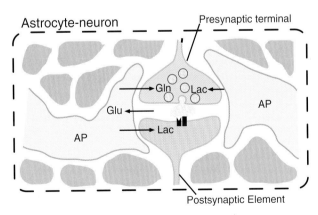

FIGURE 13.14 The astrocyte–neuron metabolic unit. Glutamatergic terminals and the astrocytic processes that surround them can be viewed as a highly specialized metabolic unit in which the activation signal (glutamate) is furnished by the neuron to the astrocyte, whereas the astrocyte provides the precursors needed to maintain the neurotransmitter pool (glutamine, lactate, alanine), as well as the energy substrate (lactate). AP, astrocyte process.

and alanine), but also the energy substrate (lactate) (Fig. 13.14). The efficacy of the predominant excitatory synapse in the brain, the glutamatergic synapse, cannot be maintained without a close astrocyte–neuron interaction.

References

Andriezen, W. L. (1893). On a system of fibre-like cells surrounding the blood vessels of the brain of man and mammals, and its physiological significance. *Int. Monatsschr. Anat. Physiol.* **10**, 532–540.

Attwell, D., and Laughlin, S. B. (2001). An energy b udget for signalling in the grey matter of the brain. *J. Cereb. Blood Flow Metab.*

Chatton, J. Y., Marquet, P., and Magistretti, P. J. (2000). A quantitative analysis of L-glutamate-regulated Na$^+$ dynamics in mouse cortical astrocytes: implications for cellular bioenergetics. *Eur. J. Neurosci.* **12**, 3843–3853.

Clarke, D. D., and Sokoloff, L. (1999). Circulation and energy metabolism of the brain. *In* "Basic Neurochemistry: Molecular, Cellular and Medical Aspects" (G. Siegel, B. Agranoff, R. W. Albers, S. K. Fisher, and M. D. Uhler, eds.), pp. 637–669. Lippincott-Raven, Philadelphia.

Danbolt, N. C. (2001). Glutamate uptake. *Prog. Neurobiol.* **65**, 1–105.

Erecinska, M. (1989). Stimulation of the Na+/K+ pump activity during electrogenic uptake of acidic amino acid transmitters by rat brain synaptosomes. *J. Neurochem.* **52**, 135–139.

Erecinska, M., and Silver, I. A. (1990). Metabolism and role of glutamate in mammalian brain. *Prog. Neurobiol.* **35**, 245–296.

Fellows, L. K., Boutelle, M. G., and Fillenz, M. (1992). Extracellular brain glucose levels reflect local neuronal activity: A microdialysis study in awake, freely moving rats. *J. Neurochem.* **59**, 2141–2147.

Fox, P. T., Raichle, M. E., Mintun, M. A., and Dence, C. (1988). Nonoxidative glucose consumption during focal physiologic neural activity. *Science* **241**, 462–464.

Frackowiak, R. S. J., Lenzi, G. L., Jones, T., and Heather, J. D. (1980). Quantitative measurement of regional cerebral blood flow and oxygen metabolism in man using 150 and positron emission tomography: Theory, procedure and normal values. *J. Comput. Assist. Tomogr.* **4**, 727–736.

Frackowiak, R. S. J., Magistretti, P. J., Shulman, R. G., and Adams, M. (2001). "Neuroenergetics: Relevance for Functional Brain Imaging." HFSP, Strasbourg.

Iadecola, C., Pelligrino, D. A., Moskowitz, M. A., and Lassen, N. A. (1994). Nitric oxide synthase inhibition and cerebrovascular regulation. *J. Cereb. Blood Flow Metab.* **14**, 175–192.

Kacem, K., Lacombe, P., Seylaz, J., and Bonvento, G. (1998). Structural organization of the perivascular astrocyte endfeet and their relationship with the endothelial glucose transporter : A confocal microscopy study. *Glia* **23**, 1–10.

Kety, S. S., and Schmidt, C. F. (1948). The nitrous oxide method for the quantitative determination of cerebral blood flow in man: Theory, procedure, and normal values. *J. Clin. Invest.* **27**, 476–483.

Magistretti, P., and Pellerin, L. (1999). Cellular mechanisms of brain energy metabolism and their relevance to functional brain imaging. *Phil. Trans. R. Soc. Lond. B* **354**, 1155–1163.

Magistretti, P. J., Pellerin, L., Rothman, D. L., and Shulman, R. G. (1999). Energy on demand. *Science* **283**, 496–497.

Magistretti, P. J., Sorg, O., and Martin, J. L. (1993). Regulation of glycogen metabolism in astrocytes: Physiological, pharmacological, and pathological aspects. *In* "Astrocytes: Pharmacology and Function" (S. Murphy, ed.), pp. 243–265. Academic Press, San Diego.

Maher, F., Vannucci, S. J., and Simpson, I. A. (1994). Glucose transporter proteins in brain. *FASEB J.* **8**, 1003–1011.

Ogawa, S., Tank, D. W., Menon, R., Ellermann, J. M., Kim, S.-G., Merkle, H., and Ugurbil, K. (1992) Intrinsic signal changes accompanying sensory stimulation: Functional brain mapping with magnetic resonance imaging. *Proc. Natl. Acad. Sci. USA* **89**, 5951–5955.

Owen, O. E., Morgan, A. P., Kemp, H. G., Sullivan, J. M., Herrera, M. G., and Cahill, G. F. J. (1967). Brain metabolism during fasting. *J. Clin. Invest.* **46**, 1589–1595.

Pellerin, L., and Magistretti, P. J. (1994). Glutamate uptake into astrocytes stimulates aerobic glycolysis: A mechanism coupling neuronal activity to glucose utilization. *Proc. Natl. Acad. Sci. USA* **91**, 10625–10629.

Phelps, M. E., Huang, S. C., Hoffman, E. J., Selin, C., Sokoloff, L., and Kuhl, D. E. (1979). Tomographic measurement of local cerebral glucose metabolic rate in humans with (F-18)2-fluoro-2-deoxy-D-glucose: Validation of method. *Ann. Neurol.* **6**, 371–388.

Pierre, K., Pellerin, L., Debernardi, R., Riederer, B. M., and Magistretti, P. J. (2000). Cell-specific localization of monocarboxylate transporters, MCT1 and MCT2 in the adult mouse brain revealed by double immunohistochemical labeling and confocal microscopy. *Neuroscience* **100**, 617–727.

Proverbio, F., and Hoffman, J. F. (1977). Membrane compartmentalized ATP and its preferential use by the Na+-K+ ATPase of human red cell ghosts. *J. Gen. Physiol.* **69**, 605–632.

Roy, C. S., and Sherrington, C. S. (1890). On the regulation of the blood supply of the brain. *J. Physiol. (Lond.)* **11**, 85–108.

Schurr, A., Miller, J. J., Payne, R. S., and Rigor, B. M. (1999). An increase in lactate output by brain tissue serves to meet the energy needs of glutamate-activated neurons. *J. Neurosci.* **19**, 34–39.

Sokoloff, L. (1981). Localization of functional activity in the central nervous system by measurement of glucose utilization with radioactive deoxyglucose. *J. Cereb. Blood Flow Metab.* **1**, 7–36.

Swanson, R. A., Morton, M. M., Sagar, S. M., and Sharp, F. R. (1992). Sensory stimulation induces local cerebral glycogenolysis: Demonstration by autoradiography. *Neuroscience* **51**, 451–461.

Takahashi, S., Driscoll, B. F., Law, M. J., and Sokoloff, L. (1995). Role of sodium and potassium ions in regulation of glucose metabolism in cultured astroglia. *Proc. Natl. Acad. Sci. USA* **92**, 4616–4620.

Tsacopoulos, M., Evequoz-Mercier, V., Perrottet, P., and Buchner, E. (1988). Honeybee retinal glial cells transform glucose and supply the neurons with metabolic substrates. *Proc. Natl. Acad. Sci. USA* **85**, 8727–8731.

Tsacopoulos, M., and Magistretti, P. J. (1996). Metabolic coupling between glia and neurons. *J. Neurosci.* **16**, 877–885.

Van den Berg, C. J., and Garfinkel, D. (1971). A simulation study of brain compartments. Metabolism of glutamate and related substances in mouse brain. *Biochem. J.* **123**, 211–218.

Villringer, A., and Dirnagl, U. (1995). Coupling of brain activity and cerebral blood flow: Basis of functional neuroimaging. *Cerebrovasc. Brain Metab. Rev.* **7**, 240–276.

Pierre J. Magistretti

NERVOUS SYSTEM DEVELOPMENT

Neural Induction and Pattern Formation

This chapter covers some of the key events that take place in the early stages of development of the vertebrate nervous system, a period during which structures such as the neural tube, placodes, and neural crest are formed, setting in place the foundations on which a functioning nervous system is subsequently built. The first part of the chapter describes how these embryonic structures are first specified by inductive tissue interactions and how they form by the process of morphogenesis. The second part of the chapter describes the extensive early developmental events required for regionalizing the nervous system along its different axes. Regionalization requires the complex processes of neural patterning that endow neural precursor cells with the ability to give rise to correct types of neuron in appropriate locations in the adult nervous system. These processes are gradual, continuous, and begin when neural tissue first forms. We describe some of the processes underlying neural patterning, beginning with how polarity along each of the neuraxes is first established and progressing to more fine levels of regional organization.

NEURAL INDUCTION

Embryonic Origins of the Nervous System

The vertebrate nervous system is a derivative of the ectoderm: one of the three major regions, or germ layers, of the blastula-stage embryo that forms during early cleavage stages (Fig. 14.1). As the embryo undergoes gastrulation, the two other germ layers, endoderm and mesoderm, invaginate inward, leaving the ectoderm on the surface and converting the embryo into three layers. Following gastrulation, cells in each of the different germ layers begin forming the anlagen that serve as the foundation on which the different organ systems are built. In the ectoderm, different tissue derivatives are generated at this stage depending on position along the dorsoventral (DV) and anteroposterior (AP) axes of the embryo. On the dorsal side of the embryo, the ectoderm thickens to form the *neural plate*, a structure the shape of a keyhole with the broad end located anteriorly. During a complex morphogenetic process called *neurulation*, cells in the neural plate give rise to the neural tube and, subsequently, the central nervous system (CNS). Cells at the edge of the neural plate come to lie at the dorsal surface of the neural tube during neurulation, form the *neural crest* and emigrate, subsequently giving rise to most of the peripheral nervous system. The area around the edge of the cranial neural plate contains a domain where various sensory structures such as the ear, nose, and cranial sensory ganglia will arise from isolated ectodermal areas called placodes. Finally, ectoderm located more ventrally gives rise to epidermis. Early stages of neural development involve processes that divide ectoderm into regions along the DV axis that then give rise to very different tissues, including the nervous system.

Neural Induction and the Organizer

Division of the ectoderm into different fates along the DV axis requires inductive interactions that were discovered in the early part of the 20th century (Harland and Gerhart, 1997). One of these interactions,

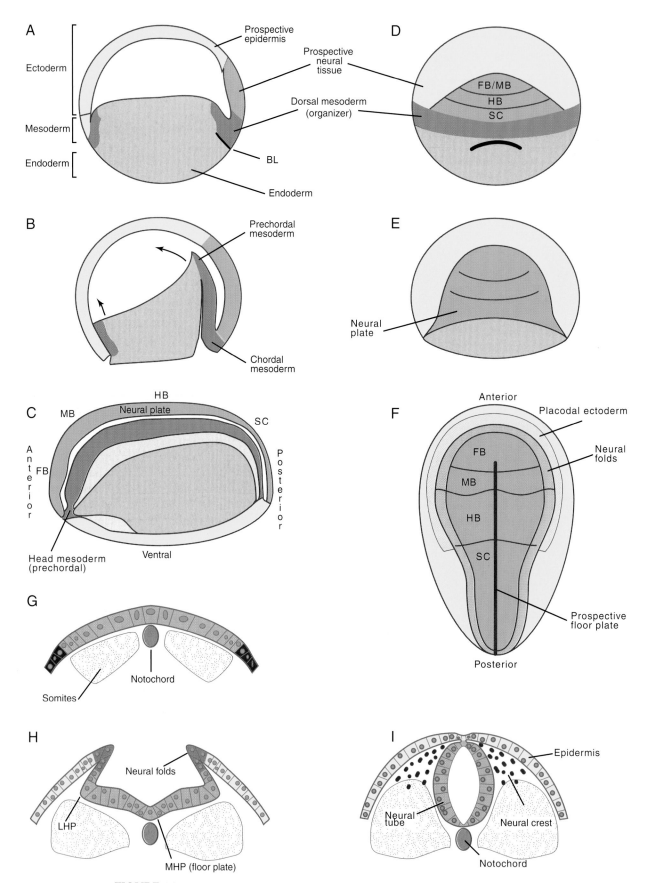

FIGURE 14.1   Blastula stage through neurulae, highlighting gastrulation and neurulation.

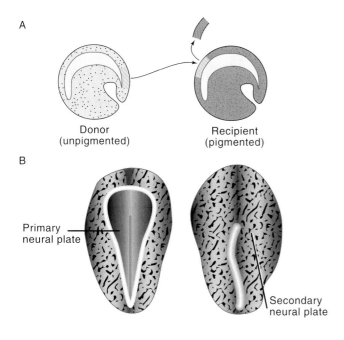

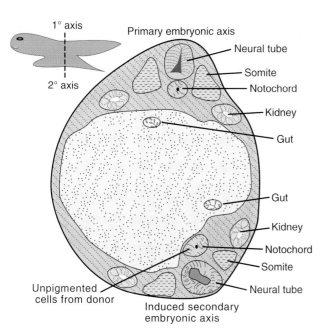

FIGURE 14.2 Organizer transplantation experiment. (A) Mangold and Spemann transplanted a small piece of tissue located just above the blastopore lip on the dorsal side of one blastula stage embryo onto the ventral side of another. (B) The graft, marked by a lack of pigmentation, was incorporated into the host embryo, which then formed a secondary dorsal axis evident as a second neural plate forming on the ventral side. (C) Tissue sections through the twinned embryo show that the graft contributes to the mesoderm, primarily the notochord, while the secondary neural tube derives from the host embryo.

called *neural induction*, was revealed at that time by a tissue-grafting experiment carried out by Mangold and Spemann on early amphibian embryos (Fig. 14.2). At the blastula stage, the amphibian embryo consists of a ball of cells with a distinct animal/vegetal axis marked by a pigmentation pattern. The pigmented animal pole, lying at the top of the embryo, is the ectoderm, the middle portion of the embryo is the mesoderm, while the vegetal pole contains the endoderm. During gastrulation, mesoderm and endoderm invaginate into the embryos while the ectoderm spreads and covers the outside. Gastrulation begins on what will be the dorsal side of the embryo, which is therefore marked by the first site of involution called the blastopore lip. When Mangold and Spemann transplanted a small piece of tissue around the dorsal blastopore lip (DBL) from one blastula-stage embryo to the ventral side of another, the host embryo responded to the grafted tissue by forming a complete secondary dorsal axis (Fig. 14.2). Importantly, the only tissues in the second dorsal axis that were formed from the transplanted DBL tissue were those that would be normally derived from dorsal mesoderm, such as the notochord. Other tissues in the secondary dorsal axes were not derived from the transplanted tissue but from the tissue in the host embryo. In particular, the secondary dorsal axis contained a complete nervous system that was derived entirely from the ventral ectoderm of the host embryo, a tissue that would have differentiated into skin in the absence of a graft. Tissue in the DBL was later termed the organizer because of its ability, when transplanted, to reprogram both ventral ectoderm and mesoderm to form dorsal tissues. Following Mangold and Spemann's lead, it was subsequently found that transplanting tissue that forms at the anterior end of the primitive streak in chick or mammalian embryos, called *Hensen's node*, also duplicates the dorsal axis and induces a secondary nervous system. Thus, all vertebrate embryos appear to contain a region, called *Spemann's organizer*, which causes ectoderm to form dorsal (neural) rather than ventral (skin) tissues.

Organizer transplantation experiments also gave the first indication that signals produced by tissues in the DBL or Hensen's node were responsible for inducing different regions of the CNS. In these experiments, the transplants used were taken from embryos at different stages of gastrulation and were smaller in size. The DBL of **younger** embryos contains the first involuting tissue that comes to lie anteriorly during gastrulation. When transplanted, the younger DBL tissue induces head structures that contained neural tissue from the anterior portions of the neuraxis. Conversely, the DBL from **older** embryos contains

BOX 14.1

TRANSGENIC MICE AND ENGINEERED MUTATIONS

Rapid and complementary advances in the fields of molecular biology and experimental embryology have combined to offer neuroscience researchers unprecedented power to manipulate the mammalian genome. The technologies used for these manipulations have been worked out primarily in the laboratory mouse and fall into two basic classes: those used for transgenic mice and embryonic stem cell chimeric mice.

Transgenic mice are created by the injection of a cloned DNA fragment into the male pronucleus of a recently fertilized mouse embryo. The fragment will integrate into the host genome and be passed through subsequent mitoses to all of the cells of the adult, including the gametes. The integrated DNA fragment, now known as a "transgene," is usually engineered to contain a promoter and associated regulatory sequences, a structural gene, and a 3' polyadenylation signal. Transgenes add to the genome. As a genetic element, the chromosomal site of integration is random, and there is no wild-type allele on the sister chromosome. As an expressed locus, the transgene message is made over and above the endogenous gene expression pattern. This technique can be used as both an analytical and an experimental tool. Used as an analytical tool, the potency of a certain genetic element to direct cell- or tissue-specific gene expression can be determined by using the element to regulate marker genes such as β-galactosidase or green fluorescent protein. The genetic elements that regulate the temporal and spatial expression pattern of *Hox* genes in hindbrain, tyrosine hydroxylase in adrenergic neurons, and L7 in Purkinje cells have all been explored by this means. Used as an experimental tool, transgenes can exploit a genetic element with known specificity to deliver a gene product to an ectopic cell site or developmental time. Thus, the PDGF promoter has been used to drive the expression of human β-amyloid precursor protein, the L7 promoter has been used to deliver diphtheria toxin to differentiating Purkinje cells, and the β-actin promoter has been used to

deliver *Hox-A1* to inappropriate sites in the developing embryo.

Embryonic stem cells (ES cells) are stable cell lines derived from the inner cell mass of the preimplantation embryo. They are totipotent, which means that if they are introduced into a host embryo, they can contribute to all cell types in the resulting chimera (including gametes). The use of homologous recombination in ES cells allows changes to be engineered in specific genetic loci in culture. By using modified cells to create chimeras, changes can be introduced into the mouse germline and propagated as new mutations. The mutations can be insertions, deletions, modifications, or any combination of the three. When the engineered insertion/deletion disables the normal allele, the resulting mutation is often referred to by the slang term "knockout." These techniques alter the genome. As a genetic element, the engineered locus replaces a specific gene locus, and there is a normal wild-type allele on the sister chromosome. Used in this way, a knockout mutation can be used to model an inherited disease. Lesch-Nyhan (HPRT-null), ataxia-telangectasia (ATM-null), and fragile-X mental retardation syndrome (FMR1-null) have all been modeled in this way. As an expressed locus, the knockout transcript is made instead of the wild-type gene product. This technique can thus be used to create a modified locus such that the targeted gene is mutated rather than destroyed. In the same way an endogenous transcript of one gene can be replaced with that of a different one. Thus, sequences encoding *Engrailed-2* have been inserted into the *Engrailed-1* locus in such a way that the *Engrailed-1* transcript is lost (a null mutation) and *Engrailed-2* is made in its place.

These are only some of the ways in which the powerful new technologies of transgenic and knockout mice are providing powerful genetic tools for use in neuroscience research.

Karl Herrup

tissue that involutes later and comes to lie more posteriorly along the embryonic axis. When transplanted, this tissue induced tail structures that contained neural tissue from just the posterior portions of the neuraxis. These observations indicated that the organizer consists of two parts, a head and tail organizer, each of which appears to be a source of signals that not only induces ectoderm to form neural rather than epidermal tissue,

but also signals that determine what region of the CNS will form. The role of the organizer tissue in the regionalization of the CNS is discussed further later.

Searching for the Elusive Neural Inducer

The transplantation experiments of Mangold and Spemann in the 1930s suggested that ectoderm is induced to form neural tissue by factors produced by the organizer. In subsequent years, identification of the neural inducer occupied the attention of several generations of scientists, thus representing one of the holy grails in developmental neurobiology. This search has also important historical significance because many of the techniques now used to study cytokines in neurobiology have their origins in the early attempts to identify neural inducers. For example, in the late 1920s, Holtfreter described culture methods for amphibian embryos, in which the ectoderm is removed from blastula-stage embryos and maintained *in vitro* in media of simple salt solutions. One important application of these early tissue culture techniques was to assay for neural inducers: isolated ectoderm grown in culture differentiates into epidermal tissue, but forms neural tissue when

exposed to a source of neural inducing signals, such as a piece of organizer tissue. With these types of assays available, the search for neural inducers was an active area of research in the 1940s and 1950s using the biochemical techniques that were available at the time. Unfortunately, the search for a bonafide neural inducer proved to be more problematic than initially expected and was frustrated by the observation that ectoderm could be neuralized when exposed to a wide variety of differentiated tissues, tissue extracts, and various purified molecules. These inducers, later termed artificial inducers, were unlikely to be physiologically relevant, but raised the possibility that neural inducers are not instructive, but permissive in their action. Indeed, this idea was supported in later years by results showing that ectodermal tissue differentiates into nerve cells when dissociated into indi-

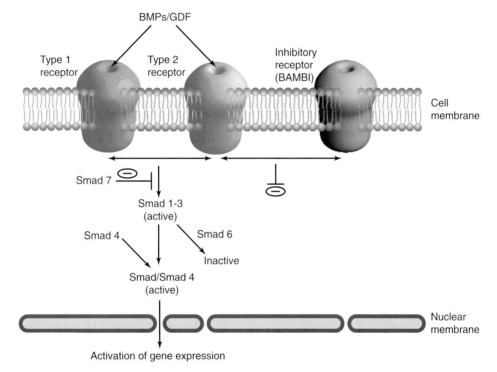

FIGURE 14.3 Signaling pathway involving BMPs. Diverse biological processes, including numerous events during neural development, are mediated by a large family of polypeptide growth factors (PGF) related to transforming growth factor-β (TGF-β). Members of the TGF-β superfamily fall into three broad groups: the BMP, activin, and GDF group members. All these ligands signal by a similar transduction pathway, although signaling by the BMP subfamily is highlighted here. Their receptors are heterodimeric, containing a type I and a type II subunit, both of which contain cytoplasmic domains with serine/threonine kinase activity. Dimerization of two receptor subunits following binding of a TGF-β-like PGF initiates a signal transduction pathway that activates a family of cytoplasmic proteins, the SMADs, which translocate to the nucleus to activate the expression of downstream target genes. Each receptor favors different members of the SMAD family, accounting in part for the diversity of biological activity by the TGF-β superfamily. Significantly, diverse types of inhibitors regulate signaling by this family of PGFs. Extracellular proteins such as chordin, tolloid, and twisted gastrulation interact with the BMP-like ligands, regulating their diffusion through the extracellular milieu and their ability to bind receptor. Cell surface proteins such as BAMBI inhibit signaling by binding up BMPs but failing to transduce a signal. Inhibitory SMADs poison the signal transduction pathway. The plethora of mechanisms that regulate signaling negatively by TGF-ß superfamily members emphasizes the importance of inhibition as a developmental regulatory mechanism.

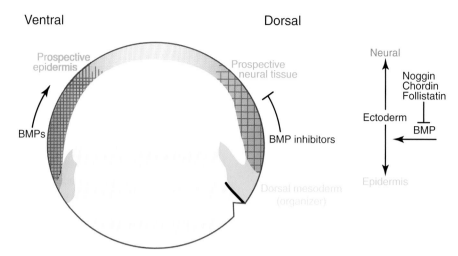

FIGURE 14.4 Default model for neural induction. BMPs are expressed in ectoderm on the ventral side of the embryo, inducing ectoderm to become epidermis. The organizer on the dorsal side releases inhibitors of the BMPs, such as noggin, chordin, and follistatin, which diffuse into the ectoderm on the dorsal side, block the effects of BMPs, and allow neural tissue to form.

vidual cells and cultured. One way to view these results is that ectodermal cells are preprogrammed to form neural tissue and need very little impetus to do so.

BMPs as Inducers of Epidermis

In the latter part of the 20th century, molecular players were discovered that act to determine whether ectodermal cells become neural or epidermal. The mechanism by which these molecules act forms the basis for the "default model" of neural induction that conceptually is very different from what the early embryologists imagined (Weinstein and Hemmati-Brivanlou, 1999). In this model, ectodermal cells are induced to be epidermal by a class of polypeptide growth factors (PGFs) called bone morphogenetic proteins (BMPs) (Fig. 14.3). Blocking BMP signaling prevents ectoderm from becoming epidermal and so it becomes neural through a default pathway (Fig. 14.4).

Critical evidence in support of the default model initially came from experiments in frog embryos, where there are simple assays for examining the role of PGF signaling pathways in the development of the ectoderm. One line of circumstantial evidence came from analyzing the spatial distribution of RNA encoding BMP ligands, in particular one called BMP4, in early embryos. BMP4 is expressed throughout the ectoderm at blastula stages, but during gastrulation is lost from the neural plate and remains high in nonneural ectoderm that forms epidermis. More direct evidence for a role of these ligands in ectoderm fate came from disrupting BMP signaling in embryos

experimentally. In these experiments, researchers altered the coding sequence of the proteins required for BMP signaling, producing mutants that are not only inactive, but can poison the activity of endogenous proteins. When such mutants for the BMP receptors, or the ligands, or components in the signal transduction pathway are introduced into frog embryos by RNA injection, they block BMP signaling and efficiently induce the ectoderm to form neural tissue. Thus, artificial inhibitors of BMP signaling mimic the neural-inducing activity of the organizer. Finally, when ectodermal cells are dissociated, they form nerve cells as described earlier, presumably because they are no longer exposed to sufficiently high levels of BMPs. Indeed, if BMP4 is added back to these cells, they revert to epidermis. The default model rests on the observations that the ectoderm produces BMPs that are potent epidermalizing agents and that blocking the expression or the activity of BMPs induces the ectoderm to form neural tissue.

Neural Induction by Natural Inhibitors of BMPs

According to the default model, one would predict that the organizer acts as a neural inducer by releasing extracellular signals that block BMP signalling. Indeed, several potent secreted inhibitors of BMP ligands have been identified, whose expression is restricted to the organizer tissue in different vertebrate embryos. For example, five secreted polypeptides—follistatin, noggin, chordin, cerberus, and nr3—are expressed in the organizer of the frog embryo. With the exception of nr3, these proteins, although unrelated in sequence, bind tightly to BMP ligands and prevent them from activating their receptors. When added to isolated ectoderm, these proteins induce the formation of neural tissue, presumably by sequestering and inhibiting endogenously produced BMPs.

Given their potent activity as inhibitors of BMP signaling and their early expression in organizer tissue, molecules such as chordin, noggin, follistatin, and cerberus are good candidates for the long-sought after neural inducers. Proving that they are neural inducers, however, depends largely on eliminating their activity in embryos by mutation and asking whether this leads to the predicted loss of neural tissue. Genetic analyses in zebrafish and mouse embryos are partially consistent with the idea that noggin and chordin are neural inducers. Mouse embryos that lack chordin and noggin activity by knockout mutations develop with a severe reduction in the size of the brain, in particular a loss of the forebrain, consistent with a reduction in the size of the neural plate. In zebrafish, a loss-of-function mutation in the chordin gene (the *chordino* mutant) reduces the size of the neural plate, whereas loss-of-function mutations in a BMP (*Swirl*) expand it. Thus, inhibition of BMP signaling by extracellular inhibitors is likely to be used by vertebrate embryos to establish a domain of dorsal ectoderm that gives rise to neural tissue.

The nervous system is reduced in size but not eliminated in embryos where the extracellular inhibitors of BMPs are absent by mutation, raising the question of whether these events are the only ones required for neural tissue to form in early embryos. One view is that other BMP inhibitors of the type exemplified by noggin and chordin have yet to be identified and these will need to be eliminated from the organizer before all BMP inhibitory activity in the early embryo is removed. However, an alternative view is that these extracellular inhibitors can only go so far in establishing a domain of ectoderm on the dorsal side where neural tissue forms (Streit and Stern, 1999). In this view, BMP antagonists can expand a neural domain by extending the border between the neural plate and the epidermis outward, but other events are required on the dorsal side to establish neural tissue, particularly early on when neural induction begins at blastula stages. Another complicating factor is that embryos of different vertebrate species differ in terms of how effectively the BMP antagonists convert ectoderm into neural tissue. For example, results obtained by implanting small beads releasing noggin and chordin into chick embryos argue against the simple idea that BMP antagonists are sufficient to generate neural tissue, particularly if they arrive too late. One possibility is that extracellular inhibitors are only partially

effective at blocking autocrine BMP signaling and that a complete shutdown of signaling in this pathway requires additional events that act directly and more effectively on the expression or activity of the components in the pathway at blastula stages or even earlier. If this were indeed the case, the nature of these additional events will be need to be illuminated further before we have a complete picture of how a region of ectoderm is set aside in the early embryo to form neural tissue.

It should be emphasized that neural tissue induced in ectoderm by simply inhibiting BMP signaling lacks many of the regional characteristics found in neural tissue induced by organizer tissues. The neural tissue induced by these inducers is forebrain-like, based on the expression of early regional gene markers such as those discussed later, but many of the regional characteristics associated with a mature nervous system are lacking. Preventing BMP signaling allows ectoderm to undergo neural rather than epidermal differentiation, but other mechanisms are required for inducing different areas of the nervous system.

Summary

The nervous system first arises in the vertebrate embryo from a region of ectoderm that is induced to form the neuroepithelium of the neural plate and tube rather than differentiating into epidermis. Classical transplantation studies have shown that dorsal ectoderm forms neural tissue in response to signals from the organizer. More recent studies have shown that ventral ectoderm undergoes epidermal differentiation in response to endogenously produced BMP4 and that neural inducers might act by inhibiting the activity of these epidermalizing signals in dorsal ectoderm. Current candidates for neural inducers include molecules such as noggin and chordin. These inhibitors, however, may be only part of the story, suggesting that additional events that prevent BMP activity in dorsal ectoderm are required.

Early Neural Morphogenesis

Among the earliest changes during the formation of the vertebrate nervous system are ones associated with morphological changes in tissue structure (Fig 14.1). At the cellular level, cells in the ectoderm lose the morphology characteristic of a simple, occluding embryonic epithelium as they take on the morphology of the pseudostratified epithelium of the neural plate and tube. During this process, the basal–apical polarity of the epithelium is maintained as discussed later. At a tissue level, the neuroepithelium of the neural plate undergoes the complex morphogenetic movements of neurulation to form the neural tube, which invaginates into the embryo, pinches off from the surrounding ectoderm and forms a separate tissue anlage. On a smaller scale, but with similar types of morphogenetic movements, anlagen for the sense organs delaminate from the ectoderm around the neural plate, following inductive interactions between particular regions of the invaginating neuroepithelium and adjacent, overlying nonneural ectoderm. These inductive interactions are not completely understood, although mechanistically they are likely to be similar to those that occur during neural induction. Placodal structures include the otocysts, which forms the ear; the lens of the eye; the olfactory placodes, which forms the nose; and neurons that contribute to most of the cranial sensory ganglia. Thus, the morphological processes that underlie formation of the neural tube and placodes share a number of common features, but how these processes are mediated at either the molecular or cellular level remains poorly understood.

Neurulation

Neurulation plays a fundamental role in the establishment of neural tissue. Failure to complete this process results in an open neural tube—a relatively common class of human birth defect called spinal bifida. In higher vertebrates, neurulation can be divided into two phases which differ in their morphological movements: a primary phase involving the brain and most of the spinal cord and a secondary phase involving more posterior regions of the spinal cord. During primary neurulation, the neural plate buckles at the midline, while the edges of the neural plate elevate and fuse at the dorsal midline to form the tube (Fig. 14.1). How these movements are achieved, however, is difficult to dissect in terms of attributing particular steps in the process of neurulation to particular cellular events within neurulating tissues. Instead, primary neurulation is probably driven by complex tissue mechanics that result from coordinated changes in cell shape and cell movements within subregions of the neuroepithelium, as well as changes in cell behavior outside of the neural plate. Within the neural plate, a furrow forms via the wedging of neuroepithelial cells along the dorsal midline of the neural plate that acts as a hinge around which the plate bends (Fig. 14.1H). This hinge point, which becomes the floor plate of the neural tube, probably contributes to the buckling of the neural plate but is apparently not necessary for neurulation to take place. Concurrently, the shape of the neural plate changes dramatically as the cells within it undergo an active rearrangement process, called convergence-extension. The extensive cell intercalation during convergence-extension narrows the neural plate along its mediolateral axis and greatly extends the plate along the AP axis of the embryo (Fig. 14.1C, F). Movements of convergence-extension, coupled with the bending of the neural plate at flexure points and cell intercalation in the surrounding ectoderm, bring the neural folds together where they fuse at the dorsal midline to create the tube that segregates from nonneural ectoderm into the embryo (Fig. 14.1I).

The morphogenetic movements that take place during neurulation also appear to be important in terms of setting up the different regions of the neuraxis. For instance, the neural tube is wider at its rostral end where the brain forms than at the caudal end, which forms the spinal cord. This difference in shape arises in part because the movements of convergent extension, which narrow the neural plate, are much more pronounced in posterior regions, presumably as a result of early patterning events along the AP axis. In addition, in some regions of the tube the neuroepithelium undergoes significant changes in shape and cell movement in order to establish a region that will form a particular portion of the nervous system. One of the most impressive examples of these more specialized regionalized movements occurs as a prerequisite to the formation of the eye. Eye formation is first evident morphologically during neurulation, when the neuroepithelium at the level of the prospective diencephalon evaginates to form the bilaterally paired eye vesicles. At the point where the neural tube and eye vesicle join, the neuroepithelium eventually pinches together to form the optic stalk. At the same time, the eye vesicle forms a cup and divides further into an inner layer that gives rise to the retina and an outer layer that will form the pigmented epithelium. Thus, eye formation starts with a specialized series of morphogenetic processes that shape the neuroepithelium into structures required for forming different parts of the eye.

Molecular Bases of Morphogenesis

Neural morphogenesis is likely to depend in part on the fact that embryonic cells adhere preferentially to their own kind. Differential cell adhesion can be demonstrated by cell aggregation assays in which the epidermis and neural tube are isolated, dissociated into single cells, and mixed together in culture. Over time in culture, neural and epidermal cells sort back out into homogeneous populations of cells.

The molecular bases of differential cell adhesion may reside within a subfamily of glycoproteins called cadherins (Redies, 2000). The cadherin superfamily consists of cell surface proteins whose extracellular domain contains multiple, tandem copies of a unique motif, referred to as the EC domain. A large number of different proteins (~80) fall into this superfamily, which can be subdivided further into subfamilies based on the structure of their intracellular domains. Classical cadherins are one cadherin subfamily whose intracellular domain binds the catenins and connects to the actin-based cytoskeletal network. Their extracellular domains bind homotypically, mediating the interaction of adjacent cells expressing the same cadherin type. Clusters of classical cadherins at points of cell–cell contact lead to the formation of adherens junctions, through which the actin-based cytoskeleton of cells within a tissue become interconnected. There are about 15 classical cadherins expressed within developing vertebrate embryos; many are expressed differentially when new tissue anlagen form and many show regionalized expression domains in the developing CNS (Redies, 2000). These different cadherin types may account for differential adhesion that arises when new tissues form or may account in part for the differences between subregions of the CNS that form during neural patterning.

Summary

Formation of the vertebrate nervous system begins with a series of striking changes in tissue morphology as the ectoderm forms the neural plate and tube. Neural tube formation involves the complex morphogenetic process of neurulation that requires coordinated changes in cell shape, cell division, cell migration, and cell–cell contacts. Changes in cell adhesion, through the expression of molecules such as the cadherins, are likely to be one factor that underlies the segregation of the ectoderm into neural and nonneural tissues. However, among the least understood aspects of early neural development are the molecular events that account for the many cellular processes underlying morphogenesis. The general sense is that these events ultimately impinge on the molecules that promote cell–cell contact or regulate the force-generating, actin-based cytoskeletal network. For example, mutations in proteins known to regulate the dynamics of cytoskeletal actin polymerization represent one distinct class of mouse mutants with neural tube defects. Much remains to be learned, however, about how changes at the molecular, cellular, and tissue level account for these morphogenetic processes.

EARLY NEURAL PATTERNING

As discussed earlier, the neural plate is a morphologically homogeneous sheet of epithelial cells derived from dorsal ectoderm, which acquires its neural potential and fate as a result of inductive signaling. As the neural plate rolls up and closes into a tube, a series of constrictions appear in its wall, subdividing the anterior end of the tube into a series of vesicles representing the anlagen of fore-, mid-, and hindbrain (c.f., Figs. 14.8 and 14.16). Further subdivision ensues, most conspicuously in the hindbrain region (rhombencephalon), where a series of segment-like swellings, rhombomeres, are formed. Caudal to the hindbrain, the neural tube forms a long narrow cylinder that is the precursor of the spinal cord. These early morphological features of the neural tube dictate the overall plan of the CNS and predict its later regional specializations. The neuroepithelium then commences with the production of a huge diversity of region-specific cell types, each having a distinct identity in terms of morphology, axonal trajectory, synaptic specificity, neurotransmitter content, and so on. Different neuronal cell types also carry distinctive surface labels that may ensure accuracy of axonal navigation and the formation of appropriate connections with other cells. Perhaps most strikingly, individual neurons or groups of similar neurons originate at predictable times and at precise positions within the various regions of the neural tube. In some cases, neurons remain in their position of origin during and following differentiation; in other cases, young neurons or their precursors are directed to migrate along stereotypic paths to settle in locations distant from their position of origin. Correct specification of this intricate spatial ordering, or *pattern*, of cells is crucial to later events in CNS development when neurons establish complex arrays of specific interconnection that constitute functional networks. Activity-dependent processes and regressive events, such as the pruning of axons and cell death, later reinforce and refine initial patterns of connectivity, but a high degree of precision is achieved from the outset, dependent on, and as a direct result of, appropriate cell patterning. How the different regions of the CNS, and the individual cell types they each contain, are assigned their identity in early development remains an outstanding problem in neurobiology.

Until recently, studies of the earliest developmental stages have been hampered severely by our inability to detect nascent pattern. However, discovery of a multitude of molecular markers that reveal subregions of the neuroepithelium has made it possible to visualize emergent heterogeneity in what was previously seen only as a "white sheet" of cells.

From its inception, the central nervous system is organized along orthogonal planar axes: longitudinal (anteroposterior or AP) and transverse. Neural tube folding and closure deflect the transverse axis from its original lateromedial orientation so that it becomes dorsoventral with respect to the body. The third axis is radial (apical–basal) and has little involvement in early patterning, as the radial organization of the tube is largely uniform throughout (with the principal exception of the cerebral and cerebellar cortices). In contrast, both the planar axes are nonuniform. Different neuronal types appear at different positions in these two dimensions as if reading their grid references on a map. Indeed, a Cartesian coordinate system of *positional information* is a useful framework with which to visualize neural pattern. As shown later, various morphogens act as *positional signals* on one or other of the planar axes, usually by establishing gradients of activity as their concentration falls with distance from a localized source. Uncommitted neural precursor cells respond to the local morphogen concentration by expressing specific transcriptional mediator genes (e.g., *homeobox* genes) that encode the *positional value* of the cell. In effect, cells measure their position by reading the strength of signals and finally adopt a specific fate that is appropriate for their grid reference in the neuroepithelium. An assigned positional value not only directs differentiation but also, for migrating neurons, translocation away from the site of origin to a new location.

Establishment of the AP Axis

The initial establishment of AP polarity along the neuraxis is coupled intimately to the establishment of the main body axis during early embryonic development. Although axis determination in the vertebrate embryo remains poorly understood, it may have conceptual similarities with the strategies used for axis determination in the *Drosophila* embryo, where genetic studies have produced a detailed understanding. In *Drosophila*, AP polarity is first established by a gradient of positional information produced by the maternal morphogen Bicoid emanating from the anterior pole of the egg. The gradient of the Bicoid transcription factor initiates a cascade of transcription factor activation that progressively subdivides the body axes further into smaller segmental units. As these repeat units are established, genes of the *Antennapedia/Bithorax* homeotic complex (HOM-C) act in a well-ordered manner to define unique segment identities. Similarly, formation of the body

axis in vertebrates is likely to involve the imposition of a crude polarity of transcription factor expression along the AP axis, which is then refined at later stages into smaller domains of gene expression.

Embryology of Early AP Patterning

Studies of neural induction have not only revealed the role of organizer tissues in inducing ectoderm to become neural, but also a role in imparting AP polarity on the developing CNS. Specifically, the organizer can be subdivided into two parts: one that induces head structures (i.e., brain) and another that induces tails (i.e., spinal cord) when transplanted into host embryos, leading Spemann and his students to propose that initial AP polarity of the CNS is established via different signals produced by head and tail organizers. These differ in their position within blastula stage embryos, their time of involution during gastrulation, and where they come to lie after gastrulation is complete (Fig. 14.5A). In amphibian and fish embryos, head organizer tissue is comprised of the mesoderm and endoderm that lie deep on the dorsal most side of the embryo (Niehrs, 1999). During gastrulation, this tissue moves anteriorly to form the prechordal mesendoderm (PME), lying underneath the anterior ectoderm that is induced to form the *prechordal* neural plate. In contrast, tail organizer tissue lies more superficially and laterally on the blastula fate map. During gastrulation, this tissue involutes later, forms derivatives of the chordal mesoderm, such as the notochord and somites, and underlies the posterior neural plate, referred to as the *epichordal* neural plate. When AP patterning signals pass between organizer tissues and the ectoderm is still a matter of debate. Signaling might occur before gastrulation by so-called planar signals, at times when inducing signals from both tail and head organizer regions only need to transmit over a short distance within the plane of the ectoderm to induce neural tissue and to impose AP patterning at late blastula stages. Alternatively, these patterning signals may not be transmitted until late stages of gastrulation, when the shortest distances between the organizer tissue and the dorsal ectoderm are vertical interactions between opposing cell layers. Both the timing of AP patterning signals and their source also differ among vertebrate species (Fig. 14.5). In the mouse embryo, for example, the head organizer includes a region of anterior visceral endoderm (AVE) that lies adjacent to the prospective prechordal neural plate, producing anteriorizing signals before the onset of gastrulation (Beddington and Robertson, 1998). Anterior neural fate in the mouse is likely to require signals from the AVE synergizing with those produced by PME cells as they come to lie underneath

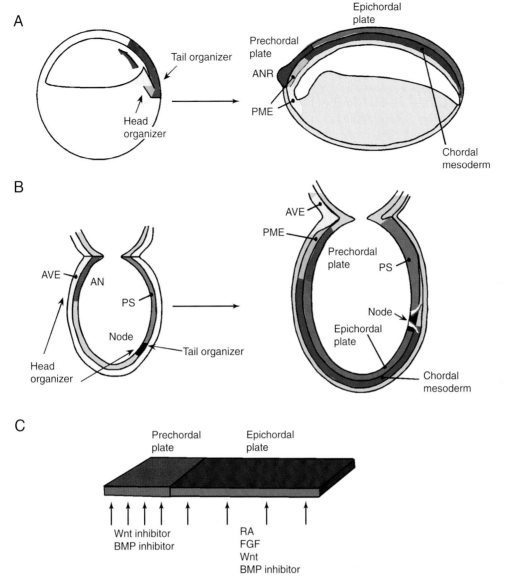

FIGURE 14.5 AP polarity of vertebrate CNS. (A) Initial AP polarity in a frog embryo is established via signals emanating from the head organizer, consisting of deep cells in endoderm (yellow) and the mesoderm (green), or from the tail organizer located in dorsal mesoderm (blue cells). Signals from these tissues may pass into the adjacent ectoderm to initiate AP patterning at blastula stages as shown on the left. Following gastrulation, as shown on the right, head organizer tissue becomes the prechordal mesendoderm (PME, yellow and green tissue) and lies anteriorly underneath the prechordal plate (forebrain), whereas tail organizer tissue becomes notochord and somites (chordal mesoderm, blue tissue) and lies underneath the epichordal neural plate. The anterior neural ridge (ANR) is also the source of signals that anteriorize the neural plate. (B) Initial AP polarity in the mouse embryos is established by signals emanating from the anterior visceral endoderm (AVE) acting on the adjacent epiblast to induce anterior neural fate (AN) before gastrulation begins, as shown on the left. During gastrulation, mesoderm (blue tissue) invaginates both anteriorly and posteriorly from the node (arrows from the node), as shown on the right. Anteriorly, the mesoderm(green) pushes underneath the epiblast coming to lie underneath the anterior neural plate (prechordal neural plate, red tissue), while posteriorly, the mesoderm comes to lie underneath the epichordal neural plate to form somites and notochord. (C) Despite the difference in tissues involved in AP patterning of the CNS, similar signals are required for inhibiting both BMP and WNTs to generate the prechordal plate, whereas posteriorizing signals in the form of WNTs, FGFs, and RA are required for generating the epichordal neural plate.

the anterior neural plate later during gastrulation. In the zebrafish embryo, the role of head organizer is transferred to the anterior ridge of the neural plate, which has potent anteriorizing activity, acting at later stages to maintain an anterior neural fate (Houart *et al.*, 1998). Thus, depending on the vertebrate species, head and tail organizer capabilities may reside in multiple tissues, although these organizer tissues may impose early AP patterning by the same mechanism, as discussed later.

The head/tail organizer model has subsequently been modified by embryologists such as Neiuwkoop based on the results obtained by treating isolated, cultured ectoderm with artificial inducers: a variety of agents can induce neural tissue, presumably because they inhibit BMP signaling. These artificial inducers, known as activators, induced ectoderm to form neural tissue with forebrain-like properties. Embryologists also identified a second class of agents, known as transforming agents, which could not induce neural tissue, but when applied along with the activators, induce neural tissue with posterior characteristics (i.e., spinal cord). These observations led to the activation/transformation model where the head and tail organizers produce different mixtures of activating signals that induce neural tissue with an anterior neural fate and transforming signals that convert anterior neural tissue into more posterior fates.

Molecular Basis of Early Anterior–Posterior Patterning

The issue of AP neural pattern has been examined more recently using molecular approaches that have been aided by techniques that allow one to visualize the expression of genes within developing embryos. As mentioned earlier, these techniques reveal the formation of a nascent neural pattern based on the expression of genes that mark different regions of neural tissue. They have also proven useful for following the production of signaling molecules by organizer tissues as they move about during gastrulation. Significantly, one insight from more recent studies is that the PME (i.e., head organizer) releases at least two classes of inhibitor molecules in order to establish an AP neural pattern. The mechanism by which these secreted proteins act is conceptually similar to the activation/transformation model proposed earlier, but with an added twist.

As described earlier, isolated ectoderm from frog embryos can be induced efficiently to be neural tissue by any means that inhibits signaling by BMPs. As predicted by the activation/transformation model, neural tissue generated by BMP inhibitors expresses anterior neural markers, such as the homeobox gene, *Otx2*, which indicates the presence of forebrain-like tissue, but fails to express more posterior neural markers indicative of the hindbrain or spinal cord. *Otx2* is not only a useful early marker for the anterior, prechordal neural plate, but is also required for its subsequent development, as revealed by the lack of anterior neural structures in the *Otx2* knockout mouse. As also predicted by the activation/transformation model, when neural tissue induced by BMP inhibitors is

treated with another class of factors, the expression of anterior neural markers is extinguished while the expression of posterior neural markers is induced. Posteriorizing agents include fibroblast growth factors (FGFs), members of the WNT family of signaling molecules, and retinoic acid. All three transforming signals are expressed by chordal mesoderm (i.e., tail organizer tissue), making them strong candidates as signals required for posteriorizing the central nervous system (Fig. 14.5C).

Based on the activation/transformation model, the PME (head organizer) should produce BMP inhibitors to induce anterior neural development. Indeed, PME expresses such BMP inhibitors as Chordin and Noggin, and mice develop anterior neural truncations if both molecules are eliminated by mutation. However, more recent studies indicate that inhibition of BMP alone is not sufficient to generate anterior neural tissue in embryos. Indeed, the PME produces a second class of secreted molecules, such as Dickkopf, Cerberus, and frzb1, which act as molecular sinks for the WNTs, inhibiting their activity as posteriorizing, transforming agents (Niehrs, 1999). The importance of WNT inhibitors was first gleaned from experiments in frog embryos, where inhibiting BMP signaling on the ventral side of the embryo experimentally produces a secondary dorsal axis, but one that contains only posterior neural tissue. However, if both BMP and WNT signaling are inhibited simultaneously in a similar experimental paradigm, a secondary head forms, containing neural tissue with both forebrain and midbrain derivatives. Subsequently, a variety of experimental approaches in frog, fish, chick, and mouse embryos have shown that WNTs are potent posteriorizing agents, whose activity needs to be inhibited anteriorly by WNT inhibitors in order to form anterior neural tissue. Dickkopf is a particularly strong candidate for a WNT inhibitor produced by the head organizer, as blocking its activity in embryos leads to anterior truncations.

Summary

AP patterning of the CNS begins during the process of neural induction as dorsal ectoderm takes on a neural fate. This process divides nascent neural tissue into prechordal (anterior) and epichordal (posterior) neural plate regions based on signals that come from adjacent head and tail organizing tissues. Formation of the prechordal plate requires two inhibitory signals produced by the head organizer: one that inhibits BMP and the other WNT signaling. Tail organizer tissue produces potent posteriorizing agents, including WNTs, FGFs, and retinoic acid. The extent of signals required for generating AP polarity, however, is not fully known and the

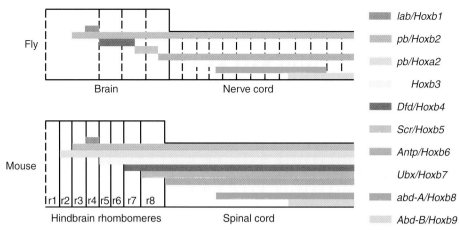

FIGURE 14.6 Hox gene expression domains in the CNS of fly and mouse. Nested domains of homeotic genes along the AP axis of the Drosophila CNS closely parallel those of their homologues in mouse. Compare, for example, the fly gene *labial* (*lab*) with its mouse homologue *Hoxb1*. *Hox* genes specify a positional value along the AP axis, which is interpreted differently in fly and mouse in terms of downstream gene activation, resulting in neural structure; what is shared between the two organisms is not the AP pattern of their respective CNS but the means of encoding the position of a cell along the AP axis. After Hirth *et al.*, (1998).

details of their action remain to be explored. Interestingly, both neural and anterior-neural are default states, requiring specific molecular activity to become nonneural (BMP) or posterior-neural (WNT).

REGIONALIZATION OF THE CENTRAL NERVOUS SYSTEM

Following the establishment of polarity along the AP axis of the embryo and the delineation of prechordal and epichordal regions of the neural plate, the AP axis becomes further regionalized into smaller and smaller domains, as revealed by the expression of developmental control genes. This process of progressive regional refinement involves two general classes of mechanism—the establishment of local organizers as sources of diffusible factors (morphogens) that inform neighboring cells about their position and fate and the partitioning of the neuroepithelium into small modules or segments in which development can proceed with a degree of autonomy. In both cases, a conspicuous and important feature is the setting up of boundaries, which position a local organizer, contain cells within a compartment, or both. We will illustrate these patterning mechanisms by reference to selected examples. Our intention is to outline general principles rather than to provide a comprehensive review of nervous system patterning, for which the reader is referred to Brown *et al.* (2001).

Definition of AP Pattern by Differential Homeobox Gene Expression

Central to the illumination of vertebrate CNS pattern formation has been the discovery that developmental control genes related to genes with a known patterning role in the Drosophila embryo are expressed in spatially restricted domains of the neural plate and tube. These regulatory genes, many of which encode homeodomain proteins, include HOM-C homologues, whose nested expression subdivides the spinal cord and the hindbrain; engrailed homologues, which define midbrain–hindbrain boundary and adjacent regions, and the homologues of *orthodenticle* and *empty spiracles*, which define midbrain and forebrain regions.

Homeotic selector (*HOM-C*) genes specify positional value along the main body axis of the fly embryo. Consistent with their also serving a function in the assignment of AP positional value, the vertebrate homologues of HOM-C, the *Hox* homeobox genes, retain a clustered chromosomal organization in which the relative position of a gene in the cluster reflects its boundary of expression along the AP axis (Fig. 14.6). Duplications during evolution of the vertebrate genome have increased the number of *Hox* genes such that mammals may possess up to four copies of genes that are represented singly in Drosophila. Divergence between these paralogous genes would be expected to increase the resolution of pattern control. *Hox* genes are expressed in overlapping, or nested, domains along the AP axis of the early embryo, with those at the 3′ ends of the clusters being expressed most anteriorly, in the hindbrain, where there is a precise correspondence between their anterior ex-

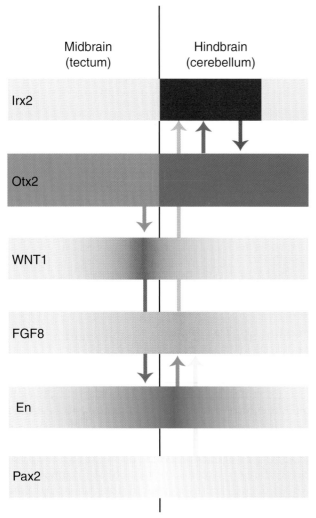

FIGURE 14.7 Genes involved in establishing the MHB organizer and regulating its function. Initial cross-repression between *Otx2* and *Gbx2* , possibly in association with *Pax2*, establishes the AP position of subsequent events at the MHB. Initially, broad domains of *Wnt1* and *Fgf8* expression are narrowed to sharp rings on either side of the boundary. WNT1 is required for the maintenance of *En* expression. *Irx2*, a relative of the *Iroquois* gene of Drosophila, establishes competence in rhombomere 1 for cerebellar development. *Pax, En, Wnt1*, and *Fgf8* later become mutually dependent, with feedback regulation ensuring that the MHB remains sharply defined.

pression borders and the boundaries between the morphological segments of the hindbrain neuroepithelium (rhombomeres; see later and Fig. 14.9).

Accumulating evidence supports the view that, by encoding positional value, *Hox* genes control the identity and phenotypic specializations of subregions of the epichordal neural tube in which they are expressed. Loss-of-function mutations of anteriorly expressed *Hox* genes result in malformations that represent a transformation of rhombomere identity. In the *Hoxb1* mutant mouse, for example, rhombomere

(r) 4 (where the gene is normally expressed at a high level) loses its r4-specific character and takes on that of r2, where the gene is not normally expressed. Similarly, overexpression of *Hoxb1* in r2 causes it to adopt phenotypic characters of r4.

Anterior to r2, the brain does not express *Hox* genes but displays a spatially restricted expression of other transcriptional control genes whose homeoboxes are divergent from the *Hox* type. These genes are also highly conserved between flies and vertebrates. Two homologues of the Drosophila segmentation gene, *engrailed* (*en*), are expressed in a broad region either side of the midbrain–hindbrain boundary (MHB), which later forms the cerebellum and the optic tectum (Fig. 14.7). Expression of the *En* genes is graded, being strongest at the MHB and declining both anteriorly and posteriorly. Morphological derivatives of the entire domain of *En* expression are deleted in *En1* knockout mice, showing that *En* function is crucially involved in the morphogenetic specification of the region (Wurst *et al.*, 1994). Transplantation studies using chick/quail chimaeras have shown that the induction and/or maintenance of *En* expression in neuroepithelial grafts correlates well with later morphological development into midbrian–hindbrain structures, whereas other studies have shown that the AP polarity of the retinotectal axon projection follows the posteriorly increasing levels of graded *En* expression in the posterior midbrain.

Homologues of the gap genes *orthodenticle* and *empty spiracles*, which function as homeotic selectors in the specification of particular head segments and brain neuromeres in Drosophila, are expressed in overlapping domains that encompass the entire rostral extremity of the AP axis with the exception of the ventral forebrain: the two *Emx* genes are forebrain specific (discussed later), whereas the two *Otx* genes have wider expression, encompassing both forebrain and midbrain. The *Otx2* knockout mouse has an extreme phenotype that shows the importance of the gene but betrays little about its function—the entire head rostral to r3 is deleted. This is explained by the fact that *Otx2* is also expressed in the visceral endoderm that lies beneath the anterior ectoderm, where it is required for the induction of anterior neural structure during gastrulation (Acampora and Simeone, 1999). However, the gastrulation phenotype can be rescued by expressing *Otx* in the visceral endoderm while the ectoderm remains functionally null for *Otx2*. This reveals the brain-specific function of the gene, which is to maintain anterior neural identity; in the absence of neuroectodermal *Otx2*, the anterior brain becomes converted into hindbrain, with an enlarged cerebellum rather than forebrain forming the anterior end of the CNS.

An important later function of *Otx2* is to set the position of the midbrain–hindbrain boundary, whose local organizer functions are discussed later. The sharp posterior border of *Otx2* expression coincides with the anterior expression border of another homeobox gene, *Gbx2*, in the anterior hindbrain. Mutual or cross-repression between the two genes stabilizes the interface, forming a boundary where specialized signaling cells are generated (Fig. 14.7). Experimentally extending the expression domain of *Otx2* into hindbrain territory causes the *Gbx2* border and MHB differentiation to retreat posteriorly, whereas extending the *Gbx2* domain into midbrain territory results in a corresponding anterior shift of the *Otx2* border (for a review, see Rhinn and Brand, 2001).

Summary

Gene expression patterns have illuminated the time course and mechanisms underlying neural patterning. Functional studies show that homeobox genes direct AP pattern formation, establishing head-to-tail regionalization. In the hindbrain, *Hox* genes encode subregional (rhombomere) identity. At the midbrain–hindbrain boundary, *Otx* and *Gbx* genes set up and position the MHB organizer, and *En* genes induced at the MHB confer AP polarity on the optic tectum, crucial to formation of the retinotopic map.

Local Organizers of AP Pattern

Homeobox genes and other classes of transcriptional mediator regulate position-specific development. How is the expression of these genes, or their upstream regulators, directed to specific domains of the AP axis? In many cases, it appears that long-range signals from local organizers are involved, directly or indirectly, in activating specific regional control elements of these genes at appropriate levels of the axis. In the case of *Hox* genes, a gradient of retinoic acid (RA) signaling has this role of positional signal (for a review, see Gavalas and Krumlauf, 2000).

RA is a biologically active derivative of vitamin A, a deficiency or excess of which causes defects that are particularly severe in the hindbrain and branchial arch region: excess RA, for example, causes a dose-dependent anterior shift of *Hox* expression domains and a corresponding anterior-to-posterior transformation of cell fate. RA exerts its effects via multiple types of RA receptors (RARs and RXRs), members of the nuclear receptor superfamily. RA receptors are ligand-dependent transcription factors that bind as heterodimers (RAR+RXR) to RA response elements in the promoters of target genes, including *Hox* genes. In the early embryo, RA is produced by the somites that lie alongside the caudal hindbrain (r7, r8) and spinal cord, through the activity of a synthetic enzyme Raldh2. Expressed anterior to the hindbrain is another enzyme, Cyp26, which degrades RA. These appear to act as source and sink for a gradient of RA activity that traverses the AP length of the hindbrain. Thus, targeted mutation of *Raldh2* in mice and treatment of chick embryos with an antagonist that specifically blocks all RARs both cause anteriorization of the hindbrain: posterior *Hox* genes are not expressed and anterior *Hox* genes are expressed only in the posteriormost hindbrain (Dupé and Lumsden, 2001).

Immediately anterior to the expression domain of *Hox* genes is a territory, r1 and midbrain, that forms the cerebellum and optic tectum. A unitary process of specification for these adjacent regions is reflected both at the molecular level and by aspects of their developmental potential: the Drosophila *engrailed* homologues, *En1* and *En2* (as mentioned previously) and the *paired* homologues, *Pax2*, *Pax5*, and *Pax8*, are expressed in this domain (Fig. 14.7). The development of midbrain and r1 is coordinated by the MHB, whose position is stabilized by the *Otx2*/*Gbx2* interface. Thus, heterotopic grafts of MHB cells locally induce *En* expression in the host and change the fate of the host neuroepithelium such that it ultimately forms tectal structures (when grafted to the posterior diencephalon) or cerebellar structures (when grafted to the posterior hindbrain). These findings provide compelling evidence that a signal emanating from the MHB is involved in local AP patterning.

There are two prominent components of this organizing activity. The first is WNT1, expressed in a transverse ring just anterior to the MHB, which acts as a mitogen and to maintain the expression of *En* but is unable to mimic the activity of MHB grafts. The second is FGF8, expressed immediately posterior to the *Wnt1* domain, which does have midbrain-inducing and polarizing abilities (Fig. 14.8). When a bead coated with recombinant FGF8 is implanted in the posterior diencephalon of chick embryos, *Fgf8*, *Wnt1*, and *En2* expression is induced in the surrounding cells. The posterior diencephalon then becomes completely transformed into the midbrain, whose AP polarity is reversed with respect to that of the normal host midbrain in accord with the gradient of induced *En* expression (Crossley *et al.*, 1996). Loss of FGF8 function in the zebrafish mutant *Ace* results in loss of the MHB, cerebellum, and part of the tectum. Thus, *Fgf8* expression at the MHB is necessary and sufficient to establish the polarized pattern of adjoining regions. Differences in competence between midbrain and r1

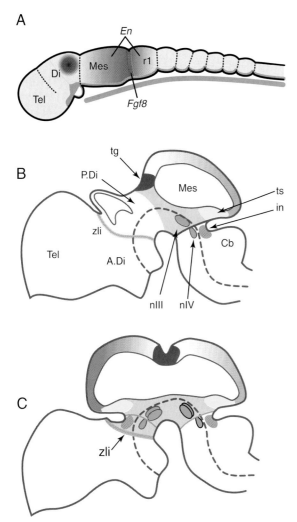

FIGURE 14.8 Role of FGF8 in mid/hindbrain patterning. (A) Implanting a bead that releases FGF8 protein (red) in the posterior diencephalon of a 1.5-day chick embryo results in the induction of *En* (blue) and the transformation of normal posterior diencephalic territory (B) into midbrain (C). In the treated embryo (C), the posterior diencephalons forms a set of midbrain structures laid out in reverse AP polarity to the normal midbrain. This is thought to be due to the induced anterior-to-posterior gradient of En protein in the diencephalon that is the mirror image of the endogenous En gradient in the midbrain (A). A.Di, anterior diencephalon; in, isthmic nuclei; Mes, midbrain; nIII, oculomotor nucleus; nIV, trochlear nucleus; P.Di, posterior diencephalon; r1, rhombomere 1; Tel, telencephalon; tg, tectal griseum; ts, torus semicircularis; zli, zona limitans intrathalamica. Data from Crossley *et al.*, (996).

presumably underlie their different developmental responses to FGF8; this may be a function of Otx2 and Gbx2 , respectively, but may also involve the differential activation of the prepattern gene *Irx2* in the cerebellar anlage (Fig. 14.7).

Summary

Mechanisms underlying the spatial expression of *Hox* and other homeobox genes, which appear to be

crucial to the delineation and subsequent development of specific subregions of the CNS, are being elucidated. Retinoic acid, produced by and diffusing from the somites, is a signaling molecule responsible for establishing the nested expression domains of the *Hox* homeobox genes in the hindbrain. The midbrain/hindbrain boundary acts as a local organizer by secreting signaling molecules affecting growth and pattern through the localized induction of other homeobox genes. FGF8, produced by cells at the MHB, is a potent factor involved in the elaboration of midbrain and cerebellar structure.

Hindbrain Segmentation

Subdivision of a tissue or large region by segmentation (metamerism) involves the allocation of defined sets of precursor cells into an axially repeated set of similar modules. A developmental strategy adopted independently by many animal phyla, segmentation offers the advantages that organizational fields remain small and specializations of cell type and pattern can be generated as individual segmental variations on the repetitive theme. In a segmented system, precise boundaries can be set for both cellular assemblies and realms of gene action.

Shortly after neural tube closure, a series of eight varicosities appear in the hindbrain region. Although transient, these *rhombomeres* are true metameric units that play a crucial role in patterning (Lumsden and Keynes, 1989). Thus, the earliest formed neurons are laid out in stripes that match the morphological repeat pattern, with neurogenesis starting within the confines of alternate, even-numbered rhombomeres, and only appearing later in odd-numbered rhombomeres—a 'two-segment repeat' pattern (Figs. 14.9A and 14.9B). Later in development, these segmental origins become obscured as specific types of interneurons become more abundant in some rhombomeres and reduced in others, while the motor nuclei condense and migrate bodily to new positions (Fig. 14.9C). Segmentation is a developmental mechanism for specifying the pattern of developing structures, not necessarily for deploying those structures in the adult.

Segmentation of the neural tube cannot proceed in the same way as for the mesoderm—through the formation of physically separate somites—because the tube has to retain epithelial continuity, not least as a conduit for extending axons. Rather, the process must involve some mechanism that restricts cell mingling. Just such a lineage restriction mechanism has been observed in the hindbrain by vital dye-marking experiments: clonal descendants of single marked cells disperse widely within the neuroepithelium, but the spreading cell clone always remains within a single rhombomere, confined at its boundaries (Fraser *et al.*, 1990). The vertebrate hindbrain thus shares with insects the phenomenon of modular construction using cell-tight developmental compartments. For rhombomeres, compartment organization prevents determined cells (i.e., with their developmental con-

trol genes activated) wandering from one rhombomere to another and blurring the resulting pattern.

What mechanism is responsible for segregating cells into compartments? One possibility is that the boundaries between rhombomeres enforce the separation, forming a mechanical barrier to cell dispersal: numerous molecular specializations that could play this role are acquired by boundaries later in develop-

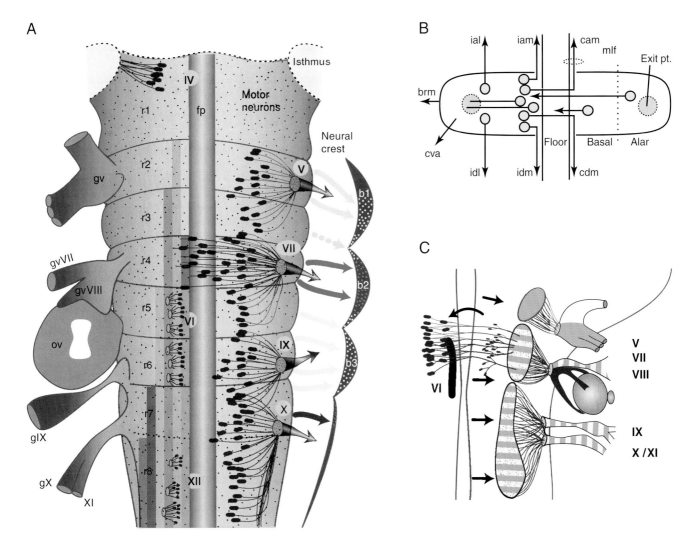

FIGURE 14.9 Distribution of neuronal types in the chick embryo hindbrain in relation to rhombomeres. (A). Shown on the right side are branchiomotor neurons, forming in r2+r3 (Vth cranial nerve, trigeminal), r4+r5 (VIIth nerve, facial), and r6+r7 (IXth nerve, glossopharyngeal), and contralaterally migrating efferent neurons of the VIIIth nerve (vestibuloacoustic), which are in the floor plate (fp) of r4 at the stage shown. Shown on the left side are somatic motor neurons, forming in r1 (IVth nerve, trochlear), r5+r6 (VIth nerve, abducens), and r8 (XIIth nerve, hypoglossal). Cranial nerve entry/exit points and sensory ganglia associated with r2 (trigeminal), r4 (geniculate, vestibuloacoustic), r6 (superior), and r7 (jugular) are shown, as is the otic vesicle (ov). Colored bars represent the AP extent of *Hox* gene expression domains; note that one of these, *Hoxb1*, is expressed at a high level only in r4. Modified from Lumsden and Keynes, (1989). (B). In addition to branchiomotor neurons, each rhombomere also contains six classes of interneuron, as defined by position and axon trajectory. r4 (as shown here) also contains contralaterally migrating vestibuloacoustic neurons (cva). (C). Later in development, branchiomotor neurons complete their laterally directed migration (arrows) and condense as defined nuclei close to their exit points. Similarly, cva neurons have completed their migration across the midline (arrow) and form a grouping in r4 and r5.

ment but none appears early enough to be implicated in lineage restriction. Alternatively, cells of adjacent rhombomeres could have a different specification state, involving the expression of surface molecules that would favor affinity between the cells within a rhombomere but reduce affinity for their neighbors. Consistent with this idea, cultured cell aggregate experiments have shown that cells from even-numbered rhombomeres mix evenly with cells from other evens (as do odds with odds), whereas odd and even cells segregate from each other. Thus, rhombomeres may partition according to an adhesion differential, obeying a two-segment repeat rule. Candidate molecules for mediating reduced intercellular affinity or adhesion at rhombomere boundaries include the Eph family of receptor tyrosine kinases and their ephrin ligands (Xu *et al.*, 1999). The receptors are expressed in odd-numbered prerhombomeres, whereas the ligands are expressed in evens. This mutually exclusive pattern means that ligand–receptor interaction can only occur at forming boundaries, where it results in sharpening of the initially fuzzy interface between the adjacent domains (Fig. 14.10).

Among the few known candidate regulators of segmental pattern in the hindbrain is zinc finger protein Krox20, an upstream transcriptional regulator of Eph receptors, which is expressed in two stripes in the neural plate that later become r3 and r5. Targeted disruption of the gene in mice results in the elimination of these rhombomeres and the fusion of r2-r4-r6 into a single region. Another class of segmentation gene, further upstream in the regulatory network that controls hindbrain segmentation, is represented by *kreisler,* a member of the the *maf* protooncogene family, which encodes a leucine zipper transcription factor. In *kreisler* mouse mutants the neural tube posterior to the r3/r4 boundary is unsegmented, a defect that is attributable to the loss of the *kreisler* expression domain, r5 and r6, as an identifiable territory. The place of r5 and r6 is taken by a region that might represent a persisting "parasegmental" (two compartment) progenitor region that has the neither their identity nor their adhesive properties. It would be expected that other as yet unidentified *maf* family members would be expressed with two-compartment periodicity in more anterior regions of the hindbrain.

One of the functions of compartment boundaries in Drosophila, notably in the wing imaginal disc, is first to generate and then to stabilize the position of specialized boundary cells that secrete signal molecules affecting the proliferation and fate of cells in the adjoining compartment territories (for a review, see Irvine and Rauskolb, 2001). Although rhombomere boundaries contain specialized cells that secrete signal molecules (e.g., FGF3, Netrin-1), this signaling function has yet to be shown.

Summary

Shortly after closure, the hindbrain neural tube becomes subdivided by transverse boundaries to form rhombomeres, a series of repetitive elements or metameres that have compartment properties. The existence of compartmental organization in the hindbrain suggests that cells become specified in segmental groups during their confinement in the ventricular zone and that they initially share a common identity, or ground state. First a row of similar boxes is formed and then the boxes are assigned individual identities according to their positional value, encoded by *Hox* genes.

AP Pattern of Spinal Nerves

Spinal nerves form a ladder-like array on either side of the spinal cord, an obvious manifestation of segmentation, but here, in contrast to the intrinsic patterning mechanism that operates in the hindbrain, segmentation occurs only in the paraxial mesoderm (somites). A serially reiterated asymmetry in the sclerotomal component of the somites allows axon to grow, and neural crest cells to migrate, preferentially within the anterior half of each somite, where neural crest cells then condense to form dorsal root ganglia (DRG). The posterior half of each somite, in contrast, expresses glycoproteins that inhibit cell migration and cause growth cone avoidance. Thus, microsurgically substituting posterior halves for anterior halves results in the local absence of peripheral nerves, whereas the converse experiment results in enlarged DRG and motor nerves. Subdivision of the paraxial mesoderm into AP-polarized somites thus ensures a positional correspondence between the segmented dermomyotome on the one hand and its sensorimotor innervation on the other (Fig. 14.11).

Although it lacks intrinsic segmentation and has a superficial uniformity of organization, the developing spinal cord does manifest distinct AP variations in cellular subtype composition, particularly with respect to motor neurons arranged in discontinuous longitudinal columns. Thus, neurons that form lateral motor columns at limb (brachial and lumbar) levels are distinct from those that form at cervical and thoracic levels, both in the identity of their peripheral targets and in the expression of different combinations of *LIM*-homeobox genes (for a review, see Pfaff and Kintner, 1998). These confer motor neuron subtype identity and targeting specificity. Furthermore, genes that lie 5' in *Hox* clusters have boundaries of expres-

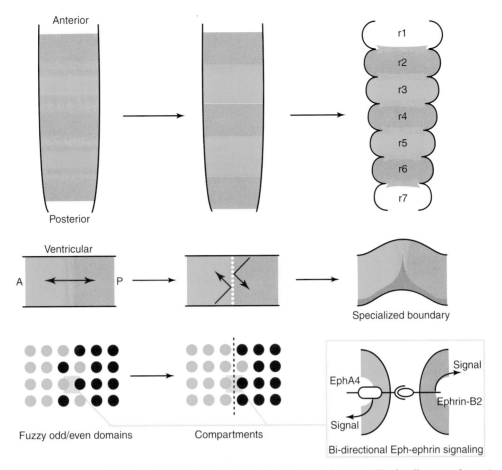

FIGURE 14.10 Stages in the compartmental organization of rhombomeres. The hindbrain is shown in plan view (top row) and longitudinal section (middle row). (Left) Genes such as *Krox20* and *EphA4* (blue) and *ephrin-B2* (pink) are expressed in alternate, fuzzy-edged stripes that correspond with presumptive rhombomeres. (Center) Subsequently, restriction to the movement of mitotic precursor cells occurs at the interfaces between newly formed rhombomeres, which are now sharply defined, and marked by increased intercellular spaces. (Right) Finally, rhombomeres are now visible morphologically by the sinuous deflection of the neuroepithelium on the ventricular–pial (apical–basal) axis and specialized cells (green) differentiate at the boundaries, which also become preferred pathways for axon growth (brown). (Bottom row) Sharpening of boundaries and cell lineage restriction occur through the interaction of Eph and ephrin molecules, both of which transduce a signal within the cell expressing them. Data from Fraser *et al.* (1990).

sion along the spinal region, suggesting, by analogy with the hindbrain, that they might underlie regional diversity as, for example, between brachial and thoracic regions. Transposition of prospective brachial and thoracic regions in chick or shifting the position of single motor neurons in zebrafish leads to changed *Hox* and *LIM*-homeobox gene coding and respecification of motor neuron identity in accord with their new positions. The most likely source of molecular signals that affect the acquisition of this regional identity is the mesoderm that flanks the neural tube.

Local Organizers of DV Pattern

The DV axis of the neural tube has a characteristic zonation, particularly prominent in the hindbrain and spinal cord, where different cell types differentiate stereotypically at different DV positions. In the ventral half of the cord, specialized glia, called floor plate cells form a narrow strip at the midline. Above the floor plate are five zones containing, in ventral to dorsal sequence, V3 interneurons, motor neurons, and three other types of interneuron, V2, V1, and V0 (Fig. 14.13). Further subtypes of interneuron differentiate in the dorsal half, whereas the dorsalmost region, represented early on by neural folds that mark the transition between cells with neural and epidermal fates, forms the migratory neural crest cells that give rise to the glia and the majority of neurons in the peripheral nervous system. Later, after the neural crest has departed, the dorsal midline is populated by nonneurogenic roof plate cells.

The patterning of neuronal cell types has been studied intensively in the spinal neural tube, such that this currently represents our closest approach to understanding how fine-grained pattern is generated in the CNS as a whole. Unlike on the AP axis, where local organizers signal position and fate to neighboring cells through single morphogen gradients, the DV axis has organizers at both dorsal and ventral poles and their respective morphogen gradients appear to counteract one another.

Ventral Organizers

Crucially involved in patterning the ventral neural tube is the notochord, a mesodermal skeletal structure that occupies the midline of the embryo directly beneath the neurectoderm. Grafting experiments in avian embryos have shown that both floor plate and

motor neuron differentiation depend on notochord signals. Early removal of the notochord results in a normal-sized spinal cord in which both of these ventral cell types are absent, with dorsal cell types and dorsal-specific markers appearing in their place. Similarly, implanting a supernumerary notochord alongside and in contact with the lateral neural plate results in formation of an additional group of floor plate cells at the point of contact, with clusters of motor neurons on either side (Fig. 14.12). These experiments show not only the power of the ventral midline signal to influence fate choice, but also the multipotent competence of responding neural tube cells at different DV positions (but not at different AP positions, see later). At a slightly later developmental stage, the floor plate itself acquires the same inductive capabilities—it can also induce motor neurons and will induce itself homeogenetically. The floor plate thus becomes an organizing center for a ventral pattern that is built into the neural tube itself.

Although it first appeared that motor neuron and floor plate induction would require different signals, one diffusible and the other contact dependent, a single molecule can account for both processes (for a review, see Briscoe and Ericson, 2001). *Sonic hedgehog*

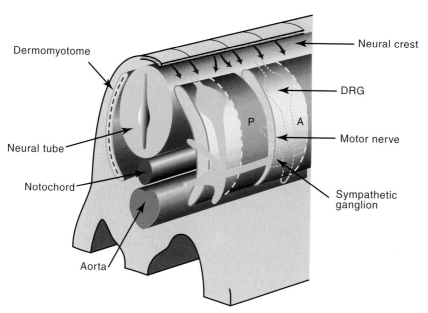

FIGURE 14.11 Segmented pathways for motor axon growth and neural crest migration in the trunk region. The AP positions at which motor axons collect to form a ventral root motor nerve and crest cell aggregate to form a dorsal root ganglion (DRG) are determined by somites. By the stage at which these constituents of the peripheral nervous system appear, the medial (sclerotomal) region of somites has dispersed and surrounds the notochord and ventral neural tube. The sclerotome is divided into anterior (light gray) and posterior (dark gray) halves, which are distinct from each other according to cell density and molecular markers. All components of the peripheral nervous system are confined to the anterior half sclerotome of each somite, which is permissive for the migration of neural crest cells (arrows), some of which condense to form DRG, and the ingrowth of motor neuron growth cones.

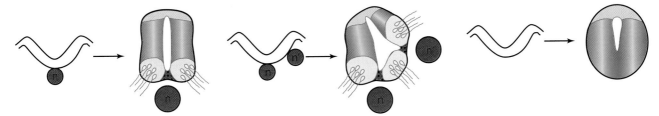

FIGURE 14.12 Influence of ventral midline signals on spinal cord pattern. Cross sections through the developing chick spinal cord at the neural plate stage (left) and later (right) showing the effect of adding or removing notochord. (Left) During normal development, the floor plate (red) develops above the notochord (n) and motor neurons (yellow) differentiate in the adjacent ventrolateral region of the neural tube. *Pax6* (blue) is expressed in more dorsal regions. (Center) Grafting a donor notochord (n′) alongside the folding neural plate results in formation of an additional floor plate and a third column of motor neurons. *Pax6* expression retreats from the transformed region. (Right) Removing the notochord from beneath the neural plate results in the permanent absence of both floor plate and motor neurons in the region of the extirpation. *Pax6* expression extends through the ventral region of the cord.

(*Shh*) is expressed first in the notochord and then in the floor plate and can elicit ectopic floor plate and motor neuron differentiation when misexpressed in the dorsal neural tube. Similarly, an activated form of Smoothened, the signal-transducing component of the SHH receptor, acts in cell autonomous fashion to produce ventral cell types ectopically. The choice of cell fate by progenitor cells in explants appears to be influenced by the concentration of the diffusible protein (SHH) to which they are exposed: threefold incremental changes in SHH concentration can result in the generation of five distinct classes of ventral neural tube cell types *in vitro*, including, at the higher end of the range, motor neurons, V3 interneurons, and floor plate cells (Fig. 14.13). Midventral neural plate cells that are contacted by the notochord are thus likely to be exposed to a high local concentration of SHH, exceeding the threshold for floor plate induction, whereas the lower levels of SHH that diffuse from floor plate are sufficient to induce motor neuron and ventral interneuron differentiation, but insufficient to induce the floor plate. Activity blocking antibodies abolish the notochord-mediated induction of ventral cell types showing that SHH is necessary as well as sufficient for establishing the ventral polarity of the neural tube.

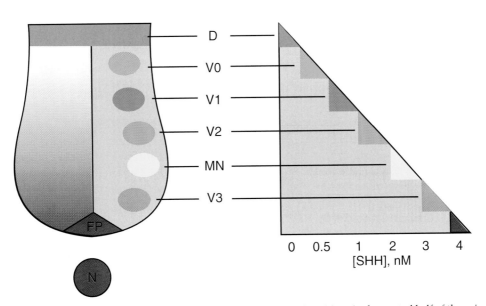

FIGURE 14.13 Formation of different cell types at different DV positions in the ventral half of the spinal cord. Sonic hedgehog (SHH) is responsible for generating neuronal diversity in the ventral half of the spinal cord. SHH protein (red), produced by the notochord (N) and floor plate (FP), acts as a graded signal, which induces different cell types at different DV positions *in vivo* (left) and at different concentrations *in vitro* (right). After Briscoe and Ericson (2001).

The ability of midline signals to influence development of the ventral neural tube is not restricted to the spinal cord. In addition to inducing motor neurons and floor plate in the hindbrain and midbrain, midline signals are also involved in the development of AP region-specific neuronal subpopulations. Serotonergic neurons of the hindbrain raphé nucleus and dopaminergic neurons of the midbrain substantia nigra both develop close to the floor plate and can be induced to form in competent neuroepithelium by the notochord, floor plate, or SHH protein. The issue of how ventral midline signaling can elicit different responses at different AP positions is considered below.

Dorsal Organizers

In genetically or surgically notochordless animals, dorsal markers are expressed in the ventral spinal cord, showing that cell pattern in the dorsal half of the spinal cord does not require notochord signals. However, dorsal cell types such as neural crest, roof plate, and dorsal interneurons do not develop by default, but are induced by an interaction between the lateral neurectoderm and the epidermal ectoderm. The latter is the source of a contact-dependent signal that induces the differentiation of both roof plate cells and neural crest cells and that is likely to be transmitted in planar fashion at the open neural plate stage, when the neural and epidermal ectoderm are contiguous. This dorsalizing signal appears to be mediated by BMPs, in particular BMP4 and BMP7 (Fig. 14.14). Both molecules are expressed in the dorsal ectoderm and both can mimic the ability of epidermal ectoderm to induce roof plate and neural crest cells. Consistent with the concept of counteracting gradients from ventral and dorsal poles, the domains of ventral neuron subtypes are expanded dorsally in zebrafish mutants lacking these BMPs. As for the ventral neural tube, where initial SHH activation is passed onto the floor plate by homeogenetic induction, so in the dorsal neural tube BMP4 and BMP7, together with other TGF-β-like proteins, are subsequently expressed in the dorsal neural tube itself. At both ventral and dorsal poles, the transfer of signal molecule expression to the neuroepithelium attends the physical separation of the neural tube from the initial source, presumably ensuring a more precise control of concentration within the tube.

Definition of DV Pattern by Differential Homeobox Gene Expression

At the time of neuronal differentiation, each of the five zones of neuronal cell types in the ventral neural

tube is defined by the combinatorial expression of homeobox genes. These genes are either induced (*Nkx2.2*, *Nkx6.1*) or repressed (*Pax6*, *Pax7*, *Dbx1*, *Dbx2*) at defined concentrations of SHH protein (Fig. 14.15). The differential responses to a graded SHH signal is thought to set up a pattern of fuzzy zones in the ventral half of the cord, which is later refined and sharpened by cross-repressive interactions between the homeobox genes themselves (see Briscoe and Ericson, 2001): the expression borders of complementary genes are seen to move following gain and loss of function of the opposing gene, as for *Otx2/Gbx2* at the MHB (see earlier discussion). Such shifts in the expression domains of these and other homeobox genes result in corresponding and predictable changes in neuronal identity, demonstrating the critical role of these homeobox genes as determinants of cell fate.

As for the AP axis, where positional determinants of identity are conserved with Drosophila, there are also striking similarities for the DV axis. For example, the homologue of *Nkx2.2*, *vnd*, is expressed close to the ventral midline of the fly embryo and is required for establishing the identity of its ventralmost neuroblasts (Cornell and von Ohlen, 2000).

Summary

Patterned cell differentiation along the DV axis of the epichordal neural tube involves the initial medial–lateral polarization of the neural plate and the later generation of distinct cell types at different DV positions under the spatial control and coordinate actions of an SHH-mediated ventralizing signal from the notochord (later from the floor plate) and a BMP-mediated dorsalizing signal from the epidermal ectoderm (later from the roof plate). SHH is both necessary and sufficient for inducing a range of ventral cell types, including floor plate cells, motor neurons and interneurons, at different concentrations—it therefore has the prime characteristic of a morphogen. Patterning along the entire DV axis involves the intersection of opposing signals emanating from the two poles: BMPs act to limit the ventralizing activity of SHH, whereas SHH acts to limit the dorsalizing activity of BMPs.

Intersection of AP and DV Patterning Mechanisms

The early inductive signals that establish DV cell fate appear to be similar along the entire epichordal neuraxis. However, at a constant DV position, there are marked differences in the identity of neurons at different AP positions, such as between oculomotor neurons and dopaminergic neurons of the midbrain and bran-

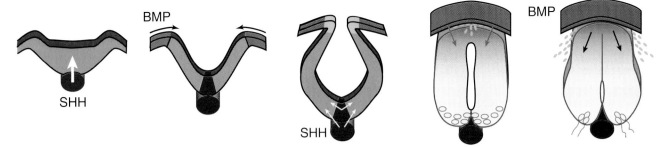

FIGURE 14.14 Stages in the formation of DV pattern in the spinal cord and hindbrain. The notochord underlies the neural plate and expresses *Shh* (red). The notochord-derived SHH protein induces differentiation of the floor plate, which also expresses *Shh*. *Bmps* (dark blue) are expressed in epidermal ectoderm adjoining the neural plate. As the neural plate closes, neural crest cells individuate (light blue) at the junction between neural and epidermal ectoderm. At the early neural tube stage, *Isl1*–expressing motor neuron precursors (yellow) appear close to the floor plate and neural crest cells leave the dorsal tube and midline ectoderm through breaks in the basal lamina. Bmp expression transfers to the dorsal neural tube Finally, motor neurons differentiate in the ventral cord. White and yellow arrows denote SHH signaling; black and purple arrows denote BMP signaling.

chiomotor neurons of the hindbrain (Fig. 14.16A). That these distinct cell types arise in response to apparently similar levels of SHH signaling suggests that the choice of fate depends on the competence of the responding tissue—SHH must act within the context of previously established AP positional cues and previously specified AP positional values. That this is indeed the case has been demonstrated experimentally by heterotopic grafts of rhombomeres, as explained in the legend to Fig. 14.16B.

REGIONALIZATION OF THE PRECHORDAL CENTRAL NERVOUS SYSTEM

Studies in mouse and chick embryos have led to the proposal that segmentation operates in the forebrain, as in the hindbrain, but the significance of the six or seven transverse subdivisions ("prosomeres") described for the forebrain remains unclear: repeat

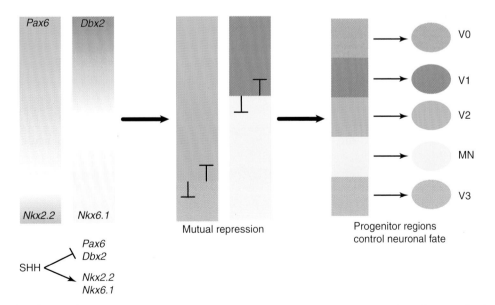

FIGURE 14.15 Model for ventral neural patterning. (Left) Graded SHH signaling from the ventral pole induces new expression of some homeobox genes (e.g., *Nkx2.2, Nkx6.1*) and represses the existing expression of others (e.g., *Pax6, Dbx2*). (Center) Cross-repressive interactions between pairs of transcription factors sharpen mutually exclusive expression domains. (Right) Profiles of homeobox gene expression define progenitor zones and control neuronal fate. After Briscoe and Ericson, (2001).

patterns of cellular organization or gene expression—repetition is the essence of segmentation—do not obviously accompany the segment-like morphology. Crucially, cell lineage tracing experiments have failed to confirm a restriction to cell mingling at the borders of these domains in the diencephalon (Larsen *et al.*, 2001). However, a number of early expressed developmental control genes are expressed in a patchwork quilt of small domains, subdividing the diencephalon and telencephalon (the main posterior and anterior subdivisions of the forebrain) into a number of transverse and longitudinal domains. Little is known about the patterning mechanisms involved in setting up these localized domains of gene expression other than that FGFs are implicated in signaling at the anterior end of the axis. Here, FGFs secreted from a putative organizer region known as the anterior neural ridge (ANR) are responsible for inducing and/or maintaining telencephalic (*Bf1*) gene expression and for maintaining telencephalic identity (Rubenstein and Beachy, 1998). Grafting the ANR of zebrafish (known as row 1) posteriorly results in the local induction of telencephalic genes, whereas ablation of these cells leads to the loss of identifiable telencephalic territory (Houart *et al.*, 1998). Earlier in development, row 1 cells secrete an antagonist to WNTs, whose activity must be reduced in order to correctly specify the anteriormost part of the nervous system (see earlier discussion).

More is known about patterning on the DV axis of the telencephalon, which is conspicuously subdivided into a dorsal pallial region, which becomes the neocortex and archicortex (hippocampus) in mammals, and a ventral subpallial region that forms the basal ganglia. Whereas the pallium remains a sheet-like roof over the lateral ventricles as it develops, proliferation in the subpallial region thickens the wall considerably, forming two swellings from which the basal ganglia arise: the lateral ganglionic eminence (LGE), which gives rise to the striatum, and the medial ganglionic eminence (MGE), which produces the globus pallidus. The pallial and subpallial moieties of the telencephalic vesicle are segregated by a longitudinal boundary, which marks the domain border of several dorsoventrally expressed developmental control genes and which may also act as a lineage restriction, at least during early stages of development.

DV Pattern in the Forebrain

The forebrain is devoid of motor neurons and, in all but the posterior diencephalon, it has no floor plate nor is it underlain by notochord. The absence of these midline structures raises the question of how the

bilateral organization of the forebrain and the differentiation of its ventral cell types are controlled. It appears, however, that even in this terminal expansion of the central nervous system a common mechanism is used for ventral patterning. SHH is expressed along the ventral midline of the forebrain and ventral forebrain cells express the transcriptional mediators *Isl1* and *Nkx2.1* in response to SHH signaling.

Genetic studies have also identified the ventral midline of the diencephalon as an organizing region for patterning the ventral diencephalon, which includes the eye field. This territory is deleted in the *Shh* knockout mouse and in a zebrafish nodal mutant (*cyclops*), which also lack *Shh* expression in ventral midline structures. The phenotype of these mutants most obviously involves fusion of the eyes around the anterior pole of the embryo. The optic stalk, a region that normally expresses *Pax2*, is diminished, whereas the retina, which normally expresses *Pax6*, extends throughout the optic territory such that the eyes are fused not by optic stalk tissue but by retina. Overexpression of *Shh* in zebrafish produces phenotypes that are reciprocal to those seen in *cyclops*.

SHH is also required for the generation of both major components of the basal ganglia. Early on, ventral telencephalic cells respond to midline SHH by expressing *Nkx2.1* and forming the MGE. Later, more dorsal cells respond to SHH by expressing LGE markers, but not *Nkx2.1* (Khotz *et al.*, 1998). The different responses of medial versus lateral regions appear to reflect a change in the competence of telencephalic cells with time, with the resulting DV pattern reflecting the delay in reception of the SHH signal rather than a difference in SHH concentration (Fig. 14.17).

Pax6 and Eye Development

Pax6 encodes a transcription factor that is expressed in the developing neural tube and the optic vesicle; later, as the eye develops, transcripts appear in the lens, retina, and cornea. A fundamental role in eye development is indicated both by the conservation of this expression pattern in all vertebrate embryos and by the absence of eyes the *Pax6* null mutant mouse—named *small eye* for its heterozygous phenotype. *Pax6* may thus lie at the head of a genetic cascade that controls development of the visual apparatus. The Drosophila homologue of *Pax6*, *eyeless*, is expressed transiently during early stages of eye disc development and is required for eye formation. *Eyeless* mutants have small or absent eyes, whereas overexpression of *eyeless* leads to the formation of eyes by

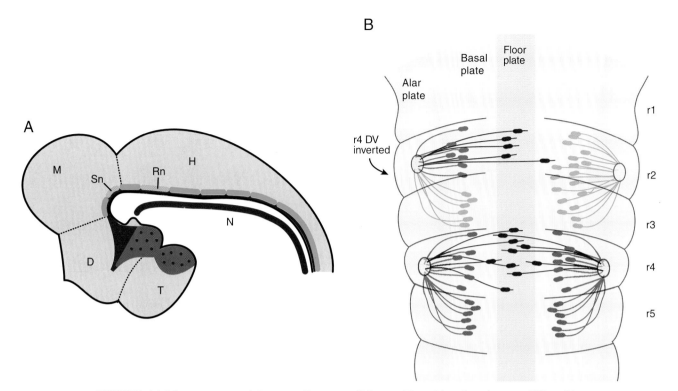

FIGURE 14.16 Formation of distinct cell types at different AP positions but the same DV position. (A) Stage in the formation of CNS pattern, seen in lateral view. The notochord (n) underlies the spinal cord, hindbrain (h), midbrain (m), and posterior part of the diencephalon (d), where its tip lies close to the infundibulum. *Shh* (red) is expressed by both notochord and midventral neural tube cells, including those of the telencephalon (t). At midbrain and hindbrain levels, *Isl1* positive motor neurons (green), serotonergic neurons (rn; orange), and dopaminergic neurons (sn; yellow) differentiate adjacent to *Shh*-expressing ventral midline cells. In the forebrain, the expanded domain of Shh expression is also associated with *Isl1*-expressing cells (blue) that are not motor neurons. (B) Positional values are established on the AP axis before the DV axis. In the hindbrain, rhombomere 4 is marked by the high-level expression of *Hoxb1* and, at the later stage shown, by the emergence of Hoxb1+ motor neurons (blue) and a unique cell group adjacent to the floor plate, the contralaterally migrating vestibuloacoustic (CVA) efferent neurons (red). When r4 is transplanted to a more anterior position (left side of diagram) it maintains *Hoxb1* expression and CVA neurons are produced, even when the graft is inverted dorsoventrally and the ventral cell types arise from what were originally dorsal cells but are now placed in contact with the floor plate. That AP-specific ventral cell types are formed ventrally, irrespective of the original DV position of their precursors, shows that precursors are multipotent at the stage of grafting but that their potency has already been restricted to a repertoire appropriate to AP position (AP regional identity). However, they are still competent to respond to ventral midline signals that only later determine cell type identity appropriate to DV position (data for B from Simon *et al.*, 1995).

other imaginal discs, including those of wing, leg and antenna (Halder *et al.*, 1995). Although the discovery of homologous genes in related developmental pathways in flies and vertebrates is no longer greeted with surprise, what is extraordinary about this gene conservation is that vertebrate and insect eyes bear no structural similarities to each other and they function in quite different ways; they have classically been regarded as analogous rather than homologous structures. Thus, the discovery of a homologous master gene is persuasive evidence that the eyes of flies and vertebrates have a common developmental origin—

perhaps in the establishment of a developmental field from which an eye develops.

Patterning the Cortex

The cerebral cortex, a brain region unique to mammals, comprises a small number of distinct subregions defined anatomically by the number of layers (e.g., the neocortex has six, whereas the hippocampus has three) and a very large number of discrete functional areas—more than 50 in the human neocortex. One difficulty in addressing the question of how the elabo-

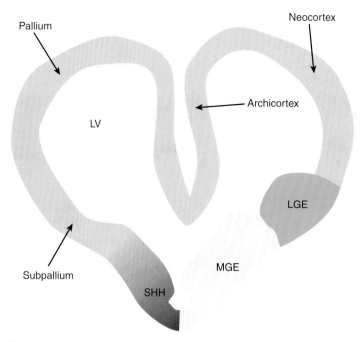

FIGURE 14.17 Regulation of DV pattern in the telencephalon by Sonic hedgehog. Cross section of mouse telencephalon at early (left side) and later (right side) stage. SHH produced in the ventral midline region controls development of the basal ganglia primordia and medial and lateral ganglionic eminences (MGE, LGE). First, ventral SHH induces MGE gene expression; SHH (partly produced by the MGE) induces LGE gene expression later.

rate areal pattern of the neocortex develops is that it is virtually uniform in structure and cytoarchitecture from one end to the other, at least in lower mammals such as mouse and rat. Furthermore, few known developmental control genes are expressed early enough to be candidate area determinants, and none of these is unique to a single prospective area. Thus, it has long been thought that the areal pattern is imposed on the neocortex by extrinsic elements, principally via the thalamic afferents that penetrate the cortex in an area-specific manner. However, it now appears that the cortical neuroepithelium acquires regional pattern prior to afferent innervation and in a manner not unlike other regions of the neural tube, with transcriptional mediators being expressed in a graded fashion in response to a local concentration of morphogens diffusing from localized sources. The homeobox gene *Emx2* and the FGF receptor *Fgfr3*, for example, are expressed in a gradient along the AP extent of the cortex, whereas transcription factor Lef1 (a mediator of WNT signaling) displays graded expression from medial to lateral. Putative signaling centers include the anterior pole, which secretes FGFs, and the posteromedial cortical hem region, which secretes WNTs and BMPs. According to a recent model (Ragsdale and Grove, 2001), areal specification may involve threshold levels of such transcription

factors rather than the presence or absence of area-specific factors (Fig. 14.18). So far, however, there is little more than provocative expression data (of but few genes) to support this model, although it is already clear that the level of *Emx2* expression can specify positional identity and that WNTs participate in cortical patterning. Thus, in contradiction to long-standing ideas, the cortical pattern is probably set up early within the parent neuroepithelium and the role of thalamic innervation is secondary reinforcing, refining or modifying this initial pattern.

CONCLUSIONS

Neural-inducing factors and modifiers produced during gastrulation have a basic role in establishing an initial crude AP regional identity in the neural plate that emerges from the dorsal surface of the embryo toward the end of this period. The nature of this early patterning information remains unclear, but mesendoderm-derived factors that deplete WNTs have been implicated in conferring forebrain identity. A number of factors cooperate to posteriorize an initially anterior neural specification state. This coarse-grained pattern is subsequently refined by the action

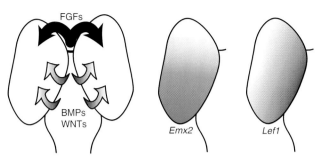

FIGURE 14.18 Model for areal patterning in the cortex. Signaling centers at the anterior pole (FGFs) and the cortical hem (BMPs, WNTs) set up graded expression of transcriptional mediators (*Emx2, Lef1*) that control regional identity. After Ragsdale and Grove (2001).

of local organizers which exert regional growth control and which induce or repress transcriptional mediators of regional fate. These, in turn, may also interact among themselves, sharpening domains of action by cross-repression. The combined processes of segmentation and compartmentation provide an alternative or perhaps additional mechanism for sharpening gene expression borders and cellular domains. These events result in the precise identification of regions and subregions. Although we tend to think of neuraxial patterning as a series of discrete steps leading to greater refinement, it is a continuous process that extends over a protracted period of development and involves a continuity of signaling systems (e.g., RA, BMPs, SHH). We also tend to think of pattern as being acquired separately on AP and DV axes, whereas it is clear that cell specification on the DV axis must intersect with and act on already existing AP positional values. It is also clear that patterning mechanisms must be integrated with those that control neurogenesis, a topic that is considered in Chapter 15.

The conservation of expression pattern and function of developmental control genes shows that a ground pattern of CNS development is shared across vertebrates. What will be interesting for the future is to discover the genetic and cellular mechanisms involved in the elaboration of this pattern in different species, such as zebrafish and mouse, whose adult brains bear little resemblance, especially in forebrain organization. What is required is insight into the major unresolved questions of how fine-grained axial distinctions in neuronal identity are specified and how genes orchestrate neuronal migration, a component of the specified state that is crucial to the correct formation of pattern. For the neocortex, an immediate prospect is the elucidation of regionalization mechanisms; here, the rapid accumulation of genetic data,

combined with genetic and embryological manipulations, will soon reveal how this, the most complex of CNS regions, acquires its rich pattern of functional areas.

References

Cornell, R. A., and von Ohlen, T. (2000). Vnd/nkx, ind/gsh, and msh/msx: Conserved regulators of dorsoventral neural patterning? *Curr. Opin. Neurobiol.* **10**, 63–71.

Crossley, P. H., *et al.* (1996). Midbrain development induced by FGF8 in the chick embryo. *Nature* **380**, 66–68.

Dupé, V., and Lumsden, A. (2001). Hindbrain patterning involves graded responses to retinoic acid signalling. *Development* **128**, 2199–2208.

Fraser, S. E., *et al.* (1990). Segmentation in the chick embryo hindbrain is defined by cell lineage restrictions. *Nature* **344**, 431–435.

Halder, G., *et al.* (1995). Induction of ectopic eyes by targeted expression of the *eyeless* gene in Drosophila. *Science* **267**, 1788–1792.

Hirth, F., *et al.* (1998). Homeotic gene action in embryonic brain development of Drosophila. *Development* **125**, 1579–1589.

Houart, C., *et al.* (1998). A small population of anterior cells patterns the forebrain during zebrafish gastrulation. *Nature* **391**, 788–792.

Khotz, J., *et al.* (1998). Regionalization within the mammalian telencephalon is mediated by changes in responsiveness to Sonic hedgehog. *Development* **125**, 5079–5089.

Larsen, C., *et al.* (2001). Boundary formation and compartition in the avian diencephalon. *J. Neurosci.*

Lumsden, A., and Keynes, R. (1989). Segmental patterns of neuronal development in the chick hindbrain. *Nature* **337**, 424–428.

Redies, C. (2000). Cadherins in the nervous system. *Prog. Neurobiol.* **61**, 611–648.

Simon, H., *et al.* (1995). Independent assignment of anteroposterior and dorsoventral positional values in the developing chick hindbrain. *Curr. Biol.* **5**, 205–214.

Streit, A., and Stern, C. D. (1999). Neural induction: A bird's eye view. *Trends Genet.* **15**, 20–24.

Wurst, W., *et al.* (1994). Multiple developmental defects in *Engrailed-1* mutant mice: An early mid-hindbrain deletion and patterning defects in forelimbs and sternum. *Development* **120**, 2065–2075.

Xu, Q., *et al.* (1999). In vivo cell sorting in complementary segmental domains mediated by Eph receptors and ephrins. *Nature* **400**, 267–271.

Suggested Readings

Briscoe, J., and Ericson, J. (2001). Specification of neuronal fates in the ventral neural tube. *Curr. Opin. Neurobiol.* **11**, 43–49.

Brown, M., *et al.* (2001). "The Developing Brain." Oxford Univ. Press, Oxford.

Gavalas, A., Krumlauf, R. (2000). Retinoid signalling and hindbrain patterning. *Curr. Opin. Genet. Dev.* **10**, 380–386.

Harland, R., and Gerhart, J. (1997). Formation and function of Spemann's organizer. *Annu. Rev. Cell Dev. Biol.* **13**, 611–667.

Irvine, K. D., and Rauskolb, C. (2001). Boundaries in development: Formation and function. *Annu. Rev. Cell Dev. Biol.* **17**, 189–214.

Pfaff, S., and Kintner, C. (1998). Neuronal diversification: Development of motor neuron subtypes. *Curr. Opin. Neurobiol.* **8**, 27–36.

Ragsdale, C. W., and Grove, E. A. (2001). Patterning the mammalian cerebral cortex. *Curr. Opin. Neurobiol.* **11**, 50–58.

Rhinn, M., and Brand, M. (2001). The midbrain-hindbrain boundary organizer. *Curr. Opin. Neurobiol.* **11**, 34–42.

Rubenstein, J. L. R., and Beachy, P. A. (1998). Patterning the embryonic forebrain. *Curr. Opin. Neurobiol.* **8**, 18–26.

Weinstein, D. C., and Hemmati-Brivanlou, A. (1999). Neural induction. *Annu. Rev. Cell Dev. Biol.* **15**, 411–33.

Andrew Lumsden and Chris Kintner

15

Neurogenesis and Migration

One of the most remarkable features of the developing nervous system is the wide-ranging migration by precursor cells. During transformation of the *neural plate* into the *brain, spinal cord,* and *peripheral ganglia,* cells migrate extensively and undergo significant rearrangements prior to differentiation into an astonishing array of neurons and glia. As described in previous chapters, soluble cues and localized transcription factors establish a set of precursor cells early in development, marking the primary zones of the brain and, in many cases, the specific types of neural progenitors in those regions. Within these regions—spinal cord, hindbrain, midbrain, forebrain—specific patterns of cell migration emerge to deploy cells into the cellular architecture characteristic of the region. This architecture in turn sets forth the functional organization of brain regions. The molecular nature of the cues guiding cell movement are only beginning to be understood and appear to differ between different regions of the nervous system. This chapter compares the strategies used to generate final cell pattern in the peripheral and central nervous systems, considering classical views of brain development that resulted from anatomical studies, as well as emerging molecular programs of neurogenesis and cell migration that have resulted from genetic and molecular genetic studies.

DEVELOPMENT OF THE PERIPHERAL NERVOUS SYSTEM

The Neural Crest is a Migratory Cell Population That Forms Multiple Derivatives

The *neural crest* is a transient population of cells, so named because they arise on the "crest" of the closing neural tube. This cell population is unique to vertebrates and forms most of the peripheral nervous system (PNS). Neural crest cells migrate extensively along characteristic pathways and give rise to diverse and numerous derivatives. All of the *dorsal root, sympathetic, parasympathetic,* and *enteric ganglia* are derived from neural crest cells. Furthermore, most *cranial sensory ganglia* receive a contribution from the neural crest, with the remaining cells derived from *ectodermal placodes.* In addition to forming neurons and glia of the peripheral nervous system, neural crest cells form melanocytes, cranial cartilage, and adrenal chromaffin cells. This wide variety of cell types arises from precursors in the neural folds and neural tube that are multipotent and have stem cell properties (Bronner-Fraser and Fraser, 1988; Stemple and Anderson, 1992) *(see Chapter 16 for a discussion of stem cells).*

The neural crest originates at the border between the neural plate and the nonneural ectoderm by an inductive interaction between these two tissues (Selleck and Bronner-Fraser, 1995) *(see Chapter 14).* Precursors with the potential to form neural crest initially are contained within the dorsal portion of the neural tube, and these premigratory neural crest cells subsequently emerge from the neural tube. Cells in the neural tube are epithelial and look much like contiguous soda cans that have a defined top (apical) and bottom (basal) side. They are closely apposed to one another and are connected by various types of adhesive junctions. In contrast, migratory cells such as neural crest cells are mesenchymal, having a fibroblast-like morphology which facilitates their movement. Thus, precursor cells within the neural tube change from an epithelial to a mesenchymal morphology as they turn into migratory neural crest cells. Such an *epithelial-to-mesenchymal conversion* is a common event in development during the formation of tissues and organs. The transcription factor Slug is expressed in premigratory and early migrating cells and represents the earliest known neural crest marker. Slug has been associated with epithelial–mesenchymal conversions in a number of cell types and its function appears to be necessary for the emigration of neural crest cells. Initiation of neural crest cell migration proceeds in a rostral-to-caudal progression along most of the neural axis, following upon the heels of the head-to-tailward closure of the neural tube. After emigration, these cells move in a highly patterned fashion through neighboring tissues and localize in diverse sites.

Initiation of Migration

As they change from epithelial to migratory mesenchymal cells, neural crest cells undergo changes in adhesive properties. While within the neuroepithelium, neural tube cells express high levels of the *cell adhesion molecules* N-cadherin and cadherin-6b. The cells downregulate these cadherins during migration and upregulate cadherin-7. Upon coalescing into ganglia and ceasing migration, cadherin-7 is downregulated and N-cadherin-6b are again upregulated (Nakagawa and Takeichi, 1998). This suggests that a shift in cell surface and adhesive properties may accompany the onset and cessation of migratory behavior. Neural crest cells also turn on RhoB during the initiation of migration.

After leaving the neural tube, neural crest cells encounter extracellular spaces that are rich in *extracellular matrix* (ECM) *molecules*, such as fibronectin, laminin, collagens, and proteoglycans. These may serve as a good migratory substrate and, indeed, the neural crest cell surface has abundant integrin receptors that mediate adhesion to ECM molecules. Furthermore, antibodies to the β_1 *subunit of integrin* cause severe perturbations in neural crest development in the head. They appear to prevent the migration of some neural crest cells from the cranial neural tube. In the trunk, function-blocking antibodies that interfere with the α_4 *subunit of integrin* cause defects in neural crest cell movement, but fail to alter the segmental pattern of migration through the somites. These results suggest that perturbing integrin function alters the properties of migratory cells, but not their overall metameric pattern of migration. Thus, cell–matrix interactions may play a permissive role in the migration of neural crest cells through the somites, but cannot play an instructive role in directing the precise patterns or pathways for crest cell migration.

Techniques for Following Migratory Neural Crest Cells

When neural crest cells emerge from the neural tube, they first enter a cell-free space in which they are easily identifiable (Fig. 15.1).

Subsequently, they invade other tissues in which they are difficult to distinguish. Therefore, it is necessary to *mark* neural crest cells in order to study their migratory patterns and derivatives. A variety of techniques have emerged for this purpose, ranging from transplantation of tissue containing premigratory neural crest cells to lineage tracers and molecular markers. *Neural tube transplantations* have provided a wealth of information about neural crest migratory pathways and, in particular, derivatives arising from this population. Although this approach was widely used in amphibians for studying numerous embryonic processes, it has been applied most successfully to the analysis of neural crest migratory pathways and derivatives in avian embryos (LeDouarin and Kalcheim, 1999). Initial experiments in birds involved transplanting a neural tube from a donor labeled with the radioactive marker [³H]thymidine into an unlabeled host (Weston, 1963). Neural crest cells generated from the labeled neural tube were also labeled and could be identified readily in the periphery. This technique yielded important information about early stages of neural crest migration, but the label became diluted with further cell division and was not useful for looking at long-term differentiation of neural crest cells into diverse derivatives.

To circumvent this problem, LeDouarin took advantage of the ability to perform grafts between

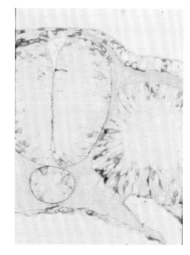

FIGURE 15.1 A transverse section through a chick embryo showing neural crest cells initiating migration from the dorsal neural tube and into an ECM-filled space. Courtesy of Jan Lofberg.

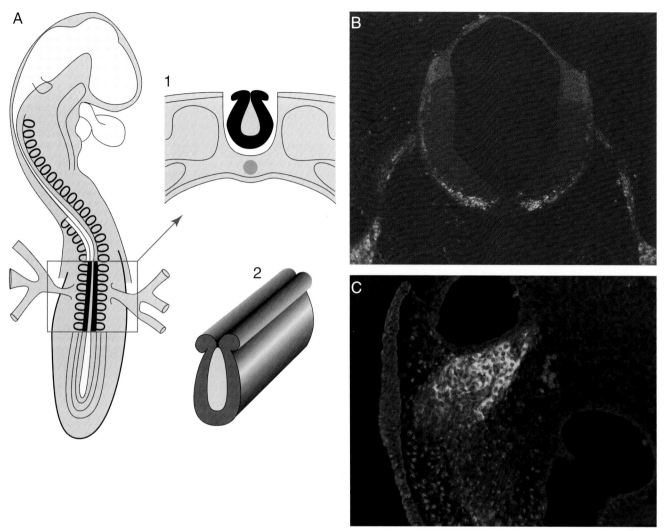

FIGURE 15.2 Procedures for grafting a fragment of the neural primordium from a donor quail into a host chicken embryo as used by LeDouarin and colleagues. (A) View of an avian embryo with anterior at the top. Neural folds are shown in black in the boxed region; this structure is removed and transplanted to a host embryo. (1) Cross section through the embryo in regions shown in the box with the neural tube (2) shown in black. From LeDouarin (1982). (B) An example of a section through an embryo after grafting of a quail neural tube into a chick host. Quail cells are recognized by a quail-specific antibody (red), whereas neurons are marked in green with a neurofilament marker. (C) A higher magnification section showing quail cells (red nuclei) incorporated into a neural crest-derived ganglion, stained green with a neurofilament antibody. Courtesy of Anne Knecht and Clare Baker.

related species of birds, such that the grafted cells were indelibly marked (Fig. 15.2). This created an interspecific "**chimera**," from the Greek meaning "fabulous monster," containing a donor quail portion of the neural tube and neural crest in an otherwise normal chick host embryo. Quail neural crest cells migrate away from the grafted neural tubes and can be recognized easily within the host chick embryo by staining for condensed heterochromatin, which characterizes the quail but not chick cells.

More recently, this technique has been facilitated greatly by the advent of quail-specific antibodies. Use of the chick–quail marking system made it possible to

demonstrate that neural crest cell populations originating from different axial levels follow distinct migratory pathways and give rise to different progeny once they reach their destinations.

In addition to grafting experiments, antibodies that recognize neural crest cells, such as HNK-1 and NC-1 antibodies, made it possible to identify early migrating neural crest cells without the necessity of performing microsurgery. The exclusive use of neural crest antibodies has several pitfalls because these antibodies are neither entirely specific nor stain the full complement of neural crest cells. However, they do provide important confirmatory information

BOX 15.1

LABELING EMBRYONIC CELLS AND THEIR PROGENY

To study the movements and fates of specific cells over time, one must label the cells in some way that distinguishes them from their neighbors. In the earliest fate-mapping studies, cells were labeled by external application of either vital dyes or colored powders. These methods enabled one to obtain information about the movements of large populations of cells, but were compromised by the tendency of the labels to either diffuse away or detach from the cells to which they were initially applied. More accurate marking was obtained with the [^{3}H]thymidine-labeling method, first developed in the late 1950s by Weston (1963) to study neural crest cell migration. In this method, the cells of interest are removed from a donor animal, incubated with [^{3}H]thymidine (which becomes incorporated into cell nuclei during DNA synthesis), and transplanted into a host animal (from which the equivalent endogenous cell population has usually been removed). Transplanted cells can be distinguished from those of the host by autoradiography. Although the thymidine label is nondiffusible, it has the disadvantage of becoming diluted over time as the labeled cells divide. In addition, autoradiographic processing is very time-consuming. In the 1980s, it was discovered that additional sensitivity and much greater ease of use could be obtained with fluorescent dyes, of which the lipophilic dye DiI has proven by far the most popular because of the intensity of its fluorescence (Honig and Hume, 1986; O'Rourke et al., 1992). However, even the DiI signal becomes diluted to undetectable levels in rapidly dividing cell populations.

To follow cells through unlimited cell divisions, one must use cellular markers that propagate as cells divide. This realization led to the use of interspecific chimeras, in which a cell population of interest is removed from a donor animal and transplanted into a host of a different species whose cells carry visible markers different from those of the donor. The most commonly used inter-specific chimeras have employed either unpigmented and pigmented species of amphibians, or quail and chick embryos. The quail/chick chimera system, developed by Le Douarin (1982), takes advantage of a heterochromatin marker found in the nuclei of quail cells but absent from chick cells. The quail/chick chimera system proved key to the accurate delineation of the migratory pathways and developmental potentials of neural crest cells, which undergo especially extensive migrations within the embryo and so are particularly difficult to track.

More recently, the application of exogenous genetic markers has permitted permanent and heritable labeling of cells in species other than avians and amphibians (Walsh and Cepko, 1988). In this method, cells are infected with a retrovirus carrying a reporter gene, such as β-galactosidase, the expression of which can be detected histochemically (Fig. 15.19), or green fluorescent protein, which can be visualized directly under fluorescence optics. The retrovirus is administered by injection into the region of interest. Following infection of cells surrounding the injection site, the reporter gene carried by the virus is incorporated into the DNA of the cell and is subsequently expressed in both infected cells and their progeny through unlimited rounds of cell division.

One encounters a special challenge when trying to trace the fates of single cells rather than cell populations. Some organisms, such as *Caenorhabditis elegans* and zebrafish, are sufficiently translucent that each of their cells can be identified individually under Nomarski optics and followed with time-lapse photography. In

---

about the pathways followed by neural crest cells. More recently, a number of other molecular markers for early neural crest populations have become available. These include the cell adhesion molecule cadherin-6b and the transcription factor Slug, expressed in the neural folds and neural crest cells during early stages of migration and Sox10, expressed in early migrating neural crest cells and later in neural crest-derived glia.

One problem with using antibodies or molecular markers to follow cell migratory patterns is that these do not represent true lineage markers. Shifts in their expression patterns could just as easily reflect up- or downregulation of these molecules as changes in cell position. Therefore, approaches for labeling small groups as well as large populations of neural crest cells have been employed to follow individual cell movements and interactions within the population. One successful approach has been to inject the *lipophilic vital dye DiI* into the neural tube or neural folds. Because the dye is hydrophobic and lipophilic, it intercalates into all cell membranes that it contacts. Injection into the neural tube marks all neural tube cells, including presumptive neural crest cells, within its dorsal aspect. Because the time and location of injection can be controlled, this provides a direct

BOX 15.1 *(cont'd)*

most organisms, however, the cells must be labeled in some way. Two methods for doing this have been developed so far. In the first method, individual cells are microinjected intracellularly with a dye, usually fluorescent (Jacolson ad Huose, 1981; Bronner-Fraser and Fraser, 1988). Dyes used are ones that cannot diffuse out of the cell or pass through gap junctions so that only the injected cell and its progeny are labeled. The limitation of this method, as with all dye-labeling methods, is dilution of the dye with cell division. This problem can be overcome through the use of retroviral labels such as those described earlier. To label only single cells rather than cell populations, one uses extremely dilute solutions of retrovirus. In theory, only a few cells within the exposed population are infected, and the distance between infected cells is greater than the distance across which progeny of any one cell (i.e., a clone) would be expected to disperse. In practice, it is difficult to be certain that adjacent labeled cells within a cluster arise from a single infected cell rather than multiple ones, especially given increasing evidence that cells within a single clone can disperse for large distances across the developing brain (Walsh and Cepko, 1992; O'Rourke *et al.*, 1995) To help get around this problem, Walsh and Cepko (1992) developed a technique in which cells are treated with retroviral solutions derived from a complex library of 100 retroviruses, each bearing a unique sequence tag. Following histochemical visualization of clones within brain sections, cells are dissected out and analyzed by polymerase chain reaction to determine what sequence tag they bear. Demonstration that two or more cells bear the same sequence tag provides strong evidence that these cells derive from a single cell infected by a single retrovirus particle. For further discus-sion of this problem, see Walsh and Cepko (1992) and Luskin *et al.* (1993).

Gabrielle G. Leblanc

References

Bronner-Fraser, M., and Fraser, S. E. (1988). Cell lineage analysis reveals multipotency of some avian neural crest cells. *Nature* **335**, 161–164.

Honig, M. G., and Hume, R. I. (1986). Fluorescent carbocyanine dyes allow living neurons of identified origin to be studied in long-term cultures. *J. Cell Biol.* **103**, 171–187.

Jacobson, M., and Hirose, G. (1981). Clonal organization of the central nervous system of the frog. II. Clones stemming from individual blastomeres of the 32- and 64-cell stages. *J. Neurosci.* **1**, 271–284.

LeDouarin, N. M. (1982). "The Neural Crest." Cambridge Univ. Press, Cambridge.

Luskin, M. B., Parnavelas, J. G., and Barfield, J. A. (1993). Neurons, astrocytes, and oligodendrocytes of the rat cerebral cortex originate from separate progenitor cells: An ultra-structural analysis of clonally related cells. *J. Neurosci.* **13**, 1730–1750.

O'Rourke, N. A., Dailey, M. E., Smith, S. J., and McConnell, S. K. (1992). Diverse migratory pathways in the developing cerebral cortex. *Science* **258**, 299–302.

O'Rourke, N. A., Sullivan, D. P., Kaznowski, C. E., Jacobs, A. A., and McConnell, S. K. (1995). Tangential migration of neurons in the developing cerebral cortex. *Development* **121**, 2165–2176.

Walsh, C., and Cepko, C. (1988). Clonally related cortical cells show several migration patterns. *Science* **241**, 1342–1345.

Walsh, C., and Cepko, C. L. (1992). Widespread dispersion of neuronal clones across functional regions of the cerebral cortex. *Science* **255**, 434–440.

Weston, J. A. (1963). A radioautographic analysis of the migration and localization of trunk neural crest cells in the chick. *Dev. Biol.* **6**, 279–310.

approach for following migratory pathways. When dye injections are made focally into neural folds, this technique can be used to label very small numbers of cells. It has the further advantage of being applicable to almost all vertebrates. A disadvantage, however, is that the dye becomes diluted with each cell division and, therefore, is not useful for examining the long-term differentiation of neural crest derivatives.

Because most studies of cell migration *in vivo* look only at the beginning and end point, little is known about the dynamics of neural crest cell movement. Advances in imaging technologies have made it possible to acquire more refined images *in ovo*. Time-lapse movies of cranial neural crest migration can be generated by injecting DiI into the lumen of the chick neural tube, and high-resolution confocal images can be made of the labeled cells over time (Fig. 15.3). These movies make it possible to visualize the migratory behavior of neural crest cells as they emerge from the cranial neural tube and migrate toward the branchial arches. As the embryo develops, it is possible to follow individual cell movements within the branchial arches, which will give rise to the bone and cartilage of the jaw. Neural crest cells move in defined streams and appear to form distinct chains in which cells are oriented along the same trajectory and remain in contact via their processes.

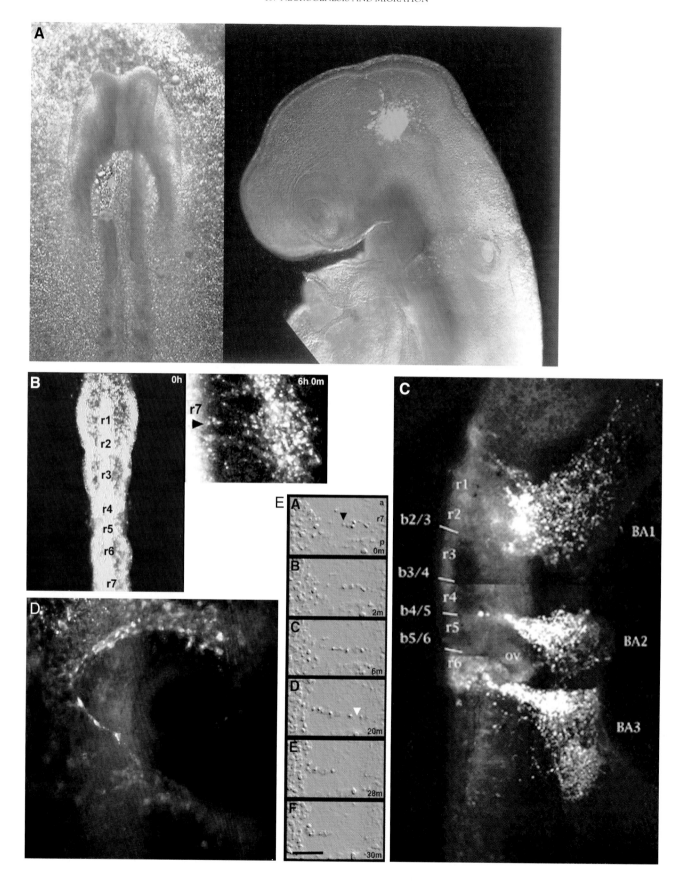

This suggests a large degree of intercommunication between migrating populations of cranial neural crest cells.

Summary

A number of different methods have proved useful for following the pathways of neural crest migration, including neural tube transplantations, vital dye labeling, and antibody staining. These have made it possible not only to establish the various routes of neural crest migration occurring at different axial levels, but also to follow the derivatives of neural crest cells arising from distinct locations.

Regionalization of the Neural Crest Along the Body Axis

Despite differences in the nature of the techniques involved, quail/chick chimeras, molecular markers, and DiI labeling have provided similar pictures of the migratory pathways followed by neural crest cells. These migratory pathways and the derivatives formed by neural crest cells are regionalized according to their original position along the anterior/posterior axis, such that cells from a given axial level give rise to a characteristic array of progeny and follow distinct pathways from those arising at other axial levels (LeDouarin and Kalcheim, 1999; Noden, 1975). The different populations of neural crest cells arising along the neural axis have been designated as cranial, vagal, trunk, and lumbosacral (Fig. 15.4). Distinct cell types differentiate from these different populations.

At cranial levels, some neural crest cells contribute to the *cranial sensory ganglia* and the *parasympathetic*

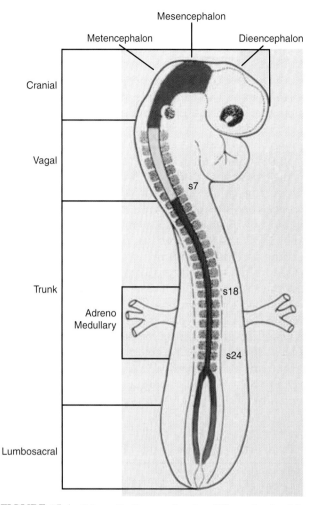

FIGURE 15.4 Schematic diagram showing different levels of the neural axis from which neural crest cells arise. From anterior to posterior, the neural axis can be divided into cranial, vagal, trunk, and lumbosacral levels. Each gives rise to distinct derivatives.

◀ **FIGURE 15.3** Labeling of neural crest cells with liphophilic tracer dyes. (A) On the left is a chick embryo viewed shortly after unilateral ablation of the neural folds of roughly half the neural tube at the level of the presumptive midbrain. A spot of DiO (green) was focally injected into the remaining neural tube, and DiI (red) was injected into the bordering intact neural folds. On the right, the same embryo after 48 h of further development. Cells that were originally in the neural tube had dispersed as migratory neural crest cells from both the green- and the red-labeled spots. (B–D) Different views of time-lapse movies of embryos in which the neural tube and premigratory neural crest cells were labeled with DiI. (B) Two views of the same embryo immediately after DiI labeling (left) and several hours after neural crest migration from the hindbrain. Rhombomeres (r1–r7) are indicated. (C) A similar embryo at a later time point by which time neural crest cells have migrated into the branchial arches (BA). (D) At higher magnification of neural crest streams in the branchial arches, cells seem to be in close contact as if following each other in narrow streams. (E) Following individual cells by time-lapse cinematography demonstrates close and maintained connections between individual cell pairs. Courtesy of Paul Kulesa and Scott Fraser.

ciliary ganglion of the eye, whereas others migrate ventrally to form many of the *cartilaginous elements of the facial skeleton*. One of the interesting things about neural crest-derived bones of the head is that these are the only skeletal elements in the body that are derived from ectoderm. Precise quail/chick grafting experiments have determined the regions of neural tube from which neural crest cells arise to contribute to cartilaginous elements and cranial ganglia (Noden, 1975). Neural crest cells originating in the midbrain migrate primarily as a broad, unsegmented sheet under the ectoderm; they contribute to derivatives ranging from the skeleton around the eye, connective tissue and membranous bones of the face, to the ciliary ganglion and trigeminal ganglia (LeDouarin and Kalcheim, 1999). Neural crest cells arising in the hindbrain migrate ventrally and enter the branchial arches to form the bones of the jaw.

Vagal neural crest cells migrate long distances to form the *enteric nervous system*, which also receives a contribution from the lumbosacral neural crest. Within the gut, the earliest generated crest cells move as a wave from anterior to posterior to populate the bowel, which they appear to populate in sequence such that the anterior portions are populated by neural crest cells first and the cells move to progressively more posterior sites. Mice bearing a "lethal spotted" mutation lack neural crest cells in a portion of their bowel. This leads to a lack of innervation in the region called aganglionic bowel. As a consequence, food waste fails to move through this portion of the bowel, leading to a disorder called "megacolon." A similar defect is observed in humans leading to "Hirschsprung's disease." This disorder arises from a defect in molecules called endothelins and their receptors. The failure of neural crest migration in the aganglionic bowel of lethal spotted mutant mice is caused by a defect in mesenchymal components of the gut, whereas the neural crest cells themselves are normal. Trunk neural crest cells follow two primary migratory pathways (Fig. 15.5): a *dorsolateral pathway* between the ectoderm and the somite and *a ventral pathway* through the rostral half of each sclerotome, the mesenchymal portion of the somite which will go on to form the vertebrae.

Cells following the dorsolateral stream give rise to *melanocytes*. Those cells following the ventral pathway give rise to the peripheral nervous system of the trunk, including the chain of *sympathetic ganglia* and *dorsal root ganglia*, as well as *chromaffin cells* of the adrenal medulla. In addition to these neurons, these cells generate *glia* of the peripheral ganglia and *Schwann cells* that ensheathe and myelinate peripheral axons.

Summary

The neural crest can be subdivided into specific subpopulations based upon their level of origin along the neural tube. Different populations follow different migratory pathways and form characteristic types of derivatives. For example, cranial bone and cartilage only arise from the cranial neural crest.

Grafting of Neural Crest Cells to New Locations—Intrinsic Versus Extrinsic Cues?

Neural crest cells that arise and migrate at different axial levels assume different fates. Thus, it is possible that they are specified at early times to take on particular fates. For example, one possibility is that neural crest cells are preprogrammed by their axial level to populate specific derivatives; alternatively, neural crest cells might be multipotent and migrate naively into available locations, where local cues provide them with instructions about their fates. To test the role of migratory pathways in choice of fate, neural tubes from particular axial levels have been grafted to new locations. This is referred to as a "**heterotopic**" graft. These experiments have revealed, for example, that when vagal neural crest cells are grafted to trunk regions, they form normal trunk derivatives (dorsal root ganglia, sympathetic ganglia, etc.) and normal vagal derivatives (enteric ganglia of the gut) (Fig. 15.6). The gut is immediately ventral to the trunk region and is connected to it by a narrow piece of tissue called the dorsal mesentery. Despite their close proximity, trunk neural crest cells normally fail to invade the gut where enteric ganglia form. When vagal neural tubes are grafted in place of trunk neural tubes, however, donor vagal neural crest cells do invade the gut and form enteric ganglia. Therefore, these cells can respond to normal trunk neural crest migratory pathways, but, in addition, some cells behave in a "uniquely vagal" fashion and migrate directionally to the gut. This indicates some intrinsic differences between the two populations. Along similar lines, when cranial neural tubes are grafted in

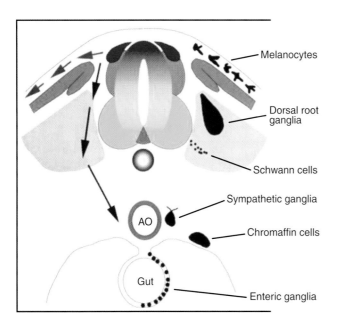

FIGURE 15.5 Schematic diagram of an idealized embryo in cross section showing pathways of neural crest migration in trunk and derivatives formed. Neural crest cells migrate along two primary pathways: dorsally under the skin or ventrally through the sclerotome. Dorsal migrating cells form pigment cells, whereas ventrally migrating cells give rise to dorsal root and sympathetic ganglia, Schwann cells, and cells of the adrenal medulla. Drawn by Mark Selleck.

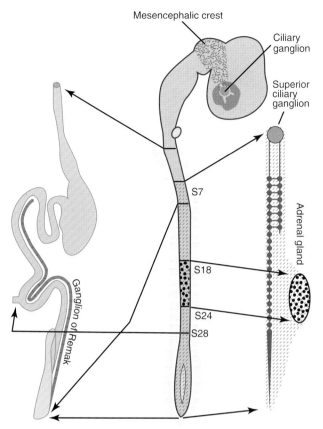

FIGURE 15.6 Neural crest cells at different levels along the anterior–posterior axis give rise to distinct autonomic and adrenomedullary derivatives in avian embryos. In the cephalic region (center), mesencephalic crest cells populate the ciliary ganglion. Ganglia of the sympathetic chain (right), including the superior ciliary ganglion, are formed from spinal neural crest cells originating caudal to somite 5. Cells of the adrenal medulla (right) originate exclusively from neural crest cells between somites 18 and 24. Vagal neural crest cells generated between somites 1 and 7 form enteric ganglia (left), whereas cells of the ganglion of Remak (left) are derived from the lumbosacral neural crest posterior to somite 28. Drawing provided by Dr. M. Bronner-Fraser.

place of the trunk neural tube, donor cranial neural crest cells form some normal derivatives in the trunk-like dorsal root and sympathetic ganglia. Other cells, however, fail to migrate and instead differentiate into ectopic cartilage. In the reciprocal experiment, avian trunk neural crest cells grafted to the head region appear unable to generate cartilage at all, although they can participate in the formation of elements of the cranial ganglia (LeDouarin and Kalcheim, 1999) (Fig. 15.6).

These experiments suggest two things: (1) environmental factors can influence neural crest cells from different axial levels to express a broader range of fates than they would normally express when left *in situ* and (2) some neural crest cells undergo their

intrinsic program even when grafted to an ectopic site. Thus, some combination of *intrinsic and extrinsic information* is likely to govern neural crest cell fate decisions. The migratory pathways taken by neural crest cells are likely to play an important regulatory role in cell fate specification. Indeed, different migratory pathways contain different distribution patterns of important inducing factors. A number of factors, including BMPs, neuregulins, and glucocorticoids, have been demonstrated to influence the choice of neural crest cells into neural, glial, or chromaffin lineages (see Chapter 16). When added to multipotent neural crest stem cells in culture, these factors can drive these cells into neural, glial, or chromaffin lineages, respectively. Accordingly, BMP-7 is present in the dorsal aorta adjacent to the location where trunk neural crest cells differentiate into sympathetic neurons. Similarly, glucocorticoids are produced by the adrenal cortex, which surrounds the adrenal medullary cells.

In addition to specific growth factors, the timing of emigration may play an important role in eventual neural crest cell fate decisions. Neural crest cells exhibit an orderly pattern in the timing of migration, with cells initally following the ventral pathway and later contributing to progressively more dorsal derivatives. Although early and late migrating cranial neural crest cells appear to have a similar developmental potential, it is likely that the cell population does undergo a change in the range of fates that the cells can assume. For example, the last emigrating trunk neural crest cells in the bird give rise to pigment cells and appear to have a limited capacity to form sympathetic neurons. However, *stem cells* appear to persist in the neural tube and retain the potential to form neural crest. Well past the normal time of neural crest cell emigration, cells with the full range of neural crest potential can be isolated from the ventricular zone of the developing spinal cord (Sharma *et al.*, 1995). In the embryo, these late-emigrating cells appear to contribute to a subpopulation of neural crest derived cells in the dorsal root ganglia.

Summary

Neural crest cells are somewhat plastic with respect to their prospective fates. When put into a new environment, they sometimes behave according to their new location. However, some cells act according to their original location and thus have some "intrinsic" information. With time, the developmental potential of neural crest populations becomes restricted, although a subpopulation of "stem cells" may remain until late stages.

Segmental Migration of Neural Crest Cells

A hallmark of the developing peripheral nervous system is its inherent *segmentation*. After neural crest cells migrate from the neural tube and through the somites, they condense to form segmentally arranged sensory and sympathetic ganglia. For each somite, a single sensory and sympathetic ganglion forms. This exquisite and reproducible pattern suggests the presence of some inherent segmental information in the embryo that is responsible for segmental migration and gangliogenesis of neural crest cells. In longitudinal sections through early embryos, it is clear that neural crest cells migrate in a metameric pattern, moving exclusively through the rostral half of each somite while failing to enter the caudal half (Fig. 15.7).

Such a segmental pattern of migration could be caused by inherent cues within the neural tube that direct neural crest cells to migrate segmentally. Alternatively, tissues through which neural crest cells migrate may contain patterning information that results in segmental migration.

The relationship between neural crest cells and their surrounding tissues has been explored by manipulating the neural tube and/or somites in a series of grafting experiments. Removal of the somites results in the formation of huge, unsegmented neural crest-derived ganglia, suggesting that somites are necessary for the segmental migration of neural crest cells. However, inversion of the segmental plate in the rostrocaudal dimension reverses the pattern of neural crest migration, such that neural crest cells migrate through the half of the rotated sclerotomes that was originally rostral but is now caudal. Motor axons, which also traverse the rostral sclerotome in normal animals, exhibit similar behavior to neural crest cells after segmental plate rotation. This suggests that the information necessary to guide neural crest cells and motor axons is intrinsic to the somites. Furthermore, these experiments show that the rostrocaudal polarity of the somites is already established at the segmental plate stage.

Other experimental manipulations demonstrate that the caudal half of each somite is inhibitory whereas the rostral half somite is permissive for neural crest migration and motor axon guidance. If somites are constructed to contain only caudal sclerotome tissue, neural crest cells and motor axons fail to migrate altogether. Conversely, an all-rostral somite results in the absence of segmentation for both neural crest cells and motor axons. Taken together, these findings demonstrate that the segmental migration of both neural crest cells and motor axons is due to cues inherent in the somite. These cues may be caused by

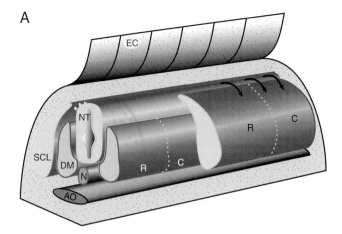

FIGURE 15.7 Trunk neural crest cells migrate in a segmental fashion. (A) Schematic diagram demonstrating that neural crest cells migrate through the sclerotomal portion of the somites, but only through the rostral half of the sclerotome. (B) In longitudinal section, neural crest cells (green) can be seen migrating selectively through the rostral half of each somitic sclerotome (S). From Bronner-Fraser (1986).

attractive cues in the rostral-half sclerotome, inhibitory cues in the caudal-half sclerotome, or a combination of both. The finding that somites containing all caudal-half sclerotomes cannot support neural crest migration strongly suggests that some of the guidance cues are inhibitory.

As in the trunk, the migration of neural crest cells in the hindbrain is also segmented. Three broad streams of migrating cells are found adjacent to rhombomere 2 (r2), r4, and r6, whereas no neural crest cells are apparent adjacent to r3 and r5. Focal injections of DiI at the levels of r3 and r5 have demonstrated that both of these rhombomeres generate neural crest cells and that the apparent segmental pattern results from the DiI-labeled cells that originated in r3 and r5 deviating rostrally or caudally and failing to enter the adjacent preotic mesoderm or otic vesicle region.

Eph receptor tyrosine kinases and their ligands display intriguing patterns of expression in the developing nervous system. Their distributions are consistent with potentially important roles in early neural patterning and in regulating the pattern of segmental migration by neural crest cells. Eph receptors are functionally divided into two subclasses: Eph A

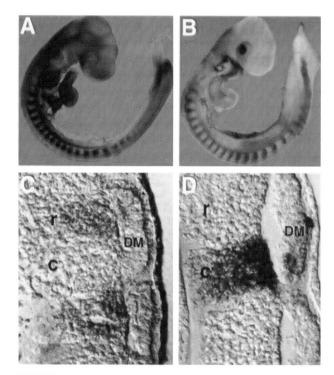

FIGURE 15.8 Distribution of Eph receptors (A and C) on neural crest cells in the rostral sclerotome and ephrin ligands in the caudal sclerotome (B and D) of chick embryos. Eph receptors are on neural crest cells in the rostral half of each somite, whereas inhibitory ephrin ligands are expressed in the caudal halves of each sclerotome. From Krull *et al.* (1997).

receptors, which interact primarily with a GPI-linked subclass of ligands, and Eph B receptors, which interact primarily with a transmembrane subclass of ligands (see Chapters 17 and 18). Eph receptor/ligand interactions have been implicated in axonal patterning events, such as the topographic organization of the retinotectal projection and regional organization of the forebrain and hindbrain (Wilkinson, 2001).

Eph receptors of the B class are expressed on neural crest cells as they migrate through the somites (Fig. 15.8). The cognate ligand for the Eph B receptor, ephrin B1, is expressed in a reciprocal pattern in the caudal portion of the sclerotome—the region through which neural crest cells fail to migrate. Adding exogenous ligand to activate the endogenous Eph B receptor in all regions of the somite results in a disruption of the segmental pattern of neural crest migration and demonstrates that the ligand is inhibitory for neural crest migration. These studies show that neural crest migration is linked intimately to both formation and segmentation of the somites. Functional interactions between Eph receptors and ligands appear to restrict neural crest cells to the rostral half sclerotomal domain. This in turn leads to their segmental migration and the subsequent metameric distribution of neural crest-derived sensory and sympathetic ganglia.

Summary

Trunk neural crest cells move in a segmental pattern, which is controlled by inhibitory molecules present in the caudal-half of each somite. Neural crest cells have Eph receptors on their surface. When they encounter ephrin ligands in the caudal somite, they are diverted from this location, leading to selective migration through only the rostral-half somite. This in turn leads to the segmental distribution of peripheral ganglia.

Cessation of Neural Crest Migration

Neural crest cells exhibit an orderly pattern in their migration. Whereas the first cells to migrate tend to move most ventrally, later migratory cells contribute to progressively more dorsal derivatives. The different destinations of neural crest derivatives are therefore populated in a sequential order during development. One possibility is that the early migrating cells "fill" the more ventral sites, effectively clogging up the pathway. Alternatively, the sites themselves may change with time so that they can no longer support migration.

Surpisingly little is known about how neural crest cells know that they have reached the appropriate destination and stop their migration. This is in marked contrast to the developing CNS, where a number of mutations affect the ability of neuroblasts to cease migrating. It is clear that cell adhesion molecules such as N-cadherin and N-CAM are up regulated after cells reach their final sites and condense to form peripheral ganglia. However, there is no evidence for a causal role for cell adhesion molecules in this process.

Neurogenesis in the PNS

Some of the factors and signaling cascades that result in neurogenesis in the developing PNS are beginning to be understood (see Chapter 16). Many neural crest cells appear to be multipotent and not yet committed to a neural fate. However, particular external factors can influence their fate decisions. For example, clonal populations of neural crest cells become neural in the presence of BMPs and glial in the presence of glial growth factor. Similarly, activation of Notch signaling promotes gliogenesis at the expense of neurogenesis in neural crest cells and their derivatives. Certain transcription factors may bias cells toward certain fates; e.g., while mash-1 is essential for sympathetic neuron formation, neurogenins are essential for sensory fates (Christiansen *et al.*, 2000).

An interesting contrast between the developing PNS and the CNS is that migrating neural crest cells proliferate rapidly as they move. In fact, even after exhibiting defined neuronal characteristics, some neural crest derivatives continue to divide. For example, in the developing sympathetic ganglia, neural crest-derived cells express neurotransmitters and other proteins characteristic of sympathetic neurons but remain actively mitotic. However, other neural crest cells such as sensory neurons appear to withdraw from the cell cycle well before they express neuronal traits.

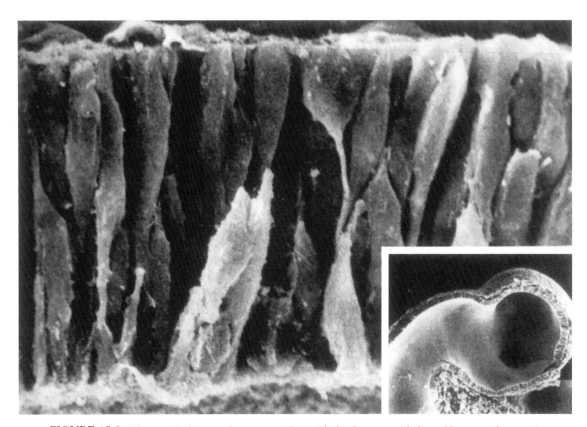

FIGURE 15.9 The ventricular zone forms a pseudostratified columnar epithelium. Here neural progenitor cells have been visualized in the cerebral vesicle of a hamster embryo using scanning electron microscopy. Neuroepithelial cells are elongated bipolar cells that, at this early stage of development (E9.25), span the entire wall of the cerebrum. Some of the cells at the ventricular surface (bottom) appear spherical; these cells have retracted their cytoplasmic processes and are presumably rounding up in preparation for mitosis. Other rounded cells at the external surface (top) may be young neurons beginning to differentiate. (Inset) A low-power view of the hamster cerebral vesicle, corresponding roughly to that of a human embryo at the end of the first month of gestation. From Sidman and Rakic (1973).

Summary

Neural crest cells migrate over long distances throughout the body to form diverse cell types, including neurons, glia, melanocytes, and cells of the adrenal gland. The migratory pathways of neural crest cells vary along the rostrocaudal body axis, and the local environments through which cells migrate and eventually differentiate play an important role in phenotypic specification. The migration of neural crest cells is guided by both positive (attractive or permissive) and inhibitory (repulsive) cues that are found in the environment.

DEVELOPMENT OF THE CENTRAL NERVOUS SYSTEM

Formation of the Basic Embryonic Zones of the Cerebral Cortex

After the neural tube closes, the forebrain vesicle consists of a *neuroepithelium* that is one cell in thickness (Fig. 15.9). Within the neuroepithelium, interphase cells extend fine processes from one side of the epithelium to the other. As the cells enter mitosis, however, the cells retract their processes and drop to the ventricular surface to divide. Following cell division, daughter cells then reextend processes, becoming bipolar again, and continue again through the cell cycle in a process known as *interkinetic nuclear migration*. As neurogenesis begins, a few daughter cells exit the cell cycle and move above the zone of dividing cells, which is called the *ventricular zone* (VZ) or the *proliferative zone* (Fig. 15.10). This first migration of postmitotic cells out of the ventricular zone is thought to occur by a simple process of translocation whereby the nucleus moves outward through the radial processes of the cell to reach the outer part of the brain rather than through a crawling motion of the cell. As rapid cell division thickens the proliferative zone, the emerging cortical structure progresses from a simple neuroepithelial sheet into a complex multilaminar system. The first step in this process involves the creation of the *preplate* (PP), a cell-sparse zone

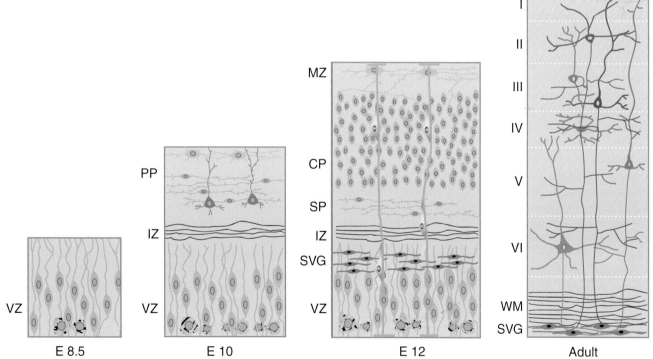

FIGURE 15.10 Development of the cerebral cortex. The ventricular zone (VZ) contains the progenitors of neurons and glia. The first neurons to be generated establish the preplate (PP); their axons, as well as ingrowing axons from the thalamus, establish the intermediate zone (IZ). The subsequently generated neurons of cortical layers II–VI establish the cortical plate (CP), which splits the preplate into the marginal zone (MZ), or future layer I, and the subplate (SP), a transient population of neurons. After the completion of neuronal migration and differentiation, six cortical layers are visible overlying the white matter (WM) and the subplate has largely disappeared. Neural precursors in the subventricular zone (SVZ) continue to generate neurons that migrate rostrally into the olfactory bulb, even during postnatal life.

from which nuclei are apparently excluded during interkinetic movements in the epithelium. Second, a zone of growing axons appears, forming an *intermediate zone* (IZ) between the ventricular zone and the preplate. In the cortex, these axons pioneer the connections in both directions between the cortex and the thalamus. The neuroepithelium thus progresses from a single layer of dividing cells to three zones, termed the *ventricular zone* (proliferating cells), *intermediate zone* (axons), and *preplate* (postmitotic neuronal precursors). Subsequently, with the onset of neurogenesis of neurons of the *cortical plate* that will comprise the cortical layers, the preplate is split into two regions: the *marginal zone* (future layer 1) at the top and the *subplate* below.

As the pace of cell proliferation continues, a secondary zone forms above the intermediate zone, termed the *subventricular zone* (SVZ). Cells within this secondary ventricular zone continue proliferation through the early postnatal period, following three different pathways of migration and patterns of differentiation. As discussed later, one population of precursor cells in the cortical SVZ forms a migratory stream toward the olfactory bulb. A second population produces a major wave of gliogenesis, with precursor cells undergoing radial migration out into the emerging cortical layers. In the final stages of neurogenesis in the SVZ, cortical interneurons are generated. It should be emphasized that these basic cell zones are unique to the embryonic brain, without direct counterparts in the adult structure. All become so altered over the progression of development as to be unrecognizable in the mature nervous system.

Thus, development of the CNS builds from a basic columnar organization of cells within the neuroepithelium of the brain vesicles. As the VZ thickens, postmitotic cells migrate away from the germinal zone, along the inner face of the neural tube, and form layers in cortical regions such as the cerebral cortex and cerebellum and mantles of cells in subcortical regions such as the thalamus. The appearance of a rich diversity of cell types within these regions and the development of the patterns of connectivity between them were studied in brilliant detail by the Spanish neuropathologist Ramon y Cajal, who provided precise information on the development and anatomy of fiber tracts and circuitry that emerge later. By examining embryos of different vertebrate species, using modifications of Golgi's staining methods, Cajal was able to discern the key features of neural development and to chronicle the growth and connectivity of the major classes of nerve cells. In his studies of cortical development, he proposed that the laminar structure of higher vertebrates is essential for the for-

mation of complex circuits and he spent much of his life describing how the complex varieties of neurons emerge within the brain.

As first documented in studies on human fetal development, and reviewed comprehensively by Sidman and Rakic (1973), the movements of precursor cells away from CNS germinal zones led to the formation of three general classes of structures: layered structures with predominantly radial migration patterns, including the cortex, the hippocampal formation, and the cerebellar cortex; layered structures formed by mixed radial and tangential migration, including the retina and spinal cord; and nonlayered structures, including the brain stem, mesencephalon, and diencephalon, where movements of multipotent precursor cells result in the formation of nuclear structures.

Within the ventricular zone, one of the first cells to express markers of differentiation is a specialized form of glial cell, called the *radial glial cell*. This cell, now recognized by its expression of the RC2 antigen, extends long processes perpendicular to the ventricular surface toward the overlying cerebral wall and continues to elongate as the brain thickens such that it spans from the ventricular surface to the pial surface throughout development. As discussed later, these radial processes presage the basic columnar plan of development, providing a scaffold "in plane" with the layer of dividing cells for young neurons to migrate away from the primary germinal matrix. This general scheme of migration sustains the early patterning of gene expression seen to set forth regional domains and sets in motion the histogenesis of the brain, namely the development of specific classes of cells and patterns of connections.

Three cortical regions of the brain have been studied intensively, providing paradigms for understanding the formation of laminar structures: the cortex, the hippocampus, and the cerebellum. Of these, the cerebellum and the hippocampus are more simple structures, having only two neuronal layers, each with one principal class of neuron. The cerebral cortex is far more complex, with six layers of cells containing multiple cell types. Although details of the development of these three regions differ, three basic steps underlie their formation: precursors proliferate in a germinal zone, postmitotic precursors migrate away from the germinal zone in the radial direction, and postmigratory cells form synaptic circuits.

Methods to mark cells undergoing cell division and cells entering specific differentiation pathways have made it possible to decipher the pattern in which different neuronal populations are generated in the embryonic brain. [³H]Thymidine labeling, discovered

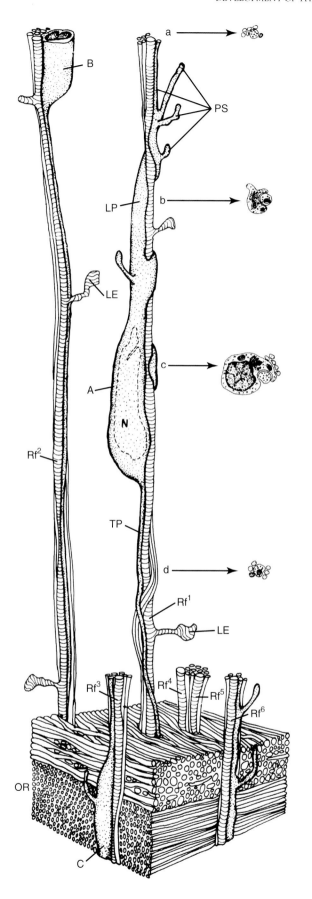

by Sidman and colleagues in the 1950s, provides a key tool for marking the "birthdate" or date of last division of any given precursor cell in the developing brain. Whereas cells that continue to divide after that day dilute the label, cells going through this penultimate division retain strong [³H]thymidine labeling. Using this labeling method, Sidman, Altman, and others showed that neurons in the layers of cortical regions of brain are generated in an "inside-out" pattern; i.e., later generations of precursor cells migrate out beyond early generations of cells to form successive layers. Thus, within the ventricular zone, specific neuronal cell populations arise in sequence and, as they emigrate out from the germinal layer along the radial fibers, begin their complex differentiation programs.

Patterns of Precursor Cell Migration from Primary Proliferative Zones

As mentioned earlier, radial glial cells are among the first cells to differentiate within the thickening cerebral wall. First described over a century ago by Kolliker, Retzius, and Ramon y Cajal, radial glia span the neural tube, providing cellular "spokes" to the radial plane of the neuroaxis. Neuroanatomical studies, including three-dimensional reconstructions of electron microscopic views (Fig. 15.11), show that postmitotic neurons are closely apposed to radial glial fibers, which led Rakic to propose that this system provides the primary substrate for the migration of cortical neurons and the emergence of superficial layers at a distance of some 3000 μm in higher vertebrates.

FIGURE 15.11 Serial section electron microscopy was used to create three-dimensional reconstructions of three migrating neurons (A–C) in the developing cerebral cortex. Migrating neurons in the intermediate zone are intimately apposed to radial glial fibers (striped vertical shafts, RF1-6), which extend short lamellate expansions (LE) at a right angle to their main axis. The lower part of the diagram depicts the numerous parallel axons of the optic radiations (OR). These axons have been deleted from the upper portion of the figure to reveal the radial glial fibers. Nuclei (N) of migrating neurons are elongated, and their leading processes (LP) are thicker and richer in organelles than their trailing processes (TP). Each leading process extends several pseudopodial endings (PS), which are thought to explore the territory through which the neuron is migrating. Several cross sections through a migrating neuron are shown (a–d), revealing that the migrating cell partially encircles the shaft of the radial glial fiber and that these intimate contacts are continuous throughout the length of the cell. From Sidman and Rakic (1973).

A role for radial glia in directed migration along the radial plane of the neuroaxis is supported by studies in the developing hippocampus, where neurons follow the undulating pathways of the radial fibers to form neural layers. Thus, the radial glial fiber system provides the primary guidance pathway for the emigration of postmitotic neurons from germinal zones and the formation of neuronal laminae in cortical brain regions.

In contrast to the cortex, the retina lacks radial glial fibers. In the absence of glial guides, clones arising from marked progenitors still organize a columnar pattern suggestive of radial movements (Fekete *et al.*, 1994; Reese and Tan, 1998). Once the cells begin to differentiate, however, single cone, horizontal, amacrine, and ganglion cells move across the columnar pattern, mixing with cells derived from different precursors. The mode of migration of young neurons in the retina is apparently by an accentuation of the interkinetic, to and fro movements of the nuclei with cells in various phases of the cell cycle, movements seen in early phases of cortical development, prior to the formation of the four embryonic layers.

Studies by Pearlman and colleagues on the cerebral cortex indicate that cells emigrating from the ventricular zone along the glial scaffold use nuclear translocation before they attach to the glial fiber system. Once on the glial scaffold, however, the neurons migrate by holding the nucleus in the posterior portion of the soma and moving stepwise along the glial guides (Rakic, 1971, 1972; Edmondson, 1987). Thus the cortex uses a system of radial glial fibers, along with the basic columnar pattern of cell division, to move cohorts of neurons out into the thickening brain. As discussed later for cerebellar granule cells, Hatten and colleagues analyzed the details of glial-guided migration in tissue culture by purifying young neurons and glia from developing brain and recombining them *in vitro*.

The Cerebellar Granule Cell and Radial Migration

The *cerebellar granule neuron* precursor cell population presents a model for CNS precursor cell generation and migration. Although granule cells undergo their final migrations in a radial pathway along glia, they present an anomaly with respect to the inside-out model pathway of migrations used by the cerebral cortex. The earliest precursors of granule cells proliferate at the edge of the neuroepithelium (rhombic lip), where there is no overlying cellular structure (Fig. 15.12). This pool of dividing precursor cells streams rostrally across the lip, onto the outer surface

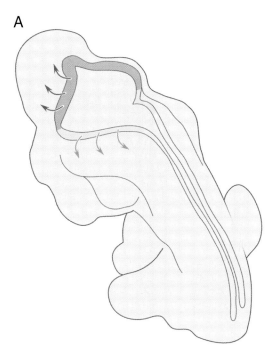

A

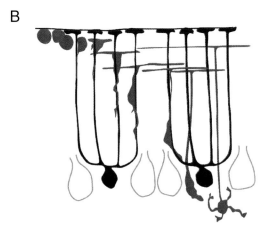

B

FIGURE 15.12 Migration of precursors of the granule neuron in the developing cerebellar cortex. The cerebellar primordium arises from the anterior portion of the IVth ventricle, with young granule cell precursors arising along the edge of the ventricle in an area called the rhombic lip (arrow). (A) An embryo is shown at embryonic day 13, with the rhombic lip highlighted in red. Cells from the posterior portion of the lip migrate ventrally to form the olivary nucleus in the brain stem. Neurons of this nucleus will project their axons to the other principal neuron of the cerebellar cortex, the Purkinje cell. As development proceeds, the granule neuron precursors first spread across the roof of the anlage, and later migrate inward to their final destination. (B) Granule neurons undergoing various steps of development are shown in red. Precursors at the outer surface undergo rapid proliferation, with cells underneath them beginning to differentiate, as evidenced by the extension of parallel fibers. After neurite extension commences, the cell body is polarized and attaches to the fibers of the Bergmann glia, which serve as a substrate for migration through the molecular layer. After migration, the granule cell extends dendrites.

of the anlage, where they establish a displaced germinal zone, the *external germinal layer* (EGL).

The continued proliferation of EGL cells generates an expansive pool of precursors that spread rostromedially across the roof of the anlage. After birth, rapid proliferation in the EGL expands the zone from a single cell layer to a layer eight cells in thickness. Precursor cell proliferation continues within the EGL until the end of the second postnatal week in the mouse, when the zone disappears due to the inward migration of postmitotic cells to form the *internal granule cell layer*. Whereas target neurons of the granule cell undergo a short period of proliferation within the ventricular zone of the cerebellar anlage, from approximately embryonic days (E) 11–E14 in the mouse, the prolonged period of clonal expansion of EGL precursor cells within the secondary germinal zone, from E13 until postnatal day (P) 15, generates a huge population of cells. In adulthood, granule neurons outnumber the other principal neuron of the cerebellar cortex, with which granule cells form the basic cerebellar circuitry, Purkinje cells by 250:1 in the mouse, a figure that rises to approximately 400:1 in humans.

Although granule cell precursors continue to proliferate and expand the pool of progenitors for a long period, a number of experiments show that their identity is set by their early position within the dorsoventral axis of the primordium. First, when early progenitors are transplanted into the postnatal EGL, these precursors become granule cells. This suggests that the precursors are specified to be granule cells and that they are competent to respond to signals for differentiating into mature neurons. One signal that is critical for the early specification of granule cells is a diffusible, local signal, the BMPs. At least three BMPs (GDF7, BMP6, and BMP7) can induce the expression of granule cell markers and can specify ventral cells toward a granule cell fate. These BMPs are expressed in the overlying roof plate. The role of the roof plate in granule cell specification and development is seen in the neurological mutant mouse *dreher* where roof plate formation fails to a great extent and granule cell development is defective. Cloning of the *dreher* gene by the Hatten laboratory shows that it encodes *Lmx1a*, a member of the LIM homeodomain gene family. The early specification of granule cell precursors by their position in the neuraxis is consistent with the emerging view of the importance of precursor cell position for the establishment of cell fate.

Over the past several years, the molecular basis of granule cell specification has begun to be understood. Very early in development, precursors of the granule cell express the bHLH transcription factor *Math1*, as well as the zinc finger proteins Ru49/Zipro1 and Zic1 and Zic3. As the cells migrate across the surface of the anlage and form the external germinal zone, the cells are still expressing these markers as well as nestin, a marker often seen in undifferentiated neurons. Once the cells exit this proliferative zone and begin to migrate down into the cortex, they shift to another bHLH gene, *NeuroD*, a sign of differentiation. Genetic studies have shown that *Math1* is essential for granule cell specification, as targeted disruption of the gene leads to a loss of the granule cell population. The role of bHLH genes in the control of precursor cell development, especially differentiation and thus migration, is an important area for future research.

In addition to bHLH genes, several gene pathways control the proliferation of EGL precursors prior to migration. This step is extremely important because it regulates the size of the granule cell population, leading to the most numerous cell population in the brain. In addition, it sets forth the ratio of granule neurons to their target cells, the Purkinje neuron, thereby controlling the establishment of the principal circuit in cerebellar cortex, that between the Purkinje cell and the granule cell. Recent work has shown that Purkinje cells release Sonic Hedgehog, which acts as a potent mitogen for granule cells. Thus, it appears that communication between these two principal neurons is essential to their development. In addition to Sonic Hedgehog, *Notch2* and its ligand *Jagged1* serve as powerful mitogens for granule cell precursors. Both Sonic Hedgehog and Notch2 appear to control cell division through the downstream transcriptional regulator *Hes1*.

As the granule cell precursors exit the cell cycle, they express genes that function in axon formation such as the axonal glycoprotein TAG1 and class III β tubulin. Several other genes have been shown to signal the progression of precursors into differentiation (Fig. 15.13), including the serine threonine kinase *Unc51.1* and the receptor tyrosine kinase *DDR1*. Once granule cells begin this program of differentiation, they bind to astroglial cells via neuron–glia adhesion systems, including astrotactin, integrins, and neuregulin, and commence their migration along the glial guides.

Dynamics of Cell Migration

To examine the dynamics of *neuronal migration* of neurons along glial fibers, Hatten and colleagues used video-enhanced differential contrast microscopy to obtain a detailed view of the morphology and behavior of migrating cerebellar neurons. The cytological features of *living*, migrating granule neurons *in vitro*

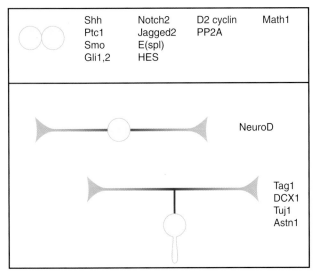

FIGURE 15.13 Changing patterns of gene expression during granule cell development. As granule cell precursors transit from proliferation (upper box) to differentiation (lower box), they express specific gene pathways. During proliferation, Sonic Hedgehog and Jagged1 serve as potent mitogens for the cells. Genes of the sonic hedgehog pathway, including *Patched (Ptc1)*, *Smoothened (Smo)* and *Gli*, are expressed in dividing precursor cells. Genes of the *Notch 2* pathway are also expressed, including *Jagged1*, *E(spl)*, and *Hes1*. In addition, the *D2 cyclin* and *PP2A phosphatase* transcripts are abundant in proliferating cells. Among genes that specify neurons, the *Math1* gene, shown to be essential for granule cell development by Zogbhi and colleagues, is expressed. As the cells begin to extend neurites, they downregulate *Math1* and begin to express another bHLH gene, *NeuroD*. In addition, they express markers of early steps in neurite extension, including the TAG1 glycoprotein, a special tubulin labeled by anit-tuj1 antibodies, and *Astrotactin (Astn)*, a neuron–glia adhesion molecule important for migration along the glia.

are remarkably similar those described by Rakic for cells assumed to be migrating *in vivo*. Migrating neurons express a highly extended bipolar shape along the glial fiber, form a close apposition with the glial process along the length of the neuronal cell soma, and extend a leading process in the direction of migration (Rakic, 1971, 1972; Edmondson, 1987) (Fig. 15.14).

Video observations on living cells were extended by correlating the behavior of migrating neurons with their cytology, as viewed in the electron microscope. In cells that were moving prior to fixation, a specialized migration junction, an "interstitial junction," is present beneath the neuronal cell soma at the site of apposition with the glial fiber. This junction consists of a widening of the intercellular space, and filamentous material in this space that spans the cleft and membranes of each cell, contiguous with cytoskeletal elements. The interstitial junction is seen only in cells that were moving along the glial process. In contrast,

in resting cells, *puncta adherentia* or attachment junctions occur where the neuron apposes the glial fiber, and unlike the migration junction, these small focal densities lack any obvious connections to the cytoskeleton of the apposing cells. Thus, migrating neurons form a "**migration junction**" along the apposition between migrating neuron and glial fiber.

Summary

The formation of neural layers in the CNS results from the proliferation of precursor cells in discrete zones along the ventricles called ventricular zones. As the cells become postmitotic, they emigrate out of this zone to form overlying layers. A system of radial glial fibers provides the primary scaffold for this form of migration, ushering young neurons from their site of

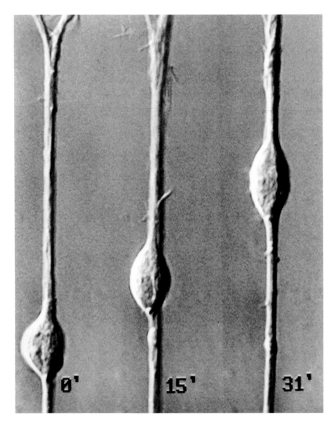

FIGURE 15.14 Hippocampal neurons migrating *in vitro* along the processes of astroglial cells from the cerebellum. Neurons are capable of migrating along a variety of radial glial fibers, even those derived from heterotypic regions. In both heterotypic and homotypic cocultures of neurons and glia, time-lapse imaging reveals that the elongated migrating neurons form close associations with glial processes as they crawl along them. The leading processes of migrating cells are highly active, extending numerous lamellipodia and filopodia. In contrast to the filopodia of axonal growth cones (see Chapter 17), filopodia extending from leading processes are short (1–5 mm in length). Time elapsed (minutes) in real time. Photo provided by Dr. M. E. Hatten.

origin out to the newly developing layers. This mode of migration places the large, output neurons within the proper layers for formation of the neural circuitry of the brain.

Genetic Studies on Migration—The Discovery of Molecular Pathways

While the cell biology of neuronal migration along glia is understood in detail, clues about the molecular

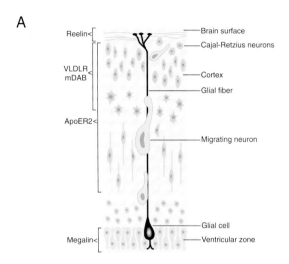

A

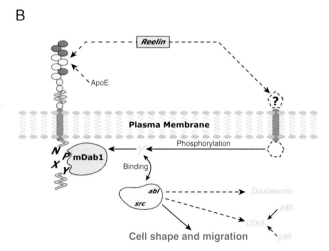

B

FIGURE 15.15 The role of the Reelin protein in cortical development. Reelin is expressed by Cajal-Retzius cells in the outer layer of the developing cortex. As neurons migrate out along the glial fibers, Reelin is proposed to organize the cortical plate. (B) A model for Reelin action is shown. Reelin binds to a receptor, VLDLR or ApoER2 in the surface membrane, which leads to downstream signaling via *Dab1*, resulting in alterations in gene expression. In addition, Cdk5 phosphorylates cytoskeletal components such as tau and neurofilaments, which may affect organization of the cytoskeleton and properties of migrating neurons.

mechanisms that guide radial migration are only beginning to emerge. A primary resource for the discovery of migration molecules is the study of mutations that disrupt migration and the formation of neuronal layers. One of these mice, called the *reeler* **mouse** because of its unsteady gait, has served as a prototype for genetic studies (Rice and Curran, 1999). In *reeler* mice, the laminar organization of both the cerebral cortex and the cerebellar cortex is severely disrupted, with cells scattered across the laminar boundaries. Another mouse called *scrambler* has a similar phenotype, i.e., scrambled layers. Molecular cloning of the *reeler* gene, by Curran and colleagues, through insertional methods revealed that *reeler* encodes a large extracellular matrix protein called reelin (D'Arcangelo *et al.*, 1995) (*Reln*). Reln is secreted by Cajal Retzius cells, the first cells to migrate away from the VZ, and its absence prevents correct formation of the cortical plate and subsequent waves of migration to form the neuronal laminae of cortex (Fig. 15.15).

The analysis of other mice with phenotypes that resembled that of reeler unexpectedly led to the elucidation of the pathway of Reln signaling. The receptor for Reln is a member of the lipid-binding receptor family, VLDLR, and the apoER2 receptor. Targeted disruptions of these genes by Herz and colleagues revealed mice with disorganized cortical lamina, suggesting that these genes act in the same pathway as Reln. Direct binding studies have confirmed the role of VLDLR and apoER2 as receptors and, more recently, of the procadherins as a second class of Reln receptor. Two other mouse mutants that exhibit migration disorders, *scrambler* and *Yotari* mice, have turned out to contain mutations in a downstream gene, *Disabled (Dabl)*, which is thought to be involved in signaling in the reelin pathway. Thus, genetic and molecular genetic studies led to the elucidation of the first described molecular control of cortical migration. The precise mechanism by which Reln functions is not yet known. One idea is that Reln is needed for neurons to halt their movements and assemble into the neuronal layers.

Analysis of the **genetics of human brain malformations** has also led to the discovery of genes that function in migration. Neurologists have described several inherited or familial syndromes involving autosomal dominant and X-linked forms of lissencephaly. In this condition, cerebral cortical neurons fail to migrate normally and form a thick, disordered layer along the brain ventricles, thus giving rise to a "smooth brain" that lacks the sulci and gyri of the normal brain. Several genes underlying this disorder have been identified and cloned. The *Lis1* gene is responsible for the autosomal dominant forms of the gene, and *Doublecortin* (DCX) is responsible for the X-linked form. In males, DCX mutations produce lissencephaly that is very similar to Lis1 phenotypes. Heterozygous individuals show a phenotype called double cortex, i.e., an extra subcortical layer of gray matter. In biochemical experiments, both Lis1 and DCX have been shown to be microtubule-binding proteins. LIS1 has been shown to form complexes with dynein, a component of the mitotic spindle, suggesting that it might be important in precursor cell division. In protein-binding studies, LIS1 binds to NudF, a homologue of an *Aspergillus* protein that interacts with the microtubule organizing center. Thus, the interaction of LIS1 and DCX with tubulin, either during migration or during mitosis, provides an exciting new avenue toward understanding the role of the cytoskeleton in the control of CNS migrations.

Genes that interact with actin components of the cytoskeleton have also been identified through studies of human brain malformations (Fig. 15.16). Human X-linked *periventricular heterotopia*, a condition where neurons fail to leave the ventricular zone, is caused by mutations in a gene encoding Filamin 1 (Flna), an actin cross-linking phosphoprotein. Flna is thought to be involved in the filopodial extension during migration. Mutations in another gene producing a similiar phenotype in mice where neurons fail

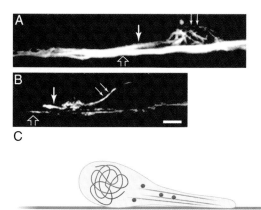

FIGURE 15.16 Cytoskeletal organization of migrating neurons. Cerebellar granule cells migrating along glial substrates were stained with antibodies against tubulin (A) or with phalloidin, an agent that labels actin (B). Staining with tubulin reveals a specialized cage like structure around the nucleus, which may function in migration. (C) A model for migration shows a specialized tubulin arrangement around the nucleus as well as in the mictotubules projecting into the leading process of the migrating cells. Evidence indicates that several proteins involved in cortical malformations, including LIS1 and Doublecortin, bind to tubulin in migrating neurons. Thus, the cytoskeleton is a crucial control element for migration.

to leave the ventricular zone is the cyclin-dependent kinase Cdk5 and its activator p35. Studies on the expression of Cdk5 and p35 suggest a role for these genes in actin regulation. Both proteins are localized in the leading edge of cortical growth cones in culture studies, and Cdk5 binds to Rac and Pak1 kinase, part of the signaling pathway that regulates actin organization in cells. The similar phenotypes of Flna and Cdk5/p35 defective brains underscore the importance of actin dynamics to cell proliferation and migration.

Summary

Studies of mutations with brain malformations have yielded exciting new information on the molecular basis of CNS migration (Hatten, 1999). So far, three groups of molecules have been discovered: adhesion systems such as Reelin, Astrotactin, Neuregulin, and Integrins α3,6; molecules that bind microtubules such as LIS1 and DCX; and those that bind actin such as Filamin1 and Cdk5/p35.

Nonradial Migrations in Brain

While the *radial pathway* provides the major route for the migration of cells from cortical ventrical zones into the neuronal layers, with 70–80% of the cells using this pathway, *nonradial pathways* are used to provide interneurons for the cortex and to form nuclei of the brain stem that communicate with the cerebellar cortex. We shall see that this class of migration occurs along the tangential axis of the emerging brain rather than the radial axis. The first suggestion of this tangential migratory pathway came from studies by McConnell and colleagues, who showed that some precursors follow a nonradial migratory pathway migrating within the intermediate zone of the developing cortex. Several lines of evidence, using retroviral markers and mouse chimeras, indicate that the two pathways of migration relate to classes of neuronal precursors, with projection neurons of the cortex being arranged radially and GABAergic interneurons being dispersed tangentially (Walsh and Cepko, 1992; Luskin, 1993; Tan, *et al.*, 1995). Surprisingly, cells that undergo tangential migration follow a ventrodorsal pathway, in this case from the basal telencephalon up into the cortex. *GABAergic neurons* arise in the *medial and lateral ganglionic eminences* (MGE and LGE) and migrate dorsally into the developing cortex. The molecular basis of this pathway has been confirmed by Rubenstein and colleagues in studies on the phenotype of mice lacking transcription factors that regulate either the regionalization (*Nkx2.1*) of forebrain or the differentiation (*Dlx1, Dlx2, Mash1*) of LGE and MGE neurons. Double mutations of Dlx1,2 have a fourfold

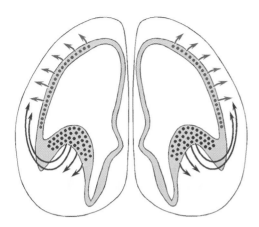

FIGURE 15.17 Migration of cortical interneurons from two major subdivisions of the developing basal telencephalon: medial and lateral ganglionic eminences (MGE and LGE). As shown by the work of Anderson and Rubenstein, early in neurogenesis, GABA-expressing cells from the MGE migrate tangentially into the cerebral cortex, primarily via the intermediate zone, whereas cells from the LGE do not. Later in neurogenesis, LGE-derived cells also migrate into the cortex, primarily through the subventricular zone (SVZ). This ventrodorsal pattern of migration thus gives rise to a large proportion of interneurons in the developing cortex.

reduction in GABAergic interneurons (Anderson *et al.*, 2001). As these neurons constitute about 20% of all cortical neurons, the migratory pathway of these cells represents a major source of cortical neurons. Their migrations occur as the primary migrations along the radial glial axis set forth the laminar patterning of the region. Studies on these different mutants suggest that MGE-derived cells migrate early, along axon tracts in the intermediate zone, whereas LGE cells migrate later, through the SVZ. Thus the cortical system uses a combination of ventrodorsal migratory pathways and radial migratory pathways. Distinct classes of neuronal progenitors arise in specific positions within the neuroepithelium and utilize specific migratory paths. The principal projection neurons migrate along radial glial cells to set forth the basic laminar plan and later derived interneurons follow a ventrodorsal pathway of migration (Fig. 15.17).

While the cerebral cortex provides an example of ventrodorsal migrations, the cerebellar cortex provides a case of a dorsoventral pathway of migration. To control aspects of motor activity, the cerebellar cortex integrates motor signals with sensory feedback signals. Six nuclei in the brain stem serve as relay centers for information coming from the cerebral cortex and the spinal cord. Although they are situated in the ventral portion of the brain stem, a combination of classical anatomical studies and new genetic studies have revealed that these cells originate very close to one another in the dorsal rhombencephalon,

within the rhombic lip area. Whereas granule cells of the cerebellar cortex migrate rostrally over the roof of the anlage, cells of these nuclei migrate ventrally to the ventral aspect of the hindbrain. The migratory stream of precursors across the surface of the hindbrain is a transient embryonic structure, called the corpus pontobulbare.

The pathway of migrations from the rhombic lip to the ventral hindbrain is reminiscent of dorsoventral pathways of migration in lower animals, including the extensive migrations seen in the worm *C. elegans*, where counterparts of the diffusible chemoattractant/chemorepulsive molecule netrin-1 and its receptor unc5 function in dorsoventral axon migration. The dorsoventral migration of the olivary precursor cells has been shown to involve the diffusible factor *netrin-1* (Alcantara *et al.*, 2000). Its receptor, a homologue of the *C. elegans* unc5-related proteins, is also expressed in the migrating olivary precursors, suggesting that netrin-1 may serve as a chemoattractant agent in the migration of these neurons toward the ventral midline.

Two types of experiments have shown the relationship of cells of the rhombic lip to cells of the precerebellar nuclei. First, chick quail marking experiments indicate that a subpopulation of cells within the upper aspect of the rhombic lip, the zone giving rise to cerebellar granule cells, gives rise to the lateral pontine nucleus. Second, using an FLP recombinase-based fate mapping approach, Rodriguez and Dymecki (2000) have provided evidence that the ventral brain stem system derives from dorsally located rhombic neuroepithelium. Moreover, by fate mapping, they uncovered an unexpected subdivision within the precerebellar primordium: embryonic expression of *Wnt1* appears to identify the class of precerebellar progenitors that will later project mossy fibers from the brain stem to the cerebellum. As cells of the olivary nucleus, derived from the lower rhombic lip, project to Purkinje cells and those of the pontine nucleus, derived from the upper rhombic lip, project to the other principal neuron, the granule cell-specific fates arise within the same domain to give rise to the cerebellar system. Moreover, directed patterns of migration—of proliferating granule cell precursors in the dorsal direction and then along Bergmann glia and of postmitotic precursors in the ventral direction and then along axon tracts—give rise to the cerebellar system. Within the system, different patterns of gene expression can be shown to specify particular cell classes, with *Math1/Zic1/Zic3/Zipro1* marking granule cell precursors and *Wnt1* marking the neurons that will project axons to these cells (Wang and Zoghbi, 2001).

Thus the cerebellar system, one of the most ancient of brain regions, combines dorsoventral patterning with radial migratory pathways. The position of neuronal precursor cell populations along the dorsoventral axis of the region establishes the different classes of progenitors—granule cells, Purkinje cells, olivary neurons, and pontine neurons—and a sequential program of migration involving an intitial dorsoventral movement and a subsequent radial migration positions the cells within the circuitry of the cerebellum. Further genetic analysis of this system should provide more detailed insights into the mechanisms that specify different cell classes and their modes of migration.

Summary

While radial migrations provide a primary pathway for CNS migrations, the recent discovery of dorsoventral and ventrodorsal pathways of migration suggests that the mammalian brain uses strategies employed in invertebrate systems as well as novel radial pathways. The combined use of these two pathways allows for the integration of cells generated in distant germinal zones to be integrated into the region, as in cortex, or for cells generated in positions proximal to their target regions to act at long distance, as in the cerebellar system.

Anterior–Posterior Migrations in Brain

During the late stages of cortical histogenesis, the *SVZ* of the cortex gives rise to several classes of cells, including oligodendrocytes and interneurons. This

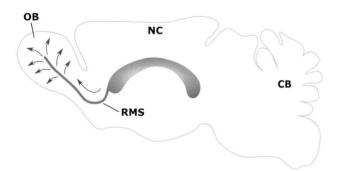

FIGURE 15.18 Migration of neurons from the subventricular zone of the cortex into the olfactory bulb. As cortical development proceeds, a subventricular zone (SVZ) of dividing precursor cells is established above the ventricular zone. Proliferating neurons in this zone migrate long distances in the posterior–anterior direction to reach the olfactory bulb. At later times in development, when the ventricular zone has disappeared, the SVZ continues to produce large numbers of neurons destined for the olfactory bulb. Indeed, this process continues into adulthood, making SVZ one of the rare sources for neuronal renewal in the adult.

zone persists even after the cortex has formed with late-arising cells destined for the olfactory system. During adulthood, the SVZ provides a steady source of new neurons for the olfactory bulb with neurons migrating from the cortical SVZ anteriorly toward the olfactory bulb to form the *rostral migratory stream* (Fig. 15.18). In addition, the cortical SVZ provides a dramatic case of neuronal stem cells in adult brain. As neurons turn over in the adult neuroepithelium and grow new axons to the olfactory bulb, the SVZ provides a constant source of new target cells. To reach the olfactory bulb, SVZ cells migrate as a broad stream in a "daisy chain"-like migration, on the interwoven bundle of their own processes, with glial cells acting to enwrap the moving strands of cells. In the case of SVZ precursor cell migration to the olfactory bulb, targeted mutational analysis indicates a functional role for polysialyated forms of N-CAM in cell movements.

The *spinal cord* combines interkinetic displacements, formation of a mantle layer, limited radial migration along glial fibers, and extensive tangential migration along axon tracts. Sanes and colleagues have used retroviral marking methods to reveal extensive intermixing of precursor cells within the germinal zone of the spinal cord (Leber and Sanes, 1995) (Fig. 15.19). The extent of precursor cell movement apparently becomes progressively restricted during development of the cord. An interesting feature of spinal cord development is the movement of cells along the anterior–posterior axis of CNS.

Summary

Precursors in the SVZ of the cortex undergo long-range posterior-to-anterior cell migrations, moving within glial sheaths, to reach the olfactory bulb. AP migrations are also seen in the spinal cord, although on a much more limited basis, where young neurons move in an anterior-to-posterior direction along emerging axon tracts.

Subcortical Structures—The Diencephalon

Within the developing *diencephalon*, a simpler plan of cell organization emerges. Precursors proliferate within the ventricular zone and then migrate short distances away from this zone using radial glial guides. Above this columnar pattern of cells, the young neurons move tangentially, forming a mantle of postmitotic cells. Cells within the mantle zone gradually aggregate into ganglion-like structures (nuclei) or sheets. Thus radial glial play a very limited role in the diencephalon. Instead, a very different and as yet elusive mode of cell assembly occurs in this

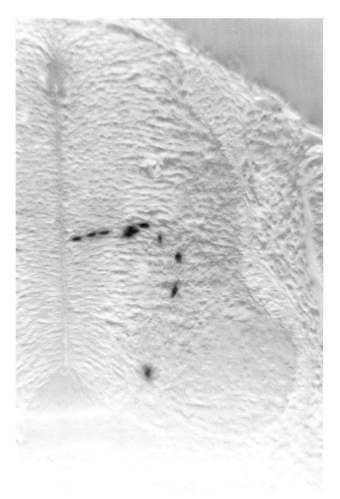

FIGURE 15.19 Lineage analysis using retroviral vectors in the embryonic chick spinal cord reveals both radial and tangential pathways for neuronal migration. A recombinant retrovirus was used to infect progenitor cells of the spinal cord with a harmless bacterial marker gene that encodes the enzyme β-galactosidase. Expression of this enzyme by progeny of the infected cell can be detected by a histochemical reaction that turns the cell blue. The clonal progeny of spinal progenitor cells initially migrate radially out of the ventricular zone. In many clones, however, some young neurons then turn orthogonally to migrate tangentially within the intermediate zone. These neurons appeared to employ circumferentially oriented axons to guide their tangential movements. From Leber and Sanes (1995).

area of brain. One finding of possible relevance to the formation of condensed groups of cells, the nuclei, is expression of the calcium-dependent cadherin adhesion molecules in nonlaminar areas of brain. Studies by Ganzler and Redies (Arndt and Redies, 1996) demonstrate that postmitotic neurons undergoing assembly in the diencephalon in developing chick brain express the cell adhesion molecule R-cadherin. In this aspect, cell assembly in the diencephalon may follow strategies used in the formation of PNS ganglia.

One interesting theme of development of the diencephalon has been its potential relationship to the development of the hindbrain. In the hindbrain, segmental units or *rhombomeres* serve to generate compartments with strict lineage restrictions. On the basis of morphology and gene expression, the diencephalon can also be divided into segemental units called *neuromeres*, or *prosomeres*. Specific patterns of gene expression, especially of transcription factors such as Dlx1,2 and Nkx2.1, have led some to subdivide the three prosomeres further. Although prosomeres appear to be counterparts of rhombomeres of the hindbrain, cell lineage restriction studies by Larsen *et al.* (2001) using dextran as a cellular label argue against this interpretation. Indeed, only a narrow stripe of cells that lie between the prospective dorsal and ventral thalami, called the zona limitans intrathalamica or zli, has cells with restricted lineages that do not mix with cells in other prosomeres. Thus the diencephalon cannot be considered a counterpart of the hindbrain.

Summary

The diencephalon has a more primitive program of cell movements than the cortex, with neurons forming a thick mantle layer and then aggregating into thalamic nuclei. Although this region is apparently organized into units called prosomeres, cells in prosomeres are not immicible, suggesting that the diencephalon does not have an overt segmental pattern.

Migration of PNS Neurons into Brain, the LHRH Cells

Although it was long assumed that all CNS cells originate from within the wall of the developing neural tube, recent experiments demonstrate that one system of neurons in the hypothalamus originates outside the brain vesicles, entering the brain through a highly unusual migratory pathway. This group of cells, *luteinizing hormone-releasing hormone* (LHRH) *neurons*, provides a key neuroendocrine system for both maturation of the immature reproductive system and maintenance of the adult reproductive system. In humans, a failure of this migration is seen in Kallman's syndrome. Experiments to trace the origin of these cells within the region of the diencephalic neuroepithelium that gives rise to the adult hypothalamus unexpectedly revealed that LHRH-expressing neurons first appear in the olfactory pit, a neural crest derivative that gives rise to the nasal epithelium. Combined use of thymidine-labeling methods, *in situ* hybridization of LHRH mRNA, and immunocytochemical localization of cells expressing the LHRH

BOX 15.2

KALLMANN SYNDROME

Although many somatic and developmental abnormalities (hearing loss, cleft lip and palate, renal aplasia, and various neurological deficits) may be present in Kallmann syndrome, the principal features are anosmia (the inability to smell) and infertility (hypogonadism and sterile gonads). A dysfunction involving smell and reproduction was originally described in 1856 by Maestre de San Juan, and Kallmann and colleagues reported the first familial cases in 1944. The symptoms associated with Kallmann syndrome remained unexplained, however, until researchers demonstrated that two key players in the dysfunction share a common developmental origin—the olfactory placode. These key players are (1) olfactory receptor neurons—primary sensory neurons for the sense of smell. Cell somata are located in the nasal epithelium, and axons terminate in glomeruli in the olfactory bulb (2) Gonadotropin-releasing hormone (GnRH) neurons are neuroendocrine cells required for reproductive maturation and competence. The cell somata are located in the forebrain, and axons terminate in the median eminence of the hypothalamus.

During normal prenatal development, olfactory receptor neurons and pheromone receptor neurons, primary sensory neurons for olfactory stimuli related to social and/or reproductive behavior, remain in the nasal cavity while their axons traverse the nasal septum to the developing brain. When they reach the brain, olfactory receptor axons induce formation of the olfactory bulb, the region in the telencephalon containing mitral cells, secondary neurons for relay of olfaction, which together with olfactory receptor axons form the functional olfactory unit (the glomeruli), while the axons of pheromone receptor neurons grows caudally into the developing accessory olfactory nucleus. In contrast to olfactory and pheromone receptor neurons, GnRH neurons reside in the brain after birth. To attain their adult-like distribution, during normal development, GnRH neurons leave the nasal cavity and migrate into the developing telencephalon, following a route across the nasal septum similar to that taken by olfactory and pheromone receptor neuron axons. However, as axons from the olfactory receptor neurons head rostrally into the developing olfactory bulb, GnRH neurons turn caudally, perhaps in association with pheromone receptor neuron axons, toward the developing diencephalon.

In Kallmann syndrome, the development of these systems is perturbed; both GnRH neuron and olfactory and pheromone receptor neuron axons migrate to the base of the cribiform plate but halt outside the brain, as seen in a fetus diagnosed prenatally with Kallmann syndrome. Kallmann syndrome is a rare disorder. The most frequent mode of transmission is X-linked, although autosomal recessive and autosomal dominant transmissions have been reported. The rarity of the syndrome is directly related to reproductive dysfunction of affected individuals, which results in deletion of the mutant gene(s) from the populations.

Cloning of the KAL gene, the deduced amino acid sequence of which suggested an extracellular matrix component (secreted protein) with antiprotease and/or cell adhesion functions, heightened anticipation that a candidate molecule guiding olfactory and pheromone receptor axons and GnRH neurons through nasal regions had been found. Unexpectedly, the KAL gene was expressed in brain by cells of the olfactory bulb but not in cells in nasal regions, i.e., in neither migrating neurons (GnRH cells) nor neurons in the nasal epithelium. Interestingly, the KAL gene has not been identified in rodents. However, based on its spatiotemporal expression pattern in humans and chickens, KAL is no longer a viable candidate for a guidance molecule directly involved in the migrational events observed in nasal regions. KAL is now proposed to have a role in the events regulating contact and maintenance of olfactory receptor axons within the olfactory bulb. How the KAL protein affects movement of GnRH neurons into the brain remains a mystery, but the current hypothesis suggests that the anosmia (due to hypoplasia or aplasia of the olfactory bulb) observed in Kallmann syndrome results from a CNS olfactory target cell defect. Effective treatment for reproductive dysfunction is available for patients with Kallmann syndrome, but early diagnosis is important; without treatment, pubertal onset does not occur. Substitution hormone therapy is necessary to induce secondary sex characteristics, and treatment with GnRH often restores fertility.

Susan Wray

References and Suggested Readings

Kallmann, F. J., Schoenfeld, W. A., and Barrera, S. E. (1944). The genetic aspects of primary eunuchoidism. *Am. J. Ment. Defic.* **48**. 203–236.

Maestre de San Juan, A. (1856). Falta total de los nervios olfactorios con anosmia en un individuo en quien exista una atrofia congenita de los testiculos y miembro viril (II). *El Siglo Medico* **131**. 211.

Wray, S. (2001). Development of luteinizing hormone releasing hormone neurons. *J. Neuroendocrinol.* **13**. 3–11.

protein subsequently proved that the 800 or so LHRH neurons of the murine hypothalamus originate in the vomeronasal area of the olfactory system. As the precursor cells exit the cycle and initiate expression of LHRH, they migrate 1–3 mm through the nasal septum and into the forebrain. The pathway of their migration follows the axon tract of the vomeronasal-nervus terminalis neurons, cells shown by DuLac and Axel to express a novel class of protein kinase receptors, pheromone receptors, thought to play a signaling role in neuroendocrine function. Although small in numbers, LHRH neurons thus provide a rare case of neuronal precursor cell immigration into developing brain, as well as a model for axon-guided neuronal migration.

Summary

Neurons of the LHRH are unique as they migrate from the PNS into the brain. Their pathway of migration is an axon tract, suggesting that axonal adhesion molecules could provide a mechanism for this unusual form of migration.

Conclusion

Development of the vertebrate nervous system progresses via a relatively simple set of neurogenic events to produce a complex multilaminate structure. The dynamics of this process, in both the extent of cell movements and the projection of specific patterns of connections, is remarkable. Whereas lower organisms have extensive dorsoventral and anterior posterior pathways of migration, the mammalian brain adds the radial component of migration dispatching young neurons over great distances to form neuronal laminae. Over the past decade, genetic and molecular genetic experiments have provided the first molecular insights into radial migration, as well as revealed new pathways of migration, primarily along the dorsoventral axis, that likely represent ancient mechanisms. Further genetic studies across the species can be anticipated to increase our understanding of the remarkable process of migrations in the CNS.

References

Arndt, K., and Redies, C. (1996). Restricted expression of R-cadherin by brain nuclei and neural circuits of the developing chicken brain. *J. Comp. Neurol.* **373**(3), 373–399.

Bronner-Fraser, M., and Fraser, S. (1988). Cell lineage analysis shows multipotentiality of some avian neural crest cells. *Nature* **335**(8), 161–164.

Christensen, J. H., Coles, E. G., and Wilkinson, D. G. (2000). Molecular control of neural crest formation, migration and differentiation. *Curr. Opin. Cell Biol.* **12**, 719–724.

Edmondson, J. C., and Hatten, M. E. (1987). Glial-guided granule neuron migration in vitro: A high-resolution time-lapse video microscopic study. *J. Neurosci.* **7**, 1928–1934.

Fekete, D. M., Perez-Miguelsanz, J., *et al.* (1994). Clonal analysis in the chicken retina reveals tangential dispersion of clonally related cells. *Dev. Biol.* **166**(2), 666–682.

Hosoda, K., Hammer, R. E., Richardson, J. A., Baynash, A. G., Cheung, J. C., Giaid, A., and Yanagisawa, M. (1994). Targeted and natural (piebald-lethal) mutations of endothelin-B receptor gene produce megacolon associated with spotted colon color in mice. *Cell* **79**, 1267–1276.

Krull, C. E., Lansford, R., Gale, N. W., Marcelle, C., Collazo, A., Yancopoulos, G., Fraser, S. E., and Bronner-Fraser, M. (1997). Interactions between Eph-related receptors and ligands confer rostrocaudal polarity to trunk neural crest migration. *Curr. Biol.* **7**, 571–580.

Larsen, C. W., Zeltser, L. M., *et al.* (2001). Boundary formation and compartition in the avian diencephalon. *J. Neurosci.* **21**(13), 4699–4711.

Leber, S. M., and Sanes, J. R. (1995). Migratory paths of neurons and glia in the embryonic chick spinal cord. *J. Neurosci.* **15**(2), 1236–1248.

LeDouarin, N. M. (1982). "The Neural Crest." Cambridge Univ. Press, New York.

LeDouarin, N. M., and Kalcheim, C. (1999). "The Neural Crest." Cambruidge Univ. Press, New York.

Nakagawa, S., and Takeichi, M. (1998). Neural crest emigration from the neural tube depends on regulated cadherin expression. *Development* **125**, 2963–2971.

Noden, D. M. (1975). An analysis of the migratory behavior of avian cephalic neural crest cells. *Devl. Biol.* **42**, 106–130.

Rakic, P. (1971). Neuron-glia relationship during granule cell migration in developing cerebellar cortex. A Golgi and electronmicroscopic study in macacus rhesus. *J. Comp. Neurol.* **141**(3), 283–312.

Rakic, P. (1972). Mode of cell migration to the superficial layers of fetal monkey cortex. *J. Comp. Neurol.* **145**, 61–84.

Reese, B. E., and Tan, S. S. (1998). Clonal boundary analysis in the developing retina using X-inactivation transgenic mosaic mice. *Semin. Cell Dev. Biol.* **9**(3), 285–292.

Rodriguez, C. I., and Dymecki, S. M. (2000). Origin of the precerebellar system. *Neuron* **27**, 475–486.

Sechrist, J., Serbedzija, G., Scherson, T., Fraser, S., and Bronner-Fraser, M. (1993). Segmental migration of the hindbrain neural crest does not arise from segmental generation. *Development* **118**, 691–703.

Selleck, M. A. J. and Bronner-Fraser, M. (1995). Origins of the avian neural crest: The role of neural plate-epidermal interactions. *Development* **121**, 526–538.

Serbedzija, G., Bronner-Fraser, M., and Fraser, S. E. (1989). Vital dye analysis of the timing and pathways of avian trunk neural crest cell migration. *Development* **106**, 806–816.

Sharma, K., Korade, Z., and Frank, E. (1995). Late-migrating neuroepithelial cells from the spinal cord differentiate into sensory ganglion cells. *Neuron* **14**, 143–152.

Sidmon and Rakic (1973). Neuronal migration with special reference to the developing human brain: A review. *Brain Res.* **62**, 1–35.

Stemple, D. L., and Anderson, D. J. (1993). Lineage diversification of the neural crest: *In vitro* investigations. *Dev. Biol.* **159**, 12–23.

Tan, S.-S., Faulkner-Jones, B., *et al.* (1995). Cell dispersion patterns in different cortical regions studied with an X-inactivated transgenic marker. *Development* **121**, 1029–1039.

Walsh, C., and Cepko, C. L. (1992). Widespread dispersion of neuronal clones across functional regions of the cerebral cortex. *Science* **255**(5043), 434–440.

Wang, H. U., and Anderson, D. J. (1997). Roles of Eph family trans-membrane ligands in repulsive guidance of trunk neural crest migration and motor axon outgrowth. *Neuron* **18**, 383–396.

Weston, J. A. (1963), A radiographic analysis of the migration and localization of trunk neural crest cells in the chick. *Dev. Biol.* **6**, 279–310.

Wilkinson, D. G. (2001). Multiple roles of EPH receptors and ephrins in neural development. *Nature Rev. Neurosci.* **2**, 155–164.

Suggested Readings

Anderson, S. A., Marin, O., *et al.* (2001). Distinct cortical migrations from the medial and lateral ganglionic eminences. *Development* **128**, 353–363.

Hatten, M. E. (1999). Central nervous system neuronal migration. *Annu. Rev. Neurosci.* **22**, 511–539.

Rice, D. S., and Curran, T., (1999). Mutant mice with scrambled brains: Understanding the signaling pathways that control cell positioning in the CNS. *Genes Dev.* **13**, 2758–2773.

Wang, V., and Zoghbi, H. (2001). Genetic regulation of cerebellar development. *Nature Rev. Neurosci.* **2**, 484–491.

Marianne Bronner-Fraser and
Mary Beth Hatten

Cellular Determination

NEURONAL PHENOTYPES AND DETERMINANTS

Neuronal Phenotypes and Fates

Neural cells express many different anatomical, physiological, and biochemical characteristics or "phenes." Some of these are developmentally transient; others are permanent and represent the phenotype, or identity, of particular neural cells. The terms *phenotype*, identity, and fate are often used interchangeably with respect to cells, but strictly speaking, *neuronal fate* refers to the future phenotype of an as yet undifferentiated neural precursor.

Neurons show an enormous variety of different phenotypes, and the differences between neurons can be dramatic. Compare, for example, a cone cell in the retina and a cerebellar Purkinje cell. They have completely different shapes, patterns of connectivity, and physiological characteristics. Phenotypic differences can also be subtle, such as between types of pyramidal cells of the cerebral cortex, which may differ only with regard to their axonal projection to different subcortical targets.

The distribution of neurons expressing different phenotypes is not random, but follows a highly invariant pattern in a given species. Thus, neurons located at a given position within the nervous system always express the same phenotype. Whereas in vertebrates, this statement is true on the level of populations of neurons (e.g., cells of layer III of the cortical area 17 are glutaminergic pyramidal cells projecting to cortical areas 18 and 19), in many invertebrates it is true even on the level of individual, uniquely

identifiable cells. This raises the question of how neuronal fate is controlled during development. Experimental studies carried out over the last few decades have provided substantial progress in answering this question. This chapter attempts to summarize some of the main insights gained into the mechanisms controlling neuronal fate.

Cues and Determinants

To investigate the mechanisms controlling the cellular fate, one assays for "cues" or activities that induce changes in this fate. For example, neural crest-derived sympathoadrenal precursors give rise to sympathetic neurons when grown in simple culture medium, but take on the fate of adrenal chromaffin cells if grown in the presence of the glucocorticoid hormone. This hormone thus possesses an activity that can influence the fate of sympathoadrenal cells. The glucocorticoid hormone constitutes a cue that influences the sympathoadrenal fate. Generally speaking, *fate-controlling cues* are present in two different realms: the external environment outside the neuron and the internal environment inside the neuron.

a. The environment into which the neuron is born and gradually differentiates provides *extrinsic cues* in the form of diffusible molecules, signals attached to the membranes of adjacent cells, and extracellular matrix bound signal molecules.

b. The neuron itself, before onset of differentiation, expresses or inherits from its precursor *intrinsic cues*. Many of these intrinsic cues, as we will see, turn out to be transcriptional activators or repressors (Fig. 16.1).

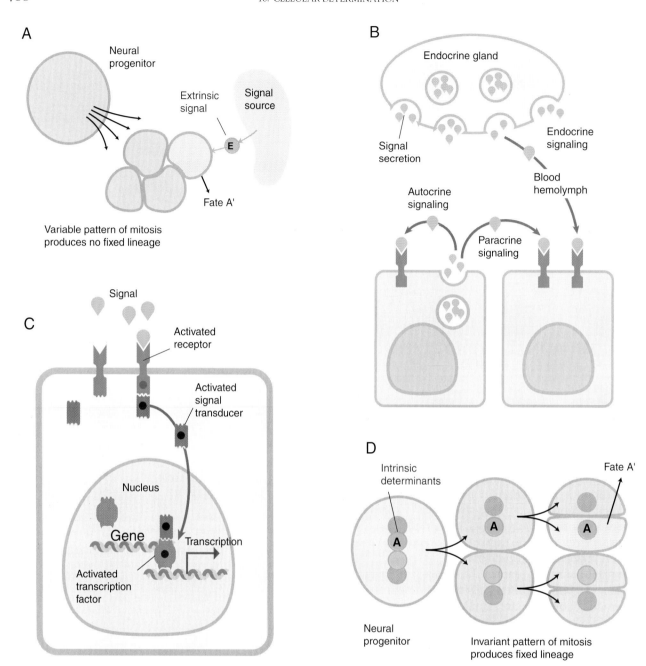

FIGURE 16.1 Neural fate is controlled by extrinsic and intrinsic determinants. (A) Extrinsic determinants, or signals, are molecules that reach a cell from an external source located in the environment of the cell and prompt the cell to express a certain fate. (B) Different sources of extrinsic signals. Endocrine signals reach a given cell from a distant tissue (endocrine gland) via the blood or hemolymph. Paracrine signals act from neighboring or nearby cells; autocrine signals are produced by the same cell that reacts to them. (C) Generic signal transduction pathway involving the activation of a membrane-bound receptor by an extracellular signal, followed by the activation of cytoplasmic signal transducers and nuclear transcription factors. (D) Intrinsic determinants are molecules that are expressed in the progenitor cell and then forwarded during an invariant pattern of mitosis to the progeny. In this example, determinant A is forwarded to the cell shaded green whose fate it determines to become A′.

Extrinsic Cues Activate Signal Transduction Cascades and Control Differential Gene Expression in the Recipient Cell

Embryonic neural precursors start out in an undetermined state and need input from their environment to become determined. Factors that act on a cell from the outside, and that originate in other embryonic cells, are called *extrinsic determinants* (Fig. 16.1A). In some cases, signaling molecules can be secreted from remote cells (hormones, growth factors); these are *endocrine* signals. In other cases, signaling molecules that are secreted from, or presented on the membranes of neighboring cells, are called *paracrine* signals (Fig. 16.1B).

Signaling molecules activate specific receptors in the membranes of cells whose fate they influence. These receptors then initiate a signal transduction cascade in the responding cell (Fig. 16.1C). Activated receptors may possess enzymatic activity: an important family of receptors falling into this category are tyrosine kinase and serine/threonine kinase receptors. Alternatively, activated receptors may interact with other membrane-bound or cytosolic proteins, which in turn have enzymatic activity. The *signal transduction cascades* activated by the receptors involve a variety of different second messenger systems that eventually act on transcription factors, proteins that bind to the regulatory sites of specific genes.

In most vertebrates, neural precursors that pass through an extended undetermined phase and become determined as a result of extrinsic signaling generally show *regulative development*, meaning that many cells can respond to the same external cues to build a normal nervous system. Thus, removing one or even several undetermined precursors does not result in any missing parts in the mature nervous system because other undetermined cells, exposed to the same signals, take on the fate of the removed ones.

Intrinsic Cues Are Cytoplasmic or Nuclear Proteins Inherited from Progenitor Cells or Present in Newborn Cells

Determinants of cell fate that reside within a cell from its birth onward are called *intrinsic determinants*. Intrinsic determinants are inherited through cell divisions (Fig. 16.1D). We can imagine a neural progenitor cell that contains a multitude of different determinants in the form of mRNAs and proteins. During its subsequent mitoses, these determinants are distributed in a reproducible fashion to the individual daughter neurons. For such a mechanism to work, embryonic cell divisions have to follow a reproducible pattern (Fig. 16.1D). Progenitors that divide in an invariant pattern are said to produce a *fixed lineage*.

Neural progenitors, called neuroblasts, of many invertebrate embryos, including annelids, molluscs, arthropods, and nematodes, follow fixed lineage patterns. Neural progenitor division in these organisms is said to be *determinative*. Determinative development in these organisms can be shown experimentally to be very different than the regulative neural development of vertebrates, as demonstrated by removing individual neural progenitor cells. As a result of cell ablation, the neurons that would normally descend from the ablated progenitor are missing in the adult.

DETERMINATION OF NEURAL PROGENITORS

Origin of Neural Progenitors in the Neurectoderm

Progenitors of the nervous system arise from specialized regions of the ectoderm called the *neurectoderm* (Fig. 16.2). In vertebrates (Figs. 16.2A–16.2D), the entire dorsal part of the ectoderm forms the neurectoderm. This region invaginates to become the elongated, dorsally located neural tube from which brain and spinal cord develop. In many invertebrate groups, particularly in arthropods (Figs. 16.2E–16.2H), a ventrally located strip of ectoderm gives rise to the ventral chain of segmental ganglia (which can be compared to the vertebrate spinal cord), and an anterior-lateral patch of ectoderm gives rise to the brain. Progenitors of the central nervous system of invertebrates are called *neuroblasts*. Neuroblasts separate from the neurectoderm and move inside the embryo as individual cells. The neighboring cells, which stay behind after the neuroblasts have migrated in, are called dermoblasts and give rise to the epidermis. After segregation from the ectoderm in both vertebrates and invertebrates, neural progenitors start to **proliferate** (Fig. 16.2G).

Invertebrate Neuroblasts and Ganglion Mother Cells

In insects and many other invertebrate groups, the mode of proliferation is peculiar: each mother neuroblast divides unequally into one large and one small daughter cell. The large cell remains as a neuroblast and continues to go on this way for a number of rounds. The small cell, called the *ganglion mother cell* (GMC), typically divides one more time and both of its daughter cells differentiate into mature neurons. Often, ganglion mother cells and immature neurons form a stack on top of the neuroblast from which they originated. Because postmitotic neurons generally do not migrate, the progeny of a neuroblast remain spa-

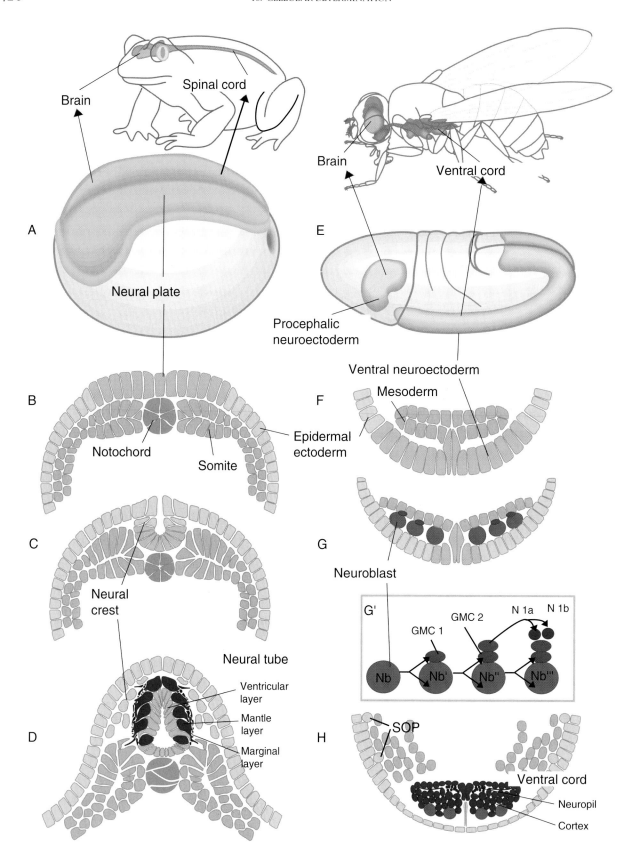

tially close to one another, with the position of each neuron dependent on the position of the neuroblast and the time at which it was born. Thereby, a two-layered cortex-neuropil architecture typical of the mature ganglion is generated (Fig. 16.2H).

Progenitors of the invertebrate peripheral nervous system, called sensillum progenitors or *sense organ progenitors (SOPs)*, originate from the neurectoderm, as well as other positions of the ectoderm, at a later stage. Formation of these cells is discussed in more detail later.

Vertebrate Neuroblasts and the Ventricular Layer

In vertebrates, neural progenitors form a continuous epithelium that lines the lumen or ventricle of the neural tube and is called the *ventricular layer* or zone (Fig. 16.2D). These progenitors first divide symmetrically in the plane of the epithelium. After variable periods of time, neuroblasts spin off postmitotic daughters. Generation of a postmitotic neuron in some parts of the vertebrate neuroepithelium, such as the cortex, has been seen to be associated with asymmetric cleavages. The cell that remains next to the ventricle continues to divide as a neuroblast, while its sibling exits the cell cycle and migrates toward the outer surface of the neural tube. Here the young neurons form dendrites and axons. At this stage, the nervous system has reached a three-layered configuration of a ventricular layer, mantle layer, and marginal layer.

The peripheral nervous system of the vertebrate nervous system consists of sensory neurons, most of which derive from the **neural crest** (Fig. 16.2D), an

elongated population of cells located on either side along the lateral border of the neural plate. As the neural plate rolls into the tube during neurulation,

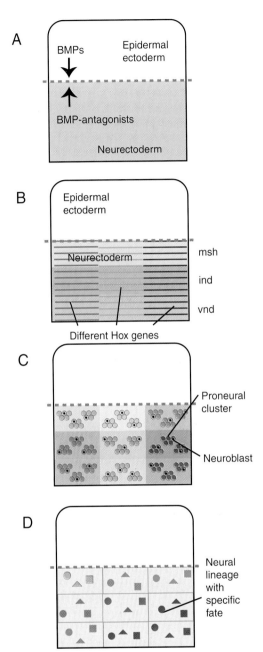

FIGURE 16.2 Synopsis of early neural development in amphibians (A–D) and insects (E–H). (A and E) Dorsolateral views of embryos at the onset of neurulation. The neurectoderm is shaded light blue. (B and F) Schematic cross sections of the embryos. (C and G) Cross sections at a later stage, when neurulation is well under way. In vertebrates, the neural plate folds in to become the neural tube. Cells at the junction between the neural tube and the epidermal ectoderm (green) form the neural crest, which gives rise to the peripheral and autonomic nervous systems. In insects, individual neural progenitors (neuroblasts; purple) delaminate from the ventral neurectoderm. They divide in a stem cell mode (G'), producing stacks of daughter cells called ganglion mother cells (GMC). Each ganglion mother cell divides into two neurons (e.g., N1a, N1b). (D and H) Cross sections of late embryos in which some neurons (red) have differentiated. In vertebrates, these neurons delaminate from the neuroepithelium and form the so-called mantle layer. Neurites gather at the outside of the neural tube (marginal layer). In insects, neuronal cell bodies form an outer layer (cortex); neurites gather in the center, forming the neuropile. Progenitors of the peripheral nervous system [sensory organ progenitors (SOPs); green] segregate from different locations in the epidermis.

FIGURE 16.3 Stepwise commitment of neural lineages. (A) BMP proteins and their antagonists delineate the boundaries of the neurectoderm. (B) Coordinate genes are expressed in transversal stripes (e.g., Hox genes) and longitudinal stripes (e.g., vnd, ind, msh). Combinations of coordinate genes provide different regions of the neurectoderm with a specific intrinsic "code" that plays an important role in determining the fate of neural lineages coming from these regions. (C) Neural progenitors are singled out from the neurectoderm by proneural and neurogenic genes. (D) Specific progenitors and their lineages differentiate by expressing different intrinsic cues in the form of transcriptional regulators.

BOX 16.1

NEURAL STEM CELLS

The proliferating progenitor cells or neuroblasts that give rise to more differentiated progeny but themselves remain in the cell cycle are called neural stem cells. Some frogs and fish continue to grow bigger throughout their lifetimes, and their brains grow with their bodies, adding new cells from localized stem cell populations. However, in most animals, including humans, most proliferating cells use themselves up during development so the sources of new neurons in an adult animal are extremely limited. This is why damage to the central neuron system (CNS) is medically much more serious than damage to the some other organs, such as the skin or liver, where stem cells that persist into adulthood can replace injured tissue. Nevertheless, it has been found that even in adult mammals, *neural stem cells* (NSCs) are found in or near ventricular layers throughout the neuraxis, and it has even been shown that peripheral cells, e.g., hematopoietic stem cells of the blood, may have the potential to become neural (Blau *et al.*, 2001). This "new view" of stem cells contrasts with the "old view"—that there is little or no neurogenesis in adulthood. Periventricular astrocytes have been identified as the possible source of these NSCs. Interestingly, one pocket of rich stem cell activity is in the hippocampus, where learning takes place (see Chapters 50 and 51). At the time of writing, there was great excitement about the potential of using these cells in a replacement strategy for brain damage due to injury, stroke, or degenerative diseases such as Parkinson's disease. One could imagine harvesting neural stem cells from the hippocampal area of a Parkinson's disease sufferer, proliferating these cells in culture under conditions where they begin to differentiate as dopaminergic neurons, and using these expanded stem cells to replace ones lost from the subtantia nigra of the patient. Indeed, mice that serve as models of Parkinson's disease have had their conditions ameliorated by transplants of neural stem cells.

Important questions abound about neural stem cells in the adult brain. Why do these cells remain undifferentiated and capable of division when their neighbors have exited the cell cycle and differentiated? What signals do these cells need in order to stimulate their proliferation and differentiation? How can their differentiation toward particular types of neurons or glia be controlled experimentally? While there is much speculation on the role of various signaling and growth factors in regulating these processes, much more work needs to be done to identify the molecules that prevent stem cells from differentiating and the signals that release their potential. Interestingly, the environment of the organism may play a key role in this process. Rats raised in complex environments containing toys and exercise wheels show more proliferation of hippocampal stem cells than rats raised in simple cages. Stress works in the other direction and seems to inhibit cell proliferation in the hippocampus. The identification of key regulatory factors might prove invaluable in treating neural or glial degenerative conditions without the need for transplants.

Another source of stem cells in mammals is the inner cell mass of the early conceptus. These are the cells that give rise to all the tissues of the embryo proper. When these *embryonic stem* (ES) *cells* are grown in culture, some of them turn into neural precursors. It seems that the lessons learned about the mechanisms of neural induction in *Xenopus* are paying off in this context, because antagonizing the BMP signaling pathway using neural inducers such as noggin and cerberus (see Chapter 14) increases the probability that ES cells will follow a neural pathway. ES cells have an advantage over neural stem cells from adults because the former cells are easier to grow and come from a stage in development when their potential fates are less restricted by the inheritance of intrinsic determinants. Clearly, the more we know about neuronal determination, the more likely we will be able to direct stem cells down appropriate developmental pathways that will be useful in treating the damaged nervous system.

William A. Harris and Volker Hartenstein

Reference

Blau, H. M. Brazelton, T. R., and Wermon, J. M. (2001). The evolving concept of a stem cell: Entity or function? *Cell* **105**, 829–841.

these cells form a solid column on the dorsal aspect of the neural tube. Some components of the cranial peripheral nervous system derive from ectodermal *placodes* located on either side of the neural plate.

Regionalization of the Neurectoderm

During the course of neurulation, the neurectoderm becomes subdivided into regions with distinct fates, such as the forebrain, hindbrain, and spinal cord in vertebrates or different neuromeres in arthropods. Regionalization of the vertebrate neural tube is discussed in detail in Chapter 14. However, because the genetic mechanism underlying neurectoderm regionalization is involved intricately in neural fate specification, we need to review this process briefly here. At the core of the regionalization gene network are two groups of genes, which, in a simplified manner of speaking, provide the neurectoderm with a system of Cartesian coordinates and are therefore referred to as *coordinate genes.*

The Medio–Lateral System

The initial signaling event that sets up the boundaries of the neurectoderm involves the antagonistic action of two secreted signals distributed in a graded fashion (Sasai and DeRobertis, 1997; Fig. 16.3A). One signal with high concentrations laterally is formed by several proteins of the Bone Morphogenetic Protein (BMP) family. A *Drosophila* BMP homologue with similar function is Decapentaplegic (Dpp). The BMP/Dpp signal promotes epidermal ectoderm and pushes the boundary of the neurectoderm medially. The opposing signal is formed by the BMP antagonist, chordin (*Drosophila* homologue: Sog), which promotes neurectodermal development.

Once the boundaries of the neurectoderm are set up, three homeobox (Hox) genes, *vnd, ind,* and *msh,* are expressed in longitudinal stripes in the neural primordium of flies and vertebrates (Cornell and Ohlen, 2000). The sequence in which they are expressed is conserved, with *vnd* demarcating the neurectoderm neuroblasts close to the midline, *msh* the lateral part of the neurectoderm, and *ind* an intermediate stripe (Fig. 16.3B). The loss or ectopic expression of these genes affects a definitive change in mediolateral neural fate. The mechanism responsible for setting up these stripes involves responses of the promoters of these genes to threshold levels of the morphogen Dpp (see earlier discussion), which forms a gradient of expression from dorsal (high) to ventral (low). In vertebrates, another morphogen, Sonic hedgehog (Shh), forms an opposite gradient (high concentrations ventrally and low concentrations dorsally) which is also critical to direct the expression of the mediolateral genes (see later). Once set up, the boundaries between the stripes of vnd, ind, and msh are sharpened by mutual repression.

The Anterior–Posterior System

The so-called Hox genes are expressed in sharply demarcated, partially overlapping anterior–posterior domains in the neural primordium in flies, vertebrates, *Caenorhabditis-elegans,* and many other invertebrates. These genes provide neural lineages with intrinsic "information" that reflects their location along the antero–posterior axis. Hox genes form a gene complex in which members expressed at a given antero–posterior level in the embryo are located at a corresponding position within the complex on the chromosome. Hox gene expression is restricted to the middle and posterior portions of the neural primordium. Anteriorly, another group of highly conserved genes called *head gap genes (which include otd/Otx, tll/Tlx, ems/Emx, and ey/Pax6)* are expressed in nested domains within the brain (Shimamura *et al.,* 1995).

In segmented arthropods, the neural primordium is subdivided into segmental units (*neuromeres*). Segment polarity genes, among them *Hedgehog (Hh), engrailed* (*en;* regulates *Hh* expression) and *wingless* (wg), control positional information within each individual segment (Bhat, 1999).

These coordinate genes in the medio–lateral and antero–posterior axis collaborate to specify a positional identity to each cell of the neural ectoderm in a developing organism. The mechanisms by which these genes are originally turned on in characteristic patterns were discussed in Chapter 14. Once they are expressed in progenitors, however, the expression pattern of a particular set of coordinate genes is usually inherited by the progeny of these cells and may act as intrinsic determinants of neuronal fate.

Specification of Neural Progenitors by the Proneural and Neurogenic Network

The neurectoderm of insects and most other invertebrates, although patterned in a positional sense, is still a mixed population of cells. Only some of these cells become neuroblasts, whereas others stay at the surface of the embryo and develop as epidermal progenitors (Fig. 16.3D). Cell–cell interactions that take place within the neurectoderm define the number and pattern of neuroblasts and SOPs. Experimental and genetic studies suggest a two-step mechanism for this process. First, discrete groups of neurectodermal cells are made competent to become neuroblasts. These groups of cells, called *proneural clusters,* represent *equivalence groups* in which all cells initiate a neural fate. In *Drosophila,* a group of *proneural genes* expressed in the proneural clusters are involved in making ectodermal cells competent to become neural progenitors (Figs 16.4A and 16.4D). In a second step, cells of the proneural cluster interact to sort out which of them will become neurons and which will fall back to become dermoblasts. In particular, nascent neuroblasts send out inhibitory signals to their neighbors,

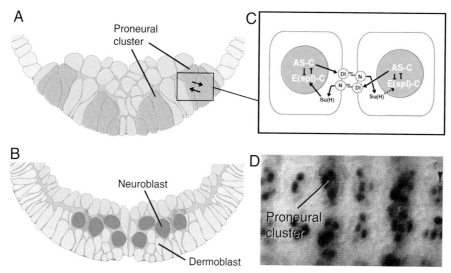

FIGURE 16.4 Control of neuroblast–dermoblast determination in *Drosophila*. (A) Section of neurecto-derm prior to the time of neuroblast formation. Proneural genes are expressed in small groups of cells called proneural clusters. (B) Section of neurectoderm after neuroblasts have separated from the dermoblast. Interactions of cells with proneural clusters result in the restriction of proneural genes in neuroblasts, which give rise to the nervous system. (C) Restriction of proneural gene expression to neuroblasts depends on Notch signaling, which is activated by the signal Delta. Notch and the signal transducer Su(H) activate the transcriptional regulator E(spl) and repress the expression of proneural genes. (D) Detail of proneural gene expression (from Skeath and Carroll, 1992).

inhibiting these cells from becoming neuroblasts. Experiments done in grasshopper embryos were the first to reveal the existence of such inhibitory inter-actions (Fig. 16.5). Shortly after the neuroblasts segre-gated, they were ablated by a laser microbeam. It was found that the ablated neuroblasts were replaced by neighboring cells, which would otherwise have developed into dermoblasts, not neuroblasts. Genetic studies in *Drosophila* led to the discovery of a group of genes, called *neurogenic genes*, which mediate this inhibitory cell–cell interaction. Both invertebrates and vertebrates use proneural and neurogenic genes in the initiation of neural determination.

Proneural Genes

Proneural genes are transcription factors of the basic helix-loop-helix (bHLH) family. In *Drosophila*, four of these genes form a complex called the *achaete-scute* complex (AS-C). Loss of proneural gene function leads to a reduction or total loss of neuroblasts and/or SOPs. Typically, cells deprived of proneural gene function do not form neural progenitors and develop as dermoblasts instead. In other cases, neural progenitors may start to form, but abort their neural development and undergo apoptosis.

Neurogenic Genes

The activity of proneural genes in the neurecto-derm would lead to a large fraction of this layer

forming the nervous system. This is prevented by the function of neurogenic genes that encode a cell com-munication mechanism used by the ectoderm cells to restrict the number of neural progenitors. Loss of function of any of the neurogenic genes results in a higher number of neural progenitors, at the expense of dermoblasts. The neurogenic genes *Notch* (**N**) and *Delta* (**Dl**) encode membrane proteins. Other neuro-genic genes, such as those in the *Enhancer of split complex* [**E(spl)-C**], code for transcription factors that may act to control the expression of proneural genes.

Proneural/neurogenic Gene Interactions

Proneural genes are expressed in all cells of a given proneural cluster. Genes activated by these transcrip-tion factors are other proneural genes as well as some neurogenic genes, particularly Dl. The activation of Dl, initially in all cells of the cluster, initiates the inhibitory process leading to the restriction of proneural gene expression and neural competence to a single cell, which will then segregate as a neural progenitor (Fig. 16.4C). The transmembrane Dl protein is a "signal" that acts on the Notch receptor. Notch is also expressed on all cells of the proneural cluster. When Dl on one cell binds Notch on another, it sets in motion a signal transduction cascade that involves another neurogenic gene called *Suppressor of Hairless* [**Su(H)**]. Activation of Notch leads to the translocation of Su(H) to the nucleus, where it activates other genes, among

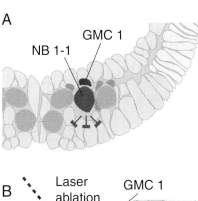

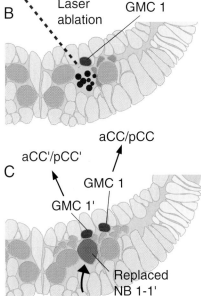

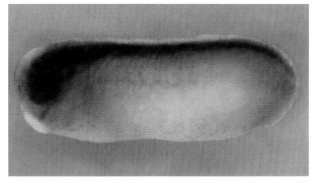

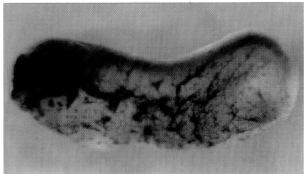

FIGURE 16.6 NeuroD turns epidermal cells into neurons. (Top) A normal *Xenopus* embryo stained for the neural marker NCAM shows no staining in epidermis. (Bottom) A neuroD-injected embryo has NCAM-stained cells with neuronal morphologies staining in the ventral epidermis.

FIGURE 16.5 Lateral inhibition in insect neuroblasts. (A) Neuroblasts (magenta) emit inhibitory signals restricting the number of neurectoderm cells (blue) that embark on a neuroblast pathway. If one neuroblast is ablated by laser microbeam (B), the inhibitory signal is relieved. As a result, the underlying neurectoderm will give rise to a "substitute" neuroblast that expresses the same fate as the original deleted neuroblast (C).

Proneural and Neurogenic Genes Play Important Roles in Vertebrates

Both proneural and neurogenic genes are used in similar ways in vertebrates. Among the proneural genes, three AS-C homologues (**ASH** genes) have been identified. Experimental studies using transgenic animals, in which genes have been mutated by homologous recombination (gene knockouts), as well as injection of active or inactive forms of the message, show that the proneural genes in vertebrates are required for the determination of certain populations of neural cells. In *Xenopus*, injection of active XASH-3 mRNA into blastomeres leads to an increased number of neural progenitor cells in the neural tube. In similar experiments, the bHLH proneural gene neuroD causes a transformation of epidermal cells into neurons (Fig. 16.6). Conversely, knockout of MASH-1 in mice leads to the absence of populations of neural cells. Homologues of the neurogenic genes N, Dl, Su(H), and E(spl)-C have also been identified in vertebrates. The most revealing insight to the function of these genes in vertebrates has been gained by experiments in *Xenopus*, where active forms of Notch-1 or Delta-1 mRNAs were injected into early blastomeres. This

them the neurogenic E(spl)-C. E(spl)-C proteins are bHLH transcription factors that repress the proneural genes completing an inhibitory feedback loop.

Fluctuations in the level of gene expression may lead to a slightly higher level of proneural genes in one cell, or a few cells, of the proneural cluster. This cell has an advantage over its neighbors because it expresses more Dl signal and thereby suppresses proneural genes in the neighboring cells. Initially, the proneural expression level is uniformly high in all cells of the proneural cluster. Subsequently, expression increases in one cell; as it does so, the neighboring cells decrease proneural gene expression.

treatment resulted in decreased formation of the earliest born primary neurons. Lack of Dl function (obtained by injecting a **dominant-negative** Dl deletion construct) has an effect opposite from that of overexpression of active Dl, i.e., increased formation of primary neurons.

SPECIFICATION OF NEURAL LINEAGES BY INTRINSIC MECHANISMS

Neuroblast Lineages in *Drosophila* and *C. elegans*

In invertebrates, many aspects of neuronal fate are determined by intrinsic factors that are already expressed at the neuroblast stage. As summarized earlier, the expression pattern of medio–lateral genes, homeobox genes, and segment polarity genes superimposes a Cartesian-like system of intrinsic determinants over the neurectoderm (Fig. 16.4B). When a neuroblast delaminates, it takes with it the particular combination of coordinate genes that were expressed in the proneural cluster from which the neuroblast is derived. Thus, coordinate genes represent the first set of intrinsic determinants that provide a neuroblast and the clone of neurons/glial cells it produces with a distinct identity (Fig. 16.4D).

Genetic analysis has shown that the absence or overexpression of coordinate genes leads to alterations of whole groups of clonally related cells. An example shown in Fig. 16.7 is the control of neuroblast lineage fate by the segment polarity gene *gooseberry* (*gsb*). In normal development, *gsb* is expressed in a complete row of neuroblasts that includes the neuroblast 5-2 (Fig. 16.7A). The lineage produced by 5-2 consists of at least 10 neurons with different phenotypes. In contrast, neuroblast MP2, which normally does not express *gsb*, exhibits a quite unusual lineage formed by two neurons: MP2d and MP2v (Fig. 16.7B). If *gsb* is expressed ectopically in MP2, its lineage is converted into a Nb5-2 lineage (Skeath *et al.*, 1995).

Drosophila neuroblasts have different identities from each other due to their unique combinations of coordinate gene expression, but all nevertheless go through a similar program of proliferation and give rise to a series of distinct GMCs. The first GMCs of a neuroblast lineage tend to lie deeper in the CNS and generate neurons with long axons, whereas the later arising GMCs stay closer to the edge of the CNS and generate neurons with short axons. Their parent neuroblasts tend to go through a temporally conserved program of transcription factor expression. In the stages when the first GMCs are generated, most

neuroblasts express *hunchback* (*hb*), and GMCs expressed at this time inherit this Hb expression. Later, the same neuroblasts turn off *hb* and express Krueppel (*Kr*) instead, and GMCs generated at this stage inherit *Kr* expression. Experiments in which *hb* or *Kr* is eliminated or expressed at the wrong time lead to predictable switches in the fates of early and later born descendants of these neuroblasts (Isshiki *et al.*, 2001). Thus, the expression of both spatially and temporally coordinated transcription factors in neuroblasts is preserved in their progeny and forms part of the increasingly rich inheritance of each developing neural progenitor. The ontogenetic roots of a neural progenitor can be read in the combination of transcription factors it expresses, and these factors in turn influence the eventual phenotype of the cell.

The nervous system of *C. elegans*, although highly determinative, is generated in a piecemeal fashion in that neurons come from a variety of very different lineages (Sengupta and Bargmann, 1996). For example, functionally related motor neurons of *C. elegans* arise during embryogenesis from 3 separate precursors, while the rest arise postembryonically from 13 different precursors. Most of our knowledge concerning the mechanisms of neuronal determination in this organism comes from mutations that interfere with this process. Many of these mutations, as might be expected, are found in genes that encode transcription factors. The nematode POU domain gene *unc-86* is a good example (Baumeister *et al.*, 1996). In the wild-type animal, a neuroblast called "Q" divides into anterior and posterior daughter cells, Ql.a and Ql.p (Fig. 16.7C). The *unc-86* gene is turned on only in the Ql.p daughter cell and its progeny. Ql.p produces two sensory neurons (PVM, SDQ), whereas Ql.a produces one central neuron (PQR) and one cell that dies. A loss of function mutation in *unc-86* results in the "transformation" of Ql.p, the cell in which it is normally expressed, into a cell that behaves like the mother cell of Ql.a and Ql.p. Thus, instead of producing the neurons PVM and SDQ, the "transformed-Q1.p" continues to divide in the pattern of its mother cell, the Q neuroblast.

The *Drosophila* homologue of *unc-86* (called *dPOU28*) is also expressed in a subset of GMCs and seems to function in a way that is closely related to its function in *C. elegans*. For example, dPOU28 is expressed in the first GMC (GMC-1) of the neuroblast 4-2 lineage (Fig. 16.7D). GMC-1 produces two identified neurons, RP2 and its sibling, which both discontinue dPOU28 expression. If dPOU28 is misexpressed experimentally by heat shock in postmitotic neurons, they both adopt the fate of their GMC-1 mother cell and divide again.

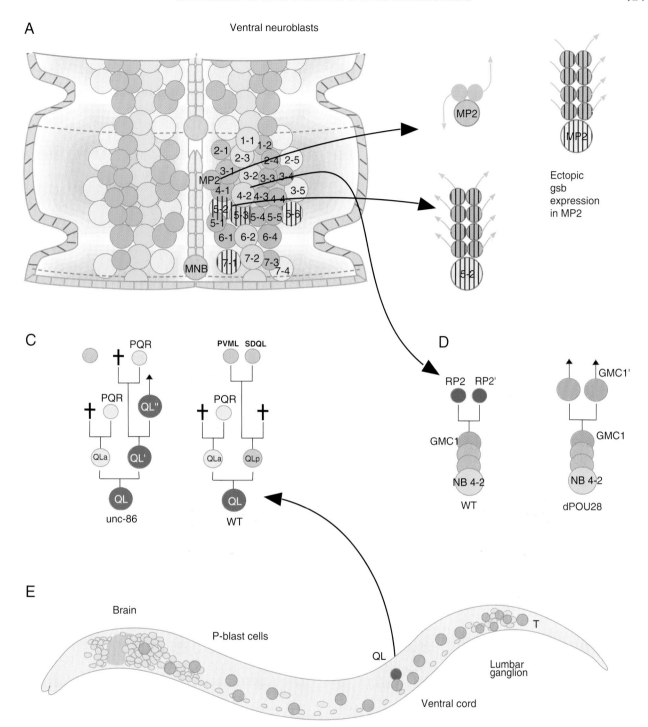

FIGURE 16.7 Specification of neuronal lineages by intrinsic mechanisms in *Drosophila* and *C. elegans*. (A) A schematized neuroblast map of *Drosophila*. All neuroblasts of one hemisegment are numbered. Different shades of blue indicate affiliation of neuroblasts to different subpopulations, distinguished by their time of birth. Purple hatching indicates a row of neuroblasts expressing the gooseberry (gsb) gene. (B) Two lineages, MP2 with 2 neurons and 5-2 with more than 10 neurons, are shown. Normally, only the 5-2 lineage expresses gsb. Ectopic expression of gsb in MP2 leads to conversion of this lineage into a 5-2 lineage. (C) unc-86, which encodes a *C. elegans* POU protein, is expressed in the neural progenitor cell QL. QLp and its sibling, QLa, derive from the QL cell. In wild-type animals (left), QLa, after one division, gives rise to a neuron (PQR) and a cell that undergoes programmed cell death (cross); QLp divides twice and produces two neurons (PVM, SDQ) and one cell that dies. In unc-86 loss-of-function mutations (right), QLp behaves like its mother, QL. (D) The *Drosophila* dPOU28 protein is expressed in a number of ganglion mother cells, among them GMC1 of neuroblast 4-2. In wild-type flies (left), this GMS produces two identified motor neurons (RP2 and its siblings). If dPOU28 is expressed under heat-shock control in these neurons (right), they behave like ganglion mother cells and continue to divide.

Asymmetric Distribution of Intrinsic Determinants during Neuroblast Proliferation

The intrinsic factors that we have looked at thus far are typically inherited by the progeny of a neuroblast and thereby regulate patterns of gene expression. However, a more intricate problem arises when "cocktails" of intrinsic determinants found in the cytoplasm of the neural progenitor are distributed differentially to its progeny. This is accomplished by *asymmetric cell division*. As soon as they leave the neurectoderm behind, insect neuroblasts start dividing asymmetrically to produce two unequally sized daughter cells, a large second order neuroblast remaining at the surface, and a small GMC lying interiorly. Two transcription factors, Numb and Prospero (Pro), are expressed in most neuroblasts. At neuroblast division, these factors become localized to the smaller daughter, the GMC, where Prospero moves into the nucleus and influences fate (Lu *et al.*, 2000; Fig. 16.8). Numb acts by inhibiting the neurogenic signaling cascade described earlier.

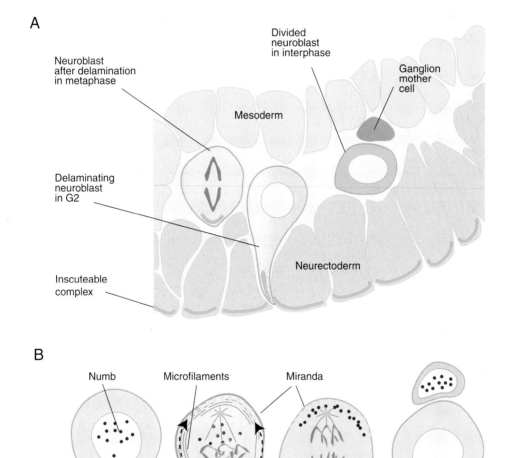

FIGURE 16.8 Control of asymmetric cell division in *Drosophila*. (A) Schematic section of neurectoderm at the stage of neuroblast delamination. The Inscuteable protein complex (*green*) is expressed apically in the neurectoderm and is carried interiorly by delaminating neuroblasts. (B) Inscuteable complex controls asymmetric distribution of intrinsic fate determinants, such as Numb (*red*), by orienting the mitotic spindle vertically and by localizing the Miranda protein (*yellow*) basally. Miranda traps Numb at the apical pole of the dividing neuroblast and thereby channels it into the ganglion mother cell.

To understand how the asymmetric localization of Pros and Numb is controlled in delaminated neuroblasts, we must turn to a group of proteins expressed in the neurectoderm prior to delamination. These proteins, among them Inscuteable (Insc) and Bazooka (Baz), form a multiprotein link (the *Insc complex*) to the apical membrane of neurectoderm cells. When neuroblasts delaminate, the Insc complex is maintained apically. As the neuroblast enters mitosis, the Insc complex anchors the centrioles in a vertical orientation, resulting in a vertical mitotic spindle. At the same time, the Insc complex, in conjunction with an actin-based cytoskeleton mechanism, drives the distribution of several key proteins along this vertical plane so that they are inherited asymmetrically. In particular, a cytoplasmic protein, Miranda (Mira),

becomes enriched at the basal neuroblast pole such that when cytokinesis separates daughter cells of the neuroblast, Mira is trapped in the GMC. It is Mira that, in turn, binds the aforementioned determinants, Numb and Pros, to the basal neuroblast pole and thus directs their localization to the GMC. Both Pros and Numb are initially present at low levels in the entire neuroblast.

It is likely that the molecular machinery that directs the mitotic spindle and distribution of intrinsic determinants in *Drosophila* neuroblasts is also active in the vertebrate nervous system, as several homologues of Numb have been identified in mouse. Mouse Numb is inherited asymmetrically in dividing neural progenitors of the cortex, neural crest, and spinal cord, where apical–basal asymmetric divisions have been noted.

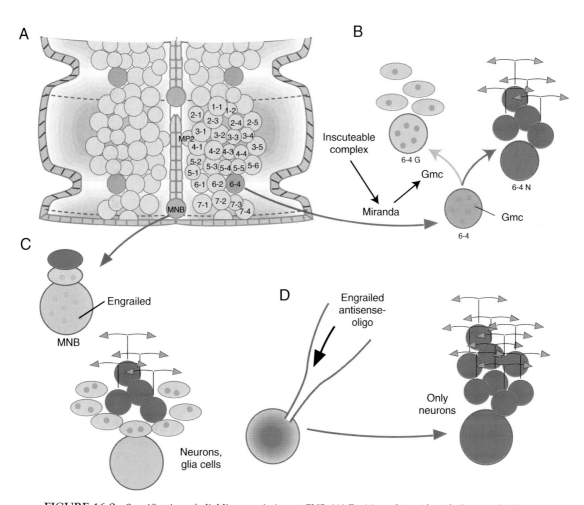

FIGURE 16.9 Specification of glial lineages in insect CNS. (A) Position of two identified neuroglioblasts in the *Drosophila* neuroblast map (see Fig 7A). (B) Separation of neuronal and glial sublineages in progenitor 6-4. The glial regulatory protein, Gmc, is expressed in 6-4. When this cell divides into two equally sized daughter cells, 6-4 G and 6-4 N, the Inscuteable complex and Miranda segregate Gmc into 6-4 G, which thereby becomes specified as glioblast. (C and D) The MNB neuroblast produces both glial cells and neurons. The *engrailed* gene, which encodes a homeodomain transcription factor, is required for glial sublineage. When *en* function is reduced by injecting antisense oligonucleotides, MNB forms only neurons (D).

Mice homozygous for a *Numb* loss-of-function allele show defects in neural tube closure and forebrain development, suggesting that this gene plays an important role in neural fate determination as well.

Determination of Neuronal versus Glial Lineages in *Drosophila*

Neurons and glia, the two main classes of cells of which the nervous system is composed, can be subdivided further into a multitude of different subtypes of cells. In both vertebrates and invertebrates, the application of lineage tracers to individual progenitors has yielded clones that contain both neurons and glia cells, suggesting that neurons and glia are generally

produced from a common progenitor called a *neuroglioblast*. How is separation between neuronal and glial cell types controlled? In *Drosophila*, intrinsic determinants of glial fate are expressed at an early stage in neuroglioblasts and become localized asymmetrically to the presumptive glial cells.

Two genes encoding transcriptional regulators, *glial cells missing* (*gcm*) and *reversed polarity* (*repo*), are expressed in most glial precursors in insects. Their crucial involvement in glial fate is attested to by the fact that ectopic expression of these genes converts neurons into glial cells and that loss-of-function mutants lack glial cells. Gcm is expressed first and seems to activate Repo by direct binding to the *repo* promoter. The directed expression of Gcm in glial pre-

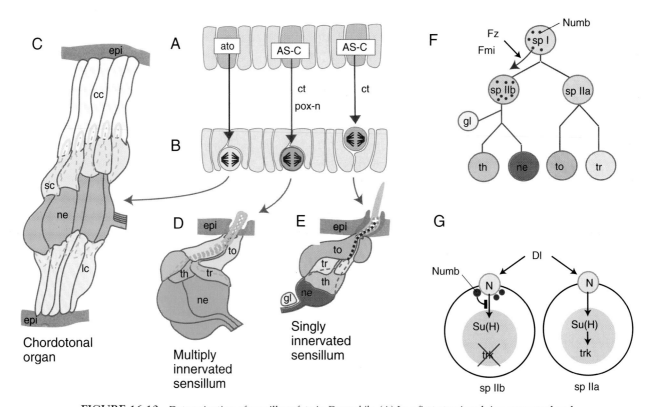

FIGURE 16.10 Determination of sensillum fate in *Drosophila*. (A) In a first step involving proneural and neurogenic genes, sensillum progenitors (SOPs) are selected from proneural clusters in the ectoderm. (B) Sensillum type-specific intrinsic determinants specify SOPs to produce different lineages. Progenitors of chordotonal organs require atonal (ato). *Pox-neuro* (*pox-n*) is required for the development of multiply innervated sensilla (which are typically chemoreceptors); *cut* (*ct*) is required for all classes of external sensilla, as opposed to chordotonal organs. (C+E) Shape and arrangement of fully differentiated sensillum cells in chordotonal organs (C), multiply innervated sensilla (D), and singly innervated, mechanoreceptive sensilla (E). All sensilla have bipolar neurons (ne) and accessory cells. In external sensilla, three accessory cells (th, thecogen cell; tr, trichogen cell; to, tormogen cell) form sheaths around the sensory dendrites and produce the stimulus-receiving bristle. In chordotonal organs, accessory cells form a ligament that attaches the neurons at two distant points of the epidermis (epi; cc, cap cell; lc, ligament cell; sc, scolopale cell). (F) Lineage of SOP (spI) giving rise to a singly innervated mechanoreceptor. SpI divides into two daughters: spIIa and spIIb. The Numb protein, an intrinsic determinant of sensory neurons, is segregated into the spIIb daughter cell. Two proteins, the cadherin Fmi and the receptor Fz, are required for the asymmetric distribution of Numb. (G) Numb acts in spIIb by suppressing Notch signaling.

cursors has been studied in a neuroglioblast called NB6-4T (Akiyama-Oda *et al.*, 2000; Fig. 16.9B). Following delamination, this progenitor cell divides into two cells of equal size (an exception to the usual rule that neuroblasts divide into a small GMC and a large second order neuroblast!). From then on, one of the NB6-4T daughters acts as a "pure" neuroblast and the other as a pure glioblast. Only the glioblast and its progeny express Gcm. Gcm expression in this daughter cell depends on the same "asymmetric division machinery" that was described earlier. Thus, during metaphase of NB6-4T mitosis, Miranda is concentrated on the medial surface of NB6-4T. Mira localizes both Pros and Gcm to that side and thus causes the medial daughter of NB6-4T to develop as glioblast.

Another well-studied neuroblast in *Drosophila* and grasshopper is the median neuroblast (MNB; Fig. 16.9C). Each segmental ganglion possesses one MNB, which gives rise to uniquely identifiable neurons and glia cells along the midline (Condron *et al.*, 1994). Three phases of MNB proliferation can be distinguished: a first phase of exclusively neuronal production, a second phase of gliogenesis, and a third phase in which neurons are produced again. The switch from neurogenesis to gliogenesis requires expression of the transcription factor *engrailed* (*en*). If the expression of *en* is inhibited by injecting *antisense* oligodeoxynucleotides into MNB, the cell fails to generate glia. Instead, supernumerary neurons (of the same type normally produced by the MNB) appear (Fig. 16.9D).

Determinants of Sensillum Lineages and Sublineages

Multiple small sensory organs called sensilla form the sensory part of the peripheral nervous system of most invertebrates. These are scattered at more or less regular intervals over the entire body surface (Fig. 16.3H). The cells that compose each sensillum are clonal descendants of a single SOP progenitor. Most *Drosophila* sensilla fall into three classes (Jan and Jan, 1993): (i) external *mechanosensilla* are formed by one neuron surrounded by three accessory cells (Fig. 16.10E); (ii) *chemoreceptors* and hygroreceptors are similar to mechanoreceptors in the composition of accessory cells; these sensilla are innervated by several (often physiologically distinct) neurons (Fig. 16.10D); and (iii) *chordotonal organs* are also formed by one neuron and three accessory cells; these structures sit beneath the epidermis and insert into the epidermis at two points, whereupon they are stimulated by stretch (Fig. 16.10C).

The first step in sensillum development, the determination of SOPs, is controlled in a manner similar to that regulating neuroblast determination. Thus, the expression of proneural genes of the AS-C defines proneural clusters in the ectoderm that are competent to form SOPs (Fig. 16.10A). At the same time, proneural genes activate inhibitory cell–cell interactions, mediated by neurogenic genes, which single out one SOP and prompt all other cells of the proneural cluster to abort neural development. The identities of individual SOPs are specified by intrinsic factors to produce the different sensillum types (Fig. 16.10B). *Cut* (*ct*) is a homeobox-containing gene expressed in precursors of all external sensilla. If *ct* is absent, external sensilla do not develop and chordotonal organs appear instead. *Poxn* is expressed in precursors of multiply innervated sensilla; in the absence of *poxn*, multiply innervated sensilla are transformed into singly innervated mechanoreceptors. *Atonal* (*ato*) is, expressed and required in the proneural clusters giving rise to chordotonal organs. Loss of *ato* function, results in the absence of these cell types; the ectopic expression of *ato* in other SOPs also induces the production of chordotonal organs.

Each specified SOP undergoes an invariant pattern of cell divisions. This division pattern has been investigated in detail for the external mechanosensory organs called bristles or *macrochaetes*. The primary SOP (spI) for each macrochaete divides into two inherently different secondary SOPs; spIIa and spIIb (Fig. 16.10F). The axis along which spIIa and spIIb are aligned is identical for all microchaetes and coincides with orientation of the later formed sensory bristle (which points posteriorly). spIIa, located posteriorly, produces the outer two accessory socket and shaft cells. The anterior daughter SpIIb divides into a neuron and a support cell, after first giving rise to a glial cell. Several intrinsic determinants, including the asymmetrically inherited *numb* (see earlier discussion), control the fate of spIIa versus spIIb (Fig. 16.10F). In this case, *numb* is distributed to spIIb on cell division. In the absence of *numb*, spIIb is transformed into spIIa; neither neurons nor support cells appear but sensilla form instead with double sockets and shafts. Neither the Insc complex nor miranda, which localizes numb in neuroblasts, plays a role in SOPs. The factors that do this job in SOPs are the signaling molecule Frizzled (Fz) and the adhesion molecule Flamingo (FMI). Loss of function of either Fz or FMI randomizes spindle orientation and numb localization (Usui *et al.*, 1999).

Sensilla in *Drosophila* are not determined solely by intrinsic mechanisms. In fact, these organs are a model system for studying the interface between intrinsic and extrinsic determinants. Sensillum cells form an equivalence group until shortly before differentiation begins. Thus, even though Numb is inherited asymmetrically, inactivating the N/Dl pathway during or after SOP division results in a lineage composed exclusively of neurons. In contrast, expressing an activated form of Notch in all SOP progeny transforms them all into socket cells. These findings imply that the expression of proneural genes in the SOP sets the SOP lineage on a neural course, from which these cells are then diverted by Notch activation. The inheritance of Numb makes a cell less sensitive to Notch signaling, thus the asymmetric distribution of Numb controls which particular cell of the SOP lineage will continue as a neuron and which will be diverted to form other cells (Lu et al., 2000; Fig. 16.10G). The mechanism by which Numb acts on Notch is direct, by binding to Notch and inactivating the transmission of a signal to the nucleus. Thus, the cell inheriting Numb (spIIb) does not react to Dl (which is expressed on both daughters), whereas spIIa does.

SPECIFICATION OF NEURAL FATES BY EXTRINSIC MECHANISMS

Neural Fate in Vertebrate Peripheral Nervous System: Specification of Sympathoadrenal (SA) Progenitors, Neurons, and Glia

The vertebrate neural crest is a transient population of cells that arises along the lateral edges of the neural plate (Chapter 14). Crest cells become localized to the dorsal part of the neural tube as it folds up and then leave the neural tube and migrate along several well-defined pathways (Fig. 16.11). Neural crest stem cells give rise to a large variety of cell types, among them skeletal tissue, melanocytes, sensory neurons and glial cells (Schwann cells) of the peripheral nervous system, adrenergic and cholinergic neurons of the autonomic nervous system, and the endocrine chromaffin cells of the adrenal medulla. As described in Chapter 15, experiments in which crest cells have been transplanted to different regions of the body axis indicate that precursors are multipotent when they start their emigration from the neural tube and acquire instructions to differentiate as distinct cell types during their migration or upon arrival at their final destination.

The commitment to a particular fate is a multistep process that involves the exposure of crest cells to a sequence of instructive environments during migration (Groves and Bronner-Fraser, 1999). One of the

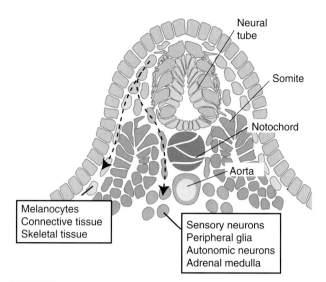

FIGURE 16.11 Neural crest lineages. Schematic cross section of vertebrate embryo in which migrating neural crest cells (green) are indicated. These cells follow two different pathways: a dorsal one (light green), giving rise to melanocytes, connective tissue, and skeletal tissue, and a ventral one, giving rise to sensory and autonomic ganglia, as well as the adrenal medulla.

first decisions that crest cells make as they leave the neural tube is whether to go down the pathway that gives rise to skeletal and connective tissue or the pathway that gives rise to neuronal, glial, and melanocyte (NGM) fates (Fig. 16.11). NGM progenitors then split into various groups such as sympatho–adrenal (SA) progenitors, which give rise in turn to neurons and glia of the sympathetic nervous system and adrenal chromaffin cells.

Sympathetic ganglia first form in the vicinity of the dorsal aorta, which expresses BMP2 (Fig. 16.12). In culture, BMP2 turns on a program of neurogenesis in SA cells by inducing expression of the proneural bHLH gene MASH1 (Fig. 16.12B). However, further cues are needed if these cells are to become neurons. SA progenitors plated on a suitable laminin-containing substrate in the absence of any growth factor form short, neuron-like processes (Fig. 16.12C). These processes are much more extensive when the growth factor FGF is added to the medium, whereas the neurotrophic factor NGF has no effect. Initially, SA progenitors are unresponsive to NGF because they do not express the NGF receptor. One of the effects of FGF is to induce the NGF receptor gene, thereby making the SA cells responsive to NGF, which stimulates their differentiation as neurons.

Some SA progenitors continue to migrate further and populate the adrenal gland, where they begin to differentiate. Here, they are exposed to glucocorticoid hormone (Fig. 16.12D). Glucocorticoids are steroid

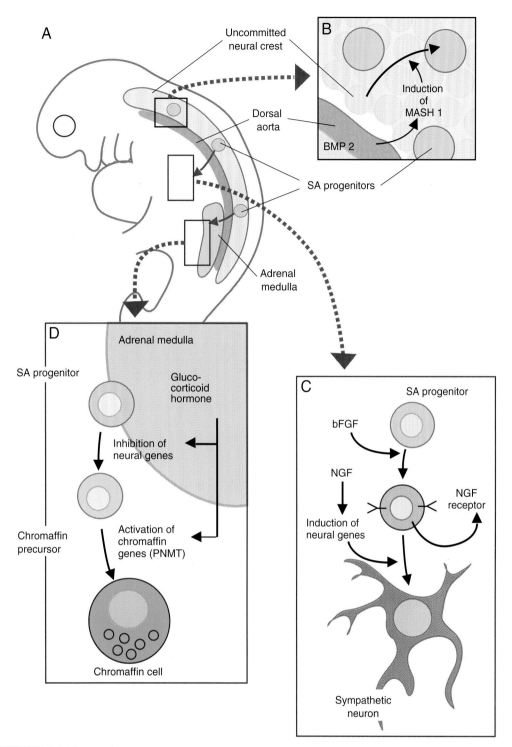

FIGURE 16.12 Cell fate determination of the SA progenitor in vertebrates. SA progenitors represent a subpopulation of neural crest cells (A). Secreted signals from the dorsal aorta, including BMP2, induce the expression of proneural genes (MASH 1) in the SA progenitors and thereby drive this cell onto a neural pathway (B). Other extrinsic cues are required for the final differentiation of the SA progenitor. The sequential action of bFGF and NGF induces differentiation of the SA progenitor as a sympathetic neuron (C). Glucocorticoids (D) sequentially evoke two different responses: (1) they inhibit neuronal differentiation by suppressing the transcription of neuron-specific genes (*peripherin*, *GAP-43*) and (2) they activate transcription of chromaffin cell-specific genes (e.g., *PNMT*).

hormones that bind to receptors that themselves can serve as regulators of gene transcription. Glucocorticoids evoke two different responses in SA progenitors in culture: (1) they inhibit neuronal differentiation by suppressing the transcription of neuron-specific genes and (2) they activate the transcription of chromaffin cell-specific genes such as PNMT. The effect of the hormone-activated glucocorticoid receptor on these genes, at least in the case of PNMT, seems to be a direct one, as binding sites for the glucocorticoid receptor have been identified in the regulatory region of the PNMT gene.

Neuregulin-1 (**Nrg-1**) is a secreted protein that induces crest cells to adopt glial fates (Fig. 16.13). Neural crest cells express Nrg-1 once they have migrated peripherally and coalesced into distinct masses, as in the dorsal root or sympathetic ganglia. Nrg-1 is expressed in those cells that have already started to exhibit a neuronal phenotype, and not in glial cells. The Nrg-1 receptor is expressed by all migrating neural crest cells, so cells are sensitive to Nrg-1 as soon as they arrive at their destination. In the absence of added Nrg-1, the majority of clones obtained from cultured neural crest cells contain both neurons and glial cells, but if Nrg-1 is applied, it suppresses the expression of a neuronal phenotype and

most clones develop as pure glia. However, if crest cells are exposed to both BMP-2 and Nrg-1 in culture, BMP-2 predominates and most cells develop as neurons. Notch activation also regulates glial determination in crest-derived cells. As neurons begin to differentiate, they express Dl, which through Notch activation on neighboring cells overrides the neuralizing influence of BMP2 and turns off proneural gene activity.

Neural Fate in Vertebrate CNS: Specification of Glia

The optic nerve, in addition to containing the axons of retinal ganglion cells, has two main types of glia: astrocytes, which make contact with blood vessels and nodes of Ranvier, and oligodendrocytes, which myelinate axons. Oligodendrocytes and astrocytes derive from distinct precursor cells: Oligodendrocyte precursor cells (OPCs) and astrocyte precursor cells (APCs; Fig. 16.4A). When OPC cells are cultured in a serum-free medium, they stop dividing and become oligodendrocytes, but when cultured in the presence of astrocytes, they continue to divide before differentiating, much as they do *in vivo*. Astrocytes secrete platelet-derived growth factor (PDGF) and neuro-

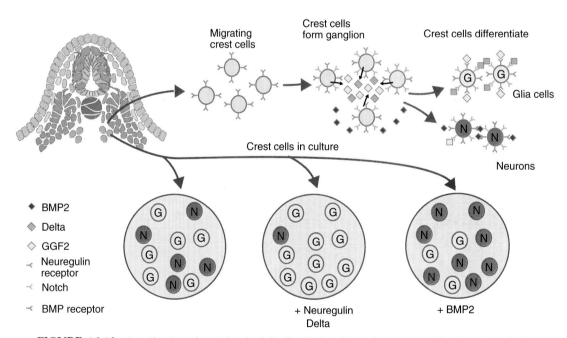

FIGURE 16.13 Specification of peripheral glial cells. If placed in culture, crest cells give rise to both neurons (N) and glial cells (G). Addition of the secreted signal neuregulin to the medium, or expressing the signal molecule Delta, enhances the proportion of glial cells developing from the culture. BMP2 has the opposite effect, increasing the number of neurons. These and other data suggest a model in which fluctuations in the level of secreted or membrane-bound signals in the local environment of neural crest cells will lead to the segregation of glial cells and neurons from an initially homogeneous cell population.

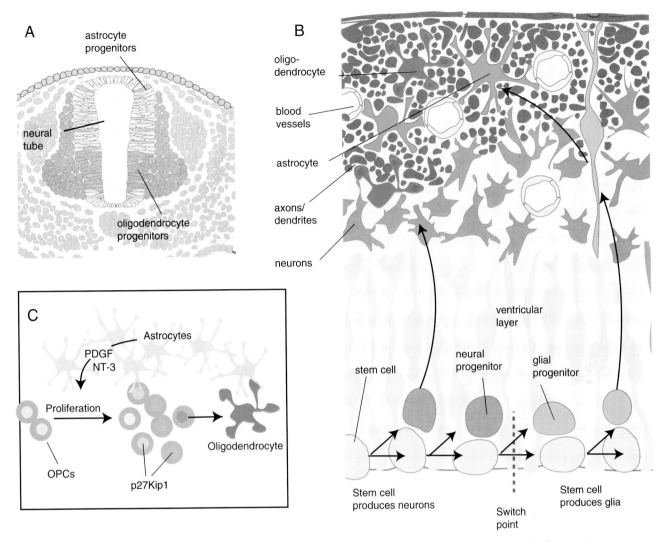

FIGURE 16.14 Glial cell development in vertebrates. Two main types of glial cells, oligodendrocytes and astrocytes, are formed in the neural tube. Astrocyte progenitors are distributed at all levels, whereas oligodendrocyte progenitors derive from the ventral neural tube (A). Oligodendrocytes form processes that wrap around axons and give rise to the myelin sheath (B). Astrocyte processes connect to capillaries and neurites. Glial progenitors and neural progenitors are derived from the same pool of stem cells that divide in the ventricular layer of the developing neural tube (bottom of B). At early stages, a stem cell generates neuroblasts. Later, it undergoes a specific asymmetric division (the "switch point") at which it changes from making neurons to making glia. (C) In a culture system of optic nerve-derived oligodendrocyte progenitors (OPC) and astrocytes, OPCs depend on secreted signals for proper proliferation and differentiation. Astroytes secrete PDGF and NT-3, which maintains cell division. In the absence of these factors, OPCs stop dividing and differentiate. The internal clock that determines when an OPG stops dividing and differentiates depends on the level of the p27Kip1 protein, a cell cycle inhibitor that increases over time with continued proliferation and finally drives the cells to exit the cell cycle.

trophin 3, which stimulate the continued division of OPCs (Fig. 16.4C). In the presence of PDGF, OPCs appear to rely on an intrinsic clock to time their differentiation. If enough PDGF is present, OPCs differentiate after a given number of cell divisions. The clock seems partially to run on the buildup of p27Kip1, a cell cycle inhibitor that increases over time with continued proliferation and finally drives the cells to exit the cell cycle.

In the central nervous system of vertebrates, multipotent stem cells give rise to glia as well as neurons. It is usually the case that neurons arise first and glia last. Time-lapse studies of these stem cells in culture show that they tend to go through several rounds of asymmetrical cell divisions, giving rise to neuroblasts, and they suddenly make a transition to symmetrical cell divisions, which give rise to glioblasts (Qian *et al.*,

2000) (Fig. 16.4B). It is not known how this transition happens, although several studies indicate that activation of the Notch signaling pathway plays an important role in gliogenesis. Transient activation of Notch promotes the differentiation of astroglia from hippocampus-derived neural stem cells. When a constitutively activated form of Notch is introduced via a viral host into the embryonic forebrain, many of the infected cells become radial glia. If a comparable experiment is performed later, around the time of birth, the infected cells become periventricular astrocytes, which are a likely source of neural stem cells (see Box 16.1). Activation of the Notch pathway suppresses the transcription of proneural bHLH transcription factor, such as neurogenin-1 (Ngn-1), which promotes neurogenesis by functioning as a transcriptional activator for genes involved in neural differentiation. Interestingly, Ngn-1 also blocks astrocyte differentiation by inhibiting transcription factors that are necessary for gliogenesis.

Cell–Cell Signaling Determines Fate in the Insect Compound Eye

The insect compound eye is built of a large number of identical facets, called ommatidia (Wolff and Ready, 1993). *Drosophila* possesses approximately 800 ommatidia in each eye. Each contains several different cell types of photoreceptors and accessory cells. There are eight identifiably unique photoreceptors in each ommatidium; six of them (R1–R6) form an outer trapezoidal array, whereas two (R7 and R8) are located in the center (Figs. 16.15 and 16.16A). Among the accessory cells are cone cells, which form the lens of each ommatidium, and pigment cells, which surround the photoreceptors and optically shield the ommatidia from one another.

Cells of the ommatidia are formed from clonally unrelated, uncommitted precursor cells that are generated from the proliferation of cells in the eye imaginal disc. This is quite different from the neuroblast-derived CNS neurons or SOP-derived peripheral sensilla described earlier, whose cells are typically produced in a fixed lineage. In the eye, cell–cell interactions between postmitotic photoreceptors and accessory cells are solely responsible for specifying cell fates. A crucial part of the mechanism relies on the fact that ommatidial cells do not appear all at once, but follow a reproducible temporal sequence (Fig. 16.6B). During late larval life, a wave of differentiation passes over the eye disc in a posterior-to-anterior direction. In front of the wave, cells are still

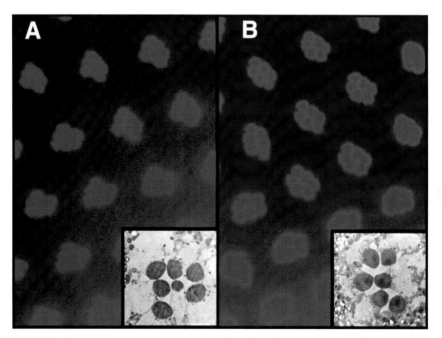

FIGURE 16.15 Photoreceptors in the eye of normal and *sevenless* mutants. (A) If a light is shined from the back of a fly's head and focused in the facets of the eye, individual photoreceptors can be seen because of their ability to pipe light. The wild-type animal has the normal pattern of seven photoreceptors visible in each facet. The small one in the center is photoreceptor R7. (B) The same technique used in a *sevenless* mutant shows only the six large photoreceptors R1–6 in each facet. R7 is missing. Insets show electron micrographs through single facets.

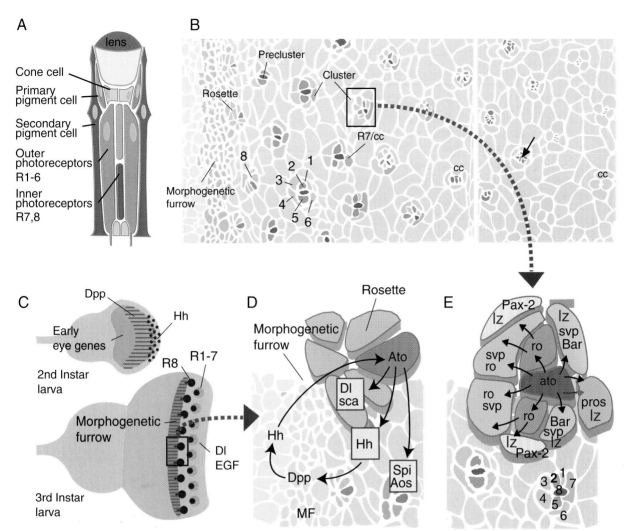

FIGURE 16.16 Determination of ommatidial cell fate in the *Drosophila* compound eye. (A) Schematic longitudinal section of ommatidium depicting cell types in different colors. (B) Diagram based on a camera lucida drawing (Wolff and Ready, 1993) showing a surface view of part of the eye imaginal disc at a stage when photoreceptor clusters become assembled in a sequential fashion. Gray profiles indicate the apical surface of undifferentiated cells; colored profiles demarcate different types of photoreceptors and cone cells. At the left margin, all cells are undifferentiated. This is followed by a phase in which eye disc cells become more closely packed and constricted at their apical pole, thereby forming the morphogenetic furrow. As they leave the furrow, cells form more or less regularly spaced rosettes (light red). Within each rosette, a single cell becomes singled out as the photoreceptor R8 (dark red). At the time when it becomes distinguishable morphologically, four other photoreceptors (R2, R5: lilac; R3, R4: blue) have joined R8. Together, these five cells form the so-called preclusters. Three more photoreceptors (R1, R6: blue; R7: orange) join the preclusters, leading up to complete photoreceptor clusters. This step is followed by the appearance of four cone cells (green) which surround the photoreceptors in a circular fashion. On the right side of the panel, photoreceptors can be seen to segregate from the surface. Their apical membranes (all shown in purple) become increasingly smaller (arrow) and finally disappear altogether. (C) Initiation of compound eye development. During midlarval stages (Top), the signal Hedgehog (Hh; red) is expressed at the posterior tip of the eye disc. Hh activates the expression of another signaling protein, Dpp (blue), which turns on several "early eye genes," which commit the undifferentiated, proliferating cells that comprise the eye disc to an eye fate. During late larval stages, Hh and other factors initiate differentiation of the first ommatidial cells, the R8 photoreceptors, by turning on the proneural gene atonal (ato). This sets in motion other signaling pathways (EGFR signaling; Notch/Delta signaling) required for the proper spacing of ommatidia and the determination of other ommatidial cell fates. (D) Determination and spacing of R8 are controlled by the proneural gene *atonal* (*ato*), as well as the inhibitory signals Delta (Dl) and Scabrous (Sca). Initially switched on in the entire morphogenetic furrow, *ato* expression then becomes restricted to a mosaic of regularly spaced cells, which subsequently differentiate as R8. Continued secretion of Hh, which signals across the MF toward the more anterior cells of the eye disc, drives the morphogenetic furrow across the eye disc. (E) Determination of photoreceptors R1–R7 and cone cells. Secretion of the TGF B homologue Spitz (Spi) from R8 stimulates cells surrounding R8 via the *Drosophila* EGF receptor homologue (DER), the Ras signaling pathway (symbolized by black arrows). In conjunction with other signaling events, including Notch/Delta, photoreceptors are induced to express specific transcription factors, which are required for their respective fates. The *lozenge (lz)* gene is expressed in R1, R6, R7, and cone cells; *seven-up (svp)* is expressed in R1, 6, 3, and 4; *rough (ro)* in R2, 3, 4, and 5; *BarI* in R1, and 6; *prospero (pros)* in R7, and *Pax-2* in cone cells.

dividing and uncommitted, whereas behind the wave front, which is visible as a depression in the disc called the *morphogenetic furrow* (MF), cells are mostly postmitotic and are beginning to differentiate. As they leave the MF, cells of the eye disc become arranged in a pattern of "rosettes" that foreshadow the regular ommatidial pattern. Soon afterward, one cell, which will become the R8 photoreceptor, is singled out in each rosette. Subsequently, signals emitted by R8 induce neighboring cells to adopt the other ommatidial cell fates. Being the first cells to differentiate, R8 cells can be considered as "crystallization centers" around which the other ommatidial cells aggregate in a stereotyped pattern. Accordingly, the mechanism controlling compound eye development can be broken down into the induction and spacing of R8 cells and the induction of other ommatidial cell types.

Induction and Spacing of R8

To grasp the intricate back-and-forth signaling processes that ultimately lead to the regular pattern of R8 cells, we need to begin at an early stage in eye disc development when the disc comprises a small pouch of proliferating cells. At this stage, a set of transcription factors, encoded by the so-called early eye genes, is expressed in the disc (Fig. 16.16C). Among the early eye genes are *sine oculis, eyes absent, eyeless,* and *dachshund* (Brennan and Moses, 2000), each of which has a homologue in vertebrates that is also involved in eye development. The role of early eye genes is to commit the undifferentiated, proliferating cells that comprise the eye disc to an eye fate. Absence of any single eye gene results in a failure of eye development. In turn, ectopic expression of an early eye gene in another undifferentiated primordium, such as that of the wing or leg, is able to induce ectopic eye development.

Cells expressing early eye genes require the expression of another gene, the proneural gene *atonal (ato),* to develop into R8 photoreceptors. *Ato* is turned on by the signaling protein Hh (a homologue of vertebrate Shh, discussed in Chapter 15), which is expressed at the posterior tip of the eye disc. Initially, *ato* comes on in a continuous band of cells within the morphogenetic furrow. Atonal, similar to proneural gene function in the ventral neurectoderm, initiates a lateral inhibition mechanism that involves N/Dl signaling (Fig. 16.16D). By this mechanism, *ato* expression becomes restricted to a mosaic of regularly spaced cells, which subsequently differentiate as R8. These cells continue emitting Hh, which signals across the MF toward the more anterior cells of the eye disc to induce the next set of R8 cells. This Hh-mediated feedback mechanism drives the wave of differentiation, i.e., the morphogenetic furrow, across the eye disc.

Induction of Other Ommatidial Cells by R8

The expression of *ato* in cells leaving the morphogenetic furrow commits cells exclusively to the R8 fate. No other cell of the ommatidium expresses this gene, indicating that *ato* is an intrinsic determinant only for R8. However, deleting *ato* results in the total failure of eye development, which indicates that R8 must play a pivotal inductive role, triggering the determination of other cells that join the ommatidial clusters in an invariant temporal sequence. The first cells to join the R8 cell shortly after its determination are R2, R3 R4, and R5 (Fig. 16.6B). Together with R8 they make up an ommatidial "precluster." The next cells to join the cluster are R1 and R6, followed by R7 and four cone cells; the last cells to join the cluster are the different types of pigment cells.

Each type of ommatidial cell expresses a unique set of intrinsic determinants. For example, *rough (ro)* is expressed in all cells of the precluster except R8 (i.e., in R2, R5, R3, R4). *BarI* appears in R1 and R6; *Seven-up (svp)* in R1, R6, R3, R4, *Prospero (pros)* in R7 and cone cells, and *Pax-2* in cone cells only (Fig. 16.16E). Each of these factors is intricately linked to the normal differentiation of the respective cells in which it is expressed, as revealed by the fact that a particular cell type fails to develop in an eye disc that lacks the corresponding gene. The main question is how the expression of the cell-type-specific sets of transcription factors are directed to the proper cells. It was originally suspected that specific signals are required to elicit the expression of particular transcription factors. However, a wealth of experimental studies carried out over the last decade has unearthed only a small number of signaling pathways. It now seems that various combinations of fairly common signaling pathways activated in precise spatiotemporal patterns are responsible for specifying the plethora of different transcription factors in the ommatidial cells.

Shortly following its own determination, R8 puts out signals that activate two different signaling pathways: Notch and Ras. The Notch pathway is activated by Dl, which we had already encountered in the previous sections as a lateral inhibitor of neurogenesis. The Ras pathway represents a highly conserved biochemical cascade of cytoplasmic kinases (Ras, Raf, MPK), which in this case are activated by the epidermal growth factor receptor (EGFR). R8 emits a signal, Spitz (Spi), that activates this receptor and another signal, Argos (Aos), that acts as an inhibitor. Activation of these signaling cascades spreads concentrically from R8 to the precluster cells (R2, R3, R4, and R5) and then the remainder of the ommatidial cells. The precise, temporally regulated activation of EGFR and Notch signaling pathways assigns distinct phenotypes to the cells that join the ommatidial clusters.

The way in which differential signaling pathway activation controls ommatidial cell fates has been studied most closely for two cell types, R7 and the cone cells, which appear at a relatively late stage when all other photoreceptors are already in place. The *Pax-2* gene specifies cone cells. To express *Pax-2*, the cone-cell-to-be depends on three inputs (Flores *et al.*, 2000): (1) the previous expression of the transcription factor *lozenge* (*lz*); (2) activation of the N/Dl pathway, and (3) activation of the EGFR signaling pathway. If any one of these prerequisites is not met, the cells will fail to express *Pax-2* and will not differentiate as cone cells. Conversely, if a set of cells that normally does not receive all three inputs is exposed to them experimentally, these cells will express *Pax-2* and become cone cells. For example, the precluster cells that normally form R3 and R4 activate both Ras and N pathways, but do not express *lz*. If *lz* expression is turned on in these cells experimentally, they develop as cone cells. Conversely, R7 normally expresses *lz*, but does not activate the N pathway. Expression of activated N in the R7 precursor will turn this cell into a cone cell.

The effect of *lz*, EGFR, and N/Dl signaling on *Pax-2* expression is a direct one. Biochemical analyses have shown that Lz, as well as the "output" transcription factors activated by EGFR signaling (Pnt) and N/Dl signaling (Su(H)), bind to and activate the *Pax-2* gene directly. It is thought that the regulation of other transcription factors required for the production of different ommatidial cell fates may also be specified directly by a temporally controlled profile of Notch and Ras activation.

Sevenless and the Induction of R7

The determination of the R7 cell deserves special mention in view of the pivotal role it has played in opening up the molecular–genetic study of signaling pathways. The important advantage of a genetic model system like *Drosophila* has to offer is that developmentally relevant molecules, such as signaling proteins, receptors, and signal transducers, can be identified by mutant screens. One of the first of such screens in the field of cell determination took advantage of the fact that only one of the photoreceptor cells of each ommatidium, R7, is sensitive to ultra violet (UV) light. Thus, mutagenizing flies and screening for offspring that are blind to UV light yielded a fly line that lacked the R7 cell in every ommatidium and was therefore aptly called *sevenless* (*sev*) (Fig. 16.5). The close study of this gene showed that it encodes a

receptor of the receptor tyrosine kinase family and that it is expressed (among other cells of the eye disc) in the cell that will become R7. Lack of the receptor causes the cell that would normally become R7 to develop as a cone cell instead. In several follow-up screens, many signal transducing molecules and transcription factors activated by the Sev receptor were identified. Among them were the *Drosophila* homologues of Ras, Raf, and MAPK. One of the most rewarding findings was the identification of the signal that binds to Sev. Given the widespread expression of Sev, it was clear that a signal emanating from a point source must exist, in order to ensure that Sev would become active only in one cell. The logical candidate to emit such signal would be R8, the only cell in broad contact with the presumptive R7. A genetic screen for R7-less flies yielded identification of a membrane bound signaling molecule, called Bride of sevenless (Boss), that is expressed specifically in R8 cells and serves as the ligand for Sev. These experiments provided an impressive demonstration of the awesome power of genetic screens combined with precise knowledge of the developing system in identifying new genes and proteins controlling development.

In light of more recent results concerning the role of the Ras signaling pathway in ommatidial development, the role of Boss and Sev may seem puzzling. As stated earlier in this section, the Ras signaling pathway, activated by the EGFR and its signal Spi, is active in all photoreceptor cells and is required for cell specification. Furthermore, Spi or EGFR can fully substitute for the Sev receptor: Flies lacking the Sev gene can be rescued by expressing active EGFR in the presumptive R7 cells. So why is there a separate signal/receptor activating the Ras pathway required in R7? As in many such seemingly enigmatic occurrences of "unnecessary" complexity in nature, one can only speculate. One possible explanation is phylogenetic: Perhaps R7, as the last appearing photoreceptor in the photoreceptor cluster, was added at a later stage of evolution and may have required a second boost in Ras signaling. The genetic control mechanism had at least two ways to accomplish this. First, control of Spi release could have been modified such that a second peak occurred at the time of R7 appearance. Second, a new signal/receptor system that acted more locally could have been recruited. Nature "chose" the second alternative.

Neuronal Fate in the Vertebrate Spinal Cord

Cell specification in vertebrate spinal cord, especially along the dorsoventral axis, is an excellent system for investigating the control of cell fates in the

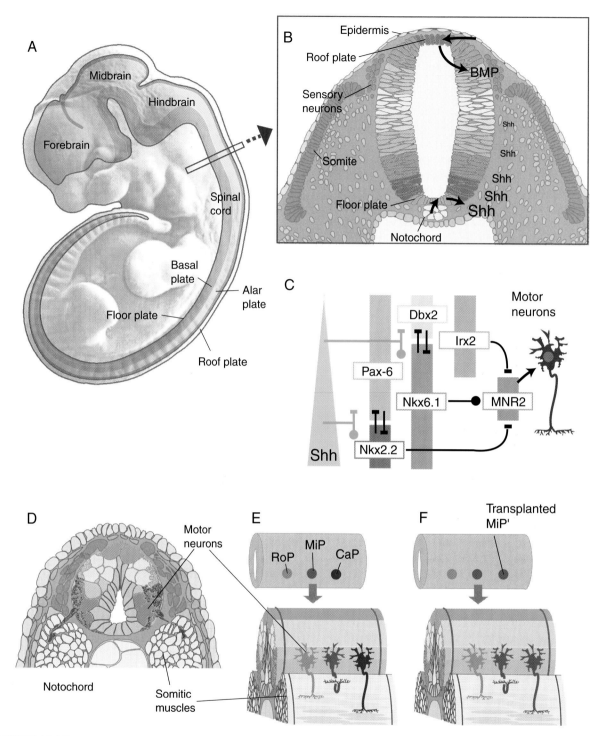

FIGURE 16.17 Specification of motor neurons in the vertebrate spinal cord. **(A)** The neural tube, shown here for a mouse, is subdivided into four longitudinal domains: the floor plate, basal plate, alar plate, and roof plate. Motor neurons are derived from the basal plate. **(B)** Schematic cross section of the neural tube. The notochord, which is located underneath the floor plate, releases the signal Sonic hedgehog (Shh). Consecutively, Shh is released from the floor plate and forms a gradient with high concentrations ventrally and low concentrations dorsally. BMP molecules released from the dorsal epidermis and dorsal neural tube form an opposing gradient. **(C)** In a concentration-dependent manner, Shh directs expression domains of the class I and class II homeodomain genes (see text for details). **(D)** Schematic cross section of a late embryonic zebrafish embryo depicting the location of primary motor neurons and somites, which give rise to axial musculature. **(E):** Each zebrafish somite is initially innervated by three primary motor neurons. RoP, MiP, and CaP. These neurons project their axons to intermediate, dorsal, and ventral axial muscles, respectively. **(F)** If MiP is transplanted to a posterior position prior to axon formation, it adapts to the new environment and projects to the ventral musculature.

CNS because there are a limited number of neural types (Jessell, 2000). The most ventral part of the cord is called the *floor plate* and dorsal to this structure are different classes of interneurons and motor neurons (Figs.16.17A and 16.17B). Transplantation experiments have shown that the floor plate is induced by a Shh signal emitted from the underlying notochord (see Chapter 14). Once induced, the floor plate serves as a secondary source of Shh. As a result of these ventral sources, a gradient of the Shh signal seems to percolate dorsally. Amazingly, at least five different neuronal types are generated progressively in response to this single gradient. The most ventral neurons require the highest doses of Shh, and successively more dorsal ones require correspondingly less. When Shh is missing or antagonized with an antibody, there is no floor plate, nor indeed any ventral neuronal type in the spinal cord.

How do cells at different dorsoventral levels interpret their differential exposure to a single molecule to acquire different fates? The readout of the Shh level is first registered by the expression of several homeodomain proteins, which are either turned on or off at particular Shh thresholds (Fig. 16.17C). Class I proteins are repressed at different Shh thresholds, whereas class II proteins are activated at particular Shh concentrations. In this way, the ventral boundaries of class I expression and the dorsal boundaries of class II expression set up several unique domains. The boundaries between these domains are sharpened through cross-repression of the two classes of genes. Thus, for example if the ventral border of the class I *Pax-6* gene overlaps the dorsal border of the class II *Nkx2.2* gene, cross-repression sets in so that only one of these genes is expressed in any particular progenitor. In each domain, then, a certain combination of homeodomain transcription factors is uniquely expressed. Note that except for the role of Shh in initiating these longitudinal stripes of homeodomain transcription factors, the mechanism is very similar to that used in setting up the mediolateral coordinate genes *vnd*, *ind*, and *msh*, in *Drosophila*. Indeed *vnd* is homologous to *Nkx2,* suggesting a conserved coordinate system.

Motor neurons arise from the domain that uniquely expresses *Nkx6.1* but not *Irx3* and *Nkx2.2*. *Nkx6.1*, unhindered by the repressive activities of these other factors, turns on another gene called *MNR2* uniquely in this domain. Once expressed, MNR2, which is itself a transcription factor, can regulate its own expression and is sufficient to drive spinal progenitor cells down a motor neuron pathway. The latter has been shown by experiments in which motor neurons arise dorsally when MNR2 is expressed ectopically in dorsal progenitors that would normally make interneurons.

Motor neurons in the spinal cord are organized into functional columns that project to different muscle groups in the mature animal. A combinatorial code of different LIM/homeodomain transcription factors uniquely defines the different motor columns. These motor columns can be further divided into pools that innervate specific muscles. In zebrafish, each spinal segment has just three primary motor neurons: RoP, MiP, and CaP (for rostral, middle, and caudal primary; Figs. 16.17D, and 16.17E). CaP innervates ventral muscle, RoP innervates lateral muscle, and MiP innervates dorsal muscle. If these motor neurons are transplanted to different positions a few hours before they begin axonogenesis, they seem to switch fate; e.g., CaP transplanted into the RoP position can innervate lateral instead of ventral muscle (Eisen, 1991; Fig. 16.17E). These results suggest that the position of the cell soma specifies the axonal projection of the different primary neurons. When these primary motor neurons change their projection pattern, they initiate a new program of LIM homeobox gene expression.

Finally, motor columns are further subdivided into motor pools that innervate individual muscles. These pools are distinguished by the expression of a distinct member of the ETS family of transcription factors. For example the ETS gene *ER81* is expressed in motor neurons that innervate the limb adductor muscle in chicks, whereas iliotrochanter motor neurons express the *PEA3* ETS gene. We will come back to these ETS genes in the last part of this chapter where we discuss target influences on the development of the neuronal phenotype.

Dorsal fates in the spinal cord depend on a BMP signal, secreted from the epidermis flanking the neural plate. Dorsal progenitors, like neural crest, appear to depend on BMPs to turn on crest markers like *slug*. BMPs also induce roof plate cells of the neural tube to express *Dorsalin*, another BMP family member. It appears that the BMP gradient emanating from the dorsal neural tube opposes the Shh, gradient emanating from the ventral regions. When spinal cord explants from the intermediate regions are exposed to Shh, they form ventral cell types, but if BMP is added, they form more dorsal cell types.

Temporal Changes in Extrinsic Cues

Histogenesis of the Cerebral Cortex

External cues can change with time. One of the best examples of this comes from the mammalian cortex. The cerebral cortex is a six-layered structure in which each layer has distinct populations of neurons that

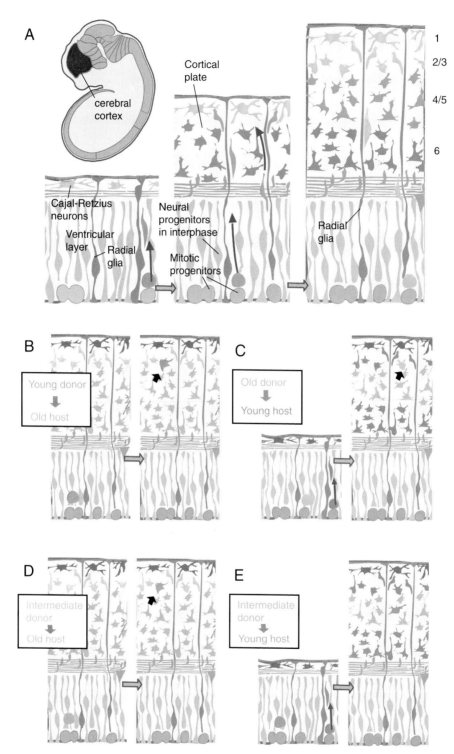

FIGURE 16.18 Laminar fate determination in the cerebral cortex. (A) Morphogenesis of the mammalian cerebral cortex. Neural precursors are born in the ventricular layer and migrate away from the ventricular surface, following tracks provided by radial glial cells. The first born cells are the Cajal-Retzius neurons (left in figure). Later born neurons accumulate in a dense matrix of cells, the cortical plate (middle of figure). In this plate, neurons are ordered by birth date in such a way that older neurons (magenta) remain in deep layers, and younger neurons (blue) migrate through the deep layers to attain a superficial position (right in figure). (B) If ventricular cells from young donors (which normally would become deep cells) are transplanted into an old host, they adapt to their new environment and develop as superficial neurons (arrow). (C) In converse heterochronic transplantation (old donor to young host), transplanted ventricular cells maintain their laminar fate and become superficial neurons. (D) Layer 4 neurons transplanted into older brains switch their fate so that it is appropriate for the upper layer neurons. (E) When layer 4 neurons are transplanted into younger hosts, they end up in layers 4 and 5, but not layer 6.

differ in size, morphology, and projection patterns. Cortical neurons arise from asymmetric divisions of progenitors or stem cells in the ventricular zone. They then migrate along radial glial processes to the forming cortical plate where they arrange themselves in an inside-out gradient, such that the earliest-generated cells inhabit deepest layers and the last-born cells are nearest the surface (Fig. 16.18A). Thus cells destined for layers 2/3 must migrate through layers 6, 5, and 4, which have already formed. In principle, cortical cells could be determined with respect to layer as they are generated or they might obtain their fate from the position they migrate into. To test these possibilities, cells generated at early times were transplanted into older hosts (McConnell, 1995) (Fig. 16.18B). Although in a normal environment their time of birth would have fated them for layer 6, many of the transplanted cells switched their fates and ended up in layers 2/3. Further experiments showed that these early generated cells are derived from multipotent cells that fix their fate according to the environment in which they complete their final cell division. The environment changes with time, thus providing distinct cues that influence cellular fate. In contrast to the earliest-born cells, cells born at much later times destined for the upper layers of cortex are restricted in their developmental potential. These cells produce upper layer cortical cells when they are transplanted into a younger animal (Fig. 16.18C), regardless of where they complete their final cell cycle. These experiments suggest that progenitors found at late stages of neurogenesis have lost the competence to produce earlier-generated phenotypes.

What about the laminar fate potential of progenitors in the middle stages of cortical development? When the progenitors of layer 4 neurons are transplanted into older brains, in which layer 2/3 was being generated, they switch their fate so that it is appropriate for the later environment and generate layer 2/3 neurons (Fig. 16.18D). However, when transplanted into a younger environment in which layer 6 neurons are being generated, they show a restricted potential, ending up in layers 4 and 5, but not 6 (Fig. 16.18E). These results suggest that environmental cues influence progenitors to produce neurons of different layers, but that the competency of these precursors becomes increasingly restricted over time so that they can respond only to a similar or older environment, but not a younger one.

Histogenesis of the Vertebrate Retina

The vertebrate retina develops from a population of pluripotent neuroepithelial progenitors, which produce a diversity of neurons and glia (Figs. 16.19 and 16.20B). Neurogenesis and determination in the retina follow a temporal but lineage-independent order (Livesy and Cepko, 2001). Thus, at any given time during retinogenesis, only a few fates are available to differentiating cells. Cells born early in mammals generally adopt fates as retinal ganglion cells (Figs. 16.20B and 16.20C). Horizontal cells and cones are also born early. Amacrine cells are produced subsequently, followed by rods, bipolars, and Müller cells. This progressive shift in cell type genesis is supported by dissociation experiments in which cells are put into culture at low density at various stages of development. It is possible to force cells to differentiate prematurely because isolation inhibits mitotic activity. Thus, if mitotic cells are isolated at the time when retinal ganglion cells (RGCs) are normally born, their progeny tend to turn into ganglion cells in culture. If mitotic cells are isolated at later stages, they become rod photoreceptors in culture.

These results are consistent with an intrinsic progression of cell fates, which could operate via a clock mechanism such that cells generated early are intrinsically fated to become RGCs and later ones to become rods. To test this idea, retinal cells were removed at the stage when RGCs are being born, labelled with BrdU, dissociated, mixed into aggregates, and cultured *in vitro* (Fig. 16.20E). The labeled cells differentiated into RGCs. However, if the same types of cells were mixed with an excess of retinal cells several days older (i.e., when photoreceptors were being generated), the labeled cells generally became photoreceptors. This work shows that individual cells have the capacity to differentiate into different cell types, and the fate they choose depends largely on the environment in which they are born. One mechanism that promotes the production of distinct fates at different times is that earlier generated cell types negatively regulate their own numbers. For example, RGCs secrete a factor that inhibits other cells from choosing an RGC fate (Fig. 16.20D). Differentiated RGCs also secrete NGF, which binds to the p75 receptor that is expressed on cells that are in the process of becoming RGCs. Activation of the p75 receptor leads to cell death (see Chapter 20). RGCs thus have two activities: one that prevents the determination of other RGCs and one that kills any potential RGCs that escape the first signal.

The Notch signaling pathway, by allowing only a certain number of cells to differentiate at any one time, is also very important in creating cellular diversity in the vertebrate retina (Dorsky *et al.*, 1997). Because the expression of specific factors that influence cell fate changes over time, the changing competence of a cell to respond to its immediate envi-

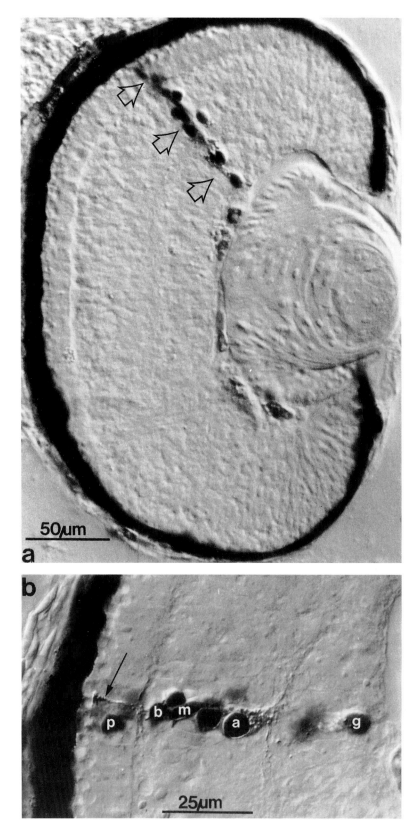

FIGURE 16.19 Clone of cells in the *Xenopus* retina. (a) Daughters of a single retina progenitor injected with horseradish peroxidase are seen to form a column that spans the retinal layers and contributes many distinct cell types, (b) p, photoreceptor; b, bipolar cell; m, Muller cell; a, amacrine cell; and g, ganglion cell.

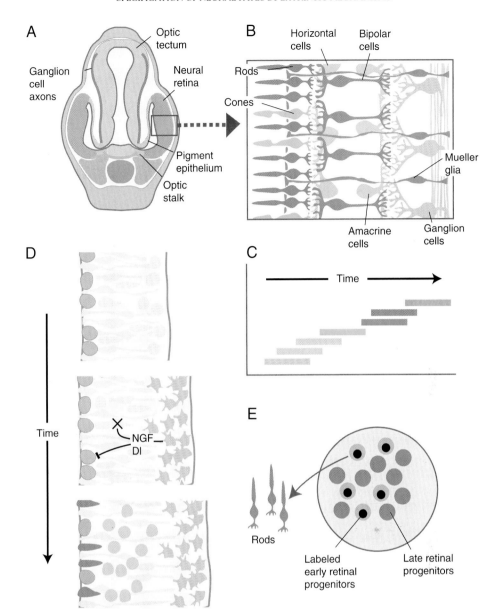

FIGURE 16.20 Vertebrate retina development. (A) The neural retina bulges out of the ventral neural tube at the level of the diencephalon. It is joined to the brain by the optic stalk along which the axons of retinal ganlion cells will course on their way to the tectum. (B) The seven major cell types in the retina coded by color. Their laminar arrangement by cell type is evident. (C) Birth dating studies in the retina show that different cell types are born in different but overlapping periods of histogenesis. (D) Differentiation inhibitors (DI) released from RGCs inhibit retinoblasts from producing RGCs. RGCs also release NGF, which can kill newly differentiating RGCs before they fully differentiate. (E) When early generated cells (labeled by a pulse of BrdU) are mixed with older cells in culture, they show an increased probability of turning into late cells, such as rods.

ronment will have a dramatic impact on its fate. Retinal cells can be forced to differentiate earlier or later than normal by manipulating the levels of Notch and Delta signaling; this in turn causes cells to assume fates that appear appropriate for the time at which they differentiate. If all cells were permitted to respond at the same instant, they might all choose the same fate! Thus the neurogenic signaling pathway in the vertebrate retina is a basic regulatory mechanism that can be used to generate neuronal diversity by affecting the timing of differentiation in a changing external environment.

Target Tissues Regulate Cell Fate

The fate of a neuron may be determined completely in many respects at the time it is born or shortly thereafter. For some neurons, however, the final fate choice comes only after the cell has established contact with its synaptic targets, showing that decisions about cell fate can stretch from early embryogenesis to the final phases of differentiation. In many neurons, a final fate choice is between survival and death, and this decision is often influenced strongly by trophic factors produced by the target. Target-dependent neuronal cell death is discussed in Chapter 19. This chapter presents examples of other dramatic decisions influenced by the target.

Transmitter Choice by Sympathetic Neurons

All neural crest cells that become sympathetic neurons start life producing the neurotransmitter noradrenalin. They receive the signal to be adrenergic as they migrate; by the time these neurons coalesce into ganglia, they are all adrenergic. Many of these neurons send out axons to smooth muscle targets; these sympathetic neurons remain adrenergic throughout life. A few sympathetic neurons, however—e.g., those that innervate sweat glands—switch their neurotransmitter phenotype late in development and secrete the neurotransmitter acetylcholine (Ach; Fig. 16.21). Neurotransmitter choice in these cells is a late aspect of cell fate that is regulated by the target (Francis and Landis, 1999). Fibres innervating sweat glands are initially entirely adrenergic, but during the second postnatal week in the rat, the neurons begin to turn off tyrosine hydroxylase and other adrenergic enzymes and begin to make choline acetyltransferase, the synthetic enzyme for ACh production. The ablation of adrenergic neurons at early stages of development completely eliminated the emergence of cholinergic innervation, indicating that the two transmitters come from the same fibers that switch transmitter phenotype rather than from distinct populations of axons that arrive at different times. Dramatic evidence for the role of the sweat glands themselves in inducing the switch in phenotypes comes from transplantation experiments. Transplanting foot pad tissue, rich in sweat glands, to areas of the body that usually receive adrenergic sympathetic innervation, such as the hairy skin of the thorax, leads to the induction of cholinergic function in the sympathetic axons that innervate the transplanted glands. Similarly, replacing footpad tissue with a noradrenergic target causes the population of sympathetic neurons that usually switch their transmitter to remain noradrenergic. Factors capable of causing an

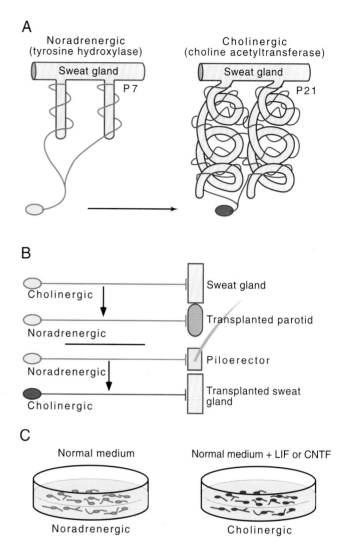

FIGURE 16.21 Transmitter switching by target-derived factors. (A) All sympathetic neurons appear to start differentiation as noradrenergic neurons. Some of these neurons—in this case, a rat—innervate the sweat glands. Noradrenergic sympathetic neurons that innervate the sweat gland invariably switch their transmitter phenotype as the sweat gland matures. These neurons stop making tyrosine hydroxylase and start making choline acetyltransferase. (B) Switching *in vivo* can be affected by transplanting different end organs to the same sympathetic neurons. Thus the adrenergic-to-cholinergic switch can be prevented by replacing sweat gland-rich targets such as the foot pad with a piece of parotid gland, usually the recipient of adrenergic innervation. Conversely, an adrenergic-to-cholinergic switch can be accomplished by transplanting foot pad tissue onto hairy skin, which is usually innervated by adrenergic sympathetic neurons. (C) Factors such as LIF and CNTF, found in target tissues such as heart muscle and food pad, can influence neurotransmitter choice in cultured sympathetic neurons causing cells that would differentiate as adrenergic neurons to become cholinergic.

adrenergic-to-cholinergic switch in phenotype have been purified from culture media, but the actual factor that operates in sweat glands to produce this effect *in vivo* has not yet been identified definitively.

Synaptic Partner Matching by Motor and Sensory Neurons

Stretch receptors in vertebrate muscles send axons into the spinal cord and synapse specifically on motor neurons that project back to that same muscle (Fig. 16.22A). This circuit controls the basic knee jerk reflex. We know that sensory afferents are not programmed autonomously to recognize these *homonymous* motor neurons: if the sensory fibers are forced to innervate other muscles, they choose new synaptic partners: motor neurons innervating those other muscles. One could imagine a mechanism by which this synaptic matchup was made on the basis of synchronized activity patterns, but blockade of activity during the period when these connections are made does not alter the specificity. Therefore, it seems that molecular cues from the periphery are transmitted to the sensory axons, and the sensory axons use this information to find the appropriate synaptic partners centrally (Frank and Weller, 1993). This idea is consistent with an experiment in which ventral limb muscles were replaced with dorsal ones. The sensory neurons that innervate the ventral muscles were thus forced to innervate ectopic dorsal muscle, and the sensory neurons synapsed with the motor neurons that went to the original dorsal musculature (Fig. 16.22B). Interestingly, after sensory neurons innervated the new muscles, they started to express the same ETS gene as the motor neurons that innervate that muscle. Limb ablation studies show that signals from the periphery, perhaps from the muscles themselves, help establish the coordinated pattern of ETS gene expression in the motor and sensory neurons that innervate particular muscle. Thus, peripherally coordinated gene expression seems to help specify this late aspect of cell determination and influence synaptic specificity.

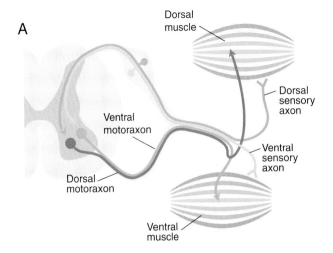

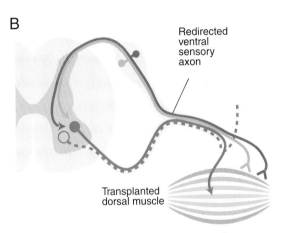

FIGURE 16.22 Sensory/motor matching. (A) A normal animal. The red motor neuron goes to a dorsal muscle while the green motor neuron innervates the ventral muscle. The stretch receptive sensory neurons that innervate these muscles synapse on the corresponding motor neurons in the spinal cord. (B) An animal in which a dorsal limb muscle was transplanted in place of a ventral one. The sensory neurons that normally innervate the ventral muscles are thus forced to innervate the dorsal muscle. As a result they change their properties and synapse in the spinal cord with the motor neurons that go to the dorsal muscle in its new position.

SUMMARY

The production of diverse neuronal and glial phenotypes is accomplished by an elaborate interplay between intrinsic cues and extrinsic signals. Intrinsic determinants include cytoplasmic factors that are inherited from the ancestor of a cell and nuclear proteins that act cell-autonomously by regulating gene expression. Cells also receive instructions from neighboring cells that influence their fates. Whether diffusible or membrane-bound, these extrinsic signals alter the expression of genes important for cell fate. The substantial progress that has been made in identifying the genes and proteins required for normal cell fate determination reveals that many of these molecular mechanisms are highly conserved between invertebrates and vertebrates.

References

Akiyama-Oda, Y., Hotta, Y., Tsukita, S., and Oda, H. (2000). Mechanism of glia-neuron cell-fate switch in the Drosophila thoracic neuroblast 6-4 lineage. *Development* **127**, 3513–3522.

Baumeister, R., Liu, Y., and Ruvkun, G. (1996). Lineage-specific regulators couple cell lineage asymmetry to the transcription of the *Caenorhabditis elegans* POU gene unc-86 during neurogenesis. *Genes Dev.* **10**, 1395–1410.

Bhat, K. M. (1999). Segment polarity genes in neuroblast formation and identity specification during Drosophila neurogenesis. *Bioessays* **21**, 472–485.

Brennan, C. A., and Moses, K. (2000). Determination of *Drosophila* photoreceptors: Timing is everything. *Cell. Mol. Life Sci.* **57**, 195–214.

Cornell, R. A., and Ohlen, T. V. (2000). Vnd/nkx, ind/gsh, and msh/msx: Conserved regulators of dorsoventral neural patterning? *Curr. Opin. Neurobiol.* **10**, 63–71.

Dorsky, R. I., Chang, W. S., Rapaport, D. H., and Harris, W. A. (1997). Regulation of neuronal diversity in the Xenopus retina by Delta signalling. *Nature 385*, 67–70.

Eisen, J. S. (1991). Determination of primary motoneuron identity in developing zebrafish embryos. *Science 252*, 569–572.

Flores, G. V., Duan, H., Yan, H., Nagaraj, R., Fu, W., Zou, Y., Noll, M., and Banerjee, U. (2000). Combinatorial signalling in the specification of unique fates. *Cell* **103**, 75–85.

Francis, N. J., and Landis, S. C. (1999). Cellular and molecular determinants of sympathetic neuron development. *Annu. Rev. Neurosci.* **22**, 541–566.

Frank, E., and Wenner, P. (1993). Environmental specification of neuronal connectivity. *Neuron 10*, 779–785.

Groves, A. K., and Bronner-Fraser, M. (1999). Neural crest diversification. *Curr. Top. Dev. Biol.* **43**, 221–258.

Isshiki, T., Pearson, B., Holbrook, S., and Doe, C. Q. (2001). Drosophila neuroblasts sequentially express transcription factors which specify the temporal identity of their neuronal progeny. *Cell* **106**, 511–521.

Jan, Y. N., and Jan, L. Y. (1993). The peripheral nervous system. *In* "The Development of *Drosophila melanogaster*," (M. Bate and A. Martinez-Arias, eds.) pp. 1207–1244. Laboratory Press, Cold Spring Habor, NY.

Jessell, T. M. (2000). Neuronal specification in the spinal cord: Inductive signals and transcriptional codes *Nature Rev. Genet.* **1**, 20–29.

Livesey, F. J., and Cepko, C. L. (2001). Vertebrate neural cell-fate determination: Lessons from the retina. *Nature Rev. Neurosci.* **2**, 109–118.

Lu, B., Jan, L., and Jan, Y. N. (2000) Control of cell divisions in the nervous system: Symmetry and asymmetry. *Annu. Rev. Neurosci.* **23**, 531–556.

McConnell, S. K. (1995). Strategies for the generation of neuronal diversity in the developing central nervous system, *J. Neurosci* **15**, 6987–6998.

Qian, X., Shen, Q., Goderie, S. K., He, W., Capela, A., Davis, A. A., and Temple, S. (2000). Timing of CNS cell generation: A programmed sequence of neuron and glial cell production from isolated murine cortical stem cells. *Neuron* **28**, 69–80.

Sasai, Y., and De Robertis, E. M. (1997). Ectodermal patterning in vertebrate embryos. *Dev. Biol.* **182**, 5–20.

Sengupta, P., and Bargmann, C. I. (1996). Cell fate specification and differentiation in the nervous system of *Caenorhabditis elegans*. *Dev. Genet.* **18**, 73–80.

Shimamura, K., Hartigan, D. J., Martinez, S., Puelles, L., and Rubenstein, J. L. (1995). Longitudinal organization of the anterior neural plate and neural tube. *Development* **121**, 3923–3933.

Skeath, J. B., Zhang, Y., Holmgren, R., Carroll, S. B., and Doe, C. Q. (1995) Specification of neuroblast identity in the Drosophila embryonic central nervous system by gooseberry-distal. *Nature* **376**, 427–430.

Usui, T., Shima, Y., Shimada, Y., Hirano, S., Burgess, R. W., Schwarz, T. L., Takeichi, M., and Uemura, T. (1999), Flamingo, a seven-pass transmembrane cadherin, regulates planar cell polarity under the control of Frizzled. *Cell* **98**, 585–595.

Wolff, T., and Ready, D. F. (1993). Pattern formation in the Drosophila retina. *In* "The Development of *Drosophila melanogaster*," (M. Bate and A. Martinez-Arias, eds.), pp. 1277–1326. Cold Spring Habor Laboratory Press, Cold Spring Harbor, NY.

William A. Harris and Volker Hartenstein

17

Growth Cones and Axon Pathfinding

Approximately 100 years ago, Ramon y Cajal described for the first time the growing tips of nerve cell axons. He named them growth cones and, in an unparalleled feat of scientific conjecture based on morphological observations of fixed material, described their behavior:

> From the functional point of view, one might say that the growth cone is like a club or battering ram endowed with exquisite chemical sensitivity, rapid ameboid movements, and a certain motive force allowing it to circumvent obstacles in its path, thus coursing between various cells until reaching its destination (Ramon y Cajal, 1890).

Decades later, Harrison developed the technique of growing living tissue in culture and demonstrated the truth of Cajal's description of a highly motile, ameboid specialization at the tips of growing axons. Shortly after, Speidel took advantage of the thinness and transparency of tadpole fins to examine living growth cones extending *in situ*. Viewed in real time, their shape changes very slowly, at a rate just detectable by an observer. Viewed with modern time-lapse techniques, however, the dynamism of their ever-changing morphology as they crawl forward is striking. The pioneering studies of Cajal, Harrison, and Speidel identified the growth cone as the key decision-making component in the elaboration of axonal pathways and inspired subsequent studies of the cell biology and behavior of growth cones *in vivo* and *in vitro*.

The growth cone at the distal tip of an axon extending in tissue culture is flattened into a thin fan-shaped sheet with many long, very thin spikes radiating forward (Fig. 17.1). The fan-shaped sheets are called lamellipodia, and the spikes are called filopodia or microspikes. Some growth cones growing *in situ* have a similar appearance, particularly when extending on basement membranes or cell surfaces (Fig. 17.2). It is not unusual, however, to observe spindle-shaped growth cones with tufts of forward-directed filopodia within axon bundles. It has been suggested that more complex growth cone shapes are characteristic of slowly extending growth cones choosing between possible routes of extension, whereas simpler morphologies are characteristic of rapidly extending growth cones coursing along permissive tracts.

GROWTH CONES ARE ACTIVELY GUIDED

Growth cones crawl forward as they elaborate the axons trailing behind them, and their extension is controlled by cues in their outside environment that ultimately direct them toward their appropriate targets. What is the nature of these guidance cues and how do they affect growth cone behavior? Several different theories were proposed to account for the ability of the nervous system to wire itself. One view, already implicit in Ramon y Cajal's writings and reinforced by Speidel's observations, held that axonal growth was highly directed, with each class of axons navigating along a distinctive prescribed pathway to reach its target. Competing with this view was the idea that axonal growth involved a certain amount of random wandering of axons throughout the embryonic environment and that connections appropriate for proper functioning of the nervous system were somehow maintained and reinforced at the expense of inappropriate connections. In the 1920s and 1930s, Paul Weiss vigorously proposed various mechanisms to explain the selective retention of appropriate connections.

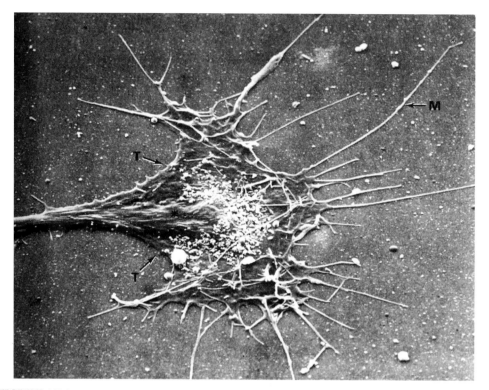

FIGURE 17.1 Scanning electron micrograph of a growth cone in culture. Growth cones extending on a flat surface are typically very thin, with broad lamellae and numerous filopodia. From Wessells and Nuttall (1973).

A number of experiments rapidly provided evidence against Weiss's ideas, which were all but refuted by the classic experiments of Sperry, started in the 1940s, which demonstrated highly specific targeting of regenerating retinal ganglion cell axons to the

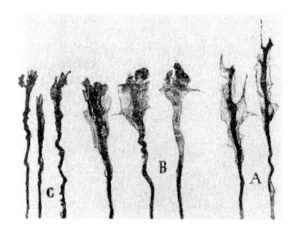

FIGURE 17.2 Growth cones are highly variable in morphology. Growth cones *in vivo* have a wide variety of shapes. This variability is partially due to the seemingly chaotic generation and withdrawal of individual lamellae and filopodia over time and partially due to the variety of surfaces over which growth cones crawl. From Ramon y Cajal (1890).

optic tectum (Sperry, 1963). Further, the application of axonal tracing techniques over the past two decades has made it possible to observe a variety of different classes of axons en route to their targets. These studies have shown that it is necessary to distinguish two phases in the establishment of connections (Goodman and Shatz, 1993). When projecting to the vicinity of their target field, axons grow along very stereotyped trajectories and make few errors of projection. The growth is highly directed, and in cases where a single axon navigates to an isolated target cell (as occurs in many places in invertebrate species), selection of the target cell is equally precise. A good example is the highly stereotyped and reproducible extension of individual axons arising from defined insect neurons as they grow within the central and peripheral nervous systems (Raper *et al.*, 1983; Caudy and Bentley, 1986). Results like these suggest that neurons are programmed to connect with specific targets even before they extend their axons, an idea supported by the finding that axons of ectopic vertebrate motoneurons reach their normal and appropriate targets even when they must traverse unusual routes to do so (Fig. 17.3) (Lance-Jones and Landmesser, 1980).

A more complex process occurs, however, when many similar axons arrive at a target field containing

A   Stage 15-16   B   Stage 28 1/2

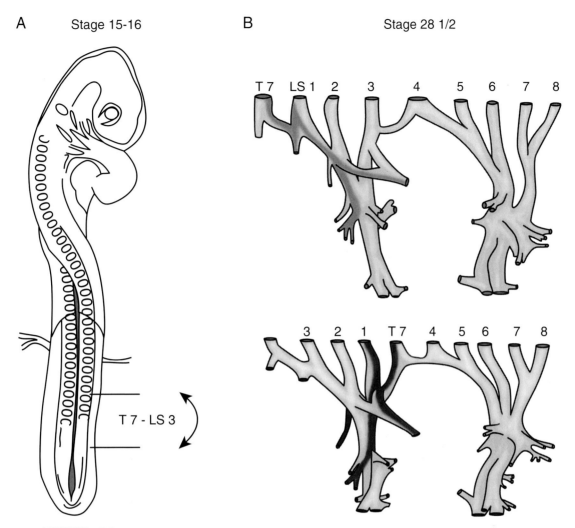

FIGURE 17.3 Neurons are specified to their targets, as shown in experiments in which the cell bodies of motoneurons are displaced by reversal of the spinal cord, yet their axons reach the appropriate target muscles. (A) The spinal cord between segments T7 and LS3 in chick embryos was reversed at a stage (Stage 15–16) before motoneurons have sent out their axons. (B) Projections of motoneurons from levels T7–LS1 were visualized 3 days later (Stage 28.5) by injection of a tracer into the cell body region of the motoneurons in the spinal cord, which diffused anterogradely down the axons. In control embryos (left), the innervation of specific muscles, including the sartorius muscle, is observed. After reversal (right), axons of the motoneurons exit the spinal cord via different nerve roots, yet the axons find their appropriate target muscles. Adapted from Lance-Jones and Landmesser (1980).

numerous similar target cells, as in the case of a group of motor axons all innervating the many muscle fibers in a single muscle. In these circumstances, individual axons arborize widely within the target field and initially contact many target cells, only later refining their pattern of connections in a process that depends on the precise patterns of electrical activity in the neurons and target cells. The rest of this chapter focuses on the first step in the formation of connections: the directed growth of axons to target fields. The selection of target cells and the role of electrical activity in this process are discussed in Chapters 18 and 20.

GUIDANCE CUES FOR DEVELOPING AXONS

How do axons succeed in navigating through the embryonic environment to targets that in some cases can be many centimeters away? The trajectories of many axons appear to be broken up into short segments, each perhaps a few hundred micrometers long. The daunting task of reaching a distant target is then reduced to the simpler task of navigating each of these successive segments. This task is well illustrated

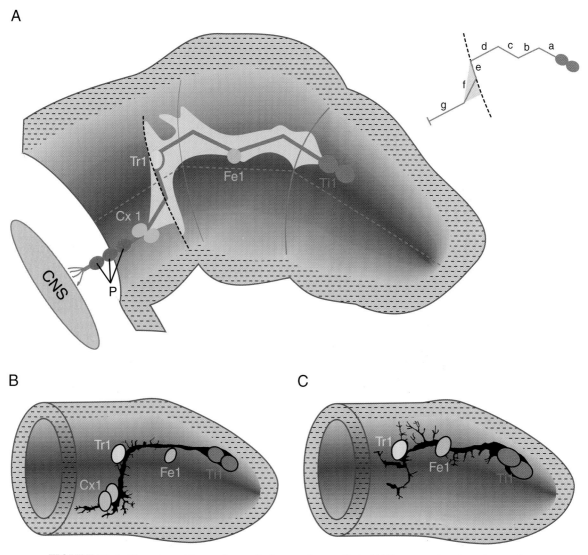

FIGURE 17.4 Stepwise guidance of axons in the grasshopper limb. (A) Summary drawing of a grasshopper limb showing the trajectory of the axons of the pair of Ti1 neurons, which take a characteristic trajectory to the central nervous system. The red line indicates the average trajectory of these axons based on analysis of several thousand axons. The stippled area indicates regions in which branches of Ti1 axons occur. The trajectory is broken into seven segments designated a–g, as shown in the diagram to the right of the drawing. Shaded regions in the diagram indicate the range of axon locations that are observed. Some of the segments end at a particular cellular landmark, such as segment b, which ends at the Fe1 neuron. Other segments end at stereotyped locations where there is no obvious landmark, such as segment a, which ends about 50 μm from the Ti1 cell bodies. Adapted from Caudy and Bentley (1986). (B and C) Segment f ends at the Cx1 cell, which is required for guidance, because axons fail to progress forward when the Cx1 cell is ablated (C). (B) Control trajectory. Adapted from Bentley and Caudy (1983).

by the central projections of sensory axons in the developing limb of the grasshopper. The pathway they follow can be divided into discrete segments, each bounded by a specific cell or group of cells that marks the end of one segment and the beginning of the next (Fig. 17.4) (Caudy and Bentley, 1986). Ablation of some of these cells with a laser microbeam results in profound misrouting of the axons when

they reach the vacant site (Fig. 17.4B and C). Evidence for the existence of such guidepost cells harboring important guidance information has in fact been obtained in a variety of species, including vertebrates.

The appreciation that axonal trajectories are formed in small segments pushes the question back one step: How do axons navigate each small segment

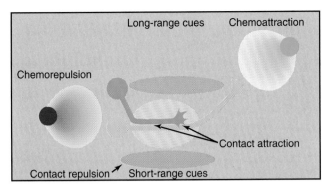

FIGURE 17.5 Axons are guided by the simultaneous and coordinate actions of four types of guidance mechanisms: contact attraction, chemoattraction, contact repulsion, and chemorepulsion. Individual growth cones might be "pushed" from behind by a chemorepellent, "pulled" from in front by a chemoattractant, and "hemmed in" by attractive and repulsive local cues (cell surface or extracellular matrix molecules). Push, pull, and hem: these forces act together to ensure accurate guidance. Adapted from Tessier-Lavigne and Goodman (1996).

of their trajectory? Axons appear to be guided along their appropriate trajectories by their responses to selectively distributed molecular signals within the developing embryo. Studies in the past decade have led to the view that axon guidance involves the coordinate action of four types of cues: short-range (or local) cues and long-range cues, each of which can be either positive (attractive) or negative (repellent) (Fig. 17.5). The operations of short- and long-range guidance mechanisms and of attraction and repulsion are not mutually exclusive. Rather, axons may generally be guided over each individual segment of their trajectories by several different types of mechanisms acting in concert to ensure reproducible and high-fidelity guidance. Many experiments have shown that axons may navigate short segments by using several and, in some cases, even all four types of cues (Fig. 17.5): a repellent from behind the axons to "push," a corridor marked by a permissive local cue and bounded by an inhibitory local cue to "hem in" the growth, and an attractant at the end of the corridor to "pull" (Tessier-Lavigne and Goodman, 1996). Push, pull, and hem: these forces working together can ensure accurate guidance.

The identification of signaling molecules that function as guidance cues has depended primarily on three experimental approaches: (1) pairing biochemistry and *in vitro* tissue culture assays to detect proteins with either attractive or repellent properties, (2) using forward genetics to identify mutations that affect axon trajectories *in vivo*, or (3) using genetic and tissue culture approaches to characterize the functions of molecules with distributions or molecular structures that make them attractive candidate guidance cues.

Four prominent families of signaling molecules are now thought to make significant contributions to axon guidance: semaphorins, netrins, slits, and ephrins (Fig. 17.6). The identification and characterization of these cues and their receptors have led to several important generalizations about guidance mechanisms (Tessier-Lavigne and Goodman, 1996; Chisholm and Tessier-Lavigne, 1999). First, guidance cues come in families, which may, in some cases, comprise both diffusible members that can function in long-range axon guidance, as well as nondiffusible members functioning at short range. Second, many guidance cues are multifunctional, attracting some axons, repelling other axons, and sometimes controlling other aspects of axonal morphogenesis such as axonal branching or arborization. Different axons may respond to the same cue differently because of differences in their complement of surface receptors or differences in their signal transduction pathways. Third, many (although not all) cues are evolutionarily conserved between vertebrates and more primitive invertebrate organisms, with species homologues performing similar roles in axon guidance. Higher vertebrates typically have many more members within a given family of guidance cues, and these cues are likely to have overlapping functions. These four families are discussed briefly to illustrate these features of wiring mechanisms.

Semaphorins

The first semaphorin to be discovered was grasshopper Semaphorin 1a. This transmembrane protein is distributed in stripes in the epidermis of the leg. Antibodies to Sema 1a perturb the trajectories of pioneer sensory axons growing in the vicinity of the Sema 1a stripes (Kolodkin *et al.*, 1992). There are currently approximately 20 known distinct semaphorin family members identified in higher vertebrates (Fig. 17.5A). Roughly a third of these are secreted molecules that have a positively charged C terminus that is likely to fasten them to cell surfaces or the extracellular matrix. One semaphorin is thought to attach to the cell surface through a phosphatidyl-inositol linkage. The remaining semaphorins are transmembrane molecules. This family of signaling proteins is therefore likely to act in the immediate vicinity of the cells that produce them. All contain the family signature semaphorin domain, a roughly 500 amino acid domain that is the key signaling element of the semaphorins. Their biological specificity is at least in part determined by a relatively short stretch of amino acids within the semaphorin domain.

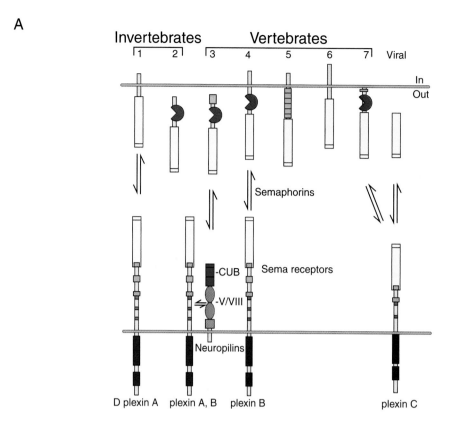

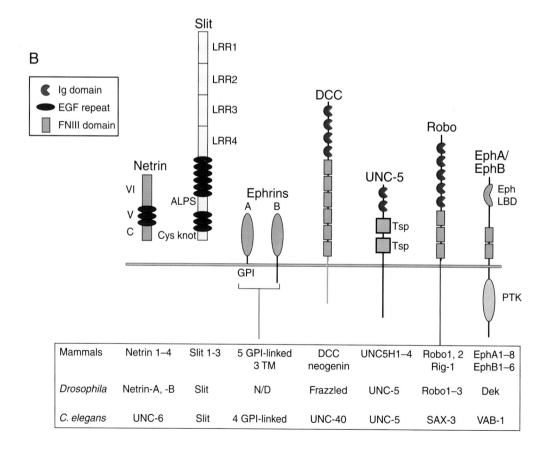

The first vertebrate semaphorin was purified biochemically from brain extracts using an *in vitro* bioassay that detects axonal repellents (Luo *et al.*, 1993). Most of the secreted and one of the transmembrane semaphorins have since been shown to repel very specific subsets of cultured axons (Raper, 2000). Two of the secreted semaphorins have been reported to act as either repellents or attractants for different sets of cultured axons. Based on information currently available, semaphorins seem more often than not to act as repellents; however, the activities of most of the transmembrane semaphorins remain untested, and only a handful of semaphorin activities have been determined *in vivo*.

The primary receptors for semaphorins are members of the plexin family, transmembrane proteins that are distant relatives of the semaphorins themselves (Fig. 17.5A) (Raper, 2000). Many transmembrane semaphorins in insects and vertebrates have been shown to bind plexins directly. Secreted vertebrate semaphorins, however, do not. Instead, they bind to a second class of receptor components, the neuropilins, which in turn complex with plexins (Fig. 17.5A); different secreted semaphorins require specific combinations of neuropilin-1 and -2 to evoke a response (Raper, 2000).

Netrins

The netrin family (Fig. 17.5B) is smaller than the semaphorin family, with about half a dozen members identified in vertebrates. The first vertebrate members were identified as proteins that can mimic a diffusible outgrowth-promoting activity for axons in the spinal cord (Tessier-Lavigne *et al.*, 1988; Serafini *et al.*, 1994) and have been shown to function in attracting subsets of axons to various targets in the spinal cord and brain, most notably to the midline of those structures

(see later). Remarkably, netrin-1 also appears to function as a long-range repellent, providing a push from behind for a group of axons in the hindbrain that grow away from the midline, thus illustrating the bifunctionality of guidance cues. Strikingly, netrins are vertebrate homologues of the UNC-6 protein of the nematode *Caenorhabditis elegans*, a protein similarly involved in both attracting some axons toward the nervous system midline and in repelling others away from it (Wadsworth *et al.*, 1996). Netrin homologues are also expressed at the midline of the nervous system of *Drosophila melanogaster*, where they contribute to attracting axons to the midline. In all of these organisms, the attractive effects of netrins on axons are mediated by receptors of the DCC family, whereas repulsive actions require receptors of the UNC5 family; both sets of receptors are members of the immunoglobulin gene superfamily (Fig. 17.5B) (Chisholm and Tessier-Lavigne, 1999). These findings on netrins and their receptors vividly illustrate the remarkable conservation of axon guidance mechanisms during evolution.

Identification of netrins as long-range guidance cues also illustrates the fact that long-range and short-range guidance mechanisms can be closely related. Although netrins are capable of long-range attraction, they are closely related in structure to one region of the archetypal nondiffusible extracellular matrix (ECM) molecule laminin-1. In fact, the extent to which netrins can diffuse in the embryo may be regulated so that, like secreted semaphorins, in some circumstances they may function as local rather than long-range cues (Serafini *et al.*, 1994; Wadsworth *et al.*, 1996). Thus, as in the distinction between attractive and repulsive cues, there may not be a hard and fast distinction between local and long-range cues.

◄ FIGURE 17.6 Structures of semaphorins, netrins, slits, ephrins, and their receptors. (A) There are seven classes of semaphorins (two invertebrate and five vertebrate). Of the ~20 mammalian semaphorins, 5 are secreted (class 3) and the others are divided into four families of transmembrane or GPI-linked proteins. Semaphorin sequences are also found in certain viral genomes (V). Semaphorin receptors include plexins (of which nine are known in mammals, divided into classes A–C) and neuropilins (two in mammals). Class 3 semaphorin signaling is mediated by complexes of neuropilins (which serve as binding moieties) and plexins (signaling moieties). Domains in these proteins include semaphorin (sema) domains, immunoglobulin-like (Ig) domains, Met-related sequence (MRS) repeats, glycine–proline-rich (GP) repeats, Sex-plexin (SP) motifs, CUB domains, and coagulation factor V/VIII homology (V/VIII) domains. Adapted from Winberg *et al.* (1998) and Chisholm and Tessier-Lavigne (1999). (B) Identities and structures of netrins, slits, ephrins, and their receptors in mammals, *Drosophila*, and *C. elegans*. Domain structures are approximately to scale. Common motifs in many axon guidance proteins include Ig-like domains, EGF repeats, and fibronectin type III (FNIII) domains. Netrin domains are laminin homology domains V and VI (containing three EGF repeats). Slit domains are LRR (leucine-rich repeat), ALPS, and cysteine knot; all species have EGF repeats 1–6, vertebrate slits have EGFs 7–9 (illustrated), whereas *C. elegans* and *Drosophila* have only EGF repeat 7. Ephrins are GPI-linked (ephrin-A) or transmembrane (ephrin-B). UNC-5 family proteins contain two thrombospondin (Tsp) domains. The N-terminal ligand-binding domain (LBD) of Eph receptors, although originally described as an Ig domain, is a novel domain. Eph receptors contain a cytoplasmic protein-tyrosine kinase (PTK) domain. The number and names of family members in *C. elegans*, *Drosophila* and mammalian species are indicated; N/D, not determined. Adapted from Chisholm and Tessier-Lavigne (1999).

Slits

Slits are large secreted proteins (Fig. 17.5C) that were implicated in axonal repulsion through genetic studies of a chemorepellent factor in *D. melanogaster* (Kidd *et al.*, 1999) and through studies of proteins that can induce repulsion of migrating axons neurons and collapse of axons in vertebrates; a single slit protein functions in axonal repulsion in *C. elegans* as well. In mammals there are three known slit proteins, which play an important role in repelling several classes of axons in the mammalian forebrain. The repulsive actions of slit proteins are mediated by receptors of the Robo family (Kidd *et al.*, 1998) (Fig. 17.5C), which, like DCC and UNC5 family netrin receptors, are also members of the immunoglobulin superfamily. In addition to repulsive actions, a mammalian slit protein has been shown to be a positive regulator of branching of some axons and dendrites (Wang *et al.*, 1999), further illustrating the multifunctionality of axon guidance cues.

Ephrins

Ephrins are a family of cell surface signaling molecules that play important roles in many developmental events including axon guidance (Holder and Klein, 1999). There are two subfamilies (Fig. 17.5D). Eight class A ephrins are tethered to the cell surface via GPI linkages, and six class B ephrins are transmembrane molecules. Ephrins must be clustered together to activate their receptors and are unlikely to be active if released from the cell surface. These ligands bind receptor tyrosine kinases of the Eph family. Class A ephrins interact with various degrees of selectivity with five class A Eph receptors, whereas class B ephrins interact with three class B Eph receptors (Fig. 17.5D). Ephrins have been shown to play an essential role in organizing topographic projections that connect, for example, retinal ganglion cells in the eye with their target cells in the appropriate portion of the optic tectum in lower vertebrates, or the lateral geniculate nucleus of the thalamus in higher vertebrates (see Chapter 18).

The following sections of this chapter explain how the guidance cues just discussed are thought to control growth cone trajectories, followed by how these cues are deployed *in vivo* to affect accurate guidance.

Summary

Four prominent families of signaling molecules—semaphorins, netrins, slits, and ephrins—are involved intimately in the guidance of growing axons. These guidance cues can function in long-range or short-range axon guidance. Many guidance cues are multifunctional and can function in attraction, in repulsion, or in regulating branch formation. Furthermore, many cues are conserved evolutionarily, both in structure and in function, between vertebrates and invertebrates. In addition to semaphorins, netrins, slits, and ephrins, members of other families of molecules are expected to play important roles in guidance decisions, although their roles for the most part are still being defined. These molecules include other members of the immunoglobulin gene superfamily, other extracellular matrix components, transmembrane phosphatases, and cadherins (Tessier-Lavigne and Goodman, 1996).

GUIDANCE CUES AND THE CONTROL OF ACTIN POLYMERIZATION

Guidance cues are signaling molecules that influence the cell biological mechanisms by which growth cones extend, turn, and retract. The forward-crawling motion of a growth cone depends on its own intrinsic motile mechanism interacting with a permissive outside environment. The extension and withdrawal of the leading edge and the filopodia are an intrinsic, autonomous property of a healthy growth cone. Once the leading edge has extended, an appropriate substratum on which it can attach and become stabilized must be present. Once attached, an inherent traction-generating mechanism within the growth cone causes tension to develop. Unattached or poorly attached processes are thereby withdrawn, whereas tension exerted against attached processes helps draw the body of the growth cone forward. The continuous repeated cycling of extension, attachment, retraction of poorly attached processes, and tension generation produces net forward extension. In principle, guidance cues could act at any one of these steps to affect the direction in which growth cones extend.

Actin Cycle and Axon Growth

One way in which guidance cues can affect the direction of growth cone advance is by controlling the actin polymerization that helps drive protrusion of the leading edge of the growth cone. A dense meshwork of fibrillar actin (F-actin) is concentrated at the leading edge of the growth cone (Fig. 17.7). New actin polymerization just behind the leading edge effectively helps push it forward, while, on average, F-actin is simultaneously depolymerized at an equal

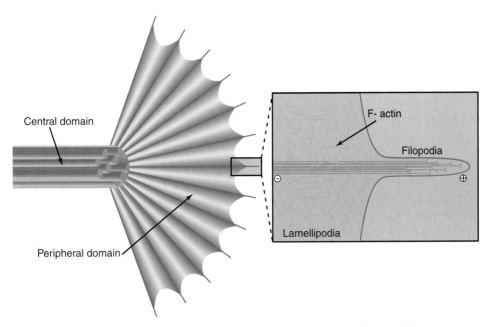

FIGURE 17.7 Distributions of microtubules and fibrillar actin in a growth cone. Microtubules are an important structural component of the axon that splay out within the proximal portion of the growth cone. All of their growing ends are pointed toward the leading edge. Actin is highly concentrated in the filopodia and in the leading edges of lamellae. Within filopodia, actin fibrils are oriented with their growing tips pointed distally. The same is true of many fibrils within lamellae, although many additional fibrils are oriented randomly and form a dense meshwork. Modified from Lin *et al.*(1994).

rate elsewhere. A second important component of growth cone motility is a continuous rearward flow of polymerized actin away from the leading edge toward the more proximal part of the growth cone. This actin flow can be visualized in cultured growth cones with the aid of a drug that blocks actin polymerization (Fig. 17.8). Actin monomers generated by depolymerization in the body of the growth cone are recycled to the front, polymerized again at the leading edge, and swept rearward, where they are depolymerized once again. This continuous rearward flow of polymerized actin generates a kind of "caterpillar tread" within the interior of the growth cone. If this caterpillar tread is linked to a permissive substratum through cell surface receptors, it advances the leading edge and withdraws the trailing edge. Most proteins selected at random do not provide a substratum on which growth cones can advance. Particular representatives of several special families of proteins have been shown to provide permissive substrata for growth cone extension. Among these are extracellular matrix molecules, such as laminin-1 (mentioned earlier) and fibronectin, or specialized cell surface molecules from either the immunoglobulin superfamily or the cadherin family. These molecules are bound by specific cell surface molecules, which include members of the integrin, immunoglobulin, and cadherin superfamilies.

Linking Cytoskeleton and Permissive Substratum Molecules

Cell surface receptors that bind permissive substratum molecules must in turn be linked to the cellular cytoskeleton (Lin *et al.*, 1994). Indirect linkages between the cytoskeleton and members of the integrin, cadherin, and immunoglobulin families can give the cytoskeleton traction on the substratum and help advance the actin caterpillar described earlier (Fig. 17.9). This traction can be modulated by the phosphorylation of specific cytoplasmic proteins. For example, activity of the nonreceptor tyrosine kinase Src reduces the strength of cadherin and integrin mediated cell adhesion. Localized activation of these kinds of signaling pathways could control the direction of growth cone advance by modulating adhesion to the substratum.

The actin caterpillar generates tension within the growth cone and causes processes that are poorly attached to the substratum to shrink or withdraw. Evidence indicates that myosin-based motors drive retrograde actin flow (Lin *et al.*, 1996). When the retrograde movement of actin is impeded by a relatively strong attachment between the actin cytoskeleton and the surface substratum, not only is the leading edge of the growth cone advanced, but microtubules tend to

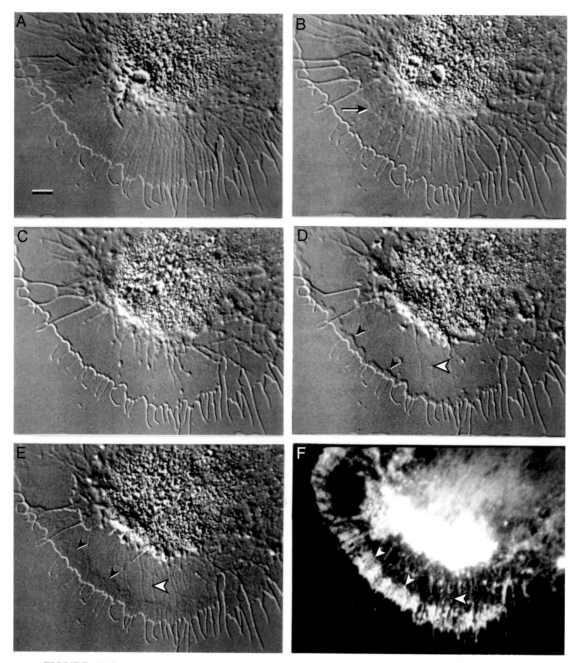

FIGURE 17.8 Actin polymerizes at the leading edge and is then translocated rearward. A growth cone on polylysine is well spread but does not advance forward (A). Fibrillar (F) actin within the growth cone can be visualized with differential interference contrast optics. (B) Addition of a drug that halts actin polymerization, cytochalasin B, first leads to the loss of actin just behind the leading edge (the most distal form of F-actin is indicated by the arrow). An F-actin-free zone grows as the remaining F-actin is translocated toward the center of the growth cone (C). F-Actin begins to polymerize at the leading edge when cytochalasin B is removed (D and E). The distribution of F-actin in (E) is shown after it was decorated with fluorescently conjugated phalloidin (F). From Forscher and Smith (1988).

be drawn forward. The strong attachment of individual filopodia to appropriate cellular targets induces additional localized actin accumulation in the contacting process, and these processes are preferentially invaded by microtubules. In this way, filopodia can act as scouts for less advanced portions of the growth cone, seizing hold of permissive substrata and reorienting subsequent process extension.

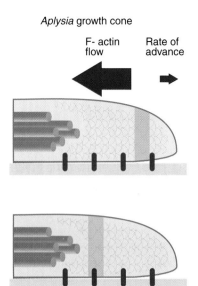

Aplysia growth cone

FIGURE 17.9 Linkage of the actin cytoskeleton to a permissive surface is required for forward advance. Actin is polymerized at the leading edge of the growth cone (right) and is swept toward the rear. If the actin meshwork is not linked to cell surface receptors that bind permissive molecules on adjacent cell surfaces, the actin cycles from front to rear but does not advance the growth cone. If the actin meshwork is attached to these receptors, the meshwork remains in place and newly polymerized actin helps advance the leading edge. Modified from Lin *et al.*(1994).

Interactions between Cytoskeleton and Guidance Receptors

How do cues such as semaphorins, netrins, slits, and ephrins tap into these mechanisms for growth cone extension to affect guidance? Attractive and repulsive signals could promote the extension of the leading edge by increasing the local rate of actin polymerization in the preferred direction or by decreasing its rate of depolymerization in other directions. Repellent signals could exert their effects by affecting actin polymerization in the opposite way. It is therefore reasonable to expect that many signaling pathways activated by guidance cues ultimately converge on actin polymerization. Studies of the receptor mechanisms for the families of guidance cues described here are beginning to bear out this prediction by showing that activation of these receptors can directly or indirectly alter the activity of small Rho family GTPases such as Rac and RhoA, which are key regulators of the actin polymerization events in cell motility in a large variety of cell types. For example, the netrin receptor DCC activates Rac (through an unknown mechanism), whereas activation of the semaphorin receptor plexin B1 favors Rho activity over Rac activity at least partly by binding and sequestering activated Rac. Activation of an Eph receptor can activate RhoA through an adaptor protein called

ephexin, which binds the receptor and stimulates exchange of GDP for GTP on the GTPase, leading to its activation (Shamah *et al.*, 2001). Activation of Robo receptors can also alter GTPase activity at least in part by the opposite mechanism, i.e., the recruitment of proteins with intrinsic GTPase-activating activity that stimulate Rho family GTPases to hydrolyze GTP and inactivate themselves (Wong *et al.*, 2001). These initial studies are showing that Rho family GTPases are important intermediates in the control of actin polymerization by axon guidance cues, although there are still considerable gaps in our understanding of the pathways from receptors to these GTPases. Our understanding of events downstream of GTPases is equally patchy. For example, semaphorin 3A-induced growth cone collapse requires the activity of LIM kinase, an enzyme that affects actin polymerization through its phosphorylation of cofilin, a protein that severs actin polymers. This and other effectors of the small GTPases are being studied intensively for their roles in linking small GTPases to the actin cytoskeleton for axon guidance.

Summary

Growing axons utilize an intrinsic, actin-based treadmilling mechanism to extend filopodia and advance the leading edge of the growth cone. Growth cone extension requires an appropriate substratum for attachment and stabilization, which allows an inherent traction-generating mechanism within the growth cone to generate tension. This tension results in the withdrawal of poorly attached processes and the growth of processes that form attachments with the substratum. Net forward extension results from repeated cycles of extension, attachment, and the retraction of poorly attached processes. Cell surface receptors that bind substratum molecules are linked indirectly to the cellular cytoskeleton, and these linkages can be modulated by the activation of signaling pathways. The binding of extracellular guidance cues to receptors on the growth cone surface likely modulates axon growth by regulating actin polymerization, with attractive cues promoting actin polymerization and repulsive cues promoting depolymerization. Many guidance receptors directly or indirectly modulate the activity of small Rho family GTPases, which are key regulators of actin polymerization.

GUIDANCE *IN VIVO*: REUSING CUES FOR DIFFERENT PURPOSES AND CHANGING RESPONSES TO CUES

How are guidance cues interpreted by growth cones *in vivo* and how do they direct the appropriate wiring together of the nervous system? The guidance of an axon from its inception through its acquisition of a target is a complex process that can be broken down into a series of discrete decisions. This section illustrates some important features of how guidance cues are used to direct particular types of guidance decisions. We first focus on how a single guidance cue, semaphorin 3A, is used in multiple different ways to affect distinct types of decisions. We then describe how multiple guidance cues and receptors cooperate closely to direct a complex series of guidance events at the nervous system midline.

Multiple Guidance Roles for Semaphorin 3A

Semaphorin 3A was originally identified as a repellent for cultured sensory axons (Luo *et al.*, 1993). Since then, its *in vivo* functions have been studied in organ culture systems, in mice in which its gene is disrupted

by homologous recombination, and through the expression of dominant negative receptors that block its function. These studies have shown roles for semaphorin 3A in initial axon and dendrite extension, in axon fasciculation, and in regulating target field invasion.

Initial Axon and Dendrite Extension

Perhaps the earliest guidance-related decision made by a neuron is the initial direction in which the primary axon should extend. One brain region in which this has been studied is the cortex. Just after pyramidal cells are born in the ventricular zone and have migrated some distance toward the pia (Chapter 15), they generally have a bipolar morphology with a process pointed toward the pia and an opposing process pointed toward the ventricular zone. The pial process will differentiate into the apical dendrite, while the opposing process differentiates into the

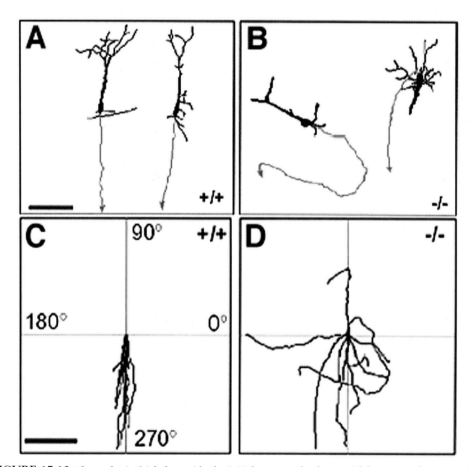

FIGURE 17.10   Semaphorin 3A helps guide the initial outgrowth of pyramidal axons in the cortex. (A) Pyramidal neurons are visualized in perinatal wild-type (+/+) mice by backfilling their projection axons with a hydrophilic dye. Their axons extend directly toward the deeper white matter (bottom) while their dendrites stretch toward the pial surface (top). (B) In semaphorin 3A mutant mice, pyramidal cells are appropriately polarized, but their axons and dendrites are not oriented correctly. (C) A summary of the axon trajectories of pyramidal cells in semaphorin 3A +/+ mice as compared to those (D) in semaphorin 3A –/– mice. From Polleux *et al.* (1998).

primary axon that grows in the deep white matter to distant targets such as the spinal cord, other areas of the cortex, or the thalamus. Semaphorin 3A has been shown to play an important role in orienting axon elongation and dendrite formation in a series of elegant organ culture assays (Polleux *et al.*, 1998). Late-stage embryonic cortical neurons were labeled and then cultured briefly on just-born cortical slices. Pyramidal cells cultured on the slice near the marginal zone beneath the pia generally grow their axons toward the ventricular surface, whereas those growing on top of deeper cortical layers well away from the marginal zone have no preferred direction. This demonstrates that layers near the marginal zone can impose a polarity on pyramidal cell growth. If the ventricular edge of one slice is jammed up against the pial margin of another, then cortical axons grow away from the marginal zone on both slices, suggesting that the marginal zone secretes an axonal repellent that drives growing axons away. This repellent activity is likely to be semaphorin 3A. Explanted aggregates of cells secreting recombinant semaphorin 3A repel pyramidal axons and can thereby mimic the orienting activity of the marginal zone. Antibodies to the semaphorin 3A receptor component neuropilin-1 neutralize the orienting effect of the marginal zone. Most importantly, the polarity of pyramidal cell growth in semaphorin 3A mutant mice is disrupted (Fig. 17.10). These experiments strongly suggest that semaphorin 3A produced and secreted near the marginal zone contributes to the orientation of pyramidal axon outgrowth by repelling the axons away from the pial surface and toward the deeper white matter.

Interestingly, semaphorin 3A helps orient the growth of apical pyramidal dendrites in a similar manner, but instead of acting as a repellent as it does for pyramidal axons, it acts as an attractant (Polleux *et al.*, 2000). One possible explanation for how semaphorin 3A can have opposing activities in different parts of the same pyramidal cell is provided by experiments using cultured *Xenopus* spinal cord neurons. In these cells, attractants such as netrin can be converted to repellents by decreasing intracellular cAMP levels, whereas repellents such as semaphorin 3A can be converted to attractants by increasing cGMP levels (Song *et al.*, 1998). The dendrites of cortical pyramidal cells have very high concentrations of guanylate cyclase that are thought to elevate the level of cGMP locally, thereby converting the activity of semaphorin 3A to that of an attractant (Polleux *et al.*, 2000). In this way, the same semaphorin gradient can be used to orient pyramidal axons toward the underlying white matter while simultaneously orienting apical dendrites in the opposite direction.

Axon Fasciculation

Once axons have begun to grow, they are often observed to extend upon the surfaces of axons that have preceded them on the same route. Thick bundles of axons called fascicles are built up over time, and many closely associated fascicles generally make up a nerve. Growth cones grow within fascicles because axons are a preferred substratum compared to the surrounding tissue. One factor determining this preference is the presence of permissive molecules, such as N-cadherin or L1, that promote axon outgrowth on the surfaces of axons. A second factor is the presence of repellents in the surrounding tissue that discourage axon outgrowth in those regions, thereby helping drive axon–axon fasciculation. Semaphorin 3A serves again as an example of this process. Semaphorin 3A is expressed widely in tissues surrounding many peripheral nerves and acts as a repellent for sensory and motor axons. Several peripheral nerves are visibly defasciculated in mice that are homozygous for mutated semaphorin 3A (Fig. 17.11) (Taniguchi *et al.*, 1997). For the most part, peripheral axons reach their appropriate targets, but some enter regions they would normally avoid. Many of the axons with abnormal and incorrect trajectories are eliminated later in development, very likely through the mechanisms described in Chapter 20.

Regulating Target Field Invasion

Projection neurons whose axons connect widely separated regions of the body are generally the first axon pathways to form in the embryo. In this way, they can make their appropriate connections while the embryo is small and before the distances between cell bodies and their targets become prohibitive. Such an early start, however, requires that these axons arrive at their targets very early, sometimes well before the targets are sufficiently differentiated to accept innervation. Early arriving axons must therefore halt their growth and wait near their target until it is ready for them. This kind of waiting period is a feature of the developing olfactory system. The first olfactory sensory axons grow from the epithelium lining the nasal passageways all the way to the telencephalon well before their target, the olfactory bulb, differentiates. Olfactory axons halt their growth at the surface of the central nervous system (CNS) for several days. Additional axons continue to arrive and they too halt at the edge of the CNS as the bulb differentiates beneath them. Olfactory axons enter en masse once the bulb is sufficiently differentiated to receive them. In chick embryos, this waiting period is at least partially enforced by semaphorin 3A expressed in the telencephalon. Expression of a dominant negative

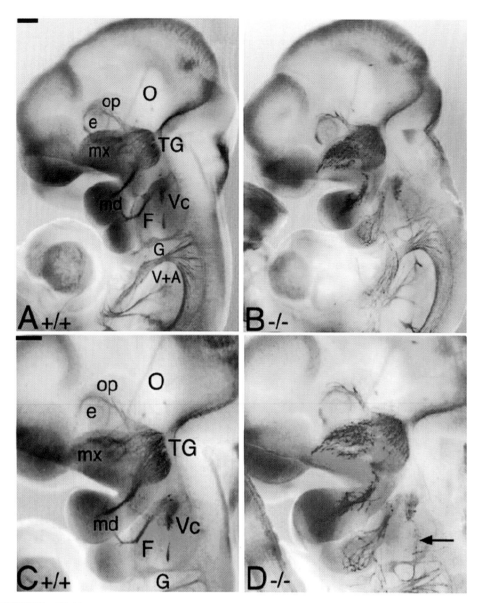

FIGURE 17.11 Semaphorin 3A helps maintain fasciculation of axons within cranial nerves. Antineurofilament staining was used to compare the trajectories of peripheral nerves in (A and C) wild-type (+/+) and (B and D) semaphorin 3A mutant mice (−/−). Normally, axons within a nerve travel together, but in the mutant animal, several nerves are loosely organized. This is most apparent in the mandibular branch of the trigeminal nerve (md) and also the facial nerve (F). Other abbreviations include ophthalmic (op) and maxillary (mx) branches of the trigeminal, glossopharyngeal (G), vestibulocochlear (Vc), oculomotor (O), vagal (V), and accessory nerves (A). Positions of the eye (e) and trigeminal ganglion (TG) are marked. Scale bars: 250 μm. From Taniguchi *et al.* (1997).

form of neuropilin-1 in olfactory sensory neurons blocks their ability to be repelled by semaphorin 3A. Olfactory sensory neurons expressing dominant negative neuropilin-1 do not observe the normal waiting period outside the CNS while the bulb differentiates, but instead, they tend to plunge into the CNS prematurely and grow past their appropriate target region (Fig. 17.12) (Renzi *et al.*, 2000). In this case, semaphorin 3A may not only be acting as a repellent that prevents the premature entry of axons into an imma-

ture target, but as a paralytic that holds axons near their target and prevents them from growing away.

Guidance at the Midline: Changing Responses to Multiple Cues

Single guidance cues probably rarely or never act by themselves, and the integration of several simultaneously active cues is required for most, if not all, guidance decisions. This can be illustrated by inter-

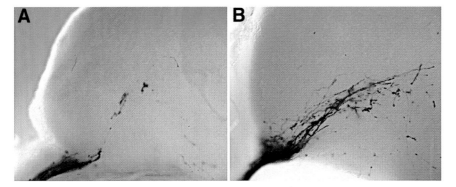

FIGURE 17.12 Semaphorins help prevent olfactory sensory axons from entering the nascent chick olfactory bulb prematurely. Olfactory axons normally wait outside the CNS for several days while the olfactory bulb differentiates beneath them. (A) Axons expressing a control construct and a neuronal tracer protein wait normally while a small number of migrating cells enter the CNS. (B) Axons expressing a dominant negative semaphorin receptor enter prematurely and overshoot their target, the olfactory bulb. From Renzi *et al.* (2000).

actions between the activities of many different guidance cues of the netrin, slit, and semaphorin families at the midline of the developing nervous systems of both invertebrates and vertebrates, which have been elucidated through genetic, biochemical, and embryological studies in rodents, in *Drosophila* and *C. elegans*.

As illustrated in Fig. 17.13 and 17.14, in both vertebrates and invertebrates the so-called commissural axons are attracted to the nervous system midline by

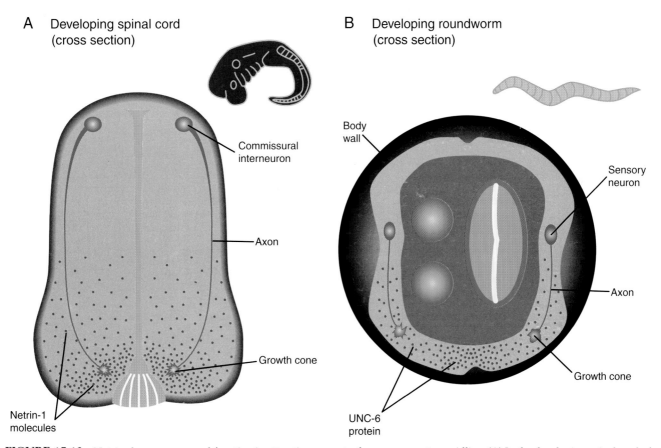

FIGURE 17.13 Netrins have a conserved function in attracting axons to the nervous system midline. (A) In the developing spinal cord of vertebrates, commissural interneurons with their cell bodies in the top (dorsal) half of the spinal cord send axons tipped by growth cones to floor plate cells at the ventral midline of the spinal cord because they are attracted by netrin-1 secreted by floor plate cells. (B) In the nematode *C. elegans*, sensory neurons similarly send axons ventrally because they are attracted by the netrin UNC-6.

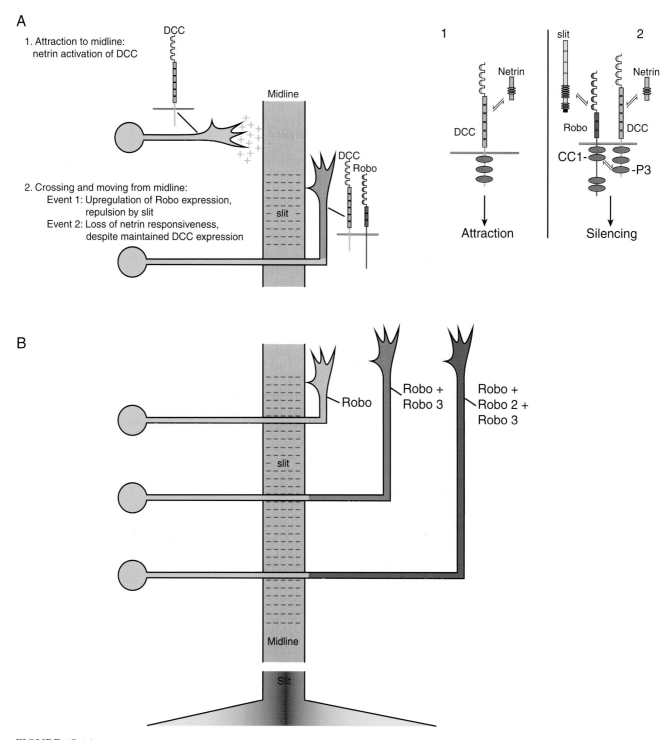

FIGURE 17.14 Robo receptors transduce a midline repulsive signal encoded in slit proteins and silence netrin-mediated attraction. (A) As shown in Fig. 17.13, commissural axons are initially attracted to the midline by netrin protein made by midline cells, which activates DCC family receptors in the axons. Commissural axons cross the midline and then turn, but normally never recross the midline because the axons upregulate expression of the Robo receptor, thereby becoming sensitive to the midline repellent slit. In addition, activation of the Robo receptor by slit silences the netrin receptor DCC through direct binding of the Robo and DCC cytoplasmic domains (diagram on right). Adapted from Stein and Tessier-Lavigne (2001). (B) The distance from the midline at which axons turn to project parallel to the midline is determined by the complement of Robo receptors made by the axons. Slit protein is present in a gradient, which is interpreted differently by the different Robo receptors. Axons expressing just Robo turn near the midline. Axons expressing both Robo and Robo3, turn further away. Axons expressing Robo, Robo3, and Robo2 turn at the greatest distance. In this way, a single gradient of slit protein can elicit graded responses of the axons. Adapted from Simpson *et al.* (2000) and Rajagopalan *et al.* (2000).

members of the netrin family, which activate receptors of the DCC family (Tessier-Lavigne and Goodman, 1996; Chisholm and Tessier-Lavigne, 1999). The midline is not, however, the final destination for these axons: upon reaching it, axons cross the midline, then they turn at right angles and project alongside the midline to other levels of the embryo, and finally they leave the midline area altogether to reach their eventual targets (Fig. 17.14). This behavior immediately raises a paradox: if the midline is such an attractive environment for the axons, how can they leave it? The answer is that midline cells, in addition to making attractive netrin proteins, also make repellents of the slit family (and, in vertebrates, of the semaphorin family) (Fig. 17.14A) (Kidd *et al.*, 1999; Zou *et al.*, 2000). Axons can approach and then cross the midline a first time because they are initially insensitive to these repellents and thus respond only to the attractive effects of the netrins. However, and quite remarkably, upon crossing the midline the axons become responsive to the repellents by increasing the expression or function of receptors for the repellents, including upregulating expression of the slit receptor Robo on their surfaces (Fig. 17.14A) (Kidd *et al.*, 1998; Zou *et al.*, 2000). What causes this dramatic change in receptor expression and function is not yet known, but its net effect is to make the axons interpret the midline as a repulsive environment, which helps expel the axons from the midline and move on to the next leg of their trajectory.

The upregulation of responsiveness to midline repellents is only half of the equation, however: to be efficiently expelled from the midline, it would be desirable for the axons to stop being attracted. Indeed, the attractive response of these axons to netrins is switched off (silenced) through a mechanism involving direct binding of the slit receptor Robo to the netrin receptor DCC: activation of the Robo receptor by slit causes a specific region of its cytoplasmic domain to bind a specific region of the DCC receptor cytoplasmic domain and to prevent it from transducing an attractive response to netrin (Fig. 17.14A) (Stein and Tessier-Lavigne, 2001). Together, these two mechanisms (upregulation of a response to midline repellents and silencing of the attractive receptor) ensure that the growth cones perceive a once attractive environment, the midline, as unambiguously repulsive. More generally, the ability illustrated here of growth cones to change their responses to guidance cues makes it possible for them to move from one intermediate target (such as the midline) to the next along their often complex and lengthy trajectories.

Guidance at the midline also illustrates another way in which more complex behaviors of axons can be directed by guidance cues. Different subpopula-

tions of commissural axons extend different distances from the midline after crossing it before they turn (Fig. 17.14B). In *Drosophila*, it has been shown that the distance at which axons turn from the midline is determined by differential responses of the axons to a single gradient of slit protein emanating from the midline and that these differential responses in turn are determined by the complement of Robo family receptors expressed by the growth cones. All commissural axons in *Drosophila* express Robo itself, but there are also two other Robo receptors—Robo 2 and Robo3—expressed by commissural axon subpopulations (Simpson *et al.*, 2001; Rajagopalan, 2001). Axons expressing just Robo turn immediately upon crossing the midline, but axons expressing all three Robos extend a sizable distance from the midline before turning, whereas those expressing Robo and Robo3 extend an intermediate distance before turning (Fig. 17.14B). That the complement of receptors determines the site of turning was demonstrated in experiments in which the set of Robo family receptors on axons was altered transgenically and the behavior of the axons changed in predicted ways (Simpson *et al.*, 2001; Rajagopalan, 2001). For example, axons that normally express Robo and Robo3 will turn immediately after crossing the midline if the Robo3 gene is deleted, whereas axons that normally only express Robo will extend the predicted distance before turning if they are forced to express other Robos (Fig. 17.14B). Although it is not yet known mechanistically how the Robo receptor complement determines graded growth cone responses, these studies nonetheless illustrate how axons can show differential responses to a graded distribution of a single cue to help build more complex circuits in the developing nervous system.

Summary

The mechanisms that guide the growth of axons *in vivo* involve the simultaneous interpretation of multiple cues. Adding to the complexity of understanding axon guidance is the fact that even the same cue can be interpreted differently by different cells, by the same cell at different times, or even at the same time but in different subcellular domains. Semaphorin 3A is an example of a single guidance cue that serves multiple roles during development: it repels the axons of cortical pyramidal neurons away from the pial surface and toward the white matter, while simultaneously attracting the growth of their apical dendrites; it regulates axon–axon fasciculation in the peripheral nervous system, and it serves as a "stop and wait" signal for the development of olfactory sensory axons. The study of the growth of commissural axons to the midline exemplifies the dynamic changes in axon responsiveness to multiple guidance cues during the process of axon growth. Before reaching the midline, commissural axons are attracted by netrins and fail to respond to repellent molecules that are also at the midline. However, upon reaching the midline, the axons acquire responsiveness to the repellent molecules (through upregulation of receptor function triggered by an unknown mechanism) and concomitantly lose their responsiveness to netrin (through a process of receptor silencing). These alterations in the competence of growth cones to respond to environmental cues enables the axon to leave an attractive intermediate target and continue on its way toward its next destination. In this manner, the strategic deployment of guidance cues and regulated changes in the response of axons to those cues enables the growth cone to sequentially sample and interpret local cues on its journey toward a target.

FUTURE DIRECTIONS

Considerable progress has been made in the past decade in identifying some of the key molecules that function to guide axons and the receptors that mediate their attractive or repulsive effects. In coming years we can expect to identify still more families of axonal guidance molecules. One of the greatest current challenges is elucidating the signal transduction pathways within growth cones that mediate attractive and repulsive responses. The dissection of these signaling pathways will be an essential first step in understanding how multiple guidance cues are integrated by the growth cone and together determine its direction of migration. We can also expect to see the identification of signals that alter growth cone responsiveness to guidance cues and thereby help reprogram them as they progress from one choice point to the next along their trajectories. A greater understanding of axon growth and guidance during development will increase our ability to control axon regrowth in the adult nervous system and is therefore likely to help in the development of therapies to regenerate axonal connections following injury in the adult.

References

Bentley, D., and Caudy, M. (1983). Pioneer axons lose directed growth after selective killing of guidepost cells. *Nature (Lond.)* **304**, 62–65.
Caudy, M., and Bentley, D. (1986). Pioneer growth cone steering along a series of neuronal and non-neuronal cues of different affinities. *J. Neurosci.* **6**, 1781–1795.
Chisholm, A., and Tessier-Lavigne, M. (1999). Conservation and divergence of axon guidance mechanisms. *Curr. Opin. Neurobiol.* **9**, 603–615.
Forscher, P., and Smith, S. J. (1988). Actions of cytochalasins on the organization of actin filaments and microtubules in a neuronal growth cone. *J. Cell Biol.* **107**, 1505–1516.
Goodman, C. S., and Shatz, C. J. (1993). Developmental mechanisms that generate precise patterns of neuronal connectivity. *Cell (Cambridge, Mass.)* **72**, 77–98.
Holder, N., and Klein, R. (1999). Eph receptors and ephrins: Effectors of morphogenesis. *Development* **126**, 2033–2044.
Kidd, T., Bland, K. S., and Goodman, C. S. (1999). Slit is the midline repellent for the robo receptor in Drosophila. *Cell* **96**(6), 785–794.
Kidd, T., Brose, K., Mitchell, K. J., Fetter, R. D., Tessier-Lavigne, M., Goodman, C. S., and Tear, G. (1998). Roundabout controls axon crossing of the CNS midline and defines a novel subfamily of evolutionarily conserved guidance receptors. *Cell* **92**, 205–215.
Kolodkin, A. L., Matthes, D. J., O'Connor, T. P., Patel, N. H., Admon, A., Bentley, D., and Goodman, C. S. (1992). Fasciclin IV: Sequence, expression, and function during growth cone guidance in the grasshopper embryo. *Neuron* **9**, 831–845.
Lance-Jones, C., and Landmesser, L. (1980). Motoneurone projection patterns in the chick hind limb following early partial reversals of the spinal cord. *J. Physiol. (Lond.)* **302**, 581–602.
Lin, C.-H., Thompson, C. A., and Forscher, P. (1994). Cytoskeletal reorganization underlying growth cone motility. *Curr. Opin. Neurobiol.* **4**, 640–647.
Luo, Y., Raible, D., and Raper, J. A. (1993). Collapsin: A protein in brain that induces the collapse and paralysis of neuronal growth cones. *Cell* **75**, 217–27.
Polleux, F., Giger, R. J., Ginty, D. D., Kolodkin, A. L., and Ghosh, A. (1998). Patterning of cortical efferent projections by semaphorin-neuropilin interactions. *Science* **282**, 1904–1906.
Polleux, F., Morrow, T., and Ghosh, A. (2000). Semaphorin 3A is a chemoattractant for cortical apical dendrites. *Nature.* **404**(6778), 567–573.
Rajagopalan, S., Vivancos, V., Nicolas, E. and Dickson, B. J. (2000). Selecting a longitudinal pathway: Robo receptors specify the lateral position of axons in the Drosophila CNS. *Cell* **103**(7), 1033–1045.
Ramon y Cajal, S. (1890). Sur l'origine et les ramifications des fibres nerveuses de la moelle embryonaire. *Anat. Anz.* **5**, 609–613. Extract from Ramon y Cajal, S. (1909). "Histology of the Nervous System" (N. Swanson and L. W. Swanson, transl.). Oxford Univ. Press, Oxford, 1995.
Raper, J. A. (2000). Semaphorins and their receptors in vertebrates and invertebrates. *Opin. Neurobiol.* **10**, 88–94.
Raper, J. A., M. Bastiani, and Goodman, C. S. (1983) Pathfinding by neuronal growth cones in grasshopper embryos. II. Selective fasciculation onto specific axonal pathways. *J. Neurosci.* **2**, 31–41.
Renzi, M. J., Wexler, T. L., and Raper, J. A. (2000). Olfactory sensory axons expressing a dominant-negative semaphorin receptor enter the CNS early and overshoot their target. *Neuron* **28**, 437–447.
Serafini, T., Kennedy, T. E., Galko, M. J., Mirzayan, C., Jessell, T. M., and Tessier-Lavigne, M. (1994). The netrins define a family of axon outgrowth-promoting proteins homologous to *C. elegans* UNC-6. *Cell (Cambridge, Mass.)* **78**, 409–424.
Shamah, S. M., Lin, M. Z., Goldberg, J. L., Estrach, S., Sahin, M., Hu, L., Bazalakova, M., Neve, R. L., Corfas, G., Debant, A., et al. (2001). EphA receptors regulate growth cone dynamics through the novel guanine nucleotide exchange factor ephexin. *Cell,* **105**(2), 233–244.
Simpson, J. H., Bland, K. S., Fetter, R. D., and Goodman, C. S. (2000). Short-range and long-range guidance by Slit and its

Robo receptors: A combinatorial code of Robo receptors controls lateral position. *Cell*, **103**(7), 1019–1032.

Sperry, R. W. (1963). Chemoaffinity in the orderly growth of nerve fiber patterns and connections. *Proc. Natl. Acad. Sci. USA* **50**, 703–710.

Song, H., Ming, G., He, Z., Lehmann, M., McKerracher, L., Tessier-Lavigne, M., and Poo, M. (1998). Conversion of neuronal growth cone responses from repulsion to attraction by cyclic nucleotides. *Science* **281**, 1515–1518.

Stein, E., and Tessier-Lavigne, M. (2001). Hierarchical organization of guidance receptors: Slit silences netrin attraction through a Robo/DCC receptor complex. *Science* **291**, 1847–2034.

Taniguchi, M., Yuasa, S., Fujisawa, H., Naruse, I., Saga, S., Mishina, M., and Yagi, T. (1997). Disruption of semaphorin III/D gene causes severe abnormality in peripheral nerve projection. *Neuron* **19**, 519–530.

Tessier-Lavigne, M., and Goodman, C. S. (1996). The molecular biology of axon guidance. *Science* **274**, 1123–1133.

Tessier-Lavigne, M., Placzek, M., Lumsden, A. G., Dodd, J., and Jessell, T. M. (1988). Chemotropic guidance of developing axons in the mammalian central nervous system. *Nature* (*Lond.*) **336**, 775–778.

Wadsworth, W. G., Bhatt, H., and Hedgecock, E. M. (1996). Neuroglia and pioneer neurons express UNC-6 to provide global and local netrin cues for guiding migrations in *C. elegans*. *Neuron* **16**, 35–46.

Wang, K. H., Brose, K., Arnott, D., Kidd, T., Goodman, C. S., Henzel, W., and Tessier-Lavigne, M. (1999). Biochemical purification of a mammalian slit protein as a positive regulator of sensory axon elongation and branching. *Cell* **96**, 771–784.

Wessells, N. K., and Nuttall, R. P. (1978). Normal branching, induced branching, and steering of cultured parasympathetic motor neurons. *Exp. Cell Res.* **115**, 111–122.

Winberg, M. L., Noordermeer, J. N., Tamagnone, L., Comoglio, P. M., Spriggs, M. K., Tessier-Lavigne, M., and Goodman, C. S. (1998). Plexin A is a neuronal semaphorin receptor that controls axon guidance. *Cell* **95**, 903–916.

Wong, K., Ren, X. R., Huang, Y. Z., Xie, Y., *et al.* (2001). Signal transduction in neuronal migration: Roles of GTPase activating proteins and the small GTPase Cdc42 in the Slit-Robo pathway. *Cell* **107**, 209–221.

Zou, Y., Stoeckli, E., Chen, H., and Tessier-Lavigne, M. (2000). Squeezing axons out of the gray matter: A role for Slit and Semaphorin proteins from midline and ventral spinal cord. *Cell* **102**, 363–365.

Jonathan Raper and Marc Tessier-Lavigne

Target Selection, Topographic Maps, and Synapse Formation

A fundamental issue in neurobiology is defining the mechanisms by which neurons recognize and innervate their targets. Formation of a proper functioning nervous system depends on the development of precise connectivity between appropriate sets of neurons or neurons with peripheral targets such as muscles, tendons, skin, and various organs. The development of appropriate synaptic connections requires a series of steps, including the specification and generation of neurons and their target cells (Chapters 14, 15, and 16), the guidance of axons to their targets (Chapter 17), the selection of appropriate targets, the formation of orderly specific projections within the target, and ultimately induction of a specialized presynaptic terminal and postsynaptic membrane (this chapter). The first section of this chapter focuses on the mechanisms and molecules that govern target selection by cortical, retinal, and spinal axons and the formation of topographically ordered connections. The second section focuses on the signaling molecules and mechanisms that induce presynaptic and postsynaptic differentiation at the neuromuscular synapse. The third section summarizes current views of how presynaptic and postsynaptic differentiation is initiated in the central nervous system (CNS).

TARGET SELECTION AND MAP FORMATION

Target Selection by Delayed Interstitial Axon Branching

As discussed in Chapter 17, the growth cone makes navigational decisions in response to axon guidance molecules. This process of pathfinding by the growth cone is crucial to bring the axon within the vicinity of its targets. The growth cone has also long been considered to be responsible for the process of target selection itself. In some vertebrate systems, especially in many of the projections studied in Drosophila and other invertebrates, the growth cone tipping the primary axon does ultimately select its target. Many neurons, though, in the vertebrate brain innervate multiple, widely separated targets by axon collaterals and therefore face a unique problem of target selection during development. It is becoming increasingly apparent that in these situations, the process of target selection is accomplished by a distinct mechanism, often referred to as delayed interstitial axon branching.

A prominent example of neurons that employ delayed interstitial branching as a mechanism of target selection is layer 5 neurons in the mammalian neocortex (Fig. 18.1). Layer 5 neurons form the major output projection of the cortex and establish connections with several targets in the midbrain, hindbrain, and spinal cord. Studies by O'Leary and colleagues show that during development, layer 5 axons extend out of the cortex along a spinally directed pathway; their growth cones ignore several potential targets as they grow past them and continue to extend caudally through the corticospinal tract. Axon collaterals extended by layer 5 axons later innervate the brain stem and spinal targets. One of the major brain stem targets is the basilar pons, a prominent nucleus that lies at the ventral surface of the anterior hindbrain, and is particularly well suited for studying this mechanism of target selection. Evidence obtained from the examination of fixed tissue sections suggests that the collaterals to the basilar pons, as well as to the other subcortical targets of layer 5 axons, develop by a delayed interstitial branching from the axon shaft

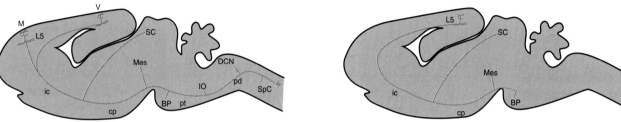

FIGURE 18.1   Area-specific subcortical projections of layer 5 neurons of the neocortex develop by delayed interstitial branching and selective axon elimination. The three main phases of this mechanism are illustrated in schematics of a sagittal view of the developing rat brain. (A) Primary axon extension. Layer 5 neurons (L5) extend a primary axon out of the cortex along a pathway that directs them toward the spinal cord (SpC) passing by their subcortical targets. (B) Delayed collateral branch formation. Subcortical targets are later contacted exclusively by axon collaterals that develop by a delayed extension of collateral branches interstitially along the spinally directed primary axon. As a population, layer 5 neurons in all areas of rat neocortex develop branches to a common set of targets. (C) Selective axon elimination. As illustrated for visual and motor cortex, specific collateral branches or segments of the primary axon are selectively eliminated to generate the mature projections functionally appropriate for the area of neocortex in which the layer 5 neuron is located. BP, basilar pons; cp, cerebral peduncle; ic, internal capsule; M, motor cortex; pd, pyramidal decussation; pt, pyramidal tract; SC, superior colliculus; V, visual cortex. Adapted from O'Leary and Koester (1993).

millimeters behind the growth cone, often days after the parent axons have grown past the target. Time-lapse imaging in hemibrain slice preparations from neonatal mice has provided further evidence that the branches form *de novo* along the portion of the axon shaft overlying the target. Evidence from collagen gel assays suggests that the target releases a diffusible activity with chemoattractant properties that induces branching along layer 5 axons, and directs the branches into the target. Thus, the axon shaft millimeters behind the growth cone is actively involved in target selection.

Examples of interstitial branching as the primary mechanism of target selection in vertebrates are accumulating. These examples include the extensive analysis by Katherine Kalil and co-workers on the development of cortical callosal projections, as well as the development of axonal projections from the hippocampal formation (i.e. the subiculum) to the mammillary bodies, dorsal root ganglion neurons to the spinal gray matter, and innervation of the dorsal lateral geniculate nucleus by retinal axons. In addition, as dis-

cussed later, the formation of topographic connections by retinal axons in the optic tectum of chicks and superior colliculus of rodents also occurs by interstitial branching along the axon shaft.

Exuberant Axonal Connections and Collateral Elimination

The development of many axonal projections in the brain is characterized by an initially exuberant, or widespread, growth of axons, followed by the elimination of functionally inappropriate axon segments and branches. For example, this mechanism is used to generate the adult patterns of callosal, intracortical, and subcortical projections of the mammalian neocortex (O'Leary and Koester, 1993). In the adult cortex, neurons that send an axon through the midline corpus callosum to the opposite cortical hemisphere, termed callosal neurons, have a limited, discontinuous distribution. Giorgio Innocenti and colleagues were the first to show that the limited adult distribution of callosal neurons emerges from an early widespread, continuous distribution of cortical neurons that send an axon through the corpus callosum. Several groups of investigators used retrograde tracers as fate markers to show that the developmental restriction in the distribution of callosal neurons is due to the loss of callosal axons rather than to the death of the parent neurons, which maintain an ipsilateral cortical connection. Collateral elimination has also been implicated in establishing the mature connections between cortical areas in the same hemisphere and in the refinement of horizontal connections within an area. For example, in adult visual cortex, layer 2/3 neurons have discrete horizontal projections to groups of other layer 2/3 cells with similar receptive field properties. However, Larry Katz and others have shown that the initial axonal outgrowth from layer 2/3 cells is very widespread in the horizontal plane, and the mature pattern of connections emerges in part through collateral elimination.

Organization of the adult neocortex into functionally specialized areas requires that each area establishes projections to specific subsets of targets in the brain stem and spinal cord. During development, though, layer 5 neurons project more broadly and form collateral projections to a larger set of layer 5 targets than they will retain in the adult (Fig. 18.1). The functionally appropriate patterns of layer 5 projections characteristic of the adult are later pruned from this initial widespread pattern through selective axon elimination. Depending on the cortical area in which the layer 5 neuron is located, it will eliminate different subsets of the initial complement of branched projections and retain only those that are functionally appropriate. For example, layer 5 neurons in motor cortex lose their collateral branch to the superior colliculus, but retain branches to other targets, including the basilar pons, dorsal column nuclei, inferior olive, and spinal gray matter. In contrast, layer 5 neurons in visual cortex lose the entire segment of their primary axon and its branches caudal to the basilar pons and retain branches to the pons and superior colliculus. Although functionally inappropriate for the proper operation of the adult brain, the eliminated collateral branches or axon segments should not be viewed as projection errors, as they seem to be elaborated according to a specific axonal growth program characteristic of that general class of neuron.

The cellular mechanisms that control axon elimination and the final patterning of cortical projections are not well understood, but available evidence indicates a role for neural activity, specifically the sensory information being relayed by thalamocortical input. Elimination of callosal axons is perturbed by a variety of peripheral manipulations of either visual or somato-

sensory input, which alters either patterns of neural activity (e.g., strabismus) or absolute levels of activity (e.g., dark-rearing, eyelid suture, or silencing of retinal activity with the sodium channel blocker, tetrodotoxin). In these instances, callosal axon elimination is abnormal, resulting in the retention of callosal connections in parts of the cortex that would normally lose them. Similar findings have been obtained for the development of layer 2/3 horizontal connections. Thus sensory input plays an important role in developing the adult pattern of callosal and intracortical connections by influencing the pattern of axon elimination.

Heterotopic transplant experiments show that collateral elimination by layer 5 neurons is also plastic during development. Developing layer 5 neurons transplanted from the visual cortex to the motor cortex permanently retain their normally transient spinal axon, whereas layer 5 neurons transplanted from the motor cortex to the visual cortex lose their normally permanent spinal axon and retain their transient axon collateral to the superior colliculus. Thus, projections retained by transplanted layer 5 neurons are appropriate for the cortical area in which the transplanted neurons develop, not where they were born.

Summary

In summary, many projections in the vertebrate brain are formed by the mechanism of delayed interstitial branching along the length of the axon shaft. During development, neurons often project to more targets than in the adult and generate their adult pattern of connections through a process of selective axon or collateral elimination. This developmental phenomenon of transiently "exuberant" axonal projections may provide a substrate for developmental plasticity. For example, alterations in axon elimination may be a source of functional sparing or recovery following neural insults during development. In addition, this mechanism may contribute to differences between species in axonal connections, as suggested by studies of the projection from the subiculum to the mammillary bodies in mammals ranging from rodents to rabbits to elephants (O'Leary, 1992).

Topographic Map Development

Once axons reach their targets, they must select appropriate target cells with which to form synaptic connections. Many axonal projections within the brain establish an orderly arrangement of connections within their target field, termed a topographic map. These maps are arranged such that the spatial order of the cells of origin is reflected in the order of their axon terminations; thus, neighboring cells project to neighboring parts of the target to form a smooth and continuous map. Topographic projections are especially evident in sensory systems, such as the somatosensory and visual. In the somatosensory system, a map of sensory receptors distributed on the body is reiterated multiple times at various levels of the neuraxis. In the visual system, the main objective is to represent the visual world in the brain, i.e., to reconstruct a topographic representation of the visual world that projects onto the retina and is remapped multiple times in the brain, initially through direct retinal projections to the dorsal thalamus and midbrain. This precise mapping requires maintenance of the spatial ordering of the axons of retinal ganglion cells (RGCs) within their central targets in a pattern that reflects their origins in the retina. The projection from the retina to its major midbrain target, the superior colliculus (SC) of mammals, or its nonmammalian homologue, the optic tectum, has been the predominant model system for understanding the development of topographic axonal connections. Initially, a coarse map is formed and then it becomes refined by axon remodeling. This refinement is driven in part by activity-dependent mechanisms that are influenced by correlations in the patterns of electrical activity between neighboring RGCs (discussed in Chapters 20 and 21). However, a large body of evidence developed since the early 1950s has shown that, independent of neural activity, the target presents guidance information to incoming axons that controls their development of topographic connections.

The Chemoaffinity Hypothesis

The mechanisms that control the establishment of topographic maps have been studied intensively for many decades, but only in recent years has the molecular control of this process begun to be defined. The chemoaffinity hypothesis, formally proposed by Roger Sperry in the early 1960s, has been a driving force in the field. Sperry designed clever experiments to address earlier theories such as that of Weiss, which posited that the specificity of neuronal connections in an adult resulted from the "functional molding" of circuits formed more or less at random; connections that are functionally appropriate are retained and others are eliminated. Sperry studied the regeneration of the retinotectal projection in newts and frogs; in these amphibians, unlike in birds or mammals, cut RGC axons are capable of regenerating to reestablish functional connections with target neurons in the tectum. In one particularly conclusive experiment, Sperry cut the optic nerve, rotated the eye in its orbit by 180°, and allowed the RGC axons to regrow to the tectum. According to earlier theories, one would predict that the axons should eventually form a novel pattern of connections that could generate appropriate behavioral responses to visual stimuli. Instead, Sperry showed that the frogs behaved as if their visual world had been rotated 180°. For instance, when a fly was presented in the upper left-hand quadrant of the visual field of the rotated eye, the frog responded by diving down to the right. This inappropriate response was retained throughout the life of the frog, even after attempts to train the animal to compensate for the rotation. These findings suggested that the regenerated RGC axons had reestablished their original pattern of connections, which was subsequently confirmed by Sperry and others using anatomical and electrophysiological analyses. These findings provided experimental evidence inconsistent with the prevailing theories of the time that the adult pattern of axonal connections is established by the selective retention of functionally appropriate connections, and eventually led to the chemoaffinity hypothesis.

FIGURE 18.2 Repellent effects of ephrin-A ligands on retinal axons in vitro. (A and B) Summary of use of the membrane stripe assay to analyze the effects of membrane-associated molecules in the optic tectum, such as ephrin-A ligands, on the guidance of retinal ganglion cell (RGC) axons. This elegant *in vitro* assay, developed by Friedrich Bonhoeffer, has been used extensively by many investigators to characterize repellent versus attractant effects of membrane-associated molecules on axon guidance. A retinal strip oriented along the nasal–temporal axis is explanted on carpets consisting of alternating 90-μm-wide lanes of membranes derived from the anterior (A) or posterior (P) third of the tectum or from heterologous cell lines (e.g., Cos or 293T cells) mock transfected or transfected with *ephrin-A2* or *ephrin-A5* cDNA . RGC axons growing out of the temporal half of the retinal strip show a strong preference to grow on anterior tectal membranes, whereas those growing out of the nasal half show no preference. In contrast, temporal axons do not show a preference for anterior membranes when posterior membranes are pretreated with heat or proteases, indicating that the preference is due to a repellent in posterior membranes. ephrin-A2 and ephrin-A5 are candidate mediators of this repellent activity, as they are enriched in posterior membranes and repel retinal axons in the stripe assay. Adapted from O'Leary *et al.* (1999). (C and D) Examples of RGC growth preferences in the stripe assay. Lanes containing *ephrin-A2*- or *ephrin-A5*-transfected cell membranes are labeled with rhodamine isothiocyanate (RITC) fluorescent beads, visualized as red lanes in the lower part of each panel. Temporal RGC axons grow predominantly on membranes from mock-transfected cells, due to ephrin-A mediated repulsion that more strongly affects temporal than nasal RGC axons. These temporal-nasal differences in ephrin-A repulsion exhibit an abrupt transition at midretina on *ephrin-A2*-transfected membranes, similar to the preferences observed on anterior and posterior tectal membranes, and in contrast to the more gradual transition in growth preferences observed on *ephrin-A5*-transfected membranes. Adapted from Monschau *et al.* (1997).

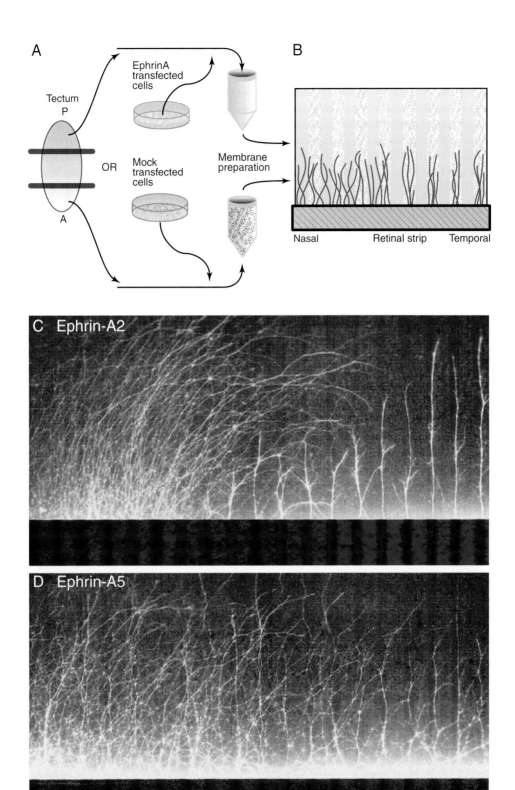

Sperry proposed that molecular tags on projecting axons and their target cells determine the specificity of axonal connections within a neural map. Further, he suggested that these molecular tags might establish topography through their distribution in complementary gradients that mark corresponding points in both sensory and target structures. Representation of the retina onto the tectum (or SC) is typically simplified to the mapping of two sets of orthogonally oriented axes: the temporal–nasal axis of the retina along the anterior–posterior (A–P) axis of the tectum and the ventral–dorsal axis of the retina along the medial–lateral (or dorsal–ventral) axis of the tectum. Based on the chemoaffinity hypothesis, each point in the tectum would have a unique molecular address determined by the graded distribution of topographic guidance molecules along the two tectal axes, and similarly each RGC would have a unique profile of receptors for those molecules that would result in a position-dependent, differential response to them by RGC axons. Over the next half century, the specificity of the projections of RGC axons to tectal cells was investigated further by the tracing of axonal projections following experimental manipulations, first in the regenerating retinotectal system and later during the development of the projection. Manipulations included rotations or transplantations of the retina, tectum, and even the optic pathway using either the whole structure or parts of it. Experiments showed that regenerating and developing RGC axons formed topographically appropriate connections even when they are experimentally deflected within the tectum or forced to enter the tectum from abnormal positions or with a reversal in the relative time of arrival of populations of RGC axons. This body of evidence supported the basic tenet of the chemoaffinity hypothesis that the establishment of topographic projections involves the recognition of positional information on the tectum.

Prior to the discovery of the ephrins (described later), arguably the most compelling evidence for topographic guidance molecules came from the work of Friedrich Bonhoeffer and co-workers using several elegant *in vitro* assays, including the membrane stripe and growth cone collapse assays. Using the membrane stripe assay, they showed that chick temporal RGC axons, given a choice between growing on alternating lanes of anterior and posterior tectal membranes, show a strong preference to grow on their topographically appropriate anterior membranes, whereas nasal RGC axons exhibit no preference (Fig. 18.2). A critical finding was that the growth preference of temporal axons was not due to an attractant or growth-promoting activity associated with anterior tectal membranes, but instead to a repellent activity associated with posterior tectal membranes. This was the first demonstration of a role for repellent activities in axon guidance. By taking advantage of the finding that posterior tectal membranes also preferentially collapse the growth cones of temporal axons, the repellent activity was isolated biochemically to a 33-kDa, GPI-anchored protein referred to as the repulsive guidance molecule (RGM); the cloning of RGM has yet to be reported.

Ephrin-As Control Mapping along the A–P Axis of the Target

A major breakthrough toward understanding the molecular control of topographic mapping came in 1995 with the cloning of two closely related genes: ephrin-A2 [originally called eph ligand family-1 (ELF-1)] by John Flanagan and colleagues and ephrin-A5 [originally called repulsive axon guidance signal (RAGS)] by Bonhoeffer, Uwe Drescher, and colleagues. These proteins, like all members of the ephrin-A family, are anchored to the cell membrane by a GPI linkage and bind with similar affinities and activate the same receptors, members of the EphA subfamily of receptor tyrosine kinases (Fig. 18.3). Based initially on their expression patterns, and subsequently on functional and genetic studies, ephrin-A2, ephrin–A5, and EphAs have been shown to control the topographic mapping of RGC axons in

FIGURE 18.3 Eph receptors and their ephrin ligands. Eph receptors comprise the largest family of receptor tyrosine kinases, currently numbering 14 members, and are divided into two subfamilies, EphA (A1 to A8) and EphB (B1 to B6), with distinct binding specificities that correlate with structural similarities. The nine known ephrins are divided into ephrin-A (A1–A6) and ephrin-B (B1–B3) subfamilies on the basis of sequence homology and their membrane anchoring: ephrin-As are anchored by a glycosyl phosphatidylinositol (GPI) linkage and ephrin-Bs by a transmembrane domain. Within each receptor–ligand subfamily, the ligands bind, albeit with different affinities, and activate, with few exceptions (e.g., EphA1 and EphB5), all of the receptors, but only a very limited interaction occurs between subfamilies (e.g., EphA4 interacts with ephrin-As and two ephrin-B proteins, and EphB2 interacts with ephrin-B and ephrin-A6). Although membrane-anchored ephrins activate Eph receptors, soluble forms of an ephrin can do so only when clustered artificially. Clustered ligand binding results in the formation of receptor multimers and activates the catalytic kinase domain on the cytoplasmic portion of the Eph receptor. In addition, ephrin-B ligands themselves can also transduce signals; thus receptor–ligand binding can result in bidirectional signaling into receptor-expressing and ligand-expressing cells. Emerging evidence suggests that ephrin-A ligands may also be capable of bidirectional signaling.

Receptors

Ligands

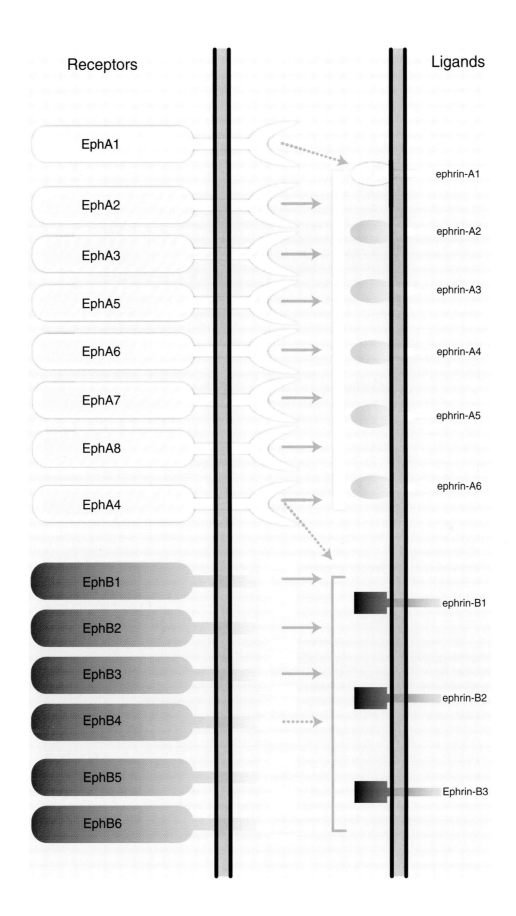

EphA1

EphA2

EphA3

EphA5

EphA6

EphA7

EphA8

EphA4

EphB1

EphB2

EphB3

EphB4

EphB5

EphB6

ephrin-A1

ephrin-A2

ephrin-A3

ephrin-A4

ephrin-A5

ephrin-A6

ephrin-B1

ephrin-B2

Ephrin-B3

their principal targets in the brain. In chick, ephrin-A2 is expressed in an increasing A–P gradient across the entire tectum, and ephrin-A5 is expressed in a steeper A–P gradient limited to posterior tectum; together they combine to form an increasing gradient across the A–P tectal axis (see Figure 18.6). RGCs express three of the seven known EphA receptors, EphA3, EphA4, and EphA5, but only EphA3 is expressed in a gradient, which is highest in temporal retina and lowest in nasal retina.

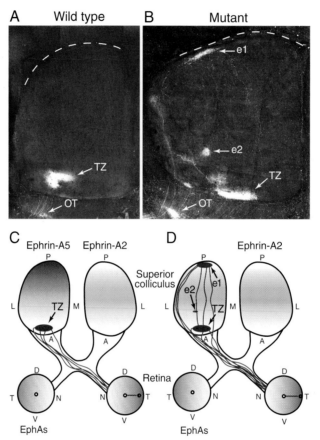

FIGURE 18.4 RGC projections in wild-type and *ephrin-A5* knockout mice related to the expression patterns of *ephrin-A5* and *ephrin-A2*. (A and B) Anterograde DiI labeling of RGC axons from peripheral temporal retina in wild-type and *ephrin-A5* knockout mice. Dorsal views of whole mounts of the superior colliculus (SC) are shown; midline is to the right, dashed lines indicate the posterior SC border. (A) In wild-type mice, temporal RGC axons end and arborize in a densely labeled termination zone (TZ) in anterior SC. The RGC projection to optic tract nuclei is also evident (OT). (B) In *ephrin-A5* null mutant mice, temporal RGC axons also end and arborize in a densely labelled TZ at the topographically appropriate site in anterior SC, temporal axons also project to and arborize at topographically inappropriate sites in far-posterior SC (e1) and anterior SC (e2). (C and D) Schematic representations summarizing temporal RGC axon mapping in wild-type and *ephrin-A5* mutant mice in relationship to the expression of *ephrin-A5* and *ephrin-A2*. (C) In wild-type mice, a focal DiI injection in peripheral temporal retina labels axons (red lines) that form a dense TZ (red oval) in the topographically correct anterior SC. *ephrin-A5* (blue shading) is expressed in a low anterior (A) to high posterior (P) gradient across the SC. *ephrin-A2* (orange shading) is expressed highest in midposterior parts of the SC and declines to low levels in more anterior and far-posterior SC. Together, ephrin-A5 and ephrin-A2 form a smooth gradient of repellent activity across the SC. EphA receptors are expressed in a high temporal (T) to low nasal (N) gradient by RGCs. (D) In *ephrin-A5* mutant mice, *ephrin-A2* (orange shading) is expressed in the same pattern as in wild type. A focal DiI injection in temporal retina labels axons that form a dense TZ in topographically correct anterior SC; in addition, aberrant terminations (e1, e2) form at topographically incorrect locations. The pattern of ectopic arbors relates to the maintained expression pattern of *ephrin-A2*: ectopic arbors are typically present in far-posterior and anterior SC where *ephrin-A2* expression is low, but are rare in mid-SC where *ephrin-A2* expression is highest. This distribution suggests that in the absence of ephrin-A5, ectopic arbors are present where the levels of repellent activity due to ephrin-A2 are too low to prevent their formation and stabilization. D, dorsal; L, lateral; M, medial; V, ventral. Adapted from Frisén *et al.* (1998).

Because temporal retina with high levels of EphA3 maps to anterior tectum with low levels of ephrin-As, and vice versa, ephrin-A2 and ephrin-A5 likely act as axon repellents that affect temporal axons more strongly than nasal. This suggestion has been confirmed by *in vitro* and *in vivo* studies (Nakamoto *et al.*, 1996; Monschau *et al.*, 1997). Experiments employing membrane stripe and growth cone collapse assays using membranes from transfected cell lines show that both ephrin-A2 and ephrin–A5 repel temporal axons preferentially, and that at the appropriate concentrations, retinal axons exhibit a graded temporal to nasal response to ephrin-A5 (Fig. 18.2). *In vivo*, temporal axons specifically avoid ectopic patches of ephrin-A2 that were overexpressed in the anterior tectum following infection with recombinant retrovirus. These studies suggest that the interaction of EphA3 with ephrin-A2 and ephrin-A5 could determine the specificity of RGC projections along the A–P tectal axis.

Although species-specific differences are apparent in the particular EphAs and ephrin-As that are expressed, or in their patterns of expression, the basic theme described earlier for chicks is constant across all vertebrate species examined. For example, as in chick tectum, ephrin-A2 and ephrin-A5 combine to form a smooth increasing A–P gradient in the mouse SC. However, their pattern of expression in the SC differs substantially from chick tectum: ephrin-A5 is expressed in an increasing A–P gradient across the SC, resembling ephrin-A2 in chick tectum, whereas ephrin-A2 is expressed at high levels in a broad domain centered on mid-posterior SC and shows a graded decline to low or no expression in the anterior third and far-posterior SC. The expression of EphA receptors by RGCs also differs between chick and mouse. In mouse, EphA3 is not expressed by RGCs, EphA4 is expressed uniformly by RGCs, and both EphA5 and EphA6 are expressed in a high temporal to low nasal gradient.

The graded expression of ephrin-As and their differential repulsion of temporal versus nasal RGC axons strongly implicate them as topographic guidance molecules, as predicted by Sperry. The first genetic test of whether they are required for proper topographic mapping came from an analysis of mice with a targeted deletion of ephrin-A5 (Frisen *et al.*, 1998) (Fig. 18.4). The mapping of RGC axons in the SC of ephrin-A5 null mice is topographically aberrant in a manner consistent with the loss of ephrin-A5 and the maintained expression of ephrin-A2. For example, temporal RGC axons form ectopic projections to far-posterior SC and within the anterior third of the SC. As expected, topographic mapping defects in ephrin-

A2/A5 double knockout mice are more severe than in either ephrin-A single knockout (Feldheim *et al.*, 2000). Surprisingly, though, temporal RGC axons do form a normal-appearing termination at the topographically correct site in anterior SC of ephrin-A5 null SC; even in ephrin-A2/A5 double knockout mice, in the complete absence of any ephrin-A expression, temporal RGC axons form a termination zone, albeit smaller, in anterior SC at the approximately correct position. These loss-of-function analyses show that ephrin-As are required for proper topographic mapping, but other molecules likely work with them to generate topographic order along the A–P axis in the SC.

Loss-of-function studies of the action of EphA receptors in the development of topographic maps in mice are complicated by potential redundancy in the roles of EphA5 and EphA6 and the fact that mice lacking EphA5 die as embryos well before topographic order emerges. An alternate gain-of-function strategy took advantage of the features that ephrin-As bind and activate with similar efficacy most EphA receptors and that EphA3 is not expressed by RGCs in mice. Mice were generated in which EphA3 was expressed ectopically in about half of the RGCs distributed uniformly across the retina, thus producing two subpopulations of RGCs, one which has the wild-type gradient of EphA receptors (EphA5 and EphA6) and one with an elevated gradient of overall EphA expression (Brown *et al.*, 2000). In these mice, projection of EphA3 RGCs is compressed to the anterior half of the SC, indicating that the level of the EphA receptor dictates the degree to which an RGC axon is repelled by ephrin-As. Surprisingly, though, the projection of the wild-type RGCs is compressed to the posterior half of the SC and is likely excluded from the anterior SC by competitive interactions with the EphA3 RGCs. Thus, mapping of the two RGC subpopulations is not determined by the absolute level of EphA receptor signaling, but instead appears to be controlled by the relative difference in EphA signaling. These findings also reveal a hierarchy in the mechanisms for generating topographic maps, showing that molecular axon guidance information, such as that signaled by ephrin-As and EphAs, dominates over activity-dependent patterning mechanisms, which are based on near-neighbor relationships and correlated activity.

Development of Topographic Maps and Implications for Actions of Guidance Molecules

Studies on the development of topographic retinotectal projections in chicks and rodents have altered our way of thinking about the mechanisms that control topographic map development. Prior to this work, most of what we know about the behavior of RGC axons during map development was based on the studies of amphibians and fish done by many investigators, including Scott Fraser, Haijme Fujisawa, Bill Harris, Christine Holt, and Claudia Steurmer. There are several reasons for this bias, including that these animals were already widely used for studies of retinotopic mapping because of their ability to regenerate retinal connections and the relative ease with which their visual systems could be studied experimentally. Throughout the life of frogs and fish, the retina adds RGCs around its entire circumference, whereas the tectum adds cells only to its posterior end. These disparate growth patterns result in a phenomenon termed "shifting connections," where retinal connections shift continually posteriorly to accommodate newly arriving temporal axons as they form connections in anterior tectum and allow the map to retain its proper topographic organization. This phenomenon is exaggerated at the initial stages in development, when axons arising from central–nasal retina and central–temporal retina both terminate at what is then the posterior end of the nascent tectum. As the tectum adds cells to its original posterior end, central–nasal axons retract their arbors and reestablish them in the newly differentiated posterior tectum, whereas the central–temporal axonal arbors remain behind. However, most RGC axons arrive to the tectum at later stages, grow directly to their topographically appropriate site, and form terminal arbors by an elaboration of the growth cone and back-branches that form at its base. Compared to chicks and mammals, frogs and fish require a properly functioning visual system at relatively early stages of neural development when the tectum is very small. Thus, early on their RGC axonal arbors are disproportionately large compared to the tectum and cover a greater percentage of its surface area than at later stages. The finer grain resolution of the adult retinotectal projection is not achieved by arbor retraction; instead, the size of individual arbors and the tectum itself increases over development, but the tectum grows at a much greater rate.

Historically, gradient models proposed to account for topographic mapping along the A–P tectal axis were designed to explain topographic targeting of growth cones and were based on adhesion mechanisms, which were in vogue to explain most cell–cell interactions during development. These models required countergradients of attractant activities along the A–P tectal axis and corresponding countergradients in the retina, which defined unique, "best-fit," combinations of adhesion for growth cones arising from different retinal locations. The demonstration that graded repellent activities, such as ephrin-As, act as topographic guidance molecules in principle simplifies the mapping solution, as a single repellent gradient could be sufficient to direct topographic growth cone targeting if the receptor–ligand interaction followed the law of mass action, where the repellent signal (or receptor–ligand complex) is determined by the product of the concentrations of EphA receptors and ephrin-A ligands. RGC growth cones would stop their posterior extension along the A–P tectal axis when they attained a threshold level of repellent signal determined by ephrin-A activation of the EphA receptors. Growth cones from progressively more temporal retina have progressively higher levels of EphA receptors and would attain their threshold level of repulsion at progressively more anterior tectum with lower levels of ephrin-As (Fig. 18.6).

Because numerous studies of frogs and fish concluded that topographic retinotectal connections develop by the direct topographic targeting of RGC axon growth cones, similar mechanisms were assumed to account for mapping in other vertebrates. However, the use of more recently introduced axon tracers that give high-resolution filling of RGC axons in chicks and mammals has revealed an unexpected and distinct picture of the development of topographic retinotectal projections in warm-blooded animals. Analyses of topographic mapping of RGC axons in chick tectum indicate that a primary role for topographic guidance molecules is to regulate topographic branching along RGC axons, a process that imposes unique requirements on the molecular control of map development (Yates et al., 2001). In chick, topographically appropriate connections are established exclusively by branches that form along the axon shaft. RGC axons initially grow past their appropriate termination site along the A–P axis of the tectum (Fig. 18.5). Branches later form along the shaft of RGC axons; in contrast to growth cone targeting, branch formation is topographically biased for the correct location along the A–P axis. Topography is enhanced through the preferential arborization of appropriately positioned branches and the elimination of the overshooting segments of the primary axons and any ectopic branches. Use of a modified membrane stripe assay shows that temporal axons preferentially branch on their topographically appropriate anterior tectal membranes and that this branching specificity is due to the inhibition of branching on posterior tectal membranes by ephrin-As. Similar analyses suggest that similar mechanisms are used in rodents to develop topography in the retinocollicular projection. These findings indicate that topo-

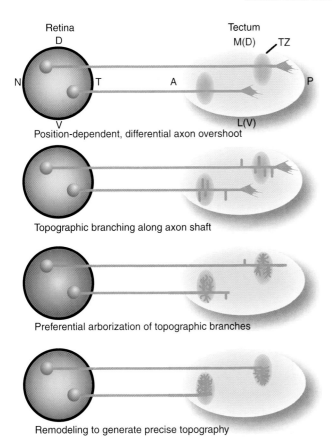

FIGURE 18.5 Development of topographic order in the chick retinotectal projection. RGC axons initially exhibit a position-dependent, differential overshoot of the topographic location of their appropriate termination zone (TZ) along the anterior (A) – posterior (P) tectal axis: temporal axons overshoot the greatest distance and nasal axons the least. In contrast, branches form along the shaft of RGC axons with a substantial degree of topographic specificity for the A–P location of their future TZ. Precise topography is established through the preferential arborization of appropriately positioned branches and elimination of ectopic branches and axon segments. D, dorsal; L, lateral; M, medial; N, nasal; T, temporal; V, ventral. Adapted from Yates *et al.* (2001).

graphic branch formation and arborization along RGC axons, rather than the initial targeting of axon growth cones, are critical events in retinotectal mapping in mammals. The level of ephrin-As posterior to their correct termination site is sufficient to inhibit branching along the overshooting segments of RGC axons, but alone cannot account for topographic branching (Fig. 18.6). Thus ephrin-As must cooperate with other, presently unidentified, molecular activities to generate appropriate mapping along the A–P tectal axis.

In addition to overshooting their termination site along the A–P tectal axis, most RGC axons also enter and extend across the tectum at positions either medial or lateral to it. Interstitial branches not only form along the shaft of RGC axons with a topographic bias along the A–P axis, but most also extend along the M–L axis in the direction that corrects the location of the axon and positions the branch at the appropriate termination site. The emerging evidence points to a role for the EphB/ephrin-B subfamily in controlling the directed extension of branches along the M–L axis. Ephrin-B1 is expressed in a high medial (dorsal) to low lateral (ventral) gradient in tectum, and four of the six EphB receptors are expressed by RGCs in both chick and mouse: EphB2, EphB3, and EphB4 are expressed in a high ventral to low dorsal gradient, and EphB1 is expressed uniformly. Because ventral retina with high levels of EphBs maps to medial tectum with high levels of ephrin-B1, and vice versa, it is likely that signaling through the graded EphB receptors promotes axon attraction—an action distinct from that of ephrin-As in RGC mapping, and the repellent effect that ephrin-B1 has on motor axons.

Role of Patterned Neural Activity in Topographic Mapping

It is well established that neural activity plays an important role in the development of axonal connections in many neural systems, including the segregation of RGC axons into eye-specific laminae in the lateral geniculate nucleus or eye-specific stripes in experimentally created three-eyed frogs (see Chapters 20 and 21). However, neural activity appears to have a limited role in the development of topography in the retinotectal projection. The first studies to address this issue were done by Bill Harris, who homotopically transplanted axolotl eyes into the California newt, a species that produces endogenous tetrodotoxin (TTX), a neurotoxin that blocks Na$^+$ channels. The transplanted axolotl RGCs were silenced by the TTX, but their projection to the tectum developed an appropriately ordered topographic map. Similarly, in other species in which the map develops by the direct topographic targeting of RGC axons, such as fish and frogs, activity blockade has little affect on topography. For example, RGC axonal arbors are unaffected in zebrafish bathed in either TTX or AP5, and blocking NMDA receptors in Xenopus results only in a slowing of map development. Even in chicks and rats, in which the early retinotectal projection is topographically more diffuse, a considerable degree of order emerges under activity blockade. In chick, both TTX and grayanotoxin, which keeps Na$^+$ channels in an open state, interfere with the elimination of only a small proportion of overshooting axon segments and aberrant branches and arbors. Similarly, in rats, chronic application to the SC of AP5, an antagonist of the NMDA class of glutamate receptor, which blocks the activation of SC neurons by RGCs (which use glu-

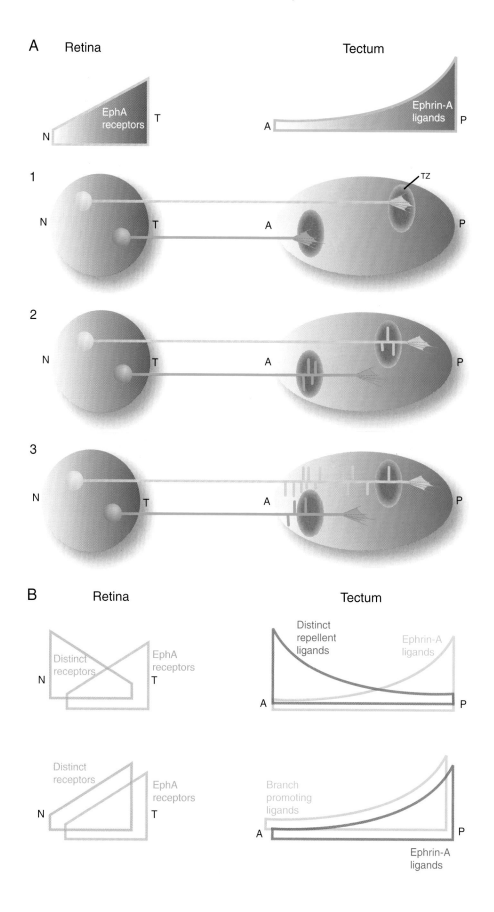

tamate as their neurotransmitter), also results in the abnormal retention of a small proportion of topographically aberrant axons and arbors. However, in both chicks and rats, activity blockade does not prevent the elimination of a large proportion of aberrantly targeted axons and arbors, nor does it prevent the development of dense arborizations of RGC axons at their topographically correct sites. In conclusion, molecular guidance mechanisms appear to be the major contributors to the development of topographic maps, and activity-dependent mechanisms serve to refine the initial map.

Summary

The formation of topographic maps involves the establishment of an initial, coarse map that is subsequently refined. Analysis of the retinotectal system in amphibians, fish, birds, and mammals shows that the initial map is formed based on positional information present in the tectum. In birds and mammals, a critical mechanism in map development is the topographic specific branching of RGC axons that overshoot their correct TZ. Topographic guidance information is encoded in the form of gradients of signaling molecules along both A-P and M-L axes of the target. Ephrin-A ligands and EphA receptors control, in part, RGC axon mapping along the A-P axis. Other receptor–ligands systems must also be involved.

Target Selection by Spinal Motor Axons

Spinal motor axons project in a topographic manner to skeletal muscles. For example, motor neurons in rostral parts of the spinal cord innervate rostral muscles, whereas those in caudal spinal cord innervate caudal muscles. The axons of motor neurons exit the spinal cord, extend across the rostral half of each developing somite at their exit level, and converge upon a plexus where they intermingle with other motor axons that will innervate different muscles. As described in Chapter 17, spinal motor axons are initially directed out of the spinal cord by repellent guidance molecules expressed by the floor plate. The segmental patterning of motor nerves appears to be due to repulsive molecules such as T-cadherin, collagen IX, ephrin-B1 and ephrin-B2, which are expressed preferentially in the caudal half of the somite, repel motor axons *in vitro*, and *in vivo* appear to restrict the path of motor axons to the rostral half of the somite. In the plexus, the growth cones begin to sort and associate with other axons that will innervate the same muscle. In the case of motor axons that will innervate a limb, after leaving the plexus, they project to either the ventral or the dorsal premuscle mass in the limb and later to the appropriate individual muscle. The projection of motor axons to their target muscles appears to be accurate from the outset, with few targeting errors.

Much of the evidence for how the axons of motor neurons select their appropriate target muscles initially came from the studies of Landmesser and colleagues on the guidance of motor axons to skeletal muscle cells in the developing chick embryo. The idea that motor axons are guided to their appropriate targets by navigational cues presented along the pathway is supported further by experiments in which

FIGURE 18.6 Actions and limitations of ephrin-As in retinotectal map development. (A) The top panel schematizes the approximate gradient profiles for EphA receptors and ephrin-A ligands in the chick retina and optic tectum, respectively. RGCs show a high temporal (T) to low nasal (N) gradient of EphA receptor expression, due mainly to EphA3. Ephrin-A2 and ephrin-A5 combine to form a low anterior (A) to high posterior (P) gradient of expression across the tectum. (A1–A3) Observed and theoretical behaviors of RGC axons. Growth cones stop at A–P positions in the tectum where they reach a threshold level of repellent activation following a mass action law of receptor–ligand interactions. Temporal growth cones, which have high levels of EphA receptors, reach threshold levels of repellent at anterior (A) positions in the tectum, with low levels of ephrin-A ligand. Growth cones from nasal retina (N), which have low levels of EphA receptors, will reach threshold levels of activation at more posterior (P) positions in the tectum. This mechanism can account for the guidance of RGC growth cones to their topographically correct TZ, as is observed in amphibians and fish (A1), as well as the position-dependent overshoot of RGC axons, as observed in chicks (A2). However, a single repellent gradient, such as that formed by ephrin-A ligands in the tectum, alone is insufficient to generate topographic branching along RGC axons observed in chick (A2). Ephrin-As can inhibit branching along the segment of the overshooting axons posterior to their correct TZ, but anterior to the correct TZ, the level of ephrin-A repellent signal would be below the threshold required to inhibit branching. Thus, if only the tectal ephrin-As regulated branching, all RGC axons should exhibit increased branching at more anterior positions in the tectum, which have the lowest levels of the ephrin-A repellent signal (A3).(B) Illustrated are two potential models, among many, that can account for topographic branching along RGC axons. Both models incorporate the graded ephrin-A repellent and a distinct graded activity that cooperates with it to generate topographic branching. In each case, the ephrin-A repellent prevents branching along the axon shaft posterior to the TZ and the distinct graded activity regulates branching along axons anterior to their TZ. One model includes a distinct repellent in a gradient that opposes the ephrin-A gradient and acts by inhibiting branching along the axon shaft anterior to the TZ. Thus, branching along the axon shaft occurs at an A–P tectal position below threshold for branch inhibition for both of the repellent signals. The other model includes a branch-promoting activity in a gradient that roughly parallels the ephrin-A gradient. In this model, branching along the axon shaft occurs at an A–P tectal position above threshold for the branch-promoting signal, but below threshold for branch inhibition by the ephrin-A repellent signal. Adapted from O'Leary *et al.* (1999).

motor neurons and/or their targets are displaced by transplantation. These studies demonstrate that axons of displaced motor neurons, which arrive at the plexus from an aberrant location, are able to reorient and emerge from the plexus to innervate their appropriate targets. The directional signals are apparently not supplied by muscle, as motor axons project accurately to the appropriate region of the developing limb even in the absence of muscle cells. Thus, mesenchymal cells in the plexus region are thought to have an important role in providing cues that guide and direct motor axons to the appropriate region of the developing limb. Evidence is beginning to emerge on the molecular control of the pathfinding decision at the limb plexus. Hepatocyte growth factor, which is expressed in the sclerotome and the limb mesenchyme, can guide motor axons *in vitro*. Other work has shown that the level of EphA4 expression by motor axons dictates in part the selection of dorsal versus ventral pathways at the hindlimb plexus, contributing to the topographic organization of motor projections (Helmbacher *et al.*, 2000). During normal hindlimb innervation, motor axons converge on the sciatic plexus, and those projecting dorsally into the limb express higher levels of EphA4 than those choosing the ventral pathway, which appears to have higher levels of ephrin-A expression. In EphA4 mutant mice, dorsal motor axons fail to enter the dorsal limb and instead project ventrally.

Axons associate, or fasciculate, with one another at certain points during pathfinding and diverge from one another as they grow to distinct targets. Thus, fasciculation and defasciculation are likely to be highly regulated and have important consequences for accurate pathfinding. Consistent with this idea, mutations of certain receptor tyrosine phosphatases (RTPs) in *Drosophila* result in poor defasciculation and an inability of motor axons to branch and readily target appropriate muscles. Thus, signaling through receptor tyrosine kinases (RTKs) and RTPs is likely to regulate adhesion between motor axons. Laminin, N-cadherin, N-CAM, polysialic acid, and fibronectin can also have a role in fasciculation. Nevertheless, these adhesion molecules alone may not have a role in directing subsets of motor axons to their appropriate pathways. Thus, it is possible that RTKs and RTPs control fasciculation and steering by regulating the strength of adhesion between motor axons or between axons and their substrates.

Motor axons enter the dorsal or ventral region of the developing limb before individual muscles have separated and taken on their unique identities; shortly after individual muscles begin to form, the main limb nerves branch as subsets of motor axons leave the main nerve to grow toward their appropriate muscles. Muscle cells may have a role in directing motor axons toward the appropriate muscle as the axons approach them, as in muscleless limbs the main limb nerves enter and form primary branches in the appropriate dorsal or ventral part of the limb, but fail to form the secondary branches that would grow to individual muscles.

Studies in *Drosophila* done by several groups, most notably Goodman and colleagues, have identified several molecules expressed by muscle cells that influence motor axon target selection. Fasciclin III is a cell surface protein expressed by a subset of motor neurons and their target muscle cells. Fasciclin III-expressing motor neurons normally innervate only fasciclin III-expressing muscle cells, but will innervate inappropriate muscle cells induced experimentally to express fasciclin III. Other adhesive molecules, such as fasciclin II and connectin, as well as repulsive molecules, such as the semaphorins, may have similar roles in regulating target selection.

In vertebrates, ephrins are involved not only in the segmental patterning of spinal motor nerves, but work done by Sanes and colleagues, as well as other groups, has shown that ephrin-As are involved in the selection by motor axons of their target muscles and in the development of topographic connections onto the muscle. Subsets of motor neurons express EphA3, EphA4, and EphA5 in patterns that relate to the expression of their ephrin-A ligands by muscles, and they respond to the ephrin-As in ways consistent with the mapping of rostral motor pools onto rostral muscles, and rostral portions of motor pools onto rostral fibers within their target muscles. In rodents, developing muscles express all five ephrin-As identified at the time, and ephrin-A1 and ephrin-A5 are expressed more highly in rostral muscles (e.g., shoulder and forelimb) than in caudal muscles (e.g., hindlimb). *In vitro*, ephrin-A5 inhibits the growth of caudal motor axons more strongly than rostral motor axons. *In vivo*, the topographic mapping of motor axons is degraded when the gluteus muscle overexpresses an ephrin-A5 transgene and in the diaphragm muscle of mutant mice lacking both ephrin-A2 and ephrin-A5. Similarly, in chick, motor neurons that innervate hindlimb muscles express EphA4, and their axons avoid parts of the limb that express ephrin-A2 and ephrin-A5, both of which inhibit the growth of these axons *in vitro*. Thus, ephrins are involved in establishing the topographic specificity of neuromuscular connections.

Summary

In summary, motor axons originating from specific subsets of motor neurons innervate specific muscles in a topographic manner. This process, which occurs with few guidance errors, involves a number of critical choice points in growth cone navigation. Ephrins act to funnel motor axons into their appropriate paths as they exit the spinal cord and navigate distally and control their appropriate topographic innervation of target muscles. Other families of molecules implicated in axon guidance and fasciculation are also involved in the control of this process.

DEVELOPMENT OF THE NEUROMUSCULAR SYNAPSE

Once axons have arrived at their appropriate target destination, synapse formation ensues. Much of our understanding about the mechanisms of synapse formation arises from studies of the neuromuscular synapse. These studies have benefited from (1) the relative ease of experimentally manipulating developing and regenerating neuromuscular synapses *in vivo*, (2) cell culture systems for both motor neurons and skeletal muscle cells, (3) the *Torpedo* electric organ, an abundant and homogeneous source of neuromuscular-like synapses, and (4) transgenic and mutant mice for studying and altering gene expression. Consequently, we have a good, although incomplete, understanding of the mechanisms that lead to the formation of the neuromuscular synapse.

Muscle differentiation and synapse formation occur concomitantly during development and require several weeks from initiation to completion. Shortly after contact between a growing motor axon and a differentiating myotube is established, signals are exchanged between nerve and muscle that stimulate the formation of a highly differentiated presynaptic nerve terminal and a highly specialized postsynaptic apparatus. Although functional synapses form within minutes to hours after contact between developing motor nerves and myotubes, mature and fully differentiated synapses are not evident, at least in mammals, until several weeks after the first contacts are made. The formation of a mature synapse requires further arborization of nerve terminals, withdrawal and editing of synaptic connections, changes in the efficiency of acetylcholine release, and modifications of the postsynaptic membrane.

An adult myofiber, a syncitial cell containing several hundred to several thousand nuclei, is innervated by a single motor axon that terminates and arborizes over ~0.1% of the muscle fiber's cell surface. The acetylcholine receptor (AChR) is localized to this small patch of the muscle fiber membrane, and its localization to synaptic sites during development is a hallmark of the inductive events of synapse forma-

tion. Although other proteins are likewise concentrated at synaptic sites, much of our knowledge about synaptic differentiation has come from studies aimed at understanding how AChRs accumulate at synaptic sites.

Substructural Organization of the Neuromuscular Synapse

The precise organization of molecules in pre- and postsynaptic membranes belies the concept that the neuromuscular synapse is a simple synapse. Rather, the substructure of pre- and postsynaptic membranes suggests that complex mechanisms are required to assemble the synapse and to coordinate pre- and postsynaptic differentiation.

Nerve terminals are situated in shallow depressions of the muscle cell membrane, which is invaginated further into deep and regular folds, termed postjunctional folds (Fig. 18.7). AChRs and additional proteins (see later) are localized to the crests of these postjunctional folds, whereas other proteins, including sodium channels, are enriched in the troughs of the postjunctional folds. The nerve terminal is likewise organized spatially, and its substructural organization reflects that of the postsynaptic membrane. Synaptic vesicles are sparse in the region of the nerve terminal underlying Schwann cells and are abundant in the region of the nerve terminal facing the muscle fiber. Moreover, synaptic vesicles are clustered adjacent to a poorly characterized specialization of the presynaptic membrane, termed active zones, which are the sites of synaptic vesicle fusion. Active zones are organized at regular intervals and are aligned precisely with the mouths of the postjunctional folds. This precise registration of active zones and postjunctional folds ensures that acetylcholine encounters a high concentration of AChRs within microseconds after release, thereby facilitating synaptic transmission. The alignment of structural specializations in pre- and postsynaptic membranes, separated by a 500-Å synaptic cleft, suggests that spatially restricted signaling between pre- and postsynaptic cells is important to coordinate pre- and postsynaptic differentiation. The mechanisms that align active zones and postjunctional folds are not understood, but $\alpha3\beta1$ integrin is concentrated at active zones and several laminins are found in the synaptic basal lamina, raising the possibility that laminin/integrin interactions have a role in positioning and organizing active zones.

The following section summarizes our current understanding of the signaling mechanisms that lead to the differentiation of nerve terminals and the post-

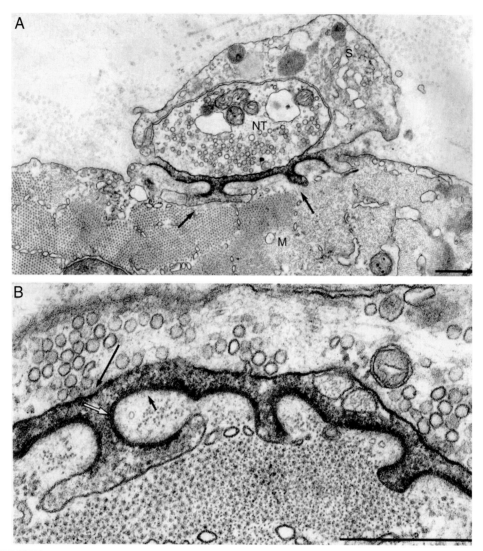

FIGURE 18.7   Pre- and postsynaptic membranes at the neuromuscular synapse are highly specialized. (A) An electron micrograph of a neuromuscular synapse shows that the nerve terminal is capped by a Schwann cell and is situated in a shallow depression of the muscle cell membrane, which is invaginated further into deep and regular folds, termed postjunctional folds (arrows). AChRs, labeled with α-bungaro-toxin coupled to horseradish peroxidase, are concentrated at the synaptic site. (B) A higher magnification view shows that AChRs are concentrated at the crests and along the sides of the postjunctional folds (white arrow). Rapsyn, NRG receptors, and MuSK are also concentrated in the postsynaptic membrane, whereas Agrin, NRG-1, Acetylcholinesterase, S-laminin, and certain isoforms of collagen are localized to the synaptic basal lamina. The postjunctional folds of the myofiber are spaced at regular intervals and are situated directly across from active zones and clusters of synaptic vesicles in the nerve terminal (arrows).

synaptic membrane. These studies indicate that signals for presynaptic and postsynaptic differentiation are localized to the synaptic basal lamina.

Motor Neurons Induce Postsynaptic Differentiation in Cell Culture

Primary myoblasts, isolated from developing embryos, or myoblast cell lines, fuse to one another to form multinucleated myotubes, which express *AChR* genes as well as a large number of other genes characteristic of adult muscle. These cultured myotubes can be innervated by cultured spinal cord neurons, and AChRs and acetylcholinesterase (AChE) become clustered at these nascent, nerve–muscle contacts. Synapses that form in cell culture, however, do not fully represent synapses that form *in vivo*, as motor axons fail to stop and form arborized nerve terminals on myotubes in cell culture; consequently, the synapses that form in cell culture resemble en passant synapses rather than bona fide end plates. Nonetheless, by monitoring the fate of AChRs labeled prior to innervation, Anderson and Cohen (1977) showed that AChRs cluster at synapses, in large part, from a reorganization of AChRs expressed on the myotube cell surface prior to innervation. These classic studies demonstrate that motor axons provide signals that reorganize and cluster AChRs at developing synapses.

The Synaptic Basal Lamina Contains Signals for Synaptic Differentiation

The idea that signals for inducing both presynaptic and postsynaptic differentiation are contained in the synaptic basal lamina arose from studies of regenerat-

ing neuromuscular synapses. Following damage to a motor axon, the distal portion of the motor axon degenerates, and the proximal end regenerates to muscle. The regenerated axon precisely reinnervates the original synaptic site and forms a synapse that is indistinguishable from the original synapse. Original synaptic sites are not thought to provide guidance cues to motor axons; rather, it is believed that the vacated perineurial tubes, containing Schwann cells and their basal lamina, provide a favorable substrate for motor axons and have a role in directing regenerating motor axons to original synaptic sites (Son and Thompson, 1995). Although motor axons precisely reinnervate original synaptic sites, there appears to be little, if any, selectivity among motor neurons or among Schwann cells in assuring accurate regeneration; indeed, both original and foreign motor neurons

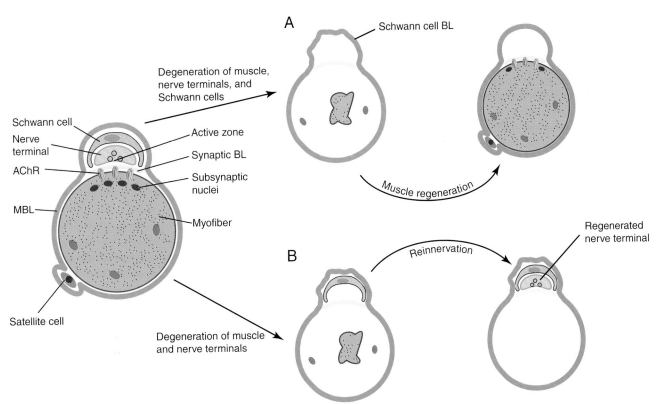

FIGURE 18.8 The synaptic basal lamina contains signals for presynaptic and postsynaptic differentiation. A cross section of normal muscle containing a nerve terminal (NT), Schwann cell, and myofiber is shown at the far left. *AChR* genes are induced in synaptic nuclei (red) and AChRs (green) are concentrated at synaptic sites. Active zones and clusters of synaptic vesicles in the nerve terminal are aligned with postjunctional folds in the myofiber. Each myofiber is ensheathed by a basal lamina (MBL), which is specialized at the synaptic site (synaptic BL) and which remains intact following degeneration of the original myofiber. The MBL serves as a scaffold for regenerating myofibers, which form from the fusion of satellite cells that proliferate following damage to the original myofiber. (A) Experiments showing that the synaptic basal lamina contains signals for clustering AChRs and activating *AChR* genes in synaptic nuclei. Following damage and degeneration of axons, Schwann cells, and myofibers, new myofibers regenerate within the basal lamina of the original myofiber in the absence of the nerve. AChRs cluster and *AChR* gene expression is reinduced at original synaptic sites in myofibers that regenerate in the absence of the nerve and other original presynaptic cells. (B) Experiments showing that the synaptic basal lamina contains signals for inducing presynaptic differentiation. Following damage and degeneration of axons and myofibers, motor axons regenerate to original synaptic sites in the absence of the myofiber and accumulate synaptic vesicles precisely across from the sites of the original postjunctional folds.

can accurately and functionally reinnervate original synaptic sites in denervated muscle.

Following damage to motor axons and muscle, nerve terminals and muscle fibers degenerate and are phagocytized, but the basal lamina of the muscle fiber remains intact. Even in the absence of nerve terminals and muscle fibers, several structures, including the terminal Schwann cells, the basal lamina of the postjunctional folds, and AChE, remain at the original synaptic site and allow for its identification.

Axons eventually regenerate into the muscle, and new myofibers regenerate within the basal lamina of the original myofiber. The regenerated motor axons form synapses with the regenerated myofibers precisely at the original synaptic sites. If axons regenerate into muscle, but muscle regeneration is prevented, axons still unerringly reinnervate the original synaptic site on the basal lamina, and active zones form in register with the basal lamina of the original postjunctional folds (Fig. 18.8) (Sanes *et al.*, 1978). Thus, the presence of the myofiber is necessary neither for precise reinnervation nor for the morphological differentiation of regenerated nerve terminals. The vacated perineurial tubes, containing Schwann cells and their basal lamina, may direct regenerating motor axons to original synaptic sites, but the induction of active zones suggests that cues in the synaptic basal lamina have a role in organizing the presynaptic terminal.

If regeneration of motor axons is prevented, but myofibers are allowed to regenerate, AChRs accumulate and membrane folds form in the regenerated myofiber precisely at the original synaptic site on the basal lamina (Burden *et al.*, 1979). Thus, in the absence of nerve terminals, myofibers, and terminal Schwann cells, information that remains at the original synaptic site instructs both presynaptic and postsynaptic differentiation. Because the synaptic basal lamina is the most prominent extracellular structure remaining at neuromuscular synapses following removal of all cells, these results indicate that the synaptic basal lamina contains signals that can induce differentiation of both nerve terminals and myofibers.

Anchoring signaling molecules to the synaptic basal lamina is likely to be critical for spatially restricting signaling and ensuring the precise arrangement of proteins in presynaptic and postsynaptic membranes at the neuromuscular synapse. In the CNS, it may likewise be important to restrict the action of signaling molecules by tethering membrane-bound signaling molecules to the cytoskeleton.

BOX 18.1

TORPEDO ELECTRIC ORGAN

The majority of proteins known to be localized to neuromuscular synapses were first identified in postsynaptic membranes isolated from the electric organ of the marine ray *Torpedo*. Indeed, this specialized tissue has been essential for the identification and purification of the AChR, AChE, Rapsyn, Syntrophin, Agrin, MuSK and several synaptic vesicle proteins. The electric organ is a particularly homogeneous and abundant source of pre- and postsynaptic membranes that are similar in structure and function to those at neuromuscular synapses. The biochemical advantages of the electric organ are evident from its anatomy. The postsynaptic cell, which differentiates initially as a syncitial skeletal muscle fiber but subsequently loses its contractile machinery, is termed an electroplaque. Each electroplaque is a thin, elongated cell (1 cm × 1 cm × 10 mm) that is so densely innervated that nearly one-half of the electrocyte membrane is studded by nerve terminals. In contrast, nerve terminals occupy less than 0.1% of the cell surface of a skeletal myofiber.

Because of this dense innervation and because the electric organ from a moderate size ray weighs several kilograms, it is possible to obtain several mg of purified postsynaptic proteins from a single electric organ.

Innervation is restricted to the ventral surface of the electroplaque, whereas the dorsal surface is enriched for the sodium/potassium ATPase which maintains the resting potential. Because the electroplaque lacks action potentials, activation of AChRs on the innervated ventral surface results in a voltage drop across the innervated but not the non-innervated membrane of the electrocyte. Since thousands of electroplaques are stacked closely one upon another, the potential difference across a single electrocyte is summated by the stack of electroplaques, resulting in a several thousand volt potential difference across the entire electric organ, a voltage that is sufficient to stun prey.

Steven J. Burden, Darwin Berg,
and Dennis D. M. O'Leary

Agrin Is a Signal for Postsynaptic Differentiation

Because clustering of AChRs, unlike the formation of active zones, can be studied readily in cell culture, it has been far simpler to identify the basal lamina signals that induce postsynaptic rather than presynaptic differentiation. Extracellular matrix from the *Torpedo* electric organ, a tissue that is homologous to muscle but more densely innervated, contains an activity that stimulates AChR clustering in cultured myotubes, and like the signal that induces clustering of AChRs at developing neuromuscular synapses, the electric organ activity causes clustering of AChRs by posttranslational mechanisms (see Box 18.1). McMahan and colleagues purified the electric organ activity, which they termed Agrin, and showed that Agrin is synthesized by motor neurons, transported in motor axons to synaptic sites, and deposited in the synaptic basal lamina. Agrin also stimulates the clustering of other synaptic proteins (see later), including AChE, Rapsyn, Utrophin, muscle-derived Neuregulin-1 (NRG-1), and NRG receptors, ErbBs (see later), indicating that Agrin has a central role in synaptic differentiation (Fig. 18.9).

cDNAs encoding Agrin have been isolated from *Torpedo* electric lobe and from the CNS of higher vertebrates. Agrin is a ~200-kDa protein containing multiple epidermal growth factor (EGF)-like signaling domains, two different laminin-like domains, and multiple follistatin-like repeats. The four EGF-like domains and three laminin G domains are contained in the carboxyl-terminal region, which is sufficient for inducing AChR clusters in cultured myotubes; sequences in the amino-terminal region are responsible for the association of Agrin with the extracellular matrix.

The *agrin* gene is expressed in a variety of cell types. Alternative splicing results in multiple Agrin isoforms that differ in their AChR clustering efficiency. The isoform that is most active in clustering AChRs is expressed in neurons, including motor neurons, whereas other Agrin isoforms are expressed in additional cell types, including skeletal muscle cells. The active, neuronal-specific isoforms of Agrin contain 8, 11, or 19 amino acids at a splice site, referred to as the Z site in rat Agrin and the B site in chick Agrin.

Two lines of evidence indicate that the local release of Agrin by motor nerve terminals is necessary for clustering AChRs at synaptic sites and for postsynaptic differentiation: (1) antibodies against Agrin block AChR clustering at nerve–muscle synapses that form in cell culture and (2) mice lacking Agrin lack normal synapses (see later) (Gautam *et al.*, 1996). Experiments with chimeric synapses between different frog species indicate that nerve-derived Agrin is present at synaptic sites from the earliest stages of synapse formation. Further, experiments with chimeric synapses between chick and rat indicate that blocking antibodies to nerve-derived but not to muscle-derived Agrin inhibit AChR clustering. Finally, mice deficient only in neural Agrin lack neuromuscular synapses (Lin *et al.*, 2001).

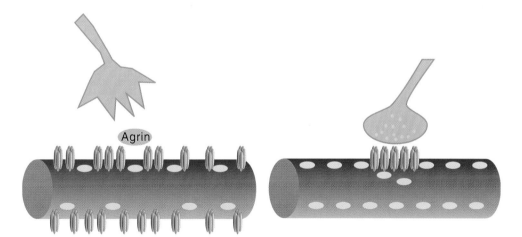

FIGURE 18.9 Agrin-mediated signaling. Motor neurons synthesize and release Agrin into the synaptic basal lamina, where it acts to maintain AChRs (yellow) at synaptic sites. A longitudinal view of a multinucleated myofiber innervated by a single nerve terminal is shown. The diagram shows that AChRs (blue) and MuSK (red) are concentrated in the postsynaptic membrane. This figure proposes that the Agrin receptor is likewise concentrated in the postsynaptic membrane. Agrin (yellow), which is concentrated in the synaptic basal lamina, is thought to bind to the Agrin receptor, concomitantly stimulating oligomerization of the Agrin receptor and MuSK and the tyrosine kinase activity of MuSK. MuSK stimulation activates a signaling pathway (arrows), which clusters AChRs at synaptic sites.

Although muscle-derived Agrin may have a subtle or later role in synaptic differentiation, these results demonstrate that muscle-derived Agrin cannot substitute for nerve-derived Agrin in clustering AChRs.

In addition to stimulating clustering of AChRs and other synaptic proteins, Agrin stimulates tyrosine phosphorylation of AChR β and δ subunits. The role of AChR tyrosine phosphorylation is not known.

MuSK Is Required for Agrin-Mediated Signaling and Synapse Formation

The mechanisms of Agrin-mediated AChR clustering are not known, but a receptor tyrosine kinase, termed MuSK, is a critical component of an Agrin receptor complex. MuSK is expressed in *Torpedo* electric organ and in skeletal muscle, where it is concentrated in the postsynaptic membrane. Mice deficient in MuSK (DeChiara *et al.*, 1996), like *agrin* mutant mice, lack normal neuromuscular synapses. Indeed, the similar phenotype of *agrin* and *MuSK* mutant mice, at least at birth, is consistent with the idea that MuSK is a component of an Agrin receptor complex. Both *agrin* and *MuSK* mutant mice are immobile, cannot breathe, and die at birth. Muscle differentiation is normal in *agrin* and *MuSK* mutant mice, but muscle fibers in *MuSK* mutant mice lack all known features of postsynaptic differentiation. Muscle-derived proteins, including AChRs and AChE, which are concentrated at synapses in normal mice, are distributed uniformly in *MuSK* mutant myofibers. In addition, *AChR* genes, which are normally transcribed selectively in synaptic nuclei of normal muscle fibers (see later), are transcribed at similar rates in synaptic and nonsynaptic nuclei of muscle fibers from *MuSK* mutant mice.

Muscle fibers in *agrin* mutant mice are similarly deficient in postsynaptic differentiation, at least at birth. Earlier in development, however, AChRs are clustered in the central region of muscle, in the absence of Agrin (Lin *et al.*, 2001). These surprising results indicate that Agrin is required neither to cluster AChRs *in vivo* nor to position these AChR clusters in the central region of the muscle (see later). Therefore, Agrin appears to be required to maintain rather than to induce AChR clusters (see later) (Lin *et al.*, 2001, Yang *et al.*, 2001).

Five lines of evidence indicate that MuSK is required for Agrin-mediated signaling and is a component of the Agrin receptor complex: (1) Agrin can be chemically cross-linked to MuSK in cultured myotubes; (2) Agrin induces rapid tyrosine phosphorylation of MuSK in cultured myotubes; (3) a recombinant, soluble extracellular fragment of MuSK inhibits

Agrin-induced AChR clustering in cultured muscle cells; (4) cultured *MuSK* mutant muscle cells, unlike normal muscle cells, do not cluster AChRs in response to Agrin; and (5) dominant-negative forms of MuSK inhibit Agrin-induced AChR clustering in cultured myotubes. MuSK itself, however, does not bind Agrin, indicating that other activities or additional proteins are required for Agrin to activate MuSK.

How does MuSK activation lead to postsynaptic differentiation? Agrin stimulates the rapid phosphorylation of MuSK, and the kinase activity of MuSK is essential for Agrin to stimulate clustering and tyrosine phosphorylation of AChRs. Well-characterized signaling pathways (e.g., MAP kinase, PI3-kinase, PLC-γ), however, are neither activated by Agrin/ MuSK signaling nor required for Agrin to stimulate AChR clustering. Signaling downstream from MuSK depends on phosphorylation of a tyrosine residue (Y553) in the juxtamembrane region of MuSK. Phosphorylation of this tyrosine is thought to be important for Agrin to fully activate MuSK kinase activity and to recruit a downstream signaling component(s) required for phosphorylation and clustering of AChRs. At present, however, little is known about proteins that are recruited to activated, phosphorylated MuSK. Evidence shows, however, that Rac and Cdc42, small GTP-binding proteins that regulate actin organization, are required for Agrin to stimulate AChR clustering. Moreover, at least one kinase acts downstream from MuSK and is recruited and/or activated by Agrin-activated MuSK, as staurosporine, a protein kinase inhibitor, inhibits Agrin-induced AChR tyrosine phosphorylation and clustering without blocking tyrosine phosphorylation of MuSK.

Rapsyn Is Required for Postsynaptic Differentiation and Is Downstream of Agrin and MuSK

A 43-kDa protein, termed Rapsyn, has an important role in Agrin-mediated signaling. Rapsyn is a myristolated, peripheral membrane protein that is present at 1:1 stoichiometry with AChRs at synaptic sites and that interacts directly with AChRs and potentially other synaptic proteins, including Dystroglycan and Dystrophin, Utrophin, Syntrophin, and Dystrobrevin, proteins that are components of a subsynaptic, cytoskeletal complex.

Agrin stimulates the clustering of Rapsyn in myotubes grown in cell culture, and clustering of Rapsyn and AChRs occurs coincidentally at developing synapses. Rapsyn is critical for synapse formation, as mice lacking Rapsyn die within hours after birth and have difficulty moving and breathing (Gautam *et al.*,

1995). Importantly, normal clustering of AChRs, NRG receptors, Utrophin, and Dystroglycan is lacking in *rapsyn* mutant mice. MuSK, however, is clustered at synaptic sites in *rapsyn* mutant mice, indicating that clustering of MuSK at synaptic sites occurs independently of Rapsyn. *AChR* expression appears normal in *rapsyn* mutant mice, as *AChR* mRNAs are enriched in the central region of the muscle. The persistence of synapse-specific gene expression (see later) in *rapsyn* mutant mice is likely to explain the enrichment of AChRs within the central region of *rapsyn* mutant muscle fibers.

Forced expression of Rapsyn in *Xenopus* oocytes or in a fibroblast/muscle-like cell line results in clustering of Rapsyn. Moreover, clustering of Rapsyn is necessary and sufficient to cluster AChRs, as well as MuSK, in these cells. Because Rapsyn is expressed at similar levels in myoblasts and myotubes, but is clustered only in myotubes, clustering of Rapsyn is normally regulated during myogenesis. Thus, it is unclear whether the Agrin/MuSK-independent clustering of Rapsyn in certain cell lines or in *Xenopus* oocytes is a result of overexpression or is stimulated by activities present in these cells and not in myoblasts.

Agrin and MuSK Are Required for Retrograde Signaling and Presynaptic Differentiation

Although pathfinding of motor axons to muscle is normal in mice lacking Agrin or MuSK, *agrin* and *MuSK* mutant mice lack normal nerve terminals. In the mutant mice, branches of the main intramuscular nerve fail to stop and differentiate and instead wander aimlessly across the muscle. Because MuSK is expressed in skeletal muscle and not in motor neurons, it seems likely that the aberrant behavior of presynaptic terminals in *MuSK* mutant mice is due to indirect actions of the Agrin/MuSK signaling system. These results indicate that Agrin, released from nerve terminals, causes the muscle cell, via MuSK activation, to reciprocally release a recognition signal back to the nerve to indicate that a functional contact has occurred. In response to this muscle-derived recognition or adhesion signal, the nerve undergoes presynaptic differentiation and stops growing. Alternatively, the lack of synaptic activity in *agrin* and *MuSK* mutant mice may result in aberrant retrograde signaling, resulting in exuberant growth of motor axons. In either case, these results demonstrate the importance of the reciprocal signaling relationship between nerve and muscle during development. (DeChiara *et al.*, 1996; Gautam *et al.*, 1996)

Certain Genes Are Expressed Selectively in Synaptic Nuclei of Myofibers

Like AChR protein, mRNAs encoding the different AChR subunits (α, β, γ, or ϵ and δ) are concentrated at synaptic sites. Studies with transgenic mice that harbor gene fusions between regulatory regions of *AChR* subunit genes and reporter genes have shown that *AChR* genes are transcribed selectively in myofiber nuclei near the synaptic site. Thus, localized transcription of *AChR* genes in synaptic nuclei is responsible, at least in part, for the accumulation of *AChR* mRNA at synaptic sites. This pathway is important for ensuring that AChRs are expressed at the required density in the postsynaptic membrane, as defects in synapse-specific gene expression of the *AChR* ϵ subunit gene are the cause of a congenital myaesthenia (see later).

Like *AChR* subunit genes, the *utrophin* gene is transcribed selectively in synaptic nuclei, resulting in an accumulation of *utrophin* mRNA and protein at synaptic sites. mRNAs encoding Rapsyn, N-CAM, MuSK, sodium channels, and the catalytic subunit of AChE are also concentrated in the synaptic region of skeletal myofibers, raising the possibility that these genes are likewise transcribed preferentially in synaptic nuclei. Thus, synapse-specific transcription may be a common and important mechanism for localizing a variety of gene products to the neuromuscular synapse.

Neuregulin-1 Is a Candidate for the Signal That Activates Gene Expression in Synaptic Nuclei

Studies of regenerating muscle have shown that a signal for synapse-specific transcription is contained in the synaptic basal lamina. Because soluble forms of Agrin do not increase *AChR* expression in cultured muscle, Agrin does not appear to be a likely candidate for the transcriptional signal in the synaptic basal lamina. Among the potential candidates for the transcriptional signal are the products of the *nrg-1* gene. The *nrg-1* gene encodes more than a dozen alternatively spliced products that have multiple activities. Although originally purified as a ligand that stimulates tyrosine phosphorylation of the *neu* oncogene, NRG-1 was purified independently from the CNS as an activity, termed AChR inducing activity (ARIA), that induces AChR synthesis and from the pituitary as an activity, termed glial growth factor (GGF), that stimulates the proliferation of Schwann cells.

NRG-1 is concentrated at neuromuscular synapses and can activate *AChR* gene expression in muscle cells grown in cell culture. NRG-1 contains a single EGF-like domain, which is necessary and sufficient for cell signaling. Motor neurons synthesize NRG-1, and NRG-1 protein is detectable in motor axons, indicating that some of the NRG-1 protein at synaptic sites is synthesized by motor neurons. Skeletal myofibers, however, also synthesize NRG-1, and some of the NRG-1 at synaptic sites is synthesized by myofibers. These findings raise the possibility that NRG-1 could act as an autocrine and/or paracrine signal at neuromuscular synapses.

ErbB3 and ErbB4, two members of the EGF receptor family, are receptors for NRG-1. Both ErbB3 and ErbB4 are concentrated in the postsynaptic membrane at neuromuscular synapses, and the colocalization of NRG-1, ErbB3, and ErbB4 at synapses supports the idea that NRG-1 is a signal that regulates synaptic differentiation (Figure 18.10). Nevertheless, because mice lacking NRG-1, ErbB2, or ErbB4 die, due to a failure of heart development, at E10.5, several days prior to neuromuscular synapse formation, examination of

these mutant mice has not helped resolve whether NRG-1-mediated signaling is required for synapse-specific gene expression.

Adult mice that are heterozygous for the Ig isoform of NRG-1 express fewer AChRs at neuromuscular synapses, supporting the idea that NRG-1, supplied by motor neurons and/or muscle, has a role in regulating AChR expression at adult synapses. Neuronal NRG-1, however, is not required for synapse-specific transcription at developing synapses, as the pattern of AChR transcription is normal in newborn mice lacking NRG-1 specifically in motor and sensory neurons (Yang et al., 2001). These experiments leave open the possibility that muscle-derived NRG-1 may be required for synapse-specific transcription. Because neural Agrin can cluster muscle-derived NRG-1 and ErbBs, it is possible that neural Agrin regulates synapse-specific transcription by defining the limits of NRG-1 and NRG receptor expression and thus restricting an autocrine NRG-1 signaling pathway to synaptic sites in muscle.

GABP Is an Ets Domain Transcription Factor That May Regulate Synapse-Specific Transcription

A binding site for Ets domain proteins in the AChR δ subunit gene is critical for synapse-specific and NRG-1-induced gene expression in mice. Importantly, mutation of an Ets-binding site in the human AChR ε subunit gene leads to a myopathy, termed congenital myasthenic syndrome, due to decreased AChR expression. This Ets site binds GABP, a complex containing GABPα, an Ets protein, and GABPβ, a protein that lacks an Ets domain but dimerizes with GABPα, suggesting that GABP may be a transcriptional regulator that responds to NRG-1 signaling and stimulates transcription of AChR genes in synaptic nuclei. NRG-1, however, does not stimulate binding of GABPα to DNA, suggesting that NRG-1 may stimulate AChR transcription by modifying GABP or by regulating the association of other transcription factors with GABP.

Electrical Activity Regulates Gene Expression

Changes in the pattern of muscle electrical activity have an important role in regulating the electrophysiological and structural properties of muscle, as well as the ability of motor axons to innervate muscle. The expression of several genes, including AChR genes, is repressed by electrical activity, and this repression, together with focal activation in synaptic nuclei, as described earlier, contributes to the disparate

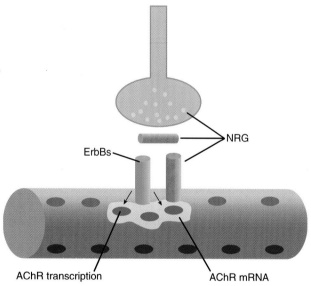

FIGURE 18.10 Synapse-specific gene expression. A longitudinal view of a multinucleated myofiber innervated by a single nerve terminal. The diagram shows that AChR subunit genes are transcribed selectively in nuclei (green) in the synaptic region of the myofiber, resulting in an accumulation of AChR mRNA (light blue) and protein (dark blue) at synaptic sites. The nerve induces this spatially restricted pattern of transcription, and the extracellular signal that triggers synapse-specific gene expression is contained in the synaptic basal lamina. NRG-1 (yellow), which is synthesized by motor neurons and skeletal muscle fibers and which is associated with both synaptic basal lamina and pre- and postsynaptic membranes, is the best candidate for the signal that induces synapse-specific transcription. NRG receptors, ErbB3 and ErbB4 (red), together with ErbB2, are concentrated in the postsynaptic membrane. This model proposes that NRG-1 stimulates a signaling pathway (arrows) that induces AChR genes in nuclei near the activated NRG receptors.

levels of AChR expression in synaptic and nonsynaptic regions of the muscle. A binding site for myogenic bHLH transcription factors, or E box, in the proximal promoter of *AChR* subunit genes is essential for electrical activity-dependent transcription, as transgenes containing a mutation in this E box, unlike wild-type transgenes, are not induced following denervation. These results suggest that electrical activity decreases the level and/or activity of E box binding proteins, leading to decreased *AChR* expression. The mechanisms that lead to decreased expression and activity of myogenic bHLH proteins are not understood, but the involvement of several protein kinases, including PKA, CAM kinase II, and PKC, has been suggested.

Muscle-Autonomous Patterning of AChR Expression

The preceding sections have emphasized the role of motor neuron-derived signals in patterning the distribution of AChR expression. Recent studies, however, have shown that AChRs are clustered in muscle in the absence of innervation and that these AChR clusters are enriched in the central region of the muscle. Likewise, *AChR* transcription is also patterned in muscle lacking innervation. These findings indicate that the pattern of AChR expression in skeletal muscles is determined, at least in part, by mechanisms that are independent of motor innervation, as suggested by earlier studies (Yang *et al.*, 2000, 2001;

Lin *et al.*, 2001). In addition, these results raise the interesting possibility that spatial cues that restrict axon growth and promote synapse formation might be provided by molecules that are also prepatterned in muscle.

These findings suggest a new model for the sequential steps involved in establishing the pattern of AChR expression on developing skeletal muscle fibers. An initial, spatially restricted pattern of AChR expression is generated in muscle independent of neurally derived Agrin, or indeed of any other neural signal. Because this prepattern is not observed in mice lacking MuSK, the emergence of this muscle AChR prepattern, nonetheless, coopts at least some of the same molecules used during normal synaptogenesis. Arrival of the nerve, and its attendant signals, converts the AChR prepattern into the more refined pattern of *AChR* transcription and AChR clustering characteristic of mature synapses. This conversion appears to be dependent on two separable nerve-dependent programs: one program appears to utilize neurally derived Agrin to maintain AChR expression at nascent synaptic sites and a second program, possibly triggered by electrical activity, extinguishes AChR expression throughout the muscle. These two programs thus ensure the stable expression of AChR clusters selectively at nascent synapses. The mechanisms that are intrinsic to muscle and responsible for establishing regional differences in muscle in the absence of innervation are not known.

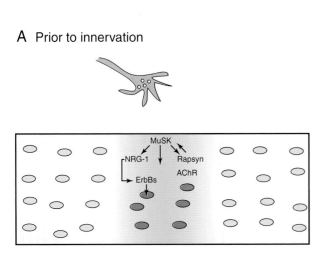

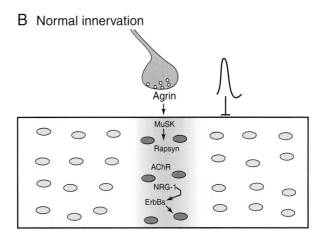

FIGURE 18.11 Model for prepatterning and refining AChR expression in skeletal muscle. (A) In the absence of innervation, AChRs are clustered and *AChR* transcription is enhanced in the central region of muscle. MuSK is necessary for patterning AChR expression, indicating that MuSK is clustered and activated, possibly by Rapsyn, in the central region of the muscle. Activated MuSK clusters ErbBs and muscle-derived NRG-1 and could thereby establish an autocrine signaling pathway that stimulates *AChR* transcription. (B) Innervation refines the prepattern by restricting AChR clusters and *AChR* transcription to synaptic sites. This refinement requires neural Agrin, which maintains *AChR* transcription and clustering at synaptic sites. This refinement also requires an Agrin-independent neuronal activity, possibly ACh-induced electrical activity, which represses *AChR* transcription and clustering in nonsynaptic regions. Neuronal NRG-1 is not required for synapse-specific transcription, as synapse-specific transcription is normal in mice lacking neuronal NRG-1.

Summary

Signals exchanged at nascent synaptic sites ensure that differentiated presynaptic terminals are aligned precisely with a highly specialized postsynaptic membrane. Agrin, supplied by motor neurons, has a key role in this process. Agrin acts by stimulating MuSK, a receptor tyrosine kinase expressed by muscle. Analysis of mice lacking innervation, however, suggests that a coarse pattern of postsynaptic differentiation is present prior to innervation and that neuronal signals, including Agrin, selectively maintain, rather than induce, postsynaptic differentiation at sites of nerve–muscle contact (Fig. 18.11).

SYNAPSE FORMATION IN THE CENTRAL NERVOUS SYSTEM

Neurons in the central nervous system typically receive thousands of synapses employing a variety of neurotransmitters. The location and capability of individual synapses can be critical for the proper integration of excitatory and inhibitory input, and they often need to incorporate plasticity as well. These requirements pose intriguing challenges for synapse formation involving the production, assembly, and sorting of numerous synaptic components targeted to distinct sites on the neuron. Cell–cell interactions are crucial for the proper pairing of pre- and postsynaptic components and for adjustment of their signaling capabilities. In contrast, the vertebrate neuromuscular junction presents a much simpler situation in which the postsynaptic muscle cell needs only to support a single large synapse and to generate components for reliable, suprathreshold transmission. Nonetheless, some of the principles elucidated at the neuromuscular junction (NMJ) are likely to have widespread applicability at CNS synapses, such as strategies for tethering components at membrane sites and transsynaptic mechanisms for coordinating pre- and postsynaptic assembly.

This section examines synapse formation between neurons and focuses on fast, chemical transmission. The postsynaptic receptors in these cases are ligand-gated ion channels (ionotropic receptors), as is true at the NMJ; slow transmission involving metabotropic receptors is not considered here. Much progress has been made in the last decade elucidating the molecular composition of both pre- and postsynaptic structures on neurons (Chapters 8 and 9). A great deal has also been learned about mechanisms underlying synaptic plasticity, and some of these are also likely to be important for synapse formation (Chapters 50 and

51). Until recently, however, little was known about the critical events initiating synapse formation between neurons or about the mechanisms controlling subsequent recruitment and assembly of pre- and postsynaptic components. Now several exciting reports have identified candidate molecules and mechanisms contributing importantly to these processes. These findings are highlighted here. Not addressed are mechanisms responsible for later stages of synaptic maturation, such as those involving the exchange of postsynaptic receptor isotypes during development.

The First Contact between Axons and Their Neuronal Targets

Cells can express both pre- and postsynaptic components prior to synapse formation (Craig and Lichtman, 2001). For example, motoneuron growth cones release packets of ACh before interacting with muscle, and muscle cells express nicotinic AChRs before contact by motor axons. Cell–cell interactions, however, are essential for the proper juxtaposition of synaptic components and for achieving the mature complement of both pre- and postsynaptic elements. Such interactions must be mediated initially by specific molecules that trigger a cascade of events in the synaptic partner.

The earliest contacts may be mediated by filopodia that extend from either growing axons or dendrites (Jontes and Smith, 2000). These tiny extensions form rapidly and reversibly (Chapter 17). Imaging studies both in culture and *in vivo* indicate that when filopodia contact potential synaptic partners, they can lose their motility and become selectively stabilized. The contacts are then thought to transform into synaptic structures either on the dendritic spine shaft or, in the case of spiny neurons, into dendritic spines (Craig and Lichtman, 2001). Indeed, synaptic specializations have been seen on filopodia themselves in such situations. Activity is likely to play an important role in regulating the behavior of filopodia: synaptic stimulation results in local increases in the number and length of filopodia, and these increases are blocked by inhibitors of NMDA receptors (Jontes and Smith, 2000). The effects of activity are likely to be complex, as the motility and morphology of dendritic spines can be regulated differentially by synaptic activity depending on the amount of stimulation and the developmental window being examined.

Inductive Events in Presynaptic Development

What molecular interactions mediate the induction of a synaptic specialization in the CNS? A striking recent discovery was the finding that the expression of neuroligin in nonneuronal cells can induce the development of presynaptic elements in axons that contact these cells (Scheiffele *et al.*, 2000). Neuroligins represent a small family of brain-specific transmembrane proteins that can bind to β-neurexins on opposing cells. Using the innervation of cerebellar granule cells by pontine axons as a model for the developing synapse, Serafini and colleagues showed that neuroligin-1 and -2 are expressed in the granule cells at the right time to influence synaptogenesis. They then demonstrated that the heterologous expression of neuroligin by nonneuronal cells in culture induces focal accumulations of the synaptic vesicle proteins synapsin, synaptotagmin, and synaptophysin (here used as synaptic markers) in pontine axons. Moreover, the presynaptic structures that formed were capable of vesicle exocytosis as evidenced by the transfer of synaptotagmin epitopes from the synaptic vesicle lumen to the axon surface upon depolarization of the axon. Neuroligin–neurexin interactions appear to be required for synapse formation between neurons as suggested by experiments in which a soluble β-neurexin fusion protein was added to cocultures of pontine explants and cerebellar granule cells. The fusion protein prevented the granule cells from inducing presynaptic specializations in the pontine axons, presumably by competitively inhibiting neuroligin from binding to neurexin receptor on pontine axons. These experiments demonstrate that neuroligin is sufficient to induce early steps in presynaptic differentiation, although whether it is also necessary for synapse formation *in vivo* remains to be addressed experimentally.

How might neuroligin on the postsynaptic cell induce presynaptic development? The extracellular portion of neuroligin is sufficient for the inductive effect: when this fragment alone is tethered in the membrane of cells artificially via a lipid linker, it still induces presynaptic specializations in adjacent pontine axons (Scheiffele *et al.*, 2000). Thus the induction does not require assistance from intracellular components in the presumptive postsynaptic cell expressing the neuroligin. The induction may be mediated by presynaptic b-neurexin acting as the neuroligin receptor and binding intracellularly to the presynaptic protein CASK/Lin-2, which links to other proteins involved in vesicle processing. On the postsynaptic side, the intracellular domain of neuroligin can bind several proteins associated with the postsynaptic machinery, including PSD-95 and other components capable of clustering NMDA receptors. This, in principle, provides a link between neuroligin–neurexin interactions and the juxtaposition of presynaptic vesicular components with the postsynaptic signal transduction machinery.

One candidate factor that might act prior to neuroligin and other such cell-adhesion molecules in synapse formation is the secreted protein WNT-7a. Using the same cerebellar system just described, Salinas and co-workers showed that exogenous WNT-7a can mimic an endogenous granule cell factor that induces the characteristic spreading of pontine mossy fiber axon terminals as they initiate synapse formation (Hall *et al.*, 2000). Antagonists of the WNT-7a signaling pathway blocked the inductive effects of the endogenous component. Normal synaptic development was delayed in WNT-7a knockout mice, resulting in reduced synapsin clustering and simplified presynaptic membrane structures. WNT-7a is known to activate a seven-transmembrane receptor protein that inhibits the microtubule phosphorylating kinase GSK-3β. Cytoskeletal changes resulting from microtubule rearrangement could shape presynaptic morphological development and facilitate the recruitment of appropriate organelles.

The number of presynaptic components required for regulated vesicular release is enormous (Chapter 8), but it has been suggested that the recruitment of such components at presynaptic sites may be much simplified by preassembly. Imaging studies on hippocampal neurons in culture after expression of GFP-tagged presynaptic vesicle proteins showed that the neurons contain large packets of presynaptic components that migrate distally along the axon (Jontes and Smith, 2000). The packets are much larger than individual synaptic vesicles and contain a variety of presynaptic proteins, including VAMP, SV2, synapsin, amphiphysin, and voltage-gated calcium channels. The packets collect at nascent points of axo-dendritic contact and subsequently display stimulus-dependent vesicle recycling. As such, the packets offer a mechanism by which preassembled presynaptic components can be efficiently captured by or recruited into a future active site, as defined by local interactions between presumptive pre- and postsynaptic neuron partners.

Control of Postsynaptic Development

In contrast to the NMJ, where postsynaptic development is relatively well characterized, little is known about the transsynaptic mechanisms that control postsynaptic development in neurons. This is all the more surprising given the vast array of postsynaptic neuronal components that have been identified and the extensive analysis of postsynaptic mechanisms contributing to synaptic plasticity. Unsolved is the question of how the postsynaptic neuron targets appropriate receptors to individual synaptic sites. Almost certainly the presynaptic neuron plays a key role in ensuring that the type of receptor found post-synaptically matches the neurotransmitter expressed by the axon. Evidence for this comes from studies in cell culture indicating that some classes of receptors cannot be induced to cluster unless the pre-synaptic terminal provides a transmitter match (Craig and Lichtman, 2001). Even this correlation is not absolute, however, suggesting that a hierarchy of overlapping signals may specify receptor distribution.

One of the best understood examples of postsynaptic receptor clustering on neurons is provided by the glycine receptor. A host of studies, including mouse knockouts, demonstrates that gephyrin, a peripheral membrane protein associated with the receptor, is essential for receptor clustering at synaptic sites on dendritic shafts (Kneussel and Betz, 2000). Gephyrin is well equipped to serve as a scaffolding protein, linking receptors to the cytoskeleton; it binds with high affinity to polymerized tubulin, the actin-binding protein profilin, and the lipid-binding protein collybistin. Receptor activation is required for clustering: the specific blockade of glycine receptors with strychnine or the general blockade of activity by TTX prevents postsynaptic accumulation of the receptors. Blockade of L-type calcium channels has a similar effect, indicating that calcium influx is essential for clustering, and several candidate downstream signaling events have been identified (Kneussel and Betz, 2000).

The organization of postsynaptic components at glutamatergic synapses is more complex. The synapses may form *in vivo* by the initial accumulation of NMDA receptors at postsynaptic sites and the subsequent addition of AMPA receptors. This view is supported both by electron microscopy using immunogold labeling and by electrophysiology in which NDMA receptor-rich "silent synapses" are identified initially in development. A strong early candidate for clustering NMDA receptors during synapse formation is the postsynaptic density protein PSD-95, which binds directly to the receptors and serves as a scaffold or linker for a variety of other components (Craig and Lichtman, 2000). Mouse knockouts, however, indicate that PSD-95 is not essential for NMDA receptor localization at synapses; perhaps other PDZ-containing proteins substitute in this situation.

While the "rapsyn/gephyrin" equivalent for NMDA receptors remains to be identified, it has been sug-gested that developing NMDA synapses may utilize a mechanism reminiscent of MuSK actions at the neuro-muscular junction. The mechanism involves EphB receptors and their cognate ligands ephrinB proteins, which can interact to promote NMDA receptor cluster-ing at synaptic sites (Dalva et al., 2000). Both EphB receptors and ephrinBs are localized at excitatory synapses in the CNS. EphB receptors coimmunoprecip-itate with NMDA receptors when solubilized from brain, and the activation by ephrinB of EphB receptors transfected into neurons in culture causes an increase in the colocalization of NMDA and EphB receptor in clusters. The coclustering depends only on the extracel-lular portions of the NMDA and EphB receptors and may reflect a direct interaction between them. Most important, EphB receptor activation by ephrinB in culture increases the number of functional synapses, as judged by FM1-43 labeling of recycling synaptic vesi-cles. As with neuroligin, these experiments demon-strate that ephrinB–EphB receptor interactions are sufficient to stimulate synapse formation but leave unanswered the question of whether they are also necessary.

A novel component capable of clustering AMPA receptors on certain types of neurons is the immediate early gene product Narp (O'Brien et al., 1999). Narp is a member of the pentraxin family, extracellular com-ponents capable of head-to-head aggregation. It was isolated initially as a hippocampal protein that is enriched by stimulation and was subsequently shown to codistribute with synaptic AMPA receptors, pri-marily on aspiny neurons in the spinal cord and in the hippocampus. Cell culture experiments indicate that Narp can act both from pre- and postsynaptic loca-tions to cluster AMPA receptors. As an extracellular component, it may interact directly with the receptors because it can be immunoprecipitated as a Narp–AMPA receptor complex. Because patterned electrical activity upregulates Narp expression, it may con-tribute to activity-dependent synapse maturation. The functional role of Narp *in vivo* has yet to be evaluated.

The Role of Activity in Glutamatergic Synapse Formation

The role of activity in the formation of glutamater-gic synapses has been the subject of intensive study. Spiny neurons largely confine excitatory glutamater-gic input to dendritic spines, and spine stability and morphology are known to be influenced by activity. Chronic NMDA receptor blockade increases NMDA receptor density at synaptic sites in culture, and a blockade of activity increases synaptic AMPA recep-tors as well. Particularly intriguing in this context is the activity of CGP15, a small extracellular GPI-linked protein initially discovered as a gene product that is upregulated by activity in adult hippocampus (Cantallops *et al.*, 2000). *In vivo* expression of CPG15 increases axonal arborization and synaptic maturation, as evidenced by a precocious increase in the ratio of AMPA/NMDA-mediated currents. Moreover, CPG15 induced a decrease in silent synapses, consistent with an early acquisition of AMPA receptors at such sites. The ability of CPG15 to increase AMPA receptors at synapses is not blocked by NMDA receptor antagonists, indicating that CPG15 acts downstream of the receptors. One model drawing these observations together is that activity may drive the initial arborization of dendrites and formation of spines, whereas activity at subsequent stages stabilizes functional contacts unless overridden by excess CPG15 (Cantallops *et al.*, 2000).

The role of activity in synapse formation in the CNS has been the subject of continuing controversy, in part because the effects of synaptic activity are likely to differ substantially with the stage of devel-

opment examined. One report suggests that synaptic activity is completely unnecessary for the initial stages of synapse formation. Thus Munc18-1 null mutants display normal brain development until relatively late stages of maturation (Verhage *et al.*, 2000). Munc18-1 is a membrane-trafficking protein that is absolutely required *in vivo* for secretion of the neurotransmitter. The null mutant fails to display spontaneous transmission and fails to release transmitter when treated with α-latrotoxin. Nonetheless, morphological development of synaptic connections appears normal until massive neuronal degeneration occurs late in development. It will be informative to examine the composition and organization of synaptic components in such mutants at the molecular level to assess how far synaptic development can proceed in the absence of synaptic transmission.

Most of the mechanisms and molecular candidates for synaptogenic agents described previously are thought to act on entire classes of synapses. Unanswered is the question of how synaptic speci-

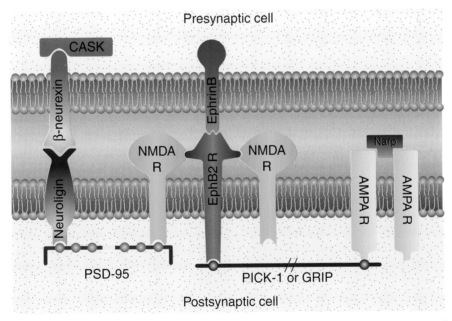

FIGURE 18.12 Model showing transsynaptic interactions that may coordinate presynaptic and postsynaptic elements at glutamatergic synapses. The PDZ-containing protein PSD-95 binds to NMDA receptors, whereas other PDZ-containing proteins, PICK-1 and GRIP, bind to AMPA receptors. Neuroligin on the postsynaptic cell binds to β-neurexin in the presynaptic membrane and, via Cask and other components, may nucleate organization of the presynaptic terminal. The ability of neuroligin to bind postsynaptically to PSD-95 and associated NMDA receptors would help align pre- and postsynaptic specializations. Similarly, presynaptic ephrinB binding to postsynaptic EphB2 receptors, which regulate the clustering of NMDA receptors, would help concentrate both EphB2 and NMDA receptors at synaptic sites. Because EphB2 receptors can also bind to PICK-1 and GRIP, EphB2 receptors may provide an indirect link between NMDA and AMPA receptors. Narp may offer yet another mechanism for clustering certain populations of AMPA receptors. Interactions among these proteins have been established by *in vitro* binding and immunoprecipitation experiments; the importance of these interactions for synapse formation *in vivo* remains to be determined.

ficity is generated within classes. The discovery of cadherin-related neuronal receptors (CNRs) and the demonstration that their genomic arrangement has remarkable parallels to the immunoglobulin family encourage speculation that such components may generate the diversity needed to help specify synaptic connections (Wu and Maniatis, 1999). By splicing different exons encoding unique extracellular domains to exons encoding a common intracellular domain, each family of CNRs offers numerous possibilities for producing distinctive recognition molecules. The fact that such molecules couple to the same intracellular effector indicates a common downstream function and encourages speculation that CNRs may provide a kind of molecular code for synapse formation. Both classical cadherins and CNRs can be found concentrated at synapses, but their significance for synaptic specificity has yet to be determined.

Summary

The diversity of synapses found in the nervous system is likely to be matched by an equally diverse array of mechanisms producing the synapses. These mechanisms are only now beginning to be elucidated.

Prime candidates at present for synaptogenic roles (Fig. 18.12) include transmembrane proteins interacting with cognate receptors on the apposing cell surface (e.g., neuroligin/β-neurexin; ephrinB/EphB receptors), diffusible molecules that instruct synaptic development in target cells (e.g., WNT-7a) or interact directly with synaptic components (e.g., Narp), membrane-attached components that act to promote maturation both pre- and postsynaptically (e.g., CPG15), and intracellular components that act locally to organize synaptic constituents (e.g., gephyrin). Testing the effects of such components *in vivo* will be a high priority in the near term. Neuronal activity is also important for certain aspects of synapse formation, but exactly how it participates and whether it employs mechanisms shared with those governing synaptic plasticity remain intriguing questions. Finally, we are only beginning to identify molecular families (e.g., CNRs) that may contribute to achieving the remarkable synaptic specificity found in the nervous system. Determining how specific components participate in and direct the continuing "handshake" of transsynaptic signals governing synapse formation is one of the many challenges for the future.

BOX 18.2

RETT SYNDROME AND RELATED DISORDERS

Rett syndrome (RTT) is a neurodevelopmental disorder first recognized as a distinct clinical entity by Andreas Rett in 1966. It is a genetic disorder caused by mutations to a gene encoding a protein involved with suppressing transcription.

Classic Rett syndrome affects approximately 1:15,000 females, first appearing after 6 to 18 months of apparently normal development. Neurodevelopment is then interrupted, and affected girls begin to regress: they lose acquired skills involving language and purposeful hand use is replaced by stereotypic hand-wringing. Other symptoms progressively appear: microcephaly, gait ataxia, apraxia, apnea and hyperpnea, seizures, scoliosis, and growth retardation.

Milder forms of the syndrome that lack certain signs, as well as very severe forms, lack the period of normal development and cause hypotonia and infantile spasms. It has also been discovered that males with methyl-CpG-binding protein 2 (MeCP2) mutations can survive beyond birth with a severe mental retardation syndrome that causes motor dysfunction as well. As more mutation analysis is performed, the classification of these different clinical entities as variants of one syndrome is now being verified at a genetic level.

How can a mutation to one causative and widely expressed gene be manifested as primarily a neurological syndrome with delayed onset?

RTT is caused by mutations in the X-linked gene encoding MeCP2. MeCP2 is a transcriptional repressor protein that binds to methylated CpG dinucleotides throughout the genome. This modifies the chromatin structure, rendering DNA inaccessible to the transcriptional machinery. Discovering which genes are misregulated in the absence of functional MeCP2 is crucial for understanding the pathogenesis of this disorder and related syndromes.

Many types of mutation commonly found in patients (nonsense, missense, and frameshift) are likely to lead to a partial loss of protein function. Interestingly, C-to-T transitions at eight different CpG dinucleotides in the gene account for almost 70% of patient mutations.

The mutation type affects disease severity, but the correlation between mutation type and phenotype is difficult to evaluate in females because of the confounding influence of X chromosome inactivation.

<hr>

BOX 18.2   *(cont'd)*

<hr>

The messenger RNA (mRNA) encoding MeCP2 is present in a wide variety of tissues, but levels are approximately six times higher in the brain; this may be a clue to the neurological manifestation of the mutations. *In situ* studies of the developing and fully differentiated mouse brain demonstrate expression throughout the brain, with elevated levels in the olfactory bulb and hippocampus. For genes that may be methylated in neurons and silenced by MeCP2, the mutated protein could allow inappropriate expression, thereby disrupting neuronal development.

Another aspect of the Rett syndrome phenotype that is difficult to reconcile with the expression pattern of MeCP2 is the delay in the onset of overt features. One possible explanation is that the genes repressed by MeCP2 do not become methylated until later in development. Several neuronal gene promoters have, in fact, been found to undergo a developmental change in methylation.

For example, *Stac*, a gene expressed primarily in brain (and at highest levels in the hippocampus, cerebellum, and inferior olive), displays a developmental change in methylation pattern in the mouse brain, and the glial fibrillary acidic protein gene undergoes methylation during neuronal maturation in the rat brain. These examples demonstrate that neuronal maturation may require changes in the expression of genes mediated by DNA methylation.

It remains to be determined why mutation of the widely expressed *MECP2* gene leads to a neuronal phenotype, what genes are regulated by *MECP2*, and how mutations in *MECP2* give rise to the characteristic features of Rett syndrome. When suitable animal models become available, addressing these perplexing issues will become possible.

Graham V. Lees

Adapted from M. D. Shahbazian, H. Y. Zoghbi (2000). Molecular genetics of Rett syndrome and clinical spectrum of MECP2 mutations. Curr Opin Neurol. **14**(2), 171–176.

References

Anderson, M. J., and Cohen, M. W. (1977). Nerve induced and spontaneous redistribution of acetylcholine receptors on culture muscle cells. *J. Physiol. (Lond.)* **268**, 757–773.

Brown, A., Yates, P. A., Burrola, P., Ortuño, D., Vaidya, A., Jessell, T. M., Pfaff, S. L, O'Leary, D. D. M., and Lemke, G. (2000). Topographic mapping from the retina to the midbrain is controlled by relative but not absolute levels of EphA receptor signaling. *Cell* **102**, 77–88.

Burden, S. J, Sargent, P. B., and McMahan, U. J. (1979). Acetylcholine receptors in regenerating muscle accumulate at the original synaptic site in the absence of the nerve. *J. Cell Biol.* **82**, 412–425.

Cantallops, I., Haas, K., and Cline, H. T. (2000). Postsynaptic CPG14 promotes synaptic maturation and presynaptic axon arbor elaboration in vivo. *Nature Neurosci.* **3**, 1004–1011.

Dalva, M. B., Takasu, M. A., Lin, M. Z., Shamah, S. M., Hu, L., Gale, N. W., and Greenberg, M. E. (2000). EphB receptors interact with NMDA receptors and regulate excitatory synapse formation. *Cell* **103**, 945–956.

DeChiara, T. M., Bowen, D. C., Valenzuela, D. M., Simmons, M. V., Poueymirou, W. T., Thomas, S., Kinetz, E., Compton, D. L., Park, J. S., Smith, C., DiStefano, P. S., Glass, D. J., Burden, S. J., and Yancopoulos, G. D. (1996). The receptor tyrosine kinase, MuSK, is required for neuromuscular junction formation in vivo. *Cell* **85**, 501–512.

Feldheim, D. A., Kim, Y. I., Bergemann, A. D., Frisen, J., Barbacid, M., and Flanagan, J. G. (2000). Genetic analysis of ephrin-A2 and ephrin-A5 shows their requirement in multiple aspects of retinocollicular mapping. *Neuron* **25**, 563–574.

Feng, G., Laskowski, M. B., Feldheim, D. A., Wang, H., Lewis, R., Frisen, J., Flanagan, J. G., Sanes, and J. R. (2000). Roles for ephrins in positionally selective synaptogenesis between motor neurons and muscle fibers. *Neuron* **25**, 295–306.

Frisen, J., Yates, P. A., McLaughlin, T., Friedman, G. C., O'Leary, D. D. M., and Barbacid, M. (1998). Ephrin-A5 (AL–1/RAGS) is essential for proper retinal axon guidance and topographic mapping in the mammalian visual system. *Neuron* **20**, 235–243.

Gautam, M., Noakes, P. G., Moscoso, L., Rupp, F., Scheller, R. H., Merlie, J. P., and Sanes, J. R. (1996). Defective neuromuscular synaptogenesis in agrin-deficient mutant mice. *Cell* **85**, 525–535.

Gautam, M., Noakes, P. G., Mudd, J., Nichol, M., Chu, G. C., Sanes, J. R., and Merlie, J. P. (1995). Failure of postsynaptic specialization to develop at neuromuscular junctions of rapsyn-deficient mice. *Nature* **377**, 232–236.

Hall, A. C., Lucas, F. R., and Salinas, P. C. (2000). Axonal remodeling and synaptic differentiation in the cerebellum is regulated by WNT–7a signaling. *Cell* **100**, 525–535.

Lin, W., Burgess, R. W., Dominguez, B., Pfaff, S. L., Sanes, J. R., and Lee, K. F. (2001). Distinct roles of nerve and muscle in postsynaptic differentiation of the neuromuscular synapse. *Nature* **410**, 1057–1064.

Monschau, B., Kremoser, C., Ohta, K., Tanaka, H., Kaneko, T., Yamada, T., Handwerker, C., Hornberger, M. R., Loschinger, J., Pasquale, E. B., Siever, D. A., Verderame, M. F., Muller, B. K., Bonhoeffer, F., and Drescher, U. (1997). Shared and distinct functions of RAGS and ELF–1 in guiding retinal axons. *EMBO. J* **16**, 1258–1267.

Nakamoto, M., Cheng, H. J., Friedman, G. C., McLaughlin, T., Hansen, M. J., Yoon, C. H., O'Leary, D. D. M., and Flanagan J. G. (1996). Topographically specific effects of ELF–1 on retinal axon guidance in vitro and retinal axon mapping in vivo. *Cell* **86**, 755–766.

O'Brien, R. J., Xu, D., Petralia, R. S., Steward, O., Huganir, R. L., and Worley, P. (1999). Synaptic clustering of AMPA receptors by the extracellular immediate-early gene product Narp. *Neuron* **23**, 309–323.

O'Leary, D. D. M. (1992). Development of connectional diversity and specificity in the mammalian brain by the pruning of collateral projections. *Curr. Opin. Neurobiol.* **2**, 70–77.

O'Leary, D. D. M., and Koester, S. E. (1993). Development of projection neuron types, axonal pathways and patterned connections of the mammalian cortex. *Neuron* 10, 991–1006.

Sanes, J. R., Marshall, L. M., and McMahan, U. J. (1978). Reinnervation of muscle fiber basal lamina by after removal of myofibers: Differentiation of regenerating axons at original synaptic sites. *J. Cell Biol.* **78**, 176–198.

Scheiffele, P., Fan, J., Choih, J., Fetter, R., and Serafini, T. (2000). Neuroligin expressed in nonneuronal cells triggers presynaptic development in contacting axons. *Cell* **101**, 657–669.

Verhage, M., Maia, A. S., Plomp, J. J., Brussaard, A. B., Heeroma, J. H., Vermeer, H., Toonen, R. F., Hammer, R. E., van den Berg, T. K., Missler, M., Geuze, H. J., and Sudhof, T. C. (2000). Synaptic assembly of the brain in the absence of neurotransmitter secretion. *Science* **287**, 864–869.

Wu, Q., and Maniatis, T. (1999). A striking organization of a large family of human neural cadherin-like cell adhesion genes. *Cell* **97**, 779–790.

Yang, S., Li, W., Prescott, E. D., Burden, S. J., and Wang, J. C. (2000). DNA topoisomerase IIbeta and neural development. *Science* **287**, 131–134.

Yang, X., Arber, S., William, C., Li, L., Tanabe, Y., Jessell, T. M., Birchmeier, C., and Burden, S. J. (2001). Patterning of muscle acetylcholine receptor gene expression in the absence of motor innervation. *Neuron* **30**, 399–410.

Yates, P. A., Roskies, A. R., McLaughlin, T., and O'Leary, D. D. M. (2001). Topographic specific axon branching controlled by ephrin-As is the critical event in retinotectal map development. *J. Neurosci.* **21**, 8548–8563.

Burden, S. J. (1998). The formation of neuromuscular synapses. *Genes Dev.* **12**, 133–148.

Craig, A. M., and Lichtman, J. W. (2001). Synapse formation and maturation. *In* "Synapses" (W. M. Cowan, T. C. Sudhof, and C. F. Stevens, eds.), pp. 571–612. Johns Hopkins University Press; Baltimore, MD.

Fischbach, G. D., and Rosen, K. M. (1997). ARIA: A neuromuscular junction neuregulin. *Annu. Rev. Neurosci.* **20**, 429–458.

Flanagan, J. G., and Vanderhaeghen, P. (1998). The ephrins and Eph receptors in neural development. *Annu. Rev. Neurosci.* **21**,309–345.

Frisen, J., Holmberg, J., and Barbacid, M. (1999). Ephrins and their Eph receptors: Multitalented directors of embryonic development. *EMBO J.* **18**, 5159–5165.

Helmbacher, F., Schneider-Maunoury, S., Topilko, P., Tiret, L., and Charnay, P. (2000). Targeting of the EphA4 tyrosine kinase receptor affects dorsal/ventral pathfinding of limb motor axons. *Development* **127**, 3313–3324.

Jontes, J. D., and Smith, S. J. (2000). Filopodia, spines, and the generation of synaptic diversity. *Neuron* **27**, 11–14.

Kneussel, M., and Betz, H. (2000). Clustering of inhibitory neurotransmitter receptors at developing postsynaptic sites: The membrane activation model. *TINS* **23**, 429–435.

Lee, S. H., and Sheng, M. (2000). Development of neuron-neuron synapses. *Curr. Opin. Neurobiol.* **10**, 125–131.

McMahan, U. J. (1990). The agrin hypothesis. *Cold Spring Harb. Symp. Quant. Biol.* **55**, 407–418.

O'Leary, D. D. M., Yates, P., and McLaughlin, T. (1999). Mapping sights and smells in the brain: Distinct mechanisms to achieve a common goal. *Cell* **96**, 255–269.

Purves, D., and Lichtman, J. W. (1985). Principles of Neural Development, Chapters 10 and 11, pp. 229–270.

Sanes, J. R., and Lichtman, J. W. (1999). Development of the vertebrate neuromuscular junction. *Annu. Rev. Neurosci.* **22**, 389–442.

Schaeffer, L., de Kerchove d'Exaerde, A., and Changeux, J. P. (2001). Targeting transcription to the neuromuscular synapse. *Neuron* **31**, 15–22.

Suggested Readings

Brown, M., Keynes, R., and Lumsden, A. (2001). "The Developing Brain," Chapter 10, pp. 261–280. Oxford Univ Press, New York.

Steven J. Burden, Darwin Berg, and
Dennis D. M. O'Leary

19

Programmed Cell Death and Neurotrophic Factors

One of the hallmarks of embryonic development is the enormous production of new cells and the acquisition of new cellular properties (phenotypes). Accordingly, in the past, a major focus of developmental neurobiologists has been the study of these progressive events, including proliferation and migration (Chapter 16), pathway formation (Chapter 18), synaptogenesis (Chapter 19), and phenotype determination (Chapters 15 and 17). In this context, the concept of significant regressive events, such as cell death, occurring during development, was initially considered counterintuitive, often relegated to a subordinate position, or even denied altogether. One of the pioneers in this field, the American embryologist John Saunders, noted nearly 40 years ago that one is intuitively uncomfortable with the notion that cell death has a place in embryonic development.

Yet we now know that cell loss and other regressive events, including synapse elimination (Chapter 19), are the rule rather than the exception. In virtually all developing tissues that have been examined, substantial cell loss occurs (Oppenheim, 1991). Genetic programs that result in cell death have been suggested as a default phenotype pathway for all cells (Raff, 1992). Neurons only escape this default fate by receiving the appropriate survival (trophic factor) signals that induce changes in transcriptional events required for cell survival and neuronal differentiation. If the notion that cells are "born to die" is correct, then the molecular mechanisms restricting cell death programs are critical. Both intercellular trophic factors and intracellular mechanisms governing cell death are important for normal development and for many pathologies that arise later in life. Aberrations in the mechanisms regulating the balance between cell proliferation and cell elimination can lead to pathologies of progressive

tissue growth and differentiation (i.e., cancer) or pathologies of abnormal neuronal death (i.e., neurodegenerative disease). Mechanisms that regulate the balance between cell death and production also serve to determine the ultimate number and maintenance of neurons in the nervous system. Genes regulating these mechanisms in turn provide an underlying substrate for evolutionary changes in shaping brain structure and adaptive behavior (Jaaro *et al.*, 2001).

Both progressive and regressive events during development are regulated by intercellular signals. Somewhat surprisingly, many of the same intercellular signals that contribute to the regulation of progressive events during nervous system development (cell proliferation, migration, differentiation, axonal and dendritic growth, synaptogenesis, synaptic plasticity) also contribute to the control of regressive events (cell death/survival, axon collateral elimination, and dendritic pruning) (Korsching, 1993). While many neurotrophic factors were originally discovered and appreciated for their activity as regulators of neuronal survival and axonal growth, other signaling peptides were first discovered as growth factors or cytokines within other organ systems and were later found to also regulate the development of selected neurons or glia. Neurotrophic factors are now appreciated for their activities in both developing and mature nervous systems (Lewin and Barde, 1996). They play important roles in the regulation of activity-dependent anatomical and functional plasticity of the nervous system, as well as the repair of the damaged nervous system throughout life.

Because neurons may die for a variety of reasons and in many different situations, it is important to describe the type of cell death observed most often in the developing nervous system. Although the loss of

TABLE 19.1   Major Events in the Discovery and Characterization of NGF and Their Importance for
Understanding Neuronal Cell Death[a]

1934   *Hamburger* discovered that removal of the limb bud in the chick embryo resulted in reduced numbers of sensory and motor neurons in the spinal cord and suggested that targets in the limb are the source of signals that control neuronal development and that travel retrogradely in axons to their respective centers

1939   *Hamburger* discovered that transplantation of an additional supernumerary limb bud resulted in increased numbers of sensory and motor neurons in the spinal cord, providing additional evidence that targets are the source of signals that control neuronal development. He proposed that targets act on innervating neurons by providing signals that recruit undifferentiated cells to develop into sensory or motor neurons

1942   *Levi-Montalcini* and *Levi* confirmed that early limb bud removal reduced the number of sensory and motor neurons but proposed that the hypothetical target-derived signals act to maintain the survival of differentiating neurons, not to recruit undifferentiated cells

1948   *Bueker*, a former student of Hamburger, implanted different mouse tumors into the region of the chick hind limb as a source of rapidly growing homogeneous peripheral "target" tissue in an attempt to identify the cellular source of normal target-derived signals. One tumor, sarcoma 180, a cell line derived from connective tissue, was found to produce a modest (30%) but significant increase in the size of limb sensory ganglia. It was without effect on motor neurons. Bueker concluded that the tumor provided a periphery with specific histochemical properties favorable to sensory but not motor innervation

1949   *Hamburger* and *Levi-Montalcini* repeated earlier limb removal experiments, and their results supported the previous interpretation of Levi-Montalcini and Levi. They also discovered that many sensory neurons undergo a period of normal or naturally occurring cell death. They proposed that the addition or removal of a limb bud acts to reduce or enhance the normal cell death process by perturbing target-derived signals that promote neuronal survival

1951   *Levi-Montalcini* and *Hamburger* repeated the Bueker experiment using sarcoma 180 and discovered an even more striking effect of the tumor on both sensory and sympathetic ganglia but again no effect on motor neurons. They concluded that the tumor cells produce specific growth-promoting agents

1953   *Levi-Montalcini* and *Hamburger* carried out additional transplantation experiments with sarcoma 180 and discovered that sympathetic and sensory ganglia remote from the tumor and not connected with it by nerve fibers were also enlarged greatly. This suggested involvement of a diffusible factor. Transplantation of tumors onto the chorioallantois, which were therefore only in communication with the embryo via the circulation, was fully effective in causing hyperplasia of ganglia, confirming that the growth-promoting activity was indeed due to a diffusible agent

1954   *Levi-Montalcini*, *Meyer*, and *Hamburger* developed an *in vitro* assay that used explanted sympathetic ganglia. Ganglia cocultured with fragments of tumor cells lacking any physical contacts between the two exhibited massive outgrowth of nerve fibers (Fig. 19.2). The extent and density of outgrowth provided a rapid quantitative bioassay for subsequent attempts to isolate and purify the tumor factor

1956   *Cohen* and *Levi-Montalcini*, in an attempt to purify the agent found in mouse sarcoma 180, used snake venom as a rich source of phosphodiesterase for the separation of nuclei acid and protein fractions in the tumor material. To their great surprise, tumor fractions containing the snake venom were several thousandfold more potent than control tumor homogenates in promoting nerve growth *in vitro* and *in vivo*. Subsequent experiments showed that the activities in the tumor and snake venom were identical.

1960   *Cohen* examined the mammalian homolog of the snake venom gland—the salivary gland—and discovered that the salivary gland of male mice was an even richer source of the same growth-promoting activity found in the tumors and venom gland. When an antiserum to the mouse factor was injected into newborn mice, all sympathetic neurons were lost

1969   *Bocchini* and *P. Angeletti* described a method for the purification of biologically active NGF from male mouse submaxillary glands. This activity is the β subunit of NGF, also known as 2.5S NGF. It has been estimated that to purify NGF from relevant target organs would have required a purification factor of 100 million, whereas a purification factor of only 100–200 was sufficient to purify NGF from the mouse salivary gland. Even more remarkable was the discovery that salivary glands from female mice or other mammals do not contain this extremely high concentration of NGF

1971   *R. Angeletti* and *Bradshaw* identified the amino acid sequence of 2.5S NGF purified from the mouse submaxillary gland

1982   *Barde* and colleagues isolated a novel neurotrophic factor from the mammalian brain (brain-derived neurotrophic factor) (BDNF). Unlike the original purification of NGF from a fortuitous rich source—the salivary gland— this factor was isolated from many brains by an amazing purification factor of several millionfold. BDNF was identified and isolated using an *in vitro* survival assay with sensory neurons, but this activity was not blocked with NGF-specific antibodies

1983   *Korsching* and *Thoenen* developed a sensitive two-site immunoassay, allowing for the first time the detection of NGF in target organs. With this method it was possible to demonstrate a strong correlation between the density of sympathetic innervation and target levels of NGF, a finding consistent with the neurotrophic theory

1986   The Nobel Prize in medicine was awarded to *Levi-Montalcini* and *Cohen* for the discovery of NGF and EGF

1989   The sequencing and molecular cloning of BDNF by *Barde* and colleagues revealed a high degree of sequence homology between the new factor and NGF. This finding resulted in the rapid molecular cloning and sequencing of other related *neurotrophins* containing the conserved regions without prior protein purification

---

[a] See Cowan (2001).

cells during normal development has been called many different things (including normal cell death, spontaneous cell death, naturally occurring cell death, and developmental cell death), this chapter uses the term programmed cell death (PCD). PCD is defined as the spatially and temporally reproducible and species-specific loss of large numbers of individual cells during development. Accidental, injury-induced, pathological, and disease-related forms of cell death are not included (even though we recognize that the biochemical and molecular mechanisms used to kill cells in these situations may overlap with those involved in developmental PCD). Additionally, because many differentiated cells in adult vertebrates undergo continuous turnover by cell death and cell division (e.g., blood cells, gut epithelium, hepatocytes in liver, olfactory epithelium, skin), this form of cell loss is also a type of PCD. However, because much of cell death during development appears to serve distinct functions related to embryogenesis, rather than to tissue homeostasis, we restrict our definition to a developmental context. This definition of PCD also makes no a priori assumptions about either the morphological or the biochemical pathways by which cells die or the stimuli that trigger cell death. The use of the word "programmed" refers to the reproducible, spatiotemporal occurrence of cell loss and is not meant to imply that the cell loss is genetically pre-determined, inherited from precursor cells, or inevitable. In fact, PCD is clearly not predetermined in most cases, but instead is critically dependent on epigenetic signals arising from cellular interactions. Finally, as discussed in more detail later, the term PCD is not synonymous with the term apoptosis, which refers to only one specific, albeit common, mode of cell death.

CELL DEATH AND THE NEUROTROPHIC HYPOTHESIS

Early embryological studies of the interactions between developing neurons and their peripheral targets laid the foundation for the discovery of cell death and neurotrophic factors (Hamburger, 1992). These studies formed the conceptual framework for the "neurotrophic"(nerve feeding) hypothesis. In retrospect, the discovery and recognition of normal cell death reflect the triumph of observation over conventional wisdom and the Zeitgeist, whereas the discovery of the first neurotrophic factor, NGF, represents a colorful history marked by a rare combination of scientific reasoning, intuition, and serendipity (see Table 19.1) (for a review, see Cowan, 2001). Although

the decision about when a discovery occurred is often arbitrary, the consensus is that the trophic theory and cell death stories began together in the mid-1930s. The notion of trophic interactions determining neuronal number began with the observations of Viktor Hamburger on the effects of early removal of the wing bud in the chick embryo on the later development of sensory and motor neurons in the spinal cord that innervate the limb. Hamburger's observations confirmed earlier controversial studies claiming that, sensory ganglia and motor nuclei were reduced greatly in size in the absence of the limb. He postulated that peripheral target fields in the limb control the development of innervating centers (sensory ganglia and motor neurons) by signals transmitted retrogradely along axons from targets to afferent neurons. These signals were originally thought to act

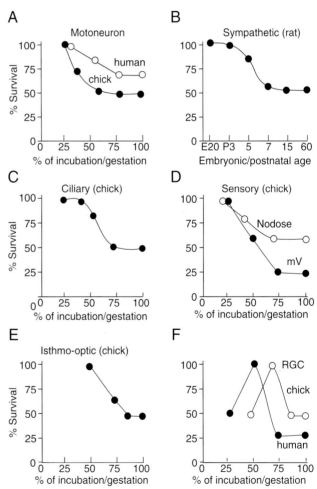

FIGURE 19.1 PCD in six different neuronal populations in chick, rat, and human embryos. mV, mesencephalic sensory nucleus of the fifth trigeminal nerve; RGC, retinal ganglion cells; ciliary, parasympathetic ciliary ganglion; sensory, spinal dorsal root ganglion; sympathetic, superior cervical ganglion.

by recruiting or inducing undifferentiated precursor cells to develop into sensory or motor neurons (Fig. 19.1). Later studies by Hamburger supported this idea by showing that when the size of the peripheral target was increased by transplantation of a supernumerary wing bud, motor nuclei and sensory ganglia were enlarged or hypertrophied (Fig. 19.2). Thus, as early as 1934 the stage was set for the search for hypothetical target-derived retrograde signals, a search that eventually led to the discovery of NGF.

Although the recruitment hypothesis provided a simple and elegant means of accounting for differences in the size of nerve centers after the deletion or addition of wing buds, it was wrong. Strikingly new ideas are seldom fully appreciated or accepted into

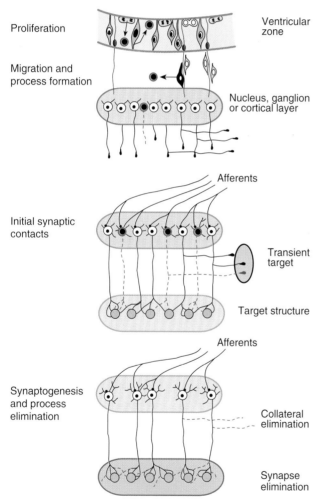

FIGURE 19.2 Stages of neuronal development when PCD occurs. PCD can occur at all stages between proliferation and synaptogenesis. Once synaptic connections are stabilized, normal PCD ceases. Following the period of PCD, axonal pathways and synaptic connections are refined by collateral and synapse elimination. Round red cells with a dark center represent cells undergoing PCD. From Burek and Oppenheim (1999).

the prevailing conceptual framework at the time they are first proposed (see Box 19.1). Neuronal cell death offers a prominent example. Ernst and Glucksmann first recognized that cell death is an integral part of normal embryonic development, but to many this concept originally seemed counterintuitive (Hamburger, 1992). By 1949, Hamburger and Rita Levi-Montalcini had provided further evidence to support the significance of normal embryonic neuronal death and postulated that target-derived signals act to regulate the number of neurons that survive embryonic development. In subsequent studies, they and their colleagues identified a specific protein (NGF) that influenced development of the same populations of neurons (sensory and sympathetic) that their earlier studies had suggested were regulated by target-derived signals (Fig. 19.3).

By 1960, the preparation of specific antibodies that block NGF activity allowed Stanley Cohen and co-investigators to demonstrate the almost total degeneration of sympathetic ganglia *in vivo* following the specific deprivation of NGF activity (Fig. 19.3). Only with this "immunosympathectomy" (the removal of the sympathetic system by antibody treatment) was NGF first considered to be an endogenous survival or maintenance factor for these neurons. Even then, it took another 20 years before the normal death of a proportion of developing sympathetic neurons was first described and shown to be regulated by NGF, and it was a few years later still before a sensitive NGF immunoassay was used to establish that NGF was synthesized (produced) in limiting trace amounts by sympathetic targets and transported retrogradely to ganglionic neurons. Accordingly, not until three decades after the original discovery that an unkown chemical substance produced by tumor cells affects the development of sensory and sympathetic neurons dramatically was it finally recognized that NGF was the hypothetical target-derived trophic signal first postulated by Hamburger and Levi-Montalcini in 1949 to be involved in regulating the number of surviving neurons in these populations during normal development. Collectively, these studies provide strong evidence supporting the foundation of the neurotrophic hypothesis.

NERVE GROWTH FACTOR: THE PROTOTYPE TARGET-DERIVED NEURONAL SURVIVAL FACTOR

Characterization of the functional role of NGF became the archetypical model for the investigation of other putative neurotrophic factors. Analysis of the

BOX 19.1

PARANEOPLASTIC NEUROLOGIC DISORDERS

Study of paraneoplastic neurologic disorders (PNDs) has provided insights into human neurodegenerative disorders, neuron-specific biology, and tumor immunology. PNDs are believed to be triggered when proteins normally expressed only within the nervous system are expressed ectopically in tumor cells. The propensity of certain types of cancer cells to coopt specific brain proteins suggests that the function of PND antigens is of particular interest to both tumor cell biology and neurobiology. Immunologically, because of the blood–brain barrier and the immune privilege of neurons, tumor cells expressing such neuronal antigens are able to be recognized by the immune system as expressing "foreign" proteins. An immune response is generated that has been shown to be similar to that seen following viral infection, including both antitumor cell antibodies and T cells. This immune response effectively suppresses tumor growth, but also becomes competent to break the immune privilege of the brain and cause severe neurodegenerative disease.

Antiserum obtained from PND patients has provided natural reagents for expression cDNA cloning and subsequent identification of brain-specific proteins associated with specific neurodegeneration. These proteins have fallen into several categories. These include two newly discovered families of neuron-specific RNA-binding proteins, cytoplasmic signaling proteins, synaptic vesicle proteins, and neurotransmitter proteins or their associated proteins. In almost every instance, the proteins identified have been found to be expressed exclusively in neurons at all developmental times, suggesting that their biology has the potential to yield insights into unique cellular properties of neurons.

Nova and Hu neuronal RNA-binding proteins are targeted in a variety of neurodegenerative disorders associated with lung or gynecologic cancers. These range from dysfunction of brain stem and spinal cord inhibitory neurotransmitter systems (Nova) to limbic encephalopathy (memory loss), sensory loss, cerebellar dysfunction, motor loss, and other disorders (Hu). Two Nova genes expressed exclusively in the CNS encode proteins harboring three KH-type RNA-binding domains. These proteins recognize specific RNA-binding motifs (UCAY) by forming pseudo Watson–Crick base pairing with RNA, as demonstrated by X-ray crystallography. Understanding the means of specific RNA recognition led to the identification of Nova as the first neuron-specific regulator of neuronal alternative splicing. Nova binds to specific intronic RNA elements in inhibitory neurotransmitter receptors and regulates their

utilization of alternatively spliced exons. It is unknown whether Nova may also regulate the expression of these or other neuronal mRNAs outside of the nucleus.

Four Hu genes have been identified: three of which are expressed exclusively in neurons and one of which is expressed outside of the nervous system. Each gene encodes proteins harboring three RRM-type RNA-binding motifs with high and low homology, respectively, to the Drosophila neurogenesis and splicing proteins elav and sex-lethal. In the nucleus, Hu proteins function as adaptors that bridge nuclear RNAs and the nuclear export machinery; in the cytoplasm, Hu proteins are implicated in the stabilization of a number of short-lived mRNAs that contain AU-rich elements. Neuronal Hu proteins are expressed very early in development, and some evidence suggests that they may play an important role in the early differentiation of postmitotic neurons.

Two families of PND antigens are cytoplasmic signaling proteins expressed in gynecologic cancers [the cdr2 (or the Yo antigen)] and small cell lung cancer (recoverin). The cdr2 antigen is targeted in patients who develop cerebellar degeneration and is expressed very specifically in cerebellar Purkinje neurons. The first third of the cdr2 protein harbors a long coiled-coil leucine zipper. This dimerization motif interacts with the c-myc protein in Purkinje neuronal cytoplasm and is believed to downregulate c-myc activity. Recoverin is targeted in patients who develop blindness and is expressed specifically in photoreceptors. Recoverin binds to calcium and activates guanlyate cyclase in photoreceptors.

The best described synaptic vesicle associated PND antigen is amphiphysin, which is targeted in breast cancer patients who develop a syndrome of motor hyperactivity termed stiff-person syndrome. Amphiphysin proteins are thought to be multiprotein adaptors that contribute to synaptic vesicle recycling by bringing together many of the proteins required for endocytosis.

Each of the PND antibodies described to date has led to the identification of neuron–specific antigens whose functions are just beginning to be understood. Neurologists continue to describe new antineuronal antibodies associated with cancer and neuronal degeneration. Study of the rare but fascinating PNDs is likely to continue to provide insight into proteins with biologic functions that distinguish neurons from other cells.

Robert B. Darnell

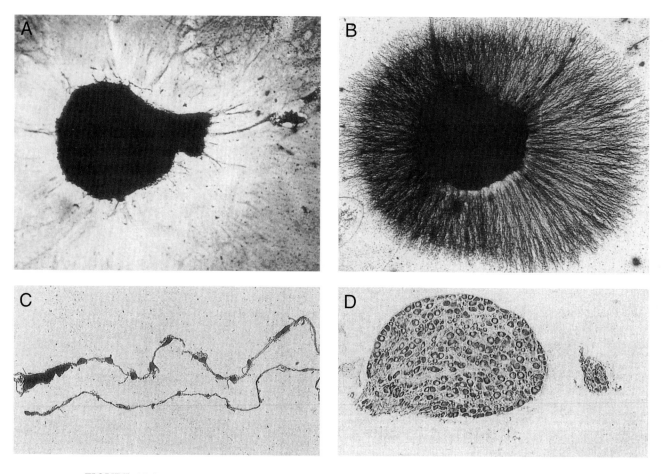

FIGURE 19.3 Biological activity of NGF. Explanted sensory and sympathetic ganglia or dissociated neurons were used in bioassays detecting neurotrophic activity. A ganglion explant assay was used to purify NGF. (A) Control ganglion 24 h in culture without NGF and (B) experimental ganglion 24 h after NGF treatment. Treatment with NGF causes the formation of a "halo" of axonal growth from sensory neurons in the ganglion (100 ng ml⁻¹). Why the factor was named is obvious. Reprinted with permission from Levi-Montalcini. (C and D) Experimental immunosympathectomy. Antibodies that selectively block NGF activity were administered to newborn mice to deprive the developing animals of endogenous factor. Sympathetic ganglia were examined several weeks after the treatment (N, normal ganglia; E, ganglia deprived of NGF for 3–5 days). Note the almost complete disappearance of the sympathetic chain ganglia (C) and the loss of neurons in individual ganglia (D).

function(s) of a putative neurotrophic factor involved several steps. Typically, the biological activities and target cell specificity of putative factors were first investigated *in vitro* to determine whether the factor acted directly on isolated neurons or whether its effects were mediated indirectly through other cell types. Primary cultures of neurons dissociated from readily dissected peripheral ganglia were ideal for these early assays. Analysis of the developmental expression of specific trophic factors and their corresponding receptors has been used to determine if both the ligand and the receptor are normally present at the appropriate time and place for the putative factor to serve in the regulation of a specific subpopulation of neurons. Treatment of embryos with excess

exogenous factor has been used to determine if the survival or differentiation of responsive neurons is restricted by either the production or the access to a limited quantity of endogenous factor. Finally, methods that inhibit the function of specific trophic factors or their receptors have allowed investigators to determine whether the pertubation of endogenous trophic factor signaling alters normal development. These factor/receptor deprivation experiments have included treatment with activity-blocking antibodies that prevent trophic signaling, treatment with soluble receptor-body antagonists that compete for and adsorb endogenous ligands, and the generation of transgenic mice with null mutations of either the factors or their receptors.

Sympathetic and sensory ganglia removed from developing animals have been shown to produce a dense halo of axonal outgrowth when treated with NGF (Fig. 19.3). In fact, this "axonal halo" assay—not a neuronal survival assay—was the original biological activity first used to purify and characterize NGF as a trophic factor. NGF was shown to be required for the survival of dissociated sympathetic and some sensory neurons when they were grown in the absence of non-neuronal cells. This demonstrated that NGF could prevent cell death by the direct activation of receptors on isolated neurons. When developing embryos were treated with excess exogenous NGF, sympathetic and sensory ganglia were enlarged significantly, and axonal growth from these neurons increased markedly. In addition, ganglia in NGF-treated embryos contain many more neurons than normal because naturally occurring cell death had been prevented. The soma was enlarged significantly by NGF treatment, and the dendritic arbors of sympathetic neurons were more complex. These studies indicated that the supply or access to endogenous NGF in sympathetic and sensory targets was likely to be rate limiting for the survival and growth of these dependent populations. The most convincing evidence that NGF is required for neuron survival has been gained from NGF deprivation experiments. Embryos treated with antibodies that selectively block NGF activity as well as the null mutation of either NGF or its trkA receptor in transgenic mice have both confirmed that sympathetic as well as some sensory neurons require NGF for survival (Fig. 19.3). NGF was localized to the peripheral targets of these neurons at the time of their normal innervation, consistent with its role as a target-derived survival factor. Further, the level of NGF synthesis was correlated with the density of target innervation, and the NGF receptor, trkA, was localized to dependent afferent neurons at the times and places appropriate for regulating normal PCD. The localization of NGF synthesis in sympathetic targets and the loss of these neurons with NGF deprivation firmly established NGF as a prototype target-derived neurotrophic factor required for the survival of sympathetic neurons and a subset of sensory neurons.

Transcription of NGF mRNA is regulated during development and can be altered in mature animals by a number of environmental stimuli, including injury, hormone levels, and changes in neural activity. NGF appears to be released from target cells that synthesize it by constitutive pathways and, in many cases, by activity-dependent mechanisms of secretion. This is especially true of central nervous system (CNS) neurons that secrete NGF on demand following membrane depolarization through the release of internal stores of Ca^{2+}. One prediction of the neurotrophic hypothesis is that access to NGF in only the distant target region is adequate to support the survival of the remote cell body. This idea has been tested by Campenot and colleagues *in vitro*. NGF has been applied restrictively only to local axon terminals in a three compartment tissue culture chamber to determine the long- and short-range effects of NGF treatment. NGF-dependent neuronal cell bodies in the central chamber survived when only their terminals were treated with the factor, indicating that target-derived NGF available only to axons can generate and retrogradely transport the signaling required for cell body survival. Axonal branches were lost rapidly and selectively in outer chambers where NGF was withdrawn, but were maintained and grew in the outer chambers where NGF was added. This important demonstration illustrates the capacity of target-derived NGF to have both direct long distance effects on the survival of neurons and direct local effects on the growth, maintenance, and sprouting of axonal branches. NGF-responsive neurons possess both a high-affinity receptor, trkA (with a dissociation constant or K_D concentration of $10^{-11}M$), and a relatively low-affinity receptor, p75 ($K_D = 10^{-9}M$) (Fig. 19.4). Many of the biological activities of NGF have been attributed to the ligand-induced transduction of trkA. Receptor-bound NGF is internalized by axon terminals within membrane-bound vesicles and is transported retrogradely to the neuronal cell body, where it is eventually degraded.

Summary

The modern study of neuronal cell death began with investigations of how synaptic targets of sensory and motor neurons regulate their development. Viktor Hamburger and Rita Levi-Montalcini, beginning in the 1930s, ultimately showed that targets promote the survival and maintenance of innervating neurons. This notion, in turn, provided a conceptual framework for the discovery of the first target-derived neurotrophic agent, nerve growth factor. From these beginnings, the neurotrophic hypothesis was formulated: neurons compete for limiting amounts of target-derived survival promoting (trophic) agents during development. NGF was established as the prototypical target-derived neurotrophic factor.

THE NEUROTROPHIN FAMILY

Only a few subpopulations of peripheral neurons, including sympathetic and some sensory neurons, are

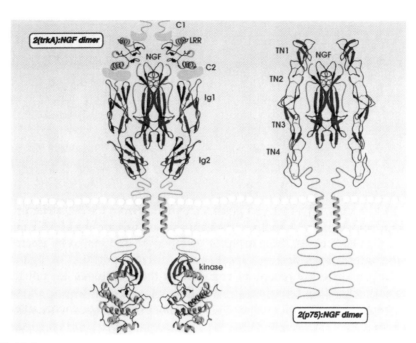

FIGURE 19.4 Models of the catalytic (full-length) trkA receptor for NGF and p75LNTR. Note the absence of a cytosolic kinase domain in p75 and the ability of one ligand (NGF) to bring together two receptor molecules to initiate signaling. From McDonald and Rust (1995).

exclusively dependent on NGF for survival during development. While some neurons in the basal forebrain are NGF responsive, the survival of CNS neurons is largely unchanged following the null mutation of NGF. Therefore, other survival factors are likely to also regulate neuron survival elsewhere in the nervous system. Extracts made from a number of tissues, as well as media containing proteins secreted by a variety of cultured neuronal and nonneuronal cells, all have been shown to support the survival of many different classes of neurons that are not NGF dependent and do not express the NGF receptor trkA. The existence of these non-NGF neurotrophic activities led to efforts to identify and purify other survival factors during the 1960s, 1970s, and 1980s. Because neurotrophic factors are made in extremely low quantities, the biochemical isolation of NGF-related molecules using conventional protein purification methods proved to be difficult.

A significant breakthrough occurred with the purification of a second NGF-related neurotrophic factor by Yves Barde and colleagues. Unlike NGF, which was purified several hundredfold from an extraordinarily rich biological source unrelated to the nervous system (see Box 19.1), endogenous brain-derived neurotrophic factor (BDNF) was purified several millionfold from adult pig brains. Each kilogram of starting material yielded only a microgram of factor which over time was eventually sequenced and cloned to produce recombinant factor. The molecular cloning

and expression of BDNF opened the door for an accelerated period of research on NGF-related factors. When the protein structure of BDNF was compared with NGF, they were both found to encode homodimers of small, very basic secreted peptide ligands with an amino acid homology of approximately 50%. Using polymerase chain reaction primers prepared from homologous domains to search for other related proteins, investigators rapidly identified additional neurotrophin family members in multiple species (Lewin and Barde, 1996). Described as neurotrophins or nerve feeding factors (i.e., NT-3 and NT-4/5, NT-6), these additional proteins were cloned and sequenced without the requirement of exhaustive protein purification.

Each neurotrophin family member is synthesized as an approximately 250 amino acid precursor that is processed into a roughly 120 amino acid protomer. Homologous regions of the several different family members are concentrated in six hydrophobic domains containing cysteine residues. The linkage formed by each homodimer ligand utilizes these regions to form a "cysteine knot" that ties the twin protomers together. The secreted dimer appears as a symmetrical twin with variable regions containing basic amino acid residues exposed on the surface (Figs. 19.4 and 19.5) (McDonald and Rust, 1995). Because all family members share this core structure, they are remarkably similar, with three-dimensional symmetry around two axes. The symmetry of this twin structure

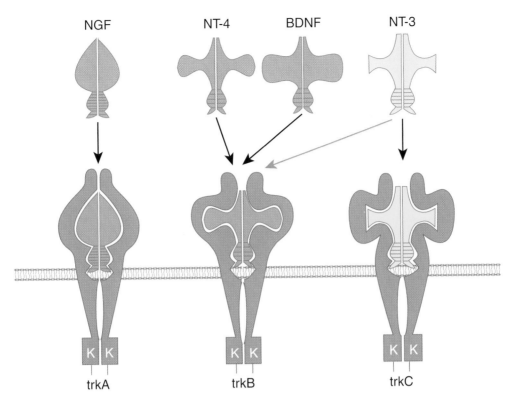

FIGURE 19.5 Ligand binding preferences of neurotrophins for each member of the trk receptor family. Not shown are the truncated (kinase deleted) isoforms of trkB and trkC. Other isoforms containing inserts and deletions also exist, providing a wide variety of receptors (see Table 19.1).

allows the neurotrophin ligand to activate receptors by binding separate receptor molecules together in the membrane for the initiation of receptor transduction (Figs. 19.5 and 19.6). The exposed outer regions that vary between neurotrophin family members are responsible for receptor-binding specificity.

Summary

The purification, molecular cloning, and expression of BDNF opened a floodgate of research on an NGF-related family of neurotrophic factors called neurotrophins or nerve feeding factors. Each neurotrophin family member is released as a homodimer with a conserved region containing a cysteine knot in the core of the molecule. The secreted factor is a symmetrical twin with duplicate sites used for bivalent receptor binding.

NEUROTROPHIN RECEPTORS

NGF binds to a relatively small number of very high-affinity-binding sites and a second set of about 10-fold more abundant, but lower affinity, binding

sites at higher concentrations (Chao, 1995). The 75-kDa protein (p75) was purified and cloned first. It is a transmembrane glycoprotein with extracellular cysteine repeat motifs that share structural homology with the tumor necrosis factor receptor family. The cytoplasmic domain of p75 lacks the kinase domain present in most growth factor receptors for intracellular signal transduction, but it can signal through ceramide pathways (Fig. 19.5). When expressed in fibroblasts, this receptor has low-affinity NGF-binding properties (ligand binding is rapidly on and off) and therefore has also been called the low-affinity NGF receptor (LNGFR). This name has proven to be a misnomer, as other neurotrophin family members also bind p75 with a similar affinity. It is therefore perhaps more appropriately named the low-affinity neurotrophin receptor (p75LNTR).

A major breakthrough in the characterization of the NGF receptors came with the fortuitous discovery and cloning of an oncogene identified in a human colon cancer. The sequence of this 140-kDa transmembrane protein contained a cytoplasmic kinase common to many growth factor receptors. Because it did not have a known ligand, it was an "orphan" receptor. The

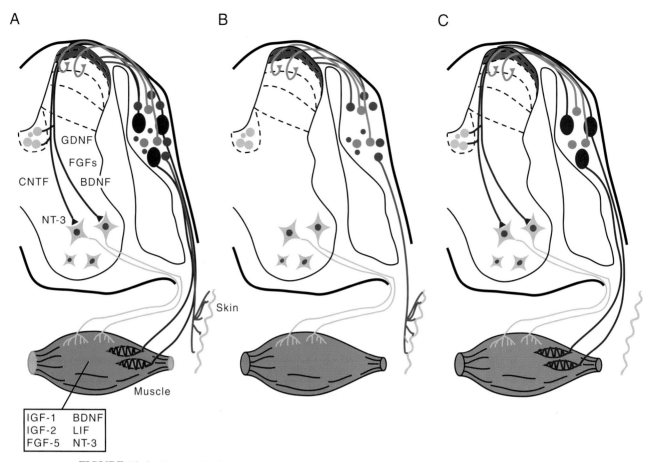

A B C

IGF-1 BDNF
IGF-2 LIF
FGF-5 NT-3

FIGURE 19.6 Phenotypic alterations in sensory motor pathways caused by null mutations in NGF/trkA and NT-3/trkC. In the DRGs of normal mice, small-diameter (red), medium-diameter (green), and large-diameter (blue) neurons are present. Many of the small-diameter neurons innervate skin, respond to temperature and pain, and have terminations in the dorsal-most laminae of the spinal cord. These neurons are lost when NGF or trkA is absent (compare A and C). Large-diameter neurons innervate muscle spindles and other proprioceptive end organs and have axon terminations in the lowest laminae of the dorsal horn and in the ventral horn. These neurons are lost when NT-3 or trkC is absent (compare A and B).

corresponding protooncogene was named trk (pronounced "track"—for tropomyosin-related kinase). It was rapidly appreciated as a member of the tyrosine kinase-containing receptor superfamily (Huang and Reichardt, 2001). Surprisingly, this trk mRNA expression was localized to neurons, in particular to NGF responsive neurons. Low-stringency screening of cDNA libraries with the original trk protooncogene probes led to the discovery of other related neurotrophin receptors. The NGF binding receptor was called trkA, whereas two additional 145-kDa members of a related protein family were named trkB and trkC (Fig. 19.5). Expression of trkA in a mouse fibroblast cell line or in frog oocytes conferred specific high-affinity NGF binding and NGF-induced receptor phosphorylation. NGF-signaling properties have been examined most extensively in the NGF responsive pheochromocytoma (PC12) cell line, derived from

adrenal medullary cells. Mutant PC12 cell lines that have lost their capacity to respond to NGF contain many p75LNTR receptors but lack trkA. Transfection of these mutant cells with trkA restores their biological responses to NGF treatment. Combined with the localization of trkA on NGF responsive neurons, these studies indicated that trkA alone is sufficient to bind NGF and mediate many of its biological activities in neurons. The most convincing evidence for the necessity of trkA comes from the analysis of transgenic mice lacking functional trk receptors (Huang and Reichardt, 2001). As expected, these mice have a phenotype that is almost identical to that of transgenic animals that have a null mutation for NGF.

The trkB receptor is specifically activated by low concentrations of BDNF or NT-4/5 and, to a lesser extent, by higher concentrations of NT-3. NT-3 activates the trkC receptor most effectively. All trk receptors contain three leucine-rich motifs, two cysteine clusters, and two immunoglobulin-like motifs in the extracellular region, a transmembrane domain and a tyrosine kinase domain in the cytosolic region (Fig. 19.5). The unusual combination of extracellular motifs makes up the ligand-binding region and places this family in a novel class of tyrosine kinase receptors. The region of highest sequence homology among family members and other growth factor receptors is in the kinase domain.

Receptor isoforms resulting from splice variants of trk mRNA transcripts exist for each family member (Table 19.2). Some isoforms contain peptide inserts in the extracellular or cytoplasmic domain that alter receptor function. Other trk isoforms contain specific deletions that truncate the receptor, including several receptors in which the entire kinase domain is deleted (trkB$_{TK-}$ and trkC$_{TK-}$). A variety of both full-length and kinase-deleted or truncated receptors are widely expressed on neurons throughout the nervous system. Truncated receptors, which are also expressed on glial cells, can bind and internalize their cognate ligand, but they cannot initiate the phosphorylation events required for receptor signal transduction (Fig. 19.6). As a result, the distribution and membrane concentration of truncated receptors could potentially modulate neurotrophin activity by restricting the availability of factors to full-length receptors.

Although trk receptors account for most of the biological responses of neurons to neurotrophins, p75LNTR can facilitate trk ligand binding and neurotrophin responses and can initiate other pathways for intracellular signaling independent of trk receptors (Chao, 1995; Huang and Reichardt, 2001). Sensory neurons from transgenic mice that lack p75LNTR require higher NGF concentrations for survival than

TABLE 19.2 The Neurotrophin Family and Its Receptors

	Receptor		
Factor	Full-length kinase-containing isoforms[a]	Nonkinase forms[b]	Example of responsive neurons[c]
NGF	trkA (trkA$_{E1}$)	p75[d]	Cholinergic forebrain neurons Sympathetic ganglia DRG nociceptive
BDNF	trkB	p75^{LNTR} trkB$_{T1}$ trkB$_{T2}$	Many CNS populations Vestibular ganglia Nodose ganglia DRG mechanoreceptors
NT-3	trkC (trkC$_{TK+14}$) (trkC$_{TK+25}$ TrkC$_{TK+39}$) trkB and trkA nonpreferred	p75^{LNTR} trkC$_{TK-158}$ trkC$_{TK-143}$ trkC$_{TK-113}$ trkC$_{TK-106}$	Many CNS populations Cochlear ganglia DRG proprioceptive
NT-4[e]	trkB	p75 trkB$_{T1}$ trkB$_{T2}$	Many CNS populations Nodose ganglia Petrosal ganglia
NT-6[f]	trkA	p75	

[a] trkA$_{E1}$ (extracellular 6 amino acid insert) is expressed primarily in neurons, whereas trkA without the insert is expressed primarily on nonneuronal cells. Avian trkB receptors include five catalytic isoforms and four catalytic receptors with inserts or deletions. trkC$_{TK+}$ represents isoforms with kinase inserts of amino acid length indicated.

[b] Mammalian trkB noncatalytic receptors include two kinase-deleted isoforms (T1 is expressed at equivalent levels as catalytic trkB without tyrosine kinase but with 23 cytoplasmic amino acids, whereas T2 has only 21 cytoplasmic amino acids). Avian trkB isoforms include five kinase-deleted isoforms. trk$_{CTK-}$ represents isoforms with kinase deletions of amino acid length indicated.

[c] Only a few examples from a long list of responsive neurons. trkB and trkC (along with BDNF and NT-3) are more widespread than trkA or NGF in CNS.

[d] p75^{LNTR} may associate with trkA to yield high-affinity binding. It can cause sphingomyelin hydrolysis and affect internalization and retrograde transport of BDNF and NT-4.

[e] NT-4 is also called NT-4/5: cloned from frog and named NT-4 and cloned from mammals and named NT-5. The most variable neurotrophin family member.

[f] NT-6 found only in teleost fish. Receptor and biological properties are not fully characterized.

sensory neurons from normal animals. Antibodies that block NGF binding to p75LTNR but not trkA reduce high-affinity NGF-binding sites, and p75LNTR has been demonstrated to enhance trkA receptor phosphorylation. Several mechanisms have been proposed to account for an accessory role of p75. The fast on and fast off kinetics of p75LNTR could maintain and increase the local concentration of neurotrophins in the neighborhood of the membrane surface and thereby increase the access of trk receptors to ligand. Alternatively, the lower affinity p75LNTR could form a transient heterodimer with trk receptors and thereby "hand off" the factor for trk binding. In addition to enhancing NGF binding to and activation of trkA, p75LNTR initiates NGF responses in cells that lack trkA. NGF binding to p75LNTR increases sphingomyelinase activity, producing the lipid second messenger molecule ceramide, and causes activation and translocation of the transcription factor nuclear factor κb (NFκb) that promotes cell survival. However, p75LNTR is structurally related to members of the tumor necrosis factor receptor (TNFR) family, many of which regulate the onset of cell death programs in the immune system and, for that reason, are termed death receptors. The cytoplasmic domain of p75LNTR contains a "death domain" sequence similar to active sequences found in the TNFR family, and the p75LNTR mechanisms of inducing PCD appear to be shared with other death receptors. Frade and colleagues have shown that under certain conditions, p75LNTR seems to mimic the death receptor function of the TNFR in the immune system. In some neuronal cells that express p75LNTR but not trkA, NGF apparently induces cell death via p75LNTR binding (Huang and Reichardt, 2001). Once bound, p75LNTR may also activate a separate PCD signaling pathway, the Jun kinase cascade. Jun kinase activation results in the production of the Fas ligand, which appears to promote PCD in neurons by the autocrine stimulation of the Fas receptor. The Jun kinase cascade also activates the transcription factor p53 with gene targets that include the proapoptotic gene BAX (see later). Ceramide produced by activation of the p75LNTR death domain can contribute to PCD in some cells by inhibiting some of the trk signaling pathways (see later). It should be noted that NGF and other trophic factors can be utilized in different cells or in different epochs of time to induce many diverse biological activities. It is noteworthy that under these specific circumstances (the absence of trk activity), a factor originally identified for the capacity to prevent PCD appears instead to be utilized to execute programs promoting neuronal death.

Summary

Many neurons have both high- and low-affinity binding sites for neurotrophins. Many biological responses are associated with high-affinity binding and rapid phosphorylation signaling events. All neurotrophins bind p75LNTR or the low-affinity neurotrophin receptor. p75LNTR lacks a cytoplasmic kinase domain but can facilitate ligand binding to and enhance signaling through trkA and independently initiate signaling. There are three tyrosine receptor kinase or trk family members: trkA, trkB, and trkC. Each binds one or more members of the neurotrophin factor family. Splice variants of trks result in isoforms that include truncated receptors lacking signaling capabilities. These truncated receptors may modulate neurotrophin activity by limiting the access of full-length receptors to factors during development. p75LNTR is related to the TNFR family of death receptors and contains a cytosolic "death domain." Activation of p75LNTR under certain conditions may serve to kill neurons or other cell types through well-established signaling pathways used to promote PCD.

CYTOKINES AND GROWTH FACTORS IN THE NERVOUS SYSTEM

Cytokines Mediate Cell Interactions Both outside and within the Nervous System

Although some aspects of communication between neurons, including synaptic transmission and neurotrophin signaling, are highly specialized and largely restricted to the nervous system, others are not. All vertebrate organs and tissues regulate growth and maintenance through diffusible signaling molecules. In many tissues, the expression of these intercellular induction factors is important for governing the proliferation and differentiation of both embryonic and adult stem cells. In addition, these factors also play an important role in the response of tissues to trauma, inflammation, infection, or tumor growth. In 1974, Stanley Cohen proposed that both lymphocyte-derived and nonlymphocyte-derived chemotactic and migration inhibitory factors be grouped into families of cytokines ("cell movement factors"). More recently, this term has been adopted as a general umbrella for many families of secreted proteins that mediate diverse biological responses including changes in the immune system (interleukins), tumor cytotoxicity (tumor necrosis factors), and inhibition of viral replication or cell growth (interferons) (see Table 19.3).

TABLE 19.3 Cytokine and Growth Factor Families

Family	Representative members	Original biological activities
Neutrophins	NGF, BDNF, NT-3, NT-4/5, NT-6	Neuronal survival and differentiation
Neuropoietic cytokines	CNTF, LIF, CT-1, oncom	Survival of ciliary neurons, leukemia inhibitory activity, increased cholinergic properties
Tissue growth factors	GDNF, TGF-α, TGF-β, FGFs, IGF-1α, IGF-1β, IGF-2, EGF, PDGF	Cell proliferation and differentiation in diverse tissues and organs, dopaminergic cell differentiation
Interleukins	IL-1α, IL-1β, IL-2 through IL-15	Immunoregulation, diverse activities in the immune system
Tumour necrosis factors	TNF-α, TNF-β	Tumor cytotoxicity
Chemokines kines	MCAF, MGSA, RANTES, NAP-1, NAP-2, MIP-1	Leukocyte chemotaxis and cell activation
Colony-stimulating factors	G-CSF, M-CSF, GM-CSF	Hematopoietic cell proliferation and differentiation
Interferons	IFN-α, IFN-β, IFN-γ	Inhibition of viral replication, cell growth, or immunoregulation

Many cytokines were originally named according to the particular biological activity that was utilized for their isolation, only to be later rediscovered or renamed as important mediators of other physiological processes. For example, some factors were isolated on the basis of their ability to enhance the survival of specific populations of neurons isolated *in vitro*. These include ciliary neurotrophic factor (CNTF), glial-derived neurotrophic factor (GDNF), and neurturin. CNTF is a member of a broader family of neuropoietic cytokines, including leukemia inhibitory factor (LIF), oncostatin M, and cardiotrophin-1, that share a common three-dimensional structure and receptor subunits. CNTF was originally isolated and named because it supports the survival of neurons cultured from parasympathetic ciliary ganglion. Other proteins that were originally identified as mitogens or chemotactic factors in nonneuronal tissues have also been shown to affect either the survival or the differentiation of neurons, including the fibroblast growth factors, insulin-like growth factors, and hepatocyte growth factor (HGF). The first neuronal function identified for LIF was the induction of cholinergic properties in cultured sympathetic neurons, but it also supports the survival of several classes of neurons and induces neural precursors to become astrocytes. LIF, which has a number of actions in the immune system and other nonneuronal tissues, shares receptor subunits with CNTF (as described later) and therefore can mimic both the survival and the cholinergic differentiation activities of CNTF observed in culture. Many cytokines important for the development or maintenance of other organs and tissues are also widely expressed within the nervous system. Their roles in the nervous system, however, remain to be defined. Likewise, factors first recognized as neuronal survival factors have mitogenic properties for either nonneuronal cells or neuronal precursors. As a result, these pleiotropic factors are grouped into families based on their protein sequences and receptor usage rather than on their biological properties. Table 19.3 summarizes only a few of the known ligands, receptors, and biological functions for the CNTF-related family of neurokines, the GDNF/TGF-related superfamily, and FGFs.

Summary

CNTF and LIF belong to a neuropoietic cytokine family. The expression and biological properties of these cytokines distinguish them from neurotrophins. They possess widespread neurotrophic activity for many different neuronal and nonneuronal populations *in vitro* and facilitate the cholinergic differentiation of sympathetic and motor neurons. GDNF and neurturin are members of the TGF-B gene family and have effects on dopaminergic and motor neurons. FGFs may play important roles during development or after injury.

NEUROTROPHIC FACTORS HAVE MULTIPLE ACTIVITIES

Neurotrophic factors that prevent neuronal death during development appear to have many other important biological activities, including effects on cell proliferation, migration, differentiation, axonal growth and sprouting, alterations in dendritic arbors, and functional plasticity of the nervous system (see

Table 19.3). Frequently, different populations of neurons respond to the same factor in distinct ways, and the same neuron may respond differently to the same factor at different developmental stages. Variations in neuronal responses to the same factor appear to depend not only on modifications of trk or p75 receptors, but also on potential differences in the intracellular context of downstream signaling pathways. The distinctive activities of a neurotrophic factor on different cells or during different epochs of development

TABLE 19.4 Percentage of Neurons Lost In Neurotrophic Factor or Receptor Deficient Mice[a]

Neurotrophic factor/receptor null mutation	Viability	Neuronal losses in PNS ganglia					Neuronal losses in CNS nuclei			
		Sensory dorsal root ganglia	Sensory trigeminal ganglia	Sensory nodose petrosal ganglia	Sensory vestibular ganglia	Sensory cochlear ganglia	Sympathetic superior cervical ganglia	Spinal moto- neurons	Facial moto- neurons	Other CNS phenotypes
TrkA[b,c]	Poor	Up to 90%[b]	−70%[b]	?	N	N	−>95%	?	?	Forebrain[b]
NGF[b]	Poor	−70%[b]	−75%[b]	?	?	N	−>95%	?	?	
TrkB[d]	Very poor	−30%[d]	−60%	−90%	−60%	−15%	?	N	?	Forebrain hindbrain
BDNF[d-f]	Moderate	−35%[d,e]	−30%	−45%	−85%	−7%	?	N	N	
NT-4[g]	Good	N	N	−40%	N	?	N	?	?	
BDNF/NT-4	Good	N	−9%	−90%	−90%	?	N	N	N	
Trk C[d,h]	Moderate	−20%	−21%	−14%	−15%	−50%	N	?	?	
NT-3[b,d,g,h,j,i]	Very poor	−60%	−60%	−30%	−20%	−85%	−50%	?	?	
TrkB/TrkC	Very poor	−41%	?	?	−100%	−65%	?	?	?	Forebrain hindbrain[i]
BDNF/NT-3	Very poor	−83%	−74%	−62%	−100%	−100%	?	?	?	
BDNF/ NT-4/NT-3	Very poor	−92%	−88%	−96%	−100%	?	−47%	−20%	−22%	
c-ret[l,n]	Good	?	?	?	?	?	Yes[m]	?	?	
CNTFRα[k,m]	Very poor	N	N	?	?	?	N	?	−40%	
LIFR	Very poor	?	?	?	?	?	?	−40%	−35%	
GFRα1[k-m]	Very poor	N	N	−15%	N	N	N	?	N	
GFRα2[k]	Poor	N	N	N	N	N	N	−24%	?	
GFRα3[n]	Good	N	N	?	?	?	Yes[m]	?	?	
GDNF[k,m]	Very Poor	−23%	?	−40%	N	?	−35%	−22%	N	
Neurturin[k]	Good	yes[n]	yes[n]	N	?	?	N	N	?	

[a] For detailed reviews of null mutation experiments, see Huang and Reichardt, (2001).

[b] Small nociceptive and thermoceptive sensory neurons lost·

[c] Marked reductions in hippocampal innervation, despite apparent normal numbers of cholinergic basal forebrain neurons.

[d] 40–60% loss of trigeminal mesencephalic neurons.

[e] Loss of slow adapting sensory neurons.

[f] Complete loss of carotid body innervation; CNS deficits in neurons expressing NPY, calbindin, and parvalbumin; cerebellum foliation defects; loss of CNS myelinated axons.

[g] Loss of D hair afferents.

[h] Loss of proprioceptive sensory neurons.

[i] Loss of mechanoreceptor sensory neurons.

[j] Increased apoptosis observed in the developing hippocampus and cerebellum.

[k] Loss of parasympathetic neurons in the ciliary, submandibular, and/or otic ganglia.

[l] Loss of trigeminal motoneurons.

[m] Loss of most enteric neurons in the stomach and/or intestines.

[n] Most superior cervical ganglion neurons are lost.

[o] Specific loss of many GFRa2 positive neurons.

reflect the intrinsic properties of differentiating neurons or a dynamic change in a trophic response due to alterations in neural activity or other signaling events. In addition to target-derived sources of neurotrophins, factors can also be delivered for release at presynaptic terminals by anterograde axonal transport or instead released locally for autocrine or paracrine activity.

As described earlier, neurotrophins have been shown repeatedly to play fundamental roles in the regulation of many peripheral neuronal populations. Null mutations of neurotrophins or their cognate trk receptors manifest specific deficits in dependent populations (see Table 19.4 and Fig. 19.6) (Huang and

Reichardt, 2001). However, relatively few changes in the number of neurons have been observed in the CNS of the neurotrophin or trk receptor null mutant mice. This observation was surprising because significant cell death occurs in the central nervous system, and neurotrophic factors and their receptors are widely expressed in the central nervous system during this period. The complexity and number of synaptic relationships established by CNS compared to those established by PNS neurons may partially explain why CNS neurons are not as sensitive to the loss of a single neurotrophin or neurotrophin receptor (Fig. 19.7). The trophic support to CNS neurons is likely to arise from multiple families of neurotrophic

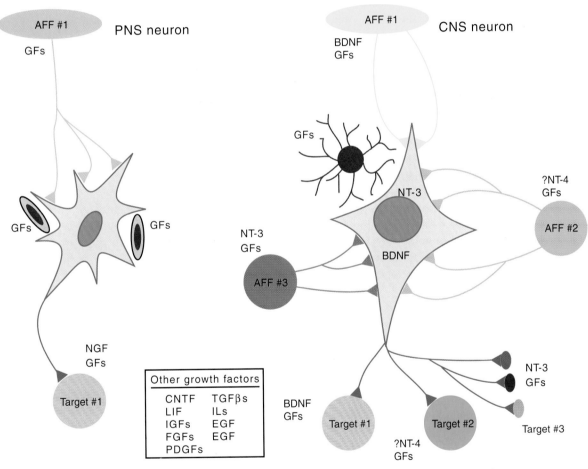

FIGURE 19.7 Possible sources of trophic support for peripheral (PNS) and central (CNS) neurons. Peripheral neurons like the sympathetic neuron in the diagram have only two sources of support: one in the periphery (target 1) and one in the ganglion (AFF 1). It is also possible that glial cells in the ganglion represented by ovoid cells adjacent to the sympathetic neuron could secrete a trophic factor(s). In contrast, central neurons like the one in the diagram receive synaptic input from many neurons (AFF 1 and 2), which could serve as a source of anterograde trophic support. The ability of neurons to synthesize and secrete neurotrophins is indicated by the presence of BDNF and NT-3 in the neuronal cell body. Central neurons may also project to several different targets (targets 1–3) which could each provide retrograde trophic support. Candidate trophic factors are indicated adjacent to these hypothetical targets. Like glial cells in the periphery, astrocytes may also produce growth factors.

factors with possible synergistic and/or compensatory effects.

The traditional view of the neurotrophic hypothesis has been that trophic support is derived from target tissues, but other sources of trophic support are now recognized. In many regions of the nervous system and during different stages of development, neurons may coexpress mRNAs encoding both the neurotrophic factor and its receptor. This coexpression is especially true for BDNF and NT-3. Interpretation of mRNA localization studies is complicated by the fact that neurotrophic factors may not simply be released locally in the region of the cell body, but may also or instead be delivered to distant regions of the nervous system by anterograde or retrograde axonal transport. Thus, although the original neurotrophic hypothesis that neurons depend on target-derived trophic factors still holds true for many neurons during critical periods of development (including sympathetic neuron dependence for target-derived NGF), other mechanisms of trophic support appear to play an important functional role in development. Some of these mechanisms are described in a later section.

Finally, although beyond the scope of the present chapter, neurotrophins and other neurotrophic factors and their receptors are also distributed throughout the mature brain, and neurotrophic factors can alter neural activity by rapid and long-term changes in synaptic transmission. Neurotrophins also play a role in modulating long-term changes in functional and anatomical plasticity in the developing and mature brain by altering long-term potentiation and synaptic connectivity.

Summary

NT-3 and BDNF are expressed in regions of neurogenesis and differentiation in both the CNS and the periphery. For example, early neuronal precursors respond by increasing cell proliferation, exiting mitosis, becoming restricted in a multipotential fate into a neuronal phenotype, and/or maintaining cells until targets are innervated. Experiments that block neurotrophic activity (by ligand- or receptor-specific antibody treatment or in transgenic mice with null mutations) demonstrate that both NT-3 and BDNF are required for the early development of neurons. Evidence for an essential role of individual factors or receptors is strongest in the peripheral nervous system, where cell numbers are reduced markedly. In the DRG, neurotrophin responsiveness can be correlated with somatosensory function. In general, small pain-sensitive neurons are dependent on NGF, some middle-size

mechanoreceptors for touch are lost in BDNF knockouts, and large proprioceptive neurons are NT-3 dependent. Sensory neurons differ in when they become neurotrophin dependent and whether they alter their neurotrophin requirements during development.

TRK RECEPTORS ARE SIMILAR TO OTHER GROWTH FACTOR RECEPTORS

Neurotrophin binding to trk receptors at the cell surface causes the formation of receptor dimers and coactivation of their tyrosine kinase activity. The homodimeric structure of the factors allows each bivalent ligand to bring two separate receptor molecules into close proximity. Aggregated receptors phosphorylate each other on specific tyrosine substrates within intracellular domains. The generation of phosphotyrosine residues in turn activates the receptor kinase and further catalyzes the formation of large signaling complexes through the recruitment of cytosolic and membrane-associated proteins (Fig. 19.8). Many of these cytosolic proteins are adaptor proteins that link the activated receptor kinase with intracellular signaling pathways shared by other receptor systems. Once activated, the receptor initiates intracellular signals both locally in the cytoplasm and by a series of enzymatic cascades that eventually produce changes in gene transcription within the nucleus (Segal and Greenberg, 1996). Receptor signal transduction involves multiple signaling pathways that can differ greatly between individual neurons or in the same neurons at different periods of time (depending on recent events). This means that the response of neurons to trophic factor stimuli is dependent on the intracellular status of the cell in a dynamic fashion. Some intracellular signaling pathways show very rapid and transient changes, whereas others produce slower and longer lasting cellular responses. The signaling machinery of the cytoplasmic catalytic domain of trk receptors is similar to that employed by many other growth factor receptors (Ip and Yancopoulos, 1996). The molecular components for these pathways are so well conserved that many of the signaling proteins are interchangeable among invertebrate and vertebrate species. Three of these pathways have been identified as the launching sites for trk signal transduction events that mediate survival as well as many other cellular responses to neurotrophins (Fig.19.8). All three pathways begin with adaptor proteins that contain a structural motif, the src homology domain 2 (SH2), which specifically recognizes the phosphotyrosine residue and flanking sequences. They are the (1) *Ras-MAP kinase activation pathway*, (2) *phospholipase C (PLC-γ) pathway*, and (3) *phosphatidylinositol-3*

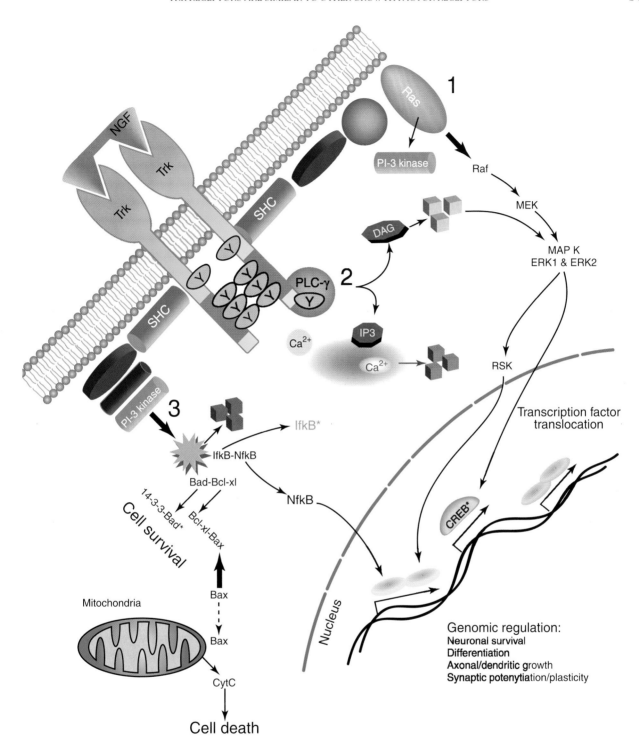

FIGURE 19.8 Trk signaling pathways. Neurotrophins (ie., NGF) are bivalent ligands binding to two trk receptor monomers. Ligand binding initiates trk receptor transduction by the phosphorylation of tyrosine residues (Y) in the cytoplasmic domains. Once activated, trk kinase further phosphorylates specific tyrosine residues forming docking sites for adaptor and linker proteins (blue figures), which in turn engage signaling cascades shared by other growth factor receptors. The three signaling pathways illustrated are the (1) Ras-MAP kinase pathway; (2) phospholipase C pathway, and (3) the PI-3 kinase pathway. See text for details.

kinase (PI-3K) pathway (Fig. 19.8). PLC-γ activity generates two distinct second messenger signals: inositol trisphosphate (IP$_3$) and diacylgycerol (DAG). IP$_3$ rapidly releases intracellular Ca^{2+} sequestered in local membrane compartments. This signal initiates the activity of local Ca^{2+} dependent enzymes (protein kinases and phosphatases). Similarly, DAG regulates the activity of DAG-dependent enzymes. Both Ras and PI-3 kinase pathways are engaged via the adapter protein Shc (SH-2 containing) and associated linker or extender proteins. One of the best known Ras-dependent signaling pathway is activation of the ERK family of MAP kinases. This cascade is composed of serine/ threonine kinases that are serially phosphorylated and activated. The initial member of this cascade is Raf, which binds directly to the active form of p21Ras and in turn becomes activated enzymatically. Raf phosphorylates and activates MEK, which in turn phosphorylates the MAP kinases (ERK1 and ERK2). Interestingly, MAP kinases can also be activated independently from Ras by DAG-dependent protein kinases via the PLC-γ pathway. Once activated, these MAP kinases in turn phosphorylate a number of cytoplasmic and nuclear effectors. Importantly, activation of MAP kinases and their substrate, the protein kinase p90Rsk, results in the translocation of these enzymes into the nucleus. In the nucleus, they phosphorylate a number of transcription factors, including several well-known immediate-early genes (i.e., c-*fos* and c-*jun*), as well as delayed response genes activated by CREB (cAMP response element-binding protein). Once activated, transcription factors cause rapid and long-lasting changes in gene expression regulating cell survival, axonal and dendritic growth, neuronal differentiation, synaptic potentiation, and plasticity.

In many different cases, this Ras-dependent pathway plays a critical role in neuronal differentiation. This includes the production of enzymes that regulate the synthesis of neurotransmitters. One paradox in understanding neurotrophin and growth factor signaling is that although many growth factor receptors also employ the Ras MAP kinase pathway, the ultimate downstream effects of growth factor receptor activation can be very different. For instance, the NGF-mediated trkA activation of Ras in PC12 cells stops cell division and induces neuronal differentiation and neurite outgrowth. Treatment of the same cells with epidermal growth factor (EGF) activates the same Ras pathway through the EGF receptor but instead results in a dramatic increase in cell proliferation. The ultimate biological response appears to be distinguished by the duration of Ras activity in response to either NGF or EGF receptor transduction. TrkA activation of Ras persists much longer compared to only a rapid and

transient Ras activation following EGF receptor transduction. These results suggest that the duration of Ras activation is a critical determinant of transcriptional activity and biological responses (Huang and Reichardt, 2001). In addition, the requirement on Ras-dependent pathways for biological responses varies among neuron types. DRG sensory neurons require Ras activation for some neurotrophin responses, whereas sympathetic neurons do not. Trk signaling pathways also employ intracellular messengers that are apparently expressed only in certain cell phenotypes. SNT (suc-associated neurotrophic factor-induced tyrosine-phosphorylated target) is phosphorylated and activated by a Ras-independent pathway only in PC12 cells and some neurons.

Neurotrophic factor receptor activation of the PI-3 kinase pathway is essential for the normal survival of many neurons. The phosphatidyl inositides made by PI-3 kinase regulate in part the activity of Akt/protein kinase B. This important protein kinase plays a critical role in controlling the biological activity of several regulatory proteins that govern normal programmed cell death (see Fig. 19.8 and sections that follow). BAD and IFκB are two of the many substrates phosphorylated by Akt. Cell death is normally promoted by the binding of BAD to a cell death inhibitor, Bcl-xl, and this default binding is inhibited by the Akt phosporylation of BAD. BAD can also be phosphorylated by MAP kinases through Ras activation. Bcl-xl blocks normal cell death by binding and inhibiting Bax, a member of the BCL-2 family that promotes the mitochondrial release of cytochrome C and PCD (see sections that follow). Once BAD is phosphorylated, it is trapped by binding proteins (14-3-3 proteins), thereby allowing free BCL-xl to dimerize and block the proapoptotic activity of Bax. Another Akt substrate, IFκB, binds the transcription factor NFκB within the cytosol. Akt phosphorylation of IFκB results in its degradation. Once released from cytosolic sequestration, NFκB is translocated to the nucleus where it enhances the transcription of genes that promote cell survival. A number of cytokine receptors and p75 appear to promote cell survival by NFκB activation. Many of the other known regulators of cell death (caspases, caspase inhibitors, BCL-2, and Apaf-1) all share the consensus site required by substrates for Akt activation. PI-3 kinase can be activated directly by ligand-bound trk receptors via the Shc adaptor protein or indirectly through Ras activation. Trk receptor activation of both the PI-3 kinase and the Ras-ERK pathways suppresses the capacity of activated p75LNTR to induce cell death programs via Jun kinase and ceramide production. In some cases, p75LNTR may therefore induce neuronal death where appropriate neurotrophin binding to trk receptors is absent. Interactions between the multiple trk receptor signaling pathways in different cell phenotypes and under a variety of dynamic receptor signaling conditions provide a rich assortment of interrelated mechanisms to govern PCD machinery.

Summary

There are three tyrosine receptor kinase or trk family members; trkA, trkB, and trkC. Signaling pathways used by the trk family members are shared with those activated by many growth factor receptors also using tyrosine kinase for receptor transduction. Neurotrophin binding to trk causes receptor dimerization and phosphorylation of cytoplasmic tyrosine residues. Phosphotyrosines recruit cytosolic adaptor proteins that couple the activated receptor with intracellular signaling pathways. The biological response of the cell to a neurotrophic factor is dependent on the intrinsic intracellular substrate environment of the specific cell phenotype and the dynamic status of the pathway that varies with recent cell history. Three of the best investigated signaling pathways are PLC-γ, Ras-ERK kinase, and PI-3K. Normal programmed cell death is governed in many neurons by PI-3 kinase activation of the protein kinase Akt. Trophic factor deprivation can lead to the release of proapoptotic mechanisms that promote cell death.

PROGRAMMED CELL DEATH OF NEURONS IS WIDESPREAD IN INVERTEBRATE AND VERTEBRATE SPECIES

Although the loss of developing cells has been reported in many vertebrate and invertebrate species, one cannot be certain that PCD is a universally conserved feature of all living animals. It appears likely that one of the driving forces in the evolution of programmed cell death was the necessity to selectively eliminate cells invaded by viruses or other pathogens. Because pathogen-driven PCD occurs in plants, prokaryotes, and eukaryotes, it seems reasonable to infer that PCD occurs in virtually all taxonomic groups (Ameisen, 1996). In contrast, the programmed death of developing cells in the nervous system could only occur once nervous systems evolved in multicellular organisms. Because a systematic taxonomic study of the evolution of cell death in the nervous system of multicellular organisms has not been undertaken, we do not know whether it occurs in coelenterates (e.g., hydra) in which the first primitive nervous systems have been identified. Nonetheless, the appearance of cell death in unicellular organisms, and of neuronal cell death in many invertebrate species, including worms, flies, and grasshoppers (Ellis et al., 1991), is consistent with the idea that some developing neurons die in virtually all organisms with a distinct nervous system.

Available evidence suggests that neuronal death involves virtually all regions and cell types in the nervous system. In fact, cell death in the nervous system has been found to occur almost everywhere that it has been looked for. Motoneurons, sensory neurons (and their peripheral receptors), autonomic neurons, and both long projection neurons and local circuit neurons in the brain and spinal cord all undergo restricted periods of PCD (Burek and Oppenheim, 1999). Although the magnitude of neuronal cell death varies from population to population, as many as one-half or more of all cells in a population will die during development (Fig. 19.1). In some special cases, such as the loss of transient neuronal structures during insect and amphibian metamorphosis (e.g., the Rohon-Beard sensory neurons in fish and frogs), most or all cells die. Cell death in the nervous system thus clearly occurs on a very large scale, indicating that it plays a fundamental and essential role in normal development.

Studies of cell death in the nervous system have focused on the loss of developing postmitotic neurons as they form synaptic connections with targets and afferents (discussed later). However, extensive PCD also occurs during neurulation and in mitotically active cells, as well as in postmitotic but undifferentiated neurons in the early neural tube (Fig. 19.2). Accordingly, PCD in the nervous system is not limited to any particular stage of development. The loss of cells at different developmental stages probably serves distinct functions and may be mediated by different mechanisms (Oppenheim et al., 2001). PCD also occurs in central and peripheral glial cells. For example, myelin-forming oligodendrocytes in the optic nerve and Schwann cells in peripheral nerves die by PCD. Their loss is thought to reflect a competition for axon-derived trophic signals, the end result of which is the survival of an appropriate number of glial cells for optimum myelination of the available axons (Fig. 19.9). Because glia have been studied much less extensively, it is not known whether the death of nonneuronal cells throughout the nervous system is as common as the death of neurons nor are the mechanisms that regulate the death and survival of glial cells as clearly known as for neurons.

Because PCD is the normal differentiated or terminal fate of many developing cells, commitment to this fate occurs in much the same way as the phenotypic fate of cells destined to survive in the embryo. Developmental biologists have identified two major

A

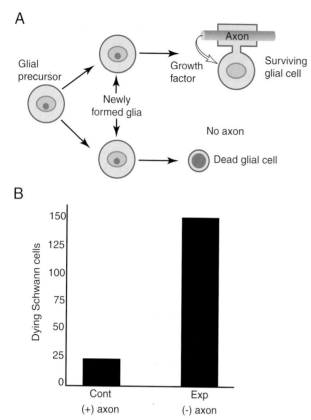

B

FIGURE 19.9   The PCD of glial cells is regulated by axonally derived signals. (A) Glial cells that fail to compete successfully for these signals undergo PCD. (B) The number of dying Schwann cells in the ventral root of the chick embryo is increased following the induced death of motor neuron axons. Control (Cont) indicates the normal ventral root and experimental (Exp) indicates ventral roots with greatly reduced motor axons. From Burek and Oppenheim (1999).

whereas most PCD in vertebrates is conditional and regulated by cell–cell interactions (Ellis *et al.*, 1991; Burek and Oppenheim, 1999). Despite this distinction, as described later, many of the genetic and molecular pathways for PCD are remarkably similar in invertebrates and vertebrates.

Summary

The programmed cell death of developing neurons appears to occur in virtually all vertebrate and invertebrate species. More generally, PCD also occurs in many different cells and tissues of plants, unicellular, and multicellular organisms and thus may have arisen early during evolution as a defense against viral infections. With few exceptions, cell death occurs in virtually all types of developing vertebrate and invertebrate neurons and can take place at stages of development from the time of proliferation until the establishment of synaptic connections. Developing glial cells also exhibit PCD. Cell death is the terminal phenotypic fate of subpopulations of developing neuronal and glial cells and, like other cell fate decisions, is controlled by epigenetic signals.

MODES OF CELL DEATH IN DEVELOPING NEURONS

The specific morphological appearance exhibited by degenerating neurons can provide insight into the cellular and molecular mechanisms by which the cells are destroyed. Historically, pathologists were the first to be interested in this issue, and they focused on distinguishing different kinds of cell and tissue degeneration following disease, injury, and trauma (Clarke and Clarke, 1996). Over 125 years ago, the term necrosis was coined to describe what today comprises the major form of accidental or pathological degeneration. For example, the pathological necrotic death of neurons following injury usually involves the degeneration of groups of contiguous cells in a region that initiates an inflammatory response that can be discerned easily in tissue sections. At about the same time that necrosis was described, however, another form of cell degeneration, spontaneous cell death, was observed in regressing ovarian follicles and mammary glands of normal adult mammals. Spontaneous cell death was thought to provide a means for counterbalancing mitosis in adult tissues in which the turnover of cells normally occurs. PCD typically involves the sporadic loss of individual cells in a population that often degenerate by a different mode from necrosis, one that does not involve inflamma-

ways in which the commitment of a cell to a particular differentiated phenotype occurs (Gilbert, 2000). The first mechanism, intrinsic or *autonomous specification*, involves the segregation of critical cytoplasmic molecules during embryonic cleavage. In this way each cell obtains a distinct set ("mosaic") of cytoplasmic determinative molecules that can act to influence cell fate without reference to signals from neighboring cells. The second mechanism of commitment involves extrinsic signals from other cells and is called *conditional specification*. Initially, the cells have the potential to follow more than one path of differentiation. As development proceeds, however, signals from other cells act to gradually limit and specify cell fate. Although all organisms use a combination of autonomous and conditional developmental strategies, as a general rule most invertebrates predominately exhibit mosaic development, whereas most vertebrates exhibit conditional development. For example, much of the PCD in invertebrates is autonomous,

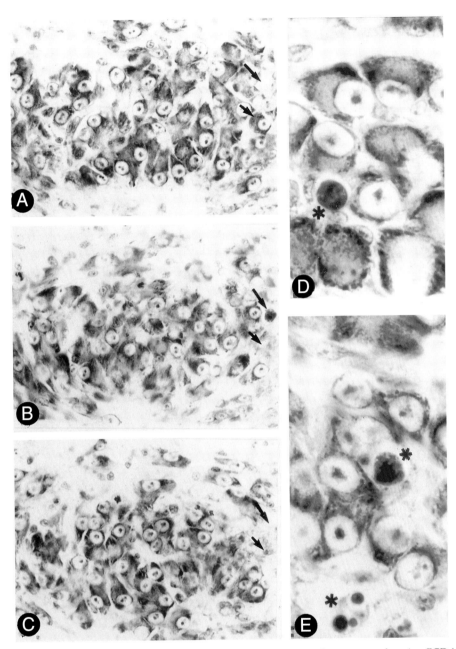

FIGURE 19.10 Examples of healthy sensory and motor neurons and neurons undergoing PCD in the spinal cord of the chick embryo. (A–C) Three adjacent 10-μm-thick serial sections of the ventral horn. Note that both healthy (short arrows) and dying (long arrows) motor neurons appear in only one of the serial sections and therefore would not erroneously be counted twice in adjacent sections. Typical sensory (D) and motor (E) neurons (asterisks) undergoing PCD can be distinguished easily from healthy surviving neurons and glia (for a detailed discussion of cell counting methods, see Clarke and Oppenheim, 1995).

tion. Early steps in the spontaneous cell death cascade leading up to when histological signs of frank degeneration first occur may take many hours or days. Once that point is reached, however, the degenerative process is rapid, with individual cells dying and being removed in minutes or a few hours. The loss of thousands of neurons over several days is the consequence of many rapid individual cell deaths that at any moment in time represent only a small minority (~1%) of all the cells in the population. Therefore, the occurrence and magnitude of even massive spontaneous cell death can (and often did) go unnoticed. To date, the most direct and commonly used method for estimating the number and timing of neurons that die *in vivo* is by counting healthy and dying neurons in serial histological sections through the entire neuronal population being studied at different stages of development (Figs. 19.1 and 19.10).

Until quite recently, the pathways of spontaneous cell degeneration in adult and developing tissues have been generally dichotomized into death by either apoptosis or necrosis, a distinction based initially on morphological differences and later on other apparent differences between the two (Fig. 19.11). Apoptosis is a Greek word indicating the seasonal piecemeal dropping of leaves from a tree and was originally coined to describe all forms of spontaneous cell death that share certain morphological characteristics. Cells dying by apoptosis shrink in size and the nuclear chromatin condenses and becomes pyknotic, whereas the cell membrane and cytoplasmic organelles tend to remain relatively intact. Eventually the cytoplasm and nucleus break up into membrane-bound apoptotic bodies that are phagocytized either by macrophages or by healthy adjacent cells. In contrast, necrosis involves an initial swelling of the cell, only modest condensation of chromatin, cytoplasmic vacuolization, breakdown of organelles, and rupture of the cell membrane allowing the release of cellular contents (causing inflammation), followed by shrinkage and loss of nuclear chromatin. Because necrotic cell death elicits an inflammatory response, macrophages derived from the immune system attack and phagocytize cellular debris. In contrast, cell death by apoptosis usually involves individual cells that are engulfed or phagocytized before they can release their cellular contents and induce an inflammatory response in adjacent tissue. Phagocytosis of apoptotic cells can involve either typical macrophages or, more often, engulfment by adjacent cells that act transiently as nonprofessional macrophages (e.g., in the nervous system, these include radial glia cells, Schwann cells, and other neurons). Phagocytes recognize dying cells by their expression of death-related cell surface signals.

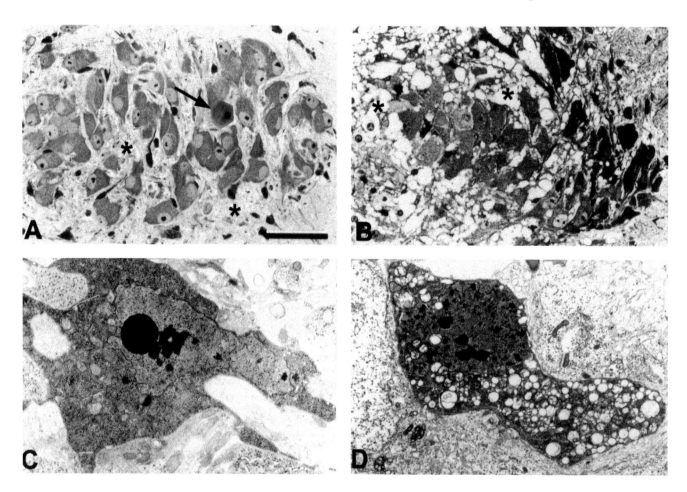

FIGURE 19.11   Spinal motoneuron in the chick embryo. (A) Ventral horn from a control embryo. Note that only one cell (arrow) is undergoing apoptotic PCD and the neuropil (*) is intact. (B) Ventral horn from an embryo following an excitotoxic (glutamate) lesion. Most neurons are undergoing a necrotic cell death (dark cells) and the neuropil is disintegrating (*). Apoptotic (C) and necrotic motoneurons (D) in the chick embryo spinal cord as seen with an electron microscope.

Another feature that has been used to distinguish between apoptotic and necrotic cell death is the occurrence of a specific form of chromosomal DNA fragmentation and degradation during early stages of apoptosis that is mediated by specific proteases. DNA digestion occurs at internucleosomal sites, producing small, double-stranded fragments of DNA that migrate in a ladder pattern in multiples of 180–200 bp after electrophoresis in agarose gels. This form of DNA fragmentation can also be visualized in tissue sections by a technique that labels the double-stranded DNA breaks associated with apoptosis.

It is widely believed that apoptosis and necrosis reflect mechanistically distinct cell death pathways that are triggered by different stimuli. However, our basic understanding of these pathways is still limited, and caution should be exercised in drawing too fine of a distinction between them. For example, a variety of toxic and traumatic stimuli, such as CNS ischemia, previously thought to only involve necrotic cell death, can also induce morphological signs of apoptosis and may be associated with changes in PCD- or apoptosis-associated genes. The PCD of developing vertebrate neurons provides a striking example of the problems encountered in attempting to rigidly classify the pathway of degeneration as being either necrotic or apoptotic (Koliatsos and Ratan, 1999; Leist and Jaatek, 2001). Developing neurons may adopt one of at least three different morphological modes during PCD: (1) apoptotic, (2) autophagic, and (3) cytoplasmic

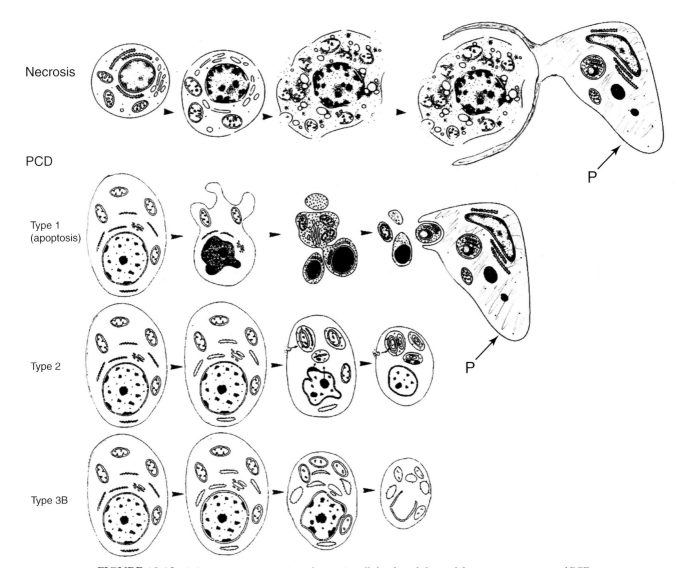

FIGURE 19.12 Schematic representation of necrotic cell death and three of the commonest types of PCD observed at the ultrastructural level (see Koliatsos and Ratan, 1999). Only type 1 PCD meets most of the criteria for defining apoptosis. The cells on the right marked P represent phagocytic cells engulfing necrotic cell corpses and apoptotic bodies. Phagocytosis also occurs in the other types of PCD but is not shown.

(Fig. 19.12). Only the first fits the classic morphological definition of apoptosis. Inhibition of the apoptotic mode of PCD often results in death of cells by alternative pathways (e.g., autophagic). The cytoplasmic type of PCD also shares several features with necrotic cell death, including an early breakdown of organelles and late lysis of the nucleus. Despite the occurrence of these different morphological types of death, it is clear that they reflect PCD, as they involve the stereotypic loss of individual cells at specific times during development without triggering an inflammatory response. Within the context of the developing nervous system, the dichotomy of apoptosis vs necrosis is an oversimplification that should be abandoned. Instead, both developing cells undergoing normal PCD and neurons dying following injury should be categorized by operational definitions that use morphological, genetic, and biochemical criteria for describing their many distinct modes of degeneration. As described in the following section, one of the major success stories since the early 1990s has been the remarkable progress made in understanding the biochemical pathways of PCD and identifying the specific genes involved (Hengartner, 2000).

Summary

Historically, degenerating cells have been categorized into two classes: death by apoptosis or death by necrosis. Although the situation is more complex than is reflected in this simple dichotomy, apoptosis in general is more characteristic of PCD, whereas necrosis is more characteristic of cells that die following injury or trauma. A variety of morphological features have been used to distinguish between these two types of cell death, and the occurrence of a specific kind of DNA fragmentation in cells characterizing apoptosis has become a major criterion for categorization. However, the occurrence of certain features of apoptosis in neurons following injury indicates that a more accurate means of identifying and defining distinct forms of PCD is needed.

THE MODE OF NEURONAL CELL DEATH REFLECTS THE ACTIVATION OF DISTINCT BIOCHEMICAL AND MOLECULAR MECHANISMS

As described previously, the normal death of cells in the developing nervous system has long been thought to be regulated by competition for neurotrophic molecules. Until quite recently, investigators

agreed that the doomed neurons, lacking a sufficient trophic factor to sustain normal metabolic events, passively degenerated by a process analogous to starvation. However, PCD of some nonneuronal cells was known previously to be an active, ATP-dependent process. For example, it has long been known that RNA or protein synthesis inhibitors prevent the programmed death of muscle cells in metamorphic insects and amphibians and also block the hormone-induced death of thymocytes in the mammalian immune system (Ellis et al., 1991). Additionally, genetic mutations in the nematode worm Caenorhabditis elegans that prevent PCD had also been described previously, thereby providing further evidence suggesting that neuronal death is a genetically regulated process in which cells may participate actively in their own demise. Beginning in the late 1980s, these various lines of evidence forced a reappraisal of the view that cell death in the nervous system is a passive process and led to the demonstration that for many types of neurons, PCD is metabolically active and is regulated by the interaction of specific genetic programs that either inhibit or induce degeneration. Neurotrophic survival molecules are thought to act as extracellular signals that when present in sufficient amounts either inhibit the expression or activity of proteins produced by cell death ("killer") genes or induce the expression or activity of "protective" gene products that block the action of cell death genes. Considerable progress has been made since the early 1990s in identifying cell death-associated genes and their pathways of action. Due to historical precedent, these have been classified as pro- and antiapoptotic genes. Although we retain this terminology, the genes involved may actually induce both apoptotic and nonapoptotic modes of degeneration (see the previous section).

Although early genetic studies of cell death in C. elegans demonstrated that PCD is regulated by specific genes, the first indication that the PCD of developing vertebrate neurons may also be controlled by similar so-called "killer" or "death" genes appeared in 1988 (Yuan and Yankner, 2000). Cultured neonatal rat sympathetic neurons, which normally require NGF for survival, remain viable following NGF removal if mRNA or protein synthesis inhibitors were added to the cultures. Subsequently, other types of developing neurons were also shown to be rescued by these drugs both in vitro and in vivo following trophic factor deprivation. These findings were interpreted as evidence that one or more steps in the neuronal PCD pathway requires the de novo transcription of genes and expression of proteins that actively destroy the cell and suggested that one important role of trophic factors is to suppress the activity of these genes. Because the genetics, cellular anatomy and cell lineages in *C. elegans* have been so well defined and because much of the genome has now been sequenced, this organism provides a particularly informative and powerful model for analyzing the molecular genetics of PCD (Wllis *et al.*, 1991). Of the approximately 1000 somatic cells generated (of which 302 are neurons and 56 are glial cells), 131 undergo embryonic PCD and most of these are neurons. In each individual, the same cells die at specific times in development and these corpses are then engulfed and degraded by neighboring cells. Despite the enormous evolutionary gap that separates the appearance of worms and vertebrates, significant homology exists in the structure and function of specific cell death pathways between these two taxonomic groups.

As summarized in Fig. 19.13, there is a sequential cascade of genes involved in PCD in *C. elegans*. Upstream of the actual execution of the death process, genes such as ces (cell death specification) and egl-1 (egg-laying-1) specify certain cell types for death while sparing others. For example, the ces-2 gene is required for the death of two pharyngeal neurosecretory motoneurons (NSM), whereas the egl-1 gene causes the death of egg-laying neurons (ELN); the death of other cells is not affected by either of these genes. Manifestation of the death fate requires expression of two other proapoptotic genes, ced-3 and ced-4 (ced, cell death), which together mediate the actual breakdown of cellular constituents. Prevention of cell death induced by ced-3 and ced-4 can occur by activation of the antiapoptotic gene ced-9. A separate gene, nuc-1 (nuclease-1), is required for the degradation of DNA in dying cells, and six additional genes, ced-1, 2, 5, 6, 7 and 10, are involved in the engulfment of dead cellular corpses by neighboring healthy cells. Evidence for the involvement of this genetic cascade in cell death and survival in *C. elegans* comes from several different approaches, most notably from genetic studies of loss-of-function mutants. For example, in the absence of ced-9, many cells that normally survive die, whereas in the absence of ced-3 or ced-4, all PCD is prevented.

Identification of the DNA sequences of the major cell death genes ced-3, ced-4, and ced-9 in the 1980s and early 1990s resulted in the subsequent discovery of vertebrate homologues that serve similar functions (Pettman and Henderson, 1998; Yuan and Yankner, 2000). Vertebrate homologues of nematode cell specification genes (ces, egl-1) have not yet been identified. However, the death receptor Fas may provide an analogous mechanism for the selection of specific cells for PCD in some populations of vertebrate neurons. In mammals, ced-3 is represented by a large family of related cysteine proteases called caspases, whereas ced-4 is represented by a single vertebrate homologue, apaf-1 (apoptosis protease activating factor), that is required for caspase activation. The survival-promoting function of ced-9 was originally represented by a single vertebrate homologue, bcl-2 (B-cell lymphoma-related gene), but subsequently other bcl-2 family members have been identified with similar functions in preventing cell death (e.g., bcl-x). Surprisingly, other bcl-2 family members have also been identified with the opposite function, namely that of promoting cell death (e.g., bax, bim). Loss-of-function mutations in mice by targeted gene deletion (gene knockout) of many of these vertebrate homologues have confirmed their role as important regulators of PCD.

The increased complexity of the genetic regulation of PCD in vertebrates vs C. *elegans*, as reflected in the multiple vertebrate ced-3 and ced-9 homologues, is further supported by the involvement of other vertebrate genes, such as cytochrome c, reactive oxygen species, nuclear transcription factors, and inhibitory apoptotic proteins (IAPs). In some situations, cell cycle genes normally involved in the regulation of mitosis, have also been shown to modulate PCD. This

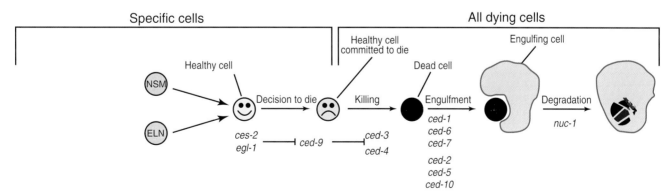

FIGURE 19.13   Schematic representation of the major steps in the developmental PCD pathway of neurons in the nematode worm *C. elegans* (for details, see text and Ellis *et al.*, 1991).

increased genetic complexity in vertebrates in general and in neurons in particular probably reflects a need for multiple levels of control of death and survival at the cellular level. It also provides for diverse pathways of PCD in different cells and tissues, at different stages of development, and in response to different death and survival signals. For example, the PCD of mitotically active and immature postmitotic neurons appears to involve some unique genetic pathways not shared by more differentiated post-mitotic neurons. In some neurons, neurotrophic factors and other extracellular

signals may induce death rather than promote survival by binding to so-called death receptors. For example, immature cells in the retina may be induced to die following activation of the low-affinity neurotrophin receptor p75 by NGF, and PCD in this situation involves intracellular pathways partly distinct from those used when neurons die following the loss of neurotrophic support (see discussion on p75LNTR; Pettmann and Henderson, 2000; Huang and Reichardt, 2001). Although the genetic and biochemical pathways that regulate PCD in the vertebrate nervous

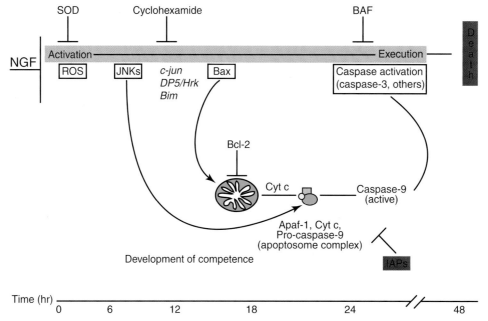

FIGURE 19.14 Temporal sequence of events during NGF deprivation-induced sympathetic neuronal death. NGF removal activates the programmed cell death pathway inducing the apoptotic death of neurons withing 24–48 hr. The sequence of events is shown in a linear pathway for simplicity; the approximate time-line of these events is also indicated. One of the events that occurs early after NGF deprivation is a transient increase in reactive oxygen species; these appear to be important for mediating sympathetic neuronal death, as microinjection of superoxide dismutase delays neuronal apoptosis. Following that, the activity of c-jun N-terminal kinases (JNKs) and phosphorylation of the c-jun protein is increased during sympathetic neuronal death. This event appears to be important because microinjection of either an anti-c-jun neutralizing anti-body or a dominant-negative c-jun construct prevents sympathetic neuronal apoptosis. Sympathetic neuronal death is blocked by macromolecular synthesis inhibitors, such as cycloheximide, and therefore is thought to require the expression of certain death-promoting genes. Expression of certain genes such as c-jun, DP5/Hrk, and Bim are increased during neuronal death. Although the expression of these genes is temporally correlated with the increase in JNK activation, their exact importance is mediating cell death remains unclear. Among Bcl-2 family proteins, Bax is essential in mediating sympathetic neuronal death; overexpression of Bcl-2 also retards apoptosis in these neurons. NGF deprivation induces the translocation of cytosolic Bax to mitochondria and the subsequent release of cytochrome c from mitochondria. The release of cytochrome c is necessary but not sufficient to induce caspase activation. NGF deprivation induces another event called the development of competence, which is needed, along with cytosolic cytochrome c, to activate caspases. The competence pathway may promote caspase activation by regulating the inhibitor of apoptosis (IAP) proteins in these neurons. Like most other cell types, caspase activation in sympathetic neurons may occur due to formation of the apoptosome complex comprising cytochrome c, Apf-1, and caspase-9. Activated caspase-9 may in turn activate other effector caspases such as caspase-3, which cleave specific cellular proteins and irreversibly commit the neurons to undergo apoptosis (for details, see Hengartner, 2000; Yuan and Yankner, 2000). In some situations, these neurons undergo a nonapoptotic type of PCD that involves a different sequence of biochemical events (see text).

system have been examined in many different neuronal cell types, at present the most detailed understanding of these mechanisms has been attained for neurons in autonomic sympathetic ganglia (Fig. 19.8).

In neonatal rodents, 40–50% of the previously generated neurons in sympathetic ganglia undergo PCD (Fig. 19.1). The neurons that die appear to be the losers in a competition for limiting amounts of target-derived NGF. Reductions in endogenous amounts of NGF *in vivo* result in increased cell death, whereas increasing NGF levels above that normally present rescues sympathetic neurons from PCD. A convenient model used to study the intracellular pathways that mediate sympathetic PCD involves depriving cultured neonatal neurons of NGF. In the absence of NGF, virtually all sympathetic neurons die by apoptosis within 48 h. By using this model to examine the biochemical and molecular changes that occur following NGF deprivation it has been possible to define a temporal cascade of intracellular events that characterize the PCD pathway (Fig. 19.14). As shown, a central integrator of cell death in this model is the mitochondrion (Yuan and Yankner, 2000). By monitoring the expression and activation of so-called pro- and antiapoptotic bcl-2 family members, the mitochondrion modulates cell survival by a regulated release of molecules (e.g., cytochrome c) that activates the downstream cell death machinery (e.g., caspases). Although most neurons appear to share the same cell death program shown in Fig. 19.8, the specific bcl-2 and caspase family members involved may differ between specific types of neurons or for neurons at different stages of development. In other cases, death receptor-induced death may occur by a pathway not requiring the mitochondrion. There is also increasing evidence that alternative, caspase-independent pathways may exist for mediating the normal PCD of some neurons. For example, although not yet demonstrated for neurons, the PCD of some nonneuronal cells involves the mitochondrial-derived apoptosis-inducing factor (AIF), which does not require caspases (Leist and Jaattela, 2001). It seems likely that the different morphological modes of neuronal PCD described in the previous section (Fig. 19.6) reflect the activation of a variety of caspase-dependent and caspase-independent biochemical pathways.

Summary

PCD is a metabolically active process that involves a specific genetic pathway(s) necessary for the cascade of events leading to degeneration. Several genes in the PCD pathway were first identified in *C. elegans* and homologues are found in vertebrates. Because the survival of developing neurons is dependent on successful competition for trophic molecules, a widely used model for the investigation of PCD signaling pathways is trophic factor deprivation. Both *in vivo* and *in vitro* models of trophic factor deprivation are being used to identify the temporal cascade of events involved in neuronal PCD. The mitochondrion is a central integrator of cell death signaling. Although all neurons appear to share common biochemical and molecular PCD pathways, morphological and biochemical evidence also suggests the presence of different mechanisms for some neurons. For example, there are both caspase-dependent and caspase-independent modes of neuronal cell death, as well as mitochondrial-dependent and -independent PCD. Because neurons are postmitotic and finite, multiple, relatively fail-safe mechanisms may be required to protect them from accidental death.

PROGRAMMED CELL DEATH IS REGULATED BY INTERACTIONS WITH TARGETS, AFFERENTS, AND NONNEURONAL CELLS

The PCD of vertebrate neurons and their precursors can occur at any stage of neuronal development from neurulation to the time of establishment of synaptic connections with targets and afferents and can involve mitotically active cells and migrating neurons, as well as undifferentiated and immature postmitotic cells (see Fig. 19.2). However, the most common and historically the best studied type of PCD of neurons involves postmitotic, differentiating cells that die while establishing synaptic connections with other neurons and target cells (Burek and Oppenheim, 1999; Pettmann and Henderson, 1998). Because massive neuronal death and its regulation were first clearly recognized in studies of neuron–target interactions, the role of targets in controlling PCD has historically received the most attention. More recently, signals derived from afferent inputs, as well as from nonneuronal cells such as central and peripheral glia and endocrine glands (e.g., steroid hormones), have been shown to be possible sources of trophic regulation of cell death and survival (Fig. 19.15).

Studies of the regulation of vertebrate neuronal PCD have shown that targets are critically involved in regulating how many cells in the innervating population survive or die. Complete or partial deletion of targets reduces survival, whereas increasing the size or number of available targets results in increased survival (Oppenheim, 1991). Although it is thought that the relationship between neuronal survival and the availability of synaptic targets is proportional and

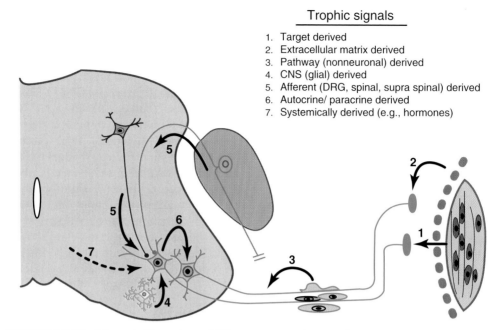

Trophic signals

1. Target derived
2. Extracellular matrix derived
3. Pathway (nonneuronal) derived
4. CNS (glial) derived
5. Afferent (DRG, spinal, supra spinal) derived
6. Autocrine/ paracrine derived
7. Systemically derived (e.g., hormones)

FIGURE 19.15   Schematic illustrations of different sources of potential trophic signals acting on motor neurons in the spinal cord. Motor neurons (green cell bodies) can receive trophic support from a number of different sources. Axon terminals of the motor neurons have access to diffusible (1) or extracellular matrix-associated (2) trophic factors produced by muscle. Schwann cells (3) in the peripheral nerve or ventral root could provide trophic support. Glial cells (4) in the spinal cord (astrocytes and/or oligodendrocytes) could influence motor neuron survival. Motor neurons receive afferent input from several sources, including descending fibers, dorsal horn, and dorsal root axons (5), which could supply trophic support. Finally, motor neurons could influence the growth and survival of themselves and their neighbors (6), as well as respond to trophic support provided by circulating hormones (7).

linear (this has been called numerical, quantitative, size, or systems matching), there may also be other ways in which the number of neurons that innervate a target can be regulated. For example, signals associated with but not derived directly from target cells (e.g., glia) may modulate PCD. Spinal motoneurons provide one of the best examples of how size matching is regulated by target-derived signals.

In the case of avian spinal motoneurons that innervate limb skeletal muscle, the number of neurons that survive the period of PCD bears a 1:1 relationship with the number of primary myotubes present in individual muscle precursors during the period of cell death, rather than being correlated with the final number of myotubes or myofibers (i.e., muscle size) present after the cessation of cell death. Accordingly, in this situation, motoneuron numbers, and therefore survival and death, are controlled in part by some factor (a neurotrophic agent?) that is limited by the number of initial primary myotubes available during the cell death period.

Although the essential factors provided by targets that mediates neuronal survival are not known for most populations of neurons, extrapolation from what is known for sensory, sympathetic, and motor neurons suggests that specific target-derived neurotrophic agents are involved. For example, as described earlier, sympathetic neurons require target-derived NGF as a survival factor, whereas distinct sub-populations of sensory neurons in peripheral ganglia require one or more of the neurotrophins, NGF, NT-3 BDNF, and NT-4/5. Target-dependent motoneuron survival is mediated by muscle-derived proteins. Several candidate motoneuron trophic factors have been identified and include BDNF, NT-45/5, IGF, HGF, CT-1, and GDNF. PCD of CNS neurons in the avian isthmo-optic nucleus (ION) and neurons in the mammalian thalamus and substantia nigra are controlled by many of the same mechanisms involved in the PCD of peripheral neurons, including a need for target-derived neurotrophic factors such as BDNF. As discussed previously, the survival of myelin-forming glial cells also involves competition, in this case, competition for trophic signals derived from axons. In both neurons and glia, the final outcome of this competitive process (Figs. 19.2 and 19.9) is the survival of optimal numbers of cells for innervation (neurons) or myelination (glia) (Oppenheim *et al.*, 2001).

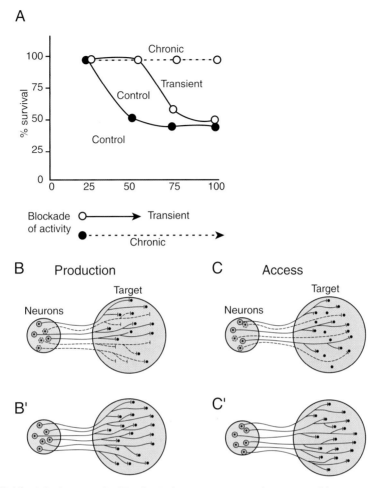

FIGURE 19.16 (A) The normal PCD of spinal motoneurons can be prevented by treatments that block efferent neuromuscular activity in the embryos, causing paralysis. Long-term (chronic) paralysis results in the maintenance of rescued neurons throughout incubation, whereas the resumption of neuromuscular activity following a transient blockade results in a delayed PCD of the rescued cells. (B) According to the production hypothesis, motoneurons in normally active embryos compete for limiting amounts of the target muscle-derived trophic factor (solid dots in the target). (B') Activity blockade increases the production of the trophic factor, thereby promoting motoneuron survival. (C) According to the access hypothesis, sufficient trophic factor is produced by target muscles of normally active embryos, but due to insufficient branching by some neurons, they are unable to access the available trophic factor and die. (C') Activity blockade increases branching, allowing more neurons access to the trophic factor, thereby promoting survival. Dashed lines indicate dying neurons (For details, see Burek and Oppenheim, 1999).

Motoneurons (and some other neuronal populations as well, including retinal ganglion cells, ION cells, and ciliary neurons) have another interesting property; their target dependency appears to be regulated by physiological synaptic interactions with their targets (Burek and Oppenheim, 1999). Following the formation of synaptic contacts between motoneurons and target muscles, the initiation of synaptic transmission activates the muscle and results in embryo movements. Chronic blockade of this activity during the cell death period with specific drugs or toxins that cause paralysis prevents the death of all motoneurons (Fig. 19.16). Although the cellular and molecular

mechanisms that mediate this effect are unknown, two major hypotheses have been proposed (Fig. 19.16): the *production hypothesis*, which predicts that the production of trophic factor by the target is regulated inversely by target muscle activity, and the *access hypothesis*, which argues that a sufficient trophic factor is initially produced by targets to maintain all motoneurons, but that activity regulates access to this factor by modulating axonal branching and the formation of neuromuscular synapses, thus restricting the uptake of the trophic factor to axons and synaptic terminals. At present, evidence favors the access hypothesis (Terrado *et al.*, 2001). Regardless of which of these two hypotheses is proven correct, however, it is clear that neuronal activity at both early and later stages of embryogenesis can make fundamental contributions to nervous system development. A recent striking example of this is the observation that in mutant embryonic and neonatal mice lacking all afferent and efferent synaptic transmission, there is a massive PCD of virtually all CNS neurons (Verhage *et al.*, 2000).

PCD is also modulated by specific perturbations of afferent inputs. Four such cases that have been examined in considerable detail are spinal motoneurons; the ION; the avian ciliary ganglion; and optic tectal neurons that are innervated by retinal ganglion cells. In all four cases, surgical removal of afferent inputs prior to or during the period of PCD results in significant increases in cell death. Because similar changes in PCD also occur after the blockade of afferent synaptic activity, the functional input provided by afferents appears to be of fundamental importance in this situation (Oppenheim *et al.*, 2001). Although the cellular mechanisms are not well established, the survival and death of newly generated neurons in the developing and adult hippocampus provide another example of how afferent activity can regulate these events. Learning, stress, motor activity, sensory input, and early experiences appear to control cell numbers in the hippocampus by activity-dependent modulation of neuronal survival (Oppenheim *et al.*, 2001; Young *et al.*, 1999). Functional afferent input may act to regulate the survival of postsynaptic neurons by several different mechanisms: (1) Depolarization by afferents can alter intracellular calcium levels in postsynaptic cells, which in turn can independently modulate survival; (2) afferent activity can regulate the expression of trophic factors and their receptors in postsynaptic cells; and (3) the release of trophic factors from terminals of afferent axons or adjacent glial cells may be regulated by activity and provide a survival signal to postsynaptic cells. At present, which, if any, of these mechanisms mediates the effects of afferent input on PCD is not clear. Because the PCD of many developing neurons may be coordinately regulated by signals derived from targets, afferents, and nonneuronal cells, an important unresolved issue is how these different sources interact to control survival. One possibility is that targets regulate the response of neurons to afferent input and that afferents regulate the response to target-derived signals. In this scheme, the relative influence of targets and afferents would have to be balanced in some way for optimal survival.

Although targets and afferents appear to be the major source of signals that regulate the survival of differentiating neurons, they are not likely to be the only such survival signals (Fig. 19.15). Other possibilities are (1) neurons themselves may produce neurotrophic factors that act by autocrine or paracrine pathways; (2) glial cells synthesize trophic factors and, in some cases, may be the source of trophic survival signals for neurons; and (3) the survival and differentiation of neurons in sexually dimorphic regions of the vertebrate nervous system depend on hormonal signals (gonadal steroids) from endocrine cells far removed from the neurons themselves. Additionally, other hormones such as thyroxine and the insect ecdysteroids can regulate the differentiation and survival of many types of neurons in both males and females; (4) the survival of many nonneuronal cells is known to depend on signals associated with adhesive interactions between the cell and its extracellular matrix. Cell adhesion molecules such as the integrins are also expressed on developing neurons and interact with receptors in the extracellular matrix (ECM). One such integrin molecule, laminin, is expressed in the nervous system and has been observed frequently to promote the survival of cultured neurons. Although *in vivo* evidence is lacking, laminin may modulate neuronal survival by promoting neuron-ECM interactions; finally (5), it also seems likely that the survival of neurons may be modulated by direct cell–cell contacts that do not involve classic trophic factors as mediators of the survival signal (e.g., by the modification of gap junctions and therefore the exchange of small signaling molecules).

Summary

During development, the fate of a cell, including PCD, can be determined by intrinsic cell-autonomous mechanisms or by extrinsic signals derived from cell–cell interactions. The survival of most developing neurons is likely to be dependent on a variety of signals, including multiple trophic factors derived from diverse sources, that serve to maintain survival and regulate differentiation in complex ways that reflect the specific requirements of neurons at each step in their development. Although developing neurons can undergo PCD at any stage of differentiation, the best studied type of PCD occurs as neurons are establishing connections with targets and afferents. Targets and afferents provide critical survival-promoting signals that prevent PCD. One major class of such signals are neurotrophic molecules. Neurons are thought to compete for limiting amounts of these trophic agents. For many populations of neurons, synaptic transmission also plays an important role in regulating survival.

FUNCTIONS OF NEURONAL PROGRAMMED CELL DEATH

Why does PCD occur? This is a reasonable question to ask because the loss of large numbers of developing neurons is counterintuitive. Why should embryos invest precious resources in generating cells and tissues only to later cast many of these aside? A satisfactory answer to this apparent paradox requires an evolutionary perspective that addresses two central aspects of the problem, First, how did the biochemical machinery (the death program) needed to actively kill cells arise? Second, why, in many tissues, are more cells generated than are apparently needed? Because PCD acts to delete these excess cells, an understanding of the overproduction is critical if one is ever to understand cell death from an evolutionary perspective.

Because all animals are under considerable selective pressure to resist the cellular spread of infection by viruses and pathogens, it is perhaps not surprising that several defense strategies have evolved to accomplish this. One such defense involves the activation of a cell death (suicide) program in which the biochemical death pathway triggered by viral infection closely resembles that seen in PCD. This program effectively removes the infected cell and prevents the spread of the virus. For example, in the absence of the proapoptotic genes ced-3 and ced-4, pathogens are more likely to kill infected worms (*C. elegans*), whereas when these genes are functional, the infected cells undergo PCD, thereby maintaining the viability of the individual organism (Aballay and Ausubel, 2001). Viruses, in turn, have evolved counterstrategies to block the activation of this suicide program. Such selective pressures acting on both the virus and their target cells could account for the evolution of the genetic and biochemical death program. An alternative model argues that PCD arose pari passu with the genetic and biochemical machinery regulating cell division. According to this view, DNA defects in mitotically active and postmitotic cells activate cell cycle genes, which in turn activate proapoptotic pathways as a means to eliminate "defective" cells. Understanding the evolution of the biochemical death program does not help answer the second question of why there is often a massive overproduction of neurons during development that are later eliminated by PCD? Two explanations have been offered (Oppenheim, 1991). First, each case of PCD may have evolved to serve a distinct biological function. For example, according to this view, in the case of spinal motoneurons, natural selection is thought to be directly responsible for both the overproduction and the subsequent death of neurons as a means for creating an optimal (adaptive) level of functional muscle innervation (e.g., size matching).

The second view is that the overproduction of neurons (or other cells) is an inevitable outcome of the imprecise kinetics of proliferation of precursor cells. Once excess cells are available, however, natural selection then acts via selective survival and death to mediate a variety of different adaptive needs. Following the loss of essential survival signals, death of excess cells could be accomplished easily by coopting the cellular death machinery that evolved to kill cells following viral infection. The major distinction between these two views is that in the first, the overproduction and later death or survival of the excess cells are believed to be directly selected for, whereas in the second, the overproduction and later death of cells are inevitable and unselected outcomes of proliferative mechanisms that alone are not able to precisely control the final, optimal number of neurons. In the well-studied case of spinal motoneurons in the chick embryo, the pre-cell death number of neurons varies little, indicating that proliferation is closely regulated. For example, at the end of the proliferative phase, there are about 24,000 (±2000) lumbar motoneurons, one-half of which subsequently undergo PCD (approximately 11,000–12,000 ± 500 will survive). Therefore, PCD is not needed to correct for imprecise, unregulated proliferation although it does appear to reduce interindividual variability in neuron numbers (i.e., there is more interindividual variability before vs after the period of cell death). Even though proliferation is tightly regulated, it may not by itself be able to reliably generate optimal numbers of cells (Oppenheim, 1991). In reality, both of the proposed mechanisms may occur. For example, it seems highly likely that the creation of transient structures that function at one stage of development but later regress and are discarded (e.g., the tail of tadpoles, larval muscles of insects, and transient neuronal structures such as sensory Rohon-Beard cells in frogs and fish) reflects the direct selection via evolution of PCD as a means for mediating adaptive regressive events. In contrast, the presence of increased numbers of neurons in limb vs those in nonlimb spinal segments of vertebrates may result from the unselected outcome of an overproduction of neurons at all spinal levels, followed by increased survival in limb compared to nonlimb regions. For chick spinal motoneurons, a combination of these factors appears to contribute to final cell numbers. Prior to the onset of cell death, fewer motoneurons are present in nonlimb than in limb-innervating regions, whereas somewhat less cell loss occurs by PCD in the limb-innervating regions. Thus, regulation of final cell numbers can occur at both cell genera-

TABLE 19.5   Some Possible Functions of PCD in the
Nervous System

Category	Examples
1. Removal of cells that appear to have no function	Death of neurons in either males or females for creating sexually dimorphic structures
2. Removal of cells of an inappropriate phenotype	Death of neuronal precursors located in regions of the spinal cord, such as the roof or floor plate, that lack neurons in the adult
3. Pattern formation and morphogenesis	Death of neural crest cells in specific segments of the hindbrain
4. Systems matching	Creation of optimal levels of innervation between interconnected groups of neurons and between neurons and their nonneuronal targets
5. Error correction	Death of neurons with inappropriate synaptic connections or aberrant pathway projections
6. Guidance	Loss of neurons or glia that guide neuronal migration or axonal growth at specific stages of development
7. Transient function	Death of sensory, motor, and CNS neurons that serve a transient physiological/behavioral function during development (e.g., Rohon-Beard sensory neurons in tadpoles)
8. Removal of harmful cells	Death of cells with defective DNA or infected by viruses
9. A means of evolutionary change	Adaptive changes in the ontogenetic death and survival of cells in response to genetic mutations (e.g., the production of excess neurons could be used for innervation of new targets made available by the evolution of limbs)

tion and survival phases of development and involves the modulation of proliferation and cell death.

Many of the circumstances in which the PCD of neurons occurs is thought to mediate distinct adaptive functions, as summarized in Table 19.5. In many of these examples, the production of excess neurons provides a substrate on which survival or PCD can then act to meet a variety of adaptive needs. Although the biological functions attributed to PCD in these situations are quite plausible, few of them have been directly demonstrated experimentally to serve a specific adaptive role. As we identify new genes that regulate PCD, and as we gain a better understanding of how cellular and molecular signals control cell death and survival, we will be presented with increased opportunities for preventing PCD *in vivo* and directly assessing whether

its occurrence is selectively advantageous. For example, the creation of genetically modified animals lacking or overexpressing specific cell death-associated genes (e.g., *caspases, bcl-2*) will provide insight into this problem by the opportunity to assess the physiological and behavioral phenotype of animals with hundreds of thousands of excess neurons in specific regions of the brain and spinal cord.

Summary

The biochemical and molecular pathways that are necessary for PCD may have evolved as a means to defend against viral infection. Once this cellular capacity arose, however, it is likely that it was coopted to serve a variety of other biological functions. In the nervous system, these functions include establishing optimal levels of connectivity between neuronal populations, eliminating aberrant cells or connections, and serving transient functional needs of the embryo.

PROGRAMMED CELL DEATH, DEVELOPMENTAL DISORDERS, AND NEURODEGENERATIONS

The widespread occurrence of PCD during normal development indicates that cell loss, together with cell production (proliferation), is a fundamental mechanism for controlling final cell numbers in many tissues. The cessation of normal PCD in most tissues late in development (e.g., in the nervous system) and the homeostatic balance between proliferation and death in other adult tissues (e.g., skin) also underscore the importance of precisely regulating cell numbers even into adulthood. Dysregulation of normal PCD could be maladaptive and pathological (Koliatsos and Ratan, 1999). For example, developmental, genetic, or congenital neurological defects may be caused by perturbations of PCD. However, there is relatively little solid evidence on this point. Although there are many genetic mutations in animals and humans that involve significant alterations in neuron numbers, whether these always reflect the loss of control of PCD or reflect other abnormalities that could also influence final cell numbers is often not known.

One developmental genetic disease in humans for which aberrant PCD has been implicated is infantile spinal muscular atrophy (SMA). The most severe form of SMA (type I SMA) is an autosomal-recessive condition in which there is an excessive loss of spinal motoneurons during late prenatal and early postnatal life, resulting in respiratory failure and death by 1 to 3 years of age (Koliatsos and Ratan, 1999). One gene involved in this disease has been mapped to chromosome 5 and has been shown to be homologous with an antiapoptotic baculovirus gene product (p35), a member of the family of IAPs, that act in the same way as bcl-2 to inhibit PCD in insects and vertebrate cells. The first two coding exons of the gene for this so-called "neuronal apoptosis inhibitory protein (NAIP)" are deleted in approximately 70% of type I SMA patients. A second gene involved in SMA has also been mapped to chromosome 5 and is mutated in 95% of all SMA patients (types I–III). This gene (spinal motor neuron, SMN) interacts normally with bcl-2 to exert synergistic effects on motoneuron survival. The specific mutations in SMN found in SMA patients appear to inhibit this synergism and render the motoneurons more vulnerable to PCD. This suggests that due to mutations in one or both genes, the failure to inhibit normal PCD of motoneurons at the appropriate time in SMA patients may be responsible for the increased cell loss.

The idea that aberrant cell death in the developing and adult nervous system may reflect a loss of normal control mechanisms for PCD is appealing in that the increased understanding of positive and negative genetic regulation of PCD provides a potentially powerful and rational approach to the development of therapeutic treatment strategies. A hopeful sign in this regard comes from reports that neuronal (or glial) death in Alzheimer, Parkinson, Huntington, Down syndrome, and ALS disease patients and in some forms of traumatic CNS injury (e.g., head trauma, ischemia, cerebral stroke, spinal cord injury, perinatal asphyxia) exhibits some characteristics of apoptosis, such as the stereotyped fragmentation of DNA and the expression of genes or gene products associated previously with developmental PCD (e.g., the bcl-2 gene family) (Koliatsos and Ratan, 1999). In some of these diseases, specific gene mutations have been identified that may directly or indirectly perturb inter- and intracellular mechanisms involved in the maintenance and survival of specific populations of neurons. Other brain pathologies in which programmed cell death may be involved include fetal alcohol syndrome, schizophrenia, major depression disorders, Shy–Drager syndrome, narcolepsy, and fetal exposure to excitotoxic drugs. Therefore, in addition to the important diverse roles of PCD during normal development and in adult tissue homeostasis, studies leading to a better understanding of the cellular and molecular mechanisms of PCD may ultimately shed new light on the causes and prevention of a variety of neurological disorders and brain pathologies that affect large numbers of the human population. As we learn more about the molecular components of the cell death pathway, there will be increased opportunities for intervention using transgenes, drugs, and neurotrophic factors. For example, caspase inhibition by pharmacological agents is currently one promising approach that is being actively pursued by many laboratories and biotechnology and drug companies. The use of stem cells for replacing lost neurons and glia is another promising therapeutic strategy, and viral vectors for expressing neurotrophic factors in neurons may provide long-term protection from injury-induced cell death.

A number of major issues will need to be resolved before realistic therapeutic strategies involving the use of neurotrophic factors, intervention of cell death pathways, or stem cells can be considered for clinical application. These issues include safe and reliable modes of treatment, targeting the therapy to the affected cells, prevention of untoward side effects, and whether the rescue of neurons from cell death leads to the long-term survival of healthy functional cells. Although none of these issues has been satisfactorily addressed for either animal models or in human disease, the last problem, that of promoting the survival of healthy, functional neurons, has received some positive support from the study of fly mutants with a form of retinal degeneration that is a model for human cases of severe retinitis pigmentosa, a leading cause of blindness involving aberrant cell death of photoreceptor cells. Overexpression of the antiapoptotic IAP gene p35—a caspase inhibitor—in the mutant fly prevents the apoptosis of photoreceptor cells, resulting in the retention of significant visual behavior and retinal function (Davidson and Stellar, 1998). This success in preventing blindness in the fly provides hope and a rationale for the eventual use of cell death prevention strategies in the treatment of human disease. Despite this hope, however, there are as yet no successful cases in which human CNS pathologies or vertebrate animal models of these conditions have been significantly ameliorated by therapies designed to prevent cell death.

Summary

Because PCD is primarily a developmental phenomenon, historically the major focus of investigation has been the normal biology of cell death in the embryo, fetus, and newborn. However, with the growing recognition that pathological cell death may share certain biochemical and molecular features with PCD, there is growing hope that a better understanding of PCD may reveal potential therapeutic strategies for the treatment of neurodegenerative disease and neuronal loss following CNS trauma.

References

Ameisen, J. C. (1996). The origin of programmed cell death. *Science* **272**, 1278–1279.

Barbacid, M. (1995). Life, and death in mice without Trk neurotrophin receptors. *In* "Life, and Death in the Nervous System" (C. F. Ibanez, T. Hokfelt, L. Olsow, K. Fuxe, M. Jornvall, and L. Ottoson, eds.), pp. 345–360. Pergamon, Oxford.

Bothwell, M. (1995). Functional interactions of Neurotrophins, and neurotrophin receptors. *Annu. Rev. Neurosci.* **18**, 223–253.

Burek, M. J., and Oppenheim, R. W. (1999). Cellular interactions that regulate programmed cell death in the developing vertebrate nervous system. *In* "Cell Death, and Diseases of the Nervous System" (V. E. Koliatsos and R. Ratan, eds.), pp. 145–180. Humana Press, Totowa, NJ.

Chao, M. V., and Hempstead, B. L. (1995). p75, and trk: A two-receptor system. *Trends Neurosci.* **18**, 321–326.

Clarke, P. G. H., and Oppenheim, R. W. (1995). Neuronal death in vertebrate development: *In vivo* methods. *Methods Cell Biol.* **46**, 277–321.

Clarke, P. G. H., and Clarke, S. (1996). Nineteenth century research on naturally occurring cell death, and related phenomena. *Anat. Embryol.* **193**, 81–99.

Cowan, W. M. (2001). Viktor Hamburger, and Rita Levi-Montalcini: The path to the discovery of nerve growth factor. *Annu. Rev. Neurosci.* **24**, 551–600.

Davidson, F. F., and Steller, H. (1998). Blocking apoptosis prevents blindness in Drosophila retinal degeneration mutants. *Nature* **391**, 587–591.

Ellis, R. E., Yuan, J., and Horvitz, H. R. (1991). Mechanisms, and functions of cell death. *Annu. Rev. Cell Biol.* **7**, 663–698.

Gilbert, S. F. (2000). "Developmental Biology." Sinauer, Sunderlund, MA.

Hamburger, V. (1992). History of the discovery of neuronal death in embryos. *J. Neurobiol.* **23**, 1116–1123.

Hengartner, M. O. (2000). The biochemistry of apoptosis. *Nature* **407**, 770–776.

Huang, E. J., and Reichardt, L. F. (2001). Neurotrophins: Roles in neuronal development and function. *Annu. Rev. Neurosci.* **24**, 677–736.

Ip, N., and Yancopoulos, G. (1996). The neurotrophins, and CNTF: Two families of collaborative neurotrophic factors. *Annu. Rev. Neurosci.* **19**, 491–515.

Jaaro, H., Beck, G., Conticello, S. G., and Fainzibler, M. (2001). Evolving better brains: a need for neurotrophins? *Trends Neurosci.* **24**, 79–85.

Koliatsos, V. E., and Ratan, R. (eds.) (1999). "Cell Death, and Disease of the Nervous System." Humana Press, Totowa, NJ.

Korsching, S. (1993). The neurotrophic factor concept: A reexamination. *J. Neurosci.* **13**, 2739–2748.

Leist, M., and Jaattela, M. (2001). Four deaths, and a funeral: From caspases to alternative mechanisms. *Nature Rev. Mol. Cell Biol.* **2**, 589–598.

Lewin, G. R., and Barde, Y. A. (1996). Physiology of the neurotrophins. *Annu. Rev. Neurosci.* **19**, 289–317.

McDonald, N. Q., and Rust, J. M. (1995). Insights into neurotrophin function from structural analysis. *In* "Life, and Death in the Nervous System" (C. F. Ibañez, T. Hokfelt, L. Olson, K. Fuxe, H. M. Jornvall, and D. Ottoson, eds.), pp. 3–18. Pergamon, Oxford.

Oppenheim, R. W. (1991). Cell death during development of the nervous system *Annu. Rev. Neurosci.* 14, 453–501.

Oppenheim, R. W., Calderó, J., Esquerda, J., and Gould, T. (2001). Target-independent programmed cell death in the developing nervous system. *In* "Brain, and Behaviour in Human Development" (A. F. Kalverboer, and A. Gramsbergen, eds.), pp. 343–407, Kluwer, Dordrecht, The Netherlands.

Pettmann, B., and Henderson, C. E. (1998). Neuronal cell death. *Neuron* **20**, 633–647.

Raff, M. C. (1992). Social controls on cell survival, and cell death. *Nature* **356**, 397–400.

Segal, R., and Greenberg, M. (1996). Intracellular signaling pathways activated by neurotrophic factors. *Annu. Rev. Neurosci.* **19**, 463–489.

Terrado, J., Burgess, R. W., DeChiara, T., Yancopoulos, G., Sanes, J. R., and Kato, A. C. (2001). Motoneuron survival is enhanced in the absence of neuromuscular junction formation in embryos. *J. Neurosci.* **21**, 3144–3150.

Verhage, M., Maia, A. S., Plomp, J. J., Brussaard, A. B., Heeroma, J. H., Vermeer, H., Toonen, R. F., Hammer, R. E., van den Berg, T. K., Missler, M., Geuze, H. J., and Südhof, T. C. (2000). Synaptic assembly of the brain in the absence of neurotransmitter secretion. *Science* **287**, 864–869.

Young, D., Lawlor, P. A., Leone, P. Dragunow, M., and During, M. J. (1999). Environmental enrichment inhibits spontaneous apoptosis, prevents seizures, and is neuroprotective. *Nature Med.* **5**, 448–453.

Yuan, J., and Yankner, B. A. (2000). Apoptosis in the nervous system. *Nature* **407**, 802–809.

Ronald W. Oppenheim and James E. Johnson

CHAPTER

20

Synapse Elimination

AN OVERVIEW OF SYNAPSE ELIMINATION

In both the developing central and peripheral nervous systems, synapse formation generates some connections that exist only transiently in development. Proof that synapses are being lost comes from the finding that in many parts of the mammalian nervous system, axons are synaptically connected to partners during development that they are no longer connected to later in life. At the neuromuscular junction this is quite obvious because at each adult neuromuscular junction (usually one per muscle fiber) there is only

one motor axon, whereas at birth almost all junctions receive convergent innervation from multiple axons. In autonomic ganglia, axons also transiently hyper-innervate ganglion cells in early neonatal life. In the developing central nervous system (CNS), several cases of *synapse elimination* are well known (Table 20.1). For example, multiple climbing fibers innervate each Purkinje cell at birth, whereas all but one is removed in early postnatal life. Perhaps the best-known examples of synapse elimination occur in the visual system. In both the thalamus (dorsal lateral geniculate nucleus) and the primary visual cortex, inputs associated with the two eyes innervate common cells and then segregate into eye-specific regions.

TABLE 20.1 Synapse Elimination in the Mammalian Nervous System

Visual cortex (layer IV)	Binocular to monocular	Postnatal monkey, cat, ferret	Hubel and Wiesel (1963); Hubel *et al.* (1977); Wiesel (1982)
Thalamus (lateral geniculate nucleus)	Binocular to monocular, >20 to ~1–2 retinal axons	Postnatal cat and rat	Shatz (1990); Chen and Regehr (2000)
Retina (retinal ganglion cells)	On/off to on or off–center receptive fields	Postnatal ferret	Wang *et al.* (2001)
Cerebellum (Purkinje cell)	>3 to 1 climbing fibers	Postnatal rat	Mariani (1983)
Parasympathetic (submandibular ganglion)	~5 to ~1 preganglionic axons	Postnatal rat	Lichtman (1977)
Sympathetic (superior cervical ganglion)	~14 to ~7 preganglionic axons	Postnatal hamster	Lichtman and Purves (1980)
Neuromuscular junction	2–6 to 1 motor axons	Postnatal rat, mouse	Redfern (1970); Brown *et al.* (1976)

Fundamental Neuroscience, Second Edition

In all these cases, synapse elimination reduces the number of axons that innervate target cells, making the term *"input elimination"* perhaps a better way of describing the phenomenon. However, in most of the developing CNS, for technical reasons it is unknown whether synapse elimination is occurring. The difficulty is that *total* numbers of synapses may not be decreasing even though the number of inputs is, and assaying for a change in the number of innervating axons requires a means of counting them or at least having a situation where distinct but overlapping pathways can be separately labeled or stimulated (such as the two eyes). For example, accurate counts of innervating axons using whole cell voltage clamp recordings of lateral geniculate neurons in slices have shown far more input elimination than anyone had imagined (Chen and Regehr, 2000). Stimulation of the optic nerve with progressively larger voltages and counting the amplitude steps in the excitatory postsynaptic currents in lateral geniculate cells reveal a dramatic change from >20 innervating axons to only 1 or 2 during the first postnatal month during the time eye opening occurs. This previously undetected elimination may mean that such massive loss is occurring in many parts of the developing brain.

Interestingly and importantly, the remaining retinogeniculate axons more than compensated for the loss of axonal convergence by increasing their efficacy by greater than 50-fold. The same trend was seen many years ago in the submandibular ganglion where the one remaining input was always far more powerful than any of the inputs at the time when five to six multiple axons converged (Lichtman, 1977). At the neuromuscular junction as well, remaining inputs increase their quantal content as other inputs are eliminated (Colman *et al.*, 1997). It thus appears that while some inputs are being removed, the survivors are potentiated. One obvious question is whether the compensation of the remaining inputs is explained by changes in the efficacy of the remaining synapses and/or the addition of new synapses elaborated by the remaining input.

In the submandibular ganglion, the simplicity of the neuropil (most synapses are axosomatic) allowed direct counts of synapse number during the period when the number of innervating axons is dropping. In this ganglion, input elimination was accompanied by concurrent synapse addition by the remaining input. In particular, over the first postnatal month, there is approximately a twofold increase in the number of synapses, whereas the number of innervating axons is reduced fivefold (Fig. 20.1). This compensation indicates that remaining axons are increasing the number of synaptic contacts by approximately a factor of 10 as other axons lose all their connections.

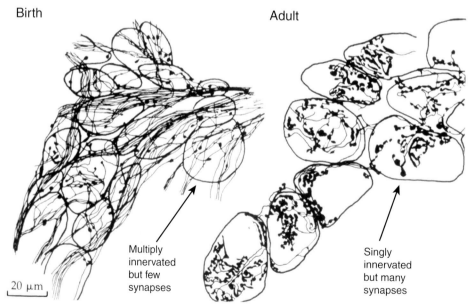

Birth

Adult

Multiply innervated but few synapses

Singly innervated but many synapses

20 μm

FIGURE 20.1 The total number of synapses on ganglion cells in the rat submandibular ganglion increases during early postnatal life. Camera lucida drawings of clusters of about 10 ganglion cells at birth (left) and in adult animals (right) that were treated with zinc iodide osmium. This reagent selectively fills terminal axons and synaptic boutons with a dense black precipitate. The number of synaptic boutons increases while the number of preganglionic axons innervating each ganglion cell by electrophysiological measures decreases, a fact confirmed by electron microscopy. Thus, remaining axons create new synapses to more than compensate for the loss of input. Modified from Lichtman (1977).

Such compensatory synaptogenesis means that assays of the total *number* of synapses at various developmental stages or following learning paradigms may belie a rather dramatic change in the *source* of the synapses.

It is also clear that in many situations the alterations occurring during this developmental reorganization are better described as a *redistribution of synapses* than as loss per se. The view is based on the fact that the total number of innervating axons is not changing (Brown *et al.*, 1976) because input elimination occurs in regions of the nervous system after the period of *naturally occurring cell death* (see Chapter 19). Thus, as the elimination process reduces the number of axons converging on postsynaptic cells, it does not entirely remove axons from the postsynaptic target but rather reduces the number of target cells innervated by each axon, i.e., it reduces the amount of axonal divergence as individual axons restrict their synapses to a smaller number of postsynaptic target cells (Fig. 20.2). In muscle, this axonal trimming has been long appreciated in an electrophysiological assay: the proportion of the total twitch tension an individual axon exerts decreases gradually over the period of synapse elimi-

nation (Brown *et al.*, 1976). Newer techniques of visualizing all the branches of single axons by transgenic expression of GFP (Feng *et al.*, 2000) has allowed this *branch retraction* to be observed directly (Fig. 20.3; Keller-Peck *et al.*, 2001).

Summary

While the number of postsynaptic cells an axon contacts decreases, the strength of the maintained connections increases. This redistribution refines synaptic circuitry by allowing an axon to strongly focus its innervation on a subset of the cells it initially contacted while at the same time each postsynaptic cell is restricted to responding to a subset of the axons that initially innervated it.

THE PURPOSE OF SYNAPSE ELIMINATION

The purpose of synapse elimination does not seem to be *error correction* because the lost connections are

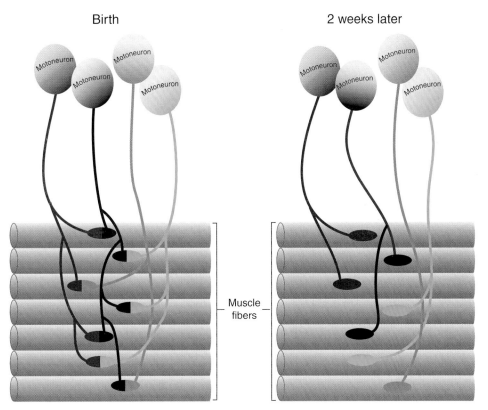

FIGURE 20.2 Diagram showing the change in innervation of individual neuromuscular junctions (ovals on muscle fibers) by axonal branch trimming. Over the first several weeks of postnatal life, rodent motor axons remove branches and, as a consequence, each neuromuscular junction undergoes a transition from innervation by multiple converging axons to innervation by only one axon. At the same time, the number of muscle fibers innervated by an axon decreases substantially.

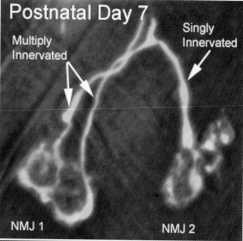

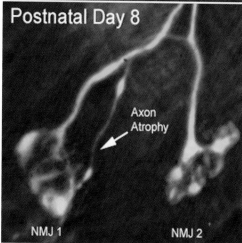

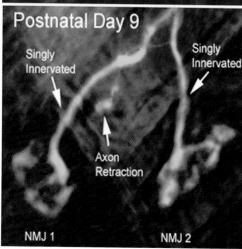

FIGURE 20.3   Time-lapse imaging of synapse elimination. Two neuromuscular junctions (NMJ1 and NMJ2) were viewed *in vivo* on postnatal days 7, 8, and 9 in a transgenic mouse that expresses YFP in its motor axons. The acetylcholine receptors at the muscle fiber membrane are labeled red with rhodamine tagged α-bungarotoxin. The transition from multiple to single innervation of NMJ1 as one axon, a sibling branch of the axon that innervates NMJ2, undergoes atrophy and appears to retract. The eliminated branch terminates in a "retraction bulb." Modified from Keller-Peck *et al.* (2001).

from the same presynaptic populations as the connections that are maintained. In some situations the outcome of synapse elimination may *sharpen specificity* based on topographic maps. It is possible, however, that the outcome of synapse elimination is biased by the same kind of cues that promote selective synapse formation rather than synapse elimination being the mechanism that achieves the specificity. Indeed, in some cases, there seems to be little evidence of intrinsic positional or other qualitative differences between axons that are maintained and those that are lost. A different idea, then, is that the loss of connections is a consequence of the extreme degree to which mammalian (and other vertebrate) nervous systems are composed of *duplicated neurons* (Lichtman and Colman, 2000). For example, pools of motor neurons that may number in the hundreds innervate individual skeletal muscles containing thousands of muscle fibers. Rather than having a single identified motor neuron innervating a single identifiable muscle fiber, as can occur in invertebrate nervous systems, in vertebrates many duplicated neurons seem to have nearly identical roles as does the large population of duplicated postsynaptic cells that constitute a muscle. It is likely that two consequences of this redundancy are increased axonal convergence and increased axonal divergence. For example, in mammalian muscles, because the many nearly identical motor neurons projecting to one muscle would all be equally appropriate presynaptic partners for each muscle fiber, it is not unexpected that multiple axons can converge on the same target cell. At the same time, the multiple duplicated muscle fibers are all equally appropriate targets for each motor neuron, causing each motor neuron to diverge to innervate many muscle fibers. Given the redundancy in both pre- and postsynaptic populations, it should therefore not be surprising that there are overlapping *converging and diverging pathways* in the developing nervous system. What is surprising, is that in at least some parts of the developing nervous system, this overlap is short lived. During development, axonal branches are pruned, causing the projection of each axon to become completely nonoverlapping and thus distinct. From a functional standpoint in muscle, for example, the removal of overlap in axon projections eliminates redundancy, and thus the recruitment of each motor axon gives rise to a substantive increase in tension of the muscle. Before input elimination is complete, the overlap makes some of the connections functionally redundant (because muscle fibers do not integrate synaptic input, once a muscle fiber is activated by one axon it cannot add additional force by the recruitment of another axon). Such *sorting of inputs* is apparently also valuable in sorting functionally homologous streams of information. Thus, depth perception (stereopsis) is thought to require removal, via input elimination, of convergence in the visual streams originating from the two eyes. In all situations studied to date, synapse elimination tends to parse a highly redundant circuitry into multiple unique functionally distinct circuits. This is likely a fundamental and essential maturational step for synaptic circuits that begin with a good deal of redundancy, such as our own nervous systems.

One line of argument that supports this view comes from a comparison of animals, such as insects, that show little evidence of neuronal redundancy and little evidence of input elimination with animals, such as mammals, with large redundant pools of neurons and extensive elimination. One interesting difference is that humans and other mammals seem quite dependent on experience for the acquisition of their behavioral repertoire, whereas invertebrate behavior is, to a greater degree, intrinsic. Compare, for example, the ease with which a newly hatched dragonfly takes wing with the protracted period necessary before a human can walk. It is possible that the neuronal redundancy found in higher vertebrates that gives rise to overlapping convergence and divergence pathways is used in the acquisition of skills by the experience-mediated *selection* of connections.

In mammals, functionally useful behavioral repertoires may emerge by the elimination of alternative synaptic circuits. This view is based on experiments showing that neural activity in one set of circuits can cause the weakening and elimination of competing circuits (see later). The invertebrate plan, however, is based on a built-in set of synaptic circuits tuned by evolution to be useful for a particular task. In invertebrates, there is no competition between circuits and the animal is designed for one set of tasks only. The advantage of selection of circuitry by experience (as opposed to natural selection) is that the nervous system of the animal is more able to adapt during its own lifetime (i.e., it allows for extensive learning). The down side is that such animals require learning and practice to choose the circuits and thus while they are developing are helpless and depend on their parents for a long period. However, because experience rather than genes plays the major role in dictating what one ultimately masters, the behavioral repertoire of the species is far more diverse. One slightly disturbing conclusion that follows from this view is that learning by selection leads to indelible change because competing inputs are removed and can no longer influence the circuits from which they are detached. The result of such elimination might be that with age, as an individual learned more, it would become increasingly set in its ways: alternative ways

of responding would be lost from its repertoire by synapse elimination, making it difficult to, among other things, teach old dogs new tricks. However, memories may be long lasting (decades) because they are indelible—once alternative inputs have been eliminated, they cannot affect the remaining connections. These speculations, if true, would place the mechanism of input elimination at center stage in the quest for the way learning and memory lead to indelible changes in synaptic circuitry, perhaps even in adults. Whatever one believes about the roles of synapse elimination for adult learning, it remains a central feature of the developmental reorganization of the nervous system.

Summary

In contrast to invertebrates, the nervous systems of terrestrial vertebrates contain reduplicated populations of neurons that serve each function. Elimination of synaptic connections during development may be an adaptation that converts highly overlapping connections of redundant neurons into unique circuits. Because this conversion may be based on neural activity, this process may tune the nervous systems of higher animals to the particular experiences of each individual animal.

A ROLE FOR INTERAXONAL COMPETITION

A number of lines of evidence suggest that the loss of synapses is the consequence of *competition*. The word "competition," however, has many different meanings. In broadest terms, competition occurs when more than one individual (in this case, axons) is capable of having the same fate (e.g., sole occupation of a neuromuscular junction) and the probability of having that fate is related inversely to the number of individuals that can have that fate. The point of defining competition so broadly is to emphasize that competition does not imply what kind of mechanism drives the outcome—even lotteries, where winners are picked by random, are competitions. Synapse elimination occurring on muscle fibers and Purkinje cells is thought to be competitive because there is always only one axon remaining at the completion of the process and therefore more than one axon cannot share the same fate. This fate is not preordained (e.g., an extensive molecular specificity that matches each motor axon to a subset of muscle fibers) because there is no evidence of stereotypy in the pattern of connections from one animal to the next. However, saying the process is a competition does not provide insight into the mechanism, i.e., what drives the competition. Competitions range from, at one extreme, mechanisms that are completely direct where the contestants interact with each other (e.g., a sumo wrestling match) to mechanisms that are completely indirect where a third party (a judge) decides the outcome and the contestants have no interactions whatsoever (e.g., competition for a Pulitzer prize).

Classic studies by Hubel and Wiesel (Hubel and Wiesel, 1963; Hubel *et al.*, 1977) showed that the two eyes initially share target fields in visual cortex but that the thalamic input from the two eyes segregates during a developmental *critical period* in early postnatal life. This segregation is in part due to the elimination of synapses such that once the critical period is over, cells in the input layer of the visual cortex no longer receive binocular innervation. During this critical period the outcome of the segregation could be radically skewed in favor of one eye if the activity of the other eye was decreased (e.g., by patching one eye). The result of such monocular deprivation implied that the eyes were *competing* for control of the postsynaptic cells they shared temporarily during development (see also later and Chapter 21). In particular, in the visual system the final pattern of connections from the two eyes seemed to be driven by disparities in the activity of the two visual streams,

one from each eye. If each eye had the same average amount of activity, each ended up with similar amounts of cortical territory. However, if there were imbalances between the eyes in terms of visual experience, the outcome tipped the segregation in favor of one eye over the other. The skewing that resulted from depriving one eye of vision was due both to additional losses in the connections driven by the inactive eye and to additional maintenance of the connections from the normally active nondeprived eye. Ordinarily, each eye's afferents relinquish its connections with approximately half of the postsynaptic cells initially shared in visual cortex. When one eye is deprived of vision, its projection to the cortex loses connections with nearly all cells, whereas the nondeprived eye's inputs are not eliminated from any of the territory they initially contacted. Furthermore, binocular eye closure during the critical period appears to have far less serious effects than monocular occlusion. These results support the idea that synapse elimination is due to an activity-mediated competitive interaction between the connections driven by the two eyes, but how might activity mediate such competition?

At the neuromuscular junction, evidence suggests that activity of the *postsynaptic cell* is a critical intermediary in the competition (in a sense a judge). Much evidence shows that synapse elimination at the neuromuscular junction is affected by activity levels

---

BOX 20.1

α-BUNGAROTOXIN

A number of different dyes, stains, and markers are useful in revealing synaptic structure and function. Some of the more powerful have been borrowed from nature. Many toxins and poisons bind to specific proteins. One example is the snake toxin α-bungarotoxin (α-btx). This toxin is a constituent of the venom of a *Krait* snake of the species *bungarus*. The lethality of α-btx is the consequence of its ability to bind to the α subunits of nicotinic AChRs in skeletal muscle cells of vertebrates (with a few notable exceptions: snakes, mongooses, and hedgehogs). Because α-btx is an irreversible competitive antagonist of the AChR, its binding thus paralyzes and suffocates the prey. Researchers have taken advantage of this snake toxin to study many aspects of the AChR. For example, α-btx was used to purify AChRs from *Torpedo* membranes. Furthermore, the toxin can be conjugated to radioactive

markers or to fluorescent molecules that can be seen in the microscope to stain receptors on muscle cells to determine their distribution, stability, and motility in the membrane. Because the toxin binds essentially irreversibly to the receptor in the muscle fiber membrane, receptors can be labeled once and then their behavior followed over time. This approach has provided substantial evidence about the stability of synaptic regions on muscle fibers, the lifetime of receptors in the membrane at the junctional sites, and how AChRs move within the plane of the membrane. For studies of synapse elimination in particular, the toxin has also been used to selectively inactivate some regions of a synapse by "puffing" it locally over a small region of a junction.

Rachel O. L Wong and Jeffrey W. Lichtman

(Thompson, 1985). However, it has been less clear how activity might mediate interaxonal competition, as conflicting evidence suggests that active and inactive axons are at an advantage. Further confusing matters is the fact that the total number of axons innervating the muscle as a whole is not changing, which implies that no individual axon's activity pattern is *the* worst because all axons maintain some neuromuscular junctions and thus all axons must outcompete other axons at some junctions at least. Indeed, because axons are trimming some of their branches, each axon is both winning and losing competitions in the muscle. To better understand the way activity might mediate interaxonal competition at a single neuromuscular junction, an experiment somewhat analogous to unilateral eye closure was accomplished by focal postsynaptic silencing at one site with α-bungarotoxin (see Box 20.1) within an otherwise normally active neuromuscular junction (Balice-Gordon and Lichtman, 1994). The result of this focal neuromuscular blockade was that there was local synapse elimination at that site. Postsynaptic silencing of an entire neuromuscular junction, however, has no such effect. These results mean that when some synaptic sites are activated, neurotransmission at those sites incites synapse elimination at sites that are not active at the same time. Because the terminal branches of one axon are more likely to be synchronously active than branches of different axons, this activity-based mechanism would tend to pit the terminals of one axon (a *synaptic "cartel"*) against the terminals of other axons that are not active at the same time. In this view, the role of activity in synapse elimination is to destabilize inactive synapses and to cause them to be eliminated, via signaling in the postsynaptic cell. One possibility is that active synapses generate two kinds of postsynaptic signals: one that protects them from the destabilizing effects of activity and the other that punishes other inputs that are not active at the same time (Fig. 20.4). This notion is unlike (actually the obverse) of the often-cited Hebb postulate in which synchronously active synapses tend to be strengthened. In this case, synchronously active inputs punish inputs that do not participate in activating the cell. It remains unclear what is the physical basis of these protective and punishment signals. Because neurotransmitter receptors are sometimes permeable to calcium and the depolarization their activity induces can raise intracellular calcium levels in other ways, one idea is that calcium signaling serves one or both of these roles.

The accessibility and relative simplicity of the neuromuscular junction have allowed some of the structural details of this competition to be explored.

These details provide a framework within which to think about the actual mechanism of synapse elimination. In mice at birth, a time when all muscle fibers are still multiply innervated, each neuromuscular junction is innervated by several axons. The inputs are highly intermingled and the extent of the areas occupied by each is similar. At birth the axon terminals overlie a relatively uniform oval-shaped cluster of AChRs. At this stage, electrophysiological evidence suggests that the multiple converging inputs at a neuromuscular junction have similar synaptic strengths. Junctions that remain multiply innervated into the second postnatal week, however, are quite different. First, many junctions are now innervated by axons that have substantially different strengths (Colman *et al.*, 1997), suggesting that the elimination process gradually alters the competitors. Second, rather than having intermingled inputs, the terminal branches of the competing axons become segregated from each other (Fig. 20.5; Gan and Lichtman, 1998). This segregation suggests that there is a spatial component to the competition; in particular, that axons *locally destabilize* other inputs in their immediate vicinity. Although the destabilizing signal is not identified, its effects on axonal branches are quite striking. Branches that are soon to be eliminated become atrophic and appear to detach from the basal lamina. This detachment implies that removal of the adhesive links between synaptic terminals and the extracellular matrix that overlies neuromuscular synapses may be an important component in the elimination process. Once detached, the atrophic axon branches gradually become shorter as if they are being resorbed back, although it is possible that some parts of the axon branch are being phagocytosed by the surrounding glia (Schwann cells). Time-lapse imaging of neuromuscular junctions in transgenic mice that express different fluorescent proteins in different axons (Feng *et al.*, 2000) has allowed the sequence of events that lead to elimination to be followed over time at individual neuromuscular junctions in living animals (Walsh and Lichtman, unpublished results). It is clear from these studies that sometimes the remaining axon grows to take over the territory occupied previously by the eliminated input. However, evidence suggests that the takeover is not the cause of synapse elimination because, in some cases, the losing axon leaves without takeover. In those cases, the underlying AChRs that are no longer occupied rapidly disappear from that synaptic site. These results argue that the signal that causes synapse elimination can operate even when the inputs are not directly in contact with each other, supporting the idea that the postsynaptic cell may mediate interaxonal competition.

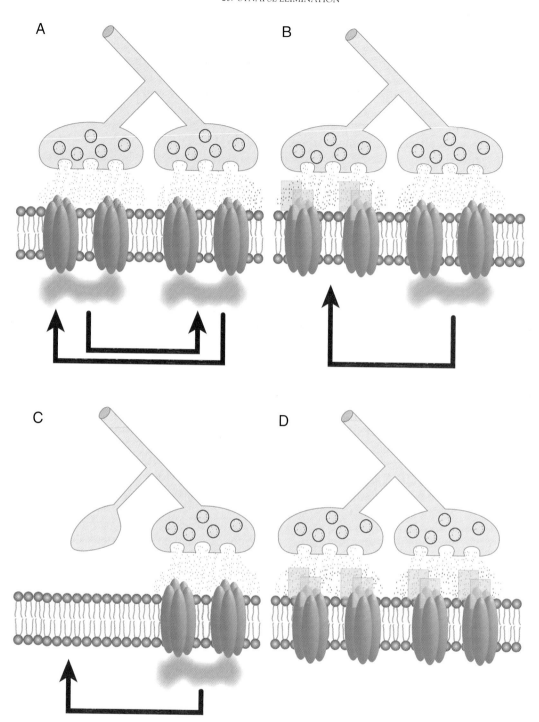

FIGURE 20.4 Experimental evidence suggests that synapse elimination results from activity-mediated signals within a postsynaptic cell. (A) Postsynaptic receptor activation may elicit two opposing signals within a muscle fiber. One consequence of receptor activation is a "punishment" signal (red arrows) that causes the loss of receptors from the postsynaptic membrane. Receptor activation may also generate a "protective" signal (blue clouds) that prohibits the punishment signals from destabilizing the postsynaptic apparatus at sites of receptor activation. When all the receptors are activated synchronously, there is no loss of receptors from the synapse (due to the blue clouds). (B) When two inputs are activated differentially, the active receptors are protected, and the inactive ones (x) are not. (C) This leads to the loss of the inactive (unprotected) receptors from the membrane and a subsequent withdrawal of the overlying nerve terminal. (D) However, when all the receptors are silent, there is no punishment signal (red arrows) and thus no synapse loss. Adapted from Jennings (1994).

Birth

Postnatal day 8

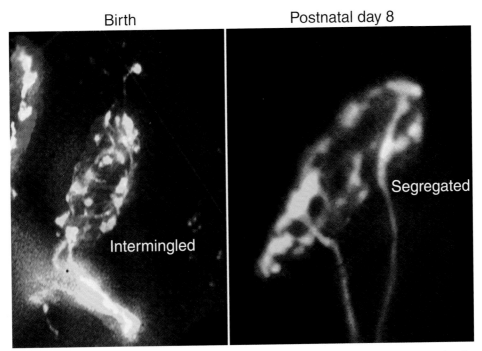

FIGURE 20.5 During synaptic competition, synapses of competing axons segregate from each other at individual neuromuscular junctions. Using mice in which different axons are labeled with different colors of fluorescent lipophilic dyes (Gan and Lichtman, 1998) or by expression of different fluorescent proteins (e.g., cyan and yellow fluorescent proteins, shown here) it is apparent that at multiply innervated junctions at birth, axon terminals of competing axons are highly intermingled (left) but at those junctions that remain multiply innervated 1 week later, the axons occupy nonoverlapping territories. This transition implies that the signals that underlie competition between axons have a spatial component. From M. Walsh and J. Lichtman, unpublished results.

Summary

Intersynaptic competition seems to be mediated by signals that pass within the postsynaptic cell between synaptic contact sites of competing axons. The identity of these signals and how they induce synapse elimination are not yet known.

SPATIAL PATTERNING OF CONNECTIVITY BY SYNAPSE ELIMINATION

Because many sensory connections in the brain are spatially organized into layers, columns, or maps during development, it is possible that synapse elimination plays a role in organizing these patterns. Competition for postsynaptic targets leading to the elimination of erroneous connections is now known to be an important means by which *patterned inputs* are established during development. The most extensively studied example of competition in the CNS is development of the *visual system*. Indeed, competition leading to synapse elimination and the refinement of connectivity is found at all levels of the visual pathway (see Fig. 20.6).

The classic work of Hubel and Wiesel in the 1960s (discussed briefly earlier) has provided important insights into how distinct patterns of visual connections are shaped during development (Wiesel, 1982). In young primates, neurons of layer IV in the visual cortex can be activated by inputs driven from both the left and the right eye, i.e., they are driven binocularly. Subsequently, however, inputs driven by each eye become strongly dominated by the right or left eye (Fig. 20.6). The cortical neurons that are activated by each eye are grouped together in a striking pattern of alternating stripes known as *ocular dominance columns* (Fig. 20.7). This pattern of innervation can be demonstrated either electrophysiologically (Hubel and Wiesel, 1963) or anatomically by injecting into one eye a radioactive tracer that is transported anterogradely to the cortex (Hubel *et al.*, 1977).

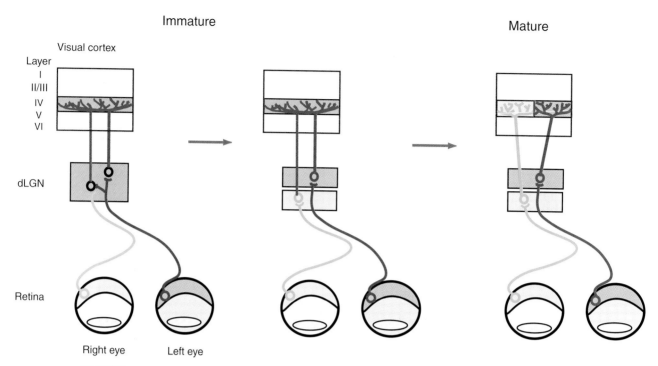

FIGURE 20.6 In the mature mammalian visual system, retinal ganglion cells from each eye (color-coded red or blue) connect to different target cells in the dorsal lateral geniculate nucleus (dLGN). Additionally, the axonal projections from each eye are organized into separate eye-specific layers in this nucleus. The axonal terminals of dLGN neurons in each eye-specific layer terminate and occupy adjacent territories, forming ocular dominance columns in layer IV of the primary visual cortex (see Fig. 20.7). Outside of layer IV, cortical neurons are binocular. Thus, pathways representing the left and right eyes are separated spatially and functionally from the retina to layer IV. These highly organized pathways in the adult emerge during development from less precise patterns of connectivity. Both dLGN neurons and layer IV cells initially receive converging eye input in the immature visual system. During development, inputs representing the two eyes segregate first in the dLGN and then in the cortex. Regions of overlap of inputs subserving the left and right eyes are in purple.

The emergence of ocular dominance columns reflects the anatomical remodeling that takes place at the level of individual axonal arbors. Thalamocortical axons projecting to layer IV are initially distributed evenly within this layer, but over the course of development, they end up with a patchy distribution, with arbors becoming restricted to one or more eye-specific columns (Fig. 20.6). Thus, the change in the width of ocular dominance columns is mediated by a change in the relative amount of synapse elimination and maintenance from the inputs of each eye. This should not be taken to mean that the total number of synapses is decreasing during this period. Just as in the peripheral nervous system (PNS), the remaining axons elaborate many new connections that more than compensate numerically for the loss of connections from the withdrawing axons. In other words, the process of ocular dominance column formation is one in which individual arbors lose, but also gain, synaptic space in the target. The critical distinction is thus related to where connections are added and lost. The elimination restricts the neuronal population that serves each eye, whereas the addition strengthens the connections that remain.

Separation of the inputs from the two eyes occurs twice in the visual system. Prior to the emergence of ocular dominance columns, eye input to the dorsal lateral geniculate nucleus (dLGN) of mammals segregates into layers, rather than into columns (Figs 20.6 and 20.7). In embryonic cats, axonal terminals of ganglion cells from the two eyes overlap extensively within the dLGN before gradually segregating to form the characteristic *eye-specific layers* by birth. As in the cortex, this refinement process involves both the retraction of axonal side branches in inappropriate regions of the geniculate nucleus and the elaboration of processes within the correct eye layer (Shatz, 1990).

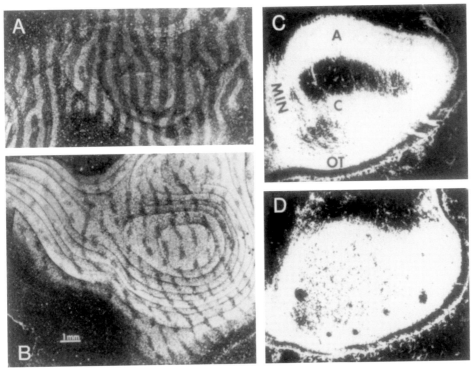

FIGURE 20.7 (A) Ocular dominance columns of the neonatal monkey primary visual cortex, at the level of layer IVC, revealed by injecting [3H]proline into the vitreous of one eye. Light stripes represent the antero-gradely transported label from the injected eye. Dark regions are occupied by axons driven by the other eye. (B) Monocular deprivation by lid suture of one eye (in this case, from 2 weeks after birth, for 18 months) results in the shrinkage of the columns representing the deprived eye and an expansion of the columns of the nondeprived eye (Hubel *et al.*, 1977). (C) Injection of another tracer, horseradish peroxidase (light regions), into one eye reveals the layer pattern of axonal terminals of ganglion cells in the dorsal lateral geniculate nucleus of the cat, shown here for an animal at embryonic day 56 (about a week before birth). OT, optic tract; MIN, medial interlaminar nucleus; A and C, layers A and C of the geniculate receive inputs from the contralateral eye. (D) Chronic infusion of tetrodotoxin into the brain between embryonic days 42 and 56 prevented the formation of the eye-specific layers. Adapted from Shatz and Stryker (1988).

Physiological studies support anatomical observations that geniculate neurons are binocularly driven initially, but maintain the input from only one eye at maturity (Shatz, 1990). In addition, the number of axonal inputs declines dramatically in early postnatal life (see also Table 20.1). The extensive loss of inputs involves not only competing inputs from cells of the two eyes; competition also takes place between functionally distinct ganglion cells from within an eye. For example, in the ferret, each eye-specific layer can be further divided into two sublaminae, each receiving inputs exclusively from retinal ganglion cells that are either depolarized (on cells) or hyperpolarized (off cells) by light stimulation. *On and Off sublaminae* emerge only after eye-specific layers are formed, with both processes occurring before vision is possible. Even in animals without distinct on and off sublamination in the geniculate nucleus, such as mice, these target neurons are only innervated by one subtype of

retinal ganglion cell at maturity. The progressive loss of retinal inputs onto geniculate neurons continues even after eye opening, during which time the receptive fields of these cells become refined spatially (Tavazoie and Reid, 2000). A summary of the progressive loss of inputs onto geniculate neurons is shown in Fig. 20.8.

The refinement of connectivity patterns by synapse elimination in the visual system is not confined to the separation of eye input but may also occur in the formation of *retinotopic maps*. These maps convey positional information concerning the image that is relayed in a topographical manner to visual centers in the brain. Retinotopic maps are found in the optic tecta of fish, amphibians, and chick and its analog, the superior colliculus, in mammals, as well as in the dorsal lateral geniculate nucleus and visual cortex of mammals. Evidence indicates that synapse elimination sharpens the relatively coarse retinotopic maps

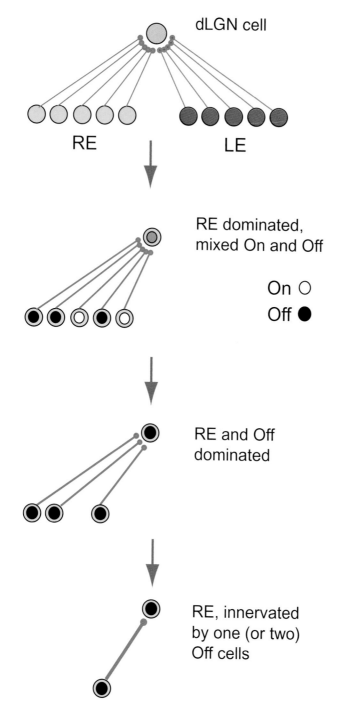

dLGN cell

RE   LE

RE dominated,
mixed On and Off

On ○
Off ●

RE and Off
dominated

RE, innervated
by one (or two)
Off cells

FIGURE 20.8 The type and number of inputs from retinal ganglion cells onto dLGN neurons are reduced progressively with development through mechanisms that require retinal activity. First, left (LE) and right (RE) eye inputs become segregated. On and off subtypes of retinal ganglion cells within an eye then compete to maintain connections with the dLGN cell. After only one subtype of cell dominates the receptive field center responses of the dLGN cell, further refinement occurs (after eye opening), whereupon the number of ganglion cells is reduced further. This final step leads to a refinement of the receptive field shape of the geniculate neuron. Note, however, that although synapses are lost, the remaining connections may become "stronger" (thicker lines) due to elaboration of more inputs from the remaining cells.

formed during development (or, in fish and amphibians, during regeneration). The mechanisms responsible for the formation of the initial map are discussed in Chapter 18. In lower vertebrates, however, a fairly precise map is laid down at the earliest stages when retinal axons first invade their targets so that this refinement is minor. In chick and rodents, however, a significant degree of axonal remodeling takes place before a fine-grain map is apparent. This is not surprising because in lower vertebrates, the problem of making a fine-grain retinotopic map is complicated by the continual addition of ganglion cells at the periphery of the retina and by the continual growth of the tectum to accommodate newly arriving retinal axons. In contrast, in the chick and rodent, much of map formation occurs when the available target space is already final (for review on map formation in different species, see Roskies *et al.* 1995).

Synapse elimination in the context of map refinement appears to occur as aberrant branches of axonal terminals are removed (Fig. 20.9). In the newborn rat, there is extensive overlap of the axonal branches and arbors of both temporal and nasal retinal axons in the superior colliculus. However, by the end of the second postnatal week, axonal arbors of temporal ganglion cells are highly restricted to the rostral end of the colliculus, whereas terminal arbors of nasal ganglion cells are positioned tightly at the caudal portion of this target. On the structural level, at least, *map refinement* in the mammalian superior colliculus, like the formation of eye-specific layers in the dLGN and ocular dominance columns in the cortex, involves both retraction of incorrectly placed arbors and elaboration of correctly positioned terminals.

How are exuberant branches removed during retinotopic map refinement? One way is the removal of incorrectly positioned arbors by cell death. Indeed, this mechanism contributes to map refinement in the rat superior colliculus (Roskies *et al.*, 1995). Likewise, cell death may also contribute to the refinement of eye input in the cat geniculate nucleus because eye-specific layers are formed during the period of naturally occurring cell death in the ganglion cell population. Although cell death appears to contribute to the removal of inaccurately placed processes, anatomical studies suggest that axonal branches within incorrect target regions retract without cell loss. Unlike the formation of ocular dominance columns or eye-specific layers, whether this loss of axonal side branches reflects the elimination of synaptic connections is not known because, to date, the patterns of connections at each stage of map formation have not been assessed physiologically.

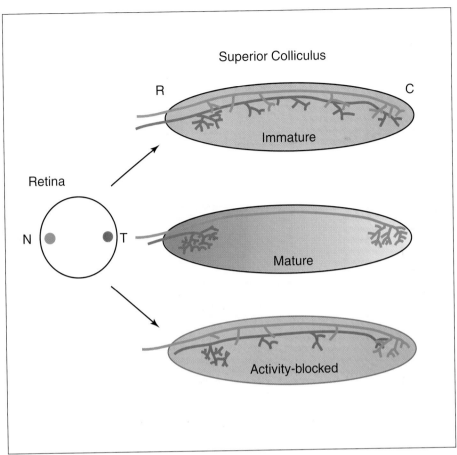

FIGURE 20.9 In the mature rat visual system, the axon terminals of temporal (T) retinal ganglion cells are highly restricted to the rostral (R) part of the superior colliculus, a subcortical target of the ganglion cells. Conversely, the terminal arbors of nasal (N) axons occupy predominantly the caudal (C) part of the colliculus. During postnatal development, however, individual temporal and nasal axons are not confined to the rostral or caudal parts of the colliculus but instead elaborate many side branches, which are eliminated with maturation. Blockade of postsynaptic activity by an *in vivo* infusion of D-APV, an NMDA receptor antagonist, prevents the elimination of side branches. Thus, sharpening of the retinotopic map requires neurotransmission.

Summary

Throughout the visual pathway, connections are not only added but are lost during development. Elimination of synapses helps shape connectivity patterns, such as ocular dominance columns and retinotopic maps, as well as refine the receptive field properties of visual neurons.

ACTIVITY IS REQUIRED FOR SYNAPSE ELIMINATION

One of the more influential experiments in the field of synaptic plasticity was the discovery by Hubel and Wiesel that axonal segregation that occurs during early postnatal life can be altered dramatically by modifying the relative activity impinging on the cortex from the two eyes (Wiesel, 1982; see also Sur and Leamey, 2001). When kittens were reared with one eye sutured closed, the ocular dominance columns subserving that eye were dramatically smaller than those associated with the open eye (Figs. 20.7 and 20.10). The large size of the columns driven by the open eye is not necessarily the result of sprouting of axonal terminals into territory normally occupied by the sutured eye. More likely, the open eye remains connected to a greater proportion of the cells that it initially contacted, whereas the sutured eye loses a greater proportion of its initial connections. There is a period of development during which the patterning of ocular dominance columns is most easily perturbed (called the critical period), but after which it becomes insensitive to manipulations of visual experience (see Chapter 21).

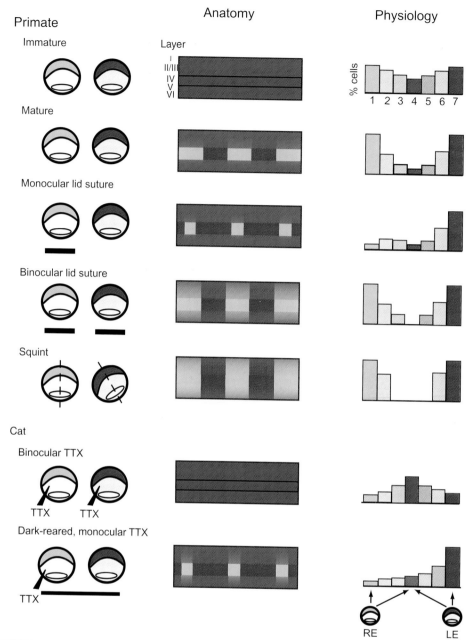

FIGURE 20.10 Summary of the development of ocular dominance columns in the primate and cat under normal and activity perturbed conditions. For each condition, the spatial patterns of left (red) and right (blue) eye geniculocortical afferents within the six layers of primary visual cortex are shown. Purple regions indicate overlap between left and right eye terminals. Physiological recordings show the distribution of cells recorded from layers II to V. Cell responses are exclusively right (bin 1) or left (bin 7) eye driven or are driven by both eyes but with preference to either right (bins 2,3) or left (bins 5,6) eyes. Cells driven equally by both eyes are represented in bin 4. Columns form in the absence of patterned vision (binocular lid suture, dark rearing) but not when all activity is abolished (binocular TTX). A relatively less active eye loses territory in comparison to the more active eye (monocular lid suture; dark-reared and monocular TTX). Disruption of patterned vision by binocular lid suture or strabismus results in a decrease in binocular cells outside of layer IV.

The "shift" in eye preference does not appear to depend on patterned vision *per se*. If the nonoccluded eye is silenced totally with an intraocular injection of *tetrodotoxin* (TTX), the cortical response is shifted toward the sutured and spontaneously active eye. Interestingly, when postsynaptic activation of cortical cells is prevented by the chronic application of GABA$_A$ receptor agonists, cortical neurons develop a preference for inputs from the closed eye (Sur and Leamey, 2001). With monocular deprivation alone, the cortical territory occupied by inputs driven by the closed eye is reduced compared to the territory occupied by the inputs of the open eye. When postsynaptic activity is blocked, axons responding to the deprived eye do not lose territory and the inputs of the open eye fail to innervate cortical regions they would otherwise have occupied if the cortical cells were responsive. These findings clearly demonstrate that postsynaptic activity is important, and furthermore, the more active input does not always win the competition if the postsynaptic cell is prevented from responding. The effect of activity blockade on the structure of geniculate arbors is rapid, occurring within a few days after the blockade. Functional suppression of the deprived eye input is accompanied closely by a remodeling of the arbor structure.

Ocular dominance columns appear, however, when both eyes are sutured from birth or when the animal is raised in the dark (Fig. 20.10; see Wiesel, 1982). Implicit in this observation is that activity required for the segregation of visual inputs does not arise only from visual stimulation through vision (photoreceptor activation). Indeed, although ocular dominance columns remain plastic for a time (during the critical period) after birth, in monkeys at least, ocular dominance columns are apparent prior to birth. In contrast, ocular dominance columns do not form at all when postnatal kittens received injections of TTX into both eyes (Fig. 20.10), which abolishes all activity from the retina. In fact, in dark-reared animals in which one eye received TTX treatment, cortical cells become biased toward the spontaneously active eye (Fig. 20.10). Collectively, these experiments imply that an imbalance of activity from the two eyes fuels the separation of eye inputs to layer IV of the primary visual cortex and that this activity first arises independent of visual stimulation. However, it should be emphasized that *patterned vision* during the critical period is important for the continual presence of ocular dominance columns in layer IV. In addition, very few binocular cells are encountered outside of layer IV in binocular lid suture or dark-reared animals, suggesting that binocularity requires synchronous activity in both eyes. This is further supported by experiments in which *strabismus* or squint is produced artificially after cutting an eye muscle (Fig. 20.10). In such cases, although both eyes receive the same amount of patterned illumination, binocular vision was not possible—cells in the retina that mapped to the same position in the cortex viewed different parts of the visual world. The result is a dramatic reduction in binocular cells in the cortex.

A role for *spontaneous activity*, rather than visual experience, in guiding the segregation of retinogeniculate connections to form eye-specific layers in the LGN is evident in cats, ferrets, and monkeys because this process occurs well before the retina is sensitive to light. Chronic infusion of TTX during prenatal life into the region of the LGN during the period of eye-specific segregation prevents the emergence of the eye-specific layers in cats (Fig. 20.7). On and off sublaminae in the ferret geniculate nucleus also appear before photoreceptors mature (Wong, 1999). Taken together, these observations suggest that the immature retina may provide spontaneously generated signals that could be suitable for the early segregation of visual inputs in the geniculate nucleus and cortex.

What information may be contained in the spontaneous activity patterns of immature retinas that lead to the refinement of connectivity in the visual system? Surprisingly, the immature retina generates a distinct spatiotemporal pattern of activity in the absence of visual stimulation (Wong, 1999). The activity of neighboring retinal ganglion cells is correlated by propagating *waves*, which have no preferred direction of propagation and which occur periodically, about once a minute (Fig. 20.11). Retinal waves contain temporal and spatial cues that could guide the activity-dependent refinement of retinogeniculate connections. For example, because waves are generated independently in each retina, activities from the two eyes are unlikely to be coincident. Asynchrony between the inputs of the two eyes could account for the segregation of inputs into different eye-specific layers in the LGN and ultimately into different ocular dominance columns. Moreover, because the waves ensure that nearby retinal ganglion cells are better synchronized than more distant cells, geniculate neurons are able to gauge neighbor relationships in the retina by their sequential activation. This feature could be useful for refinement of the retinotopic map. Retinal waves may also provide the means by which the terminals of on and off ganglion cells segregate because the temporal patterns of on and off cells become distinct during the period of on–off segregation in the LGN. Pharmacological blockade of retinal waves during the period of eye-specific segregation in the ferret dLGN prevents the emergence of these layers, suggesting that activity from the retinas is involved (Wong, 1999). However, whether it is patterned activity rather just its presence, or whether retinal waves drive other developmental processes *in vivo* remains to be tested by altering, rather than abolishing, the spontaneous activity patterns of the ganglion cells. Although activity from retinas contributes to driving the segregation of retinogeniculate projections, this activity alone is unlikely to be sufficient for specifying which layer in the LGN should subserve the left or right eye or, in the ferret, on or off cells. The stereotyped representation of contralateral and ipsilateral inputs in the lateral geniculate nucleus from animal to animal suggests that mechanisms other than that

arising from activity-driven competition influences the patterning of retinogeniculate projections. Future investigations defining the early patterns of convergence and divergence of connections from the two eyes at the level of single geniculate neurons are needed to reveal whether the "direction" of synapse elimination is biased by the initial innervation patterns and what mechanisms establish these initial biases. Furthermore, correlated spontaneous activity independent of retinal drive also exists in thalamocortical and intracortical circuits—how activity at these higher levels shapes connectivity between the LGN and the cortex, and within the cortex, remains to be elucidated (Sur and Leamey, 2001).

Experiments in ferrets have also refocused attention on discerning the relative roles of activity-dependent versus activity-independent mechanisms in setting up ocular dominance columns (Crowley and Katz, 2000), i.e., whether experience or intrinsic molecular templates are primarily responsible for establishing ocular dominance columns. Stripe-like patterns are seen in the visual cortex of the ferret even when the eyes are removed before geniculate axons reach the cortex. This raises the possibility that geniculocortical projections may be more specific in their initial innervation patterns than previously thought. Indeed, physiological recordings showing convergence of left and right eye input to immature cortical cells are quite limited, mainly because these cells respond poorly to light stimulation. Moreover, the exact extent of overlap between immature geniculocortical axons subserving the two eyes is difficult to ascertain with monocular injections of tritiated proline because of spillover of this tracer across eye layers in the immature geniculate (LeVay et al., 1978). However, several key experiments suggest that visual projections undergo transition from an intermixed to a segregated state.

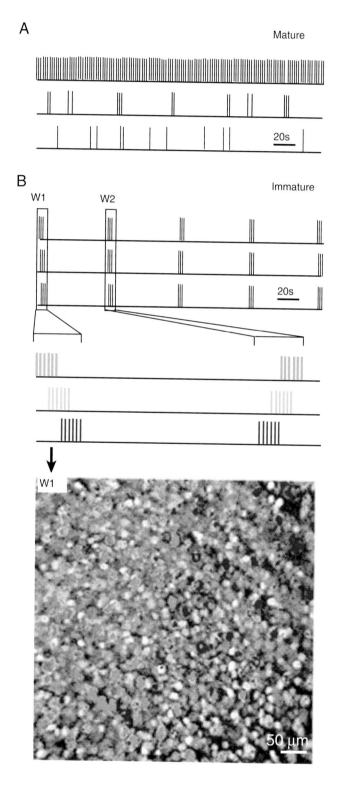

FIGURE 20.11 Immature retinas generate waves of spontaneous activity prior to vision. (A) In the mature retina, retinal ganglion cells show diverse and uncorrelated patterns of action potential activity. Action potentials (vertical lines) of three cells are schematized here. (B) Before eye opening, retinal ganglion cells generate rhythmic bursts of action potentials that are synchronized between neighboring cells. The synchrony is not perfect, as shown by the colored spikes at an expanded time scale. This is because the activity propagates across the retina, during which some ganglion cells are activated before others. A wave of activity (W1) is evident when calcium indicator dyes are used to monitor spike activity (colored image). In this example, the wave propagated from green to yellow to red cells (images obtained once every second). Cells that did not participate in this wave are not pseudocolored. Waves can propagate in any direction; e.g., the green-colored cell fired first in wave 1 (W1), whereas it fired last at W2.

Deafferentation of inputs to the auditory thalamus results in innervation of this region by retinal axons whose terminals initially overlap, but segregate over time to form eye-dominant clusters (Sur and Leamey, 2001). The segregation of left and right eye axonal terminals in targets that normally do not receive visual input strongly suggests that competitive mechanisms are involved (Wong, 1999). Another experiment demonstrating competitive interactions resulting in segregated eye inputs is the *three-eyed frog* experiment (Constantine-Paton and Law, 1978). Transplanting a third eye into the frog embryo results in the formation of ocular dominance stripes in the optic tectum where they are normally absent. Segregation does not occur if electrical activity is blocked. Finally, observations from a mutant strain of Belgian sheep dog support the idea that normally, competitive interactions occur to segregate the projections of the two eyes (Willams *et al.*, 1994). These animals lack an optic chiasm such that each geniculate nucleus is monocular. Although layers are present in the dLGN, an interlaminar zone is missing at the retinotopic position where retinal ganglion cells on either side of the vertical meridian project. Normally, these ganglion cells are located in different eyes, but in the achiasmastic dog, they are neighbors projecting from the same eye. If retinal waves are present (Fig. 20.11), the most likely explanation is that asynchronously active afferents normally segregate from each other, but in the achiasmastic dog, the activity of ganglion cells on either side of the vertical meridian would be synchronized. Thus, the interlaminar zone may emerge as a consequence of activity-mediated competition.

Not all visual maps appear to undergo refinement by activity-dependent synapse elimination. Cortical neurons that respond with similar preference to the orientation of a moving stimulus are clustered together and systematically form a map of orientation preference in the primary visual cortex (Sur and Leamey, 2001). These *orientation maps* are present before eye opening in cat, and thereafter appear unchanged even when visual stimulation is perturbed. However, because the presence and organization of orientation maps can at present only be assessed by physiological methods requiring visual stimulation, it remains unclear whether there is precision in the formation of these maps from the onset. It is clear, however, that orientation tuning of individual cortical neurons becomes sharper with development and that this process requires retinal activity. This suggests that remodeling of inputs takes place at the functional level, but how neighboring cells come to share the same or similar orientation preference remains unknown. Indeed, it is intriguing to find that

fairly good orientation maps can be "recreated" in the auditory cortex when visual input is rerouted to the auditory thalamus during development. These findings imply that the emergence of systematic representations of the visual world depends at least, in part, on the characteristics and possibly competitive events involving presynaptic inputs during development (Sur and Leamey, 2001).

Summary

Neural activity is necessary for driving synapse elimination during the refinement of immature visual connections. Vision is necessary for maintaining the early patterns of connections that are sculpted by spontaneous retinal activity.

HOW WIDESPREAD IS ACTIVITY-DRIVEN SYNAPSE ELIMINATION?

A clear example of synapse elimination in the developing CNS outside of the visual system is the *climbing fiber input* onto cerebellar Purkinje cells (Crepel, 1982). The proximal tree of Purkinje cells is initially multiply innervated by climbing fibers arising from the inferior olive of the medulla. Upon maturation, these neurons become singly innervated (Box 20.2). The loss of climbing fiber inputs depends on the presence of parallel fiber innervation of the distal part of the Purkinje cell arbor (Box 20.2). Elimination of granule cell (parallel fiber) inputs to Purkinje cells by X irradiation or in mutants such as *leaner*, *weaver*, and *staggerer* mice results in a higher incidence of Purkinje cells that are multiply innervated by climbing fibers at adulthood. Removal of the parallel fiber input, however, does not necessarily argue that activity is important. Studies that address this issue more directly include perturbation of activity along the parallel fiber—Purkinje cell pathway in mGluR1 knockout mice and when NMDA receptor antagonists are introduced *in vivo*. In both cases, the elimination of climbing fibers is prevented in a proportion of Purkinje cells. Thus, while it appears that the activity of parallel fibers affects the outcome of the climbing fiber input, it remains unclear how important activity in both parallel and climbing fiber pathways acts to eliminate inputs from climbing fibers. What is intriguing, however, is that the loss of one type of input (climbing fiber) is influenced by interactions of the target Purkinje cell with a completely separate and physiologically distinct set of input (parallel fibers).

BOX 20.2

DIFFERENT MECHANISMS OF CNS SYNAPSE ELIMINATION

Synapses are eliminated in the developing CNS by axonal and dendritic remodeling. (A) A common mechanism involves the loss of axonal terminals from presynaptic cells that initially contact a target neuron. A clear example of this is the climbing fiber (CF) connections onto Purkinje cells (PC) in the cerebellum. The loss of climbing fiber input is dependent on interactions that involve parallel fibers from granule cells (GC). (B) A second, less studied mechanism involves spatial reorga-

nization of the dendritic arbor of the postsynaptic cell. This is well documented for on and off retinal ganglion cells (RGCs). While presynaptic bipolar (BP) cell axonal terminals that contact retinal ganglion cells are stratified on differentiation, on and off retinal ganglion cells lose dendrites before elaborating exclusively in one sublamina of the inner plexiform layer (IPL).

Rachel O. L. Wong and Jeffrey W. Lichtman

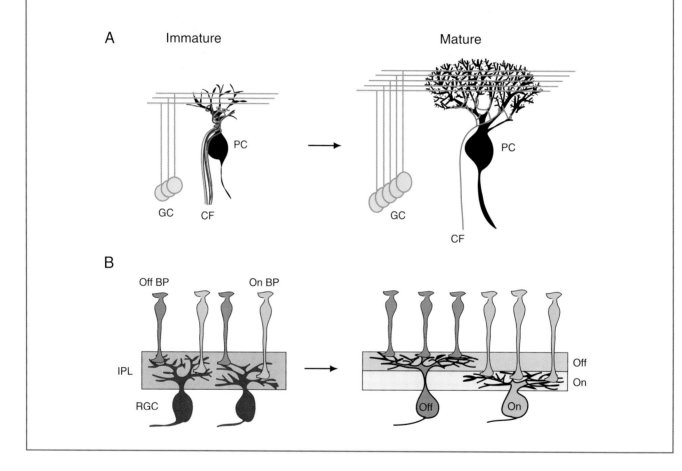

A notable example outside the visual system in which the precise distribution of inputs appears to form in the absence of activity is the unique spatial pattern of connectivity found in the rodent *somatosensory system* (O'Leary *et al.*, 1994). The whiskers or vibrissae of rodents are innervated by separate vibrissal nerves, which are activated by movement of the whiskers. The vibrissal fibers terminate principally in two regions of the brain stem, the trigeminal

nucleus and nucleus oralis, which send projections in turn to the ventroposterior thalamus and to region S1 of the somatosensory cortex. The arrangement of the whiskers on the face is reflected topographically in a distribution of discrete functional units, called *barrels*, in S1 (Fig. 20.12). Such distinct arrangements of connections have encouraged neurobiologists to examine how this pattern forms and to draw similarities with the development of ocular dominance columns.

Experiments that manipulate activity in the somatosensory system, however, have produced unexpected and conflicting results. Early experiments in which activity was blocked by the chronic infusion of TTX to the infraorbital nerve or to S1, or the application of NMDA receptor antagonists to S1, did not prevent the emergence or arrangement of the barrels during development. However, in mice lacking the NR1 subunit of the NMDA receptor, barrelettes are absent in the trigeminal nucleus (brain stem; Fig 20.12). Pharmacological blockade of the NMDA receptor from birth, in contrast, did not prevent barrellete formation. These results may conflict because barrelette formation is slowed in NR-1 knockout mice (because they die shortly after birth, it is not possible to test this hypothesis), or the pharmacological blockade from birth

occurred too late, as barrelettes are normally present by this age. When barrel formation is assessed by examining the distribution of cortical cells or the afferent arbor structures by anatomical means, results suggest that activity plays no role in the development of this topographical arrangement. However, more recent studies using physiological approaches indicate that activity is necessary. Normally, short latency responses for each vibrissa are confined within a single barrel in S1, but in glutamate receptor antagonist-treated animals, these responses were detected in surrounding barrels as well (Fox *et al.*, 1996). Whether synaptic connections are eliminated during barrel formation and activity plays a role in such a process remains an open question. Transplantation studies, however, show that barrels

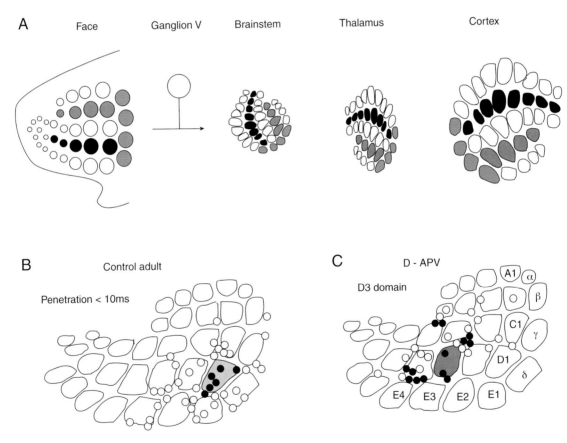

FIGURE 20.12 (A) Patterns of functional units in the somatosensory system of rodents. Each mystacial vibrissa on the face is represented in a one-to-one functional relationship with groups of target neurons along the somatosensory system, ultimately representing barrels in the S1 region of the cortex. (B) Blockade of postsynaptic activity by the NMDA receptor antagonist D-APV during neonatal development does not prevent the emergence of barrels in S1. However, although the anatomical arrangement appears unaffected by this treatment, physiological analysis indicates otherwise. Short latency responses (black dots, direct monosynaptic excitation from thalamic afferents) of layer IV neurons in S1 to vibrissa stimulation are normally confined to the appropriate barrel (see control adult). Long latency responses are shown by open circles; these extend across adjacent barrels. However, in the D-APV-treated cortex (C), short latency responses are found not only within but also outside the boundaries of the appropriate barrel (Fox *et al.*, 1996).

are unlikely to be an intrinsic feature of the somatosensory cortex because these structures still form when S1 is replaced by a piece of embryonic visual cortex (O'Leary *et al.*, 1994).

Summary

A clear case of synapse elimination in the CNS is the loss of climbing fiber input onto Purkinje cells during development. Elimination of climbing fiber input is dependent in part on activity-mediated interactions involving the parallel fiber input from granule cells. A role for activity-dependent synapse elimination in determining patterned connectivity in the CNS is not so apparent in the somatosensory barrel cortex.

HOW ARE SYNAPTIC CONNECTIONS ALTERED?

In general, there are a number of ways by which the overall synaptic input is altered during competition for targets. First, existing connectivity can be changed by mechanisms that alter the number of contacts via elimination or synaptogenesis. Elimination could be achieved by cell death. However, synapse elimination continues long after the period of naturally occurring cell death. Elimination of inputs has thus largely been attributed to the *retraction of axonal terminals* (Box 20.2). However, structural reorganization of the *dendritic arbor* also contributes significantly to the remodeling of connectivity. This is particularly evident for retinal ganglion cells, which remodel their dendritic trees during development such that at maturity, their dendrites stratify in either the on or the off sublaminae of the inner plexiform layer (Box 20.2). Because of the highly dynamic behavior of axons and dendrites during the period of synaptogenesis, there is now much focus on understanding how interactions between axons and dendrites lead to the formation, loss, and maintenance of inputs over time.

Rather than a physical withdrawal of contact, existing synapses may be "altered" by changes in their strength or efficacy via the mechanisms of *long-term potentiation* (LTP) or *long-term depression* (LTD). Both these possibilities have experimental support, and segregation of visual inputs probably occurs by a combination of gross removal and depression of synapses. Evidence also indicates that changes in synaptic efficacy may be the forerunner to elimination or may occur in parallel to synapse loss serving to strengthen (or weaken) competing inputs. For example, synaptic enhancement involving LTP-like modifications and

NMDA receptors may play a role in segregation. LTP occurs in primary visual cortex, it is easier to elicit in younger animals than in adults, and rearing animals in the dark prolongs the period during which it can be elicited (Sur and Leamey, 2001). Experiments that disrupt LTP in the developing visual cortex by infusing the NMDA receptor blocker APV, however, have yielded results that are difficult to interpret. In particular, although segregation into ocular dominance columns was disrupted, APV apparently blocked all neural activity, much like TTX. Blockade of NMDA receptors in visual targets also prevents refinement of the retinotopic map in frogs and the formation of on and off sublaminae in the ferret LGN. In all these cases, however, whether the disruption of normal segregation events is the result of decreased LTP or decreased activity in general remains unclear.

How does activity affect arbor size and distribution and, presumably, patterns of inputs? Accumulating evidence shows that neurons not only require specific growth factors for survival, as described in Chapter 19, but also depend on the same factors for their maintenance. Interest in the role of *neurotrophic molecules* in synaptic competition has been sparked by the discovery of the developmental expression of neurotrophins and their receptors in the developing brain. Nerve growth factor (NGF) has been implicated in the normal segregation of ocular dominance columns in visual cortex of rats, whereas NT-4 and BDNF are thought to play a role in synaptic rearrangement in visual cortex of cats. These trophic molecules appear to act both pre- and postsynaptically. Application of BDNF on cortical layer IV cells in culture promotes dendritic growth, whereas continuous infusion of NT-4 and BDNF in the visual cortex prevents the formation of ocular dominance columns. Presumably the geniculate arbors either fail to refine or grow excessively. The activity of neurons appears to be correlated with their response to trophic molecules. Although none of the present experiments conclusively demonstrates that neurotrophins are involved directly in synapse elimination at the cortex, the current findings do suggest that these molecules can be involved intimately in the establishment of synaptic connections in the developing visual system (Sur and Leamey, 2001).

Summary

The molecular and cellular changes that underlie synapse elimination are not yet understood. In particular, how changes in "synaptic strength" relate to the maintenance or loss of connectivity have yet to be ascertained.

IS SYNAPSE ELIMINATION STRICTLY A DEVELOPMENTAL PHENOMENON?

Synapse elimination is generally thought to be a developmental phenomenon, occurring mostly during a discrete period of time. In the developing visual system, the period during which synaptic rearrangement, including synapse elimination, occurs is referred to as the *critical period*. For example, the effects of monocular deprivation can be partially reversed if the period of deprivation does not exceed the critical period (Wiesel, 1982). Beyond the critical period, ocular dominance columns can no longer be adjusted even when one eye is no longer used for decades (see Chapter 21).

What signifies the end of the critical period? One possibility is that the end is related to a change in the milieu of developmental signals that control synaptic plasticity. An example of this could be the developmental regulation of the expression patterns of trophic factors or their receptors in the CNS. In many cases, however, the disappearance or downregulation of trophic factors and their receptors does not coincide with the end of the critical period. A second possibility is that at the end of the critical period, synaptic competition no longer can occur because the inputs of the competitors have segregated, and the remaining inputs are all synchronously (or mostly synchronously) active. If this scenario occurs, then desynchronization of preserved inputs should result in further synaptic remodeling. This remodeling could be manifest as loss of some of the desynchronized connections, or strengthening of other connections, but not addition of new connections. Evidence to support this mechanism comes from experiments in both the PNS and the CNS. At the adult neuromuscular junction, blockade of postsynaptic AChRs in part of a junction results in synapse elimination in the inactive region. In the CNS, focal binocular retinal lesions lead to the loss of visually driven activity in cortical cells subserving that part of the visual field. However, these cortical cells eventually become visually active, with receptive fields that are expanded and located in regions bordering the *retinal scotoma* (Gilbert, 1998). This rearrangement in receptive field organization has been explained by the strengthening of normally silent projections from adjacent retinal regions through the elaboration of new synapses. Finally, experiments using mutant mice in which GABAergic inhibition is much reduced suggest that the maturation of inhibitory circuits terminate the period within which monocular deprivation exerts its effects (Sur and Leamey, 2001).

Even though competition can reemerge under conditions in which the activity of existing inputs becomes asynchronous, the system must ultimately reach a state in which no more competition can occur because all possible competitors have been eliminated. Memory formation requires plasticity, but memory storage requires stability in the face of ongoing experience. This apparent dichotomy is mechanistically consistent with the experience-induced loss of synaptic connections. In this view, the formation of memories requires that a subset of connections is selected while others are eliminated, and that once connections are eliminated, those inputs can no longer influence the circuits that have been established. Thus, new experiences are unable to overwrite the memories already laid down. Because losses induced during synapse elimination are permanent and activity mediated, such losses could potentially be a way in which alterations in the brain synaptic circuitry could occur and be maintained indefinitely.

Summary

Synapse elimination occurs during development, mostly within a discrete period, the critical period, within which connections are modified easily. However, the representation of sensory surfaces in the brain can be altered even in mature animals. Whether such changes in the adult involve synapse rearrangement is unclear.

References

Balice-Gordon, R. J., and Lichtman, J. W. (1994). Long-term synapse loss induced by focal blockade of postsynaptic receptors. *Nature* **372**, 519–524.

Brown, M. C., Jansen, J. K., and Van Essen, D. (1976). Polyneuronal innervation of skeletal muscle in newborn rats and its elimination during maturation. *J. Physiol.* **261**, 387–422.

Chen, C., and Regehr, W. G. (2000). Developmental remodeling of the retinogeniculate synapse. *Neuron* **28**, 955–966.

Colman, H., Nabekura J., and Lichtman J. W. (1997). Alterations in synaptic strength preceding axon withdrawal. *Science* **275**, 356–361.

Constantine-Paton, M., and Law, M. I. (1978). Eye-specific termination bands in tecta of three-eyed frogs. *Science* **202**, 639–641.

Crowley, J. C.,and Katz. L. C. (2000). Early development of ocular dominance columns. *Science* **290**, 1321–1324.

Feng, G., Mellor, R. H., Bernstein, M., Keller-Peck, C., Nguyen, Q. T., Wallace, M., Nerbonne, J. M., Lichtman, J. W., and Sanes, J. R. (2000). Imaging neuronal subsets in transgenic mice expressing multiple spectral variants of GFP. *Neuron.* **28**, 41–51.

Gan, W. B., and Lichtman, J. W. (1998). Synaptic segregation at the developing neuromuscular junction. *Science* **282**, 1508–1511.

Hubel, D. H., and Wiesel, T. N. (1963). Receptive fields of cells in striate cortex of very young, visually inexperienced kittens. *J. Neurophysiol.* **26**, 994–1002.

Hubel, D. H., Wiesel, T. N., and LeVay, S. (1977). Plasticity of ocular dominance columns in the monkey striate cortex. *Philos. Trans. R. Soc. Lon.* **278**, 377–409.

Jennings, C. (1994). Death of a synapse. *Nature* **372**, 498–499.

Keller-Peck, C. R., Walsh, M. K., Gan, W. B., Feng ,G., Sanes, J. R., and Lichtman, J. W. (2001). Asynchronous synapse elimination in neonatal motor units: Studies using GFP transgenic mice. *Neuron* **31**, 381–394.

LeVay, S., Stryker, M., and Shatz, C. J. (1978). Ocular dominance columns and their development in layer IV of the cat's visual cortex: A quantitative study. *J. Comp. Neurol.* **179**, 223–244.

Lichtman, J. W. (1977). The reorganization of synaptic connexions in the rat submandibular ganglion during post-natal development. *J. Physiol.* **273**, 155–177.

Lichtman, J. W., and Purves, D. (1980). The elimination of redundant preganglionic innervation to hamster sympathetic ganglion cells in early post-natal life. *J. Physiol.* **1301**, 213–228.

Redfern, P. A. (1970). Neuromuscular transmission in new-born rats. *J. Physiol.* **209**, 701–709.

Shatz, C. J., and Stryker, M. P. (1988). Prenatal tetrodotoxin infusion blocks segregation of retinogeniculate afferents. *Science* **242**, 87–89.

Tavazoie, S. F., and Reid, R. C. (2000). Diverse receptive fields in the lateral geniculate nucleus during thalamocortical development. *Nature Neursci.* **3**, 608–616.

Wang, G. Y., Liets, L. C., and Chalupa, L. M. (2001). Unique functional properties of on and off pathways in the developing mammalian retina. *J. Neurosci.* **21**, 4310–4317.

Williams, R. W., Hogan, D., and Garraghthy, P. E. (1994). Target recognition and visual maps in the thalamus of achiasmatic dogs. *Nature* **367**, 637–639.

Suggested Readings

Crepel, F. (1982). Regression of functional synapses in the immature mammalian cerebellum. *Trends Neurosci.* **5**, 266–269.

Gilbert, C. D. (1998). Adult cortical dynamics. *Physiol Rev.* **78**, 467–485.

Lichtman, J. W., and Colman, H. (2000). Synapse elimination and indelible memory. *Neuron* **25**, 269–278.

Mariani, J. (1983). Elimination of synapses during the development of the central nervous system. *Prog. Brain Res.* **58**, 383–392.

O'Leary, D. D. M., Ruff, N. L., and Duck, R. H. (1994). Development, critical period plasticity, and adult reorganizations of mammalian somatosensory systems. *Curr. Opin. Neurobiol.* **4**, 535–544.

Roskies, A., Friedman, G. C., and O'Leary, D. D. M. (1995). Mechanisms and molecules controlling the development of retinal maps. *Perspect. Dev. Neurobiol.* **3**, 63–75.

Shatz, C. J. (1990). Competitive interactions between retinal ganglion cells during prenatal development. *J. Neurobiol.* **21**, 197–211.

Sur, M., and Leamey, C. A. (2001). Development and plasticity of cortical areas and networks. *Nature Rev. Neurosci.* **2**, 251–262.

Thompson, W. J. (1985). Activity and synapse elimination at the neuromuscular junction. *Cell Mol. Neurobiol.* **5**, 167–182.

Yuste, R., and Sur, S. (1999). Development and plasticity of the cerebral cortex: From Molecules to maps. *J. Neurobiol.* **41**, 1–6.

Wiesel, T. N. (1982). Postnatal development of the visual cortex and the influence of environment. *Nature* **299**, 583–591.

Wong, R. O. L. (1999). Retinal waves and visual system development. *Annu. Rev. Neurosci.* **22**, 29–47.

Rachel O. L. Wong and
Jeffrey W. Lichtman

CHAPTER

21

Early Experience and Critical Periods

The nervous system has evolved to cope with an environment that is in many ways largely predictable. Therefore, much of the structure and function of the brain can be specified by genetic determinants that reflect the common experience of previous generations. Most of this circuitry is established prenatally, guided by genetically determined molecular mechanisms and shaped by patterns of spontaneous impulse activity that propagate through the central nervous system (CNS) in unborn animals, as discussed in Chapters 17–20.

Not all aspects of an animal's world are certain, however: Details of an animal's physical characteristics vary, as do habitats and social conditions. To deal with such uncertainties, the CNS maintains the capacity to modify its connections based on the interactions of an animal with its environment. Through adaptive adjustment based on use or quality of performance, the developing nervous system customizes its connections to the individual animal with a precision that does not need to be, and sometimes cannot be, encoded in the genome.

Although the patterns and strengths of synaptic connections in the nervous system are capable of some degree of adaptive adjustment throughout the lifetime of an animal, many connections pass through a period during early life when the capacity for adjustment in response to experience is substantially greater than it is in adulthood. This period is referred to as a sensitive or critical period. A sensitive period is a developmental stage during which neurons select their permanent repertoire of inputs from a wider array of possible inputs. Tested behaviorally, it is a period during which the properties of

neurons are particularly sensitive to modification by experience.

An extreme form of a sensitive period is referred to as a critical period, a stage when appropriate experience is essential for the normal development of a pathway or a set of connections. During a critical period, a pathway awaits specific instructional information in order to continue developing normally. This information causes the pathway to commit irreversibly to one of a number of possible patterns of connectivity. If appropriate experience is not gained during the critical period, the pathway never attains the ability to process information in a normal fashion and, as a result, perception or behavior is impaired permanently. For example, there are critical periods for the development of form vision and stereopsis in primates (Riesen,1961; Jampolsky, 1978); for the development of appropriate social and emotional responses to members of the same species, referred to as "imprinting," in birds and mammals (Immelmann, 1972; Hess, 1973; Leidermen, 1981); and for the development of language skills in humans (Newport *et al.*, 2001).

Many experimental models are currently being explored in an attempt to understand how early experience transforms the initial wiring plan of the nervous system into the exquisitely precise patterns of connectivity that are required to mediate the behavior of an individual. This chapter discusses four model systems that have been relatively well studied. None of these systems is understood in satisfying detail. Together, however, they illustrate a number of important principles, not the least of which is the profound influence that early experience can exert on the development of the brain and behavior.

SOUND LOCALIZATION: CALIBRATED BY EARLY EXPERIENCE IN THE OWL

A model system that is highly modifiable during development is the sound localization pathway that creates a map of auditory space in the midbrain of the barn owl (Fig. 21.1). This pathway transforms a representation of auditory spatial cues that exists in the central nucleus of the inferior colliculus (ICC; Chapter 26) into a topographic representation of space in the external nucleus of the inferior colliculus (ICX). The auditory map of space is then sent on to the optic tectum, the avian analog of the mammalian superior colliculus, where it aligns with and is integrated with a visual map of space. The function of this pathway is to extract spatial information that can be used to direct orienting movements of the eyes and head toward auditory stimuli (Chapter 33).

The pathway derives the location of a sound source by evaluating spatial cues that are present in the auditory signals at the two ears. For owls, as for most animals, the most important cues for sound localization are interaural timing differences (ITDs) and interaural level differences (ILDs). ITDs arise when one ear is closer than the other to the source of a sound. They are due to the difference in the path length that sound must travel to reach the near versus the far ear. Because the ears are on the sides of the head, ITD varies systematically with the horizontal (azimuthal) location of a sound source (Fig. 21.2A). ILDs result from the fact that each ear is most sensitive to sound coming from certain directions. Consequently, a sound from a particular direction will usually produce a higher sound level in one ear than the other. ILD varies both with the azimuthal and with the elevational location of a sound source in spatial patterns that depend on sound frequency.

In creating the map of auditory space, the nervous system can only roughly anticipate the relationship between encoded values of ITD and ILD and the locations of sound sources that produce them. The correspondence of ITDs and ILDs with locations in space changes with the size and shape of the head and ears, features that vary across individuals, as well as for a given individual during growth. Moreover, the encoded values of sound timing and level that are transmitted to the CNS depend on the relative sensitivity and transduction properties of each ear, which can differ between the two ears. Therefore, to establish and maintain an accurate map of space in the optic tectum, this midbrain pathway must learn the exact relationship between the encoded cue values and the locations of sound sources in space.

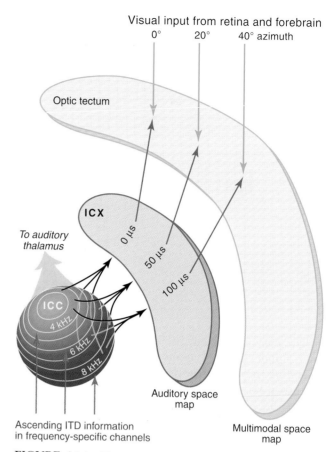

FIGURE 21.1 The ascending auditory pathway to the optic tectum in the barn owl. Auditory inputs enter the optic tectum from the brain stem (bottom arrows); these inputs already encode frequency-specific information about interaural time difference (ITD). These inputs project into the central nucleus of the inferior colliculus (ICC), where they are organized topographically by frequency. Bands in the ICC represent these frequencies (e.g., 4, 6, 8 kHz). Neurons in the ICC convey information both to the auditory thalamus (the primary pathway) and to the external nucleus of the inferior colliculus (ICX). In the ICX, ITD information is combined across frequency channels to synthesize a map of auditory space. For example, an ITD of 0 μs is generated by sound stimuli directly in front of the animal, such that sound reaches the two ears at exactly the same time. At the position marked 0 μs in the ICX are neurons that respond maximally to sounds with an ITD value of 0 μs and thus respond selectively to sounds originating in front of the animal. Sounds originating, for example, from positions that are further to the left-hand side will reach the ears with progressively greater left ear-leading ITDs and thus stimulate neurons with progressively larger best ITDs. From the ICX, the auditory map of space is conveyed via a topographic projection to the optic tectum. Here the auditory map is aligned and merged with a visual map of space (top arrows, representing inputs from the retina and the forebrain) to produce a multimodal space map.

The influence of early experience on the owl's auditory space map has been demonstrated using a variety of techniques that change the relationship between cue values and locations in space: For

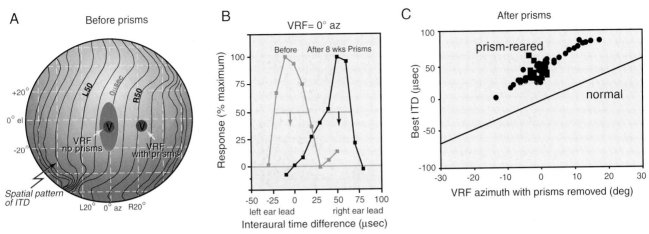

FIGURE 21.2 Rearing owls with laterally displacing, optical prisms causes an adaptive shift in the tuning of neurons in the optic tectum for ITD. (A) This map represents the space in front of the owl, showing both the elevation and the azimuth of a stimulus in space. Contour lines indicate the correspondence of ITD values (in microseconds) with particular locations in space. The point at which the 0° axes intersect represents the point in space directly in front of the owl's head. The auditory (A) and visual (V) receptive fields of one tectal neuron are shown in the center of the map. This neuron responds optimally when the stimulus is directly in front of the animal. Normally, the auditory and visual receptive fields are aligned. Optical prisms induce a horizontal displacement of the neuron's visual receptive field (VRF), resulting in a misalignment between A and V. (B) Tuning for ITD is shifted by prism experience. These ITD tuning curves were recorded from similar sites in the optic tectum before (blue) and after (purple) 8 weeks of prism experience. Both sites had a VRF at 0° azimuth. After 8 weeks of experience, the neuron is tuned for the ITD produced by an acoustic stimulus at the location of the optically displaced VRF, as shown in A. Arrows indicate the best ITD for each site; the best ITD is defined as the center of the range of ITDs to which the neuron responded with more than 50% of its maximum response. (C) The relationship between best ITD and VRF azimuth is shifted systematically from normal in prism-reared owls. The black line indicates the regression of best ITD on VRF azimuth that is observed in normal owls. Dots represent individual sites in a prism-reared owl. The map of ITD is shifted systematically relative to the visual map of space.

example, the external ears have been altered drastically or the auditory canal of one ear has been plugged chronically (Knudsen *et al.*, 1994; Knudsen, 1999). The midbrain pathway responds adaptively to such manipulations by adjusting the tuning of neurons in the ICX and optic tectum to ITDs and ILDs that restore an accurate map of space. In young animals, this plasticity enables the recovery of a substantially normal auditory map even after severe disruptions of hearing. In adult animals, plasticity is far more limited in extent.

An instructive signal that adjusts the tuning of ICX and tectal neurons is provided by the visual system. The instructive role of vision in guiding the tuning of ICX and tectal neurons has been demonstrated in experiments in which owls wear optical displacing prisms that chronically shift the visual field (Knudsen, 1999). Owls cannot counterrotate their eyes (as humans do) to compensate for the prisms. Therefore, to maintain the alignment of the auditory and visual maps of space in the optic tectum, the midbrain pathway learns new associations between auditory cue values and locations in the visual field.

The effect of experience with displacing prisms on auditory spatial tuning is most apparent in the optic tectum, where the visual receptive field of each neuron indicates the location in auditory space to which that neuron should normally be tuned. When prisms that displace the visual field horizontally are placed in front of the eyes, the visual receptive field of a tectal neuron is shifted horizontally and out of alignment with the auditory receptive field of the neuron (Fig. 22.2A). In juvenile birds, continuous experience with such prisms over a period of 6 to 8 weeks causes the auditory receptive fields of tectal neurons to realign with their visual receptive fields: Tectal neurons become tuned to the values of auditory cues that correspond with an auditory stimulus at the location of their optically displaced visual receptive fields (Figs. 21.2B and 21.2C). As a result, the auditory map of space is shifted across the optic tectum to match the optically shifted visual map. This adjustment is adaptive because, by making it, the animal alters its orientation toward sounds so that it sees the source of the sound through the prisms.

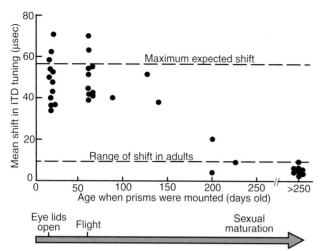

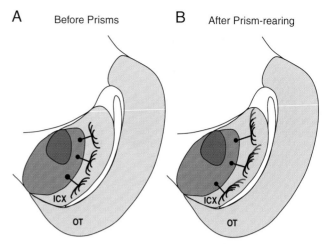

FIGURE 21.3 The sensitive period for visual calibration of neuronal ITD tuning in the optic tectum. Each dot represents data from a single owl. The large arrow below is a time line, indicating important developmental stages in an owl's life. Each owl experienced a 23° displacement of the visual field for at least 60 days. ITD tuning was then measured at 15 to 23 sites in the optic tectum. The difference between the best ITD measured and the best ITD expected normally, based on the location of the site's VRF (see Fig. 21.2C), was taken as the "shift in ITD tuning." The mean shift in ITD tuning for the population of sampled sites as a function of the age of the owl when prisms were first mounted is plotted.

FIGURE 21.4 Schematic model of the change in the pattern of axonal projections from the ICC to the ICX that accompanies the shift in the map of ITD in the ICX. Based on DeBello and Knudsen (2001). (A) The initial state of the projection before prism experience. (B) After prism experience, axonal projections from the ICC to the ICX are shifted systematically as indicated by the red arbors.

This adaptive auditory plasticity is regulated developmentally. The magnitude of the shift in neuronal ITD tuning that can be induced by a prismatic displacement of the visual field depends greatly on the developmental stage of the animal (Fig. 21.3). Large shifts in ITD tuning, of up to 70 μs, occur only in juvenile owls. In adult owls, experience with prisms rarely shifts best ITDs (the ITDs that elicit a maximal neuronal response) by more than 10 μs, even after many months of prism experience. The stage during which prism experience induces large-scale changes in ITD tuning, the sensitive period, ends as the owls approach sexual maturity, at about 200–250 days old.

Although an experience-dependent shift in ITD tuning is observed most easily in the optic tectum (due to the physiological reference provided by the visual receptive field of the neuron), the site in the pathway where the plasticity actually takes place is in the ICX: The maps of ITD in the ICX and in the optic tectum are shifted by equivalent amounts in prism-reared owls, whereas the representation of ITD in the ICC remains unaltered.

The shift of the space map in the ICX is associated with an anatomical change in the pattern of axonal projections from the ICC to the ICX (DeBello *et al.*, 2001). A topographic projection from the ICC to the ICX brings ITD information to the appropriate site in the ICX, where the information is integrated across frequency channels to create spatial receptive fields (Fig. 21.1). A topographic projection is established early in development, before prism experience exerts its effects (Fig. 21.4A). Prism experience causes neurons in the portion of the ICC that represents the shifted values of ITD to project strongly to novel regions of the ICX that then become tuned to those abnormal values of ITD. This novel projection coexists with the normal projection in owls with shifted space maps (Fig. 21.4B). Thus, experience induces the elaboration of axons at sites where they support appropriate responses in the ICX.

The newly learned responses that result from prism experience are mediated differentially by a special class of glutamate receptor, the *n*-methyl-*D*-aspartate receptor (NMDA) receptor. Drugs that specifically block this receptor, such as AP5, eliminate or severely reduce the responses of ICX neurons to the newly learned value of ITD while having substantially less effect on their responses to the normal value. Thus, the expression of newly learned responses in this pathway depends heavily on the activation of NMDA receptors. As shown later, the NMDA receptor plays a critical role in many other examples of experience-dependent plasticity as well.

As mentioned earlier, large shifts in ITD tuning in response to visual field displacement occur only in juvenile owls during a sensitive period. In contrast, removal of prisms from adult owls that have been raised from the day of eye opening wearing prisms results in a shift of the map of ITD back to normal. Thus, the genetically programmed, normal pattern of connectivity persists into adulthood even without validation by experience. In owls that have been raised with prisms, the adult circuit is able to switch back and forth, over a period of weeks, from the abnormal representation of ITD to the normal representation of ITD and *vice versa*, depending on the visual world the animal experiences. In this case, patterns of connectivity learned during the sensitive period, together with the genetically programmed pattern of connectivity, establish the range of connectional states that the circuit can assume later in adult life.

Summary

The location of a sound source is derived by evaluating spatial cues that are present in the auditory signals at the two ears. Interaural timing differences and interaural level differences are used to determine the position of a sound in space. In owls, this information is used to create a map of auditory space, which is aligned closely with a visual map of space in the optic tectum. The process by which these two maps are aligned relies on early experience during a sensitive period in development. The process can be altered by rearing owls with prisms, to shift the position of the visual field, or with ear plugs, which change the relationship between auditory cues and the locations of sound sources in space. Plasticity during the sensitive period involves anatomical changes in axonal projections and requires the func-

tion of the NMDA subtype of glutamate receptor, a molecule that plays a critical role in other examples of experience-dependent plasticity.

BIRDSONG: LEARNED BY EXPERIENCE

The song of most song birds, like human language, is learned early in life during a critical period (Konishi, 1985; Doupe and Kuhl, 1999). Birdsong is a special form of vocal communication used by certain species of birds to identify neighbors, defend territories, and attract mates. Songs are distinguished from other communication sounds by their length, spectral complexity, and periodic structure—properties that give birdsong its melodic quality. The songs sung by birds are characteristic of the species ("conspecific song"); dialects of the species' song often reflect the geographical area in which the bird was raised (Fig. 21.5A).

Songs are passed on from one generation to the next by a combination of genetic instruction and learning. In a few species of song birds, the influence of genetic instruction is strong and learning plays a relatively minor role. In most, however, the role of learning is paramount. Some of these species learn new songs each year ("seasonal learners"), whereas others learn their songs only once during an early critical period.

White-crowned sparrows and zebra finches are model species that learn their songs during a critical period (Immelmann, 1972; Konishi, 1985). The extent of the critical period in each species has been deter-

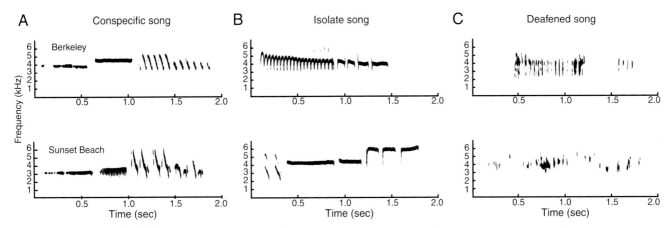

FIGURE 21.5 Songs of white-crowned sparrows. These are sonograms (time–frequency sound spectrograms) of songs from birds with different kinds of early experience. Sound energy in each frequency band is indicated by the darkness of the trace. (A) Song dialects. Birds raised in different areas sing slightly different songs. These dialects are stable for many years and are transmitted by learning. (B) Isolate songs. These simpler songs develop in birds raised in acoustic isolation or in birds that fail to copy a tutor song. (C) Songs of deafened birds. These kinds of songs develop in birds that are deafened after the critical period for song memorization but before the period of vocal learning. The birds need to hear their own voice to develop normal song. From Konishi (1985).

mined by raising birds in acoustic isolation and then exposing them to conspecific song for brief periods in development. The effect of this experience on song learning is assessed by observing the song that the male eventually sings (in these species, only the male sings). Birds raised in acoustic isolation throughout the critical period sing an "isolate" song (Fig. 21.5B) that lacks the spectral and temporal complexity typical of normal song. When baby birds are allowed to hear conspecific song even for a few days during the critical period, however, they memorize that particular song and reproduce it accurately when they later learn to sing.

Song learning in these species illustrates an important principle that pertains to most critical period learning: The nervous system is genetically predisposed to accept only a limited range of potential stimuli as appropriate for learning (Doupe and Kuhl, 1999). For example, baby birds that are allowed to hear only alien songs that differ substantially from their conspecific song develop isolate song, indicating that they reject these distinctly alien songs as models for learning. Even within the range of songs that a bird will learn, it strongly prefers a conspecific song when given a choice of several similar song types. Moreover, babies learn a conspecific song rapidly, whereas they learn slightly different alien songs only after much longer periods of experience. Thus, the pathway responsible for song memorization contains genetically determined filters that require certain spectral and temporal features before the stimulus is accepted as appropriate, and within the range of stimuli that is deemed acceptable, some song patterns are preferred over others.

Song learning involves two components: song memorization and vocal learning. In white-crowned sparrows, these components are separated by many months, whereas in zebra finches, which develop much more rapidly, they overlap. During the critical period for song memorization, according to a current hypothesis, high-order sensory neurons become tuned to respond selectively to the acoustic patterns of the songs that the bird memorizes. During the period of vocal learning, these high-order neurons act as templates for evaluating the bird's own song, guiding the development of song so that it eventually matches the previously memorized song pattern.

A Critical Period Exists for Song Memorization

The critical period for song memorization begins at about 2 weeks of age and lasts for about 8 weeks in both zebra finches and white-crowned sparrows (Immelmann, 1972; Doupe and Kuhl, 1999). Baby birds

that are exposed to a conspecific song before the critical period opens do not learn the song, even though they can hear at this early age. This suggests that the neuronal substrate for song memorization is not yet ready to be shaped by experience. Similarly, babies that do not hear a normal song until after 3–4 months of age do not learn to sing a normal song. Apparently, by this age the influence of experience on the neuronal substrate for song memorization has become reduced greatly.

The time at which the critical period for song memorization closes for a given individual is determined by the individual's own experience. Once the critical period has opened, exposure of a baby bird to normal song for 1 week is sufficient for the bird to learn the song, and subsequent exposure to other songs does not affect the song that the bird comes to sing. For this bird, the critical period closed after a week of experience. If, however, a baby bird is kept in acoustic isolation (or hears only songs that are suboptimal as models for learning) for many weeks past the opening of the critical period and then hears normal song, it learns the normal song. Thus, during the critical period the nervous system waits in a receptive state for appropriate experience-dependent instruction. Once this instruction is received, the nervous system presumably establishes a particular pattern of connectivity that is irreversible, thus closing the critical period.

When a baby bird is deprived continuously of appropriate auditory experience, its capacity to memorize song eventually diminishes with age. Under these conditions, the critical period closes gradually because of additional factors (discussed later) that reduce the plasticity of the relevant pathway. As a bird approaches this age, experience with appropriate stimuli must be richer in order to have an effect. For example, white-crowned sparrows raised in acoustic isolation until 50 days of age no longer memorize songs presented from loudspeakers, but do memorize songs presented by live tutors. Thus, enrichment of the sensory experience provided by social interactions with the tutor overcomes the decline in the facility of the pathway for song learning.

Vocal Learning

Learning to sing requires a combination of vocal practice and auditory feedback. A young bird that is deafened after song memorization but before the onset of vocal learning, and is thereby prevented from hearing its own voice, will not develop a normal song (Fig. 21.5C). Clearly, auditory feedback is essential for shaping the patterns of connectivity in the vocal motor pathway while the bird is learning to sing. Presumably, auditory feedback is necessary for the bird both to learn how motor system commands correspond with the sounds that it produces and to compare the sounds it produces with its memorized song template.

A Neural Pathway Exists for Song Learning

The neural mechanisms that underlie song memorization are being explored in many laboratories but, as yet, we know little about this aspect of song learning. In contrast, a great deal is known about the neural mechanisms that underlie song production. The pathway for song production was identified by its sexual dimorphism in species in which only males sing. In these species, there is a conspicuous network of hypertrophied nuclei, referred to as the song system, that is found only in males (Fig. 21.6). The song system consists of two distinct groups of nuclei: one group in the posterior forebrain that is responsible for song production and another in the anterior forebrain that is critical for vocal learning.

The posterior, vocal motor pathway consists of three serially connected nuclei: the higher vocal center (HVC) and the robust nucleus of the archistriatum (RA) in the forebrain and the hypoglossal nucleus in the brain stem (Fig. 21.6). As a bird prepares to sing, a wave of neural activity spreads from the HVC to the

RA, and finally to the hypoglossal nucleus, which contains the motor neurons that control the vocal musculature. Bilateral lesions of the HVC or the RA leave birds permanently incapable of producing song, although they still can make other kinds of unlearned vocalizations.

The anterior pathway (Fig. 21.6) consists of area X, a thalamic nucleus (DLM), and the lateral portion of the magnocellular nucleus of the anterior neostriatum (LMAN), and is essential for experience-dependent adjustments of song (Brainard and Doupe, 2000). Lesions made in the LMAN of a young bird that is just learning to sing cause a dramatic cessation of song development, freezing the bird's song in an immature state. This freezing of song resembles song crystallization. In adult birds, LMAN lesions result in birds that sing normal songs, but can no longer maintain their songs based on experience.

The anterior pathway apparently provides information to the vocal motor pathway for the purpose of vocal learning. According to one hypothesis, the anterior pathway compares auditory feedback about the song that a bird produces with a stored template of the memorized song. The result of this comparison is then used to instruct the development and maintenance of connections in the vocal motor pathway. Consistent with this hypothesis, area X and the LMAN in the anterior pathway contain neurons that respond maximally to the sound of the bird's own song (Fig. 21.7). During development, axons from the LMAN are the first to innervate the RA in the vocal motor pathway. Information transmitted by the LMAN-RA pathway is mediated predominantly by NMDA receptors, a class of glutamate receptors that, when activated, is known in other systems to induce synaptic plasticity. As birds begin learning to sing, a second set of axons enters the RA from the HVC in the vocal motor pathway and begins making glutamatergic synapses. These later connections may be guided by the activity of the preexisting, LMAN-RA synapses.

Hormonal Regulation of Learning

The period of vocal learning closes as birds reach sexual maturity and circulating levels of steroid hormones rise. Evidence indicates that the abrupt increase in androgen hormones triggers the termination of the period of vocal learning. Exposure of a juvenile bird to high levels of testosterone causes its song to "crystallize" (become stable) prematurely in an abnormal state (Konishi, 1985). Conversely, juvenile birds that are castrated before they learn to sing produce inconsistent song patterns throughout life.

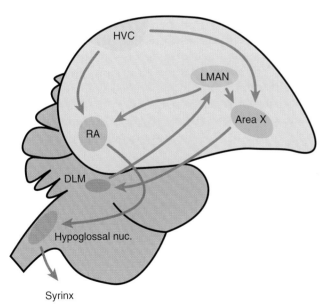

FIGURE 21.6   The song system in songbirds. This is a schematic diagram of a side view of the brain of a songbird. The vocal motor pathway, shown in red, consists of the higher vocal center (HVC), the robust nucleus of the archistriatum (RA), and the hypoglossal nucleus. The anterior pathway, shown in blue, consists of area X, the medial portion of the dorsolateral nucleus of the thalamus (DLM), and the lateral portion of the magnocellular nucleus of the anterior neostriatum (LMAN).

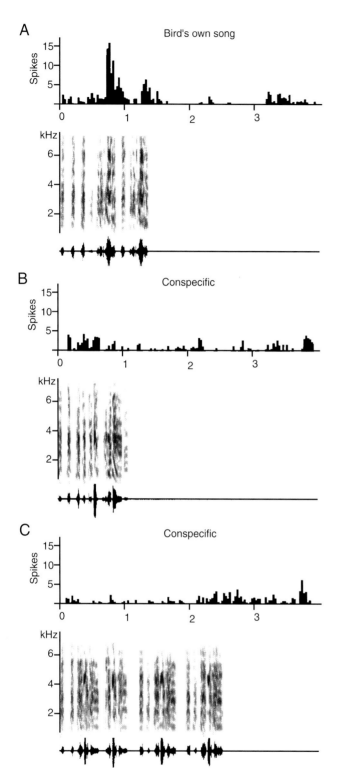

FIGURE 21.7 Selectivity of an LMAN neuron for the bird's own song. In each panel, the upper plot is a peristimulus histogram of spike responses of the neuron to the song stimulus; the middle plot is the sonogram (see Fig. 21.5) of the song; the lower plot is an oscillogram (amplitude waveform) of the song. (A) Strong responses to the bird's own song. (B) This conspecific song elicits a weak response. (C) This conspecific song suppresses the baseline activity of the neuron. From Doupe (1997).

A cellular link between sex hormones and song plasticity has been found in the LMAN. Neurons in the LMAN, as well as in the HVC, RA, and hypoglossal nuclei, bind and accumulate androgens. As the period of vocal learning closes, the density of dendritic spines on LMAN neurons decreases dramatically, suggesting that synaptic selection has taken place. In addition, the total volume of the LMAN regresses precipitously and the influence of LMAN activity on the song motor nuclei declines (Wallhausser-Franke et al., 1995). Thus, the close of the period for vocal learning may be due to synaptic selection and stabilization in the LMAN, triggered by a rise in steroid hormone levels.

Seasonal song learners, such as canaries, appear to recapitulate the process of song memorization and vocal learning each year. This relearning is linked with, and could result from, the waxing and waning of steroid hormone levels. This raises the intriguing possibility that this critical period can be opened and closed by hormonal or environmental factors.

Summary

Song is a learned form of vocal communication used by certain species of birds to attract mates, defend their territories, and identify their neighbors. Songs are learned in two phases: the first is song memorization, in which a song is heard and memorized during a critical period; the second is vocal learning, in which vocal practice and auditory feedback shape the final form of the song during a later period. The neural pathway for song production is sexually dimorphic in many species in which only males sing. A separate pathway, in the anterior forebrain, plays a special role in vocal learning, guiding adjustments in the song production pathway as the bird learns to sing.

FILIAL IMPRINTING: BABIES LEARN TO RECOGNIZE THEIR PARENTS

For many species of birds and mammals, including ducks, geese, mice, and monkeys, parental care is essential for the survival of the young. The young of these species learn rapidly to distinguish their parents from all other individuals and form a unique and close relationship with their parents from that point on—a process referred to as filial imprinting (Hess, 1973). Filial imprinting can involve the learning of visual, auditory, olfactory, and gustatory cues that identify a parent. The learning of these cues takes

A

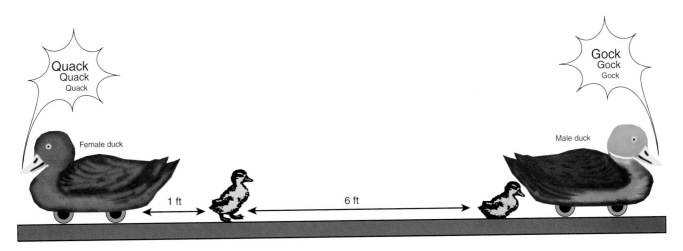

B

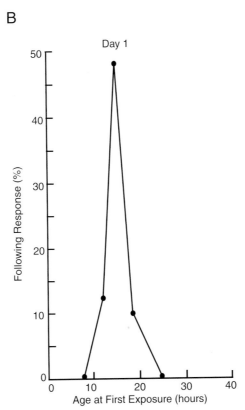

FIGURE 21.8 Filial imprinting. The critical period for imprinting in ducklings occurs during a few hours in the first day of life. Ducklings were exposed once, for 10 min, to one of several models of a male duck. Imprinting was assessed 5 to 70 h later by offering the ducklings a choice between the previously presented model and a model of a female duck and noting which of the models the ducklings followed. (A) This is one of the four different tests that were applied. In this test, the model of the male duck was located much further away than the model of the female duck. This test demonstrated that the duckling would respond to the imprinting object even though the female model was closer and louder. (B) The plot indicates the percentage of ducklings that scored perfectly in the assessment of their following responses to the imprinting model. From Ramsay and Hess (1954).

place during short, well-defined critical periods early in postnatal life.

The visual component of the learning process is usually preceded by auditory, olfactory, and/or gustatory components. In many species, the babies learn to recognize the vocalizations of the mother based on experience that begins before or soon after the animal is born. In addition, babies may learn the odor and/or taste of the mother from the odors and tastes experienced immediately after birth. The recognition of the parent based on acoustic and/or chemical cues helps the young select the correct individual for visual imprinting, once the eyes and nervous system are capable of adequate form vision.

The critical periods for filial imprinting are relatively discrete and can be as short as a few hours in some species (Fig. 21.8). If a baby is deprived of a suitable object for imprinting throughout the critical period, it never learns to respond appropriately to the social signals offered later by a member of its species. If a baby is in contact throughout the critical period only with an individual of another species, as often occurs when animals are raised by humans, the baby will imprint on that individual and may, from then on, ignore members of its own species. In the classic experiments by Konrad Lorenz, for example, baby geese that had been raised by Lorenz from the time of hatching followed him about as if he were their mother.

As in the previous examples of developmental learning, young animals exhibit an innate preference to imprint on normal stimuli. When given a choice, babies in the process of imprinting attend preferentially to images that more closely resemble members of their own species. Thus, when baby ducks are given the choice of imprinting on geese or on people, they imprint on the (duck-like) geese. This predilection is based on genetically programmed preferences for simple, conspicuous features, referred to as sign stimuli by ethologists, that tend to distinguish the species from all others. This implies that the neural circuitry involved in filial imprinting, like that involved in song learning, contains genetically determined neuronal filters that help identify stimuli that are appropriate models for learning. As imprinting proceeds, learning causes these filters to become more selective until ultimately the young are capable of discriminating one individual from all others.

Filial Imprinting Has a Neural Correlate

In one model system, the guinea fowl, changes in neuronal morphology correlate with auditory imprinting. In this species, auditory imprinting causes

neurons in a particular region of the anterior forebrain, the medial neo- and hyperstriatum (MNH), to be activated strongly and specifically by the imprinted acoustic stimulus (Scheich, 1987). In birds that are imprinted, the dendrites of large principal neurons in the MNH exhibit about half the density of spines as do the same class of neurons in animals that are not imprinted on an auditory stimulus. This effect, which is reminiscent of the effect of song learning on the dendrites of LMAN neurons, suggests that, in this pathway, experience during the critical period causes a selective elimination of inputs from a large initial repertoire of inputs. The inputs that are eliminated are presumably those that do not contribute to the representation of the imprinted auditory stimulus.

Summary

Young animals of many species learn rapidly to distinguish their parents from other individuals, a process known as filial imprinting. During a brief, early critical period, animals learn to identify a parent's vocalizations, odor, taste, and/or appearance. Young animals exhibit an innate preference to imprint on stimuli that are characteristic of their own species. This implies that the neural circuitry involved in filial imprinting contains genetically determined neuronal filters that help identify stimuli that are appropriate models for learning.

BINOCULAR VISION

Animals that have eyes oriented forward see a large portion of frontal space with both eyes. Normally, the views of frontal space that are provided by each eye are combined ("fused") into a single binocular percept. Binocular fusion improves the ability to detect weak signals under adverse conditions and enables the ability to see depth on the basis of small disparities in the images on the two retinas, referred to as "stereoscopic vision."

Binocular fusion and stereoscopic vision develop only in animals that experience normal binocular vision during early life (Jampolsky, 1978). Binocular fusion requires that the eyes be aligned properly and that signals from corresponding points on the two retinas (e.g., centers of the foveas) activate the same neurons in the visual cortex. The alignment of the eyes and the convergence of visual inputs onto neurons in the cortex are guided by early experience. For binocular fusion to develop, matched visual inputs from the two eyes must persist throughout a critical period. When this does not occur, as when the eyes are not aligned properly or when the visual input from one eye is substantially degraded relative to that from the other eye, the capacity for binocular fusion may be permanently lost. Under these conditions, animals suppress information coming from one (the weaker) eye, a condition referred to as amblyopia, and they perceive the world in front of them based on inputs from only one eye.

There Is a Critical Period for Binocular Fusion

The critical period for binocular fusion has been explored in monkeys and cats using a variety of manipulations that deprive baby animals of binocular vision. One manipulation, which mimics the effects of a monocular cataract, is suturing closed the lids of one eye (monocular deprivation). Based on the effects of this manipulation, the critical period for binocular fusion in kittens lasts approximately the first 3 months of postnatal life. If a kitten experiences monocular deprivation for just a few weeks during this period, visually guided behaviors mediated by the deprived eye are impaired severely and permanently. In con-

trast, an equivalent visual impairment experienced after the end of the critical period has no apparent effect on binocular fusion. Similar critical periods occur in monkeys and humans.

Experience Shapes Ocular Representation in the Visual Cortex

In the mammalian nervous system, visual information from the two eyes first comes together at the level of the primary visual cortex (Chapter 27). Visual experience during a critical period determines how much of the visual cortex is devoted to processing input from each eye and the degree to which binocular inputs are combined (Hubel and Wiesel, 1970; Hubel *et al.*, 1977).

Early in ontogeny, and in many species before birth, afferents that provide inputs from the left and right eyes, respectively, begin to cluster in separate, interleaved areas in layer 4 of the visual cortex. This early clustering of eye-specific inputs from the lateral geniculate nucleus (LGN) is driven by a combination of molecular mechanisms and patterns of spontaneous neuronal activity, as described in Chapter 20.

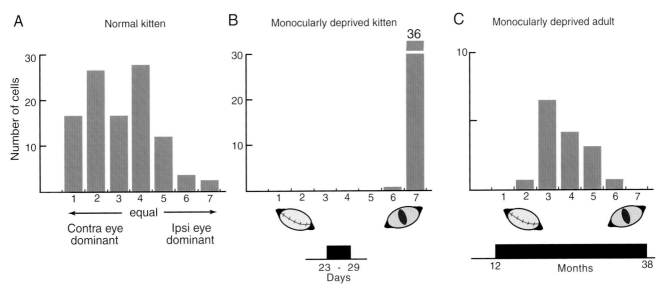

FIGURE 21.9 Effect of chronic closure of one eye on the responsiveness of visual cortical neurons to input from each eye. (A) Ocular dominance distribution in the primary visual cortex of two normal kittens, 3 to 4 weeks old. Cells in group 1 were driven only by the contralateral eye; for group 2, the contralateral eye was markedly dominant; for group 3, the contralateral eye was slightly dominant; for group 4, there was no apparent difference in the drive from the two eyes; for group 5, the ipsilateral eye dominated slightly; for group 6, it dominated markedly; and for group 7, cells were driven only by the ipsilateral eye. (B) Ocular dominance distribution was altered dramatically in a kitten exposed to contralateral eye closure for 1 week (from 23 to 29 days of age). (C) Ocular dominance distribution was essentially normal in an adult cat exposed to contralateral eye closure for 26 months. From Hubel and Wiesel (1970).

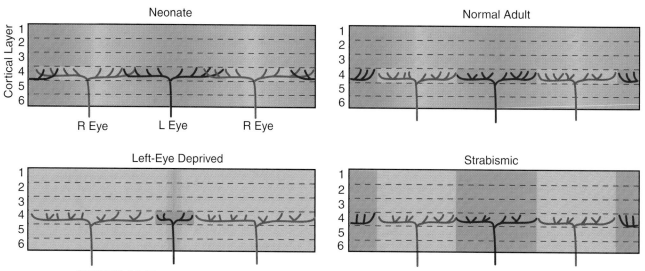

FIGURE 21.10 Schematic diagram of the effects of visual experience on ocular representation in the primary visual cortex of monkeys. Right eye input is represented as red; left eye input is represented as dark purple. Neonate: LGN afferents representing the left and right eyes, respectively, terminate in layer 4 in alternating zones that overlap slightly at the beginning of a critical period when visual experience influences ocular representation in the primary visual cortex. Neurons in the upper and lower layers of the cortex are driven by input from either eye, with the relative strength of the left eye and right eye inputs varying systematically across the cortex. Normal adult: With normal visual experience throughout a critical period, columnar representations of the left and right eyes are sharpened and stabilized. Left eye deprived: After chronic closure of the left eye during this critical period, the termination zones of LGN afferents from the left eye have decreased, whereas those of LGN afferents from the right eye have expanded. Most neurons in the upper and lower layers are driven by input from the right eye. Strabismic: After chronic misalignment of the eyes during this critical period, the termination zones of LGN afferents from the left and right eyes have become completely segregated from each other and equal in size. Neurons in all cortical layers are driven by input from only one eye or the other.

Soon after birth, a critical period opens during which visual experience influences the competition among LGN afferents for territory in layer 4. As long as the eyes are coordinated and used equally, the normal final state, consisting of equally wide ocular dominance columns, is achieved (Figs. 21.9A and 21.10). If, however, vision is impaired in one eye, due to monocular lid closure in an experimental animal or to a cataract in a human, for example, the balance between LGN afferents in their competition for layer 4 territory is disrupted: LGN afferents that convey input from the impaired eye lose the ability to drive layer 4 neurons in an abnormally large region of the cortex, whereas LGN afferents that convey input from the normal eye gain the ability to drive layer 4 neurons in an abnormally large portion of the cortex. As a consequence, activity throughout most of the visual cortex becomes driven by LGN afferents from the normal eye (Figs. 21.9B and 21.10).

The competition between LGN afferents for the control of layer 4 neurons is in a state of dynamic equilibrium throughout the critical period. Afferents from a previously deprived eye can regain territory in layer 4 if the lids of the deprived eye are opened and the lids of the previously open eye are sutured closed, a procedure referred to as "reverse suture."

Anatomical correlates of the functional takeover of layer 4 neurons by inputs from one eye are found in the patterns of LGN afferent terminations in layer 4. In animals that experience monocular impairment during the critical period, layer 4 termination zones for afferents from the deprived eye shrink whereas those from the nondeprived eye expand. At the cellular level, axons conveying input from the deprived eye decrease in total length and branch less in layer 4 compared to normal, whereas axons conveying input from the nondeprived eye branch even more profusely than normal (Fig. 21.10).

Most neurons in the layers above and below layer 4 are normally driven binocularly, with the relative dominance of left eye versus right eye inputs varying systematically across the cortex (Fig. 21.10). Ocular

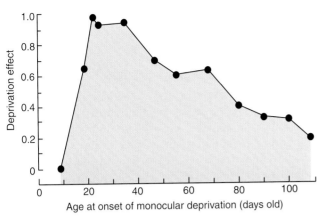

FIGURE 21.11 The critical period for ocular representation in the primary visual cortex of the cat. The degree of functional disconnection of cortical neurons from the deprived eye is quantified and plotted as a function of the kitten's age at the time of monocular closure. Chronic monocular closure lasted 10 to 12 days. Each point represents data from a single animal. Functional disconnection was based on the ocular dominance distribution (see Fig. 21.9) and indicated the degree to which the influence of the closed eye was weakened or lost. The index was defined such that the mean value for normal cats was 0, whereas total disconnection resulted in a value of 1. From Olson and Freeman (1980).

dominance in these upper and lower layers is determined not only by the relative amounts of activity originating from the left and right eyes but also by the temporal correlation of that activity. Misalignment of the eyes (strabismus), which can be induced experimentally by cutting the medial rectus muscles, leads to equal visual stimulation of the two eyes, but a loss of synchrony of activity from the two eyes that results from the animal viewing the same objects with both eyes. If the eyes are strabismic during the critical period, cortical ocular dominance columns develop and are of normal width, but binocular responses in the upper and lower layers are lost permanently (Fig. 21.10). The crucial role of synchronous binocular activity in the development of cortical binocular responses has been demonstrated directly in kittens by blocking neural activity from both eyes (by injecting the eyes with tetrodotoxin) and by imposing various patterns of activity on the optic nerves by electrical stimulation (Lein and Shatz, 2001). When both optic nerves are stimulated synchronously, neurons in the cortex remain binocularly driven. In contrast, when the left and right optic nerves are stimulated equally but asynchronously, neurons in the cortex become monocularly driven with approximately equal numbers of neurons responding to each eye.

Cellular mechanisms by which the amount and synchrony of synaptic activity might shape the func-

tional and anatomical architecture of the visual cortex are described in Chapter 20. In brief, they include the adjustment of synaptic strength, by both long-term potentiation and long-term depression, through a process that depends on the activation of NMDA receptors in the cortex. In addition, the anatomical remodeling of LGN axons, which underlies ocular dominance column formation in layer 4, depends on the availability of neurotrophins—BDNF and NT-4—as well as on the expression of their cognate receptor, TrkB (Lein and Shatz, 2001).

A Critical Period for Ocular Representation Exists in the Visual Cortex

The critical period for ocular representation in the visual cortex has been studied particularly carefully in cats by measuring the age dependence of the effects of monocular lid closure (Fig. 21.11). The onset of the critical period is rapid, beginning at about 3 weeks in cats. By 4 to 6 weeks of age, the cortex is maximally sensitive to monocular deprivation: A few days of monocular deprivation causes a complete shift in ocular dominance, leaving the cortex almost entirely driven by input from the nondeprived eye. Beyond 6 weeks of age, the critical period gradually closes: Over the next 10 months, the rate at which ocular dominance can be shifted by monocular deprivation and the degree to which it can be shifted both decrease. Once a cat is about 1 year old, monocular deprivation even for months no longer affects ocular dominance in the cortex. Similar critical periods, but extending later in life, exist for the visual cortex in monkeys and humans.

The close of the critical period in cats can be delayed substantially by raising animals in complete darkness. At the beginning of the critical period, most cortical neurons respond to inputs from either eye, but the responses tend to be weak (Fig. 21.10). In cats that are raised in the dark until well past the end of the critical period (as defined by monocular occlusion), cortical neurons continue to be driven binocularly and their responses remain weak. When these animals are finally allowed visual experience, the responses of these neurons gradually increase in strength and the relative representation of left eye and right eye inputs in the cortex is shaped by the animal's experience: In monocularly deprived cats, nondeprived eye inputs become predominant in the cortex, and in cats that experience binocular vision, normal ocular dominance columns develop. This indicates that the critical period has remained open. Thus, without experience-driven input, the mecha-

BOX 21.1

CRITICAL PERIODS IN HUMANS

Many human capabilities depend critically on experience gained during early life. These capabilities range from fundamental capacities, such as stereoscopic vision, visual acuity, and binocular coordination, to high-level capacities, such as social behavior, language, and the ability to perceive forms and faces. In each case, normal experience during a restricted period in early life is essential for the normal development of the capacity. The rules that govern these critical periods appear to be the same as those that govern critical periods in other animals, as described in the text.

The best known and most thoroughly studied critical period in humans is for language (Newport *et al.*, 2001). A clear relationship exists between the age of exposure to a language and the level of proficiency achieved in that language. This relationship holds for the learning of both first and second languages. Acquisition of a first language has been assessed in children who have been raised in the absence of any language (feral or abused children) or, more frequently, in congenitally deaf children who have been raised without the aid of sign language. Much more data are available for people who began learning a second language at different ages. For both first and second languages, a thorough command of the language is attained by those who learn the language before 7 years of age. The degree of language proficiency that is eventually achieved decreases progressively with age of exposure and reaches adult levels by the end of adolescence.

Only certain aspects of language are affected by learning during critical periods (Newport *et al.*, 2001; Kuhl, 2000). Full proficiency with grammar (the classes of words, their functions and relations in a sentence), syntax (the way in which words are put together in a sentence), and the production and comprehension of phonetics (the speech sounds of a language) are each dependent on early exposure to language. In contrast, semantics (word meaning) and size of vocabulary are not affected by the age of exposure. Thus, critical periods seem to affect the formal and subtle aspects of language, whereas the capacity to learn new words and their meanings continues unabated throughout life.

Physiological measures reveal an age dependence in the way in which language is processed and represented in the brain (Weber-Fox and Neville, 1996; Dehaena *et al.*, 1997). Various techniques have been used to assess brain activity while human subjects make perceptual judgements in language tasks. These techniques include functional magnetic resonance imaging, position emission

tomography, and event-related potentials. In normal adults, language is processed in specific areas, primarily in the left or "dominant" hemisphere. In people who have learned a second language pior to the age of 7 years, the brain areas that are involved in processing the first and second languages overlap extensively. In contrast, in people who have learned a second language later in life, the areas of the brain that are activated by the second language do not overlap, or they overlap little, with those that are activated by the first language: brain areas activated by language are less lateralized to the left hemisphere and are more variable across subjects. The effect of age at the time of learning on the brain areas activated by language is far more conspicuous for tasks requiring grammatical and phonic judgements than for tasks requiring semantic judgements. Thus, consistent with the behavioral observations, described earlier, of the age dependence for learning grammar and phonetics, the regions of the brain that contribute to the processing of grammar and phonetics are shaped in a unique way during critical periods.

Detailed knowledge of the mechanisms that control critical periods and of the plasticity that occurs during critical periods will provide a basis for formulating optimal therapeutic procedures to help minimize long-term harmful effects of early abnormal experience, associated with neonatal and childhood disabilities, for example, and maximize the acquisition of normal function once normal conditions are restored. Such knowledge may also lead to improved methods of rearing and teaching normal children that take advantage of the full capacity of the central nervous system to learn from experience.

Eric I. Knudsen

References

Dehaena, S., Doupoux, E., Mehler, J., Cohen, L., Perani, D., van de Moortele, P.-F., Leherici, S., and Le Bihan, D. (1997). Anatomical variability in the cortical representation of first and second languages. *Neuroreport* **17**, 3809–3815.

Kuhl, P. K. (2000). A new view of language acquisition. *Proc. Natl. Acad. Sci. USA* **97**,d 11850–11857.

Newport, E. L., Bavelier, D., and Neville, H. J. (2001). Critical thinking about critical periods: Perspectives on a critical period for language acquisition. *In* "Language, Brain and Cognitive Development: Essays in Honor of Jacques Mehler" (E. Doupoux, ed.), pp. 481–502. MIT Press, Cambridge, MA.

Weber-Fox, and Neville, H. J. (1996). Maturarional constraints on functional specializations for luanguage processing: ERP and behavioral evidence in bilingual speakers. *J. Cognit. Neurosci.* **8**, 231–256.

nisms that control ocular representation in the cortex remain in an uncommitted state, waiting for instruction for a prolonged, if not indefinite, period of time.

The critical period for ocular representation in the cortex is atypical in one respect: There is no predisposition to establish a normal pattern of connectivity based on normal experience. Even after baby cats or monkeys have experienced normal binocular vision for several weeks, monocular deprivation still causes the responses in the cortex to become dominated by the nondeprived eye. Moreover, once the responses in the cortex become dominated by one eye, reinstating normal visual input to the previously deprived eye does not restore normal binocular responses in the cortex (Fig. 21.9B). Instead, the nondeprived eye continues to dominate the responses of cortical neurons for as long as animals have been studied (up to 5 years after restoration of binocular input). Thus, unlike in the cases of bird song learning and filial imprinting, the pattern of neural connectivity that supports normal function in the visual cortex is not stabilized immediately by exposure to normal binocular input. Instead, normal binocular vision must persist throughout the entire critical period to prevent the cortex from becoming dominated by monocular responses. An adaptive advantage of this characteristic of the binocular pathway has yet to be recognized.

Summary

Binocular fusion occurs when signals from corresponding points on the two retinas activate the same neurons in visual cortex, a process that is guided by early experience. During prenatal development and before the onset of vision, inputs from the left and right eyes segregate from each other to form ocular dominance columns of roughly equal width in the visual cortex. Soon after birth, a critical period opens during which the visual experience of the animal has a dramatic effect on the representation of the eyes in the cortex. If vision is normal, the established patterns of ocular representation are consolidated and refined. If vision is impaired in one eye, due perhaps to a cataract, inputs carrying information from the deprived eye shrink and those from the normal eye expand. If synchronous visual stimulation of the two eyes is disrupted, as in strabismus, ocular dominance columns develop and are of normal width, but neurons in the upper and lower layers fail to develop binocular responses. The end of the critical period can be delayed by rearing animals in complete darkness.

PRINCIPLES OF DEVELOPMENTAL LEARNING

During the later stages in the development of neural pathways, patterns of neuronal activity, driven by stimuli or the animal's behavior, shape the strength and patterns of connections that are being formed between neurons. From a range of possible patterns of connectivity, the shaping process selects a pattern that is appropriate for the individual's experience.

For some pathways, the influence of experience-driven activity is not critical; it simply adjusts and fine-tunes connections that are largely genetically determined. This is the case with the owl's auditory space processing pathway, which can return to a genetically programmed, normal pattern of connectivity throughout the animal's life, once the animal experiences normal sensory input.

For other pathways, however, genetic programming is less specific or persistent, and experience is essential for the selection of one particular set of connections over all others. Such pathways, which include the song pathway in birds and the pathways that subserve filial imprinting and binocular vision, depend on specific instruction during a critical period to make a commitment to a pattern of connectivity that is appropriate for the individual.

Such developmental learning is distinguished from learning that can occur in adults by the magnitude and the permanence of the changes. Developmental learning can cause large-scale changes in the anatomy and/or functional response properties of neurons—well beyond the range of changes that occur in adults. Moreover, changes that result from early experience often persist throughout the lifetime of an animal.

Developmental learning is influenced heavily by genetic predisposition. Only a limited range of stimuli is allowed to operate as an instructive influence for a particular pathway; within this acceptable range, some stimuli are preferred over others. The predisposition of the nervous system to be instructed by "normal" experience probably originates in the selectivity of the response properties, genetically determined as well as shaped by experience, of the neurons that provide input to the sites in the pathway where the adjustments take place. As learning progresses, the selectivity of the pathway for acceptable input becomes progressively higher.

Whether a particular pathway passes through a critical period can vary across species. For example, some songbirds, such as canaries and mockingbirds, learn new songs seasonally throughout life, whereas others, such as white-crowned sparrows and zebra finches, learn their songs only during a critical period. Such species differences may provide a useful tool for uncovering the mechanisms that are responsible for critical periods.

The magnitude of changes that may result from experience-driven adjustments varies greatly across pathways and across species. The magnitude of changes depends on the degree of genetic specification of the inputs to the site of change. When the selection of appropriate inputs is from a large potential range of inputs, the effect of experience can have a profound influence on a pathway. Conversely, when the range of potential inputs is highly restricted by genetic specification, the effect of experience is correspondingly small.

The duration of different critical periods also varies greatly. At one end of the spectrum are the critical periods for imprinting, which may open and close within hours (Fig. 21.8). At the other end are critical periods for acquiring complex cognitive capabilities, such as language (described in Chapter 52), which may involve several component critical periods. These are highly variable across individuals and may last for many years.

Deprivation Prolongs Critical Periods

Critical periods close once an animal receives adequate experience. When the animal is deprived of appropriate experience, the critical period is prolonged. For example, raising songbirds in acoustic isolation extends the critical period for song memorization, and raising cats in complete darkness extends the critical period for ocular representation in the visual cortex. This characteristic of critical periods indicates that the event that triggers critical period adjustments is the powerful and repeated activation of neurons at the site where changes take place. Without the vigorous activation of these neurons, the pathway remains in an uncommitted state and capable of adjusting in response to experience when it becomes available. This characteristic suggests that for young animals (including humans) suffering from a peripheral or central abnormality, no input is better than abnormal input. This implies that the optimal therapeutic strategy for such individuals is to deprive them of relevant sensory input until the abnormality can be corrected. Otherwise, an abnormal sensory experience may close the critical period, resulting in a commitment to an abnormal pattern of connectivity that cannot later be reversed.

Developmental Learning Has a Cellular Basis

Experience-driven changes in neural connectivity can involve the remodeling of axons and dendrites, the elaboration of new synapses, and/or the regulation of synaptic efficacy. Neuronal remodeling and the establishment of new synapses could be guided by the same mechanisms that control synaptogenesis during ontogeny (Chapter 18). Neurotrophins (described in Chapter 19), for example, could regulate axonal elaboration based on experience-driven activity if they were secreted by highly active postsynaptic neurons and were taken up selectively by recently active, presynaptic axonal arbors. Uptake of neurotrophins by active arbors would induce them to grow and elaborate new synaptic connections, whereas inactive arbors would regress due to inadequate trophic support. Evidence for this hypothesis has been found in the visual cortex (Lein and Shatz, 2001).

Changes in connectivity patterns could also involve the regulation of synaptic efficacy within the preexisting synaptic repertoire of a neuron. The mechanisms that regulate synaptic strength include those that underlie synaptic plasticity in the adult nervous system (Chapter 50). Long-term potentiation (LTP) and long-term depression (LTD), for example, have been shown to operate in many models of developmental learning. Moreover, the ubiquitous presence of NMDA receptors, which are known to participate in LTP and LTD, at sites of change in the various models of developmental learning indicates that this class of glutamate receptor plays a key role in adjusting patterns of connectivity during sensitive periods.

Opening of Critical Periods Depends on Neuronal Maturation

Critical periods cannot open until the relevant neural pathways have developed to a point where they can support plasticity. An inability to support plasticity may be caused by the absence of adequate neuronal connectivity, neurotransmitters, receptors, or second-messenger systems. In addition, critical periods cannot open until the nervous system is capable of conveying the information that will be used to shape the patterns of connectivity. For example, critical periods that involve form vision cannot open until afferent activity encodes visual spatial information in adequate detail. This dependence implies that critical periods for regions of the brain that process high-level information cannot open until relevant information from lower level areas is sufficiently precise and reliable. The reliable encoding of low-level information may, in turn, depend on earlier critical period experience. Thus, the development of complex capabilities may involve cascades of critical periods affecting different levels of processing at different ages.

The Closing of Critical Periods May Involve Several Mechanisms

Critical periods end once an individual has received adequate experience and the relevant pathway is irreversibly committed to a particular pattern of connectivity. The factors that render the commitment irreversible are not known. Many factors may play a role and the factors that are most important may differ across different pathways.

One factor is that the molecular mechanisms that support changes in synaptic efficacy (described in Chapter 50), such as LTP and LTD, may be altered permanently as a consequence of adequate experience or age. Evidence supporting this possibility comes again from the visual cortex. As the critical period for ocular representation in layer 4 ends, the abundance of NMDA receptors decreases sharply in layer 4 and the kinetic properties of NMDA receptors change, making them less effective in modifying synaptic efficacy. In addition, the effect of stimulating metabotropic glutamate receptors, which also play a role in regulating synaptic efficacy, changes markedly as the critical period closes.

A second factor is that the capacity for large-scale neuronal growth may be lost as the critical period closes. In those pathways in which axonal elaboration is a necessary component of experience-based changes in connectivity, loss of the mechanisms that support axonal growth would end the critical period. In the visual cortex of cats, for example, levels of the growth-associated protein GAP-43, which is thought to be necessary for axonal growth, decrease precipitously during the critical period. A loss of responsiveness of presynaptic axonal arbors to neurotrophins secreted by postsynaptic neurons would also diminish the capacity for axonal elaboration. Indeed, in the visual cortex of ferrets, receptors for neurotrophins that mediate axonal remodeling are transformed from an active into an inactive form as the critical period ends (Lein and Shatz, 2001).

A third factor is the sharpening of functional tuning that results from experience. Initially in development, neuronal responses are relatively weak and broadly tuned. Experience causes selective changes in anatomical connections and synaptic efficacy, as described earlier, that refine the patterns of both excitatory and inhibitory connectivity. These changes are self-reinforcing due to the action of self-organizational mechanisms that operate by Hebbian principles (Chapter 50). As a result, once a circuit has been shaped to process information in a certain way, it becomes far more difficult for altered experience to induce new patterns of connectivity.

Each of the aforementioned mechanisms could be enabled by the repeated, vigorous activation of postsynaptic neurons. Hence, they could explain the resistance of a pathway to further change following exposure to adequate experience. In addition, these mechanisms could be enabled as a function of the animal's age.

A host of other factors impede anatomical and/or functional change that accompany the aging process and, therefore, could contribute to the irreversibility of critical period learning: the myelination of axons, preventing them from growing or retracting; the stabilization of synapses by the extracellular matrix or by proteoglycans; the appearance of molecules that prevent growth; and the disappearance of molecules that enable growth. Also, the action of inhibitory circuits, which become effective relatively late in development, can either enable or impede plasticity.

Attention and arousal also influence critical period plasticity. Without adequate attention to the stimulus or arousal from the experience, experience-dependent changes do not take place. Even after a critical period has ended under standard conditions, heightening an animal's attention or arousal can still trigger learning, as exemplified by birdsong learning from live tutors after learning from tape-recorded songs no longer takes place. Therefore, an age-dependent decrease in the release of the neuromodulators norepinephrine (NE) and acetylcholine (ACh), which mediate the effects of arousal and attention, or in the responsiveness of neurons to these molecules could diminish the capacity of experience to induce changes. In the cat visual cortex, depletion of NE and ACh has been shown to decrease ocular dominance plasticity. Conversely, administration of NE to the visual cortex of adult cats increases its modifiability.

Finally, an increase in sex hormones may, directly or indirectly, bring developmental learning to an end independent of experience. In many examples of developmental learning, the capacity for change declines abruptly when animals reach sexual maturity. This is the case for adjustments in the auditory space map in owls and for song learning in birds. Steroid hormones, particularly, estrogen, are known to regulate the density of synapses and various neurotransmitter receptors, the kinetics of NMDA receptors, and the responsiveness of neurons to sensory stimulation. An increase in steroid hormone levels or the expression of hormone receptors on neurons could trigger mechanisms in neurons that make them resistant to further large-scale changes.

Summary

Developmental learning occurs at all levels in the nervous system to shape the functional properties of pathways in response to the experience of the individual. In pathways that pass through a sensitive period, experience-driven activity has the opportunity to specify, from a range of possible patterns of connectivity, the pattern that is optimal for the individual's experience. For many pathways, information gained from this experience is essential for guiding the normal development of the pathway. In such cases, this highly plastic period is referred to as a critical period.

Learning that occurs during a critical period is distinguishable from learning that occurs in adult animals in several respects. First, the changes occur readily only during a restricted period in the lifetime of the animal. Second, critical period learning involves the selection of a particular pattern of connectivity from a range of possible patterns. For example, a baby imprints on a particular individual as its parent, or a songbird selects particular songs to learn to sing. Third, changes in the nervous system that occur during critical periods persist throughout life.

Critical periods vary in timing and duration across pathways and across species; some last only a few hours, whereas others last until the individual reaches sexual maturity. Critical periods open once the information conveyed to a pathway is sufficiently precise and the pathway is competent to support plastic change. The signal that induces change is probably the repeated, vigorous activation of postsynaptic neurons by presynaptic activity representing the occurrence of an appropriate stimulus or the execution of adaptive behavior. The range of stimuli that are effective in driving plastic change is specified by genetic preprogramming, with most pathways biased heavily to prefer normal patterns of stimulation. Critical periods close once an irreversible commitment to a pattern of connectivity has been made. This commitment can be triggered by the experience itself or it can occur eventually as a consequence of age.

Closure of a critical period is defined by a dramatic decrease in the plasticity of a system. The mechanisms that close a critical period probably vary for different pathways. When experience-induced changes require anatomical remodeling, the end of the critical period may be controlled by factors that regulate cell growth. Alternatively, when the induced changes require adjustments in synaptic efficacy, the critical period will be controlled by factors that influence the capacity of synapses to modify their efficacy. At this time, however, the specific mechanisms that are responsible for closing a particular critical period remain unknown.

References

Brainard, M. S., and Doupe, A. J. (2000). Auditory feedback in learning and maintenance of vocal behaviour. *Nature Rev. Neurosci.* **1**, 31–40.

DeBello, W. M., Feldman, D. E., and Knudsen, E. I. (2001). Adaptive axonal remodeling in the midbrain auditory space map. *J. Neurosci.* **21**, 3161–3174

Doupe, A. J. (1997). Song- and order-selective neurons in the songbird anterior forebrain and their emergence during vocal development. *J. Neurosci.* **17**, 1147–1167.

Doupe, A. J., and Kuhl, P. K. (1999). Birdsong and human speech: Common themes and mechanisms. *Annu. Rev. Neurosci.* **22**, 567–631.

Hess, E. H. (1973). "Imprinting: Early Experience and the Developmental Psychobiology of Attachment." Van Nostrand-Reinhold, New York.

Hubel, D. H., and Wiesel, T. N. (1970). The period of susceptibility to the physiological effects of unilateral eye closure in kittens. *J. Physiol.* (*Lond.*) **206**, 419–436.

Hubel, D., Wiesel, T., and LeVay, S. (1977). Plasticity of ocular dominance columns in the monkey striate cortex. *Philos. Trans. R. Soc. Lond. Ser. B* **278**, 377–409.

Immelmann, K. (1972). Sexual imprinting in birds. *Adv. Study Behav.* **4**, 147–174.

Jampolsky, A. (1978). Unequal visual inputs and strabismus management: A comparison of human and animal strabismus. In Symposium on Strabismus. *Trans. New Orleans Acad. Ophthalmol.* **26**, 358–492.

Knudsen, E. I. (1999). Mechanisms of experience-dependent plasticity in the auditory localization pathway of the barn owl. *J. Comp. Physiol. A* **185**, 305–321.

Knudsen, E. I., Esterly, S. D., and Olsen, J. F. (1994). Adaptive plasticity of the auditory space map in the optic tectum of adult and baby barn owls in response to external ear modification. *J. Neurophysiol.* **71**, 79–94.

Konishi, M. (1985). Birdsong: From behavior to neuron. *Annu. Rev. Neurosci.* **8**, 125–170.

Leiderman, P. (1981). Human mother-infant social bonding: Is there a sensitive phase? *In* "Behavioral Development" (K. Immelmann, G. W. Barlow, L. Petrinovich, and M. Main, eds.), pp. 454–468. Cambridge Univ. Press, Cambridge.

Lein, E. S., and Shatz, C. J. (2001). Neurotrophins and refinement of visual circuitry. *In* "Synapses" (W. M. Cowan, T. C. Sudhog, and C. F. Stevens, eds.), pp. 613–649. Johns Hopkins Univ. Press, Baltimore, MD.

Newport, E. L., Bavelier, D., and Neville, H. J. (2001). Critical thinking about critical periods: Perspectives on a critical period for language acquisition. *In* "Language, Brain and Cognitive Development: Essays in Honor of Jacques Mehler" (E. Doupoux, ed.), pp. 481–502. MIT Press, Cambridge, MA.

Olson, C. R., and Freeman, R. D. (1980). Profile of the sensitive period for monocular deprivation in kittens. *Exp. Brain Res.* **39**, 17–21.

Ramsay, A. O., and Hess, E. H. (1954). A laboratory approach to the study of imprinting. *Wilson Bull.* **66**, 196–206.

Riesen, A. (1961). Stimulation as a requirement for growth and function in behavioral development. *In* "Functions of Varied Experience" (D. W. Fiske and S. R. Maddi, eds.), pp. 57–105. Dorsey Press, Homewood, IL.

Scheich, H. (1987). Neural correlates of auditory filial imprinting. *J. Comp. Physiol. A* **161**, 605–619.

Wallhausser-Franke, E., Nixdorf-Bergweiler, B. E., and DeVoogd, T. J. (1995). Song isolation is associated with maintaining high spine frequencies on zebra finch LMAN neurons. *Neurobiol. Learn. Mem.* **64**, 25–35.

Eric I. Knudsen

SENSORY SYSTEMS

Fundamentals of Sensory Systems

In bringing information about the world to an individual, sensory systems perform a series of common functions. At its most basic, each system responds with some specificity to a stimulus and each employs specialized cells—the peripheral receptors—to translate the stimulus into a signal that all neurons can use. Because of their physical or chemical specialization, the many types of receptors transduce the energy in light, sound, mechanical, or thermal stimulation into a change in membrane potential. That initial electrical event begins the process by which the central nervous system (CNS) constructs an orderly representation of the body and of things visible or audible. To bridge the distance between peripheral transduction and central representation, messages are carried along lines dedicated to telling the CNS what has taken place in the external world and where it has happened. Such precision requires that labor be divided among neurons so that not only different stimulus energies (light vs sound vs mechanical deformation of skin or hair) but also different stimulus qualities (e.g., low-frequency flutter vs high-frequency vibration in the somatosensory system) are analyzed by separate groups of neurons.

In addition to their organization along labeled lines, sensory systems perform common types of operations. Foremost among these is the ability of each system to compare events that occur simultaneously at different receptors, a process that serves to bring out the greatest response where the difference in stimulus strength (contrast) is greatest. At late stages in sensory processing, systems make comparisons with past events and with sensations received by other sensory systems. These comparisons are the fundamental bases of perception, recognition, and comprehension.

This chapter gives an overview of the functional attributes and patterns of organization displayed by the somatosensory, auditory, and visual systems and outlines the physiological and anatomical principles common to all sensory systems. When variations on a common theme exist, they are discussed with the goal of bringing the general pattern into sharper focus.

SENSATION AND PERCEPTION

The Function of Each Sensory System Is to Provide the CNS with a Representation of the External World

Because of the changes that occur around an individual, each sensory system has the task of providing a constantly updated representation of the external world. Accomplishing this task is no simple feat because it requires a close interaction between ascending or stimulus-driven mechanisms and descending or goal-directed mechanisms. Together these two mechanisms evoke sensations, give rise to perceptions, and activate stored memories to form the basis of conscious experience. Ascending mechanisms begin with the activity of peripheral receptors, which together form an initial neural representation of the external world. Descending mechanisms work to sort out from the large amount of sensory input those events that require immediate attention. In doing so, the descending mechanisms alter ascending inputs in ways that optimize perception.

Perception of a sensory experience can change even though the input remains the same. A classic example is seen in the image of a vase that can also be perceived as two faces, pointed nose to nose (Fig. 22.1).

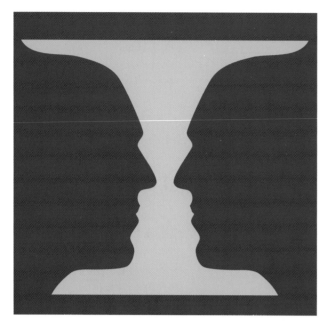

FIGURE 22.1 An example of a figure that can elicit different perceptions (faces or vase) even though stimulus and sensation remain constant. The mind can "see" purple figures against a blue background or a blue figure against a purple background.

In this case the image remains the same—the sensory input remains constant—but the perception of what is being viewed changes as the goal of the viewer changes or as his or her attention wanders. Using this example, it is apparent that detection of a stimulus and recognition that an event has occurred are usually called sensation; interpretation and appreciation of that event constitute perception.

Psychophysics Is the Quantitative Study of Sensory Performance

A psychophysical experiment determines the quantitative relationship between a stimulus and a sensation in order to establish the limits of sensory performance (Stevens, 1957). Such an experiment relies on reports from a subject who is asked to judge quantitatively the presence or magnitude of a stimulus as careful adjustments in the physical attributes are made. One example of threshold detection is the *two-point limen*, in which two blunt probes, separated by a distance that is progressively enlarged or reduced over a series of trials, are applied to the skin surface. The minimum separation distance at which a subject reports two stimuli half the time and one stimulus the other half is taken as the detection threshold. That distance can be measured accurately and is found to vary markedly across the body surface; the two-point limen is smallest for the fingertips and

largest for the skin of the back. Other studies, such as those exploring the detection of relative magnitudes of stimuli, can include assessments of object heaviness, loudness of sound, or brightness of light. Studies of this sort have been combined with neurophysiological experiments to compare reports from subjects (sensory behavior) with the responses of single cells (neuronal physiology). Through this procedure the neural mechanisms underlying sensory perception can be examined.

RECEPTORS

Receptors Are Specific for a Narrow Range of Input

Neurons of the brain and spinal cord do not respond when they are touched or when they are exposed to sound or light. Each of these forms of energy must be first transduced by specialized cells,

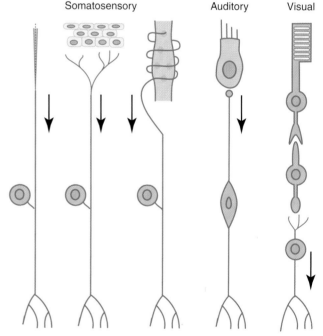

FIGURE 22.2 Receptor morphology and relationship to ganglion cells in the somatosensory, auditory, and visual systems. Receptors are specialized structures that adopt different shapes depending on their function. In the somatosensory system the receptor is a specialized peripheral element that is associated with the peripheral process of a sensory neuron. In the auditory and visual systems, a distinct type of receptor cell is present. In the auditory system, the receptor (hair cell) synapses directly on the ganglion cell, whereas in the visual system, an interneuron receives synapses from the photoreceptor and in turn synapses on the retinal ganglion cell. Adapted from Bodian (1967).

thereby converting the stimulus into a signal that produces a neuronal response. In every sensory system, cells that perform such a transduction are called *receptors* (Fig. 22.2). For each of the fundamental types of stimuli (mechanical or thermal energy, sound, or light) there is a separate population of receptors selective for the particular form of energy. Even within a single sensory system, there are classes of receptors that are particularly sensitive to one stimulus (e.g., heat or cold) and not another (muscle stretch). This specificity in the receptor response is a direct function of differences in receptor structure and chemistry.

Receptor Types Vary across Sensory Systems

Systems differ in the number of distinct receptor types they incorporate, and a correlation exists between the number of receptor types displayed by a system and the types of stimuli that system is able to detect. In the somatosensory system, there is a large number of receptor types and an ability to detect many types of stimuli. Separate receptors exist to transduce a variety of mechanical stimuli, including light touching of hairless skin, deformation of hair, vibration, increased or decreased skin temperature, tissue destruction, and stretch of muscles or tendons (Fig. 22.2). In the auditory system, two classes of receptor—the inner and outer hair cells of the cochlea—transduce mechanical energy of the basilar membrane, which is set in motion by sound (Dallos,1996). Here, the motility of outer hair cells is thought to provide an additional amplification of the basilar membrane motion to increase sensitivity and allow sharp tuning to sound frequency. The inner hair cells respond to the amplified vibrations and excite the large population of neurons upon which they synapse. Thus the two types of receptors act in concert to transduce a single type of stimulus, sound. In the visual system, transduction is performed by two broad classes of receptor in the retina: rods and cones. The number of cone types varies from one type in some species to two types in many species to three types in a few species, but cones in general serve to allow sensitivity to wavelengths of light, enabling color vision. Rods are more sensitive to light and enable vision when light levels are dim.

Receptors Perform a Common Function in Unique Fashion

All receptors transduce the energy to which they are sensitive into a change in membrane voltage. The task of the receptor is to transmit that voltage change by one route or another to a class of neurons—universally referred to as ganglion cells—that send their axons into the brain or spinal cord (Fig. 22.2). Systems vary in the mechanism whereby receptors and ganglion cells interact. Most receptors in the somatosensory system are part of multicellular organs, the neural components of which are the terminal specializations of dorsal root ganglion cell axons. An appropriate stimulus applied to a somatosensory receptor produces a generator potential—a graded change in membrane voltage (Katz, 1950)—that, when large enough, leads to action potentials that can be carried over a considerable distance into the central nervous system.

Receptors of the auditory and visual systems are separate, specialized cells that transduce a stimulus and then transmit the resulting signal to the nearby process of a neuron. Because the distances between receptor and target neuron are short, auditory hair cells and photoreceptors do not generate action potentials but signal their response by a passive flow of current. Auditory and visual systems differ in the path between receptor and ganglion cell. In the cochlea, auditory receptors form chemical synapses directly with the processes of ganglion cells so that the response properties of inner hair cells are conveyed directly to the ganglion cells on which they synapse. That is not the case in the retina, where photoreceptors relay their response through populations of interneurons interposed between them and retinal ganglion cells (Dowling, 1987) (Fig. 22.2). Because of this additional synapse and the opportunity it affords for summation and comparison of receptor signals, the retinal ganglion cell response differs appreciably from that of photoreceptors.

The mechanisms whereby receptors transduce and transmit signals are known in greater or lesser detail for each system. Visual transduction is a well-understood, rapid process in which a weak signal (a single photon) can be amplified greatly through a biochemical cascade, leading to the closure of thousands of Na^+ channels and a hyperpolarizing response (Yau and Baylor, 1989). For auditory hair cells and somatosensory mechanoreceptors, the mechanical deformation of a part of the cell is transduced into a change in membrane voltage (Hudspeth, 1985). The response of mechanoreceptors is similar to that of photoreceptors in being of one sign only, but it is a sign opposite to that of photoreceptors, as an appropriate tactile stimulus leads to the opening of Na^+ channels and a depolarizing response. This requirement for depolarization may result from the demands placed on the somatosensory ganglion cell to generate action potentials and transmit information over long distances. In contrast, auditory receptors can generate a biphasic response. When protruding villi of the hair cell, called stereocilia, are deflected in one direction, transducer channels open and the cell is depolarized. Yet with deflection of stereocilia in the opposite direction, the same channels close and the cell is hyperpolarized, although to a lesser extent (Hudspeth, 1985). Because sound usually produces a back-and-forth deflection of stereocilia, the result is a back-and-forth movement of the receptor potential—at least for low and moderate frequencies of sound. Thus, the receptor output contains temporal information about the waveform of an acoustic stimulus.

Receptors Have Characteristic Patterns of Position and Density

Receptors are not scattered randomly across the sensory surface. An orderly arrangement of receptors exists along the skin, the basilar membrane, and the retina. In the retina, for example, photoreceptors adopt a hexagonal packing array (Wassle and Boycott, 1991), and in the cochlea, a single row of inner hair cells lines up parallel to three rows of outer hair cells (Dallos, 1996). The arrangement of receptors in the skin is less orderly. However a nonrandom distribution is immediately evident in a comparison of the density of cutaneous receptors across the skin surface. By far the greatest density of receptor terminals is found at the fingertips and the mouth, whereas receptors along the surface of the back are at least an order of magnitude less frequent. Such differences in peripheral innervation density are tightly correlated with spatial acuity.

Receptors Are the Sites of Convergence and Divergence

The relationship between receptor and ganglion cell is seldom exclusive. Most commonly, a single ganglion cell receives input from several receptors and, in many cases, a single receptor sends information to two or more ganglion cells. *Convergence* and *divergence* go hand in hand for the somatosensory system as an individual receptor is often innervated by axons of several ganglion cells while at the same time the axon of a single ganglion cell can branch to end as part of several receptor organs. In the somatosensory system, however, the amount of divergence and convergence varies with the class of receptor involved (e.g., thermal receptor vs mechanoreceptor) and the location of the receptor on the body surface (e.g., shoulder vs fingertip). Similar features are seen in the visual system, as divergence and convergence dominate different parts of the retina populated by different receptor types. In the cone-rich central retina, each cone provides as many as four ganglion cells with their main visual drive, whereas in the rod-rich periphery, a few dozen rods supply each gan-

glion cell with its visual input. In its precision and in its implications for sensory processing, nothing approaches the divergence seen in the cochlea, where a single inner hair cell can be the source of all input received by 20 ganglion cells. Thus, what emerges from a comparison across systems is that convergence and divergence from receptor to ganglion cell vary directly with the demands placed on the system at the specific location. When spatial resolution is a requirement, the convergence of receptor inputs onto individual ganglion cells is low. When detection of weak signals is necessary, convergence is high. When receptor input is used for a complex function or for multiple functions, divergence of input from a single receptor onto many ganglion cells occurs.

Receptors Vary in Their Embryonic Origin

For auditory and somatosensory systems, the various classes of receptors and ganglion cells are part of the peripheral nervous system, generated as progeny of neuroblasts located in neural crests and sensory placodes. That is not the case for photoreceptors and retinal ganglion cells. The retina is generated as a protrusion of the embryonic diencephalon and thus all its neurons and supporting cells are CNS derivatives of neural tube origin. As a result of their origin, receptors and ganglion cells of the auditory and somatosensory system are supported by classes of nonneuronal cells (modified epithelial supporting cells and Schwann cells), whereas photoreceptors and retinal ganglion cells are supported by CNS neuroglial cells. Most dramatic of all the consequences resulting from this difference in origin is the ability of axons in somatosensory peripheral nerves to regenerate and reinnervate targets after they are damaged, as opposed to the complete and permanent loss of visual function when optic nerves are cut or crushed.

PERIPHERAL ORGANIZATION AND PROCESSING

Sensory Information Is Transmitted along Labeled Lines

A long-appreciated principle that unites structure and function in a sensory system is the doctrine of specific energy, or the *labeled line* principle. This principle states that when a particular population of neurons is active, the conscious perception is of a specific stimulus (Fig. 22.3). For example, in one particular population of somatosensory neurons (colored orange on Fig. 22.3), activity is always interpreted by

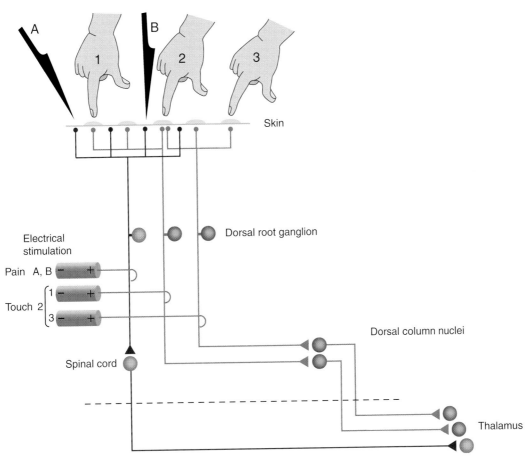

FIGURE 22.3 Example of labeled lines in the somatosensory system. Two dorsal root ganglion (DRG) cells (blue) send peripheral axons to be part of a touch receptor, whereas a third cell (red) is a pain receptor. By activating the neurons of touch receptors, direct touching of the skin or electrical stimulation of an appropriate axon produces the sensation of light touch at a defined location. The small receptive fields of touch receptors in body areas such as the fingertips permit distinguishing the point at which the body is touched (e.g., position 1 vs position 2). In addition, convergence of two DRG axons onto a single touch receptor on the skin permits touch stimulus 2 to be localized precisely. Electrical stimulation of both axons produces the same sensation, although localized to somewhat different places in the skin. Sharp stimuli (A,B) applied to nearby skin regions selectively activate the third ganglion cell, eliciting the sensation of pain. Electrical stimulation of that ganglion cell or of any cell along that pathway also produces a sensation of pain along that region of skin. Stimulus A and B, however, cannot be localized separately with the pain receptor circuit that is drawn. As the labeled lines project centrally, they cross the midline (decussate) and project to separate centers in the thalamus.

the CNS as a painful stimulus, no matter whether the stimulus is natural (a sharp instrument jabbed into the skin) or artificial (electrical stimulation of the appropriate axons). An entirely separate population of neurons (colored blue on Fig. 22.3) would signal light touch. Why this is so can be seen from the fact that receptors are selective not only in what drives them, but also in the postsynaptic targets with which they communicate. Each ganglion cell transmits its activity into a well-defined region of the CNS, after which a strictly organized series of synaptic connections relays information in a sequence that eventually leads to the thalamus and then to the cerebral cortex (Darian-Smith *et al.*, 1996). It is this orderly relay from receptor to ganglion cell to

central neurons at each of several stations that makes up a labeled line. All sensory information arising from a single class of receptors is referred to as a *modality* (e.g., the sensations of pain and light touch involve distinct modalities). Thus, the existence of labeled lines means that neurons in sensory systems carry specific modalities.

Topographic Projections Dominate the Anatomy and Physiology of Sensory Systems

Receptors in the retina and body surface are organized as two-dimensional sheets, and those of the cochlea form a one-dimensional line along the cochlear length. Receptors in these organs communicate with ganglion cells and those ganglion cells with central neurons in a strictly ordered fashion, such that relationships with neighbors are maintained throughout. This type of pattern, in which neurons positioned side by side in one region communicate with neurons so positioned in the next region, is called a *topographic pattern*. As an example, the two touch-sensitive neurons in Fig. 22.3 innervate somewhat different positions in the skin. Thus, light touch at position 3 will activate the right-most ganglion cell in the dorsal root ganglion, whereas touch at position 1 will activate the neighboring ganglion cell. The central projections of these cells are kept separate and activate different targets in the thalamus and above. The end result is a map of the sensory surface of the skin. This topography of all sensory systems shows that in any sensory region each neuron is specific for the place at which a stimulus occurred as well as the modality of that stimulus.

Neural Signaling Is by a Combination of Rate and Temporal Codes

A great deal of research has been aimed at determining the codes by which neurons signal the presence and the intensity of a stimulus. Certainly, one code is which receptors are activated, as discussed earlier for the principle of labeled lines and receptor topography. Within a given receptor, the firing rate or frequency of action potentials signals the strength of the sensory input. The perceived intensity arises from an interaction between this firing rates and the number of neurons activated by a stimulus. There is also a temporal code in some systems. For instance, the phase-locking ability of auditory neurons extends to sound frequencies up to several thousand cycles per second (kHz), and this code is likely to be important in the perception of the pitch of sounds. In addition, all sensory systems must deal with the fact that stimuli can move, as with vibratory stimuli on the

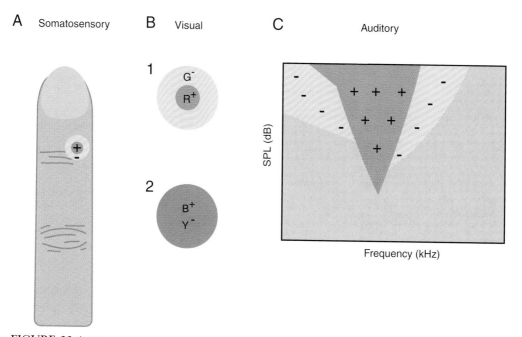

FIGURE 22.4 Center/surround organization of receptive fields is common in sensory systems. In this organization, a stimulus in the center of the receptive field produces one effect, usually excitation, whereas a stimulus in the surround area has the opposite effect, usually inhibition. (A) In the somatosensory system, receptive fields display antagonistic centers and surrounds because of skin mechanics. (B) In the retina and visual thalamus, a common type of receptive field is antagonistic for location and for wavelength. Receptive field 1 is excited by turning on red light (R) at its center and is inhibited by turning on green light (G) in its surround. Receptive field 2 is less common and is antagonistic for wavelength (blue vs yellow) without being antagonistic for the location of the stimuli. Both are generated by neural processing in the retina. (C) In the auditory system, primary neurons are excited by single tones. The outline of this excitatory area is known as the tuning curve. When the neuron is excited by a tone in this area, the introduction of a second tone in flanking areas usually diminishes the response. This "two-tone suppression" is also generated mechanically, as is seen in motion of the basilar membrane of the cochlea. All of these center/surround organizations serve to sharpen responses over that which would be achieved by excitation alone.

skin. This temporal information in a stimulus is carried by the time-varying pattern of activity in small groups of receptors and central neurons.

Lateral Mechanisms Enhance Sensitivity to Contrast

A hallmark of all sensory systems is the ability of neurons at even the earliest stages of central processing to integrate the activity of more than one receptor. The most common and easily understood of these mechanisms is *lateral* (or surround) *inhibition*

(Fig. 22.4). By this mechanism, a sensory neuron displays a receptive field with an excitatory center and an inhibitory surround (Kuffler, 1953). Such a mechanism serves to enhance contrast: each neuron responds optimally to a stimulus that occupies most of its center but little of its surround. In some cases the comparisons involve receptors of different types so that the center and surround differ not only in sign (excitation vs inhibition, On vs Off), but also in the stimulus quality to which they respond. One such example occurs in visual neurons that possess centers and surrounds responsive to stimulation of different

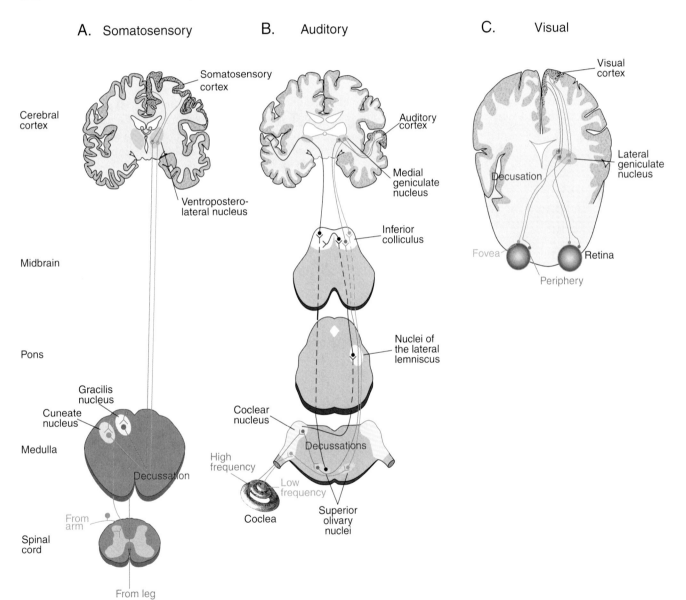

FIGURE 22.5 Comparison of central pathways of sensory systems. In every case, soon after peripheral input arrives in the brain, decussations result in one hemifield being represented primarily by the brain on the opposite side. Each pathway has a unique nucleus in the thalamus and several unique fields in the cerebral cortex. Within each of these areas, the organized mapping that is established by receptors in the periphery is preserved.

types of cones. These cells display a combination of spatial contrast (the difference in the location of cones that produce center and surround) and chromatic contrast (the difference in the visible wavelengths to which these cones respond best). Similar types of responses are evident in the somatosensory system, where the difference between center and surround is the location on the skin from which each is activated. In this case, skin mechanics produce receptive fields with a central hot spot of activity and a surrounding inactive zone. In the auditory system, lateral suppressive areas (Fig. 22.4) are also produced by mechanics, in this case the mechanics of the basilar membrane of the cochlea. These two-tone suppression areas are demonstrated by exciting the auditory nerve fiber with a tone in the central excitatory area and observing the response decrease caused by a second tone in flanking areas (Sachs and Kiang, 1968). In all these sensory systems, center/surround organization serves to sharpen the selectivity of a neuron either for the position of the stimulus or for its exact quality by subtracting responses to stimuli of a general or diffuse nature.

CENTRAL PATHWAYS AND PROCESSING

Axons in Each System Cross the Midline on Their Way to the Thalamus

Axons of ganglion cells entering the CNS form the initial stage in a pathway through the thalamus to the cerebral cortex (Fig. 22.5). Axons in all three systems cross the midline—they *decussate*—prior to reaching the thalamus. A single, incomplete decussation occurs in the visual system of primates, where slightly more than half the axons of the optic nerve cross the midline at the optic chiasm. Decussation in the somatosensory system is nearly total, as all but a small group of axons cross the midline in the spinal cord or brain stem. These decussations serve the broad functions of bringing together all axons carrying visual information from half the visual world or of bringing somatosensory information into alignment with motor output, which is itself a largely crossed system. In contrast, multiple decussations occur in the auditory system, prior to the thalamus, as comparison of input from the two ears is the dominant requirement of sound source localization. Nevertheless, at high levels in the auditory system, one side of the brain is concerned mainly with processing information about sound sources located toward the opposite side of the body, as demonstrated by lesion/behavioral studies of sound localization. In all of these ascending

systems, a common pattern exists in which a prominent, heavily myelinated (lemniscal) tract carries rapidly transmitted messages into the thalamus.

Specific Thalamic Nuclei Exist for Each Sensory System

Information from each of the sensory systems must be relayed through the thalamus on its way to the cerebral cortex (Fig. 22.5). This relay involves either a single large nucleus or, in the case of the somatosensory systems, two nuclei: one for the body and one for the face. In each nucleus, synaptic circuits are said to be "secure" because activity in presynaptic axons usually leads to a postsynaptic response. Within the thalamic nuclei, neurons performing one function (e.g., relay of discriminative touch) are segregated from those performing another (e.g., relay of pain and temperature). Even within one function, mappings of neurons are preserved so that there is separation of neurons providing for touch information from the arm vs from the leg and of neurons responding to low vs high sound frequencies (Fig. 22.5). Usually, for each thalamic nucleus, there is a population of large neurons and one or two populations of small neurons (Jones, 1981). In each case the larger neurons carry the most rapidly transmitted signals from the periphery to the cortex.

Multiple Maps and Parallel Pathways

Nuclei in the central pathways often contain multiple maps. For instance, in the auditory system, axons of spiral ganglion cells divide into branches as they enter the CNS and terminate in three subdivisions of the cochlear nucleus. Each division contains its own map of sound frequency (tonotopic map) that was originally established by the cochlea. The greatest number of maps generated from ganglion cell input is found in the visual system of primates, in which as many as six separate retinotopic maps are stacked on top of one another in the lateral geniculate nucleus (LGN, in the thalamus), which receives direct input from the retina (Kaas *et al.*, 1972). Such a large number of distinct maps in the LGN is indicative of inputs from ganglion cells that vary in location, structure, and function. For vision, one idea is that surface features such as color and form are carried along a path separate from the one that handles three-dimensional features of motion and stereopsis. The functional significance of multiple maps in general, however, remains to be clarified. Perhaps the need for multiple parallel paths exists because of the relatively slow speed and the limited capacity of single neurons. So rather than have the same group of neurons perform

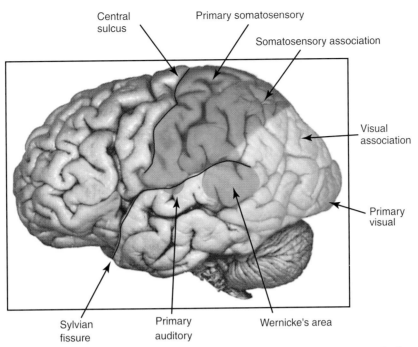

FIGURE 22.6   The location of primary sensory and association areas of the human cerebral cortex. The primary auditory cortex is mostly hidden from view within the Sylvian fissure. From Guyton (1987).

different functions in serial order, each of several parallel groups performs a separate function. This leads eventually to the problem of binding together all features of a stimulus into a coherent percept, the neural basis for which may be the synchronized activity of neurons across several areas of the cerebral cortex (Singer, 1995).

SENSORY CORTEX

Sensory Cortex Includes Primary and Association Areas

Axons of sensory relay nuclei of the thalamus project to a single area or a collection of neighboring areas of the cerebral cortex, thereby providing them with a precise topographic map of the sensory periphery. These parts of cortex are frequently referred to as *primary sensory areas* (Fig. 22.6). Neighboring areas with which the primary areas communicate directly or by a single intervening relay area are sensory *association areas*.

Response Mappings and Plasticity

Each area of sensory cortex shares with its subcortical components a map of at least part of the sensory periphery. Thus, retinotopic, somatotopic, and tono-

topic maps are evident in the relevant areas of cortex. The retina and skin are two-dimensional sheets so the map of the sensory periphery on the surface of the cortex is a simple transformation of the peripheral representation onto the cortex. In the auditory periphery, there is a one-dimensional mapping of frequency. This tonotopic mapping is faithfully represented along one dimension of cortical distance, and

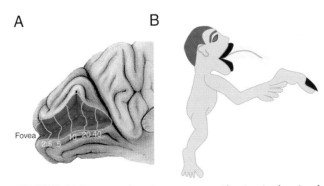

FIGURE 22.7   Examples of sensory magnification in the visual and somatosensory systems. (A) Determination of a visual field map in the human primary visual cortex shows that more than half this area is devoted to the central 10° of the visual field. Very little is devoted to the visual periphery beyond 40°. From Horton and Hoyt (1991). (B) Figure of how the human body would appear if the body surface were a perfect reflection of the map in the first somatosensory cortex. The mouth and tongue and the tip of the index finger enjoy a greatly enlarged representation in the thalamus and cortex.

the orthogonal direction may map a second, as yet undiscovered, property.

In the periphery, the distribution of somatosensory and visual receptors is uneven. The site of central vision in primate retina—the fovea or macula—and the fingertips of the hand in primates are regions that possess a high density of receptors with small recep-

tive fields. Such an uneven distribution of neurons devoted to a structure is further amplified in the CNS so that a greater percentage of neural machinery subserves the representation of the retinal fovea or the fingertips than the representation of other regions of the retina or body surface (Fig. 22.7). This expansion of a representation in the CNS, referred to as a

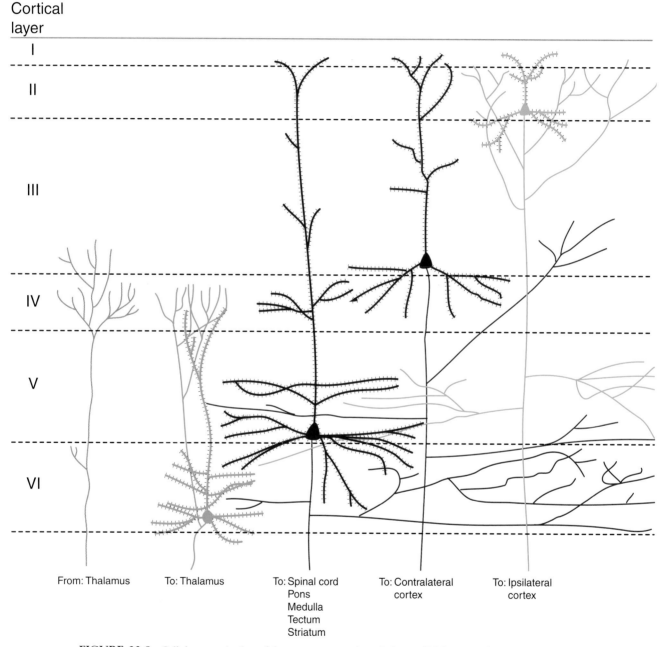

FIGURE 22.8 Cellular organization of the sensory cortex into six layers (I–VI). Inputs from the thalamus terminate mainly in layers III and IV. The main output neurons of the cortex are pyramidal cells, which are distributed in different layers according to their projections. Descending projections are to the thalamus (neurons in layer VI) or to the spinal cord, pons and medulla, tectum, or striatum (neurons at various levels in layer V). Ascending projections to other "higher" cortical centers are often from neurons located above layer IV; some of these projections are to the same hemisphere (layer II) or to the opposite hemisphere (layer III). Adapted from Jones (1985).

magnification factor, appears particularly impressive in humans, in whom a very large part of primary visual cortex is devoted to the couple of millimeters of retina in and around the fovea. In the auditory cortex, such magnification of frequency representation is uncommon, but occurs in bats that use constant frequencies in their echolocating signals.

It is now clear that mappings of sensory cortex are not fixed and immutable but rather plastic. In the somatosensory system, if input from a restricted area of the body surface is removed by severing a nerve or by amputation of a digit, that portion of the cortex that was previously responsive to that region of the body surface becomes responsive to neighboring regions (Merzenich *et al.*, 1984). In the auditory system, following high-frequency hearing loss, the portion of cortex previously responsive to high frequencies becomes responsive to middle frequencies. Such plasticity of cortical maps requires some time to be established and could result from strengthening of already established lateral connections or from growth of new connections. It is likely but not firmly established that the same types of mechanisms cause cortical changes during the processes of learning and memory.

A Common Structure Exists for Sensory Cortex

Neurons in areas of the sensory cortex (and most other areas of the cerebral cortex) are organized into six layers. The middle layers (III and IV) are the main site of termination of axons from the thalamus (Fig. 22.8). In the primary sensory cortices, these middle layers are enlarged and contain many small neurons. Because the small cells resemble grains of sand in standard histological preparations, the sensory areas are themselves referred to as granular areas of cortex.

Columnar Organization

Properties other than place in the periphery are mapped in primary sensory areas of the cortex. The third spatial dimension of the cortex, that of depth, arranges neurons in adjacent 0.5- to 1-mm-wide regions, referred to as *columns* (Mountcastle, 1997). In these columns, neurons stacked above and below one another are fundamentally similar but differ significantly from neurons on either side of them. One example of columns with a clear anatomical correlate is the division of the primary visual cortex of most primates and some carnivores into a series of alternating regions dominated by the right and left retinas. Each ocular dominance column contains cells driven exclusively or predominantly by one eye; adjacent

columns are dominated by the other eye. Other properties, such as selectivity for the orientation of a visual stimulus and the contrast between it and the surround, are also arranged in columns of primary visual cortex (Hubel, 1988). Similar types of columns are evident in the somatosensory system, as regions of modality and place specificity. In the auditory system, neurons within a column generally share the same best frequency and the same type of binaural interaction characteristic: either one ear excites the neurons and the other inhibits or suppresses the response to the first ear (suppression column) or one ear excites and the other ear also excites or facilitates the response to the first ear (summation column). Moreover, in areas of nonprimary cortex, the feature displayed most commonly by neurons of a particular area is one that often comes to occupy columns. A good example is found in the middle temporal area (MT) of visual association cortex, where neurons are tuned for the direction of a moving visual stimulus. Neurons selective for one particular direction of visual stimulus movement are organized into columns through the depth of MT; these are flanked by columns of neurons tuned for other directions of movement (Albright *et al.*, 1984). So consistent are these findings among sensory, motor, and association areas that columnar organization is viewed as a principal organizing feature for all of the cerebral cortex (Mountcastle, 1997).

Stereotyped Connections Exist for Areas of Sensory Cortex

Neurons of the cerebral cortex send axons to subcortical regions throughout the neuraxis and to other areas of the cortex (Fig. 22.8). Subcortical projections are to those nuclei in the thalamus and brain stem that provide ascending sensory information. By far the most prominent of these is to the thalamus: the neurons of a primary sensory cortex project back to the same thalamic nucleus that provides input to the cortex. This system of descending connections is truly impressive, as the number of descending corticothalamic axons greatly exceeds the number of ascending thalamocortical axons. These connections permit a particular sensory cortex to control the activity of the very neurons that relay information to it. One role for descending control of thalamic and brain stem centers is likely to be the focusing of activity so that relay neurons most activated by a sensory stimulus are more strongly driven and those in surrounding less well activated regions are further suppressed.

The overwhelming majority of cortical neurons project to other areas of cortex (Fig. 22.8). Cortico-cortical projections link primary and association areas of the sensory cortex and establish parallel paths so that different aspects of vision, audition, and somatic sensation come to be handled by different areas of cortex. These connections establish a hierarchy within a system, such that "ascending" or "forward" connections begin with neurons from superficial cortical layers (I–III) and end with axonal terminations mainly in layers III and IV of higher cortical regions. Similarly, the ascending projection from the thalamus terminates mainly in these layers in primary sensory cortices. Corresponding descending projections from higher to lower cortical regions begin in the deep or superficial cortical layers and project to layers outside of III and IV. In addition to projections to the ipsilateral hemisphere of cortex, there are also projections to the contralateral hemisphere via the corpus callosum and other commissures. In visual and somatosensory systems, these commissural connections are restricted in origin and termination; they exist to unite the representation of midline structures into a coherent percept (Hubel, 1988).

Response Complexity of Cortical Neurons

Responses of cortical neurons in primary sensory cortices are more complex than those seen for neurons in the periphery. One example is seen in the primary visual area of the cerebral cortex, where neurons are responsive to stimuli that are not concentric circles (center and surround) but elongated lines possessing a specific orientation. Comparable synthesis of simpler inputs to reconstruct more complex features of stimulus is apparent at higher levels in the visual system (Logothetis and Sheinberg, 1996) and in the somatosensory and auditory areas of the cerebral cortex.

Physiologically, processing and selectivity for stimulus features become progressively more complex within the hierarchically organized pathways that connect primary with association areas of the cortex (Gallant and Van Essen, 1994). In the visual system, separate "streams" involved in visuosensory and eventually visuomotor functions have been described; one is responsible for using visual cues to drive appropriate eye movements and the other for dealing with the tasks of visual perception (Gallant and Van Essen, 1994). In the somatosensory system, separate motor and limbic paths exist to perform much the same functions for the entire body, supplying sensory input to coordinate and adjust motor output and using complex input from many receptor types to match the shape of a tactual stimulus with one already stored in memory (Johnson and Hsiao, 1992). In the association pathways of the human auditory

system, a specialized area of cortex, Wernicke's area, plays a fundamental role in processing speech and language information and in communicating with Broca's area to form a speech motor response. These streams are not separate, as traditionally viewed "motor" areas such as Broca's are now known to become activated in comprehension tasks. Apparent from this pattern in association areas of the cortex is the continued pressure for a division of labor within each sensory system; not one that produces separate paths for analyzing elemental features of a stimulus but one that combines those features either to elicit appropriate movements or to match a stimulus with an internal representation of the world.

SUMMARY

The functional organization of sensory systems shares common themes of transduction, relay, organized mappings, parallel processing, and central modification. It is no surprise that a case has been made for a common phylogenetic origin of sensory systems. Differences among the systems, however, demonstrate that each has existed and operated independently for as long as there have been vertebrates. What remains in overview is a well-ordered basic plan from periphery to perception that has been modified in its details as variations in niche have led to specializations in function.

References

Albright, T. D., Desimone, R., and Gross, C. G. (1984). Columnar organization of directionally selective cells in visual area MT of the macaque. *J. Neurophysiol.* **51**, 16–31.

Gallant, J. L., and Van Essen, D. C. (1994). Neural mechanisms of form and motion processing in the primate visual system. *Neuron* **13**, 1–10.

Hudspeth, A. J. (1985). The cellular basis of hearing: The biophysics of hair cells. *Science* **230**, 745–752.

Johnson, K. O., and Hsiao, S. S. (1992). Tactual form and texture perception. *Annu. Rev. Neurosci.* **15**, 227–250.

Jones, E. G. (1981). Functional subdivision and synaptic organization of the mammalian thalamus. *Int. Rev. Physiol.* **25**, 173–245.

Kaas, J. H. Guillery, R. W., and Allman, J. M. (1972). Some principles of organization in the dorsal lateral geniculate nucleus. *Brain Behav. Evol.* **6**, 253–299.

Katz, B. (1950). Depolarization of sensory terminals and the initiation of impulses in the muscle spindle. *J. Physiol. (Lond.)* **111**, 261–282.

Kuffler, S. W. (1953). Discharge patterns and functional organization of mammalian retina. *J. Neurophysiol.* **16**, 37–68.

Logothetis, N. K., and Sheinberg, D. L. (1996). Visual object recognition. *Annu. Rev. Neurosci.* **19**, 577–621.

Merzenich, M. M., Nelson, R. J., Stryker, M. P., Cynader, M. S., Schoppmann, A., and Zook, M. (1984). Somatosensory cortical map changes following digit amputation in adult monkeys. *J. Comp. Neurol.* **224**, 591–605.

Sachs, M. B., and Kiang, N. Y. S. (1968). Two-tone inhibition in auditory-nerve fibers. *J. Acoust. Soc. Am.* **43**, 1120–1128.

Singer, W. (1995). Time as coding space in neocortical processing: A hypothesis. *In* "The Cognitive Neurosciences" (M. S. Gazzaniga, ed.), pp. 91–104. MIT Press, Cambridge, MA.

Stevens, S. S. (1957). On the psychophysical law. *Psychol. Rev.* **64**, 153–181.

Wassle, H., and Boycott, B. B. (1991). Functional architecture of the mammalian retina. *Physiol. Rev.* **71**, 447–480.

Yau, K.-W., and Baylor, D. A. (1989). Cyclic GMP-activated conductance of retinal photoreceptor cells. *Annu. Rev. Neurosci.* **12**, 289–328.

Suggested Readings

Dallos, P. (1996). Overview: Cochlear neurobiology. *In* "The Cochlea" (P. Dallos, A. N. Popper, and R. R. Fay, eds.), pp. 1–43. Springer-Verlag, New York.

Darian-Smith, I., Galea, M. P., Darian-Smith, C., Sugitani, M., Tan, A., and Burman, K. (1996). The anatomy of manual dexterity: The new connectivity of the primate sensorimotor thalamus and cerebral cortex. *Adv. Anat. Cell Biol.* **133**, 1–142.

Dowling, J. E. (1987). "The Retina: An Approachable Part of the Brain." Belknap Press, Cambridge, MA.

Hubel, D. H. (1988). "Eye, Brain and Vision." Freeman, New York.

Mountcastle, V. B. (1997). The columnar organization of the neocortex. *Brain* **120**, 701–722.

Stewart H. Hendry, Steven S. Hsiao, and
M. Christian Brown

23

Sensory Transduction

Since the early 19th century, the prevailing understanding of sensory perception has been based on the idea that each sensory modality has its own type of receptor cell. Modern research is replacing this with the view that each modality has its own particular combination of molecular and cellular properties involved in membrane signal transduction. In this view, sensory transduction of each modality represents a distinct adaptation of membrane signaling mechanisms.

Some of the receptor cells and their signaling mechanisms are summarized in Fig. 23.1. It is clear that the diversity of mechanisms is encompassed within an overall framework of membrane receptors and second messenger systems. Within this framework, each sensory modality has its unique series of molecular steps, from the initial interaction of the stimulus energy with its receptor to the final generation of the electrical response by the receptor cell membrane channels. This common language of signaling mechanisms unites the study of sensory transduction, which in turn is part of the much larger study of membrane signaling mechanisms in cells throughout the body. This framework of sensory signaling mechanisms applies across phyla, to both vertebrate and invertebrate species. It looks forward to the eventual emergence of a molecular biology of sensory perception.

This chapter focuses on four of the main types of sensory receptors and shows how these principles apply.

PHOTOTRANSDUCTION

Vision in vertebrates is subserved by two types of photoreceptors: rods and cones. Rods consist of three principal compartments (Fig. 23.2): (1) The outer segment is composed of a stack of flattened discs, surrounded by the plasma membrane, that act to increase the sensory membrane area. The visual pigment rhodopsin is densely packed in the disc membrane but is also found to a lesser degree in the plasma membrane. (2) The inner segment is attached to the outer segment via a connecting cilium and contains a region of densely packed mitochondria called the myoid region. (3) The cell body contains the nucleus and perinuclear assortment of organelles involved in macromolecular synthesis and metabolism. A fine axon-like process connects the cell body to the rod output terminal (spherule), which contains ribbons and associated vesicles involved in neurotransmitter storage and release.

The cone outer segment differs from that of the rod in that increased surface area is achieved by repeated infolding of the plasma membrane. As in the rod, the inner segment contains a dense array of mitochondria and connects to the cell body, which contains the nucleus and macromolecular synthesizing organelles. The axon-like process connecting the cell body to the cone pedicle differs considerably in length among species. In the human, the connecting fiber at the fovea is called the fiber of Henle and can measure up to several hundred micrometers in length because of the lateral displacement of the output terminals (pedicles) from the fovea. The cone pedicle contains ribbons and vesicles involved in neurotransmitter storage and release.

Light Hyperpolarizes the Photoreceptor Membrane

Intracellular recording from fish cones in the 1960s (Tomita, 1965) first showed that light absorption leads

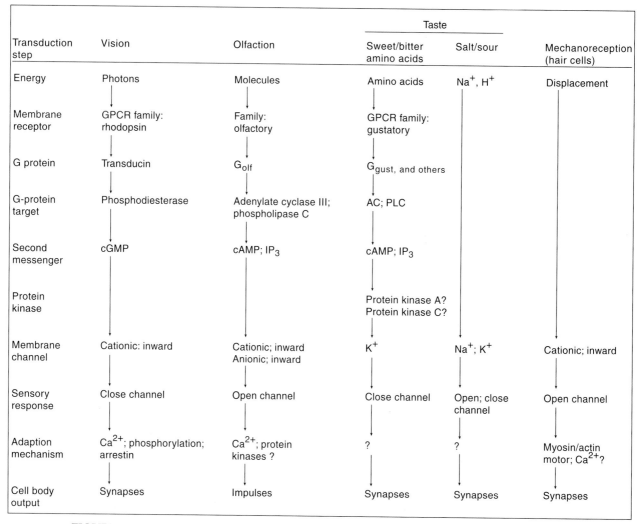

FIGURE 23.1 Summary of second-messenger pathways underlying sensory transduction in different sensory receptor cells GPCR, G-protein receptor family. Modified from Shepherd (1994).

to hyperpolarization of the membrane of vertebrate photoreceptors. The original observation came as a surprise because the adequate stimulus for known sense organs at that time, such as stretch receptors, led to depolarization and excitation. Rods from many species have also been found to hyperpolarize in response to light. Rods and cones do not normally generate action potentials but rather respond to light with slow, graded hyperpolarizations (Fig. 23.3A). The ionic basis of hyperpolarization was found to be suppression of an inward current carried mainly by sodium ions (Hagins *et al.*, 1970)

The amplitude of the current is decreased transiently by dim flashes or steps of light and reduced to zero by bright light (Fig. 23.3B). For dark-adapted rods, the absorption of approximately 30 photons is estimated to cause a 50% reduction in the amplitude of the light-regulated current, and 100 photons are

sufficient for total suppression. In dark-adapted humans, the behavioral perception of light is achieved when a small number (5-7) of photons generated by a brief flash arrive at a restricted area of retina. Under these conditions the probability of two photons arriving at the same single cell is very low. Isolated rods from amphibians produce detectable responses to single photons. The single-photon response has an amplitude of about 1 mV and 1 pA, corresponding to the suppression of 10^6 monovalent cations at the dark resting potential; it lasts for several seconds and has a peak approximately 1 s after light absorption.

The light-regulated current decreases in amplitude when external sodium ions are partially withdrawn and disappears altogether when sodium is replaced completely by an impermeant ion (Hagins *et al.*, 1970). The simplest interpretation of these results is that the light-regulated current is carried mainly by sodium

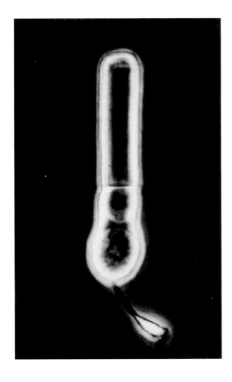
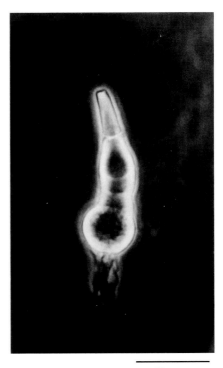

20 μm

FIGURE 23.2 Phase-contrast micrographs of freshly dissociated rod (left) and cone (right) photoreceptor cells from the tiger salamander retina. Cells were obtained after papain treatment and mechanical disruption of tissue. From MacLeish *et al.* (1984).

ions, but more complex explanations involving other ions cannot be ruled out. Suppression of an inward sodium current by light explains the hyperpolarization of the membrane observed with intracellular voltage recording. The reversal potential of the light response is in the range of 0 to 10 mV, thereby suggesting the additional involvement of ions other than sodium because the equilibrium potential for sodium ions is considered to occur at a more positive potential. Ion selectivity studies have shown that other monovalent (e.g., potassium) and divalent (e.g., calcium) ions can permeate the light-regulated conductance mechanism in the outer segment. In fact, calcium is more permeant than sodium, but the large sodium current arises from the higher concentration of sodium in the bathing medium. The total suppression of the light-regulated current by the removal of sodium has been explained by proposing that the conductance mechanism requires the presence of sodium for its activation.

Phototransduction Involves an Internal Messenger

Several lines of evidence support the claim for an internal messenger. In the case of rods, the bulk of rhodopsin is stored in the flattened discs in the outer segment, and the discs are isolated from the plasma membrane of the outer segment in which the light-regulated current is present. Also, the time course of the single-photon response is on the order of seconds, which is much longer than the open time of known membrane conductance mechanisms. It is easy to explain the time course by assuming that light activates a process with effective molecular intermediates that lasts seconds.

Ion substitution experiments indicate that reducing the concentration of external calcium increases the amplitude of light-regulated current dramatically (Hagins *et al.*, 1970) and led originally to the reasonable hypothesis that calcium is the internal messenger. A counter view was provided when a light-activated cGMP phosphodiesterase was discovered (Yee and Liebman, 1978) along with a fall in the amount of extractable cGMP in light. According to the cGMP hypothesis, an effect of light is to decrease the level of cGMP, which in turn leads to suppression of the inward current.

Biochemical studies have indicated that the level of extractable cGMP increases as the activity of calcium ions decreases in the external solution. This result pointed to an interrelationship between calcium and

A

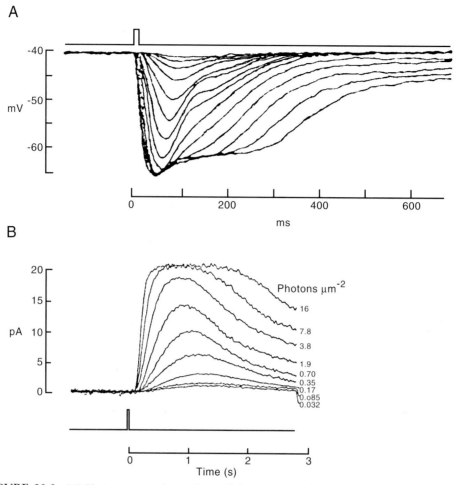

B

FIGURE 23.3 (A) Photoresponse of cone. Intracellular recordings from cone in the intact turtle retina showing superimposed responses to brief flashes of light of increasing intensity. Responses are slow, graded hyperpolarizations that show amplitude saturation to bright flashes. The responses of rods share essential features but are slower and rods are more sensitive to light. From Baylor (1987). (B) Light-suppressed rod currents vs light intensity Traces are superimposed responses showing the transient suppres sion by light of the current entering the outer segment. From Baylot *et al.* (1979).

cGMP and highlighted the difficulty in establishing causality when changes in the level of one or the other of these two agents were seen to have an effect.

Using the patch-clamp technique, Fesenko and colleagues (1985) were the first to show that cGMP increases the conductance of inside-out patches of outer segment membrane when applied from the cytoplasmic side (Fig. 23.4A). The action of cGMP is direct and does not require the presence of ATP and therefore does not seem to involve cGMP-dependent protein kinases and protein phosphorylation. Activation of the cGMP-gated conductance by cGMP shows cooperativity (Fig. 23.4B), suggesting that three to four cGMP molecules are required for channel activation. In addition, the channel does not desensitize to cGMP, a property expected because the levels of cGMP are high in the dark.

Calcium ions, in the presence of magnesium, were ineffective in controlling membrane conductance from the cytoplasmic side. This finding led to the establishment of cGMP as the internal messenger and to the rejection of the calcium hypothesis.

Rhodopsin Is a Member of a Superfamily of Signaling Molecules

The rhodopsin molecule is composed of a protein component, opsin, and an organic molecule, 11-*cis*-retinal. Opsin is a member of the seven transmembrane domain family of molecules that modify their interaction with G proteins in response to the binding of effectors. Other members of this family include olfactory receptors and likely some taste receptors (see

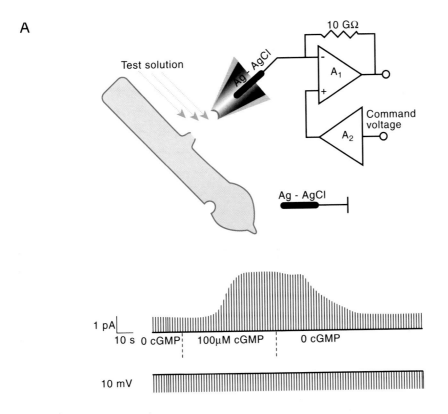

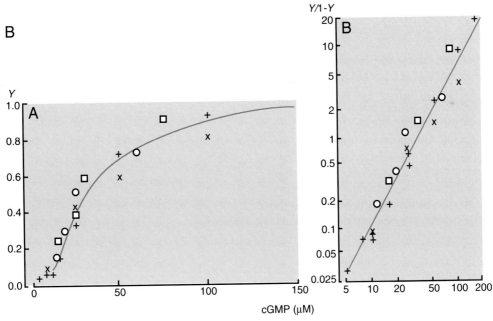

FIGURE 23.4 (A) Sensitivity of rod outer segment excised patch to cGMP. The top electrical trace shows the current through an excised patch of outer segment membrane in response to 10-mV voltage pulses in the presence or absence of cGMP. The application of cGMP to the cytoplasmic side of the excised patch was accompanied by an increase in current indicating the activation of a conductance mechanism by cGMP. From Fesenko *et al.* (1985). (B) Dose response of the cGMP-induced current in an excised patch of ROS. (Left) The normalized response as a function of the concentration of cGMP is shown on the left. (Right) The slope of the curve on the right gives an estimate of the Hill coefficient for the activation reaction and suggests that two, or possibly three, molecules of cGMP are required to activate the conductance mechanism. From Fesenko *et al.* (1985).

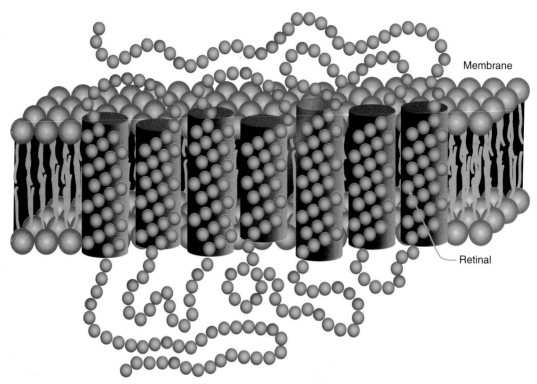

FIGURE 23.5 Proposed arrangement of a rhodopsin molecule within the plasma membrane of a rod. There are seven transmembrane domains and three cytoplasmic and three extracellular loops. The carboxy terminus faces the cytoplasm. From Hargrave and McDowell (1992).

later). Opsin is a single polypeptide made up of 348 amino acids (Fig. 23.5). The transmembrane domains form α helices that are connected by shorter linear sequences. 11-*cis*-Retinal sits in a pocket formed by the transmembrane α helices and, on absorption of a photon, is converted to the all-*trans* isomer. A number of intermediates of rhodopsin have been identified following light absorption. Based on its time of appearance, metarhodopsin II is thought to be the active intermediate in phototransduction. Following further conformational changes in the protein, the all-*trans*-retinal dissociates from opsin and is transported to the retinal pigment epithelium for reisomerization to 11-*cis*-retinal before retransport to the photoreceptor.

The Biochemical Cascade Involves Transducin, a G Protein

Several biochemical studies contributed to the model described by Fung, Hurley, and Stryer in 1981 (Fig. 23.6). In that model, photoactivated opsin, R*, interacts with a photoreceptor-specific G protein called transducin (T), which exists as the heterotrimeric complex $T\alpha\beta\gamma$, with GDP bound to the α subunit. Interaction with R* leads to an exchange of GDP for GTP and a dissociation of the T complex to

form $T\alpha$-GTP and $T\beta\gamma$ subunits. A single R* may generate several hundred $T\alpha$-GTP molecules, providing amplification or gain in the pathway. The $T\alpha$-GTP

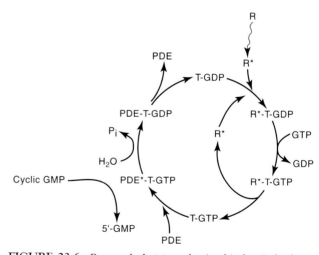

FIGURE 23.6 Proposed phototransduction biochemical scheme. Light causes the conversion of rhodopsin (R) to photolyzed rhodopsin (R*), which eventually leads to the hydrolysis of cGMP by the activation of phosphodiesterase. The proposed scheme contains two amplification steps whereby a single R* generates hundreds of T–GTP molecules and a single activated phosphodiesterase molecule hydrolyzes hundreds of cGMP molecules. From Fung *et al.* (1981).

subunit binds to an inactive form of a cGMP phosphodiesterase, which itself exists in the heterotrimeric complex $\alpha\beta\gamma$-phosphodiesterase (PDE). Activation of PDE is achieved by removing an inhibitory action brought about by the binding of the γ subunit of PDE to Tα-GTP. The $\alpha\beta$-PDE complex contains the PDE activity; several hundred cGMP molecules are hydrolyzed per activated PDE, thereby providing a second amplification step in the transduction pathway.

Restoration of the System Involves Several Molecular Events

The presence of GTPase in the outer segment converts Ta-GTP to Tα-GDP, which leads to a dissociation of Tα-GDP from the PDE-$\alpha\beta$ subunit. The PDE-γ subunit then reassociates with the PDE-$\alpha\beta$ subunits and inhibits PDE activity. In addition, R* undergoes phosphorylation by rhodopsin kinase, which is thought to diminish the ability of R* to interact with transducin. Finally, arrestin, a 48-kDa protein of the outer segment, is proposed to interact with R* to prevent interaction with transducin.

The GMP-Gated Channel Is an Integral Membrane Protein

The functional cGMP-gated channel complex is thought to be composed of an as yet undetermined number of 63-kDa subunit polypeptides. Hydropathicity plots suggest four or six putative transmembrane segments. The cGMP-binding region is situated near the carboxy terminus on the cytoplasmic surface of the membrane. In excised patches from rod outer segments, application of 10 μM 1-cis-diltiazem reversibly and completely blocks the current induced by 90 mM cyclic GMP when both agents are applied from the cytoplasmic side. Channels expressed in oocytes are blocked by higher concentrations of 1-cis-diltiazem, and reconstituted channels are reported to show little or no 1-cis-diltiazem sensitivity. The composition of lipids in the bilayer is thought to influence the ability of 1-cis-diltiazem to block the action of cGMP.

A Small Fraction of Available cGMP Channels Are Open in the Dark

Under physiological conditions, the maximal light response of amphibian rods is in the range of 40–60 pA. However when high levels of cGMP are injected into the cell, light responses of 1500 pA are observed (MacLeish *et al.*, 1984). This finding indicates that under normal conditions the vast majority, 190% and as high as 99%, of the cGMP-gated channels in the

outer segment are already closed in the dark. The reason for the large reservoir of cGMP channels is not clear, but a consequence of working at the foot of the dose–response curve is relative linearity in the relationship between conductance induced by cGMP and the concentration of cGMP. Using the size of the cGMP current as a calibrator of the levels of cGMP, researchers have estimated that the free cGMP concentration in the dark is 1–5 μM. The extractable amounts of cGMP are considerably higher, indicating that a substantial fraction of the extractable cGMP is actually bound within the cells. A number of binding sites, including sites on the enzyme, PDE, and others on cGMP-gated channels, have been suggested.

cGMP-Gated Channels Have Properties Critical for Phototransduction

In the presence of normal levels of external calcium, single channel activity is not discernible; power spectrum analyses provide estimates of the single

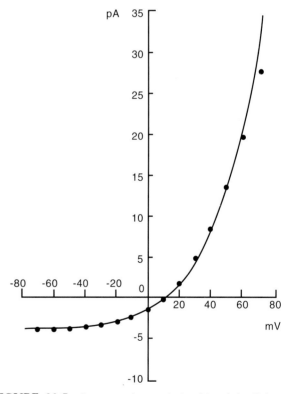

FIGURE 23.7 Current–voltage relationship of the light-suppressed rod current. The curve shows how the light-suppressed current varies with the membrane potential. In the assumed normal operating range (–35 to –60 mV), the size of the current is fairly constant. As the membrane potential approaches 0 to + 10 mV, the current approaches zero. As the inside of the cell is made progressively more positive, the current rises rapidly as shown. From Yau (1994).

channel conductance in the range of 100 fS and a mean open time of 1–2 ms (Fesenko *et al.*, 1985). Single channel activity becomes discernible when external calcium is reduced. The absence of channel noise with normal levels of calcium provides a good background for detecting small photoresponses.

Under physiological conditions, the cGMP conductance mechanism shows outward rectification (Fig. 23.7). In the normal operating range of –35 to –60 mV, the current–voltage curve is relatively flat, producing a constant current region. On approaching 0 mV, the I–V curve changes slope, crosses the voltage axis near 0 mV, and increases rapidly as the inside is made positive. The constant current region in the normal operating range ensures that changes in the light-regulated current arise from transduction events and not from changes in the voltage in response to light. That is, the current in open channels during a light response does not change due to the change in voltage.

Early sodium replacement experiments showed that the removal of sodium ions leads to the abolition of the light response. Subsequent experiments using excised plasma membrane patches from the outer segment revealed that a variety of cations are capable of permeating the conductance mechanism. The rank order is Ca:Na:K = 12:1:0.7. At rest, the fraction of current carried by sodium is largest because sodium is the most abundant ion present.

Extrusion Mechanisms Restore Ionic Balance

Two mechanisms of ion extrusion are prominent in rods. The first is an energy-dependent Na,K-ATPase located in the inner segment. This mechanism pumps sodium ions out and potassium ions into the cell,

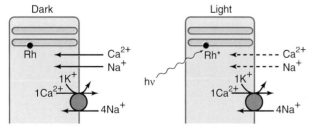

FIGURE 23.8 Calcium flux and the Na–K–Ca rod outer segment exchanger. In the dark (left), both sodium and calcium ions enter the interior of the rod outer segment (Ras) through the cGMP-gated conductance mechanism. To maintain a balance, calcium ions are extruded via an exchange mechanism, with the stoichiometry as shown, that utilizes the energy in the sodium and potassium gradients. In bright light (right), the calcium influx is eliminated but the calcium extrusion process continues, thereby reducing the concentration of free calcium in the ROS. From Yau (1994).

particularly in the dark when the inward sodium current is highest. The second mechanism is a Na-K-Ca exchanger that is found in the outer segment (Fig. 23.8). This mechanism seems to regulate internal calcium levels in the face of calcium entry through cGMP-gated channels. During the light response, when the inward sodium current through cGMP-gated channels is reduced, the activity of the exchanger is maintained, serving to lower intracellular-free calcium. This lowering of intracellular-free calcium has been proposed to increase the activity of the guanylate cyclase, which boosts the return of cGMP levels and returns the cell to the prelight condition.

Phototransduction Shows Adaptation to Light

Photoreceptors adapt to steady background light by decreasing their sensitivity to light. The presence of adaptation increases the dynamic range of rods to cover roughly three orders of magnitude of light intensity. This means that flash intensities that give saturating responses in fully dark-adapted cells give submaximal responses in the presence of steady illumination. The adaptation is fairly rapid and is thought to involve a number of steps in the phototransduction pathway. Research is centered on the role that lowered intracellular calcium might play in mediating light adaptation. The intracellular activity of calcium falls in the presence of light because the influx of calcium is reduced by the suppression of the light-regulated current, but calcium efflux is maintained through the activity of the Na-K-Ca exchanger. A well-established effect of the fall in intracellular activity is an increase in the activity of guanylate cyclase, which acts to restore the level of cGMP that was reduced by light.

Invertebrate Phototransduction Takes Place in Microvillar Photoreceptor Cells

A variety of model systems have been used to study invertebrate phototransduction. These systems include cells from *Limulus*, barnacle, squid, and flies. Despite the great morphological variety in invertebrate photoreceptors, the following features appear common to most. The soma contains organelles specialized for phototransduction, as well as the nucleus and biosynthetic apparatus found in most cells. The visual pigment is stored in a microvillar-rich compartment called a rhabdomere. Microvilli are formed from plasma membrane extensions. In close association with the rhabdomere is an intracellular compartment called the submicrovillar cisternae, which is thought

Light Depolarizes the Photoreceptor Membrane in Invertebrates

Invertebrate photoreceptors respond to light with depolarization (e.g., *Limulus*). Depolarization arises from a conductance increase and an increase in the current carried by sodium ions. Potassium ions also permeate the conductance mechanism, but the permeability change to potassium is estimated to be about half that to sodium, and at the resting potential of –50 mV, the sodium current is considerably larger than the potassium current.

Intracellular recordings from invertebrate photoreceptors reveal small transient depolarizations, called bumps, that are observed in the dark or in response to dim light. The amplitude, latency, and duration of the bumps vary from response to response. In *Limulus*, where bumps have been studied best, the mean amplitude is 0.4 nA, the mean latency is 150 ms, and the mean duration is 80 ms. Background illumination (i.e., light adaptation) leads to a decrease in the amplitude of the bumps as well as to a decrease in mean latency and duration. Decreases in the concentration of bathing calcium lead to increases in the amplitude, latency, and duration of the bumps.

There is overwhelming evidence, arising mainly from statistical analyses of responses to dim lights, that bumps arise from the absorption of single photons of light. From the average size and duration of a bump, it has been estimated that 108 monovalent ions are translocated across the membrane. To account for the charge movement, thousands of channels are presumed to open more or less simultaneously, thereby evoking the production of a diffusible messenger(s) in the phototransduction process to account for the amplification step.

The responses to bright light are thought to arise from the summation of elementary bumps. Mean duration and latency of the response to bright light are shorter than those of a population of bumps. The shorter duration can be accounted for by considering that the later occurring bumps in the response are in effect somewhat light adapted, and the decreased latency can be accounted for qualitatively by considering that within the population of evoked bumps there will be a number with short latencies. A complete explanation of the differences observed in the responses of individual bumps and the macroscopic response is not currently available.

Phototransduction in Invertebrates Involves an Internal Messenger

On the basis of the amplification step in the generation of bumps and on evidence to be presented later, the existence of an internal messenger(s) in the phototransduction pathway has been proposed. The following scheme is widely accepted. Light absorption by the visual pigment leads to activation of the enzyme phospholipase C (PLC) through the involvement of a G protein. The activated PLC causes the release of inositol trisphosphate (IP_3) from phosphoinositol 4,5-bisphosphate, which in turn stimulates the release of calcium from intracellular stores. The rise in free calcium is then proposed to lead to the activation of cation-selective channels in the plasma membrane through an unidentified intermediate (Ranganathan *et al.*, 1994). The movements of calcium are complex and poorly understood. Measurements of extracellular calcium suggest that considerable amounts of calcium leave the cell in response to light. This calcium is probably derived from intracellular stores that must be replenished for proper continued transduction. A maintained rise in intracellular calcium in response to steady light is further proposed to be the signal for light adaptation, as a result of which the sensitivity to light and bump size decreases. cGMP has been proposed as an internal messenger based on reports that cGMP is able to activate a conductance in excised patches of *Limulus* photoreceptors, but no biochemical evidence has been reported to substantiate this physiological finding.

Supportive evidence for this scheme is provided by the following findings.

1. The norpA (no receptor potential) mutants of *Drosophila*, which are defective in PLC, are also defective in phototransduction.

2. Injection of IP_3 leads to a depolarization and bursting activity resembling bumps. The reversal potential of the IP_3-induced response is the same as that induced by light. Also, injection of IP_3 leads to a decrease in the light response and the response to a repeated injection of IP_3.

3. In a number of species, illumination leads to an increase in labeled IP_3 following incubation with labeled inositol.

4. Illumination leads to the activity of a GTPase, which has been shown to be a termination step in the mobilization of the G protein.

5. Light-dependent and IP_3-dependent rises in intracellular free calcium have been reported.

6. Injection of the hydrolysis-resistant GTP analog GTPγS leads to persistent activation of the phototransduction pathway and thereby mimics light.

Rhodopsin and Metarhodopsin Are Interconvertible by Light

A striking difference between the molecular mechanisms in vertebrate and invertebrate transduction is the behavior of the chromophore in response to light. In vertebrates, the 11-*cis* isomer of vitamin A aldehyde is isomerized to the all-*trans* isomer, which then dissociates from the protein moiety, opsin, over a time course of seconds to minutes. The all-*trans* isomer diffuses out of the cell, whereupon it is transported to the retinal pigment epithelium for reisomerization to the 11-*cis* isomer and retransport to the photoreceptor. In invertebrates, the chromophore remains linked covalently to the protein moiety and the interconversion from rhodopsin to metarhodopsin is driven by light. Blue light (<490 nm) drives the reaction from rhodopsin to metarhodopsin, whereas longer wavelength light (1580 nm) drives the reaction from metarhodopsin back to rhodopsin. Slower mechanisms have been described whereby metarhodopsin is converted to rhodopsin in the dark.

Invertebrates Have a Prolonged Depolarizing Afterpotential

Many invertebrate photoreceptors demonstrate a prolonged depolarizing afterpotential (PDA) when a substantial amount of rhodopsin is converted to metarhodopsin by light. The duration of the PDA can be terminated by the application of long wavelength light, which converts metarhodopsin to rhodopsin. A number of similarities have been reported between PDA and a prolongation of the light-suppressed current in vertebrates observed in response to bright flashes. A specific molecular explanation for the PDA involves the inability to phosphorylate metarhodopsin formed by light. The implication is that unphosphorylated metarhodopsin leads to persistent activation of the phototransduction cascade, and upon phosphorylation or reconversion to rhodopsin the PDA is terminated. A number of mutants have been isolated on the basis of the effect on the PDA.

The Study of Mutants Can Provide Insight into Transduction Mechanisms

One of the advantages of working with insects, in particular *Drosophila*, is their short life span and the increased opportunities to generate and study specific mutations within the visual system. A number of mutations involve degeneration of specific photoreceptor cells, whereas others affect aspects of the

electrical signaling that can be used to shed light on the biochemical cascade of events in transduction. Several mutants exhibit photoreceptor degeneration.

The mutant ninaE was selected on the basis of an electrical phenotype. The response to blue light showed neither inactivation nor an afterpotential, hence the name nina. Mutations in the ninaE locus show defects in the visual pigment rhodopsin, which is contained in the R1–R6 photoreceptors of *Drosophila*. The result of this mutation is degeneration of the R1–R6 photoreceptors.

The rdgB (retinal degeneration B) mutant of *Drosophila* is a conditional mutation that requires the presence of light for the degeneration of R1–R6 photoreceptors. In darkness, virtually no degeneration occurs. Treatment with hydrolysis-resistant analogs of GTP, GTPγS, or Gpp(NH)p, as well as with fluoride ions, causes degeneration in the dark presumably by activating the transduction pathway at an early stage. Interestingly, the double mutant rdgB and norpA does not show degeneration.

The phenotype of homozygotes ranges from unresponsive cells to cells with only modest response to light. The norpA gene (no receptor potential) is expressed in photoreceptors and codes for a phospholipase C enzyme. The existence of the norpA mutation strongly implicates PLC in the phototransduction cascade. Neither the rhodopsin content nor the conversion of rhodopsin to metarhodopsin measured spectrophotometrically seems defective in norpA mutants.

The phenotype of the *trp* (*transient receptor potential*) mutation in *Drosophila* is evident in the response to bright lights. The responses to dim light appear normal except for bright steps, the responses relax to values close to baseline in the mutant, and there is a maintained or plateau value for wild-type cells. The electrical response is similar to that seen when the calcium blocker lanthanum is applied, suggesting that the trp mutation leads to a decrease in calcium entry. One suggestion is that the trp gene codes for a type of calcium channel expressed in the plasma membrane of invertebrate photoreceptors. The entry of calcium is thought to be essential in the maintenance of calcium stores inside the photoreceptors. The bump size is unaffected by the mutation, but the frequency of occurrence is reduced severely following the initial response to light. Also, the response latency in the presence of background light is reduced in the mutant. These results indicate that different mechanisms control bump size and the frequency of occurrence. The trp mutation in *Drosophila* is similar to the nss (no steady state) mutation in the blowfly *Lucilia*.

Summary

Diurnal vertebrates have two classes of photo-receptors: rods and cones. Rods are very sensitive to light and subserve vision under scotopic conditions. Cones are less sensitive and subserve vision under photopic conditions. The conversion of light to an electrical signal depends on the presence of visual pigment molecules that are concentrated in the outer segment of rods and cones. These molecules are composed of a seven transmembrane protein component and the 11-*cis*-retinal isomer of vitamin A. Light absorption by the visual pigment causes the isomerization of the 11-*cis*-retinal to all-*trans*-retinal. This is the only light-sensitive step in the light response pathway.

The isomerization of vitamin A triggers a cascade of biochemical reactions and results in the activation of cyclic GMP phosphodiesterase. Activated cyclic GMP phosphodiesterase hydrolyzes cyclic GMP, which causes a decrease in a depolarizing cationic current. The result is membrane hyperpolarization.

The cascade of biochemical reactions contains amplification steps. The electrical response to light is slow and graded. Invertebrate photoreceptors depolarize in response to light. Several mutants are available for possible deciphering of the biochemical steps in the light response of invertebrates.

OLFACTORY TRANSDUCTION

In most species, odor signals play critical roles in feeding, mating, reproduction, and social organization. These behaviors require the fundamental operations of odor detection and odor discrimination. The mechanisms underlying these operations have been the subject of increasing study, and some of the basic principles are beginning to emerge. The principles have come mainly from work on the olfactory receptors of salamanders and rodents among vertebrates and lobsters and insects among invertebrates. Parallel studies are beginning to reveal equivalent signaling mechanisms in the receptor cells of the vomeronasal organ in vertebrates and in the chemosensory cells of nematodes.

Odor Stimuli Consist of a Wide Range of Small Signal Molecules

Odor signals are low molecular weight molecules that fall into several broad classes. In aquatic animals, the molecules tend to be water soluble and include various amino acids that are important for food recognition. Bile salts are also effective stimuli for species such as fish and may function as alarm signals to warn of the presence of predators.

In terrestrial animals, the molecules tend to be small (under 200 Da) and volatile so that they can vaporize readily and be carried in the air; they also tend to be lipid soluble. Some of these are acids, alcohols, and esters found in various plant and animal foods. Some are essential oils. Others are aromatic compounds given off by flowering plants. They may function for long-distance signaling of the presence of food objects in the environment, of the organisms as well as for the palatability of those objects during eating.

An important category consists of molecules used in reproductive activities, including signals used in attracting mates, identifying them, copulating, blocking pregnancy, facilitating nipple attachment by infants, and infant identification. Some of these activities are mediated by complex mixtures of acids, esters, and other types of common molecules; others by individual larger and more complex molecules such as musks; and still others by specific types of molecules for conspecific signaling known as *pheromones*.

Many types of odor molecules have molecular weights and geometrical sizes and shapes that are in the same range as common neurotransmitters such as acetylcholine, glutamate, γ-aminobutyric acid, and glycine. Thus it is not surprising that their receptors may be related.

In order to organize this great variety of molecular types in a rational way, an approach has been developed using as stimuli homologous chemical series (see Box 23.1). This approach has given rise to the concept that a given receptor protein or olfactory cell has a *molecular receptive range* (MRR). This is analogous to the wave length spectrum of a cone pigment or the spatial receptive field of a cell in the visual pathway.

Odor Molecules Are Transduced by Olfactory Receptor Neurons

Most vertebrate animals sense odor molecules by means of olfactory receptor neurons (ORNs) located in a pseudostratified epithelium within the nasal cavity. These are bipolar neurons; a thin dendrite arises from one pole, ending in a knob from which arise 6–12 cilia (Fig. 23.9). These contain the 9 + 2 pairs of microtubules characteristic of true cilia in other cells of the body. The cilia are thin (0.2 mm in diameter near the knob, tapering to 0.1 mm near their tips) and vary in length in different species, from 5–10 mm in humans to 200 mm in frogs. They contain no other organelles. The knobs and cilia are embedded in the mucus overlying the epithelium. The cilia

---

BOX 23.1

HOMOLOGOUS CHEMICAL SERIES OF ODOR COMPOUNDS

Aliphatic (straight chain)
Alkanes: C-C
Alkenes: C=C

<Alcohols: C-C-OH>

Aldehydes: C-C=O
Ketones: C-C=O -C
Carboxylic acids: C-C=O -OH
Esters: C-C=O -O-C
Amines: C-C-NH2

Aromatic (cyclic)
Benzenes: B-C
Phenols: C-OH
Sensory Transduction

The use of these homologous series has provided a systematic method for establishing the molecular receptive range of a cell in the olfactory pathway (see text and Chapter 25).

Peter R. MacLeish,
Gordon M. Shepherd,
Sue C. Kinnamon, and
Joseph Santos-Sacchi

---

greatly increase the surface area containing the olfactory receptors. The large number of cilia form a dense mat within the mucus layer that provides an effective device for capturing odor molecules that are absorbed from the air into the mucus. The mucus is viscous (secreted by the supporting cells) except for a watery surface layer (secreted by Bowman's glands). From the other pole of the neuron, a thin unmyelinated axon arises and joins other axons in the submucosa to form bundles that connect to the olfactory bulb.

Invertebrates such as lobsters and insects also have bipolar olfactory sensory neurons. These generally have longer and more numerous cilia surrounded by lymph and are encased in antennal hairs. The cilia may contain microtubules. In insects, odor molecules access the cilia through pores in the hair, which empty into small spaces called "kettles," where the molecules are absorbed and diffuse to the ciliary membrane. In the nematode, sensory cells have elongated dendrites that end in cilia within pore structures in the snout.

Odor-Binding Proteins May Link Odor Molecules to Odor Receptors

The hydrophobic nature of most odor molecules important for terrestrial animals has implied that special mechanisms may be needed to transport the odor molecules through the lymph or mucus to receptive sites on the cilia. These are referred to as odor-binding proteins (OBP). The best evidence is for a pheromone-binding protein (PBP) in the insect (Vogt and Riddiford, 1981). It is postulated that the PBP binds the pheromone molecules, thereby solubilizing them, and transports them to the cilia receptors; an esterase in the lymph could be involved in inactivating the pheromone molecules. OBPs are predominantly helical proteins with relatively high and narrow specificities for their ligands. By means of photo-affinity labeling of bacterially expressed recombinant PBP, specific amino acid residues that form the binding site for the pheromone ligand have been identified. PBPs may present a combined binding protein–pheromone surface to the odor receptor, similar to the manner in which MHC molecules are involved in presenting antigens to antibodies. It is also possible that PBPs may be involved in both presentation and inactivation of pheromone components.

Putative OBPs have also been found in the vertebrate, where they are secreted by nasal glands into the mucus covering respiratory as well as olfactory nasal epithelium. The vertebrate OBPs are small (ca. 20 kDa), soluble proteins. Cloned and sequenced vertebrate OBPs have an eight-stranded barrel structure that is unrelated to the residue sequence and helical structure

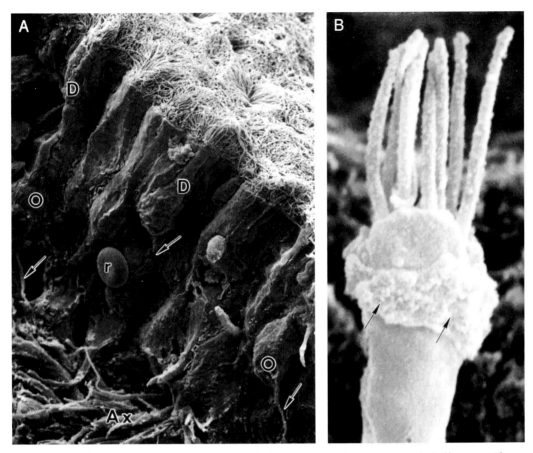

FIGURE 23.9 Olfactory receptor neurons are bipolar cells within the pseudostratified olfactory epithelium. (A): Scanning electron micrograph of the human olfactory epithelium, showing cell bodies of the olfactory receptor neurons (O) with their dendrites (D) ending in cilia that form a mat within the mucus layer overlying the epithelium. From the deeper aspect an axon (arrows) arises, forming bundles (Ax) in the submucosa. Red blood cells (r). (B) High magnification view of the distal dendritic knob giving rise to olfactory cilia. The terminal web is visible encircling the know (arrows). From Morrison and Costanzo (1990).

of the insect OBPs. Vertebrate OBPs have broad odor–ligand affinities, in contrast to the narrower binding affinities of insect OBPs.

To date, no direct physiological evidence has been reported for functions of vertebrate OBPs. Patch recordings from freshly isolated salamander olfactory neurons bathed in artificial medium show responses to odors, suggesting that the mucus, including OBPs, is not necessary for odor molecules to stimulate ORNs. It is speculated that vertebrate OBPs normally may enhance odor responses by concentrating odor molecules in the mucus, presenting them to the receptors, and facilitating their inactivation and removal.

G-Protein-Coupled Receptors Are the Initial Site of Odor Transduction in Mammals

Given their lipid solubility, odor molecules could act at several receptor sites: on or within the membrane or within the cytoplasm. The consensus site at present is a family of G-protein-coupled (GPC) membrane receptors. These were anticipated in 1985 with the demonstration that odors stimulate the cAMP second messenger system in isolated cilia preparations and were finally demonstrated by Buck and Axel (1991). This family of seven transmembrane G-protein-coupled receptors is believed to be the largest gene family in the genome, accounting for up to 3% of the genome in mammals. Numerous members of this gene family have been identified in a variety of species; the count thus far is 33 different species. They have also been identified in large numbers in testes and in small numbers in 30 other tissues of the body. Equivalent olfactory receptors have been identified in insects, although they bear little sequence similarity. A large chemoreceptor family in nematodes accounts for an even larger share of the nematode genome. Some of this information is summarized in Box 23.2.

BOX 23.2

THE LARGEST FAMILY IN THE GENOME

The OR family in the vertebrate ranges in number from catfish (in which a few dozen to 100 are expressed) to mice and rats (up to 1000 members expressed). With the completion of the Human Genome Project, the number of human olfactory genes has been determined to be 900, of which 350 are functional genes and 550 are pseudogenes. The Mouse Genome Project has reported some 900 OR genes, of which nearly all are functional. Chromosome mapping shows that olfactory receptor genes are found commonly in clusters and are distributed broadly in different chromosomes.

This very large gene family presents special problems for developing a rational nomenclature and integrating the sequence information with other types of data. To support this effort, an Olfactory Receptor Database (ORDB) has been built and is accessible over the web

(*senselab.med.yale.edu/ordb*). It contains related data, such as molecular models of receptor–odor ligand interactions, and links to a database of Odor Molecules (odordb), which contains their preferential interactions with ORs that have been expressed and analyzed.

Cloning and sequencing of genes for other types of chemical receptors have continued apace. At the present writing, these include vomeronasal receptors and bitter taste receptors in the vertebrate, olfactory receptors in *Drosophila*, and chemoreceptors in the nematode. These are also archived together with related information at senselab.

Peter R. MacLeish,
Gordon M. Shepherd,
Sue C. Kinnamon, and
Joseph Santos-Sacchi

Determinants on Odor Molecules Interact with Residue Subsites in a Binding Pocket in Olfactory Receptors

The key question in odor transduction is: How is the information contained in different odor molecules transferred to different olfactory receptors? This corresponds to the question in vision: how is the information contained in different wave lengths of light transferred to different visual pigment molecules?

It was predicted early that there would be a large number of olfactory receptors and that each would have a region of high sequence variation where selective interactions with different odor molecules could occur in a combinatorial fashion. With the cloning of the receptors, it was recognized that the high degree of sequence diversity in transmembrane domains IV, V, and VI could serve this function. Computer models were constructed to test the hypothesis that odor ligands bind in a pocket (Fig. 23.10A) similar to that formed by the β-adrenergic receptor (another member of the GPC receptor superfamily) to interact with its neurotransmitter ligand (epinephrine; Fig. 23.10B). Specific sites within the pocket are hypothesized to determine the molecular receptive range of each receptor (Fig. 23.10C).

Experimental analysis of this hypothesis is difficult. First, expressing the receptors in heterologous systems has turned out to be very difficult. Second, in contrast

to most G-protein-coupled receptors, which have narrow affinities for known ligands, olfactory receptors are likely to have broad MRRs. Finally, because there may be thousands of odor ligands, defining the full MRR for a given receptor may turn out to be impossible.

Zhao and colleagues (1998) used a strategy of transfection with a recombinant adenovirus to overexpress a given receptor in the olfactory epithelium of the rat. They tested the electro-olfactogram (EOG) responses of the epithelium to a battery of odors that included several homologous series as well as various other odorous compounds. Among some 80 compounds tested, only longer chain aldehydes gave increased responses over controls, of these, octyl aldehyde gave the peak response, with lesser responses for flanking members of the series (Fig. 23.11A). These experiments provided the first direct evidence that a member of the large gene family of GPC receptors is specifically sensitive to odor stimuli and provided the first evidence of its MRR. Interactions between different odors could be characterized in terms of agonists and antagonists (Fig. 23.11B), suggesting that a pharmacology of olfactory receptors may emerge to permit a rigorous exploration of the range of odor ligands and their interactions at the receptor level.

Insight into the molecular mechanisms for the preferential binding of octanal by receptor I7 was provided by computational modeling of the receptor. The rank order of the specificities in experiment and

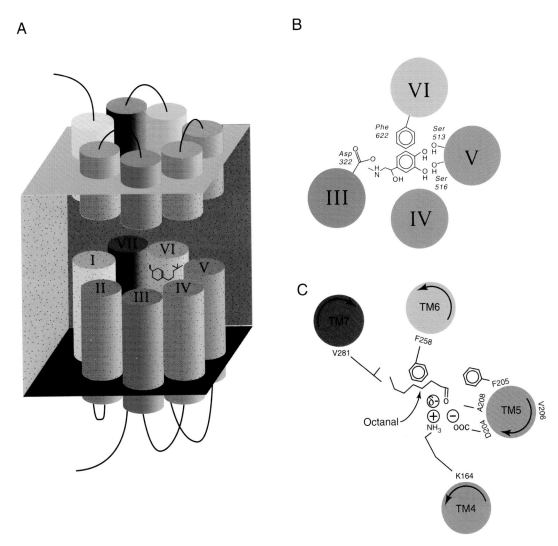

FIGURE 23.10 Molecular modeling analysis provides evidence that odor molecules activate olfactory receptors within a binding pocket similar to that formed by the transmembrane domains (TMs) in β-adrenergic receptors. (A) Schematic model shows how an odor molecule, lyral, may interact with its receptor at a depth within the membrane similar to that at which epinephrine interacts with the β-adrenergic receptor. (B) Specific determinants on the epinephrine molecule are believed to interact with specific amino acid residues in the b-adrenergic receptor. Interactions include coulombic interactions between the cationic amine group of epinephrine and aspartate on TM III; aryl–aryl interactions between the phenyl group and phenylalanine on TM IV; and sterospecific hydrogen bonds between the catechol hydroxyl groups and dual series on TM V. (C) Residue sites shown by molecular modeling to be especially significant in interacting with octal aldehyde in the rat I7 receptor. Sites on TM IV bearing N-rich residues appear to be particularly characteristic of olfactory receptors. Other important sites forming the binding pocket are as indicated. Based on Shepherd and Firestein (1991) and Singer (2000).

model for C6-C9 compounds was similar (Fig. 23.11A). The strongest interaction is between the OH group of octanal and the nitrogen of a lysine residue in the binding pocket (Fig. 23.11C). The differing affinities of the rat I7 receptor for the aldehydes from I6 to I9 appear to reflect physical constraints of other residues forming the binding pocket (see Fig. 23.11C). Modeling of the differing shapes of the aldehydes has given

further insight into the interactions between ligands and binding pocket (Fig. 23.11D). These models may be studied further at senselab.med.yale.edu/ordb. The response spectra of isolated ORNs have been determined, and polymerase chain reaction has been used to identify the receptors. Computational models were able to replicate the rank ordering of preferred ligands showed by a given receptor and pointed

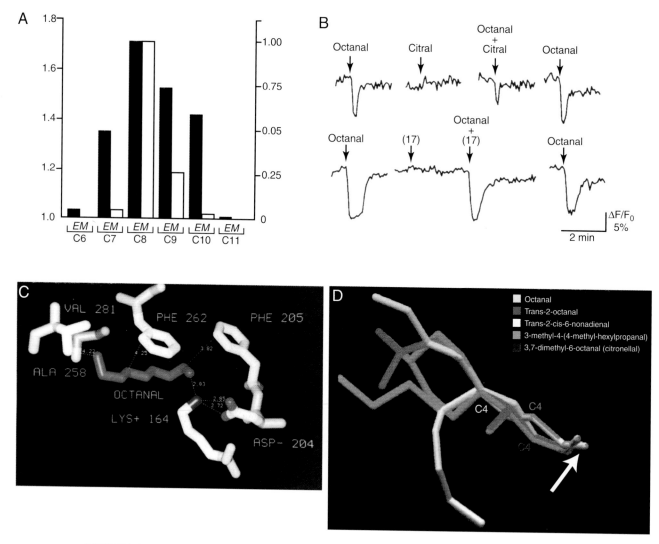

FIGURE 23.11 Detailed analysis of odor binding. (A) Computational (open bars) preferences for aliphatic aldehydes from C6 to C9 have the same rank order as experimental (filled bars). (B) Analysis of I7 responses showing that citral, with no effect of its own, nonetheless reduces the response to citral (acting as a pharmacological antagonist), whereas 2,5,5-trimethyl-2-octenal (17) had little effect on the octanal response. (C) High-resolution analysis of modeled interactions between octanal and key residue sites in the I7 binding pocket. Note how the aldehyde ligand is tethered to the lysine residue through strong OH⁻N⁺ interactions, with weaker interactions determining the preferred shape and length. (D) High-resolution analysis of the conformation of octanal and related molecules showing how the different ligands share conformation at the functional group but differ at the tail ends, giving less favorable fits with the binding pocket. A combines Zhao *et al.* (1998) and Singer (2000); B,D from Araneda *et al.* (2000); B from Singer (2000).

again to a binding pocket where the differential interactions between ligands and receptors take place.

In summary, odor transduction begins with the interactions of a limited number of determinants on odor molecules with a limited number of residue subsites in a binding pocket in olfactory receptor proteins in a combinatorial fashion. Terminology for the interacting entities on the odor molecules has not yet been agreed upon (see Box 23.3). The differential binding

of different odor molecules is the basis for the ability to discriminate between many different odors (see Chapter 24).

cAMP and IP3 Are Second Messengers in Mediating Odor Responses

The finding that olfactory cilia contain an adenylate cyclase that is sensitive to odor stimuli led

---

BOX 23.3

WHAT IS IN A NAME?

The distinguishing features of an odor molecule have been called determinants or, alternatively, epitopes. Epitope is a term from the immune system, where it typically refers to a large reactive site formed by 6–10 amino acids, in contrast to odor compounds of the size of single amino acids, whose determinants are at the atomic level; other terms, such as odortype or odotope, may be therefore be more appropriate. The similarity with the pharmacophores of molecules that bind other members of the G-protein-coupled receptor family suggests that the set of determinants on an odor ligand may be also referred

to as an olfactophore. Theoretical studies suggest that odor ligands commonly comprise three to four determinants, which interact with two to six receptor subsites. Using these estimates, theoretical and computational models can account for the ability of up to 1000 receptors in the mammal to discriminate many more different odors.

Peter R. MacLeish,
Gordon M. Shepherd,
Sue C. Kinnamon, and
Joseph Santos-Sacchi

---

quickly to the molecular cloning and sequencing of all of the components of this second messenger system (Fig. 23.12). These include an olfactory-specific G_s protein (G_{olf}) and an adenylate cyclase type III. This pathway shows interesting adaptations for olfactory transduction. Cyclic AMP production is rapid; in rapid stop-flow experiments, exposure of an isolated cilia preparation to brief olfactory stimuli elicits an abrupt rise in cAMP within 50 ms, with a transient return to baseline.

Evidence for the involvement of a phosphotidylinositol pathway in odor transduction in some species has also been adduced. In stop-flow experiments on preparations of cockroach antennae and rat cilia, odor stimulation elicits short latency transient IP_3 production similar to that shown by cAMP. An important question is whether different odors are associated with the different pathways. In the stop-flow experiments on isolated cilia, it has been reported that odors are associated with either the cAMP or the IP_3 pathway, but not both. However, in cultured olfactory cells, coactivation of the pathways by several different types of odors has been reported. In lobster olfactory neurons, both pathways are present; odor stimulation of a cell leads either to depolarization or to hyperpolarization through the activation of several types of membrane conductances (see Fig. 23.12 and later in this chapter).

A Cyclic Nucleotide-Gated Channel Similar to That in Photoreceptors Is Involved in the Odor Response

Patch recordings from the cilia have shown that in inside-out configurations, cAMP directly activates a

membrane conductance. In single channel recordings in the attached patch mode, the same channels are activated by both cAMP and odors, showing that this is indeed the sensory conductance. The channel has high sequence similarity with the cyclic nucleotide-gated (CNG) channel in photoreceptors. Surprisingly, the native olfactory channel has a higher affinity (K_D 4 mM) for cGMP (the natural ligand in the photoreceptor) than for cAMP (K_D 20 mM). A similar difference has been found in cloned channels. The role of cGMP may be related to gaseous second messengers in the odor response. A Hill coefficient of approximately 2, for both cAMP and cGMP, indicates that channel opening is cooperative, requiring the simultaneous binding of at least two ligand molecules. Selective mutation analysis has identified the nucleotide-binding sites that are specific for the rod photoreceptor channel and the olfactory receptor cell channel (Fig. 23.13).

Like the photoreceptor channel, the olfactory CNG channel is nonselective for cations. Unlike the photoreceptor, the olfactory channel is closed in the absence of sensory stimulation. When odor molecules bind to the receptor and lead to the production of cAMP, the cAMP activates the channel, causing a net inflow of cations that depolarizes the membrane toward an equilibrium potential around zero. Calcium entering through the channel acts as a second messenger activating a chloride channel to increase the outflow of chloride down its gradient from a high internal concentration; this amplifies the depolarization, thereby maximizing the amount of depolarizing sensory current while minimizing calcium inflow that would be harmful to the cilia. In addition, the chloride channel has a very small unitary conductance (less

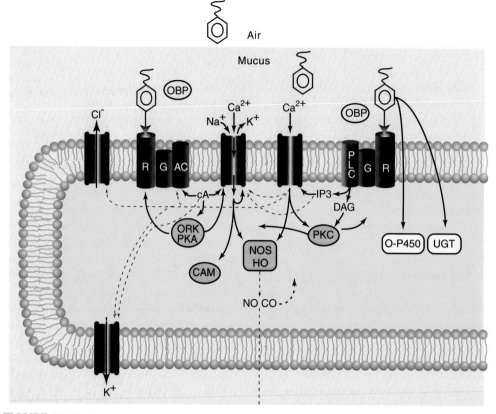

FIGURE 23.12 Sensory transduction of odor molecules involves complex second messenger pathways. Odor molecules are initially absorbed into the olfactory mucus, where they may bind to olfactory-binding protein (OBP), which carries them to the olfactory cilia. The main transduction mechanism in many species is the cyclic AMP pathway, which involves the activation by odor molecules of a receptor (currently believed to be represented mainly by the large gene family of olfactory receptors), a GTP-binding protein (G); an adenylate cyclase (AC), which produces cyclic AMP (cA); and a nonspecific cationic cyclic nucleotide-gated (CNG) channel. The CNG channel is also gated by cyclic GMP (not shown). In some species, evidence exists for activation of a phospholipase (PLC)–inositol trisphosphate pathway that acts on a plasma membrane Ca channel. Ca also gates a Cl conductance that contributes substantially to the sensory current in many species. Ca^{2+} and cA also gate K currents in some species to produce suppressive responses, especially in invertebrates. Solid lines show pathways that have been demonstrated in the rat; dashed lines show pathways demonstrated in other species, including lobster, insect, catfish, mudpuppy, salamander, frog and toad. Second messenger pathways through nitric oxide synthase (NOS) and heme oxygenase (HO) producing the gaseous messengers NO and CO, respectively, are also indicated by dashed lines. Pathways for desensitization and other types of modulation include olfactory receptor kinase (ORK), phosphokinase A (PKA), and C (PKC), diacyl glycerol (DAG), and Ca–calmodulin (CAM). Clearing of odors and other exogenous molecules may take place by olfactory cytochrome P450 (O-P450) and uridyl glucuronic transferase (UGT). Based on many authors; adapted from Shepherd.

than 1 pS), and hence amplification is achieved with minimal noise.

The combined sensory current causes a depolarization that spreads through the cilia and dendritic knob through the dendrite to the cell body and axon hillock, activating voltage-gated channels that generate action potentials. In this way, the amplitude and time course of the graded sensory potentials generated by odor stimuli are transduced into a frequency code of impulses that propagate through the axon to its terminals in the olfactory bulb.

Olfactory Neurons Are Complex Integrative Units

In some species, such as the salamander, transduction involves mainly the depolarizing conductance gated by cAMP together with a depolarizing calcium-gated chloride conductance (see Fig. 23.1). In other species there has been evidence for an IP_3-gated calcium conductance in the plasma membrane, but this is controversial in the rat because G_{olf} knockout mice, presumably specific for the cAMP pathway,

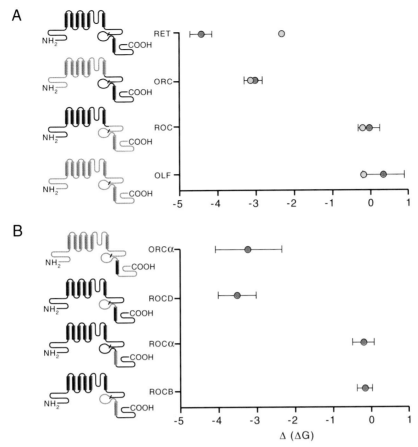

FIGURE 23.13 Chimeras of the retinal and olfactory cyclic nucleotide-gated (CNG) channels show the segments responsible for differing cyclic nucleotide selectivity. (A) The differing affinities of the wild-type retinal (RET) and olfactory (OLF) channels are little affected by substitutions of the transmembrane domains. (B) Localization of the site of CNG selectivity to the C-terminal intracellular helix. ROCB, RET channel that contains the 132 amino acid residues of the putative OLF CNG-binding domain. ROCD, similar to ROCB, but retains the RET C helix. ORC*ga and ROC *ga, only the 24 amino acid residues of the C helices have been exchanged. Graphs show ratio of free energy change of cyclic AMP binding according to the del Castillo and Katz scheme (red circles and standard deviations) and the Monod–Wyman–Changeux model (gray circles). From Goulding *et al.* (1994).

show no other responses as measured by the EOG. Still other species, such as the lobster, have potassium conductances that are modulated either by cAMP or by calcium. These conductances tend to move the membrane potential toward the equilibrium potential for potassium, hyperpolarizing the membrane and opposing the generation of impulses. The interplay of depolarizing and hyperpolarizing sensory potentials is similar to the interplay of excitatory and inhibitory synaptic potentials in central neurons. ORNs thus function as complex integrative units in processing their odor stimuli.

Olfactory neurons vary widely in their responsiveness to different odors, presumably reflecting the differing affinities of their receptors. This means that cells differ in both their threshold and their range of responsiveness to different odors. However, any given cell shows a limited concentration range to a given odor, usually only one to two orders of magnitude. This limited range has been found both in extracellular recordings of receptor neuron responses to square odor pulses (Fig. 23.14A) and in patch recordings of responses of isolated receptor cells to rapid pulses delivered in a bath (Fig. 23.14B). Thus, the total concentration range to which the organism is sensitive is due to parallel processing through different subsets of sensory neurons.

The different concentration ranges of different ORNs for a given odor reflect the relative affinities of olfactory receptors in different ORN subsets for that odor ligand.

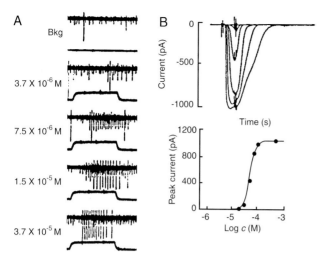

FIGURE 23.14 Olfactory receptor neurons show narrow response ranges of odor concentration. (A) A single salamander olfactory receptor cell responds with increasing impulse discharge to increasing concentrations of amyl acetate odor (the highest concentration of 3.7×10^{-5} was near maximal for the frequency of the impulse response before a spike decrement was observed). From Getchell and Shepherd (1978). (B) Patch recordings show membrane current responses to increasing odor concentration. (Top) Membrane current responses to increasing concentrations of isoamyl acetate. Small spikes are artifacts showing the onset and offset of the odor pulse. (Bottom) Graph of peak current versus odor concentration shows the narrow concentration range of this cell covering less than one log step from threshold to maximum response. From Firestein *et al.* (1993).

Olfactory Adaptation Occurs in Several Stages

The decline of a sensory response during sustained stimulation is referred to as adaptation. In olfactory sensory neurons, adaptation proceeds in several stages. Experimental studies have quickly identified calcium as a key player. The first stage (step 5 in Fig. 23.15), of decline from the initial peak in the sensory response, is associated with the action of calcium; in the absence of calcium there is no decline, and patch recordings show continued channel activity with no desensitization. Single channel analysis has shown that an increase in internal calcium reduces the channel open probability. This effect appears to be mediated by an intermediate calcium-binding protein, possibly calcium–calmodulin, which binds to the channel protein to reduce its affinity for cyclic nucleotides. Increases in intracellular calcium following odor stimulation have also been documented using calcium-sensitive dyes. The calcium increase caused by odor stimuli in individual cilia can be visualized by confocal microscopy. Such analysis at the level of the individual cilium is comparable to the imaging of calcium changes in individual cilia of hair cells.

The second stage of adaptation is called short-term adaptation (STA). This occurs in response to the action of caged cAMP alone and suggests a feedback pathway from calcium and involves continued desensitization of the response by calcium/calmodulin-dependent protein kinase II acting on adenylate cyclase (step 6 in Fig. 23.15). This is followed by long term adaptation (LTA), which involves the activation of guanylate cyclase and the production of cyclic GMP (step 7 in Fig. 23.15). Another longer term contributor is a Na/Ca exchanger, which restores the ion balance (step 8 in fig. 23.15).

Calcium ions also act externally to reduce the conductance of the channel. In the absence of calcium, the channel has a unitary conductance of some 45 pS; in normal extracellular calcium, calcium entering the channel induces a "flicker block," reducing the conductance to less than 1 pS. This block is removed by depolarizing the membrane, suggesting that in normal calcium, olfactory sensory neurons act as coincidence detectors for cyclic nucleotide production plus membrane depolarization. In normal calcium and at normal resting potential, most of the channels appear to be in the blocked state. This mechanism may enhance the signal-to-noise ratio of the sensory response, as in photoreceptors.

Odor Responses Encode Odor Molecules by Their Sensory Currents

The outcome of these transduction steps is the generation of a sensory current by the CNG channels. In response to stimulation with a particular odor, the amplitudes and time courses of this sensory current vary in different neurons, reflecting the differing affinities of the receptors and the properties of the second messenger pathways. These differences across the whole population of sensory neurons provide the basis for encoding the information carried in particular odor molecules. However, a single cell cannot encode independent properties of the stimulus by itself. For this, parallel inputs from other cells responding differentially to those independent properties are needed; this is why there are many receptor cells. These inputs need to go to a processing station where they can be compared and processed for further transmission to higher centers. This is the function of the olfactory bulb (see Chapter 24).

Transduction Mechanisms in the Vomeronasal Organ Are Similar and Different

In addition to the main olfactory epithelium, a second site of chemical messenger transduction exists

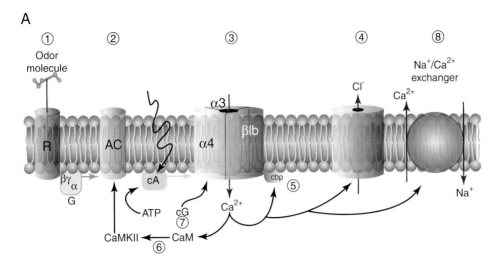

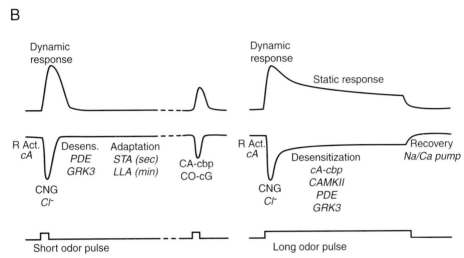

FIGURE 23.15 Olfactory adaptation occurs in successive stages. (A) Schematic diagram of the sensory transduction components in the cilia in greater detail. Steps 1–3 generate the initial sensory response. Step 4: calcium activates a chloride conductance, which amplifies the sensory response. Step 5: Ca^{2+} activates a calcium binding protein (cbp), which produces immediate adaptation from the initial dynamic response peak. Step 6: Ca^{2+} activates a calcium/calmodulin-dependent protein kinase II, which produces short-term adaptation (LTA). Step 7: Ca^{2+} activates a cyclic GMP second messenger pathway which activates CO, which acts on the CNG channel to produce long-term adaptation (LTA). Step 8: a Ca/Na exchanger restores ion balance. Abbreviations, see text. Based on Menini (1999); Zufall and Leinders-Zufall (2000), and others.

in vertebrates. This site is Jacobson's organ, also known as the vomeronasal organ (VNO; see Chapter 24). It is present in a variety of vertebrate species and appears to be specialized for transmitting signals from less volatile or nonvolatile odorous compounds. Phylogenetically, it is first differentiated clearly in snakes, where it is involved in several functions, including mating behavior and responses to prey odors that are sampled from the tongue as it is drawn over the inlet to the organ. In rodents, the organ is well developed and is believed to be stimulated by sexually active substances that access the inlet to the organ as a male directly investigates the female's vaginal opening.

In ungulates such as deer and horses, the inlet is exposed by a nasal movement called a flehmen reaction, in which the male investigates the urine of the female to determine her mating receptivity.

Two families of genes encoding putative receptor proteins have been isolated from the vomeronasal organ in rats. First was a family of seven transmembrane, G-coupled receptors that is distinct from the OR gene family in the main olfactory epithelium. A second family in the rat and mouse has a very long N-terminal extracellular domain and shares sequence similarity with calcium sensory receptors and metabotropic glutamate receptors.

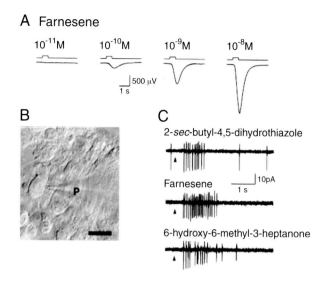

A Farnesene

10^{-11}M 10^{-10}M 10^{-9}M 10^{-8}M

500 μV
1 s

B

P

C

2-*sec*-butyl-4,5-dihydrothiazole

Farnesene   10pA
                          1 s

6-hydroxy-6-methyl-3-heptanone

D

Name	Chemical structure	Origen	Possible chemosignalling function in femail mice	Detection threshold EVG response
2,5-dimethylpyrazine		Female urine	Puberty delay	10^{-8} - 10^{-7}M
2-*sec*-butyl-4,5-dihydrothiazole		Male bladder urine	Oestrus synchronizzation puberty acceleration	10^{-10} - 10^{-9}M
2,3-dedydro-*exo*-brevicomin		Male bladder urine	Oestrus synchronizzation puberty acceleration	10^{-10} - 10^{-9}M
α-and β-farnesenes		Male preputial gland	Puberty acceleration	10^{-11} - 10^{-10}M
2-heptanone		Female or male urine	Oestrus extension	10^{-11} - 10^{-10}M
6-hydroxy-6-methyl-3-heptanone		Male bladder urine	Puberty acceleration	10^{-8} - 10^{-7}M

FIGURE 23.16 VNO receptor cells are narrowly tuned and extremely sensitive to pheromone-like molecules. A. Patch recordings of membrane currents elicited by farnesene (15 carbon) at increasing concentrations. (B) Photomicrograph of recording pipette patched on a cell. (C) Impulse discharges of different cells responding to three different substances. (D) Chemical structures of the putative pheromone molecules tested. From Leinders-Zufall *et al.* (2000).

It is widely believed that these proteins function as pheromone receptors. Paradoxically, the best behavioral evidence for a pheromone in mammals, is androstenedione in pigs, which mediates its effects through the main olfactory pathway rather than the VNO. The receptor functions of these proteins thus await further study.

Strong clues have been obtained by recording the receptor currents of VNO cells in response to stimulation with candidate pheromone-like molecules in the urine or sexual glands. It has been shown that VNO cells can respond to extremely low concentrations of these molecules, down to 10^{-11} dilution (Leinders-Zufall *et al.*, 2000) (Fig. 23.16). A given substance activated only approximately 1% of cells tested (similar to the percent of cells expressing a given VNO receptor). Responsive cells were highly selective for a single substance (i.e. they behaved like insect pheromone specialists) at all concentrations. These experiments thus open the way to systematic comparison of the selective properties of ORNs in the main olfactory epithelium and the VNO.

Summary

The olfactory receptor cell is a complex neuron, in which one of a large number of possible broad affinity receptors activates multiple second messenger and desensitization systems to transduce the information carried in odor molecule determinants into sensory currents, which are then converted into impulse discharges. Sensitive detection depends on the amplification in the second messenger systems within a single cell and the summation that occurs over the large population of receptor cells. Discrimination between odors cannot be accomplished by a single cell because it cannot distinguish odor type from odor intensity. Discrimination between odors therefore depends initially on the ensemble of differentially responding cells with their overlapping response spectra. Discrimination further requires an ordered map of projections of the ensemble and circuits to read the parallel pathways. The sensory responses are therefore carried in the frequency of impulse discharge to the olfactory bulb, where circuits compare the parallel inputs comprising an orderly map and discriminate odor type and odor intensity. The resulting integrated ensemble is the basis for further processing that gives rise to the perception of smell (Chapter 24).

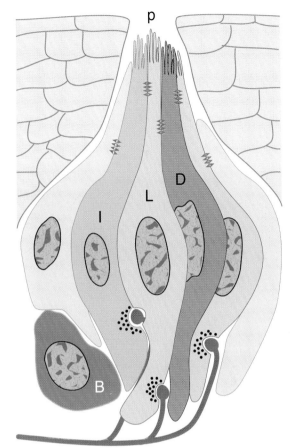

FIGURE 23.17 Diagram of a taste bud showing basal stem cells (B) and taste receptor cells. Most taste buds contain dark (D), light (L), and intermediate (I) taste cells. The apical tips of the taste cells contain microvilli that protrude through the taste pore (p) into the oral environment, whereas the basolateral membrane forms chemical synapses with afferent nerve fibers. A typical taste bud contains 50–150 taste receptor cells.

TASTE

Taste Stimuli Are Transduced by Taste Receptor Cells

The sense of taste is mediated by taste receptor cells, which are organized into tiny onion-shaped end organs called taste buds. Taste buds are found primarily within papillae of the lingual epithelium, although in mammals, some taste buds are found in other parts of the oral cavity and in fish they are also abundant on the barbels and over much of the body surface. A typical taste bud contains 50–150 spindle-shaped receptor cells (taste cells) that extend from the basal lamina to the mucosal surface of the tongue (Fig. 23.17). The apical tip of each receptor cell contains microvilli that project into the mucus of the oral

environment. The basolateral membrane of taste cells forms chemical synapses with primary gustatory nerve fibers that enter the base of the taste bud. These sensory fibers travel in the facial, glossopharyngeal, or vagus nerves to gustatory nuclei in the brain stem.

In contrast to odorants, taste stimuli generally are water-soluble, nonvolatile compounds encountered at relatively high concentrations. Four or five primary taste qualities—salty, sweet, sour, bitter, and umami (the savory taste of monosodium glutamate and some nucleotides)—describe most gustatory sensations in humans. This classification scheme is based on electrophysiological and psychophysical studies showing that adaptation to any one of the primary taste qualities has no effect on the others. For example, when a bitter-tasting compound is placed on the tongue, the response to subsequent presentations of bitter stimuli

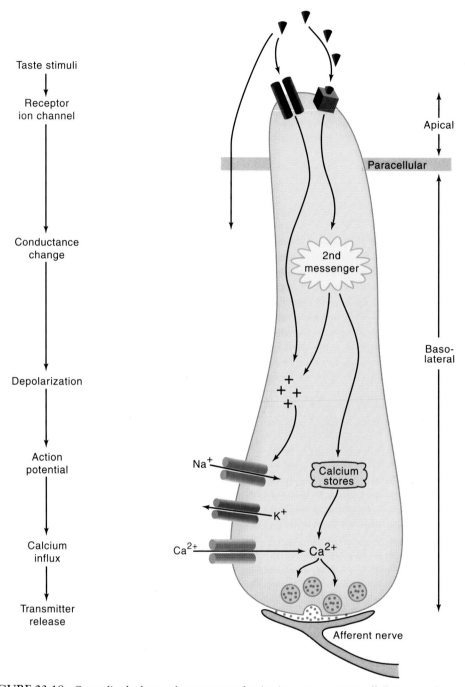

FIGURE 23.18 Generalized scheme of sensory transduction in a taste receptor cell. Taste stimuli interact with the apical membrane, either by binding to specific membrane receptors or by modulating apically located ion channels. The interaction usually leads to membrane conductance change, membrane depolarization, action potentials, Ca^{2+} influx, and transmitter release. Some taste stimuli activate second messenger pathways that trigger the release of Ca^{2+} from intracellular stores. Whether Ca^{2+} release is sufficient to cause release of neurotransmitter is not known.

will be reduced due to adaptation, but the taste of sweet compounds will be unaffected. Whether umami is clearly a primary taste quality is still controversial. Most taste stimuli are hydrophilic molecules, including Na^+ salt (salty), divalent salts, and KCl (salty and

bitter), acids (sour), sugars (sweet), amino acids (sweet, bitter, and umami), and proteins (sweet and bitter). Some taste stimuli are lipophilic, including the bitter-tasting alkaloids and many synthetic sweeteners. Because diffusion through the aqueous saliva is slow for lipophilic compounds, carrier proteins analogous to odorant-binding protein may transport such molecules to the apical microvilli.

Taste transduction is initiated when sapid molecules interact with sites on the apical microvilli of taste receptor cells. The interaction leads to a membrane conductance change, depolarization, and transmitter release from the taste cell onto gustatory fibers (Fig. 23.18). Although taste cells were once thought to be passive transducers, it is now clear that they possess voltage-gated sodium, calcium, and potassium channels and regularly generate action potentials in response to most taste stimuli. The precise role of the action potential in the transduction process is not known, although it may be involved in activation of the calcium channels underlying transmitter release and in the coding of stimulus intensity. Because the chemical structures of different taste stimuli differ greatly from one another, it is not surprising that taste cells use a diversity of mechanisms for signal transduction. Such mechanisms include direct interaction of taste stimuli with apically located ion channels, G-protein-coupled receptors, and ligand-gated ion chan-

nels. How these mechanisms are utilized by taste receptor cells to transduce the different taste qualities is considered next.

Sodium Ions Permeate Apically Located Na⁺ Channels to Depolarize Taste Cells

Evidence suggests that the sodium salt taste, at least in rodents, is transduced by the epithelial sodium channel ENaC (Lindemann et al., 1999). This channel, which is responsible for sodium transport in a variety of epithelial tissues, is expressed on the apical membrane of salt-sensitive taste cells, where it mediates the passive influx of sodium (Fig. 23.19). Sodium simply diffuses through the open channels to depolarize taste cells; presumably the sodium is pumped out by a NaK-ATPase on the basolateral membrane. The first evidence for a role of ENaC in taste came from experiments showing that the gustatory nerve response to NaCl was inhibited by amiloride, a diuretic drug known to block these channels in other transporting epithelial tissues. More recently, patch-clamp recordings have demonstrated directly the presence of amiloride-sensitive sodium channels in taste cell membranes. These channels have a high selectivity for sodium, a low single-channel conductance (5 pS), and are regulated by hormones such as vasopressin and aldosterone.

It appears that ENaC is used to detect sodium primarily in species that have a deficiency of sodium in their diet, including rodents and other herbivores. Behavioral studies with these species have shown that in the presence of amiloride, NaCl cannot be distinguished from KCl. In other species, including humans, different mechanisms for sodium detection are likely. One of these mechanisms is paracellular, involving the diffusion of NaCl through tight junctions at the apex of the taste bud, thereby increasing sodium concentrations in the extracellular space along the basolateral membranes of taste cells. Presumably, this sodium enters the taste cells to depolarize them, but the channels or transport proteins involved have not been identified.

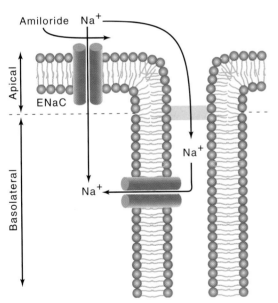

FIGURE 23.19 Sodium salt transduction. Sodium permeates apically located amiloride-sensitive Na⁺ channels; the Na⁺ simply flows down its electrochemical gradient to depolarize the taste cell. Data suggest that the epithelial Na⁺ channel ENaC is the channel that mediates Na⁺ transduction, at least in rodents. Some Na⁺ also penetrates the tight junctions at the apex of the taste bud. This Na⁺ likely enters the cell via Na⁺-permeable channels on the basolateral membrane (the paracellular pathway). Whether these basolateral channels are the same amiloride-sensitive channels that are expressed on the apical membrane is not known. Sodium that enters the cell is pumped out by a Na⁺, K+-ATPase on the basolateral membrane (not shown).

Acids Depolarize Taste Cells by Modulating Ion Channels Sensitive to Changes in Proton Concentration

Another taste quality that does not require specific membrane receptors for transduction is sour taste. Sour taste is produced by acids, and the degree of sourness depends primarily on proton concentration. Patch-clamp studies suggest that several different ion channels may participate in sour transduction, which

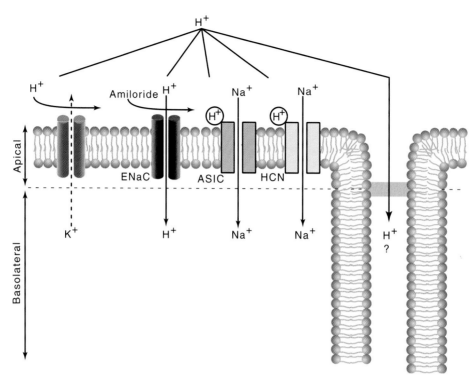

FIGURE 23.20 Acid (sour) transduction. Protons utilize several mechanisms for transduction. One mechanism involves proton permeation of the amiloride-sensitive Na$^+$ channel ENaC. Other mechanisms include the proton-gated, acid sensing ion channels (ASICs) and the proton-modulated, hyperpolarizing cation channel HCN. In addition, protons block apically located K$^+$ channels to depolarize taste cells. Protons probably also permeate the paracellular pathway, but the effects of protons on basolateral channels have not been determined.

is not surprising because protons are capable of modulating most ion channels (Fig. 23.20). One channel that has been found to transduce protons in hamster taste cells is the amiloride-sensitive sodium channel ENaC, the same channel that transduces sodium salt. Both loose patch recordings from taste buds *in situ* and whole cell recordings from isolated taste cells showed that, in the absence of sodium, proton influx through amiloride-sensitive sodium channels depolarized taste cells and contributed to the detection of acids. Because sodium salt can be distinguished easily from the taste of acids, additional mechanisms must exist for the detection of protons. One of these mechanisms may involve acid-sensing ion channels (ASICs), proton-gated cation channels found in brain and sensory ganglia that mediate pain in response to tissue acidosis. At least one ASIC subunit has been identified in taste cells, but its role in sour taste has not been determined. Other channels that have been proposed to participate in sour transduction in mammalian taste cells include hyperpolarization-activated channels, chloride channels, and proton channels. The

relative roles of these different channels in sour taste transduction have not been determined.

Specific Membrane Receptors for Complex Taste Stimuli

In contrast to the ionic taste stimuli just described, specific membrane receptors appear to be required for the transduction of sugars, synthetic sweeteners, amino acids, and many bitter-tasting compounds. Several different receptors are likely to be involved with taste transduction, and recently several putative G-protein-linked taste receptors have been cloned (Fig. 23.21). A novel variant of the metabotropic glutamate receptor mGluR4 has been identified in taste cells, and this receptor appears to underlie the transduction of glutamate (umami) taste (Chaudhari *et al.*, 2000). This receptor is discussed in more detail in the section on amino acids.

Two different families of G-protein-linked taste receptors have been cloned as a result of the genetic sequencing of mouse and human genomes. The T1R

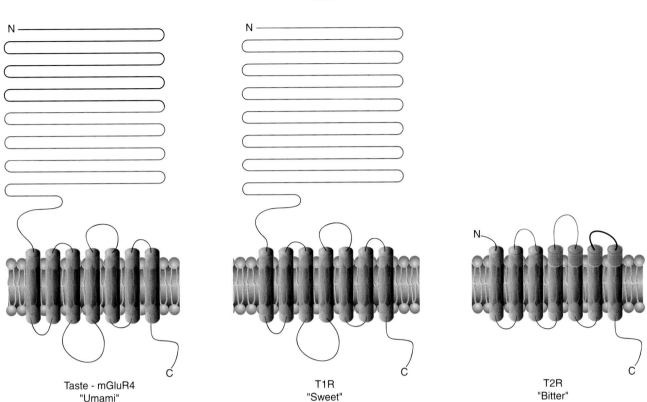

Taste - mGluR4   T1R   T2R
"Umami"   "Sweet"   "Bitter"

FIGURE 23.21 Complex stimuli utilize G protein-coupled receptors for transduction. Three families of taste receptors have been cloned. Taste–mGluR4, a candidate umami receptor, is a truncated variant of the brain form of the receptor. The T1R family consists of three members, one of which (T1R3) was cloned from the sweet-responsive locus SAC, suggesting that it is a sweet receptor. The T2R family of receptors was cloned from the human bitter-sensitive locus PROP. This family consists of approximately 30 different receptors, 3 of which have been expressed in heterologous cells and shown to respond to bitter stimuli.

receptor family has three members, T1R1–T1R3. These receptors bear structural homology to the metabotropic glutamate receptors, with a large N-terminal region believed to house the ligand-binding domain. Although none of these receptors has been expressed, T1R3 was identified in the "SAC" locus, a locus known to be associated with sweet taste deficits in mice. Importantly, several amino acid residues differ in the putative ligand binding domains of the receptor in taster and nontaster mice, suggesting that T1R3 is a sweet taste receptor (Montmayeur *et al.*, 2001).

A second, much larger family of G-protein-linked taste receptors, the T2Rs, was cloned from a locus in humans that is linked to the bitter taste perception of propylthiouracil (PROP) (Adler *et al.*, 2000). The T2R receptor family is believed to comprise over a hundred receptors, two of which have been expressed in heterologous cells and shown to respond specifically to bitter taste stimuli. Unlike T1R receptors, the T2R

receptors have a short N-terminal sequence and bear structural homology to the olfactory receptors. The specific role of these receptors in bitter transduction is considered in more detail later.

Sweet Taste Involves Receptors Linked to the cAMP and IP₃ Second Messenger Pathways

Receptors for sugars are thought to be coupled to G_S, the GTP-binding protein that stimulates adenylate cyclase. Taste cell depolarization is thought to involve a cyclic nucleotide-dependent closure of potassium channels (Fig. 23.22). The first evidence for a role of cyclic nucleotides in sweet transduction came from biochemical studies in which sucrose stimulated adenylate cyclase in a preparation of rat taste buds. The increase in cAMP required GTP, suggesting the involvement of G-protein-coupled receptors. The involvement of potassium channels in the transduc-

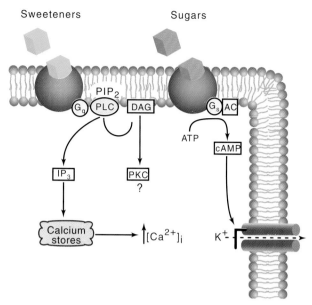

FIGURE 23.22 Sweet transduction. Sugars have been found to activate adenylate cyclase (AC), resulting in a cAMP-dependent closure of K^+ channels and membrane depolarization. Synthetic sweeteners activate phospholipase C (PLC), producing the second messengers IP_3 and diacylglycerol (DAG). IP_3 causes the release of Ca^{2+} from intracellular stores, whereas DAG activates protein kinase C (PKC). Whether PKC is involved in the transduction of synthetic sweeteners is not known, but additional steps are likely, as sweeteners elicit trains of action potentials in taste cells.

tion cascade comes from electrophysiological studies showing that sweet stimuli depolarize taste cells by decreasing potassium conductance. The effect is mimicked by membrane-permeant analogs of cAMP and cGMP. Whether the cAMP blocks the potassium channels directly or whether activation of cAMP-dependent protein kinase is required has not been resolved.

Biochemical and calcium imaging studies have indicated that synthetic sweeteners may use a pathway for transduction different from that engaged by sugars. Evidence comes from biochemical assays showing that synthetic sweeteners stimulate IP_3 and DAG rather than cAMP in rat taste buds (Fig. 23.22). Calcium imaging studies using fura-2 are consistent with these findings; stimulation of taste cells with synthetic sweeteners causes release of calcium from intracellular stores, whereas sucrose stimulation causes calcium influx in the same taste cells (Bernhardt *et al.*, 1996). How release of IP_3 and DAG lead to transmitter release in taste cells is not known. Studies suggest that DAG activates protein kinase C to depolarize taste cells, but the precise mechanisms involved have not been elucidated.

Bitter Taste Involves Both G-Protein-Coupled Receptors and Apically Located Ion Channels

The large number of bitter-tasting compounds and the diversity of their molecular structures suggest that bitter taste involves multiple mechanisms of transduction. Indeed, several mechanisms have been proposed, and several components of bitter signaling pathways have been identified (Fig. 23.23). The best understood mechanism involves binding of bitter compounds to the T2R family of bitter taste receptors. Two receptors have been functionally expressed in heterologous cells and found to be narrowly tuned to particular bitter compounds:- mT2R5 responds specifically to cyclohexamide, whereas mT2R8 responds strongly to denatonium and weakly to PROP.

These receptors are linked to a heterotrimeric G protein consisting of α-gustducin and its partners, $\beta 3$ and $\gamma 13$ (Huang *et al.*, 1999). α-Gustducin has considerable sequence homology to the transducins, G proteins that activate phosphodiesterase in the photoreceptor transduction cascade. Activation of α-gustducin activates phosphodiesterase to decrease cyclic nucleotide concentrations in taste cells, while the $\beta\gamma$ partners of gustducin stimulate phospholipase C$\beta 2$ to produce IP_3 and DAG. While the physiological significance of the decrease in cyclic nucleotides is still unclear, IP_3 binds to type III IP_3 receptors on smooth endoplasmic reticulum, causing a release of Ca^{2+} from intracellular stores. Whether the Ca^{2+} released from intracellular stores is sufficient to trigger transmitter release is still unknown. Transgenic mice lacking the α-gustducin protein have been produced. These gustducin "knockout" mice are less sensitive than normal mice to bitter compounds, confirming that gustducin plays an important role in bitter transduction. However, gustducin knockout mice are also less sensitive to sweet stimuli so further experiments will be required to elucidate the role of gustducin in taste.

Some bitter compounds are lipophilic and likely activate intracellular signaling mechanisms directly. These include caffeine and theophylline, which increase intracellular cGMP levels by the direct inhibition of phosphodiesterases. Specific membrane receptors do not appear to be required for the transduction of these compounds. Other bitter compounds that do not require specific membrane receptors for transduction are bitter salts, including KCl and divalent salts. In *Necturus* taste cells, apically located potassium channels mediate their transduction. Divalent salts directly block a resting efflux of potassium, depolarizing the taste cells, whereas potassium salts depolarize cells by the passive influx of potassuim through the channels. Whether apical potassium channels con-

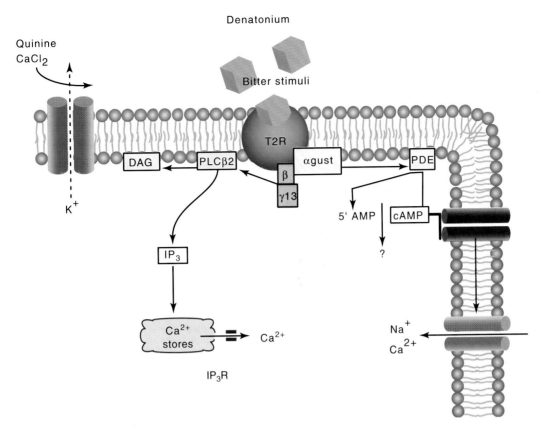

FIGURE 23.23 Bitter transduction. The bitter stimulus denatonium binds to a T2R taste receptor, resulting in activation of a heterotrimeric G protein consisting of α-gustducin and its two partners, $\beta 3$ and $\gamma 13$. α-Gustducin activates phosphodiesterase (PDE) to decrease cAMP, whereas $\beta 3/\gamma 13$ activates phospholipase C $\beta 2$ (PLC $\beta 2$) to produce IP_3 and diacylglycerol (DAG). IP_3 binds to IP_3 receptors on the smooth endoplasmic reticulum to cause the release of calcium from intracellular stores. The ion channels that respond to the decrease in cAMP have not been identified, but direct cyclic nucleotide-blocked cation channels may be involved. In this case, denatonium would depolarize taste cells by removing the cAMP block of the cation channels, allowing an influx of cations. Another mechanism for bitter transduction involves a direct block of apically located K^+ channels by quinine and divalent salts. Block of K^+ channels causes a reduced efflux of K^+, resulting in membrane depolarization.

tribute significantly to bitter transduction in mammals remains to be seen.

Amino Acids Utilize Ligand-Gated Channels and G-Protein-Coupled Receptors for Transduction

Mechanisms involved in the transduction of amino acids are illustrated in Fig. 23.24. Amino acids have been studied extensively in catfish, where barbels contain a high density of taste buds and the taste cells are extremely sensitive to amino acids. Biochemical and electrophysiological studies indicate that L-arginine and L-proline are transduced by ligand-gated cation channels on the apical membrane of taste cells.

Membrane vesicles from catfish taste epithelia have been incorporated into bilayers on the tips of patch pipettes to study the properties of these channels. Both L-arginine and L-proline activate nonselective cation channels in these bilayers, suggesting that the channels are coupled directly to their receptors.

The L-argine-gated channel has a conductance of 45 pS and is activated maximally by 100–200 mM L-arginine. The L-proline-gated channel has a conductance of 49 pS and is activated maximally by 2–4 mM L-proline. These values are consistent with the binding affinities and electrophysiological responses to these amino acids.

The only amino acid that has been studied extensively as a taste stimulus in mammalian taste cells is

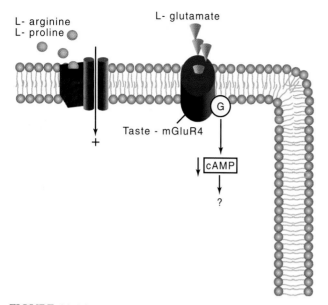

FIGURE 23.24 Amino acid transduction. Taste cells located in catfish barbels are extremely sensitive to particular amino acids. Both L-arginine and L-proline directly activate ligand-gated cation channels to depolarize taste cells. In contrast, in mammalian taste cells, L-glutamate likely activates the metabotropic glutamate receptor taste– mGluR4, resulting in a decrease in cAMP. How the decrease in cAMP leads to membrane depolarization is not understood.

L-glutamate, which is believed to elicit the "umami" sensation. As noted earlier, a recent study demonstrated a novel variant of the metabotropic glutamate receptor mGluR4 from taste-derived mRNA. Taste–mGluR4, which has a truncated N-terminal region compared with the brain form of the receptor (Fig. 23.22), has been functionally expressed in heterologous cells. Taste–mGluR4 responds to glutamate at the expected concentration range for glutamate taste and leads to decreases in intracellular cAMP. *In situ* hybridization has shown that taste–mGluR4 is expressed in taste buds, but not in the surrounding nongustatory epithelium. Evidence suggesting that this receptor has a role in glutamate taste comes from studies showing that L-AP4, the specific ligand for mGluR4, evokes behaviors in rats that are similar to those evoked by L-glutamate. Electrophysiological studies are required to confirm the role of taste–mGluR4 in taste transduction.

Current research interests are focused on identifying the molecular components involved in the different transduction pathways, as well as how the different components are segregated into different cells. For example, do cells that express the T2R bitter taste receptors respond only to bitter compounds or do these cells also respond to other taste modalities? A considerable effort is focused on identifying the specific role of α-gustducin in taste transduction.

Summary

Taste cells use a diversity of mechanisms for transduction. Ionic stimuli (e.g., salts and acids) interact directly with ion channels to depolarize taste cells, whereas more complex stimuli (e.g., sugars and amino acids) bind to receptor proteins that are coupled either to G proteins and second messengers or directly to ion channels. Transduction ultimately results in an increase in intracellular calcium and a release of transmitter from the taste cell onto gustatory afferent fibers.

MECHANORECEPTION

Organisms are capable of detecting both remotely generated mechanical perturbations in the environment (sound and vibration) and self-generated mechanical perturbations induced by body movement. The organ system responsible for this capability is known as the acoustico (or octavo)-lateralis system, and it uses as its basic sensory unit a modified epithelial cell—the hair cell. Hair cells are located in a variety of specialized sensory organs. For example, in the mammal, the organ of Corti detects sound, and the vestibular sensory structures detect angular and linear acceleration through space. The lateral line system in fishes and amphibia detects water-borne vibrations.

Hair Cells Transduce Mechanical Energy Directly into Electrical Energy

Hair cells are polarized epithelial cells whose major functions are partitioned into apical and basal cellular compartments (Fig. 23.25). The apical end of the cell is specialized for the reception and translation of mechanical energy into receptor currents, whereas the basal end is specialized for the transmission of information to the central nervous system via synaptic contacts with the primary afferent neuron. Stereocilia are modified microvilli, a fraction of a micrometer in width, that project from the cell apex and contain an abundant supply of tightly packed actin filaments, bound by fimbrin, coursing along their length. Depending on which specific organ the hair cells reside in, the number of these stiff, rod-like stereocilia ranges from about 10 to 300, and their lengths range from a fraction to tens of micrometers. The stereocilia, which are bundled together by extracellular filamentous linkages, taper rapidly as they insert into the cuticular plate, an actin-rich apical cytoplasmic structure. Because the stereocilia are stiff, they pivot at their insertion when deflected. All hair cells, at one point in their differentiation, possess an additional

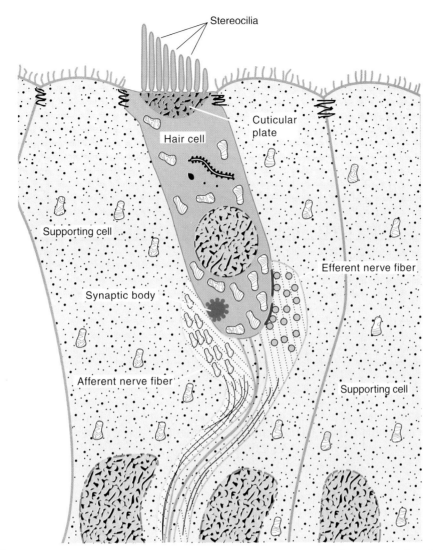

FIGURE 23.25 Schematic of a hair cell with supporting cells. Reprinted with permission from Hillman (1976).

apical protrusion, the kinocilium. This is a true cilium and contains the characteristic 9 + 2 microtubule doublets. In the organ of Corti, mature hair cells have lost this kinocilium and possess only stereocilia. The stereocilia of all hair cells are arranged hexagonally in rows and graded in height, with the tallest stereocilia row adjacent to the kinocilium or, in cells lacking the kinocilium, adjacent to its residual basal body. This characteristic morphologic polarization of the stereocilia bundle identifies the orientation of the bundle's responsiveness to mechanical deflection.

Through a variety of accessory mechanisms specific to each sensory organ, mechanical sensory stimuli ultimately cause a deflection of the hair bundle. When the bundle is deflected toward the tallest stereocilia row, a depolarization of the cell from its normal negative resting potential occurs, resulting

in an increase in neurotransmitter release and excitation of the afferent nerve fiber (see Fig. 23.26). When the deflection is in the opposite direction, hyperpolarization occurs, resulting in a decrease in transmitter release and inhibition of fiber activity.

Receptor Potentials Are Evoked by Mechanically Gated Ion Channels within Stereocilia

With the stereocilia bundle in its resting, unperturbed position, a standing inward current exists through a small proportion (10–25%) of mechanically activated channels thought to be located within each stereocilium. Because these channels are nonselective for cations, this inward, positively charged flux tends

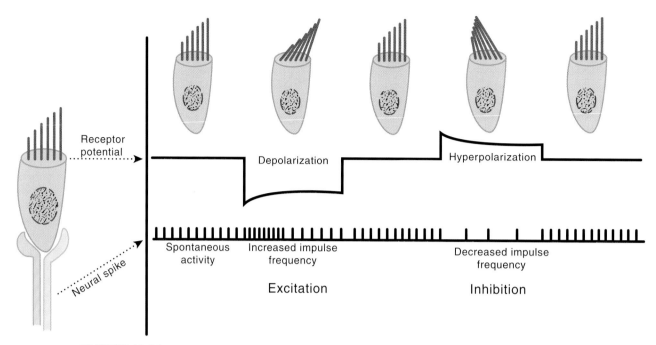

FIGURE 23.26 Illustration of hair cell stimulation, receptor potential response, and afferent fiber discharge. From Flock.

to depolarize the hair cells. In many hair cell sensory systems, including the organ of Corti, the ionic milieu surrounding the hair bundle is richest in potassium; thus, the major charge carrier for the transduction current is potassium. However, small amounts of calcium are also required to sustain stereociliar channel activity. Several lines of evidence indicate that the flow of transduction current into hair cells occurs near the top of the hair bundle, i.e., channels are located near the tips of the stereocilia. As implied earlier, displacement of the bundle toward the tallest stereocilium increases the proportion of open channels, thereby producing an increase above the inward

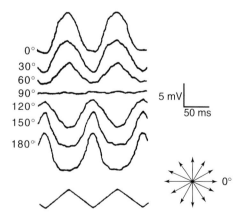

FIGURE 23.27 Evaluation of stereocilia directional sensitivity. Maximal sensitivity occurs when displacements are toward or away from the tallest steeociliar row. From Shotwell (1981).

resting current. The subsequent flow of current across the basolateral membrane produces a depolarizing voltage change, a receptor potential, capable of activating a variety of voltage-dependent conductances in that membrane. Conversely, closure of transduction channels during bundle movement away from the tallest stereociliar row reduces the inward current, effectively hyperpolarizing the basolateral membrane. Maximum sensitivity to deflection is achieved only along this axis; orthogonal deflection produces no response, whereas intermediate angles of deflection produce responses whose magnitude depends on the size of the vectoral component along the most sensitive axis (Fig. 23.27). The degree of bundle deflection, corresponding to the intensity of the mechanical stimulus, produces graded changes in the magnitude of the receptor potential. However, the relation between degree of bundle deflection and receptor potential magnitude is neither linear nor symmetric. Bundle displacements in the depolarizing direction are more effective than equal displacements in the opposite direction. The displacement–response function is sigmoidal and shifted from its midpoint (Fig. 23.28), with saturating electrical responses evoked by deflections as small as 300 nm. Thus, symmetrical sinuoidal deflections of the bundle (as might occur with acoustic stimuli) will produce both sinusoidal (ac) and superimposed depolarizing steady-state (dc) changes in membrane potential. Maximal transducer conductance changes up to about 10 nS have been

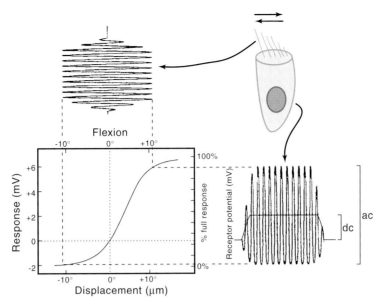

FIGURE 23.28 Sigmoidal input-output function of hair cell. Symmetrical sinusoidal displacement of stereocilia produces ac and dc receptor potential components. From Hudspeth and Corey (1977).

observed, and single unit conductances on the order of 20–100 pS have been either measured or estimated. From such measures, the number of channels per stereocilium has been computed to be one to two.

Extracellular Stereocilia Tip Links May Underlie Transducer Gating

The molecular basis of the hair bundle's response polarity appears to reside in specialized structural attachments at the tips of stereocilia (Fig. 23.29). These "tip links" are elastic filaments ("springs") that link the top of each stereocilium with a dense membranous plaque on the upper side of the adjacent taller stereocilium and occur in line with the axis of maximal bundle sensitivity. They are believed to provide the tension required to open transduction channels during bundle deflection, with one end of the filament being anchored and the other pulling on the channel gate. As the hair bundle tilts during deflection in the excitatory direction, adjacent stereocilia shear against one another, stretching and increasing the tension of tip links, thereby increasing the probability that transducer channels will open. When the deflection is in the hyperpolarizing direction, tip link tension slackens and the channels tend to close. In line with tip link or gating spring hypothesis, destruction of the tip links by enzymatic (elastase) or chemical (calcium chelators) treatments can abolish mechanical transduction. In addition, if tip link tension accounts for much of the bundle's stiffness, as expected, bundle compliance varies with the extent of

deflection. The deflection versus bundle compliance function is bell shaped, with maximum compliance occurring when half the transduction channels are open. Furthermore, compliance changes are abolished by blocking stereociliar transduction channels with aminoglycoside antibiotics.

Hair Bundle Sensitivity Resets during Static Deflection

In hair cells from a variety of organs, the induced receptor current does not remain constant when a hair bundle is statically deflected, but decays with a time constant of a few tens of milliseconds to about 20% of its initial value. This adaptation, which is calcium dependent, results from a shift in the bundle's sigmoidal displacement–response function along the displacement axis in the direction of the deflection (Fig. 23.30). If adaptation did not occur, then superimposed deflections would produce little response during a static deflection. Essentially, this adaptation shift may be viewed as a functional return of the bundle toward its resting position, where bundle deflections are most efficient in transducing mechanical stimuli. Necessarily, however, under constant bundle deflection, the reestablishment of high sensitivity must occur at the level of the channel-gating process itself.

Adaptation is lacking in the absence of extracellular calcium and in the presence of intracellular calcium chelators. As calcium levels increase, adaptation occurs more rapidly and to a greater extent. The adap-

A

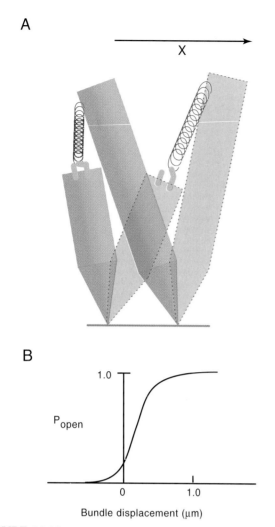

FIGURE 23.29 Gating spring model of hair cell transduction. (A) Tip links connecting channel gate to adjacent taller stereocilium tense during displacement toward the taller stereocilium, thus increasing the probability that the channel will open (B). From Pickles and Corey (1992).

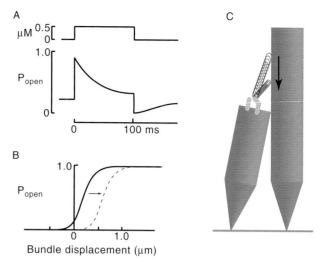

FIGURE 23.30 Hair cell response adaptation. (A) When a constant displacement stimulus is delivered to the bundle, the response (open probability) declines over time. (B) During this time the sigmoidal input-output function is shifted along the displacement axis (open probability) declines over time. (B) During this time the sigmoidal input-output function is shifted along the displacement axis closure during the constant displacement. From Pickles and Corey (1992).

tation process may be related to direct actions of calcium on the transduction channels themselves or on a mechanism responsible for tip link tension control. The latter hypothesis envisions a molecular motor (perhaps myosin I) that maintains a resting tension on the tip link by constantly attempting to move the tip link's upper insertional plaque up the length of the stereocilium. During bundle deflection in the excitatory direction, tip links are initially further tensed, thereby opening transduction channels that permit the influx of calcium ions. Calcium ions are believed to cause the molecular motor to slip during its climb up the stereocilium, thereby slackening the link's tension and allowing the channel's gate to close under constant bundle deflection. Reestablishment of resting

tip link tension follows because the motor renews its climb as calcium influx is halted and the ion is buffered intracellularly. With this restablishment of resting tip link tension, the hair cell is prepared to signal efficiently small mechanical perturbations superimposed on the initial static one. Static deflections in the inhibitory direction also evoke adaptation; as a consequence of reduced calcium influx, the motor will attempt to reinstate resting tip link tension by climbing. However, adaptation occurs to a greater extent for deflections in the excitatory direction.

Adaptation is a relatively slow process and may be useful for maintaining high sensitivity in sensory organs responding to relatively slow or static deflections of stereocilia, such as the vestibular organs. In turtle auditory hair cells, however, adaptation time constants have been measured below 0.5 ms, a speed that may warrant reevaluation of the myosin adaptation hypothesis or may indicate dual adaptation processes. Nevertheless, the usefulness of adaptation in auditory sensory organs is not obvious because acoustic stimuli, being rapid and balanced about zero in nature, produce no static displacements. Thus, even though adaptation to static bundle deflection has been demonstrated in mammalian auditory hair cells, acoustically evoked receptor potentials (both ac and dc) of these hair cells do not normally decrease in magnitude over the time course of stimulation. However, other membrane characteristics, principally

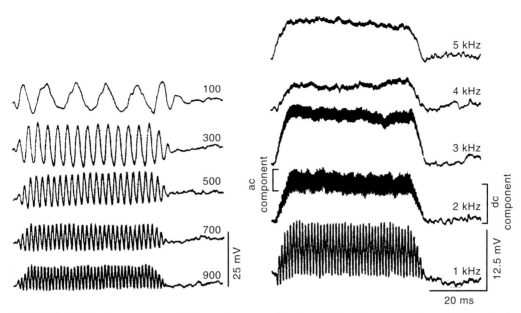

FIGURE 23.31 Receptor potentials from the mammalian inner hair cell in response to acoustic bursts of increasing frequency. Because of the cell's *RC* time constant, the ac component diminishes as frequency increases. However, the dc component remains intact. From Russell and Sellick (1983).

those of the basolateral membrane, can significantly affect the magnitude of receptor potentials during stimulation across the acoustic spectrum.

Electrical Properties of the Basolateral Membrane Shape Receptor Potentials

The speed of the hair cell transduction process is incredibly fast compared to transduction in other sensory systems, such as vision, olfaction, and the taste modalities of sweet and bitter. The delay between a bundle deflection and the onset of receptor current is estimated to be about 10 μs at 37°C. This rapid response is a consequence of direct gating of transduction channels, and such speed is essential for auditory hair cells to detect acoustically evoked bundle deflections in the kilohertz (thousand per second) range. Humans can detect frequencies up to about 20–30 kHz, and some mammals, such as bats, can hear above 100 kHz. Although receptor currents may be generated without attenuation across frequency, receptor potentials, which ultimately are responsible for the release of neurotransmitter at the hair cell synapse, are susceptible to the RC filter characteristics of the basolateral membrane. The RC time constant of auditory hair cells ranges from a fraction of a millisecond to a few milliseconds, at the resting potential. This translates in the frequency domain to a low-pass filter whose cutoff frequency (fc, the frequency at which the response energy is halved) ranges from tens of hertz to about 1 kHz. As detailed

earlier, both ac and dc receptor potentials are generated by sinusoidal stimulation of the hair cell bundle. The ac potentials are susceptible to the membrane filter, such that as the frequency of constant amplitude stimulation increases above fc, the receptor potential magnitude will halve for every octave increase (Fig. 23.31). Ultimately, at very high frequencies, ac responses will be negligible, but the dc component will remain unperturbed—a process termed rectification. It is this depolarizing dc component of the receptor potential, arising from the asymmetrical nature of the transduction process, that drives the release of neurotransmitter during high-frequency stimulation. The actual cutoff frequency may be considered dynamic because receptor potentials themselves may activate voltage-dependent ionic conductances in the basolateral membrane that will modify the resistive component of the RC product (Kros *et al.*, 1998). In outer hair cells from the organ of Corti, the capacitance of the basolateral membrane is also highly voltage dependent (Santos-Sacchi, 1991), and therefore in this cell type variations in both resistive and capacitive components may influence the membrane filter.

Frequency Selective Sensitivity Is Achieved by Hair Cells through a Variety of Mechanisms

Hair cells in auditory organs typically respond best to a particular frequency of stimulation, referred to as the characteristic frequency. In the intact animal, hair

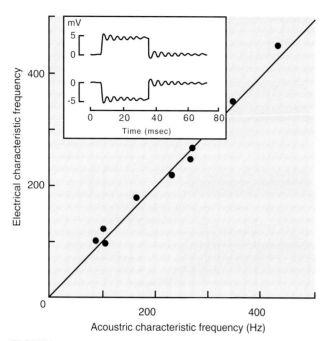

FIGURE 23.32 Electrical tuning in turtle hair cells. When a current pulse is injected into a hair cell, a damped oscillation is observed at stimulus onset and offset (inset). The frequency of the electrically induced oscillation corresponds to the acoustically determined best frequency of that cell. From Crawford and Fettiplace (1981).

cells are spatially arrayed along the length of the sensory epithelium according to increasing characteristic frequency; i.e.) they are organized tonotopically. The mechanism underlying such frequency selectivity may reside within the hair cell itself or arise from accessory structures that selectively enhance a particular stimulus frequency prior to detection by the hair cell. In hair cells of some lower vertebrate auditory or vibration-sensing organs, when the bundles are deflected sinusoidally across a range of stimulus frequencies, the ac receptor potential may not be governed simply by the attenuation effects of a low-pass membrane filter. The activation and interaction of voltage-dependent ionic conductances in the basolateral membrane, namely calcium-activated potassium and calcium conductances, can, under certain conditions, promote the amplification of the response to a particular stimulus frequency, the resonant frequency of the cell. To illustrate, when a depolarizing current pulse, which is a wide band stimulus, is injected via an electrode into a hair cell from the turtle's basilar papilla, the membrane potential demonstrates a damped oscillation or ringing (Crawford and Fettiplace, 1981; Fig. 23.32). The frequency of the oscillation corresponds to the acoustically determined characteristic frequency that

the hair cell would have had in the intact epithelium. Blocking the basolateral ionic conductances of the cell abolishes the ringing phenomenon. The particular frequency that is enhanced in cells exhibiting ringing appears to be governed by the kinetics of the potassium channels residing in the basolateral membrane. Cells tuned to high frequencies have channels that gate at faster rates than those responsible for low-frequency tuning. Although the electrical resonant frequency observed in hair cells from a variety of acoustic and vibration sensitive organs corresponds roughly to the range of characteristic frequencies determined by natural stimuli in the intact animal, the occurrence of such electrical tuning does not necessarily compel the cell to utilize this process in the intact organ. Indeed, hair cells with *in vivo* characteristic frequencies in the kilohertz range may exhibit electrical resonances an order of magnitude lower, but this discrepancy may relate to the detrimental effects of dissociating single cells from the intact organ. In any event, electrical tuning has not been measured and probably cannot be sustained at frequencies above 500 Hz due to the limitations of channel kinetics. Other mechanisms must be invoked to account for selectivity at high frequencies.

In most auditory organs, systematic variations in hair cell structure occur along the tonotopic axis of the epithelium. In particular, the height of stereocilia bundles increases toward the low-frequency region of the organ. This systematic change in bundle height underlies a systematic change in the mechanical resonance of the bundles, similar to the variation of pitch conferred by variation of string length in a harp. Cells with tall bundles have low characteristic frequencies because the bundles preferentially oscillate at low frequencies. Short-bundled cells have high characteristic frequencies. This pretransduction mechanism appears to account satisfactorily for frequency selectivity in some lower vertebrates; however, in higher vertebrates, especially mammals, more elaborate mechanical tuning mechanisms exist.

The mammalian organ of Corti rests upon an acellular basilar membrane (BM) that extends along the coiled cochlea. Two types of hair cells, inner hair cells (IHC) and outer hair cells (OHC), reside within the organ. Cells at the basal end of the coiled BM have high characteristic frequencies, whereas those at the apex have low ones. Von Bekesy, who won the Nobel prize in 1968, discovered that different regions of the BM are tuned to particular frequencies; low-frequency tones cause maximal vibrations of the BM near the apex, whereas high-frequency tones are most effective at the base. Characteristic frequencies are distributed tonotopically and are derived from the passive

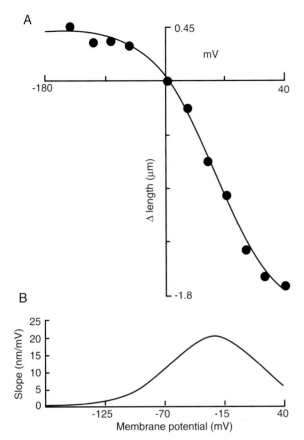

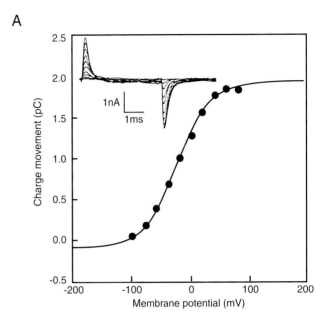

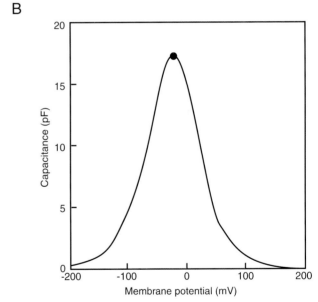

energetic boost to BM motion, provide an enhanced stimulus to the IHCs, which are the cells predominantly innervated by auditory nerve afferents.

FIGURE 23.33 Mechanical response of mammalian outer hair cell (OMC) under voltage clamp. The OHC changes its length when the cell is held at different membrane potentials (A). The slope of the sigmoidal input-output function defines the cell's sensitivity to membrane potential change (B). From Santos-Sacchi (1992). Used with permission.

FIGURE 23.34 Gating charge associated with OHC motility voltage sensor. When the membrane potential is stepped with increasingly larger depolarizing voltages from a negative holding potential, nonlinear capacitive currents are generated and are obvious after linear capacitive currents are subtracted (inset). Integrating the onset currents, a measure of the amount of charge moved within the membrane can be obtained (A). The function is sigmoidal and has characteristics similar to the mechanical response. The first derivative of the charge with respect to membrane voltage defines the cell's nonlinear capacitance (B). From Santos-Sacchi (1991).

mechanical characteristics of the BM. The vibration of the BM induces bending of the stereocilia bundles, consequently, hair cells located at a particular location along the BM respond best to that frequency determined by BM tuning. However, the intrinsic frequency selectivity afforded by passive BM tuning is not great enough to account for the very selective responses observed in hair cells and eighth nerve fibers. OHCs, probably through a mechanical feedback scheme, are required to boost BM motion and enhance frequency selectivity, a process termed the "cochlea amplifier." In the absence of OHCs or under conditions in which OHCs are selectively impaired, frequency selectivity is likewise impaired. OHCs are unique because they function as both receptors and effectors, transducing mechanical stimuli via hair bundle displacement and changing length and other mechanical properties in response to the generated receptor potentials. These mechanical events, via an

Active Mechanical Properties of the Outer Hair Cell Drive the Mammalian Cochlea Amplifier

OHCs are cylindrically shaped and increase in length by a factor of about four from the high-frequency to the low-frequency region of the cochlea. When an isolated OHC is stimulated electrically, it responds by altering its length. No other auditory cell type responds in this manner. The mechanical response is voltage dependent; depolarizing stimuli induce contractions and hyperpolarizing stimuli induce elongations. The length change versus voltage (dL vs dV) function (Fig. 23.33A) is sigmoidal, and like the stereocilia transducer function, it is operatively offset from its midpoint; the midpoint voltage is near -30 mV and the OHC resting potential is near -70 mV. The slope of the function (dL/dV; Fig. 23.33B) indicates the sensitivity of the mechanical response to voltage change, and responses as large as 30 nm/mV have been found. *In vitro*, at least, this maximum sensitivity or gain resides at a voltage that is depolarized relative to the resting potential of the cell. The mechanical activity of the cell is not akin to any other known form of cellular motility and is governed directly by voltage-dependent, integral membrane protein motors, recently identified as the gene product of Prestin (Zheng *et al.*, 2000), one of a family of sulfate transporter genes.

Through a variety of experimental approaches, motor activity has been shown to be restricted to the lateral membrane of the OHC. As might be expected for a voltage-dependent process that resides within the membrane, a charged voltage sensor must exist, just as voltage-dependent ion channels have voltage sensors. The existence of an OHC motility voltage sensor is confirmed by measuring gating charge movements (capacitive-like currents) under voltage clamp while blocking ionic conductances. These gating currents represent the restricted movement of the charged voltage sensor within the plane of the lateral membrane; increasing voltage will move more charge (thus activating more motors) according to Boltzmann statistics. Maximum charge moved is about 7500 e/μm^2. This value is also believed to characterize the density of motor molecules in the lateral plasma membrane. The plot of charge versus voltage (Q/V) is sigmoidal (Fig. 23.34A) and has the same shape and characteristics as the dL versus dV function. The slope of the Q/V function is defined as capacitance, and thus the capacitance of OHC is a bell-shaped function of voltage (Fig. 23.34B). This nonlinear capacitance rides atop the cell's intrinsic linear membrane capacitance of 1 μF/cm^2. Thus, in an OHC of about 70 μm in length, at the point where motile gain is maximum (i.e., where half the motors are activated), the capacitance peaks at about double the cell's linear capacitance. As mentioned earlier, such nonlinear capacitance may have significant effects on membrane-filtering characteristics.

Although the mechanical response is voltage dependent and is not evoked by activation of any particular voltage-dependent ionic conductance, the activity of the voltage sensor requires intracellular chloride, and in intact OHCs a stretch-activated chloride conductance appears crucial for maintaining and modulating motor activity.

On a system level, the effects of OHCs on auditory performance may be considered nonstatic. This results from the susceptibility of OHC motor function to a variety of physiological factors, including modulation of membrane tension, resting membrane potential, and phosphorylation. Each of these can modify the voltage dependence of motor function.

Because hearing sensitivity and frequency selectivity in mammals span the kilohertz range, any mechanism designed to augment hearing must function at these rates. Indeed, OHC motility has been demonstrated, *in vitro*, to extend well into the tens of kilohertz range. Nevertheless, because the mechanical response is voltage dependent, it will be affected by the RC time constant of the OHC. In this scenario, at high frequencies, transmembrane ac receptor potentials, which presumably drive the mechanical response *in vivo*, will be attenuated greatly. Consequently, a current debate focuses on the relative contribution of lateral membrane activity and stereocilia activity, each of which is capable of force production, to the cochlea amplifier. Active mechanical responses of the stereocilia bundle may be driven by calcium influx through calcium-sensitive, mechanically activated stereocilia channels, and thus may not be limited by the membrane filter (Martin and Hudspeth, 1999). Of course, identification of important role of chloride in the function of prestin and its mechanically activated flux through the lateral plasma membrane may underlie a similar voltage independence. In this way the OHCs of the mammalian inner ear may have overcome the limiting effects of the membrane filter at high-frequency acoustic stimulation.

Summary

Hair cells are modified epithelial cells that function to transduce mechanical energy from the environment into electrical energy. The gating of mechanically sensitive nonselective cationic channels within apical membrane specializations, termed stereocilia, induces modulation of a standing inward receptor current. In turn, this current evokes a change in membrane potential, a receptor potential, across the basolateral membrane. The receptor potential, which is shaped by basolateral membrane conductances, ultimately controls the release of hair cell neurotransmitter and afferent spike activity. Frequency specificity can arise from many mechanisms intrinsic and extrinsic to the hair cell. In the mammal, mechanical tuning of the sensory epithelium enhanced by active mechanical feedback from the outer hair cell provides for the exquisite ability to resolve frequency information.

References

Adler, E., Hoon, M. A., Mueller, K. L., Chandrashekar, J., Ryba, N. J. and Zuker, C. S. (2000). A novel family of mammalian taste receptors. *Cell* **100**, 693–702.

Araneda, R. C., Kint, A. D., and Firestein, S. (2000). The molecular receptive range of an odorant receptor. *Nature Neurosci.* **3**, 1248–1254.

Buck, L. D., and Axel, R. (1991). A novel multigene family may encode odorant receptors: A molecular basis for odorant recognition. *Cell* **65**, 175–187.

Chaudhari, N., Landin, A. M., and Roper, S. D. (2000). A metabotropic glutamate receptor variant functions as a taste receptor. *Nature Neurosci.* **3**, 113–119.

Crawford, A. C., and Fettiplace, R. (1981). An electrical tuning mechanism in turtle cochlear hair cells. *J. Physiol. (Lond)* **312**, 377–412.

Fesenko, E. E., Kolesnikov, S. S., and Lyubarsky, A. L. (1985). Induction by cyclic GMP of cationic conductance in plasma membrane of retinal rod outer segment. *Nature* **313**, 310–313.

Hagins, W. A., Penn, R. D., and Yoshikami, S. (1970). Dark current and photocurrent in retinal rods. *Biophys. J.* **10**, 380–412.

Hildebrand, J. G. (1995). Analysis of chemical signals by nervous systems. *Proc. Natl. Acad. Sci. USA* **92**, 67–74.

Hillman, D. E. (1976). "Frog Neurobiology" (R. Llinas and W. Precht, eds.), p. 452. Springer-Verlag, Berlin.

Huang, L., Shanker, Y. G., Dubauskaite, J., Zheng, J. Z., Yan, W., Rosenzweig, S., Spielman, A. I., Max, M., and Margolskee, R. F. (1999). Ggamma13 colocalizes with gastducin in taste receptor cells and mediates IP$_3$ responses to bitter denatornium. *Nature Neurosci.* **2**, 1055–1062.

Kros, C. J., Ruppersberg, J. P., and Rusch, A. (1998). Expression of a potassium current in inner hair cells during development of hearing in mice. *Nature* **394**, 281–284

Leinders-Zufall, T., Lane, A. P., Puche, A. C., Ma, W., Novotny, M. V., Shipley, M. T., and Zufall, F. (2000). Ultrasensitive pheromone detection by mammalian vomeronasal neurons. *Nature* **405**, 792–796.

Lindemann, B., Gilbertson, T. A., and Kinnamon, S. C. (1999). Amiloride-sensitive sodium channels in taste. *In* "Current Topics in Membranes" (D. Benos, ed.), pp. 315–36. Academic Press, San Diego.

MacLeish, P. R., Schwartz, E. A., and Tachibana, M. (1984). Control of the generator current in solitary rods of the *Ambystoma tigrinum* retina. *J. Physiol.* **348**, 645–664.

Martin, P., and Hudspeth, A. J. (1999). Active hair-bundle movements can amplify a hair cell's response to oscillatory mechanical stimuli. *Proc. Natl. Acad. Sci. USA.* **96**, 14306–14311.

Montmayeur, J. P., Liberles, S. D., Matsunami, H., and Buck, L. B. (2001). *Nature Neurosci.* **4**, 492–498.

Ranganathan, R., Backsai, B. J., Tsien, R. Y., and Zuker, C. S. (1994). Cytosolic calcium transients: Spatial localization and role in *Drosophila* photoreceptor cell function. *Neuron* **13**, 837–848.

Santos-Sacchi, J. (1992). On the frequency limit and phase of outer hair cell motility: Effects of the membrane filter. *J. Neurosci.* **12**, 1906–1916.

Tomita, T. (1965). Electrophysiological study of the mechanisms subserving color coding in the fish retina. *Cold Spring Harb. Symp. Quant. Biol.* **30**, 559–566.

Vogt, R., and Riddiford, L. M. (1981). Pheromone binding and inactivation by moth antennae. *Nature* **293**, 161–163.

Wes, P. D., and Bargmann, C. I. (2001) *C. elegans* odour discrimination requires asymmetric diversity in olfactory neurons. *Nature* **410**, 698–701.

Yee, R., and Liebman, P. A. (1978). Light-activated phosphodiesterase of the rod outer segment. *J. Biol. Chem.* **253**, 8902–8909.

Zheng, J., Shen, W., He, D. Z., Long, K. B., Madison, L. D., and Dallos, P. (2000). Prestin is the motor protein of cochlear outer hair cells. *Nature* **405**, 149–155.

Suggested Readings

Jahn, A., and Santos-Sacchi, J. (eds.) (2001). "Physiology of the Ear," 2nd Ed. Singular Press.

Kinnamon, S. C., and Margolskee, R. F. (1996). Mechanisms of taste transduction. *Curr. Opin. Neurobiol.* **6**, 506–513.

Reed, R. R. (1994). The molecular basis of sensitivity and specificity in olfaction. *Sem. Cell. Biol.* **5**, 33–38.

Shepherd, G. M. (1994). Discrimination of molecular signals by the olfactory receptor neuron. *Neuron* **13**, 771–790.

Simon, S. A., and Roper, S. D. (1993). "Mechanisms of Taste Transduction." CRC Press, Boca Raton, FL.

Von Bekesy, G. (1960). "Experiments in Hearing." McGraw-Hill, New York.

Yau, K.W. (1994). Phototransduction mechanism in retinal rods and cones. The Friedenwald Lecture. *Invest. Ophthal. Vis. Sci.* **35**, 9–32.

Zuker, C.S. (1996). The biology of phototransduction in *Drosophila*. *Proc. Natl. Acad. Sci. USA* **93**, 571–576.

*Peter R. MacLeish, Gordon M. Shepherd,
Sue C. Kinnamon, and Joseph Santos-Sacchi*

Chemical Senses: Taste and Olfaction

The chemical senses of taste and olfaction have several elements in common, but differ in a number of significant ways. The taste and olfactory systems are both concerned with extracting information from chemical stimuli in the environment. Both respond to a wide array of chemicals and both use G-protein-coupled receptors, although some taste stimuli interact directly with ion channels (see Chapter 23). Both taste and olfactory receptors undergo continual turnover and replacement throughout life. Taste receptors, however, are modified epithelial cells, whereas olfactory receptors are neurons. More is known about the coding of taste quality than of odor quality, partly due to relative agreement on the existence of four elementary gustatory sensations; olfactory stimuli give rise to many sensations and there is less agreement on what constitutes basic odor qualities. Topographic arrangements are more important in the representation of odor information than in the coding of taste quality, where they have little influence. Both of these systems appear to utilize the responses of populations of neurons to code stimulus information. Taste and olfactory inputs are important for the survival of the organism and the species. Both systems play a major role in food selection and in avoiding the ingestion of toxins. Olfactory stimuli provide important social cues, especially those used in reproductive behavior and mother–infant relationships.

TASTE

The sense of taste provides a gateway for monitoring and controlling the ingestion of food. It responds to chemical substances in the oral cavity and helps regulate the interaction between ingestive behavior

and the internal milieu. The term "taste" often refers to the complex of sensations known as flavor perception, which includes sensory information from the olfactory, gustatory, and trigeminal systems. More strictly defined, taste refers to the sensations arising from the stimulation of gustatory receptors. Throughout this chapter, the terms "taste" and "gustation" are used interchangeably to refer to the gustatory system.

The transduction of specific chemical stimuli (e.g., sodium ions, sugars, acids, or alkaloids) by taste receptor cells gives rise to activity in several types of gustatory nerve fibers. Understanding the neural coding of taste information begins with knowledge about how chemical sensitivities, represented by specific receptor transduction mechanisms (see Chapter 23), are distributed and organized among peripheral and central gustatory neurons. The role of an individual neuron in the coding of taste quality must be considered in the context of the multiple sensitivities of these cells. In addition to producing taste sensations (salty, sweet, sour, or bitter), chemical stimulation of gustatory receptors provides critical input for several somatic and visceral responses related to food ingestion and rejection. Viewing taste as an oral component of the visceral afferent system provides an important perspective on the involvement of gustatory information in the control of taste-mediated behaviors.

Taste Receptors Are Situated within Taste Buds Located in Several Distinct Subpopulations

Taste is mediated through chemical stimulation of gustatory receptor cells, which are located in taste buds distributed within the oral, pharyngeal, and laryngeal mucosa. Taste buds on the tongue are con-

631

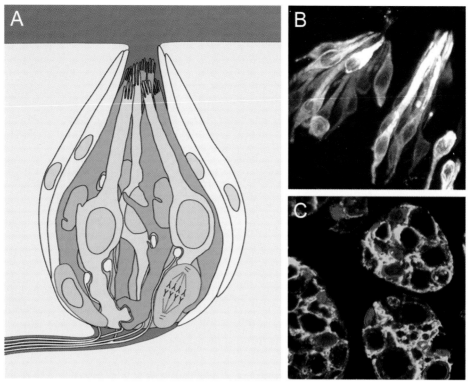

FIGURE 24.1 Cell types in mammalian taste buds. (A) The taste bud is a barrel-shaped structure containing different cell types, including basal cells, dark cells, and light cells. These epithelial receptor cells make synaptic contact with distal processes of cranial nerves VII, IX, or X, whose cell bodies lie within the cranial nerve ganglia. Microvilli of the taste receptor cells project into an opening in the epithelium, the taste pore, where they make contact with gustatory stimuli. (B) The characteristic spindle shape of taste receptor cells is revealed when a subset of light cells is immunoreacted to an antibody against α-gustducin, a gustatory G protein. (C) When sectioned transversely, light cells appear round in cross section, as shown by α-gustducin immunoreactivity (red), whereas the characteristic shape of dark cells produced by their thin cytoplasmic projections enveloping neighboring light cells is revealed with an antibody against the H blood group antigen (green).

tained within distinct papillae; those in other areas are distributed across the surface of the epithelium. At the ultrastructural level, at least two kinds of cells can be discerned within the taste bud (Fig. 24.1). They are termed dark cells and light cells on the basis of their ultrastructural characteristics. Subsets of these basic types are also suggested based on both ultrastructural and immunocytochemical properties. Cells within a taste bud are arranged in a concentric columnar fashion, with their apical microvilli projecting toward a pore that opens through the epithelium into the oral cavity (Figs. 24.1A and 24.1B); gustatory stimuli interact with receptors and ion channels on these apical microvilli (Chapter 23). The base of the taste bud is penetrated by terminal branches of the afferent nerve, which make synaptic contact with the receptor cells (Fig. 24.1A). A single nerve fiber may innervate cells in more than one taste bud, each of which is innervated by several different afferent fibers.

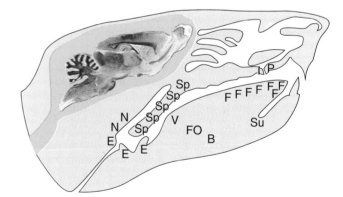

FIGURE 24.2 Diagram of a parasaggittal section through the hamster oral cavity showing the distribution of various taste bud populations, which are found in the fungiform (F) papillae on the anterior tongue, the vallate (V) and foliate (FO) papillae on the posterior tongue, the soft palate (SP), the incisive papillae (IP) on the hard palate, and the laryngeal surface of the epiglottis (E). Small numbers of taste buds are also found on the buccal wall (B), the sublingual organ (Su), and the nasopharynx (N). These taste buds are innervated by branches of the VIIth, IXth, and Xth cranial nerves (see text).

Taste receptors in mammals are distributed within several subpopulations of taste buds, as illustrated for the hamster (Fig. 24.2). About 18% of the hamster's taste buds are located in the fungiform papillae (F) on the anterior portion of the tongue, 32% are within the foliate papillae (FO) on the posterior sides of the tongue, 23% are in the single midline vallate papilla (V) on the posterior tongue, about 14% are on the palate—distributed between the nasoincisive papillae (IP; 2%) and the soft palate (SP; 12%)—and about 10% are on the laryngeal surface of the epiglottis (E) and the aryepiglottal folds. A small number of taste buds are also within the sublingual organ (Su), the buccal walls (B), the nasopharynx (N), and the upper reaches of the esophagus. Similar distributions occur in rats and other mammalian species that have been examined, including humans.

Turnover and Replacement of Taste Bud Cells Are Continuous Processes

Taste receptor cells arise continually from an underlying population of basal epithelial cells. Whether the cell types identifiable on structural grounds are different cell types or a single type at different stages of maturation has been a subject of debate. In rats, the life span of a taste cell in a fungiform papilla is approximately 10 days. The afferent nerve maintains a trophic influence over the taste buds, which degenerate when their nerve supply is removed. Although innervation by gustatory nerve fibers is necessary to maintain the

structural integrity of the taste bud, the gustatory sensitivities of the receptor cells appear to be determined by the epithelium itself (see Box 24.1). Interestingly, the several branches of a chorda tympani (CT) axon that innervate different fungiform papillae have similar profiles of sensitivity. Combined with the fact that the sensitivity of a given receptor field appears to be determined by the epithelium, this suggests that during cell turnover the nerve fibers are guided to make contact with particular types of receptor cells.

Although taste cells are modified epithelial cells, they possess many characteristics of neurons. Several recent investigations have demonstrated the presence of a variety of cell surface molecules and other neural antigens on cells in mammalian taste buds. The neural cell adhesion molecule (NCAM) is expressed on a subset of vallate taste bud cells in the rat and mouse and also on the innervating fibers of the glossopharyngeal nerve. Transection of the nerve results in a loss of NCAM expression as the taste buds degenerate. Reinnervation of the vallate papilla following bilateral nerve crush is accompanied by NCAM expression in the nerve, followed by differentiation of the epithelium and the subsequent expression of NCAM in the differentiated taste cells. A similar temporal sequence is seen during taste bud development in the mouse. A number of other molecules, including several of the human blood group antigens (A, B, H and Lewis[b]), α-gustducin (a gustatory G protein), serotonin, vasoactive intestinal polypeptide (VIP), several cytokeratins, and neuron-specific enolase

---

BOX 24.1

TASTE RECEPTOR CELL SENSITIVITY IS DETERMINED BY THE EPITHELIUM

The formation and maintenance of taste buds are dependent on their innervation by gustatory nerve fibers, but the nerve itself does not dictate the sensory responsiveness of the taste buds. In a now classic experiment, Bruce Oakley showed that altering the innervation of the taste buds had no influence on their response characteristics. In this experiment, Oakley (1967) transected the chorda tympani (CT) and glossopharyngeal (IXth) nerves of the rat and cross-anastomosed one to the other, resulting in either fungiform taste buds being reinnervated by the IXth nerve or vallate taste buds being reinnervated by the CT nerve following regeneration. Electrophysiological recording experiments then showed that when the IXth nerve had been rerouted

to the anterior tongue, its fibers responded better to sodium chloride than to quinine, like those of the normal CT nerve. Similarly, when CT fibers had been routed to the posterior tongue, they responded more to quinine than to sodium chloride, like those of the normal IXth nerve. This experiment demonstrates that the receptor phenotype is a property of the target epithelium rather than the innervating nerve; thus, the trophic influence of the nerve over taste bud differentiation and maintenance does not extend to the receptor expression within the taste cells.

David V. Smith

(NSE) are also expressed by subsets of taste cells. Many of these molecules could play a role in either the structural integrity of the taste bud or mediation of axon-taste cell recognition. Some taste cell markers are restricted to separate or overlapping subsets of light cells (e.g., α-gustducin, NCAM, serotonin, and the Lewis[b] and A blood group antigens), whereas others appear to be expressed by most, if not all, dark cells (H and B blood group antigens, 2B8 carbohydrate epitope; Fig. 24.1C).

Gustatory Inputs to the Brain Stem Are Distributed Differently across Several Cranial Nerves

Taste buds in the fungiform papillae on the anterior portion of the tongue and in the more rostral of the foliate papillae on the sides of the tongue are innervated by the chorda tympani branch of the facial (VIIth) nerve. Axons of the CT travel to the anterior tongue along with the lingual nerve (a branch of the mandibular division of the Vth nerve), which carries somatosensory innervation from the same area. The greater superficial petrosal (GSP) branch of the VIIth cranial nerve innervates taste buds on the soft palate via the lesser palatine nerve and in the nasoincisor ducts via the nasopalatine nerve. Neurons giving rise to the gustatory fibers of the CT and GSP are located within the geniculate ganglion of the facial nerve. These two branches of the VIIth nerve carry gustatory information to the rostral pole of the nucleus of the solitary tract (NST), where their afferent terminations are largely coextensive.

Vallate and foliate papillae on the posterior tongue contain taste buds innervated by the lingual-tonsillar branch of the glossopharyngeal (IXth) nerve, which also supplies taste fibers to the nasopharynx and general somatosensory fibers to the posterior third of the tongue. In rodents, over half of all the taste buds are distributed within vallate and foliate papillae. Afferent gustatory fibers of the IXth nerve, the cell bodies of which lie in the petrosal ganglion, project into the medulla and terminate within the NST somewhat caudal to, but overlapping with, the termination of the VIIth nerve.

Taste buds distributed on the laryngeal surface of the epiglottis, on the aryepiglottal folds, and in the upper reaches of the esophagus are innervated by the internal branch of the superior laryngeal nerve (SLN), which is a branch of the vagus (Xth) nerve. This nerve also carries somatosensory innervation from the supraglottic portion of the laryngeal mucosa. Chemosensitive fibers of the SLN, whose cell bodies lie within the nodose ganglion of the vagus nerve,

project into the NST caudal to those of the VIIth and IXth cranial nerves.

The various populations of taste buds differ in their sensitivities and contribute different kinds of afferent information to the brain stem. Although there are species differences in the distributions of some of these sensitivities, the general conclusion is that the various taste bud populations provide different kinds and amounts of gustatory information. It is likely that these variable inputs are important for different kinds of taste-mediated behavior. A summary of the responsiveness of hamster CT, IXth, and SLN taste fibers depicts the mean response profiles of fibers in these nerves (Fig. 24.3). Receptors on the anterior tongue (CT) and palate (GSP) provide relatively more information about NaCl and sucrose than receptors on the posterior tongue (IXth) or in the larynx (SLN). Sensitivity to HCl is relatively similar in every gustatory nerve; quinine–HCl (QHCl) clearly has its greatest relative effect in the IXth nerve. Only the SLN responds to water. The GSP nerve, which is not shown because no single fiber data are available, is relatively more responsive to sucrose than the CT nerve. The differential information arising from these various gustatory nerves projects into the NST, where appropriate connections provide for the reflexive control of ingestive and protective responses that are triggered by taste stimulation.

Behavioral studies have begun to define taste quality for a number of mammalian species, includ-

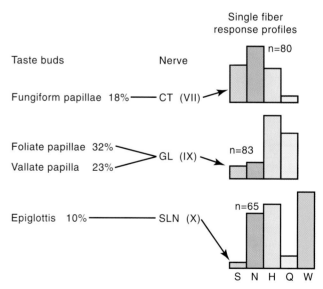

FIGURE 24.3 Profiles of mean response of single fibers in the hamster chorda tympani (CT), glossopharyngeal (GL), and superior laryngeal (SLN) nerves to four representative taste stimuli and distilled water applied to the fungiform, foliate, vallate, or epiglottal taste buds. Stimuli: S, sucrose; N, sodium chloride; H, hydrochloric acid; Q, quinine hydrochloride; W, distilled water.

ing rats and hamsters. These rodents discriminate easily among sucrose, NaCl, HCl, and QHCl. They group the tastes of other sugars and sodium saccharin with sucrose, other acids and nonsodium salts such as NH_4Cl with HCl, other sodium salts with NaCl, and some bitter-tasting salts such as $MgSO_4$ with QHCl. Input from the VIIth nerve is sufficient to allow neural and behavioral discrimination among sugars, sodium salts, acids, and bitter substances. For example, behavioral discrimination between NaCl and KCl or between KCl and QHCl appears to require the VIIth nerve; this discrimination is disrupted in rats by bilateral transection of the CT and/or GSP nerves. Cutting the IXth nerve has no effect on these discrimination tasks. These kinds of experiments suggest that taste input from the facial nerve is critical for taste discrimination. However, the glossopharyngeal nerve may be more important in brain stem taste mechanisms, as suggested by the reduction in quinine-elicited gapes following IXth nerve damage in rats. Fibers of the SLN innervating laryngeal chemoreceptors, however, do not distinguish among stimuli with different taste qualities. Chemosensitive fibers of the SLN appear to be suited to a role in airway protection by signaling deviations from the normal pH and ionic milieu of the larynx rather than in the discrimination among gustatory qualities.

Gustatory Afferent Information Flows into Two Major Ascending Pathways

Afferent fibers of the VIIth, IXth, and Xth cranial nerves carry gustatory information to the NST—the medullary relay for the gustatory and visceral afferent systems (Fig. 24.4). These fibers terminate in the rostral pole of the NST (VIIth nerve) and at intermediate (IXth nerve) and more caudal (Xth nerve) levels. There is some overlap in their terminal fields within the NST, which lie predominantly rostral to the projection of general visceral afferent fibers of the vagus. From the NST, ascending fibers project in most species to third-order cells within the parabrachial nuclei (PbN) of the pons, more or less parallel to the projection of general visceral sensation from the caudal NST. A thalamocortical projection arises from the PbN to carry taste information to the parvicellular portion of the ventroposteromedial nucleus of the thalamus (VPMpc) and on to the gustatory neocortex (GN), located in rodents within the agranular insular cortex. In primates, taste fibers bypass the pontine relay and project directly to the VPMpc.

Arising in parallel with the thalamocortical projection is a second projection that carries gustatory afferent information into limbic forebrain areas

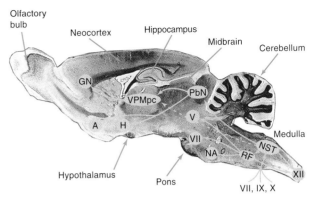

FIGURE 24.4 Schematic diagram of the ascending gustatory pathway; descending projections are not shown. Connections of the rodent gustatory system within the CNS are shown by solid lines; the projection from NST to VPMpc in primates is indicated by a dashed line. NST, nucleus of the solitary tract; PbN, parabrachial nuclei; VPMpc, venteroposteromedial nucleus (parvi cellularis) of the thalamus; GN, gustatory neocortex; A, amygdala; H, hypothalamus; NA, nucleus ambiguus; RF, reticular formation; V, VII, and XII, trigeminal, facial, and hypoglossal motor nuclei; VII, IX, and X, axons of peripheral gustatory fibers in the facial, glossopharyngeal, and vagal cranial nerves.

involved in feeding and autonomic regulation, including the lateral hypothalamus, the central nucleus of the amygdala, and the bed nucleus of the stria terminalis. Descending axons within the gustatory system arise from the insular cortex and several ventral forebrain areas and project to the PbN and NST. There are also numerous local connections among neurons within the NST and with cells of the oral, facial, and pharyngeal motor nuclei (V, VII, ambiguus, and XII), either directly (as with XII) or via interneurons in the reticular formation. These hindbrain systems form the substrate for many taste-mediated somatic and visceral responses related to ingestion and rejection of tastants.

Gustatory Afferent Neurons Extract Several Types of Sensory Information

The gustatory system extracts three types of information from chemical stimuli: quality, intensity, and hedonic value. Most researchers agree that in the absence of olfactory or somatosensory cues, much of taste experience can be described by the sweet, salty, sour, and bitter qualities. However, considerable debate continues over whether some other qualities (e.g., umami—the taste of glutamate) should be included or whether any qualities are unique categories of taste perception. Intensity is a dimension common to all sensory systems, reflecting the magnitude of the evoked sensation. Hedonic value, the perceived pleasantness or unpleasantness of a taste sensation, is based on genetic, physiologic, and experiential factors, as well as on the characteristics of the stimulus. Taste is an inherently hedonic sense, relating strongly to motivated behavior. Although these stimulus dimensions can be assessed separately, they are not independent. For example, the perceived qualities of many taste stimuli change with stimulus concentration. Moreover, the hedonic value of a stimulus is largely determined by its quality and intensity. Many omnivorous mammals share concentration-dependent preferences for substances humans describe as tasting sweet or salty and aversions to substances humans term sour or bitter. Presumably, these predispositions reflect evolutionary pressures related to the ingestional consequences (i.e., nutritional or toxic) of potential foods.

Organization of the gustatory system is determined largely by genetic and developmental factors. However, there are also mechanisms allowing experience and physiologic state to influence gustatory neural processing and perception. Species-specific predispositions toward the hedonic value of a stimulus can be overcome in acquired preferences or aversions or in

response to metabolic or pharmacologic manipulations. Evidence also indicates that such factors can influence the neural processing of gustatory information. Thus, gustatory afferent input provides at least three types of information that are interrelated in complex ways. How taste intensity, quality, and hedonic value are represented in the nervous system is the problem of gustatory neural coding.

At the outset, two features of this system may be noted to have important implications for gustatory coding. First, both peripheral and central gustatory neurons typically respond to more than one of the stimuli representing the salty, sweet, sour, or bitter taste qualities, often to as many as three or four. A broadly tuned neuron in the rostral NST of the hamster was excited by sodium and nonsodium salts, by acids, and by the bitter stimulus QHCl (Fig. 24.5). It was inhibited by sucrose and DL-alanine, both of which taste sweet to humans. Because the responses of such taste neurons can be modulated by both quality and intensity, the response of any one neuron alone is entirely ambiguous with respect to either parameter. In addition, gustatory neurons are often responsive to thermal and tactile stimuli. Thus,

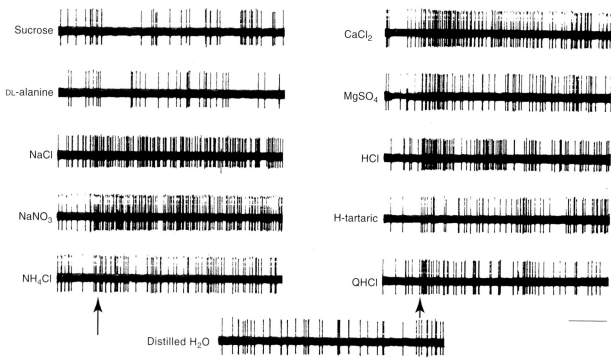

FIGURE 24.5 Responses of a neuron in the nucleus of the solitary tract of the hamster to several taste stimuli applied to the fungiform papillae. Arrows indicate the onset of the response, of which about 5 s are shown, preceded by about 1 s of response to distilled water. The concentrations of the stimuli are those that produce a half-maximal response to these chemicals in the hamster's chorda tympani nerve. This cell shows a positive excitatory response to all of these stimuli except sucrose and DL-alanine, which produce an inhibition of ongoing activity. From Smith *et al.* (1979).

impulse traffic in a single neuron may be related to several stimulus parameters, making the unambiguous interpretation of that signal impossible without comparing it to activity in other cells. Therefore, in thinking about how sensory information is coded in the gustatory system, it is important to remember that cells at all levels of the pathway are broadly responsive to stimuli that vary in perceptual quality, are more broadly responsive at high than at low intensities, and are often sensitive to other modalities, such as touch and temperature.

Another important feature of the taste system is that, unlike most other sensory systems, it has no distinct topographic arrangement in its central neural organization. This lack of topography is not surprising because neither the molecules that constitute taste stimuli nor the perceptions of sweet, salty, sour, or bitter correspond to any continuous dimension of matter, space, or energy. There is some segregation of peripheral nerve terminations within the NST, and the taste bud subpopulations innervated by these nerves display somewhat different patterns of chemical sensitivity (Fig. 24.3). This differential sensitivity results in rough topographic differences in responsiveness within the NST. This segregation continues throughout the gustatory pathway to the cortex, where there are separate terminal fields for VIIth and IXth nerve inputs. Although this spatial separation has been proposed to be important in the neural coding of taste quality, central taste neurons at all levels have broadly tuned response characteristics and many have receptive fields in two or more receptor populations. At present, there is little evidence that taste quality is represented by a topographic code.

It is generally assumed, if not explicitly stated, that gustatory stimulus intensity is coded by neural impulse frequency and increased numbers of responding neurons. All neurons responsive to taste stimuli show some modulation by stimulus concentration; there is no evidence that only a specific subset of cells is responsible for coding stimulus intensity. These cells also vary in their threshold sensitivities to stimulus concentration. Unlike gustatory intensity and quality, the issue of hedonic coding has not been addressed systematically in neurobiological studies of the taste system, probably because hedonic value is not independent of either quality or intensity and can be modified by both experience and physiologic state. Evidence, however, has shown that some taste-responsive neurons in ventral forebrain areas, such as the amygdala, are tuned to the hedonic value of the stimulus rather than to taste quality. This hedonic dimension is critically important in the control of many taste-mediated responses related to food ingestion and rejection.

Taste Neurons Are Broadly Tuned across Qualities

Since the earliest electrophysiological studies of single peripheral taste fibers, it has been recognized that individual gustatory neurons are responsive to stimuli representing more than one of the four taste qualities. Nevertheless, neurons within the taste pathway can be grouped into classes based on their relative sensitivities. For example, when the stimuli 0.1 M sucrose, 0.03 M NaCl, 3 mM HCl, and 1 mM QHCl are ordered hedonically from most to least preferred, the response profiles of hamster CT and/or IXth nerve fibers show a single peak as sucrose-, NaCl-, HCl-, or QHCl-best fibers. Thus, peripheral taste fibers have an organization to their sensitivities; three neuron classes are defined by their sensitivities to four basic stimuli applied to the anterior portion of the tongue: sucrose-, NaCl-, and HCl-best fibers; a QHCl-best class is evident in the IXth nerve.

The grouping of taste neurons into classes can be appreciated by examining the responses of 31 neurons of the hamster PbN to an array of 18 stimuli applied to the anterior tongue (Fig. 24.6). The neurons are arranged according to their response profiles, with cells 1–10 being most responsive to sweet stimuli, 11–20 to sodium salts, and 21–31 to acids and nonsodium salts or QHCl (neuron 31). The green bars in Fig. 24.6 represent responses to four prototypical stimuli: sucrose (sweet), NaCl (salty), HCl (sour), and QHCl (bitter). The blue bars in Fig. 24.6 represent responses to other stimuli, shown along the abscissa. Although the response profiles within a group are not identical, there appear to be essential similarities among profiles of neurons within a group and striking differences between profiles in different groups.

These response profiles were subjected to a hierarchical cluster analysis, which addressed whether it is reasonable to assume that they were sampled from distinct subpopulations rather than from a single population. In this analysis, the most similar pairs of profiles are clustered together first, followed by the clustering of profiles that are more dissimilar, generating a dendrogram depicting the hierarchical arrangement of this clustering (Fig. 24.7). The analysis segregated the neuron profiles into three major clusters, members of which are connected by solid lines. This conclusion is based on a regular, stepwise increase in the intercluster distance as the linking proceeds, until, in moving from three clusters to two, a dramatic increase in the intercluster distance occurs. The neuron classes defined by the cluster analysis are labeled S, H, and N (Fig. 24.7), corresponding to the neurons responding most to sucrose (S) and other

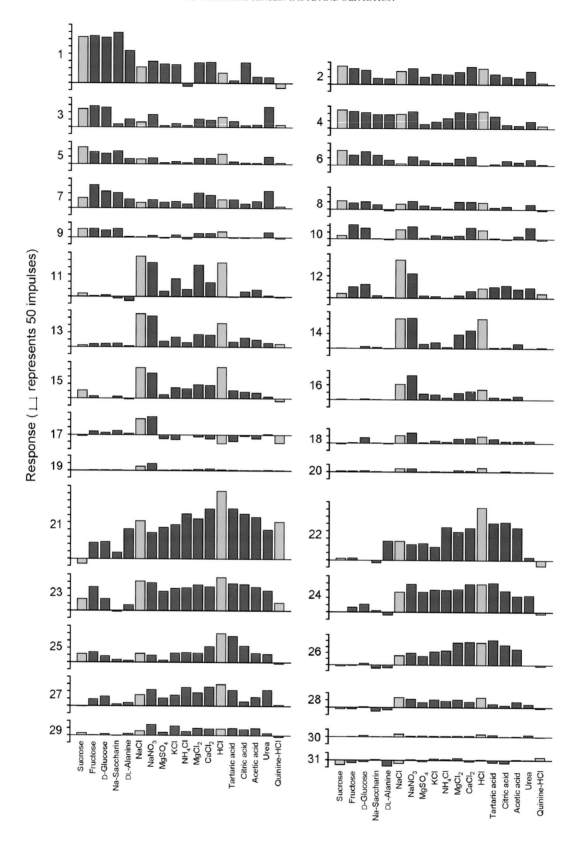

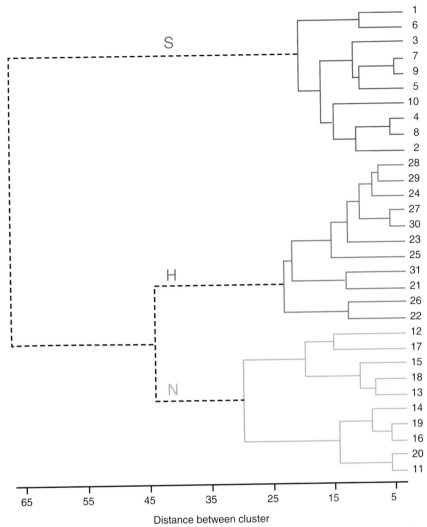

65   55   45   35   25   15   5

Distance between cluster

FIGURE 24.7 Cluster analysis of hamster PbN neural response profiles. The parallel horizontal lines of the dendrogram represent profiles, or groups of profiles, of neurons indicated at the right and numbered as in Fig. 24.6. The major profile clusters (S, H, N) are identified to the left of the defining vertical lines. Distances between profiles (or groups of profiles) are obtained by projecting the vertical lines to the distance scale along the abscissa. Modified from Smith *et al.* (1983a), with permission of the American Physiological Society.

sweet stimuli, HCl (H) and other acids, and NaCl (N) and NaNO₃, respectively. Similar classes emerge from hierarchical clustering of peripheral fibers and medullary neurons in the hamster when as few as 3 or as many as 18 stimuli are applied to the anterior portion of the tongue. The stimulus array must, however, include at least one example of three stimulus classes: (1) sweeteners, (2) sodium salts, and (3) nonsodium salts and acids. A QHCl-best class of neurons only emerges following anterior tongue stimulation when the concentration of QHCl is considerably greater than 1 mM.

FIGURE 24.6 Response profiles of hamster PbN neurons. Numbers to the left of each profile identify the neurons. The left-hand column shows profiles for odd-numbered neurons, and the right-hand column shows profiles for even-numbered neurons (and neuron 31). Neurons 1–10 are most responsive to sweet-tasting stimuli, neurons 11–20 are most responsive to sodium salts, and neurons 21–31 are most responsive to acids and nonsodium salts or quinine (neuron 31). Test stimuli are listed along the abscissa, beneath bars whose heights represent response rates for 5 s. Each tick mark represents 50 impulses per 5 s above the spontaneous rate. Response rates that are lower than the spontaneous rate are seen as bars extending below the horizontal zero line. Green bars represent responses to prototypical stimuli (sucrose, NaCl, HCl, and QHCl), and blue bars represent responses to other stimuli. Data from Smith *et al.* (1983a).

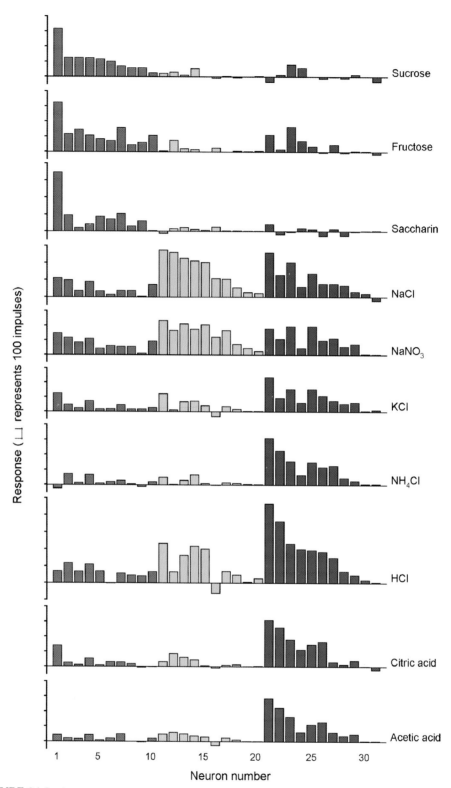

FIGURE 24.8 Across neuron patterns for hamster PbN neurons (replot of data from Fig. 24.6). Response rates elicited for 5 s in PbN neurons 1–31 are represented by consecutive filled bars from left to right. Each row depicts the pattern elicited by stimuli listed at the right. S neurons (1–10, as defined by the cluster analysis of Fig. 24.7) are shown in red, N neurons (11–20) in green, and H neurons (21–31) in blue. Neuron numbers are indicated along the abscissa. Each tick mark represents 100 nerve impulses in a 5-s period. Bars extending below the zero line indicate response rates lower than the spontaneous rate. Data from Smith *et al.* (1983a).

When this array of 18 stimuli was applied to the hamster's fungiform papillae, the responses of neurons in the PbN reflected the perceptual similarities and differences among the stimuli, as determined by studies of behavioral generalization among taste stimuli by hamsters. Stimuli with similar taste quality produce patterns of activity across taste neurons that are highly correlated. The responses of all 31 neurons to 10 of these stimuli indicate that stimuli with similar tastes produce similar patterns of activity (Fig. 24.8). The correlation between the patterns produced by sucrose and sodium saccharin is 0.85, between NaCl and NaNO$_3$ is 0.91, and between citric and acetic acid is 0.95. Stimuli with different tastes, however, do not correlate (e.g., sucrose and NaCl, $r = -0.09$; fructose and HCl, $r = 0.06$) or correlate much less strongly (e.g., NaNO$_3$ and citric acid, $r = 0.41$). Within this stimulus array, three distinctly different patterns are seen. One is elicited by sucrose, fructose, and sodium saccharin. NaCl and NaNO$_3$ elicit a second pattern, whereas a third pattern is evoked by acids and non-sodium salts. Within these patterns, the most responsive neurons for a particular group of stimuli tend to fall within one of the neuron clusters. For example, for the patterns evoked by sucrose, fructose, and sodium-saccharin, neurons in the S cluster (neurons 1–10) are the most responsive. For the sodium salts, the N cluster (neurons 11–20) is most responsive; however, the H neurons are often quite responsive as well. For nonsodium salts and acids, the H cluster (neurons 21–31) is most responsive, although HCl also activates N neurons. Thus, within the activity elicited

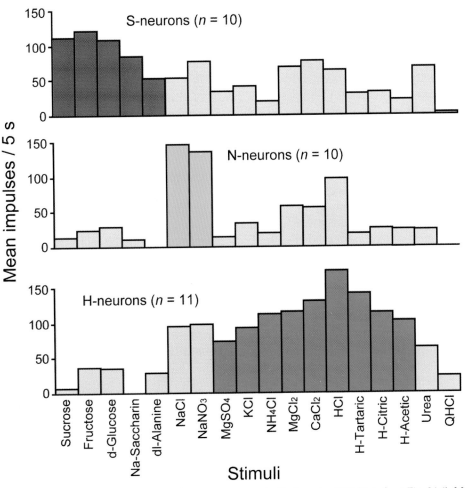

FIGURE 24.9 Mean responses of the three neuron types in the hamster PbN (data from Fig. 24.6). Mean response rates elicited for 5 s in PbN neurons by each of the 18 stimuli are depicted by bars from left to right. Within each mean profile, the stimulus class that is most effective in driving that neuron type is indicated by colored bars (red, sweet stimuli; green, sodium salts; blue, nonsodium salts and acids); all other stimuli are depicted by gray bars. Stimuli are indicated along the abscissa. Modified from Smith *et al.* (1983b), with permission of the American Physiological Society.

in the hamster PbN, the responses of particular sets of neurons (S, N, or H) typically dominate the patterns evoked by particular sets of stimuli (sweet-tasting, sodium salts, or nonsodium salts and acids).

Inspection of these neural response profiles (Fig. 24.6) reveals that neurons in the hamster PbN are relatively broadly tuned across stimuli that differ in quality. Mean response profiles for the three neuron types in the hamster PbN (Fig. 24.9) show that these neuron types, although defined by similarities and differences in their response profiles and to a large extent by which of the basic taste stimuli (sucrose, NaCl, or HCl) they respond to best, are responsive to most of these stimuli to some extent. Often these cells respond quite vigorously to two or more stimuli that are known to be clearly behaviorally discriminable, such as Na-saccharin and CaCl₂ or urea (S neurons), NaCl or HCl (N neurons), or NaCl and KCl (H neurons).

Mechanisms of Taste Quality Coding Are Controversial

The nature of the neural coding in this system has been debated vigorously for many years, with considerable disagreement about whether taste quality is represented by activity in specific neural channels (a labeled line code) or by the relative activity across the responsive neurons (a population code). Even the existence of four basic taste qualities is not universally accepted, with some authors insisting on additional qualities and others arguing that taste experience is a continuum upon which the familiar qualities are merely arbitrary points. The multiple sensitivity of taste-sensitive neurons makes a strict labeled line hypothesis difficult to accept, although there is compelling evidence for taste neuron types based on similarities in their profiles of sensitivity (Figs. 25.6–25.8).

Prior to the development of neurophysiological recording methods, a long tradition of human psychophysical research provided considerable support for the notion that taste experience could be reduced to a few basic qualities, although not necessarily the traditional four. This idea, combined with Mueller's doctrine of specific nerve energies, led to the expectation that the perception of taste quality would arise from the activation of one of a few neuron types, each coding a single taste quality. Early neurophysiological recordings showing that peripheral taste fibers in several species are responsive to stimuli representing more than one taste quality discounted this strict "labeled line" theory. As a result, an "across neuron pattern" theory suggesting that taste quality is coded by the relative activity across a population of neurons was proposed. Such a population code accommodates

the multiple sensitivity of taste neurons and requires neither specific neuron types nor taste primaries. However, the persisting view of the importance of taste primaries later led to a modification of the labeled line theory proposing that taste quality is coded by the activity in a few "best stimulus" channels, i.e., by neurons that respond best, but not specifically, to one of the basic taste qualities.

Accumulating evidence suggests that there are functional classes of neurons that correspond in some way to primary taste qualities. However, analyses show that no single class of neurons in isolation can discriminate well between different taste qualities. The neural coding problem essentially rests on whether the activity in a given taste neuron is an unambiguous representation of the quality of the stimulus applied to its receptors or whether this activity is meaningful only in the context of activity in other afferent neurons. This section reviews relevant neurophysiological data that bear on this issue and suggests that taste quality is coded in the relative rates of activity across several neuron types.

Population Coding of Taste Quality

Multiple sensitivity of fibers in the CT nerve (reviewed in Box 24.2) first led Pfaffmann (1955) to propose that taste quality is coded by the pattern of activity across taste fibers. With this coding hypothesis, taste quality remains invariant with increased intensity even though any single neuron may increase its breadth of responsiveness. The pattern of activity generated across the entire array of taste neurons at a higher concentration is similar in shape but varies in amplitude, whereas activity in any one cell cannot unambiguously represent both stimulus quality and intensity. The patterns of activity to several stimuli evoked across hamster PbN neurons reveal that stimuli with similar tastes, such as the three sweeteners or the two sodium salts, generate highly correlated patterns of activity across these cells (Fig. 24.8). Several behavioral investigations have shown that experimental animals judge stimuli that evoke well-correlated neural patterns to have similar tastes. This population approach to quality coding makes the multiple sensitivity of gustatory neurons an essential part of the neural code for taste quality; it stresses that the code for quality is given in the response of the entire population of cells, placing little or no emphasis on the role of an individual neuron. Erickson (1968) has argued that such a coding mechanism could operate for many sensory systems, particularly for nontopographic modalities employing neurons that are broadly tuned across their stimulus array.

BOX 24.2

THE EARLIEST RECORDINGS OF SINGLE PERIPHERAL TASTE FIBERS REVEALED MULTIPLE SENSITIVITIES

The earliest electrophysiological recordings of afferent taste fiber activity were made by Carl Pfaffmann (1955), who recorded the activity of single chorda tympani (CT) nerve fibers in the rat, cat, and rabbit. At that time, he was expecting to find individual nerve fibers that responded specifically to stimuli representing each of the basic human taste qualities of salty, sweet, sour, and bitter. To his surprise, most single fibers in the CT nerve responded to stimuli representing more than one taste quality, often as many as three or four. This led Pfaffmann to propose that taste quality must be represented by the relative amounts of activity across a number of afferent fibers, an idea that came to be known as the "across fiber pattern theory" of taste quality coding. This notion accounted well for the multiple sensitivity of taste afferent neurons at all levels of the gustatory system. Although there has been considerable ensuing controversy over the nature of taste quality coding, the basic idea of a pattern code, in which taste quality is represented in the population response, is still the most viable explanation for the neural coding of taste quality.

David V. Smith

When across neuron correlations are calculated for an array of gustatory stimuli, those with similar tastes correlate highly and those with different tastes correlate less (see Fig. 24.8). Almost every neurophysiological study that has taken this approach to analyzing the responses of gustatory cells has shown that such neural patterns reflect the qualitative similarities among taste stimuli. Often the across neuron correlations serve as input to a multivariate statistical procedure to generate a "taste space" that represents the similarities and differences among the stimuli within the neural population. A three-dimensional taste space for 18 stimuli was generated using multidimensional scaling of the across neuron correlations among all 18 stimuli (Fig. 24.10). Proximity within the space represents similarity in the population response. Within this space, sweet-tasting stimuli (red circles), sodium salts (green squares), nonsodium salts and acids (blue circles), and the two bitter-tasting stimuli (yellow squares) are clearly separated. This arrangement of stimuli based on similarities among their across neuron patterns suggests that the information within these patterns is sufficient to discriminate among these four groups of stimuli, even though any one cell in the hamster PbN is very likely to respond to stimuli of more than one group (as seen in Fig. 24.6).

Labeled Lines

Although mammalian taste neurons are broadly tuned, many investigators have attempted to group them into functionally meaningful categories, typically on the basis of their best stimulus or their response profiles. The implication that distinct neuron types may play a role in the coding of taste quality began with the categorization of hamster CT fibers into best-stimulus groups. This categorization became the focus of an ensuing controversy over the neural representation of taste quality when Pfaffmann (1974) proposed that these fiber types code taste quality in a labeled line fashion. This hypothesis suggests that "sweetness" is coded by activity in sucrose-best neurons, "saltiness" by activity in NaCl-best neurons, and so forth. In this scheme, activity in a given cell type provides complete information on the quality of the stimulus. In contrast to a population approach to taste coding, this labeled line position advocates a "feature extraction" approach, in which particular neurons (or groups of neurons) play specific roles in the representation of taste quality.

Gustatory Neuron Types Define the Population Response to Taste Stimuli

A labeled line code requires the existence of neuron types, whereas a population code does not. The number of labeled lines would equal the number of discrete taste qualities, which would each be signaled by activity in separate afferent channels. Consequently, the existence of gustatory neuron types has been sharply contested on the assumption that their existence somehow implicates them as labeled lines. However, the mere existence of neuron types (defined by their best stimulus, similarities in their profiles, or other criteria) does not necessarily imply that these classes of cells comprise labeled lines. A classic

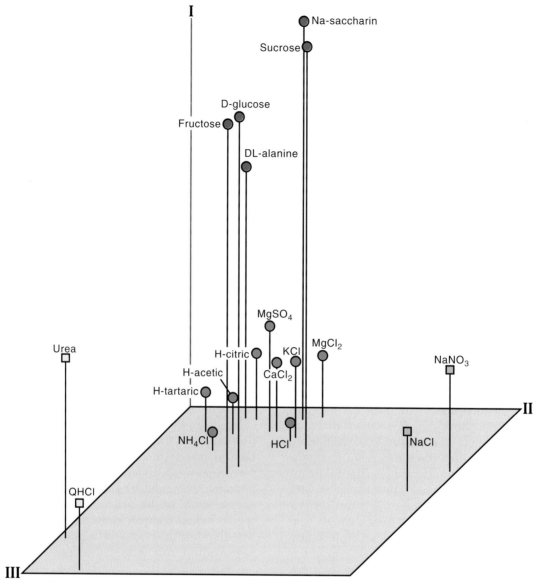

FIGURE 24.10 Three-dimensional "taste space" showing similarities and differences in the response patterns of PbN neurons elicited by 18 stimuli delivered to the hamster's anterior tongue. This space was derived from multidimensional scaling of the across neuron correlations among these stimuli recorded from neurons in the PbN of the hamster (data shown in Fig. 24.6). Proximity within the space represents similar population responses, whereas distance represents dissimilar patterns of evoked activity. Four groups of stimuli are indicated by different symbols (sweet stimuli, red circles; sodium salts, green squares; non-sodium salts and acids, blue circles; bitter stimuli, yellow squares). Modified from Smith *et al.* (1983b), with permission of the American Physiological Society.

example in which receptor types are evident but there is general agreement about the existence of a population code is in vertebrate color vision, as discussed later.

As seen earlier, neuron types are readily distinguishable within the hamster PbN based on the relative similarities and differences among their response profiles. Although the recognition of neuron types depends on the strictness of one's criteria when examining a cluster dendrogram, the dendrogram for the

hamster PbN (Fig. 24.7) strongly suggests neuron types. This hierarchical arrangement is also seen in hamster CT and IXth nerve fibers. At all levels of the hamster gustatory system that have been examined, there is strong evidence that taste sensitivities are organized into relatively distinct sets of fibers and neurons. Of course, the real issue with respect to sensory coding is what role these neuron types play in the neural code for taste quality.

The roles played by neuron types in the hamster brain stem in the definitions of across neuron patterns have been examined (Smith *et al.*, 1983b). This study led to the conclusion that the neural distinction among stimuli with different tastes (such as sodium and nonsodium salts) depends on comparisons of the activity in different neuron types (such as NaCl- and

HCl-best cells) and that one neuron type alone was insufficient to discriminate between stimuli with different taste qualities. Further, the responses of particular groups of neurons dominated and essentially defined the similarities among stimuli of a particular quality (Fig. 24.8). That is, each neuron type is essential to the representation of a particular taste quality,

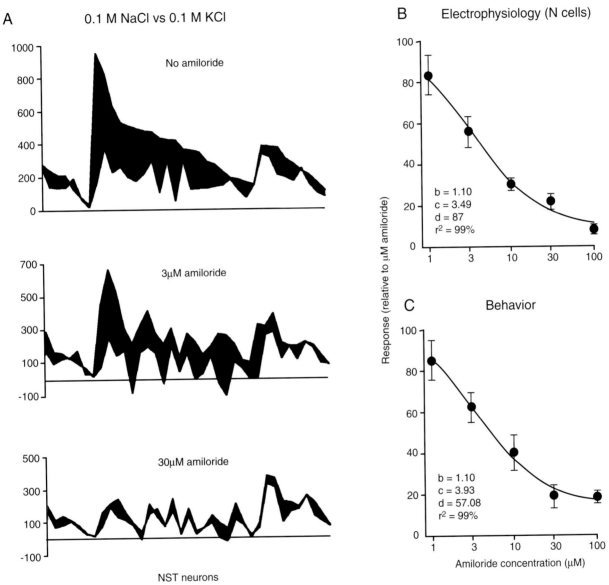

FIGURE 24.11 The effects of blocking taste receptor cell activity with amiloride on neural and behavioral responses to NaCl and KCl in rats. (A) Across neuron patterns in cells of the rat NST for 0.1 *M* NaCl and KCl in three conditions: without amiloride, mixed with 3 μ*M* amiloride, and mixed with 30 μM amiloride. Neurons are arranged along the abscissa by neuron type (S, then N, then H) and within each type by decreasing response to 0.1 *M* NaCl; the arrangement of neurons is the same in each graph. The area between the two patterns is shaded to highlight the difference between them, which is eliminated by amiloride in a concentration-dependent manner. (B) Dose–response effect of amiloride on the firing rate of N neurons in the rat NST. Net responses in 10-s trials were standardized to responses in the no amiloride condition. (C) Performance of rats in a two-lever discrimination task (data from Spector *et al.*, 1996) standardized to the percentage of correct responses in the no amiloride condition. Three-parameter sigmoidal curves were fit to both dose–response data sets (in B and C); values for slope (b) and half-maximum amiloride concentration (c) were virtually identical for both neural and behavioral data. Modified from St. John and Smith (2000), with permission of the American Physiological Society.

but cannot serve in isolation as a labeled line. This coding mechanism is similar to the coding of a stimulus wavelength by the vertebrate visual system, where three types of broadly sensitive photoreceptor pigments are involved. The color of the wavelength of light falling on the retina can be encoded accurately by considering the relative activity in these three photoreceptors, i.e., by a pattern. Deficiencies in one or more of the photoreceptor pigments result in various forms of visual chromatic deficiency or "color blindness." Data on color-blind individuals show that the absence of any one of the three photoreceptor types results in the inability to discriminate among particular sets of wavelengths.

Experiments on the rat NST reveal a gustatory analog to visual color blindness. Following a block of the amiloride-sensitive sodium channel (see Chapter 23) with amiloride, rats cannot behaviorally discrimi-

nate NaCl from KCl (Spector *et al.*, 1996). Likewise, after amiloride treatment of the tongue, cells in the NST cannot distinguish between sodium and non-sodium salts; i.e., the across neuron patterns evoked by these stimuli become highly similar (St. John and Smith, 2000). This effect is restricted to salt responses in S and N neuron types; H neuron responses are unaffected by amiloride. The result is that the neural patterns evoked by NaCl and KCl become highly correlated (Fig. 24.11A), as these two salts stimulate H neurons similarly (see also Fig. 24.8). The population response to a sodium salt can be distinguished from that to a nonsodium salt or acid only if the activities of both N and H cells contribute differentially to the patterns; amiloride makes the patterns similar by removing the differential contribution of S and N neurons. Amiloride has corresponding effects on NST neurons and on behavioral discriminability (Figs. 11B

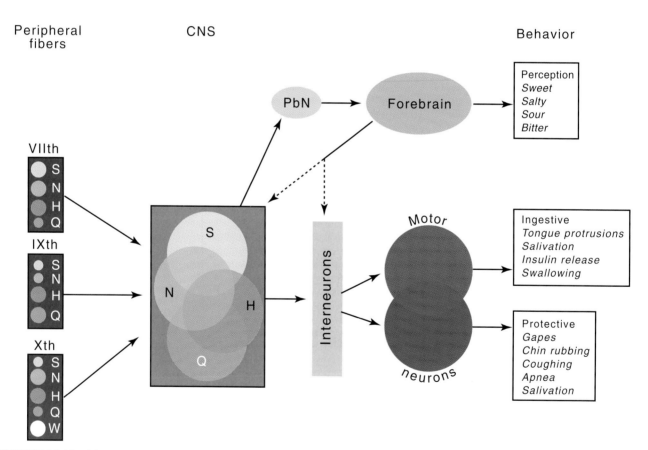

FIGURE 24.12 Schematic diagram of the chemosensory inputs of three cranial nerves to the taste responsive portion of the nucleus of the solitary tract (NST) and their putative roles in taste-mediated behaviors. The size of the filled circles for each of the peripheral nerves (VIIth, IXth, and Xth) depicts the relative responsiveness of these nerves to sucrose (S), NaCl (N), HCl (H), QHCl (Q), and water (W). Sensitivities of NST cells are largely overlapping, with each cell type somewhat responsive to two or three of the basic stimuli. Sucrose and QHCl stimulate few of the same NST cells, however. Output from the NST ascends in the classic taste pathway to give rise to perceptions of sweetness, saltiness, sourness, and bitterness and to hedonic tone (not shown). Local reflex circuits within the brain stem control ingestive and protective responses evoked by taste stimulation. Behavioral data suggest that both ingestive and protective responses can be triggered in parallel, depending on the quality of the stimulus. Reprinted with permission from Smith and Frank (1993). Copyright CRC Press, Boca Raton, Florida.

and 11C). These experiments show that all neuron types are necessary for the gustatory system to sort out different groups of stimuli (sweeteners, sodium salts, non-sodium salts and acids, and bitter substances) based on their across neuron patterns. Taste quality discrimination depends on a comparison of activity across broadly tuned neuron types, comparable to the coding of color vision by broadly tuned photoreceptors.

Taste Information Plays a Role in Ingestive Behavior

Taste physiologists have focused largely on the role of gustatory neurons in taste quality perception, but a number of taste-mediated somatic and visceral responses, ranging from tongue movements to salivation to preabsorptive insulin release, have their neuronal substrate within the brain stem. The VIIth, IXth, and Xth nerves have differential sensitivities and make different contributions to taste-mediated behaviors (Fig. 24.12).

Taste may be considered the oral component of the visceral afferent system, which includes gustatory, respiratory, cardiovascular, and gastrointestinal functions. As noted earlier, taste buds innervated by the VIIth, IXth, and Xth nerves contribute somewhat differentially to this visceral continuum. Peripheral nerve fibers activated by sucrose project into the NST, where sucrose-sensitive cells also respond to NaCl and to HCl, but are often inhibited by QHCl. Ultimately, the output of these second-order neurons ascends to the forebrain to give rise to the perception of sweetness (Fig. 24.12). Simultaneously, these cells provide input to somatic and visceral motor systems that drive the ingestive components of feeding behavior, including mouth and tongue movements, salivation, insulin release, and swallowing. Conversely, QHCl-sensitive fibers project into the NST, where they drive cells that are also responsive to HCl and NaCl but not to sucrose. Quinine-sensitive cells of the NST send ascending projections to the forebrain to give rise to sensations of bitterness (Fig. 24.12), but they also provide input to motor systems that drive behaviors associated with rejection. The superior laryngeal branch of the Xth nerve is involved in swallowing, airway protection, and a number of other visceral reflexes. In addition to its obvious role in regulating ingestive behavior, taste triggers a number of metabolic responses, including salivary, gastric, and pancreatic secretions. Thus, in addition to their mediation of gustatory sensation, taste buds may have a number of roles related to gustatory–visceral regulation, depending on their peripheral distribution and innervation.

Measures of Taste Reactivity Reflect the Hedonic Aspects of Taste

In addition to evoking the perception of taste quality, gustatory stimuli trigger several reflexive response sequences that are related to the ingestion and rejection of food substances. These behavioral sequences range from ingestive and protective somatic motor responses to visceral motor activity associated with gastrointestinal function. A number of overt motor responses to taste stimulation can be quantified and measured; these responses have been termed "taste reactivity" and are useful indexes of the hedonic value of a gustatory stimulus.

Taste reactivity in the rat consists of sequences of ingestive or protective behaviors that reflect the palatability (i.e., hedonic value) of a gustatory stimulus (Grill and Norgren, 1978). Ingestive responses begin with rhythmic mouth movements, followed by midline tongue protrusions, lateral tongue protrusions, and swallowing; this sequence is triggered by sucrose and other hedonically positive (appetitive) stimuli. Protective responses include oral gapes and a number of somatic motor sequences such as head shaking, chin rubbing, forelimb flailing, paw pushing, face washing, and increased locomotion, all elicited by quinine and other hedonically negative (aversive) stimuli. Results from taste reactivity tests typically correspond with other short-term palatability measures such as lick rate tests. Sucrose and quinine produce opposite patterns of ingestive and protective taste reactivity, and mixtures of sucrose and quinine can trigger a combination of these behaviors. Sodium salts and acids produce patterns consisting of combinations of both ingestive and protective behaviors. The taste quality of the stimulus is directly related to the specific pattern of taste reactivity.

Decerebrate rats are able to exhibit normal patterns of taste reactivity to stimuli infused into their mouths. Both ingestive and aversive oral and somatic motor responses are elicited by gustatory stimulation in these animals, suggesting that the neural substrate important for discriminating among taste stimuli is intact within the hindbrain. Similarly, anencephalic human neonates produce normal facial expressions in response to gustatory stimuli. Thus, information arising from the peripheral gustatory apparatus projects into the brain stem and makes connections at that level to produce the appropriate response sequences. To produce ingestive responses, peripheral fibers carrying information about sweet stimuli, which are numerous in the CT and GSP nerves, must ultimately provide input to a specific set of motor neurons that control tongue protrusions, lateral tongue movements, and swallowing (Fig. 24.12). Similarly, the oral and somatic motor outputs characteristic of the responses to quinine must arise from motor neurons that receive input arriving at the NST from peripheral taste fibers carrying information about bitter stimuli, which are most numerous in the IXth nerve. Second-order gustatory cells in the NST project indirectly through interneurons in the reticular formation to brain stem motor nuclei that control oromotor responses.

One can view ingestive and protective motor sequences as parallel processes that can be driven one at a time, as by sucrose or quinine, or simultaneously, as by sucrose–quinine mixtures. Because most peripheral gustatory fibers and brain stem neurons have multiple sensitivities to different taste qualities, many of the cells contributing to each of these output systems may respond to several stimuli; thus, a stimulus such as NaCl or HCl might evoke output in both systems. These multiple sensitivities, however, do not extend to sucrose and quinine, which generally do not stimulate the same cells and which are often mutually inhibitory in brain stem cells. Thus, sweet and bitter stimuli produce relatively independent afferent inputs and are characterized by opposite patterns of motor output. These motor patterns can be generated by other stimuli to varying degrees and can be modified in the intact animal by conditioning, presumably via descending influences from the forebrain.

Taste Activity in the Medulla Is Modulated by Descending Pathways

Responses of brain stem cells to gustatory stimulation are subject to several modulatory influences. For example, systemically administered glucose, insulin, and pancreatic glucagon alter the responses of cells in the rat NST to tongue stimulation with glucose. The mechanisms underlying these inhibitory effects are unknown; they may involve a direct effect of the increased availability of glucose on the recorded cells or an inhibitory synaptic influence descending from the forebrain. That descending pathways can exert a modulatory influence over brain stem taste cells was first demonstrated by electrophysiological studies on decerebrate rats. There are direct descending projections from gustatory areas of the ventral forebrain to both PbN and NST. Inputs from the gustatory cortex, the central nucleus of the amygdala, and the lateral hypothalamus have all been shown to both excite and inhibit the activity of cells of the rostral NST; inhibitory responses produced by cortical activation are blocked by the $GABA_A$ receptor antagonist bicuculline.

Studies have begun to reveal mechanisms of synaptic transmission within the gustatory region of the NST (Bradley et al., 1996). The inhibitory neurotransmitter GABA has been shown to play a role in the processing of respiratory, cardiovascular, and other information in the visceral portion of the NST. Many small ovoid interneurons within the gustatory NST express GABA or its degradative enzymes.

Electrophysiological recordings from cells in the rostral NST in in vitro slices from both rats and hamsters have shown that GABA produces inhibition of activity in these cells, which is mediated predominantly by the $GABA_A$ receptor subtype. These studies suggest that the gustatory portion of the NST is under the influence of a tonic GABAergic inhibitory network. The inhibitory action of GABA on taste-elicited responses of cells in the NST (and its reversal by bicuculline) has been demonstrated by extracellular recording in vivo combined with local micropressure injection of these agents into the nucleus. These latter data and those recorded in vitro strongly implicate GABAergic inhibitory mechanisms in the processing of gustatory information through the NST.

The responses of cells in the gustatory zone of the NST can be blocked by glutamate antagonists. Excitatory postsynaptic potentials (EPSPs) recorded from rat NST cells in vitro in response to electrical stimulation of the solitary tract are reduced by both CNQX and APV, antagonists to the AMPA-kainate and NMDA glutamate receptors, respectively. Both of these agents also reversibly block or reduce the responses to chemical stimulation of the anterior tongue in hamster NST cells recorded in vivo. All cells responsive to taste stimulation are blocked by CNQX, regardless of their profiles of sensitivity; there is no evidence that the neurotransmitter is different for cells of different types (i.e., sucrose vs NaCl best). Therefore, it is very likely that glutamate acts as a neurotransmitter between gustatory afferent fibers and taste-responsive cells in the NST.

Evidence also indicates that taste-responsive cells in the NST are excited by substance P (SP) and are inhibited by met-enkephalin. Immunocytochemical studies have shown that SP- and enkephalin-containing neurons are present within the gustatory zone of the NST and that SP-containing fibers enter this nucleus from a number of yet unknown sources. In vitro experiments on rat brain stem slices have shown that bath application of SP excites a number of cells in the gustatory zone of the NST. The role of these SP-responsive NST cells in gustatory processing has been demonstrated in the hamster NST in vivo, where responses to anterior tongue stimulation with NaCl or sucrose are enhanced by local microinjection of SP. In vivo experiments also show that a subset of taste-responsive neurons in the NST are inhibited by met-enkephalin.

Summary

Taste receptors respond to a variety of chemical compounds to give rise to a limited number of sensations (saltiness, sweetness, sourness, bitterness, and, perhaps, umami). The transduction mechanisms for taste stimuli are located on receptor cells within taste buds distributed in several subpopulations, innervated by one of four different peripheral nerves. These nerves project into the nucleus of the solitary tract in the medulla and contain different distributions of gustatory neuron types. From there, projections arise to the parabrachial nuclei in the pons and then to the thalamus and gustatory neocortex. A parallel pathway carries taste information into the ventral forebrain to areas involved in autonomic regulation. Facial nerve fibers respond predominantly to sweet-tasting stimuli and sodium salts, whereas those of the glossopharyngeal nerve are predominantly responsive to aversive stimuli such as bitter-tasting stimuli and acids. The gustatory system extracts information about taste intensity and quality and about the hedonic value of the stimuli. Gustatory neurons are broadly tuned to stimuli of different quality and often respond to tactile and temperature stimulation as well. Although researchers traditionally have disagreed about the nature of taste quality coding, there is good evidence that taste quality is represented by the relative activity across several well-defined neuron types in both peripheral and central nervous systems. Taste information plays a key role in the control of ingestive behavior, and the consequences of ingestion and experience can feed back onto the gustatory system via both excitatory and inhibitory mechanisms to alter taste sensitivity.

OLFACTION

The olfactory system must provide several operations that are essential for the survival of most animal species. These include the ability to detect and discriminate the considerable range of signal molecules that mediate instinctive behaviors involved in prey–

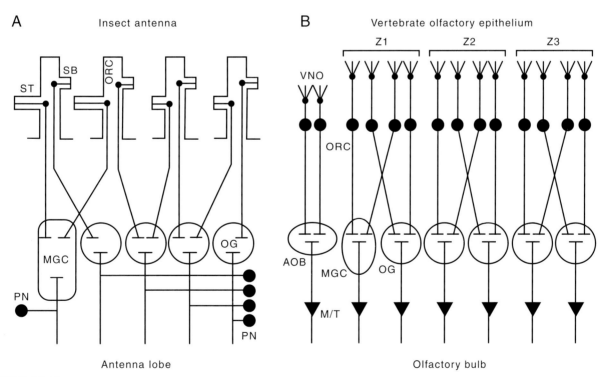

FIGURE 24.13 Comparison between the olfactory pathways of invertebrates and vertebrates. (A) Insect: SB, sensillum basiconica; ST, sensillum trichodea; ORC, olfactory receptor cells; MGC, macroglomerular complex; OG, ordinary glomeruli; PN, principal neuron. Not shown are local interneurons involved in intraglomerular processing between ORC terminals and PN dendrites. (B) Vertebrate: VNO, vomeronasal organ; Z1–Z3, expression zones for different olfactory receptor proteins; ORC, olfactory receptor cells; AOB, accessory olfactory bulb; MGC, modified glomerular complex; M/T, mitral/tufted cells. Not shown are local interneurons (periglomerular cells and granule cells) involved in intrabulbar processing at glomerular and M/T cell body levels. From Hildebrand and Shepherd (1997).

predator interactions, food selection, mating and reproduction, and social organization, and it must be able to do this for novel odors that may enter the environment unpredictably and be significant for one or more of these behaviors.

To meet these criteria, animals have evolved olfactory systems that share a number of features. The conservation of mechanisms across phyla is fundamental to understanding the neural basis of olfaction. There are several common features of the receptor cells and the first relay station: the antennal lobe in insects and the olfactory bulb in mammals (Fig. 24.13). Critical mechanisms for odor detection and discrimination

will be described within this integrated framework. The main theme will be that these represent adaptations of fundamental membrane and cellular mechanisms for the particular demands of the molecular stimuli that are unique for olfaction.

Odor Stimuli Consist of a Wide Range of Small Signal Molecules

Odor stimuli fall into several broad classes (see Chapter 23). Odor-generating compounds in aquatic species tend to be amino acids or bile salts. In terrestrial animals, there is a great diversity of acids,

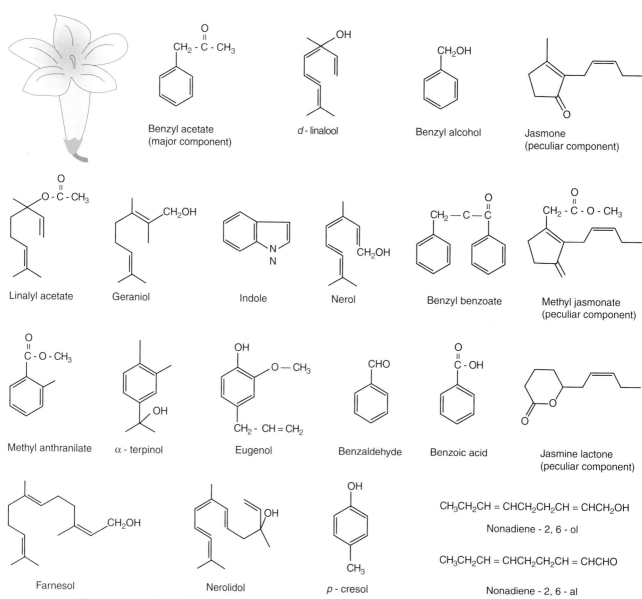

FIGURE 24.14 Odor molecules given off by the jasmine flower that constitute the smell of jasmine as an odor object (Mori and Yoshihara, 1995).

alcohols, esters, and aromatic compounds, as well as longer chain fatty acids and more complex molecules, such as musks and steroids, some of which act as components of pheromones.

Experimental and theoretical analyses of the mechanisms of odor stimulation and odor processing are usually carried out using single odor types, much as the analysis of visual processing rested initially on the use of simple spots and edges of light. However, in nature, behaviorally significant objects are more complex. The visual system is very good at identifying complex patterns such as faces. Similarly, with the olfactory system, animals are very good at identifying the complex odors that identify individuals of a species. In analogy with vision, complex odors may be referred to as *odor objects*. In most cases, an odor object is signaled by a blend of two or more compounds (Fig. 24.14). The task of the olfactory system is thus to identify not just a single odor molecule, but a complex blend representing an odor object of behavioral significance to the organism.

Olfactory Receptor Cells Respond to Odors as Specialists or Generalists

As described in Chapter 23, the responses of olfactory receptor cells to different odors reflect the response spectra of the olfactory receptor proteins that they express. The analysis of those transduction mechanisms has depended on *in vitro* analysis; the goal is now to understand the response spectra of *in vivo* olfactory receptor neurons (ORNs). These have traditionally been studied using extracellular unitary recordings from cells exposed to pulses of odor. The best stimulus control is achieved in insects, where the recording electrode samples the activity of a receptor cell in an individual antennal hair while it is subjected to quantitatively controlled odor pulses.

The classical studies of Dietrich Schneider and colleagues (Boeckh *et al.*, 1966) in the silk moth showed that ORNs can be classified into two groups. Cells called *specialists* are in one group that responds narrowly to only one type of molecule or at most a small number of closely related types. These types consist mainly of the sex attractant pheromone molecules used by females to attract males during mating. In contrast, cells called *generalists* respond to a wide range of different types of molecules, such as the alcohols or esters, that are associated with different types of food objects in the environment. Some in-between categories of cells may respond somewhat more broadly to related types of molecules (broad specialists) or somewhat more narrowly to broad classes of

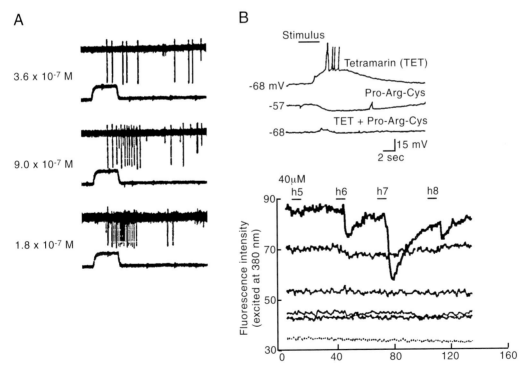

FIGURE 24.15 Examples of odor responses of different types of olfactory receptor neurons in different types of experimental preparations. (A) Extracellular unit recordings of excitatory single cell responses (upper traces) to increasing odor concentrations (lower traces) in the *in vivo* salamander olfactory epithelium. From Duchamp-Viret *et al.* (1999). (B) Lobster receptor neurons respond to different types of stimuli with either excitatory or inhibitory responses. From McClintock and Ache (1989).

odors (food specialists). Note that insect ORNs can respond to odors with either excitation or suppression, indicating the presence of relatively complex transduction cascades in the cilia.

In vertebrates, the classical studies of Robert Gesteland and colleagues (1965) revealed that ORNs in the frog tend to respond to a broad range of odor stimuli with a variety of patterns of impulse discharges. From that time, researchers have assumed that vertebrate ORNs are all generalists (Fig. 24.15). By careful control of the stimulus, it has been ascertained that vertebrate ORNs give mostly excitatory responses to odor stimuli. However, suppressive responses may also be present in some species due to second messenger pathways that reduce the depolarizing cAMP-mediated response (see Chapter 23).

BOX 24.3

BROAD SPECTRA ARE THE BASIS FOR SPECIFIC ODOR DISCRIMINATION

The finding that many olfactory receptor cells display broad overlapping response spectra to different odors is often thought by students to be inconsistent with the ability of animals to make exquisite discriminations between similar odors. It seems more intuitive that responses should be narrowly tuned and distinctive for each odor rather than broadly tuned with much overlap. The corresponding question has been the subject of considerable controversy in the taste system; the current consensus is that taste cells tend to respond best to one of the submodalities but with lesser overlapping responses to the other submodalities.

Another instructive comparison is with the color system in vision, which is based on three subsets of cones, each expressing a receptor differentially tuned to wavelengths of light. Although these cones are called red, green, and blue, these names refer only to the wavelength of the peak response of the cone; all have broad flanks of lesser responsiveness that cover most of the visible light spectrum. It is well recognized (see Chapter 23) that by itself a given type of cone gives no intrinsic information about wavelength; in fact, it is unable to distinguish between the wavelength and the intensity of a given light source. It is only through the differential overlapping responses of the cone types across the visible spectrum, and through downstream neural circuits that compare the responses, that wavelength is distinguished independently of intensity and that color perception is possible. This involves synaptic interactions among the pathways originating in the three cone subsets, interactions that heighten the contrast among the responses and are therefore called color opponent mechanisms.

To what extent can these principles apply to odor discrimination? The principles are particularly clearly understood in color vision because the stimulus varies only along one dimension, wavelength. In olfaction, a given series of chemical compounds can be arranged similarly in one dimension, such as in straight chains of 2 to 10 or so carbon atoms (aliphatic compounds) ending in the same functional group (e.g., alcohols). However, intersecting with this series are a countless number of other series with different side groups (chains, rings, etc.) and functional groups. Typically, odors change systematically with increasing numbers of carbon atoms in a series up to a point, but then change dramatically, presumably reflecting the intersection with other series with different properties.

Because of the many different types of chemical compounds involved, odor space is termed multidimensional. It is therefore vastly larger and more complicated than color space. Nonetheless, it is a reasonable working hypothesis that some of the same principles should apply: spectra of receptor molecules and the receptor cells that contain them are likely to overlap considerably, and the microcircuits at the first stages of synaptic processing in the olfactory bulb are likely to be involved in the interactions necessary for distinguishing odor ligand properties from odor intensity.

Further evidence in support of these principles is provided by work on artificial noses. In one prototype, polymer matrices with different physicochemical properties are dipped in a fluorescent indicator dye. The tips give different fluorescence to different vapor stimuli; the fiber optic responses are then read by an artificial neural network that compares and contrasts them. The device readily distinguishes the stimulus compounds on the basis of their overlapping responses to the different types of tips. The principles are thus similar to those explained earlier. The authors point out that the responses need not have any common or systematic molecular basis; all that is required is that the responses are different and that they overlap.

Gordon M. Shepherd

These same experiments show that increasing odor concentration elicits an increasing frequency of impulse discharge, indicating that odor concentration can be encoded by single ORNs. However, the dynamic range is only an order of magnitude, suggesting that recruitment of ORNs with different thresholds for a given odor may also contribute to concentration encoding, which is discussed further later.

Specialist cells have not been found in the main olfactory pathway of vertebrates for pheromones or pheromone-like substances, despite the range of vertebrate behaviors, such as mating preferences and territorial marking. One hypothesis is that in many vertebrates the pheromones may be special blends (i.e., complex odor objects) of different types of molecules (e.g., acids and ketones), which implies that many cells may be able to respond to any one type, but only a few may respond maximally to the blend. Another is that specialist ORNs tuned to specific vertebrate pheromones do exist and are waiting to be found. Specialist cells have been found in the vomeronasal organ.

As discussed in Chapter 23, experimental and computational analysis of expressed olfactory receptor genes has shown that individual ORNs are able to discriminate structural features, called determinants, of odor molecules, which include functional groups, hydrocarbon length, electrical charge, and stereoscopic shape. This information in the molecular domain is transduced into the electrical response of the sensory neuron. The different overlapping response spectra of the receptor proteins and their ORNs constitute the basis for further processing by the circuits of the olfactory pathway (Box 24.3).

What Is the Spatial Organization of ORNs in the Olfactory Epithelium?

In mammals the olfactory epithelium is distributed over the medial septal wall and the lateral turbinates toward the back of the nasal cavity. The ORNs that express a given receptor gene are located within one of roughly four zones that run anterior to posterior in the epithelium.

It has been commonly believed that the organization of ORNs within a zone is random. However, summed potential recordings of the electro-olfactogram (EOG) indicate that there are hot spots in different parts of a zone for different odors, and calcium imaging of single cells within swatches of the olfactory epithelium shows that there are clusters of ORNs responding to the same odor within a given zone. These clusters may reflect the migrations of ORNs

from stem cells in the basal part of the olfactory epithelium (OE). There is much fundamental interest for further analysis of the spatial organization of ORNs within the OE.

Is Olfactory Projection Organized Topographically?

In most other sensory systems (visual, auditory, somatosensory) there is a topographical organization of the output from the sensory receptors to the brain. This might not be expected in the olfactory system because of the nonspatial character of the odor stimulus and the zonal organization of the olfactory epithelium. The lack of spatial localization of the odor stimulus has suggested that space is available in the olfactory pathway to process other aspects of the odor stimuli, i.e., determinants on the odor molecules.

The classical studies of Edgar Adrian (1950) showed that different odor stimuli elicit different gradations of activity along the extent of the olfactory bulb, suggesting that at least a crude topographical organization of the olfactory receptor cells and their projections from the olfactory epithelium to the olfactory bulb may be present. At the same time, anatomical evidence for this organization was obtained by le Gros Clark. Tract-tracing methods, including fiber degeneration stains, radioactively labeled amino acid transport, horseradish peroxidase (HRP) transport, and monoclonal antibody staining, have provided a wealth of evidence for the topographical organization of the olfactory epithelium and its projection to the bulb in mammals.

In situ hybridization and gene-targeting methods showed that the subset of ORNs expressing a given receptor protein converge onto one or a few glomeruli in the olfactory bulb (Fig. 24.16). The picture that has emerged is that a given glomerulus or small number (2–3) of neighboring glomeruli receives its input from sensory cells arranged within anterior–posterior strips of cells within one epithelial zone. These experiments thus provide strong experimental evidence for the concept that subsets of ORNs expressing a single receptor gene project their axons as a labeled line onto one or a few target glomeruli. However, as physiological and metabolic data suggest, this labeled line is complex and broadly tuned, overlapping in specificity with many others (see later).

Studies of fish and amphibians have provided little evidence of topographical organization between epithelium and bulb. This seeming inconsistency appears to have been resolved by comparing the sizes of the systems: fish and amphibia have relatively small numbers of receptor cells (of the order of 10^6 on

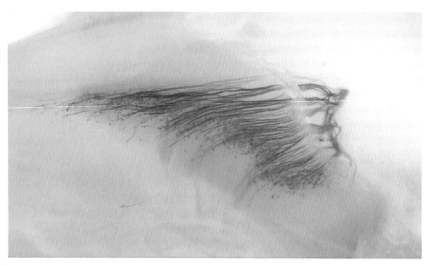

FIGURE 24.16   Whole mount of the nose of a rat shows olfactory receptor axons converging on a single glomerulus. This subset of cells is stained for a lacZ reporter linked to mRNA for one type of olfactory receptor and the microtubule-associated protein tau. From Mombaerts *et al.* (1996).

a side) contained in correspondingly small patches of olfactory epithelium, whereas most mammals have large numbers of receptor cells (e.g., 15×10^6 in rat; 50×10^6 in rabbit) spread over large extents of epithelium. The scaling rule therefore seems to be that a small system, such as that of a fish or frog, is equivalent to a small part of a large system, such as that of a mammal. This interpretation is supported by the *in situ* hybridization studies of receptors. Comparisons with insects need to take into account the complex organization of the olfactory glomeruli (see later).

Within the olfactory bulb the receptor cell axons terminate in the rounded regions of neuropil termed glomeruli. Anatomical studies from the time of Ramon y Cajal have shown that the glomerulus is an anatomical unit for the convergence of axons from many ORNs. In rats, the 15 million receptors converge onto some 1500 glomeruli, giving an average overall convergence of some 10,000:1.

Olfactory Glomeruli Are Anatomical Units for Processing Specific Odor Information

The olfactory glomerulus is the universal anatomical and functional unit for olfactory processing (Fig. 24.13). In mammals, the glomerulus is a spheroidal region of neuropil consisting of the preterminal axons and terminal boutons of olfactory receptor cell axons and the distal dendritic tufts of mitral (M), tufted (T), and periglomerular (PG) cells. The border of the glomerulus is demarcated by several layers of glial processes and by a ring of cell bodies of PG cells. In mammals, a glomerulus ranges from 50–100 μm in

diameter in mouse to 150–200 μm in rabbit and is thus comparable in size to a barrel in rat somatosensory cortex or an orientation column in visual cortex. In amphibia and fish, the glomeruli are smaller, 20–50 μm in diameter, and much less distinct, partly due to a paucity of surrounding PG cells.

In insects, glomeruli are formed by preterminal axons and terminals of the olfactory receptor neurons, which make synapses on the terminal neurites of the principal neurons and local interneurons of the antennal lobe. The large size and reproducible positions of the glomeruli have made it possible to demonstrate unique identities and to provide detailed glomerular maps of several species of insects.

Olfactory Glomeruli are Functional Units That Form Spatial Images of Odor Molecules

The functional significance of glomerular units, or glomerular modules as they are often called, is seen when an animal is exposed to an odor and the activity patterns in the olfactory bulb are observed. The key observation is that different odors evoke different patterns of active glomeruli located in distinct domains within the olfactory bulb. Thus, the focal glomerular activity elicited by the odor of amyl acetate is localized in two broad zones, one medial and one lateral, within the olfactory bulb glomerular sheet (Fig. 24.17). In contrast, the activity elicited by camphor is distributed in a curving line of smaller glomerular patches. Although the two domains overlap, their overall patterns are distinct and different. These results suggest that each type of odor elicits a characteristic pattern of glomerular

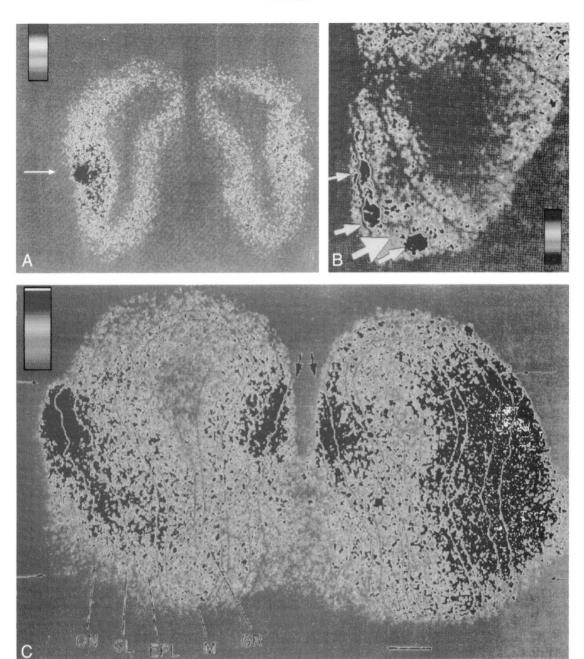

FIGURE 24.17   The 2-deoxylucose (2DG) method reveals the functional organization of the olfactory glomerular sheet. (A) Patterns of 2-deoxyglucose utilization in an X-ray film autoradiograph of a frontal section through the ofactory bulb of a rat exposed to a low concentration of the odor of amyl acetate. A single focus associated with one glomerulus or a small group of neighboring glomeruli is seen in one of the olfactory bulbs. (B) With a moderate concentration of amyl acetate, the activity induced in the glomerular layer is characterized by activation of several glomeruli or groups of glomeruli (white lines outline the histological layers). (C) With a high concentration of odor of amyl acetate, the induced activity consists of broad regions of increased 2DG uptake, centered on the glomerular layer in medial and lateral regions of the olfactory bulb, that are roughly bilaterally symmetrical.

activation in the olfactory bulb. The patterns may be considered to constitute odor images in neural space.

These maps were obtained with the original 2-deoxyglucose (2DG) mapping method, which has been confirmed and extended by other techniques

(Table 24.1). Each method has its advantages and disadvantages. Two main categories are optical methods and activity mapping methods. Optical methods give high resolution at the level of single glomeruli. Many of these studies have focused on the local architecture

TABLE 24.1   Methods for Odor Mapping
in the Olfactory Bulb

Single unit recordings

Focal field potential recordings

2-Deoxyglucose

c-fos RNA or protein

Voltage sensitive dyes

Intrinsic imaging

Calcium imaging

fMRI (functional magnetic resonance imaging)

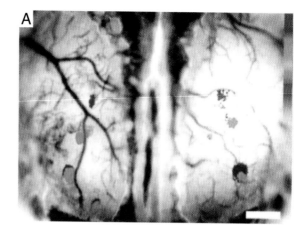

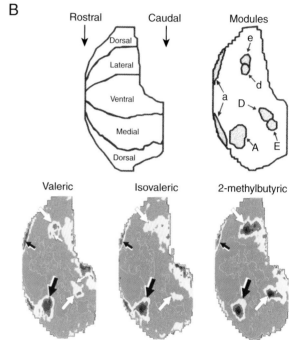

FIGURE 24.18   Odor maps. (A) Visualization of odor-elicited activity in glomeruli of the dorsal olfactory bulb by intrinsic imaging. From Belluscio and Katz (2001). (B) Global maps of odor-elicited activity patterns in the glomerular layer by 2-deoxyglucose. From Johnson and Leon (2000).

of relations between individual glomeruli activated by odors with related molecular structures (Fig. 24.18A). This is key for understanding what one may call the "rules of molecular relatedness," which govern how determinants on related odor molecules are represented by the relatedness between activated glomeruli in the glomerular odor maps. However, these methods image only a small portion of the total (10–15%) in the dorsal region. Global activity mapping methods such as 2DG are complementary in that they image the entire glomerular sheet, including areas in the 85% of the bulb not accessible to optical methods (Fig. 24.18B).

In some cases the elicited activity can be correlated with histologically defined glomeruli; one such example is the modified glomerular complex (MGC) that is active in suckling rat pups (Figs. 24.13; see also below). This set of glomeruli was the first to be characterized by both its anatomical identity and its functional specificity. It appears to belong to a set of so-called "necklace glomeruli" that are arranged around the accessory olfactory bulb and that receive input from a special set of ORNs. Injections of HRP into the MGC show labeling of cells primarily within a strip along the septal epithelium and in smaller strips over the turbinates. Studies in the insect using calcium imaging have given results similar in basic properties to those in the vertebrate, i.e., different overlapping glomerular patterns activated by different odors, and increasing extent of activated glomeruli with increasing odor concentration.

A different methodological approach has been to focus on the time course of the electrophysiological responses of olfactory cells. These studies (Laurent *et al.*, 1996) have suggested that the temporal spiking patterns contain information that itself could encode the identity of the stimulating odor molecule. This approach is still in its early stages and more information is needed, such as where in the odor maps are the responses recorded; how do the temporal patterns relate to the spatial maps; and how long does it take in the temporal response for

the response pattern to transmit decipherable information? This approach has thus stimulated the field with new questions requiring further study.

Individual ORN Axons May Use Local Cues to Find Their Glomerular Targets

How does an ORN expressing a given olfactory receptor type make a connection to the appropriate glomerulus in the olfactory bulb? Anatomical studies give evidence that axons and axon fascicles follow local cues in arriving at specific glomeruli and intraglomerular compartments. An intriguing possibility may be present in the receptors themselves. Computational studies have identified amino acid residues that form a binding pocket where interaction with odor molecule determinants takes place (Chapter 23). These studies have also identified residues in the external loops of the receptors that are correlated with specific residues in the binding pocket. These external residues therefore serve as markers for the binding specificity of the pocket. This would enable any receptors expressed in the axon and axon terminals to take part in cell–cell interactions mediating axonal guidance and target recognition for the establishment of appropriate synapses in the glomeruli.

One possibility is that impulse activity in the axons is necessary during development for the axons to find their target glomeruli. The answer to this specific hypothesis has been controversial, with some favoring and some opposed. Another approach has been to use sophisticated gene targeting methods to swap olfactory receptor genes to test whether the subset expressing the swapped gene would connect to the old or the new glomerulus. The results thus far are that the axons, defying the biologists' simple rules, go somewhere in between. The targets themselves do not seem necessary; transgenic mice lacking mitral and periglomerular cells form normal-appearing glomeruli.

Odor Processing by Olfactory Glomeruli Is Mediated by Excitatory and Inhibitory Microcircuits

The olfactory bulb provides the first stage of synaptic processing of the sensory information in the olfactory pathway. It is thus analogous in position to the retina in the initial processing of visual information (Box 24.4; Fig. 24.19). Within the bulb are two stages of processing: one involving glomeruli and the other involving granule cells.

Within a glomerulus, olfactory axons make glutamatergic excitatory synapses onto the dendrites of the principal neurons (M/T cells), as well as the dendrites of a type of short axon cell, the PG cell, in most species (Fig. 24.20). The M/T dendrites are glutamatergic onto PG cell dendrites, and there are both GABAergic and DAergic synapses from dendrites of PG cell populations onto M/T cell dendrites. These connections are believed to mediate numerous types of interactions; they include serial excitatory synapses (which spread excitation widely within a glomerulus), recurrent and lateral inhibitory synaptic circuits, and disinhibitory synaptic interactions. Feedback excitation is mediated by autoreceptors for glutamate, and feedback amplification is mediated by voltage-gated Na channels in the dendritic membranes.

The excitatory mechanisms presumably amplify the EPSPs in the M/T dendritic tufts and thus enhance the signal-to-noise ratio, which together with the amplification in the transduction mechanisms (Chapter 23) and the high convergence ratios described ealier underlie the high sensitivity of odor detection. These mechanisms are discussed further later. The interactions can be carried out within compartments within a given glomerulus; they may also allow activity to spread throughout a glomerulus. A glomerulus may therefore be a complex anatomical and functional unit containing several levels of organization.

In addition to intraglomerular processing, there is interglomerular processing through the axons of the PG cells, which make type II (presumably GABAergic

---

BOX 24.4

THE OLFACTORY BULB AND RETINA HAVE SIMILAR BASIC PLANS

Although the olfactory bulb and the retina have distinctive types of cells and circuits, they are similar in their overall plan and in many aspects of their microcircuit organization. Each has straight-through pathways for direct transmission of the sensory information (Fig. 24.19). In addition, both regions provide two levels of lateral processing: one at the level of sensory input and the other at the control of output. The significance of these two levels is best understood in the retina, where the lateral interactions can be clearly related to such obvious properties as enhancement of spatial contrast. Similar microcircuits for feedback and lateral inhibition exist at both levels in the olfactory bulb. These microcircuits may be involved in contrast enhancement between molecular stimuli. Research provides strong support for this function (see text).

Gordon M. Shepherd

A

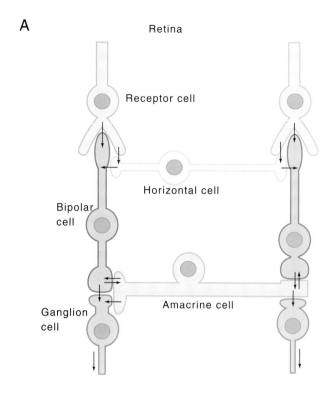

Retina

B

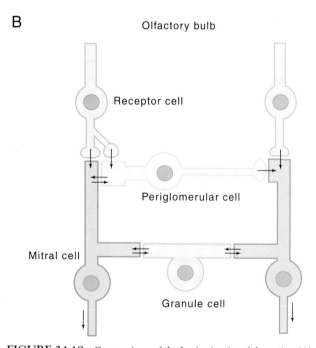

Olfactory bulb

FIGURE 24.19 Comparison of the basic circuits of the retina (A) and the olfactory bulb (B). Although these regions process distinctly different types of sensory information, the overall similarity of their organization and the detailed similarity of some of their local circuits indicate conserved principles in the neural mechanisms for processing both types of information.

inhibitory) synapses on PG cells related to neighboring glomeruli and on the dendritic shafts of M/T cells as they emerge from the glomeruli. One action of these synapses may be to inhibit PG cells and M/T dendrites, thus providing contrast enhancement between neighboring glomeruli. Another possibility is that the action could be excitatory by means of a network of presynaptic PG cell inhibitory actions and by GABAergic synapses acting through a reversed chloride gradient.

Insect Glomeruli Appear to Mediate Complex Processing

As noted earlier, in the insect, olfactory axons commonly terminate on interneuronal neurites so that there are complex sequences of synaptic connections between the olfactory input and the output of the principal neurons. The synaptic connections within the glomeruli of the insect antennal lobe thus may provide for more complex processing of afferent information than in the glomeruli of vertebrates. This scheme would be in accord with the general principle in the invertebrate of delegating more processing to more peripheral structures. An analogy in this respect is the complex retina of submammalian species, characterized by multiple layers of synaptic processing through the neurites of amacrine cells. Similar multiple sequences of processing within the glomeruli of insects would account for the ability of those creatures to accomplish complex odor discrimination despite the relatively few glomeruli in their olfactory centers compared with those of mammals.

In addition to ordinary glomeruli, the antennal lobes of males of certain species of insects contain an enlarged, sexually dimorphic glomerular structure. In the cockroach, this structure is called the *macroglomerulus*, and in the tobacco worm, it is called the *macroglomerular complex* (**MGC**) (reviewed in Hildebrand, 1995). These structures constitute a male-specific olfactory-labeled line dedicated to detection and sensory analysis of the female's species-specific sex pheromone. In tobacco worm, the MGC is the site of primary synaptic processing of afferent inputs of antennal ORNs narrowly tuned to respond to components A and B and at least one other component of the female's sex pheromone.

Granule Cells Mediate Contextual Molecular Contrast Enhancement

The second level of synaptic processing in the olfactory bulb depends mainly on one type of micro-

Intraglomerular　　　　　Interglomerular

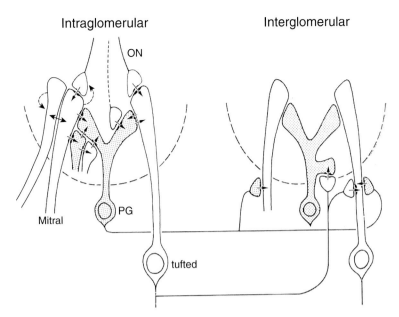

FIGURE 24.20 Diagram summarizing the synaptic organization of the glomerular layer. Note the separation into intraglomerular and interglomerular fields. Synaptic polarities and morphologies (symmetric and asymmetric) are indicated. Open profiles indicate presumed excitatory synaptic action of glutamate on AMPA and NMDA receptors; shaded profiles indicate presumed inhibitory action of GABA on GABA$_A$ receptors.

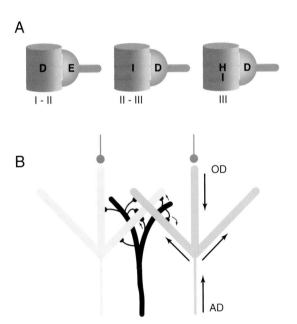

FIGURE 24.21 (A) Model for the action of the dendrodendritic synaptic pathway between mitral (pink profiles) and granule (blue profiles) cells during successive time periods I, II, and III following generation of the impulse at the soma. D, depolarization; H, hyperpolarization; E, excitation; I, inhibition. (B) Diagram of the circuit connections between mitral and granule cell dendrites that mediate self- and lateral inhibition of the mitral cells. OD, orthodromic activation; AD, antidromic activation. Adapted from Rall and Shepherd (1968).

circuit, composed of reciprocal dendrodendritic synapses that mediate M/T-to-granule excitation and granule-to-M/T inhibition (Fig. 24.21). Through this means, activated M/T cells mediate feedback inhibition on themselves and lateral inhibition on their neighbors. These inhibitory interactions control the frequency of impulse output from the M/T cells and thus are the basis of the temporal encoding of odor information that is of increasing interest. Lateral inhibition is activated by retrograde spread of the impulse into the secondary dendrites so it directly reflects the output of the neuron. This was an early example of the type of impulse backpropagation that is of current interest in the functional organization of many types of central neuron (see Chapter 12). The secondary dendrites are relatively long, thus providing for lateral inhibition onto a large population of neighboring cells that belong to neighboring glomerular units. It has been postulated that this inhibition contributes a more complex, more contextual type of contrast enhancement between cells belonging to different glomerular modules. Formations of single and higher order odor-opponent cells may be present at both levels, in analogy with color processing in the retina, to maintain odor constancy, despite different odor concentrations and different odor combinations.

Odor-driven responses

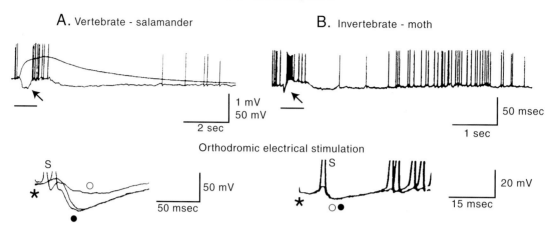

FIGURE 24.22 Electrophysiological recordings of odor responses of a vertebrate mitral cell (A) and an invertebrate principal neuron (B) showing similarities in their response properties. See text for explanation. (A) From Hamilton and Kauer (1989), (B) from Christensen *et al.* (1993).

Odor Stimuli Elicit Excitatory–Inhibitory Responses among Bulbar Cells

The responses of ORNs to odor stimulation vary in their specificity and intensity coding (cf. Fig. 24.15), and the responses of ORN subsets are fed to the glomeruli that are the basis for processing by the olfactory bulb circuits. What can be learned about these processing mechanisms?

The responses in the olfactory bulb are complex, but some patterns are emerging. In the salamander, responses of a M/T cell to an odor pulse may show one of several clearly defined types (Fig. 24.22): no response; excitation at threshold odor concentration, replaced by a brief excitatory burst followed by suppression at higher concentrations; or only suppression at all levels of concentration. The excitatory responses are usually preceded by a brief hyperpolarization. The output cells in the antennal lobe of insects show a similar pattern, including a similar initial hyperpolarization. Mammals show similar categories of response, but with more variations on these simple patterns.

The excitatory responses are presumably due to factors discussed earlier: convergence of excitatory ORN inputs and positive feedback mechanisms through recurrent synaptic excitation, synaptic disinhibition, or GABAergic inputs affecting reversed chloride gradients (Fig. 24.20). The subsequent suppression could reflect synaptic inhibition at the glomerular level (either intra- or extraglomerular actions) or granule cell level. Responses that are

inhibitory at all concentration levels might reflect the actions of interglomerular inputs from more active glomeruli, or granule cells. The initial brief hyperpolarization may be caused by an initial action of granule cells.

The excitatory mechanisms dig the signals out of the noise from competing activity in neighboring glomerular units. The inhibitory mechanisms contribute to mechanisms for feature enhancement. Simultaneous recordings from pairs of mitral cells have shown that cells close together (within 40 μm), and therefore more likely to be connected to the same or a neighboring glomerulus, respond similarly to a given odor, whereas cells farther apart (more than 150 μm) tend to show opposite types of responses. This result, together with other studies, has supported the idea that a main function of the dendrodendritic synapses present at both the glomerular and granule cell levels is to mediate lateral inhibition and that the role of this lateral inhibition is to enhance contrast between different odors. It has been hypothesized that PG cell inhibition between glomerular units may be involved in the discrimination of odors that are closely related in structure.

In addition to M/T cells, PG cells are also driven by olfactory neuron (ON) synaptic inputs. Electrophysiological recordings show that they may give single spike or burst responses to single ON volleys, which may contribute both to excitatory boosting of the glomerular response within their glomerulus of origin and to inhibitory contrast mechanisms between different glomeruli (Fig. 24.20).

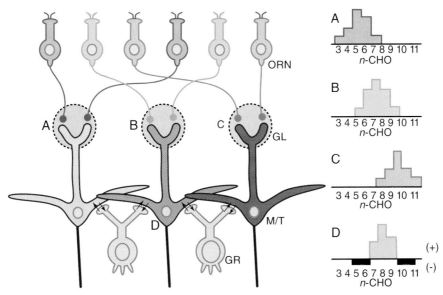

FIGURE 24.23 Summary of physiological evidence for molecular contrast enhancement through lateral inhibitory microcircuits in the olfactory bulb. Diagram of the functional organization underlying contrast enhancement between the responses of mitral cells to neighboring members of a homologous series (n-CHO) of odor molecules. The broad responses mediated from an ORN subset through glomerulus (GL) B are sharpened in the mitral/tufted (M-T) cell D by inhibitory interactions mediated by reciprocal dendro-dendritic synaptic circuits through granule cells (GR). See text for details. From Yokoi *et al* (1995).

Bulbar Circuits Underlie Odor Discrimination

Lateral inhibition mediated by granule cells is extensive because it is mediated mainly through the secondary dendrites, which reach across many glomerular units. The role of this inhibition has been tested in experiments in which multiple electrode penetrations have been made in the olfactory bulbs of rabbits stimulated with different types of odor molecules. Recordings have shown that M/T cells preferentially responsive to specific classes of odor molecules (e.g., acids, alcohols, esters) are located in specific domains of the olfactory bulb, as suggested by 2DG studies. Within a region, M/T cells tend to show narrow specificities for two or three neighboring members of a particular carbon series (Fig. 24.23). These narrow specificities are also seen for corresponding members of parallel carbon series (e.g., for corresponding acids, alcohols, or esters). Contributing to this narrow specificity is inhibition of responses to closely related molecules. This type of surround inhibition mediates contrast enhancement between odor ligands with closely related determinants as described earlier. Pharmacological analysis suggests that this inhibition is mediated by the dendrodendritic circuit between M/T and granule cells. However, more work is needed to identify the contribution made by PG cells.

Membrane Properties Underlying Olfactory Bulb Circuits Are Becoming Known

Because of its layered structure and distinct cell types, the mammalian olfactory bulb has been an attractive subject for analysis of membrane properties for many years. Some of the neurotransmitters and voltage-gated currents present in bulbar cells have been identified in relation to the key functional properties involved in odor processing (Fig. 24.24).

Current research is aimed at several critical questions concerning the contributions of olfactory bulb dendrites to olfactory circuits. First, both patch recordings and computational modeling indicate that action potential initiation shifts within the mitral cell dendrites, from the axon initial segment with weak excitatory inputs to the distal primary dendrite with strong input. This is believed to extend the range of mitral cell responsiveness in the face of increasing inhibition by the granule cells. Second, the extent of action potential invasion of the secondary dendrites is critical for determining the extent of activation of the inhibitory surround from the granule cells. Evidence shows that the invasion involves active propagation that enhances this spread. Finally, GABA release from the spines of the granule cells can be activated by calcium entering through the NMDA receptors on the spines, independently of voltage-gated channels as in

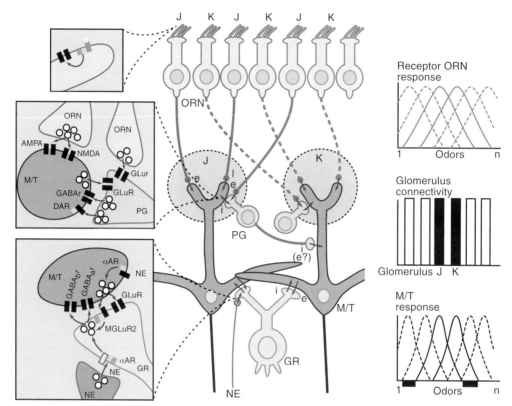

FIGURE 24.24 Summary of several of the key types of synaptic receptors and their involvement in olfactory bulb microcircuits underlying odor processing and odor memory. See text for explanation. From Shepherd and Greer (1998).

the classical model. Current experiments are aimed at determining the conditions in which this may occur naturally.

Many Systems Modulate the Behavioral State of the Olfactory Bulb

Like most sensory pathways, the olfactory pathway is under control by intrinsic modulators and by centrifugal fibers from centers in the brain. In fact, the wealth of peptidergic and centrifugal inputs probably puts it under more modulatory control by more different behavioral states than any other brain system.

A moment's reflection gives a reason: The sense of smell is crucial to the two basic behaviors—feeding and mating—that are at the core of most animal life. In each case the significance of a given smell in eliciting a given behavior depends closely on the behavioral state of the animal. For example, the smell of food is attractive when an animal is hungry but not when full. The neural basis of this has been tested in rats; recordings from mitral cells in rats exposed to food odors showed strong responses when the

rats were hungry but suppression when they were sated.

Within the olfactory bulb, dopamine D2 receptors have been localized to the glomerular and olfactory nerve layer and are possible sites of action by dopamine-containing PG cells. Although the role of dopamine (DA) remains unclear, several studies have indicated that DA has a role in olfactory processing. For example, the dopamine receptor agonist apomorphine blocks a 2DG pattern of glomerular activity induced by odor stimulation; this effect is prevented by pretreatment with the DA receptor antagonist haloperidol. Odor learning increases dopamine levels in the olfactory bulb, whereas odor deprivation increases D2 receptor density present on olfactory nerve terminals. These studies suggest that DA exerts a neuromodulatory action on sensory input.

Two centrifugal systems arise in the brain stem: the noradrenergic (NA) system, originating in the locus coeruleus, and the serotonergic system, arising in the dorsal raphe. NA is probably involved in modulating the olfactory system at both bulbar and olfactory cortical levels at different stages of development. NA reduces granule cell inhibition of mitral cells;

experiments on cultured cells suggest that this is due to the reduction of glutamate release from mitral cells through a presynaptic α-adrenergic inhibition of high threshold calcium currents, and possibly also a presynaptic reduction in GABA release from granule cells. This NA mechanism could mediate some forms of olfactory learning. Another important centrifugal system consists of cholinergic fibers arising from the basal forebrain.

Stem Cells and Olfactory Function

There is much current interest in stem cells and the possibilities they raise for maintaining or repairing brain function. The olfactory system is unique in the brain in being supplied in the adult by two sources of stem cells.

First is the olfactory epithelium, where new ORNs arise from basal stem cells during development and throughout the adult life of the animal. During development, new ORNs expressing specific ORs differentiate from basal cells in the olfactory placode. During early life the process of neurogenesis begins to be activated by dying ORNs, leading to a constant turnover of ORNs. The mechanisms include commitment of a progenitor cell to its particular OR, exclusion of all but the expressed gene allele, assembly of the second messenger components, and, as described earlier, the axon guidance to the target glomerulus. The mechanisms must match the specificity of the OR binding pocket for its odor ligand determinants with the appropriate glomerular site in the odor map that represents the relatedness between the determinants.

The second example is the anterior migratory stream. Stem cells in the ventricular epithelium of the basal forebrain give rise to neural progenitor cells, which migrate anteriorly to the olfactory bulb, where they differentiate and become incorporated into the populations of granule cells and periglomerular cells. This process also occurs throughout adult life. Migration involves homotypic interactions between migrating cells, rather than migration along radial glia as in the cerebral cortex. Fate determination apparently does not occur until the migrating cells enter the olfactory bulb. Current studies are aimed at understanding how the new cells are incorporated into the processing circuits of the bulb.

Almost nothing is known about the mechanisms controlling these processes. Further work is thus needed to understand the relevance of these mechanisms to olfactory processing, as well as gaining insights into the fundamental problems of stem cell functions in the brain.

The Vomeronasal–Accessory Bulb System Mediates Specific Odor Information in Parallel

In addition to the main olfactory pathway, a parallel pathway exists for transmitting signals from less volatile or nonvolatile odorous compounds. This pathway originates in the vomeronasal organ (VNO), also referred to as Jacobson's organ (Fig. 24.13). It is present in a variety of vertebrate species. Phylogenetically, it is first differentiated clearly in snakes, where it is involved in several functions, including mating behavior and responses to prey odors that are sampled from the tongue as it is drawn over the inlet to the organ. In rodents, the organ is well developed and is believed to be stimulated by sexually active substances that access the inlet to the organ as a male directly investigates the female's vaginal opening. In ungulates such as deer and horses, the inlet is exposed by a nasal movement called a flehmen reaction in which the male investigates the urine of the female to determine her mating receptivity.

The VNO projects to a structure called the accessory olfactory bulb (AOB). In rodents, this bulb is located at the posterior dorsal surface of the main olfactory bulb (MOB). It contains the same types of cells and the same laminae as the main olfactory bulb, although they are differentiated less clearly. The AOB and MOB are anatomically distinct, and this separation continues also in their central pathways. Memory mechanisms involving the dendrodendritic interactions in the accessory olfactory bulb are discussed in Chapter 12.

Signal transduction in VNO receptor cells is described in Chapter 23. Two classes of putative receptors are associated with different G proteins which define separate anatomical subsystems. By *in situ* hybridization and immunocytochemical staining, $G_i\alpha2$ was found to be present in receptor neurons whose cell bodies are located in the middle layer of the VNO and project to the anterior part of the AOB. In contrast, $G_o\alpha$ is expressed in receptor neurons whose cell bodies are located in the basal layer of the VNO and whose axons project to the posterior part of the AOB.

It is widely believed that VNO receptors function only as pheromone receptors, and pheromone receptors are restricted to the VNO, but neither of these assumptions is justified by the evidence. The best-documented pheromone in mammals, androstenedione in pigs, mediates its effects through the main olfactory pathway rather than through the VNO. Meredith (2001) has provided a thorough and balanced review of this problem.

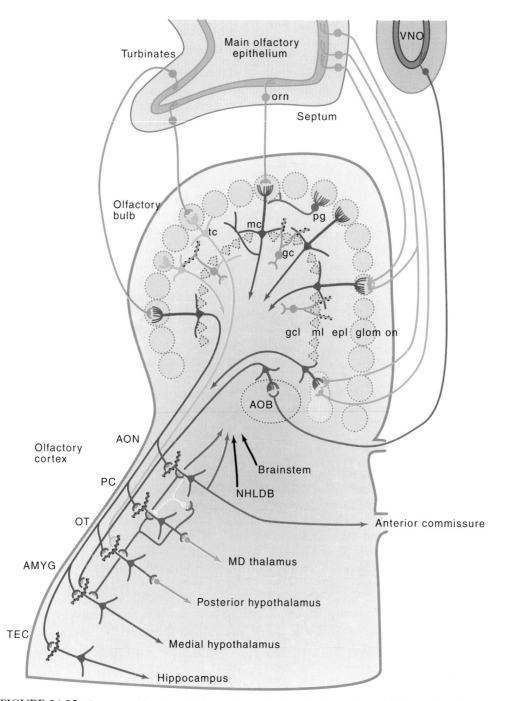

FIGURE 24.25 Summary of main projection pathways in the olfactory system. AON, anterior olfactory nucleus; PC, pyriform cortex; OT, olfactory tubercle; AMYG, amygdala; TEC, transitional entorhinal cortex; NHLDB, nucleus of horizontal limb of diagonal band; MD, mediodorsal.

Olfactory Bulb Output Goes Directly to Olfactory Cortex

The output of the olfactory bulb is carried by the axons of mitral cells and their smaller counterparts, the tufted cells (Fig. 24.25). These axons project directly to olfactory cortex in the forebrain, the only sensory system to have this immediate access to the forebrain (all other sensory systems project first to the spinal cord, brain stem, or diencephalon, as noted in other chapters). The olfactory cortex has a three-layer structure that represents the primitive anlage of forebrain cortex found in fish, amphibia, and reptiles (Fig. 24.25). The principal neuron is the pyramidal cell, with apical and basal dendrites bearing spines and recurrent collaterals connecting both to inhibitory interneurons and directly to other pyramidal cells. M/T axons make excitatory connections to spines on the distal apical dendrites. Processing in the cortex takes place by means of the intrinsic excitatory and inhibitory synaptic circuits. Together these neural elements and their connections constitute a basic, canonical circuit. This type of circuit is present in other types of cortex, such as the hippocampus and neocortex, suggesting that it represents the simplest type of cortical circuit, which is adapted and elaborated in the other types to carry out different or more complex types of functional operations.

Like cortical regions in other systems, the olfactory cortex is differentiated into several different areas. The main area is the pyriform (sometimes called the prepyriform) cortex. This area receives input from both M and T cells. It projects to the mediodorsal thalamus, which in turn projects to medial and lateral orbitofrontal areas of the neocortex. It is at this level that conscious perception of odors presumably takes place. Second is the olfactory tubercle, which receives input mainly from T cells. In the primate, this is called the anterior perforated substance because of the numerous blood vessels that penetrate its surface at the base of the brain. Its structure is modified by the accumulations of small cells, called islets of Calleja,

which contain high densities of dopaminergic nerve terminals. Third is the cortico-medial group of amygdalar nuclei, which receive specific input from the accessory olfactory bulb. Fourth is the lateral entorhinal area, which projects to the hippocampus. Last is the anterior olfactory nucleus, a sheet of cells just posterior to the olfactory bulb in subprimates.

In insects, output neurons from the antennal lobe project to higher centers, chief of which is the mushroom body. Here higher processing of the olfactory stimuli and integration with other sensory modalities take place, which control the animal's behavior.

Summary

The olfactory system must detect and discriminate between expected and unexpected odors. The neural mechanisms underlying olfactory discrimination involve synaptic circuits that extract and compare the signals processed in glomeruli (Box 24.5). Information within the glomeruli is processed through a series of excitatory and inhibitory signals mediated by different neurotransmitters and second messengers. The excitatory circuits amplify the signal; inhibitory circuits serve to discriminate between the stimuli. Animals are very good at recognizing the complex

---

BOX 24.5

PRINCIPLES OF ODOR MAPS

Odor stimulation gives rise to spatial patterns of activity in the glomerular layer of the olfactory bulb due to the differential activation of glomeruli.

The glomerulus is the basic molecular, anatomical, developmental, and functional unit for odor mapping and odor processing.

The pattern of activated glomeruli for a given odor is relatively constant across animals for equivalent odor stimulation conditions. However, the pattern can change under different experimental conditions (e.g., anesthesia, adaptation).

The pattern for a given odor characteristically includes sites in the medial and lateral bulb, reflecting the pattern of projections of olfactory sensory neuron subsets. The patterns are characteristically bilaterally symmetrical, dependent on equivalent stimulating conditions on the two sides of the nose.

Identified glomeruli can be correlated with specific odors. This is true of the modified glomerular complex in mammals, and particularly true of identifiable glomeruli in the insect.

Different odors elicit activity in different, often overlapping, patterns. It is hypothesized that processing of the differing patterns by olfactory bulb circuits provides the basis for olfactory discrimination.

A given homologous chemical series (such as alcohols, acids, aldehydes) activates overlapping shifted patterns, reflecting similarities of chemical structure in the series.

At a weak concentration, an odor elicits activity in the single or small group of glomeruli receiving input from the olfactory receptor neuron subset whose receptor type is most sensitive to that odor. Higher odor concentrations activate increasing numbers of glomeruli. Changes in odor pattern with increasing concentration may be correlated with perceptual changes. It is therefore hypothesized that the odor patterns are also involved in the encoding of odor concentration. For references, see Xu *et al.* (2000).

Gordon M. Shepherd

odors that identify individuals of the species. This is usually signaled by a blend of two or more compounds representing an odor object of behavioral significance to the organism. Many cells may be able to respond to one molecular type but only a few may respond maximally to the blend. Anatomically, the olfactory system is organized topographically. Actual perception of odors is believed to occur in the frontal cortex of mammals and in higher brain centers called mushroom bodies in insects. In addition to the main olfactory pathway in vertebrates, a parallel accessory pathway exists for transmitting signals from less volatile odorous compounds. This is important in reptiles and mammals for detecting odors that stimulate behavioral responses.

References

Adler, E., Hoon, M. A., Mueller, K. L., Chandrashekar, J., Ryba, N. J. P., and Zuker, C. S. (2000). A novel family of mammalian taste receptors. *Cell* **100**, 693–702.

Adrian, E. D. (1950). The electrical activity of the mammalian olfactory bulb. *Electroencephalogr. Clin. Neurophysiol.* **2**, 377–388.

Belluscio, L., and Katz, L. C. (2001). Symmetry, stereotypy, and topography of odorant representations in mouse olfactory bulbs. *J. Neurosci.* **21**, 2113–2122.

Boeckh, J., Kaissling, K. E., and Schneider, D. (1965). Insect olfactory receptors. *Cold Spring Harb. Symp. Quant. Biol.* **30**, 263–280.

Bradley, R. M., King, M. S., Wang, L., and Shu, X. (1996). Neurotransmitter and neuromodulator activity in the gustatory zone of the nucleus tractus solitarius. *Chem. Senses* **21**, 377–385.

Chaudhari, N., Landin, A. M., and Roper, S. D. (2000). A metabotropic glutamate receptor variant functions as a taste receptor. *Nature Neurosci.* **3**, 113–119.

Christensen, T. A., Waldrop, B. R., Harrow, I. D., and Hildebrand, J. G. (1993). Local interneurons and information processing in the olfactory glomeruli of the moth. *Manduca sexta. J. Comp. Physiol. A* **173**, 385–399.

Duchamp-Viret, P., Chaput, M. A, and Duchamp, A. (1999). Odor response properties of rat olfactory receptor neurons. *Science* **284**, 2171–2174.

Erickson, R. P. (1968). Stimulus coding in topographic and nontopographic afferent modalities: On the significance of the activity of individual sensory neurons. *Psychol. Rev.* **75**, 447–465.

Gesteland, R. C., Lettvin, J. Y., and Pitts, W. H. (1965). Chemical transmission in the nose of the frog. *J. Physiol. (Lond.)* **181**, 525–559.

Grill, H. J., and Norgren, R. (1978). The taste reactivity test. I. Mimetic responses to gustatory stimuli in neurologically normal rats. *Brain Res.* **143**, 263–280.

Hamilton, K., and Kauer, J. S. (1989). Patterns of intracellular potentials in salamander mitral tufted cells in response to odor stimulation. *J. Neurophysiol.* **62**, 609–625.

Hildebrand, J. G., and Shepherd, G. M. (1997). Molecular mechanisms of olfactory discrimination: Converging evidence for common principles across phyla. *Annu. Rev. Neurosci.* **20**, 595–631.

Johnson, B. A., and Leon, M. (2000). Modular representations of odorants in the glomerular layer of the rat olfactory bulb and the effects of stimulus concentration. *J. Comp. Neurol.* **422**, 496–509.

Laurent, G., Wehr, M., and Davidowitz, H. (1996). Temporal representations of odors in an olfactory network. *J. Neurosci.* **16**, 3837–3847.

McClintock, T. S., and Ache, B. W. (1989). Hyperpolarizing receptor potentials in lobster olfactory receptor cells: Implications for transduction and mixture suppression. *Chem. Senses* **14**, 637–647.

Meredith, M. (2001). Human vomeronasal organ function: A critical review of best and worst cases. *Chem. Senses* **26**, 433–445.

Mombaerts, P., Wang, F., Dulac, C., Chao, S. K., Nemes, A., Mendelsohn, M., Edmondson, J., and Axel, R. (1996). Visualizing an olfactory sensory map. *Cell* **87**, 675–686.

Mori, K., and Yoshihara, Y. (1995). Molecular recognition and olfactory processing in the mammalian olfactory system. *Prog. Neurobiol.* **45**, 585–619.

Oakley, B. (1967). Altered taste responses from cross-regenerated taste nerves in the rat. *In* "Olfaction and Taste II" (T. Hayashi, ed.), pp. 535–547. Pergamon, London.

Pfaffmann, C. (1955). Gustatory nerve impulses in rat, cat and rabbit. *J. Neurophysiol.* **18**, 429–440.

Pfaffmann, C. (1974). Specificity of the sweet receptors of the squirrel monkey. *Chem. Sens. Flav.* **1**, 61–67.

Rall, W., and Shepherd, G. M. (1968). Theoretical reconstruction of field potentials and dendrodendritic synaptic interactions in olfactory bulb. *J. Neurophysiol.* **31**, 884–915.

Shepherd, G. M., and Greer, C. A. (1998). Olfactory bulb. *In* "The Synaptic Organization of the Brain" (G. M. Shepherd, ed.), 4th Ed., pp. 159–203. Oxford Univ. Press, New York.

Smith, D. V., Van Buskirk, R. L., Travers, J. B., and Bieber, S. L. (1983a). Gustatory neuron types in the hamster brainstem. *J. Neurophysiol.* **50**, 522–540.

Smith, D. V., and Frank, M. E. (1993). Sensory coding by peripheral taste fibers. *In* "Mechanisms of Taste Transduction" (S. A. Simon and S. D. Roper, eds.), pp. 295–338. CRC Press, Boca Raton, FL.

Smith, D. V., Van Buskirk, R. L., Travers, J. B., and Bieber, S. L. (1983b). Coding of taste stimuli by hamster brainstem neurons. *J. Neurophysiol.* **50**, 541–558.

Spector, A. C., Guagliardo, N. A., and St. John, S.J. (1996). Amiloride disrupts NaCl versus KCl discrimination performance: Implications for salt taste coding in rats. *J. Neurosci.* **16**, 8115–8122.

St. John, S. J., and Smith, D. V. (2000). Neural representation of salts in the rat solitary nucleus: brainstem correlates of taste discrimination. *J. Neurophysiol.* **84**, 628–638.

Xu, F. Q., Greer, C. A., and Shepherd, G.M. (2000). Odor maps in the olfactory bulb. *J. Comp. Neurol.* **422**, 489–495.

Yokoi, M., Mori, K., and Nakanishi, S. (1995). Refinement of odor molecule tuning by dendrodendritic synaptic inhibition in the olfactory bulb. *Proc. Natl. Acad. Sci. U.S.A.* **92**, 3371–3375.

Suggested Readings

Axel, R. (1995). The molecular logic of smell. *Sci. Am.* 154–159.

Gilbertson, T. A., Damak, S., and Margolskee, R. F. (2000). The molecular physiology of taste transduction. *Curr. Opin. Neurobiol.* **10**, 519–527.

Hildebrand, J. G. (1995). Analysis of chemical signals by nervous systems. *Proc. Natl. Acad. Sci. USA* **92**, 67–74.

Shepherd, G. M. (1994). Discrimination of molecular signals by the olfactory receptor neuron. *Neuron* **13**, 771–790.

Smith, D. V., and Margolskee, R. F. (2000). Making sense of taste. *Sci. Am.* **284**, 32–39.

Smith, D. V., St. John, S. J. (1999). Neural coding of gustatory information. *Curr. Opin. Neurobiol.* **9**, 427–435.

David V. Smith and Gordon M. Shepherd

The Somatosensory System

Sensory systems provide a continuous representation of the external world in a way that makes sense for the organism. This task is difficult because the capacity of an individual neuron to carry information is small, whereas the amount of information the system carries is huge. The somatosensory system solves this problem by breaking down each sensory event into well-defined modalities that are carried forward along paths reserved for each modality. In this way, the organization of the somatosensory system resembles that of the auditory and visual systems. The somatosensory system differs qualitatively from other sensory systems in its multiple roles, as it provides the central nervous system (CNS) with a continuous representation of the external and the internal state of the body, thereby serving both sensory and motor functions. The many roles played by the somatosensory system can be divided into three essential functions.

Exteroceptive functions include the sensations of touch, temperature and pain and tell an animal about environmental stimuli. These are further divided into three modalities: (1) mechanoreception, through which all nonpainful mechanical stimuli are sensed; (2) thermoreception, composed of heat and cold; and (3) nociception, the sensation of both burning pain and sharp pain.

Proprioceptive functions include the kinesthetic senses of position and movement. They rely on input from muscles, tendons and joints to provide information about relative location of the body and limbs and the direction, force, and speed of their movement.

Interoceptive functions arise from sensory receptors in the internal viscera and provide information about the health and well-being of the viscera. Included in these functions is some information that reaches consciousness and some that does not.

Each of the broad somatosensory modalities is furthered divided into submodalities. For example, mechanoreception includes fine touch, skin stretch, flutter, and vibration. At its most fundamental, a submodality is the sensation produced when a single primary sensory axon is active. This definition demonstrates the principles of receptor specificity and modality segregation by which stimulation of a single receptor produces activity along a select path of neurons in the CNS. This information permits the organism to accurately determine both the kind and the location of a stimulus.

This chapter reviews the way in which each of the somatosensory modalities is sensed by the peripheral nervous system, carried into the CNS, and processed to produce a conscious perception. Beginning with a discussion of peripheral mechanisms of somesthesis and moving progressively through the CNS toward a merger of sensory systems with the motor system, the function of the somatosensory system can be appreciated from the physiology of individual neurons and their anatomical relationships with one another. In this discussion, three themes are repeated: (1) *modality segregation*, meaning the grouping together of neurons and axons that carry one type of information and their separation from neurons and axons that carry other types; (2) *somatotopy*, or the orderly mapping of the body surface throughout the CNS; and (3) *neural coding*, which deals with the relationship between the activity of the neuron and the behavior of the animal. Studies of neural coding compare quantitative measures of neuronal response (electrophysiology) with behavior (psychophysics) to determine which groups of cells might be responsible for an observed behavior and how neural activity mediates that behavior. Because they are complex and involve large numbers of neurons, the codes underlying only some aspects of tactile perception have been discovered. These are discussed at greatest length.

PERIPHERAL MECHANISMS OF SOMATIC SENSATION

Psychophysics of Mechanoreception

Form Perception

One example of tactile form discrimination is the ability of a subject to detect when two points along the skin are stimulated. This test involves the application of two blunt points to the skin at a known separation during which a subject is asked whether the sensation is that of one point or two. When the separation between the two points is small, a single point is perceived, but as the separation increases, the sensation changes to that of two points. The minimal separation between two points that permits both to be perceived, referred to as the *two-point limen*, is a simple measure of spatial acuity. This acuity varies across the skin surface (Fig. 25.1). Locations of highest acuity, such as at the fingertips and around the mouth (two-point limens of 0.9 and 0.5 mm), are at least two

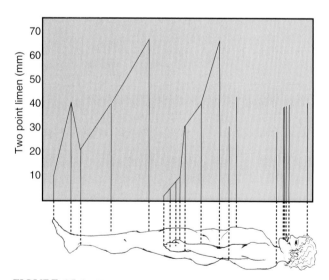

FIGURE 25.1 Variation in two-point limen (threshold) across the body surface. The graph plots the distance necessary for a human subject to detect two blunt probes as separate stimuli. That distance is lowest for the fingertips and mouth (approximately 10 mm) and highest for the legs, shoulders, and back (as much as 70 mm). From Patton, H. D., Sundsten, J. W., Crill, W. E., and Swanson, P. D. (eds.) (1976). "Introduction to Basic Neurology," p. 160. Saunders, Philadelphia.

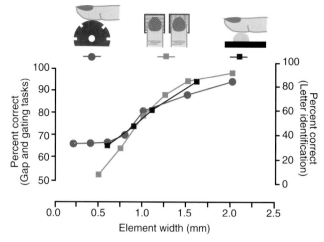

FIGURE 25.2 Results of psychophysical experiment illustrating that the threshold for tactile acuity on the finger pad is about 1 mm. In the experiments, subjects were required to correctly identify the presence of gaps that varied in width, the orientation of gratings that varied in spacing, or the letter embossed onto an otherwise smooth surface. An increase in stimulus dimension (width of the gap, spacing between gratings, or height of the letter) produced an increase in psychophysical performance in all three tasks.

orders of magnitude more sensitive than the region of lowest acuity, the back (60–70 mm). Other means of measuring spatial acuity, such as the detection of embossed letters that vary in height or of bars that vary in spacing and orientation, demonstrate that tactile spatial acuity depends on the innervation density of the skin (Fig. 25.2). The greater the density, the higher the acuity. Further, the ability of human subjects to read Braille characters at rates of 100 characters/minute demonstrates that the somatosensory system is capable not only of high spatial resolution, but also of high temporal resolution.

Texture Perception

Whereas form is easy to describe and to define in quantitative terms, texture is neither easily definable nor quantitatively accessible. Surfaces of different texture can be subjectively divided into groups that include slippery, rough, leathery, and wet, but little is known of the number and character of elemental features in texture perception.

Vibration Perception

The tactile system easily discriminates mechanical vibrations transmitted through objects grasped by the hand. From these vibrations arise the human ability to use and manipulate objects and to make sense of what is occurring at the working ends of tools. As an example, a driver can easily tell how smooth a road surface is by the vibrations transmitted through the steering wheel to the hands. Perceptually divided into two separate sensations—flutter, at frequencies of less than 40 Hz, and vibration at higher frequencies—the dual sense of flutter/vibration spans the range of frequencies from 5 to 400 Hz, with a definite maximal sensitivity around 200 Hz. Detection threshold, or the amount of skin indentation that produces a detectable stimulus, is a U-shaped curve with 50-μm indentations required at 10 Hz, only 1 μm at 200 Hz, and more than 65 μm at 400 Hz. Once the detection threshold is exceeded, any further increase in stimulus amplitude produces a perception that the strength of the stimulus has increased.

Structure and Function of Peripheral Receptors

Mechanoreceptors

The body surface is covered by hairy skin and hairless or glabrous skin, in which are embedded four types of mechanoreceptors responsible for the detection of light mechanical stimuli. At the heart of each mechanoreceptor's function is the ability to transduce a particular mechanical stimulus into a change in membrane potential. What differs among the various receptor types and what makes them uniquely sensitive to particular stimuli are the location in the skin and the form of the capsule that surrounds the axon terminal (Table 25.1).

Transduction of mechanical stimuli into neuronal activity begins with four well-characterized peripheral receptors in glabrous skin, two of which

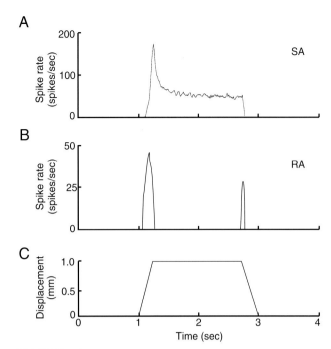

FIGURE 25.3 Response of slowly adapting (SA) and rapidly adapting (RA) peripheral afferents to a sustained indentation of the skin surface. SA afferents (A) respond with an early peak in activity and a lowered but sustained discharge that persists as long as the indentation continues (C). In contrast, RA afferents (B) respond to the onset and termination of the stimulus and not to the continued indentation.

occupy superficial regions of the skin and two others deeper tissue. In each position, one type of receptor fires only briefly with onset and offset of the stimulus and is therefore referred to as rapidly adapting (RA).

TABLE 25.1 Summary of Primary Afferent Fibers and Their Roles

Modality	Submodality	Receptor	Fiber type	Conduction velocity (m s⁻¹)	Role in perception
Mechanoreception	SAI	Merkel cell	Aβ	42–72	Pressure, form, texture
	RA	Meissner corpuscle	Aβ	42–72	Flutter, motion
	SAII	Ruffini corpuscle	Aβ	42–72	Unknown, possibly skin stretch
	PC	Pacinian corpuscle	Aβ	42–72	Vibration
Thermoreception	Warm	Bare nerve endings	C	0.5–1.2	Warmth
	Cold	Bare nerve endings	Aδ	12–36	Cold
Nociception	Small, myelinated	Bare nerve endings	Aδ	12–36	Sharp pain
	Unmyelinated	Bare nerve endings	C	0.5–1.2	Burning pain
Proprioception	Joint afferents	Ruffini-like and paciniform-like endings, bare nerve endings	Aβ	42–72	Protective function against hyperextension
	Golgi tendon organs	Golgi endings	Aα	72–120	Muscle tension
	Muscle spindles	Type I	Aα	72–120	Muscle length and velocity
		Type II	Aβ	42–72	Muscle length
	SAII	Ruffini endings	Aβ	42–72	Joint angle?

In contrast, two other types of receptors (one deep and one superficial) maintain their activity so long as a stimulus persists and therefore is referred to as slowly adapting (SA) (Fig. 25.3). As outlined later, these two subdivisions, deep vs cutaneous and rapidly adapting vs slowly adapting, are fundamental to the roles these receptors play in the discrimination and localization of mechanical stimuli.

Cutaneous receptors   For superficial or cutaneous receptors, responding to low-energy mechanical stimuli delivered to the skin, RA responses are characteristic of *Meissner corpuscles* and slowly adapting type I (SAI) responses are typical of *Merkel disks* (Fig. 25.4).

RA axons terminating in Meissner corpuscles are responsible for the perception of movement along the skin, most noticeably as somatosensory feedback when objects are grasped. Comparisons of human psychophysics and physiology of single peripheral fibers demonstrate that RA afferents are responsible for the ability of humans to detect low-frequency vibration, a sensation referred to as flutter.

Sensory information from Meissner corpuscles and RA afferents leads to adjustment of grip force when

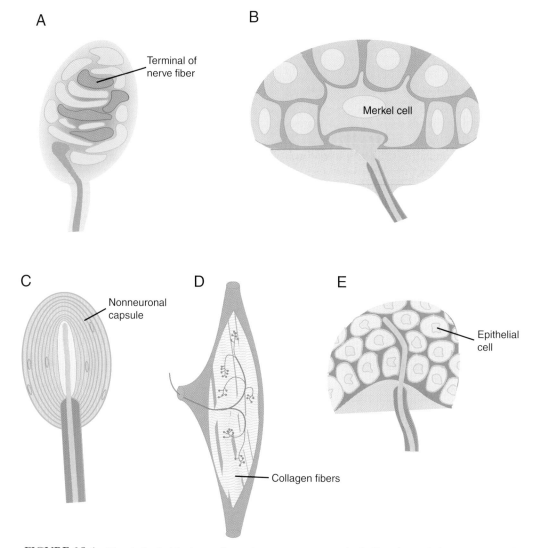

FIGURE 25.4 Morphological features of somatosensory receptors, including the variation in nonneural components. (A) Meissner corpuscles are composed of axonal loops, separated by nonneuronal, supporting cells. (B) Merkel disks are characterized by the close association between afferent axons and Merkel cells. Because of their shape and role in fine cutaneous discrimination, they are often referred to as "touch domes." (C) Pacinian corpuscles include a central sensory axon, surrounded by a fluid-filled capsule that filters out all sustained stimuli. (D) Ruffini endings are driven by skin stretch because of the termination of primary afferents among collagen fibrils of the skin. (E) Free nerve endings, characteristic of nociceptors, are left unprotected from chemicals that are secreted or applied to the skin.

objects are lifted. These afferents respond with a brief burst of action potentials when objects move a small distance during the early stages of lifting. In response to RA afferent activity, muscle force increases reflexively until the gripped object no longer moves. Such a rapid response to a tactile stimulus is a clear indication of the role played by somatosensory neurons in motor activity.

The second type of cutaneous receptor, Merkel disks, and the SAI axons terminating in them are responsible for form and texture perception. As would be expected for receptors mediating form perception, Merkel disks are present at high density in the digits and around the mouth ($50/mm^2$ of skin surface), at lower density in other glabrous surfaces, and at very low density in hairy skin. This innervation density shrinks progressively with the passage of time so that by the age of 50, the density in human digits is reduced to $10/mm^2$.

SAI axons contacted by Merkel cells display slowly adapting, low threshold responses to cutaneous stimuli. Unlike RA axons, SAI fibers respond not only to the initial indentation of skin, but also to a sustained indentation up to several seconds in duration. Receptive fields of single SAI axons include multiple points of maximal sensitivity ("hot spots") that are particularly sensitive to the edges of objects pressed into the skin.

Deep mechanoreceptors Two separate classes of peripheral receptors in deep tissue produce rapidly and slowly adapting responses to somatosensory stimuli. The Pacinian corpuscles are rapidly adapting receptors and Ruffini endings are slowly adapting.

1. **Pacinian corpuscles** Pacinian afferents operate at the extremes of sensory function by being exquisitely sensitive to minute vibrations on the skin, with a threshold of 10 nm at 200 Hz. At the same time these afferents have very large receptive fields that usually cover several digits and, in some cases, an entire hand. They are the receptors responsible for the sensation of high frequency vibration.

2. **Ruffini corpuscles.** Sensory axons at the core of Ruffini corpuscles (referred to as SAII axons) display slowly adapting responses to the lateral movement or stretching of skin, usually in one direction only. Their receptive fields are large and diffuse, producing responses to movements of limbs and digits. Because direct stimulation of SAII axons produces no conscious sensation in humans, their role in somatosensory perception is unknown.

Much of the selectivity of each of these receptors for a particular submodality is a product of its structure (Figs. 25.4 and 25.5). Meissner corpuscles are

Meissner corpuscles (RA)

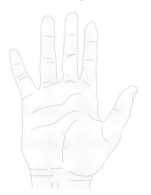

Merkel receptors (SAI)

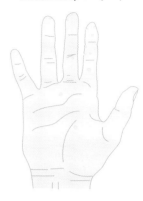

Pacinian corpuscles (PC)

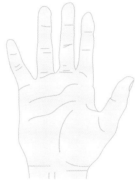

Ruffini corpuscles (SAII)

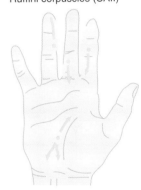

FIGURE 25.5 Map of receptive fields on the human hand displayed by the various receptor types. Receptive fields vary in overall size from punctate zones displayed by RA and SAI afferent to broad regions of the palm or entire fingers with Pacinians. SAII afferents respond to stimuli that produce skin stretch and are often selective for the direction of stretch.

encapsulated nerve endings tethered to specialized skin cells by collagen fibers, thereby making RA axons very sensitive to skin stretch. Moreover, the ability to localize small movements over large areas of skin surface results from the innervation of many widely displaced (3–4 mm) Meissner corpuscles by a single RA axon. Merkel disks have a structure much simpler than that of Meissner corpuscles, as a single SAI axon terminal ends in close apposition to a single Merkel cell. Such a one-to-one correspondence allows for maximum spatial resolution (Box 25.1).

With respect to deep receptors, Pacinian afferents derive their RA properties from the structure of the corpuscle that surrounds the axon terminal. Surrounded by capsules of supporting cells and fluid-filled spaces that filter out the contribution of sustained stresses, the central Pacinian axon terminal is left to respond only to high-frequency indentation of the skin surface. In contrast, each Ruffini corpuscle is innervated by a core axon that breaks up into thin fibers, arranged so that

BOX 25.1

NEURAL CODING

The contribution of each receptor type to perception of spatial form and texture can be compared in an experiment in which Braille characters are used as a stimulus. Spatial details of the characters are well preserved in the response of Merkel cell/SAI afferents, are less well preserved for Meissner corpuscle/RA afferents, and are absent entirely in the response of Pacinian afferents or Ruffini/SAII afferents. These findings indicate that SAI afferents are the source of the information by which Braille characters are perceived. Pacinian and SAII afferents are useless for this task, not only because they fail to resolve the details of a tactile stimulus, but also because their innervation density is far too low to support a coherent image. Responses typical for each member of the four receptor classes (Fig. 25.6) indicate that SAI afferents provide information about the fine spatial structure of a stimulus pressed into the skin. Moreover, SAI afferents appear to convey information about texture, specifically about the roughness and possibly the hardness of an object. In fact, the code for roughness exists in the difference in firing rates between adjacent SAI afferents: similar firing rates in a group of neighboring afferents would signal a smooth stimulus (e.g., glass), whereas marked spatial variation in firing would be interpreted as a rough stimulus (e.g., sandpaper). The coarser the grain of the sandpaper, the greater the difference in firing rates among adjacent SAI receptors.

Stewart H. Hendry and Steven S. Hsiao

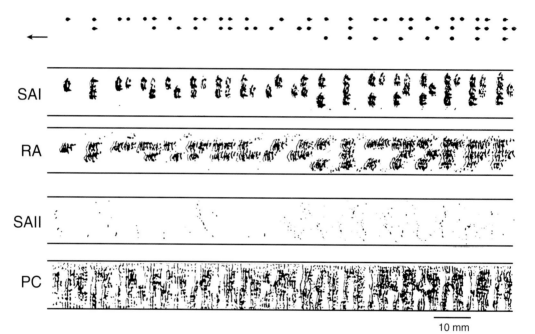

10 mm

FIGURE 25.6 Response of peripheral axons to a Braille pattern of dots scanned over the surface of a human fingertip at a rate of 60 mm/s. with 200-μm shifts in position after each pass. Dots represent individual action potentials. Only the response of the SAI afferents (Merkel disk receptors) follows the Braille pattern faithfully, whereas RA afferents and Pacinians (PC) produce a response that distorts the input. SAIIs display little response to this stimulus. Adapted from Phillips *et al.* (1990).

physical stretching of the corpuscle leads to deformation of the axon itself. Much the same structural arrangement is used for a similar purpose by a type of proprioceptor, the Golgi tendon organ.

Innervation of hairs Hairs are innervated by mechanoreceptors that also occur in dermis and epidermis, such as Merkel disks and Meissner corpuscles. Two additional types of mechanoreceptors,

Lanceolate endings and pilo-Ruffini receptors, innervate only hairs.

Lanceolate endings are made up of long axon terminals running parallel to the hair shaft and surrounded by a thin layer of supporting cells. These rapidly adapting receptors are sensitive to minute movements of hairs and encode the velocity of a stimulus by increasing action potential frequency as stimulus velocity increases.

Pilo-Ruffini receptors closely resemble true Ruffini corpuscles, but possess no capsule. As seen for true Ruffini corpuscles, pilo-Ruffini receptors depolarize when they are deformed.

Nociceptors

As for somatosensory modalities, the perception of pain is mediated by specialized receptors that activate neurons in specific regions of the CNS devoted to processing pain. Yet there is an affective component to pain that leads to different perceptions and interpretations, depending on the subject's mood, attentiveness, personality, and past experience. The role played by pain's affective component is clear from the observation that pain during childbirth is objectively more intense than that associated with solid malignant tumors but subjectively far less unpleasant. Furthermore, the unpleasantness of pain can be reduced with training, even though

the intensity remains at an undiminished level. These considerations have led to the idea that each painful experience can be mapped along two axes; one that includes purely discriminative properties, such as location and intensity, and the other that includes behavioral expectations and reactions.

Many psychophysical studies of pain have shown that thresholds vary among individuals and among body sites on an individual. So whereas a single grain of sand under the eyelid is very painful, many grains of sand under the feet evoke no pain sensations. For this reason the use of mechanical stimuli is avoided in psychophysical studies and thermal stimuli, which are much less variable, are commonly used. These studies have found that the normal threshold for thermal pain is 45°C, the temperature at which heat produces tissue damage.

Specific nociceptors exist in cutaneous and deep tissues and in the viscera. They differ fundamentally from mechanoreceptors, which show no change in their firing rate or in their spike rhythm when a stimulus goes from innocuous to noxious. Nociceptors can be divided into two functionally distinct groups: those responsive to intense mechanical stimuli only and those responsive to a variety of noxious stimuli. These differ little between glabrous and hairy skin and are similar across mammalian species.

BOX 25.2

CLASSIFICATION OF PERIPHERAL NERVE AXONS

The peripheral processes of dorsal root ganglion cells run in peripheral nerves as they extend to the skin surface or other peripheral target. These axons vary in diameter in a manner that is consistent with the morphology and function of their terminal receptors by a commonly used letter code.

Aα fibers are the largest (15–20 mm) and most heavily myelinated ones that conduct action potentials most rapidly (approximately 100 m/s); they are exclusively the axons of muscle spindles and Golgi tendon organs.

Aβ fibers are medium-sized (5–15 μm) and well-myelinated axons of Pacinian and Meissner corpuscles and of Merkel disks, with conduction velocities near 50 m/s.

Aδ fibers are thin (1–5 μm), poorly myelinated axons of mechanical nociceptors, thermal receptors, and mechanoreceptors with large receptive fields; axon potential conduction velocities range from less than 10 to slightly more than 30 m/s).

C fibers are very thin (less than 1 mm in diameter), poorly conducting axons (as slow as 0.4 m/s) that terminate without capsules or other types of end organs in skin. They include thermonociceptors, some thermal receptors, and C mechanoreceptors. C fibers dominate the contents of a cutaneous nerve, as they make up 80% of axons terminating in skin. As a class, they most frequently terminate at the junction of the dermis and the epidermis.

Intermixing of axons from different peripheral nerves near the spinal cord produces spinal nerves. Segregation of motor axons produces ventral roots, whose cell bodies are found in the ventral horn of the spinal cord. Sensory axons enter the capsule of the dorsal root gangli and mix with the central processes given off by the dorsal root ganglion cell. Central processes then enter the spinal cord as dorsal roots.

Stewart H. Hendry and Steven S. Hsiao

Mechanical nociceptors Axons responding to a mechanical stimulus only if it is very intense (i.e., high-threshold mechanoreceptors) have a broad range of conduction velocities, from less than 10 m/s to more than 50 m/s. Most are in the Aδ range (15–30 m/s) (see Box 25.2 for notation) and possess receptive fields consisting of 5–20 small spots (approximately 2–3 mm in diameter), widely distributed in tissue that is otherwise unresponsive to noxious stimuli. In many cases, only those stimuli sufficient to produce tissue damage lead to well-defined responses.

Mechanical nociceptors are notable for their very high threshold to thermal stimulation when it is first applied. When heat is applied repeatedly, however, stimulus threshold is reduced greatly and the response to suprathreshold stimuli is increased. This phenomenon, referred to as *sensitization*, does not extend to mechanical stimulation; i.e., repeated application of heat does not increase the sensitivity or response of the nociceptor to aversive mechanical stimuli.

Polymodal nociceptors Almost half of the unmyelinated axons of a peripheral nerve respond well not only to intense mechanical stimuli, but also to heat and noxious chemicals. Axons of these polymodal nociceptors make up the majority of very slowly conducting (<1 m/s) C fibers in a peripheral nerve. Their receptors respond to minute punctures of the epithelium, with a response magnitude that depends on the degree of tissue deformation. They also repond to temperatures in the range of 40–60°C and change their response rates as a linear function of warming when temperatures exceed 46°C (in contrast with the saturating responses displayed by nonnoxious thermoreceptors at these high temperatures). Mechanical and thermal receptive fields of the polymodal receptors overlap extensively and both enlarge predictably with increased stimulus intensity.

The axonal terminals of nociceptive axons possess no connective tissue sheaths and, for that reason, are often referred to as free nerve endings. Because they are not protected by physical barriers, nociceptor terminals are sensitive to chemical agents, including substances produced and released at the site of injury and toxins injected by other organisms. The most powerful among these is the peptide bradykinin. It and other agents diffuse over distances of several millimeters and can initiate or modulate the activity of many nociceptors. Protein receptors inserted into the membrane of nociceptor axons are the means by which diffusable agents, intense mechanical stimuli, and thermal stimuli are all effective in eliciting pain. Best studied among them are vanilloid receptors, which lead to nociceptor depolarization in the presence of capsaicin (an extract of chili peppers), the application of heat, and the intense deformation of skin.

Pain qualities carried by the two fiber types The relatively rapidly conducting Aδ and the slowly conducting C fiber nociceptors are responsible for two very different qualities to pain. The rapidly transmitted signal, often with high spatial resolution, is called *first pain* or cutaneous pricking pain. Not only is it well localized, it is also easily tolerated even if it is accompanied by a reflexive withdrawal response. This relatively fast signal is transmitted by mechanical nociceptors and their Aδ axons. The much slower, highly affective component is called *second pain* or burning pain. Because second pain is carried by slowly conducting C fibers, second pain follows pricking pain by a signficant delay (e.g., 1 s for pain at the fingertips or the toes). This pain is poorly localized and very poorly tolerated.

Some sources describe the presence of a third or deep pain, arising from viscera, musculature, and other deep tissues, such as joints. Deep pain is poorly localized, can be chronic, and is often associated with referred pain, in which tissue damage at one site is interpreted as occurring at a second site. Because of the extreme affective component to deep pain, it is tolerated very poorly and is thus not well studied and understood.

Thermoreceptors

Specific thermoreceptors respond with a sustained response over a narrow range of skin temperatures but do not respond to skin indentation. Thermoreceptors can be divided into warm and cold receptors, both of which end in dermis or deep epidermis as unencapsulated terminals. Axons of warm receptors are unmyelinated, slowly conducting C fibers that make up a significant fraction of axons in a typical peripheral nerve, whereas axons of cold receptors are lightly myelinated, more quickly conducting Aδ fibers and constitute at least a quarter of the axons in a peripheral nerve.

Receptive fields of thermoreceptors are very small spots, 1 mm in diameter in glabrous skin and 3–5 mm in hairy skin, three or four of which are innervated by a single primary axon. At a temperature of 30–35°C, both warm and cold spots discharge, but as temperatures increase, cold spots reduce their firing frequency whereas warm spots increase firing. Reductions in temperature produce the opposite result (Fig. 25.7).

A simple experiment illustrates the fact that cold and warm spots respond in opposite directions to a

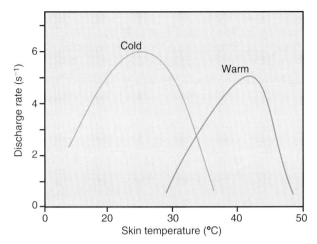

FIGURE 25.7 Rate of firing of thermoreceptors in monkey hand with variation in skin temperature. Cold receptors are most responsive to temperatures at or slightly above 20°C, whereas warm receptors show a peak response at or above 40°C. Fluctuations near body temperature produce modulations in the response of both receptors.

change in temperature and signal that change to the CNS. If one hand is submerged in frigid water and the other is in very warm water and then both are plunged into tepid water (30–35°C), the previously chilled hand will feel warm and the previously heated hand will feel cold. This result shows that thermoreceptors are very poor indicators of absolute temperature but are very sensitive to changes in skin temperature.

Thermoreceptors are extremely sensitive to localized changes in temperature and can signal very small changes if they are applied rapidly (5° C per minute). In contrast, slow changes of 0.5° C/min produce no change in receptor activity and no report by human subjects of a change in perceived temperature. When the thermal stimulus is applied by touching a hot or cold object to the skin, localization is extremely precise because of the tactile component of the stimulus. However, when temperature changes are imposed by a radiant heat source, localization is extremely imprecise with very gross misplacement (e.g., front versus back) on the trunk (Box 25.3).

Proprioceptors

One component of somatic sensation is directly related to the state of the body itself rather than to its relationship with the external environment. This proprioceptive or kinesthetic sense is related to the capacity to sense the position of joints, to sense their direction and velocity of movement, and to determine the effort needed to grasp and lift objects. Because proprioception is involved with movements of the joints and limbs, it is generally considered to be closely associated with the motor system. It is also

---

BOX 25.3

HYPERALGESIA AND ALLODYNIA

Unlike other somatosensory modalities, which show adaptation to the continuous presentation of a stimulus, the sensation of pain becomes greater when a painful stimulus is presented repeatedly. Thresholds for both mechanical nociceptors and thermal nociceptors can be lowered greatly by a prior, painful stimulus. This process, called hyperalgesia, includes a primary effect at the site of injury and a secondary effect in undamaged tissue surrounding the wound. Primary hyperalgesia includes a lowered threshold for both mechanical and thermal stimuli and probably occurs through the local release of one or more chemical agents. A particularly strong case can be made for bradykinin as the chemical mediator of primary hyperalgesia. It is not clear whether this effect is mediated by C fiber polymodal nociceptors or by mechanical nociceptors.

In contrast to primary hyperalgesia, secondary hyperalgesia exists with a lowered threshold only for subsequent mechanical stimuli. This secondary effect is associated with an area of erythema or flare that is smaller than the more diffuse region of hyperalgesia. Studies using local stimulation and local anesthetics have shown secondary hyperalgesia to be of neural origin, most likely produced when primary afferent axons are activated. A CNS component to secondary hyperalgesia is inferred from the observation that the lowered threshold to nociceptive stimuli extends over too great a distance to be accounted for by strictly peripheral mechanisms.

Allodynia is a related phenomenon in which nonnoxious stimuli produce painful responses. Perhaps the most common example of allodynia is pain produced by lightly touching burned skin. Changes in both the skin and the spinal cord have been implicated in allodynia.

Stewart H. Hendry and Steven S. Hsiao

true that because signals for voluntary movements are generated by commands originating in regions of the forebrain, the CNS is able to sense the position of limbs by keeping track of these commands. This process is usually referred to as *efferent copy* or corollary discharge. One clear indication of this process is seen in the fact that objects appear heavier when muscles fatigue and more motor output is required to lift them, even though sensory input does not change.

Despite the existence of CNS-generated signals of position, sensory input from the periphery is required for movements imposed upon a limb and to ensure that limbs have been moved to the intended location. Such sensory input can be visual for visually guided movements, or even auditory as limbs come in contact with the external world. However, humans have a high capacity to discriminate both position and movement of limbs without visual or auditory feedback and can do so for changes in proximal joints of as little as 0.2°.

The sense of limb position at rest and the sense of limb movement or kinesthesia are the products of inputs from cutaneous mechanoreceptors, joint receptors, and two specialized proprioceptors, muscle spindles and Golgi tendon organs.

Mechanoreceptors Of the cutaneous mechanoreceptors described earlier, only Ruffini/SAII afferents could encode joint position, as by responding to skin stretch in a directionally selective manner they are capable of detecting the direction in which joints are moved. Experiments in which SAIIs are blocked by local anesthesia indicate that their role depends on their location. When skin around the knee is anesthetized, subjects experience no change in the capacity to determine joint position, yet when the skin around the mouth, hands, and feet is anesthetized, subjects show a greatly reduced ability to use these stuctures or detect their passive movement. For some body parts, then, SAII afferents appear to play an active part in proprioception.

Joint receptors Several types of receptors are located in the joint capsule and respond to the bending of joints. These include slowly adapting responses in the joint capsule, arising from Ruffini-type endings and from paciniform corpuscles (small, elongated Pacinian corpuscles). Because humans who have had joint capsules anesthetized or removed surgicaly experience no loss of limb position sense, it is clear that these receptors are not involved in coding joint position. Instead, they play primarily a protective role by signalling and thereby preventing hyperextension or hyperflexion of the joint.

Muscle spindles These most complex peripheral receptors are a type of encapsulated ending, as much as 10 mm in length, each of which includes a single, large diameter (group Ia) primary sensory axon and a single thinner (group II) secondary sensory axon. The sensory axons terminate as tightly wound coils around the central, noncontractile regions of muscle fibers, called intrafusal fibers. Sensory axons around intrafusal fibers are sensitive to elongation of the muscle and to the subsequent recovery from stretch.

Diversity in the structure of intrafusal muscle fibers and of sensory axons permits muscle spindles to sense both dynamic and static components of muscle stretch. Primary axons and the intrafusal fibers they innervate are particularly sensitive to the earliest, most rapid change in muscle length and fire at a rate that varies with the velocity of change. In contrast, secondary axons and their intrafusal fibers are more sensitive to new static positions of the muscle produced by sustained stretching or contraction.

One function of muscle spindles can be seen in the patellar tendon or knee jerk reflex. To elicit this reflex, intrafusal muscle fibers of leg flexors are stretched tonically by crossing the leg and then are lengthened quickly by a sharp tap of the patellar tendon. This process of making the spindle afferents respond to lengthening of the muscle is referred to as "loading" the muscle spindle. A very rapid contraction of the flexor muscles follows. Because muscle contraction occurs through physical shortening of extrafusal fibers, intrafusal fibers are also shortened and the spindles are said to be "unloaded." Thus, one major function of the spindles is to provide the sensory component of a spinal reflex. Muscle spindle afferents also convey nonreflexive sensory information to higher stations in the somatosensory system (see later), which permits an animal to appreciate where its limbs are in space and, thus, to coordinate a rich variety of movements of body and limbs.

Golgi tendon organs These receptor organs are located in the fibrous tendons of muscles, where 10–20 individual muscle fibers join the ends of collagen fibers. Axons of group 1b afferents terminate in and among the collagen fibers so that when the tendon is stretched, the axons and terminals are compressed, causing them to discharge. By this arrangement, contraction of the muscle and the consequent pull on the collagen fibers of the organ cause the sensory axon to respond (Fig. 25.8).

The most easily demonstrated effect of Ib afferent activity is relaxation of the muscle of which the Golgi tendon organ is a part. This effect, known as *autogenic inhibition*, is produced by a simple spinal cord circuit,

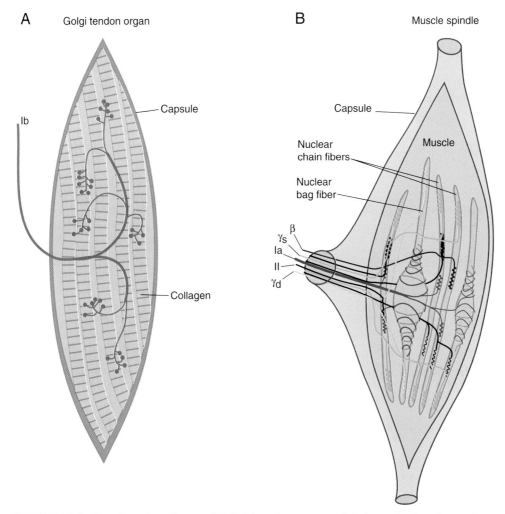

A Golgi tendon organ

Ib

Capsule

Collagen

B Muscle spindle

Capsule

Nuclear
chain fibers

Nuclear
bag fiber

Muscle

β
γs
Ia
II
γd

FIGURE 25.8 Proprioceptive afferents. (A) Golgi tendon organs and their termination along collagen fibers of the tendon capsule. These afferents respond when the entire capsule is stretched, usually by overvigorous contraction of the muscle. (B) Muscle spindle afferents (Ia and II) terminate on the noncontractile portions of intrafusal muscle fibers. They are arranged in parallel with work muscle fibers and respond to stretch of the entire muscle. Specialized motoneurons (γ) provide the motor innervation of the intrafusal muscle fibers and control the overall sensitivity of the muscle spindle.

through which contraction forces that threaten to pull the muscle away from its tendon are inhibited. As far as their proprioceptive functions are concerned, Golgi tendon organs do not respond to passively maintained limb position or to imposed changes in that position. There is reason to suspect that they are partially responsible for position sense, however, perhaps by sending information to the CNS about mechanics outside the muscle, thereby correcting muscle spindle activity for the contribution made by tendon length and compliance.

Dorsal Root Ganglion Cells

Each of the receptor types described earlier is innervated by primary sensory axons arising from

dorsal root ganglion (DRG) cells or, in the case of the neck and head, trigeminal ganglion cells. These cells are organized as collections of neurons in the peripheral nervous system, referred to as *ganglia*, and form two parallel chains along either side of the spinal cord.

All DRG neurons obey a simple morphological plan: they give rise to no dendrites and receive no synapses. Each cell contributes an axon that bifurcates close to the soma, sending one process out to the periphery and a second into the CNS. These peripheral and central processes serve as parts of a continuous cable carrying action potentials from their peripheral terminal sites in the skin, muscles, and tendons to their central terminal sites in the spinal cord or brain stem.

The peripheral axons of any individual dorsal root innervate a region of skin that is common across subjects within a certain expected variability. So, for example, the dorsal root ganglion at the 4th thoracic level innervates the region around the nipples, whereas the ganglion at the 10th thoracic level innervates the region around the umbilicus. Each of these regions is called a *dermatome*, and because of the stereotyped pattern of their organization, a dermatomal map can be generated (Fig. 25.9). Missing from most maps is the fact that the boundaries between dermatomes are not rigid, as somata in adjacent dorsal roots send axons to partially overlapping regions of skin. Nonetheless, dermatomal maps are

valuable in evaluating injuries or infections restricted to a small number of doral root ganglia, as careful testing with a fine probe applied to the skin can reveal the extent of damage or inflammation.

Dorsal root ganglion cells can be grouped into different classes by variations in the common morphological plan, specifically by variations in the size of somata, the diameter of axons, the morphology of peripheral terminals, and the site of central terminations. A division into two classes, one with large somata and the other with smaller somata, has a clear functional correlate, as large DRG cells are responsible for transduction and relay of low threshold mechanical stimuli and proprioceptive stimuli, whereas small

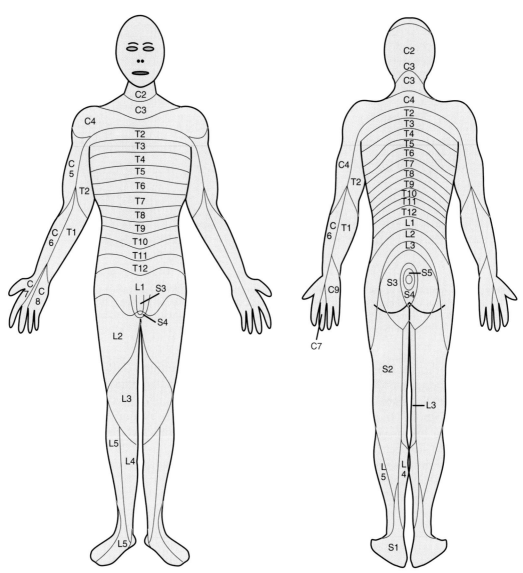

FIGURE 25.9 Classic dermatomal map showing the distribution of spinal nerves and the segments from which they arise. Despite extensive overlap between nerves arising from adjacent segments, this map permits localization of injuries and other conditions that give rise to restricted sensory deficits.

DRG cells are responsible for nociception and thermo-reception.

Summary

Peripheral receptors begin the division of labor that characterizes the somatosensory system. Because they are the peripheral terminals of different classes of dorsal root ganglion cells, each of which has its own sites of termination in the CNS, receptors are the basis for parallel processing at the earliest stages in somatic sensation. Experimental studies that compare the physiology of receptors with the behavior of humans and other primates establish the role that various types of receptors play in the perception of specific stimuli. The rest of the somatosensory system selects which peripheral information is relevant to make it useful for motor behavior and bring it to consciousness.

SPINAL AND BRAIN STEM COMPONENTS OF THE SOMATOSENSORY SYSTEM

Separate Paths for Mechanoreception and Nociception/Thermoreception

A basic principle of somatosensory functional organization draws strict correlation between the physiological properties and morphology of the peripheral axon of a DRG and the site at which its central axon terminates; i. e., information from each class of mechanoreceptor, nociceptor, and thermoreceptor reaches a unique group of neurons in the CNS. This principle of organization, referred to as modality segregation, is the mechanism whereby neurons responsible for conveying different sensations form separate pathways into and through the CNS. Such a division begins in the peripheral nerves and continues as dorsal root axons enter the spinal cord (Fig. 25.10; Box 25.4). There the central processes of DRGs take two different routes (Fig. 25.11).

Path of Small-Diameter Fibers Carrying Pain and Temperature

Most small-diameter, lightly myelinated and unmyelinated axons that carry information about pain and temperature enter the dorsal horn in a lateral division of fibers, turn to ascend or descend in a bundle of axons called Lissauer's tract for one to three segments, and terminate in layers I and IIa of the dorsal horn and in layers V, VI, and X of the intermediate horn (Fig. 25.11B; Box 25.4). By this arrange-ment, Lissauer's tract is made up principally of DRG axons, with only 20–25% of its axons arising from neighboring segments of the spinal cord (referred to as propriospinal axons).

Path of Larger Fibers Carrying Discriminative Inputs

Medium- and large-diameter axons that carry discriminative touch and proprioception enter in the medial division of the dorsal root and either terminate in layers IIb and III or turn to ascend in the gracile and cuneate fasciculi (dorsal columns). Axons in the dorsal columns include not only primary, dorsal root axons, but also axons of cells in layer III, referred to as postsynaptic dorsal column axons. These axons relay information from the layer III neurons similar to that carried by medial-division fibers of the dorsal root.

Although identical, so far as the sizes of axons they contain and the sensory modalities they carry, gracile and cuneate fasciculi differ in the parts of the body from which they convey somatosensory information. The gracile fasciculus exists through the full length of the cord. Its axons include the central processes of dorsal root ganglion and axons of spinal neurons from the lower half of the spinal cord, including thoracic segments 7 though 12 (T7–T12), all six lumbar segments (L1–L6), and the single coccygeal segment. As a result, this fasciculus carries somato-sensory input from the feet, legs, and lower trunk. The cuneate fasciculus is found only from the middle of the thoracic cord to the medulla because it is made up of ganglion cell central processes and spinal axons from only the upper thoracic segments (T1–T6) and all eight cervical segments (C1–C8). These axons carry information from the hands, arms, and upper body. In both gracile and cuneate fasciculi, axons are arranged so that those entering from more posterior spinal seg-ments occupy more medial positions in the tracts. This pattern, in which axons ascend in dermatomal fashion, is subtly rearranged near the site of termina-tion in the dorsal column nuclei. There, axons of dif-ferent dermatomes but of adjacent skin regions come together to form a topographic map (see later).

Outline of Central Somatosensory Pathways

By way of the dorsal columns, discriminative somatosensory inputs are carried to gracile and cuneate nuclei (dorsal column nuclei) of the lower medulla. In turn, neurons in the dorsal column nuclei give rise to axons that cross the midline of the medulla and ascend in a fiber bundle called the medial lemniscus. These terminate in the lateral division of the ventro-posterior nucleus (VPL) in the dorsal thalamus (Fig. 25.11A). In contrast, axons of nociceptors and

BOX 25.4

ANATOMY OF THE SPINAL CORD

As in any region of the CNS, groups of cell bodies and bundles of axons occupy different domains in the spinal cord. In a reversal from what is seen in other prominent regions of the CNS, axonal bundles (referred to as tracts or fasciculi) occupy the perimeter of the spinal cord, whereas cell bodies occupy its central core.

Those tracts directly relevant to somatic sensation are ones that carry sensory information to the brain (ascending tracts) and those that carry regulatory influences from the brain to spinal neurons (descending tracts). Ascending tracts include axons that are the central processes of dorsal root ganglion cells, as well as axons of spinal neurons. They synapse in several nuclei in a pattern that is characteristic for each tract. Descending axons originate in the cerebral cortex and in subcortical regions, and terminate on neurons of the cord. These include many axons that control voluntary movements, others that regulate the tonic sensitivity of motoneurons, and some that serve as part of a system that relays somatosensory information from higher levels onto neurons at lower levels.

The entry of dorsal root axons, the exit of ventral root axons, and the midline split the white matter of the spinal cord into three large divisions: dorsal, lateral, and ventral funiculi. The dorsal funiculus is a purely sensory division with ascending axons in most mammals, including monkeys and humans. It is composed of two large fiber tracts, the gracile and cuneate fasciculus, that together make up the dorsal columns. The ventral funiculus consists principally of several descending tracts that provide tonic regulatory input to spinal cord neurons, especially motor neurons and associated interneurons of the spinal cord. Both sensory and motor tracts are found in the lateral funiculus, the latter including the large lateral corticospinal tracts in primates and most other mammals.

For the purpose of carrying ascending information, the lateral funiculus can be divided in half. At the periphery of the more dorsal half (i.e., the dorsolateral funiculus) are axons carrying proprioceptive information to the cerebellum, whereas at the periphery of the ventral or anterior half (the anterolateral system) are axons carrying thermoreceptor and nociceptor inputs and some mechanoreceptor information.

Neurons of the cord occupy three large regions, in which they are arranged in groups that resemble layers but are properly thought of as nuclei (see Fig. 25.10).

1. The dorsal horn (layers I–V) contains neurons that receive input from the dorsal root ganglia and relay somatosensory information to other neurons of the CNS. It is composed of three broad groups of neurons, arranged as layers. These are lamina I (nucleus posteromarginalis), lamina II (substantia gelatinosa), and laminae III–V (nucleus proprius). Many studies have documented a fundamental subdivision of substantia gelatinosa into laminae IIa, containing cells that respond to nociceptive stimuli, and laminae IIb, in which neurons innervated by cutaneous mechanoreceptors are located.

2. The intermediate horn (laminae VI–VIII) consists of many propriospinal neurons (those whose axons do not leave the spinal cord but which may terminate in segments above or below their parent somata) and others that relay somatosensory information to higher levels of the CNS both for conscious appreciation of sensory inputs and for coordination of movements.

3. The ventral horn (lamina IX and X) contains motor neurons that provide the direct innervation of muscles and interneurons that modulate motor neuron activity.

Stewart H. Hendry and Steven S. Hsiao

---

thermoreceptors terminate in the spinal cord itself (i.e., in lamina I, lamina V of nucleus proprius, and laminae VI–VIII of the intermediate horn). These spinal neurons then send their axons across the midline of the spinal cord and ascend as the *anterolateral system* to terminate either in the brain stem or in several nuclei of the dorsal thalamus.

Functional Organization of the Dorsal Column/Medial Lemniscal System

Physiological Properties

Synaptic inputs reaching the dorsal column nuclei and outputs from it are notable for the strength of the connections they form, the modality specificity

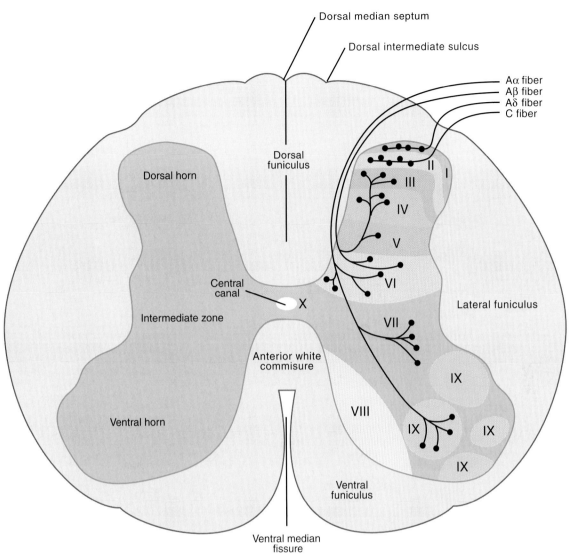

FIGURE 25.10 Anatomy of the spinal cord at a cervical level. Gray matter can be divided into groups of neurons that form layers in both dorsal (sensory) and ventral (motor) horns. Termination of large (Aα and Aβ) and small (Aδ and C) afferent axons in the cord vary by depth. The two groups enter the cord separately and terminate in regions that overlap very little.

imposed upon the neurons in the system, and for the precise body map observed across the entire population of neurons. These are the cardinal properties of the dorsal column-medial lemniscal system that recur in the ventrobasal complex of the thalamus and in the first somatosensory area of the cerebral cortex.

Beginning in the dorsal column nuclei and continuing at all subsequent stages in the somatosensory system is an intrinsic processing that imposes an inhibitory region around the central excitatory region of the receptive field of a neuron. This *lateral or surround inhibition* is generated in gracile and cuneate nuclei by populations of inhibitory interneurons that receive their inputs from primary sensory axons. The

key to lateral inhibition is the spatial organization of excitatory and inhibitory inputs: both are maximal at the center of the receptive field of the cell but whereas the excitation is sharply focused at the center, inhibition is more widely spread and thus dominant in the receptive field periphery. As a result, individual neurons in the dorsal column nuclei exhibit lower response rates and maximal discharges from smaller regions than the primary sensory afferents. Stimulus contrast is enhanced by this mechanism, providing for finer spatial discrimination.

It is important to reiterate that lateral inhibition, generated by intrinsic inhibitory circuits, is a characteristic not only of dorsal column nuclei but also of

A

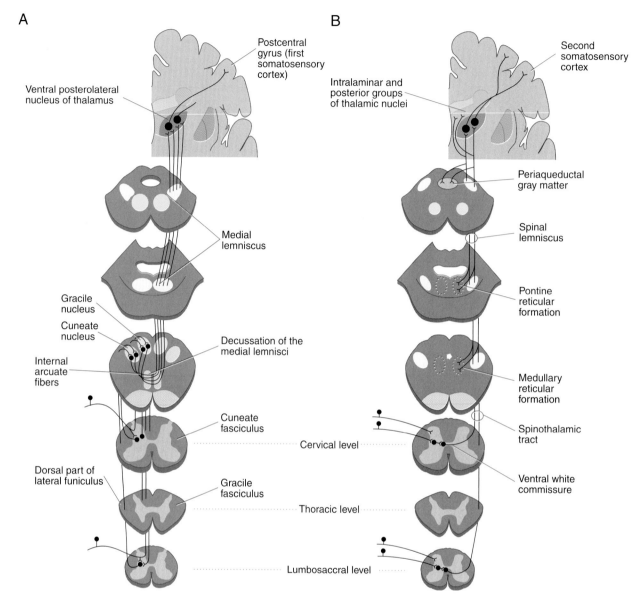

FIGURE 25.11 Anatomy of ascending somatosensory paths. (A) Organization of the dorsal column-medial lemniscal system from entry of large-diameter afferents into the spinal cord to the termination of thalamocortical axons in the first somatosensory area of the cerebral cortex. An obligatory synapse occurs in the gracile and cuneate nuclei, from which second-order axons cross the midline and ascend to the ventral posterolateral nucleus of the thalamus (VPL) by way of the medial lemniscus. (B) Organization of the spinothalamic tract and the remainder of the anterolateral system. Primary axons terminate the spinal cord itself. Second-order axons cross the midline and ascend through the spinal cord and brain stem to terminate in VPL and other nuclei of the thalamus. Collaterals of these axons terminate in the reticular formation of the pons and medulla.

the ventrobasal complex and of somatosensory areas of the cerebral cortex so that similar refinement and feature selectivity of receptive fields are characteristic of those regions as well.

Dorsal Column Nuclei

During their ascent to gracile and cuneate nuclei, axons of the dorsal columns are sorted by place and

modality. Somatotopic sorting takes place as those axons entering each of the dorsal columns earliest are displaced medially, whereas later entering axons form sheets or lamellae more laterally. Modality sorting also takes place, at least for the gracile fasciculus, as only RA inputs remain in that tract prior to its termination in the gracile nucleus. SA inputs reach the gracile nucleus but do so through other spinal pathways, such as those of the spinocervicothalamic system (see later).

Gracile and cuneate nuclei are organized into functionally distinct groups. A *reticular region* composed of scattered neurons that occupy the entire rostral one-third and the deep part of the caudal two-thirds of each nucleus is innervated by primary sensory axons and by postsynaptic dorsal column fibers. Well-defined *cell clusters* in the superficial portion of the caudal two-thirds of each nucleus receive input only from primary sensory axons and possess receptive fields no larger than those of the primary fibers that innervate them. Most neurons in this region display RA responses to cutaneous mechanical stimuli, similar to those of peripheral RA afferents. Receptive fields in the reticular region tend to be larger than those of afferent axons, suggesting that convergence of inputs from different axons takes place. However, that convergence displays a strong tendency to occur among fibers of the same modality, with Pacinian and SA responses predominating. Even here, a segregation of different functional types takes place as Pacinian-like responses are found in neurons of the posterior reticular region and slowly adapting responses in neurons of the anterior one-third of the nucleus.

A second level of functional organization is seen in the body map contained within the two dorsal column nuclei. The human somatosensory brain stem contains a body map of a "small man" or homunculus (analogous "small rats," "small cats," and "small monkeys" exist in the same regions of these species). Similar body maps are present in the subsequent stages of somatosensory processing so that at least one homunculus can be detected in regions of the human brain. Somatotopy in dorsal column nuclei is the result of a topographic projection of primary sensory axons and of postsynaptic dorsal column fibers onto neurons of these nuclei. This and higher order projections in the somatosensory system are said to be topographic when adjacent points in one nucleus project to adjacent regions of a second nucleus. As a result of these projections, a map of the lower body is imposed upon the gracile nucleus and the upper body on the cuneate nucleus. Such maps are distorted largely because of the greater number of receptors on some parts of the skin surface (the fingertips) than on others (the back and shoulders), but partly because of a true expansion in CNS machinery devoted to certain parts of the body.

When the somatotopic map is assembled for gracile and cuneate nuclei, it resembles an animal lying on its back with its limbs extended upward. Distal regions, such as the digits or tips of the paws, are mapped along the dorsal surface of each nucleus, whereas axial regions are mapped ventrally. Lateral to the cuneate nucleus is the spinal trigeminal nucleus, providing a representation of the face and completing the body map.

Spinocervicothalamic Pathway

Because of its resemblance to the postsynaptic dorsal column fibers and because its axons eventually merge with those of the medial lemniscus, the spinocervicothalamic pathway can be considered a part of the lemniscal system. The spinocervicothalamic system is a major component of the ascending somatosensory system in carnivores, but appears much diminished in primates. In humans the pathway and the neurons that give rise to it are highly variable, as they are reportedly nonexistent in some individuals and quite robust in others.

The focal point of the spinocervicothalamic pathway is the *lateral cervical nucleus*, a cluster of cell bodies in the lateral funiculus at the first and second cervical segments of the spinal cord. This nucleus receives inputs from small groups of neurons in lamina IV–VII (nucleus proprius) of the spinal cord that are responsive to low threshold stimulation of hair follicle afferents. Second order axons from nucleus proprius neurons ascend in the ipsilateral dorsal columns, exit at high cervical levels and terminate in the lateral cervical nucleus.

Neuronal receptive fields in the lateral cervical nucleus are organized somatotopically but tend to be larger than the fields of the innervating axons, suggesting a moderate degree of convergence from afferent fibers onto single lateral cervical neurons. Such convergence occurs within rather than across functional classes of axons, as cervicothalamic neurons respond to stimuli of single modalities. To reach the next stage of somatosensory processing (the thalamic ventrobasal complex), axons of the lateral cervical nucleus cross the midline in the cervical spinal cord, ascend to merge with the axons of the medial lemniscus, and terminate in the ventroposterolateral nucleus (VPL).

The Anterolateral System

Origin of the Anterolateral System

Neurons in layer I, layer V, and layers VI–VIII of the spinal cord give rise to axons that terminate in the dorsal thalamus, the midbrain, and the reticular formation of the pons and medulla. Because each group of axons crosses the midline and ascends in the anterolateral quadrant of the spinal cord, they are referred to collectively as the anterolateral system.

Spinal neurons of the anterolateral system are innervated by axons of the lateral division of the dorsal roots, and thus respond to mechanical nociceptive stimuli, thermal stimuli (whether nociceptive or innocuous), and innocuous mechanical stimuli carried by mechanoreceptors with large receptive fields (i.e., crude touch).

Dorsal Horn Circuitry and the Anterolateral System

Spinal circuits that appear specific for nociception include two classes of interneurons.

a. **Islet cells** are classical local circuit neurons with narrowly restricted axons and dendrites. Their dendrites receive inputs from all classes of primary sensory axons and, in turn, form synapses with those axons, thereby providing inhibition of slower Aδ and C fiber inputs by the more rapid Aβ fiber inputs. Through circuitry of this type, nociceptive input is suppressed by the simultaneous natural stimulation of mechanoreceptors or by artifical stimulation of their axons.

b. **Stalk cells** receive both nociceptive and non-nociceptive input and, in turn, relay information to spinothalamic neurons in lamina I. Thus, they are a key component to the transmission of nociception to higher levels of the CNS.

From the termination of primary sensory axons onto stalk cells and other classes of spinal neurons, two classes of nociceptive neurons have been described: those with nociceptive-specific responses, found in lamina I, and multisensory neurons that occupy deeper layers of the cord. Multisensory neurons respond to nonnoxious mechanical stimuli at low spike frequencies and to overtly noxious stimuli at high frequencies and are thus referred to as "**wide dynamic range**" cells. Only nociceptive-specific cells and not wide dynamic range cells provide higher centers with information about the existence, location, and intensity of painful stimuli.

Termination of Anterolateral Axons

Fibers of the anterolateral system terminate at three levels in the CNS. A sizable fraction terminates in the medulla and pons upon loosely organized groups of neurons interspersed among thin bundles of criss-crossing axons in a region referred to as the *reticular formation*. This ascending system is the *spinoreticular* pathway, which serves to provide pain inputs that produce forebrain arousal and affective response rather than discriminating the location of the stimulus. Spinoreticular axons arise predominantly from the cervical cord, where approximately the same number of cells contribute to it as provide axons for the spinothalamic tract.

A smaller group of anterolateral axons terminates in the superior colliculus of the midbrain and in the region surrounding the cerebral aqueduct [periaqueductal gray region (PAG)]. These *spino-mesencephalic* axons carry purely nociceptive information and include, in part, collaterals of axons innervating the dorsal thalamus. Axons terminating in the PAG are implicated in descending mechanisms of controlling pain (Fig. 25.12) (see later).

The bulk of the anterolateral system is composed of axons terminating in the dorsal thalamus. These

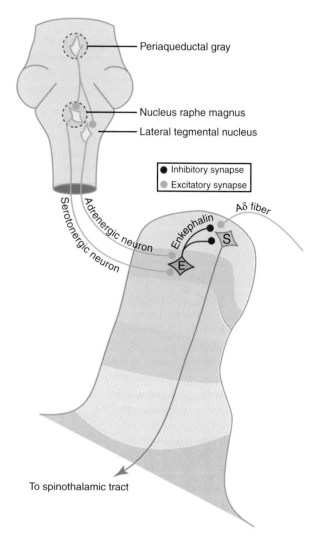

FIGURE 25.12 Descending control of pain. Serotoninergic axons arise from neurons in the nucleus raphe magnus and adrenergic axons from neurons in the lateral tegmental nucleus. Neurons in each nucleus are innervated by neurons of the periaqueductal gray area and both form excitatory synapses onto spinal interneurons (E). Those interneurons use opiate-like peptides (enkephalins) as neurotransmitters; release of enkephalins inhibits both the incoming nociceptive axons and the spinothalamic neurons (S) on which they synapse.

spinothalamic axons are present in all mammals and are particularly robust in primates. They terminate in three thalamic nuclei.

Ventroposterolateral nucleus (VPL) This is the principal relay nucleus of discriminative somatosensory information and receives both spinothalamic and medial lemniscal inputs. As outlined later, however, the two systems of input axons do not converge onto single VPL neurons but innervate different collections of cells in this nucleus. Spinothalamic neurons innervating VPL are found in layers I and V of the monkey spinal cord and include separate groups of cells with nociceptive, thermoreceptive, and mechanoreceptive properties.

The medial nucleus of the posterior complex (POm) Neurons terminating in this nucleus carry a nondiscriminative, affective component of a painful stimulus. Receptive fields of POm cells are usually large and include separate, noncontiguous regions on both sides of the body. In most cases, only nociceptive inputs succeed in driving POm neurons, although responses of individual neurons are insecure and change markedly with variations in skin temperature or anesthetic state.

Central lateral nucleus (CL) This intralaminar thalamic nucleus is part of a general system for cortical activation, and its neurons innervate many areas of the cerebral cortex. Studies of humans show that spinothalamic innervation of CL is not part of a discriminative pathway because the stimulation of intralaminar nuclei produces reports of burning sensations over most of the body.

Descending Control of the Anterolateral System

Two brain stem regions, the PAG of the midbrain and the rostroventromedial medulla (RVM), provide descending control of nociceptive neurons in the anterolateral system. Activity in PAG is routed through brain stem nuclei that terminate in the spinal cord. Neurons in these nuclei release either serotonin or norepinephrine onto interneurons in the spinal cord, which in turn directly inhibit nociceptive afferent axons. Opioid peptides and exogenously administered opiates work at two major locations in this circuit. These include neurons of the PAG, which express opiate receptors, and the spinal cord, where the inhibitory interneurons synthesize and release opioid peptides and nociceptive axons display opiate receptors.

The Trigeminal System

Parallels with the Spinal Somatosensory System

Much as sensory axons for the trunk and limbs are processes of DRG cells and form parts of peripheral nerves, axons conveying somatosensory inputs from the face and head are processes of neurons of the trigeminal ganglion and make up the afferent component of the trigeminal or fifth (V) cranial nerve. The trigeminal nerve divides into three large branches, hence its name: they are ophthalmic, maxillary, and mandibular nerves. These nerves innervate the skin in nonoverlapping regions of the face, and in doing so end as mechanoreceptors, thermoreceptors, and nociceptors in a manner precisely analogous to that of a dorsal root ganglion.

Central processes of trigeminal ganglion cells enter the CNS at the middle of the pons and adopt a path for discriminative touch that is distinct from the path for pain and temperature. Large-diameter axons carrying fine tactile inputs terminate near the level of the trigeminal nerve's entry, in the main sensory nucleus (Fig. 25.13A). Most axons given off by the main nucleus cross the midline, ascend as trigeminothalamic axons, join with the medial lemniscus caudal to the thalamus, and terminate in the ventroposteromedial nucleus (VPM). In most regards, then, this is the trigeminal equivalent of the dorsal column/medial lemiscal system. In contrast, small lightly myelinated and unmyelinated axons entering the trigeminal nerve descend in the spinal trigeminal tract to terminate in the spinal trigeminal nucleus (Fig. 25.13B). This nucleus is composed of three subdivisions, pars oralis, interpolaris, and caudalis, which together form a long chain of contiguous neurons that extends from the caudal border of the main nucleus to the second cervical segment. Pars caudalis is the region that most closely resembles the anterolateral system in its structure and function. It is the site of termination for nociceptors and thermoreceptors, and neurons in pars caudalis give off crossed and uncrossed axons that terminate in the thalamus.

Unique Features of the Trigeminal System

The trigeminal system contains specialized neuronal populations and displays some functional properties that are unlike those of the spinal somatosensory system. The most obvious of these is the displacement of ganglion cells that innervate spindles of the muscles of mastication. Although of similar neural crest origin as neurons of the trigeminal ganglion and of DRGs, these cells do not occupy a position in the ganglion itself or in any part of the peripheral nervous system. Instead the neurons make up a distinct nucleus in the

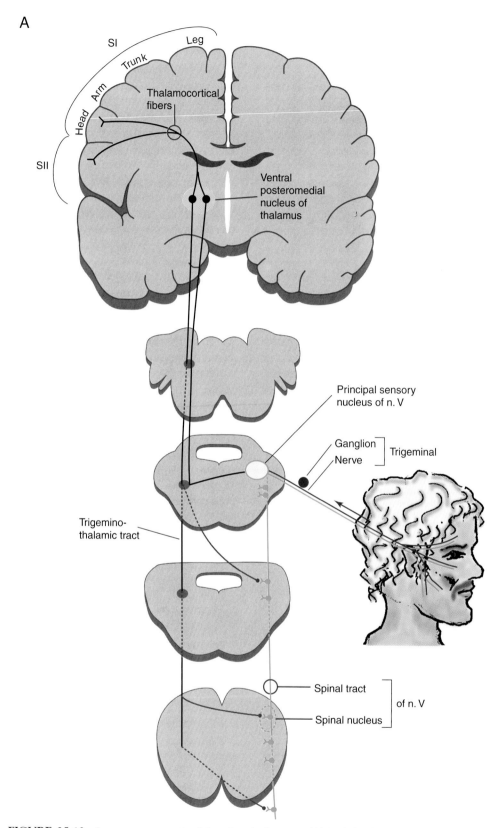

FIGURE 25.13 Sensory components of the trigeminal system. (A) Path for discriminative touch. Large-diameter afferents from the face innervate second-order neurons in the spinal trigeminal nucleus (pars oralis) and the principal sensory nucleus. Neurons in these nuclei give rise to axons that cross the midline, ascend in the trigeminothalamic tract, and terminate in the ventral posteromedial (VPM) nucleus of the thalamus.

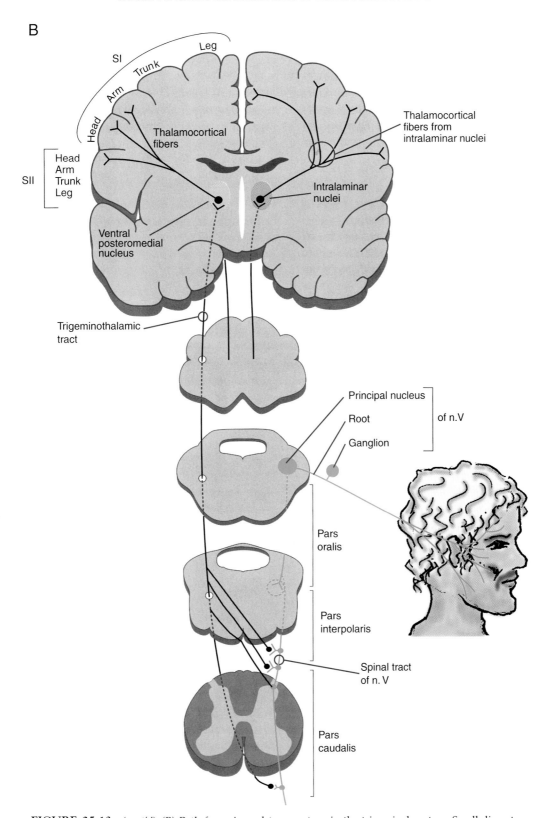

FIGURE 25.13 (*cont'd*) (B) Path for pain and temperature in the trigeminal system. Small-diameter afferent axons descend in the spinal trigeminal tract and terminate in the pars caudalis of the spinal nucleus. Second-order axons cross the midline and ascend to the thalamus.

midbrain called the trigeminal mesencephalic nucleus and, as such, are the only documented example of CNS neurons derived from neural crest rather than neural tube. Analogous to the situation with muscle spindle afferents in the spinal cord, a small population of axons from the mesencephalic nucleus terminates directly in the trigeminal motor nucleus, thereby providing a monosynaptic relay from stretch receptor to motoneuron.

A second feature unique to the trigeminal system is the innervation of specialized structures. Most prominent among these is tooth pulp, which are thought to be innervated solely by C and Aδ nociceptors. Experimental studies indicate that the majority of these axons terminate in pars interpolaris of the spinal nucleus. In some species, such as rodents, the most highly specialized structures innervated by the trigeminal nerve are the mystacial vibrissae or whiskers. Nuclei in the rodent trigeminal system contain neuronal aggregates dedicated to each whisker. Such aggregates in the main sensory nucleus of V, in VPM, and in the somatosensory cortex are even grouped into rows to produce a complete and isomorphic representation of the whisker pad. Given the name "barrels" in cortex, barreloids in VPM, and barrelets in the principal sensory nucleus, these neuronal aggregates have provided one of the most easily exploited model systems for studying somatosensory structure, function, and development.

Summary

Parallel paths exist in both the spinal somatosensory and trigeminal systems. Separate paths exist to process and relay discriminative sensations, such as fine touch, and the more poorly localized sensations of pain and temperature. These different modalities are carried by different groups of neurons, whose axons occupy separate parts of the spinal cord and brain stem until they converge in the ventrobasal complex.

THE THALAMIC VENTROBASAL COMPLEX

Definition of the Ventrobasal Complex

The ventrobasal complex includes the two divisions of the ventroposterior nucleus that receive somatosensory input from the body and head. Axons of both the medial lemiscus and the spinothalamic tract terminate in the lateral subdivision of the VPL; trigeminothalamic fibers from the principal sensory nucleus and from the spinal trigeminal nucleus inner-

vate the medial subdivision of VP (VPM). A third nucleus can be included in the VB of primates. This ventroposterior inferior nucleus (VPI) has a unique cell architecture, with neurons smaller than those in the rest of VB. However, the cortical projection of VPI serves to best distinguish it from VPL and VPM, for neurons in VPI innervate exclusively the second somatosensory cortex (SII).

From the convergence of lemniscal and anterolateral fibers, one might expect a convergence of discriminative, mechanoreceptive inputs with pain and temperature information in both VPL and VPM. Such convergence does not occur, as inputs from discriminative pathways and pain/temperature pathways terminate on different groups of neurons, producing neurons specific for single modalities.

Somatotopic Organization in VB

VPL and VPM are organized somatotopically so that neurons responding to stimulation of one region of the contralateral body surface are segregated from those responding to other regions. In the body map for the ventrobasal complex, representation of the mouth is most medial and the neck most lateral in VPM, whereas the hand is most medial and the feet are most lateral in VPL. Each part of the body is represented in a sheet of cells, called lamellae, that take a curved path from dorsal to ventral in the VB. All neurons in a particular lamella respond to stimulation of the same region on the surface of the body or face. As the stimulus is moved along the body surface, activity in the VB moves from one lamella to its immediate neighbor.

Functional Subdivisions in VB

The termination of medial lemniscal axons in VPL divides it into functional subdivisions. At a coarse level, the nucleus is divided into a core region that receives predominantly cutaneous inputs and a shell region that receives predominantly deep tissue inputs. At a finer level, lemniscal axons terminate in narrow elongated rods (200–300 µm in diameter) that provide a group of thalamocortical neurons with their somatosensory input. These neurons, in turn, project to a zone in the cerebral cortex less than 1 mm in diameter.

Receptive Field Properties of Neurons in VB

Lemniscal Properties

Extreme synaptic security is a property characteristic of VB neurons innervated by the medial lemniscus, as they possess the ability to follow activity in presynaptic axons up to rates of more than 100 Hz. Separate populations of VB neurons display rapidly and slowly adapting reponses to cutaneous simulation and rapidly adapting responses to pressure, all of which suggest that they are driven indirectly by SAI, RA, and Pacinian afferents. These findings accent the relay properties of VB and suggest that much of the circuitry in this nucleus is devoted to transferring a faithful replica of medial lemniscal and trigemino-thalamic inputs to the cortex.

Anterolateral Inputs

Neurons in VB driven by inputs from the antero-lateral system include both nociceptive-sensitive and thermosensitive cells. Anterolateral fibers terminate most densely in the shell region of VPL and do so as rods, similar to the pattern of lemniscal terminations. Anatomical evidence indicates that anterolateral and lemniscal rods do not overlap. Nonetheless, populations of nociceptive and thermoreceptive neurons in VPL exhibit a much greater degree of convergence from mechanoreceptors than is evident in spinothalamic neurons, and both receptive field sizes and stimulus intensities suggest that these cells can perform well in precisely locating painful stimuli.

Summary

Variations in function and structure divide the ventrobasal complex into several parts. Separate nuclei, VPL and VPM, receive and process inputs from the body and head, respectively. Each nucleus is, itself, subdivided into regions, the physiology of which is dominated either by discriminative senseations or by pain and temperature.

SOMATOSENSORY AREAS OF THE CEREBRAL CORTEX

Definition of the Somatosensory Cortex

Areas of cerebral cortex are defined by three properties: structure, function, and connectivity. Connectivity and function are a matter of cause and effect, as the physiology of somatosensory areas of cortex arises principally from their connections, and particularly from inputs from VB and areas of cerebral cortex. Correlations between structure and connectivity are also evident across the cortex.

In the somatosensory system, two areas of cerebral cortex receive direct synaptic inputs from VB: the first somatosensory area (SI) in monkey and humans is in the posterior bank of the central sulcus and on the crown of the postcentral gyrus, and the second somatosensory area (SII) is on the lip and upper bank of the lateral fissure. These two are innervated not only by axons from VB, but also from one another, as a dense reciprocal projection exists between the two. Together, they then send axons to areas adjacent to them in the parietal lobe and insula, all of which can be considered part of the somatosensory system, and to areas of the motor cortex.

First Somatic Sensory Area (SI)

Modern studies have identified four physiologically and anatomically distinct areas in SI, analogous to the areas of human cortex originally designated areas 3a, 3b, 1, and 2. Each area contains neurons responsive to somatic stimuli and each receives direct axonal terminations from VB (Fig. 25.14); however, the precise source of those inputs varies, as few VB neurons send collaterals to two areas in SI. As a result, the physiological properties of neurons in one area differ appreciably from those of other areas.

Function of SI

At their most basic, cortical areas in SI perform different functions. Neurons in areas 3b and 1 are responsive to cutaneous inputs, both rapidly adapting and slowly adapting. In contrast, areas 3a and 2 respond to deep stimuli, with area 3a particularly responsive to muscle afferents and area 2 to joints. In each area, receptive fields are larger than those displayed by primary sensory axons but are nonetheless specifically RA-like, SA-like, or Pacinian-like. Thus, SI most clearly shows the division of labor that began in the periphery with the elaboration of different receptor types and the preservation of their selectivity for stimulus quality. This is the hallmark of the labeled line concept for somatic sensation.

Lesion studies indicate that area 3b is critical for the performance of tactile discrimination based on the shape or texture of a stimulus. Removal or inactivation of this area leads to a lack of appreciation of the quality or even the existence of tactile stimuli. Lesions of area 1 disrupt performance based on texture but leave intact performance based on stimulus size, whereas lesions in area 2 produce the opposite result. These findings indicate that area 3b is a conduit for all cutaneous sensibility, that area 1 is specialized for the analysis of SAI and RA inputs, and that area 2 integrates positional information with edge detection to form an accurate impression of the shape of an object.

A complete map of the body surface exists in each of the four areas of SI in Old World monkeys and thus it is assumed that four homunculi exist in human SI.

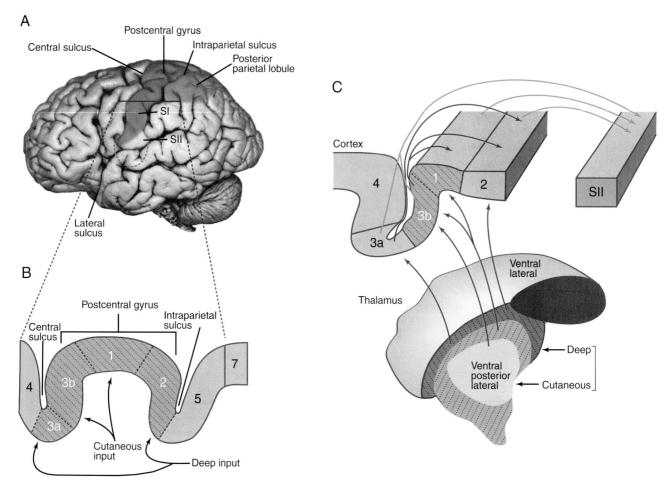

FIGURE 25.14 Functional organization of the ventrobasal complex and first somatosensory cortex (SI). (A) Location of SI in the postcentral gyrus and its relationship to SII and the somatosensory association cortex in the posterior parietal lobe. (B) Cross section through the postcentral gyrus, cut orthogonal to the central sulcus. SI is divided into four anatomically and functionally distinct areas. They are bordered by area 4 of the precentral motor cortex and by area 5 of the parietal association cortex. (C) Relationship between regions of cutaneous and deep input to VPL and the termination of thalamocortical axons in SI. The serial processing of somatosensory inputs is also indicated by the projections from one area of SI to others and from all areas in SI to the second somatosensory area (SII). Adapted from Jones and Friedman (1982).

Although complete, body maps contain many distortions, the most dramatic of which are the greatly enlarged representations of the hand, particularly the digits, and of the face. Representation of the digits occupies more than 100 times the cortical surface area devoted to the trunk (Fig. 25.15). By this relative enlargement in cortical representation, the digits and lips are said to be magnified, and the degree of over-representation is called the *magnification factor*.

Structure, Connections, and Physiological Properties

Area 3b is most densely innervated by axons of the core region in VB and displays the typical granular cytoarchitecture of primary sensory areas (Fig. 25.14). In fact, a compelling argument has been made that area 3b in Old World monkeys is equivalent to the entire SI of other mammals. The adjacent area 3a

varies in structure along the length of the central sulcus, but can be seen as a region of hybrid structure, with many small cells, typical of area 3b, but also groups of larger cells, typical of the bordering precentral motor cortex. Areas 1 and 2 display the homotypical six-layered pattern characteristic of most areas of cerebral cortex. So similar is their structure that determining where area 1 ends and area 2 begins can be extremely difficult.

In each area, responses to peripheral stimuli are recorded for neurons from just below the pial surface of the cortex, in layer II, to just above the white matter, in layer VI. A consistent feature of the cortex is the basic similarity in physiological properties displayed by neurons in a radial traverse through the cortex so that cells in layers II–VI along a true radial path in SI respond to the same stimulus applied to the same part

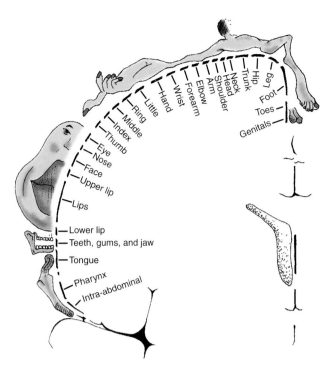

FIGURE 25.15 Somatotopic organization of human SI. The body map produces a homunculus with foot representation most medial and face representation most lateral. Note the expanded representation of some structures, such as the mouth and hand. Reprinted with permission from Penfield and Rasmussen (1950), copyright renewed 1978.

of the body surface. Thus neurons exhibiting place and modality specific responses are organized as radial arrays or *columns*. These columns originate from the patchy termination of thalamocortical, intracortical, and callosal axons in areas of SI and are carried to all

neurons in a column by radially organized axons that arise from neurons in one layer and terminate upon neurons in another layer.

Seven out of 10 neurons in monkey VB send their axons to area 3b, where they terminate in the middle layers (layers III and IV). Neurons in layers II and III of area 3b then relay inputs to layer IV of the other areas in SI. This pattern in which layer III neurons in one area send axons to layer IV of another is typical of a pattern referred to as "feed forward" because the connections occur for a primary sensory area communicating with a higher order area. In this sense, areas 1 and 2 can be considered a second cortical step in the analysis of somatosensory inputs. These patterns of thalamocortical and cortico-cortical connections suggest that overlaid upon the parallel processing of cutaneous vs deep inputs in SI is the serial processing of information. For example, the function of area 3b inputs to areas 2 is to contribute information from cutaneous receptors to an area dominated by deep inputs, providing a unified representation of a stimulating object.

Differences in the receptive field properties of neurons in the areas of SI subscribe to a certain logic given the varying sources of somatosensory inputs. In the VB-dominated area 3b, neurons display very small, simple receptive fields, with neurons in layer IV of area 3b possessing receptive fields most similar to those of peripheral afferents. Neurons in overlying layers (II and III) display more complex responses (e.g., the presence of distinct excitatory and inhibitory subregions) over larger areas of the body surface. Those large, complex receptive fields are then donated

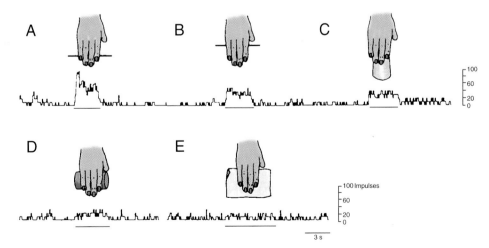

FIGURE 25.16 Response of neurons in monkey SI to the active grasping of objects. Variations in the position and shape of complex objects elicit responses of different strengths from neurons in this region of cortex. Most effective for this particular neuron is an edge applied to the tips of the fingers (A). Least effective is a flat sheet of paper (E).

by layer II–III neurons to area 1, where convergence and processing of inputs produce receptive fields with properties such as selectivity for the direction of a moving stimulus (Fig. 25.16).

It is in area 3a that knowledge of thalamocortical and cortico-cortical connections has been most useful in interpreting an area's unique role. Positioned as it is between the precentral motor area (area 4) and the granular area 3b of SI, area 3a could easily be seen as a sensory area with a motor function. Consistent with this potential are this area's cell structure and connectivity: thalamocortical inputs are predominantly from neurons in VB that are themselves responsive to proprioceptive stimuli, whereas densest intracortical inputs are from the parietal association cortex and the supplementary motor area, cortical areas that also innervate the precentral motor area. That neurons in area 3a respond to proprioceptive stimuli arising from muscles makes sense for an area that appears to represent a path whereby sensory information reaches motor cortex. However, neurons of area 3a do not directly innervate areas of motor cortex but project instead to area 2 and to an area of parietal association cortex (area 5). From both of these areas, sensory information does reach the precentral motor and premotor areas, but by a path that is considerably more indirect than might have been predicted. Area 3a then is not a direct conduit for proprioceptive input to motor cortex, but is an intermediate stage of somatosensory processing, one whose output is combined with others before that information is sent to areas of motor cortex. Moreover, there is recent and compelling evidence of the role played by area 3a in a decidedly nonproprioceptive function, namely the reception and processing of painful stimuli. These findings indicate that at least two distinct somatosensory modalities employ area 3a as part of a circuit to influence motor activity.

From their innervation of motor and association areas, areas of SI can be seen to integrate somatosensory information and to relay such information to areas that control and coordinate body and limb movements. Other regions receiving information from SI include SII and the cortical areas around it and a series of subcortical nuclei. Most of the latter are, themselves, part of the somatosensory system, including VB, the dorsal column nuclei, and the dorsal and intermediate horns of the spinal cord. Much speculation and some clever experimentation have gone into determining what the descending control of somatosensory relay nuclei might accomplish. The clearest idea at this time seems to be that descending output from the cortex serves to selectively activate neurons that are processing information from a specific body location and modality. Much of this descending pro-

jection can be seen as the anatomical substrate for the influence of attention on somatosensory processing. Attentional mechanisms help limit the amount of information that the CNS needs to process simultaneously and ensures that irrelevant stimuli, such as the constant sensation of clothes in contact with the skin, does not unduly occupy the limited resources available for cortical processing. Predictably, the response of neurons in SI, particularly in SII, is affected greatly by the attentional state of an animal.

Receptive Field Plasticity

Fundamental changes take place in the somatosensory cortex when peripheral receptors or their axons are damaged. Because there is a limit to the time in development during which manipulations produce the most robust changes in cortical anatomy and physiology (a time referred to as the *critical period*), the general impression had grown that SI was largely immutable in adult life. Research over the past decade has shown repeatedly that this impression is mistaken. Manipulations such as digit amputation or nerve section that eliminate input from a part of the body surface lead to a rearrangement of the body map in SI. Through this process, a part of SI normally responsive to one body region, such as the first digit, comes to respond to adjacent regions (neighboring digits). This type of somatosensory rearrangement can be extremely rapid, occurring within minutes of a manipulation, and thus depends on the ability of pre-existing but ineffectual synaptic contacts in the cortex to now drive cortical neurons. Moreover, body map rearrangements can occur without the production of trauma anywhere in the somatosensory system, but with only subtle manipulations such as a coordinated stimulation of body regions and classical conditioning of cortical responses. A search for the mechanism of plasticity indicates that for SI, itself, enhancement of connections formed by thalamocortical and intracortical axons permits a limited rearrangement in the body map, one that spans a distance of 2–3 mm. Thus, the ability of inputs from one finger to capture cortical territory previously driven by another finger can be seen as a strictly intracortical event driven by changes in intracortical excitation and inhibition. For much larger expansions that occur over several millimeters of SI, such as those that occur following limb amputation or the sectioning of several dorsal roots, rearrangement in the body map includes expansion in body maps not only in SI but also in the dorsal column nuclei and VB. So extensive is this rearrangement that parts of SI previously responsive to the hand and arm come to respond to stimulation of the face and head.

Second Somatosensory Area (SII)

SII is the area of cerebral cortex in the upper bank of the lateral fissure that receives direct inputs from VB and whose neurons respond robustly to cutaneous stimulation of low intensity. By this definition, SII is approximately one-fourth the size of SI in surface area and contains at least one and probably two complete representations of the body (Fig. 25.17). Complete destruction of SII leaves a monkey permanently incapable of discriminating objects on the basis of their texture and permanently impaired in discriminating among objects of different sizes.

SII is the first stage of cortical somatosensory processing in which both sides of the body surface are represented in a sizable proportion of neurons. Inputs from the ipsilateral body surface reach SII predominantly from the contralateral hemisphere by way of axons in the corpus callosum, although a minor input

is relayed through neurons in VB that are innervated by medial lemniscal axons ascending and terminating ipsilaterally. The transcallosal input to SII serves the obvious function of midline fusion. By this process, receptive fields along the body midline are generated in SII that extend for some distance into each half of the body, thus forming a coherent percept of a single body map. A less obvious function of the callosal input to SII is seen in studies of humans and non-human primates. To learn a tactile discrimination task with one hand and to perform it with the other is an ability accomplished easily and quickly by an intact human or monkey. However, it is a task that is lost when the corpus callosum is cut or SII is removed surgically, thereby demonstrating a major role for SII in the interhemispheric transfer of tactile discrimination.

In this context of midline fusion and interhemispheric transfer, three types of SII neurons stand out in monkeys: those with bilaterally symmetric receptive fields of distal extremities (e.g., responsive to stimulation of the third digit on both hands), those with continuous receptive fields along the midline, and those with exclusively contralateral receptive fields. So far as their receptive field properties are concerned, individual neurons in SII display a complex physiology, including multidigit receptive fields that often extend to three or more digits of the same hand, as well as to digits of the contralateral hand. Many neurons in SII (more than 80%) are affected directly by the attentional state, with approximately half the responsive population showing enhanced responses when a stimulating object is attended to and half showing suppressed responses to the same condition. These responses, being more complex than the ones sampled in any area of SI, have raised the strong possibility that SII is a higher order stage in a hierarchy of somatosensory areas. Evidence for such a hierarchy has come from studies of rhesus monkeys in which the somatosensory receptive fields of SII neurons were eliminated after the surgical removal of SI. Contrasting data show, however, that SII of at least one species of monkey is on an equivalent hierarchical plane as SI and that ablation of SII has as great an effect on SI neurons as the ablation of SI has on SII neurons. If there is any general lesson to this, it is most likely that areas of somatosensory cortex are neither strictly hierarchical in organization nor entirely parallel.

In primates, SII is the recipient of inputs from all four areas of SI, and in each case, intracortical axons terminate densely in layer IV of SII. Neurons of SII, in turn, give rise to axons that innervate two neighboring areas of insular cortex and from there somatosensory information reaches the amygdala and hippocampus

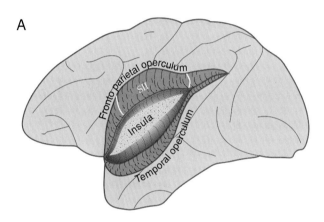

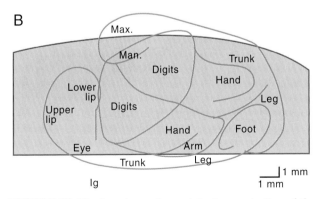

FIGURE 25.17 Location and somatotopic organization of the second somatosensory area in rhesus monkeys. (A) Partially unfolded view of the cortex in the lateral sulcus. SII is located in the upper bank of that sulcus; its borders are indicated by the yellow lines. (B) Map of the body surface in SII indicating the presence of two separate maps in this area and the relative expansion of the hand and digit representation.

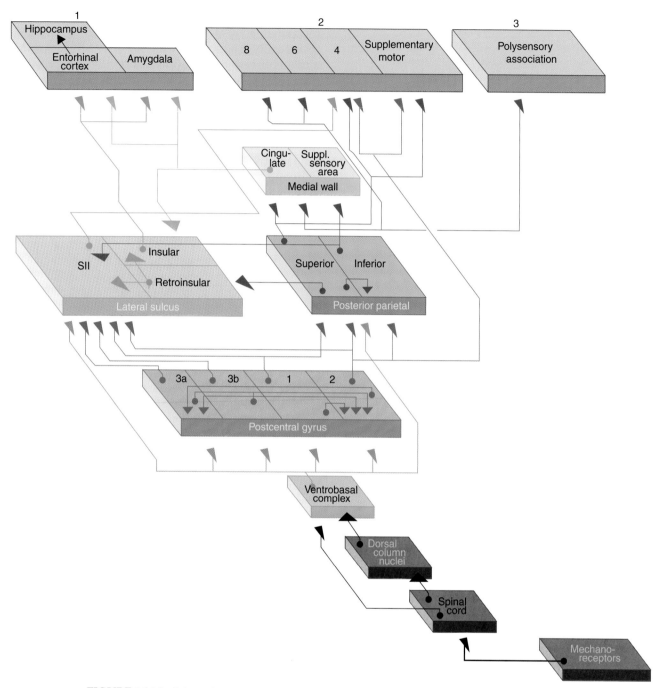

FIGURE 25.18 Schematic representation of the path taken by mechanoreceptor input to eventually reach three cortical targets. All relevant information reaches the ventrobasal complex and most is relayed to the areas of SI. From there, by steps through SII and the posterior parietal areas, somatosensory information reaches (1) the limbic system (entorhinal cortex and hippocampus), as a means for becoming part of or gaining access to stored memories; (2) the motor system (primary and supplementary motor cortex), where the continuous sensory feedback onto motor system occurs; and (3) the polysensory cortex in the superior temporal gyrus, in which creation of a complete and abstract sensory map of the external world is thought to occur. Adapted from Wall (1988), with permission.

(Fig. 25.18). Thus, SII in rhesus monkeys and presumably in other primates can be seen as a funnel for the relay of somatosensory information into the limbic system. By this scheme, SII is vital as the obligatory

route taken by sensory inputs mediating tactual learning and memory.

A second major role for SII apparent from its intracortical connectivity is that of sensorymotor integration. One of the central components of coordinated movements is a continuous somatosensory feedback that permits changes in a motor program to occur. For example, the act of precisely grasping an object requires strict coordination between somatosensory feedback and motor program and, as indicated from studies in which lesions are placed within the CNS, that feedback makes its way to the brain stem through the dorsal columns. Finding that neurons in areas of motor cortex display relatively low threshold somatosensory responses is not surprising in this context, and the conclusion had been that such responses are a function of the input to motor areas from SI. Such responses survive complete removal of SI, however, showing the connections from this area to motor cortex to be neither necessary nor sufficient. Cutaneous and deep responses in motor areas cannot arise from thalamocortical inputs because these inputs originate in thalamic nuclei other than VB, whose somatosensory responses are weak and require very strong stimuli. One remaining and obvious source of somatosensory input to the motor cortex is SII.

Posterior Parietal Areas

Various descriptors and definitions are used for the areas of parietal cortex posterior to area 2. If cortico-cortical inputs are combined with a traditional scheme for numbering areas of cortex, then two cortical areas (areas 5 and 7) with two subdivisions each (a and b) may be considered part of the somatosensory system.

The rostral half of the posterior parietal cortex is made up of areas 5a and 7b. These are the areas directly innervated by area 2 in monkeys and in which somatosensory responses to low threshold stimuli can be mapped easily. Their output to the precentral motor area indicates that they play a role in integrating somatosensory information with motor behavior. Specifically, they are implicated in the attentional and motivational control of movements that are related to tactile stimuli.

The caudal half of the posterior parietal cortex, especially area 7a, is a site for convergence of somatosensory and visual inputs. It is a region implicated very strongly in visual functions of localizing a stimulus and of directing attention to that stimulus. These caudal parietal regions, in the bank of the intraparietal sulcus of Old World monkeys, are clearly involved in directing eye movements and are thus at a pivot point in somatosensory, visual, and motor systems. Although neurons are responsive to both somatosensory and visual stimuli in this area, it

cannot be said that neurons display receptive fields in the same sense that neurons in SI do. Instead, responses can be elicited from any place in the sensory periphery but in a manner that depends on the context of the stimulus.

Both halves of the posterior parietal cortex appear to function as stations for the higher order analysis and relay of somatosensory inputs to areas of motor control. Unilateral damage to these areas produces confounding results among primates. In monkeys, such damage leads to few somatosensory deficits, amounting to only a partial neglect of tactile stimuli delivered to the contralateral body surface. Neglect in humans, however, is strictly lateralized and dramatic. Strokes or missile wounds that destroy the posterior parietal cortex of the nondominant hemisphere produce a near-complete tactile neglect syndrome, but one that is restricted to the ipsilateral side of the body. These findings are an example of extreme specialization among areas of the human cerebral cortex.

Parallel and Hierarchical Processing in Somesthesis

As outlined earlier, a major issue left to be resolved is the organization of somatosensory areas into parallel and hierarchical systems. In the former, two or more collections of areas operate independently to perform different functions. In the latter, areas line up in a bottom-to-top arrangement in which simple processing in early areas leads to progressively more complex processing at later stages. The two are not mutually exclusive, as areas may be divided first into parallel tracks and then, within those tracks, arranged as a hierarchy. Parallel processing of somatosensory information is apparent in the broadest sense, as a dorsal stream leads from SI to eventually reach motor and premotor areas of the frontal lobe, whereas a ventral stream includes limbic and prefrontal areas. One is tied to the somatosensory control of motor behavior, and the other to the discrimination of objects. At a finer level, however, there is the question of whether intermediate stages of processing fit into strict parallel or hierarchical schemes. Two very different functions, the perception of painful stimuli and the discrimination of tactile shape, can be used to explore this issue.

The appreciation of pain involves a discriminative and an affective component, as discussed previously. A parallel processing model suggests that separate areas of the cerebral cortex deal with the two components. Studies that record from neurons in monkey somatosensory areas or image the functional activity in human cerebral cortex indicate that both SI and SII are part of a discriminative path, whereas areas of the cingulate and insular cortex are parts of an affective path. There is still some argument, however, about the discriminative function of SI and increasing doubt about the role of SII. For example, the timing of neural activation in the human cortex suggests that SII may be involved primarily with recognition of a stimulus as painful and direction of attention to that stimulus. SII may be seen most properly as a place in which sensorimotor and discriminative functions coexist, either as parts of a common circuit or as separate entities within a broadly defined region. Evidence of at least two body representations in SII, located in zones of distinct intracortical connections, favors the idea of separate functional entities in this area.

For tactile shape processing in humans, a strongly hierarchical system has been proposed in which discrimination of an object's shape relies on a progressively finer selectivity of features in going from SI to areas of frontal and parietal cortex. By this scheme, activity in SI would serve as a very coarse filter for the possible shapes that could stimulate a hand whereas neurons in other areas, selective for more complex features, would encode a more restricted range of shapes in their response. Considerable data show, however, that many aspects of distinguishing one stimulus from another are found in the response of neurons distributed across several areas. Crosstalk in the connections among areas of somatosensory cortex certainly supports the idea of a distributed network. Perhaps a maturing view of somatosensory and related motor areas is that each participates in a variety of tasks and together form functional ensembles that are neither strictly parallel nor arranged in a clear hierarchy.

Summary

Over the course of the past few decades the early concepts of somatosensory system function and organization have been challenged, only to be reaffirmed by further work. Thus, the specificity of function that begins with the several classes of peripheral receptor had been challenged by ideas that in the firing rate and pattern of a neuron existed critical information about modality. Those challenges have been largely refuted, and the concept of labeled lines beginning in the periphery and continuing centrally has been established more firmly. Similarly, the broad division of the somatosensory system into lemniscal and anterolateral groups remains as one of the earliest appreciated and most clearly documented functional divisions of a sensory system into parallel paths. Perhaps the greatest single advance has come from

the application of simultaneous psychophysical and neurophysiological approaches of studying somatic sensation in alert, trained monkeys. By that approach the contribution of single neurons to the perception of form and texture has been demonstrated and the dynamic processing of tactile information has been accented. It is the latter, dynamic aspects of somatosensory function, where the future of somatosensory research lies. From studies of rearrangements in somatotopy following peripheral manipulations to those documenting the role of attention on the response properties of neurons, the static image of the somatosensory system is being replaced by one in which the context of a stimulus is a key component of a neuron's response.

References

Apkarian, A. V. (1995). Functional imaging of pain: New insights regarding the role of the cerebral cortex in human pain perception. *Semin. Neurobiol.* **7**, 279–293.

Bodegård, A., Geyer, S., Grefkes, C., Zilles, K., and Roland, P. E. (2001). Hierarchical processing of tactile shape in human brain. *Neuron* **31**, 317–328.

Campbell, J. N., Raja, S. N., Cohen, R. H., Manning, D. C, Khan, A. A, and Meyer, R. A. (1989). Peripheral neural mechanisms of nociception. *In* "Textbook of Pain" (P. D. Wall and R. Melzack eds.), p 22–45. Churchill Livingstone, New York.

Caterina, M. J., Julius, D. (2001). The vanilloid receptor: A molecular gateway to the pain pathway. *Annu. Rev. Neurosci.* **24**, 487–518.

Craig, A. D. (1995). Pain, temperature and the sense of the body. *In* "Somethesis and the Neurobiology of Somatosensory Cortex" (O. Franzen, ed.). Birkhauser, Boston.

Darian-Smith, I. (1984). The sense of touch: Performance and peripheral neural processes. *In* "Handbook of Physiology," Vol. 3, pp. 739–788.

Darian-Smith, I. (1984). Thermal sensibility. *In* "Handbook of Physiology," Vol. 3, p. 879–913.

Fitzgerald, M. (1989). Peripheral neural mechanisms of nociception. *In* "Textbook of Pain" (P. D. Wall and R. Melzack, eds.), p. 46–62. Churchill Livingstone, New York,

Hoffbauer, R. K., Rainville, P., Duncan, G. H., Bushnell, M. C. (2001). Cortical representation of the sensory dimension of pain. *J. Neurophysiol.* **86**, 402–411.

Jessell, M., and Dodd, J. (1989). Peripheral neural mechanisms of nociception. *In* "Textbook of Pain" (P. D. Wall and R. Melzack, eds.), pp. 82–101. Churchill Livingstone, New York

Jones, E. G. (1984). The Thalamus. Plenum Press, New York.

Kaas, J. H. (2000). The reorganization of somatosensory and motor cortex after peripheral nerve or spinal cord injury in primates. *Prog. Brain Res.* **125**, 173–179.

Melzack, R., Casey, K. L. (1968). Sensory, motivational and central control determinants of pain: A new conceptual model. *In* "The Skin Senses," (D. R., Kenshalo, ed., pp. 423–443) Thomas, Springfield, IL.

Shoham, D., and Grinvald, A. (2001). The cortical representation of the hand in macaque and human area S-I: High resolution optical imaging. *J. Neurosci.* **21**, 6820–6835.

Timmerman, L., Ploner, M., Haucke, K., Schmitz, F., Baltissen, R., and Schnitzler, A. (2001). Differential coding of pain intensity in the human primary and secondary somatosensory cortex. *J. Neurophysiol.* **86**, 1499–1503.

Vallbo, A. B. (1995). Single-afferent neurons and somatic sensation in humans. *In* "The Cognitive Neurosciences" (M. S. Gazzaniga, ed.), pp. 237–252. MIT Press, Cambridge, MA.

Wall, J. T. (1988). *Trends Neurosci.* **11**, 549–557.

Willis, W. D. (1989). Peripheral neural mechanisms of nociception. *In* "Textbook of Pain" (P. D. Wall and R. Melzack, eds.), pp. 112–127. Churchill Livingstone, New York.

Zelena, J (1994). Nerves and Mechanoreceptors. Chapman Hall, London 355 pp.

Zhang, H. Q., Murray, G. M., Coleman, G. T., Turman, A. B., Zhang, S. P., and M. J. Rowe (2001). Functional characteristics of the parallel SI- and SII-projecting neurons of the thalamic ventral posterior nucleus in the marmoset. *J. Neurophysiol.* **85**, 1805–18222.

Millan, M. J. (1999). The induction of pain: An integrative review. *Prog. Neurobiol.* **57**, 1–164.

Mountcastle, V. B. (1984). Central nervous mechanisms in mechanoreceptive sensibility. *In* "Handbook of Physiology," Vol. 3, pp. 789–878.

Perl, E. R. (1984). Pain and nociception. *In* "Handbook of Physiology," Vol. 3, pp. 915–975.

Romo, R., and Salinas, R. (2001). Touch and go: Decision-making mechanisms in somatosensation. *Annu. Rev. Neurosci.* **24**, 107–137.

Wall, P. D. (1989). Peripheral neural mechanisms of nociception. *In* "Textbook of Pain" (P. D. Wall and R. Melzack, eds.), pp. 102–111, Churchill Livingstone, New York.

Suggested Readings

Dubner, R., and Bennett, G. J. (1983). Spinal and trigeminal mechanisms of nociception. *Annu. Rev. Neurosci.* **6**, 381–418.

Stewart H. Hendry and Steven S. Hsiao

CHAPTER

26

Audition

The auditory system detects sound and uses acoustic cues to identify and locate sounds in the environment. The auditory system shares functional and evolutionary similarities with other mechanoreceptive systems, such as the vestibular system and the lateral line system of lower vertebrates. All of these systems use the same type of receptor cell—the hair cell—and all are specialized to detect an external stimulus that eventually causes the stereocilia of the hair cells to be displaced. Unlike other mechanoreceptive systems, the auditory system is sensitive to sound. This chapter explores the characteristics of the auditory system that make it sensitive to sound and that make it sensitive to the location of a sound source. The generalized mammalian auditory system is emphasized, but examples are also taken from studies of animals with specialized auditory systems, such as those of bats and owls, which have advanced our knowledge of audition greatly.

A major difference between the auditory system and other sensory systems is the fast time scale on which the auditory system works. Sounds are oscillations of air pressure that vary rapidly with time, often thousands of oscillations per second (Fig. 26.1). These oscillations are mimicked by the receptor potentials of the hair cells and are then transformed into a spike code by the auditory nerve and transmitted to the brain. Within the brain, specialized auditory neurons extract information from the spike code. Such information can, for example, determine that a sound source is located to one side of the head using interaural time differences as small as 10 µs. This impressive time sensitivity is mentioned often in this chapter and is a unique characteristic of the auditory system.

AMPLITUDE AND FREQUENCY RANGES OF HEARING

Sound is quantified by specifying its amplitude and frequency content (Fig. 26.1) (reviewed by Geisler, 1998). Amplitude of sound pressure is usually specified by a scale of sound pressure level (SPL, in decibels or dB), which logarithmically compresses the huge differences between the pressures that are just audible and those that are very loud. The range of levels over which hearing is possible begins at about 0 dB, the threshold of human hearing in the most sensitive frequency range. As an example of the exquisite sensitivity of hearing, at 0 dB, the amplitude of air particle movements are about 0.01 nm in extent! The upper limit of hearing is about 120 dB, where sounds cause damage to the ear, and where a sensation called auditory feeling or pain begins.

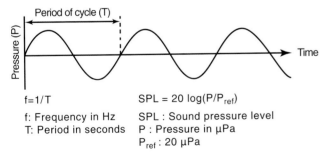

FIGURE 26.1 Sound pressure as a function of time for the sinusoidal pressure of a pure tone. The two important characteristics of this sound are its frequency (f, in Hz) and its sound pressure level (SPL, in dB). As shown, frequency is the reciprocal of the period of the cycle. Periods of sound waves in the audible range are very fast: the period of a 1000 Hz tone is 1 ms. SPL is a logarithmic function of acoustic pressure and is related to sound pressure by the equation shown.

Sound frequency is the number of oscillations of air pressure per second, measured in Hertz (Fig. 26.1). Humans are sensitive to frequencies from about 20 to 20,000 Hz, with the most sensitive range being 1000 to 4000 Hz (1 to 4 kHz). Most energy in human speech is between about 0.25 and 3 kHz. Smaller animals have frequency ranges that are higher than humans. For instance, mice and bats are able to hear sound frequencies higher than 50 kHz at the expense of relatively poor sensitivity at low frequencies. Although auditory experiments often use pure tone stimuli that contain a single frequency (Fig. 26.1), most naturally occurring stimuli are complex and contain a multitude of frequencies, each having a different amplitude and time course. Complicated stimuli can be broken down into their simple components by Fourier analysis. Because of nonlinear behavior of the auditory system, however, its responses to a complex stimulus are not always predictable from the sum of the responses to its individual components.

EXTERNAL AND MIDDLE EAR

The peripheral auditory system is divided into the external, middle, and inner ears (Fig. 26.2). The external ear is composed of the pinna and external auditory canal. These structures convey sound to the middle ear, but not without influencing it. This influence emphasizes and de-emphasizes certain sound frequencies, resulting in peaks and notches in the sound spectrum. Because positions of the peaks and notches depend on the location of the sound source, they provide information about location, even when using only one ear (monaural sound localization). Such information may be especially important for determining the elevation of a sound source because spectral peaks and notches are one of the few cues that depend strongly on the elevation of a sound source

Mechanosensitive organs in lower vertebrates, such as the lateral line of fish, are sensitive to

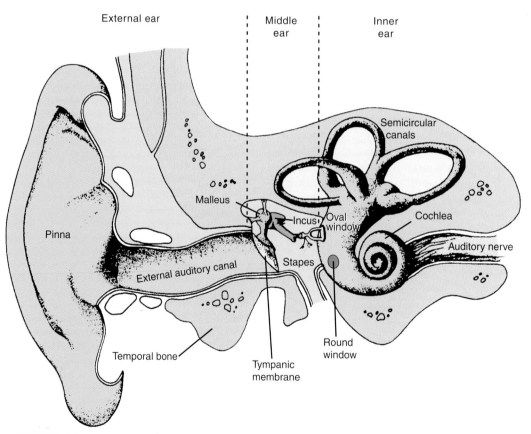

FIGURE 26.2 Drawing of the auditory periphery within the human head. The external ear (pinna and external auditory canal) and the middle ear (tympanic membrane or eardrum, and the three middle ear ossicles: malleus, incus, and stapes) are indicated . Also shown is the inner ear, which includes the cochlea of the auditory system and the semicircular canals of the vestibular system. There are two cochlear windows: oval and round. The oval window is the window through which the stapes conveys sound vibrations to the inner ear fluids. From Lindsey and Norman (1972).

vibrations in aquatic environments. When vertebrates evolved onto land, they faced the problem of converting sound in air to sound in fluid, as the inner ear of vertebrates remains fluid filled. Sound at an air–fluid interface is almost completely reflected back into the air, rather than being transmitted into the fluid. The function of the middle ear is to ensure efficient transmission of sound from air into the fluid of the inner ear (reviewed by Geisler, 1998). The middle ear begins at the tympanic membrane (eardrum), continues with the three middle ear ossicles (malleus, incus, and stapes), and ends at the footplate of the stapes, which contacts the inner ear fluids at the oval window of the cochlea (Fig. 26.2). The middle ear also has air spaces and two middle ear muscles. There are several ways in which the middle ear increases the transmission of sound into the inner ear. Most importantly, because the area of the eardrum is larger (by about 35 times) than the area of the stapes footplate, there is a corresponding increase in pressure from the eardrum to the stapes footplate. Additionally, there may be small contributions from a lever action of the ossicles and a buckling motion of the tympanic membrane, both increasing the force applied to the footplate. Together, these mechanisms provide a pressure gain of about 25 to 30 dB in the middle frequencies over what would be achieved by sound striking the oval window directly. This amount of gain means that for middle frequencies, most of the acoustic energy that strikes the eardrum is transmitted into the middle ear. For lower and higher frequencies, however, energy is lost. When sound conduction through the middle ear is compromised, a patient has a conductive hearing loss. One disease that causes a conductive hearing loss is otosclerosis, in which bony growths around the stapes cause it to adhere to surrounding bone and lessen its transmission of vibration. A surgical procedure called a stapedectomy usually restores hearing by replacing the native stapes with a prosthetic one.

THE COCHLEA

The inner ear is located deep within the head (Fig. 26.2). The inner ear contains the cochlea, which is the sensory endorgan for the auditory system. It also contains the utricle, saccule, and cristae of the three semicircular canals, which are the sensory endorgans for the vestibular system (see Chapter 33). The word cochlea comes from the Greek word *kokhlias*, meaning "snail," as the cochlea is coiled like the shell of a snail. In most species, the long spiraled tube of the cochlea has two to four turns, which are visible in cross-section (Fig. 26.3A). The sensory organ, the

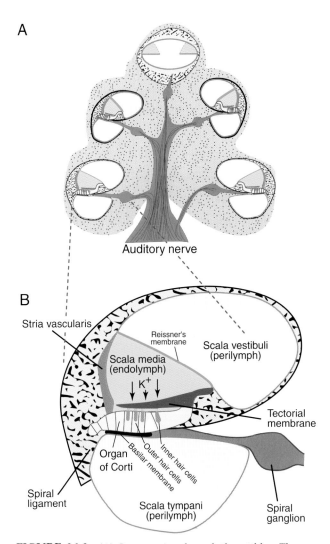

FIGURE 26.3 (A) Cross section through the cochlea. The cross section shows that there are approximately three turns in this human cochlea and that they spiral around a central core (modiolus) that contains the auditory nerve. (B) Cross section through one cochlear turn to illustrate important cell groups (organ of Corti, spiral ligament, stria vascularis, and spiral ganglion) and the main fluid compartments [scala vestibuli, scala media (shaded orange), and scala tympani]. Within the organ of Corti, sensory cells (inner and outer hair cells) are shaded dark blue and are situated between the basilar and tectorial membranes, which move when sound stimulates the cochlea. When these membranes cause motion of the stereocilia of the hair cell, the receptor current, a potassium (K^+) current, flows into the hair cells from the endolymph. The high K^+ concentration and high electrical potential of the endolymph are created by the stria vascularis, and these factors increase the driving force for the receptor current. Supporting cells in the organ of Corti are shaded light blue; these cells form a network that is coupled by gap junctions and may recycle K^+ back to the stria vascularis. Also shown is the spiral ganglion, which contains cell bodies of the auditory nerve fibers.

organ of Corti, contains the receptor cells (hair cells) and supporting cells. The organ of Corti rests on the basilar membrane and is covered by the tectorial membrane (Fig. 26.3B). Hair cells are of two types:

inner hair cells and outer hair cells. Their names are derived from the position of the hair cells along the cochlear spiral: inner hair cells are located innermost along the spiral and outer hair cells are located outermost. There is one row of inner hair cells and usually three rows of outer hair cells. In the human cochlea, there are about 3500 inner hair cells and about 14,000 outer hair cells.

Outer Hair Cells Contribute to Auditory Sensitivity

Sound-induced vibrations of the middle ear are transmitted into the cochlear fluids and then to the basilar membrane and organ of Corti. Early experiments by Georg von Békésy determined that the pattern of basilar membrane motion was a traveling wave that begins at the base of the cochlea and pro-

ceeds apically. Furthermore, the pattern was different for different sound frequencies, with high frequencies causing maximal motion at the base of the cochlea and lower frequencies causing motion more apically. This difference is likely caused by the fact that the basilar membrane is narrower and stiffer at the base of the cochlea and becomes wider and less stiff at the apex. Modern methods (reviewed by Dallos *et al.*, 1996; Geisler, 1998) have determined that the motion of the basilar membrane is (1) extremely sensitive in that it responds at very low sound pressures and (2) very sharply tuned to sound frequency. This sensitivity and tuning are dependent on the health of the cochlea and are especially susceptible to injury of the outer hair cells. For instance, in experimental animals in which outer hair cells have been selectively lesioned with aminoglycoside antibiotics, the high sensitivity and sharp tuning disappear. Outer hair cells may contrib-

---

BOX 26.1

OTOACOUSTIC EMISSIONS

In 1978, David Kemp made a surprising discovery: the ear can sometimes *emit* sounds. These "otoacoustic emissions" are now the focus of much interest because basic researchers can use them to study the function of the ear and because clinicians can use them as tests of hearing. Emissions are almost always so low in level that they are inaudible unless the individual is in an exceptionally quiet environment. Thus, measurement of emissions requires a sensitive, low-noise microphone that is placed in the external ear canal. Many studies indicate that the cochlea (inner ear) is the source of emissions. Within the cochlea, the outer hair cells are likely to be the generators of emissions, as these cells are motile and probably generate movements of the basilar membrane and cochlear fluids via this motility. After these movements are generated, they travel in reverse of the normal pathway for sound into the inner ear: the emissions propagate from their point of generation along the basilar membrane to the oval window, then through the middle ear via the ossicles, and finally they move the tympanic membrane to result in airborne sound.

There are two main types of emissions—spontaneous and evoked—the latter are evoked in response to an externally presented sound. Spontaneous emissions are detected from the ears of about one-third of normal hearing humans, but these emissions are rare in laboratory animals. They are almost always pure tones.

Transient-evoked emissions are evoked by a short sound such as a click and appear several to tens of milliseconds later. These emissions were first called the "cochlear echo," but they are not a real echo because more energy appears in the emission than was present in the evoking sound. Distortion product-evoked emissions (Fig. 26.4) are evoked by two tones ("primaries" of frequencies f_1 and f_2) and occur at combinations of the primary frequencies (such as at frequency $2f_1–f_2$). The two primary tones each produce traveling waves along the basilar membrane, and a likely point of generation of the emission is where these waves overlap maximally.

Otoacoustic emissions can be used clinically as a screening tool in hearing tests, as subjects with sensory hearing losses greater that 30 dB typically lack emissions. Transient-evoked or distortion product-evoked emissions are used in such tests. Emission-based tests are especially valuable for individuals such as infants who are otherwise hard to test by conventional audiometry. Otoacoustic emissions only rarely are the cause of tinnitus, the sensation of ringing in one's ears. Most individuals who have tinnitus do not have emissions corresponding to the tinnitus. Thus, tinnitus arises by some other mechanism, almost certainly within the nervous system.

M. Christian Brown

ute to basilar membrane motion because they themselves can be motile. They shorten and lengthen when depolarized and hyperpolarized *in vitro* (reviewed in Chapter 23). *In vivo*, these cells are depolarized and hyperpolarized by the receptor potentials that they produce in response to sound. Their contribution to boost the response of the basilar membrane has led investigators to designate outer hair cells as a "cochlear amplifier" of basilar membrane motion. This amplification is a key functional role for outer hair cells. The motility and amplification of outer hair cells are the likely causes of sounds that are emitted by the ear, "otoacoustic emissions" (Box 26.1).

Hair cells transduce the mechanical energy of sound into electrical receptor potentials when hair cell stereocila are displaced (reviewed in Chapter 23 and Pickles, 1988; Dallos *et al.*, 1996). In the sound-stimulated cochlea, stereocilia are deflected when the tectorial membrane, which overlies the stereocilia, moves differently than the bodies of the hair cells in the organ of Corti on top of the basilar membrane. The tips of outer hair cell stereocilia may contact the tectorial membrane directly, whereas the tips of inner hair cell stereocila may end just beneath the tectorial membrane and be displaced by fluid movements caused by motion of the tectorial membrane. When stereocilia are displaced toward the taller rows of stereocilia, the cell is depolarized, which causes the hair cell to release an excitatory neurotransmitter. When stereocilia are displaced in the other direction, the cell is hyperpolarized and the release of transmitter is decreased. Although the identity of the transmitter is not known with certainty, it interacts with a receptor, likely to be one of the glutamate receptors, on the auditory nerve terminals. The terminals are then depolarized and generate impulses that are conducted to the brain.

Endolymph Increases Auditory Sensitivity

An increase in the sensitivity of hair cells is made possible by the unique composition of the inner ear fluids. Within the inner ear, fluids are contained in three compartments known as scalae: scala tympani, scala media, and scala vestibuli (Fig. 26.3B). These scalae extend in parallel along the length of the cochlea from the base to the apex. Scala tympani and scala vestibuli contain perilymph, which is high in Na^+ and low in K^+, similar to other extracellular fluids. Scala media contains endolymph, a specialized fluid with a low concentration of Na^+ and a high concentration of K^+ (about 160 mM). The endolymph is also unusual because it has a positive electrical potential (about 90 mV), observable even in the absence of sound. The high K^+ concentration and positive electrical potential of the endolymph are not found elsewhere in the body. The organ of Corti, which contains the hair cells, is located at the junction between endolymph and perilymph (Fig. 26.3B). Stereocilia are surrounded by endolymph, whereas the remainder of the hair cell is surrounded by perilymph. The endolymph increases the sensitivity of the hair cells because it increases the transduction current, a K^+ current that flows from the endolymph into the hair cells (Fig. 26.3B). The endolymph increases this current because (1) the high concentration of K^+ in endolymph forms a concentration gradient that favors K^+ flow into the cells and (2) the positive potential of the endolymph forms a large electrical gradient that also favors K^+ flow into the hair cells. Without the endolymph, these driving forces would decrease, the transduction current would decrease, and the sensitivity of hearing would decrease.

Once the chemical and electrical properties of the endolymph are established and sound stimulates the cochlea, K^+ flows into the hair cells with little energy expenditure by the hair cells, as K^+ is flowing down its electrochemical gradient. The K^+ leaves the hair cells through channels in their basal–lateral surfaces, again without energy expenditure by the hair cells, because of the low K^+ concentration in the perilymph surrounding the basal–lateral surfaces. In this cycle for K^+ flow, hair cells can be considered simply as "gates," turning on and off the flow of the transduction current when sound deflects the stereocilia (of course, this simple view overlooks important hair cell

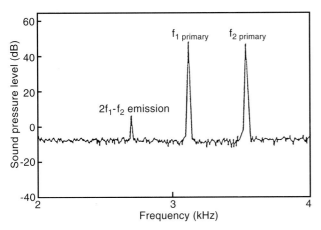

FIGURE 26.4 Distortion product otoacoustic emission from a human subject measured with a microphone placed in the ear canal. The microphone records the sound pressure of the two primary tones (frequencies f_1=3.164 kHz and f_2=3.828 kHz, each 50 dB SPL) that were used to evoke the emission and the emission at $2f_1$-f_2 (2.5 kHz at 12 dB SPL). From Lonsbury-Martin and Martin (1990).

processes, such as motility). The K$^+$ cycle depends on the electrochemical characteristics of the endolymph, which are generated by a tissue in the lateral edge of the cochlea, the stria vascularis (Fig. 26.3B). The marginal cells of the stria have a high concentration of Na$^+$,K$^+$-ATPase, an enzyme that probably helps in the accumulation of K$^+$ in the scala media and in the generation of the endolymphatic potential. The energy requirements for generation of the endolymph are placed on the stria vascularis, which has a high metabolic rate, is richly endowed with blood vessels, and is remote from the organ of Corti in the lateral part of the cochlea. This placement results in lower energy demands on the hair cells so that they do not require a high blood flow that might bring noise to the organ of Corti, interfering with sound reception. In fact, there are only a few blood vessels near the organ of Corti.

Sensorineural Hearing Loss Often Results from Damage to Hair Cells

Sensorineural hearing loss results from damage to hair cells or, less commonly, from damage to afferent nerve fibers (reviewed by Schuknecht, 1993). Hair cells can be destroyed by intense sounds, which can also damage stereocilia. Damaging sounds are generated by guns, jet engines, or personal stereos operated at high sound levels. Hair cell loss is permanent in the mammalian cochlea, but in the bird cochlea, hair cells are regenerated from nearby supporting cells (Corwin

---

BOX 26.2

COCHLEAR IMPLANTS

The cochlear implant is one of the most successful prostheses used to stimulate the nervous system (Tyler, 1993). The cochlear implant can provide partial restoration of hearing for individuals with sensorineural hearing loss. In sensorineural hearing loss, there is usually a partial or complete loss of the sensory cells (hair cells) in the inner ear (cochlea). Hair cells normally transduce the mechanical energy of sound into the electrical energy of receptor potentials. They synapse on primary auditory nerve fibers, which send information to the brain. Hair cells can be damaged irreversibly by intense sound, ototoxic drugs, or the aging process. Once lost, hair cells are not regenerated in mammals. Often, however, individuals with hair cell loss retain a significant complement of auditory nerve fibers. It is these fibers that are stimulated by the cochlear implant.

The cochlear implant consists of a microphone to record sound, an electronic "processor" that transforms the sound waveform into a code of electrical stimuli, and an array of stimulating electrodes in the cochlea. The electrode array (Fig. 26.5) is inserted through the round window into scala tympani where it lies close to the peripheral axons of primary auditory neurons. Usually, the implant consists of about a dozen electrodes that begin in the base and are spaced apically along the cochlear spiral. Those electrodes in the most basal regions are positioned to stimulate nerve fibers that originally responded to high frequencies and those in more apical regions are positioned to stimulate fibers that originally responded to lower frequencies.

In some individuals that have received implants, comprehension of speech is possible, even when there are no other cues such as lip reading. These individuals can carry on a normal conversation, even via telephone. In other individuals, however, full speech comprehension is not restored but the implant, together with lip-reading ability, assists with spoken conversation. It also provides for the detection of important sounds such as the ring of a telephone and the approach of a vehicle. Variability in the success of the implant from patient to patient probably depends on the number of surviving primary auditory neurons, the exact orientation of the electrodes with respect to the neurons, and the coding scheme of the processor that is used. The individual's motivation and the assistance received from clinicians are also likely to be important factors. Finally, individuals who have become deaf after the acquisition of spoken language reacquire language ability more easily than prelingually deafened individuals, almost certainly because of differences in the central nervous system. Cochlear implant research is focused on making improved designs for the processor and electrodes so that in the future implant users may be able to more fully comprehend speech.

M. Christian Brown

Reference

Tyler, R. S. (ed.) (1993) "Cochlear Implants: Audiological Foundations." Singular, San Diego.

and Cotanche, 1988). Damage from intense sounds can be minimized by (1) decreasing the duration of the sound exposure and (2) decreasing the level of the sound at the tympanic membrane (by wearing protectors such as earmuffs or earplugs). Hair cells can also be destroyed by chemical agents like aminoglycoside antibiotics (e.g., streptomycin, kanamycin). These agents block the transduction channels, but their mechanism of hair cell destruction is unknown. In individuals with sensorineural hearing loss, some hearing can be restored with a cochlear implant (Box 26.2).

Summary

Current research on the cochlea is centered on the mechanisms of outer hair cell motility and how this motility contributes to basilar membrane motion. The identity of the hair cell neurotransmitter remains an open question. Substantial interest focuses on the processes and factors involved in hair cell regeneration, with the eventual hope that regeneration can be encouraged to take place in mammalian cochleas. The improvement of cochlear implants is also a very active area of clinical research.

THE AUDITORY NERVE

Hair cells receive their afferent innervation from neurons of the spiral ganglion, located in the central core, or modiolus, of the cochlea (Figs. 26.3 and 26.5). These primary auditory neurons send peripheral axons to the hair cells and central axons into the brain by way of the auditory nerve, a subdivision of the

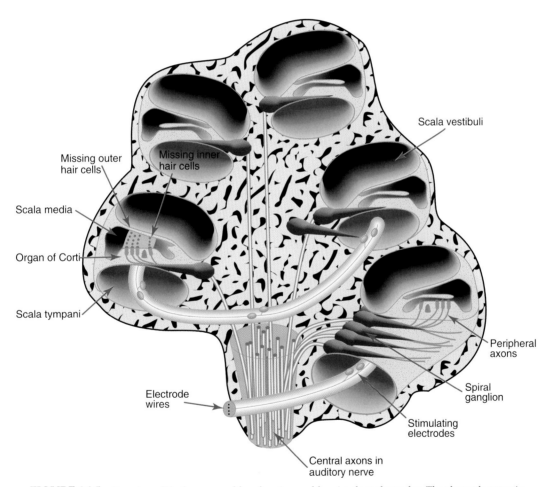

FIGURE 26.5 Drawing of the human cochlea showing cochlear implant electrodes. The electrode array is inserted through the round window of the cochlea into the fluid-filled space called scala tympani. It stimulates peripheral axons of the primary auditory neurons, which send messages via the auditory nerve into the brain. In the normal cochlea, frequency is mapped along the cochlear spiral, with the lowest frequencies at the apex of the cochlea (at the top of the figure). The different electrodes of the cochlear implant are designed to stimulate different groups of nerve fibers that originally responded to different frequencies, although because of spatial constraints the implant is not inserted all the way to the cochlear apex. From Loeb, (1985).

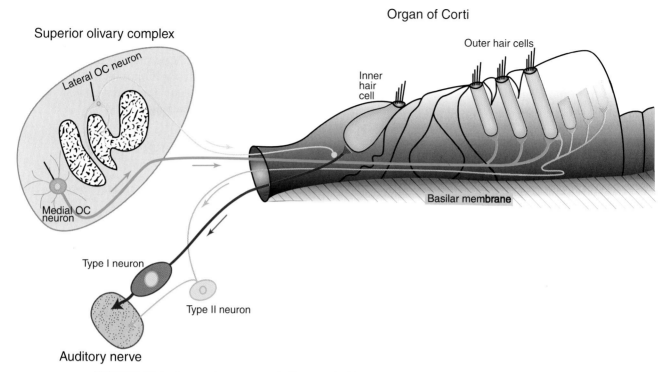

Superior olivary complex

Organ of Corti

Outer hair cells

Inner
hair
cell

Lateral OC neuron

Medial OC
neuron

Basilar membrane

Type I neuron

Type II neuron

Auditory nerve

FIGURE 26.6   Innervation patterns of afferent and efferent neurons in the organ of Corti. Afferent innervation is provided by ganglion cells of the spiral ganglion in the cochlea, which have central axons that form the auditory nerve. There are two types of afferent neurons: (1) type I neurons, which receive synapses from inner hair cells, and (2) type II neurons, which receive synapses from outer hair cells. The central axons of these ganglion cells form the auditory nerve. Efferent innervation is provided by a subgroup of neurons in the superior olivary complex that send axons to the cochlea and are hence called olivocochlear (OC) neurons. There are two types of OC neurons: (1) lateral OC neurons, which innervate type I dendrites near inner hair cells, and (2) medial OC neurons, which innervate outer hair cells. Lateral OC neurons are distributed mainly ipsilateral to the innervated cochlea, whereas medial OC neurons are distributed bilaterally to the innervated cochlea, with approximately two-thirds from the contralateral side (not illustrated) and one-third from the ipsilateral side of the brain. From Warr *et al.* (1986).

eighth cranial nerve. Two types of afferent neurons separately innervate the inner and outer hair cells (Fig. 26.6). The first type (the type I neuron) sends processes to contact inner hair cells, almost always contacting a single hair cell, whereas the second type (the type II neuron) sends processes to contact from 5 to 100 outer hair cells. Fibers from type I neurons are relatively large in diameter and myelinated; thus their information reaches the brain quickly, within a few tenths of a millisecond. Fibers from type II neurons are thin and unmyelinated and transmit information much more slowly. Both types of afferent fibers project centrally into the cochlear nucleus in the brain stem, with overlapping terminations in the main body of the nucleus, and additional type II projections into granule cell regions. Interestingly, type I neurons total about 95% of the afferent population (about 30,000 in humans), whereas type II neurons total only about 5%. Thus, outer hair cells, which number over three-quarters of the receptor cell population, are innervated by only a small minority of the afferent neurons. This innervation

plan strongly suggests that the functional role for inner hair cells and type I neurons is to serve as the main channel for sound-evoked information flow into the brain. The functional role for outer hair cells was mentioned earlier: to serve as the cochlear amplifier and enhance basilar membrane sensitivity and tuning and to increase the sensitivity of inner hair cell and type I responses. Thus, outer hair cells do make a large contribution to information sent to the brain, and this contribution is via the inner hair cells and type I neurons. Outer hair cells may also transmit information via their type II afferent neurons. What type of information these type II neurons transmit is unknown; their responses have not been determined due to the difficulty of recording from the small number of the thin type II fibers.

Responses Are Sharply Tuned to Frequency

Auditory nerve fibers respond to sound and transmit these responses to the brain via discrete action

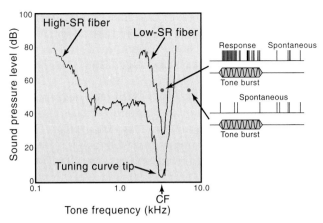

FIGURE 26.7 Tuning curves of two type I auditory nerve fibers. These curves plot the sound pressure level necessary to cause a response as a function of sound frequency. Within the tuning curve, the fiber responds to sound, whereas outside the tuning curve, there is only spontaneous firing (insets at right). The lowest point on the tuning curve is called the characteristic frequency (CF); it is the point of maximal sensitivity. The sharply tuned region near the CF is called the tuning curve tip. The sharp tuning and high sensitivity of this region are generated by the mechanical properties of the outer hair cells. Tuning curves from two fibers are shown, one from a high SR (spontaneous rate) fiber and another from a low SR fiber. As is typical, the high SR fiber has the highest sensitivity. From Kiang (1984).

labeling (Liberman, 1982). The distance to the point of innervation along the length of the cochlea is logarithmically related to fiber CF. Fibers with the lowest CFs innervate the apex of the cochlea, and fibers with progressively higher CFs innervate progressively more basal positions, as expected from the pattern of basilar membrane vibration. This precise mapping of frequency to position is known as tonotopic mapping. It is preserved as the auditory nerve projects centrally into the cochlear nucleus and for much of the central pathway. This observation strongly suggests that frequency is coded in the auditory pathway via a place code, with neurons at different places coding for different frequencies.

Phase Locking of Responses Is a Property of Auditory Nerve Fibers

Responses of auditory nerve fibers can show time-locked discharges at particular phases within the cycle of the sound waveform, a property known as phase locking (Fig. 26.8). Although locked to a particular phase, there is generally not a spike for every

potentials. The brain must extract information from these spikes and process this information to eventually form a percept of the sound that is heard. The information available to the brain via the auditory nerve is determined by which nerve fibers are responding and the rate and time pattern of the spikes in each fiber. The information sent to the brain via the auditory nerve has been studied extensively by recording the sound-evoked responses of single type I auditory nerve fibers (reviewed by Ruggero, 1992; Geisler, 1998). Graphs of minimum sound pressure level for a neural response are known as tuning curves (Fig. 26.7). The lowest point on the tuning curve is the characteristic frequency (CF). This is the frequency that evokes a response at the lowest sound pressure level; at CF, auditory nerve fibers can respond to sound levels as low as 0 dB in the most sensitive range of hearing. At low sound levels, the tuning curve is impressively narrow, indicating that the fiber responds only to a narrow band of frequencies near CF. This sharply tuned "tip" region (Fig. 26.7) is likely generated by the active motility of the outer hair cells. At high sound levels, the tuning curve becomes much wider, especially for frequencies below CF. This response to a broad range of frequencies likely reflects the passive mechanical characteristics of basilar membrane motion with little contribution from outer hair cells.

The relationship between CF and its point of innervation in a type I fiber has been studied by single unit

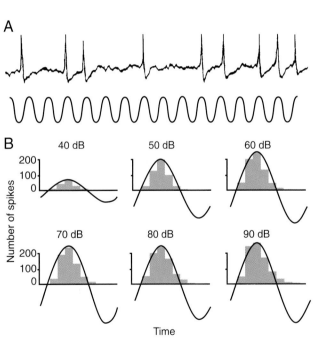

FIGURE 26.8 (A) Preferential firing of an auditory nerve fiber at a certain phase of the sound waveform. This pattern is called "phase locked," although the firing is not on every cycle of the waveform. Stimulus frequency was 0.3 kHz. (B) Histograms that quantify the time of firing plotted within one cycle of the sound waveform for many repeated cycles of the stimulus. Response of the fiber is phase locked at the moderate and high SPLs shown, even on this very fast time scale (time for one period was about 0.9 ms, given the stimulus frequency of 1.1 kHz). (A) From Evans (1975); (B) From Rose *et al.* (1971).

waveform peak. Phase locking in nerve fibers results from the fact that in inner hair cells, the AC component of the receptor potential mimics the sound waveform (see Chapter 23). Presumably, during each depolarization of the waveform, there is an increased probability of transmitter release to the auditory nerve, resulting in an increased probability of neural discharge during this phase. Phase locking decreases for frequencies above 1 to 3 kHz, mainly because of

the decline in AC receptor potential at high frequencies. For low frequencies, phase-locked information is carried by auditory nerve fibers to the brain stem. There, information may be extracted from these phase-locked patterns about the frequency of a sound. Such a temporal code for sound frequency may be important for low sound frequencies where phase locking is robust. It is less important for high frequencies where phase locking is diminished, and where coding for sound frequency is almost certainly via a place code.

Response Is a Function of Sound Level and Spontaneous Activity

The response of a single auditory nerve fiber increases with sound level until a point at which the rate of the fiber no longer increases and is saturated (Fig. 26.9A, solid line). The dynamic range over which the rate of most fibers increases is generally between 20 and 30 dB, with some fibers showing somewhat greater dynamic ranges. How then can the auditory nerve signal the large range in level of audible sound from 0 to 100 dB? First, it is likely that as the level of a tone increases, more and more fibers that are tuned to other CFs begin to respond, because tuning curves become broader at higher sound levels (Fig. 26.7). Second, auditory nerve fibers vary in their sensitivity to sound, and as sound level is increased, the less sensitive fibers begin to respond. Sensitivity of fibers at a given CF varies by as much as 70 dB. The sensi-

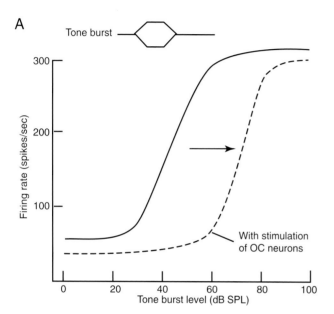

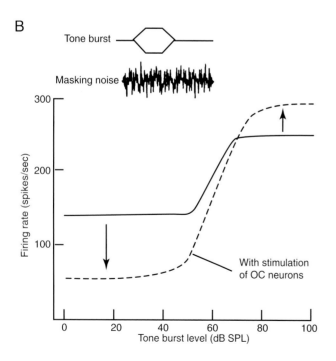

FIGURE 26.9 Rate level function for an auditory nerve fiber in response to tone bursts without (solid lines) and with (dashed lines) electrical stimulation of olivocochlear (OC) neurons. (A) With tone bursts alone, the discharge rate rises with sound level until it reaches a maximum and no longer increases (saturation). Stimulation of the OC neurons shifts the function to the right toward higher tone burst levels (arrow). This shift adjusts the dynamic range of the fiber so that it can signal changes in the tone burst level even for high sound levels; this is likely to be an important function of OC neurons. (B) When the tone bursts are accompanied by continuous masking noise (insets at top), the function in response to tone bursts is changed (solid curve). At low levels of tone bursts, the fiber has a significant firing rate because it is responding mainly to the noise. Even at high levels of tone bursts, the fiber is still responding to the noise in between tone bursts, which causes adaptation, and the fiber responds less to the tone burst than with tone bursts alone. In this case, stimulation of OC neurons (dashed line) decreases the response to the noise, thus decreasing the rate of the fiber at low levels of tone bursts (left arrow). Because the fiber is responding less to the noise, it is less adapted and has a greater response at high levels of the tone burst (right arrow). The fiber now has a greater ability to signal changes in level of the tone burst; this effect has been called "antimasking" and is likely to be another important function of the OC system. Adapted from Winslow and Sachs (1987).

tivity of response has been correlated with the rate of spontaneous firing, which is the rate of firing when there is no stimulus or when the stimulus is outside the tuning curve (Fig. 26.7). These spontaneous rates (SRs) vary from one fiber to another over the range of 0 to 100 spikes/s. Although there may be a continuum of SR, three main groups of fibers have been defined (low SR: <0.5 spikes/s; medium SR: 0.5 to 17.5 spikes/s; high SR: >17.5 spikes/s), and these groups predict many physiological and anatomical characteristics of auditory nerve fibers. The high SR fibers have higher sensitivities than medium and low SR fibers (Fig. 26.7). Low and medium SR fibers give off the largest number of terminals in the cochlear nucleus of the brain stem and preferentially innervate certain regions, such as the peripheral cap of small cells, suggesting that information carried by the different SR groups may be kept somewhat separate in the brain stem. Low SR fibers may be less sensitive, but they likely play important roles in detecting changes in sounds at high sound levels. Low SR fibers can signal changes at high sound levels because their low sensitivity causes them to respond mostly at higher sound levels and because they have less tendency to saturate, as their response often grows more slowly with sound level.

Masking Involves Adaptation and Suppression

The auditory nerve response to one stimulus may be masked, or hidden, by the presence of other stimuli. Masking involves properties of auditory nerve response such as adaptation and two-tone suppression, and possibly refractory properties. In adaptation, firing to a tone burst is high initially and then lessens, or adapts, to a steady state over time (Fig. 26.10). Adaptation probably takes place at the hair cell/nerve fiber synapse, as there is little adaptation in receptor potentials of hair cells for these short times (see Chapter 23). Because of adaptation to one stimulus, the fiber is less likely to respond to a second stimulus; i.e., the first stimulus masks the second stimulus. Masking by continuous noise changes the responses to tone bursts greatly. With tone bursts alone (Fig. 26.9A, solid line), there is a moderate dynamic range and a large difference in firing rate from low to high tone burst levels. With tone bursts in masking noise (Fig. 26.9B, solid line), there is a substantial rate at low tone burst levels because the fiber is now responding to the masking noise. At high tone burst levels, the rate is decreased because the fiber is adapted by the noise and is less likely to respond to the tone burst. Thus, with masking noise, there is much less difference in the rate of the fiber as a function of tone burst level as well as a lower dynamic range: these effects decrease the ability of the fiber to signal changes in the tone burst level.

An additional type of masking, referred to as suppressive masking, involves a phenomenon called two-tone suppression. In two-tone suppression, one tone lowers the response to a second tone even though the first tone does not excite the auditory nerve fiber. Two-tone suppression is present in the motion of the basilar membrane. It may help control the amount of gain provided by the cochlear amplifier, because as stimuli composed of several frequencies increase in sound level, two-tone suppression decreases the response of the nerve fiber so that it does not saturate. Whether there is adaptive masking or suppressive masking depends on the frequencies and levels of signals relative to the response area of the fiber. Masking is important in the auditory system because many auditory processes, such as speech comprehension, are affected greatly by maskers and because background or masking signals are common in many everyday situations.

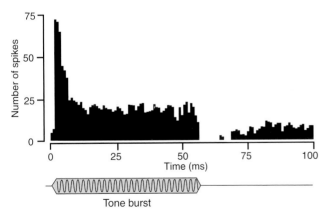

FIGURE 26.10 Poststimulus time (PST) histogram from an auditory nerve fiber in response to a tone burst (outline indicated below). A PST histogram is constructed by repeatedly presenting a stimulus while counting the number of action potentials that fall into bins of time during and after the stimulus. The histogram can be thought of as the probability of firing as a function of time. This function has an initial peak and then a decrease in firing (adaptation) during the burst. After the burst ends, spontaneous firing is lessened but then returns gradually.

Summary

Although the function of type I auditory fibers is fairly well understood, we do not yet know how afferent fibers of the outer hair cells, the type II auditory nerve fibers, function in the hearing process. Future experiments will provide insight into the roles played by different spontaneous rate groups of type I auditory nerve fibers. More work is needed to identify the mechanisms used to prevent the degradation of signals by masking noise. These mechanisms could potentially be applied clinically in the design of hearing aids and cochlear implants.

DESCENDING SYSTEMS TO THE PERIPHERY

Efferent neurons send information from the brain to the periphery. Three systems of efferent neurons send information to the auditory periphery: (1) olivocochlear efferents, which send fibers to the organ of Corti; (2) middle ear muscle motorneurons, which send fibers to the middle ear muscles; and (3) inner ear sympathetics, which send fibers to cochlear blood vessels and possibly other targets. Because little is known about the function of the sympathetics, they are not discussed. The other two systems are composed of neurons that originate in the brain stem and project to the periphery in order to control incoming information.

Olivocochlear Efferents Alter the Responses of Hair Cells and Nerve Fibers

Almost all hair cell systems have abundant efferent innervations of the sensory endorgans. The cochlear efferent neurons have cell bodies in the superior olivary complex of the brain stem and project to the cochlea and hence are called olivocochlear (OC) neurons (reviewed by Warr, 1992; Guinan, 1996). There are two groups of OC neurons—medial OC and lateral OC neurons (Fig. 26.6)—named according to the positions of their cell bodies in the superior olive. As for afferent fibers, olivocochlear fibers separately innervate the two types of hair cells in the base of the cochlea, although probably not in the apex. Medial OC neurons innervate outer hair cells, whereas lateral OC neurons innervate the inner hair cell region by synapsing on dendrites of type I auditory nerve fibers. Little is known about the lateral OC neurons, as their very thin axons are difficult to study; medial OC neurons are described below.

Activation of medial OC neurons by electrical stimulation causes them to release the neurotransmitter acetylcholine. At the outer hair cell, acetylcholine acts on a nicotinic receptor that allows Ca^{2+} influx, which then opens Ca^{2+}-activated K^+ channels, allowing K^+ efflux that hyperpolarizes the cell. Hyperpolarization probably reduces the electromotility of the outer hair cell, decreases basilar membrane motion, and reduces the responses of inner hair cells and auditory nerve fibers. These decreases shift responses of auditory nerve fibers to higher sound levels (Fig. 26.9A, dashed line). This shift means that sound levels that previously saturated the discharge rates are now within the increasing portion of the rate level curve of the fiber, so the fiber can now signal changes in sound level even at higher sound levels. Thus, one function of medial OC neurons may be to provide control of the gain of the auditory system to prevent saturation of responses. This function is accomplished via synapses on outer hair cells to control the gain of the cochlear amplifier.

Medial OC neurons may also reduce the effects of masking noise on the responses of auditory nerve fibers. Decreases in responses by maskers can occur by adaptation and suppression. The effect of OC stimulation on masked responses to tone bursts can be to *enhance* the response (Fig. 26.9B, dashed line). Responses at low tone burst levels are decreased because the response of the fiber to the noise is decreased (left arrow on Fig. 26.9B); responses at high tone burst levels are increased because there is less noise-induced adaptation and a greater response to the tone bursts (right arrow on Fig. 26.9B). The fiber now has a greater ability to signal changes in level of the tone burst; this effect has been called anti-masking and may be an important function of the OC system. An additional function of medial OC neurons may be to protect hair cells in the cochlea from damage due to intense sounds via their large synaptic endings.

The aforementioned functions for medial OC neurons (shifting the gain of the cochlear amplifier, anti-masking, and protecting the cochlea from damage) would require that the OC system have its most important effects at high levels of sound. Studies of OC neurons have shown that they do respond to sound, and in fact their responses are highest at high sound levels. Indeed, some OC neurons have rate level functions that show little tendency to saturate over large ranges of sound level. About two-thirds of OC neurons are best activated by sounds presented to the innervated ear, whereas the other third are best activated by sounds presented to the opposite ear. The OC reflex could thus be described as consensual because a stimulus applied to only one ear will evoke the reflex going to the contralateral as well as the ipsilateral side. An individual OC neuron has the opportunity to control information in a relatively restricted frequency band, as a single neuron projects to a restricted band of outer hair cells not more than an octave distance along the cochlea. The OC innervation of outer hair cells is mainly to the base and middle of the cochlea, where high and middle frequencies are represented.

Middle Ear Muscles Decrease Transmission through the Middle Ear

Two muscles are attached via tendons to the middle ear ossicles: the tensor tympani to the malleus and the stapedius to the stapes. The tensor tympani is innervated by motorneurons from the trigeminal or Vth cranial nerve, whereas the stapedius is innervated by motorneurons from the facial or VIIth cranial nerve. These muscles are abundantly innervated by motorneurons, receiving almost one motorneuron per muscle fiber. High ratios such as this are only found in other muscles where a high degree of control is necessary, such as the muscles that control the position of the eye. Like the OC reflex, the middle ear muscle reflex is consensual, with contractions in response to high-level sound in either ear and the largest contractions for binaural sound. Contractions of middle ear muscles decrease the transmission of sound through the middle ear. The effect is to decrease transmission broadly over all low frequencies (<1 kHz), where decreases are as much as 25 dB. This broad, low-frequency pattern is different from the effects of the OC system, which may be narrow and are mainly at high and middle frequencies. Functions of the middle ear muscles have been postulated mostly for the stapedius muscle. Like the OC system, the stapedius may prevent damage due to intense sounds and, by attenuating low frequencies, may prevent these frequencies from masking responses of high frequencies, thus improving speech discrimination in noise. The middle ear muscles may also decrease responses to self-generated stimuli such as speech because they contract during vocalization.

Summary

Auditory information from the ear is affected by efferent signals from the brain to the periphery. Most is known about medial olivocochlear (OC) neurons innervating the outer hair cells. Activation of these neurons shifts the response of the hair cells so that they operate at higher sound levels. Another function may be to allow discrimination of sounds that are masked by noise ("antimasking") and protect the cochlea from damage by intense sounds. Of course, the signal from OC neurons feeding back on the auditory system is generated by sound incident upon either the ipsilateral or the contralateral ear. The auditory system also enjoys the benefit of protection through the control of muscles attached to the middle ear ossicles. These muscles offer protection, as well as enhanced discrimination of sounds, through suppression of the subject's own vocalizations.

CENTRAL NERVOUS SYSTEM

Auditory Pathways Are Tonotopically Organized

The auditory nerve terminates centrally in the cochlear nucleus, which in turn projects to the other auditory nuclei of the brain stem: the superior olivary complex, nuclei of the lateral lemniscus, and inferior colliculus (Fig. 26.11). These multiple brain stem nuclei are important for determination of the location

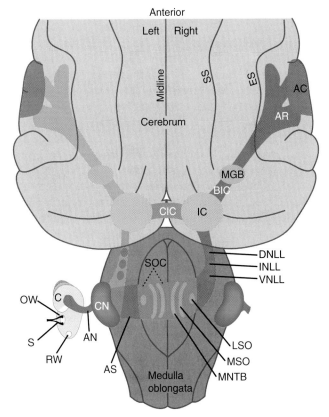

FIGURE 26.11 Simplified schematic of the pathways of the ascending auditory system of a generalized mammal. The pathway begins at the lower left with the inner ear and cochlea and ends at top right with the auditory cortex. The large band crossing the midline indicates that the bulk of the pathway is crossed by the level of the inferior colliculus. Some ipsilateral pathways and frequent commissural pathways explain the responses of some units at higher centers to ipsilateral sound. AC, auditory cortex; AN, auditory nerve; AR, auditory radiations; BIC, brachium of the inferior colliculus; C, cochlea; CIC, commisure of the inferior colliculus; CN, cochlear nucleus; DNLL, dorsal nucleus of the lateral lemniscus; ES, ectosylvian sulcus; IC, inferior colliculus; INLL; inferior nucleus of the lateral lemniscus; LSO, lateral superior olive; MGB, medial geniculate body; MNTB, medial nucleus of the trapezoid body; MSO, medial superior olive; OW, oval window; RW, round window; S, stapes; SOC, superior olivary complex; SS, suprasylvian sulcus; VNLL, ventral nucleus of the lateral lemniscus. From Kiang and Peake (1988).

of a sound source (see discussion later). The external location of a sound source is not represented directly along the receptor organ of the auditory system in contrast to other systems such as the somatosensory system, where position of a stimulus is mapped by sensory endings along the body surface. Instead, the cochlea maps frequency. Thus, locational information must then be determined by neural processing that compares interaural differences in responses; this processing is accomplished mainly in the brain stem. Above the brain stem, auditory information proceeds to the thalamus and cortex, analogous to other sensory systems. At these highest stages of the auditory pathway are the medial geniculate body of the thalamus and the auditory fields of cerebral cortex (Fig. 26.11). In addition to the ascending pathways shown in Fig. 26.11, descending systems link "higher" to "lower" centers in the auditory pathway. The functions of these descending systems have not been well explored, except for the olivocochlear and middle ear muscle systems (see earlier discussion).

An important characteristic of most central auditory nuclei is tonotopic organization, the mapping of neural CF onto position (reviewed by Webster *et al.*, 1992; Popper and Fay, 1995; Ehret and Romand, 1997). This tonotopy is established by the basilar membrane and is relayed into the central nervous system by the auditory nerve. Such inputs result in isofrequency laminae, sheets of tissue in which neurons have the same CF. These observations support a place code for sound frequency in much of the auditory central nervous system. This is especially true in higher nuclei because these neurons have a decreased ability to phase lock to the sound waveform, and thus a temporal code does not seem to be as robust. In most auditory nuclei there are not large overrepresentations of certain frequencies, although, as noted later, a given nucleus may be more devoted to low frequencies (e.g., medial superior olive) or to high frequencies (e.g., lateral superior olive). An important exception is the case of echolocating bats that use a constant frequency in their echolocating pulse; in these species, there is an over-representation of one of the constant frequencies. This over-representation begins in the cochlea and is preserved in the cortex (e.g., Fig. 26.20C). In these bats much cortical area is devoted to the constant frequency, analogous to the large somatosensory cortical areas devoted to important areas such as the hands and face.

Under certain conditions, tonotopic mappings have been shown to be capable of plastic changes (Robertson and Irvine, 1989; reviewed by Buonomano and Merzenich, 1998). After peripheral hearing loss, tonotopic mapping of the auditory cortex is altered such that a region that originally processed frequencies within the hearing loss begins to respond to adjacent frequencies. For instance, when the cochlea is damaged so that it no longer responds to high frequencies, the high frequency portion of the cortex does not stay unresponsive, but over time becomes responsive to middle frequencies where hearing is still normal. Plasticity is of interest to humans because of a common condition called presbycusis, which is hearing loss with advanced age. Presbycusis generally begins with a loss at high frequencies and spreads to lower frequencies with advancing age. While presbycusis is likely caused by peripheral changes, it may result in plastic changes in the central pathways that change the way sound is processed in the brain.

Units are Classified by their Responses to Sound

Classification by PST Histograms

The cochlear nucleus is the auditory center that is understood best at the cellular level (reviewed by Rhode and Greenberg, 1992). Cochlear nucleus neurons have been well classified both anatomically and physiologically, and structure–function correlations can be made between these classifications. Physiologically, excitation of cochlear nucleus neurons arises from their auditory nerve inputs. Single-unit recordings from cochlear nucleus neurons reveal that the auditory nerve spike pattern is changed to many new patterns. The patterns may be used to classify units on the basis of the shape of the poststimulus time (PST) histogram, which plots the spike pattern of the unit as a function of time for short-duration tone bursts. Unit types are called "pauser," "onset," "primary-like with notch," "chopper," and "primary-like" (Fig. 26.12). A correspondence has been established between these unit types and anatomical cell types of the cochlear nucleus. The correspondence was first suggested by the regional distributions of unit and cell types; e.g., there is a region of the cochlear nucleus in which one finds mostly "octopus" cells and from which mostly onset units are recorded. Direct correspondence has been made by single-unit labeling, in which a single unit is first classified physiologically according to PST type and subsequently injected with a neural tracer (e.g., horseradish peroxidase) that fills the neuron and its processes. The anatomical cell type can then be determined from postexperiment histology. These types of experiments are difficult and low yielding, but they firmly establish the structure–function correspondences, at least for neurons large enough to record and label *in vivo*.

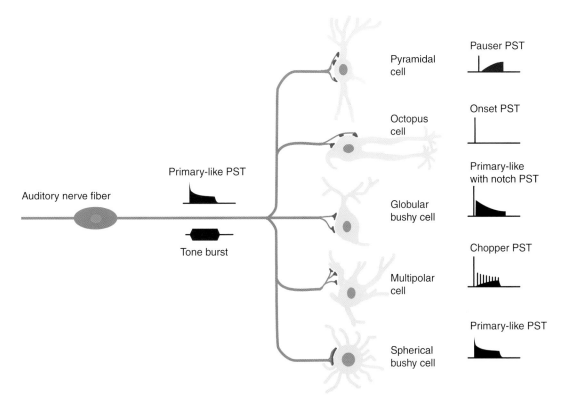

FIGURE 26.12 Schematic of the main anatomical cell types of the cochlear nucleus and their corresponding poststimulus time (PST) histograms. (Left) An auditory nerve fiber is shown with its typical response, a primary-like PST histogram (shown in Fig. 26.10). (Center) The auditory nerve fiber divides to innervate the main cochlear nucleus cell types. (Right) PST histograms corresponding to these cell types are shown. In their PST histograms, pauser units fire an initial spike and then have a distinct pause before a slow resumption of activity. Onset units fire mainly at the tone burst onset. Primary-like units get their name from the similarity of their PSTs to those of primary auditory nerve fibers, but the primary-like with notch type additionally has a brief notch following the initial spike. Chopper units have regular interspike intervals that result in regular peaks in the PST. Most of these patterns are very different from the primary-like PST and irregular interspike intervals of the auditory nerve fibers. For histograms, the sound stimulus is typically a 25-ms tone burst with frequency at the CF of the neuron and sound level at 30 dB above threshold. From Kiang (1975).

For instance, a major cell type in the ventral subdivision of the cochlear nucleus, "spherical bushy" cells, corresponds to a major unit type, the "primary-like" units (Fig. 26.12).

Use of PST histograms is helpful not only in classifying units, but also reveals functional properties of the neurons. Let us consider the example of primary-like units. The primary-like pattern reveals that the spherical bushy cell has faithfully preserved the temporal properties of the auditory nerve fiber response and implies that these units receive endbulbs from nerve fibers (see Box 26.3). In contrast, other types of cochlear nucleus neurons alter the spike patterns of the auditory nerve fibers and presumably have distinct functions. For instance, onset units respond mainly at the onset of a short tone burst (Fig. 26.12). One subclass of onset units can increase its response over a large range of SPL and might be involved in signaling sound level. Relative to mammals, tests of such hypotheses are easier in birds, where there is much more regional segregation of neurons by anatomical and physiological type in the cochlear nucleus. In birds, bushy cells are segregated in one region (nucleus magnocellularis), whereas other cell types, such as multipolar cells, are confined to a second region (nucleus angularis). The bushy cells in nucleus magnocellularis have excellent phase locking, but a poor dynamic range of response when sound level is increased. Multipolar neurons in nucleus angularis have complementary properties: poor phase locking, but excellent dynamic ranges. Overall, these results suggest that in the auditory system of diverse animal species there are separate neural pathways for time coding vs sound level coding as well as for other types of coding. Thus, the cochlear nucleus is the level where parallel pathways in the auditory system begin.

BOX 26.3

GIANT SYNAPTIC TERMINALS: ENDBULBS AND CALYCES

The largest synaptic terminals in the brain are contained in the central auditory pathway. There are two types of these giant synaptic terminals: (1) endbulbs of Held, which are found in the ventral cochlear nucleus (Fig. 26.13A), and (2) calyceal endings, which are found in the medial nucleus of the trapezoid body. Calyces are so large that it is possible to use patch electrodes to record and clamp the presynaptic terminal while simultaneously doing the same with their postsynaptic target in *in vitro* preparations (Forsythe, 1994). This type of study has given insight into presynaptic and postsynaptic regulation of transmitter release at this glutamatergic synapse.

Endbulbs and calyces enable secure transmission of information to their postsynaptic neurons. Endbulbs of Held are formed by primary auditory nerve fibers; each nerve fiber forms one or sometimes two endbulbs. The endbulbs contact and completely encircle their postsynaptic target, the spherical bushy cells of the cochlear nucleus (Fig. 26.13A). The endbulb probably forms hundreds of synapses directly onto the soma of the spherical bushy cell. In single-unit recordings near bushy cells, a metal microelectrode records a complex waveform that differs from recordings in other regions of the brain (Fig. 26.13B). The waveform consists of a prepotential followed about 0.5 ms later by a spike. The prepotential is likely from the presynaptic endbulb and the spike is from the postsynaptic bushy cell. The delay between the two events is the synaptic delay. This unusual synapse has several important properties. First, the prepotential is almost always followed by a spike, indicating that the discharge in the endbulb is securely followed by a discharge in the bushy cell. Second, the delay between the prepotential and the spike is almost always the same, indicating that the synapse has a low jitter, or variability in time (Fig. 26.13C).

The large influence of the endbulb would, for most neurons, last many milliseconds so that two closely spaced presynaptic spikes would produce only one postsynaptic spike or a second spike that was delayed, thus smearing in time the pattern of input spikes. However, the bushy cell membrane potential recovers quickly because its membrane contains specialized K$^+$ channels that allow the cell to repolarize after firing an impulse so it is "reset" and ready to fire again (Manis and Marx, 1991). The overall effect of endbulb–bushy cell specializations are to replicate the spike pattern of the auditory

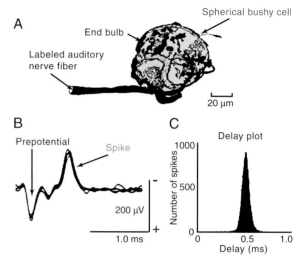

FIGURE 26.13 (A) Drawing of a labeled auditory nerve fiber forming an endbulb of Held that completely envelops a spherical bushy cell in the anteroventral cochlear nucleus. From Rouiller *et al.* (1986). (B) Superimposed waveforms recorded by an extracellular metal electrode in the anteroventral cochlear nucleus. The endbulb is such a large synaptic ending that it generates a prepotential, which is followed after a synaptic delay by the spike from the bushy cell. At this synapse, prepotentials are almost never seen unaccompanied by spikes, demonstrating the reliability of the synapse. From Pfeiffer (1966). (C) Histogram of the delay time between prepotential and spike. This represents the synaptic delay between endbulb and bushy cell. The delay of this synapse has an exceptionally low jitter in time. From Molnar and Pfeiffer (1968).

nerve fiber, producing a PST histogram and phase-locking pattern like that of an auditory nerve fiber. These characteristics are important because the end bulb–bushy cell synapse is the only central synapse in the pathway to the medial superior olivary nucleus, a nucleus where timing information from the two ears is compared in order to localize sound sources (Fig. 26.16A).

M. Christian Brown

References

Forsythe, I. D. (1994). Direct patch readings from identified presynaptic terminals mediating glutamatergic EPSCs in the rat CNS, *in vitro. J. Physiol.* **479**, 381–387.

Manis, P. B., and Marx , S. D. (1991). Outward currents in isolated ventral cochlear nucleus neurons. *J. Neurosci.* **11**, 2865–2880.

Classification by Response Map

Another important way to classify neurons in the cochlear nucleus, as well as throughout the auditory nervous system, is by the response map of a neuron (Fig. 26.14). Response maps are plotted on graphs of sound level vs frequency; like tuning curves, these maps show areas of excitation but they additionally show areas of inhibition. They are especially valuable where inhibitory influences play a role in shaping responses, such as in the dorsal subdivision of the cochlear nucleus, the inferior colliculus, and at higher stages of the auditory system. In the dorsal cochlear nucleus, five response types have been defined (Fig. 26.14). Type I neurons have excitatory tuning curves similar to those of the auditory nerve (Fig. 26.7) and have no inhibitory areas. Other response types have progressively larger inhibitory areas; e.g., type IV neurons have only a small excitatory area near CF and a narrow, knife-sharp excitatory area above CF, with the rest of their area dominated by inhibition. This inhibition is generated by inhibitory circuits within the dorsal cochlear nucleus, most likely from type II neurons. Type IV neurons correspond to the main projection neurons of the dorsal cochlear nucleus, the pyramidal neurons, whereas type II neurons are likely to be inhibitory interneurons. One hypothesis for the functional role of type IV neurons is that their sharp borders between excitatory and inhibitory areas serve to detect the spectral notches that result from the acoustic characteristics of the external ear, especially the pinna. These notches could be used for sound localization, as their frequencies depend on sound source location. The notches also depend on position of the pinna; in fact, type IV neurons receive input from brain stem somatosensory

nuclei that may inform the type IV neurons about the position of the animal's moveable pinna. Animals that lack a moveable pinna, such as humans and cetaceans (whales and porpoises), have a dorsal cochlear nucleus that differs greatly from that of other mammals by being unlayered and possibly lacking in several cell types (granule and cartwheel cells).

Classification by Laterality of Response: The Response to the Contralateral versus Ipsilateral Ear

A final important way to classify neurons is by their laterality of response, which is defined as whether the neuron responds to the contralateral or ipsilateral ear and whether the response is excitatory or inhibitory (reviewed by Irvine, 1986). Many neurons in central auditory nuclei above the cochlear nucleus are binaural and can be influenced by sound presented to either ear. A predominant pattern, however, is for the neuron to be excited by sound in the contralateral ear (the side opposite to where the neuron is located). The influence of the ipsilateral ear can be excitatory, inhibitory, or mixed. The contralateral response results from the fact that many central auditory pathways cross to the opposite side of the brain (Fig. 26.11). There are also uncrossed pathways; these pathways generate the response to the ipsilateral ear. Despite an influence of the ipsilateral ear, lesion studies indicate the functional importance of excitation from the contralateral ear. For instance, damage to the inferior colliculus or auditory cortex on one side decreases the ability to localize sounds on the opposite side. Thus, as in other sensory and in motor systems, one side of the brain is primarily concerned with function on the opposite side of the body.

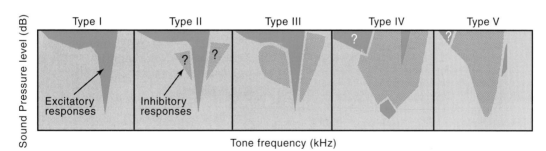

FIGURE 26.14 Unit classification by "response area." Shown are response areas for the five response types (types I–V) typically found in the cochlear nucleus. Response types are distinguished by the positions of their response areas: excitatory (green shading) and inhibitory (pink shading). Question marks show variable or uncertain areas. Type I neurons have excitatory response areas similar to the tuning curves of auditory nerve fibers. Type II neurons have similar excitatory areas and are inferred to have inhibitory flanking areas because they have little response to broad-band signals like noise. Type III neurons have similar excitatory areas and definite inhibitory areas on either side. Type IV neurons have a small excitatory area at low levels (near the characteristic frequency), as well as a knife-sharp excitatory area at higher frequencies. Inhibition dominates much of the remainder of their response area. Type V neurons are similar to type IV neurons but lack a low-level excitatory area. From Young (1984).

A   Interaural time differences

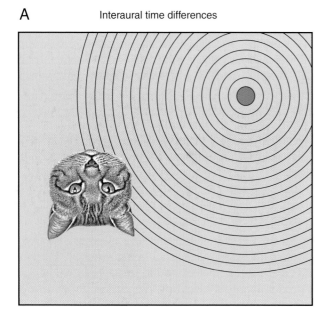

B   Interaural level differences

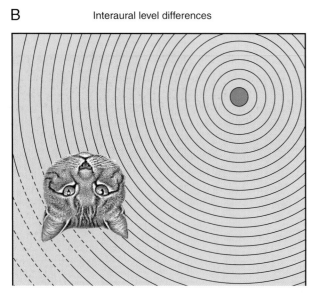

FIGURE 26.15   The two cues for binaural localization of sound. A sound source is shown as a solid dot to the right of the animal's head and sound waves are shown as concentric lines. (A) Interaural time differences result from the longer time it takes sound to travel from the source to the ear away from the source. (B) Interaural level differences result from the head forming a "sound shadow," reducing the level of sound at the ear away from the source.

The Auditory Brain Stem Uses Binaural Cues to Determine Sound Location

An important function of the auditory system is to determine the location of sound sources in space. Binaural sound localization occurs when cues from both ears are used to locate sounds (reviewed by Wightman and Kistler, 1993). This is the predominant type of localization for determining the azimuthal position of a sound source. Binaural localization uses two cues: interaural time differences (ITDs) and interaural level differences (ILDs) (Fig. 26.15). ITDs result because sound reaches the ear closest to the source sooner than the ear farther from the source (Fig. 26.15A). ITDs are a good cue for localization because they depend greatly on the azimuth of the source. For ongoing sounds, such as pure tones, they can be translated into phase differences in the sound waveforms at the two ears. These phase differences are useful at low frequencies, but become ambiguous for frequencies above about 1.5 kHz because by the time sound reaches the ear away from the source, the waveform has repeated by a cycle or more. Auditory neurons can phase lock to the sound waveform, as noted earlier. The decline in phase locking for frequencies above 1 to 3 kHz is a second reason that phase differences are less important for localizing sounds at high frequencies.

Interaural level differences (ILDs) result when the head forms a "sound shadow," reducing the level of sound at the ear away from the source (Fig. 26.15B). ILDs vary greatly with sound-source azimuth, but due to the directional characteristics of sound, ILDs are significantly large only at high frequencies and are much smaller at low frequencies. Thus, for sound localization at low frequencies (<1 kHz), ITDs are the major cues, but for localization at high frequencies (>3 kHz), ILDs are the major cues. For human performance using pure tones, the accuracy of azimuthal localization is good at low frequencies and at high frequencies, but somewhat less accurate at middle frequencies, perhaps because the cues are more ambiguous in this range. In psychophysical experiments in humans under optimal conditions, the minimum discriminable angle for localization of a sound source approaches one degree of azimuth. The physical cues corresponding to this angle are about 10 μs in ITD or 1 dB in ILD. When experiments are conducted with headphones to manipulate the ITDs and ILDs, such interaural differences are indeed discriminable in human subjects.

Mechanisms of Interaural Time Sensitivity

Two neural circuits that provide sensitivity to ITD or ILD are within the superior olivary complex (Fig. 26.16, Irvine, 1986; Yin and Chan, 1990). The neural mechanisms that generate sensitivity to ITDs are impressive given the small sizes of the differences. For instance, the central nervous system must be able to detect ITDs of 10 μs by comparing spikes coming in from the neural channels of the two sides that differ in time by 10 μs. However, 10 μs is less than the rise time of neural spikes, making the incoming spikes

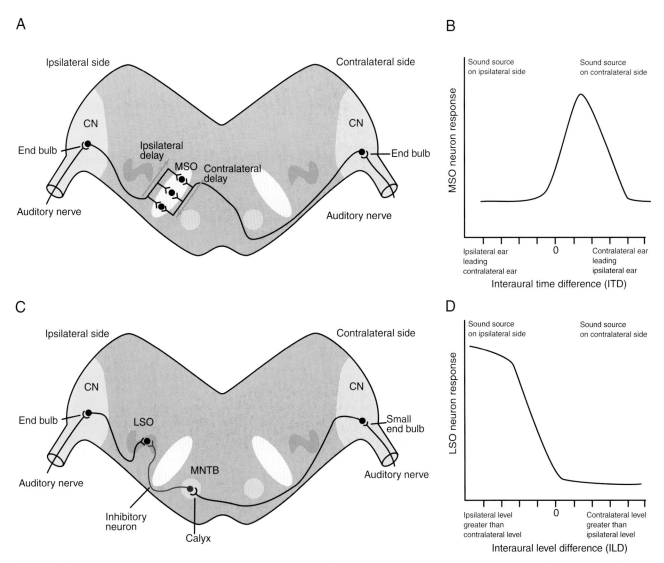

FIGURE 26.16 Innervation schematics and responses of two circuits in the lower brain stem that are important in binaural sound localization. Neuronal cell bodies are shown as dots, and fiber pathways are shown as lines; positions of large synaptic terminals (endbulbs and calyces) are indicated. (A) Circuit of the medial superior olive (MSO), which is sensitive to interaural time differences (ITD). Input to the cochlear nucleus (CN) from the auditory nerve terminates at the large endbulbs of Held that synapse onto spherical bushy cells (see Box 26.3). Bushy cells project bilaterally such that a single MSO receives input from both sides. Bushy cell inputs form delay lines such that ITD is mapped along the MSO. Data suggest that the delay line is oriented rostrocaudally and that only contralateral inputs are delayed. (B) Response of an MSO neuron as a function of ITD. Neurons within the MSO respond when spikes from their two inputs arrive at the same time. The response plotted is of a neuron in the lower part of the MSO drawn in part A; there is a large response when the ipsilateral input lags so that early contralateral input has time to proceed down the axonal delay line to reach the neuron at the same time as the lagging ipsilateral input. This type of lagging ipsilateral input would be produced by a sound source located on the contralateral side, as would be the case for a MSO on the left side of the animal shown in Fig. 26.15. (C) Circuit of the lateral superior olive (LSO), which is sensitive to interaural level differences (ILD). Excitatory input arises from the ipsilateral CN. Inhibitory input (red line) from the contralateral side is through the medial nucleus of the trapezoid body (MNTB), a nucleus of inhibitory neurons. The large synaptic ending in the MNTB is called a calyx (see Box 26.3). (D) Response of an LSO neuron as a function of ILD. There is a large response when sound is of higher level on the ipsilateral side and no response when sound is of higher level on the contralateral side. Thus, a response is produced by a sound source located on the ipsilateral side.

almost identical. The neural circuit that is sensitive to ITDs in the mammal is the medial superior olive (MSO) and its inputs (Fig. 26.16A); a similar circuit is present in birds in nucleus laminaris. The MSO inputs are from primary-like units (spherical bushy cells) of

left and right cochlear nuclei. These inputs preserve the phase-locking and timing characteristics of the auditory nerve because of the low jitter in the end bulb/bushy cell synapse (see Box 26.3). For a low frequency sound with an ITD, phase-locked spikes from

BOX 26.4

INTRAOPERATIVE NEUROPHYSIOLOGIC MONITORING

Intraoperative recordings of evoked potentials can provide early warning about surgically induced injuries to specific parts of the nervous system. Evoked potentials reflect function, and changes in function often occur before an injury becomes so severe that it results in permanent neurologic deficits. Such early warning can therefore make it possible for the surgeon to intervene and reverse an injury in time to avoid permanent neurologic deficits. The use of intraoperative monitoring can also often give surgeons an increased feeling of security because they know that the function of the parts of the nervous system that may be subject to surgical injuries are being monitored continuously. Sometimes intraoperative monitoring makes it possible to perform an operation in a shorter time. Intraoperative neurophysiologic recordings make it possible to monitor the function of specific neural systems continuously during an operation, which no other method offers. Imaging techniques, widely used for diagnostics, only provide information about structure, and present imaging techniques are not suitable for continuous monitoring in the operating room.

Brain stem auditory-evoked potentials (BAEP) and evoked potentials recorded directly from exposed structures of the auditory nervous system are now used routinely to monitor the auditory system in operations where the auditory nerve or other parts of the auditory system are at risk. Monitoring of auditory-evoked potentials can also make it possible to detect injuries to the brain stem from surgical manipulations before any other signs become manifest. Intraoperative neurophysiologic monitoring has helped decrease surgically-induced hearing deficits from injuries to the auditory nerve, and it has been an effective early warning for brain stem injuries.

The introduction of neurophysiologic methods in the neurosurgical operating room has opened the possibility for studies not previously possible. Thus, the ability to place recording electrodes directly on specific parts of the ascending auditory pathway during neurosurgical operations has provided a wealth of information about the auditory nervous system. It has specifically contributed to understanding how far-field auditory-evoked potential such as the BAEP are generated. Recordings of evoked potentials directly from exposed structures of the auditory nervous system have identified important differences between the human auditory system and that of animals used commonly in studies of the physiology of the auditory system. Intraoperative studies have also provided information about pathologies such as tinnitus and certain cochlear injuries that could not have been obtained in conventional studies in human or animals.

Aage R. Møller

From Møller, A. R. (1995). "Intraoperative Neurophysiologic Monitoring." Harwood Academic, Luxembourg.

---

one side will have a time difference relative to the other side. Phase-locked spikes will repeat this time difference many times during the many waveforms of a continuous sound. Neural delay lines that "make up" for this time difference are formed by axons for both contralateral and ipsilateral inputs, in the model originally proposed by Lloyd Jeffress (Fig. 26.16A) however, recent observations suggest that only contralateral inputs are delayed. An axon forms a delay line simply because it takes time for an impulse to travel along the axon. Within the MSO, neurons respond best when they receive coincident input from the two sides; thus a neuron in the middle of the drawing of the MSO in Fig. 26.16A would respond best if the delays were about equal. A neuron at the bottom of the drawing has a long contralateral axonal delay that makes up for stimuli coming in later from the ipsilateral side. Thus, this neuron would respond best if the sound to the con-

tralateral ear were leading, which occurs for a sound source located on the contralateral side (Fig. 26.16B). Medial superior olive neurons are thus tuned to a particular ITD and respond less to other ITDs. There appears to be a mapping of best ITD along the anterior–posterior dimension, with neurons sensitive to zero ITD located anteriorly and those sensitive to greater lead of the contralateral stimulus located more posteriorly. Thus, MSO neurons on one side respond mainly to sound sources located on the contralateral side of the head. As mentioned earlier, ITDs are most important for sound localization at low frequencies and the MSO has a tonotopic organization that is composed predominantly of neurons with low characteristic frequencies. In fact, the MSO is small or nonexistent in animals that hear poorly at low frequencies, and these animals are usually unable to localize low frequency sounds.

Mechanisms of Interaural Level Sensitivity

A second neural circuit in the brain stem, within the lateral superior olive (LSO), generates responses that are sensitive to ILDs (Fig. 26.16C). Input to the LSO from the ipsilateral side is excitatory by way of spherical bushy cells of the cochlear nucleus. Input from the contralateral side is inhibitory. This input originates from globular bushy cells of the cochlear nucleus and synapses by way of giant calyceal endings on neurons in the medial nucleus of the trapezoid body (MNTB, Fig. 26.16C). Many of the neurons in the medial nucleus of the trapezoid body are inhibitory and use the neurotransmitter glycine, which is a common inhibitory transmitter throughout the auditory brain stem. These inhibitory neurons then project to the LSO. Because of these inputs, LSO neurons compare the difference in levels of the sound at the two ears: they are excited when sound in the ipsilateral ear is of higher level, but are inhibited when sound in the contralateral ear is of higher level (Fig. 26.16D). When the sound is of equal level in the two ears, the strong contralateral inhibition usually dominates and there is little response. These neurons are thus excited by sound sources located on the ipsilateral side of the head. As the lateral superior olive projects centrally, this ipsilateral-side response is transformed to a contralateral-side response by crossing to the inferior colliculus on the opposite side. (There is also an uncrossed projection, but it is inhibitory.) As mentioned earlier, ILDs are most important for sound localization at high frequencies and the LSO has a tonotopic organization that is composed predominantly of neurons with high characteristic frequencies.

Inferior Colliculus

Ascending input from lower brain stem centers converges at the inferior colliculus, which is an obligatory synaptic station for almost all ascending neurons. The inferior colliculus consists of several subdivisions, the best studied of which is the large, laminated, central nucleus. In the central nucleus, direct input from the cochlear nucleus interacts with binaurally responsive input from the MSO and LSO. Terminals from the MSO and LSO may have limited spatial overlap, however, as the central nucleus is organized tonotopically. Low CF input (including that from the MSO) projects to the dorsolateral part of the colliculus and high CF input (including that from the LSO) projects to the ventromedial part. Many low CF collicular neurons are sensitive to ITDs, like their MSO inputs, whereas many high CF collicular neurons are sensitive to ILDs, like their LSO inputs. Interestingly, large lesions of the superior olivary

complex do not completely disrupt ILD sensitivity in the colliculus; this is evidence that ILD sensitivity is created anew at levels above the LSO. ILD sensitivity may be created in part by the dorsal nucleus of the lateral lemniscus, a nucleus within the lateral lemniscus that sends a large inhibitory projection to the colliculus. ILD sensitivity may also be created anew by inhibitory mechanisms within the colliculus. Additional circuits for the generation of ITD sensitivity have not been identified, thus the colliculus appears to be sensitive to ITD because of its inputs from the MSO.

An important question is whether the colliculus uses its inputs to form a "space map"—a mapping of sound source location to position within the brain. Such a mapping has not been reported in the mammalian inferior colliculus, but it has been observed in the deep layers of the superior colliculus, where it is in register with a mapping of the visual field. These deep layers of the superior colliculus have sensorimotor functions concerning orientation movements of the head, eyes, and pinnae. Another auditory space map has been observed in the barn owl, which hunts for prey in darkness using acoustic cues (reviewed by Cohen and Knudsen, 1999). In the owl, the mapping has been observed within a nucleus homologous to the external nucleus of the inferior colliculus (nucleus mesencephalicus lateralis dorsalis). Here, spatial receptive fields of neurons are narrow in both azimuth and elevation. These receptive fields are arranged such that there is a mapping of sound source location within the brain. This mapping demonstrates that space maps do exist, but they do not appear to be a common feature of the auditory system of nonspecialized mammals.

The Medial Geniculate and Auditory Cortex are the Highest Stages of the Auditory Pathway

The medial geniculate and auditory cortex contain subdivisions that have clear tonotopic organization, as well as subdivisions with less obvious tonotopy (reviewed by Clarey et al., 1992; de Ribaupierre, 1996). For instance, in the cortex of the cat, there are four fields that have clear tonotopic mappings (fields AI, A, P, VP), but other fields that do not (Fig. 26.17). The tonotopic axis of field AI runs from high frequencies rostrally to low frequencies caudally; other adjacent fields (such as A) have mirror-image tonotopy (Fig. 26.17B). The major ascending pathway that connects tonotopic areas at the highest levels of the pathway begins in the central nucleus of the inferior colliculus, forms synapses in the laminated ventral

A

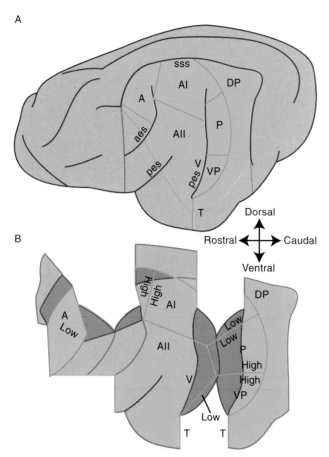

FIGURE 26.17 Auditory cortical fields in the temporal cortex of the cat. (A) Lateral view. (B) Lateral view that is "unfolded" to show the part of the fields that are normally hidden within the sulci (orange shading), as well as the high- and low-frequency limits of the tonotopic fields. The four tonotopic fields are the anterior (A), primary (AI), posterior (P), and ventroposterior (VP). Positions of the lowest and highest CFs in these fields are indicated in B. Note that at the boundaries of the tonotopic fields, the direction of tonotopy is reversed so that adjacent fields have "mirror-image" tonotopy. Other cortical fields have less rigidly organized tonotopy or little tonotopy. These fields are secondary (AII), ventral (V), temporal (T), and dorsoposterior (DP). Also indicated are suprasylvian sulcus (sss) and anterior and posterior ectosylvian sulci (aes, pes). From Imig and Reale (1980).

division of the geniculate and then continues to most of the tonotopic cortical fields. Other parallel pathways exist. A parallel pathway connecting less tonotopic areas begins in the dorsal cortex of the colliculus, forms synapses in the dorsal division of the medial geniculate and projects mainly to cortical field AII. Finally, a polysensory pathway begins in the external and dorsal nuclei of the colliculus and projects via the medial division of the geniculate to almost all the auditory cortical fields.

In general, the physiology of tonotopic areas has been explored better than that of other areas. Units from the tonotopic areas, such as the ventral division

of the geniculate and cortical field AI, tend to have short latencies and sharply tuned tuning curves. Neurons in areas with less obvious tonotopy tend to have longer latencies, broader tuning curves and responses that can habituate or stop responding after multiple presentations of the stimulus, especially in anesthetized preparations. In humans, the primary auditory cortex is located on Heschl's gyrus, which is on the superior surface of the temporal lobe (Fig. 26.11). Electrophysiological data have been obtained from this region in human patients undergoing surgery for epilepsy. In these regions, there are large evoked potentials in response to sound and auditory sensations are reported after electrical stimulation. In normal subjects, sound-evoked activation is seen in this region of the temporal cortex using imaging techniques such as positron emission tomography (PET) and functional magnetic resonance imaging (fMRI).

The medial geniculate exerts its influence on ascending information, but it does so with extensive influence from the cortex. The medial geniculate receives extensive projections from the auditory cortex: it probably receives more input from auditory cortex than from lower centers. One large projection is from the tonotopic cortical fields AI and A to the tonotopic ventral division of the medial geniculate. Apparently, however, the geniculate mediates some functions that do not require the cortex. For example, fear conditioning is a behavior that can be established by pairing a sound with a painful electric shock in rats. After conditioning is established, conditioned responses such as an increase in blood pressure can be elicited by sound alone. Work by Joseph LeDoux has shown that lesions of the auditory pathway up to and including the geniculate have a large effect on such conditioning; however, lesions of the auditory cortex do not produce large alterations. Pathways directly from the geniculate to the amygdala mediate such conditioned responses. Cortical neuron responses are also changed by conditioning; e.g., the pairing of an acoustic stimulus with a noxious stimulus greatly alters the response of cortical neurons. Such observations indicate that responses at these high levels of the auditory pathway are context dependent.

Cortical Columns

A fundamental feature of cortical organization is the cortical column, which is oriented normal to the cortical surface and runs across all six of the cortical layers. In the cortex, neurons within a column tend to have similar response characteristics. For instance, in the auditory cortex, neurons within a given column generally have similar CFs. Neurons also tend to have similar types of responses to binaural sounds; these binaural interaction characteristics are tested in preparations in which each ear is stimulated with a separate sound source. Usually one ear, the main ear, excites a cortical neuron; most often this ear is the contralateral ear. The effect of the opposite ear can be either to excite by itself or to facilitate the main ear response of the neuron (summation interaction) or to inhibit by itself or to suppress the main ear response (suppression interaction). Typically, either summation interactions or suppression interactions are found for neurons within a column. For the high CF part of AI, summation and suppression columns show some organization, although not nearly as rigid as a checkerboard pattern, with CF on one axis and alternating summation or suppression columns on the perpendicular axis. The binaural interaction classification is useful, but oversimplified, as some neurons can show both summation and suppression, depending on factors such as sound level. However, one finding that supports summation/ suppression columns as an organizational plan is the pattern of projections from a column in one hemisphere to the opposite cortical hemisphere. Neurons within a summation column tend to have large projections to the opposite hemisphere. Suppression columns tend to have few projections (with the exception of less common columns in which the contralateral ear is inhibitory and the ipsilateral ear is excitatory). These findings support binaural interaction characteristics as an important property of cortical columns.

Cortical Field AI and Sound Localization

Physiological studies suggest a role for cortical field AI in sound localization. In AI, many neurons are sensitive to interaural time and level differences, much as for neurons at lower stages of the pathway. When tested with a sound source in space, the response of many neurons depends on the azimuth of the source (Fig. 26.18). Of course, when a sound source in space is used, the receptive fields of cortical neurons will depend on the directional characteristics of the external ear, as well as neural mechanisms at all stages of the auditory pathway. As expected from the fact that auditory pathways are predominantly crossed, a large number of cortical neurons respond to sound sources centered on the contralateral side, although some are centered on the ipsilateral side. The receptive fields for many neurons occupy much of the azimuth on the contralateral side (Fig. 26.18A) and some have even wider fields that encompass both sides (omnidirectional fields). Other neurons, however, have receptive fields that are very narrow

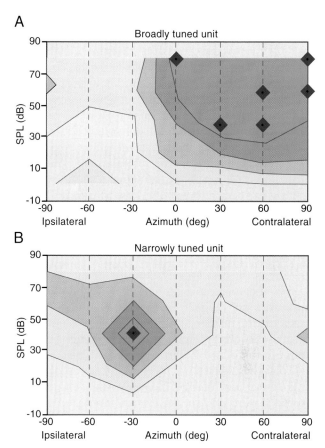

FIGURE 26.18 Receptive fields of two auditory cortex neurons plotted as a function of SPL and azimuth in the frontal hemifield. Noise bursts were used as stimuli. Small diamonds show points of maximal response, and progressively lighter shading shows regions of progressively smaller response. Zero degrees azimuth refers to directly ahead, and positive azimuths refer to points in the contralateral hemifield. From Clarey *et al.* (1994).

(Fig. 26.18B). Units within a given column tend to have receptive fields that are similar, probably because of the similar binaural interaction characteristics within a column. It is easy to imagine that neurons with summation characteristics would tend to have receptive fields that would be large and encompass both contralateral and ipsilateral sides because of their bilateral excitatory input. Units with suppression characteristics, however, would tend to have narrower fields located mainly on one side because they receive inhibitory input from the other side. Finally, the auditory cortex has not yet been shown to have an organized space map of a sound's position in external space onto a dimension within the cortex.

Behavioral studies also indicate a strong role of AI in sound localization (Jenkins and Merzenich, 1984). Cats with lesions of AI on one side have a deficit for localizing sounds on the contralateral side. Lesions of other fields that spare AI do not produce deficits.

Furthermore, the deficit is frequency specific: if the lesion is in areas of AI tuned to certain frequencies, the deficit is observed only for those frequencies. The deficit is most pronounced when the task is for a subject to move toward the sound source and is less obvious when the task is simply to lateralize the sound, i.e., to press a bar on the right or left side corresponding to the side of the sound source. This finding suggests that the simpler lateralization task is processed at a subcortical location, but the more difficult task of forming an image of a sound source's position in space and moving toward that position is processed at the cortex.

Coding of Sound Level

For auditory nerve fibers and for many other neurons in the auditory system, the firing rate of the neuron increases monotonically with sound level until saturation (Fig. 26.19, monotonic units). At high stages of the auditory pathway, however, more neurons are encountered with rate level functions that are nonmonotonic and have a prominent peak with a well-defined "best level" (Fig. 26.19, nonmonotonic units). For some neurons, the rate at high sound levels returns to zero and tuning curves can be "closed" at high sound levels rather than being open like auditory nerve fibers (Fig. 26.7). Nonmonotonic neurons can be seen in the dorsal subdivision of the cochlear nucleus and the inferior colliculus and are especially common in cortical field P. Such nonmonotonicities likely result from inhibitory influences, which, at higher stages of the auditory pathway, are often mediated by the inhibitory transmitter γ-aminobutyric acid

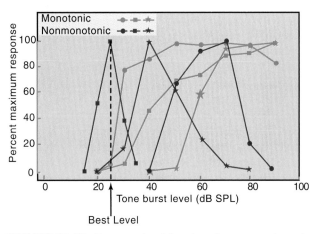

FIGURE 26.19 Response-level functions for neurons from the auditory cortex. Functions for three "monotonic" neurons (green curves) have an increasing response until saturation, whereas functions for three "nonmonotonic" neurons (red curves) have an increasing response until a certain intensity ("best level"), after which the response falls. From Phillips *et al.* (1985).

(GABA). Possibly because of these inhibitory influences, nonmonotonic units tend to have narrower response areas for sounds in space. For instance, the *y* axis of Fig. 26.18 plots the response of the neuron as a function of sound level. The broadly tuned unit (Fig. 26.18A) has a monotonic level function, whereas the narrowly tuned unit (Fig. 26.18B) has a nonmonotonic level function. Hypothetically, the best level could be an organizing principle for central auditory nuclei, but so far, organized mappings of best level have not been reported in most species, with the exception of echolocating bats.

Coding of Complex Signals in the Cortex

Animals emit a variety of vocal signals. These signals make possible a wide range of behaviors, including communication and even echolocation in bats (Box 26.5). Are there specific "call detectors" in the auditory cortices of these animals? This area is relatively unexplored; however, available evidence suggests that this type of detector may exist only rarely and that the response to vocalizations is probably represented by spatially dispersed, synchronized assemblies of cortical neurons rather than by individual neurons. However, cortical neurons do show selectivity to complex sounds such as noise bands and species-specific calls over what would be predicted from their pure tone frequency selectivity (Rauschecker *et al.*, 1995). For instance, a neuron that responds well to a particular type of call does not usually respond as well to the call played backward in time even though it has an identical frequency content. Similar results in response to speech stimuli have been found in recordings of units from auditory areas in the superior temporal gyrus of human patients undergoing surgery for epilepsy.

A number of studies using lesions of the auditory cortex indicate a strong role of the cortex in processing complex acoustic signals. After bilateral lesions of the auditory cortex, experimental animals cannot discriminate between different temporal patterns of sounds, such as a sequence in which the sound frequency pattern is a repeated "low–high–low" and a sequence in which the pattern is a repeated "high–low–high." In primates, lesions of the cortex impair discrimination of species-specific vocalizations. This impairment is more pronounced after lesion of the left cortex, indicating lateralization of processing of these vocalizations at the cortical level. Human speech is an especially complex acoustical signal; its intelligibility and production can be decreased greatly by a stroke that creates a lesion of the cortex in humans. Although there is great variability in the extent and effect of such lesions, language processing is most

BOX 26.5

BAT ECHOLOCATION

Bats offer unique opportunities for researchers studying the auditory system (reviewed by Popper and Fay, 1995). Echolocating bats emit high-frequency pulses of sound and use the return echoes to locate and capture their flying insect prey. These pulses are above the upper frequency limit of human hearing. They were discovered in the 1940s by Donald Griffin, who was then an undergraduate student at Harvard University. The echolocation performance of the bat is impressive: bats are adept enough to find a mosquito above a golf course at night. Indeed, Griffin demonstrated that bats can avoid wires as thin as 0.3 mm diameter while flying in a darkened room.

There are more than 800 species of echolocating bats, all within the suborder Microchiroptera. One of the best-studied bats is the mustached bat, *Pteronotus parnellii*. It emits echolocating pulses that have an initial part of constant frequency, followed by a part of decreasing frequency (frequency modulated). This bat is thus called a CF-FM bat (Fig. 26.20B). Some other species of bats emit only the FM portion and are called FM bats. Bats use differences between the emitted pulse and the returned echo to locate targets. Relative to the pulse, the returned echo is delayed because of the sound's round-trip travel time from the bat to the target. The delay between the pulse and echo can thus be used as a measure of target range. The echo can also be changed in frequency, or Doppler-shifted, because the bat is moving relative to the reflecting surface. Bats that are moving toward a reflecting surface will have an echo that is Doppler-shifted toward higher frequency. Most background surfaces will be Doppler shifted about the same. However, targets that are moving differently from the background will generate different Doppler shifts. For instance, a moth with moving wings will reflect an echo with a moving Doppler shift that is quite different from the stationary background. Such differences are presumably used by the CF-FM bat to locate moving targets. Insects are not always passive in the face of such predatory behavior.

For instance, some moths have good ultrasonic hearing and take evasive flight maneuvers when exposed to a bat's pulse.

Research on the auditory system of bats has been greatly aided by knowledge of the "relevant" stimulus, since much of the time the bat hears an emitted pulse followed a short time later by an echo. Pioneering work by Suga (1990) has demonstrated that the auditory cortex of the mustached bat contains many specialized areas (Fig. 26.20C). One large area (DSCF area) is devoted to processing the Doppler-shifted echo for the strongest harmonic of the pulse, near 60 kHz. These frequencies also have large representations throughout the bat's auditory system beginning at the cochlea. Within the DSCF area, there is a mapping of neuronal best level as well as characteristic frequency. In other cortical regions, there are neurons whose response properties cause them to detect various features of the pulse and echo. For instance, neurons in the FM-FM region respond preferentially to two FM pulses separated by a specific delay. The best delays for these neurons range from 0.4 to 18 ms, which would correspond to target ranges of 7 to 310 cm. Furthermore, these best delays are mapped along cortical distance. Work on the bat cortex has resulted in specific hypotheses about the function of most of their auditory cortical fields. Our state of knowledge of the cortical fields in other animals is by contrast much more primitive.

M. Christian Brown

References

Popper, A. N., and Fay, R. R. (eds.) (1992). "The Mammalian Auditory Pathway: Neurophysiology." Springer-Verlag, New York.

Suga, N. (1990). Biosonar and neural computation in bats. *Sci. Am.* June: 60–68.

interrupted by lesions of perisylvian cortex regions, especially in Wernicke's area and Broca's area (see Chapter 52). Wernicke's area is especially close to auditory cortex and can be considered an auditory association area. Lesions lateralized in the left hemisphere in right-handed individuals are most disruptive of speech comprehension and production. The lateralization of language processing in one hemisphere is a unique finding of asymmetry in brain

function, very different from the symmetry of subcortical nuclei and primary auditory cortical fields.

Imaging studies (PET, fMRI) in normal subjects suggest acoustic stimuli such as noise and modulated tones activate primary auditory cortical fields, but do not activate surrounding areas. These surrounding areas, including Wernicke's and Broca's areas, can be activated by speech stimuli. Furthermore, the activation by speech stimuli is usually lateralized to the

A

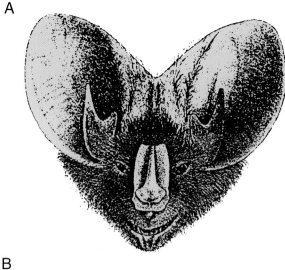

B

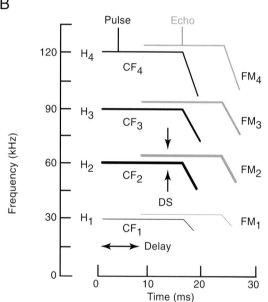

left hemisphere of right-handed individuals. Taken together, the lesion and imaging studies suggest a hierarchical pattern of cortical activation with simple stimuli being processed in the primary cortical fields and more complex stimuli, such as speech, processed in association areas that are lateralized in one hemisphere. Further imaging studies will be very useful in showing more specifically the functions of the auditory areas in the cortex.

Summary

Much about the central auditory pathways remains to be explored. Although these pathways are mapped tonotopically, whether there are other mappings in orthogonal dimensions is unknown. Much current research is focused on the plasticity of central auditory responses with auditory experience and after hearing loss and whether this plasticity is generally present at the many subcortical auditory centers. The fact that there are descending systems at many levels of the pathways is known, but research is necessary to show how these systems alter the processing of auditory information. Finally, the medial geniculate and auditory cortex are likely to play a role in sound localization, but the specifics of this role and their functions in many of the other hearing processes remain to be discovered.

C

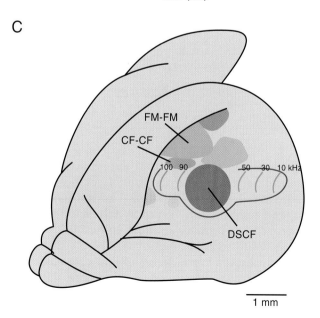

FIGURE 26.20 (A) Close-up view of an echolocating bat, *Megaderma lyra*. Like many echolocating bats, this bat has an enlarged nose leaf that probably focuses the echolocating pulse ahead. Also like many echolocating bats, this bat has enlarged external ears that make the bat more sensitive to echoes coming from ahead. From Griffin (1958). (B) Schematic of emitted pulse and returned echo of the mustached bat, *Pteronotus parnellii*. The emitted pulse consists of four harmonics (H_1–H_4), the strongest of which is H_2 at about 60 kHz. Each harmonic has an initial part of constant frequency (CF) and a later part of changing frequency (frequency modulation, FM). The echoes are returned after a travel time that causes a delay relative to the pulse. Additionally, if the target is moving relative to the bat, the echo is returned with a Doppler shift (DS) in frequency. (C) Dorsolateral view of the auditory cortex of the mustached bat showing several of the areas specialized for processing the echolocation signals. The primary auditory cortex, AI, is delineated by a red line and its isofrequency contours are indicated in kHz. It contains a region called the Doppler-shifted CF region (DSCF), which is a greatly expanded region devoted to the most prominent component of the Doppler-shifted echo (60 to 63 kHz). Other shaded regions contain neurons that are combination sensitive and respond to combinations of the pulse and echo, often at certain delays. Neurons that respond to pulse/echo CF portions are in the CF/CF region. Those that respond to pulse/echo FM portions are in the FM/FM region. From Fitzpatrick *et al.* (1993).

References

Buonomano, D. V., and Merzenich, M. M. (1998). Cortical plasticity: From synapses to maps. *Annu. Rev. Neurosci.* **21**, 149–186.

Clarey, J. C., Barone, P., and Imig, T. J. (1992). Physiology of thalamus and cortex. *In* "The Mammalian Auditory Pathway: Neurophysiology" (A. N. Popper and R. R. Fay, eds.) pp. 232–334. Springer-Verlag, New York.

Clarey J. C., Barone P., and Imig T. J. (1994). Functional organization of sound direction and sound pressure level in auditory cortex of the cat. *J. Neurophysiol.* **72**, 2383–2405.

Cohen, Y. E., and Knudsen, E. I. (1999). Maps versus clusters: Different representations of auditory space in the midbrain and forebrain. *Trends Neurosci.* **12**, 128–135.

Corwin, J. T., and Cotanche, D. A. (1988). Regeneration of sensory hair cells after acoustic trauma. *Science* **240**, 1772–1774.

de Ribaupierre, F. (1997). Acoustical information processing in the auditory thalamus and cerebral cortex. *In* "The Central Auditory System" (G. Ehret and R. Romand, eds.) pp. 317–397. Oxford Univ. Press, New York.

Evans, E. F. (1975). Cochlear nerve and cochlear nucleus. *In* "Handbook of Sensory Physiology" Vol. 5, part 2 (Keidel and Neff, eds.). Vol. 5, part 2, pp. 1–108, Springer Verlag, Berlin.

Fitzpatrick, D. C., Kanwai, J. S., Butman, J. A., and Suga, N. (1993). Combination-sensitive neurons in the primary auditory cortex of the mustached bat. *J. Neurosci.* **13**, 931–940.

Forsythe, I. D. (1994). Direct patch recording from identified presynaptic terminals mediating glutamatergic EPSCs in the rat CNS, *in vitro. J. Physiol.* **479**, 381–387.

Griffin, D. R. (1958). "Listening in the Dark. "Yale University Press, New Haven.

Guinan, J. J., Jr. (1996). The physiology of olivocochlear efferents. *In* "The Cochlea," (P. Dallos, A. N. Popper, and R. R. Fay, eds.) pp. 435–502. Springer-Verlag, New York.

Imig, T. J., and Reale, R. A. (1980). Patterns of cortico-cortical connections related to tonotopic maps in cat auditory cortex. *J. Comp. Neurol.* **192**, 293–332.

Jenkins, W. M., and Merzenich, R. B. (1984). Role of cat primary auditory cortex for sound localization behavior. *J. Neurophysiol.* **52**, 819–847.

Kiang, N. Y. S. (1975). Stimulus representation in the discharge pattern of auditory neurons. *In* "The Nervous System: Human Communication and its Disorders" (D. B. Tower, ed.) pp. 81–96, Raven Press, New York.

Kiang, N. Y. S. (1984). Peripheral Neural Processing of Auditory Information. *In* "Handbook of Physiology" (Brookhart and Mountcastle, eds.) pp. 639–674, American Physiological Society, Bethesda, MD.

Kiang, N. Y. S. and Peake, W. T. (1988). Physics and physiology of hearing. *In* "Handbook of Experimental Psychophysics" (Atkinson, R. J. Herrnstein, G. Lindzey, and R. C. Luce, eds.) pp. 277–326, Wiley, New York.

Liberman, M. C. (1982). The cochlear frequency map for the cat, Labeling auditory-nerve fibers of known characteristic frequency. *J. Acoust. Soc. Am.* **72**, 1441–1449.

Lindsey, P. H., and Norman, D. A. (1972). "Human Information Processing." Academic Press, New York.

Loeb, G. E. (1985). The functional replacement of the ear. *Sci. Am.* **252**, 104–111.

Lonsbury-Martin, B. L., and Martin, G. K. (1990). Distortion-product emissions. *Ear and Hearing* **11**, 144–154.

Manis, P. B., and Marx, S. O. (1991). Outward currents in isolated ventral cochlear nucleus neurons. *J. Neurosci.* **11**, 2865–2880.

Molnar, C. E., and Pfeiffer, R. R. (1968). Interpretation of spontaneous spike discharge patterns of neurons in the cochlear nucleus. *Proc. IEEE* **56**, 993–1004.

Pfeiffer, R. R. (1966). Anteroventral cochlear nucleus: Wave forms of extracellularly recorded spike potentials. *Science* **154**, 667–668.

Phillips, D. P., Orman, S. S., Musicant, A. D., and Wilson, G. F. (1985). Neurons in the cat's primary auditory cortex distinguished by their responses to tones and wide-spectrum noise. *Hearing Res.* **18**, 73–86.

Rauschecker, J. P., Tian, B., and Hauser, M. (1995). Processing of complex sounds in the macaque nonprimary auditory cortex. *Science* **268**, 111–114.

Rhode, W. S., and Greenberg, S. (1992). Physiology of the cochlear nuclei. In "The Mammalian Auditory Pathway, Neurophysiology" (A. N. Popper and R. R. Fay, eds.). pp. 94–152. Springer-Verlag, New York.

Robertson, D., and Irvine, D. R. F. (1989). Plasticity of frequency organization in auditory cortex of guinea pigs with partial unilateral deafness. *J. Comp. Neurol.* **282**, 456–471.

Rose, J. E., Hind, J., and Anderson, D. J. (1971). Some effects of stimulus intensity on response of auditory nerve fibers in the squirrel monkey. *J. Neurophysiol.* **34,** 685–699.

Rouiller, E. M., Cronin-Schreiber, R., Fekete, D. M., and Ryugo, D. K. (1986). The central projections of intracellularly labeled auditory nerve fibers in cats: An analysis of terminal morphology. *J. Comp. Neurol.* **249**, 261–278.

Ruggero, M. A. (1992). Physiology and coding of sound in the auditory nerve. *In* "The Mammalian Auditory Pathway, Neurophysiology" (A. N. Popper and R. R. Fay, eds.) pp. 34–93. Springer-Verlag, New York.

Warr, W. B. (1992). Organization of olivocochlear efferent systems in mammals. *In* "The Mammalian Auditory Pathway, Neuroanatomy"(D. B. Webster, A. N. Popper, and R. R. Fay, eds.) pp. 410–448. Springer-Verlag, New York.

Warr, W. B., Guinan, J. J. Jr., and White, J. S. (1986). Organization of the efferent fibers: The lateral and medial olivocochlear systems. *In* "Neurobiology of Hearing" (R. A. Altschuler, D. W. Hoffman, and R. P. Bobbin, eds.) pp. 333–348, Raven Press, New York.

Wightman, F. L., and Kistler, D. J. (1993). Sound localization. *In* "Human Psychophysics" (W. A. Yost, A. N. Popper, and R. R. Fay, eds.) pp. 155–192. Springer-Verlag, New York.

Yin, T. C. T., and Chan, J. C. K. (1990). Interaural time sensitivity in medial superior olive of cat. *J. Neurophysiol.* **64**, 465–488.

Young, E. D. (1984). Response characteristics of neurons of the cochlear nuclei. *In* "Hearing Science: Recent Advances." (C. I. Berlin, ed.) pp. 423–460, San Diego: College-Hill Press, San Diego.

Suggested Readings

Dallos, P., Popper, A. N., and Fay, R. R. (eds.) (1996). "The Cochlea." Springer-Verlag, New York.

Ehret, G., and Romand, R. (eds.). (1997). "The Central Auditory System." Oxford Univ. Press, New York.

Geisler, C. D. (1998). "From Sound to Synapse." Oxford Univ. Press, Oxford.

Irvine, D. R. F. (1986). "The Auditory Brainstem," Vol. 7. Springer-Verlag, Berlin.

Jahn, A. F., and Santos-Sacchi, J. (eds.) (2001). "Physiology of the Ear," 2nd Ed. Raven Press, New York.

Pickles, J. O. (1988). "An Introduction to the Physiology of Hearing," 2nd Ed. Academic Press, London.

Popper, A. N., and Fay, R. R. (eds.) (1992). "The Mammalian Auditory Pathway: Neurophysiology." Springer-Verlag, New York.

Schuknecht, H. F. (1993). "Pathology of the Ear," 2nd Ed. Lea & Febiger, Philadelphia.

Webster, D. B., Popper, A. N., and Fay, R. R. (eds.) (1992). "The Mammalian Auditory Pathway: Neuroanatomy." Springer-Verlag, New York.

M. Christian Brown

27

Vision

OVERVIEW

Vision is the most studied and perhaps the best understood topic in sensory neuroscience. This chapter is concerned primarily with vision in mammals and focuses on the pathway in the visual system that has to do with perception: from the retina to the lateral geniculate nucleus of the thalamus (LGN) and on to the multiple areas of visual cortex. Other regions of the brain that receive visual input (such as the superior colliculus) are dealt with briefly in this chapter and more extensively in the chapter on eye movements (Chapter 36).

Studying vision provides the opportunity to explore the brain at many different levels, from the physical and biochemical mechanisms of phototransduction (Chapter 24) to the boundary between psychology and physiology (Chapters 52 and 53). At each of these levels, the visual system has evolved to solve a number of difficult problems. In terms of the physical stimulus, vision operates over extremely wide ranges of illumination. The visual system detects single photons in the dark but can also see clearly in bright sunlight, when the retina is bombarded with over 10^{14} photons per second. At a much higher level of complexity, ensembles of neurons in the cerebral cortex are able to solve extremely difficult problems, such as extracting the three-dimensional motion of an object from two-dimensional retinal images.

At every moment, the visual system is confronted with the vast amount of information present in visual scenes. The complex circuitry of the retina has evolved so that much of this information is extensively processed and relayed to the rest of the central nervous system, both efficiently and with great fidelity. Vision, however, has not evolved to treat all of this information equally; instead, it appears to be best suited to extract the sort of information that may be useful to animals, including humans, in a natural environment. Vision allows animals to navigate in the world; to judge the speed and distance of objects; and to identify food, members of other species and familiar or unfamiliar members of the same species.

In many animals, primates in particular, more of the brain is devoted to vision than to any other sensory function. This is perhaps because of the extreme complexity of the task required of vision: to classify and to interpret the wide range of visual stimuli in the physical world. At the highest levels of processing, the cerebral cortex extracts from the world the diverse qualities experienced as visual perception: from motion, color, texture and depth to the grouping of objects, defined by the combination of simple features.

The Receptive Field Is the Fundamental Concept in Visual Physiology

The strategies that the brain uses to solve the problems of vision can be understood at a very intuitive level. The most useful concept to aid this intuition is that of the *receptive field*, which is the cornerstone of visual physiology. As defined by H. K. Hartline in 1938 (Ratliff, 1974, p. 167), a visual receptive field is the "region of the retina which must be illuminated in order to obtain a response in any given fiber." In this case, "fiber" refers to the axon of a retinal neuron, but any visual neuron, from a photoreceptor to a visual cortical neuron, has a receptive field. The definition was later extended to include not only the region of the retina that excited a neuron, but also the specific properties of the stimulus that evoked the strongest response. Visual neurons can respond preferentially to the turning on or turning off of a light stimulus— termed *on*-and-*off* responses—or to more complex features, such as color or the direction of motion. Any of these preferences can be expressed as attributes of the receptive field.

Sensory Systems Detect Contrast or Change

In the 1930s and 1940s, Hartline developed the concept of the receptive field with studies of the axons of individual neurons that project from the lateral eye of the horseshoe crab (*Limulus*) and from the frog's eye (Ratliff, 1974). The lateral eye of the *Limulus* is a compound eye made up of about 300 *ommatidia* arranged in a roughly hexagonal array. Each ommatidium contains optical elements, photoreceptors and a single neuron whose axon joins the optic nerve. Hartline found that when an isolated ommatidium was illuminated, the firing rate of its axon increased. More surprisingly, the firing of the same axon was decreased by a light stimulus in any adjacent ommatidium. This form of antagonistic behavior, known as *lateral inhibition*, serves to enhance responses to edges while reducing responses to constant surfaces. Without it, visual neurons would be just as sensitive to a featureless stimulus, such as a clean white wall, as to stimuli defined by edges, such as a white square on a black wall. Similar spatially antagonistic visual responses were found in mammals, as first demonstrated by Kuffler (1953) in the retina of the cat (Box 27.1).

Lateral inhibition represents the classic example of a general principle: most neurons in sensory systems are best adapted for detecting changes in the external environment. This principle can be explained in behavioral terms. As a rule, it is change that has the greatest significance for an animal, e.g., the edge of an extended object or a static object beginning to move. This principle can also be explained in terms of information processing. Given a world that is filled with constants—with uniform objects, with objects that move only rarely—it is most efficient to respond only to changes.

Several types of visual responses can be discussed in terms of the detection of change, or of *contrast:* defined as the fractional difference in luminance between two stimuli. There are several forms of contrast. The first is spatial contrast, the detection of which is enhanced by neurons in the retina that have lateral inhibition (center-surround organization, see Box 27.1). Next, there is temporal contrast, or change over time. Starting in the retina, visual neurons are affected very little by slow changes in illumination,

but are extremely sensitive to more rapid changes. Finally, there is motion, which is distinguished by characteristic changes in a stimulus over both space and time. Many neurons in the visual system are excited selectively by objects that have a certain rate or direction of motion. In summary, contrast sensitivity can take on at least three forms: sensitivity to spatial variations in a stimulus (spatial contrast), sensitivity to changes over time (temporal contrast) and sensitivity to changes in both space and time (motion; see Box 27.4).

Receptive Fields Encode Increasingly High-Order Features of the Visual World

From the photoreceptors to the multiple visual cortical areas, the visual system is hierarchical. One level provides input to the next in a feedforward progression, although lateral interactions and feedback are almost always present as well. As a general rule, receptive fields at successive stages of processing (from photoreceptors, bipolar cells, ganglion cells and geniculate neurons, through neurons in multiple visual cortical areas) encode increasingly high-level features of the visual stimulus. The outer segment of a photoreceptor, which contains the visual pigment, is influenced only by a small point in visual space. It is therefore almost entirely insensitive to the spatial structure of a stimulus. At the opposite extreme, neurons in the inferior parietal region of visual cortex seem to respond best when the animal is viewing a specific face (see Chapter 55).

These two extremes of visual responses illustrate the visual system's dual task: to maintain generality— the ability to respond to any stimulus—while also being able to represent specific, environmentally important classes of stimuli. High-level neurons classify visual stimuli by integrating information that is present in the earlier stages of processing, but also by ignoring information that is independent of that classification. For instance, motion-sensitive neurons in area MT of the cerebral cortex (see later) are exquisitely sensitive to the direction and rate of motion of an object, but very poor at distinguishing the object's color or its position. This lack of localization is quite common in high-level neurons: receptive fields become larger as the features they represent become increasingly complex. Thus, for instance, neurons that respond to faces typically have receptive fields that cover most of visual space. For these cells, large receptive fields have a distinct advantage: the preferred stimulus can be identified no matter where it is located on the retina.

Summary

The mammalian visual system is a complex, hierarchical system that can be studied from a number of different viewpoints. This chapter concentrates on the physiology of visual neurons, which is based on the study of receptive fields. Originally, receptive fields were defined as the area of the retina that could evoke responses in a visual neuron. The concept has evolved to include the stimulus attributes that lead to a neural response, such as color, motion, or even the complex features of a specific physical object. Within the hierarchy of the visual system—from retina to the multiple areas of the visual cortex—neurons are selective for increasingly complex or high-order features.

THE EYE AND THE RETINA

The Optics of the Eye Project an Inverted Visual Image on the Retina

The study of vision begins with the eye (Fig. 27.1), whose refractive properties are determined by the curvature of the cornea and the lens behind it. These optical elements act to focus an inverted image on the retina, where the first stages of neural visual processing take place. The curvature of the cornea is fixed, but the curvature of the lens is adjusted by smooth muscles that flatten the lens when they contract, thus bringing more distant objects into focus. The amount of light that reaches the retina is controlled by the iris, whose aperture is the pupil. The iris, which is situated between the cornea and the lens in the *anterior chamber* of the eye, contracts at high light levels and expands in the dark. It is thus partially responsible for the ability to see over a broad range of light levels, but this ability is primarily due to light and dark adaptation, two complex processes that take place in the retina (see Chapter 24).

The Retina Is a Three-layered Structure with Five Types of Neurons

The anatomy of the retina has an almost crystalline beauty, a beauty that is enhanced by the clear relationships between form and function (Dowling, 1997). It is composed of five principal layers: three layers of cell bodies separated by two layers of neural pro-

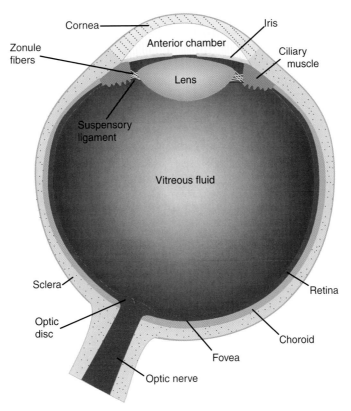

FIGURE 27.1   Schematic diagram of the human eye.

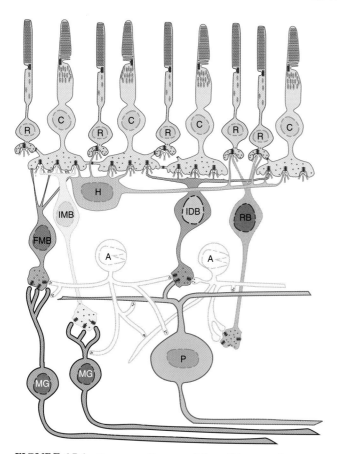

The retina is one of the few circuits in the nervous system simple enough that cell types and connections can be learned without great effort. This is made even easier since the role of each of the five cell types can be placed within a simple functional scheme. The two main attributes of the output of the retina—the point-to-point representation of the visual image and the spatially antagonistic center-surround interactions in the receptive field (see Box 27.1)—can be understood in terms of the anatomy. The direct pathway, photoreceptor → bipolar cell → ganglion cell, is the substrate for the center of the receptive field of the ganglion cell and thus for its spatial resolution. Lateral interactions in the retina, most notably the center-surround antagonism, or lateral inhibition, are mediated by horizontal cells and amacrine cells.

FIGURE 27.2 Summary diagram of the cell types and connections in the primate retina. R, rod; C, cone; H, horizontal cell; FMB, flat midget bipolar; IMB, invaginating midget bipolar; IDB, invaginating diffuse bipolar; RB, rod bipolar; A, amacrine cell; MG, midget ganglion cell; P, parasol cell. Adapted from Dowling (1997).

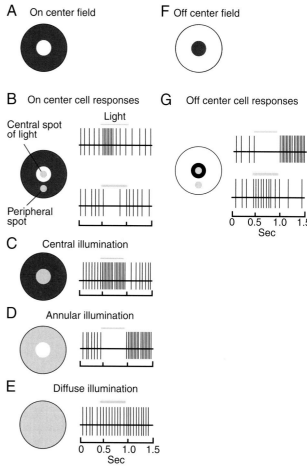

FIGURE 27.3 Visual responses of *on*-center (white) and *off*-center (dark gray) retinal ganglion cells. Visual stimuli are indicated in yellow, and the responses to these stimuli are shown to the right. See text for details.

cesses, dendrites and axons (Fig. 27.2). The vertebrate retina is oriented within the eye so that light must travel through the entire thickness of the neuropil to reach the photoreceptors. Of the three cell layers, the first is farthest from the center of the eye and is thus called the *outer nuclear layer*. It contains the cell bodies of the photoreceptors, the rods and cones (Chapter 24). The next cell layer is the *inner nuclear layer*, which contains the cell bodies of the interneurons of the retina, both excitatory and inhibitory. These include horizontal cells, bipolar cells, and amacrine cells. Finally, the *ganglion cell layer* is home to the retinal neurons whose axons form the optic nerve, the sole pathway from the retina to the rest of the central nervous system. Interposed between the cell body layers are two layers of cell processes: *inner* and *outer plexiform layers*. The two plexiform layers are the sites of all interactions between the neurons of the retina.

Photoreceptors Are Hyperpolarized by Light

Photoreceptors have been discussed at length elsewhere (Chapter 24). Here it is important to note that unlike most cells in the nervous system, the majority of cells in the retina—photoreceptors, bipolar cells, horizontal cells, and, arguably, most amacrine cells—do not normally fire action potentials. Instead, they have continuously graded membrane potentials that are modulated around a mean level. Photoreceptor cells have a tonic level of depolarization and of neurotransmitter release. They are hyperpolarized by an increment in light via a cGMP-gated process that closes sodium channels. This light-induced hyperpolarization acts to decrease the amount of neurotransmitter released by photoreceptors.

Bipolar Cells Can Be Hyperpolarized or Depolarized by Light

Bipolar cells are divided into two broad classes, termed *on* and *off* bipolars, that respond to light stimuli with depolarization and hyperpolarization, respectively. *On* bipolars are also known as *invaginating bipolars*, and *off* bipolars are known as *flat bipolars* because of the shape of the synaptic contacts they receive from photoreceptors (Fig. 27.2). Because all photoreceptors use glutamate as their neurotransmitter, these opposite responses require that *on-and-off* bipolar cells respond to the same neurotransmitter in opposite ways (Wu, 1994). Glutamate, typically an excitatory transmitter, is inhibitory for *on* bipolars. It acts by closing a cGMP-gated sodium channel, similar to that seen in photoreceptors. The depolarization of

---

BOX 27.1

KUFFLER'S STUDY OF CENTER-SURROUND RETINAL GANGLION CELLS

The classic experiments that Kuffler (1953) performed on retinal ganglion cells have formed the foundations for much of the subsequent physiological analysis of the mammalian visual system. Even beyond the study of vision, they represent a model for understanding the neurobiology of sensory systems. These experiments were performed *in vivo* in anesthetized cats. The first step in this sort of experiment is the careful placement of a fine microelectrode close to a single neuron so that action potentials can be recorded extracellularly. An oscilloscope trace of the firing pattern of this neuron is important, but the sound of action potentials on an audio monitor is even more critical. This immediate feedback allows the researcher to search for visual stimuli that excite or inhibit the neuron. Kuffler's first finding was that there were two categories of ganglion cells, as Hartline had seen in the retina of the frog. The cells were either *on,* i.e., excited by light increment, or *off,* i.e., excited by light decrement.

One of Kuffler's most important contributions was the careful mapping of lateral interactions in the retina, or what he termed the *center-surround* structure of the receptive field. When an *on* ganglion cell was being studied, a small light spot placed in the center of its receptive field would cause an immediate increase in firing rate of the cell (Fig. 27.3B, top). The center of the receptive field of an *on* ganglion cell was defined as all positions where the small spot evoked an *on* excitatory response. When the same spot was placed just beyond the center, in the region termed the *surround,* the neuron decreased its firing rate

(Fig. 27.3B, bottom). Kuffler mapped the spatial extent of the regions that evoked excitation or inhibition simply by listening to the responses to spots flashed at many different locations. Alternatively, Kuffler studied receptive fields by searching for an optimal stimulus—one that increased the firing of a ganglion cell most effectively. The strongest stimulus for an *on* center cell was a spot of light that filled the receptive field center entirely (Fig. 27.3C). Similarly, the most effective inhibitory stimulus was a bright annulus shown to the surround alone. Following such strong inhibition, the cell had an excitatory response when the stimulus was turned off (Fig. 27.3D). Finally, Kuffler studied interactions between receptive field subregions. A large bright stimulus that covered both center and surround was found to evoke a much weaker response than a smaller spot confined to the center; the surround inhibition weakened or altogether eliminated the central excitation (Fig. 27.3E).

Kuffler's early experiments, along with those of Hartline, established the technical and conceptual foundations for the field of visual physiology. Almost all subsequent work in this field can be seen as falling into three broad categories of experiments, exemplified by Kuffler's 1953 study: (1) the mapping of responses with isolated, suboptimal stimuli, (2) the search for an optimal stimulus, and (3) the study of interactions between responses evoked by two or more stimuli.

R. Clay Reid

on bipolars by light results not from excitation, but from the removal of inhibition, which occurs when photoreceptors are hyperpolarized by light. *Off* bipolars are excited by glutamate via more typical kainate receptors (named for the pharmacological agent that selectively activates them; see Chapter 10). When these cells are inhibited by light, the inhibition is in fact due to the removal of tonic excitation, which again occurs when the photoreceptors are hyperpolarized.

The functional importance of the *on* and the *off* pathways can best be understood in terms of contrast. From the bipolar cells onward, i.e., once *on*-and-*off* pathways have been established, visual neurons respond best to spatial and temporal contrast rather than to absolute light levels. Objects in the world are visible by the light they reflect; their borders are discerned usually because of different degrees of reflectance, which leads to contrast (changes in illumination, except for shadows, tend to be much more

---

BOX 27.2

QUANTITATIVE METHODS IN THE STUDY OF VISUAL NEURONS: CLASSIFICATION OF RETINAL GANGLION CELLS

Although neuroscientists have learned a tremendous amount about the visual system using the tools developed by Kuffler, researchers have been following a parallel line of studies of the visual system by asking different sorts of questions with the aid of more quantitative methods. In Kuffler's experiments and, most notably, many of Hubel and Wiesel's (see later), easily produced stimuli (such as spots, edges, and bars) were used to stimulate visual neurons. Action potentials were detected primarily with an oscilloscope and audio monitor. In the more quantitative studies of visual physiology, stimuli are shown primarily on video monitors and data are recorded with computers. The quantitative study of visual physiology constitutes a large field, which stems from the work of Hartline, Ratliff, Campbell, Barlow, and others (see Ratliff, 1974; Wandell, 1993). Analysis of the receptive fields of retinal ganglion cells in the cat performed by Enroth-Cugell and Robson (1966) represents an early and influential example of this line of research.

Stimuli used by Enroth-Cugell and Robson, and in many studies that followed theirs, consisted of *gratings*: light and dark bands whose luminance varied in a sinusoidal fashion across a screen. Gratings were not designed to be the most effective stimuli for visual neurons. The broad goal of this sort of experiment is to study not just what makes neurons respond best, but to study how they would respond to *any* stimulus and to probe what mechanisms they use to produce these responses. The analytical framework that goes along with these experiments is called *systems theory*, the study of input–output (or stimulus–response) systems. *Linear systems,* those that simply add up all of their inputs to produce an output, constitute an important part of this theory.

Enroth-Cugell and Robson used a simple test of linearity in their study of retinal ganglion cells in the cat. A grating was presented at different positions (called phases), and the responses to its introduction and removal were recorded. Two questions were addressed for each cell studied: (1) If a certain phase (whose bars were arranged white, black, and white; as in Fig. 27.4, 0°) excited the cell, did the opposite grating (black, white, and black; Fig. 27.4, 180°) inhibit it? (2) More importantly, were there null positions for the grating that evoked no response, as excitation and inhibition were perfectly balanced (Fig. 27.4, 90 and 270°)?

One class of ganglion cells, called *X cells*, passed these tests for linear spatial summation (Fig. 27.4, left) A second class of cells, *Y cells*, behaved differently. Like X cells, these cells also had a center-surround receptive field when mapped with spots and annuli. When studied with two opposite gratings, however, the responses evoked were not equal and opposite. Instead, the introduction and removal of the gratings at all positions resulted in two peaks of excitation, and no null position could be found (Fig. 27.4, right).

The use of systems theory and quantitative techniques in the study of the visual system has had a number of notable successes. It has helped in the classification of different families of visual neurons, such as X and Y cells. Further, it has been used to elucidate some of the mechanisms responsible for the responses of visual neurons (such as directionally selective cells, see Box 27.4). Perhaps most importantly, along with a large body psychophysical experiments that employ the same stimuli, it has helped create a common framework in which the responses of neurons can be related to perception.

R. Clay Reid

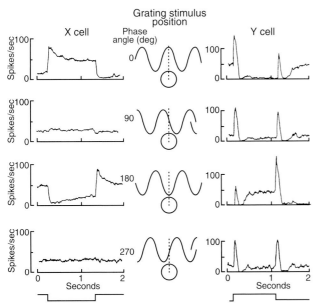

FIGURE 27.4 Visual responses of X and Y cells to contrast-reversing sine-wave gratings at different spatial phases (different positions, indicated schematically in the middle column). Visual responses, in spikes per second, are shown as poststimulus time histograms synchronized to the repetitive stimulus. Upward deflection of the lowest trace indicates introduction of the grating pattern (contrast on), and downward deflection indicates removal of the pattern (contrast off, but no change in mean luminance). Adapted from Enroth-Cugell and Robson (1966).

gradual). Because the visual system is adapted for seeing objects that can be either brighter or darker than their backgrounds, it is not too surprising that it is equally sensitive to positive and negative contrast steps.

Most ganglion cells, the output cells of the retina, receive their main excitatory input from bipolar cells. Thus these ganglion cells also have either *on* or *off* responses in the center of their receptive fields, according to which class of bipolar cells provide their input (see Box 27.1). Other ganglion cells, known as *on–off* cells, respond to both light onset and to light offset. These latter cells receive input from both classes of bipolar cells. Many of these cells respond preferentially to stimuli moving in a particular direction of motion (see Box 27.4).

Horizontal and Amacrine Cells Mediate Lateral Interactions in the Retina

There is a complex three-way synaptic relationship among the terminals of the photoreceptors, the processes of horizontal cells and the dendrites of bipolar cells (Fig. 27.2). Horizontal cells are inhibitory (GABAergic) and, as the name implies, they contact photoreceptors over a much larger horizontal extent of retina than bipolar cells. Thus, because they are the only neurons that sample over a sufficiently large area in the outer plexiform layer, horizontal cells are thought to be responsible for the antagonistic surround seen in the receptive fields of bipolar cells.

The second family of lateral interneurons in the retina, the amacrine cells (literally, cells with no axons), is a diverse class of cells that exhibits a wide range of morphologies. As is true of horizontal cells, all processing takes place on the dendrites of amacrine cells (in the inner plexiform layer), which contain both pre- and postsynaptic elements (Fig. 27.2). Most amacrine cells use GABA, glycine, or both acetylcholine and GABA as neurotransmitters, but it is thought that virtually every transmitter found in the brain is used by some amacrine cell. The functions of most of these diverse subclasses remain poorly understood. In addition to a possible role in the creation of the antagonistic surround, it has been proposed that some amacrine cells are responsible for the nonlinear responses in Y cells of the cat (see Box 27.2) or for the direction selectivity seen in the rabbit retina (see Box 27.4).

Retinal Ganglion Cells Provide the Output of the Retina

Visual information leaves the eye via the optic nerve, which is composed of the axons of all of the different classes of ganglion cells. The optic nerve begins at the *optic disc* (see Fig. 27.1). Because there are no photoreceptors at the optic disc, this circular region constitutes a blind spot in the retina. The routing of ganglion cell axons to different parts of the brain provides a number of interesting problems for developmental neurobiology (Chapters 19 and 22). The routing of axons is both macroscopic—different types of ganglion cells project to different regions of the brain—and microscopic: within any given target region, axons are sorted out in a precise manner. In each of two principal targets of retinal axons, the superior colliculus and lateral geniculate nucleus of the thalamus (LGN), a topographical map of visual space is created in which spatial relations are maintained between neighboring neurons.

This chapter is concerned primarily with the classes of retinal ganglion cells that project to LGN neurons, which in turn project to the primary visual (striate) cortex. Although cells in the LGN are more than mere relays of information from the retina, their receptive fields are quite similar to those of their ganglion cell inputs. The following discussion of retinal receptive fields, therefore, can serve equally well to describe receptive fields in the LGN.

Parallel Pathways Are Composed of Distinct Classes of Retinal Ganglion Cells in the Cat

Kuffler found that retinal ganglion cells in the cat have a stereotyped center-surround organization. Similar cells (both *on* and *off*) were found at every position across the entire retina. Researchers later discovered, however, that there are in fact several different functional classes of ganglion cells, each with distinct response properties. Although different cell classes have been found in different species, in none is the retina composed of a single mosaic of identical cells. The fact that there are multiple types of output from the retina has had a profound effect on the study of visual processing in the brain. The degree to which these *parallel pathways* (Livingstone and Hubel, 1984; Merigan and Maunsell, 1994) are combined or kept separate has been a major theme in the study of central visual pathways, particularly the visual cortex.

The idea that there are parallel sensory pathways into the brain is not new. At the beginning of the 19th century, both Bell and Müller argued for what Müller termed the "specific energy of nerves." This term is a precursor of the idea that axon sensory neurons are "labeled lines," each of which conveys distinct signals to the brain. A surprisingly modern version of this idea was given in 1860 by Helmholtz in the *"Handbook of Physiological Optics"* (2000) in which he expressed Thomas Young's theory of color vision (1807) in the following manner: "The eye is provided with three distinct sets of nervous fibers. Stimulation of the first excites the sensation of red, stimulation of the second the sensation of green, and stimulation of the third the sensation of violet."

In one of the earlier studies using a quantitative approach to receptive field mapping (see Box 27.2), Enroth-Cugell and Robson (1966) found that cat retinal ganglion cells could be classified into two categories: X and Y (more categories have been found subsequently). This classification was based on a simple criterion: did ganglion cells simply add together all of their excitatory and inhibitory inputs (linear summation) or were the interactions between inputs more complicated (nonlinear summation)? The linear/nonlinear distinction between X and Y cells (see Box 27.2) may seem fairly abstract, but these cells turned out to be different in a number of other ways. Most notably, Y cell receptive fields are, on average, three times larger than those of neighboring X cells. X cells are therefore far more numerous, because many

more X cell receptive fields are needed to effectively tile, or cover, the retina. One view is that the large, nonlinear receptive fields of Y cells make them well suited to detect change, at the cost of their ability to signal the exact location or nature of the stimulus; similarly, X cells are better at localizing more specific stimulus features, but less sensitive in detecting change.

Primate Ganglion Cells Project to Three Subdivisions of the Lateral Geniculate Nucleus: Parvocellular, Magnocellular, and Koniocellular

Primates have a number of different classes of retinal ganglion cells, each with distinct cellular morphology, projection patterns, and visual response properties. This discussion focuses on ganglion cells that project to the lateral geniculate nucleus (LGN). There are many differences among primate species (nocturnal versus diurnal, Old World versus New World); this section concentrates on the macaque; a diurnal, Old World primate. The macaque visual system has been studied extensively with anatomical, physiological, and behavioral methods. Most importantly, macaque vision is very similar to human vision.

The most numerous class of ganglion cells in the macaque retina are sometimes referred to as *P cells*, so called because they project to the dorsal-most layers of the LGN, the *parvocellular layers* (small cells; Fig. 27.9). *M cells*, which project to the two ventral layers of the LGN, the *magnocellular layers* (large cells), constitute a second class of retinal neurons. P and M cells have distinct morphologies (Fig. 27.2). P cells (also known as $P\beta$ or, in the central retina, midget ganglion cells) have very small dendritic fields. M cells (also known as $P\alpha$ or parasol cells) have much larger dendritic fields. Finally, members of a third class of retinal cells project to the *intercalated layers* between principal parvocellular and magnocellular layers. These intercalated layers are also termed *koniocellular* (dust-like, or tiny cells). There are roughly 1,000,000 P cells in the retina and parvocellular neurons in the LGN; there are 100,000 M and magnocellular neurons. Although the intercalated layers appear quite sparse and thin in standard histological sections (Fig. 27.9), there are as many intercalated cells as there are magnocellular cells. Due to their size and location, intercalated cells have been difficult to study and little is known about them in the macaque. Therefore the following section discusses only the functional properties of P and M pathways.

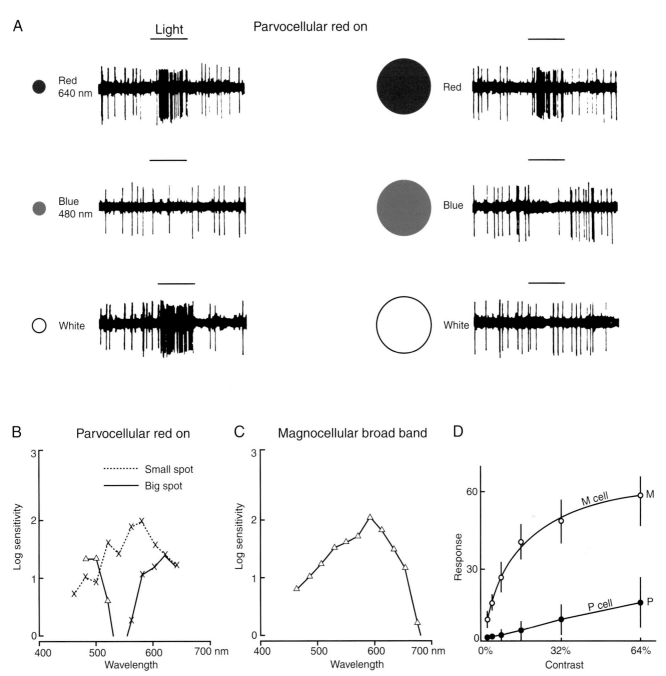

FIGURE 27.5 Visual responses of magnocellular and parvocellular neurons in the macaque. (A) Responses of a color-opponent (red-*on*/green-*off*) parvocellular neuron to small and large stimuli. For small spots, roughly the size of the receptive field center, the neuron was excited by both red and white and was weakly inhibited by blue. The responses to large spots were more selective. Red was excitatory, blue was strongly inhibitory, and white stimuli were ineffective. (B) Responses of the same red-*on*/green-*off* parvocellular neuron to different wavelengths of light. For small spots, the neuron was excited (X) for a broad range of wavelengths. For big spots, it was excited above 550 nm, from yellow to red, and inhibited (D) below 550 nm, from blue to green. (C) Responses of a magnocellular neuron to different wavelengths of light presented in the receptive field center. The neuron had *off* (D) responses at all wavelengths, i.e., no wavelength specificity was found. (D) Average contrast response functions of P (•) and M (o) cells measured in spikes per second. P cells respond poorly to low contrasts and do not saturate at high contrasts. M cells respond better to low contrasts, but saturate by 20–30%. A–C: from Wiesel and Hubel (1966). D: from Kaplan and Shapley (1986).

P and M Pathways Have Different Response Properties

As noted earlier, the receptive field properties of the LGN relay cells match closely those of their retinal afferents, but the two parallel pathways, P→ parvocellular and M→ magnocellular, are quite different. Five main characteristics distinguish the responses of P cells and M cells (see Figs. 27.5 and 27.6). (1) P cell

receptive fields are smaller than M cell receptive fields at the same retinal position. (2) M cell axons conduct impulses faster than P cell axons. (3) The responses of P cells to a prolonged visual stimulus, particularly a color stimulus, can be very sustained, whereas M cells tend to respond more transiently. (4) Most P cells are sensitive to the color of a stimulus; M cells are not (Figs. 27.5A–27.5C). (5) M cells are much more sensitive than P cells to low-contrast, black-and-white stimuli (Fig. 27.5D). These last two differences, which have strong implications for the functional role of these pathways, are discussed next.

Color-Selective Responses in the P Pathway Are Derived from Antagonistic Inputs from L and M cones

Color vision depends on the distinct sensitivities of the three classes of cone photoreceptors to different wavelengths of light (the rods are active only under low light levels and are not involved in color vision). Although fine distinctions can be made between different wavelengths, it is important to emphasize that each of the light-sensitive pigments in the three cone classes is sensitive to a broad range of wavelengths. The spectral sensitivities of these pigments overlap considerably (Fig. 27.6A). Consequently, the names sometimes used for these pigments—red, green, and blue sensitive—are inaccurate. For instance, the "red" pigment is most sensitive to light whose wavelength is 564 nm, or yellow, although it is more sensitive than the other pigments to red light. A more accurate terminology, one that identifies the relative sensitivities of the three cone absorption spectra, is usually employed: long, middle, and short wavelength sensitive (or L, M, and S).

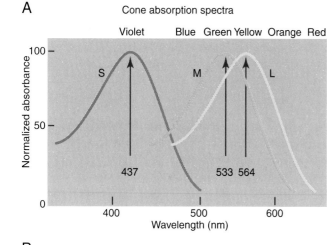

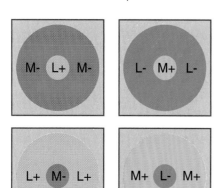

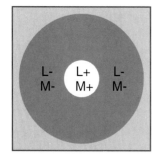 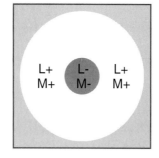

FIGURE 27.6 Aspects of color vision. (A) Absorption spectra of the three cone photoreceptors in humans: long, middle and short wavelength sensitive (L, M, and S). L and M cones in particular are sensitive to overlapping ranges of wavelengths. (B) Receptive field of the four types of red–green parvocellular cells in the macaque (labeled L+ and M+ or L- and M- according to their on-or-off centers, respectively). Classically, these small receptive fields have been described as receiving antagonistic input from L cones in their centers and M cones in their surrounds, or vice versa. When probed with color stimuli, L-*off* center and M-*off* center cells are excited by red and inhibited by green (and some blues: see Fig. 27.5 A). M-*on* and L-*off* cells are excited by green and inhibited by red. When probed with small white spots, L-on and M-on cells are excited when the stimulus is turned on; L-*off* and M-*off* cells are excited when the stimulus is turned off. (C) Receptive fields of the two main types of magnocellular cells. These larger receptive fields receive mixed L and M input to both center and surround. There are two types: *on* center (M+L+) and *off* center (L-M-).

BOX 27.3

INHERITED AND ACQUIRED DEFECTS OF COLOR VISION: RETINAL AND CORTICAL MECHANISMS

Inherited defects of color vision have been studied for over 200 years, originally with psychophysical methods but more recently with the tools of molecular genetics. Normal color vision is *trichromatic* (literally, three colored) because there are three different classes of cone photoreceptors. In the most common form of color vision defect, there are three pigments, but one of them is abnormal, or anomalous. More severe defects are found in *dichromats*, who lack a single cone type entirely. The current terminology for the three types of dichromacy was proposed by von Kries in 1897: *protanopia* (literally, the first type of blindness, or "red-blindness"), *deuteranopia* (second type, or "green-blindness"), and *tritanopia* (third type, or "blue-blindness"). While dichromats are unable to make certain color distinctions, only the very rare *monochromats*—people with one cone type or only rods—are truly color blind.

The genetics of red–green defects have long been known to be X linked: they are inherited from the mother and are fairly common in men, but they are uncommon in women. Roughly 2% of European white males are protanopes or deuteranopes and, depending on the population, between 2 and 6% are trichromats with a single anomalous pigment (either protanomalous or, more commonly, deuteranomalous). In contrast, only 0.4% of women in similar populations have red–green defects. Tritanopia, found equally in men and women, is significantly rarer. It is inherited as an autosomal-dominant trait thought to occur at low frequencies, estimated variously between 1 in 500 and 1 in over 10,000.

Because of the overlap in cone pigments, inherited color vision defects are not as simple as terms such as "red blindness" might suggest. In broad terms, protanopes and deuteranopes are unable to make specific discriminations along the red–green axis. Depending on the defect, they are unable to distinguish certain reds and greens from gray or from each other. Tritanopes are unable to discriminate between colors with and without a short wavelength component, such as between gray and certain shades of violet or yellow.

In the 1980s, Nathans, Hogness, and colleagues cloned and sequenced the three cone pigment genes and related them to color defects in humans. The cloning strategy was based on the pigments predicted close homology to rhodopsin (Fig. 27.7B). As expected from the genetics of protanopia and deuteranopia, two very similar genes for L and M pigments were found on the X chromosome. The third gene, which codes for the S pigment, was found on chromosome 7. In subsequent work by this group and others, molecular genetics of the inherited color defects, including anomalous trichromacy, have been studied in great detail.

While the inherited color deficiencies are fairly simple and well understood, acquired defects in color vision—found in a number of ocular, neurological, and systemic diseases—are far more varied. One such syndrome, *cerebral achromatopsia*, was described in the neurological literature in the 1880s. In rare patients with certain cortical lesions, the discrimination of colors and the naming of colors were severely impaired. In the majority of cases, there were other associated deficits—either an area of complete blindness (a scotoma) or an inability to recognize faces (prosopagnosia)—but in some cases, vision was otherwise quite normal. From the location of the lesions, some neurologists early on inferred the existence of a region of cortex required for color, vision, near the inferior border of the primary visual cortex.

The literature of cerebral achromatopsia, quite developed in the late 19th century, fell into eclipse for the first half of the 20th century when highly specific functional divisions of the cortex were questioned. With the discovery in the 1970s of multiple visual areas in primate cerebral cortex (Felleman and Van Essen, 1993), however, the existence of a cortical region devoted to color in humans seemed less farfetched. With recent advances in noninvasive brain imaging there is little doubt that such regions exist in humans, although their homology to brain regions in non-human primates remains controversial.

R. Clay Reid

Because green light will excite both long and middle wavelength cones, the color green can be distinguished only by the fact that it excites middle wavelength cones more strongly than it excites long wavelength cones. This distinction can be made by neurons that are sensitive to the difference between the signals from two cone classes, or neurons that are *color opponent*. In the retina and LGN, there are two categories of color-opponent cells: red–green and blue–yellow (yellow is made of the sum of long and middle wavelength cone signals; Dacey, 2000). These are sometimes also termed red-minus-green cells and blue-minus-yellow cells. The

A

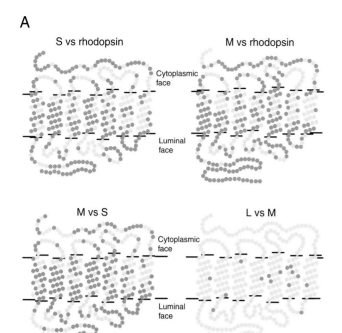

S vs rhodopsin   M vs rhodopsin

Cytoplasmic
face

Luminal
face

M vs S   L vs M

Cytoplasmic
face

Luminal
face

B

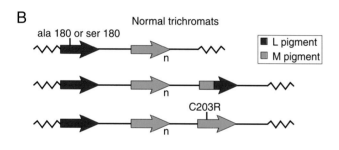

Normal trichromats

ala 180 or ser 180

| ■ L pigment |
| ■ M pigment |

n

n

C203R

n

Dichromats and anomalous trichromats

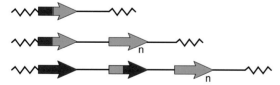

n

n

FIGURE 27.7 Molecular biology of photopigment genes. (A) Transmembrane model of cone photopigments. Homologies between the different photopigments are shown, with differences between proteins highlighted. The amino acid sequences of M and S cone pigments and rhodopsin are all approximately 40% identical (and 75% homologous), whereas L and M pigments are 96% identical (99% homologous). (B) Structure of the portion of the X chromosome coding for L and M pigments. Normally, there is one L pigment gene and several M pigment genes. Because not all of these genes are expressed, different variants can result in normal color vision (top). Many different patterns of recombination and deletion can be associated with a defect in red–green vision: either dichromacy or anomalous trichromacy (bottom). A: from Nathans *et al.*, 1986; B: from Nathans (1994).

most numerous color-opponent neurons in the primate retina are red–green opponent P cells. These cells receive antagonistic input from long and middle wavelength-sensitive (L and M) cones.

Near the fovea, the center of the retina, a P cell receives input from only one bipolar cell. This *midget bipolar* in turn receives input from a single cone (Fig. 27.2). This arrangement ensures not only that the center of the ganglion cell's receptive field is as small as possible, but also that the center receives input from only one cone type: L or M. Classically, the antagonistic surround of these P cells (or their counterparts in the LGN) has been thought to be dominated by the other main cone class, M or L, respectively (Wiesel and Hubel, 1966). Although the exact nature of the surround in red–green P cells has been somewhat controversial in recent years (Dacey, 2000), this classical view is shown in Fig. 27.6B.

There are four different types of red–green opponent P cells in the retina (Fig. 27.6B), and hence parvocellular neurons in the LGN. L-*on* center and M-*off* center cells are excited by red and inhibited by green (and some blues; see Fig. 27.5A). M-*on* and L-*off* cells are excited by green and inhibited by red. As Wiesel and Hubel showed (1966), parvocellular neurons in the LGN are sensitive to small bright spots presented in their receptive field centers, but they are most selective for the color of the stimulus when larger stimuli are used (see Figs. 27.5A and 27.5B). This is because only larger stimuli are effective in stimulating simultaneously the color-opponent center and surround. Because they absorb a broad range of wavelengths (Fig. 27.6), single cones are not very color selective. Parvocellular neurons are most color selective when the stimulus evokes antagonistic influences from two cone classes: one found in the center and the other found only in the surround.

M Cells Are Highly Sensitive to Contrast

Because of their marked color sensitivity and small receptive fields, P cells have long been thought to be involved with the ability to make color discriminations and to see the finest details. When tested with black-and-white stimuli, however, P cells responded to low contrast very poorly compared to M cells. In a study that used the quantitative methodology similar to Enroth-Cugell and Robson's (see Box 27.2), Kaplan and Shapley (1986) measured the responses of P and M cells to sine-wave gratings of various contrasts (Fig. 27.5D). Perceptually, stimuli can be detected that have less than 1% contrast (i.e., 1% luminance deviation from the mean). Kaplan and Shapley (1986) found that M cells often responded well to contrasts of under

5% and that they gave their strongest responses at contrasts as low as 20%. P cells tended to respond poorly to contrasts below 10%, a stimulus that is quite salient, and rarely reached their strongest responses below 64%. From this, Kaplan and Shapley concluded that the ability to see low contrasts is due primarily to the M cell system.

The relatively poor sensitivity of P cells to low-contrast stimuli is not well understood, but it may be partially the result of two factors: receptive-field centers receive input from a very small region of the retina, and the inputs from different cone classes are subtracted from each other, rather than added together. Whatever the reason, the poor performance of the P pathway in detecting low contrast implies an important role for M cells in the detection of the form of objects (which is robust at low contrasts), in addition to their role in the motion pathway (discussed later).

Summary

The retina, part of the central nervous system, is a self-contained neuronal circuit whose anatomy and physiology have been studied in great detail. There are five types of cells in the retina. Photoreceptors, bipolar cells, and ganglion cells constitute the direct, feed-forward pathway. Horizontal cells and amacrine cells subserve lateral interactions within the retina. Photoreceptors are all hyperpolarized by light, but bipolar cells can be either hyperpolarized (*off* cells) or depolarized by light (*on* cells). There is a great variety of retinal ganglion cells, but most have an antagonistic center-surround organization. In the primate, the two best studied classes of ganglion cells are P cells and M cells, which project to the parvocellular and magnocellular layers of the LGN, respectively. P cells have small receptive fields, are sensitive to the color of a stimulus, and are relatively insensitive to low contrasts. M cells have larger receptive fields, are insensitive to color, and are very sensitive to low contrasts.

THE RETINOGENICULOCORTICAL PATHWAY

Visual Information Is Relayed to the Cortex via the Lateral Geniculate Nucleus

In mammals with forward-facing eyes, such as most carnivores and the primates, retinal axons are routed so that visual information from the same points in space coming from the two eyes can be com-

bined. From both eyes, ganglion cells whose receptive fields are in one half of the visual field project to the opposite cerebral hemisphere (Fig. 27.8). This cross-routing occurs at the optic chiasm (from the Greek letter *chi*, χ). Here, axons from the medial (nasal, or nearer the nose) half of one retina cross over to join the axons from the lateral (temporal, or nearer the temples) half of the other retina. In other words, the temporal retina projects to the *ipsilateral* (same-side) hemisphere and the nasal retina projects to the *contralateral* (opposite-side) hemisphere. Unlike somatic sensation, which is entirely crossed (see Chapter 26), only half of the retinal axons cross. Like somatic sensation, however, the crossing of retinal axons results in each half of the external visual field being represented in the opposite cerebral hemisphere.

The LGN Is a Layered Structure That Receives Segregated Input from the Two Eyes

As they leave the optic chiasm, retinal axons from the two eyes travel together in the optic tract, which terminates in the LGN (Fig. 27.8). The LGN is com-

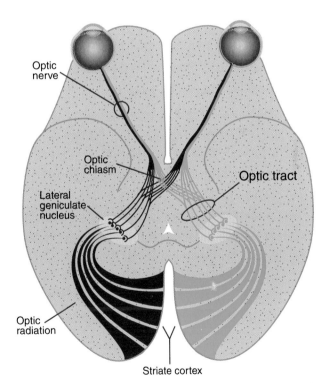

FIGURE 27.8 The retino-geniculo-cortical pathway in the human. Optic nerve axons from the nasal retina cross at the optic chiasm and join axons from the temporal retina of the other eye. Together, these contralateral and ipsilateral axons make up the optic tract, which projects to the LGN. Each of the six layers of the LGN receives input from only one eye. Axons from the LGN make up the optic radiations, which project to the striate cortex. Adapted from Polyak (1941).

posed of layers, each of which receives input from only one eye, although the number varies between species. In the macaque, the six principal layers contain most of the relay cells to primary visual cortex (Fig. 27.9). The four parvocellular layers are found dorsally. They receive P cell input from the contralateral and ipsilateral eye in the order of contra, ipsi, contra, and ipsi. The magnocellular layers are found more ventrally. They receive M cell input in the order of ipsi and contra. Interposed between these principal layers are the intercalated layers, populated by koniocellular neurons.

In the cat, the LGN has only two principal layers, called A and A1, which receive input from the contralateral and ipsilateral retinas, respectively. The neurons are again quite similar to either the retinal X cells or the Y cells that innervate them.

The Primary Visual Cortex in the Cat Is an Example of a Functional Hierarchy

Cat primary visual cortex (area 17) is perhaps the best understood neocortical area in any species. The first studies of Hubel and Wiesel (1962) form the foun-

dation of this understanding. Hubel and Wiesel found cells whose responses differed dramatically from those in the retina and thalamus. Many of these cells could be excited by stimuli presented to either eye. The primary visual cortex thus represents the first level of the visual system at which binocular interactions could form a substrate for depth perception. Most strikingly, Hubel and Wiesel found that the vast majority of cortical cells respond best to elongated stimuli at a specific orientation and give no response at the orthogonal orientation. This is in sharp contrast to cells in the retina and LGN, which are not selective for orientation.

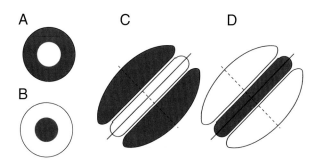

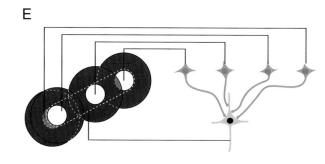

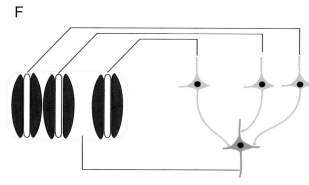

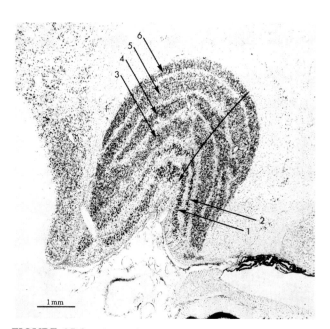

FIGURE 27.9 The six-layered LGN of the macaque monkey. The top four parvocellular layers (6, 5, 4, and 3) receive input from the ispilateral and contralateral eye in the order of contra, ipsi, contra, and ipsi. The bottom two magnocellular layers (2 and 1) receive ipsi and contra input, respectively. In between these principal layers are intercalated or koniocellular layers. The arrow from layer 6 to 1 indicates organization of the precisely aligned retinotopic maps of the six layers. The receptive fields of neurons found along this line are located at the same position in visual space. From Hubel and Wiesel (1977).

FIGURE 27.10 Hubel and Wiesel's original models of visual cortical hierarchy. (A and B) Receptive field maps of center-surround receptive fields in LGN. White: *on* responses; dark gray: *off* responses. (C and D) Receptive field maps of simple cells. (E) Model of convergent input from LGN neurons onto the cortical simple cell. (F) Model of convergent input from simple cells onto complex cells. Adapted from Hubel and Wiesel (1962).

Hubel and Wiesel described two broad classes of neurons in area 17: *simple cells* and *complex cells*. The receptive fields of simple cells were segmented into oriented *on-and-off* subregions (Figs. 27.10C and 27.10D) and were therefore most sensitive to similarly oriented stimuli. In these receptive field subregions, responses were evoked by turning a light stimulus *on* or *off*, but not by both. Given these well-defined *on-and-off* subregions in simple cells, Hubel and Wiesel suggested a straightforward hierarchical model to explain orientation selectivity: neurons in the lateral geniculate nucleus whose receptive fields are arranged in a row could all converge to excite a specific simple cell (Fig. 27.10E). Although this model has generated much controversy over the ensuing years, many of its elements have been demonstrated directly (Reid and Alonso, 1995; Ferster *et al.*, 1996).

The second class of cortical neurons, complex cells, also responded best to oriented stimuli, but their receptive fields were not elongated along a preferred orientation, nor were they divided into distinct *on-and-off* subregions. It would therefore be difficult to imagine how the responses of these neurons could be constructed directly from the center/surround receptive fields in the thalamus. Given the properties of simple cells, Hubel and Wiesel proposed a hierarchical scheme. Complex cells receive their orientation selectivity from convergent input from simple cells whose receptive fields have the same orientation preference, but have slightly different spatial locations (Fig. 27.10F).

This original model is hierarchical or serial; information flows from one level to the next in a well-defined series. In contrast to this hierarchical model

A

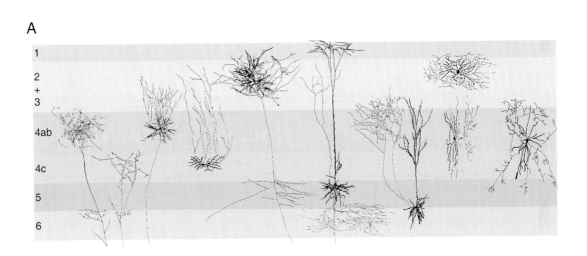

B

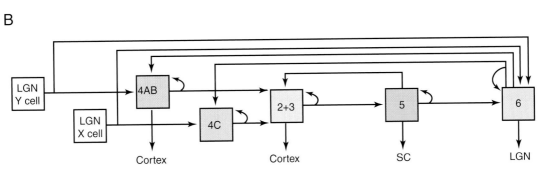

FIGURE 27.11 Circuitry of cat cortical area 17. (A) Morphology of individual cells stained with horseradish peroxidase. Thick lines: dendrites; thin lines: axons. (B) Schematic diagram of connections. Most thalamic (LGN) input is concentrated in layer 4 and, to a lesser degree, in layer 6. Y cells tend to project more superficially in layer 4 than X cells (note that sublayers 4ab and 4c are not strictly analogous to 4A, 4B, and 4C in the macaque). There is a fairly strict hierarchical pathway from layers 4 Æ 2+3 Æ 5 Æ 6 with feedback connections from 5 Æ 2+3 and 6 Æ 4. There are also many lateral connections between neurons within the same layer. Adapted from Gilbert and Wiesel (1985).

of cortical processing, it has also been proposed that each region of the cerebral cortex is made up of several different streams of information that are all processed in parallel. As with most dichotomies, elements of both hierarchical and parallel processing have been found in the visual cortex of all mammals studied. For simplicity, an outline of the organization of visual cortex in the cat is discussed here in terms of a hierarchical model. Parallel processing will be illustrated with the example of a primate visual cortex.

The hierarchical scheme has received support from several correlations between anatomy and physiology of area 17. In broad terms, simple cells are more common in the layers of cortex that receive direct input from the thalamus (layer 4 and, to a lesser extent, layer 6). Complex cells are found more frequently in layers that are more distant from the thalamic input in layers 2+3, which receive input primarily from layer 4, and in layer 5, which receives most of its input from layers 2+3 (Gilbert and Wiesel, 1985; Fig. 27.11).

In terms of their probable function in perception, the receptive fields of complex cells furnish an early example of what was meant in the introduction by a higher order representation. Complex cells convey information about orientation to later stages of processing, but that information has been combined and generalized. A simple cell responds to an oriented stimulus of a specific configuration and a specific location; in particular, it has separate *on*-and-*off* subregions. A complex cell also responds to stimuli at one orientation, but the receptive field is not segregated into *on*-and-*off* subregions. Instead, it can respond to a light or dark stimulus of the correct orientation, independent of the exact location of the stimulus within the receptive field. This sort of generalization is a recurrent theme in the cortical processing of visual information.

Several Parallel Streams Are Found in the Macaque Primary Visual Cortex

In the macaque primary visual cortex (V1, or striate cortex), a hierarchical organization is certainly present, but it is also clearly composed of several parallel streams. As discussed earlier, at least three types of inputs to visual cortex (parvocellular, magnocellular, and koniocellular) are first segregated within the LGN. Each class of neurons projects to a specific subdivision of primary visual cortex. Most thalamic afferents terminate in layer 4C, which is split into two divisions. 4Cα receives its input from magnocellular neurons and 4Cβ from parvocellular neurons. Intercalated, or koniocellular, geniculate neurons project to

layers 2+3, specifically to regions known as "blobs" (discussed later) that stain densely for the enzyme cytochrome oxidase (Livingstone and Hubel, 1984)

Thus visual information from functionally and anatomically distinct M and P retinal neurons are kept separate through the LGN and at least up to the cortical neurons that receive direct thalamic input. The degree to which these pathways—as well as the more poorly understood koniocellular pathway—are kept separate within visual cortex remains an area of active research (see Fig. 27.15).

Functional Architecture Can Be Seen in the Columnar Structure of the Visual Cortex

So far, the physiology of the visual cortex has been considered in terms of individual neurons and their response properties. Another major contribution of Hubel and Wiesel was their demonstration that cells with similar receptive field properties tend to be found near each other in the cortex. Further, they found that physiological response properties, such as orientation selectivity, are organized in an orderly fashion across the cortical surface. They termed the relationship between anatomy and physiology the *functional architecture* of visual cortex.

Hubel and Wiesel's key observation in this arena was that when an electrode is advanced through the cortex perpendicular to its surface, all neurons encountered have similar response properties. If a cell near the surface has a specific orientation and is dominated by input from one eye, then cells below it share these preferences. This finding is consistent with the idea, proposed by Lorente de Nó, that the fundamental unit in cortical architecture is a vertically oriented *column* of neurons. Hubel and Wiesel proposed that a cortical column is both a physiological and an anatomical unit, as had Mountcastle in his study of somatosensory cortex (see Chapter 26). A second observation was that the property of orientation preference varies smoothly over the cortical surface. If an electrode takes a tangential path through the cortex through many different columns, the orientation preference generally changes in a steady clockwise or counterclockwise progression, although occasionally there are discontinuous jumps (Fig. 27.12A).

In addition to orientation, at least two other parameters are mapped smoothly across the cortical surface. Cells in the visual cortex receive inputs from the two eyes in varying proportion, a property that Hubel and Wiesel termed *ocular dominance*. In tangential microelectrode penetrations, cells are found that are dominated first by input from one eye and then the other. This provides evidence for *ocular dominance columns*,

A

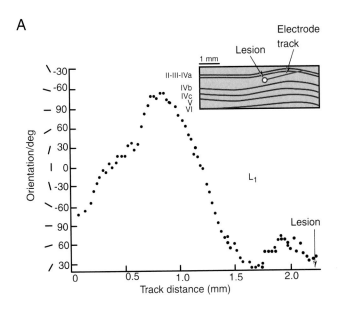

B

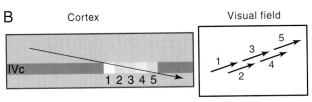

FIGURE 27.12 Two aspects of the functional architecture of the macaque primary visual cortex. (A) Graph of the preferred orientation of neurons encountered in a long microelectrode penetration through layers 2+3 (inset). There was an steady, slow progression of preferred orientations, although there were a few positions where the orientations changed more abruptly. (B) Schematic diagram of an electrode penetration through layer 4C (left) and the retinotopic positions of receptive fields (right). Numbers (1–5) indicate regions dominated by input from alternating eyes. At the border between ocular dominance columns (e.g., instance between 1 and 2), the location of receptive fields jumps back to a point represented near the middle of the previous ocular dominance column. There is a complete representation of visual space in columns dominated by each eye (1,3,5 or 2,4) and these representations are spatially interleaved. Adapted from Hubel and Wiesel (1977).

which have subsequently been demonstrated anatomically as well as physiologically. Second, prior to Hubel and Wiesel's work, a precise map of visual space across the surface of the cortex had been demonstrated. For any cortical column, receptive fields are all located at roughly the same position on the retina. Nearby columns represent nearby points in visual space in a precise and orderly arrangement. The position of a stimulus on the retina is termed its *retinotopy;* thus a region of the brain (such as the superior colliculus, LGN, or the visual cortex) that maintains the relations between adjacent retinal regions is said to have a *retinotopic map.*

Given the existence of multiple functional maps, the obvious question is: How do these maps relate to

each other? This question has been answered most definitively for the relationship between retinotopy and ocular dominance. Layer 4 in the primate is ideal for studying this question, as the receptive fields are quite small and the borders between ocular dominance columns are well defined. By making long, tangential penetrations through layer 4 of the striate cortex, Hubel and Wiesel found a precise interdigitating map from each eye. When eye dominance shifts, the receptive field location shifts to a point corresponding to the middle of the previous ocular dominance column (Fig. 27.12B). Thus there is a 50% overlap in the spatial locations represented by adjacent ocular dominance columns. In this manner, a complete representation of space is attained for both eyes while ensuring that cells that respond to overlapping points in visual space are always nearby within the cortex.

Ocular Dominance and Orientation Columns Can Be Revealed with Optical Imaging

The technique of optical imaging has proven extremely useful in the study of the functional architecture of the visual cortex. Optical imaging allows direct visualization of the relative activity of small cortical ensembles rather than relying on inferences made from single-unit studies (Blasdel and Salama, 1986; Grinvald *et al.*, 1986). The technique uses dyes that change their optical properties with neural activity. Even if no dyes are used, brain activity can be mapped with an intrinsic signal, caused primarily by changes in blood flow and blood oxygenation.

A typical optical imaging experiment works as follows (Fig. 27.13A). First, a series of digitized images is taken of a region of visual cortex (Fig. 27.13B) while the animal is presented with visual stimuli through the left eye. Next, a similar series is captured during right eye stimulation. When the right eye images are subtracted digitally from the left eye images, a striking picture is created that reveals the functional architecture of ocular dominance (Fig. 27.13C). Previously, anatomical methods had been used to produce maps of ocular dominance, and these maps appear similar to those found with optical imaging, but an important feature of optical imaging is that multiple images can be obtained from the same region of the cortex. For instance, in addition to ocular dominance, maps of the preferred orientation can also be made. A useful way to present these data is in terms of a color code, in which each color represents a different preferred orientation (Fig. 27.13D). The orientation columns revealed by optical imaging were consistent with earlier microelectrode studies (compare Fig. 27.13E

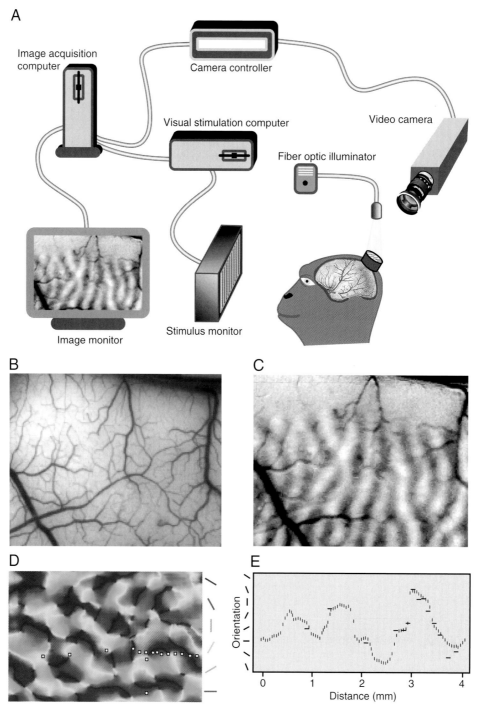

FIGURE 27.13 Optical imaging of functional architecture in the primate visual cortex. (A) Schematic diagram of the experimental setup for optical imaging. Digitized images of a region of visual cortex (as in B) are taken with a CCD camera while the anesthetized, paralyzed animal is viewing a visual stimulus. These images are stored on a second computer for further analysis. (B) Individual image (9 by 6 mm) of a region of V1 and a portion of V2 taken with a special filter so that blood vessels stand out. (C) Ocular dominance map. Images of the brain during right-eye stimulation were subtracted digitally from images taken during left-eye stimulation. (D) Orientation map. Images of the brain were taken during stimulation at 12 different angles. The orientation of stimuli that produced the strongest signal at each pixel is color coded, as indicated to the right. The key at the right gives the correspondence between color and the optimal orientation. (E) Comparison of the preferred orientation of single neurons with the optical image. At each of the locations indicated by squares in D, single neurons were recorded with microelectrodes. The preferred orientations of the neurons (dashes) were compared with the preferred orientations measured in the optical image, sampled along the line connecting the recording sites (dots). A: adapted From Grinvald *et al.* (1988); B and C: adapted from Ts'o *et al.* (1990); D and E: adapted From Blasdel and Salama (1986).

with Fig. 27.12A), but the images for the first time gave a detailed picture of the layout of orientation across the cortical surface. Details of these orientation maps—and their relationships with ocular dominance—were entirely new and had not been demonstrated with previous techniques.

Cytochrome Oxidase Staining Reveals Blobs and Stripes in Cortical Areas V1 and V2

In the primate, there is a fourth feature of the functional architecture of visual cortex in addition to retinotopy, orientation, and ocular dominance columns. When stained for the enzyme cytochrome oxidase (a metabolic enzyme whose presence indicates high activity), histological sections of V1 revealed a regular pattern of patches, or blobs (Fig. 27.14). In layers 2+3, these blobs were reported to contain neurons whose receptive fields are color selective, poorly oriented, and monocular (Livingstone and Hubel, 1984).

In V2, the second visual area in the cerebral cortex (see later), cytochrome oxidase staining reveals regions of high and low activity arranged in parallel stripes (Fig. 27.14, along the top). The anatomical connections between V1 and V2 are strongly constrained by the subdivisions revealed by cytochrome oxidase staining. Layer 4B of V1 projects to thick stained stripes; in layers 2+3, the interblob areas project to unstained stripes and blobs project to thin stained stripes.

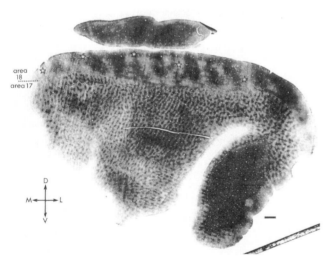

FIGURE 27.14 Macaque visual cortex stained for the metabolic enzyme, cytochrome oxidase. A tangential section through layers 2+3 of V1 (below) and V2 (above) is shown. In V1, blobs are seen in a regular array with a spacing of 400 mm. In V2, there are cytochrome oxidase-rich stripes with much coarser spacing. The distinction between thick and thin stripes (see text) is seen less readily in the macaque than in the owl monkey. Scale bar: 1 mm. From Livingstone and Hubel (1984).

The anatomy and physiology of the regions defined by cytochrome oxidase staining in V1 and V2 have been the objects of much research since the 1980s, and of much controversy. It is agreed that blobs in layers 2+3 are the sites of termination of the koniocellular thalamic afferents, but the relationship between cytochrome oxidase staining and magnocellular and parvocellular pathways, originally thought to be straightforward, is still an open question (reviewed in Merigan and Maunsell, 1994). Consensus has been reached on one point, however: magnocellular inputs dominate the pathway from 4Cα to 4B in V1; 4B then projects, both directly and indirectly (via the thick stripes in V2), to regions of the brain that process visual motion signals. Magnocellular neurons, with their rapidly conducting axons and high sensitivity to luminance contrast, are well suited to providing input to the motion-sensitive neurons in cortical areas MT and MST (see later).

Many Extrastriate Visual Areas Perform Different Functions

In early studies of the cytoarchitecture of cerebral cortex, the visual cortex was divided into three areas according to Brodmann's classification: areas 17, 18, and 19. These divisions were based on differences in cell cytoarchitecture, or differences in the size, morphology, and distributions of cells within the six cortical laminae. Area 17 is primary visual cortex, or striate cortex, so named because of a heavily myelinated sublamina within layer 4 (4Cα), prominently visible as a stripe in transverse section. Areas 18 and 19 were known simply as the visual association cortex. An assumption behind these designations was that areas defined by anatomical criteria would ultimately prove to be functionally specialized.

The demonstration of multiple visual cortical areas has been one of the important discoveries of the past quarter century in the field of sensory neurobiology. A vast expanse of cerebral cortex—greater than 50% of the total in many primate species—is involved primarily or exclusively in the processing of visual information. The extrastriate cortex now includes areas 18 and 19, as well as large regions of the temporal and parietal lobes (see Fig. 27.15 for a diagram of the four main regions of cerebral cortex: occipital, parietal, temporal, and frontal). It is composed of some 30 subdivisions that can be distinguished by their physiology, cytoarchitecture, histochemistry, and/or connections with other areas (Felleman and Van Essen, 1991). Each of these extrastriate visual areas is thought to make unique functional contributions to visual perception and visually guided behavior.

A

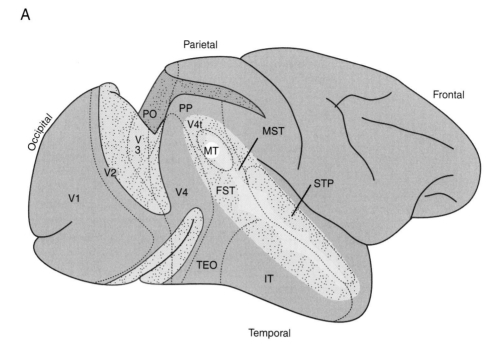

B

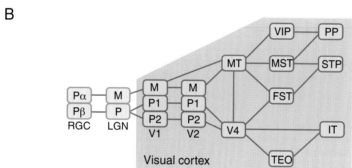

FIGURE 27.15 Extrastriate cortical regions. (A) Lateral view of the macaque brain, with the sulci partially opened to expose the areas within them. Shown are the rough outlines of the main visual areas, which take up all of the occipital cortex and much of the parietal and temporal cortex. (B) Partial diagram of the connections between visual areas. Emphasis is placed on the hierarchical organization of the connections and on the partially segregated P parvocellular and M magnocellular pathways. Adapted from Albright (1993).

As a testament to the increasing complexity of the field, the naming of visual areas (see Fig. 27.15) has progressed from the use of simple labels—V1 through V4—to the use of more complex terms specifying anatomical location of each new area, such as MT (medial temporal, or V5), MST (medial superior temporal), or IT (inferotemporal, itself made up of several distinct areas).

The dual themes of parallel and hierarchical processing are central to the understanding of the extrastriate cortex. Figure 27.15 is a vastly simplified version of a wiring diagram between visual areas (Felleman and Van Essen, 1991). Several criteria have been used to define new visual cortical areas. First, extrastriate regions have retinotopic maps of the

visual world that can be demonstrated by physiological recordings. Second, a clear hierarchy between many cortical areas can be demonstrated anatomically. There is a stereotyped pattern of projections from one visual area to the next. Where strong connections between two areas exist, these connections tend to be bidirectional. The feedforward and feedback connections are distinguished by the layers that send and receive the connections. In such a manner, a clear hierarchy can be traced, for instance, along the pathway V1→ V2→ V3→ MT→ MST (with several shortcuts, such as V1→ MT).

While physiological studies of cortical areas revealed profound differences between them, a series of studies by Ungerleider and Mishkin (1982) uncovered a higher order dichotomy between two types of processing in the extrastriate cortex. Using behavioral analyses of animals with anatomically defined cortical lesions, Ungerleider and Mishkin found a strong dissociation between the types of deficits exhibited by animals with lesions in either their parietal cortex or their temporal cortex (see Fig. 27.15). Animals with temporal lesions were often much worse at recognizing objects visually, although lower level visual function, such as acuity, was not appreciably lessened. Parietal lesions led to little or no deficit in object recognition, but visuospatial tasks, such as visually

---

BOX 27.4

THREE TYPES OF SELECTIVITY FOR MOTION

Motion is one of the most important aspects of the visual world. It is a powerful cue for navigating in the world, for segregating figures from their background, and for predicting the trajectory of objects. It is not surprising, therefore, that sensitivity to motion is a highly developed feature of the mammalian visual system. At the lowest level, a class of neurons in the retina respond best to stimuli moving in a specific direction (Barlow *et al.*, 1964). These neurons give *on–off* responses to flashed lights (denoted ± in Fig. 27.16 A), but are best excited by the motion of an object anywhere in their receptive fields. They can signal that motion in a particular range of directions is present, but because their receptive fields are relatively large and have both *on-and-off* responses, they cannot resolve the details of an object. Directionally selective retinal neurons do not project to the LGN so directional neurons found in the visual cortex (Hubel and Wiesel, 1962) create their selectivity independently and with a different mechanism.

Unlike directionally selective ganglion cells, which signal that motion is present somewhere within a large region, directionally selective simple cells in the visual cortex maintain detailed spatial information as well. A moving stimulus, such as a light bar moving to the left (Fig. 27.16B, left), is described by its trajectory in space over time. If the trajectory is plotted in space versus time, the slope represents the direction and velocity of the object. For instance, a bar moving to the right traces an oblique trajectory (up and to the left) in such a space–time plot (Fig. 27.16B, middle). When represented in a similar plot, the receptive fields of directionally selective simple cells can show a similar orientation (Fig. 27.16B, right). This plot is exactly analogous to Kuffler's maps of ganglion cell receptive fields. It represents the responses of the cell to a bright or dark bar at different positions, but it includes the time course of the responses as well. The *on* responses of this receptive field (the responses to a bright bar) are indicated with solid contour lines and are shown in white for added emphasis; *off* flanks (the responses to dark bars) are indicated with dotted contour lines.

For directionally selective simple cells, the timing of the response is directly related to the position of the stimulus. In the illustration, the cell is sensitive to a bright bar at a range of positions, but the timing of the peak response changes with position. These responses to flashed bars explain the responses to moving stimuli. Just as *on-center/off*-surround ganglion cells respond best to a bright spot on a dark background (Fig. 27.3C), a directionally selective simple cell responds best to a bar moving in a specific direction. A moving bar is the stimulus that best matches the template formed by its receptive field. In this manner, simple cell receptive fields can be strongly direction selective, but their responses preserve precise information about the position and structure of the stimulus.

A third kind of directionally selective cell is found in cortical area MT of the macaque. Receptive fields of individual neurons in MT integrate motion information over large regions of visual space. By comparison, receptive fields in the retina, LGN, and V1 can be thought of as viewing the world through much smaller apertures. If the goal of vision is to extract the properties of objects, rather than isolated features, then the existence of small receptive fields can lead to what is known as the *aperture problem*. As illustrated in Figure 27.16C, two objects moving in different directions can appear to have the same direction of motion when viewed through an aperture. In a dual study of perception in humans and of MT neurons in macaques, Movshon and colleagues (1985) analyzed the responses to complex stimuli whose components moved in different directions (such as the edges of the square in the bottom half of Fig. 27.16C), but which were perceived as coherent patterns moving in an intermediate "pattern direction." Unlike neurons in V1, many neurons in MT responded to the pattern direction rather than to the components. This would imply that these MT neurons combine their inputs in a complex manner to achieve a selectivity for the motion of extended objects rather than primitive features.

R. Clay Reid

A

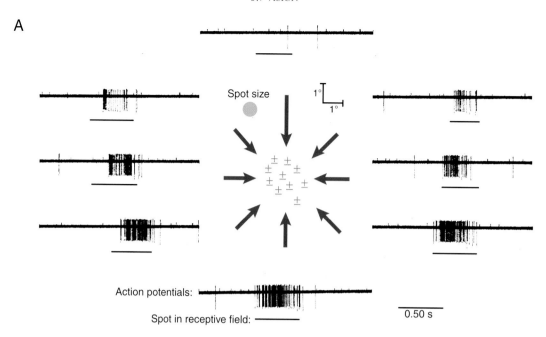

Action potentials: ⊢

Spot in receptive field: ────────

0.50 s

B

Moving bar   Simple cell receptive field

Space–Space   Space–Time   Space–Time

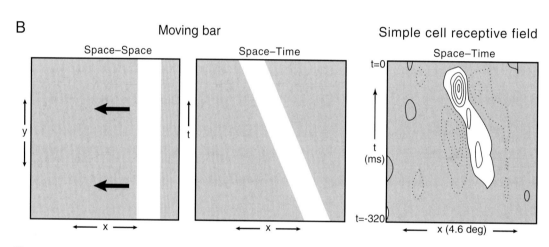

C

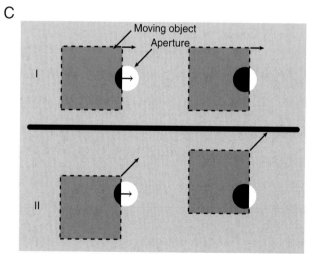

guided behavior, were impaired profoundly. From these studies and the growing body of physiological evidence, two distinct streams were postulated: a *temporal* or *ventral stream* devoted to object recognition and a *parietal* or *dorsal stream* devoted to action or spatial tasks. Ungerleider and Mishkin termed these the "what" and "where" pathways.

The temporal stream, V1→ V2→ V3→ V4→ IT ..., is discussed elsewhere (Chapter 55). This chapter considers only the parietal stream, V1→ V2→ MT→ MST .... The parietal stream is dominated by magnocellular cells and the temporal stream by parvocellular inputs, although the segregation is far from strict (Merigan and Maunsell, 1994).

In the Parietal Cortex, Neurons Are Selective for Higher Order Motion Cues

MT, or V5, is perhaps the best understood of the extrastriate visual areas. It has held particular interest ever since its was discovered in 1971 (Allman and Kaas, 1971; Dubner and Zeki, 1971), primarily because it was the first area found that was strongly dominated by one visual function. Fully 95% of the neurons in MT are highly selective for the direction of motion of a stimulus (Dubner and Zeki, 1971). In V1, a significant fraction of neurons are selective for the direction of motion, but the optimal speed may vary depending on the spatial structure of the object that is moving. In MT, speed tuning is less dependent on other stimulus attributes. Receptive fields of individual neurons in MT integrate motion information over large regions of visual space and are qualitatively less selective than neurons in the primary visual cortex. This generalization of motion signals can be achieved in a simple manner, such as by adding together inputs over space or, in a complex manner, by combining two component motions in different directions into a single coherent motion (see Box 27.4). Of even greater interest, neurons in MT (and, to a greater extent, those in MST) appear to be sensitive to more complex aspects of visual motion, such as the motion of extended objects rather than isolated features (Albright, 1993).

The range of stimuli that a given MT neuron can respond to is impressively broad—the attributes, or form cues, that define a figure can be luminance, texture, or relative motion—but the preferred direction and speed are always the same for that neuron (Albright, 1993). This is an extreme example of what were termed high-order responses in the introduction to this chapter. Neurons at lower levels in the visual system are sensitive to isolated and specific features in visual scenes. Higher visual areas respond to very specific attributes, but these attributes are increasingly remote from the physical stimulus. Instead, they represent increasingly complex concepts, such the motion of an extended object or the identity of a face.

Summary

The lateral geniculate nucleus of the thalamus is a layered structure that receives segregated input from the two eyes and projects to the primary visual cortex (V1). Geniculate neurons have center-surround receptive fields that are similar to those of their retinal inputs. In contrast, most neurons in the primary visual cortex are sensitive to the orientation of a stimulus. In mammalian species, there are elements of both hierarchical and parallel processing in the primary visual cortex. This section has emphasized that the visual cortical circuit in the cat can be seen as a functional hierarchy that transforms geniculate input into simple and then complex receptive fields. In the macaque monkey the focus has been on the parallel pathways that are kept relatively separate in the striate and extrastriate cortex.

The visual cortex has an orderly functional architecture. Neurons within a cortical column have similar receptive field attributes, such as orientation selectivity, ocular dominance, and receptive field location. Each of these receptive field attributes varies smoothly

◄ **FIGURE 27.16** Three types of direction selectivity. (A) Receptive field map of a directionally selective ganglion cell in the rabbit (± indicates where neuron responded in an *on–off* manner). Surrounding it are individual responses to stimuli moving in eight different directions. The smooth traces below each train of action potentials correspond to the position of the stimulus as it moves in the indicated direction. Horizontal bars indicate when the spot was in the receptive field. (B) Direction selectivity in cortical simple cells of the cat. A bar moving to the left (shown in a space–time plot in the middle panel) matches the template formed by a directionally selective simple receptive field (shown in a space–time plot at right). The vertical time axis in the right-hand panel corresponds to the stimulus location 0 to 320 ms *before* the neuron fired. Bright regions in the receptive field correspond to the best location for a bright stimulus at each delay between stimulus and response. (C) The ambiguous motion of an extended object when viewed through a small aperture—known as the aperture problem—is partially resolved by some neurons in macaque cortical area MT. The squares in I and II (each shown at two successive time points) are moving in different directions, but they appear identical when viewed through a small aperture. A: adapted from Barlow *et al.* (1964); B: far right adapted from McLean *et al.* (1994).

over the cortical surface. The organization of ocular dominance columns and orientation columns across the cortical surface can be visualized with optical imaging.

Finally, in the macaque monkey, there are more than 30 extrastriate visual cortical regions, each of which performs different functions. These extrastriate regions can be divided into two pathways: the temporal stream, devoted to form recognition, and the parietal stream, devoted to action or to spatial tasks. Areas in each stream form a functional and anatomical hierarchy. Neurons in successive visual areas respond to increasingly high-order or abstract features of the visual world.

References

Albright, T. D. (1993). Cortical processing of visual motion. *In* "Visual Motion and Its Role in the Stabilization of Gaze" (F. A. Miles and J. Wallman, eds.), pp. 177–201. Elsevier Science, Amsterdam.

Allman , J. M., and Kaas, J. H. (1971). A representation of the visual field in the caudal third of the middle temporal gyrus of the owl monkey (*Aotus trivirgatus*). *Brain Res.* **31**, 85–105.

Barlow, H. B., Hill, R. M., and Levick, W. R. (1964). Retinal ganglion cells responding selectively to direction and speed of image motion in the rabbit. *J. Physiol.* **173**, 377–407.

Blasdel, G. G., and Salama, G. (1986). Voltage-sensitive dyes reveal a modular organization in monkey striate cortex. *Nature* **321**, 579–585.

Dacey, D. M. (2000). Parallel pathways for spectral coding in primate retina. *Annu. Rev. Neurosci.* **23**, 743–775.

Dowling, J. E. (1997). Retina. *In* "Encyclopedia of Human Biology," 2nd Ed, Vol. 7, pp. 571–587. Academic Press, New York.

Dubner, R., and Zeki, S. M. (1971). Response properties and receptive fields of cells in an anatomically defined region of the superior temporal sulcus in the monkey. *Brain Res.* **35**, 528–532.

Enroth-Cugell, C., and Robson, J. G. (1966). The contrast sensitivity of retinal ganglion cells of the cat. *J. Physiol.* **187**, 517–552.

Felleman, D. J., and van Essen, D. C. (1991). Distributed hierarchical processing in the primate cerebral cortex. *Cerebral Cortex* **1**, 1–47.

Ferster, D., Chung, S., and Wheat, H. (1996). Orientation selectivity of thalamic input to simple cells of cat visual cortex. *Nature* **380**, 249–252

Gilbert, C. D., and Wiesel, T. N. (1985). Intrinsic connectivity and receptive field properties in visual cortex. *Vision Res.* **25**, 365–374.

Grinvald, A., Lieke, E., Frostig, R. D, Gilbert, C. D., and Wiesel, T. N. (1986). Functional architecture of cortex revealed by optical imaging of intrinsic signals. *Nature* **324**, 361–364.

Helmholtz, H. (2000). "Handbook of Physiological Optics" (J. P. C. Southall, ed.), Vol. 2, p. 143. Thoemmes Press, Bristol, UK.

Hubel, D. H., and Wiesel, T. N. (1962). Receptive fields, binocular interaction and functional architecture in the cat's visual cortex. *J. Physiol.* **160**, 106–154.

Kaplan, E., and Shapley, R. M. (1986). The primate retina contains two types of ganglion cells, with high and low contrast sensitivity. *Proc. Natl. Acad. Sci. USA* **83**, 2755–2757.

Kuffler, S. W. (1953). Discharge patterns and functional organization of the mammalian retina. *J. Neurophysiol.* **16**, 37–68.

Livingstone, M. S., and Hubel, D. H. (1984). Anatomy and physiology of a color system in the primate visual cortex. *J. Neurosci.* **4**, 309–356.

McLean, J., Raab, S., and Palmer, L. A. (1994). Contribution of linear mechanisms to the specification of local motion by simple cells in areas 17 and 18 of the cat. *Visual Neurosci.* **11**, 271–294.

Merigan, W. H., and Maunsell, J. H. R. (1994). How parallel are the primate visual pathways? *Annu. Rev. Neurosci.* **16**, 369–402.

Movshon, J. A., Adelson, E. H., Gizzi, M., and Newsome, W. T. (1985). The analysis of moving visual patterns. *In* "Pattern Recognition Mechanisms" (C. Chagas, R. Gattass, and C. G. Gross, eds.), pp. 117–151. Vatican Press, Rome.

Nathans, J., Thomas, D., and Hogness, D. S. (1986). Molecular genetics of human color vision: The genes encoding blue, green, and red pigments. *Science* **232**, 193–202.

Ratliff, F. (1974). "Studies on Excitation and Inhibition in the Retina. A Collection of Papers from the Laboratories of H. Keffer Hartline." Rockefeller Univ. Press, New York.

Reid, R. C., and Alonso, J. M. (1995). Specificity of monosynaptic connections from thalamus to visual cortex. *Nature* **378**, 281–284.

Ts'o, D. Y., Frostig, R. D, Lieke, E. E., and Grinvald, A. (1990). Functional organization of primate visual cortex revealed by high resolution optical imaging. *Science* **249**, 417–420.

Ungerleider, L. G., and Mishkin, M. (1982). Two cortical visual systems. *In* "Analysis of Visual Behavior" (D. J. Ingle, M. A. Goodale, and R. J. W. Mansfield, eds.), pp. 549–586. MIT Press, Cambridge, MA.

Wandell, B. A. (1993). "Foundations of Vision." Sinauer, Sunderland, MA.

Wiesel, T. N., and Hubel, D. H. (1966). Spatial and chromatic interactions in the lateral geniculate body of the rhesus monkey. *J. Neurophysiol.* **29**, 1115–1156.

Wu, S. M. (1994). Synaptic transmission in the outer retina. *Annu. Rev. Physiol.* **56**, 141–168.

Suggested Readings

Boynton, R. M., and Kaiser, P. K. (1996). "Human Color Vision," 2nd Ed. Optical Society of America, Washington, DC.

Hubel, D. H. (1988). "Eye, Brain, and Vision." Freeman, New York.

Marr, D. (1982). "Vision: A Computational Investigation into the Human Representation and Processing of Visual Information." Freeman, New York.

R. Clay Reid

MOTOR SYSTEMS

28

Fundamentals of Motor Systems

"All mankind can do is to move things…
whether whispering a syllable or felling a forest"
(Sherrington)

This brief quote is a reminder of the basic fact that all interactions with the surrounding world are through the actions of the motor system. When a human baby is born it is a sweet but very immature survival machine, with a limited behavioral repertoire. It is able to breathe and has searching and sucking reflexes so that it can be fed from the mother's breast. It can swallow, vomit and process

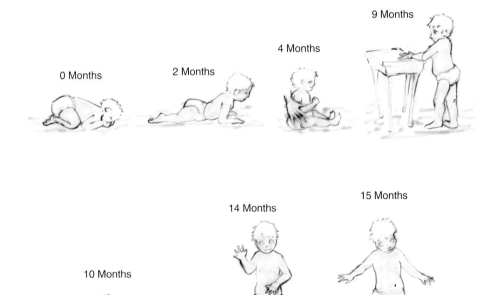

FIGURE 28.1 Motor development of the infant and young child. The pattern of maturation of the motor system follows a characteristic evolution. Two months after birth a child can lift its head, at 4 months it sits with support, and subsequently it is able to stand with support; later it crawls, stands without support, and finally walks independently. The approximate time at which a child is able to perform these different motor tasks is indicated above each figure. The variability in the maturation process is substantial. Modified from M. M. Shirley.

food, and cry to call upon attention if something is wrong. A baby also has a variety of protective reflexes that mediate coughing, sneezing, and touch avoidance. These different patterns of motor behavior are thus available at birth and are due to innate motor programs (Fig. 28.1).

During roughly the first 15 years of life the motor system continues to develop through maturation of neuronal circuitry and by learning through different motor activities. Playing represents an important element both in children and in young mammals such as kittens and pups. During the first year of life the human infant matures progressively. It can balance its head at 2–3 months, is able to sit at around 6–7 months, and stand with support at approximately 9–12 months. The coordination of different types of posture, such as standing, is a complex motor task to master, with hundreds of different muscles taking part in a coordinated fashion. Sensory information contributes importantly, in particular from the vestibular apparatus, eyes, muscle, and skin receptors located at the soles of the feet. This development represents to a large degree a maturation process following a given sequence, but with individual variability among different children. When the postural system has evolved to a sufficient degree, a child is able to start walking, which requires that the body posture is maintained while the points of support are changing

by the alternating movements of the two legs. In common language the child is said to "learn" to walk, but in reality a progressive maturation of the nervous system is taking place. Identical twins start to walk essentially at the same time, even if one has been subjected to training and the other has not. At this point the motor pattern is still very immature. Proper walking coordination followed by running appears later, and the basic motor pattern actually continues to develop until puberty. The fine details of the motor pattern are adapted to the surrounding world, but also to modification by will. The basic motor coordination underlying reaching and the fine control of hands and fingers undergo a similar characteristic maturation process over many years.

While the newborn human infant is comparatively immature, other mammals, such as horses and deer, represent another extreme. The gnu, an African buffalo-like antelope, needs to run away in order to survive attacks of predators such as lions. The young calf of the gnu can stand and run directly after birth and has been reported to be able to gallop ahead 10 min after delivery, tracking the running mother (Fig. 28.2). Clearly the neural networks underlying locomotion, equilibrium control, and steering must be sufficiently mature and available at birth, needing minimal calibration. This is astounding. A similar range of maturity is present in birds. To get out of the egg, a chick

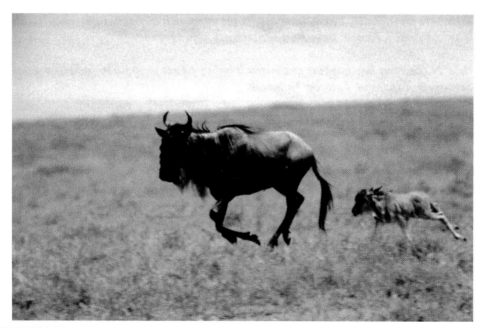

FIGURE 28.2   Some animals are comparatively mature when they are born. Ten minutes after the calf of the gnu, a buffalo-like antelope, is born it is able to track its mother in a gallop. This means that the postural and locomotor systems are sufficiently mature to allow the young calf to generate these complex patterns of motor coordination at birth. There is thus little time to calibrate the motor system after birth and obviously no time for learning. Courtesy of Erik Tallmark.

makes coordinated hatching movements to open up the eggshell to subsequently lift off the top of the egg and to stand up to walk away on two legs following the mother hen and start picking at food grains. Most birds are more immature when hatching, but after a few weeks they leave the nest flying rather successfully, for the first time in their life, and thus without any previous experience.

In addition to the basic motor skills such as standing, walking, and chewing, humans also develop skilled motor coordination, allowing delicate hand and finger movements to be used in handwriting or playing an instrument or utilizing the air flow and shape of the oral cavity to produce sound as in speech or singing. The neural substrates allowing learning and execution of these complex motor sequences are expressed genetically. What is learned, however, such as which language one speaks or the type of letters one writes, is obviously a function of the cultural environment.

BASIC COMPONENTS OF THE MOTOR SYSTEM

Motoneurons and Motor Units

The motoneurons that control different muscles are located in different motor nuclei along the spinal cord and in the brain stem. Each motoneuron sends its axon to one muscle and innervates a limited number of muscle fibers. A motoneuron with its muscle fibers is referred to as a motor unit. The muscle fibers of each motor unit have similar contractile properties and metabolic profile. The muscle fibers in different muscles are composed of three main types specialized for different demands, such as a continuous effort as in long-distance running (slow motor units) or fast explosive movements, such as lifting a heavy object [fast motor units (two subtypes)].

Motoneurons are activated by interneurons of different motor programs or reflex centers and by descending tracts from the forebrain and the brain stem. Thus motoneurons supplying different muscles can be activated with great precision by these different sources that together determine the degree of activation, as well as the exact timing of the motoneurons of a given muscle.

Sensory Receptors Are Important in Movement Control

Signals from sensory receptors are used by the motor system in a number of ways.

1. Sensory signals can trigger behaviorally meaningful motor acts such as withdrawal, coughing, or swallowing reflexes.

2. Sensory receptors may contribute to the control of an ongoing motor pattern and influence the switch from one phase of movement to another. For instance, in the case of breathing, sensory signals from lung volume receptors control when inspiration is terminated. In walking, sensory signals related to hip position and load on the limb help regulate the duration of the support and swing phases of the step cycle and correct for perturbations.

3. Sensory signals may also be more specific and influence only the level of activity of one muscle or a group of close synergists. Muscle receptors play a particularly important role in this context. They are of two types: (i) Golgi tendon organs that sense the degree of contraction in a muscle (located in series with the muscle fibers at their insertion into the tendon) and (ii) muscle spindles that signal the length of a muscle (located in parallel to the muscle fibers), as well as the speed of changes in length. Moreover, the sensitivity of muscle spindles can be regulated actively through a separate set of small motoneurons, referred to as γ-motoneurons (in contrast to the larger α-motoneurons that control muscle contraction). These two muscle receptors have fast conducting afferent axons that provide rapid feedback to the spinal cord and take part in the autoregulation of the motor output to a given muscle. Fast muscle spindle afferents provide direct monosynaptic excitation to the α-motoneurons that control the muscle in which the muscle spindle is located. Thus, lengthening a muscle will lead to excitation of its motoneurons, counteracting the lengthening. This stretch reflex thus involves negative feedback. This reflex arc also provides the basis of the muscle contraction elicited by a brief tendon tap, which is used as a clinical test to investigate whether responsiveness of the motoneuronal pool is normal (the tendon reflex) (Fig. 28.3).

4. Sensory signals from a number of different receptor systems help detect and counteract any disturbance of body posture during standing or maintenance of another body position. Skin and muscle receptors and receptors signaling joint position, as well as vestibular receptors and vision, contribute to different aspects of the dynamic and static control of body position.

5. When an object is held by the fingers, skin receptors at the contact points at the fingertips play an important role. If the object tends to slip, the skin receptors become activated and signal rapidly to the nervous system that there is a need for extra muscle force.

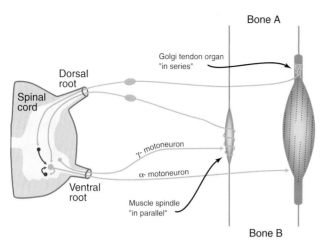

FIGURE 28.3 Feedback from muscle receptors to motoneurons: the stretch reflex. In a muscle connected between two bones, the Golgi tendon organ is located at the transition between muscle and tendon. It senses any active tension produced by the muscle fibers, being in series between muscle and tendon. The muscle spindle is located in parallel with the muscle fibers. It signals the muscle length and dynamic changes in muscle length. Both the muscle spindle and the Golgi tendon organ have fast conducting afferent nerve fibers in the range of ~100 m/s. The muscle spindle activates α-motoneurons directly, which causes the muscle fibers to contract. The sensitivity of the muscle spindle can be actively regulated by γ-motoneurons, which are more slowly conducting. The muscle spindle provides negative feedback. If the muscle with its muscle spindle is lengthened, the afferent activity from the muscle spindle increases, exciting the α-motoneurons and leading to an increased muscle contraction, which in turn counteracts the lengthening. This is called the stretch reflex. The Golgi tendon organ provides force feedback. The more the muscle contracts, the more the Golgi tendon organ and its afferent are activated. In the diagram the intercalated interneuron between afferent nerve fiber and motoneuron is inhibitory. Thus increased muscle force leads to inhibition of the α-motoneuron, which results in a decrease of muscle force. The efficacy of length and force feedback can be regulated independently in the spinal cord and via γ-motoneurons. Thus their respective contributions can vary considerably between different patterns of motor behavior.

6. A great variety of sensory signals provide information about the position of different parts of the body in relation to each other and to the external world. Such information is critical when initiating a voluntary movement. For example, to move a hand toward a given object, it is important to know the initial position of the arm and the hand in space. Depending on whether the hand is located to the left or the right of the object, different types of motor commands must be given to bring the hand to the target. Sensory information about the initial position of the hand (or any other body part) in relation to the rest of the body, as well as the target for the movement, is thus important for eliciting an effective neural command signal.

To summarize, the sensory contribution to motor control is very important in many different contexts. If sensory control is incapacitated, motor performance will in most cases be degraded. Without sensory information in different forms, movements can usually still be executed, but as a rule with much less perfection.

Feedback and Feed Forward Control

If a perturbation occurs when an object is held in the hand, or when standing in a moving bus, it will be detected by different sensory receptors. This sensory signal will be fed back to the nervous system and be used to counteract the perturbation rapidly. This represents feedback control that is a correction of the actual perturbation after it has occurred. A limiting factor for the efficacy of feedback control in biological systems is the delay involved. A sensory afferent signal must first be elicited in the receptors concerned. It then has to be conducted to the central nervous system and be processed there to determine the proper response. The correction signal must subsequently be sent back to the appropriate muscle(s) and make the muscle fibers build up the contractile force required. In large animals, including humans, the delays involved can be substantial, and during fast movement sequences there may be little or no time for feedback corrections. In less demanding, more static situations, such as standing, sensory feedback is of critical importance.

In many cases a perturbation is anticipated before it is initiated, and correction begins before it has actually occurred. This type of control is often called feed forward control in contrast to feedback. Such anticipatory control mechanisms are often automatic and involuntary, and are part of an inherent control strategy. For example, when standing on two legs and planning to lift up one leg to stand on the other, the body position begins to shift over to the supporting leg before the other leg is lifted. The projection of the center of gravity will fall between the two feet initially and will have to shift over to a projection through the supporting limb. In most instances, movement commands are designed so that the corrections of body posture required for a stable movement occur before the particular movement has started, as when lifting a heavy object. If the converse situation occurred, and body position was corrected only after a perturbation had taken place, movements would become much less precise than with feed forward control.

MOTOR PROGRAMS COORDINATE BASIC MOTOR PATTERNS

Both vertebrates and invertebrates have preformed microcircuits—neuronal networks that contain the

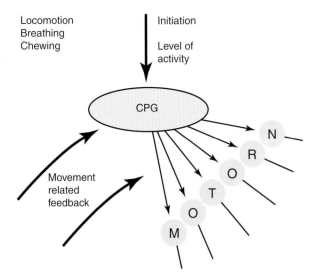

FIGURE 28.4 Motor coordination through interneuronal networks: central pattern generators. The brain stem and spinal cord contain a number of networks that are designed to control different basic patterns of the motor repertoire, such as breathing, walking, chewing, or swallowing. These networks are often referred to as central pattern generator networks (CPGs). CPGs contain the necessary information to activate different motoneurons and muscles in the appropriate sequence. Some CPGs are active under resting conditions, such as that for breathing, but most are actively turned on from the brain stem or the frontal lobes. For instance, the CPG coordinating locomotor movements is turned on from specific areas in the brain stem, referred to as locomotor centers. These descending control signals not only turn on the locomotor CPG, but also determine the level of activity in the CPG and whether slow or fast locomotor activity will occur. In order to have the motor pattern well adjusted to external conditions and different perturbations, sensory feedback acts on the CPG and can modify the duration of different phases of the activity cycle, providing feedback onto motoneurons. Although vertebrates as well as invertebrates have CPGs for a great variety of motor functions, the intrinsic operation of these networks of interneurons constituting the CPG is unclear in most cases. In invertebrates, a few CPG networks have been studied in great detail, such as the stomatogastric system of the lobster and networks coordinating the activity of the heart and locomotion in the leech. In vertebrates detailed information concerning locomotor networks is only available in lower forms, such as the frog embryo and the lamprey.

necessary information to coordinate a specific motor pattern such as swallowing, walking, or breathing. When a given neuronal network is activated, the particular behavior it controls will be expressed. A typical network consists of a group of interneurons that activate a specific group of motoneurons in a certain sequence and inhibit other motoneurons that may counteract the intended movement. Such a group of interneurons is often referred to as a central pattern generator (CPG) or motor program. This CPG can be activated by will, as at the start of walking, or be triggered by sensory stimuli, as in a protective reflex

or swallowing. In most types of motor behavior, sensory feedback may also form an integral part of the motor control circuit and may determine the duration of the motor activity such as the inspiratory phase of breathing (Fig. 28.4).

There are several different types of motor coordination.

Motor Patterns Triggered as a Reflex Response

1. Protective skin reflexes lead to withdrawal of the stimulated part of the body from a stimulus that may cause pain or tissue damage. The central program consists in this case of a group of interneurons that activate motoneurons and muscles, giving rise to an appropriate withdrawal movement. Motoneurons to antagonistic muscles are inhibited (reciprocal inhibition). The withdrawal reflexes of the limbs are often referred to as flexion reflexes, but in reality they represent a family of specific reflexes, each of which is designed to remove the specific skin region involved from the painful stimulus.

2. Coughing and sneezing reflexes remove an irritant from the nasal or tracheal mucosa by inducing a brief pulse of air flow at very high velocity (at storm or hurricane speeds). This is caused by an almost synchronized activation of abdominal and respiratory muscles, coordinated by a CPG, the activity of which is triggered by afferents activated by the irritant.

3. Swallowing reflexes are activated when food is brought in contact with mucosal receptors near the pharynx. This leads to a coordinated motor act with sequential activation of different muscles that propel the food bolus through the pharynx down the esophagus to the stomach. In this case the CPG is able to coordinate the motor act over several seconds, in contrast to the previous motor acts in which the activity occurs almost simultaneously.

Rhythmic Movements

1. Walking movements (or locomotor behaviors in general) are produced by CPGs in the spinal cord (or ganglia of invertebrates). These spinal CPGs are turned on by descending control signals from particular areas in the brain stem (locomotor areas), which also determine the level of locomotor activity (e.g., slow walking versus trot or gallop). The CPG then sequentially activates motoneurons/muscles that support the limb during the support phase and then move it forward during the swing phase. Sensory stimuli from the moving limb also contribute importantly to regulate the duration of the support phase

and the degree of activation of different muscles that are sequentially activated in each step cycle. The relative importance of the sensory component varies between species and with the speed of locomotion. During very fast movements, there is actually no time for sensory feedback to act, and adjustments need instead to be performed in a predictive mode.

2. Chewing movements are controlled by brain stem circuits that in principle are designed in a similar manner to those of locomotion and generate alternating activity between jaw-opener and -closer muscles.

3. Breathing movements are continuously active from the instant of birth to the time of death, except for short voluntary interventions when speaking, singing, or choosing not to breathe for some other reason, like diving. The level of respiration (depth and frequency) is driven by metabolic demands (e.g., pCO_2) detected by chemosensors in the brain stem where the respiratory CPG is also located. Sensory stimuli from lung volume receptors contribute by setting the level at which the inspiration is terminated and expiration takes over.

Eye Movements

Fast saccadic eye movements are used when looking rapidly from one object to another and are represented with a much more complex organization in the superior colliculus (mesencephalon) than the motor patterns discussed earlier. Saccadic eye movements with different directions and amplitudes can be generated by the stimulation of different microregions in the superior colliculus, according to a well-defined topographical map. Each microregion is responsible for activating a subset of brain stem interneurons, which in turn activates the appropriate combination of eye motoneurons in order to move the two eyes in a coordinated fashion from one position to another. The purpose is to bring the visual object of interest into the foveal region so that it can be scrutinized in the greatest detail. To recruit a saccadic eye movement to a specific site, cortical or subcortical areas have to access the appropriate microregions within the superior colliculus to trigger the specific eye movement desired.

Other types of eye movement control are used when tracking an object that is moving, as when watching a game of tennis. These tracking movements are represented in the cerebral cortex and the brain stem.

Posture

Animals, including humans, have the ability to position the body in a variety of postures. The most stable position is lying horizontally in bed, which requires little activity from the nervous system. The situation is very different when standing and even more so when supporting oneself on one leg. This requires a very structured command to handle the activation of different muscles in the legs, trunk, shoulders, and neck. The nervous system issues this complex motor command to achieve a certain position. The ability to maintain a stable position standing on one leg is then critically dependent on feedback from a variety of sensory receptors that detect falling to one side or the other. These receptors activate reflex circuits that try to counteract the impending loss of balance. Of great importance are the vestibular receptors located in the head, which sense head movements in the different directions. Vestibular reflexes act on the neck muscles to correct the position of the head, and vestibulospinal reflexes act on the trunk and the extensor muscles of the limbs. In addition, vestibular effects are also mediated indirectly by the reticulospinal system. Muscle receptors in neck and limb muscles are of equal importance. They also play a critical role in detecting and compensating for postural perturbations, in particular around the ankle, where skin receptors on the bottoms of the feet are activated. Finally, visual feedback may contribute as when one is standing on a moving surface such as the deck of a boat.

The body can be arranged in a number of ways, sitting in a relaxed way on a sofa, stiffly on an uncomfortable chair, or standing with the body and the legs held in a range of postures. In one sense the postural system is essentially automatic in that there is no conscious thought about how to achieve a given position. However, one can decide at will what posture to assume. In that sense it is a voluntary motor act organized to a large extent on the brain stem level but is also affected by areas in the frontal lobe located just in front of the motor cortex.

ROLES OF DIFFERENT PARTS OF THE NERVOUS SYSTEM IN THE CONTROL OF MOVEMENT

The different basic motor patterns are present in different forms in most vertebrates and invertebrates. In the former, the underlying neural networks are located either in the brain stem or in the spinal cord, and in the latter, in the chain of ganglia. In vertebrates, from fish to mammals the basic organization of the nervous system is similar with regard to the spinal cord, brain stem (medulla oblongata and mesencephalon), and diencephalon. Each species and

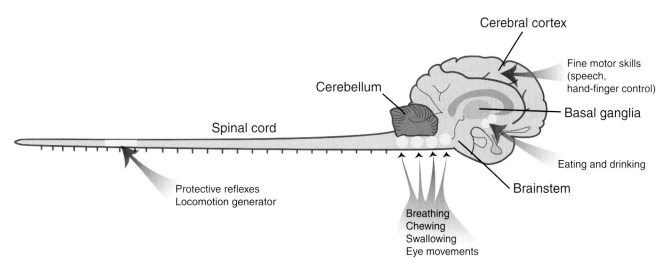

FIGURE 28.5 Location of different networks (CPGs) that coordinate different motor patterns in vertebrates. The spinal cord contains CPGs for locomotion and protective reflexes, whereas the brain stem contains CPGs for breathing, chewing, swallowing, and saccadic eye movements. The hypothalamus in the forebrain contains centers that regulate eating and drinking. These areas can coordinate the sequence of activation of different CPGs. For instance, if the fluid intake area is activated, the animal starts looking around for water, walks toward the water, positions itself to be able to drink, and finally starts drinking. The animal will continue to drink as long as the stimulation of the hypothalamic area is sustained. This is an example of recruitment of different CPGs in a behaviorally relevant order. The cerebral cortex is important, particularly for fine motor coordination involving hands and fingers and for speech.

larger group of vertebrates may have specializations related to particular types of functions, and complexity increases during evolution. The cerebral cortex, with its distinct lamination, is present in mammals and most highly developed in primates, including humans (Fig. 28.5).

Basic Motor Programs Are Located at the Brainstem—Spinal Cord Level

The brainstem—spinal cord is, to a large extent, responsible for the coordination of different basic motor patterns. The spinal cord contains the motor programs (CPGs) for protective reflexes and locomotion, whereas those for swallowing, chewing, breathing, and fast saccadic eye movements are located in the brain stem (mesencephalon and medulla oblongata). In most cases, however, both the brain stem and the spinal cord are involved to some degree. In mammals as well as lower vertebrates, the brain stem – spinal cord, isolated from the forebrain (di- and telencephalon), is able to produce breathing movements and swallowing, as well as walking and standing. These brain stem – spinal cord animals (referred to as decerebrate models) can thus be made to walk, trot, and gallop with respiration adapted to the intensity of the movements and to swallow when food is put in their mouth. However, they perform these maneuvers in a stereotyped fashion, such as a robot or a reflex

machine. The movements are thus not goal directed nor adapted to the surrounding environment, but are nevertheless coordinated in an appropriate way.

Diencephalon and Subcortical Areas of Telencephalon Are Involved in Goal-Directed Behavior—Hypothalamus and Basal Ganglia

Mammals that are devoid of the cerebral cortex but have the remaining parts of the nervous system intact have been used to investigate the importance of these areas. Such animals display a more advanced behavioral repertoire when compared to the brain stem animals described earlier. At first glance, these decorticate animals look surprisingly normal. They move around spontaneously in a big room and can avoid obstacles to some extent. They eat and drink spontaneously and can learn where to obtain food and search for food when supposedly hungry. They may also display emotions such as rage and attack other animals; however, they appear unable to interact in a normal way with other individuals of the same species. Even without the cerebral cortex, a surprisingly large part of the normal motor repertoire can be performed, including some aspects of goal-directed behavior. Thus the cerebral cortex is not required to achieve this level of complex motor behavior (however, see later discussion).

The diencephalon and subcortical areas of the telencephalon of the forebrain contain two major structures that are important in this context: the hypothalamus and the basal ganglia. The hypothalamus is composed of a number of nuclei that control different autonomic functions, including temperature regulation and intake of fluid and food. The latter nuclei become activated when the osmolality is increased (fluid is needed) or the glucose levels become low (food is required). Stimulation of the paraventricular nucleus involved in the control of fluid intake results in a sequence of motor acts involving a number of different motor programs. Continuous activation of this nucleus by electrical stimulation or local ejection of a hyperosmolalic physiological solution leads to an alerting reaction. The animal first starts looking for water (perhaps experiencing a feeling of thirst). It then starts walking toward the water, positions itself at the water basin, bends forwards, and starts drinking. The animal will continue drinking as long as the nucleus is stimulated. These hypothalamic structures are thus able to recruit a sequence of motor acts that appear in a logical order. Other parts of this region can elicit rage and attack behavior, as was first described by the Nobel laureate Walter Hess.

Basal ganglia constitute a second major structure. They are present in all vertebrates and are of critical importance for the normal initiation of motor behavior. They are subdivided into an input region (the dorsal and ventral striatum) activated by the cerebral cortex, thalamus, and the brain stem and an output region (the pallidum). The output neurons are inhibitory and have a very high level of activity at rest. They inhibit a number of different motor centers in the di- and mesencephalon and also influence the motor areas of the cerebral cortex via the thalamus. The input stage of the striatum determines the level of activity in the different pallidal output neurons. When a motor pattern, such as a saccadic eye movement, is going to be initiated, the pallidal output neurons that are involved in eye motor control become inhibited by the striatum. This means that the tonic inhibition produced by these neurons at rest is removed, and the saccadic motor centers in mesencephalon (superior colliculus) are relieved from tonic inhibition and become free to operate and induce an eye saccade to a new visual target.

The level of activity in the striatum is strongly modulated by dopaminergic neurons in the substantia nigra and associated nuclei. If the level of dopamine activity is reduced, as in Parkinson's disease, it becomes very difficult to initiate and carry out most types of movements. This is a severe handicap characterized by paucity of movement (hypokinesia). The

converse condition with enhanced levels of dopamine in the basal ganglia (which can occur as a side effect of medication) results instead in a richness of movements, and even in unintended movements (hyperkinesias). These movements may be well coordinated, but without a purpose, and occur without the conscious involvement of the patient. Dopamine neurons are thus of critical importance for the operation of the striatum and they regulate the responsiveness of the striatal circuitry to input from the cerebral cortex and thalamus.

The Cerebral Cortex and Descending Motor Control

In the frontal lobe there are several major regions that are involved directly in the execution of different complex motor tasks, such as the skilled movements used to control hands and fingers when writing, drawing, or playing an instrument. Another skilled type of motor coordination is that underlying speech, which is served by Broca's area. These different regions are organized in a somatotopic fashion. In the largest area, referred to as the primary motor cortex or M1 in the precentral gyrus, the legs and feet are represented most medially and the trunk, arm, neck, and head are represented progressively more laterally. Areas taken up by the hands and the oral cavity are very large in humans, and are much larger than that for the trunk. This is explained by the fact that speech and hand motor control require a greater precision and thus a larger cortical processing area than the trunk. The latter is important for postural control but is less involved in the type of skilled movement controlled by the motor cortex (Fig. 28.6).

The large pyramidal cells in the motor cortex send their axons to the contralateral side of the spinal cord and are able to activate their target motoneurons directly, but a number of interneurons in the brain stem or spinal cord are also influenced. These long projection neurons are called corticospinal neurons. Corticospinal neurons of the arm region in M1 thus project to arm motoneurons in the spinal cord, as well as interneurons involved in the control of arm, hand, and fingers. In addition to M1, other areas in the frontal lobe, such as the supplementary motor area and prefrontal areas, are involved in other aspects of motor coordination (Fig. 28.7).

The cortical control of movement is executed in part by the direct corticospinal neurons but also by cortical fibers that project to brain stem nuclei, which in turn contain neurons that project to spinal motor centers such as the fast rubrospinal, vestibulospinal, and reticulospinal pathways. The brain stem contains

Gyrus precentralis (M)

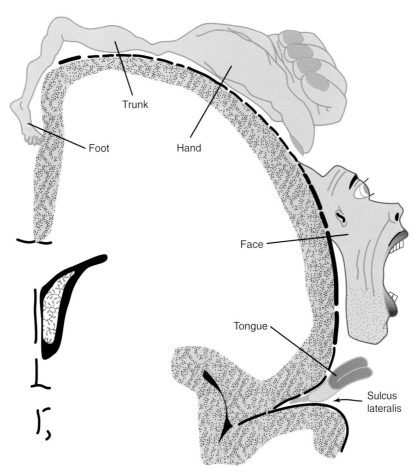

FIGURE 28.6 Organization of the primary motor cortex (M1). The different parts of the body are represented in a somatotopic fashion in M1, with the legs represented most medially, arms and hand more laterally, and the oral cavity and face even more so. Note that the two areas that are represented with disproportionally large regions are the hand with fingers and the oral cavity. They are represented in this way due to the fine control required in speech and fine manipulation of objects with the fingers. Adapted from Penfield and Rasmussen (1950).

a large number of descending pathways that can initiate movements and correct motor performance, or provide more subtle modulation of the spinal circuitry. The former act rapidly in the millisecond time frame that is required in motor control. Examples of the latter are the slow-conducting and slow-acting noradrenergic and serotonergic pathways. These pathways set the responsiveness of different types of neurons, synapses, and spinal circuits. In addition, there are direct projections from the cerebral cortex to the input area of the basal ganglia, the striatum. The cortical control of motor coordination is thus achieved through both direct action on spinal and brain stem motor centers but also to a significant degree by parallel action on a variety of brain stem nuclei. The execution of movements that are initiated from the cortex

is, to a large degree, a collaborative effort of many parts of the nervous system. The reticulospinal and vestibulospinal pathways mediate the control of posture, and the former take part in the initiation of locomotion, via the CPG located in the spinal cord (Fig. 28.8).

Judging from experiments on mammals and primates, and patients that have suffered focal lesions of the frontal lobe, the cortical control of movement is of particular importance for dexterous and flexible motor coordination, such as the fine manipulatory skills of fingers and hands and also for speech. It is very difficult for a casual observer to see the difference between a normal monkey moving around in a natural habitat and a monkey that is lacking the corticospinal direct projections to the spinal cord but has

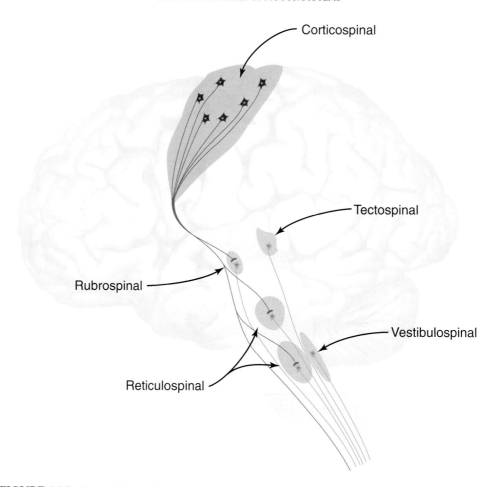

FIGURE 28.7 Descending pathways projecting from the brain that mediate motor actions to the spinal cord. From the cerebral cortex, including M1, a number of neurons project directly to the spinal cord to both motoneurons and interneurons. In addition, they also project to different motor centers in the brain stem, which in turn send direct projections to the spinal cord. One of these centers is the red (rubrospinal) nucleus, which influences the spinal cord via the rubrospinal pathway. Corticospinal and rubrospinal pathways act on the contralateral side of the spinal cord and have somewhat overlapping functions. They are sometimes referred to as the lateral system, as most of the fibers descend in the lateral funiculus of the spinal cord. Vestibulospinal and reticulospinal pathways are important both for regulating posture and for correcting perturbations, and mediate commands initiating locomotion. The different reticulo- and vestibulospinal pathways are sometimes lumped together as the medial system, as most of the axons project in the medial funiculus of the spinal cord.

all other cortical circuits intact. They are able to move around, climb, and locomote as normal monkeys. It is only when special tests are performed that one can see that delicate independent movements of the individual fingers are incapacitated. This is a type of motor coordination that is needed in monkeys and other primates for skilled manipulations of the environment, such as picking fine food objects from small holes.

The most flexible types of motor coordination, such as the skilled movements of the fingers and hands or in speech, involve the frontal lobes. These types of movements are often referred to as voluntary because they are performed at will. This terminology is some-

what ambiguous in that more basic types of motor coordination, such as the ones used when walking, chewing, or positioning ourselves in a relaxed posture, are also controlled by will, although motor coordination is handled to a larger degree by motor programs located at the brain stem—spinal cord level. Thus it appears important not to draw a clear-cut dividing line between the different types of movements, at least with respect to the voluntary aspect of their control.

It is also useful to realize that, to some degree, simple reflexes can also be modulated by will. For instance, the simple skin avoidance reflex (flexion reflex) that causes rapid withdrawal of a finger after

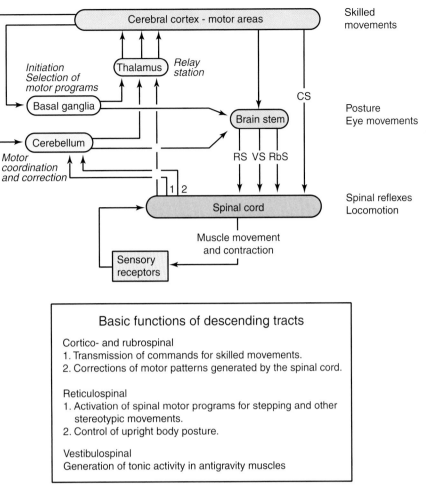

FIGURE 28.8 Summarizing scheme of the interaction between different motor centers. The different major compartments of the motor system and their main pathways for interaction are indicated. The basic functions of the different compartments and descending tracks are summarized on and below the scheme. CS, corticospinal; RbS, rubrospinal; VS, vestibulospinal; RS, reticulospinal.

touching something painful is subject to such control. Knowledge that the object will be sufficiently hot to be somewhat painful enables this modulation if it is important. If, however, the object is touched without knowing that it is hot, the hand will be withdrawn with the shortest possible latency. Thus, in the entire motor apparatus from the simplest reflex to a skilled movement, there is the possibility for modulation and flexibility. The human nervous system allows a remarkable combination of movements, adapted to different situations. This flexibility is perhaps greater for primates and humans than for any other species. However, other species may perform much better in particular types of specialized movements. A cheetah runs faster, a hawk catches prey at higher speeds, and a fly walks upside down on the ceiling.

Visuomotor Coordination—Reaction Time

Visuomotor coordination is very demanding and requires complex processing. When visualizing an approaching object like a ball, a rapid calculation provides information to bring the arms to the appropriate spot to grasp the ball at just the right time. This is an amazing achievement considering the necessity of predicting where and when the ball will arrive, the details about joint angles from hand to head that need to be considered to elicit the appropriate commands to the different muscles involved, and the time constraints. There are extensive projections to the frontal lobes from the areas in the parietal lobe processing visual information about movement.

It is clear that in order to arrive at an accurate and precise motor command, a large amount of informa-

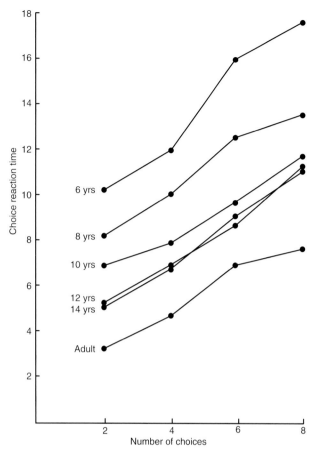

FIGURE 28.9 Reaction time tasks of different complexity and in different age groups. The choice reaction time is plotted versus the number of choices the subject is exposed to for six different age groups. A simple experimental situation with two choices takes an adult 0.3 s to initiate, but a 6 year old needs around 1.0 s. A 10 year old falls in between at around 0.7 s. An increase in the number of choices causes a marked increase in reaction time. From a practical standpoint, this provides important information when one considers the possibility for a child to cope with different demanding situations, such as moving around in a modern city. Data replotted from Conolly.

tion of different types needs to be processed about the dynamic and static conditions of the different parts of the body in relation to each other and the surrounding world. The processing time under different conditions has been investigated experimentally by having a subject respond to a signal and perform a movement, such as pressing a button when a light goes on. The delay is around 0.1–0.2 s and is called the reaction time. It represents a minimal delay for a given test situation that cannot be shortened by training (Fig. 28.9).

The more complex the situation is, the longer the reaction time. If a choice is involved, such as responding by pressing different buttons to light stimuli of different colors, the time delays become much longer than in the simple reaction time task. The choice reaction task time increases in proportion to the level of complexity and the number of choices (Fig. 28.9). When young children are tested, their reaction times are much longer than in adults. The simple reaction time for a 6 year old can be three times that of 14 year old, and the difference with choice reaction times may be even larger. This condition may have severe consequences in everyday life. In an unexpected traffic situation, a 6 year old requires at least three times longer time to interpret what he or she sees, such as an approaching car. While an adult may have sufficient time to respond, a child may have no chance. This is the basis for recommending that children below 11 years of age not bicycle in open traffic. It is noteworthy that this is a gradual maturation process and that training cannot shorten the reaction time. During aging the choice reaction time tends to increase again, a factor that can be important when driving a car.

Cerebellum

The cerebellum is a structure that is also involved in the coordination of movement. Although the cerebellum is smaller than the cerebral cortex in volume, it contains as many nerve cells as the latter. It is characterized by a very stereotyped neuronal organization with two types of inputs from mossy and from climbing fibers. These inputs not only carry information from the spinal cord about ongoing movements in all different parts of the body, but also information from the different motor centers about planned movements even before a movement has been executed. The cerebellum also interacts with practically all parts of the cerebral cortex. This means that it is updated continuously about what goes on in all parts of the body with regard to movement and also about the movements that are planned in the immediate future. Lesions of the cerebellum lead initially to great problems with postural stability and with the accuracy of different types of movements. It is noteworthy that movements in general can be carried out, but their quality is reduced drastically. Therefore, the cerebellum was originally thought to be involved exclusively in the coordination of movement. In addition to motor control, evidence has accumulated that the lateral parts of cerebellum may also be involved in different cognitive tasks.

The cerebellum is subdivided into a great number of different regions that process different kinds of information. These different regions respond via their output neurons, called Purkinje cells. The cerebellar cortex contains only inhibitory interneurons, and the two input systems, climbing fibers and mossy fibers, provide the excitatory components. All Purkinje cells are inhibitory and project to the cerebellar nuclei, which in turn are excitatory and project to different motor centers in the brain stem and to the cortex via the thalamus.

Through the interaction of climbing fibers with the mossy fiber input via granule cells, the synaptic efficacy of the input of the latter synapse onto the Purkinje cell can be regulated (depressed). This change in efficacy can last over many hours and possibly much longer and is therefore referred to as long-term depression (LTD). It is generally thought that this LTD can contribute to motor learning (see later). With regard to basic movements such as posture, walking, and the much studied eye blink reflex, the cerebellum is clearly involved through each movement phase. It is likely that the fine tuning and modification of movements that are required in different behavioral contexts involve the cerebellum. With regard to the eye blink reflex, motor learning has been demonstrated in terms of associating an unconditioned stimulus with a conditioned one. It requires that the cerebellar cortex is intact, which strongly suggests that the cerebellar cortex contributes importantly to this type of motor learning. The cerebellum is clearly of importance for the long term adaptation of different patterns of basic motor coordination.

There is still, however, much to learn about the actual processing that goes on in the cerebellum, a structure that regulates the quality of motor performance and appears to be involved in one form of motor learning. A variety of complex motor tasks, including speech and handwriting, can still be performed, but with less accuracy. Thus, the motor programs for these learned tasks cannot be stored exclusively in the cerebellum. When new types of movements are learned, such as riding a bicycle, playing an instrument, or typing at a keyboard, the new stored programs for sequences of motor acts must also involve other structures in the brain, most likely the basal ganglia and the cerebral cortex.

Motor Learning

All vertebrate and invertebrate species with a nervous system have a motor infrastructure that is determined evolutionarily. In the case of primates including humans, there are preformed circuits (e.g., CPGs) that allow performance of a basic movement repertoire (e.g., locomotion, posture, breathing, eye movements), as well as basic circuits that underlie reaching, hand and finger movements, and sound production as in speech. This constitutes the motor infrastructure that is available to a given individual, after maturation of the nervous system has occurred.

The motor system is in addition characterized by its ability to learn, in what is referred to as motor or procedural learning. For instance, one can learn how to play an instrument like the flute. The particular finger settings that produce a given tone can be retained in memory, along with the sequence of tones that produce a certain melody. Thus particular muscle combinations that produce a sequence of well-timed motor patterns are stored. Similarly, when learning to pronounce different sounds (phonemes) and combine them in words, muscle activation patterns are stored. A simpler case occurs when learning to recombine basic movement patterns to be able to maintain equilibrium while bicycling. There are a large number of examples involving different types of motor learning and parts of the body.

It is characteristic of a given learned motor program that one can "call" upon it to perform a given motor act over and over again. Despite this, there is generally little awareness of the way in which the movement is actually performed in terms of the muscles involved and their timing. Information has thus been stored in the nervous system with regard to which parts of the infrastructure of the motor system should be used to produce a given learned motor pattern, as well as the exact timing between the different components. However, the details of the complex storage process are not yet fully understood. The cerebellum clearly has a role to play, along with basal ganglia and the cerebral cortex.

CONCLUSION

After this overview of the motor control system, it should be apparent that biological evolution has succeeded in refining remarkable sensorimotor machinery capable of executing the motor tasks required for the full behavior of a given species. The degree of difficulty involved is apparent when watching the clumsiness and lack of flexibility in robots, characteristic of even the most advanced models that have been developed. Details of the different neural subsystems involved in motor control are dealt with in the following chapters.

References

Georgopoulos, A. P. (1999). News in motor cortical physiology. *News Physiol. Sci.* **14**, 64–68.

Grillner, S. (1996). Neural networks for vertebrate locomotion. *Sci. Am.* (January), 64–69.

Hikosaka, O., Takikawa, Y., and Kawagoe, R. (2000). Role of the basal ganglia in the control of purposive saccadic eye movements. *Physiol. Rev.* **80**, 953–978.

Ito, M. (2001). Cerebellar long-term depression: Characterization, signal transduction, and functional roles. *Physiol. Rev.* **81**, 1143–1195.

Lawrence, D. G., and Kyupers, H. G. J. M. (1968). The functional organization of the motor system in the monkey. I. The effects of lesions of the descending brainstem pathways. *Brain* **91**, 15–36.

Marder, E. (1998). From biophysics to models of network function. *Annu. Rev. Neurosci.* **21**, 25–45.

Matthews, P. B. C. (ed.) (1972). "Mammalian Muscle Receptors and Their Central Actions." Edward Arnold, London.

Orlovsky, G. N., Deliagina, T. G., and Grillner, S. (eds.) (1999). "Neuronal Control of Locomotion: From Mollusc to Man." Oxford Univ. Press, Oxford.

Pearson, K. G. (1993). Common principles of motor control in vertebrates and invertebrates. *Annu. Rev. Neurosci.* **16**, 265–297.

Rossignol, S. (1996). Neural control of stereotypic limb movements. *In* "Handbook of Physiology" (L. B. Rowell and J. T. Sheperd eds.), pp. 173–216. Oxford Univ. Press, New York.

Sten Grillner

The Spinal Cord, Muscle, and Locomotion

Movement occurs when muscles and external forces, such as gravity, act on the skeleton or soft tissues of the body. Most coordinated movements use several muscles, each with complex patterns of activation during the movement. The motor neurons that innervate each muscle must fire in the appropriate pattern to produce the right amount of force. Furthermore, the action of each muscle must be precisely timed in relation to the contraction or relaxation of other muscles. Coordination between pools of motor neurons that innervate different muscles is carried out, in part, by interneurons in the spinal cord. Spinal interneurons have a wide variety of inputs and outputs and are interconnected in networks that help coordinate the basic aspects of many movements. Some interneurons also receive sensory feedback that they integrate with descending motor commands. A working knowledge of these elements—muscles, motor neurons, spinal interneurons, and sensory afferents—is necessary to understand how neural commands are finally translated into physical movement. This chapter concentrates on mammals, but variations that occur in other vertebrates and in invertebrates are highlighted in Box 29.1.

MUSCLES AND THEIR CONTROL

Muscle Contraction and Neuromuscular Transmission

Muscles transform signals originating in the nervous system into mechanical actions. A typical muscle is made up of many thousands of muscle fibers, each only a few centimeters long. Muscle fibers are grouped into bundles called fascicles that are encased in connec-tive tissue and insert into tendons or bone. The individual muscle fibers are multinucleated cells that form during development from the fusion of myoblasts. Skeletal muscle fibers contain an orderly arrangement of contractile proteins that give them a striped or striated appearance. The term striated muscle is often used to distinguish skeletal muscle from cardiac or smooth muscle. Muscle fibers also contain a number of cellular specializations, e.g., the sarcoplasmic reticulum (SR), a membranous organelle that stores and release calcium in the vicinity of the contractile proteins. (Fig. 29.1)

In adult mammals, each muscle fiber is innervated by the axon of only one motor neuron. The axon contacts the muscle at the neuromuscular junction, a specialized region near the midpoint of the muscle fiber. The muscle fiber membrane at the neuromuscular junction has a number of infoldings called junctional folds. Nicotinic acetylcholine receptors (AChRs) cluster on the crests of the folds, opposite the vesicle release sites on the motor axon terminal. When a motor neuron action potential invades the presynaptic terminal, vesicles release acetylcholine (ACh), which diffuses across the cleft and binds to the AChRs. An influx of cations through the AChRs produces an end plate potential, a localized depolarization of the muscle at the neuromuscular junction. The end plate potential depolarizes the muscle sufficiently to activate voltage-gated sodium channels in the adjacent muscle fiber membrane, initiating the all-or-none action potential. The action of ACh is terminated when it is broken down in the cleft by acetylcholinesterase. Normally, the amount of ACh released and the density of AChRs ensure that every action potential in the motor neuron produces an action potential in the muscle fiber. (Box 29.2; Fig. 29.2)

BOX 29.1

DIVERSITY OF MUSCLES AND THEIR CONTROL

Most of this chapter focuses on the way that mammals coordinate muscular activity. Variations on the mammalian pattern occur in other vertebrates. Major differences are found in invertebrates, which have often evolved particular adaptations that suit their movement patterns or the constraints imposed by their environments.

The structure of the muscle itself is one area of differences. Some invertebrates require muscles that generate great force or provide extreme resistance to stretch. Organisms such as the mussel and the nematode *C. elegans* incorporate molecules of paramyosin into their thick filaments to provide additional sites for cross-bridge formation. The "catch" property is another adaptation in some invertebrate muscles. "Catch" is a state in which the muscle sustains high tension over long periods of time with little energy expenditure, remaining tightly bound until actively released. The catch state is achieved when the transmitter acetylcholine induces phosphorylation of as yet unknown muscle proteins, and catch is released through the action of neurotransmitters such as serotonin that activate adenylate cyclase. Another feature of certain invertebrates is that they move slowly. In some cases, slow movement is achieved by having longer sarcomeres, in which Ca^{2+} diffusion throughout the sarcomere takes longer. Crustacean muscles have sarcomeres that range from 2 to 25 mm in length. In mammals, longer sarcomeres are occasionally found in muscles that stiffen but do not twitch, such as the tensor tympani muscle of the cat eardrum. Whereas mammalian muscles usually contain a mixture of fiber types, some fish, such as trout, have distinct red muscles, consisting entirely of slow twitch fibers, that are used for sustained swimming and white muscles that are used for leaping and rapid bursts of speed.

Acetylcholine, the transmitter at the vertebrate neuromuscular junction, is not used by all invertebrates. Although *C. elegans* uses acetylcholine, glutamate is the transmitter used at the neuromuscular junction of many arthropods, such as the fruit fly *Drosophila*, the locust, and at the excitatory neuromuscular synapse in crayfish. Innervation patterns of the muscle are highly diverse in invertebrates. In mammals, most muscle fibers are innervated by only one motor neuron, with a few exceptions. Laryngeal muscles and spindles have dual end plates from the same motor neuron. In other organisms, polyneuronal innervation is commonly seen. In these animals, the motor neurons may merely have an additive function, as in *Drosophila*, where the recruitment of motor neurons produces graded contractions of the muscle. In other animals, motor neurons may play distinct roles. The locust jumping muscle has a dual arrangement, with one motor neuron that produces a rapid and powerful excitation and one that produces a graded excitation and contraction. Crustacean muscles are unique in their innervation by both excitatory and inhibitory neurons, with presynaptic inhibition of motor terminals. Finally, there are great differences in the central control of motor neuron activity among different animals. The distributed structure of invertebrate systems is favorable to the action of pattern generating circuits. Invertebrate neurons have structural specialties, such as electrical synapses, that can allow greater speed, as well as biophysical properties that promote rhythmic firing.

Mary Kay Floeter

The muscle fiber action potential propagates in both directions along the length of the muscle fiber and down the numerous infoldings of the surface membrane called transverse or T tubules. The action potential activates voltage-gated calcium channels in the T tubule membrane. Calcium channels in the T tubules lie in close apposition to calcium release proteins in the SR. Conformational changes in T tubule calcium channels induced by depolarization are transmitted by a direct protein–protein interaction to the SR calcium release protein, triggering the release of calcium from the SR into the muscle cytoplasm. The rise in intracellular calcium activates contractile proteins. Relaxation occurs with the reuptake of calcium into the SR.

The arrays of contractile proteins in the muscle fiber are called myofibrils. Myofibrils contain thick and thin filaments arranged longitudinally in units called sarcomeres. Thin filaments consist of actin filaments entwined by the protein tropomyosin (Fig. 29.3). Thick filaments consist of myosin, which has a head region that can bind to actin and can break down ATP. In the resting state, the myosin heads are loosely attached to actin. In the presence of calcium, myosin binds strongly to actin, forming a crossbridge. Once bound, myosin hydrolyzes ATP, and the

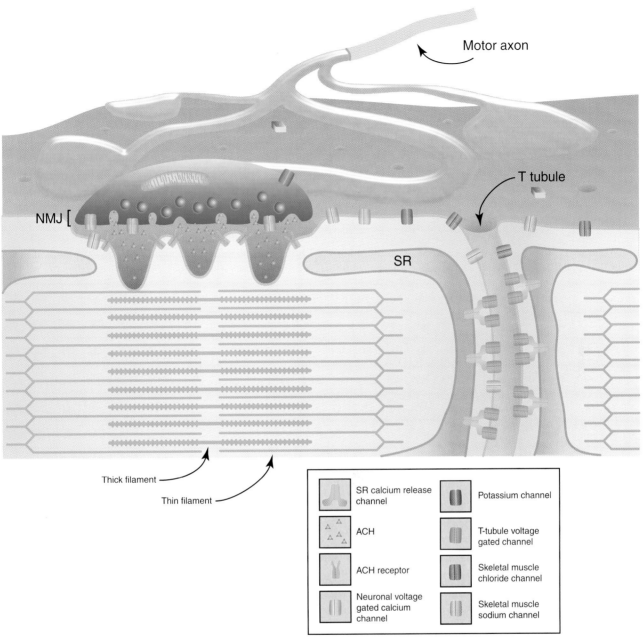

FIGURE 29.1 Diagram of the structure of the muscle showing the relationship among myofibrils (thick and thin filaments), sarcoplasmic reticulum (SR), and various ion channels of the motor axon and muscle. With permission, modified from Cooper and Jan (1999).

head swivels along the actin filament to the next binding site. The repetition of this swiveling movement in the presence of calcium and ATP causes thick and thin filaments to slide along each other, shortening the sarcomeres.

There Are Three Basic Muscle Fiber Types

Contractile and metabolic properties can be used to differentiate three different types of skeletal muscle fibers. Most muscles contain a mixture of the fiber types, but the proportions vary in each muscle according to its typical usage. In addition to histochemical and physiological measures, the patterns of skeletal muscle gene expression can be used to distinguish muscle fiber types (Table 29.1) Each muscle fiber expresses a constellation of muscle-specific genes, including myosin heavy and light chains, troponins, and creatine kinase, many of which have common transcriptional regulation (Bottinelli and Reggiani, 2000). In addition, the cellular machinery, such as the density of sarcoplasmic reticulum and mitochondria,

---

BOX 29.2

MYASTHENIC DISORDERS

Normally, neuromuscular transmission has a high safety factor, and every spike in the motor axon produces a muscle fiber action potential. This occurs because both the amount of transmitter released from the presynaptic motor axon terminal and the density of AChRs on the postsynaptic muscle fiber exceed that needed to produce an end plate potential (EPP) large enough to initiate a muscle fiber action potential. Genetic or acquired diseases that reduce the safety factor of neuromuscular transmission are called myasthenic disorders (Fig. 29.2). Myasthenic disorders cause weakness that fluctuates with use of the muscle. The most common is the acquired autoimmune disorder myasthenia gravis, caused by antibodies that bind to AChRs at the neuromuscular junction. The antibodies interfere with ACh binding and lead to internalization of AChRs and, ultimately, the loss of junctional folds. The reduced numbers of functioning AChRs produce a smaller EPP that fails intermittently to trigger a muscle fiber action potential. However, in myasthenia gravis the presynaptic terminal remains normal, such that a short burst of stimulation will produce facilitation of transmitter release, increasing the concentration of ACh in the cleft and transiently improving neurotransmission. Acetylcholinesterase inhibitors provide symptomatic improvement by blocking the breakdown of ACh, allowing a longer effect on residual receptors. Another autoimmune myasthenic disorder, Lambert–Eaton myasthenic syndrome, is caused by antibodies that bind to presynaptic voltage-gated calcium channels. Less ACh is released at the neuromuscular junction, producing small EPPs that fail to trigger

action potentials.

Congenital myasthenic syndromes (CMS) are extremely rare, but provide important insights into the function of components of the neuromuscular junction. Postsynaptic CMS stem from a deficiency and/or altered kinetic properties of the AChR. More than 40 different mutations in subunits of the AChR have been described. Most mutations decrease subunit expression or prevent subunit assembly or glycosylation, leading to reduced numbers of functioning AChRs and thereby smaller EPPs. In fast channel CMS, mutations produce decreased binding affinity for ACh, leading to a smaller quantal response and miniature EPP amplitude, without reducing the numbers of AChRs. In contrast, the slow channel CMS stem from mutations that prolong the channel opening episodes. Slow channel mutations cause depolarization block due to temporal summation of the prolonged EPPs. In the long term, cationic overloading of the postsynaptic region leads to destruction of the junctional folds and loss of AChRs. Presynaptic CMS are less common. They are caused by mutations that lead to a paucity of synaptic vesicles or defects in ACh resynthesis or vesicular packaging. As a result, fewer vesicles are released or fewer ACh molecules are contained in each vesicle, and EPPs are smaller. Identifying CMS as involving pre- or postsynaptic components and understanding how these alterations affect neuromuscular transmission are necessary for developing rational therapies for these disorders.

Mary Kay Floeter

---

varies in specific ways for muscle fiber types. Myosin heavy chain genes are the most critical for determining the contractile speed of the muscle fiber. Four main myosin heavy chain genes are expressed in adult limb muscles, and others are expressed transiently during development, in low concentrations, or in specific types of specialized muscles.

Slow twitch muscle fibers are called type 1 fibers, and fast twitch fibers are called type 2 fibers. Type 1 fibers express a myosin isoform with a relatively slow rate of ATP hydrolysis. Type 1 fibers have a slow twitch time and a slow rate of relaxation. The slow relaxation is due to slower reuptake of calcium and a lower density of sarcoplasmic reticulum. Type 1 fibers generate small amounts of a specific force. However,

they are highly vascularized, have abundant mitochondria, and contain myoglobin, a protein that binds oxygen and gives the fiber a red color. Type 1 fibers are optimized for operating aerobically for long periods without fatigue.

Fast twitch type 2 fibers express isoforms of myosin that have faster ATPase rates. Type 2 fibers have a faster twitch and faster rates of relaxation. They produce high specific forces compared to type 1 fibers. Type 2 fibers can be further subdivided according to their metabolic capacities. Type 2a fibers have moderate numbers of mitochondria and are able to use both aerobic metabolism and glycolysis to generate energy and are relatively resistant to fatigue. Type 2b fibers are pale colored, with sparse mitochondria. Type 2b

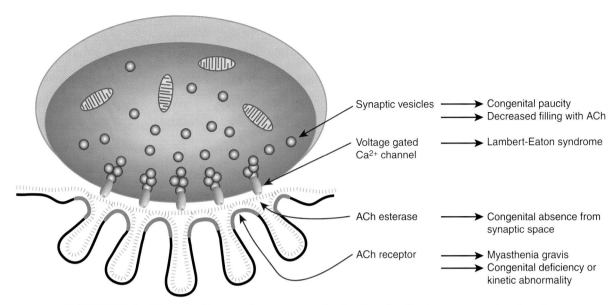

FIGURE 29.2 Schematic diagram of a neuromuscular junction showing key components subserving neuromuscular transmission and the myasthenic disorders associated with these components.

fibers use glycolysis to provide energy and therefore are highly fatigable.

The Motor Unit Is the Smallest Unit of Motor Control

In mammals, each skeletal muscle fiber is innervated by only one motor neuron, but that motor neuron innervates many muscle fibers. The axon from one motor neuron branches to innervate as many as several thousand muscle fibers. However, all muscle fibers innervated by one motor neuron normally consist of the same fiber type. One motor neuron and all of the muscle fibers it innervates is defined as the "motor unit." The muscle fibers of a single motor unit are scattered in the muscle among fibers belonging to other motor units in a mosaic pattern (Fig. 29.4) The

physiological properties of the motor unit are coherent: the physiological properties of the motor neuron are matched to fit the physiology of its target muscle fibers. Although there is a continuum of physiologic properties among motor neurons, the twitch properties and the fatigability of the motor unit can be used to classify them into three basic types.

Motor units are classified as either slow (S) or fast (F) according to their twitch contraction time, defined as the time for a motor unit to develop peak force following a single spike (Fig. 29.5A). The speed of the twitch and the rate of relaxation depend on the muscle fiber types of the motor unit and their geometry within the muscle. In general, the time required for the

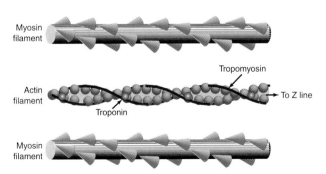

FIGURE 29.3 Thick and thin filaments. Intertwined arrays of actin, troponin, and tropomyosin make up thin filaments. Multiple myosin monomers assemble into thick filaments. From Squire (1983).

TABLE 29.1 Markers for Identifying Muscle Fiber Types

	Type 1	Type 2a	Type 2b
Histochemical staining			
ATPase pH 4.3	Strong	Weak	Weak
ATPase pH 9.4	Weak		Strong
Succinic dehydrogenase	Strong	Strong	Weak
NADH reductase	Strong	Intermediate	Weak
Glycogen stores	Low	High	High
Myophosphorylase	Low	High	High
Myoglobin	High	High	Low
Lipid globules	Many	Many	Few
SR ATPase fast	Weak	Strong	Strong
SR ATPase slow	Strong	Weak	Weak
Muscle proteins expressed			
Myosin heavy chain type	1	2A	2X or 2C
Troponin T	Slow	Fast	fast
Tropomyosin	Slow	Fast	fast

twitch force of a motor unit to decline to half its peak force is about two to three times longer than the twitch contraction time. In most movements, motor neurons fire a series of action potentials in a semirhythmic pattern rather than just a single spike. The interval between successive action potentials is shorter than the motor unit relaxation time, allowing tension generated by successive twitches to summate (Fig. 29.5B). When the motor neuron fires at intervals close to the twitch time, the individual twitches fuse to generate a steady level of force or tetanus (Figs. 29.5C and 29.5D). The optimal firing rate to develop a fused tetanus depends on the twitch time and the relaxation rate of the motor unit. Type S motor neurons innervate type 1 muscle fibers. Type S units reach peak tension most slowly, but also relax slowly. They achieve fused tetanus at relatively low firing rates, e.g., 15–25 Hz in man. Type F motor units innervate type 2 muscle fibers and have faster twitch contraction times, as well as shorter relaxation times. Slightly higher firing rates are needed to produce fusion of their twitches, e.g., 40–60 Hz in man.

Fatigue resistance is the other property used to further classify motor units. Fatigue is quantified by comparing the peak twitch force produced by a motor neuron before and after several minutes of steady firing (Fig. 29.6). Type S motor units are highly resistant to fatigue, producing the same peak force before and after a few minutes of firing. Type F motor units are further classified into a fast, fatigue-resistant type (FR) and a fast, fatigable type (FF). Type FR motor units maintain twitch force relatively well over 1 or 2

min of firing. In contrast, type FF units are unable to sustain twitch force during repeated firing. Type FR motor neuron innervate type 2a muscle fibers, and type FF motor neuron innervate type 2b muscle fibers.

The Size Principle Aids Orderly Recruitment of Motor Units

Each muscle is innervated by a pool of α motor neurons that lie either in an elongated column in the

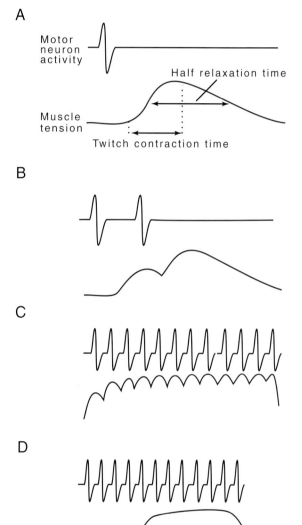

FIGURE 29.5   Muscle tension increases with motor neuron firing rate. (A) Single twitch. The twitch contraction time is defined as latency to reach the peak force, relaxation time is measured at half-maximal peak force. (B) Summation of tension with two twitches. (C) Summation of multiple twitches to produce unfused tetanus. (D) Fused tetanus with high motor neuron frequency firing.

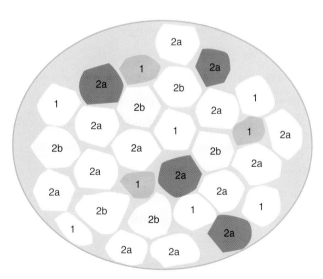

FIGURE 29.4   Cross section through a muscle fascicle showing the mosaic pattern of different muscle fiber types (1, 2a, and 2b) and how the muscle fibers innervated by three individual motor units (indicated by three different colors) are intermingled among fibers innervated by other motor units.

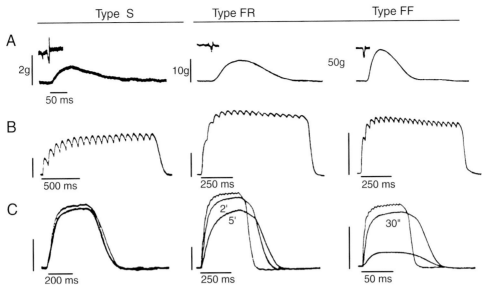

FIGURE 29.6 Contractile properties and fatigability of different motor unit types (S, FR, and FF). (A) Single twitches. Note that peak twitch is shown with different time scales and amplitude calibrations. (B) Summation of twitches in an unfused tetanus. The "sag" property, a dropping off of tension during maintained stimulation, is seen in FR and FF units. (C) Fatigability is demonstrated by a drop in the tension produced by a single twitch after short periods of activation, as noted. Note that S units show little fatigue, whereas FF units fatigue within 30 s. Reproduced with permission from Burke *et al.* (1973).

ventral horn of the spinal cord or in a brain stem nucleus (Fig. 29.7). The pool typically contains a hundred or more motor neurons, with varying proportions of type S and type F motor neurons. Because most movements consist of muscle contractions that are less than the muscle's maximal force only a fraction of the motor neuron pool will be used to produce

the desired amount of force. Motor units within the pool are activated in a characteristic sequence to produce contractions of increasing strength. Henneman (1957) first reported that this orderly sequence was based on the "size" of the motor neuron. Motor neurons that produce the smallest amounts of force are the first to begin firing, and larger motor neurons are activated later, as needed to produce greater force. His formulation has been termed the size principle. A number of anatomical and physiological properties of motor unit types correlate with measures of size. These size related properties, described later and in Table 29.2, favor

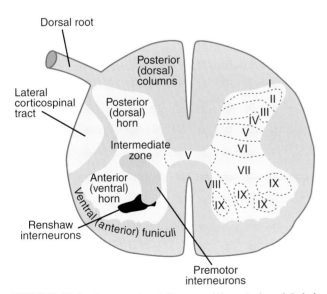

FIGURE 29.7 Cross-sectional diagram of the spinal cord. Labels on the right side indicate layers within the central gray matter, and the left side shows cellular regions and white matter tracts involved in movement control.

TABLE 29.2 Size-Related Properties of Motor Neurons

Properties that increase with size	Properties that decrease with size
Diameter of soma and axon	Resistance to fatigue
Conduction velocity	Ia EPSP amplitude
Complexity of axonal collaterals	Input resistance
Membrane area, dendritic extent	Membrane resistance
Rheobase	Time constant
Muscle fiber diameter	Duration of afterhyperpolarization
Maximum force output	Twitch contraction time Twitch relaxation time

activation of motor unit types in the following order: type S → type FR → type FF.

Type S motor neurons are the smallest of the α motor neurons, with the smallest diameter cell bodies, small dendritic arbors, and the thinnest diameter axons. This compact anatomy influences their passive electrical properties: they have a high membrane resistance, and the current required to produce firing (rheobase) is low. Synaptic inputs will produce relatively large postsynaptic potentials, according to Ohm's law. Postsynaptic potentials decay more slowly because of the longer time constants of type S motor neurons. Type S motor neurons also have long afterhyperpolarizations (AHPs) following each spike, approximately as long as the relaxation time of the motor unit. Long AHPs tend to limit the rate of repetitive firing. Thus type S motor neurons can be excited easily to reach their firing threshold and will sustain relatively slower rates of steady firing. These physiological properties of the type S motor neurons are a good match for the slow twitch properties of their type 1 muscle fiber targets. Type S motor units individually contribute small amounts of force to each contraction, but they typically make up a large proportion of the motor units in the pool, and they can sustain their force for long periods of time. Type S motor neurons also have the slowest conduction velocities.

Type FR and FF motor units overlap in many of their anatomical and electrical properties. They have similarly sized large cell bodies and dendritic trees and have large-diameter axons with the fastest conduction velocities. Type FR motor units have a lower membrane resistance and a higher rheobase than type S units and are more excitable than type FF motor neurons. Type FF are the last motor neurons in the pool to reach excitation thresholds, but also have the shortest AHPs, allowing more rapid rates of firing once activated. The two subtypes of type F units differ most in their force output and fatigue resistance, properties that are affected greatly by their target muscle fiber types. Type FF units produce the highest twitch forces, which can be 5- to 10-fold greater than that of type FR units. Type FF units are thought to be used infrequently, recruited only in movements that require the maximal muscle strength.

Although many of the properties that produce orderly activation by size are intrinsic to the motor neuron, synaptic inputs distributed uniformly to the motor neuron pool will also reinforce the orderly activation of motor units. A synaptic current of the same magnitude will produce a larger postsynaptic potential in type S motor units compared to type F motor units. Many synaptic inputs are distributed uniformly to the motor pool, and therefore the EPSP or IPSP amplitude will correlate with measures related to the motor unit size. An example is the EPSP produced by primary muscle spindle (Ia) afferents. Each Ia afferent of a muscle synapses on almost every motor neuron in the pool innervating the same muscle (homonymous motor neurons). Ia EPSPs are largest in type S motor neurons and the smallest in type FF motor neurons. Similarly, recurrent IPSPs produced by Renshaw interneurons are larger in type S motor units than in type F motor neurons. When synaptic inputs reinforce orderly recruitment, the transformation between the input and the output of the motor pool is simplified, and the behavior of individual motor units is predictable based on their recruitment order. Conversely, for a movement to occur in which motor units are recruited in an alternative sequence, the synaptic input that produces the movement must be distributed to the motor pool in a manner that opposes the size principle, as intrinsic motor neuron properties are stable from moment to moment. One example is cutaneous stimulation, which tends to produce polysynaptic IPSPs in small type S motor neurons and EPSPs in large motor neurons.

Recruitment and Rate Modulation Act Cooperatively to Control Muscle Force

To produce a muscle contraction of gradually increasing strength, the animal can recruit additional motor units or increase the firing rates of motor neurons that have already begun firing at low rates. Normally, both mechanisms, recruitment and firing rate modulation, will be used to produce stronger contractions, although the relative use varies according to the muscle and the level of force. Some muscles, such as the small hand muscles, recruit several motor units at low levels of force, and fine gradations of force are controlled by firing rate modulation. For other muscles, recruitment and rate coding occur in a more balanced fashion throughout the working force range. Recruitment is determined by the spacing of thresholds among the pool of motor neurons, whereas rate modulation is determined by the input–output relationship of individual motor neurons. The relationship between firing frequency (F) and excitatory inputs (I) of a neuron is often linear over a primary range of firing frequencies. When F–I curves are linear and the thresholds are evenly spaced, recruitment and rate modulation act in parallel on the motor neuron pool. The spacing of thresholds and F–I curves are adjustable parameters, however, changing with activity and in response to neuromodulators. Nonlinearity of F–I curves, for example, is induced when plateau potentials are acti-

BOX 29.3

PLATEAU POTENTIALS

Plateau potentials are membrane depolarizations that are maintained without synaptic inputs. The existence of plateau potentials in invertebrate neurons has been known for decades, but they were only recognized in vertebrate motor neurons in the late 1980s. Plateau potentials can be turned on when a motor neuron receives a barrage of pure excitatory inputs while under monoaminergic tone. The barrage of excitatory inputs depolarizes the motor neuron sufficiently to activate voltage-gated channels that, because of the action of monoamines, remain open until terminated by hyperpolarization. As long as the plateau depolarization exceeds the firing threshold, the motor neuron will maintain steady firing, despite the absence of continuing synaptic input.

The conductances underlying plateau potentials have been studied most carefully in turtle motor neurons. In turtles, serotonin acts through G-protein-coupled receptors on motor neurons to reduce afterhyperpolarization of the motor neuron. As a result, the motor neuron is able to build up a slight depolarization following a series of action potentials. This depolarization opens voltage-gated Ca^{2+} channels, and the resulting calcium currents maintain plateau depolarization. In cat motor neurons, the plateau current appears to be a mixed cation flux with a significant contribution from sodium ions, possi-

bly through a noninactivating sodium channel. The best evidence indicates that channels are located on the dendrites of cat motor neurons. Plateau potentials are demonstrated most easily in low threshold (type S) motor units.

The role of plateau potentials in normal movement, or a pathological role in neurological disorders, is speculative. One suggestion is that plateau potentials are used for the activation of muscles used to maintain postures, offering an energetically efficient way to sustain long bouts of motor neuron firing. Another suggestion is that the channels that produce plateau potentials act in a local, graded fashion to amplify excitatory inputs on motor neuron dendrites (Lee and Heckman, 2000). The monoaminergic pathways required for activation of plateau potentials originate in the brain stem. Plateau potentials are likely to be impaired in neurological conditions that disrupt descending monoaminergic tracts.

Mary Kay Floeter

Reference

Lee, R. H., and Heckman, C. J. (2000). Adjustable amplification of synaptic input in the dendrites of spinal motor neurons *in vivo. J. Neurosci.* **20**, 6734–6740.

vated (Box 29.3) or by sustained firing activity that produces spike frequency adaptation.

Summary

Muscle contraction is produced by an orderly sequence of electrical and chemical events, beginning with an action potential originating at the neuromuscular junction. Skeletal muscle fibers translate the electrical signal from ion channels on the plasma membrane and on the sarcoplasmic reticulum into a mechanical movement generated by muscle contractile proteins. Three basic muscle fiber types can be distinguished on the basis of differences in their contractile proteins and metabolic abilities. The properties of motor neurons are matched to the muscle fibers they innervate. A motor unit, defined as one motor neuron and all its muscle fibers, can be categorized as one of three types: slow twitch, fast twitch with fatigue resistance, or fast twitch and fatigable. Motor units are generally activated in an orderly sequence—type

S → FR → FF—known as the size principle. This orderly pattern of recruitment, in which motor units are activated in order of increasing force, ensures that movements have a smooth force profile. The size principle stems from size-related passive electrical properties and the distribution of synaptic inputs on motor neuron. During movements, motor neurons fire repetitively to produce summation of muscle twitches. Firing rate modulation and recruitment are both used to regulate how much force the muscle produces during a movement.

SPINAL NETWORKS AND THE SEGMENTAL MOTOR SYSTEM

Interneurons Play an Integrative Role in the Spinal Segmental Motor System

Each motor neuron receives thousands of synapses. The sources of its synapses are spinal interneurons, sensory afferents and descending axons from the brain stem and cerebral cortex. However, most of the synapses on motor neurons originate from various spinal interneurons, some with cell bodies residing in the same spinal segment as their target motor neurons and others, called propriospinal interneurons, with cell bodies that reside in distant spinal segments and axons that travel in the spinal white matter. Interneurons of the spinal cord have three important functions for motor control: they relay sensory inputs that allow adjustment of the motor neuron output; they relay and modulate the signal conveyed by descending inputs, and they are connected in networks that can produce patterned rhythmic outputs. Some interneurons participate in all three functions, switching from one role to another during specific movements, or carrying on two roles simultaneously. As of this writing there is no systematic nomenclature for different classes of interneurons. Some are named according to their pattern of connections, some from the reflex they mediate, some from the location of their cell bodies, and others by their activation in a particular movement. Although an interneuron may be named for one function, it is important to realize that interneurons are multifunctional and can play several roles.

A key feature of interneurons in the mammalian spinal cord is that they have many convergent and divergent connections. This connectivity allows them to integrate signals from different sources. Interneurons that receive both supraspinal and sensory inputs, for example, can relay a signal to motor neurons that combines descending commands for limb movement with sensory feedback from the moving limb. Different classes of interneurons receive distinct assortments of inputs, but almost all receive inputs from multiple sources. On the output side, most interneurons have axons that branch to connect with several different targets, including other interneurons. Those that synapse on motor neurons are called last-order interneurons: their axons can be targeted to a specific motor neuron pool or to several pools innervating muscles with synergistic functions.

Interneurons, like motor neurons, reside in pools that can be partially activated by an input. The activation of two convergent inputs may produce a greater output than the sum of the individual inputs. This can occur when a portion of the pool (the subliminal fringe) receives subthreshold excitation from the first input and thus is activated more easily by a second convergent input (spatial facilitation) or a repetition of the first input (temporal facilitation). Once the interneuron pool is maximally activated, further inputs have no additional effect (occlusion). Interneuronal linkages provide a high degree of flexibility, although outputs are less constant than a monosynaptic connection. Many descending inputs to motor neurons have parallel monosynaptic and interneuronal connections.

Central Pattern Generators: An Introduction

In the early 1900s, Graham Brown found that cats with a spinal cord transection could walk on a treadmill even after the dorsal roots were severed. Because no sensory feedback or descending input could be responsible for evoking the leg movements in these animals, he suggested that a motor program within the spinal cord itself encoded the movement. He proposed that this program consisted of two mutually inhibitory "half-centers," both under tonic excitation: one half-center drove muscles that flexed the legs and the other drove muscles that extended the legs. Mutual inhibition between the two centers would cause activity to oscillate between them, producing an alternation between flexion and extension of the limb.

This early demonstration of spinal central pattern generating circuits (CPGs) provided a contrast to a leading idea of the time, that rhythmic coordinated movements were created through a series of reflexes—stereotyped motor behaviors evoked by the sensory feedback from each preceding movement. Nevertheless, over the next several decades, investigations of CPGs dwindled, perhaps because the development of intracellular recording techniques placed a greater focus on the physiology and synaptic connections of individual neurons than on the actions by groups of neurons. Those intracellular studies were carried out in anesthetized animals in which CPGs and motor neurons are quiescent. Some work on spinal CPGs continued, however, particularly in Russia and Sweden. Modern interest in mammalian CPGs was rekindled by work of Anders Lundberg and colleagues, who studied the circuits underlying late reflexes in spinalized cats. Lundberg's formulation of the multisensory control of reflexes in different pharmacological states provided a link between spinal interneurons and CPGs (Lundberg, 1979). This work, and the growing knowledge of invertebrate pattern generating circuits, provided a foundation for studies of mammalian CPGs in the last decade.

CPGs provide a framework for understanding rhythmic movements that are performed relatively automatically, such as breathing, chewing, scratching, and walking. These movements rely heavily on spinal interneuron networks to coordinate the timing and sequence of activation and inhibition between motor neuron pools innervating different muscles. The participation of spinal pattern generators varies according to the nature of the movement. Many movements have at least components of rhythmicity, and spinal networks can be used to greater or lesser degrees by supraspinal systems. Individuated finger movements, for example, depend heavily on patterned corticospinal drive, rather than spinal CPG circuitry. Breathing, however, relies heavily on brain stem and spinal CPGs , although supraspinal inputs have the ability to override CPGs. Reaching movements probably lie somewhere in between in their use of spinal CPG circuits.

Locomotion Can Be Characterized as a Cycle

Locomotion is the action of moving from place to place, whether it be swimming, walking, or flight. All modes of locomotion use a rhythmic repetition of a sequence of muscle activity and can be described by the phase relationships between limbs, sides, or body segments. Non-limbed vertebrates such as lamprey and fish swim by generating a propulsive wave by alternately contracting and relaxing trunk muscles on opposite sides with a phase lag between segments.

Birds, however, activate wings synchronously in flight, with no phase lag.

Stepping, the major form of mammalian locomotion, is a cycle with two phases: stance, the extension phase, and swing, the flexion phase. As the upper portion of Fig. 29.8 shows for human locomotion, the stance phase begins when the heel strikes the ground and begins to bear weight. Throughout stance, the weight is gradually shifted forward, rolling from the heel to the ball of the foot. The swing phase begins when the toe leaves the ground and the limb moves forward. To accomplish this sequence of movements, muscles moving the hip, knee, and ankle joints are activated in characteristic patterns, as diagrammed in the middle portion of Fig. 29.8. Although flexor muscles are generally more active in swing and extensors in stance, the activation patterns of individual muscles can be more elaborate and finely graded. Some muscles are activated twice per cycle, whereas others are activated during only a portion of one phase (Fig. 29.9).

Several features are used to describe gait: the duration of each cycle, the relative proportion of the cycle spent in swing and stance phases, and the phase

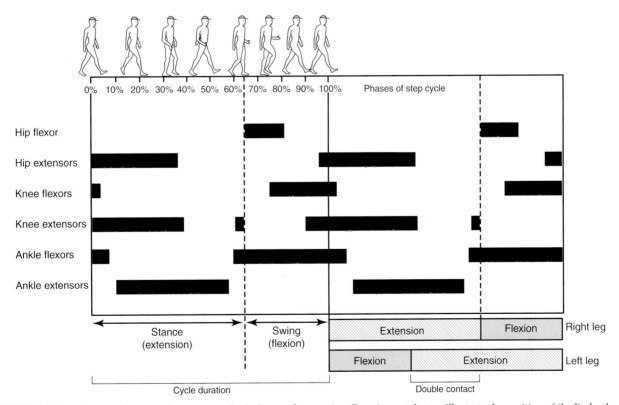

FIGURE 29.8 Schematic diagram of two step cycles in human locomotion. Drawings at the top illustrate the position of the limbs during one cycle. Dark horizontal bars below the drawings show the timing of activity in flexor and extensor muscles of the right leg. The division of each step cycle into stance (extension) and swing (flexion) phases is indicated at the bottom of the figure. During walking, the stance phases of the two legs overlap, with both feet in contact with the ground.

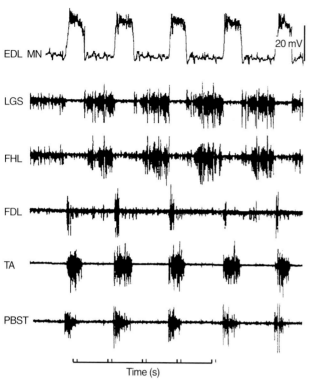

FIGURE 29.9 Five step cycles of fictive locomotion in a decerebrate cat. The upper trace (EDL MN) shows an intracellular recording from a motor neuron that innervates the extensor digitorum longus muscle, a toe, and ankle dorsiflexor. A rhythmic excitatory locomotor drive potential (LDP) is present. Lower traces are muscle nerve recordings from two ankle and foot extensors (LGS and FHL), one toe extensor (FDL), one ankle flexor (TA), and the hamstring (PBST). Activation patterns differ for each muscle. During the flexion phase, the EDL motor neuron is depolarized by approximately 20 mV and there is activity in the recording TA nerve. Briefer bursts of activity are seen at the onset of the flexion phase in FDL and PBST. LGS and FHL are active throughout most of the extension phase. Courtesy of R. E. Burke.

energy consumption. Switching from one gait to another occurs naturally as an animal changes speed, and the rate of oxygen consumption increases linearly with speed. If a gait is performed at speeds artificially lower or higher than the usual range of speeds, energy consumption rises dramatically. In stepping, most of the work consists of shifting the center of gravity to allow the body to fall forward over the foot in stance. The kinetic energy of the fall is partly conserved by contracting the knee extensor muscles isometrically at the end of the swing phase to stiffen the limb and provide resistance on impact. Isometric activation of the extensor muscles minimizes the metabolic cost associated with the formation and breaking of actin–myosin cross-bridges. The momentum of the fall is stored in the elasticity of muscles and tendons and is used to power the following step. The contribution of elastic recoil is considerable, as is obvious when walking on a sandy beach or other surface that absorbs and damps the energy of recoil.

Models of Locomotor CPGs Provide the Framework for Experimental Questions

CPGs are made up of networks of neurons that, by the nature of their interconnections and their cellular properties, are able to generate rhythmic firing (Box 29.4). For each animal, organization of the locomotor CPG circuitry reflects the body structure and the mode of locomotion. For example, in the lamprey, a limbless vertebrate, the CPG produces swimming by alternating the activation of muscles on the two sides of the body at each level. The basic rhythm generating circuitry is repeated in each segment of the lamprey spinal cord. Projections of some neurons cross spinal segments, coordinating the phase lag needed to produce a wave of contraction along the body segment. It has been possible to record from lamprey spinal interneurons during fictive swimming and determine the roles that many of the interneurons play in the CPG network. For this reason, lamprey swimming CPG is one of the best understood vertebrate CPGs. Models of the lamprey CPG incorporate many of the experimentally discovered connections and biophysical properties of these neurons (Box 29.5). The CPG has also been modeled purely mathematically as a series of coupled oscillators.

In limbed vertebrates, the CPG circuitry must coordinate movement between and within limbs. A precise timing among the movements of the hip, knee, and ankle joints is needed to produce different gaits. The leading model for the organization of CPGs for walking is an extension of the half-center model proposed by Brown (1911). Brown had proposed that the

relationships between limbs. At slow or moderate walking speeds (i.e., long cycle durations), extension is prolonged and the extension phases of opposite legs overlap. At these speeds, both feet are in simultaneous contact with the ground for some period of time during each cycle (Fig. 29.8, lower right). As the rate of walking increases, the step cycle shortens mainly by shortening the extension phase, with briefer periods of simultaneous foot contact. At high speeds, there is no overlap of extension phases, and the gait switches recognizably from walking to running. Quadrupedal animals have a greater variety of gaits—trot, canter, and gallop—each with characteristic phase relationships among the four limbs.

During locomotion, animals assume the most efficient locomotor patterns for the desired speed, and muscles are used in a way that appears to minimize

BOX 29.4

BUILDING BLOCKS OF CPGS

Patterned neuronal firing is the result of an interplay between the intrinsic membrane properties of neurons and the network connections between them. Certain patterns of anatomical connections contribute to distinct firing patterns; e.g., mutually excitatory connections between cells promote synchronous firing, whereas mutually inhibitory connections tend to produce oscillation. Membrane properties, arising from the receptors and ion channels expressed by individual neurons, can be used flexibly to produce rhythmic activity because their efficacy can be modulated by synaptic activity. Pattern generating circuits can be constructed in a variety of ways. However, a few common principles have emerged from the studies of invertebrate pattern generators

- At least some neurons in the network will have the capacity to generate bursts of spikes, prolonged depolarizations, or endogenous oscillations. This generally occurs because these neurons, which may serve as pacemakers, express ion channels with voltage or activity-dependent expression, some of which are noted in Table 29.3.

- The expression of such active properties usually requires modulatory input from central or peripheral sources.

- Circuits tend to be more complex than minimally necessary: several seemingly redundant mechanisms reinforce particular network activity patterns.

- Pattern generation emerges as the total activity of the components of the network: the same network may produce different rhythms through combinations or functional "reconfiguration" of the components.

TABLE 29.3 Ion Channels Used as Building Blocks for Intrinsic Rhythmic Activity

Channel	Action	Role in generating rhythm
I_{Nap}	Slowly inactivating or persistent sodium current	Contributes to slow bursting and plateau potentials
I_{Ca}	Voltage-gated calcium current	Contributes to burst initiation and plateau potentials
I_A	Transient potassium current activated by depolarization	Slows depolarization or produces delay before firing
I_h	Potassium current activated by hyperpolarization	Limits time that cell remains hyperpolarized and may initiate postinhibitory rebound
$I_{K_{Ca}}$	Slow potassium current activated by calcium	Produces medium afterhyperpolarization after spikes. Summation of AHPs can terminate bursts of firing. Modulated by neurotransmitters acting through G proteins

Mary Kay Floeter

CPG for walking was composed of two half-centers, one driving flexors and another driving extensors, and that reciprocal inhibition produced oscillation of activity between the two halves. Grillner (1985) proposed three important modifications: (1) that at each joint, movement in one direction was produced by a "burst generator" unit, a half-center capable of independent rhythmic activity; (2) as in Brown's model, that flexion and extension at each joint were controlled by reciprocally connected burst generators; and (3) that multijoint coordination was achieved by loose or adjustable coupling between the mosaic of burst generators controlling each of the joints (Fig. 29.12). The advantage of this model was that locomotor CPGs could be reduced to a small number of functional units.

The model of coupled burst generators is a pretty good approximation that explains most of the experimental locomotor data in cats, neonatal rats, and people. Nevertheless, its scope does not extend to details of circuitry underlying the unit burst generators. Clues to the internal organization of the CPG came from studies assessing how various perturbations affect walking. Some perturbations and inputs changed the phase or timing of the step cycle, whereas others changed only the amplitude of the flexor or extensor bursts without interrupting the rhythm. These data, together with mapping studies of

BOX 29.5

SWIMMING IN LAMPREYS

The pattern generator for swimming in the lamprey is one of the best understood CPGs in vertebrates. The lamprey swims by propagating a wave of muscular contraction along its length. The contraction of muscles on one side of this primitive vertebrate is coupled with the relaxation of muscles of the opposite side. As the wave spreads from head to tail, there is a slight delay in muscle activation from segment to segment. The delay decreases with swimming speed, producing a constant phase lag of about 1% over a wide range of speeds.

Pieces of spinal cord containing only a few spinal segments can sustain a basic swimming rhythm, which suggests that the pattern generating circuitry underlying swimming is repeated in each spinal segment. Intracellular recording during fictive swimming has allowed many of the connections between spinal neurons and their biophysical properties to be revealed. Using these features, Grillner and colleagues proposed a model in which each segment contains a half-center circuit made by interconnections among three sets of interneurons on each side of the spinal cord: excitatory, lateral, and contralaterally projecting interneurons (Fig. 29.10). The excitatory interneurons drive ipsilateral motor neurons, as well as the other two sets of interneurons. The contralaterally projecting interneurons inhibit all three classes of interneurons on the contralateral side of the cord, causing activity to alternate from side to side. All of the excitatory connections of this circuit, including the inputs from descending reticu-

lospinal axons that initiate swimming, are glutamatergic, whereas the inhibitory connections are glycinergic. In this network model, the rhythm can be modulated by sensory or other inputs.

Grillner and Matsushima (1991) created a computer simulation model incorporating the known connections and physiological properties of the three types of interneurons, including voltage- and neurotransmitter-modulated conductances. The output generated by their simulation resembled the normal swim pattern in many ways. In addition, their model correctly predicted the changes expected from modulators such as serotonin (Fig. 29.11). Subsequent studies suggest that intersegmental coordination, needed to convey information about swimming speed, is mediated by collaterals of excitatory interneurons that may extend up to 20 segments rostrally and several segments caudally. These collaterals are hypothesized to convey signals of increased excitability in one segment to the adjacent segments to regulate phase lag and adjust the swimming speed.

Mary Kay Floeter

Reference

Grillner, S., and Matsushima, T. (1991). The neural network underlying locomotion in lamprey: Synaptic and cellular mechanisms. *Neuron* **7**, 1–15.

rhythmically active interneurons, led to the hypothesis that distinct subsets of interneurons formed the "rhythm generator" component of the CPG, which sets the timing for the step cycle, and that different sets of interneurons control the amplitudes of the flexor and extensor bursts. Afferents that signal extension of the hip, for example, play a key role in triggering the transition from extension to flexion and therefore must access the rhythm generator component of the CPG. Interneurons controlling the burst amplitudes are recipients of inputs from the rhythm generating interneurons and from other inputs that bypass the rhythm generator networks. This separation of the CPG into a timing layer and a burst generating layer best explains the step-to-step modification of gait that occurs in response to changes in walking surfaces, inclines, or other sensory cues.

Locomotor CPGs in Mammals Are Distributed among Several Spinal Segments

In recent years, the isolated neonatal rat spinal cord has proven to be a very useful preparation for studying organization of the locomotor CPG. In this preparation, the CPG appears to be distributed among several spinal segments. The upper and midlumbar segments seem to be most important for rhythm generation. Caudal lumbar segments are less rhythmogenic, although the sacral cord may have a separate CPG for control of the tail (Kremer and Lev-Tov, 2000). The importance of the upper and midlumbar cord for rhythm generation has also been observed in the spinalized cat (Rossignol *et al.*, 1999) and is consistent with case reports in humans noting that irritative lesions of the upper lumbar cord produce

Brainstem

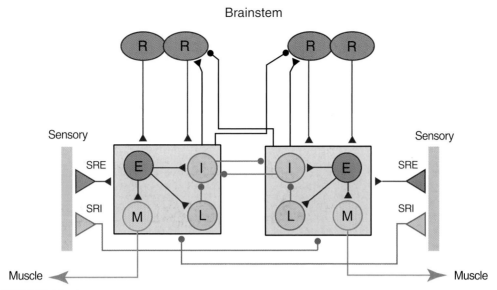

FIGURE 29.10 Model of the oscillator for swimming within each segment of the lamprey spinal cord. E, excitatory interneuron; I, contralaterally projecting interneuron; L, lateral interneuron; M, motor neuron; R, reticulospinal neuron; SRE, excitatory sensory input; SRI, inhibitory sensory input. Excitatory connections are represented by triangles and inhibitory connections by circles. Reproduced with permission from Grillner *et al.* (1995).

stepping movements (Calancie *et al.*, 1994). Identifying interneurons that form the rhythm generating network is an area of active research. One experimental approach has been to seek neurons with appropriate activation patterns during locomotion and to study their connections with microelectrodes. Activity-dependent markers, such as fluorescent calcium- and voltage-sensitive dyes, offer a different approach that reveals populations of active cells in slices or in *in vitro* preparations of the spinal

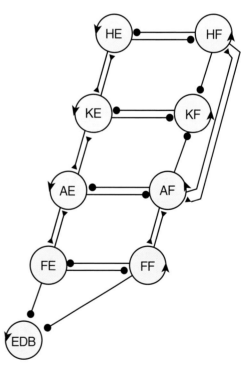

FIGURE 29.12 Scheme for multijoint coordination within a single limb using a mosaic of oscillators. Individual burst generators control movement in one direction with oscillation between units controlling extension and flexion at the hip (HE, HF), knee (KE, KF), ankle (AE, AF), and foot (FE, FF), as well as dorsiflexion of the toe by an intrinsic foot muscle (EDB). Changes in the strength of the interconnections between oscillators allow a variety of gaits. Excitatory connections are represented by triangles and inhibitory connections by filled circles. Reproduced with permission from Grillner (1985).

A   B

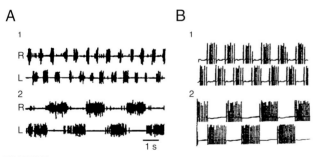

FIGURE 29.11 Real and simulated swimming motor patterns in the lamprey spinal cord. (A) Alternating motor output on the right (R) and left (L) sides of the cord produces the characteristic swimming rhythm in normal saline (1) and in the presence of 1 mM citalopram (2), a drug that increases serotonergic action. In the animal, citalopram slows the rhythm and prolongs the bursts. (B) The computer model simulates the basic rhythm in normal saline (1). When the effect of serotonin is added to the simulation (2), the model produces an output that resembles the real swimming rhythm in citalopram. Reproduced with permission from Grillner and Matsushima (1991).

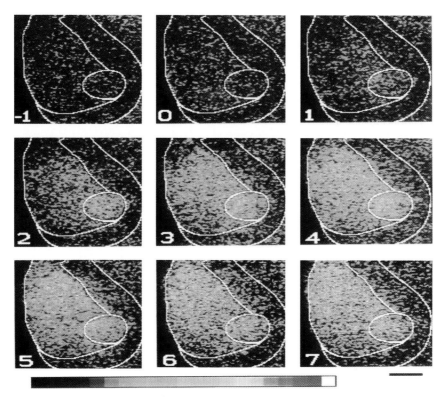

FIGURE 29.13   Optical recording of the sequence of neuronal activity in the embryonic chick spinal cord during spontaneous movement . A calcium-sensitive vital dye is used to view neuronal activity, which begins in the ventral gray matter (1 and 2) and then spreads to more dorsal areas of the cord (3–6). Calcium concentrations are indicated by changes in color. Reproduced with permission from O'Donovan et al. (1994).

cord during pharmacologically induced rhythms (Fig 29.13). A third approach has been to label neurons during locomotion with markers that are accumulated only by active neurons. Several studies identify interneurons in the ventromedial region of the spinal gray matter as candidates for the rhythm generator interneurons. *In vitro* , these cells have intrinsic properties, such as the capacity for oscillatory membrane potentials when exposed to NMDA, that would enhance rhymogenicity (Hochman *et al.*, 1994). NMDA application can induce locomotor rhythms in the isolated neonatal rat cord. Glycinergic interneurons that project to rhythmically active interneurons on the contralateral side have also been identified, and these are candidates for interlimb coordination.

Motor neurons are not thought to contribute directly to pattern generation in adult mammals. During locomotion, motor neurons receive alternating excitatory and inhibitory synaptic input, called the locomotor drive potential (LDP). A wide variety of excitatory and inhibitory last-order interneurons have been identified that are driven rhythmically by the CPG. These interneurons, found throughout the lumbar segments, are candidates for those CPG inter-

neurons that control burst amplitudes during locomotion and that transmit the LDP to motor neurons. Many also receive peripheral and descending inputs. Separate populations of last-order interneurons are needed to transmit the LDP to flexor and extensor motor neurons and to relay excitatory and inhibitory signals. Pharmacological studies of LDPs in the cat and neonatal rat indicate that glutamate is likely to be the transmitter underlying excitatory LDPs. NMDA receptors on motor neurons produce enhancement of the LDP when depolarized, contributing to plateau-like depolarizations (Fig. 29.9). According to the model outlined earlier, interneurons that make up the burst generating layer of the CPG receive certain inputs that do not connect with interneurons of the timing generator layer of CPG. This arrangement would allow certain peripheral and descending inputs to adjust muscle contraction within a step cycle without changing the pattern of gait. Some of the interneurons that are activated by peripheral afferents and the locomotor CPG network are discussed later in the context of their reflex actions.

Neurons that form a CPG network for one motor behavior are shared with CPG networks for other

BOX 29.6

TRAINING LOCOMOTOR CPGS

Much interest has focused on whether CPGs in the spinal cord can be used to produce movements in humans following spinal injury. An important aspect of this question is to determine whether peripheral inputs are able to access and activate CPG circuitry. Sensory inputs are known to play a key role in inducing plastic changes in the brain with the acquisition of motor skills. A degree of plasticity in locomotor circuitry would seem essential when learning to walk or to adapt gait patterns after injury to a limb. Can the spinal cord also undergo plastic changes and be "retrained" to walk after spinal injury? Rossignol and colleagues (1999) noted that training spinalized cats to walk on a treadmill improved their recovery of locomotor abilities. The sensory feedback of the locomotor movements was thought to play a key role in the recovery of walking abilities. Treatment with clonidine, an α-adrenergic agonist, enhanced the training. A similar training strategy has been applied to people with incomplete spinal cord injury. Initially, when patients are still unable to make any movements, a harness is used to support their body weight while their legs are passively moved along a treadmill. With daily training over several weeks, the leg muscles generate a pattern of alternation between flexors and extensor muscles that produces stepping. As their locomotor patterns recover, the support supplied by the harness is gradually lessened.

The movement that is learned is specific to the training paradigm: patients who are trained to stand and bear weight do not regain stepping (Edgerton et al., 2001). What are the mechanisms of this recovery? Conditioning and increased strength of leg muscles form a small part of the picture. Some evidence suggests that training alters the synthesis of GABA by inhibitory spinal interneurons (Edgerton et al., 2001). The more important mechanism is thought to be an increased excitability of spinal CPGs brought on by repetitive sensory inputs, enhanced by pharmacological treatments that increase norepinephrine and serotonin. To date, locomotor training has only been successful in patients with partial spinal cord injury. Sparing or regeneration of a small number of descending fibers may prove to be critical for training to be successful. More research is needed to fully understand how training works and the minimal requirements for specific descending connection or descending neuromodulatory influences. The combination of regeneration or repair, locomotor training, pharmacological treatments, and prosthetic devices is likely to be needed for developing a strategy for the recovery of locomotion after spinal injury.

Mary Kay Floeter

Reference

Rossignol, S., Drew, T., Brustein, E., and Janing, W. (1999). Locomotor performance and adaptation of the partial or complete spinal cord lesions in the cat. *Prog Brain Res.* **123**, 349–365.

behaviors. Networks can be "reconfigured"—subsets of neurons change their activity patterns and the efficacy of synaptic connections so that the network produces a different output. This process of reconfiguration probably acts through neuromodulators that set the excitability of key interneurons in the network or determine their set of active conductances. Reconfiguring an existing network is particularly efficient when neurons of both networks would need to receive input from common sources and act on common sets of motor neurons. For example, cats use their hindlimbs for scratching as well as locomotion, two behaviors that require alternating flexion and extension of muscles that act across the ankle. When the cat raises the hindlimb to scratch, it stops walking and holds the contralateral leg in tonic extension. Scratching and walking are behaviors not easily performed simultaneously, and it is likely that CPGs

share at least some common neurons. This does not mean that scratch is produced merely by using the locomotor CPG at a faster speed. The timing and combinations of contracting muscles differ in the two behaviors. An example is the differential behavior of the two long toe flexor muscles, FHL and FDL, which are active in alternate phases during walking (Fig. 29.9) but are coactive in scratch to unsheathe the claws. Descending pathways play a key role in the selection of CPGs by altering the functional interactions between neurons and setting the excitability of subsets of interneurons.

Brain Stem Structures Relay Descending Control of Spinal CPGs

Conscious decisions about initiating and maintaining walking are made in the cerebral cortex or, in lower vertebrates, in the forebrain. Brain stem structures, however, probably serve as an intermediary between the forebrain and the spinal circuits producing locomotion. In decerebrate animals, electrical stimulation of a brain stem area called the mesencephalic locomotor region (MLR) produces stepping that persists even for a short time after the stimulation ends. The MLR and the related pedunculopontine nucleus have few or no direct spinal projections, but project heavily to neurons in the pontomedullary reticular formation. Most of the reticulospinal axons involved in this region travel in the ventral and ventrolateral tracts of the spinal cord. Because lesions of the ventrolateral funiculus disrupt the ability to initiate and maintain locomotion, these reticulospinal tracts are thought to play a key role in activating the CPG neurons for locomotion (Rossignol *et al.*, 1999). Sparing of at least some fibers in the ventrolateral funiculus markedly improves locomotor recovery after spinal lesions in cats and could be necessary for the recovery of locomotor movements after spinal injury in humans (see Box 29.6).

In cats, a second descending pathway in the dorsolateral funiculus has some capacity for activating locomotor CPGs after bilateral lesions in the ventrolateral funiculi. The identity of the axons mediating locomotor recovery after such lesions has not been established. Corticospinal and rubrospinal tracts travel in the dorsolateral funiculus, as do reticulospinal tracts that modulate flexor reflexes. Isolated lesions of the dorsolateral funiculus impair the ability to support weight and produce a foot drop in cats.

Summary

Interneurons of the spinal cord have diverse connections that allow them to relay and modulate signals from peripheral afferents and descending motor pathways. Spinal interneurons are interconnected to form networks that can produce patterned rhythmic outputs. These networks, known as central pattern generators, play a role in carrying out rhythmic movements that are performed relatively automatically, such as breathing, chewing, scratching, and walking. CPGs are able to coordinate the timing and sequence of activation and inhibition between motor neuron pools innervating different muscles. Locomotion is one example of a rhythmic movement that is coordinated by CPGs. Mammalian locomotion is a cycle with alternation of limb flexion extension. Flexor and extensor motor neurons receive alternating excitatory and inhibitory synaptic inputs. Current models of locomotor CPG organization propose that activity oscillates between networks controlling the timing of the flexor and the extensor bursts. Feedback from peripheral afferents or descending inputs can adjust the timing of the locomotor cycle or the intensity of the bursts. Descending reticulospinal tracts are critical for activating the locomotor CPG neurons residing in the lumbar cord.

SENSORY MODULATION

There Are Two Major Classes of Muscle Afferents

Although spinal CPGs may be able to produce a basic sequence of muscle activity for rhythmic movements such as locomotion, the final pattern reflects fine-tuning by descending and peripheral inputs. Brown recognized the necessity for afferent inputs in his earliest description of spinal pattern generators:

> A purely central mechanism of progression ungraded by proprioceptive stimuli would clearly be inefficient in determining the passage of an animal through an uneven environment. Across a plane of perfect evenness the central mechanism itself might drive an animal with precision. Or it might be efficient, for instance, in the case of an elephant charging over ground of moderate unevenness. But it alone would make impossible the fine stalking of a cat over rough ground. In such a case each step may be somewhat different to all others, and each must be graded to its condition if the whole progression of the animal is to be efficient.... This grading can only be brought about by peripheral stimuli. (Brown, 1911)

Among the most potent peripheral stimuli that influence motor activity are inputs that arise from muscle afferents.

Muscles contain two types of specialized sensory receptors that provide feedback to the central nervous system. Muscle spindles sense muscle stretch, and Golgi tendon organs (GTOs) sense the load upon the muscle (Fig. 29.14). The muscle spindle consists of an encapsulated bundle of specialized muscle fibers called intrafusal fibers. The spindle lies within the muscle in parallel to the skeletal muscle fibers. Each spindle contains two types of intrafusal fibers—nuclear bag fibers and nuclear chain fibers—which differ in the positioning of their nuclei, the continuity of their myofibrils, and their dynamic sensitivity. The spindle receives both sensory and motor innervation. Sensory innervation is supplied by one primary afferent, the Ia fiber, and several secondary, group II afferents. Ia and group II afferents signal different features of stretch. Ia afferents are activated briefly by small stretches, such as a tap or vibration, and signal dynamic aspects of stretch. Group II secondary spindle afferents are sensitive to the level of sus-

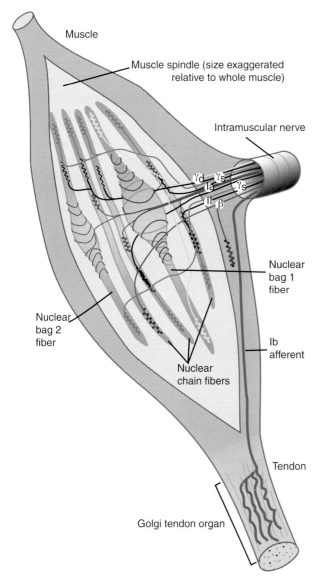

FIGURE 29.14 Structure and innervation of muscle spindles and Golgi tendon organs. The sensory innervation of the spindle is through primary (Ia) spindle afferents that innervate both nuclear bag and nuclear chain intrafusal muscle fibers and secondary (II) afferents that innervate nuclear chain fibers. Motor innervation of the spindle is supplied by static and dynamic γ motor neurons (γs and $\gamma \delta$) and by motor neurons.

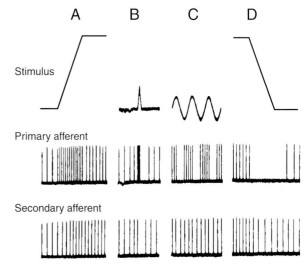

FIGURE 29.15 Responses of cat primary and secondary afferents to linear stretch (A), tap (B), vibration (C), and release from stretch (D). Reproduced with permission from Matthews (1964).

fusimotor neurons. There are two types. γ motor neurons only innervate intrafusal fibers, whereas β motor neurons innervate both intrafusal fibers and skeletal muscle fibers. β motor neurons, which are common in amphibians, are less common in mammals, although by some estimates, a third or more of mammalian intrafusal fibers may be innervated by β motor neurons.

During most voluntary movements, α and γ motor neurons are coactivated so that the sensitivity of the spindle is maintained during muscle shortening. Nevertheless, the separate innervation of intrafusal muscle fibers by γ motor neurons and skeletal muscle fibers by α motor neurons permits independent control of a movement and the gain of its sensory feedback. γ motor neurons receive positive feedback from group II spindle afferents. γ motor neurons can adjust the tone of the fusimotor system so that the spindle sensitivity differs during different types of movement. Fully independent activity of γ motor neurons has not been found in humans, but a relative dissociation between α and γ activation has been demonstrated in monkeys and other animals during very slow movements.

Golgi tendon organs consist of nerve endings interdigitated among collagen bundles of the muscle tendons. Thus the GTO lies in series with the skeletal muscle fibers. GTOs are sensitive to the load on the muscle, particularly the forces on the tendon generated by skeletal muscle fiber contraction. Each GTO senses the force generated by a small number of motor units that insert onto a local region of the tendon. The centrally projecting axons of the GTOs are called Ib

tained stretch and have firing rates proportional to the muscle length (Fig. 29.15).

Motor innervation of intrafusal fibers can compensate for changes in muscle length by adjusting the tension of the spindle. When a muscle contracts and shortens, the spindle within that muscle can become slack, causing a momentary pause in spindle afferent firing. This occurs, for example, after tapping on the tendon of a muscle to elicit a stretch reflex. Motor neurons that innervate intrafusal fibers are called afferents. Like Ia afferents, they are large myelinated axons with fast conduction velocities. Unlike spindles, GTOs do not have motor innervation.

Skeletal muscles are also innervated by smaller diameter afferents, group III and IV afferents, that respond to extracellular compounds, such as those released during muscle fatigue. These afferents relay the sense of muscle pain and soreness and produce reflex actions with a relatively slow time course.

Reflexes: An Introduction

Muscle, joint, and skin afferents provide proprioceptive and cutaneous information to the spinal cord as well as to supraspinal regions. These afferents will each be activated in a quite distinct way during a movement, signaling the displacement of particular joints, pressure on particular regions of the skin, or stretch of particular muscles. Such "multisensory" signals normally generated during movement are thought to reinforce activity in circuits that produce those selected movements. However, sometimes perturbations occur as a movement proceeds, and the sensory signal that is relayed evokes a reflex response that changes the motor output. Although reflexes are stereotyped, they are far from invariant and are typically modulated when they occur during a movement. At times, the distinction between reflexes and normal sensory feedback during a movement can be hard to discern.

Stretch Reflexes

The stretch reflex is the simplest of all the spinal reflexes and is brought into play in many movements. The circuitry underlying the stretch reflex is simple:

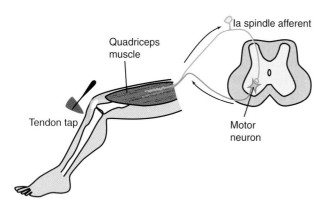

FIGURE 29.16 Basic circuitry underlying the knee-jerk stretch reflex. Ia spindle afferents from the quadriceps muscle make monosynaptic, excitatory connections on α motor neurons that innervate the quadriceps.

stretch of a muscle causes firing of spindle afferents, which synapse on α motor neurons innervating that muscle (Fig. 21.16). Ia afferents synapse monosynaptically on motor neurons that innervate the same muscle in which the spindle lies, so-called homonymous motor neurons, to produce a potent and robust EPSP. Ia afferents also synapse to a lesser extent on heteronymous motor neurons that innervate other muscles, particularly synergist muscles that produce a similar movement. The stretch reflex has a brief, phasic component, evoked by the Ia afferents at the onset of stretch, and a tonic component, which is more variable, mediated through polysynaptic pathways or group II afferents.

The Ia afferent uses the neurotransmitter glutamate. Its synapses are located on the main dendrites of motor neurons. Although monosynaptic, the stretch reflex is subject to modulation by presynaptic inhibition. The terminals of Ia afferents receive synapses from GABAergic spinal interneurons. GABAergic interneurons are activated by antagonist muscle Ia afferents, corticospinal, reticulospinal, and CPG inputs. Transmission at the GABAergic axo-axonic synapse reduces the amount of transmitter released, reducing the size of the Ia EPSP on the motor neuron. Presynaptic inhibition is a mechanism that allows modulation of the strength of the Ia input without affecting the response of a motor neuron to other inputs. During locomotion, CPGs activate presynaptic inhibitory interneurons rhythmically, gating the strength of Ia afferent feedback throughout the step cycle. During voluntary movements, descending inputs activate selected subsets of presynaptic inhibitory interneurons to reduce the strength of Ia afferents from antagonist muscles and facilitate Ia afferent inputs from the muscle about to be used.

Interneurons in Reflex Pathways

Historically, most of the work that identified different classes of interneurons came from studies of spinal reflexes: stereotyped motor actions evoked by specific sensory stimuli. With the exception of the monosynaptic stretch reflex, most reflexes are mediated by polysynaptic interneuron circuits (Table 29.4). Reflexes have been useful for reliably identifying specific interneurons, particularly last-order interneurons, and to investigate their connectivity in the laboratory (Burke, 1999). In recent years, however, it has been recognized that some of the classic reflexes depend on the "state" of the animal and can even be reversed between resting and active states. Defining these different states and understanding the mechanisms used to switch between states are active areas

TABLE 29.4 Characteristics of Selected Spinal Interneurons

Interneuron	Transmitter	Anatomy/physiology	Inputs	Outputs
IaIN	Glycine	Lamina VII; synapses on motor neuron soma; fires single spike to input volley	Corticospinal, vestibulo-spinal, rubrospinal, antagonist IaINs, Renshaw cells, locomotor networks	Antagonist motor neurons, antagonist IaINs
Ia presynaptic inhibitory (first order)	Unknown	Intermediate zone?	Corticospinal, vestibulospinal, rubrospinal, cutaneous afferents	Last-order Ia presynaptic inhibitory interneurons
Ia presynaptic inhibitory (last order)	GABA	Intermediate nucleus	Reticulospinal, locomotor networks?	Antagonist Ia afferents
Group II (excitatory)	Unknown	Intermediate zone?	Ia and/or Ib, propriospinal, descending?	Flexor motor neurons (excitatory)
Group II (inhibitory)	Unknown	Intermediate zone?	Ia and/or Ib, propriospinal, descending?	Extensor motor neurons (inhibitory)
Renshaw cell	Glycine (GABA sub-population?)	Ventral horn, medial to motor neuron pools; synapses on motor neuron dendrites; fires in high-frequency bursts	Motor neurons, Renshaw cells, corticospinal, rubrospinal, descending monoaminergic, locomotor networks, cutaneous?	Alpha motor neurons (esp. synergists), gamma motor neurons Renshaw cells, IaINs
IbIN	Glycine?	Intermediate zone; no tonic firing; single spikes when activated	Ib (extensor > flexor), Ia, and cutaneous afferents (all excitatory); corticospinal, rubrospinal, reticulospinal (all inhibitory)	Motor neurons (esp. extensor), IbINs, neuron Clarke's column (subgroup)

of current research. This section describes some of the interneurons mediating the classical reflexes. Most of these reflexes, and their underlying circuits, were originally characterized in anesthetized animals. Information on other reflexes and their interneuron circuits are covered in articles referenced at the end of the chapter.

Reciprocal Inhibition

Contraction of a muscle produces a reflex relaxation of its antagonist muscle, a phenomenon called reciprocal inhibition. Several different spinal circuits produce reciprocal inhibition. The shortest circuit produces an IPSP at disynaptic latency, with only one interneuron interposed. This interneuron is named the Ia inhibitory interneuron (IaIN) because it is excited by Ia afferents and inhibits motor neurons. The IaIN uses glycine as its transmitter. It synapses on the somas and main dendrites of motor neurons, producing a fast, potent IPSP that lasts for several milliseconds. Most inputs that activate a motor neuron also activate IaINs that project to antagonist motor neurons. Thus, IaINs receive input from descending pathways, including the corticospinal tract, and from segmental CPGs. These latter inputs use IaINs to relay inhibitory signals to motor neurons that oppose the planned movement. Because of its many convergent inputs, the strength of IaIN inhibition is highly flexible and can be overridden for those movements that require cocontraction of antagonist muscles.

Recurrent Inhibition

Recurrent inhibition provides a negative feedback mechanism to motor neurons. It is mediated by a population of inhibitory interneurons, known as Renshaw cells or recurrent interneurons, that are activated by recurrent axons of homonymous and synergist motor neurons. Early pharmacological studies showed that Renshaw cells used glycine as their transmitter, but later work provided evidence for an additional GABAergic component of recurrent inhibition. Some recurrent interneurons contain both glycine and GABA during development, probably within the same synaptic vesicle, as both use the same vesicular transporter protein. It is not known whether coexpression is maintained in adult animals or whether separate populations of GABAergic and glycinergic recurrent interneurons emerge. The role of recurrent inhibition in movement is not known, but one suggestion is that recurrent inhibition provides a type of "lateral inhibition" among synergists, leading to an enhanced contrast between activated and quiescent motoneurons.

Group I Nonreciprocal Inhibition

Nonreciprocal, or autogenic, inhibition was first described as an inhibitory reflex that was the inverse of the stretch reflex, producing relaxation of homonymous and synergist motor neurons when Ib afferents were activated. It was originally believed to be a protective reflex that occurred only when muscles were subject to injurious levels of stretch. It is now known that the interneurons that produce this reflex also receive inputs from Ia afferents, low threshold joint afferents, and cutaneous afferents. For this reason, the term group I nonreciprocal inhibition is now preferred. In anesthetized animals, stimulation of group I afferents produces inhibition of extensor motor neurons. During active movement, however, the inhibitory interneurons mediating this reflex are completely suppressed. Thus there is a state dependence of the inhibitory effects of group I muscle afferents.

Group I Excitatory Interneurons

As noted earlier, stimulation of group I afferents produces an inhibitory reflex in anesthetized or resting animals. In contrast, group I afferent stimulation causes excitation in extensor motor neurons of animals that are actively engaged in locomotion. Stimulation of group I afferents will enhance or prolong extension if the animal is in the stance phase of stepping or will reset the rhythm, switching to stance if the leg is in the swing phase (Fig. 29.17). Because the group I sensory receptors—spindles and GTOs—are exquisitely sensitive to changes in muscle stretch and load that occur during active movement, the group I excitatory pathway is likely to be potent in providing sensory feedback to regulate locomotion on a step-to-step basis. The last-order interneurons in the group I excita-

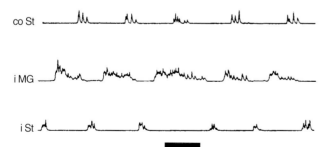

FIGURE 29.17 Recordings from three muscle nerves in a decerebrate cat exhibiting spontaneous fictive locomotion. Stimulation of group I afferents (dark bar) prolongs the extensor phase of locomotion, as seen in the ankle extensor muscle neurogram (i MG). Activity in the ipsilateral knee flexor muscle neurogram (i St) is delayed until stimulation ends. Activity of the contralateral knee flexor muscle nerve (co St) shows only a modest change. Reproduced with permission from Whelan *et al.* (1995).

tory circuit have not been identified definitively, but the voltage-dependent behavior of the EPSPs they produce in target motor neurons suggests that glutamate is their neurotransmitter. EPSPs produced by group I excitatory interneurons are larger when motor neurons are depolarized, an effect often produced by the activation of NMDA receptors. This voltage-dependent amplification of EPSPs ensures that the effects of the group I excitatory pathway are greatest in those motor neurons that receive coincident excitatory inputs. Expression of the group I excitatory pathway is state dependent and only apparent during active movement. The mechanisms for switching between the group I excitatory interneuron pathway and the inhibitory interneuron pathway in different behavioral states are unknown.

Presynaptic Inhibition

The reflex effects of group I afferents are also modulated by presynaptic inhibition. The presynaptic terminals of most sensory afferents are subject to presynaptic inhibition, in contrast to descending axons from supraspinal regions that mostly lack presynaptic inhibition. Presynaptic inhibition reduces the amount of transmitter released by the afferent fiber. Different classes of interneurons mediate presynaptic inhibition of Ia, Ib, cutaneous, and group II muscle afferents, and each class of interneurons has a characteristic pattern of descending and peripheral inputs. The existence of separate circuitry for presynaptic inhibition of Ia and Ib afferents allows independent control of the gain of feedback from muscle spindles and GTOs. This flexibility could allow the central nervous system to switch between operating modes that respond to length (Ia) feedback and those that respond to tension (Ib) feedback.

Flexor Reflexes

The simplest flexor reflex consists of hip, knee, and ankle flexion, combined with extensor muscle relaxation, in response to stimulation of the skin or a mixed nerve. A variety of peripheral afferents elicit flexor reflexes: group II and III muscle afferents, joint afferents, and high- and low-threshold cutaneous afferents. Because they can elicit a common action, these afferents are sometimes grouped together under the label "flexor reflex afferents" (FRAs). The flexor reflex is widely distributed to many muscles and has short latency and long latency components. Several polysynaptic circuits underlie the flexor reflex, and different subgroups of interneurons are thought to produce the early and late components. The late components of flexor reflexes are enhanced in spinalized animals treated with L-dopa. It has been suggested that the subgroup of interneurons producing the late components of the flexor reflex could function as the flexor half-center for the locomotor CPG.

Cutaneous Reflexes

In contrast to the widely distributed flexor reflex, stimulation of small areas of skin can result in reflex actions limited to a few muscles. One example of a local cutaneous reflex is the stumbling corrective reaction. When the skin on the top of the foot is stimulated during walking, the foot is lifted higher, as if to step over an obstacle. The stumbling corrective reaction is phase dependent, occurring only when the limb is in the swing phase of the step cycle. This and several other local cutaneous reflexes are oligosynaptic, involving only a few interneurons. The last-order interneurons in these cutaneous reflexes connect with relatively limited sets of motor neurons. It has been proposed that such interneurons offer a means to control or alter activity of specific muscles during movement without involving CPG neurons.

Pharmacology of Spinal States and Reflex Reversals

Although it is not known what defines different states of the spinal cord, it is clear that pharmacological agents can induce differences in reflexes or rhythmic activity similar to those observed in different states of activity. Agents that mimic the action of endogenous neuromodulatory transmitters, notably serotonin and norepinephrine, are the best known. These drugs are known to act through G proteins and second messenger systems to modify receptors and ion channel activity in certain neurons. Which spinal neurons these drugs, or their endogenous counterparts, normally target to switch between states is unknown. There are likely to be key interneurons whose excitability or firing properties determine the predominance of different CPG configurations; relatively little is known about the effects of neuromodulators on the active membrane properties in specific populations of interneurons.

Systemically administered drugs have differing effects on intact and spinalized animals and on isolated spinal cord preparations; effects also differ at local sites within the cord; species differences are present as well. In spinalized cats, drugs that activate α-adrenergic receptors, such as clonidine or tizanidine, enhance the ability to initiate walking on a treadmill. These drugs increase the duration of electromyogram bursts and the length of individual steps in cats. Clonidine or tizanidine also improves treadmill walking in humans with partial spinal cord injury (SCI), but has no effect with complete spinal injuries

(Box 29.6). Clonidine may produce its effects by dampening cutaneous reflexes that are disadvantageous for locomotion. Administration of L-dopa, a noradrenergic precursor, has been shown to suppress short latency flexor reflexes and enhance long latency flexor reflexes without changing stretch reflexes in acutely spinalized cats. Its effects on the different sensory reflexes are thus quite selective. Administration of glutamate or NMDA can also produce state changes in spinal cord preparations, inducing locomotor rhythms in the isolated cord preparations of lampreys and neonatal rats, and even reversing the effects of Ia afferents on disynaptic pathways.

Summary

Muscle, joint, and skin afferents provide feedback during movement that can modulate motor output, as well as produce a reflex response to an unexpected perturbation. Muscle has two kinds of specialized sensory receptors: spindles, which signal muscle stretch, and Golgi tendon organs, which signal the tension on the muscle. These are referred to as group I afferents. Sensory transmission from spindles and GTOs is subject to presynaptic modulation. Spindle afferents produce the monosynaptic stretch reflex, as well as longer latency reflexes, such as reciprocal inhibition of antagonist motor neurons, that are mediated through spinal interneurons. Cutaneous inputs produce broadly distributed reflexes, such as the flexor reflex, and local reflexes, such as the stumbling corrective reflex, which are limited to a few muscles. The interneurons in reflex pathways receive many convergent inputs from descending pathways and segmental interneurons that modulate their excitability to peripheral inputs. Interneurons in reflex pathways also function as last-order output neurons for spinal pattern generators and descending axons. The reflex effects produced by a given sensory stimulus can differ during resting and active states of motor activity. Different states of the spinal cord are probably induced by neuromodulatory transmitters, but much remains to be learned.

References

Brown, T. G. (1911). The intrinsic factors in the act of progression in the mammal. *Proc. R. Soc. London.* **84**, 308–319.

Bottinelli, R., and Reggiani, C. (2000). Human skeletal muscle fibres: Molecular and functional diversity. *Prog. Biophys. Mol. Biol.* **73**, 195–262.

Burke, R. E., Levine, D. N., Tsairis, P., and Zajac, F. E. (1973). Physiological types and histochemical profiles in motor units of the cat gastrocnemius. *J. Physiol. (Lond.)* **234**, 723–748.

Calancie, B., Needham-Shropshire, B., Jacobs, P., Willer, K., Zych, G., and Green, B.A. (1994). Involuntary stepping after chronic spinal cord injury. Evidence for a central rhythm generator for locomotion in man. *Brain* **117**, 1143–1159.

Cooper, E. C., and Jan, L. Y. (1999). Ion channel genes and human neurological diseases: Recent progress, prospects, and challenges, *Proc. Natl. Acad. Sci. USA.* **96**, 4759–4766.

Edgerton, V. R., de Leon, R. D., Harkema, S., Hodgson, J. A., London, N., Reinkensmeyer, D. J., Roy, R. R., Talmadge, R. J., Tillakaratne, N. J., Timoszyk, W., and Tobin, A. (2001). Retraining the injured spinal cord. *J. Physiol. (Lond.)* **533**, 15–22.

Grillner, S. (1985). Neurobiological bases of rhythmic motor acts in vertebrates. *Science* **228**, 143–149.

Grillner, S., Deliagina, T., Eckberg, O., Manira, A. E., Hill, R. H., Lansner, A., Orlovsky, G. N., and Wallen, P. (1995). Neural networks that coordinate locomotion and body orientation in lamprey. *Trends Neurosci.* **18**, 270–279.

Grillner, S., and Matsushima, T. (1991). The neural network underlying locomotion in lamprey: Synaptic and cellular mechanisms. *Neuron* **7**, 1–15.

Henneman, E. (1957). Relation between size of neurons and their susceptibility to discharge. *Science* **126**, 1345–1347.

Hochman, S., Jordan, L. M., and MacDonald, J. F. (1994). N-methyl-D-aspartate receptor-mediated voltage oscillations in neurons surrounding the central canal in slices of rat spinal cord. *J. Neurophysiol.* **72**, 565–577.

Kremer, E., and Lev-Tov, A. (1997). Localization of the spinal network associated with generation of hindlimb locomotion in the neonatal rat and organization of its transverse coupling system. *J. Neurophysiol.* **77**, 1155–1170.

Lee, R. H., and Heckman, C. J. (2000). Adjustable amplification of synaptic input in the dendrites of spinal motoneurons *in vivo*. *J. Neurosci.* **20**, 6734–6740.

Lundberg, A. (1979). Multisensory control of spinal reflex pathways. *Prog. Brain Res.* **50**, 11–28.

Matthews, P. B. C. (1964). Muscle spindles and their motor control. *Physiol. Res.* **44**, 219–288.

O'Donovan, M., Ito, S., and Yee, W. (1994). Calcium imaging of rhythmic network activity with developing spinal cord of the chick embryo. *J. Neurosci.* **14**, 6354–6369.

Rossignol, S., Drew, T., Brustein, E., and Jaing, W. (1999). Locomotor performance and adaptation after partial or complete spinal cord lesions in the cat. *Prog. Brain Res.* **123**, 349–365.

Squire, J. M. (1983). Molecular mechanisms in muscular contraction. *Trends Neurosci.* **10**, 409–413.

Whelan, P .J., Hiebert, G. W., and Pearson, K. G. (1995). Stimulation of the group I extensor afferents prolongs the stance phase in walling cats. *Exp. Brain Res.* **103**, 10–30.

Suggested Readings

Barbeau, H., McCrea, D. A., O'Donovan, M. J., Rossignol, S., Grill W. M., and Lemay, M. A. (1999) Tapping into spinal circuits to restore motor function. *Brain Res. Rev.* **30**, 27–51.

Burke, R. E. (1999). The use of state dependent modulation of spinal reflexes as a tool to investigate the organization of spinal interneurons. *Exp. Brain Res.* **128**, 263–277.

Engel, A. G., Ohno, K., Milone, M., and Sine S. M. (1998). Congenital myasthenic syndromes: New insights from molecular genetic and patch-clamp studies. *Ann. N. Y. Acad. Sci.* **841**, 140–156.

Hultborn, H. (2001). State-dependent modulation of sensory feedback. *J. Physiol. (Lond.)* **533**, 5–13.

Jankowska, E. (1992). Interneuronal relays in spinal pathways from proprioceptors. *Prog. Neurobiol.* **38**, 335–378.

Kiehn, O., and Eken, T. (1998) Functional role of plateau potentials in vertebrate motor neurons. *Curr. Opin. Neurobiol.* **8**, 746–752.

Pearson, K. G. (2000). Neural adaptation in the generation of rhythmic behavior. *Annu. Rev. Physiol.* **62**, 723–753.

Pette, D. (2001) Historical perspectives: Plasticity of mammalian skeletal muscle. *J. Appl. Physiol.* **90**, 1119–1124.

Prochazka, A., Clarac, F., Loeb, G., Rothwell, J. C., and Wolpaw, J. R. (2000). What do reflex and voluntary mean? Modern views on an ancient debate. *Exp. Brain Res.* **130**, 417–432.

Stuart, D. G. (1999). The segmental motor system: Advances, issues, possibilities. *Prog. Brain Res.* **123**, 3–27.

Mary Kay Floeter

30

Descending Control of Movement

Four major pathways descend from the brain to the spinal cord to control muscles that move the skeleton. These pathways arise in the vestibular nuclei (vestibulospinal), in the brain stem reticular formation (reticulospinal), in the red nucleus (rubrospinal), and in the cerebral cortex (corticospinal). While these four descending pathways work together to provide seamless control of movements from postural reflexes to delicate manipulation, they can be separated broadly into two main systems. Vestibulospinal and reticulospinal pathways can be grouped together as a medial system: their axons descend through the brain stem and spinal cord close to the midline, and chiefly innervate axial and proximal limb musculature whose motoneurons lie medially in the ventral horn. The corticospinal and rubrospinal pathways together can

be considered a lateral system: their axons descend in the lateral column of the spinal cord and chiefly innervate limb musculature, particularly distal musculature, whose motoneurons lie laterally in the ventral horn. More that just an anatomical distinction, the medial and lateral systems have different principal functions. The medial system provides postural control (Box 30.1). Monkeys with medial system lesions fall over when they attempt to ambulate and climb, but when supported, they can use their hands and fingers adeptly in retrieving food pieces from narrow holes (Lawrence and Kuypers, 1968b). The lateral system provides fine control of voluntary movement. Monkeys with lateral system lesions rapidly recover the use of all four extremities in activities such as ambulation and climbing, but they are

---

BOX 30.1

NEUROTRANSMITTERS AND POSTURE

Although most of the work on postural reflexes has concerned mammalian responses and neurophysiological mechanisms, invertebrate studies offer simpler systems that may be more directly manipulated, especially by neuropharmacological agents. The work of Kravitz and colleagues exemplifies this approach. They found that systemic administration of the aminergic neurotransmitter serotonin (see Chapter 7) causes a lobster to assume a flexed posture characteristic of defensive responses. Octopamine, in contrast, causes the animal to lie flat with its legs extended. These responses are not due to the direct action of serotonin and octopamine on muscles; both

agents stimulate muscular contraction. However, serotonin and octopamine have opposite effects on extensor and flexor motor neurons: serotonin excites flexor motor neurons and is selectively localized in a subset of interneurons. The conclusion is that serotonin acts on the lobster central nervous system to trigger the flexion posture, wheres octopamine triggers extension. In mammals, axons descending from the reticular formation release neurotransmitters, including serotonin, that have analogous modulatory functions.

Marc H. Schieber and James F. Baker

791

unable to make the fine finger movements needed to extract small pieces of food from narrow holes (Lawrence and Kuypers, 1968a). This chapter examines the contributions of first the medial and then the lateral descending systems to control of movement.

THE MEDIAL POSTURAL SYSTEM

Vestibular and Reticular Nuclei Control Posture and Reflex Behaviors

One of the important advances in neuroscience in the 19th century was the use of ablation and transection of the brain to study the localization of central nervous system function, and one of the earliest applications was to localize the level of postural control along the neuraxis. It had become clear by the beginning of the 20th century that lower portions of the mammalian brain were capable of autonomous performance of simple behaviors (Clarke and O'Malley, 1996). Sir Charles Sherrington made extensive study of the spinal reflexes and the phenomenon of decerebrate rigidity produced by brain transection.

Sherrington found that complete separation of the neuraxis near the level of the pons resulted in tonic contraction of the limb antigravity extensors in quadrupeds (Fig. 30.1). The result was an exaggerated standing posture, although the posture of these low-level decerebrate animals was not much more stable than that of an animal that has been stuffed by a taxidermist. Brain transection removed the influences of higher brain centers on brain stem nuclei, including vestibular nuclei and scattered nuclei collectively termed the reticular formation.

While the decerebrate animal does not exhibit effective stabilizing postural responses to perturbations, it does respond in a more organized fashion than spinalized animals. Depending on the level of transection and the duration of survival after transection, various degrees of evidence of a "righting reaction" can be observed. Chronic bulbospinal cats, those with medulla and spinal cord below the transection, show evidence of a righting reaction when placed on one side. The upper forelimb is flexed with gripping claws while the lower forelimb is extended under the body as if to push the body up off its side. In chronically surviving animals subjected to transection that

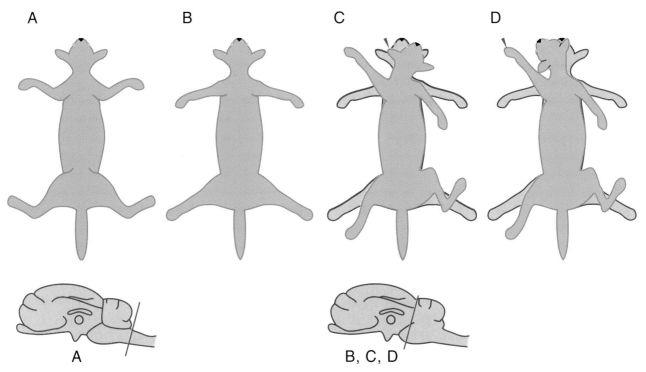

FIGURE 30.1 Posture following transection of the neuraxis. (A) The limp posture of a cat immediately after separation of the spinal cord from the brain. Limbs are neither flexed nor extended. The level of transection is shown below in a sagittal view. (B) The rigid posture of the decerebrate quadruped. All four limbs are extended. The transection, shown below, has been made through the pons. (C) Adjustment of the posture of the decerebrate preparation in response to stimulation of the pinna. All four limbs and the head alter their posture. (D) Adjustment of decerebrate posture in response to stimulation of the forepaw. Again, limbs and neck adjust. In this case the head turns toward the stimulus. Based on reports by Sherrington.

leaves the mesencephalon intact below the level of the cut, effective righting may be observed. As the level of transection is raised, posture and balance become progressively closer to normal. The decorticate animal produced by the ablation of cerebral cortical tissue has many apparently normal postural reactions, lacking only certain placing and stepping reactions. Progressively higher brain transections enable more of the vestibular (balance) and proprioceptive (muscle and position sense) circuitry that participates in postural control, as well as improving the overall balance between excitatory and inhibitory neurons in vestibular and reticular nuclei.

We now know that nuclei of the reticular formation with intact spinal projections after high brain stem transection, which are released from descending inhibition, include the locus ceruleus and raphe nuclei. These nuclei are the origins of descending noradrenergic and serotonergic neuromodulatory axonal projections that alter excitability of neurons in the spinal

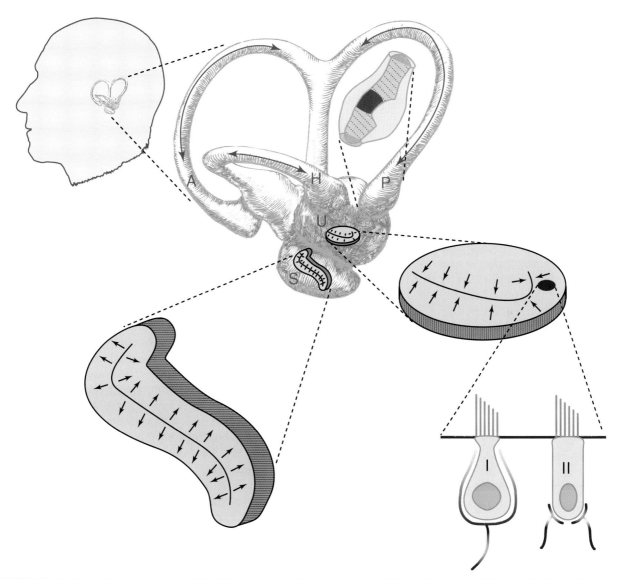

FIGURE 30.2 Vestibular canals and otoliths. The position and orientation of the labyrinth (not to scale) in the head are shown at the upper left of the figure. An enlarged view of the labyrinth shows the directions of head rotation and endolymph flow (red arrows) that excite each of the three semicircular canals. The horizontal orientation of the utricular macula and vertical orientation of the saccular macula are shown schematically. More highly magnified views of the receptor regions of a canal and of the otolith organs are shown with the cupula of the canal colored dark gray and the best directions for excitation of otolith hair cells marked by black arrows. At the lower right are two anatomical types of hair cell: the calyx or type I and bouton-ending or type II receptor. The tallest cilial extension on each cell is the kinocilium. A, anterior semicircular canal; H, horizontal semicircular canal; P, posterior semicircular canal; S, saccule containing saccular macula; U, utricule containing utricular macula; I, type I receptor; II, type II receptor. Based on studies reviewed by Wilson and Melvill-Jones.

cord, as discussed in the preceding chapter. Parts of the raphe nuclei also have a role in circadian rhythms (Chapters 41 and 42), and projections of the locus ceruleus are involved in attention (Chapter 49) and internal reward (Chapter 43). Other areas of the reticular formation involved in motor control have specific functions in generation of the locomotor rhythm (MLR, mesencephalic locomotor region, Chapter 29) and rapid eye movements (PPRF and MRF, Chapter 33). Nuclei of the reticular formation are most often studied from the perspective of their contributions to specific functional systems described in other chapters and through the actions of their monoamine neuromodulators noradrenalin (norepinephrine) and serotonin. Vestibular nuclei are studied for their contributions to postural reflexes.

The Vestibular Apparatus Senses Head Rotation and Tilt

The sensory inputs most important for postural responses are vision, proprioception, and vestibular sense. Vestibular sensory signals from the labyrinth of the inner ear provide direct information about rotations of the head and its orientation with respect to gravity. Two types of vestibular transducer organs—semicircular canals and otolithic maculae—are located within the labyrinth of the ear and respond to accelerations of the head in space. The three semicircular canals and the two otolithic maculae are stimulated by rotational and linear acceleration, respectively. The mechanical structure of the sense organ determines the nature of the effective stimulus (Wilson and Melvill-Jones, 1979).

The labyrinth (Fig. 30.2) is outlined by the bony labyrinth, a set of passages in the skull. The bony labyrinth is lined with membranes that contain endolymph (Chapter 24) and which make up the membranous labyrinth. The membranous labyrinth has a large central vessel called the utricle, another vessel called the saccule, and three narrow passages that emerge from the utricle and loop around to rejoin it. These three loops form circular passages for endolymph and are known as semicircular canals. The canals are oriented orthogonal to one another: there is a lateral or horizontal canal, an anterior or superior canal, and a posterior canal. The membranous passages of the vestibular labyrinth are joined with those of the auditory labyrinth by a thin tube, the ductus reuniens.

Each semicircular canal contains a sensory end organ ridge or crest, the crista, that rests in a swelling near one end of the canal, the ampulla. Hair cells extend cilia from the ampullary crest into a gelatinous

mass, the cupula, that occludes the canal passage. These hair cells are like other hair cell receptors, for example, in the auditory system. They have many stereocilia and one kinocilium; deflection of the hairs toward the kinocilium is excitatory. Pressure of the endolymph on the cupula acts to deflect the cilia and excite the hair cells, which make synaptic contact with the VIIIth nerve vestibular afferents. Rotational acceleration of the head can build pressure on one side of the cupula, resulting in vestibular transduction. The hair cell receptors in a given canal will be stimulated when the rotational acceleration is in a direction that builds pressure on one side of the cupula and inhibited by acceleration in the opposite direction, but will not be stimulated if the rotational acceleration pushes the fluid to the sides of the canal walls instead of along their length. Thus, the three canals have different effective directions for stimulation that depend on canal orientation in the labyrinth. In general, canals in the left inner ear are excited by leftward rotation and right ear canals by rightward rotation, with the anterior canal in each ear excited by accelerations with a forward component and posterior canals excited by backward rotations.

Given that a rotational acceleration has a component in the plane of a canal, endolymph will press on the cupula. There are, however, complicating mechanical factors. The canal passages are narrow, and the endolymph has a certain viscosity. In addition, the cupula is not a perfectly rigid pressure transducer and bends in response to the inertia of the endolymph. It is, of course, this bending that allows hair cell depolarization. These factors combine to "smooth out" the rotational acceleration signal, in effect performing a mechanical integration that converts the external acceleration stimulus into a hair cell stimulus that is now largely a rotational velocity signal. Thus, canal afferents fire action potentials at a rate approximately proportional to the velocity of head rotation.

There are two otolith organs in mammals, the utricle (utriculus) and saccule (sacculus). The names apply to the fluid chambers in which they lie, and the specific locations of the receptors are called the maculae. The two maculae are small regions that contain hair cell afferents innervated by vestibular afferents. Like canal hair cells, bending of the hairs toward the kinocilium is the excitatory stimulus for macular hair cells, and the cilia are imbedded in a gelatinous mass above the cell bodies. Unlike canal hair cells, the otolithic hair cell maculae rest in large chambers, in which fluid motion is thought to exert little or no dynamic force on the hairs. Instead, the gelatinous mass holding the cilia contains dense crystals, the otoconia or statoconia, and the entire mass above the hair cells of a macula is acted on by gravity or linear acceleration because of its higher density than the endolymph. When the head tilts, the otoconial mass sags in the direction of the tilt. This sagging, or the equivalent lagging of the mass behind a linear acceleration, provides the natural stimulus for otoliths.

The utricular macula lies on the floor of its cavity. Thus, when the body is not accelerated and the head is held approximately erect with respect to gravity, there is no stimulus to this organ, but tilts from the erect posture will excite utricular afferents. Microscopic examination of the utricular macula shows that the hair cells are not all oriented with their kinocilia in the same direction, and different directions of tilt excite different populations of utricular afferents. The direction of the hair cell indicated by its kinocilium is called its morphological polarization vector and corresponds to the best direction of tilt for exciting the receptor. The saccular macula is on the side of the saccule, approximately in a parasagittal plane, although the surface curves somewhat. Thus, there is a strong acceleration stimulus to the saccular macula when the head is erect and little or no stimulus when the head is lying on either side. Saccular hair cells also have a variety of morphological polarization vectors. The result of the many studies of primary vestibular afferents is that two types of vestibular signals are available to assist balance: rotational head velocity is signaled by the semicircular canals and head tilt or linear acceleration is signaled by the otoliths.

Vestibulocervical and Vestibulospinal Reflexes Stabilize Head and Body Posture

Vestibulocervical (neck or collic reflexes) and vestibulospinal reflexes make use of canal and otolith signals to stabilize the posture of the head and body. These reflexes are thought to serve two functions, both as stabilizing, or "negative feedback" systems (Schor et al., 1988). When the head and body rotate or tilt in any direction, the vestibular stimulus excites pathways that contract neck and limb muscles that oppose the motion so that the undesired movement is reduced or corrected. Also, the biomechanical components of the head have a characteristic resonant frequency of around 2 to 3 Hz at which oscillation is especially likely to occur, and the vestibulocervical reflex effectively dampens this tendency for oscillatory motion. The importance of vestibulocervical and vestibulospinal reflexes is demonstrated by damage to the labyrinth, section of the VIIIth nerve, or mechanical blockage of the semicircular canal passages. Unilateral labyrinthectomy causes an initial postural disability, with leaning or falling toward the side of the lesion.

Bilaterally symmetric semicircular canal plugging, which removes head velocity signals with little loss or imbalance in tonic vestibular nerve activity, produces head instability with oscillations that may persist for several days. Note that the vestibulocervical reflex, although discussed separately, is as much a vestibulospinal reflex as vestibular limb reflexes, the difference being primary action at the cervical versus lumbar spinal levels.

The neuroanatomical pathways that contribute to the vestibulocervical and other vestibulospinal reflex responses (Fig. 30.3) have been elucidated primarily

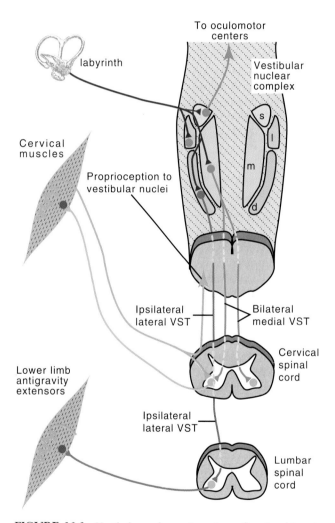

FIGURE 30.3 Vestibular and proprioceptive reflex signal inputs and major pathways from the brain stem vestibular nuclei. The medial vestibulospinal tract projects bilaterally to the cervical spinal cord to mediate the vestibulocollic reflex. The lateral vestibulospinal tract descends to lumbar levels of the spinal cord to influence limb extensors involved in balance. Neck muscle proprioceptors send signals to vestibular nuclei to participate in cervicocollic reflexes and interactions among reflexes. d, descending vestibular nucleus; l, lateral vestibular nucleus; m, medial vestibular nucleus; s, superior vestibular nucleus; VST, vestibulospinal tract.

through the use of electrical stimulation and other physiological methods. Of the four brain stem vestibular nuclei that receive the VIIIth nerve, the medial, lateral (Deiters' nucleus), and descending (inferior nucleus) contribute to the medial and lateral vestibulospinal tracts that provide direct vestibular influence on the spinal cord. The superior vestibular nucleus is primarily concerned with vestibulo-ocular reflexes (Chapter 33). Electrical activation of vestibular nucleus neuron axons from spinal cord stimulating electrodes and from stimulation of vestibular structures shows that vestibulocervical reflexes are mediated primarily by excitatory and inhibitory connections of the bilaterally projecting medial vestibulospinal tract and that ipsilateral excitation of limb extensors is carried via the lateral vestibulospinal tract. The bulk of the lateral vestibulospinal tract projects from the lateral vestibular nucleus as far as the lumbar spinal cord for vestibulospinal reflex control. Vestibular nuclei also project heavily to reticular nuclei, and only lesions that impinge on both vestibulospinal and reticulospinal pathways substantially reduce the strength of vestibular reflex responses.

Initial quantitative studies of the vestibulocervical reflex used sinusoidal stimuli and concentrated on the timing or response dynamics of the reflex head torques or the electromyographic activity that accompanied neck muscle contractions, just as response dynamics had been the focus in studies of vestibular primary afferents. The conclusion from these studies was that vestibulocervical reflex circuitry in the vestibular nuclei introduces central neural processing with two important features.

First, there is a phase-lagging element operative at low frequencies so that the velocity signal from the semicircular canals is converted to a head position signal, appropriate for repositioning the head in response to a slow change in head angle. Second, at high frequencies, vestibulocervical reflex circuitry appears to introduce a phase lead, which works in conjunction with the high-frequency phase lead of primary canal afferents to make two 90° phase leads so that the behavioral output of the reflex corresponds to opposing head angular acceleration, as would be appropriate if the inertia of the head were an important factor to be overcome for compensation during rapid head motion. Because the phase-lagging elements residing in the mechanics of the semicircular canals and in the brain stem are, in engineering terms, called "poles" and the two phase lead elements are called "zeroes," the complete model of the vestibulocervical reflex has been termed a two-pole, two-zero description. One pole and one zero are located in the periphery, due to the mechanics of the canals, and the

other pole and zero are generated by the central neural circuitry of the vestibulocervical reflex. The mechanisms by which neurons in the brain stem accomplish these functions are unknown.

Work of this kind established that the timing of vestibulocervical responses is reasonable given the function of the reflex and the mechanical properties of the load presented by the head. The mechanical properties of the multijoint system of the limbs and trunk are far more complex, and it is correspondingly more difficult to predict what the dynamics of the controlling neural signals should be. Electromyographic recordings during vestibulospinal reflexes in decerebrated animals have shown that limb extensors at low frequencies of oscillation are excited in phase with the position of the head. For example, when the head rolls slowly to the left, the left forelimb extends as if to brace against further displacement. The likely source of signals exciting these responses is the otolith organs. As the frequency of head oscillation approaches 1 Hz, the phase of vestibulospinal responses advances toward a peak in phase with head velocity. The value of this timing is debatable, but the implication is that semicircular canal signals begin to predominate over otolith signals in vestibulospinal responses at higher frequencies.

A major focus of work on both vestibulocervical and vestibulospinal reflexes is the spatial organization of the responses and the possible interaction of spatial properties and dynamics (Baker *et al.*, 1985). Early studies had concentrated on left-to-right yaw motion (as in nodding "no") for vestibulocervical reflex studies and on left ear down to right ear down rolling motion for vestibulospinal limb reflex studies. (To produce rolling motion, tilt the top of your head to the left and then right while looking straight ahead.) Of course, the vestibular reflexes work to compensate for motion in any direction. The problem of producing the correct direction of reflex response to any direction of disturbance has been considered thoroughly for the case of the vestibulo-ocular reflex that stabilizes the eyes (Chapter 33), but vestibulospinal reflexes present a more difficult situation.

In the case of the vestibulocervical reflex, there are any number of ways that the more than 30 muscles of the neck could be used to compensate for a particular direction of head rotation. What synergies or coordinations of muscle groups are used by the brain to generate compensatory vestibulocervical responses? The principles underlying the brain's pattern of coordinated activation of neck muscles to compensate for head rotation are unknown, although some features of spatial organization have been elucidated. Each of the major neck muscles exhibits a characteristic directionality of excitation in response to vestibular stimulation by rotation in many different directions, but that direction does not match the directional sensitivity of any single semicircular canal. Instead, the responses to rapid motions reflect a weighted sum of canal inputs, and various proposals attempt to account for the particular weightings observed. A complicating feature of vestibulocervical spatial organization is the dependence in some cases of the dynamics (more specifically, the phase) of vestibulo-cervical neuron or neck muscle activation upon the direction of the vestibular stimulus. This dependence has been termed spatial-temporal convergence and may reflect canal and otolith signal addition to match a varying mechanical load presented by the head for different directions of rotation. Another difficulty in the analysis of vestibulocervical responses is the presence of signals related to the velocity of eye movement or the direction in which the eyes are pointed ithin their orbits. Add to this the visual and proprioceptive signals present in vestibulospinal neural circuitry, discussed in the following sections, and the overall picture is one of a rich and complex control system that we are only beginning to understand. Comparable information on the spatial organization of vestibulospinal control of the limbs displays a similar complexity, paralleled by complex neuro-anatomical interconnections, which include ascending as well as descending axon collaterals.

The Cervicocervical Reflex Stabilizes the Head by Opposing Lengthening of Neck Muscles

The proprioceptive contribution to reflex stabilization of the head and body has been examined in many of the same ways as vestibular contributions (Peterson *et al.*, 1985). The sensory situation for proprioceptive signals is more complicated than for vestibular signals, as any of the muscles of the neck, trunk, or limbs could provide an input to influence any other muscle or synergistic group of muscles. Only the signals from neck proprioception that activate neck muscles, i.e., the neck stretch reflex or cervicocervical reflex, also called the cervicocollic reflex, are considered here. Like the stretch reflex for limb extensors, the cervicocervical reflex opposes lengthening of the muscles concerned and so is a negative feedback compensatory system. Other proprioceptive systems are often considered postural reactions rather than simple reflexes and are described in turn.

Frequency domain analysis of the cervicocervical reflex has been done by rotating the trunk of a decerebrated cat while holding its head fixed in space. This stimulates neck proprioceptors without any vestibular input. For trunk rotation frequencies below about 1 Hz, neck muscle electromyographic activity is in phase with the extent of neck stretch, which is termed a position response. At higher frequencies, responses increase rapidly in gain and advance in phase toward an acceleration response, thus the cervicocervical reflex has been described as having two phase lead terms or "zeros." It has been argued that this type of responsiveness directly reflects the properties of the muscle spindle afferents that provide the input, meaning that the brain stem does little processing of inputs from neck muscle proprioceptors. Spatial organization of the cervicocervical reflex appears to more directly parallel that of vestibulocervical responses than do the dynamics. Although attempts to elicit the cervicocervical reflex in alert animals have not been entirely successful, in decerebrate preparations the directionality of neck muscle responses to stretch matches that of vestibulocervical responses fairly well. Common directionality implies that signals for vestibular and stretch reflexes to neck muscles share some central circuitry. Not only does this directionality not match that of any single semicircular canal, it also does not appear to match the direction of pulling actions of the neck muscles under study. We are left to speculate on the principles of central organization of these reflexes. The central pathways mediating the cervicocervical reflex are more varied still, and less well mapped, than those for vestibulocervical reflex responses. There are homonymous monosynaptic stretch reflex connections, heteronymous connections to a muscle from other muscles, and longer pathways that may involve connections through medial, lateral, and descending vestibular nuclei as well as reticulo-spinal neurons.

The Brain Stem Controls Coordinated Postural Reactions

A variety of reflexes contribute to the maintenance of overall body posture. All benefit from the integrity of connections with the brain stem, and in some cases higher centers, but not all are characterized as readily by objective measures as the vestibulocervical, vestibulospinal, and cervicocervical reflexes already discussed. The tonic neck or cervicospinal reflexes are the best known of these, but the supporting reactions, placing reactions, righting reactions, hopping or stepping reactions, and others are useful parts of the neural control of posture.

The tonic neck reflex (or reflexes, as all four limbs are affected) adjusts the extension of the limbs in response to the angle of the head on the trunk. The pattern of responses was originally described by

Neck Stretch   +   Vestibular   =   Combined
reflexes alone   reflexes alone   reflexes

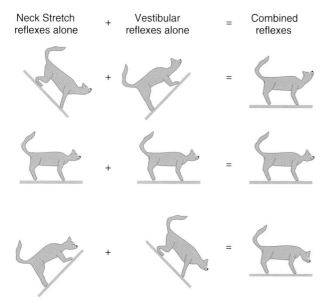

FIGURE 30.4 Operation of the tonic neck reflex in quadrupeds. The left column shows the operation of neck-to-limb proprioceptive reflexes (cervicospinal reflexes), the center column the static vestibulospinal reflexes, and the right column the antagonistic nature of their summed responses. A straight limb orthogonal to the trunk indicates a neutral posture, as in the middle row and right column of stick figures. A limb extended away from the center of the stick figure represents reflex extension (e.g., forelimb in upper left stick figure), and a reflexively flexed limb is shown in two segments (e.g., hindlimb in upper left stick figure). Based on work by Roberts.

Magnus and later refined by Roberts (1967). Newborns, humans with cerebral or vestibular damage, and decerebrate experimental animals most clearly display the tonic neck reflex, which interacts with the vestibulospinal reflex. This interaction is shown by a "Roberts diagram." Roberts tested the tonic neck reflex with roll rotations of the spine in decerebrate cats, keeping the posture of the head fixed in space to avoid vestibular stimulation. He showed that stretching the neck by rolling the spine to one side elicited flexion and extension of the forelimbs, as if the support surface had been tilted to produce the rotation. Figure 30.4 illustrates reflex responses to pitch rotation. When the spine is rotated without moving the head (left column of Fig. 30.4), a rotation that brings the head and forelimbs together causes a flexion of both forelimbs, a tonic neck reflex (lower left of Fig. 30.4). Tilting the whole body and head downward together causes a vestibulospinal reflex extension of the forelimbs (lower drawing in center column of Fig. 30.4). Normally, the tonic neck reflex is opposed by the vestibulospinal reflex, and tilting the head downward on a level body does not alter limb posture (right column in Fig. 30.4).

The placement of a limb on the ground initiates a set of reflex reactions that stiffen the limb into a supporting pillar. This response is called the "positive supporting reaction" and depends on the integrity of the brain stem. As discussed earlier, righting reactions also depend on the brain stem, and "optical righting reflexes" mediated by vision require an intact cerebral cortex. Stable posture requires that the feet be not only rigid but placed correctly on a supporting surface, and the placing reactions of quadrupeds contribute to this by moving the feet toward a visible surface (visual placing reaction) or onto a surface that has tactile contact with the top of the foot, chin, or whiskers (tactile placing reactions). Although a tactile placing reaction may be evoked in primitive form in a spinalized animal, it is generally held that at least the lower brain stem must be intact for tactile placing to occur in an effective form. Finally, if balance reactions are insufficient to maintain stable posture, as when the support surface is moved beneath the foot, the limb may hop to a new position where stable posture is possible (hopping reaction). The action of the righting reflex of cats during falling is familiar to all. Humans show a similar reaction to an unexpected drop, measurable as a short latency electromyographic response in the gastrocnemius muscle. In cats, this response survives blockage of the semicircular canals, but not total labyrinthectomy, and so appears to be otolith mediated. The action of these many postural reactions in the context of maintenance of posture and balance in intact humans has been the focus of several studies utilizing movable posture platforms.

Balance Depends on Context-Dependent Postural Strategies

How then do these descending pathways from the brain stem coordinate to produce the postural behaviors of intact animals? The basic problem of standing posture is keeping the center of mass of the body, also called center of gravity, positioned over the base of support provided by the feet so that the body does not topple. The ranges of body positions that rest over the base of support define the limits of stability. When the extremes of body sway extend beyond those limits, the body must reduce them, take a step, or fall. An important tool for exploring body stability is the posture platform, a base on which subjects can stand and be subjected to displacements of the underlying supporting surface. The posture platform is used with body position sensors and electromyography to evaluate standing posture (Nashner, 1982; Horak and Nashner, 1986; Horak and Shupert, 1994). Even on a perfectly stable support surface with vision, somesthesis, and vestibular sense all active, a standing person will sway slightly. This sway will increase as the context is altered by distorting or removing sensory input, showing the importance of the multiple avenues of balance information but also showing the adequacy of limited sensory input in maintaining upright posture. When the eyes are closed (the Romberg test used in clinical evaluation), sway is greater. When the visual surround is linked to the subject's head position in the condition called "sway referencing of vision," visual information is misleading and sway is increased. When the support surface is compliant, proprioceptive feedback is much less useful, and sway is greater. When the support surface tilts along with the body in the condition called "sway referencing of the support surface," proprioceptive information is misleading and sway is increased. When the preceding conditions are combined, sway is greater still but normal subjects can maintain upright posture through the use of vestibular information.

Sudden displacement of the platform on which a subject stands allows measurement of the latencies and patterns of electromyographic activity in the postural muscles of the legs. When the subject is standing on a large platform that is displaced forward or backward, the leg muscles contract in sequence from ankle to thigh to hip, and motion occurs primarily about the ankle joint. When the platform displacement is forward, the ankle flexor tibialis anterior on the front of the calf is first to be excited (flexion is the toe-up direction), at about 80–100 ms after the displacement. This is followed about 20 ms later by contraction of the quadriceps thigh muscles and then later still by contraction of trunk musculature. Backward displacement first elicits excitation of the gactrocnemius muscle at the back of the calf to extend the ankle, followed by excitation of thigh and trunk muscles antagonistic to those excited by forward displacement (Fig. 30.5). The overall postural reaction of distal-to-proximal excitation has been termed an "ankle strategy" for maintaining balance.

Although the ankle strategy was confirmed in all subjects tested with simple forward–backward displacement, the ankle strategy is not the only one available, and postural reactions have been shown to adapt to alterations in the support surface or sensory inputs. Displacement of a support surface that is short compared to the foot, or rotation of the support instead of displacement, demands a different postural response. A second strategy that can be adopted when ankle strategy is contraindicated is the hip strategy, in which the body is bent at the hips so that the lower half of the body moves in the same direction as it does during ankle strategy reactions while the upper body moves in the opposite direction. Thus, during a forward, front downward tilt of a supporting platform, the hips move backward and the head forward. This shifts the center of gravity, which has moved forward due to the displacement, backward so that it is placed over the support again. Other work has questioned the prevalence of ankle strategy and documented a stiffening strategy of muscle cocontraction in response to base rotation and a multilink strategy that includes ankle, hip, and neck joint motions in response to translation. Stiffening, ankle, and hip or multilink strategies are applicable to the sway that occurs during normal standing on commonly encountered kinds of surfaces and may represent basic units of postural reaction.

Like simple reflexes, these postural reactions represent neuronally mediated negative feedback responses. However, postural reactions differ from ordinary reflex responses in the degree of their dependence on context and recent experience. It also appears that the postural strategies are not mutually exclusive, but are more like additive units or building blocks. When Horak and Nashner placed subjects on

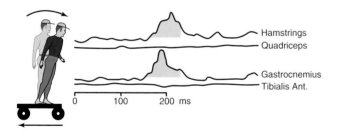

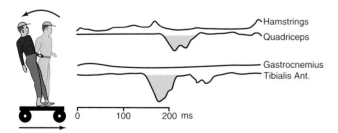

FIGURE 30.5 Sequencing of muscle activation in response to displacement of a supporting platform. When the supporting surface is displaced backward (at 0 ms), flexor muscles are excited first in the distal lower limb segments (gastrocnemius, about 80 ms latency) and then in the proximal segment (hamstrings, about 100 ms latency). Forward displacement of the platform activates lower limb extensors, again in a distal (tibialis anterior) to proximal (quadriceps) sequence. Black arrows mark the first detected electromyographic response to displacement. Based on studies by Horak and Nashner.

support surfaces intermediate in length between the long surfaces associated with ankle strategy and the short surfaces associated with hip strategy, they found that subjects adopted complex strategies that they believed represented combinations of ankle and hip strategies with different magnitudes and temporal relations. In addition, they found that during the first few trials after switching from one length of support surface to another, the subjects' responses in part reflected the previous surface, only gradually shifting from one strategy to another over several trials.

Postural responses are also elicited under feedforward control in anticipation of upcoming disturbances and in coordination with the overall motor program to be executed. This is demonstrated by asking standing subjects to grip a handle that they are asked to pull (or occasionally push), or that may pull their arm. The subjects are standing on a platform that may be displaced to elicit postural reactions. When a tone signal is used to cue the subject to pull a rigid handle, the first recorded electromyographic activity is in the postural muscles of the legs, not in the biceps arm muscle used to flex the elbow. The same order of muscle activation accompanies untriggered self-initiated handle pulls, making it unlikely that the tone somehow triggered a postural response. Rather, the postural adjustment was in anticipation of the loss of balance that would occur if the pull was unopposed by a shift in stance. Even when the handle was pulled away from the subject while in the subject's grasp, the earliest strong response was not a biceps stretch reflex, but a 60- to 70-ms latency postural response of the gastrocnemius muscle. These findings support a view of postural responses as one component of coordinated movement, often the initial component, as a stable platform is needed as a base for voluntary movements.

The range of postural reactions recorded from standing human subjects argues for a complexity beyond that observed in the vestibulocervical or vestibulospinal reflexes studied during rotation or tilting of animal subjects, but it is not yet clear whether this complexity reflects the rich variety of strategies that can achieve the single goal of balance or whether there are strong constraints on postural responses that arise from the complicated biomechanics of the multijoint system of the body. Balance is subject not only to the static requirement for location of the center of mass over the support provided by the feet, but also to dynamic factors that accompany the rapid movement of massive body parts. Inertia, viscosity, and elasticity act at each of the major joints, and the task of measuring or modeling these factors and their interactions has barely begun.

Experimental animals can also be placed on posture platforms, which in the case of quadrupeds can consist of four small pads for the limbs (Macpherson and Ingliss, 1993). Among other findings, these experiments confirm the disability of animals with spinal transection in maintaining erect posture. A surprising finding from these animal studies is that even though vestibular information from head motion accompanying body displacement is vigorous and early enough to guide reflex responses, cats are able to maintain apparently good quadrupedal standing posture and responses to unexpected motion after total labyrinthectomy. Clearly, we have a great deal to learn about the management by the brain of the many systems that contribute to posture and balance: (see Box 30.2).

BOX 30.2

VESTIBULAR PLASTICITY

The experience of sailors getting their "sea legs" suggests that, in addition to the role of context and choice of strategies we have discussed, postural reflexes and balance are adapted gradually over time for better performance in new circumstances. Clear evidence for this general phenomenon comes from the study of postural control in astronauts. After a space flight, astronauts initially rely more heavily than before on visual cues for postural orientation, and they show degraded performance in their responses to disturbances generated by a posture platform. Sway during standing is increased dramatically when visual cues are removed, and the body segments move in a less coordinated manner than before space flight. Still, the performance of astronauts after the experience of space flight is quite remarkable; they are able to balance adequately within hours of landing and regain their preflight postural performance within a few days.

Marc H. Schieber and James F. Baker

Vestibular Damage Results in Disorders of Postural Control

Control of posture involves many levels within the nervous system, and it is not surprising that disorders of posture can result from damage to the sensory periphery or to telencephalic, cerebellar, brain stem, or spinal centers. The striking motor consequences of lesions of the basal ganglia may include profound effects on posture, such as the rigidity and general poverty of movement associated with Parkinson's disease (Chapter 31), but these usually are considered in the context of the movement disorders that characterize and provide clues to the localization of basal ganglia damage. Damage to the anterior vermis of the cerebellum can exaggerate decerebrate rigidity, and cerebellar patients show poorer performance in posture platform situations, with less adaptive modification of responses, as might be expected from our knowledge of cerebellar function (Chapter 32).

Many of the more plainly visible postural disorders stem from damage to the vestibular system. Diseases of the vestibular system that affect posture (and generally also cause dizziness) include vestibular neuritis, peripheral or central tumors or infarction, and Meniere's syndrome (Baloh and Honrubia, 1990) (see Box 30.3). Bilateral involvement and acute, episodic, or chronic time courses can occur in many vestibular disorders. The most obvious form of vestibular system damage is unilateral labyrinthectomy, performed

---

BOX 30.3

MENIERE SYNDROME

The typical patient with Meniere syndrome develops a sensation of fullness and pressure along with decreased hearing and tinnitus in one ear. Vertigo follows rapidly, reaching a maximum intensity within minutes and then slowly subsiding over several hours. Often the patient is left with a sense of unsteadiness and nonspecific dizziness that can go on for days after the acute vertiginous spell. In the early stages, hearing loss is completely reversible, but as the disease progresses, residual hearing loss becomes a prominent feature. The tinnitus is typically described as a roaring sound similar to the sound of the ocean. These episodes occur at irregular intervals over years, with periods of remission unpredictably intermixed. Eventually, most patients reach the so-called "burnt out phase," where the episodic vertigo disappears and severe permanent hearing loss remains.

The clinical syndrome was first described by Prosper Meniere in 1861, but Hallpike and Cairns made the initial clinical–pathological correlation with hydrops of the labyrinth in 1938. Patients with Meniere syndrome invariably show an increase in volume of endolymph associated with distention of the entire endolymphatic system. Herniations and ruptures in the membranous labyrinth commonly occur, which may explain the episodes of hearing loss and vertigo.

Delayed endolymphatic hydrops occurs in an ear that has been damaged years before, usually by infection. With this disorder, the patient reports a long history of hearing loss, typically since childhood, followed many years later by episodic vertigo but without the typical auditory symptoms. The pathologic findings are remark-

ably similar to idiopathic Meniere syndrome, suggesting a common etiology. A subclinical viral infection could damage the resorptive mechanism of the inner ear, leading to an eventual decompensation in the balance between secretion and resorption of endolymph.

The key to the diagnosis of Meniere syndrome is to document fluctuating hearing levels in a patient with the characteristic clinical history. In the early stages, the sensorineural hearing loss is usually greater in the low frequencies. Some patients with Meniere syndrome develop abrupt episodes of falling to the ground without loss of consciousness or associated neurologic symptoms. These episodes have been called "otolithic catastrophes" because they are thought to result from a sudden mechanical deformation of the otolith receptor organ. Patients often report feeling as though they were pushed to the ground by some external force.

Because the cause of Meniere syndrome is usually unknown, treatment is empiric. Medical management consists of symptomatic treatment with antivertiginous drugs and long-term prophylaxis with salt restriction and diuretics. Many different surgical procedures have been tried but none has been consistently effective. Shunt operations to decrease the endolymph pressure have not been successful because the implanted drain devices are encapsulated rapidly by fibrous tissue. Destructive surgeries (removing the labyrinth or cutting the vestibular nerve), can stop the episodes of vertigo but do not change the tinnitus and progressive hearing loss.

Robert W. Baloh

either experimentally in animals or as the result of disease or surgical intervention against disease in humans. The postural symptoms immediately following loss of vestibular input to one side of the brain vary across species, with nonmammalian and "lower" mammalian species typically showing a more prominent tilting of the head and body toward the side of damage. Vestibular afferents have a high level of resting activity, and leaning toward the side of lost vestibular signals makes sense in that the spontaneous or resting activity of the remaining vestibular apparatus is signaling, in effect, motion toward the intact side because it is not balanced by equal resting activity from the lesioned side. To counter this neural stimulus, the affected individual tilts away from the directions of apparent motion. This static postural effect of unilateral labyrinthectomy is accompanied by dynamic postural deficits, seen in experimental animals as weakened ipsilateral limb extensor responses and delayed responses to sudden drops. Compensation for unilateral labyrinthectomy occurs over a period of a few weeks, during which there is considerable recovery.

Translating or tilting platforms provide a means for quantitative assessment of vestibular damage from unilateral labyrinthectomy or other sources, including those that result in total vestibular loss. Patients with long-standing bilateral loss may perform well on posture platforms when visual and somatosensory cues are present, but fail completely to maintain upright stance when the support surface and visual surround both sway with the patient so that only vestibular information is accurate. Patients with recent bilateral vestibular loss or who have not yet compensated for vestibular loss also do poorly when vision and support surface are unreliable, but these patients perform poorly if only one sense, be it vision or somatic sense, is made an unreliable indicator of balance.

Summary

Axons from vestibular and reticular nuclei in the brain stem descend in pathways located ventromedially in the spinal cord to provide postural tone and balance. Balance is maintained by negative feedback reflexes that are stimulated by the vestibular canals and otoliths. The vestibulocervical reflex excites neck muscles via the medial vestibulospinal tract to oppose head tilt, and vestibulospinal reflexes carried by the lateral vestibulospinal tract excite ipsilateral limb extensors to oppose body tilt. Vestibular, muscle stretch, and other reflexes work together to coordinate posture and balance, and the medial system adopts different strategies for balance control depending on

the body support surface and information from sensory inputs. The medial postural system can adapt to different postural situations, but its actions can be compromised by central neural damage or unbalanced by peripheral vestibular loss. The reflexive control of body stability and posture by the medial descending system allows the lateral descending system to specialize in execution of precise voluntary movements of the extremities.

THE LATERAL VOLUNTARY SYSTEM

While the medial system thus provides underlying postural control for stance, ambulation, and orientation of the head, the lateral system superimposes the ability to make more sophisticated, voluntary movements in response to complex features of the external environment (perceived through the senses) and internal state (stored memories, knowledge, and emotion). Much of this control is mediated by specialized regions of the cerebral cortex. Outflow from this motor cortex dominates the lateral descending system, particularly in primates and humans.

Components of the Lateral Voluntary System

The Corticospinal Projection is the Most Direct Pathway from the Cerebral Cortex to Spinal Motor Neurons

For more than a century, electrical stimulation of a limited portion of the frontal lobe of the cerebral cortex has been known to evoke movements. Electrical stimulation of this "excitable cortex" evokes movements readily because this region has relatively direct connections to spinal motor neurons. In primates with a central sulcus (Rolandic fissure) in the neocortex, cortical neurons with axons projecting to the spinal cord are found most densely in the anterior bank of the central sulcus. The density of such neurons decreases from there rostrally to the precentral sulcus (posterior bank of the arcuate sulcus in macaque monkeys) and medially to the cingulate sulcus (Fig. 30.6). This territory corresponds to cytoarchitectonic areas 4 and 6 of Brodmann. Additional corticospinal neurons in areas 1, 2, 3, 5, and 7 of the parietal lobe project to the dorsal horn of the spinal cord to regulate sensory inflow.

The axons of neurons that project from the cerebral cortex to the spinal cord constitute the corticospinal tract. Corticospinal neurons have large pyramid-shaped somata in cortical layer Vb. Their axons leave the cortex, pass through the centrum semiovale, and enter the internal capsule, along with many other

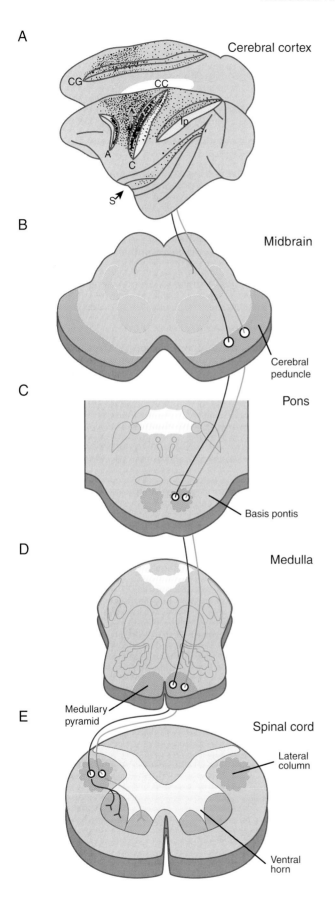

A
Cerebral cortex

CG
CC

Ip

A
C

S

B
Midbrain

Cerebral
peduncle

C
Pons

Basis pontis

D
Medulla

Medullary
pyramid

E
Spinal cord

Lateral
column

Ventral
horn

axons from other cortical areas. The corticospinal axons are concentrated most heavily in the middle third of the posterior limb of the internal capsule. As axons descend from the internal capsule below the thalamus, they come to lie on the ventral surface of the brain stem. Here, they form the cerebral peduncle of the midbrain, where the corticospinal axons are concentrated in the middle third. The axons of the peduncle become intermixed with pontine nuclear neurons in the base of the pons (basis pontis). Most of these axons synapse on pontine neurons and end here, providing input from the cerebral cortex to the cerebellum. The continuing corticospinal axons collect to form the medullary pyramid (Box 30.4). As the medulla blends into the spinal cord, the vast majority of corticospinal axons cross the midline and enter the lateral column of white matter on the opposite side of the spinal cord. Because of this decussation of the pyramidal tract, the left motor cortex controls movements on the right side of the body and vice versa. A small minority of corticospinal axons remain uncrossed and continue caudally as the ventral (or anterior) corticospinal tract near the ventral midline of the spinal cord.

As descending corticospinal axons reach their target levels in the spinal cord, they enter the spinal gray matter, where they ramify and synapse. Whereas the majority of corticospinal axons synapse on premotor interneurons in the intermediate zone (Rexed's laminae VII and VIII), a minority of these axons synapse directly on motor neurons in Rexed's lamina IX. The somata of most corticospinal neurons that make such monosynaptic connections to motor neurons lie posteriorly in area 4, and their monosynaptic connections are made on the motor neurons of distal limb muscles, whose somata are clustered in the dorsolateral ventral horn. Corticospinal axons from neurons located more anteriorly typically synapse in the ventromedial portion of the ventral horn, where the motor neurons of proximal

FIGURE 30.6 The corticospinal projection in the macaque monkey. (A) The density of corticospinal neuronal somata is shown by stippling in this lateral view of the left cerebral hemisphere; the superior medial surface of the hemisphere is also shown (above) as if reflected in a mirror. The central sulcus (C), arcuate sulcus (A), cingulate sulcus (Cg), intraparietal sulcus (Ip), and Sylvian fissure (S) are drawn as if pulled open to reveal the neurons in their banks. Two schematic corticospinal neurons, one relatively posterior and the other relatively anterior in area 4, send their axons down through the midbrain (B), pons (C), medulla (D), and spinal cord (E), which are drawn in cross section. In the spinal cord, the former corticospinal axon leaves the lateral column to terminate in the dorsolateral ventral horn, whereas the latter axon terminates in the ventromedial ventral horn.

limb muscles and axial muscles are located. Some corticospinal axons cross the midline spinal gray matter to reach the ventromedial ventral horn ipsilateral to their origin; such doubly decussating corticospinal axons, along with the uncrossed ventral corticospinal tract, may be partly responsible for the relative preservation of trunk and proximal limb movements after unilateral damage to the cortex.

Indirect Pathways to the Spinal Cord Involve Centers in the Brain Stem

The corticospinal tract is not the only output pathway through which the cerebral cortex contributes to motor control (Kuypers, 1987). The presence of other, indirect pathways in the macaque has been demonstrated by cutting the medullary pyramid on one side. Stimulation of the cortex on that side still evoked contralateral movements. The somatotopic organization of the cortex in the operated animals was similar to that in normal macaques, although the thresholds for stimulation were raised and distal movements were evoked less often.

Intermixed with corticospinal neurons in layer V of areas 4 and 6 are corticorubral neurons, whose axons project to the red nucleus (RN). Some corticospinal axons also send collaterals to the RN. In addition to cortical inputs, the RN also receives considerable input from the cerebellum (Chapter 32). Many RN neurons, particularly those in the caudal, magnocellular portion, in turn send their axons across the midline and into the lateral column of the spinal cord, terminating most heavily in the dorsolateral region of the ventral horn. These descending axons from the RN constitute the rubrospinal tract. An indirect pathway thus exists from the cortex to the RN to the spinal cord. Although the rubrospinal tract is less prominent in humans than in nonhuman primates and carnivores, the activity of rubrospinal neurons indicates that they also play a significant role during voluntary movements of the arm, hand, and fingers. The rubrospinal pathway thus works synergistically with the corticospinal pathway in controlling limb movements

A second indirect pathway involves neurons scattered in the medial reticular formation of the pons and medulla. The medial reticular formation receives input from cortical motor areas and projects via the ventral column of the spinal cord to the ventral horn, chiefly its ventromedial portion. The axons that make this projection constitute the reticulospinal tract. Although the reticulospinal tract is also part of the medial descending system, cortical inputs to the reticulospinal system may help integrate fine distal and coarse proximal movements.

Organization of the Motor Cortex

The original "motor cortex" is now appreciated to be comprised of several cortical areas. These areas are considered "motor" because (1) they project to other motor structures, (2) their ablation causes deficits in movement, and (3) their stimulation evokes or alters movements.

The Motor Cortex is Subdivided into Multiple Cortical Motor Areas

In addition to its descending projections to spinal motor neurons, the motor cortex has cytoarchitectonic features that distinguish it from other regions of the cerebral cortex. The somata of many pyramidal neurons in layer V, the output layer, are exceptionally large (Betz cells). In addition, the neurons of layer IV, the granular layer that receives thalamic input, are very sparse compared to other areas of the neocortex, and hence the motor cortex has been described as dysgranular (area 6) or agranular (area 4) cortex. Based on cytoarchitectonics, myeloarchitectonics, and histochemical features, the motor cortex of macaque monkeys can be subdivided into the cortical motor areas shown in Fig. 30.7. In general, these subdivisions show three mediolaterally oriented strips of cortex, with the primary motor cortex (M1) most posterior and two premotor strips progressively more anterior. Each of these premotor strips has a subdivision on the medial wall of the hemisphere, a second subdivision on the dorsal convexity, and a third on the ventral convexity. In addition to these subdivisions of Brodmann's areas 4 and 6, areas 23 and 24 in the banks of the cingulate sulcus and on the medial surface of the hemisphere in the cingulate gyrus are now known to contain at least two additional cortical motor areas. Cortical motor areas differ, not only in their intrinsic composition, but also in their interconnections with other parts of the central nervous system.

Cortical motor areas differ in their connections with the thalamus. M1, PMv, and SMA, for example, connect primarily with VPLo/VLc, area X, and VLo in the thalamus, respectively. These differences are significant because thalamic nuclei VPLo/VLc and area X receive major inputs from the cerebellum, whereas VLo receives major input from the basal ganglia. Thus, information processed by the cerebellum is directed largely to M1 and PMv, whereas information from the basal ganglia is sent largely to SMA.

Cortical motor areas also differ in their connections with one another and with other regions of the cortex (Fig. 30.7). For example, when horseradish peroxidase (HRP) is injected into the hand region of M1, separate pockets of retrogradely labeled neuronal somata are found in PMv, PMd, SMA, CGc, and CGr, indicating that each of these areas sends a separate projection to the hand region of M1. In contrast, PMvr, PMdr, and pre-SMA do not project directly to M1. Instead, PMvr projects to PMvc, PMdr projects to PMdc, and pre-SMA projects to PMvr.

Different cortical motor areas also receive input from different cortical sensory and association areas: M1 receives input from the primary somatosensory area (S1), PMv receives input from visual association area 7b, and PMd receives input from somatosensory association area 5. Because of these inputs, many

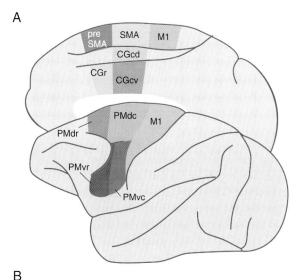

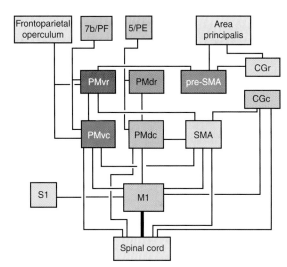

FIGURE 30.7 Cortical motor areas. (A) Diagram of a macaque brain showing current parcellation of cortical motor areas in the frontal lobe. Modified from Matelli *et al.* (1991). (B) Connections of the cortical motor areas. Most corticocortical connections are reciprocal. CGc,-cingulate motor area, caudal; CGr,-cingulate motor area, rostral; M1, primary motor cortex; PMdc, premotor cortex, dorsal caudal; PMdr, premotor cortex, dorsal, rostral; PMvc, premotor cortex, ventral, caudal; PMvr, premotor cortex, ventral, rostral; Pre-SMA, presupplementary motor area; SMA supplementary motor area proper. Thin lines to the spinal cord from PMvc, PMdc, SMA, and CGc indicate that corticospinal projections from these areas are not as strong as that from M1.

motor cortex neurons have somatosensory receptive fields. Neurons located caudally in M1 tend to respond to cutaneous modalities, whereas neurons located rostrally in M1 tend to respond to deep modalities. The somatosensory input of an M1 neuron is generally related to the output function of that neuron. For example, caudally located M1 neurons that control fingers may have cutaneous receptive fields on the fingers (Fig. 30.8A), whereas more rostrally located M1 neurons that control the biceps or triceps may have deep receptive fields in those muscles.

Somatosensory inputs to M1 also help mediate long loop responses, i.e., muscular responses that occur too slowly to be mediated by the monosynaptic stretch reflex (Chapter 29) but too quickly to be considered voluntary reactions. For example, when a subject holds a handle that suddenly jerks away, extending the elbow and stretching the biceps, three distinguishable waves of contraction may be recorded in the biceps. The first wave is the monosynaptic reflex produced by stretching the muscle; the third wave is the subject voluntarily pulling back on the handle. The middle wave occurs at a latency consistent with the conduction of impulses from muscle afferents to the cortex and then almost directly back from M1 to spinal motor neurons. Many biceps-related M1 neurons discharge a burst of impulses at a time appropriate to contribute to this long loop response. Interestingly, the strength of the long loop response may be increased if the subject plans to pull on the handle by contracting the biceps and decreased if the subject plans to push on the handle by relaxing the biceps; parallel changes may occur in the bursts of the M1 neurons. Thus, long loop responses are affected by the motor plans of the subject.

PMv receives both somatosensory and visual input via area 7b. Both the somatosensory and the visual receptive fields of PMv neurons tend to be large, and when single PMv neurons receive both types of sensory information, the fields tend to be related (Fig. 30.8B). A neuron with a somatosensory receptive field covering the forearm, for instance, may respond to visual stimuli moving near the forearm. Interestingly, if the forearm is moved to a different position, the visual receptive field of the PMv neuron moves with the forearm.

Somatotopic Organization in the Motor Cortex Is Not a One-to-One Map of Body Parts, Muscles, or Movements

The organization of the primary motor cortex, M1, has been studied more extensively than that of other

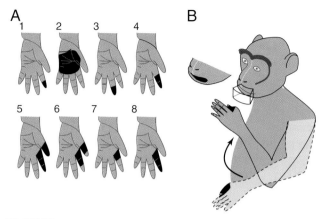

FIGURE 30.8   Sensory receptive fields in M1 and PMv. (A) Black regions show the tactile receptive fields of eight M1 neurons recorded at loci where intracortical microstimulation evoked flexion of the monkey's index and middle fingers. Other neurons at the same loci responded to passive extension of those fingers. From Rosen and Asanuma (1972) (B) A single PMv neuron responded to visual stimuli moving near the mouth, to tactile stimulation of the lips and of the skin between the thumb and the index finger, and to flexion of the elbow. From Rizzolatti *et al.* (1981).

cortical motor areas. Within the M1 of primates, the face is represented laterally, the lower extremity (or hindlimb and tail) medially, and the upper extremity (or forelimb) in between (Fig. 30.9). This overall organization of M1 according to major body parts is termed somatotopic. The somatotopic organization of M1 becomes evident in clinical neurology. Lesions on the lateral convexity of human M1 cause weakness or paralysis of the contralateral face, more medial lesions on the convexity affect the contralateral hand and arm, and lesions on the medial wall of the hemisphere affect the leg and foot.

Moreover, distal parts of the extremities and acral parts of the face (lips and tongue) are most heavily represented caudally, whereas proximal parts of the extremities and axial movements are most heavily represented rostrally. Those parts of the body that are used for fine manipulative movements (such as lips, tongue, and fingers in primates) are generally represented over a wider cortical territory than body parts used in gross movements such as ambulation.

FIGURE 30.9   Somatotopic maps in M1. (A) Map by Woolsey and co-workers (1952) in which each figurine represents in black and gray the body parts that moved a lot or a little, respectively, when the cortical surface at that site was stimulated. In addition to the primary representation on the convexity, their map shows a secondary representation on the medial surface of the hemisphere, called the supplementary motor area (SMA). As defined in this study, M1 and SMA each included several of the currently defined cortical motor areas. (B) Intracortical microstimulation of M1 in an owl monkey produced this map, consisting of a complex mosaic of different body parts. In this species, the central sulcus is only a shallow dimple, and M1 is entirely on the surface of the hemisphere. Each dot represents a stimulated locus, and lines surround adjacent loci from which movement of the same body part was evoked. Note that the forepaw digits (purple) and the hindpaw digits (green) are represented in multiple areas separated by areas representing nearby body parts. Modified from Gould *et al.* (1986). In both A and B, the inset at the top indicates the region of the frontal lobe enlarged below.

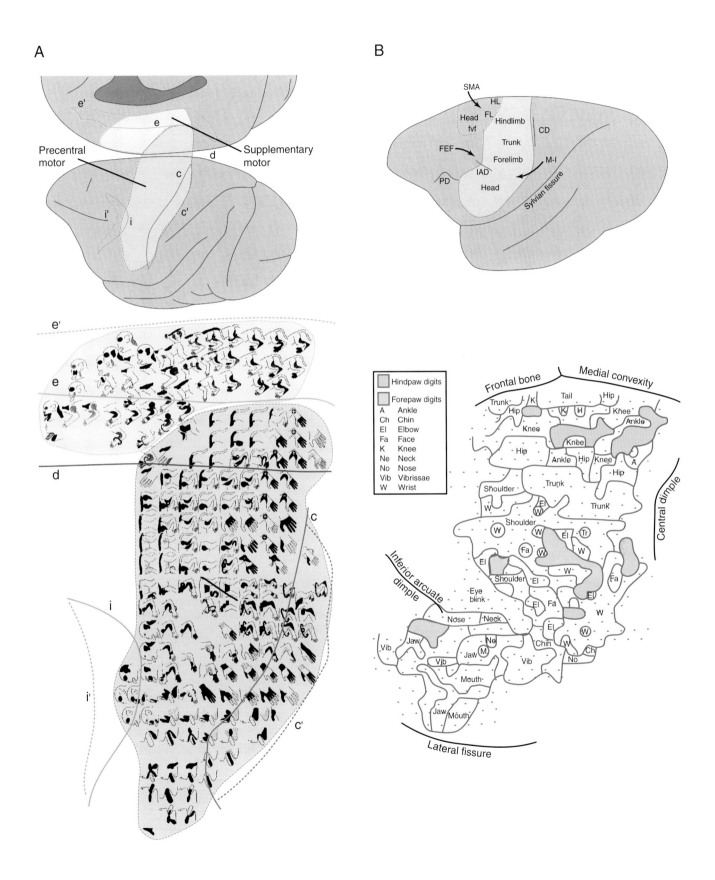

Penfield, in his cartoon of the motor homunculus (little man), and Woolsey, in his cartoon of the motor simiusculus (little monkey), conveyed this apparent magnification of certain body parts with respect to cortical territory by distorting the size of body parts relative to their normal proportions.

The somatotopic organization of M1 is not, however, a one-to-one mapping of body parts, muscles, or movements. Within the arm representation, for example, the cortical territory representing any particular part of the arm overlaps considerably with the territory representing nearby parts. This overlap results from three features of M1's organization: convergence, divergence, and horizontal interconnection.

M1 outputs arising from a wide cortical territory converge on the spinal motor neuron pool of single muscles. Convergence of M1 outputs has been shown by delivering intracortical microstimulation while observing the body for evoked movements and/or recording electromyographic (EMG) activity from multiple muscles. Maps of which body parts move or which muscles contract upon threshold stimulation at different cortical sites look like a complex mosaic (Fig. 30.10A). As the stimulation current is increased, the mosaic pieces representing a given muscle coalesce into a larger and larger territory that overlaps more and more with the territories of other muscles. These findings indicate that any given muscle is controlled by a large territory in M1 and that the territories for different muscles overlap (Fig. 30.10B).

A second factor contributing to the overlap of territories in M1 is the divergence of output from single cortical neurons to multiple motor neuron pools. Intracellular staining has shown that a single corticospinal axon may have terminal ramifications within the motor neuron pools of multiple muscles over several segmental levels of the spinal cord (Fig. 30.11A). Moreover, spike-triggered averaging of EMG activity has demonstrated that single M1 neurons can have relatively direct effects on the motoneuron pools of multiple muscles (Fig. 30.11B). These findings indicate that single M1 neurons have output connections to the spinal motoneuron pools of multiple muscles (Fig. 30.11C).

A third factor contributing to overlapping representation is the horizontal interconnectivity intrinsic to M1. Although most horizontal axon collaterals of neurons in layer V extend only 1–2 mm, some extend across the upper extremity representation, interconnecting even the territories of proximal and distal muscles

Because of convergence, divergence, and horizontal interconnections, neuronal activity is widely distributed in M1 during natural movements, even

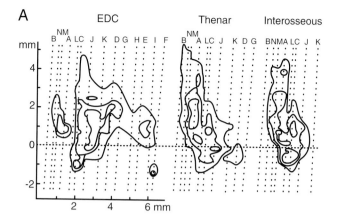
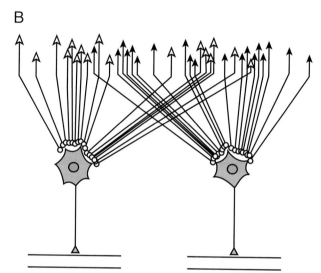

FIGURE 30.10 Convergence of M1 outputs to single muscles. (A) Isothreshold contours show the points at which EMG responses were evoked in three different muscles—extensor digitorum communis (EDC), thenar, and first dorsal interosseus—by intracortical microstimulation in the anterior bank of the central sulcus. (B) Data shown in A indicate that the cortical input to the motor neurons of any muscle originates from a wide territory in M1 and that the cortical territory providing input to a given muscle overlaps extensively with the cortical territory providing input to other muscles in the same part of the body. Modified from Andersen et al. (1975).

discrete movements of single body parts. In monkeys trained to perform individuated movements of each finger, single M1 neurons are active during movements of multiple fingers, and neurons throughout the M1 hand area are active during movements of any given finger. Likewise, in humans performing movements of different fingers, activity is distributed over the entire M1 hand representation whether the subject is moving a single finger or the whole hand. Although the entire hand representation may be activated for movement of any given finger, monkey and human studies have shown a tendency for the center of activation during movements of the thumb to be located

A

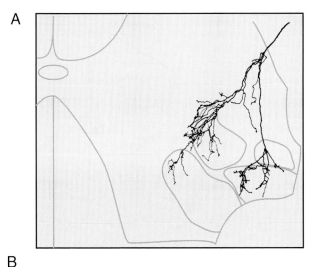

B

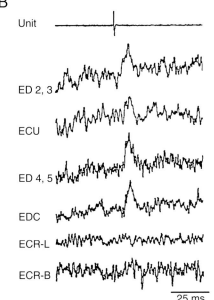

C

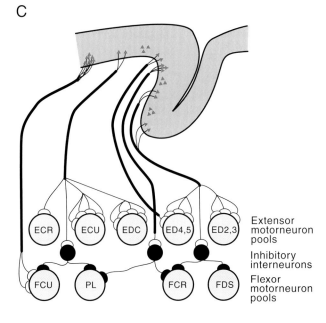

Extensor
motorneuron
pools

Inhibitory
interneurons

Flexor
motorneuron
pools

laterally to that for movements of other fingers, consistent with the somatotopic orientation of the hand in the classic simiusculus and homunculus.

The somatotopic representation in M1, like that in the primary somatosensory cortex, has a certain degree of plasticity. The cortical territory representing a given muscle can enlarge when nearby body parts are denervated experimentally. Threshold stimulation in the cortical territory that had represented a denervated body part then comes to evoke movements in nearby body parts. Enlargement of a given muscle's cortical territory occurs as well when that muscle is stretched passively or used intensely for a prolonged period. Furthermore, in normal humans who are actively practicing a complex sequence of finger movements, the cortical territory representing a given finger muscle enlarges as the subjects become skilled at performing the sequence. Because such changes can occur within several minutes, they probably are mediated by long-term potentiation and/or depression at existing synapses. This ability of the M1 cortex to reorganize may in part underlie motor recovery seen in humans after damage to M1 or the corticospinal tract.

Control of Voluntary Movements by the Motor Cortex

Several methods have enabled investigators to explore how cortical motor areas contribute to the production and control of voluntary movement in awake, behaving subjects. Whereas microelectrodes record the action potentials of single neurons, measurements made by functional imaging or by recording surface potentials reflect the net activity of thousands of cortical neurons and millions of synapses.

Multiple Cortical Areas Are Active When the Brain Generates a Voluntary Movement

These different methodologies now make it clear that many cortical areas in addition to the primary

FIGURE 30.11 Divergence of M1 outputs to multiple muscles. (A) Tracing of a single corticospinal axon ramifying in the ventral horn of the spinal cord shows terminal fields in the motor neuron pools of four forearm muscles. From Shinoda *et al.* (1981). (B) Action potentials in a cortical neuron (top trace) are followed at a fixed latency by peaks of postspike facilitation in EMGs recorded from four of six recorded forearm muscles (lower traces), consistent with monosynaptic excitation of all four motor neuron pools by that cortical neuron. The EMGs are rectified and averaged responses to 7051 action potentials in the cortical neuron. From Fetz and Cheney (1980). (C) These anatomic and physiologic findings indicate that the output of single corticospinal neurons often diverges to influence multiple muscles. From Cheney *et al.* (1985).

motor cortex are active during the planning and execution of voluntary movements. During performance of either a simple keypress or a complex movement sequence, for example, functional imaging studies in humans have shown bilateral activation of the primary sensorimotor hand representation, the supplementary motor area, and the ventrolateral premotor cortex, plus contralateral activation of the dorsolateral premotor cortex and the medial cortex rostral to the SMA. Whereas such techniques provide information on the parts of the cortex that are active in a given situation, studies of electrical potentials provide information on the time course of activation. For simple self-paced movements, cortical electrical potentials over the SMA and M1 begin to change as early as 1 s prior to the movement. As the time of movement onset approaches, the amplitude of these bilateral electrical potential shifts increases (the Bereitschaft potential). At the time of the movement, a further increase in amplitude occurs over the somatotopically appropriate region of M1 contralateral to the moving body part. Given that many cortical areas are active in controlling movement raises the question: What does each area contribute to control?

M1 Neurons Control Movement Kinematics and Dynamics

In one of the earliest studies of single neuron activity in awake behaving animals, Evarts recorded the activity of M1 pyramidal tract neurons in monkeys trained to raise and lower weights using flexion and extension wrist movements (Fig. 30.12). The discharge frequency of many M1 neurons changed systematically in temporal relation to either flexion or extension. A typical flexion-related neuron, for example, began to discharge several hundred milliseconds before flexion began. As the onset of a flexion movement approached, the discharge frequency of the neuron increased, accelerating still more as the flexion movement was made. The neuron was silent during extension. The time course of these movement-related changes in single neuron activity parallels the time course of cortical electrical potential shifts.

Evarts went on to demonstrate that the discharge frequency of M1 pyramidal tract neurons (PTNs) varied in relation to a number of mechanical parameters of the movement the monkey was making. By changing the weights the monkey had to lift, Evarts showed that PTN discharge frequency varied with the force the monkey exerted. Comparison of PTN discharge with simultaneous force recordings revealed that bursts of PTN firing were correlated with sudden increases in the exerted force, indicating a relationship between firing frequency and the rate of change of

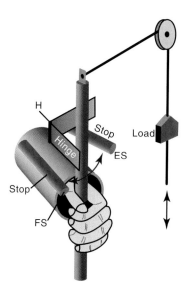

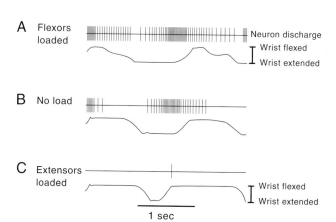

FIGURE 30.12 Discharge of a single M1 neuron in a monkey making flexion and extension wrist movements with wrist flexors loaded (A) and unloaded (B) and with wrist extensors loaded (C). The discharge rate of this neuron was greatest when the monkey used its wrist flexor muscles against a load. Modified from Evarts (1968).

force. Subsequent studies have confirmed these findings and have also shown that the discharge of M1 neurons can be related to the direction of movement, the position of a particular joint, or the velocity of movement. Cortical neurons whose firing is related to kinematic and dynamic parameters of movement are not found only in M1. Many neurons in the SMA, PMd, and parietal area 5 (which projects to SMA and PMd) fire in relation to movement direction, and some PMv neurons fire in relation to movement force. Therefore, neurons in several nonprimary cortical motor areas participate with those in M1 to control movement parameters such as direction, force, position, and velocity.

Although very strong correlations can be found between the discharge frequency of a given neuron and a particular movement parameter, every discharge of a M1 neuron does not simply encode a single parameter. Rather, single M1 neurons show various degrees of correlation with direction, force, position, and velocity. Thus, the discharge of a single neuron in the motor cortex may influence several movement parameters.

Conversely, any given parameter or other feature of a movement is represented not by the discharge of a single M1 neuron, but by the ensemble activity of a large population of cortical neurons. Although single M1 neurons discharge during movements in several directions, e.g., when the activity of many M1 neurons is summed, the resultant population may represent movement direction with considerable precision (Fig. 30.13). Researchers have correlated the force, rate of change of force, position, and velocity of flexion and extension wrist movements more accurately with the summed, weighted activity of a number of simultaneously recorded M1 neurons than with the discharge of any single neuron.

Cortical Motor Areas Prepare Voluntary Movements Based on a Variety of Cues

Cortical areas outside the primary motor cortex seem to be especially concerned with using a wide variety of sensory and other information as "cues" to select and guide movements. Insight into these cortical processes has been obtained by separating in time a cue instructing which movement to make from a second cue to execute the instructed movement. This creates a period between the two cues during which the subject knows what movement to make, but is not making the movement per se. During such an instructed delay period, many neurons in M1, SMA, and PMd discharge at their highest rate while the subject waits to move in a particular direction (Fig. 30.14). Such directional delay period activity is more common in PMd and SMA than in M1, where activity during movement execution predominates. During the delay between instruction and trigger, PMd, SMA, and other areas appear to store information on the direction of the impending movement. Indeed, neurons sometimes discharge in error during the delay, as if the monkey has seen a cue other than the one actually given and is preparing to move in the wrong direction. When such error discharges occur, the monkey often does make the wrong movement. The delay period discharge of such neurons thus represents stored information, not about which cue the monkey has seen, but rather about what movement the monkey will make.

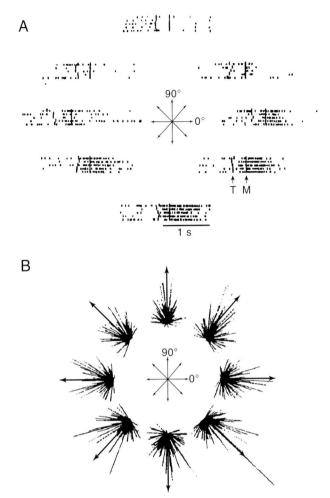

FIGURE 30.13 (A) Discharge of a single M1 neuron before and during arm movements in a monkey. Movements (represented by arrows) started from the same central point and ended at eight different points on a circle. The eight rasters show that the activity of this neuron was related to movements in four of the eight directions. The neuron discharged most intensely for movements down and to the right and was inhibited during movements up and to the left. (B) For each of the eight movements, the discharge of each M1 neuron is shown as a line pointing in the preferred direction of the neuron. Each line starts at the movement end point, and its length is proportional to the intensity of the discharge of that neuron during movement in that direction. Although the discharge of single neurons rarely identified any single movement direction with accuracy, the population vectors (arrows) summing the discharge of an ensemble of M1 neurons adequately specify each of the eight movement directions. From Georgopoulos (1988).

The direction instructed usually is the same as the direction of the actual movement. To pick up a pencil, for example, you look at the pencil and then move your hand to the same place. Somehow your brain transforms the visual location of the pencil into the location to which your hand is moved. Insight into how cue direction is transformed into movement direction has come from tasks in which these two

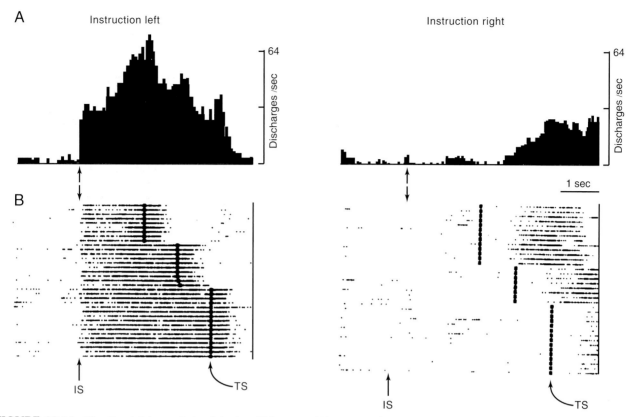

FIGURE 30.14 Directional delay period activity in a PM neuron. (A) As a monkey performed a delayed-reaction paradigm, this neuron began to discharge shortly after receiving instructions (IS) to perform a leftward movement. Discharge continued until after the monkey had subsequently received a separate triggering signal (TS, which occurred at three different time intervals after the IS) and performed the movement. During the delay between IS and TS, while the monkey did not move, the discharge of the neuron encoded the direction of the instruction, the direction of the impending movement, or both. (B) When the instruction was for rightward movement, this neuron did not discharge until after the movement had been made, presumably as the monkey was then preparing to move back to its original position. From Wise and Strick (1996).

features were experimentally dissociated, as if you looked at a pencil in a mirror and then reached to pick up the real pencil instead of the mirror image. To dissociate cue direction and movement direction experimentally, researchers have trained monkeys to perform mental rotation tasks in which a cue at one location instructs a movement to a different location.

Investigators have used such tasks to study neurons in the area principalis of the dorsolateral frontal lobe, in PMd, in SMA and in M1. In each of these cortical areas, the activity of some neurons correlates best with the direction of the instructional cue, whereas the activity of other neurons correlates best with the direction of the actual movement. In general, from the area principalis, through the PMd and SMA to M1, the percentage of cue-related neurons decreases and the percentage of movement-related neurons increases. Moreover, as time progresses from the appearance of the instructional cue-to the execution of the movement, the discharge of the neuronal populations encode cue direction initially and move-

ment direction subsequently. The transformation of cue direction into movement direction thus involves many cortical motor areas and progresses throughout the reaction time of the subject.

Some Cortical Motor Areas Are Involved in Movements in Response to Either Internal or External Cues

Another aspect of movement preparation that differentially involves certain cortical motor areas has to do with whether the instructions about what to do come from internally remembered or externally delivered cues. In one experiment, for example, monkeys were trained to touch three of four pads in randomly selected sequences that were cued when the pads were lit in sequence. Once a monkey was accustomed to a given sequence, the lights were gradually dimmed until the monkey was performing the correct sequence based only on internally remembered cues. After several of these remembered trials, the pads were lit in a different sequence for several trials. Whereas neurons in M1 showed similar discharge rates during the internally remembered and externally cued trials for a given sequence, SMA neurons were generally more active during the internally remembered trials, and PMv neurons were generally more active during the externally cued trials (Fig. 30.15).

Summary

Axons from the cerebral cortex and from the red nucleus in the brain stem descend in pathways located dorsolaterally in the spinal cord to control voluntary movements. In addition to corticospinal and rubrospinal pathways, the motor cortex also sends projections to the red nucleus and to the pontomedullary reticular formation, providing indirect pathways for voluntary control. Multiple cortical motor areas—distinguished by their inputs, their cytoarchitecture, and their interconnections with other cortical areas and with the thalamus—make different contributions to the control of voluntary movements. The most detailed motor map is found in the primary motor cortex, M1, but the somatotopic organization is limited by convergence and divergence in the corticospinal projection. Populations of M1 neurons are also in most direct control of movement kinematics and dynamics. Other cortical motor areas participate differentially in the selection of, and preparation for, voluntary movements based on a variety of internal and external cues.

SUMMARY

The motor cortex, the red nucleus, the pontomedullary reticular formation, and the vestibular nuclei each send major axonal projections descending from the brain to the spinal cord to control bodily movements. Although these pathways normally provide seamless movement control, different contributions of the medial and lateral descending pathways have been identified experimentally.

The medial system—vestibulospinal and reticulospinal—receives sensory input from the vestibular apparatus and mediates postural responses that keep the head and body stabilized for stance and gait. Additional visual and proprioceptive inputs that reach the vestibular and reticular nuclei via brain stem pathways or after processing in the cerebellum (Chapter 32) also influence postural control. Context-dependent strategies established via centers including the cerebellum and motor cortex further adapt postural responses to the needs of particular complex situations.

The lateral system—corticospinal and rubrospinal—receives, in addition to somatosensory inputs, information processed by the cerebellum (Chapter 32), the basal ganglia (Chapter 31), and association cortical areas to

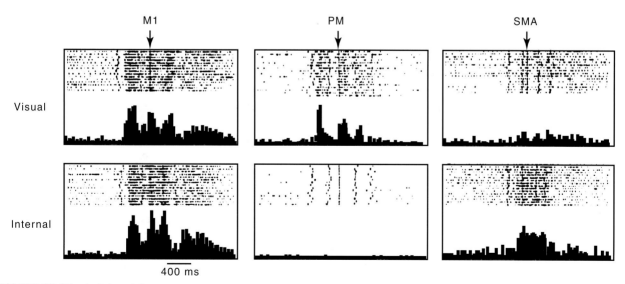

FIGURE 30.15 Activity of three neurons—one in M1, one in PM, and one in SMA—recorded as a monkey pressed three buttons in sequence. The sequence was first cued visually by lighting the buttons and was then cued internally. The M1 neuron showed similar activity whether the monkey performed from visual or internal cues. The PM neuron, however, was much more active in response to visual than internal cues, whereas the opposite was true for the SMA neuron. Modified from Mushiake et al. (1991).

mediate voluntary movements of the face and extremities. Different cortical motor areas receive different portions of these inputs and therefore make different contributions to controlling voluntary movements. The most elaborate somatotopic representation is found in the primary motor cortex, M1. While the convergence, divergence and horizontal interconnections of the intrinsic organization of M1 result in considerably distributed activation during voluntary movements, the same substrates enable substantial plasticity. Whereas M1 neurons most directly control the kinematics and dynamics of movement execution, other cortical motor areas participate in selecting which movement(s) to make on the basis of external cues and internal states.

References

Andersen, P., Hagan, P. J., Phillips, C. G., and Powell, T. P. (1975). Mapping by microstimulation of overlapping projections from area 4 to motor units of the baboon's hand. *Proc. R. Soci. Lond. Seri. B Biol. Sci.* **188**, 31–36.

Baker, J., Goldberg, J., and Peterson, B. (1985) Spatial and temporal response properties of the vestibulocollic reflex in decerebrate cats. *J. Neurophysiol.* **54**, 735–756.

Baloh, R., and Honrubia, V. (1990). "Clinical Neurophysiology of the Vestibular System," 2nd Ed. F. A. Davis, Philadelphia.

Cheney, P. D., Fetz, E. E., and Palmer, S. S. (1985). Patterns of facilitation and suppression of antagonist forelimb muscles from motor cortex sites in the awake monkey. *J. Neurophysiol.* **53**, 805–820.

Clarke, E., and O'Malley, C. D. (1996). "The Human Brain and Spinal Cord," 2nd Ed. Norman Publishing, San Francisco.

Evarts, E. V. (1968). Relation of pyramidal tract activity to force exerted during voluntary movement. *J. Neurophysiol.* **31**, 14–27.

Fetz, E. E., and Cheney, P. D. (1980). Postspike facilitation of forelimb muscle activity by primate corticomotoneuronal cells. *J. Neurophysiol.* **44**, 751–772.

Georgopoulos, A. P. (1988). Neural integration of movement: Role of motor cortex in reaching. *FASEB J.* **2**, 2849–2857.

Gould, H. J., Cusick, C. G., Pons, T. P., and Kaas, J. H. (1986). The relationship of corpus callosum connections to electrical stimulation maps of motor, supplementary motor, and the frontal eye fields in owl monkeys. *J. Comp. Neurol.* **247**, 297–325.

Horak, F., and Nashner, L. (1986). Central programming of postural movements: Adaptation to altered support-surface configurations. *J. Neurophysiol.* **55**, 1369–1381.

Horak, F., and Shupert, C. (1994). Role of the vestibular system in postural control. *In* "Vestibular Rehabilitation," (S. Herdman, ed.). F. A. Davis, Philadelphia.

Kuypers, H. G. (1987). Some aspects of the organization of the output of the motor cortex. *Ciba Found. Symp.* **132**, 63–82.

Lawrence, D. G., and Kuypers, H. G. (1968a) The functional organization of the motor system in the monkey. I. The effects of bilateral pyramidal lesions. *Brain* **91**, 1–14.

Lawrence, D. G., and Kuypers, H. G. (1968b). The functional organization of the motor system in the monkey. II. The effects of lesions of the descending brain-stem pathways. *Brain* **91**, 15–36.

Macpherson, J., and Inglis, J. (1993) Stance and balance following bilateral labyrinthectomy. *Prog. Brain Res.* **97**, 219–228.

Matelli, M., Luppino, G., and Rizzolatti, G. (1991). Architecture of superior and mesial area 6 and the adjacent cingulate cortex in the macaque monkey. *J. Comp. Neurol.* **311**, 445–462.

Mushiake, H., Inase, M., and Tanji, J. (1991). Neuronal activity in the primate premotor, supplementary, and precentral motor cortex during visually guided and internally determined sequential movements. *J. Neurophysiol.* **66**, 705–718.

Nashner, L. (1982). Adaptation of human movement to altered environments. *Trends Neurosci.* **5**, 358–361.

Paloski, W., Black, F., Reschke, M., Calkins, D., and Shupert, C. (1993). Vestibular ataxia following shuttle flights: Effects of microgravity on otolith-mediated sensorimotor control of posture. *Am. J. Otol.* **14**, 9–17.

Peterson, B., Goldberg, J., Bilotto, G., and Fuller, J. (1985). Cervicocollic reflex: Its dynamic properties and interaction with vestibular reflexes. *J. Neurophysiol.* **54**, 90–109.

Rizzolatti, G., Scandolara, C., Matelli, M., and Gentilucci, M. (1981). Afferent properties of periarcuate neurons in macaque monkeys. II. Visual responses. *Behav. Brain Res.* **2**, 147–163.

Roberts, T. (1967). "Neurophysiology of Postural Mechanisms." Plenum Press, New York.

Rosen, I., and Asanuma, H. (1972). Peripheral afferent inputs to the forelimb area of the monkey motor cortex: Input-output relations. *Exp. Brain. Res.* **14**, 257–273.

Schor, R., Kearney, R., and Dieringer, N. (1988). Reflex stabilization of the head. *In* "Control of Head Movement" (B. Peterson and F. Richmond, eds.). Oxford Univ. Press, New York.

Shinoda, Y., Yokota, J., and Futami, T. (1981). Divergent projection of individual corticospinal axons to motoneurons of multiple muscles in the monkey. *Neurosci. Lett.* **23**, 7–12.

Wilson, V., and Melvill-Jones, G. (1979). "Mammalian Vestibular Physiology." Plenum Press, New York.

Wise, S. P., and Strick P. L. (1996). Anatomical and physiological organization of the non-primary motor cortex. *TINS* **7**, 442–446.

Woolsey, C. N., Settlage, P. H., Meyer, D. R., Sencer, W., Hamuy, T. P., and Travis, A. M. (1952). Patterns of localization in precentral and "supplementary" motor areas and their relation to the concept of a premotor area. *Res. Pub. Assoc. Res. Nerv. Ment. Dis.* **30**, 238–264.

Marc H. Schieber and James F. Baker

CHAPTER

31

The Basal Ganglia

Two large subcortical motor systems send output via the thalamus to the cortical motor systems. These are the basal ganglia and the cerebellum. Although they appear to influence the same cortical areas, their connections are through private connections to separate areas of the thalamus. Furthermore, they have opposite effects: the basal ganglia output is inhibitory and the cerebellar output is excitatory. In addition to the well-established motor function of the basal ganglia and cerebellum, there is increasing evidence that both systems play roles in nonmotor behavior, including cognition, emotion, and possibly others. The basal ganglia are considered in this chapter and the cerebellum in the next (Chapter 32).

Basal ganglia are large subcortical structures comprising several interconnected nuclei in the forebrain, midbrain, and diencephalon (Fig. 31.1). Because of certain features, it is generally agreed that basal ganglia participate in the control of movement. The largest portion of basal ganglia inputs and outputs are connected with motor areas. Second, the discharge of many basal ganglia neurons correlates with movement. Third, basal ganglia lesions cause severe movement abnormalities. In addition to their role in motor control, the connections and lesion effects of the basal ganglia suggest that they may also participate in some cognitive aspects of behavior.

This chapter concentrates on the motor functions of the basal ganglia, but participation of the basal ganglia in cognition is discussed after the basic framework of basal ganglia function is presented for motor control. The anatomy of the basal ganglia is be discussed first, as it is the anatomy that provides the infrastructure for the physiology. Next we consider the activity of the individual components of the basal

ganglia during movement. Then we discuss the effect of placing a lesion in one component while leaving the rest of the nervous system intact. The combined strategy of measuring the activity of a structure

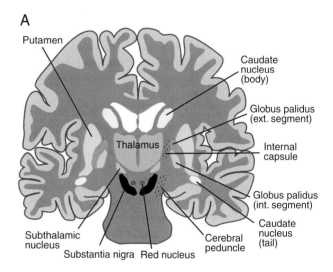

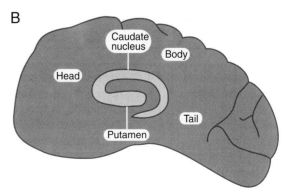

FIGURE 31.1 Location of basal ganglia in the human brain. (A) Coronal section. (B) Parasagittal section.

Fundamental Neuroscience, Second Edition

during movement and then determining the effect a selective lesion on that movement has been fruitful in studying the function of the motor system. After presentation of current models of basal ganglia motor function, the chapter concludes with a discussion of basal ganglia participation in cognitive function.

ANATOMY OF BASAL GANGLIA

The basal ganglia receive a broad spectrum of cortical inputs. The information conveyed to the basal ganglia is processed to produce a focused output to areas of the frontal lobes and brain stem that are involved in the planning and production of movement. The basal ganglia output is inhibitory, which means that an *increase* in basal ganglia output leads to a *reduction* in the activity of its targets. The fact that the basal ganglia output is inhibitory to other motor mechanisms is important to understanding its normal function.

At first glance, the anatomy of the basal ganglia may seem confusing. There are several component nuclei at different levels in the brain, and two of the nuclei [substantia nigra (SN) and globus pallidus] are divided into functionally different components. The names of some structures are different in primates than in other mammals. Furthermore, the terminology has changed over the years so that historically an individual structure may be known by more than one name. However, with consistent use of modern terminology and a functional context in which to place the anatomy, the organization of basal ganglia can be learned readily. Moreover, once learned, many aspects of its normal function and of the response to injury become much easier to understand.

The basal ganglia include the striatum (caudate, putamen, nucleus accumbens), the subthalamic nucleus (STN), the globus pallidus (internal segment or GPi; external segment or GPe; and ventral pallidum), and the substantia nigra (pars compacta or SNpc and pars reticulata or SNpr) (Fig. 31.2). The tum) and nucleus accumbens (ventral striatum). This section focuses on the neostriatum (see Box 31.3 and Chapters 43 and 44 for a discussion of the ventral system of the basal ganglia). Embryologically, the striatum develops from a basal region of the lateral telencephalic vesicle. It is named the striatum because axon fibers passing through the striatum give it a striped appearance. In rodents, the caudate and putamen are a single structure with fibers of the internal capsule coursing through, but in carnivores and primates, the caudate and putamen are separated by the internal capsule. The caudate and putamen

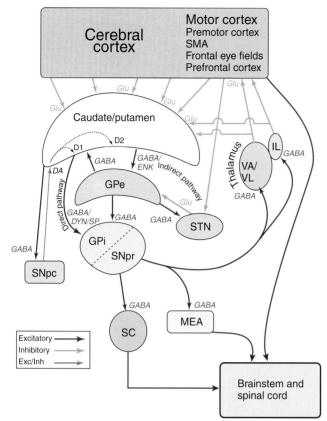

FIGURE 31.2 Simplified wiring diagram of basal ganglia circuits. Simplified schematic diagram of basal ganglia circuitry. Excitatory connections are indicated by green arrows, inhibitory connections by red arrows, and the modulatory dopamine projection is indicated by a red and green arrow. GPe, globus pallidus, external segment; GPi, globus pallidus, internal segment; IL, intralaminar thalamic nuclei; MD, mediodorsal thalamic nucleus; MEA, midbrain extrapyramidal area; SC, superior colliculus; SNpc, substantia nigra pars compacta; SNpr, substantia nigra, pars reticulata; STN, subthalamic nucleus; VA, ventral anterior thalamic nucleus; VL, ventral lateral thalamic nucleus; DA, dopamine (with D_1 and D_2 receptor subtypes); Dyn, dynorphin; Enk, enkephalin; GABA, γ-aminobutyric acid; Glu, glutamate; SP, substance P.

striatum and STN receive the majority of inputs from outside of the basal ganglia. Most of those inputs come from the cerebral cortex, but thalamic nuclei also provide strong inputs to striatum. There are no direct inputs from peripheral sensory or motor systems. The bulk of outputs from basal ganglia arises from GPi and SNpr and is inhibitory to thalamic nuclei and to brain stem. There are no direct outputs from basal ganglia to spinal motor circuitry.

The Striatum Receives Most of the Inputs to the Basal Ganglia

The striatum is located in the forebrain and comprises the caudate nucleus and putamen (neostria-

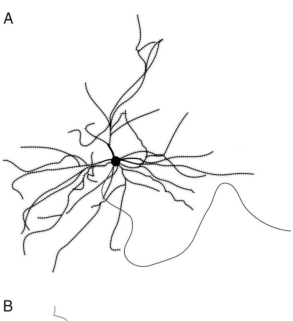
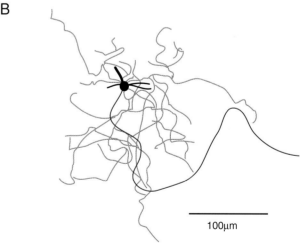

FIGURE 31.3 Two representations of a striatal medium spiny neuron that has been filled with HRP. (A) The soma and dendritic tree with numerous dendritic spines. The thin process is the axon, which has been drawn without its collaterals. (B) The same neuron drawn to show the axonal collaterals, which branch extensively within the same field as the dendritic tree. From Wilson and Groves (1980).

receive input from the neocortex, and the size of these nuclei parallels the size of the neocortex throughout phylogeny.

Four major types of neurons have been described in the striatum. The typing is based on the size of the cell body, presence or absence of dendritic spines in individual neurons that have been stained with the Golgi technique or filled with horseradish peroxidase, and other staining properties. The first and by far the most numerous neuron type is the *medium spiny neuron* (Fig. 31.3). Medium spiny neurons make up 95% of the total number of striatal neurons. They utilize γ-aminobutyric acid (GABA) as a transmitter and constitute the output of the striatum, sending axonal projections to the GP and SN. Medium spiny neurons have large dendritic trees that span 200 to 500 μm (Wilson and Groves, 1980). They also have extensive local axon collaterals that may inhibit neighboring striatal neurons. The medium spiny neurons are morphologically homogeneous, but chemically heterogeneous, as discussed later. Second, *large aspiny neurons* make up 1–2% of the striatal population. They are interneurons and are thought to use acetylcholine (ACh) as a neurotransmitter. They have extensive axon collaterals in the striatum that terminate on medium spiny neurons. The third type of neuron is the *medium aspiny cell*. These are also interneurons and are thought to use somatostatin as a neurotransmitter. The fourth type of neuron is a *small aspiny cell* that stains for parvalbumin. These are interneurons that use GABA as a neurotransmitter.

The striatum receives excitatory input from nearly all of the cerebral cortex. The cortical input uses glutamate as its neurotransmitter and terminates largely on the heads of the dendritic spines of medium spiny neurons (Fig. 31.4). The projection from the cerebral cortex to the striatum has a roughly topographical organization. For example, the somatosensory and motor cortex project to the posterior putamen and the prefrontal cortex projects to the anterior caudate. Within the somatosensory and motor projection to the striatum, there is a preservation of somatotopy. It has been suggested that the topographic relationship between the cerebral cortex and the striatum provides a basis for the segregation of functionally different circuits in the basal ganglia (Alexander *et al.*, 1986) (Fig. 31.5). These circuits include somatomotor, oculomotor, cognitive, and limbic connections. Within each circuit there appear to be subcircuits such that the primary motor cortex and premotor cortex have non-identical connections with basal ganglia structures. Likewise, dorsolateral and orbitofrontal circuits have distinct connectivity patterns.

Although the topography and somatotopy imply a certain degree of parallel organization, there is also convergence and divergence in the corticostriatal pro-

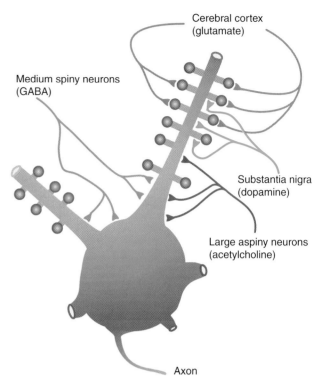

FIGURE 31.4 Pattern of termination of afferents on a medium spiny neuron. The soma and the proximal dendrites with their spines are shown.

jection. The large dendritic fields of medium spiny neurons allow them to receive input from adjacent projections, which arise from different areas of cortex. Inputs from more than one cortical area overlap (Flaherty and Graybiel, 1991), and input from a single cortical area projects divergently to multiple striatal zones (Fig. 31.6). This convergent and divergent organization provides an anatomical framework for the integration and transformation of information from several areas of the cerebral cortex.

In addition to cortical input, medium spiny striatal neurons receive a number of other inputs, including (1) excitatory and presumed glutamatergic inputs from intralaminar and ventrolateral nuclei of the thalamus; (2) cholinergic input from large aspiny neurons; (3) GABA, substance P, and enkephalin input from adjacent medium spiny striatal neurons; (4) GABA input from small interneurons; and (5) a large input from dopamine (DA)-containing neurons in the SNpc. The DA input is of particular interest because of its role in Parkinson's disease (PD, see later).

The DA input to the striatum terminates largely on the shafts of the dendritic spines of medium spiny neurons (Fig. 31.4). The location of dopaminergic terminals puts them in a position to modulate transmission from the cerebral cortex to the striatum. The action of DA on striatal neurons depends on the type

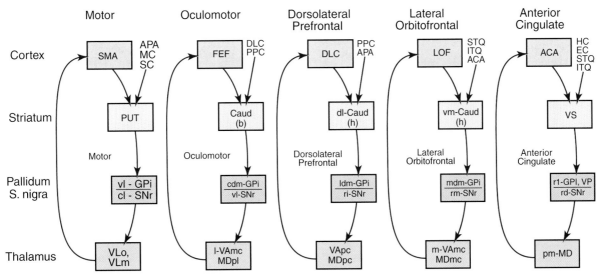

FIGURE 31.5 Hypothetical parallel segregated circuits connecting the basal ganglia, thalamus, and cerebral cortex. The five circuits are named according to the primary cortical target of the output from the basal ganglia: motor, oculornotor, dorsolateral prefrontal, lateral orbitofrontal, and anterior cingulate. ACA, anterior cingulate area; APA, arcuate premotor area; CAUD, caudate; b, body; h, head; DLC, dorsolateral prefrontal cortex; EC, entorhinal cortex; FEF, frontal eye fields; GPi, internal segment of globus pallidus; HC, hippocampal cortex; ITG, inferior temporal gyrus; LOF, lateral orbitofrontal cortex; MC, motor cortex; MDpl, mediulis dorsalis pars paralarnellaris; MDme, medialis dorsalis pars magnocellularis; MDpc, medialis dorsalis pars parvocellularis; PPC, posterior parietal cortex; PUT, putamen; SC, somatosensory cortex; SMA, supplementary motor area; SNr, substantia nigra pars reticulate; STG, superior temporal gyrus; VAmc, ventralis anterior pars magnocellularis; Vapc, ventralis anterior pars parvocellularis; VLm, ventralis lateralis pars medialis; VLo, ventralis lateralis pars oralis; VP, ventral pallidum; VS, ventral striatum, cl, caudolateral; cdm, caudal dorsomedial; dl, dorsolateral; 1, lateral; ldm, lateral dorsomedial; m, medial; mdm, medial dorsomedial; pm, posteromedial; rd, rostrodorsal; rl, rostrolateral; rm, rostromedial; vm, ventromedial; vl, ventrolateral.

of DA receptor involved. Five types of G protein-coupled DA receptors have been described (D1–D5). These have been grouped into two families based on their response to agonists. The D1 family includes D1 and D5 receptors, and the D2 family includes D2, D3, and D4 receptors. D1 receptors stimulate adenylate cyclase activity and may potentiate the effect of cortical input to striatal neurons. D2 receptors inhibit adenylate cyclase activity and may decrease the effect of cortical input to striatal neurons (see Chapters 8 and 9).

Medium spiny neurons contain the inhibitory neurotransmitter GABA. In addition, medium spiny neurons have peptide neurotransmitters that are colocalized with GABA. Based on both the type of neurotransmitters and the type of DA receptor they contain, medium spiny neurons can be divided into two populations. One population contains GABA, dynorphin, and substance P and primarily expresses D1 receptors. These neurons send axons to GPi and to SNpr. Although substance P is generally thought to be an excitatory neurotransmitter, the predominant effect of these neurons is inhibition of their targets. The second population contains GABA and enkephalin and primarily expresses D2 receptors. These neurons project to GPe and are

inhibitory. The two populations of medium spiny neurons are morphologically indistinguishable and are not segregated topographically within the striatum (Fig. 31.7). This comingling of neurons suggests that they receive similar input and thus they may convey similar information to their respective targets. However, the different targets and transmitter types of the two populations provides the substrate for one level of functional segregation within the striatum.

Although there are no apparent regional differences in the striatum based on cell morphology, an intricate internal organization has been revealed with special stains. When the striatum is stained for acetylcholinesterase (AChE), the enzyme that inactivates acetylcholine (see Chapter 8), there is a patchy distribution of lightly staining regions within more heavily stained regions. The AChE-poor patches have been called *striosomes* and the AChE-rich areas have been called the extrastriosomal *matrix*. The matrix forms the bulk of the striatal volume and receives input from most areas of the cerebral cortex. Within the matrix are clusters of neurons with similar inputs that have been termed *matrisomes*. The bulk of the output from cells in the matrix is to both segments of the GP

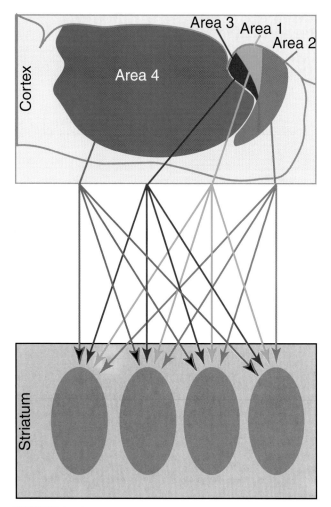

FIGURE 31.6 Schematic representation of the sensorimotor cortical projection to the striatum from arm areas in the somatosensory cortex (areas 1, 2, and 3) and motor cortex (area 4). Note that each cortical area projects to several striatal zones and several functionally related cortical areas project to a single striatal zone. After Flaherty and Graybiel (1991).

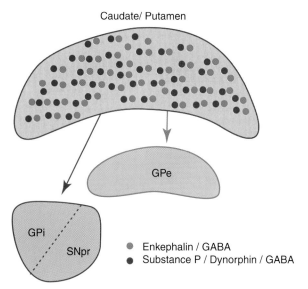

FIGURE 31.7 The two chemically different populations of striatal medium spiny neurons are intermixed. One population (blue) projects to the globus pallidus external segment (GPe) and contains GABA and enkephalin. The other population (red) projects to the globus pallidus internal segment (GPi) and substantia nigra pars reticulata (SNpr) and contains GABA, dynorphin, and substance P (red).

and to SNpr. The striosomes receive input from the prefrontal cortex and send output to SNpc. Immunohistochemical techniques have demonstrated that many substances, such as substance P, dynorphin, and enkephalin, have a patchy distribution that may be partly or wholly in register with the striosomes (Graybiel *et al.*, 1981). The striosome–matrix organization provides the substrate for another level of functional segregation within the striatum.

The STN Receives Inputs from the Frontal Lobe

The STN is located at the junction of the diencephalon and midbrain, ventral to the thalamus and rostral and lateral to the red nucleus. Embryologically,

it develops from the lateral hypothalamic cell column. Phylogenetically, it increases in size in proportion to the neocortex. The STN receives an excitatory, glutamatergic input from the frontal cortex with large contributions from motor areas, including the primary motor cortex (area 4), premotor and supplementary motor cortex (area 6), and frontal eye fields (area 8). The STN also receives an inhibitory GABA input from GPe. The output from the STN is excitatory and glutamatergic. STN projects to GPi and SNpr as well, projecting back to GPe.

Although the STN receives input from the neocortex and projects to both segments of GP and to SNpr, it is different from striatum in several ways. Unlike striatum, the cortical input to the STN is from the frontal lobe only. The output from STN is excitatory, whereas the output from striatum is inhibitory. Of the two routes from the cortex to GPi, GPe, and SNpr, the excitatory route through STN (5–8 ms) is faster than the inhibitory route through striatum (15–20 ms).

GPi Is the Basal Ganglia Output for Limb Movements

GP lies medial to the putamen and rostral to the hypothalamus. Embryologically, it arises from the lateral hypothalamic cell column. In primates, GP is separated into an internal segment and an external segment by a fiber tract called the internal medullary lamina. In rodents and carnivores, the internal segment lies within the internal capsule and is called the entopeduncular nucleus. GPe is not a principal source of output from the basal ganglia and it is considered later.

The GPi is composed primarily of large neurons that project outside of the basal ganglia. The dendritic trees of GPi neurons radiate from the cell body in a disc-like distribution and are oriented so that the faces of the disc are perpendicular to incoming axons from the striatum. The dendrites of an individual GPi cell can span up to 1 mm in diameter and therefore GPi neurons have the potential to receive a large number of converging inputs.

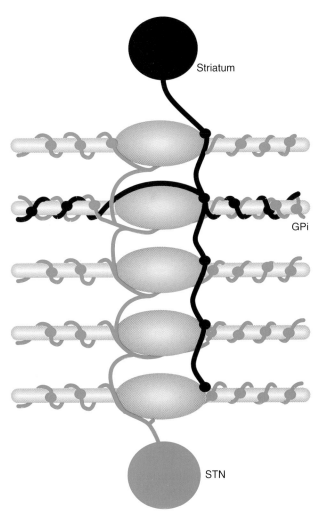

FIGURE 31.8 The two primary inputs to globus pallidus internal segment (GPi) have different patterns of termination. Axons from the subthalamic nucleus (green) are excitatory and terminate extensively on multiple GPi neurons. Axons from the striatum (red) contact several GPi neurons weakly in passing before terminating densely on a single neuron.

The principal inputs to GPi are from striatum and the STN. These two types of inputs differ in the neurotransmitters used, in their physiological action, and in their pattern of termination. As noted earlier, neurons projecting from striatum to GPi contain GABA, substance P, and dynorphin and are inhibitory. Each axon from the striatum enters GPi and sparsely contacts several neurons in passing before ensheathing a single neuron with a dense termination. This pathway has been called the "direct" striatopallidal pathway (Fig. 30.2). The excitatory, glutamate projection from STN to GPi is highly divergent such that each axon from the STN ensheathes many GPi neurons (Figure 31.8). The striatal projection to GPi is about 10–15 msec slower than the STN projection to GPi. Thus, the striatal and STN inputs to GPi form a pattern of fast, widespread, divergent excitation from STN and slower, focused, convergent inhibition from striatum.

The output from GPi is inhibitory and, like the input to this structure from striatum, uses GABA as its neurotransmitter. The majority (70%) of the GPi output is sent via collaterals to both the thalamus and the brain stem. In the thalamus, axons from GPi terminate in the oral part of the ventrolateral nucleus (VLo) and in the principal part of the ventral anterior nucleus (VApc). In turn, these thalamic nuclei project to the motor, premotor, supplementary motor, and prefrontal cortex. They also project back to striatum in a potential feedback loop. Some evidence suggests that an individual GPi neuron sends output via the thalamus to just one area of the cortex (Hoover and Strick, 1993). In other words, GPi neurons that project to the motor cortex are adjacent to, but separate from, those that project to the premotor cortex. Thus, just as there are parallel inputs from the cortex to striatum, there appear to be potential functionally parallel outputs from GPi.

Collaterals of the axons projecting from GPi to the thalamus project to an area at the junction of the midbrain and pons near the pedunculopontine nucleus, which has been termed the "midbrain extrapyramidal area." The midbrain extrapyramidal area projects in turn to the reticulospinal motor system. Other GPi neurons (20%) project to intralaminar nuclei of the thalamus or to the lateral habenula. The specific role of these projections is not known.

Substantia Nigra Pars Reticulata Is the Basal Ganglia Output for Eye Movements

Like the GP, the SN is divided into two segments. One is a densely cellular region called the pars compacta (SNpc) and the other is more sparsely cellular and is called the pars reticulata (SNpr). The pars compacta contains DA cells and is not a principal output nucleus of the basal ganglia. It is considered later. SNpr is similar to GPi in many ways, including cell size, histochemistry, and connectional anatomy.

Like GPi, the SNpr contains large neurons that project outside of the basal ganglia. The dendritic trees are less disc-like than those of GPi neurons, but like GPi neurons they extend up to 1 mm and thus receive a wide field of inputs. As in the case of GPi, the SNpr receives inhibitory inputs from striatum that contain GABA, SP, and dynorphin and excitatory inputs from STN that contain glutamate and provides inhibitory, GABAergic outputs. In the case of SNpr, these outputs are to the medial part of the ventro-lateral thalamus (VLm) and the magnocellular part of the ventral anterior thalamus (VAmc). These thalamic areas in turn project to the premotor and prefrontal cortex. Like the GPi output, SNpr sends collaterals to the midbrain extrapyramidal area and also has a projection to intralaminar nuclei of the thalamus. The primary difference in the outputs of GPi and SNpr is that the lateral portion of SNpr sends an inhibitory projection to the superior colliculus and to the para-laminar part of the medial dorsal thalamus (MDpl). MDpl projects in turn to the frontal eye fields. Thus, the lateral portion of SNpr is connected with cortical and brain stem areas that control eye movements.

GPe Is Connected to Several Other Basal Ganglia Nuclei

The GPe is one of two nuclei that may be viewed as intrinsic nuclei of the basal ganglia. The other is the SNpc, which is considered in the next section. Both GPe and SNpc receive the bulk of their input from and send the bulk of their output to other basal ganglia nuclei.

The GPe is similar in some ways to GPi. Its inputs are an inhibitory projection from the striatum and an excitatory one from STN. The patterns of termination of the striatal and STN afferents are similar in that the striatal input is focused and convergent while the STN input is divergent (Parent and Hazrati, 1993). As noted earlier, GPe and GPi receive input from neighboring striatal neurons and thereby are likely to receive similar information. Unlike GPi, the striatal projection to GPe contains GABA and enkephalin but not substance P. The functional implications of this distinction are unknown. However, the pathway taken by output of GPe is also quite different from that taken by the output of GPi, which undoubtedly has profound functional implications. The majority of the output of GPe projects to STN. The connections

from striatum to GPe, from GPe to STN, and from STN to GPi thus are referred to as the "indirect" striatopallidal pathway to GPi to distinguish it from the "direct" striatopallidal pathway that runs from striatum to GPi (Alexander and Crutcher, 1990). In addition, there is a monosynaptic GABAergic inhibitory output from GPe directly to GPi and to SNpr and a recently described GABAergic projection back to striatum. Thus, GPe neurons are in a position to provide feedback inhibition to neurons in striatum and STN and feed-forward inhibition to neurons in GPi and SNpr. This circuitry suggests that GPe may act to oppose, limit, or focus the effect of the striatal and STN projections to GPi and SNpr, as well as focus activity in these output nuclei.

SNpc Provides DA Input to the Striatum

The SNpc is perhaps the most studied structure in the basal ganglia. The SNpc is made up of large DA-containing cells and it is these neurons that degenerate in PD, which is characterized by abnormal movement (see later). DA neurons contain a substance called neuromelanin, which is a dark pigment that gives the SNpc a blackish appearance and appears to represent an oxidation product of DA. This is the basis for its name (substantia nigra = black substance). SNpc receives input from the striatum, specifically from the striosomes. This input is GABAergic and inhibitory. Other inputs to SNpc have been difficult to assess because the dendrites of SNpc and SNpr neurons overlap. Thus it is not always clear whether axons ending in the SN terminate on SNpc neurons, SNpr neurons, or both. The SNpc DA neurons project to all of caudate and putamen in a topographic manner. However, nigral DA neurons receive inputs from one striatal circuit and project back to the same and to adjacent circuits (Haber et al., 2000). Thus, they appear to be in a position to modulate activity across circuits. The action of DA depends on the receptors located on target neurons, as was discussed earlier.

Summary

Now that the anatomy of the individual components of the basal ganglia has been described, let us step back and summarize the relationships among basal ganglia nuclei and connections of the basal ganglia to the rest of the brain.

1. The striatum receives input from nearly all of the cerebral cortex such that several functionally related cortical areas project to overlapping striatal zones and that an individual cortical area projects to

several striatal zones. Cortical areas that are not functionally related project to separate zones of the striatum, although there may be some interaction between adjacent zones.

2. The striatum sends a focused and convergent inhibitory projection to the basal ganglia output nuclei, GPi and SNpr.

3. The STN receives input from the frontal lobe, especially from the motor, premotor, and supplementary motor cortex and from the frontal eye fields.

4. The STN sends a fast divergent excitatory projection to GPi and SNpr.

5. There are reciprocal and loop-like connections among basal ganglia nuclei that may play a negative or positive feedback role or may result in focusing of signals.

6. The output from the basal ganglia (GPi and SNpr) is inhibitory and projects to motor areas in the brain stem and thalamus.

7. There are no direct connections between the basal ganglia and the spinal sensory motor apparatus.

There is some disagreement among basal ganglia experts whether to view the overall anatomic organization of the basal ganglia as convergent or as multiple parallel segregated loops through the basal ganglia, each with a separate output. In support of convergence are (1) the reduction of the number of neurons at each level from the cortex to striatum to GPi and SNpr, (2) the large number of synapses on each striatal neuron, (3) the large dendritic trees of striatal, GPi, and SNpr neurons, and (4) interaction across circuits mediated by SNpc and GPe neurons. In support of parallel segregated loops are (1) the preserved somatotopy with separate representations of the face, arm, and leg in the cortex, striatum, and GPi/SNpr, (2) the relative preservation of topography through the basal ganglia, e.g., the prefrontal cortex to caudate to SNpr to VA thalamus to the prefrontal cortex and motor cortex to putamen to GPi to VLo thalamus to motor cortex, and (3) the finding that separate groups of GPi neurons project via the thalamus to separate motor areas of the cortex. It appears that there is local convergence and global parallelism, but it remains unknown whether the parallel pathways are functionally segregated or to what degree there is interaction at the interfaces between functionally different pathways.

SIGNALING IN BASAL GANGLIA

Although the anatomic organization may provide some clues as to what might be the function of basal

ganglia circuits, inference of function from anatomy is speculative. One approach to studying the function of an area of the central nervous system is to record the electrical activity of individual neurons with an extracellular electrode in awake, behaving animals. Other approaches involve inferences of neuronal signaling from imaging studies of blood flow and metabolism, or of changes in gene expression. By sampling the signal of a part of the brain during behavior, we can gain some insight into what role that part might play in behavior. Neurons within different basal ganglia nuclei have characteristic baseline discharge patterns that change with movement. If an animal is trained to perform a task consistently, the activity of single neurons can be correlated with individual aspects of the task performance. Furthermore, the timing of neural activity in one part can be compared to the timing of another and to the timing of the movement. This section emphasizes signals in the basal ganglia that are correlated with movement or the preparation for movement.

The Striatum Has Low Spontaneous Activity That Increases during Movement

In awake animals, the majority of striatal neurons (80–90%) have low baseline discharge rates of 0.1 to 1 Hz (Fig. 31.9). These neurons project outside of the striatum and therefore are probably medium spiny neurons. In general, the activity of these neurons reflects the activity of areas of cerebral cortex from which they receive inputs, but striatal neurons are less modality specific. Thus, neurons in areas of the putamen that receive input from the somatosensory

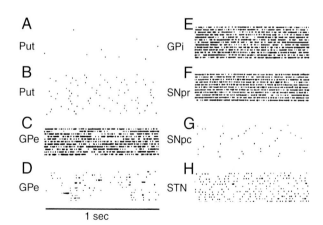

FIGURE 31.9 Representative neural discharge patterns from several basal ganglia nuclei. In the raster displays, each dot indicates the occurrence of an action potential. Each horizontal raster line represents a 1-s period of discharge. Several such periods are arranged vertically for each nucleus.

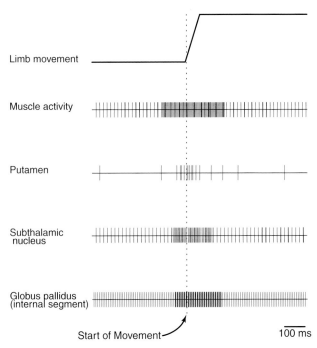

FIGURE 31.10 Schematic representation of the timing of neuronal activity in three nuclei of the basal ganglia in relation to limb movement and the muscle activity used to make the movement.

and motor cortex have activity correlated with active and passive movement, but not with specific tactile modalities such as light touch, vibration, or joint position. The activity of movement-related putamen neurons is different from corticospinal neurons in the motor cortex, but is similar to the activity of corticostriatal neurons.

Striatal neurons related to movement have a distinct somatotopy with the face represented ventromedially and the leg dorsolaterally. They tend to occur in clusters of neurons with similar discharge characteristics. These clusters of physiologically similar neurons may correspond to the anatomically defined matrisomes described earlier. Movement-related activity changes are seen as increases above the very low baseline. On average, movement-related striatal neurons fire 20 msec prior to movement (Fig. 31.10). About half of these neurons fire in relation to the direction of movement. Some neurons fire in relation to the start of movement and others in relation to the stop. Some neurons in the putamen fire in relation to self-initiated movements, some in relation to stimulus-triggered movements, and some in relation to both (Romo et al., 1992). Some neurons in the anterior part of the putamen and in the caudate nucleus that receive input from the premotor or prefrontal cortex have activity during the preparation for movement. This activity is time locked to instructional cues but not to the move-

ment itself. Some signals correlate with the instruction of whether to move ("set"). Other signals correlate with the signal to move ("go"). Although some individual neurons have signals that differentially relate to specific tasks or task parameters, as a whole the striatum is not exclusively active in relation to any of these tasks or parameters.

Striatal neurons active in relation to eye movements are located in a longitudinal zone in the central part of the caudate nucleus. This region receives input from the frontal and supplementary eye fields in the cortex. Similar to striatal neurons related to limb movements, striatal neurons related to eye movements may discharge during preparation for the movement or during the movement.

The timing of neuronal activity related to limb or eye movements is important to understanding the function of those neurons in the production of movement. In the putamen, most movement-related activity is late, occurring on average after the onset of muscle activity responsible for producing the movement. When compared to activity in the cerebral cortex, movement-related putamen neurons fire after those in the motor cortex and supplementary motor area. Putamen neurons related to movement preparation also fire substantially later than cortical neurons involved in movement preparation. Caudate neurons related to eye movements fire late relative to oculomotor areas of cortex. The late timing of striatal discharge during movement and movement preparation relative to discharge in cortical areas suggests that the striatum is not involved primarily in the initiation of movement. Instead, it receives information from cortical areas that are responsible for movement generation and may use that information for facilitation, gating, or scaling of cortically initiated movement.

A subset of striatal neurons (10%) is tonically active with discharge rates of 2 to 10 Hz. These neurons are distributed throughout the striatum and their discharge bears no specific relation to movement. These tonically active neurons (TANs) fire in relation to certain sensory stimuli that are associated with reward. For example, a TAN will fire in relation to a clicking sound if the click precedes a fruit juice reward but will not fire to the click alone or to the reward alone (Aosaki et al., 1994). It has been suggested that these neurons signal aspects of tasks that are related to learning and reinforcement. TANs are not activated by electrical stimulation of the GP and thus are probably not projection neurons. It is thought that TANs are cholinergic large aspiny interneurons that innervate the medium spiny neurons (see earlier discussions), which would place them in a position to modify the sensitivity of the medium spiny neurons to cortical input in relation to specific behavioral contexts.

STN Has Moderate Spontaneous Activity That Increases during Movement

Neurons in the STN are tonically active with average baseline discharge rates of about 20 Hz (Fig. 31.9). They are organized somatotopically and change activity in relation to eye or limb movement. For 90% of these neurons the change is an increase, occurring on average 50 msec prior to the movement (Fig. 31.10). The majority of movement-related neurons in STN have signals related to movement direction, but little is known about whether they discharge in relation to movement parameters such as amplitude or velocity.

GPi and SNpr Have High Spontaneous Activity That Increases or Decreases after Movement Initiation

As described earlier, GPi and SNpr form the output of the basal ganglia. Just as they are similar anatomically, they are also similar physiologically. Neurons in these output structures are tonically active with average firing rates of 60 to 80 Hz (Fig. 31.9). They are organized somatotopically with the leg and arm in GPi and the face and eyes in SNpr. Due to the somatotopy, studies of limb movements have focused on GPi and studies of eye movements have focused on SNpr. Because limb and eye movements are controlled differently, these studies are discussed separately.

The discharge of many GPi neurons is related to the direction of limb movement, but most GPi activity is not correlated with other physical parameters of movement, including joint position, force production, movement amplitude, or movement velocity. Few GPi neurons have activity correlated with the pattern of muscle activity. Like striatum, some GPi neurons have activity related to movement preparation. During a reaching movement, 25% of GPi neurons are related to movement preparation and 50% are related to movement, but many neurons have more than one type of response. Approximately 70% of arm movement-related GPi neurons increase activity and 30% decrease activity from this tonic baseline during movement. Because the output from GPi is inhibitory, the large proportion of activity increases during movement translates to broad inhibition of thalamic and brain stem targets with more restricted facilitation during movement.

The timing of movement-related GPi activity is late compared to the activation of agonist muscles. The average onset of GPi activity is after the onset of EMG but before the onset of movement (Fig. 31.10). There is a tendency for GPi movement-related increases to occur earlier than decreases, which probably reflects the faster speed of the excitatory pathway from the cortex to GPi via STN compared with the slower inhibitory pathway from the cortex to GPi via striatum. The late timing of GPi movement-related activity suggests that the output of the basal ganglia is unlikely to initiate movement.

Like GPi neurons, SNpr neurons are tonically active. SNpr is the principal basal ganglia output for the control of eye movements, and most studies of SNpr activity have been in eye movement tasks (Hikosaka *et al.*, 2000). Most saccade-related SNpr neurons fire in relation to the direction of the eye movements. Unlike GPi neurons during limb movements, virtually all saccade-related SNpr neurons decrease activity during the saccade. It is not known whether the fact that most GPi limb movement neurons increase and most SNpr saccade neurons decrease indicates a fundamental difference between eye and limb movement control or if it reflects task differences. Other differences between GPi limb movement neurons and SNpr saccade neurons have been noted. While GPi limb movement neurons have weak sensory responses, some SNpr neurons have strong responses to visual stimuli. For the visually responsive SNpr neurons, the spatial location of the stimulus seems to be the most salient feature.

Some SNpr neurons have their strongest relation to saccades made to remembered targets. Thus, if a visual target is presented and then removed and a monkey is trained to look to where the target had been, some SNpr cells will fire more in this condition as compared to when a saccade is made to a visible target. Some SNpr neurons have activity related to the preparation for eye movement. One-third of SNpr cells have activity related to saccades to a visual target. Another third of SNpr cells have activity related to saccades to a remembered target location. During saccades, the time of SNpr activity change is after that in the superior colliculus, a structure that is known to be involved in the initiation of saccades. Thus, for eye movements, as well as limb movements, the basal ganglia output acts after structures that initiate movement.

GPe Has Irregular Activity That Increases or Decreases after Movement Initiation

Two types of neurons have been described in GPe based on their baseline activity patterns. Most fire at a high frequency (70 Hz) that is interrupted by long pauses. A smaller number fire at a low frequency (10 Hz on average) and have frequent spontaneous bursts of activity. Both types of neurons change activity in relation to limb movement and, for the majority, these changes are increases in activity. As has been described for GPi, GPe neurons weakly and inconsistently code for movement amplitude, velocity, muscle length, or force. Like the other structures of the basal ganglia, the activity of movement-related activity is late.

SNpc Has Low Spontaneous Activity That Does Not Change with Movement, but Changes with Significant Environmental Stimuli

The activity of single neurons in the SNpc of trained animals is different from the activity of single neurons in the other basal ganglia structures. At baseline, SNpc neurons fire at a low rate (2 Hz on average). The activity of these neurons is not related to movement itself and there is no apparent somatotopy in SNpc. The neurons carry little specific information regarding sensory modality or spatial properties. The activity of SNpc neurons does change in relation to behaviorally significant events such as reward or the presentation of instructional cues. The responses to stimuli only occur if the stimulus is presented in the context of a movement task. Furthermore, the activity changes with conditioning. As an example, consider an SNpc neuron that fires in relation to an unexpected reward. If one records from this neuron over several trials while the reward is paired with a tone that precedes the reward, the SNpc neuron will gradually stop firing in relation to the reward and instead will begin to fire in relation to the tone that predicts the reward.

Thus, it appears that SNpc DA neurons can predict the occurrence of a behavioral event. In this way, SNpc neurons are similar to the TANs neurons described earlier. Remember that SNpc neurons also synapse extensively on medium spiny striatal neurons and that DA terminals are on the shafts of dendritic spines. It has been suggested that the DA input changes the sensitivity of striatal neurons to cortical inputs that terminate on the heads of dendritic spines. If so, the activity of SNpc neurons could modify the response of striatal neurons to cortical input that occurs in a specific behavioral context. Such influences may be related to the apparent ability of DA to mediate both long-term potentiation and long-term depression in striatal neurons, which in turn is likely to be an important mediator of learning and plasticity in the striatum (see Chapters 50 and 51).

Summary

Several general statements about basal ganglia movement-related neuronal discharge can be made.

1. Movement-related neurons in the striatum, STN, GP, and SNpr are arranged somatotopically.
2. Neurons in the striatum are quiet at rest and increase during movement. Neurons in STN are tonically active and increase during movement. Recalling the anatomy, this means that GPi neurons receive a widespread, tonically active excitatory input and a focused, intermittent inhibitory input.
3. Neurons in both GPe and GPi are tonically active. Most increase activity, but up to one-third decrease activity during limb movement.
4. Neurons in SNpr are also tonically active. Those that are related to saccadic eye movements decrease activity during the movement.
5. Neurons in SNpc discharge in relation to rewards and behaviorally relevant stimuli, but not to movement. They are likely to play a critical role in some types of motor learning.
6. Changes in the activity of basal ganglia occur at the onset of movement but after the muscles are already active. Thus, they are unlikely to initiate movement.

THE EFFECT OF BASAL GANGLIA DAMAGE ON BEHAVIOR

Valuable clues to the function of the basal ganglia have come from recording the activity of single neurons during behavior. However, correlation of neural activity with an aspect of behavior does not necessarily mean that neural activity causes that aspect of behavior. To better determine the role of the basal ganglia in behavior, one would want to selectively remove a specific component from an otherwise intact system. Certain human neurological diseases involve the degeneration of neurons in the basal ganglia. Historically, these diseases fueled great interest and have provided some insight into basal ganglia function. The movement disorders that result from basal ganglia damage are often dramatic. Depending on the site of the pathology, some basal ganglia diseases cause extreme slowness of movement and rigidity and others cause uncontrollable involuntary movements. Although human diseases are of great interest, they often affect more than one structure. This necessarily limits the power of functional models derived from the study of human basal ganglia diseases. In experimental animals, more selective lesions can be made, but until recently it was difficult to reproduce the movement disorders associated with human basal ganglia disease.

Experimental lesions can be made in a number of ways. Permanent lesions can be made by passing electric current through an electrode to destroy both cell bodies and axons in the area surrounding the electrode. This has the disadvantage of destroying axon fibers that are passing through the area but which are not necessarily part of the structure of interest. Injection of a small amount of certain toxic chemicals into the brain (e.g., kainic acid or ibotenic acid) results in the focal death of neurons with cell bodies in the area of the injection but axons passing through the area are spared. Agonists and antagonists of the GABA have been injected into to the brain to cause temporary, focal inactivation or disinhibition of neurons. The effect of these chemicals lasts for several hours followed by complete return to the normal state. Later we discuss the use of toxins to produce a third type of lesion, one that can remove a particular type of neurons, while leaving others intact. This section reviews the results of selective basal ganglia lesions in animals produced by a variety of techniques. We discuss human basal ganglia diseases in the context of these experiments.

Damage to the Striatum Causes Slow Voluntary Movements or Involuntary Postures and Movements

Lesions in the striatum produce variable results that depend on the location of the lesion, the lesion method, and what is measured. Many studies of unilateral striatal lesions have described only minimal deficits. If the putamen is inactivated pharmacologically with the GABA agonist muscimol unilaterally, the result is slightly slow movement of the contralateral limb. The slowed movement is associated with an increased activity of antagonist muscles. Although movement is slow after putamen lesions, reaction time is generally normal, indicating movement initiation is intact. Large bilateral electrolytic lesions result in the paucity of movement, severe slowness of movement bilaterally, and postural abnormalities. In other studies, there appears to be little effect of bilateral electrolytic putamen lesions. The reason for this discrepancy is not clear, but it may be due to differences in lesion size.

Huntington's disease (HD) is a genetically based, degenerative disease in humans that results in disabling involuntary movements. These movements are called chorea (Greek for "dance"). They are frequent, brief, sudden, random twitch-like movements that involve all parts of the body and resemble fragments of normal voluntary movement. As the disease progresses, muscular rigidity appears. Despite the excessive involuntary movements, the voluntary movements of patients with HD are slower than normal. The pathologic hallmark of HD is a marked loss of neurons in the striatum. Studies have shown that not all striatal neurons are equally affected in HD (Albin et al., 1989). In early adult-onset HD, the enkephalin-containing neurons that project to GPe are lost first. Clinically, this is associated with the presence of chorea. In late adult-onset and in juvenile-onset HD, both the enkephalin-containing and the substance P-containing striatal neurons that project to GPi and SNpr are lost. Clinically, this loss is associated with the presence of rigidity and dystonia (sustained, abnormal postures). Interestingly, experimental destructive lesions of the striatum in monkeys do not result in chorea. This is probably due to the nonselective destruction of both GPe- and GPi projecting striatal neurons. More selective disruption of the striatal–GPe pathway with a GABA antagonist administered into the GPe does produce chorea. The suggested mechanism for chorea is that disinhibition of GPe neurons (pharmacologically, or as a result of selective striatal cell death) causes inhibition of STN and GPi. This results in abnormal overactivity of motor cortical and brain stem mechanisms, resulting in chorea.

Damage to STN Causes Large-Scale Involuntary Movements

In monkeys and humans, electrolytic or pharmacological lesions in the STN cause dramatic involuntary flinging movements of the contralateral arm and leg. These movements have been called hemiballismus. They resemble chorea in their brief, random, and sudden nature, but they tend to be much larger in amplitude. After a lesion in STN, the hemiballism lasts for days to weeks before gradually resolving. Animals and humans with hemiballism can still make voluntary movements and often the voluntary movements appear to be quite normal. It has been suggested that the mechanism underlying the hemiballism is a loss of excitatory input to GPi, resulting in decreased GPi activity and ultimately in the disinhibition of cortical and brain stem motor mechanisms (Albin et al., 1989). Several lines of evidence support this. First, blocking the excitatory transmission from STN to GPi with a glutamate antagonist administered into GPi causes involuntary movements. Second, metabolic activity patterns as shown with 2-deoxyglucose uptake indicate decreased GPi output in hemiballism. Third, neuronal recording during stereotaxic surgical treatment of movement disorders has shown decreased GPi activity in patients with chorea or hemiballism. However, it is likely that chorea or hemiballism is due to abnormal patterns of basal ganglia output signals and not just tonically decreased activity. Thus, if hemiballism or chorea is produced by an STN lesion in monkeys, a second lesion placed in GPi abolishes the involuntary movements. Furthermore, in monkeys with STN lesions, the level of GPi activity is reduced even after the involuntary movements resolve. Finally, destruction of GPi in humans with hemiballism or chorea abolishes the involuntary movements and experimental lesions of GPi in monkeys but do not cause chorea. Therefore, it seems likely that chorea and hemiballism reflect an abnormal fluctuating or bursting output from the basal ganglia rather than a simple reduction of output.

Damage to GP Causes Slow Voluntary Movements and Involuntary Postures and Does Not Delay Movement Initiation

Lesions of the GPi result in slowing of movement but normal movement initiation. Because of their close proximity to each other, it is difficult to lesion GPi without including part of GPe or vice versa. Therefore, caution must be used in interpreting results of GP lesions. However, in most cases, combined GPe and GPi lesions have a similar effect to the lesion of GPi alone. Unilateral lesions of GPe and GPi result in slowness of movement, with abnormal cocontraction of agonist and antagonist muscles, but normal initiation of movement. Bilateral lesions of GPe and GPi result in even more severely abnormal flexed postures with an apparent inability to move out of them. Electrolytic lesions producing this severe abnormality have tended to be large, involving both GPe and GPi and part of the internal capsule. Similar abnormalities are seen with carbon monoxide or carbon disulfide poisoning, which results in neuron death in GPi and SNpr.

Lesions restricted to GPi result in slowness of movement of the contralateral limbs. After GPi lesions, reaction time is normal, which indicates that mechanisms involved in the initiation of movement are intact. In some studies, the slowness of movement is accompanied by a cocontraction of agonist and antagonist muscles, which results in rigidity. In most cases, there is relatively more activity of flexor muscles that is reflected in a tendency of the limbs to assume an abnormally flexed posture. Monkeys with GPi lesions are more impaired when movements are

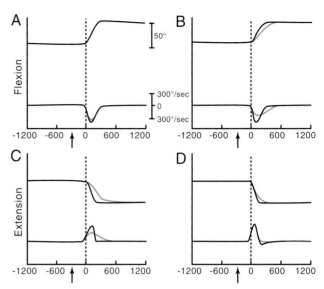

FIGURE 31.11 Wrist position and velocity in visually guided wrist movements before (black traces) and after (blue traces) a lesion of the globus pallidus internal segment. In each graph, the top traces represent wrist position, the lower traces represent wrist velocity. (A) Flexion with the flexor muscles loaded (movement made by further activating the loaded muscles). (B) Flexion with extensor muscles loaded (movement made by turning off the loaded muscles). (C) Extension with flexor muscles loaded (movement made by turning off the loaded muscles). (D) Extension with extensor muscles loaded (movement made by further activating the loaded muscles). After the lesion, the peak velocity was slower when the movements were made by decreasing the activity of the loaded muscle than when made by increasing the activity of the loaded muscle. From Mink and Thach (1991).

made by turning off active muscles than when movements are made by further turning on active muscles (Mink and Thach, 1991) (Fig. 31.11). Thus, lesions that remove the inhibitory output of the basal ganglia appear to interfere with the ability to turn off unwanted muscle activity.

Damage to SNpr Causes Involuntary Eye Movements

Due to its proximity to SNpc, it is difficult to produce electrolytic lesions exclusively in SNpr. However, with the use of the GABA agonist muscimol, it has been possible to inactivate neurons focally in SNpr. Injection of muscimol into the lateral SNpr inactivates neurons that are normally involved in saccadic eye movements. Inactivation in this area results in an inability to maintain visual fixation because of involuntary saccades (Fig. 31.12). The inability to suppress involuntary saccades appears to result from disinhibition of the superior colliculus. Injection of the GABA antagonist bicuculline into the superior colliculus

A

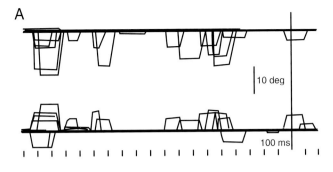

B

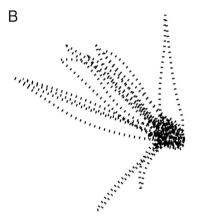

FIGURE 31.12 After inactivation of substantia nigra pars reticulata, monkeys are unable to maintain fixation of gaze because of involuntary contraction of the eye muscles. (A) The top line represents vertical eye position, and the bottom line represents horizontal eye position during attempted visual fixation. (B) Lines represent the trajectory of the involuntary eye movement when the monkey was instructed to maintain its gaze in the center dot. From Hikosaka and Wurtz (1985).

mimics the effects of muscimol in SNpr. Thus, just as GPi inactivation results in abnormal excess limb and trunk muscle activity, SNpr inactivation results in abnormal excess eye movements.

Damage to SNpc Causes Symptoms of Parkinson's Disease

Lesions of SNpc are of particular interest because the DA neurons in this nucleus die in Parkinson's disease (PD). PD is a neurological disease that affects older adults. The main symptoms of PD are (1) tremor at rest that decreases during movement, (2) slowness of movement (bradykinesia), (3) paucity of movement (akinesia), (4) muscular rigidity, and (5) unstable posture. The primary pathology in PD is a progressive degeneration of neurons in the SNpc. Additionally, there is some degree of loss of DA neurons in the ventral tegmental area and of norepinephrine neurons in the locus coeruleus. Although PD has been recognized for over a century, it has only been since the

early 1980s that a complete animal model has been available. As noted earlier, the interdigitation of SNpc and SNpr has made selective electrolytic lesions of SNpc or SNpr difficult to produce. In the 1960s, it was found that 6-hydroxydopamine (6-OHDA) produces specific lesions of catecholamine neurons. Therefore, injection of 6-OHDA into the rat SN bilaterally produces a selective loss of SNpc DA neurons. Lesions made in this way result in some of the abnormalities of PD, namely the slowness of movement and rigidity, but they did not produce tremor. In the 1980s, a street drug contaminant called MPTP (see Box 31.3) was found to produce all of the symptoms of PD in humans and in certain species of monkeys. The MPTP monkey has proven an extremely valuable model with which to explore this disease.

Despite extensive investigation, the fundamental mechanism of the tremor in PD is not known. Some evidence suggests that it results from abnormal bursting of neurons in the thalamus. The slowness of movement in PD has been associated with a reduced magnitude and duration of muscle activity during movement. In monkeys that have been given 6-OHDA or MPTP, the activity of motor cortex neurons during arm movements is also reduced compared with normal monkeys. In the MPTP monkey model of PD, some animals have abnormally increased activity of STN and GPi and decreased activity of GPi. GPi neurons in the MPTP monkey have abnormal bursting activity and abnormally increased responses to somatosensory stimuli. It has been suggested that the increased activity of GPi causes an excess inhibition of motor mechanisms in the cortex and brain stem and that this excess inhibition causes movements to be slow (Albin et al., 1989). However, it has been argued that the abnormal patterns of GPi activity may be more important than the more modest increase in tonic activity.

The rigidity of PD has been attributed in part to hyperactivity of the transcortical stretch reflex. Normally, the transcortical stretch reflex is active to resist displacement from an actively held posture. It is inhibited when subjects are instructed not to resist the displacement. People with PD have abnormally increased transcortical stretch reflexes and are unable to suppress them in response to instruction. The inability to inhibit long-loop reflexes may also account for the postural instability of PD. Patients with PD have an inappropriate cocontraction of leg and back muscles in response to perturbation from an upright stance. When the same subjects perturbed from a sitting position, they are not able to inhibit the postural reflexes that were active during stance. This suggests that the mechanism of rigidity and postural

BOX 31.2

PARKINSON'S DISEASE

Parkinson's disease (PD) is the second most common progressive neurodegenerative disorder. Patients with PD experience slowness of movement, rigidity, a low-frequency rest tremor, and difficulty with balance. These major motoric features of PD are due to the degeneration of dopamine (DA) containing neurons in the substantia nigra pars compacta (SNC) with an accompanying loss of DA and its metabolites in the striatum. PD patients may exhibit other symptoms, including cognitive dysfunction, depression, anxiety, autonomic problems, and disturbances of sleep, which may be due to the degeneration of non-DA-containing neurons. PD is characterized pathologically by the cytoplasmic accumulation of aggregated proteins with a halo of radiating fibrils and a less defined core known as Lewy bodies. Measures of increased oxidative stress are also seen, including glutathione depletion, iron deposition, increased markers of lipid peroxidation, oxidative DNA damage and protein oxidation, and decreased expression and activity of mitochondrial complex 1 in the SNC. This mitochondrial complex 1 defect is specific to the SNC, as it has not been observed in other neurodegenerative diseases. Thus, in sporadic PD, oxidative stress and mitochondrial dysfunction appear to play prominent roles in the death of DA neurons. The majority of PD appears to be sporadic in nature, however, an estimated 10% of cases are familial, with specific genetic defects. The identification of these rare genes and their functions has provided tremendous insight into the pathogenesis of PD and opened up new areas of investigation.

Two genes have been clearly linked to PD: α-synuclein and parkin. α-Synuclein is a presynaptic protein and a primary component of Lewy bodies. Very rare missense mutations at A53T and A30P cause autosomal-dominant PD. How derangements in α-synuclein lead to dysfunction and death of neurons is not known. However, aggregation and fibrillization are thought to play a central role, perhaps leading to a dysfunction in protein handling by inhibiting the proteasome. The second "PD gene" parkin is an E3 ligase for the ubiquitination of proteins. Mutations in parkin include exonic deletions, insertions, and several missense mutations and result in autosomal recessive PD. Parkin mutations are now considered to be one of the major causes of familial PD. Substrates for parkin include the synaptic vesicle-associated protein CDCrel-1, which may regulate synaptic vesicle release in the nervous system. Whether CDCrel-1 is involved in the release of dopamine is not yet known. Synphilin-1 is a protein of unknown function that was identified as an α-synuclein

interacting protein. It is a synaptic vesicle-enriched protein and is present in Lewy bodies. Synphilin-1 is a target of parkin, and expression of synphilin-1 with α-synuclein results in the formation of Lewy body-like aggregates that are ubiquitinated in the presence of parkin. Parkin is upregulated by unfolded protein stress, and expression of parkin suppresses unfolded protein stress-induced toxicity. The unfolded putative G-protein-coupled transmembrane receptor, the parkin-associated, endothelial-like receptor (Pael-R), is a parkin substrate. When overexpressed, Pael-R becomes unfolded, insoluble, and causes unfolded protein-induced cell death. Parkin ubiquitinates Pael-R, and coexpression of parkin results in protection against Pael-R-induced cell toxicity. Pael-R accumulates in the brains of autosomal-recessive Parkinson's disease patients and thus may be an important parkin substrate.

Ultimately, it would be of interest to link all the multiple genes and the sporadic causes of PD into a common pathogenic biochemical pathway. Derangements in protein handling seem to be central in the pathogenesis of familial PD. Oxidative stress seems to play a prominent role in sporadic PD, and oxidative stress leads to synuclein aggregation and/or proteasomal dysfunction. Data suggest that there may be selective derangements in the proteasomal system in the substantia nigra of sporadic PD. Thus, protein mishandling may be central to the pathogenesis of PD.

In contrast to most other neurodegenerative disorders, there is effective temporary symptomatic treatment for PD consisting of DA replacement with levodopa or DA agonists and adjunctive medications or surgical approaches. Because the neurodegeneration in PD is progressive and there is no proven preventative, restorative, or regenerative therapy, patients eventually become quite disabled. Ultimately, to affect a true cure, the underlying mechanisms of neuronal cell death need to be understood, strategies for enhancing neuronal survival and regrowth need to be developed, and consideration needs to be made toward the replacement of cells lost during the degenerative process. If these goals can be obtained, a full recovery could be achieved.

Valina L. Dawson and Ted M. Dawson

Adapted from Dawson T. M. (2000). "New Animal Models for Parkinson's Disease." *Cell* **101**(2), 115–118.
Adapted from Zhang Y., Dawson V. L., Dawson T. M., "Oxidative Stress and Genetics in the Pathogenesis of Parkinson's Disease." *Neurobiol. Dis.* **7**(4), 240–250.

THE MPTP STORY

Up until the early 1980s, the quest for a complete animal model of Parkinson's disease (PD) was largely unsuccessful. Although some of the abnormalities of PD could be cause by electrolytic lesion of SNpc or by injecting the neurotoxin 6-hydroxydopamine into SNpc, neither of these methods produced the full syndrome of PD. Then, in 1982 an unfortunate, but fortuitous, accident happened. Four young drug users in northern California developed symptoms of PD. Because PD is highly unusual in young adults, the neurologists caring for these patients began a search for the cause (Langston *et al.*, 1983). They discovered that each of the patients had recently obtained a "new" synthetic heroin. This "new heroin" contained an analog of the arcotic meperidine, 1-methyl-4-phenyl-proprionoxy-piperidine (MPPP), and a contaminant, 1-methyl-4-phenyl-1,2,5,6-tetrahydropyridine (MPTP). It turned out that MPTP was the agent responsible for the parkinsonism. MPTP is oxidized in the brain to MPP^+ by monoamine oxidase. MPP^+ is taken up by DA neurons where it inhibits oxidative metabolism in the mitochondria and ultimately leads to cell death.

Subsequently, it has been found that MPTP produces a Parkinson's-like syndrome in several species of monkeys. Unlike previous models, monkeys given MPTP had not only slowness of movement, paucity of movement, and rigidity, but also tremor. The Parkinson's-like syndrome in monkeys given MPTP is associated with a nearly complete degeneration of DA neurons in SNpc and the ventral tegmental area and variable degeneration in the locus coeruleus. MPTP monkeys improve when given the DA precursor L-DOPA and have side effects of chorea when they are given too much L-DOPA, similar to what happens in people with PD. Hence, by behavioral, pharmacological, and pathological measures, the MPTP monkey is an excellent model of human PD. It is currently used to study the pathophysiology and pharmacology of PD and it has lead to new ideas about possible causes of PD. One such idea is that environmental toxins may play a role in the etiology of PD. In this regard, it is important to note that paraquat and rotenone, two compounds that are used commonly as pesticides and/or herbicides, both have MPTP-like structures and have also been shown to damage DA neurons.

Jonathan W. Mink

Reference

Langston, J. W., Ballard, P., *et al.* (1983). Chronic parkinsonism in humans due to a product of meperidine-analog synthesis. *Science* **219**, 979–980.

instability may be similar and that they reflect an inability to suppress unwanted reflex activity.

Paradoxically, it is known that lesions of GPi or STN can ameliorate many or all of the signs and symptoms of PD without producing the abnormalities associated with lesions in these areas in normal animals or humans. This is particularly paradoxical for GPi lesions that can produce the signs of PD (flexed posture, slow movement, rigidity) in normal monkeys and in some rare human diseases, but can reduce or eliminate those signs in monkeys and humans with preexisting lesions of the DA system. Why this is the case is not known, but it may relate to long-term changes in basal ganglia physiology that result from chronic DA depletion. Chronic, high-frequency stimulation of the STN or GPi has been found to be effective for the treatment of symptoms in advanced PD. This has been called deep brain stimulation (DBS). The mechanisms by which DBS works are not well understood, but it is thought that high-frequency stimulation disrupts neural transmission and thus mimics a lesion in the stimulated area. The growth of neurosurgical treatment of PD is a direct result of knowledge about basal ganglia circuitry.

Summary

1. Damage to any basal ganglia structure may cause slowness of voluntary movement, involuntary movements, involuntary postures, or a combination of these.
2. Damage to the striatum causes voluntary movements to be slow and may produce involuntary movements or postures depending on the mechanism of damage.
3. Damage to the STN causes large amplitude involuntary limb movements.
4. Damage to the GP causes slowness of movement, abnormal postures, and difficulty relaxing muscles, but does not delay movement initiation.

5. Damage to SNpr causes abnormal eye movements, but does not delay the initiation of eye movements.

6. Damage to SNpc causes tremor at rest, slowness of movement, rigidity, and postural instability, which are the main features of PD.

FUNDAMENTAL PRINCIPLES OF BASAL GANGLIA OPERATION FOR MOTOR CONTROL

How do the basal ganglia participate in motor control? Several hypotheses have been advanced over the past century, many of which have been mutually contradictory. This has been due in part to models that infer normal function from the abnormalities resulting from basal ganglia disease. There is growing consensus that models based on human disease states may not be sufficient to explain normal basal ganglia function. Regardless, the models based on human disease have been useful in developing new treatments for movement disorders and for the development of testable hypotheses relating to basal ganglia function.

An old model of basal ganglia function is that the basal ganglia initiate movement. This model was based in large part on the manifestation of basal ganglia diseases. The paucity and slowness of movement in PD were attributed to an inability to initiate movements, whereas the involuntary movements of chorea and hemiballism were attributed to a release of normal motor systems from basal ganglia control. This model gained support from the fact that much of the output from the basal ganglia goes to parts of the thalamus that project to the premotor and motor cortex. It was argued that motor programs are stored in the basal ganglia and are called up and sent to the motor cortex for execution. This model is no longer widely accepted because it is now apparent that basal ganglia are active relatively late in relation to movement and to the activation of those brain mechanisms that are known to be involved in initiation. Furthermore, lesions of basal ganglia output do not delay the initiation of movement.

If basal ganglia do not initiate movement, what do they do? We consider three current hypotheses. One hypothesis states that although basal ganglia do not initiate movement, they contribute to the automatic execution of movement sequences. This hypothesis suggests that other mechanisms initiate the first component in a sequence, but that basal ganglia contain the programs for completion of the sequence. The second hypothesis states that the basal ganglia circuitry is made up of opposing parallel pathways that

adjust the magnitude of the inhibitory GPi output in order to increase or decrease movement. According to this hypothesis, increased GPi output slows movements and decreased GPi output increases movement. The third hypothesis states that basal ganglia act to permit desired movements and to inhibit unwanted competing movements.

Do Basal Ganglia Automatically Generate Learned Movement Sequences?

A popular hypothesis states that basal ganglia are responsible for the automatic execution of learned movement sequences (Marsden, 1987). It has been pointed out that patients with PD have difficulty moving several body parts simultaneously or sequentially, and that this difficulty is more than one would expect from a simple addition of the deficits of each component of the movement. An example of an apparent problem with sequential movements in PD is the phenomenon of micrographia (or small writing). A patient begins to write a sentence with nearly normal-sized writing, but within several letters, the writing begins to get smaller so that by the end of the sentence, it may be illegible. It has been emphasized that the early components of the sequence are larger and faster than are the subsequent components. One experiment compared the performance of elbow flexion and hand grip individually or in sequence (Benecke et al., 1986). Patients with PD performed each movement more slowly than normal subjects. However, when the movement was part of a sequence, it was slowed to an even greater degree than when it was performed separately. Another experiment involved recording the activity of GPi neurons in monkeys trained to perform two successive prompt wrist movements. It was found that some GPi neurons fired after the first component of the movement but before the second component (Brotchie et al., 1991). Proponents of the sequencing hypothesis speculate that the loss of this GPi output signal in PD is responsible for the relatively greater difficulty in producing sequential movements than in producing individual movements.

Do Basal Ganglia Produce or Prevent Movement by Using Opposing Direct and Indirect Parallel Pathways?

This hypothesis emphasizes the two major paths of information flow from the striatum to GPi and SNpr that were described earlier (Fig 31.13) (Alexander and Crutcher, 1990). To recapitulate, one is an inhibitory "direct" pathway from striatum to GPi/SNpr and the other is a net excitatory "indirect" pathway from stria-

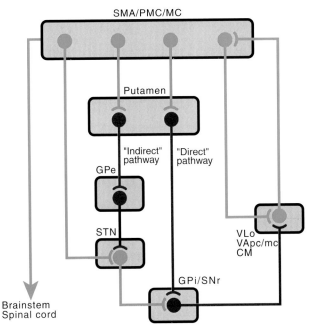

FIGURE 31.13 Schematic of proposed "direct" and "indirect" pathways from putamen to GPi. See the text for a description. Red symbols represent inhibitory pathways, and green symbols represent excitatory pathways. From Alexander and Crutcher (1990).

tum to GPe (inhibitory), from GPe to STN (inhibitory), and from STN to GPi/SNpr (excitatory). In this hypothesis, the two pathways are in balance in such a way that increased activity in the "direct" pathway causes decreased GPi/SNpr output and increased activity in the "indirect" pathway causes increased GPi/SNpr output. By adjusting the balance, cortical targets of the basal ganglia can be facilitated or inhibited. The hypothesis predicts that abnormally decreased output results in excessive movements (chorea) and abnormally increased output results in a decreased movement (PD). The "direct/indirect pathway" model has been useful for understanding and developing certain treatments of movement disorders, but it has several shortcomings when it comes to explaining normal basal ganglia function and the mechanism of treatments for involuntary movements. Despite the shortcomings, this has been a central hypothesis in the field of basal ganglia research for over 20 years. If the success of a model can be measured by the amount of research it stimulates, this one has been highly successful.

Do Basal Ganglia Select and Inhibit Competing Motor Patterns?

The output of the basal ganglia is inhibitory to posture and movement pattern generators in the cerebral cortex (via thalamus) and in the brain stem. The inhibitory output neurons fire tonically at high fre-

quencies. In this hypothesis, the motor output of the basal ganglia is analogous to a brake (Mink, 1996). The hypothesis states that when a movement is initiated by a particular motor pattern generator, GPi neurons projecting to that generator decrease their discharge, thereby removing tonic inhibition and

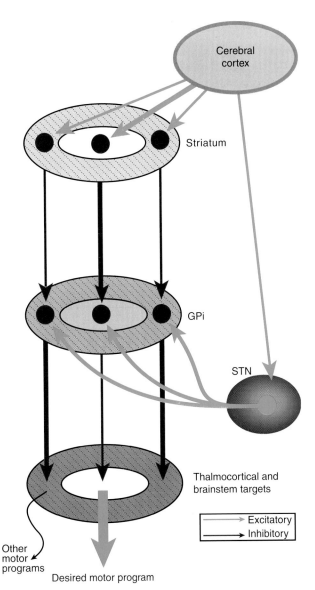

FIGURE 31.14 Relationship of proposed center-surround organization of GPi to inputs from the striatum and subthalamic nucleus. During voluntary movement, excitatory subthalamo-pallidal neurons increase the activity of the pallidal neurons in the surround territory. Inhibitory striatopallidal neurons inhibit the functional center in a focused manner. Pallidal activity changes are conveyed to the targets in the thalamus and midbrain brain stem, causing disinhibition of neurons involved in the desired motor program and inhibition of surrounding neurons involved in competing motor programs. Excitatory projections are indicated with green arrows; inhibitory projections are indicated with red arrows. The relative magnitude of activity is represented by line thickness.

"releasing the brake" on that generator. GPi neurons projecting to other movement pattern generators increase their firing rate, thereby increasing inhibition and applying a "brake" on those generators. Thus, other postures and movements are prevented from interfering with the one selected.

How might this mechanism work (Fig 31.14)? When one makes a voluntary movement, that movement is initiated by the prefrontal, premotor, and motor cortex and by the cerebellum. The premotor and motor cortex send a corollary signal to STN, exciting it. STN projects to GPi in a widespread pattern and excites GPi. In parallel, signals are sent from the cortex to the striatum, which inhibits GPi focally via a direct pathway. Striatum can also disinhibit GPi via two indirect pathways (striatum → GPe → GPi and striatum → GPe → STN → GPi). The indirect pathways further focus the effects of the fast excitatory cortico-STN pathway and the slower inhibitory cortico-striatal pathway to GPi. The net result is to release the "brake" from the selected voluntary movement pattern generator and to apply the "brake" to potentially competing posture-holding pattern generators (transcortical, vestibular, tonic neck, and other postural reflexes). The result is the focused selection of desired motor patterns and surround inhibition of competing patterns.

BASAL GANGLIA PARTICIPATION IN NONMOTOR FUNCTIONS

Although the focus of this chapter has been on motor control, it has become increasingly clear that the basal ganglia participate in a variety of nonmotor functions. These include functions of the limbic system (see Box 31.3 and Chapters 44 and 45) and cognitive functions. The anatomy of basal ganglia circuits has revealed outputs going to all areas of frontal cortex, placing the basal ganglia in a position to influence a wide variety of behaviors. As discussed earlier, specific areas of the basal ganglia are connected preferentially with specific areas of the cerebral cortex. This provides the anatomic substrate for the localization of different functions in the basal ganglia circuits. It is known that focal lesions of the striatum tend to produce deficits similar to those seen after lesions of afferent areas of the cortex. Thus, lesions of posterior putamen cause movement deficits, lesions of inferior caudate produce deficits similar to lesions of the orbitofrontal cortex, and lesions of the dorsolateral caudate produce deficits similar to lesions of dorsolateral prefrontal cortex. The basal ganglia have been implicated in a variety of nonmotor disorders, including depression, obsessive-compulsive disorder (see Box 31.4), attention deficit hyperactivity disorder, and schizophrenia. Regardless of the type of function, it is becoming clear that the basic underlying principles of basal ganglia function are similar. Thus, the intrinsic circuitry is the same for cognitive and motor parts of the basal ganglia, the basic neurophysiology appears to be the same, and the effects of lesions are analogous. For example, chorea is characterized by excessive involuntary movements, and obsessive-compulsive disorder is characterized by excessive involuntary thoughts and complex behaviors. The hypothesis of focused selec-

---

BOX 31.4

VENTRAL SYSTEM OF THE BASAL GANGLIA

There are nuclei in the brain that historically have not been included with the basal ganglia, but that are analogous to the traditional components. These lie ventral to the neostriatum and GP and are called the ventral striatum (nucleus accumbens and olfactory tubercle) and the ventral pallidum. The ventral striatum receives input from limbic and olfactory areas of the cortex, including the amygdala and hippocampus. Like the neostriatum, the ventral striatum receives a *DA* input, but it is from the ventral tegmental area (VTA), which lies medial to the SN. The ventral striatum sends a projection back to VTA and to the adjacent SNpr. The ventral pallidum is analogous to both GPe and GPi. It receives input from the ventral striatum and possibly from STN. Unlike the GP, the ventral pallidum receives direct input from the amygdala. The output of the ventral pallidum projects to the dorsomedial nucleus of the thalamus (DM) and from there to limbic areas of the cortex. By virtue of its inputs and outputs, the ventral system is closely linked to the limbic system. This linkage has led to the suggestion that the ventral system is involved to some degree in motivation and emotion (see Chapter 43). The exact nature of this role is not known, but it may be analogous to the motor role of the basal ganglia, with the inhibitory output of the ventral pallidum acting to suppress or select potentially competing limbic mechanisms.

Lesions of the ventral pallidum lead to an inability to inhibit incorrect responses in an odor discrimination task, supporting the hypothesis.

Jonathan W. Mink

BOX 31.5

HUNTINGTON'S DISEASE

Huntington's disease (HD) is an inherited progressive neurodegenerative disorder that affects about 1 in 10,000 people. Symptoms include abnormal movements (comprising both involuntary movements termed chorea or dystonia and motor incoordination), cognitive difficulties, and emotional difficulties, including depression, apathy, and irritability. Onset is usually in midlife, but can range between childhood and old age. HD is generally fatal within 15 to 20 years after onset. The disease is caused by an expanded CAG repeat coding for polyglutamine in the HD gene product, termed the "huntingtin" protein. CAG repeat lengths between about 10 and 25 are normal, whereas those above 36 cause HD. Within the expanded range, the longer the repeat, the earlier the age of onset. The normal function of huntingtin is poorly understood, but it may be involved with cytoskeletal function, or cellular transport.

Pathologically, HD is characterized by selective neuronal vulnerability. The caudate and putamen of the corpus striatum are most affected in early stages, but as the disease progresses, other areas of the brain also become affected. Within the striatum, medium spiny GABA neurons are severely affected, with up to 95% loss in advanced cases, whereas large interneurons are relatively spared. In addition, there are intranuclear inclusion bodies and perinuclear and neuritic aggregates of huntingtin in HD neurons.

The pathogenesis of HD is still incompletely understood and represents a challenge for neuroscience. The huntingtin protein is widely expressed throughout the brain and is expressed at lower levels in other regions of the body as well. HD, like other neurodegenerative diseases, involves abnormal protein folding and aggregation. The inclusions themselves appear not to be directly toxic, but they likely represent a late stage of an abnormal process, whose earlier steps are pathogenic. The study of the disease has been facilitated by the generation of cell models, invertebrate models, and mouse models. Chaperone proteins can ameliorate the pathology, perhaps by refolding abnormally folded huntingtin. Huntingtin may normally be degraded by intracellular proteolytic machinery, termed the proteasome, and inhibition of the proteosome may be one of the toxic effects of the abnormally expanded polyglutamine.

A number of lines of evidence have pointed to a possible role for abnormal gene transcription in HD. Several studies have suggested that targeting of huntingtin to the nucleus enhances toxicity. Huntingtin may normally have a role in regulation of gene transcription, although this is poorly understood. Expression array studies show that mouse and cell models have an alteration of normal gene expression patterns. Abnormal intereactions with coactivator and corepressor complexes may contribute.

Whatever the initial mechanisms, symptoms appear to be caused by both cell dysfunction and cell death, with cell death correlating best with functional disability. Thus, preventing cell death is a major goal of experimental therapeutics in HD and other neurodegenerative disorders. Cell death may partly involve apoptotic mechanisms with activation of caspases and may also involve mechanisms such as excitotoxicity, metabolic, or free radical stress. Therapeutic strategies under investigation include protection of neurons with neurotrophins, altering abnormal gene transcription patterns, and reducing cell death with inhibitors of caspase activation or blockers of excitotoxicity.

Christopher A. Ross

tion and surround inhibition has been applied to nonmotor basal ganglia functions (Redgrave *et al.*, 1999) and data support each hypothesis from cognitive science and psychiatric research.

There is increasing evidence for a role of the basal ganglia in procedural learning. Much of the research has focused on the learning of tasks or of sequential behavior. There is evidence for a role of the basal ganglia in procedural learning that leads to the formation of habits and the performance of behavioral routines once they are learned (Jog *et al.*, 1999). As described earlier, TANs and SNpc DA neurons fire in relation to behaviorally significant events. The activity patterns of these neurons change as the task becomes learned and when novel stimuli or events are introduced. There is also growing evidence for DA-mediated long-term potentiation and long-term depression in striatal neurons that is likely to play an important role in learning. It has been shown that non-TAN striatal neurons also change activity in relation to learning. In rats performing a T-maze task, striatal neurons changed activity patterns as the task became learned and more automatic (Jog *et al.*, 1999). In monkeys performing a discrimination learning task, striatal

BOX 31.6

OBSESSIVE-COMPULSIVE DISORDER

Obsessive-compulsive disorder (OCD) is a chronic disorder characterized by recurrent intrusive thoughts and ritualistic behaviors that consume much of the afflicted individual's attentional and goal-directed processes. Among the more agonizing illnesses in clinical medicine, OCD is classified as an anxiety disorder because of the marked tension and distress produced by resisting the obsessions and compulsions. Common obsessions involve thoughts of harming oneself or others, of being afflicted by various illnesses, or of being contaminated by germs. Compulsions may be a response to obsessive thoughts (e.g., repetitive handwashing following skin contact with any object due to obsessive worries of having contacted germs) or may instead reflect cognitive-behavioral rituals performed according to stereotyped rules (e.g., counting one's footsteps to avoid ending on certain numbers). Although individuals with OCD recognize that such thoughts and behaviors are irrational, they feel irresistibly compelled to engage in them.

The onset of OCD usually occurs between late childhood and early adulthood. Without treatment, OCD is often disabling. However, chronic treatment with drugs that potently inhibit serotonin reuptake can reduce the amount of time engaged in obsessions and compulsions and the magnitude of the associated anxiety. In addition, behavioral therapy involving repeated *in vivo* exposure and response prevention (e.g., having patients touch a toilet seat and subsequently preventing them from hand washing) may facilitate extinction of the anxiety responses generated by resisting obsessive thoughts and compulsive behaviors.

The etiology and pathophysiology of OCD are unknown. Converging evidence from analysis of the lesions that result in obsessive-compulsive symptoms, functional neuroimaging studies of OCD, and observations regarding the neurosurgical interventions that can ameliorate OCD implicate prefrontal cortical-striatal circuits in the pathogenesis of obsessions and compulsions. The neurological conditions associated with the development of secondary obsessions and compulsions include lesions of the globus pallidus and putamen, Sydenham chorea (a poststreptococcal autoimmune disorder associated with neuronal atrophy in the caudate and putamen), Tourette disorder (an idiopathic syndrome characterized by motoric and phonic tics that may have a genetic relationship with OCD, see Box 31.7), chronic motor tic disorder, and lesions of the ventromedial prefrontal cortex. Several of these conditions are associated with complex motor tics (repetitive,

coordinated, involuntary movements occurring in patterned sequences in a spontaneous, unpredictable, and transient manner). Complex tics and obsessive thoughts may thus both reflect aberrant neural processes originating in distinct portions of the cortical-striatal-pallidal-thalamic circuitry that are manifested within the motor and cognitive-behavioral domains, respectively. Compatible with this hypothesis, neurosurgical procedures that interrupt the white matter tracts carrying projections between the frontal lobe, basal ganglia, and thalamus are effective at reducing obsessive-compulsive symptoms in OCD cases that prove intractable to other treatments.

Functional neuroimaging studies have also implicated prefrontal cortical-striatal circuits in the pathophysiology of OCD. In primary OCD, "resting" cerebral blood flow and metabolism are increased abnormally in the orbitofrontal cortex and the caudate nucleus, and increase further during symptom provocation in these areas, as well as in the putamen, thalamus, and anterior cingulate cortex. During effective pharmacotherapy, orbital metabolism decreases toward normal, and both drug treatment and behavioral therapy are associated with a reduction of caudate metabolism. In contrast, imaging studies of obsessive-compulsive syndromes arising in the setting of Tourette syndrome or basal ganglia lesions have found reduced metabolism in the orbital cortex in such subjects relative to controls. Differences in the functional anatomical correlates of primary versus secondary OCD suggest that dysfunction arising at multiple points within the ventral prefrontal cortical-striatal-pallidal-thalamic circuitry may result in pathological obsessions and compulsions.

This circuitry in general appears to be involved in the organization of internally guided behavior toward a reward, switching of response strategies, habit formation, and stereotypic behavior. Electrophysiological and lesion analysis studies indicating that parts of the orbitofrontal cortex are specifically involved in the correction of behavioral responses that become inappropriate as reinforcement contingencies change. Such functions could potentially become disturbed at the level of this cortex itself or within the circuits conveying projections from the ventral PFC through the basal ganglia, conceivably giving rise to the perseverative patterns of nonreinforced thought and behavior that characterize the cognitive-behavioral state of OCD.

Wayne C. Drevets

BOX 31.6 (cont'd)

Suggested Readings

Baxter, L. R. (1995), Neuroimaging studies of human anxiety disorders. In "Psychopharmacology: The Fourth Generation of Progress" (F. E. Bloom and D. J. Kupfer, eds.), Chap. 80, pp. 921–932. Raven Press, New York.

LaPlane, D., et al. (1989). Obsessive-compulsive and other behavioural changes with bilateral basal ganglia lesions. Brain 112, 69–725.

McDougle, C. J. (1999) The neurobiology and treatment of obsessive-compulsive disorder. In "Neurobiology of Mental Illness" (D. S. Charney, E. J. Nestler, B. J. Bunney, eds.), pp. 518–533. Oxford Univ. Press, New York.

BOX 31.7

TOURETTE SYNDROME (TS)

A "tic" is a sudden, rapid, recurrent, nonrhythmic, stereotyped movement or sound. Individuals with TS exhibit prominent and persistent motor tics and at least one phonic tic, beginning in childhood. Current estimates of TS prevalence range between 0.1 and 1.0%, with a 3.51 male:female ratio. Symptoms wax and wane; roughly half of all TS patients experience a significant symptom decline in their early 20s, whereas others experience lifelong symptoms.

Tics differ in complexity (simple, complex) and domain of expression (motor, phonic). In addition to their outward manifestations, a variety of sensory and mental states are associated with tics. "Simple" sensory tics are rapid, recurrent, and stereotyped, and are sensations at or near the skin. "Premonitory urges" are more complex phenomena, which often include both sensory and psychic discomfort that may be momentarily relieved by a tic. The full elaboration of tics, therefore, can include a sequence: (1) a sensory event or premonitory urge, (2) a complex state of inner conflict over if and when to yield to the urge, (3) the motor or phonic production, and (4) a transient sensation of relief.

Functional impairment in TS often results from co-morbid conditions. More than 40% of individuals with TS experience symptoms of obsessive-compulsive disorder (OCD), and a comparable number have symptoms of attentional deficits and hyperactivity (ADHD).

Limited neuropathological evidence suggests four locations of potential pathology within cortico-striato-pallido-thalamic (CSPT) circuitry in TS: (1) intrinsic striatal neurons (increased neuronal packing density);

(2) diminished striato-pallidal "direct" output (reduced dynorphin-like immunoreactivity in the lenticular nuclei); (3) increased dopaminergic innervation of the striatum (increased density of dopamine transporter sites); and (4) reduced glutamatergic output from the STN (reduced lenticular glutamate content).

Volumetric neuroimaging studies report an enlarged corpus callosum, reduced caudate volume, or diminished striatal and lenticular asymmetry; these changes are subtle and are not replicated uniformly. Metabolic neuroimaging studies in TS report a reduced glucose uptake in the orbitofrontal cortex, caudate, parahippocampus, and midbrain regions and reduced blood flow in the caudate nucleus, anterior cingulate cortex, and temporal lobes. Regional glucose uptake patterns suggest distributed CSPT dysfunction, based on covariate relationships between reduced glucose uptake in striatal, pallidal, thalamic, and hippocampal regions. Tic suppression is associated with increased right caudate activation, measured by functional MRI, and by bilaterally diminished activity in the putamen, globus pallidus, and thalamus. Neurochemical imaging studies have reported relatively subtle abnormalities in the levels of dopamine receptors, dopamine release, DOPA decarboxylase, and dopamine transporter in the striatum of some individuals with TS. A report of greater caudate D2 receptor binding among more symptomatic TS identical twins may be relevant to factors contributing to heterogeneity of the TS phenotype.

There are a number of reported subtle abnormalities in the levels of major neurotransmitters, precursors, meta-

---

BOX 31.7 *(cont'd)*

bolites, biogenic amines, and hormones in blood, cerebrospinal fluid (CSF), and urine of TS subjects compared to controls. One qualitatively different finding is that of approximately 40% elevations of serum antiputamen antibodies in TS children. This finding may have particular importance, based on growing evidence for autoimmune contributions to at least some forms of TS.

Converging evidence for CSPT pathology in TS comes from neuropsychological and psychophysiological studies. Some forms of TS appear to be accompanied by abnormalities in sensorimotor gating, oculomotor, functions, and visuospatial priming consistent with mild cortico-striatal dysfunction.

The mode of TS inheritance remains elusive. First-degree relatives of TS probands are 20–150 times more likely to develop TS compared to unrelated individuals. Concordance rates for TS among monozygotic twins approach 90%, if the phenotypic boundaries include chronic motor or vocal tics, versus 10–25% concordance for dizygotic twins across the same boundaries. One affected sib-pair study with a total of 110 sib-pairs yielded a multipoint maximum-likelihood scores (MLS) for two regions (4q and 8p) suggestive of high sharing (MLS >2.0). Four additional regions also gave multipoint MLS scores between 1.0 and 2.0.

Treatments for TS focus on education, comorbid conditions, and direct tic suppression. Education is a critically important intervention for both family members and affected individuals. Treatments for comorbid conditions, particularly OCD and ADHD, are highly effective and can provide significant relief. Dopamine antagonists, particularly high potency, D2 preferential blockers, are the most potent and rapid acting tic-suppressing agents, but have important, undesirable side effects. Newer,

"atypical" antipsychotics are better tolerated, and some are effective in suppressing tics. The DA depleter tetrabenazine also offers significant tic suppression, but is not yet approved for use in the USA. α_2-Adrenergic agonists are often used as antitic agents; compared to dopamine antagonists, these drugs have relatively weaker antitic abilities and their benefit generally evolves more gradually. New therapeutic avenues for TS are being explored in controlled studies, including dopamine agonists such as pergolide, nicotinic manipulations, and Δ^9-tetrahydrocannabinol. Intractable, localized tics have also been treated successfully with injections of botulinum toxic. An effective nonpharmacologic therapy, habit reversal therapy, involves the application of cognitive and behavioral therapy principles to TS, analogous to the successful use of these therapies in the treatment of OCD.

Neal R. Swendlow

Suggested Readings

Cohen, D. J., Leckman, J. F., and Pauls, D. (1997). Neuropsychiatric disorders of childhood: Tourette's syndrome as a model. *Acta Paediatr.* **422**, 106–111.

Kurlan, R. (1997). Treatment of tics. *Neuro. Clin. North. Am.* **15**, 403–409.

Leckman, J. F., Walker, D. E., and Cohen, D. J. (1993). Premonitory urges in Tourette's syndrome. *Am. J. Psychiat.* **150**, 98–102.

Swerdlow, N. R., and Young, A. B. (1999). Neuropathology in Tourette syndrome. *CNS Spectrums* **4**, 65–74.

The Tourette Syndrome Association International Consortium for Genetics (1999). A complete genome screen in sib pairs affected by Gilles de la Tourette syndrome. *Am. J. Hum. Gen.* **65**, 1428–1436.

---

neurons changed activity as the animal learned new associations between stimuli and reward (Tremblay *et al.*, 1998). Functional imaging studies have also shown basal ganglia activity correlated with the learning of new tasks. Striatal lesions or focal striatal DA depletion impairs the learning of new movement sequences, and procedural learning has been shown to be impaired in people with PD. These findings together support a role for the basal ganglia in certain types of procedural learning. However, other brain structures have also been implicated in procedural learning, including the cerebellum (see Chapter 51). Just as the cerebellum and basal ganglia play different

roles in motor control, they are likely to play different, but complementary, roles in procedural learning. The exact nature of those different roles is the subject of current research.

Summary

It is appropriate to consider the basal ganglia as part of the motor system because the largest portion of the basal ganglia is devoted to motor control and the most prominent deficits resulting from basal ganglia damage are motor. However, it has become clear that the basal ganglia play substantial roles in nonmotor function and in more cognitive aspects of movement. These roles are the subject of active research. Ultimately there may be a unifying theory of basal ganglia function that will encompass all of the subdivisions, but at this point one can only say that it is likely that the different circuits employ similar mechanisms.

References

Albin, R. L., Young, A. B., et al. (1989). The functional anatomy of basal ganglia disorders. Trends Neurosci. 12(10), 366–375.

Alexander, G. E., and Crutcher, M. D. (1990). Functional architecture of basal ganglia circuits: Neural substrates of parallel processing. Trends Neurosci. 13(7), 266–271.

Alexander, G. E., DeLong, M. R., et al. (1986). Parallel organization of functionally segregated circuits linking basal ganglia and cortex. Annu. Rev. Neurosci. 9, 357–381.

Aosaki, T., Tsubokawa, H., et al. (1994). Responses of tonically active neurons in the primate's striatum undergo systematic changes during behavioral sensorimotor conditioning. J. Neurosci. 14(6), 3969–3984.

Benecke, R., Rothwell, J. C., et al. (1986). Performance of simultaneous movements in patients with Parkinson's disease. Brain 109, 739–757.

Brotchie, P., Iansek, R., et al. (1991). Motor function of the monkey globus pallidus. 2. Cognitive aspects of movement and phasic neuronal activity. Brain 114, 1685–1702.

Flaherty, A. W., and Graybiel, A. M. (1991). Corticostriatal transformations in the primate somatosensory system: Projections from phsyiologically mapped body-part representations. J. Neurophysiol. 66(4), 1249–1263.

Graybiel, A. M., Ragsdale, C. W., et al. (1981). An immunohistochemical study of enkephalins and other neuropeptides in the striatum of the cat with evidence that the opiate peptides are arranged to form mosaic pattes in register with striosomal compartments visible with acetylcholinesterase staining. Neuroscience 6, 377–397.

Haber, S. N., Fudge, J. L., et al. (2000). Striatonigrostriatal pathways in primates form an ascending spiral from the shell to the dorsolateral striatum. J. Neurosci. 20, 2369–2382.

Hoover, J. E., and Strick, P. L. (1993). Multiple output channels in the basal ganglia. Science 259, 819–821.

Jog, M., Kubota, Y., et al. (1999). Building neural representations of habits. Science 286, 1745–1749.

Langston, J. W., Ballard, P., et al. (1983). Chronic parkinsonism in humans due to a product of meperidine-analog synthesis. Science 219, 979–980.

Marsden, C. D. (1987). What do the basal ganglia tell premotor cortical areas? Ciba Found. Symp. 132, 282–300.

Mink, J. W., and Thach, W. T. (1991). Basal ganglia motor control. III. Pallidal ablation: Normal reaction time, muscle cocontraction, and slow movement. J. Neurophysiol. 65(2), 330–351.

Parent, A. and Hazrati, L.-N. (1993). Anatomical aspects of information processing in primate basal ganglia. Trends Neurosci. 16(3), 111–116.

Redgrave, P., Prescott, T., et al. (1999). The basal ganglia: A vertebrate solution to the selection problem? Neuroscience 89, 1009–1023.

Romo, R., Scarnati, E., et al. (1992). Role of primate basal ganglia and frontal cortex in the internal generation of movements. II. Movement-rlated activity in the anterior striatum. Exp. Brain Res. 91, 385–395.

Tremblay, L., Hollerman, J., et al. (1998). Modifications of reward expectation-related neuronal activity during learning in primate striatum. J. Neurophysiol. 80, 964–977.

Wilson, C. J., and Groves, P. M. (1980). Fine structure and synaptic connections of the common spiny neuron of the rat neostriatum: A study employing intracellular injection of horseradish peroxidase. J. Comp. Neurol. 194, 599–614.

Wilson, S. A. K. (1928). "Modern Problems in Neurology." Arnold, London.

Suggested Readings

Bolam, J. P., Hanley, J. J., et al. (2000). Synaptic organisation of the basal ganglia. J. Anat. 196, 527–542.

Graybiel, A. (1998). The basal ganglia and chunking of action repertoires. Neurobiol. Learn. Mem. 70, 119–136.

Hikosaka, O., Takikawa, Y., et al. (2000). Role of the basal ganglia in the control of purposive saccadic eye movements. Physiol. Rev. 80, 953–978.

Houk, J. C., Davis, J. L., et al., (eds.) (1995). Models of Information Processing in the Basal Ganglia: Computational Neuroscience. MIT Press, Cambridge, MA.

Middleton, F., and Strick, P. (2000). Basal ganglia output and cognition: Evidence from anatomical, behavioral, and clinical studies. Brain Cogn. 42, 183–200.

Mink, J. W. (1996). The basal ganglia: Focused selection and inhibition of competing motor programs. Prog. Neurobiol. 50, 381–425.

Penney, J. B., and Young, A. B. (1983). Speculations on the functional anatomy of basal ganglia disorders. Annul. Rev. Neurosci. 6, 73–94.

Watts, R. L., and Koller, W. C. (1997). "Movement Disorders: Neurologic Principles and Practice." McGraw-Hill, New York.

Jonathan W. Mink

CHAPTER

32

Cerebellum

The cerebellum (Latin for "little brain") is a strategic part of the nervous system. It contains more neurons and circuitry than all the remainder of the brain, and it packs this into only 10% of total brain weight. It covers the dorsal surface of the brain stem and comprises the largest part of the hindbrain. The important function of the cerebellum is to regulate neural signals in other parts of the brain, and it does this through loops of interaction. Currently, we know most about its regulatory actions on the populations of neurons that command movement and posture. Although the cerebellum is not necessary for the initiation of motion, movements become erratic in their size and direction when it is damaged—a symptom that clinicians call *dysmetria*. The cerebellum is an important site of motor learning, in addition to movement execution. The size of the cerebellum in mammals parallels the evolution of the cerebral cortex, and the newest regions of the cerebellum appear to regulate higher cerebral processes for motor planning, cognition, and problem solving.

OVERVIEW

The Cerebellum Has Lobes and Lobules

The cerebellum consists of three paired longitudinal subdivisions: the medial (or vermal) zone, the intermediate zone, and the lateral (or hemispheral) zones. The *vermis* (from the Latin worm) is a narrow structure that straddles the midline. On the cerebellar surface (Fig. 32.1A), the borders between the vermis and the *hemispheres* are demarcated by shallow indentations occupied by small veins. The medial part of the hemispheres bordering the vermis are called the *intermediate zones*. These zones are distinguished from the rest of the hemispheres primarily by their fiber connections.

Deep transverse fissures subdivide the cerebellum rostrocaudally into three lobes: *anterior, posterior,* and *flocculonodular* (Figs. 32.1B and 32.6). The anterior and posterior lobes together form the *corpus cerebelli*. In contrast to cerebral lobes, cerebellar lobes are continuous across the midline. Shallow fissures subdivide further cerebellar lobes into lobules. Each lobule consists of thin parallel folds called *folia* (leaves), which run roughly transverse to the long axis of the body. The lobules that appear in sagittal section are summarized in Box 32.1.

The number of folia in different lobules varies, but each folium contains a white matter core. In sagittal section, the core appears as arboreal branches departing from the roof of the fourth ventricle (Fig. 32.1C). Embedded into the deep white matter core on each side of the midline are cerebellar nuclei (CN)—the *medial nucleus*, which projects mainly to nuclei in the lower brain stem and the spinal cord; the *interpositus nucleus*, which targets the midbrain; and the *lateral nucleus*, which projects to the thalamus and onto the cerebral cortex. The interpositus nucleus consists of two subdivisions, which are usually referred to as anterior and posterior interpositus nuclei. In the human cerebellum, the corresponding four nuclei (Fig. 32.1A) are classically termed *fastigial, globose, emboliform,* and *dentate* because of their morphological appearance. These nomenclatures are sometimes used interchangeably. Beneath the cerebellum is the vestibular nuclear complex, some divisions of which receive input from the cerebellar cortex and therefore bear analogy with the CN.

Fundamental Neuroscience, Second Edition

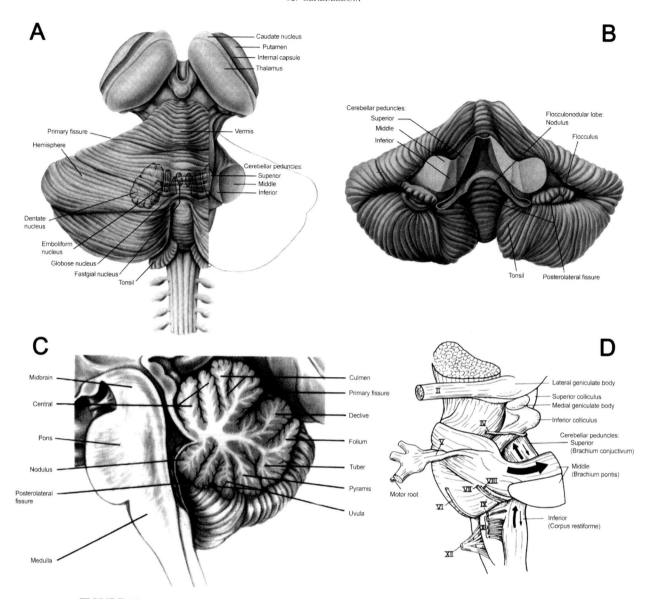

FIGURE 32.1 Gross features of the human cerebellum. (A) Dorsal view of the cerebellum and brain stem. Part of the right hemisphere has been cut out to show the cerebellar peduncles. Profiles of the four cerebellar nuclei are projected onto the cerebellar surface to indicate their position. (B) Ventral view of the cerebellum detached from the brain stem. (C) Midsagittal cut through the cerebellum and brain stem showing white matter entering the vermal lobules. (D) Left side view of the lower part of the brain stem after removal of the cerebellum to highlight routes of efferent and afferent inputs. Direction and thickness of arrows indicate directions and relative numbers of fibers in the three cerebellar peduncles. Cranial nerves are indicated by Roman numerals. (A–C) Adapted from Kandel *et al.* (2000), with permission. (D) Adapted from Brodal (1981), with permission.

The cerebellum is connected to the brain stem bilaterally by three cerebellar peduncles (Fig. 32.1D)—*superior, middle,* and *inferior* (classically termed *brachium conjunctivum, brachium pontis,* and *corpus restiforme*)—that carry information to and from the cerebellum. The superior cerebellar peduncle is mostly efferent and contains fibers from the CN to brain stem, red nucleus, hypothalamus, and thalamus; the middle cerebellar peduncle contains exclusively afferents from the contralateral pontine nuclei; and the inferior cerebellar peduncle contains afferent fibers from the brain stem and the spinal cord, as well as cerebellar efferent fibers to the vestibular nuclei.

In humans, fibers of the superior, middle, and inferior cerebellar peduncles number approximately 0.8, 20, and 0.5 million, respectively. Interestingly, the number of fibers in the massive middle cerebellar peduncle (cerebrocerebellar afferents or pontocerebellar afferents) roughly equals that of the cerebral peduncle, which carries the input of the cerebral

NOMENCLATURE FOR CEREBELLAR LOBULUES

In the classical literature, cerebellar lobules were designated by descriptive Latin names, denoting their features in humans and other mammals. Although the Latin nomenclature is still in use, a later, practical Roman numeral system has facilitated comparative neurology. According to this system, **lobules are numbered I–X** beginning at the inferior anterior vermis and ending at the inferior posterior vermis. In most mammals, each lobule contains a number of folia. The anterior lobe consists of lobules I–V, the posterior lobe of lobules IV–IX, and the flocculonodular lobe of lobulus X. Lobulation is fairly consistent across individuals of the same species and extends with few exceptions across all mammalian species, despite great variation in hemispheric development (Brodal, 1969).

Reference

Brodal, A. (1981). "Neurological Anatomy in Relation to Clinical Medicine." Oxford Univ. Press, New York.

James C. Houk and Enrico Mugnaini

cortex to the brain stem and spinal cord and, via pons, back to the cerebellum.

The Microcircuitry Is Largely Homogeneous across the Surface

The cerebellar cortex is a three-layered, folded sheet of gray matter, only 1 mm thick and largely homogeneous throughout the whole cerebellum. Its unique anisotropic layout can be appreciated by comparing the simplified transverse and sagittal views of the microcircuitry provided in Figs. 32.2 and 32.3. [The full three-dimensional complexity is elaborated later (Fig. 32.9).] The three layers of this cortex are named—beginning from the pial surface—the *molecular layer*, the *Purkinje cell layer*, and the *granular layer*. The cerebellar cortex contains (1) a single type of efferent neuron, the Purkinje cells (PCs), which are inhibitory and project to the cerebellar nucleus (CN) and to the vestibular nucleus, and (2) five main classes of interneuron, three of which are inhibitory (stellate cells, basket cells, and Golgi cells) and two of

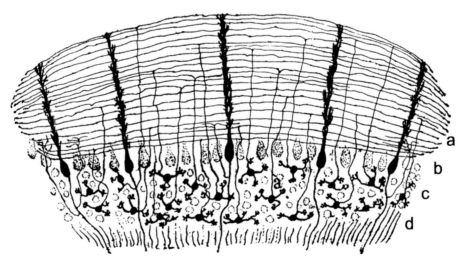

FIGURE 32.2 Transverse view of microcircuity. Schematic section of an ideal short cerebellar folium cut parallel to its course based on the Golgi impregnation method. (a) Molecular layer with parallel fibers (PFs); (b) Purkinje cell (PC) layer; (c) granular layer and (d) white matter. Stained Purkine cell dendrites, which are oriented flat perpendicularly to the direction of the folium, appear as cypress trees. PFs, which are formed by granule cell axons after a T division, synapse with a large number of PC dendrites, which they traverse along their course. Mossy fiber terminals, which provide input to granule cells, are not shown. Adapted from Cajal (1995).

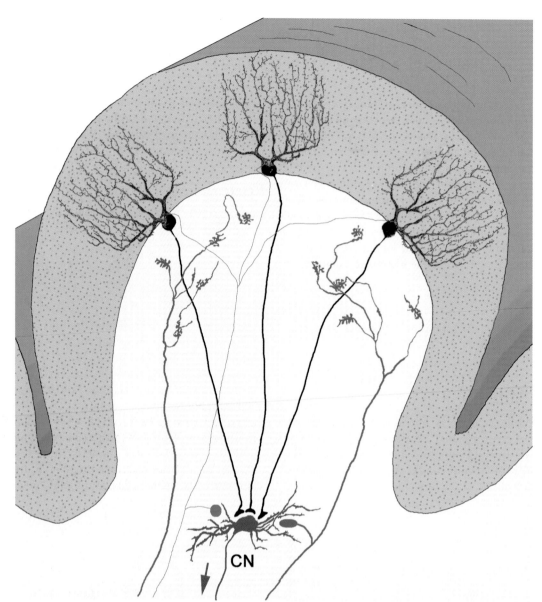

FIGURE 32.3 Saggital view of microcircuitry. Schematic illustration of a folium in parasaggittal section, with three PCs (black) illustrated in S. Ramon y Cajal's fashion. PCs send their inhibitory axon to a single excitatory cerebellar nucleus (CN) neuron and are innervated by branches of a single climbing fiber (CF) (red). Two mossy fibers (MFs) (purple) branch in the granular layer, forming terminals that innervate granule cells within glomeruli (not shown, but see Fig. 32.9). PFs, which run parallel to the direction of the folium, are represented by purple dots. The CF and one of the MFs give off collaterals, which form terminals (red and purple knobs) synapsing with the CN neuron. The CN neuron projects its axon (red arrow) to targets outside the cerebellum. Illustration by E. Mugnaini and G. Sekerkova.

which are excitatory (granule cells and unipolar brush cells). The cortex receives two main types of afferents (illustrated in color in Fig. 32.3): mossy fibers (MFs), shown as blue, and climbing fibers (CFs), shown as red, are both excitatory. The molecular layer (labeled a in Fig. 32.2) is cell poor; it contains primarily PC dendrites and their afferents—parallel fibers (PFs) and climbing fibers (but also the inhibitory stellate and basket cells that are left out of Figs. 32.2 and 32.3). The Purkinje cell layer is only one cell thick, but it is well marked by its large PCs (>50 μm in large mammals). The granular layer is extremely cell rich. It receives MFs, which form excitatory glutamatergic synapses on granule cells, unipolar brush cells, and Golgi cells.

The dendritic tree of the PC arises from the apex of the cell body and branches profusely in the molecular layer (Fig. 32.3). It is fan shaped (compare the appearance of PCs in transverse and sagittal views), like a tree trained to grow flat against a railing, and extends in a plane perpendicular to the main axis of the folium (usually the parasagittal plane). The proximal branches of the Purkinje cell dendrite appear smooth, although they are provided with scattered spines (all in contact with a single CF). In contrast, distal dendritic branches are covered with spines (spiny branchlets), most of which establish contact with PFs running perpendicular to the Purkinje tree (along the course of the folium as illustrated by the horizontal lines in Fig. 32.2). In large mammals, each Purkinje tree bears over 200,000 synaptic spines. The PC axon, after giving off some recurrent collaterals, enters the white matter and terminates in one of the cerebellar nuclei, or in the vestibular nucleus. Although PCs display some chemical heterogeneity, they all release the inhibitory neurotransmitter GABA. The output of the cerebellar cortex is purely inhibitory (Ito, 1984). This output is regulated by two prominent excitatory influences, the MF → PF pathway and direct CF inputs. PCs also receive feed-forward inhibition from basket and stellate cells and neuromodulatory inputs from noradrenergic, cholinergic, and serotonergic neurons in the brain stem.

The granular layer contains an enormous number (billions) of granule cells, which are the smallest neurons found in the brain (Fig. 32.2). Their spherical cell bodies form densely packed clusters, which are separated by islands of neuropil termed cerebellar glomeruli. It is often stated that cerebellar granule cells outnumber the sum of all the other neurons in the central nervous system. The granule cell emits four or five thin dendrites that terminate in claw-like protrusions into the glomeruli. Their axons ascend into the molecular layer where they bifurcate to form PFs, which may reach a length of 6–8 mm. The granule cell axon is provided with presynaptic varicosities along its full course. Varicosities of the ascending granule cell axon terminate on Golgi cells in the granular layer and on PC spiny branchlets in the molecular layer. Most of the varicosities are along the PF and innervate the spiny branchlets of the PCs and dendrites of the cerebellar interneurons that the PF passes along its course.

Neural Signals Are Processed According to a Modular Scheme

From the signal processing perspective, the two main divisions of the cerebellum are cerebellar cortex

and cerebellar nucleus (Fig. 32.4). The cerebellar cortex is specialized for processing extremely large amounts of information about the states of body parts, of objects around us, and of ongoing brain activities. This variety of *state information* is conveyed to the cerebellum by its numerous MF inputs. The state of body parts comes from our kinesthetic receptors, which signal the forces, lengths, and velocities of the many muscles throughout the body and the strain and motion of the skeletal joints. The state of the world is monitored by our tactile receptors, which sense contact forces, shears, and locations of nearby

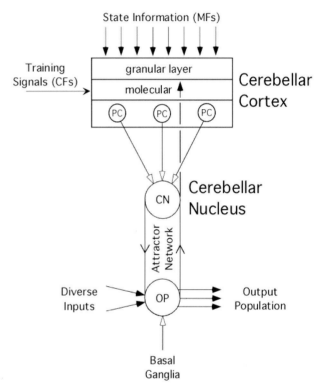

FIGURE 32.4 Modular signal processing scheme. A variety of state information arrives to this schematized module of the cerebellum via its MFs. These signals are diversified further in the granular layer to present (in the molecular layer) enormous arrays of potential PF input to many PCs (only three of which are illustrated). Under the training influence of CFs, PCs learn to detect specific patterns when they occur in their MF → PF input. The inhibitory PC → CN projections then function to regulate the spatiotemporal pattern of activity in an attractor network formed by a group of cells in CN that connect reciprocally with an output population (OP) of neurons in another part of the brain. State transitions of the attractor network, eg. from relative quiescence to intense activity, can be initiated by one of the diverse inputs to the OP under the regulatory influence of the inhibitory projection sent from the basal ganglia. When the attractor network is in its active state, the cerebellar cortex can shape OP activity into a useful spatiotemporal pattern of output. In a nutshell, a cerebellar module learns to use its complex state-related input to control the dynamics of the output population that it targets. Illustration by J.C. Houk.

objects, and by our visual and auditory systems, which analyze the properties of more distant objects in the world around us. The internal state of our brain is monitored by projections from neurons in brain areas that deal with perceptions, goals, motor commands, and problem solving. The large array of state information is called a *MF state vector* (vector is simply a concise way of referring to a set of variables).

The MF state vector is diversified further by the interneuronal circuit in the granular layer so as to produce a *PF state vector*, which functions as an enormous, highly diverse array of potential input to a large number of PCs. Under the influence of training signals conveyed by CFs to the molecular layer (Fig. 32.4), PCs learn to detect specific patterns in their state vectors. This allows PCs to classify the many patterns of state that occur at different times and under different contexts. This specialized neuronal architecture functions as a remarkable learning machine.

The pattern classifications detected by PCs are transmitted to CN neurons via inhibitory projections (open arrows in Fig. 32.4). As a consequence of the PC to CN projections being inhibitory, the cerebellar cortex is not well suited for initiating nuclear cell activity directly. However, the inhibitory input from PCs is indeed potent and is highly effective in regulating the spatial and temporal patterns of CN discharge promoted by

other causes. CN discharge is promoted both by the intrinsic properties of neurons and by excitatory synaptic input, especially that coming from collaterals of select MFs. The CN serves as the final common output from the cerebellum. The CN projects to neuronal output populations that are located in different regions of the brain, and these output neurons send collaterals that loop back onto the same region of the cerebellum (part of this loop is labeled attractor network in Fig. 32.4). These loops effectively bind populations of neurons that are located in many other parts of the brain to the regulatory operations of the cerebellum.

The signal processing scheme outlined earlier is organized in a modular fashion. Different zones of the CN receive their PC input from different parasaggital zones in the cerebellar cortex. Zones in the vermis and flocculus regulate the accuracy of trunk, leg, head, and eye movements—movements that are critical for the control of posture, locomotion, and gaze (Chapter 30). Intermediate zones regulate the accuracy of movements that we call voluntary—the reaching and grasping movements that we use to obtain and manipulate objects with our hands and arms (Chapter 30). The most lateral zones, in the hemispheres, regulate higher aspects of behavior. The enormously expanded hemispheres in humans plan complex movements, regulate cognition, and engage in problem solving.

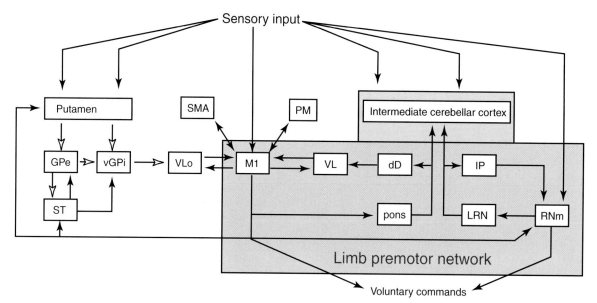

FIGURE 32.5 Application of the modular signal processing scheme to the limb premotor network. Diverse sensory inputs, or inputs from the supplementary motor area (SMA) or the premotor cortex (PM), can activate neurons in the motor cortex (M1) or magnocellular red nucleus (RNm). The spread of this activity through the limb premotor network is regulated by inhibitory input from PCs in the intermediate cerebellar cortex so as to produce a composite voluntary motor command appropriate for controlling the motion of the limb. Closed arrows designate predominantly excitatory projections whereas open arrows designate predominantly inhibitory projections; IP, interpositus nucleus; dD, dorsal zone of dentate nucleus; VL, ventrolateral thalamus; LRN, lateral reticular nucleus; VLo, pars oralis of VL; vGPi, ventral zone of globus pallidus pars interna; GPe, globus pallidus pars externa; ST, subthalamic nucleus. Adapted from J. C. Houk (2001).

Voluntary Motor Commands Exemplify Modular Signal Processing

To illustrate modular signal processing more specifically, we focus on the intermediate cerebellum and its regulation of voluntary movement commands (Fig. 32.5), as this is a relatively well-understood example of the generic modular processing diagrammed in Fig. 32.4 (Houk, 2001). In Fig. 32.5, the module regulating voluntary motor commands is highlighted, both in blue (intermediate cerebellar cortex) and in red (the limb premotor network). The limb premotor network is an example of the attractor network diagrammed in Fig. 32.4. It is composed of an elaborate set of interconnections among the CN, red nucleus, and motor cortex. Interpositus neurons project to the red nucleus directly and some project on to the motor cortex by way of the ventral thalamus. Most of the input to the motor cortex, via the thala-

mus, derives from CN neurons in a relatively small dorsal zone of dentate. Both the red nucleus and the motor cortex transmit voluntary movement commands to motor neurons in the spinal cord and brain stem via their output fibers (Chapter 30), but they also send collaterals to precerebellar nuclei, the pons and the lateral reticular nucleus (LRN), that originate MFs, which loop back to the intermediate cerebellum. These copies of motor commands (efference copy signals) inform both the cerebellar cortex and the CN about actions currently being commanded. Fig. 32.5 also illustrates connectivity with other areas of the cerebral cortex and basal ganglia.

The MF collaterals that loop back to intermediate nuclear cells close the recurrent pathways of the *attractor network* that was illustrated generically in Fig. 32.4; the concept of attractor neural networks is elaborated in Box 32.2. The resultant positive feedback in the limb premotor version of an attractor

---

BOX 32.2

ATTRACTOR NEURAL NETWORKS

Our quest to identify and understand the brain mechanisms responsible for the complex dynamics observed in neuronal assemblies has found a powerful tool in the use of neural network models. These models are based on relatively simple nonlinear units that capture only the most basic properties of individual neurons, such as the synaptic integration of inputs and nonlinear modulation of the firing rate. The rich dynamical behavior observed at the network level is due to a high degree of connectivity, and it is through the organization of this connectivity in specific circuits that functionally and computationally useful dynamical properties can be selected and stabilized. Complexity is thus a collective property whose source is to be found in connectivity.

Two basic types of network connectivity are to be distinguished: layered and recurrent. Layered networks, based on forward maps between subsequent layers, implement arbitrarily complex input–output maps. Recurrent networks, of particular interest here, incorporate feedback loops to sustain iterative dynamical processes based on the continuous update of network state. For a recurrent network composed of N neurons, the state of the network is specified through an array of N numbers representing the firing rates of the N neurons. The state of the network at any time can be visualized as a point in an N-dimensional space, where each coordinate axis corresponds to the firing rate of a specific neuron. As the state of each

neuron changes with time, the point that represents the state of the network moves in this N-dimensional space of firing rates. The trajectory described by this multidimensional point allows us to visualize the dynamic evolution of the network.

Trajectories that keep on moving about and visit more and more regions of network state space, never settling anywhere, correspond to a type of dynamical behavior called *ergodic*. More interesting dynamical behavior, associated with persistence, arises when trajectories are attracted to special regions of state space. These regions are labeled as *attractors*, and the recurrent networks whose dynamics converge to them are called *attractor neural networks*. The attractors are of three types: *fixed points*, *limit cycles*, and *strange attractors*. Here we are interested in fixed point attractors. Each one of these special points controls a specific region of state space, its *basin of attraction*. If a trajectory starts at any point within this basin, it will go toward the corresponding fixed point, where it will settle. The basin of attraction thus defines a set of network states that will evolve dynamically until they reach the attractor state. The attractor is called a fixed point because once the network reaches this special state, it remains there. The fixed point is stable because network states that are close to it flow into it. It is as if the point that represents the state of the network were a ball frictionally gliding on a landscape

BOX 32.2 (cont'd)

of hills and valleys. The ball will move toward lower points until it reaches the bottom of the valley that is strictly downhill from its initial position. Once the ball reaches this minimum, it will stay there. Attractor fixed points thus correspond to the network states at the bottom of the valleys.

Fixed point attractors provide a mechanism for the implementation of a set of motor commands in the limb premotor network (Fig. 32.5). The cerebello-thalamo-cortical-ponto-cerebellar excitatory loop acts as a recurrent network. A computational model (Hua and Houk, 1997) has established that pathways around the loop provide a mechanism for each one of these modules to develop effective lateral connections, which, in the case of the cerebellar nucleus and the thalamo-cortical circuits, take the form of a banded diagonal excitatory matrix. This type of connectivity leads to dynamical behavior controlled by the existence of two fixed points: a low activity state in which all neurons fire at very low baseline rates and a high activity state in which all neurons would fire at very high rates. In the absence of further inputs, the low activity state is an unstable fixed point and the high activity state is the stable fixed point, the attractor. However, the activity of cerebellar nucleus neurons is strongly modulated by inhibitory projections from cerebellar Purkinje cells. This modulation introduces two important modifications in the dynamical behavior of the recurrent network. First, the low activity state is stabilized by the concerted inhibitory action of the Purkinje cells. When all of them are firing, activity in the loop is suppressed. The low activity state thus acquires a small basin of attraction. Second, and crucial to the ability of the limb premotor neuron to encode a variety of motor commands, the high activity state is not

a uniform state in which all units fire at high frequency: the disinhibition of a subset of cerebellar nucleus neurons selected through the inactivation of specific Purkinje cells results in a specific pattern of activity that involves the thalamo-cortical circuits and the pons. The recurrent network sustains the high-frequency firing of a subset of neurons, whereas the others remain quiescent or fire at low-frequency, baseline levels.

The precise location of the high activity attractor in network state space depends on the inputs to the cerebellar nucleus provided by the Purkinje cells. Different attractor locations represent different subpopulations of neurons involved in high-frequency firing; each of these patterns of network activity encodes for a specific motion as it gets exported from the motor cortex into the spinal cord and the brain stem. Motion initiation requires a transition from the low-activity attractor to the high-activity attractor; the mechanism for this transition is the activation of a subset of motor cortical neurons due to sensory input from other cortical areas. The activity of the cerebello-thalamocortical-ponto-cerebellar loop can thus be understood as resulting from the competition between a low-activity fixed point with a small basin of attraction and a high-activity fixed point with a large basin of attraction. The precise network state associated with the high-activity fixed point is selected by the Purkinje cells projections onto the cerebellar nucleus; different patterns of activity encode different sets of motor commands.

Sara A. Solla

Reference

Hua, S. E., and Houk, J. C. (1997). Cerebellar guidance of premotor network development and sensorimotor learning. *Learn. Memory* **4**, 63–76.

network (red in Fig. 32.5) appears to be an important driving force for the *amplification* of motor command generation. Additional neurons need to be recruited, whereas the activity in already recruited neurons needs to be amplified in intensity and in duration so as to create the population of intense burst discharge that comprises a *composite voluntary motor command*. When positive feedback is sufficiently strong, it promotes the regenerative activity that is needed for amplification and for sustaining discharge in nuclear cells in the face of the potent inhibition sent from PCs. This regenerative activity can be *initiated* by any of the diverse inputs

(Fig. 32.4) sent to the motor cortex or to the red nucleus, such as the inputs produced by sensory cues. This raises the question of how the initiation process is regulated. Initiation of motor commands appears to be regulated by inhibitory inputs sent from the basal ganglia (Chapter 31), as shown on the left side of Fig. 32.5. This influence amounts to a disinhibition in the motor cortex, which allows other cortical inputs to initiate regenerative activity in the cortical-cerebellar loop.

Amplification in the limb premotor attractor network ensures that sufficient motor neuron activity is ultimately achieved so as to move the limb in appropriate directions and to open the hand in preparation for closing around an object that needs to be manipulated. Of course the composite voluntary command needs also to be shaped appropriately so that the individual commands contribute to the overall accuracy of reach and grasp. To achieve this, the individual commands need to have appropriate intensities and durations of discharge, which is the critical *refinement* function of well-controlled and well-coordinated arrays of potent PC inhibitory input to the limb premotor attractor network (Miller *et al.*, 2002).

How does the cerebellar cortex learn to perform this complex regulatory function? There is a growing body of evidence, reviewed in a later section, that PCs learn under the guidance of an array of training signals that are transmitted to the cerebellar cortex by CFs. Our presently limited information about climbing fibers is generally consistent with the concept that they transmit relatively specific error information to those PCs that are capable of reducing particular movement errors (Houk et al., 1996; Simpson et al., 1996). Because each PC is innervated by only a single CF, its training information can be quite specific. In contrast, the PC receives about 200,000 inputs conveying state information from its MF → PF system. The PF synapses that were activating the PC just before the climbing fiber discharged are weakened. This learning rule utilizes a special mechanism for synaptic plasticity that is discussed in a later section.

Computational models have demonstrated that the learning paradigm outlined earlier is capable of training PCs to control complex movements accurately, even in the presence of the substantial time delays that occur in the neural pathways that control and monitor a movement (Barto *et al.*, 1999). Because the capacity for overcoming time delays requires an ability to predict, one can surmise that the intermediate cerebellum may be capable of functioning as a predictive controller of the spatiotemporal patterns of neural activity in the limb premotor network. Similarly, other parts of the cerebellum should be capable of predictively controlling other output populations. Predictive regulation of neuronal populations is an extremely valuable tool for the postural, gaze, and locomotor functions of the medial cerebellum, for the voluntary movement functions of the intermediate cerebellum, and for the movement planning and cognitive functions of the cerebellar hemispheres.

Summary

The cerebellum is divided into many regional zones. Although each zone receives different inputs and projects to neuronal populations in different parts

of the brain, the microcircuitry is similar across the entire cerebellum, suggesting that signal processing operations are modular. The cerebellar contribution to the regulation of voluntary motor commands was used here to introduce modular signal processing principles.

ORGANIZATION OF SIGNAL PROCESSING MODULES

Mossy Fibers Bring Different Kinds of State Information to Different Modules

Mossy fibers originate from (i) centers, termed *precerebellar nuclei*, that project exclusively or nearly exclusively to the cerebellum and (ii) centers that send collaterals to the cerebellum in addition to having major projections outside the cerebellum. Major precerebellar nuclei are basilar pontine nuclei, the lateral reticular nucleus, and the reticular tegmental pontine nucleus, and the other major centers are vestibular nuclei, the external cuneate nucleus, and groups of cells in lamina VII of the spinal cord (Clarke's column and border cells). MFs carry diverse state information about the periphery and other brain centers. Because MFs generally originate from second-order sensory neurons, some processing of afferent information occurs before that information is sent to the cerebellum.

MFs carrying state information from different parts of the nervous system project to different parts of the cerebellum (Fig. 32.6). The anterior and posterior portions of the vermis and the adjacent hemispheral regions are innervated primarily by fibers from the spinal cord and are termed the *spinocerebellum*. The lateral portions of the hemispheres and the central folia of the vermis (the visual vermal area: folium and tuber vermis) are innervated primarily by fibers from basilar pontine nuclei and are termed the *pontocerebellum* or *cerebrocerebellum*. The pontine nucleus has an elaborate representation of input from widespread areas of the cerebral cortex (Brodal and Bjaalie, 1992). The flocculonodular lobe is innervated primarily by fibers from the vestibular ganglion and from vestibular nuclei and is termed the *vestibulocerebellum*. Important MF systems, arising in the reticular formation and the nucleus reticularis tegmenti pontis, provide the vestibulocerebellum with optokinetic information. The distribution of spinal, basilar pontine, and vestibular MF systems is in accord with functional subdivisions of the feline and primate cerebellum based on different behavioral abnormalities that result when each was each part is damaged or

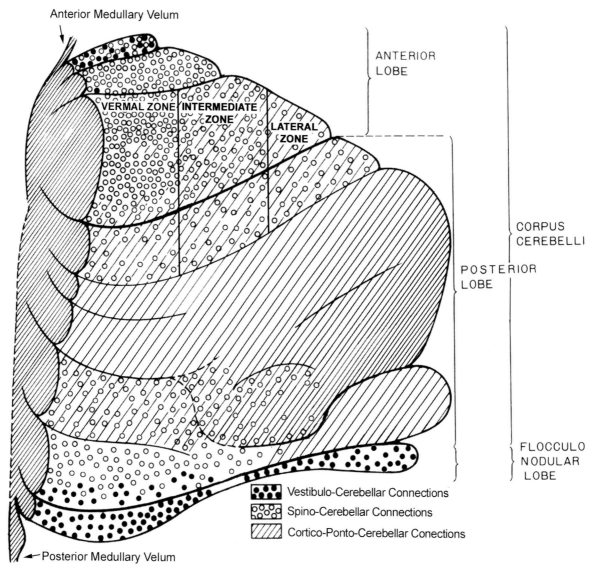

FIGURE 32.6 Organization of mossy fiber input. Schematic representation of the mossy fiber input to the anterior, posterior, and flocculonodular cerebellar lobes, which roughly define the spinocerebellar, cerebrocerebellar (pontocerebellar), and vestibulocerebellar regions. Adapted from Dow (1942).

subjected to pharmacological blockade (Voogd and Glickstein, 1998).

Upon reaching the cerebellum, MFs branch extensively. They generally distribute bilaterally, with either an ipsilateral or a contralateral predominance. They terminate either in multiple, symmetrically arranged, parasagittal zones or in patches. The few studies of the subject indicate that different mossy fiber systems remain segregated in the granular layer. A detailed study in the rat showed that each patch contains a representation of a small body part, but the same body part can have multiple representations (Bower et al., 1981). Neighboring patches can have representation of different body parts that are functionally related, e.g., perioral region and paw. The

patchy pattern is called *fractured somatotopy*. Because the mossy fiber–granule cell–Purkinje cell pathway is a widely divergent system, which may influence Purkinje cells belonging to different zones in different regions of the cerebellum more or less simultaneously, each Purkinje cell may receive information about sensory conditions, internal states, external states, and the plans of the organism.

Climbing Fibers Are Organized in Parasagittal Zones

All CFs arise from the *inferior olive*, which is a complex of larger and smaller subnuclei located in the ventral medulla oblongata (Fig. 32.7). The largest of these subnuclei, the principal olive, is expanded greatly in humans and is configured as a folded sheet of cells, resembling the expanded and folded lateral cerebellar nucleus with which it is connected. The olivocerebellar projection is strictly modular (Armstrong and Hawkes, 2000; Voogd and Glickstein, 1998). Subdivisions of the inferior olive project to specific subdivisions of the cerebellar and vestibular nuclei that underlie 0.5 mm-wide, parasagittally oriented zones of the cerebellar cortex. The same subdivisions of the cerebellar and vestibular nuclei loop back to the subnuclei of the inferior olive from which

the olivocerebellar projection originated (note the matching colors in Fig. 32.7). Moreover, projections from the cerebellar cortex to the cerebellar and vestibular nuclei and projections from the cerebellar and vestibular nuclei to the inferior olive form closely corresponding loops.

Specialized zones of CF projection to the cerebellar cortex have been identified across mammals. The vermal cerebellar cortical zone comprises three parasagittal projection zones, termed A, X, and B; the intermediate zone comprises parasagittal zones C_1, C_2, and C_3; and the hemispheral zone comprises parasagittal zones D_1 and D_2. Several subnuclei of the inferior olive contain a detailed somatotopic map, and this somatotopy is reproduced in the corresponding climbing fiber zone as a pattern of so-called microzones. The receptive fields of PC responses to MF input appear to be specifically influenced by the receptive fields of their CFs (Ekerot and Jörntell, 2001). Contrary to the systematic divergence in the MF-PF system, the climbing fiber system is highly focused onto microzones, and each microzone projects to a small cluster of nuclear neurons.

Olivary axons cross the midline in the ventral medulla at the level of their site of origin. After entering the cerebellum, an individual climbing fiber leaves collaterals in the cerebellar nucleus that provide the reciprocal nucleo-olivary projection to the parent olivary neuron and then ascends toward the cortex branching repeatedly in the sagittal plane to make contact with up to 10 Purkinje cells. Each Purkinje cell, however, receives input from only one

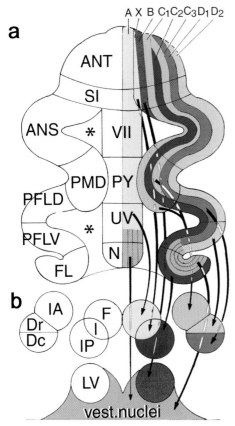

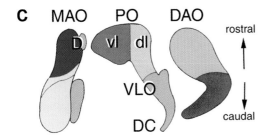

FIGURE 32.7 Organization of climbing fiber input and cerebellar output zones. Diagram of the zonal organization in the corticonuclear and olivocerebellar projections in the cat. (a) The flattened cerebellar cortex with the parasagittal zones, (b) cerebellar and vestibular nuclei, and (c) profile of the inferior olive in the horizontal plane. The longitudinal corticonuclear and olivocerebellar projection zones are indicated with capitals (A, X, B, C1–3, D1, 2). The zones, their target nuclei, and subnuclei of the inferior olive, which project to these zones, are indicated with the same colors. The diagram applies equally to the monkey cerebellum, with the exception of the floccular zones, the most medial one of which is lacking in the monkey. Asterisks: areas without cortex. ANS, ansiform lobule; ANT, anterior lobe; D, dorsomedial cell column; Dc, caudal dentate nucleus; DC, dorsal cap; dl, dorsal leaf of principal olive; FLO, flocculus; I, intermediate cell group; IA, anterior interpositus nucleus; IP, posterior interpositus nucleus; LV, lateral vestibular nucleus; MAO, medial accessory olive; N, nodulus; PFLD, dorsal paraflocculus; PFLV, ventral paraflocculus; PMD, paramedian lobule; PO, principal nucleus of the inferior olive; PY, pyramis; SI, lobulus simplex; UV, uvula; vl, ventral leaf of principal olive; VLO, ventrolateral outgrowth; VII, lobule VII. Courtesy of J. Voogd (2001).

climbing fiber. With more than a 1000 synapses of a single fiber with an individual cell, the climbing fiber–Purkinje cell pathway represents an example of a giant synapse and has powerful excitatory and metabolic effects.

The inferior olive shows several unifying structural features: (1) it contains a homogeneous population of spiny projection neurons and rare interneurons; (2) within a subnucleus, all projection neurons are coupled electrically to each other by gap junctions, most of which link together dendritic spines and may serve to share postsynaptic currents; (3) all olivary projection neurons use glutamate as a neurotransmitter and corticotropin-releasing factor (CRF) as a modulatory neuropeptide; (4) all olivary projection neurons receive excitatory and inhibitory inputs, mostly on the spines and stems of peripheral dendrites; and (5) all olivary subnuclei receive a strong GABAergic innervation. CRF is generally expressed by neurons involved in stress signaling throughout the brain.

Outflow Engages Motor, Autonomic, and Cognitive Parts of the Brain

The cerebellar outflow ultimately reaches all motor nuclei (Brodal, 1998), structures within the autonomic nervous system (Dietrichs *et al.*, 1994), and many areas of the cerebral cortex (Middleton and Strick, 1998), with topically organized connections. The outflow from neurons occupying discrete subdivisions of the cerebellar nuclei targets specific neuronal populations in the thalamus, hypothalamus, red nucleus, tectum, pons, medulla, and cervical spinal cord. The outflow also loops back to the cerebellum via several nuclei, primarily the pontine tegmental reticular nucleus, the basilar pontine nuclei, the lateral reticular nucleus, and the inferior olive.

Individual excitatory neurons residing in each cerebellar nucleus have axons that form discrete patches of synaptic terminals in a primary target nucleus, and the axons also often send collaterals to other target nuclei. Collaterals of the individual cerebellar nuclear neurons are hypothesized to terminate on functionally congruent groups of neurons in the target nuclei. The functional congruency would be achieved by the stabilization of effectual connections during maturation of the sensory motor circuits. The small inhibitory neurons of the cerebellar nuclei have axons projecting in a similarly discrete manner, but they do not collateralize; they project to specific regions of the inferior olive, the source of all CF input to PCs. It is generally assumed, therefore, that cerebellar connections are organized in a complex, but detailed topical order.

The zonal organization of cortical maps is well correlated with physiological findings. In the vestibulo-cerebellum, different zones exert a plane-specific control of the external muscles of the eye. A similar specification may be present in the zones of the corpus cerebelli, with the A zone regulating inhibitory vestibulospinal tracts, the B zone regulating the excitatory lateral vestibulospinal tract, and the intermediate C1, C2, and C3 zones regulating the rubrospinal system . A portion of the A zone in the central vermis (visual vermis: folium and tuber) is able to adapt the amplitude of saccades. Functions of the D_1 and D_2 and other as yet undefined hemispheral zones are not as well known. D_1 and D_2 zones probably regulate movements of individual digits, and other regions may regulate visual smooth-pursuit tracking, eye–hand coordination, and higher aspects of motor planning and cognitive function.

For many years, the cerebellum was thought to be involved only in the generation of movement. This belief was based on the fact that cerebellar projections had been traced only to motor areas and that cerebel-

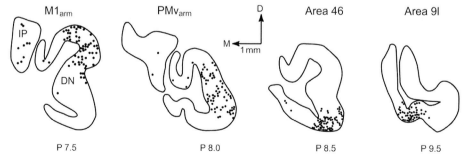

FIGURE 32.8 Output channels to four areas of cerebral cortex. Anatomical arrangement of separate output channels in the monkey dentate (DN) and interpositus (IP) nuclei, after virus injections into different cortical areas (M1$_{arm}$, PMv$_{arm}$, area 46, area 9l). Solid dots indicate neurons that were labeled by virus retrogradely transported from the cortex in three adjacent sections at the antero-posterior location indicated below each nuclear outline (P7.5, P8.0, P8.5, P9.5). D, dorsal; M, medial.
Reproduced from Middleton and Strick (1998), with permission.

lar lesions in humans seemed to cause only motor deficits. Initial suggestions that the cerebellum participates in cognition arose from anatomic connections that were postulated to exist due to the parallel expansion of the frontal lobe, lateral cerebellum, and dentate nucleus. Then retrograde transneuronal transport of special virus strains in monkeys demonstrated many specifics of these connections (Middleton and Strick, 1998). These transneuronal studies have suggested the following general principles: (1) cerebral cortical areas that project to the cerebellum (motor, premotor, and lateral intraparietal areas) and some of the nonmotor areas of the prefrontal cortex are targets of cerebellar output; (2) cerebral cortical areas that do not project to the cerebellum are themselves not the target of cerebellar output; and (3) the cerebellar output channels to different cortical areas are topically distinct zones of the dentate nucleus (Fig. 32.8).

Summary

Organization of the mossy and climbing fiber input to the cerebellum is appropriate for regulating neuronal populations in other parts of the brain that control movement, autonomic function, and cognitive operations.

NEURONS AND THEIR SIGNALS

The purpose of this section is to relate the cellular properties of cerebellar neurons to their signal processing operations. The diverse constellation of neurons in the cerebellar cortex is summarized in Fig. 32.9, which is a perspective drawing of a folium that integrates the transverse and saggital views of the cerebellar cortex given earlier (Figs. 32.2 and 32.3). The three-dimensional perspective highlights the orthogonal relationship between the flattened PC dendritic trees and the sheet of parallel fibers providing convergent input. Fig. 32.9 also illustrates the arrangement of the three types of inhibitory interneuron (Golgi, stellate, and basket cells) and other factors within this matrix.

Purkinje Cells Shape the Spatiotemporal Patterns of Cerebellar Outflow

The most remarkable neurons of the cerebellum are the Purkinje cells. The innervation of a PC by an individual climbing fiber is quite exceptional, virtually climbing all over the proximal dendrites and making

multiple excitatory synapses (Fig. 32.10). Except for the fact that CFs fire at very low rates, this would dominate the discharge of the PC. Instead, PCs have two characteristic types of discharge that can be observed with either extracellular or intracellular recording electrodes, namely the repetitive simple spikes that are mediated by PF input and the occasional complex spikes that are mediated by CF input (Thach, 1998). Recorded near the cell body under quite stable conditions, complex spikes appear as high-frequency wavelets (Fig. 32.11C2), but they are also recorded as a large spike followed by a wave that lasts for a few milliseconds.

The vast majority of the action potentials generated by PCs are the large negative–positive potentials shown in Fig. 32.11C1, called simple spikes. Simple spikes are produced by PF input to the PC. They repeat, with occasional pauses, at relatively high spontaneous rates. The simple spikes recorded from the intermediate cerebellum in the awake animal show either bursts or pauses in association with movement, and the intensities of the responses correlate with the velocity and direction of movement (Ebner, 1998). To set the stage for further discussion of the cellular neurobiology of the cerebellum, we present a simplified overview of PC and CN signals in the intermediate cerebellum and how they relate to the control of an arm movement.

Fig. 35.12 shows schematically four microscopic modules that regulate the activity of four motor cortical neurons. Microscopic modules are loops between small clusters of cortical and CN neurons, a whole array of which comprise the macroscopic module illustrated in Fig. 32.5. Each of the numbered neurons is assumed to command movement in one of four directions—motor cortical neuron 1 commands upward movement, 2 rightward, 3 downward, and 4 leftward. Each of the output neurons is reciprocally connected (via thalamic and pontine neurons) to a CN neuron that is regulated by inhibitory input from a PC (actually a parasaggital row of about 300 PCs). Adjacent to each module are two waveforms meant to represent the discharge over time of an associated Purkinje cell (upper trace) and the nuclear neuron (lower trace) to which it projects. The lower traces also represent the motor cortical neurons linked to the CNs, as they will be caused to burst simultaneously by the reciprocal cortical-cerebellar loop of the module.

Divergence of fibers within the limb premotor network (arrows between modules) allows activation to spread laterally among adjacent modules. A sensory stimulus (flash of light, or a tone) might produce just a tiny burst of activity in neuron 1. This small activation, while insufficient to drive movement, can

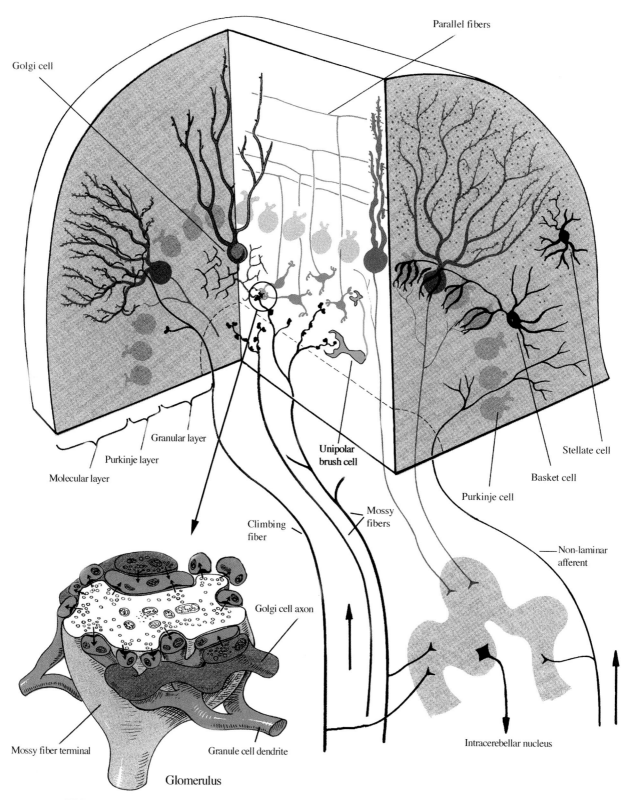

FIGURE 32.9 Cells and circuitry of the cerebellar cortex. This three-dimensional representation integrates the simplified transverse and sagittal views of a cerebellar folium shown earlier in Figs. 32.2 and 32.3. Adapted from Heimer (1995).

initiate an amplification process. Because the PC inhibition of the loop is turned off, activity can reverberate around this loop. Positive feedback would enhance the intensity and extend the duration of this reverberating activity, producing a substantial command signal for transmission to an agonist muscle for upward movement. Activity would also tend to spread to the modules controlling neurons 2 and 4, as their PCs are only producing moderate inhibition. This would command a cocontraction of right and left muscles, which would serve to stabilize the limb. In contrast, activity would not spread to the module controlling neuron 3, as its PC is bursting and is producing strong inhibition. Therefore, muscles that tend to move the limb downward would be relaxed. In a more realistic model, there would be many more such microscopic modules, each controlling movements in intermediate directions that are distributed throughout the workspace.

This example assumes that the PCs have been programmed to discharge with an appropriate time course. The upward movement command is a strong burst because its PC paused completely for the duration of the movement command. There is no down-

ward movement command because its PC fired a strong burst during the period when positive feedback was present in other loops of the limb premotor attractor network. Rightward and leftward movement commands are intermediate in intensity because their PCs do not stray much from their spontaneous level of activity. While these assumed patterns of PC activity are compatible with current neurophysiological data, the field is still lacking definitive experiments showing that correct PCs in the cerebellar cortex generate the most appropriate patterns. The motor learning mechanisms discussed at several points in this chapter should be capable of ensuring this, but the experimental evidence remains incomplete.

There is also increasing evidence that the cerebellum, motor cortex, and red nucleus are organized not in terms of preferred directions of hand movement, but rather in terms of functionally useful groups of muscles (Miller *et al.*, 2002). It is easy to see how such a system of *preferred muscle synergies* could be controlled by interconnected groups of cortical-cerebellar processing modules such as the ones discussed earlier. Arrays of modules controlling grasp

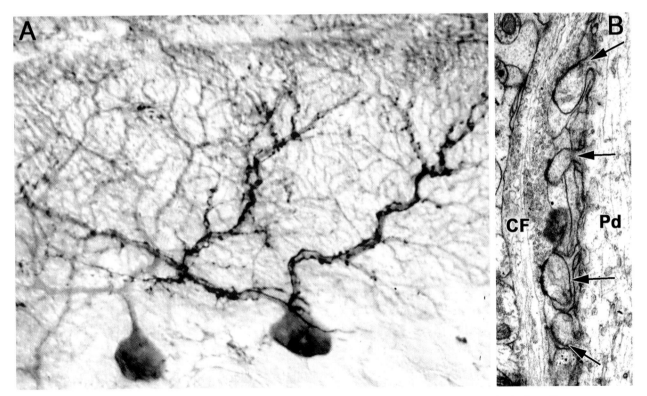

FIGURE 32.10 (A) Climbing fiber-to-purkinje cell pathway. Varicose branches of a single climbing fiber (labeled blue with a lectin) cling to the proximal dendritic domain of an individual Purkinje cell arbor (labeled brown with antiserum to calbindin). Courtesy of Rossi *et al.* (1993). (B) Climbing fiber–Purkinje cell synapses. A climbing fiber varicosity (CF) in synaptic contact with spines (arrows) of the proximal dendritic domain of the Purkine cell arbor (Pd) is shown. Courtesy of E. Mugnaini (adapted from Larsell and Jansen, 1972).

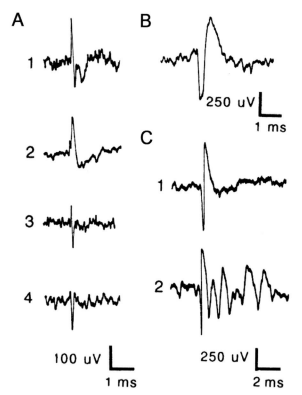

FIGURE 32.11 Spike waveshapes recorded in the awake monkey. (A) Examples of fast action potentials attributed to mossy fibers. (A1) Biphasic potential with a negative afterwave (glomerular potential). (A2) Predominantly positive potential. (A3) Biphasic potential without a negative afterwave. (A4) Triphasic potential. (B) Example of a slow negative–positive potential attributed to a Golgi cell. (C) "Simple" (C1) and "complex" (C2) spikes recorded from a Purkinje cell. Adapted from Van Kan *et al.* (1993).

muscles might be adjacent to, and partially interconnected with, modules controlling limb extension muscles. Postural responses could be coordinated by similar interconnections with modules controlling muscles of the neck, trunk and legs.

Granule, Golgi, and Brush Cells Process Excitatory Mossy Fiber Input

The MF signals that convey state information to the cerebellum excite granule cells within giant synaptic structures called glomeruli. The expanded drawing of a glomerulus in Fig. 32.9 shows that its core ingredient is a large expansion of the mossy fiber, which occurs along its branches or at the terminals. The glomerulus is packed with synaptic vesicles and with mitochondria that fuel the manufacturing of the vesicles. The dendrites of nearby granule cells send claw-like protrusions into the glomerulus where they form multiple small synaptic junctions (Fig. 32.13). Because of the large size

and glial surround of the glomerulus, extracellular electrodes are able to record the signals transmitted by MFs in one of the several ways illustrated in Fig. 32.11A. The full-fledged glomerular potential (A1) has a biphasic presynaptic component, produced when the action potential invades the glomerulus, followed by a slower negative wave, produced when excitatory postsynaptic current flows through the numerous excitatory synaptic junctions. When the negative wave is missing, the presynaptic component takes on one of the three other configurations shown in Figs. 32.11A2, 32.11A3, and 32.11A4. MFs in the intermediate cerebellum discharge at frequencies that are graded over a broad range, and different fibers signal a variety of sensory and efference copy information.

While MF activation of a glomerulus can be recorded in awake-behaving animals with extracellular microelectrodes, our knowledge of synaptic integration by the granule cell depends mostly on intracellular recordings from brain slices (Hansel *et al.*, 2001) due to the fact that the small extracellular spikes produced by their tiny axons are obscured by electrical noise. MF input activates both AMPA and NMDA receptors and, due to the latter, exhibits excellent temporal summation. Excitatory transmission is moderated by the GABAergic inhibition sent to the glomerulus by Golgi cells. The latter neurons produce slower and larger extracellular action potentials than MFs (Fig. 32.11B). Their dendrites branch broadly, mainly in the molecular layer, and they discharge at relatively steady rates that reflect the overall level of PF activity in the overlying molecular layer.

The computational ideas originated by Marr and Albus in the 1970s appear to be reasonably valid (Houk *et al.*, 1996). Golgi cell inhibition appears to function like an automatic gain control, normalizing the amount of PF input so as not to overwhelm PCs, but at the same time allowing the PF state vector to express many diverse patterns, which can then be detected selectively by individual PCs. Because the granule cells receive input from about four different MFs, the MF–granule cell system should create an expanded representation of state that is kept sparse by Golgi inhibition.

Unipolar brush cells (Fig. 32.9) are found in the granular layer of the vermal and in intermediate zones and the vestibulocerebellum (Nunzi *et al.*, 2001). They are strongly excited by individual MF inputs, or by other brush cells, and they strongly excite nearby granule cells. This circuit serves to amplify the intensity and duration of MF input. This is probably important for the enhancement and short-term storage of state information about the orientation of the organism that is characteristic of the vestibulocerebellum.

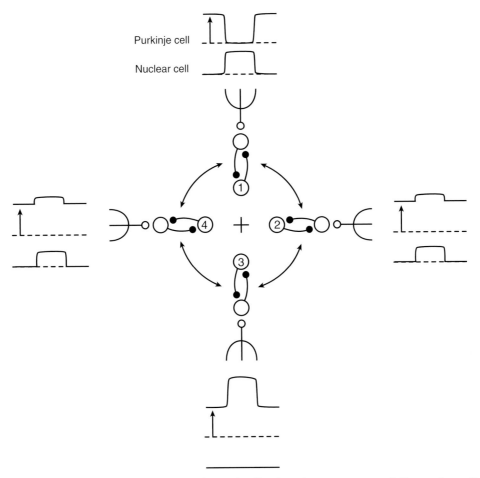

Purkinje cell

Nuclear cell

FIGURE 32.12 Signals and circuits regulating the direction of an arm movement. Four motor cortical cells, labeled 1–4, that move the arm upward (1), rightward (2), downward (3), or leftward (4). Each is reciprocally connected with a different microzone of the cerebellum, so as to form a microscopic module. Traces next to each module illustrate how pauses and bursts in Purkinje cell discharge would regulate the nuclear (and motor cortical) activity of the cell. Note the high spontaneous discharge of the Purkinje cells (dashed lines reference no discharge). Adapted from Houk and Miller (2001).

Climbing Fibers Transmit Training Information via the Inferior Olive

The CF pathway originates in the inferior olive of the brain stem. These cells display electrical activity analogous to that present in the heart—action potentials with long plateaus followed by long refractory periods—causing CFs to fire at very low rates (irregular at about 1/s). Many olivary neurons detect sensory events, but are inhibited by GABAergic inputs from the CN. This combined excitatory and inhibitory input helps signal the occurrences of errors. When the same sensory event occurs in a context that does not signify error, the small CN neurons can inhibit their responses. Olivary cells are coupled to each other electrotonically and show a slight tendency to oscillate at approximately 10 Hz (Welsh *et al.*, 1995). The diversity of the receptive fields of olivary neurons

ensures a relatively private training signal that is then transmitted to parasaggital rows of about 10 PCs. The best current examples of error detection are CFs that project to PCs in the flocculonodular lobe. They signal the slip of visual information across the retina, which is indicative of an improperly regulated eye movement command (Simpson *et al.*, 1996).

Nonlaminar Afferents Bring Neuromodulatory Influences

In addition to MFs and CFs, the cerebellum receives several types of afferents that have non-laminar distributions of their terminals. These non-laminar afferents orginate from neurons in the locus ceruleus, the raphe nuclei, or from widely distributed choline acetyltransferase(ChAT)-positive brain stem neurons, and from the hypothalamus. These afferents

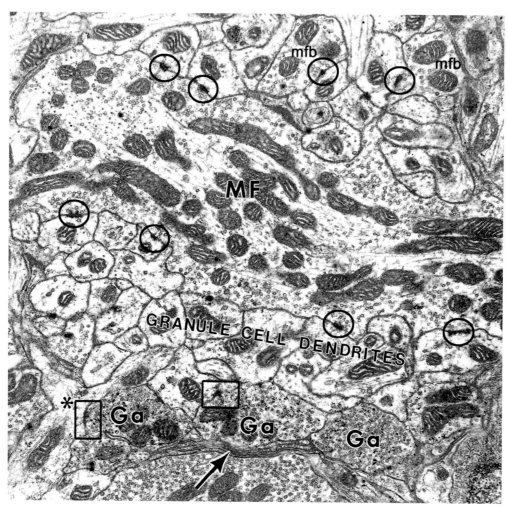

FIGURE 32.13 Mossy fiber-to-granule cell synapses in a cerebellar glomerulus. The central mossy fiber terminal (MF) forming asymmetric synaptic junctions (circled) with surrounding granule cell dendrites is shown. Granule cell dendrites form symmetric synaptic junctions (boxed) with terminals of the Golgi cell axon (Ga), which are labeled by immunogold particles (small solid dots) using antiserum to GABA. Arrow indicates astrocytic lamellar processes forming the peripheral glial sheath. Asterisk marks the shaft of a granule cell dendrite entering the glomerulus. Courtesy of E. Mugnaini (adapted from Heimer, 1995).

innervate the cerebellar nuclei and all layers of the cerebellar cortex, with some preference for the molecular layer. Afferent fibers from the locus ceruleus arrive via the superior cerebellar peduncle and release norepinephrine in the cerebellar cortex, fibers from the raphe nuclei release serotonin (5HT), fibers from ChAT-positive neurons release acetylcholine (ACh), and fibers from the hypothalamus are in part histaminergic. The nonlaminar fiber systems modulate the excitability of PCs and other cerebellar neurons. Nonlaminar afferents and their synapses are best identified with the help of cytochemical markers and tract tracing molecules. These afferents have active zones and postsynaptic densities, although it is likely that they may also release their transmitters at nonspecialized regions of their terminal branches.

Molecular Layer Interneurons Dampen Purkinje Cell Excitability

Stellate and basket cells in the molecular layer inhibit PCs via GABAergic synapses. Stellate cells, which are scattered throughout the molecular layer, provide a moderating influence that dampens large fluctuations of excitatory PF input. The dendrites of basket cells are oriented longitudinally and their axonal trees innervate parasaggital rows of PCs, forming basket-like terminations that surround the PC bodies and form paintbrush extensions around their initial axon segments. Because PCs have high spontaneous discharge rates, specializations of the basket cell seem appropriate for initiating the pauses that punctuate their spontaneous activity. The extracellular potentials of basket cells have not yet been definitively identified in awake animals, but the biphasic potentials recorded just above the PC layer are appropriate candidates. These units show bursts and pauses analogous to those recorded from PCs. Basket and stellate cells have dendrites carrying a low density of spines and receive most of the excitatory synapses on their cell bodies and dendritic shafts from both PFs and collaterals of CFs. These contacts are intermixed with inhibitory synapses from other basket and stellate cells. Basket cells are also inhibited by recurrent collaterals of PC axons.

Purkinje Cells Have Special Computational Features

The ionic currents that influence PC discharge are numerous. However, the calcium P currents underlying plateau potentials in PC dendrites (Llinás and Sugimori, 1980) are especially important from two functional perspectives: (1) promoted by excitatory input from PFs, P current-mediated plateau potentials are responsible for the relatively high spontaneous firing rates ($\approx$50 imp/s) of PCs and (2) the influx of calcium resulting from these currents is one of the factors that contributes to the motor learning mediated by the synaptic plasticity of PF $\rightarrow$ PC synapses, as is elaborated in the following section.

PC dendrites are forced, by the balance between their excitatory and inhibitory synaptic input, to make transitions in their internal state—transitions back and forth between a hyperpolarized state of low excitability and a depolarized plateau state of high excitability (Houk *et al.*, 1996). Inhibitory synaptic input from molecular layer interneurons can initiate transitions from the depolarized to the hyperpolarized state. Such transitions are important because they generate the pauses in PC discharge that remove the spontaneous inhibition of CN neurons that exists spontaneously in the cerebellum. This permits the CNs that they target to fire at very high frequencies (100–600 imp/s). This succession of events accounts for the buildup of intense activity in the reciprocal loop of module 1 illustrated in Fig. 32.12. The high CN firing rate amplifies the agonist movement command that was initiated in the motor cortex by, for example, a sensory cue.

A little later, after the movement is underway, we speculate that the PC module 1 detects the occurrence of a critical pattern in its PF state vector, signifying that the moment has arrived to terminate the movement command. Then, after conduction delays in the neuromuscular system, the movement can come to a graceful termination, at the desired end point. If the corresponding PF $\rightarrow$ PC synapses have learned to recognize this truly critical state, the PC dendrite will receive appropriately strong excitatory input at the critical moment, thus promoting the transition back to the plateau state of dendritic depolarization, which causes the PC to resume its moderately high spontaneous firing rate. The resumption of potent inhibitory input to the CN neuron turns off its intense firing, thus terminating the movement command of the module.

A different succession of events may account for the suppression of motor commands to antagonist motor neurons. PCs that regulate module 3 in Fig. 32.12 are shown to substantially increase their discharge at about the same time that the agonist-connected PC in module 1 pauses. The antagonist-connected PC is assumed to have detected the occurrence of a pattern in its state vector calling for the initiation of a movement opposite to the one it promotes if it pauses. Instead, it bursts, which helps suppress the generation of an antagonist command. Presumably some of its dendrites were sitting in their hyperpolarized states, and some of the corresponding PF $\rightarrow$ PC synapses detected the initiation of movement commands in the agonist muscles of the movement. This promotes transitions to depolarized states, which promote intense firing of that PC. The intense firing inhibits the CN to which the PC projects, preventing it from amplifying discharge in the output neuron(s) that it targets. This helps suppress movement commands to the antagonist motor neurons.

Modules 2 and 4 in Fig. 32.12 are regulated in a less intense fashion. Their PCs exhibit a modest increase in firing at movement onset, which slightly increases the inhibition sent to their CNs. This tends to dampen the buildup of positive feedback in their reciprocal loops, while not entirely inhibiting it. This is because the overall activity of the limb premotor network is strongly enhanced, which brings an excitatory influence to those loops.

By tracing through the logic of this simplified example, one can begin to appreciate the critical role played by the large array of Purkinje cells in the intermediate cerebellar cortex. The spatiotemporal pattern in this PC array plays a critical role in regulating the buildup of positive feedback in the limb premotor network, shaping it into a composite movement command that moves the limb toward an object that the organism wants to manipulate. Although all of this activity of the PC array is important, a particularly critical feature is the detection of PF states indicating that the time has come to terminate the composite movement command. If this did not happen, the resultant movement would be hypermetric. In fact, the immediate effect of lesions confined to the cerebellar cortex is hypermetria. However, over the course of functional recovery, other circuitry in the brain (e.g., intracortical circuitry and/or the loop through the basal ganglia shown in Fig. 32.5) evidently adapts in a manner that suppresses the buildup of positive feedback in the limb premotor network.

Long-Term Depression Mediates Motor Learning

The strategic role of PF → PC plasticity in motor learning has been mentioned several times earlier in this chapter. Long-term depression (LTD) is the name given to the synaptic plasticity of PF → PC synapses (Ito, 1984; Fig. 32.14). While other types of plasticity have also been found in the cerebellum (Hansel *et al.*, 2001), LTD is particularly important. Cerebellar LTD appears to differ from the long-term potentiation (LTP) present in cortical neurons (Chapter 50) in

several significant respects: (i) it desensitizes postsynaptic receptors instead of sensitizing them (depression instead of potentiation), (ii) it uses a different set of second messengers, and (iii) it appears to be a three-factor learning rule instead of the predominantly two-factor Hebbian rule associated with LTP at most other sites in the CNS (Houk and Alford, 1996). The two factors in the Hebbian rule are activity of a particular synapse and activity of the postsynaptic neuron. The three factors associated with cerebellar LTD are discussed later, and Fig. 32.15 summarizes some of the salient steps in this synaptic modification process.

Factor 1

When a PF releases glutamate at a particular synaptic spine, like the one illustrated in Figs. 32.14 and 32.15, it activates two types of glutamatergic receptor: AMPA and mGluR1. Activation of the AMPA receptors of the spine opens channels that permit depolarizing currents to flow into the spine and out into the dendrite, influencing the postsynap-

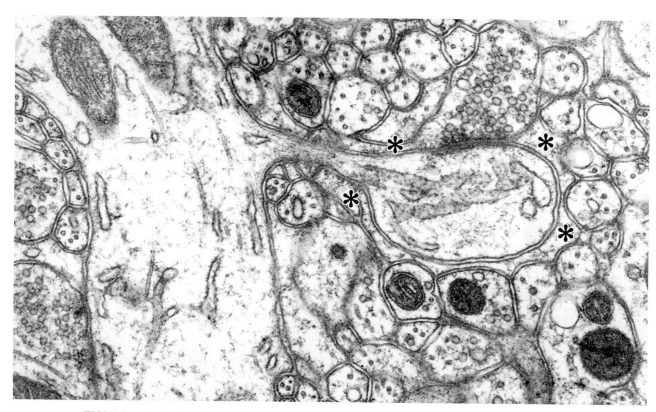

FIGURE 32.14 A dendritic spine arising from a spiny branchlet of the Purkinje cell arbor. The spine forms an asymmetric synapse with a parallel fiber varicosity. Actin forms a lattice in the spine head and parallel microfilaments in the spine neck. Dense spots on the membrane of the endoplasmic reticulum of the spine represent the large cytoplasmic domains of inositol 1,4,5-trisphosphate ($InsP_3$) receptors. These function as Ca^{2+} channels and are extremely abundant in Purkinje cells. Side branches of the astrocytic Bergmann glia fibers (asterisks) surround the synaptic profiles, with the exception of the synaptic apposition. Courtesy of E. Mugnaini (adapted from De Camilli *et al.*, 2001).

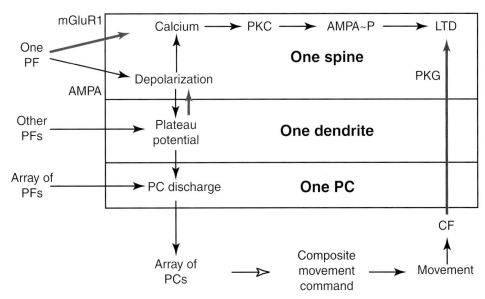

FIGURE 32.15 Multilevel principles appropriate for driving motor learning in the cerebellum. Red arrows mark three important factors in the learning rule. At the level of an individual *spine*, the glutamate released by a PF causes both a depolarizing current, mediated by AMPA receptors, and a metabotropic activation, mediated by mGluR1 receptors. The latter is a spine-specific factor. Depolarizing currents produced by several spines along the *dendrite* may summate sufficiently to produce a plateau potential. This factor signifies the PC dendrite actively participated in a movement. Metabotropic activation of individual spines combines with dendritic depolarization to activate PKC, which then phosphorylates the AMPA receptor to produce a *trace* of prior coincident synaptic and dendritic activity. Meanwhile, many dendrites and many PCs regulate the composite movement command that, after some time delay, produces a movement. If an error is then detected, the CF fires, which can activate PKG to consolidate any trace of LTD that is present in the spine.

tic depolarization of that dendrite, and the activity of the entire PC. In combination with the currents produced by many other activated spines, this synaptic activation contributes to the internal state of the dendrite and may initiate a plateau potential. If so, depolarization of the dendrite spreads back into the spine (factor 1, shown by a red arrow in Fig. 32.15) to augment spine depolarization. The activity of all of the dendrites of PC combines to control PC discharge.

Factor 2

In contrast, activation of the mGluR1 receptors of the spine initiates chemical changes that are confined to that particular synaptic spine, as summarized in Fig. 32.15. The localization of factor 2 to one spine (shown by another red arrow in Fig. 32.15) ensures that LTD will be synapse specific (Wang *et al.*, 2000). Only the synaptic weight of this particular PF → PC synapse is made eligible for modification by the learning rule. If the synapse is excited at nearly the same time that the dendrite is in its plateau state, factors 1 and 2 synergize. Through second messenger pathways, there is a local increase in the level of calcium in the spine. Then, through relatively slow second messen-

ger pathways, this phosphorylates the AMPA receptors of the spine, causing them to become desensitized. To summarize this from a computational standpoint, there is a nearly immediate activation of the dendrite and the PC, and a slow phosphorylation of the AMPA receptors of the spine. The slowness of the latter process provides a biological basis for a slow rise and decay of an *eligibility trace* signifying that this synapse is eligible for LTD (Barto *et al.*, 1999). It became eligible because it was just active and because the dendrite participated (although slightly) in helping to terminate the movement command that this PC helps to regulate.

Factor 3

Meanwhile, a composite motor command is being formulated by the regulatory actions of the array of PCs that shape activity in thousands of the microscopic modules analogous to the ones exemplified in Fig. 32.12. The thousands of elemental movement commands, transmitted by thousands of neurons comprising the output population, function in grand combination to collectively control the actual movement that is eventually made. Only then can this action be evaluated by its sensory consequences so as to provide a *training signal* transmitted by CFs (third red arrow in Fig. 32.15). The corresponding CFs are presumed to detect cases in which there are errors in the end point of the movement. Thus, after a time delay of up to a few hundred milliseconds, a particular CF either fires or remains silent. Its firing signifies that a faulty action is being produced, and an adjustment in synaptic efficacy is needed to make the error less likely in the future. Although the precise mechanism is still being investigated, evidence shows that CF firing leads to an activation of protein kinase G (PKG in Fig. 32.15). Activated PKG prevents the dephosphorylation of recently phosphorylated AMPA receptors. Thus, if the eligibility trace mentioned in the previous paragraph has not yet decayed, this CF discharge could consolidate the desensitization of the AMPA receptors, resulting in a sustained decrement in synaptic weight, which is the definition of LTD.

All three factors need to be satisfied to produce a computationally appropriate learning rule (Houk and Alford, 1996). Factor 1 (a postsynaptic factor) signifies that the dendrite and PC participated actively in the impending action. Factor 2 (a synapse-specific factor) signifies that this particular PF → PC synapse helped the PC to participate in the action. Factor 3 (a training signal) signifies that the action in which the synapse and PC participated resulted, after a substantial time delay, in an error. The slow eligibility trace helps compensate for the time delay.

We have only considered processes that depress synaptic efficacy. Learning rules need to work in both directions to train a network effectively. There is evidence for a reversal of LTD when CFs fail to detect errors, but the mechanisms have yet to receive the attention that they deserve. Another important topic is the morphological consolidation of PF → PC synaptic plasticity that occurs with long-term training (Kleim *et al.*, 1998).

Cerebellar Nuclear Cells Are of Two Types

Cells of the cerebellar nuclei consist of large excitatory neurons (*glutamatergic*) and small inhibitory neurons (*GABAergic* and/or *glycinergic*) (Mugnaini, 2000). Large nuclear neurons are induced to fire at high frequencies, apparently when activated by MF collaterals, and their firing frequency is reduced when PCs burst intensely (Miller *et al.*, 2002). Nuclear cells also exhibit some spontaneous firing under isolated conditions, which results from a tonic cation current mediated mainly by sodium influx (Raman *et al.*, 2000). Less is known about the electrophysiology of the small nuclear cells. However, their discharge should inhibit the olivary neurons to which they project, and this

mechanism appears to cancel out sensory responses during certain phases of behavior, which probably serves to refine the training signals transmitted by CFs.

Classical Conditioning Depends on the Cerebellum

One of the first forms of learning to be analyzed neurobiologically is the classically conditioned reflex (Thompson, 1986). It was discovered that the intermediate cerebellum is crucial for expression of the conditioned eyeblink reflex (Chapter 51). To comprehend how these findings relate to the neurophysiology of the cerebellum, it is helpful to relate the modular concept of cerebellar signal processing (Fig. 32.4) to the neural circuitry that is believed to mediate the conditioned eyeblink movement (Houk *et al.*, 1996; Raymond *et al.*, 1996). Conditioned eyeblinks appear to involve the intermediate cerebellum, parts of it that generate the motor commands that are sent to brain stem networks that control eyelid muscles. When the associated circuitry is labeled with an activity-dependent marker, one can visualize two separate networks (Keifer *et al.*, 1995). One links the intermediate cerebellum with the red nucleus—it is required for well coordinated conditioned reflex responses but not for the basic unconditioned reflex. The latter is controlled by a brain stem network that is required for both conditioned and unconditioned responses.

Plasticity in the cerebellum is probably only responsible for adjusting the metrics of the motor responses (Welsh and Harvey, 1989) and not for making the associative link between the conditioned and the unconditioned stimulus. The conditioned stimulus functions as a sensory cue (one of the diverse inputs in Fig. 32.4) for initiating a transition to the active state of the rubrocerebellar attractor network (Fig. 32.5), so the acquisition of a new cue is more likely to be regulated by pathways that pass through the basal ganglia.

Summary

Neurons of the cerebellum have diverse anatomic and physiologic specializations that appear to facilitate (1) the creation of input diversity in arrays of parallel fibers, (2) the detection by Purkinje cells of salient patterns that are present in these arrays, and (3) the use of these detection outcomes to regulate the temporal pattern of activity in the cerebellar nuclear neurons to which they project. Purkinje cells learn to do this through a unique form of synaptic plasticity that couples efficacy to regulatory performance, as monitored by climbing fibers.

ACTIVATION AND INACTIVATION STUDIES

We can also learn about the functions of the cerebellum by studying what happens when parts of it are activated or inactivated. Activation of the cerebellum results naturally when we use our brain networks in the course of appropriately complex behaviors, and particular regions of the cerebellum can be activated artificially by electrical stimulation. Inactivation of the cerebellum can be produced with lesions, which cause permanent changes, or with reversible inactivations produced by microinjections of pharmacological agents. This section summarizes what has been learned about cerebellar function from activation and inactivation studies.

Activation Studies Reveal Diverse Functions

For many years, the cerebellum was thought to be involved only in the execution of movement, but this appears to be wrong. Human brain imaging studies indicate that the cerebellum also participates in the planning of complex movements and in a variety of cognitive and problem-solving functions (Frackowiak *et al.*, 1997). For example, the cerebellum is activated when subjects make sequential movements and even when they imagine or passively observe movement without making movements themselves. Furthermore, the lateral cerebellum is activated in a language task in which subjects are asked to generate appropriate verbs for visually presented nouns. The observed activity is over and above the activation that occurs when nouns are simply read, indicating that the cerebellum somehow contributes to the generation of appropriate verbs. Interestingly, once a verb generation task has been rehearsed, cerebellar activation diminishes (van Mier *et al.*, 1998). As an additional example, the ventral dentate is activated bilaterally when subjects work to solve a difficult pegboard puzzle, and this activation is three to four times greater in magnitude than during simple peg movements (Kim *et al.*, 1994). Overall, these studies indicate that the newer parts of the cerebellum, the hemispheres and the dentate nucleus, are activated in ways well beyond those required for the execution of movements.

Behavioral observations of humans with cerebellar damage support the conclusion that the cerebellum participates in nonmotor aspects of cognition. In one case study, a cerebellar patient showed impaired performance on the verb generation task described earlier; he was unable to detect errors in his performance of the task and did not exhibit normal practice-related learning. Interestingly, this patient performed normally on standard intelligence and memory tests. In another study, cerebellar patients had deficits in both the production and the perception of a timing task. Lateral cerebellar regions contribute to the perception of time intervals, whereas medial cerebellar regions help mediate the timing of implemented responses.

An older method that was used to activate the cerebellum is electrical stimulation. In the absence of anesthesia, either contractions or relaxations of muscles, and resultant movements, can be elicited by electrical stimulation. The movements affected are diverse and depend, as expected, on the zone of the cerebellum that is stimulated. Sometimes the movements elicited are relatively complex sequences, consistent with the complex motor planning functions mentioned earlier.

Humans with Cerebellar Damage Exhibit Motor Deficits

In the early 1900s, Gordon Holmes described the movement deficits associated with discrete cerebellar lesions in humans that were caused by gunshot wounds. His descriptions provide the basis for classifying clinical cerebellar syndromes according to seven basic deficits.

1. *Ataxia* is a condition that involves lack of coordination between movements of body parts. The term is often used in reference to gait or movement of a specific body part, as in *ataxic arm movements*.

2. *Dysmetria* is an inability to make a movement of the appropriate distance or direction. *Hypometria* is undershooting a target, and *hypermetria* is overshooting a target. Patients with cerebellar damage tend to make hypermetric movements when they move rapidly and hypometric movements when they move more slowly and wish to be accurate.

3. *Dysdiadochokinesia* is an inability to make rapid, alternating movements of a limb. It appears to reflect abnormal agonist–antagonist control.

4. *Asynergia* is an inability to combine the movements of individual limb segments into a coordinated, multisegmental movement.

5. *Hypotonia* is an abnormally decreased muscle tone. It is manifest as a decreased resistance to passive movement so that a limb swings freely upon external perturbation. Often, hypotonia is not present in cerebellar patients or is present only during the acute phase of cerebellar disease.

6. *Nystagmus* is an involuntary and rhythmic eye movement that usually consists of a slow drift and a

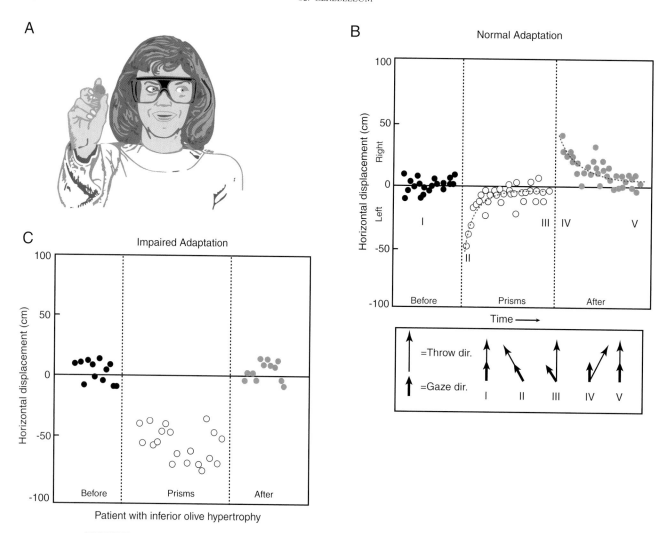

FIGURE 32.16 Prism adaptation test. (A) Eye–hand positions after adaptation to base-right prisms in a control subject. The optic path is bent to the subject's right, giving a larger view of the right side of her face. Her gaze is shifted left along the bent light path to foveate the target in front of her. Her hand position is ready for a throw at the target in front of her. (B) Horizontal locations of throw hits displayed sequentially by trial number. Deviations to the left are negative values; deviations to the right are positive. While the subject is wearing the prisms (gaze shifted to the left), the first hit is displaced 60 cm left of center. Thereafter, hits tend toward 0. After the prisms are removed, the first hit is 50 cm right of center. Thereafter, hits tend toward 0. Data during and after prism use have been fitted with exponential curves. The decay constant is a measure of the rate of adaptation. The standard deviation of the last eight preprism throws is a measure of performance. Gaze and throw directions are schematized with arrows. Inferred gaze (eye and head) direction assumes the subject is foveating the target. Roman numerals beneath the arrows indicate times during the prism adaptation experiment (see B). (C) Failure of adaptation in a patient with bilateral infarctions in the territory of the posterior inferior cerebellar artery. Adapted from Martin *et al.* (1996).

fast resetting phase. After unilateral cerebellar lesion, the fast phase of nystagmus is toward the side of the lesion.

7. *Action tremor*, or *intention tremor*, is an involuntary oscillation that occurs during limb movement and disappears when the limb is at rest. Cerebellar action tremor is generally at a low frequency (3–5 Hz). *Titubation* is a tremor of the entire trunk during stance and gait.

Cerebellar damage also causes deficits in motor learning. Studies of prism adaptation have shown that some patients with cerebellar damage are unable to adapt their hand–eye coordination to the visual displacement produced by the prism (Fig. 32.16). Most of these symptoms can be explained as a basic problem of learning to control the direction and amplitude of a movement (dysmetria), making it necessary to use multiple corrective submovements (action tremor).

Localized Inactivations Produce Modular Deficits

Damage to the cerebellar nuclei causes unique behavioral deficits (Thach, 1998). Ablations of the fastigial nucleus in cat and monkey impair movements dramatically requiring control of equilibrium, such as unsupported sitting, stance, and gait. Longitudinal splitting of the cerebellum along the midline also produces very significant and long-lasting disturbances of equilibrium. In humans, lesions in the anterior vermis preferentially impair movements requiring equilibrium control (Timmann and Horak, 1995). Much of the fastigial nucleus seems to be involved preferentially in movements like stance and gait.

Ablations of the interpositus nucleus in monkeys cause action tremor as the animals reach for food. Temporary inactivation of the interpositus nucleus and adjacent regions of dentate with cooling probes elicits tremor that is dependent on proprioceptive feedback but is uninfluenced by vision. Focal pharmacological inactivations within the intermediate region disrupt the use of particular synergies related to hand use and limb positioning (Mason *et al.*, 1998). Damage to the cortex and the inferior olive prevents many kinds of motor adaptation, including the acquisition of new and novel muscle synergies. These studies support the ideas reviewed earlier in this chapter, namely that the intermediate cerebellum regulates the composite motor commands that control the metrics of coordinated upper and lower extremity limb movements. Damage to the posterior vermis and flocculonodular lobe produces analogous disorders of eye movements (Chapter 33).

Summary

Activation and inactivation studies of the cerebellum are consistent with the concepts promoted earlier in this chapter. The cerebellum learns how to regulate neuronal populations in different parts of the brain that control different kinds of movement, autonomic function, and cognitive signal processing.

PHYLOGENETIC AND ONTOGENETIC DEVELOPMENT

There are two kinds of development: phylogenetic, in the course of evolution, and ontogenetic, from the embryo to the adult animal. Both involve an enlargement of the cerebellum that parallels the enlargement of other parts of the brain, but there are many exceptions to the concept that ontogeny recapitulates phylogeny.

The Cerebellum Reflects the Course of Vertebrate Evolution

The cerebellum is present in all vertebrates from the primitive agnathans up through the advanced pri-

---

BOX 32.3

THE GIGANTOCEREBELLUM OF MORMYRID FISH

Weakly electric fish of the family Mormyridae have an enormous cerebellum that covers their brain like our cerebral cortex covers our brain. This gigantocerebellum explains why these fish have a large brain-to-body ratio of 0.03 and why their brain uses 60% of the oxygen that they take in. For comparison, our brain-to-body ratio is only 0.02 and our brain uses only 20% of the oxygen we take in. The gigantocerebellum is composed of a ribbon of Purkinje cells 0.3 mm high and 1.0 m long that is folded back on itself repeatedly to fit within the skull. Different regions of the cerebellum receive electrosensory, auditory, and lateral line input from midbrain structures homologous to the mammalian inferior colliculus. These cerebellar regions project back to the same midbrain sensory structures from which they receive their input. Thus, this cerebellum is more involved in process-ing sensory input than in generating motor output. Although the type of processing that is done by the cerebellum of the fish is still unknown, cerebellum-like structures in another part of these fish brains, the electrosensory lobe and the dorsal octaval nucleus, generate memory-like expectations of sensory input by means of plastic changes at synapses between parallel fibers and Purkinje-like cells (Bell, 2001), analogous to what probably occurs in the cerebellum itself.

Curtis C. Bell

Reference

Bell, C. C. (2001). Memory based expectations in electrosensory systems. *Curr. Opin Neurobio.* **11**, 481–487.

mates, although its parts show considerable species variation. In the lamprey (agnathans), the cerebellum is a rudimentary structure that assists the functions of the well-developed vestibuloocular, vestibulospinal, and reticulospinal systems and is equated to the flocculonodular lobe. The cerebellum is much larger in fishes, where a corpus cerebelli distinctly appears. In electric fish (Box 32.3), the cerebellum is extraordinarily developed and includes lobes not present in other vertebrates. The cerebellum increases further in reptiles and birds, although it consists nearly exclusively of the vermal zone of the corpus cerebelli and the flocculonodular lobe. Well-developed glomeruli are present in reptiles and birds. Basket cells, however, are absent in reptiles and are well developed in birds, pointing to evolutionary sophistication of inhibitory interneural connections. In birds, the vermis is distinctly foliated, and lobules I through X are clearly apparent, but the basilar pontine nuclei are rudimentary and project to small, flattened lateral zones. In mammals, the lateral cerebellar zone expands to form the cerebellar hemispheres, in register with the development of the pontine nuclei and the cerebral cortex.

In evolution, the size of the cerebellar cortex increases more distinctly than that of the cerebellar nuclei, reflecting a greater emphasis on the computational aspects of information processing. While lobulation, in principle, is fairly consistent across mammals, despite great variation in hemispheric development, foliation shows great interspecies variation and also substantial intraspecies differences. For example, different mouse strains may show different folial patterns. In aquatic mammals, the vermal and the intermediate zones and the underlying fastigial and posterior interpositus nuclei are large, and the lateral zones relatively small. The vermal and hemispheral portions of the posterior lobe that receive pontine afferents appear mostly expanded in primates, and especially the human. The cortico-ponto-cerebellar input loops back to many areas of the cerebral cortex. In human, fibers of the middle cerebellar peduncle vastly outnumber all of the other connections.

In the Embryo, Outputs Develop First

Cerebellar neurons develop at different times from two different germinative matrices: the ventricular epithelium of the *cerebellar anlage* and the cells of the *rhombic lip* (Fig. 32.17). The cerebellar anlage, or primordium, begins as bilateral elevations of the dorsal aspect of the primitive hindbrain and caudal midbrain that grow toward the midline and ultimately fuse (Liu and Joyner, 2001). The ventricular epithe-

lium of this anlage gives rise to all cerebellar neurons, except granule cells, by a process of outward directed migration. The rhombic lip is an elevation of the rostral hindbrain that extends from the first to the eighth rhombomeres. It gives rise to the external granular layer precursors, from which granule cells originate by inward migration. The first cells to be formed in the ventricular zone of the cerebellar anlage are neurons of the cerebellar nuclei. They are followed soon after by Purkinje cells, which migrate past the developing cerebellar nuclei to their ultimate location in the cortex. Precursors committed to differentiate into unipolar brush cells, Golgi cells, basket cells, stellate cells, and glial cells, which are produced in later waves, migrate to their final positions after migration of the Purkinje cells and continue to proliferate on

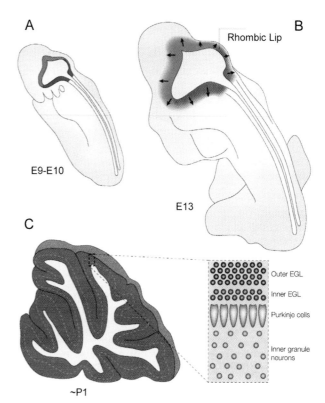

FIGURE 32.17 Early development of mouse cerebellum. (A) At embryonic day E9–E10, the rhombic lip (blue and orange) is a zone of proliferation at the level of the fourth ventricle. Cells in the blue region give rise to cerebellar granule neurons and pontine nuclei, whereas cells in the orange region give rise to other rhombic lip derivatives, such as the inferior olivary nucleus. (B) At E13, cells from the rhombic lip migrate outward to cover the cerebellar primordium forming the extrenal granular layer. (C) At early postnatal stages (P1 and further), these committed granule cell precursors continue to proliferate in the outer external granular layer (EGL), then become postmitotic and form the inner EGL, and finally migrate from the inner EGL past the Purkinje cells and into the inner granular layer, where they differentiate into granule cells establishing synaptic connections with mossy fiber terminals. From Wang and Zoghbi (2001).

their way to the cortex. At an early stage, small cells migrate from the rhombic lip over the entire external surface of the cerebellum, forming the so-called "external granular layer," where they remain quiescent until much later in development.

Cerebellar Input Structures Develop Next

After the Purkinje cells have reached the cortical plate, climbing fibers enter the cerebellum from the inferior olive and begin to innervate the Purkinje cells (Fig. 32.18), with each Purkinje cell receiving input from several climbing fibers. Much later, after the Purkinje cells have begun to receive synapses from parallel fibers, most of the climbing fiber contacts with Purkinje cells will be eliminated, leaving a private line of one climbing fiber per Purkinje cell. Mossy fibers also enter the cerebellum and grow to the level just below the Purkinje cell layer. They will ultimately synapse on granule cells, which have yet to arrive.

Shortly before and after birth, cells in the external granular layer form two contiguous strata over the developing cerebellum: the proliferative outer external granular layer and the postmitotic, premigratory inner external granular layer (Fig. 32.17). Cells of the inner layer emit axons at opposite poles that run in the coronal plane (the future parallel fibers) and then form a third process that extends toward the underlying Purkinje cells utilizing the radial Bergmann fibers as a scaffold. The third process extends progressively past the Purkinje cell layer, and the cell nucleus translocates into the process and reaches the prospective granular layer, leaving the elongating parallel fiber in place (Fig. 32.19). Normally, all external granule cells abandon the external granular layer. After this surface-to-depth migratory process, the differentiating granule cell emits short processes, or protodendrites, that search the developing mossy fiber terminals to establish connections. Successively, some of the protodendrites are pruned, while three to five of them

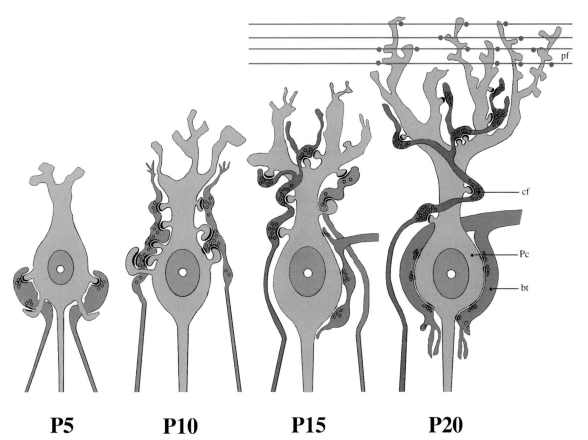

P5   **P10**   **P15**   **P20**

FIGURE 32.18   Development of the climbing fiber–purkinje cell pathway. After the Purkinje cell becomes synaptically competent at postnatal day 5 (P5), branches from two or more climbing fibers establish contact with short processes arising from the soma and successively grow to occupy first the apical dendritic stem (P10) and then the entire proximal compartment of the dendritic tree (P15). During formation of the spiny branchlets and parallel fiber synapses, supranumerary climbing fibers branches retract, leaving only one climbing fiber branch per Purkinje cell (P20). Illustration by E. Mugnaini and G. Sekerkova (based on Crepel *et al.*, 1976).

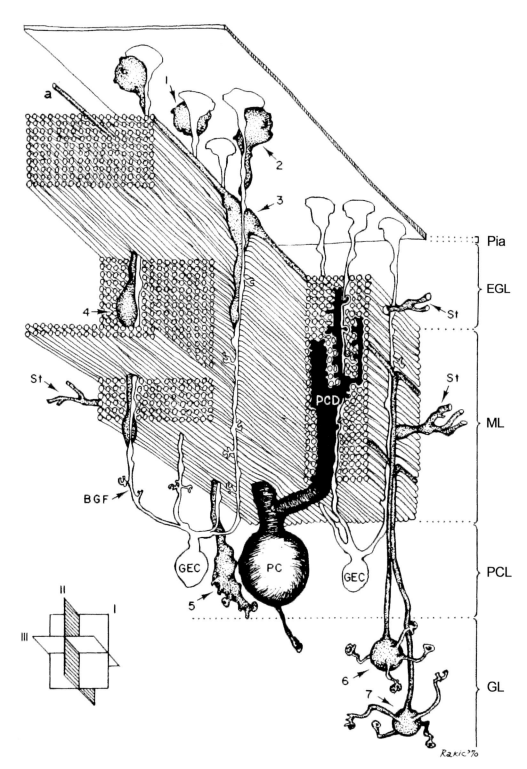

FIGURE 32.19 "Four dimensional" (time and space) developmental reconstruction of the targets of the mossy fiber–parallel fiber–Purkinje cell pathway. Granule cell precursors (arrows 1–7) migrate from the external granular layer to the definitive granular layer along radially oriented Bergmann glial fibers (BGF), leaving in place parallel fibers (a, stacked thin rods) in a process of appositional growth. Bergman glia fibers are processes of astrocytic Golgi epithelial cells (GEC) situated in the Purkinje cell (PC) layer. PCD, proximal Purkinje cell dendrite forming spiny branchlets. St, stellate cells oriented perpendicular to the parallel fibers. Pia, pial membrane; EGL, external granular layer; ML, molecular layer; PCL, Purkinje cell layer; GL, granular layer. From Rakic (1971), with permission.

progressively mature into adult granule cell dendrites. At the same time, mossy fiber terminals enlarge to accommodate the optimal number of dendritic claws. Concomitantly, Golgi cell axons establish their synapses at the base of the claws. Ensheathing of the glomeruli by lamellar processes of astrocytes becomes progressively more complete. In rodents, this process of glomerular development takes about 6 weeks.

It is interesting that the "motor" side of the cerebellar circuit (the deep nuclear cells and Purkinje cells) forms first, the "sensory" side (MFs and CFs) then arrives in place, and the "matrix" that connects the two (the granule cells and intrinsic inhibitory neurons) is the last to develop.

Human Cerebellar Development Is Not Complete at Birth

In humans, the first cerebellar structures develop at approximately 32 days after fertilization, and development is not completed until long after birth. The cere-bellar cortex of the early embryo has six distinct layers, but this number is ultimately reduced to three. The cortex begins to differentiate slightly earlier in the vermis, flocculus, and median sections of the hemi-spheres than in the lateral hemispheres. By 7 months after fertilization, cerebellar nuclei have attained the shape and location they will have in the adult. At birth, the cerebellar cortex consists of four uneven layers, and Purkinje cells and basket cells are weakly developed. The fourth layer (the external granule cell layer) disap-pears within the first postnatal year. In humans, full myelination of cerebellar connections is not complete until the second year of life.

Summary

Comparative anatomy indicates that the cerebellum develops in parallel with both the motor apparatus and the sensory input to the brain and, in mammals, becomes linked with the cerebral cortex. Ontogenetic development begins with the output neurons, proceeds

---

BOX 32.4

GENES CONTROLLING CEREBELLAR DEVELOPMENT

Work on mouse mutant strains with cerebellar abnor-malities (e.g., weaver, reeler, staggerer, rostral cerebellar malformation) and genetic studies on formation of the hindbrain have uncovered a multitude of genes and sig-naling pathways that govern development of the brain stem and cerebellum (Wang and Zoghbi, 2001). Moreover, classes of cerebellar neurons, especially Purkinje and granule cells, have been shown to interact during cerebellar development in regulating cell number and compartmentalization.

The complex interplay of several patterning genes (primarily Otx2, Gbx2, and Fgf8) sets up the isthmus organizer. This region of the early neural tube, situated at the junction between the mesencephalon and the meten-cephalon, regulates the rostrocaudal patterning of the midbrain–hindbrain and formation of the cerebellar pri-mordium. Other sets of intracellular and secreted gene products control discrete steps in cerebellar develop-ment. Math1 and genes coding numerous zinc finger proteins play major roles in generation, proliferation, and movement of granule cell precursors in the germi-nal matrix of the rhombic lip. Semaphorins, slits, netrins, and TAG1 regulate dorsoventral migration from the rhombic lip and the formation of precerebellar nuclei and pathways. Cyclin D2 and Unc5h3 regulate the prolif-eration and rostral arrest of the external granular layer, respectively. Migration of differentiating granule cells along the glial fibers of the molecular layer is set up by several molecules, including cell cycle inhibitors, tubulin-associated proteins, trombospondin, astrotactin, and neuroregulin. Genes controlling the proliferation of Purkinje cell precursors are poorly known, whereas genes of the reelin signaling pathway and netrin receptors regulate Purkinje cell migration. Genetic mechanisms that control the anterior–posterior compart-mentalization and foliation of the cerebellum are begin-ning to be defined, whereas little is known about developmental regulation of the parasagittal zones. Several molecules promoting Purkinje cell and granule cell sur-vival have been identified. These include growth factors, ion channels, and neurotransmitters. Genes regulatng pro-liferation, migration, and survival of the precursors of Golgi cells, unipolar brush cells, and stellate/basket cells are still scarcely known.

James C. Houk and Enrico Mugnaini

Reference

Wang, V. Y., and Zoghbi, H. Y. (2001). Genetic regulation of cere-bellar development. *Nature Rev.* **2**, 484–491.

BOX 32.5

CEREBELLUM — THE TRUE THINKING MACHINE

It no longer seems reasonable to consider the function of the cerebellum as being confined to the control of voluntary movement, speech, and equilibrium. Considerable evidence suggests that the cerebellum is critical also for thought, behavior, and emotion. Anatomical studies demonstrate that the cerebellum is an important part of the distributed neural circuitry that subserves cognitive processing. The association and paralimbic cerebral cortices known to subserve higher order functions are linked with the cerebellum in a precisely organized system of feedforward and feedback loops, and physiological studies indicate that these pathways are functionally relevant. Cerebellar ablation and stimulation experiments in animals have demonstrated cerebellar influences on many nonmotor functions, including classical conditioning, navigational skills, cognitive flexibility, sham rage, predatory attack, and aggression. Functional neuroimaging investigations of the morphologic correlates of cognitive processing using PET and fMRI in humans have revealed sites of activation in the cerebellum in a number of cognitive tasks. These include linguistic processing, verbal working memory, shifting attention, mental imagery, classical conditioning, motor learning, sensory processing, and modulation of emotion. Furthermore, there appears to be a topographic organization of the sites within the cerebellum activated by these different cognitive processes.

Clinical investigations of adults and children with diseases confined to the cerebellum have defined a cerebellar cognitive affective syndrome characterized by impairments of executive processing, working memory, visual spatial reasoning, language disturbances (ranging from mutism to agrammatism), and a flattened or inappropriate affect. The net effect of these deficits is a lowering of overall intellectual ability. The posterior lobe of the cerebellum appears particularly important in the generation of this syndrome, and the vermis is consistently involved when the affective component is pronounced. Elements of this clinical syndrome have also been noted in patients with developmental cerebellar anomalies, cerebellar degeneration, autism, and fragile X syndrome. In addition, cerebellar abnormalities, particularly in the vermis, have been observed in patients with schizophrenia.

The mechanisms whereby the cerebellum influences higher function are still debated. The organization of the cerebellar corticonuclear microcomplex and the interactions between the mossy and climbing fiber systems prompted the hypothesis that the cerebellum provides an error detection mechanism for the motor system. This mechanism may also be relevant for mental operations.

The relationship between the cerebellum and nonmotor function has been conceptualized as follows.

1. The cerebellum is able to subserve cognitive functions because it is anatomically interconnected with the associative and paralimbic cortices.
2. Cognitive and behavioral functions are organized topographically within the cerebellum.
3. The convergence of inputs from multiple associative cerebral regions to adjacent areas within the cerebellum facilitates cerebellar regulation of supramodal functions.
4. The cerebellar contribution to cognition is one of modulation rather than generation.
5. The cerebellum performs computations for cognitive functions similar to those for the sensorimotor system—but the information being modulated is different.
6. The disruption of the cerebellar influences on higher functions leads to dysmetria of thought, impairment of mental agility that manifests, at least in part, as the cerebellar cognitive affective syndrome.

The potential for further discovery in this field places the cerebellum, previously thought of as a motor control device, in the forefront of current behavioral neuroscience research.

Jeremy D. Schmahmann

---

to the inputs, and culminates with the interneuronal matrix.

OVERALL SUMMARY

Despite its deceptively simple circuitry, the cerebellum appears to be the most sophisticated signal processing structure in the brain. Instead of new functions being localized there, this neural machinery is used to regulate functions that are localized in other parts of the brain. Through its many mossy fibers and granule cells, Purkinje cells are presented with an enormously diverse input that reflects the state of the body, the state of the environment, and the internal state of the brain. Through the training influence of its climbing fibers,

Purkinje cells then learn to detect the occurrences of complex patterns of state, which mark the times at which they need to use their powerful inhibition to shape cerebellar nuclear output in order to regulate populations of neurons in other parts of the brain. The oldest modules of the cerebellum regulate the motor commands that orient the eyes and head toward interesting objects in the world around us. Other modules regulate the motor commands for locomotion, and yet others the command signals for voluntarily manipulating objects. The newest modules in the cerebellum, located in the hemispheres, regulate signals in the cerebral cortex that plan, perceive, and solve problems. All of these functions are complex operations, and we still have much to learn about the mechanisms that support the many signal processing operations of the cerebellum.

References

Armstrong, C. L., and Hawkes, R. (2000). Pattern formation in the cerebellar cortex. *Biochem. Cell Biol.* **78**(5), 551–62.

Barto, A. G., Fagg, A. H., Sitkoff, N., and Houk, J. C. (1999). A cerebellar model of timing and prediction in the control of reaching. *Neural Comput.* **11**, 565–94.

Bower, J. M., Beermann, D. H., Gibson, J. M., Shambes, G. M., and Welker, W. (1981). Principles of organization of a cerebro-cerebellar circuit: Micromapping the projections from cerebral (SI) to cerebellar (granule cell layer) tactile areas of rats. *Brain Behav. Evol.* **18**(1–2), 1–18.

Brodal, A. (1981). "Neurological Anatomy in Relation to Clinical Medicine." Oxford University Press, New York.

Brodal, P. (1998). "The Central Nervous System," pp. 393–418. Oxford University Press, New York.

Brodal, P., and Bjaalie, J. G. (1992). Organization of the pontine nuclei. *Neurosci. Res.* **13**, 83–118.

Cajal, S. Ramón Y (1995). "Histology of the Nervous System of Man and Vertebrates" (translated by N. Swanson and L. W. Swanson). Oxford University Press, New York.

Crepel, F., Mariani, J., and Delhaye-Bouchaud, N. (1976). Evidence for a multiple innervation of Purkinje cells by climbing fibers in the immature rat cerebellum. *J. Neuobiology* **7**, 567–578.

De Camilli, P., Haucke, V., Takei, K., and Mugnaini, E. (2001). Structure of synapses. *In* "Synapses." (W. M. Cowan, T. C. Südhof, and C. T. Stevens, eds.), pp. 89–133. Johns Hopkins University Press, Baltimore.

Dietrichs, E., Haines, D. E., Roste, G. K., and Roste, L. S. (1994). Hypothalamocerebellar and cerebellohypothalamic projections—circuits for regulating nonsomatic cerebellar activity. *Histol. Histopathol.* **9**, 603–14.

Dow, R. S. (1942). The evolution and anatomy of the cerebellum, *Biol. Rev.* **17**, 179–220.

Ebner, T. J. (1998). A role for the cerebellum in the control of limb movement velocity. *Curr. Opin Neurobiol.* **8**, 762–9.

Ekerot, C.-F., and Jörntell, H. (2001). Parallel fibre receptive fields of purkinje cells and interneurons are climbing fibre-specific. *Eur. J. Neurosci.* **13**, 1303–10.

Hansel, C., Linden, D. J., and D'Angelo, E. (2001). Beyond parallel fiber LTD: The diversity synaptic and non-synaptic plasticity in the cerebellum. *Nature Neurosci.* **4**(5), 467–75.

Heimer, L. (1995). Human Brain and Spinal Cord. Springer-Verlag, New York.

Houk, J. C., and Alford, S. (1996). Computational significance of the cellular mechanisms for synaptic plasticity in Purkinje cells. *Behav. Brain Sci.* **19**, 457–61.

Houk, J. C., and Miller, L. E. (2001). Cerebellum: Movement Regulation and Cognitive Functions. *In* "Encyclopedia of Life Sciences." Nature Publishing Group/www.els.net.

Kandel, E. R., Schwartz, J. H., and Jessel, T. M. (2000). "Principles of Neural Science." McGraw Hill, New York.

Kim, S.-G., Ugurbil, K., and Strick, P. L. (1994). Activation of a cerebellar output nucleus during cognitive processing. *Science* **265**, 949–51.

Keifer, J., Armstrong, K. E., and Houk, J. C. (1995). In vitro classical conditioning of abducens nerve discharge in turtles. *J. Neurosci.* **15**, 5036–48.

Kleim, J. A., Swain, R. A., Armstrong, K. A., Napper, R. M. A., Jones, T. A., and Greenough, W. T. (1998). Selective synaptic plasticity within the cerebellar cortex following complex motor skill learning. *Neurobiol. Learn. Memory* **69**, 274–89.

Larsell, O., and Jansen, J. (eds.) (1972). The Cerebellum. Minnesota Univ. Press, Minneapolis.

Llinás, R., and Sugimori, M. (1980). Electrophysiological properties of in vitro Purkinje cell somata in mammalian cerebellar slices. *J. Physiol. Lond.* **305**, 171–95.

Martin, T. A., Keating, J. G., Goodkin, H. P., Bastian, A. J., and Thach, W. T. (1996). Throwing while looking through prisms. I. Focal olivocerebellar lesions impair adaptation. *Brain* **119**, 1183–98.

Mason, C. R., Miller, L. E., Baker, J. F., and Houk, J. C. (1998). Organization of reaching and grasping movements in the primate cerebellar nuclei as revealed by focal muscimol inactivations. *J. Neurophysiol.* **79**, 537–54.

Miller, L. E., Holdefer, R. N., and Houk, J. C. (2002). The role of the cerebellum in modulating voluntary limb movement commands. *Archi. Itali. Biol.*

Nunzi, M. G., Birnstiel, S., Bhattacharyya, B. J., Slater, N. T., and Mugnaini, E. (2001). Unipolar brush cells form a glutamatergic projection system within the mouse cerebellar cortex. *J. Comp. Neuro.* **434**, 329–41.

Rakic, P. (1971). Neuron-glia relationship during cell migration in developing cerebellar cortex: A Golgi and electron microscopic study in *Macacas rhesus. J. Comp. Neurol.* **141**, 283–312.

Raman, I. M., Gustafson, A. E., and Padgett, D. (2000). Ionic currents and spontaneous firing in neurons isolated from the cerebellar nuclei. *J. Neurosci.* **20**(24), 9004–16.

Raymond, J. L., Lisberger, S. G., and Mauk, M. D. (1996). The cerebellum: A neuronal learning machine? *Science* **272**, 1126–31.

Simpson, J. I., Wylie, D. R., and de Zeeuw, C. I. (1996). On climbing fiber signals and their consequence(s). *Behav. Brain Sci.* **19**, 384–98.

Timmann, D., and Horak, F. B. (1995). Perturbed step initiation in cerebellar subjects. 2 Modification of anticipatory postural adjustments. *Exp. Brain Res.* **141**, 110–20.

Van Kan, P. L. E., Gibson, A. R., and Houk, J. C. (1993). Movement-related inputs to intermediate cerebellum of the monkey. *J. Neurophysiology* **69**, 74–94.

van Mier, H., Tempel, L. W., Perlmutter, J. S., Raichle, M. E., and Petersen, S. E. (1998). Changes in brain activity during motor learning measured with PET: Effects of hand of performance and practice. *J. Neurophysiol.* **80**, 2177–99.

Wang, S. S.–H, Denk, W., and Hausser, M. (2000). Coincidence detection in single dendritic spines mediated by calcium. *Nature Neurosci.* **3**, 1266–73.

Welsh, J. P., and Harvey, J. A. (1989). Cerebellar lesions and the nictitating membrane reflex: performance deficits of the conditioned and unconditioned response. *J. Neurosci.* **9**, 299–311.

Welsh, J. P., Lang, E. J., Sughihara, I., and Llinas, R. (1995). Dynamic organization of motor control within the olivocerebellar system. *Nature* **374**, 453–7.

Suggested Readings

Frackowiak, R. S. J., Friston, K. J., Frith, C. D., Dolan, R. J. and Mazziotta, J. C. (1997). Functional organisation of the motor system. *In* "Human Brain Function," pp 243–274, Academic Press.

Houk, J. (2001). Neurophysiology of frontal-subcortical loops. *In* "Frontal-Subcortical Circuits in Psychiatry and Neurology" (D. G. Lichter and J. L. Cummings, eds.), 92–113, Guilford, New York.

Houk, J. C., Buckingham, J. T. and Barto, A. G. (1996). Models of the cerebellum and motor learning. *Behav Brain Sci* **19**, 368–383.

Ito, M. (1984). "The Cerebellum and Neural Control." Raven Press, New York.

Liu A., and Joyner A. L. (2001). Early anterior/posterior patterning of the midbrain and cerebellum. *Annu Rev Neurosci* **24**, 869–896.

Middleton, F. A., and Strick, P. L. (1998). Cerebellar output: Motor and cognitive channels. *Trends Cogn Sci* **2**, 348–354.

Mugnaini, E. (2000). GABAergic inhibition in the cerebellar system. *In* "GABA in the Nervous System: The View at Fifty Years" (D. L. Martin and R. W. Olsen, eds.), pp. 383–407.

Thach, W. T. (1998). What is the role of the cerebellum in motor learning and cognition? *Trends Cogni Sci* **2**(9), 331–337.

Thompson, R. F. (1986). The neurobiology of learning and memory. *Science* **233**, 941–947.

Voogd, J., and Glickstein, M. (1998). The anatomy of the cerebellum. *TINS* **21**(9), 370–375.

James C. Houk and Enrico Mugnaini

Eye Movements

THERE ARE FIVE TYPES OF EYE MOVEMENTS

As shown in Chapter 27, the vertebrate photoreceptor mosaic of the retina transduces light energy in the form of photons into neural activity, ultimately in the form of action potentials. The spatial resolution of this transduction system is limited by the resolution of the photoreceptor mosaic, but only if the eye can be kept stationary with regard to the objects in the external world that are the subjects of visual analysis. Thus, stabilizing the retina with regard to the outside world and aligning the retina with moving or stationary targets is a critical challenge to effective vision. Evolutionary pressures have shaped the eye movement systems of all animals to meet this challenge in ways that are tailored to the visual structures and environmental needs of each species. An analysis of the neural and behavioral systems employed by vertebrates to achieve effective retinal stabilization reveals two principal classes of mechanisms: one class responsible specifically for *gaze stabilization* and a second class responsible for *gaze shifting*. While *gaze stabilization* mechanisms are found in all animals with visual systems, *gaze-shifting* mechanisms are observed only in animals that have retinal specializations, such as the primate fovea, which can be used to examine a limited region of visual space at higher acuity.

Gaze-Stabilization Mechanisms

A completely stationary animal, whose photoreceptors were anchored to the earth, would always be able to resolve stationary stimuli to the resolution limits of its retina, but when any animal moves it risks degrad-

ing its visual acuity. Rotation of the *line of sight* by movement of the head, for example, will cause a point of light fixed in the environment to streak across the retina, appearing as a line or curve to the visual system. Gaze-stabilization mechanisms are movement systems that have evolved to counteract this effect of self-motion on visual acuity. These mechanisms coordinate movements of the eye, with regard to the head, which precisely compensate for self-motion, thus stabilizing the visual world on the retina.

Gaze-stabilization mechanisms are generally described as falling into two subclasses: **vestibulo-ocular** systems and **optokinetic** systems. The vestibulo-ocular systems of vertebrates rely upon the semi-circular canals to determine the precise rate at which the head is rotated in any direction. The optokinetic system relies on the photoreceptors themselves to compute the speed and direction at which the visual world is shifting across the retina. These neural systems then precisely compensate for this rotation by activating the **extra-ocular muscles** (or eye movement muscles) to produce a perfectly matched counterrotation of the eyes. The result is that despite movements of the head, the line of sight remains constant with regard to the environment. As we will learn, the optokinetic system operates most efficiently at low velocities of rotation where the photoreceptors can be used to determine accurately the speed and direction of image motion, whereas the vestibulo-ocular system is most efficient at higher speeds of rotation where the vestibular apparatus most accurately measures head velocity. Together, these sensory motor systems have the ability to use different types of sensory data to activate a common muscular system. This common muscular system stabilizes retinal images during self-motion at velocities that range from the minimum velocities which degrade retinal acuity, up to the maximum velocities of self-motion that an animal can produce.

Gaze-Shifting Mechanisms

Versional Movements Shift the Line of Gaze with Regard to the Visual World

While essentially all vertebrates have gaze-stabilization systems, several groups within the vertebrates have evolved specialized retinas that can only be effectively employed by animals capable of shifting the direction of their gaze. Primates, for example, have evolved a highly specialized central region of the retina known as the fovea. In this region, that can gather information from only 1° of the visual world, the photoreceptor mosaic is packed at much higher density, permitting much higher resolution. This higher resolution would be useless, however, unless it could be specifically directed to areas of interest in the visual world and stabilized with regard to those stimuli. To accomplish this, essentially all vertebrates with retinal subregions specialized for higher acuity have evolved gaze-shifting systems that employ the extraocular muscles. Gaze-shifting mechanisms can be broken into two main groups: the **saccadic** system, that rapidly shifts gaze from one point to another, and the **smooth pursuit** system, which allows the fovea to track a moving target as it slides across a stationary background. It should come as no surprise that the smooth pursuit system is believed to have evolved from the optokinetic system. Both systems move the eyes to limit the velocity with that stimuli move across the retina, although one is concerned with movements of small targets while the other is concerned with movements of the entire visual world. In a similar manner, the saccadic system appears to have developed from a neurobiological mechanism shared by the optokinetic and vestibulo-ocular systems, which is discussed later. The saccadic and pursuit systems together are often referred to as **versional** systems.

Vergence Movements Shift the Lines of Gaze of the Two Eyes with Regard to Each Other

A third class of gaze-shifting eye movements have evolved in an even smaller subset of vertebrates, those with both fovea-like specializations and binocular vision. These animals have the ability to scrutinize a single visual target with both eyes and have evolved special eye movement system to control the angle formed by the lines of gaze of the two eyes. Consider a situation in which the lines of gaze from both eyes intersect with an infinitely distant target. Under these conditions the lines of gaze projecting from the two foveas are parallel. As targets for foveal vision move closer, however, the lines of gaze must *converge*. Animals who employ *binocular vision* must therefore have an eye movement system that can keep both eyes aligned with visual targets as those targets vary in depth. This binocular convergence is accomplished by adding, for each eye, a different gaze control signal to the shared saccadic or pursuit signal. This concept, that an equal saccadic or pursuit signal is sent to both eyes and that vergence signals, for each eye, are added to this common signal is known as **Hering's law of equal innervation**.

Summary

All eye movements belong to one or more of these five classes: the vestibulo-ocular, optokinetic, saccadic, smooth pursuit, and vergence systems. While each of these systems is a largely distinct neural entity, they all engage a common set of motor neurons and thus a common set of muscles. This shared motor circuitry imposes some interesting commonalities on the systems. For this reason, we first discuss the common muscular system before we examine the five eye movement systems.

OCULOMOTOR NUCLEI AND EXTRAOCULAR MUSCLES

Six Muscles Move Each Eye

In primates all eye movements are produced by the contraction or relaxation of the six extraocular muscles. These six muscles surround each eye and can produce rotations of that eye in any direction. As can be seen in Fig. 33.1 the muscles are arranged in three antagonistic pairs, much like the antagonistic pairs observed in the skeletomuscular system. The **medial** and **lateral rectus** muscles, for example, form an antagonistic pair, that controls the horizontal position of each eye. Contraction of the lateral rectus (and commensurate relaxation of the medial rectus) causes an eye to rotate outward, shifting the direction of gaze laterally. It should be noted that because the two eyes move together, contraction of the medial rectus of one eye will be accompanied by contraction of the lateral rectus of the other eye, thus rotating both eyes similarly. The **superior** and **inferior recti** are a second pair of muscles and their principal function is to control the up-and-down rotations of the eyes. Finally, the **superior** and **inferior obliques** make up the third muscle pair. Oblique muscles serve an unusual function, they control rotation of the eye about the line of sight, a type of rotation referred to as *torsion*. These two muscles also

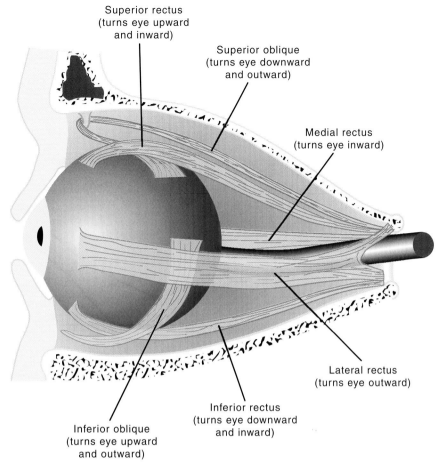

Superior rectus
(turns eye upward
and inward)

Superior oblique
(turns eye downward
and outward)

Medial rectus
(turns eye inward)

Lateral rectus
(turns eye outward)

Inferior rectus
(turns eye downward
and inward)

Inferior oblique
(turns eye upward
and outward)

FIGURE 33.1 Muscles of the eye. Six muscles, arranged in three pairs, control the movements of the eye as shown here in a cutaway view of the eye in its socket, or orbit.

make a small contribution to pulling the eye up or down. Because the superior and inferior rectus muscles also generate some torsion of the eye, the obliques are particularly important for guaranteeing that the eye, as it moves around the orbit, maintains its characteristic vertical orientation.

Three Cranial Nerves Control Eye Movement Muscles

The six extraocular muscles are innervated by three of the bilaterally paired cranial nerves. The oculomotor nerve (cranial nerve III) innervates the medial rectus, the superior and inferior rectus, and the inferior oblique on one side of the head. The cell bodies for these motor neurons thus lie in the third cranial nerve nucleus. The trochlear nerve (IV) innervates the superior oblique muscle, and the abducens nerve (VI) innervates the lateral rectus. These three pairs of nuclei, distributed through the brain stem, contain all of the **oculomotor motor neurons** and are heavily interconnected by a pathway called the **medial longi-**

tudinal fasciculus. This interconnection is important because it permits the precise coordination of the extraocular muscles that is necessary for the control of eye movements.

Eye Movements Are Produced by a Combination of Static and Dynamic Forces

In order to understand how muscle forces control the position and movement of the eyes, it is first necessary to know a little more about what resistance to movement the tissues and muscles of the orbit produce. In simplest form, the eye in the orbit can be thought of as a sphere held in place by a system of springs that tend to draw the eye into a central position. To hold the eye at a noncentral position, it is necessary for the muscles to produce a force adequate to counteract the spring tensions trying to draw the eye back to its resting central position. Movement of the eye from one eccentric location to another requires an additional, or *dynamic*, force. This is because movement of the eye is further opposed by what can be thought of as friction.

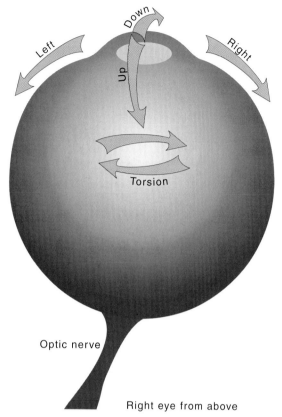

FIGURE 33.2 Axes of eye rotations. The eye muscles can rotate the eye along three axes: horizontal, vertical, and torsional.

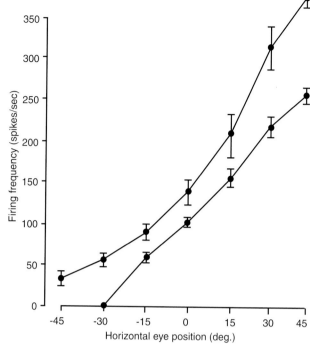

FIGURE 33.3 Rate–position curves for abducens motor neurons. Plots of the motor neuron firing rate as a function of eye position when the eye is stationary demonstrate that the motor neuron firing rate is linearly related to static eyse position. After Fuchs and Lushei (1970).

This "friction," or resistance to movement, means that if the static forces are simply changed from one moment to the next, the eye will move very slowly from its initial position to the new position specified by the new muscle tensions. To overcome this resistance, additional force is required during each movement. Thus eye movements require two sets of muscle forces, a transient dynamic force to overcome the resistance of the orbit to motion (accelerating the eye) and a second force that is precisely selected to hold the eye at its new orbital position. The holding, or *static*, force must of course be maintained as long as the eye is stationary, whereas the dynamic force need only be applied as a pulse during the actual movement of the eye.

Oculomotor muscle force is controlled directly by the firing rates of the oculomotor motor neurons. When studying oculomotor motor neurons, one can largely separate these forces by studying motor neuron firing rates either when the eye is stationary or by studying the motor neuron firing rates when the eye is in motion. In a series of classic experiments, a number of researchers conducted single neuron recording studies of motor neurons while the eye was stationary at different positions in the orbit (Fuchs and Lushei, 1970). What these scientists observed was that eye position

was a linear function of firing rate (see Fig. 33.3) *while the eye was stationary*. Each motor neuron was found to have a recruitment point, (the eye position at which the motor neuron began firing) and a characteristic slope (the number of action potentials per second in the motor neuron that was associated with a $1°$ shift of the eye toward the pulling direction of the innervated muscle). These data revealed that under static conditions, the firing rate in all oculomotor neurons is proportional to position.

Studying the responses of motor neurons during movements revealed that all of these neurons also fired a high frequency *pulse* of activity during much of the high-velocity phase of eye movements. This high-frequency pulse was of course followed by the sustained increment in firing rate associated with the new static position of the eye. From these data it was concluded that the high-frequency pulse of activity in these motor neurons generated the dynamic force required during an eye movement while the sustained change in rate produced the required static forces.

The preceding discussion describes the behavior of oculomotor motor neurons when their muscles are pulling the eye. For every eye movement, however, one muscle of each antagonistic pair must relax whenever the other contracts. During movements in which the muscle under study relaxes: motor neurons pause during the movement.

Perhaps the most interesting aspect of these observations is that all oculomotor motor neurons have this precise pattern of behavior, encoding in their rate *both* static and dynamic components of the force structure of each movement. This has two important implications: it means that all muscle fibers contribute to both movement and position holding (because all motor neurons do so) and it means that the combined *pulse/step structure* of all eye movements is computed at or before the level of the oculomotor motor neurons. As shown in the following sections, a principle task of the oculomotor system is to compute these pulse/step muscle force patterns. The challenge faced by the system is to achieve either gaze stabilization or gaze shifting by converting sensory information from many modalities—visual, vestibular, auditory, and somatosensory—into the common language of these pulse/step muscle forces.

Summary

The simplicity of the oculomotor system derives from the simplicity of its mechanics, the simplicity of its muscular and neural control, and the compactness of the brain stem circuitry that computes the fundamental neural signals required to drive it.

THE VESTIBULO-OCULAR REFLEX

The vestibulo-ocular reflex (VOR) is the neural system by which rotations of the head are detected using the semicircular canals of the vestibular organs, and the eyes are counterrotated in their sockets an equal amount in the opposite direction to stabilize the line of sight. This reflex is in constant use. Whenever you walk, for example, the VOR is engaged, compensating for the small visually disruptive movements of the head that are produced during locomotion. The VOR is also highly precise. Try rotating your head back and forth from left to right while reading this page. The head can be moved quite quickly before the text becomes unreadable.

To compensate for head rotation, the VOR rotates the eyes. When the head rotates 40°, 80°, or even 180°, it should be obvious that the eyes cannot simply continue to counterrotate or they would eventually be pointed backward in the orbit. To overcome this limitation, the eye is often reset to a central position in the orbit during a vestibular eye movement. After this reset is complete, the compensatory eye rotation resumes. Figure 33.4 plots the horizontal position of

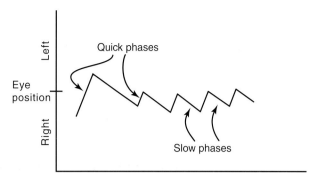

FIGURE 33.4 Nystagmus. This plot of horizontal eye position as a function of time reveals that the eye is moving slowly to the right and then shifts abruptly to the left before resuming its rightward movement. This pattern of movement is referred to as nystagmus.

the eye in the head during a long continuous rotation of the subject. Notice the comparatively slow (shallow sloped) compensatory movements followed by quick (steep sloped) resetting movements. These two classes of movements, that together make up the VOR, are called quick phases and slow phases. This characteristic pattern of alternating quick and slow phases is called **nystagmus**. (A leftward nystagmus is one in that the quick phases shift gaze to the left.) Note that only the slow phase compensates for head rotation; the quick phase simply returns the eye to the center of the orbit. The following discussion focuses on how inputs from the semicircular canals structure the compensatory slow phases of the VOR.

Semicircular Canals

Figure 33.5 shows a side view of the vestibular organ. Each of these bilaterally symmetrical organs

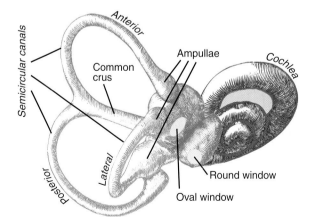

FIGURE 33.5 Semicircular canals. The bony labyrinth of the inner ear includes the semicircular canals. These three circular bony tubes are oriented to detect rotational motion in any of the three dimensions of space.

contains three circular canals, each oriented at roughly 90° to one another. Each canal consists of a very thin circular tube, filled with fluid. As the tube rotates, the fluid inside lags behind due to its inertia. The rotational motion of the tube can therefore be determined by measuring the rate at which the fluid moves relative to the tube. The vestibular organ accomplishes this by stretching a thin elastic membrane across the canal known as the **cupula**. Rotations of a canal result in deflections of the cupula, and by measuring the state of the cupula, the nervous system can monitor the rotational motion of the head. Deflection of the cupula is, in turn, monitored neurally via hair cells like those employed in the cochlea (Chapter 26). Obviously, a system of this type is most sensitive to rotations aligned precisely in the plane of the canal. Put more exactly, a given canal can only measure that portion of the rotational velocity that is in its plane. In order to completely measure the rotational velocity of the head in three dimensions, it is thus necessary to employ three separate canals, each oriented in a different plane. Together, these three canals can describe any rotation in three-dimensional space. In fact, vertebrates employ a total of six canals, three on each side, arranged in three coplanar pairs. Rotation of the head to the left, for example, activates the two canals that lie in the horizontal plane. One will be excited by this rotation as its cupula deflects hair cells in their preferred direction and the other will be inhibited, to an equal extent, as its cupula, moving in the opposite direction relative to the mirror symmetrical canal, deflects its hair cells in the opposite direction. Single unit recording studies made of canal afferent fibers during rotations show that this system does accurately code rotational velocity (Dickman and Correia, 1989). Figure 33.6 shows how a typical canal afferent fires quite quickly during each movement of the cupula in its preferred direction and more slowly during movement in its nonpreferred direction.

Vestibular Nucleus

Canal afferents synapse on neurons of the vestibular nuclei, many of which have a firing rate that is related linearly to rotational velocity in one of the canal planes (Groen *et al.*, 1952). How can this sensory measure of the rotational velocity of each canal be used to compute a matched velocity of eye rotation? Because each of the canal pairs is roughly aligned with one of the extraocular muscle pairs, the velocity signal associated with each canal could, in principle, be used to control the eye velocity governed by the aligned pair of extraocular muscles. Anatomical con-

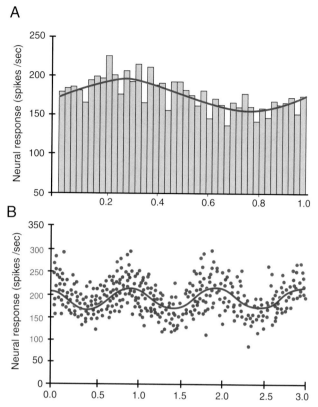

FIGURE 33.6 Hair cell response to movement of the cupula. (A) The average spike rate for a hair cell as a function of cupular position. Note that the hair cell firing rate varies sinusoidally as the cupula is deflected in and then out in a single cycle. (B) The instantaneous firing rate for one hair cell as it is deflected in and then out over three consecutive cycles. After Dickman and Correia (1989).

nections have been observed that project from the vestibular nuclei directly to the oculomotor nuclei. The canal-derived velocity signal could therefore account for the velocity of the eye, the *dynamic* component of the VOR eye movement (Fig. 33.7).

However, once the velocity of the head dropped to zero, then we might expect the eye to return to an initial, pre-VOR position. This is because the static force necessary to hold the eye at a new position in the orbit must be changed each time the velocity of the eye carries it to a new orbital position. As we learned in the preceding section, it is the static, or step, force that must persist after each eye movement is complete. If the sensory signals in the vestibular nucleus are the source of the dynamic phase of each VOR eye movement, what is the source of the accompanying change in static force? Because velocity is the first derivative of position, the step force, that we learned is responsible for static eye position, could be computed by taking the mathematical integral of the velocity signal supplied by the vestibular nuclei. A system of this type was first proposed by Robinson

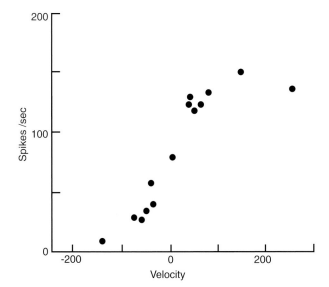

FIGURE 33.7 The firing rate of canal afferents codes velocity. This figure plots the firing rate of a canal afferent as a function of step changes in rotational velocity. Over a range of almost 300°/s the firing rate is a linear function of velocity. After Groen *et al.*, (1952).

(1975), who developed a simple model of the horizontal VOR presented in Fig. 33.8. In this model, signals proportional to velocity are generated by the horizontal semicircular canals. Those signals are then passed to the vestibular nucleus and from there to the motor neurons of the lateral and medial rectus muscles that control the horizontal position of the eye. Because medial and lateral recti are an antagonistic pair of muscles, they must receive copies of the horizontal canal output having different signs, causing one to relax while the other contracts. To supply the step of force that holds the eye in place, the Robinson model integrates the output of the horizontal canal afferents,

adding any change in step intensity to the pre-VOR step intensity and passing that signal to the oculomotor nuclei along with the dynamic velocity signal. In this way, a simple sensory signal encoding velocity is transformed into both a static and a dynamic force pair tailored to the needs of the extraocular muscle system.

The VOR Is Plastic

The preceding section described how the VOR appears to operate in general. To operate well, this system must be able to calibrate given levels of canal activation to given velocities of eye rotation. Changes in the strength or efficiency of the extraocular muscles, for example, would require that the strength of the linkage between the vestibular signal and the muscle contraction would have to be adjusted. A number of investigators have demonstrated this flexibility in the VOR by examining manipulations that change the strength of the coupling between the vestibular and muscular systems. This coupling is usually referred to as *gain* and is expressed as a fraction: the magnitude of the induced eye rotation divided by the magnitude of the vestibular rotation. Thus a gain of 1 is a circumstance in which eye and head rotations are perfectly matched, a gain of 0.5 undercompensates for head rotation by half, and a gain of 2 overcompensates by twice. To examine the limits of this adaptability, or **plasticity**, of VOR gain, human subjects were instructed to wear magnifying lenses. Like a telescope, magnifying lenses expand the view of a small region of visual space. Under these conditions, eye movements produce smaller displacements of the visual image on the retina. For example, 3× lenses would require that a subject make an eye

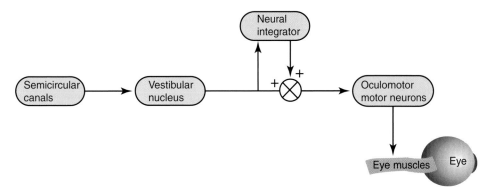

FIGURE 33.8 A model of the vestibulo-ocular reflex. Semicircular canals send a signal proportional to head velocity to the vestibular nuclei. This signal is then relayed to the oculomotor motor neurons where it controls eye velocity. A copy of this signal is also passed to the neural integrator where it is integrated to compute a signal proportional to eye position, and hence the force necessary to hold the eye stationary at its current position.

movement three times as large to compensate for a given head rotation. In one classic experiment, 2× magnifying lenses were placed on a subject, and after a period of days it was observed that the gain of the VOR had adapted to 1.8, almost compensating for the 2× magnification of the lenses (Miles and Eighmy, 1980). This experiment, and others like it, demonstrated that the VOR could be adapted. Other experiments showed that while the cerebellum was critically important for this adaptation, it could be removed after the adaptation was complete without changing the state of the VOR. This led researcher Steven Lisberger to propose a revised version of David Robinson's original model of the VOR, one in which the cerebellum uses visual information (the slippage of an image on the retina during a head movement) to determine if the current VOR gain effectively cancels out the effects of head movements. It then uses this information, often referred to as an *error signal*, to modulate the strength of an extracerebellar circuit that can increase or decrease the gain of the VOR (Lisberger, 1986).

The VOR Is Velocity Limited

Many researchers have analyzed the gain of the VOR during sinusoidal rotations of humans and animals. In these experiments, subjects are rotated back and forth at a fixed frequency, thus completing oscillation after oscillation in a fixed period of time. In these experiments, the gain of the VOR is determined at a wide range of oscillation frequencies and is plotted against frequency. These experiments are, of course, conducted in the dark so that visual stimuli, and hence optokinetic-related responses, cannot be responsible

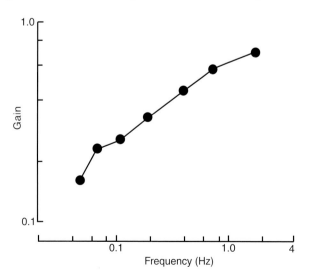

FIGURE 33.9 Gain of the vestibulo-ocular reflex as a function of frequency. After Baarsma and Collewijn (1974).

for eye movements. The rationale for this approach is that for some types of systems, those referred to as *linear*, it is possible to calculate the gain (or response) of the system to any stimulus if one knows the response of the system to all cases of single frequency stimulation. As Fig. 33.9 indicates (Baarsma and Collewijn, 1974), the VOR does counterrotate the eye almost perfectly at frequencies over 1 Hz, but the VOR is inadequate when a subject is rotated so slowly that a single back-and-forth rotation requires 10 s (0.1 Hz). This lower limit on the VOR is of particular interest because it is at those velocities that the visual system can be used to stabilize gaze. As shown in the next section, the optokinetic system does just that, efficiently compensating for very low speed movements of the head. At higher speeds, however, *it* shows a reduced gain, a gain exactly compensated for by the VOR.

Summary

The vestibulo-ocular reflex is a good paradigm for understanding motor control in general. The behavioral goals are clear-cut, the mechanics of the movements and the neuromuscular controls are straightforward, and all of the computation needed for holding and moving the eye is performed by a compact and relatively well-described circuitry within the brain stem, all driven by input signals from the semicircular canals.

THE OPTOKINETIC SYSTEM

Like the VOR, the optokinetic system uses the oculomotor musculature to stabilize gaze during rotations of the head. Unlike the VOR, the optokinetic system uses a different type of sensory data: visual information. Specifically, the optokinetic system extracts from the global pattern of visual stimulation a measure of how fast, and in what direction, the visual world is moving across the retina. This movement of the visual world, often called *retinal slip*, is then used to generate an eye movement equal in velocity and opposite in direction to the retinal slippage, thus stabilizing the visual world on the retina. Like the VOR, this optokinetic response is characterized by a slow phase (during which the eyes compensate for movement of the visual world) followed by a quick phase (which moves the eyes back from the limits of their orbital rotation to a more central position). To study optokinetic nystagmus, scientists typically present subjects with a display of vertical stripes or randomly arranged dots, which rotate uniformly around the center of the subject's head. In this environment, subjects generate a *nystagmus* with a slow phase, which compensates for the induced movement of the visual world. Because subjects are stationary in these experiments, we know that the vestibular system cannot be responsible for generating the nystagmus, which must therefore be the product of the movement of the visual stimulus.

Midbrain Circuits Translate Visual-Sensory Signals into Velocity Signals

In most vertebrates (including humans), the retina projects directly to a midbrain area just rostral to the superior colliculus called the pretectum. Many neurons in this area have been shown to become active when the visual world *slips* in a particular direction. As the velocity of this slippage increases (up to a point), the firing rate of these neurons increases. Neurons of the pretectal area encode the *velocity* and direction of retinal slip. It should come as only a slight surprise then that these visually derived midbrain velocity signals make their way directly to the vestibular nuclei via pontine and medullary relays. In fact, many vestibular neurons have been identified that become active, coding desired eye velocity, not just for vestibular stimuli (rotations of the head in the dark) but for visual (optokinetic) stimuli as well (Henn *et al.*, 1974). Thus, optokinetic stimuli and vestibular stimuli are presumed to access a common circuitry for eye velocity control because they are combined at the level of the vestibular nuclei. This common motor circuitry, which can receive input from either visual or vestibular modalities, is presumed to mathematically integrate the optokinetic velocity signals to derive the amplitude of the static force necessary to hold the eye at its new orbital position. These signals are then combined and employed to control both eye velocity and eye position.

Optokinetic Response Has Gain

Like the vestibulo-ocular response, the gain of the optokinetic system can be measured. In this case, gain is the ratio of eye rotational speed to "visual world" rotational speed. A ratio of 1.0 indicates that the eye perfectly counterrotates, completely stabilizing the visual world. A ratio of less than 1.0 indicates that the eye lags behind the visual world, only partly compensating for retinal slip. Measurements of optokinetic gain have been made as a function of frequency just as they have been made for the VOR. In this case, frequency refers to the rate at which an animal is sinusoidally oscillated in front of an illuminated and stationary visual environment after its semicircular

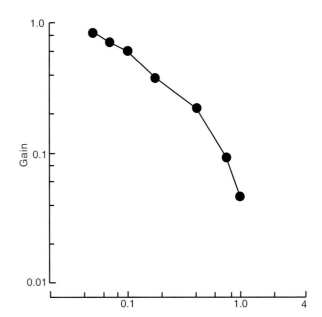

FIGURE 33.10 Gain of the optokinetic response as a function of frequency. After Baarsma and Collewijn (1974).

canals have been removed surgically (Baarsma and Collewijn, 1974). Fig. 33.10 plots gain as a function of frequency for optokinesis. Notice that the gain of the optokinetic response falls off at higher frequencies. Comparing this graph with Fig. 33.9, it should be clear that together, the optokinetic and vestibulo-ocular systems, which translate two types of signals into a common motor framework, can effectively stabilize gaze over a very wide range of image/head velocities. In many ways, these two systems can be thought of as interlocking, together achieving gaze stabilization under a wider range of conditions than either could achieve alone.

Summary

The optokinetic system complements the vestibulo-ocular reflex. Both maintain stability of gaze despite head movement and both employ simple and shared control components. Although neither system working alone can completely stabilize vision, the combined vestibulo-ocular and optokinetic systems achieve nearly perfect stabilization across a broad range of head movement velocities.

THE SACCADIC SYSTEM

Saccadic eye movements, the high-velocity gaze-shifting responses that can rotate the line of sight as quickly as 800°/s, are perhaps the most successfully studied mammalian motor system. While we still know very little about why a human or animal chooses to shift her gaze to a particular target, we are now beginning to understand how that gaze shift is accomplished. Like the gaze-holding systems already examined, the saccadic system must accomplish two goals: it must generate a dynamic force pulse that accelerates the eye to a high velocity and it must generate an increment in the static holding force to keep the eye at its new orbital position once that saccadic goal has been reached. As we will see, the saccadic system accomplishes this by using sensory data, which can come from visual, somatosensory, or auditory stimuli, to compute the eye rotation necessary to align the line of sight with a visual target. The magnitude and direction of this desired change in eye position, or *motor error*, are relayed to a set of brain stem control circuits, which compute the static and dynamic forces necessary for the selected eye rotation.

The Saccadic Brain Stem

As mentioned earlier, the eye muscles are controlled by three bilaterally symmetrical pairs of cranial nerve nuclei. Lying between these nuclei, straddling the midline of the brain stem, is the **paramedian pontine reticular formation** (PPRF). In classic experiments, it was established by a number of researchers (Keller, 1974) that the PPRF, among other things, contains neurons known as **burst neurons** and neurons known as **omnipause neurons**. Burst neurons fire a vigorous volley of action potentials beginning about 8–12 ms before each eye movement. The pattern of spikes in this burst is correlated precisely with the horizontal amplitude of the saccade. A small rotation of the eyes to the left is preceded by a small burst of activity from the left preferring burst neurons. A medium-sized rotation directly to the left is preceded by a larger burst, which codes the larger leftward component of the movement. Activity of this type could be used to generate the dynamic force pulse needed to accelerate the eye during a saccade, and commensurate with this hypothesis burst neurons often project directly into the oculomotor nuclei (Strassman *et al.*, 1986). A similar group of neurons have also been discovered just in front of the oculomotor nuclei, which seem to code vertical motor error in an identical manner.

These data suggest that the dynamic phase of a saccadic eye movement is coded by pontine burst neuron activity. This hypothesis, however, necessarily raises two questions. First, how does the saccadic system know when to terminate this dynamic burst of activity? Second, if this dynamic pulse of force were generated alone, then the viscoelastic springs that pull the eye back toward the center of the orbit would slowly return the eye to its presaccadic position. How does the saccadic system generate a change in the step, or static holding, force which is precisely adequate to hold the eye at its new position at the end of the saccade? David Robinson suggested related solutions to both of these problems. If, once again, the action potentials that make up this burst of activity were integrated mathematically, this would produce a signal proportional to the distance the eye had been moved by the burst. A feedback system could then compare the distance that the eye had been moved by the burst with the desired end point of the saccade. When these two were equivalent, the saccadic system could terminate the saccade, automatically placing the line of sight on target. This estimate of how far the eye has traveled could also be used to generate the step increment in muscle force necessary to hold the eye in place against the viscoelastic springs of the orbit. In this way, the saccadic brain stem would be largely autonomous; it would only have to receive one pair of signals, signals that specified horizontal and vertical motor error. The feedback loop would then regulate the saccade causing it to end on target and the integral of the burst could be used to compute the required step in hold force. One prediction of this hypothesis is that some location in the brain must perform the mathematical integration and that in the absence of that structure the eye would relax back toward its presaccadic position after each high-velocity saccade was complete. Cannon and Robinson (1987) were actually able to produce this result when they lesioned the prepositus nucleus of the hypoglossal nerve, suggesting that at least a portion of the proposed neural integrator does lie there.

Lying just rostral and ventral to the burst neurons, omnipause neurons were found to be a tonically active group of cells that stop firing action potentials shortly before the burst neurons become active (Keller, 1974). Unlike burst neurons, all omnipause neurons become silent immediately before all saccades. The duration of this silent period, or pause, is correlated tightly with the duration of the saccade. Further, it has been demonstrated that electrical stimulation of the omnipause region prevents all saccades from occurring. These observation suggests that the omnipause neuron pause may be a critical saccade *trigger*. Activity in these neurons acts to inhibit saccade initiation. The pause could thus serve to initiate saccades regardless of the particular motor error signals that specify the amplitude and duration of that saccade.

Where does the oculomotor brain stem receive its motor error signals? Two principle structures seem to serve that role: the superior colliculus and the frontal eye fields. We will begin our examination of the way in which motor error signals are generated with an examination of the superior colliculus.

The Superior Colliculus

The superior colliculus is a laminated structure lying above the cerebral aqueduct in the midbrain. At the end of the Nineteenth century it was discovered that electrical stimulation of this structure in animals produced high-velocity movements of the eyes similar to natural saccades. However, it was not until the early 1970s that two groups of researchers were able to reexamine this structure and provide fundamental insights into how eye movements are controlled. Robinson (1972) made an essential contribution when he repeated the classic collicular stimulation experiments of the preceeding century. In Robinson's experiments, an electrode was lowered into the colliculus and a small stimulating current was delivered through the electrode tip. What he observed was that about 20 ms after the stimulating electrode was activated, a saccadic eye movement began. The eye movement had a characteristic amplitude and direction, and once the eye had moved that characteristic amount, it stopped. If stimulation was continued for a long period, a second saccade of identical amplitude and direction would eventually be made from the end point of the last saccade. If Robinson then moved his electrode to a new location in the colliculus, he produced a similar pattern of results, but the movement amplitude and direction were different. By systematically moving his electrode, Robinson was able to map the movement amplitudes and directions produced by stimulation throughout the colliculus, and he discovered that movements were mapped topographically. Adjacent sites on the colliculus would, when stimulated, produce movements that shifted gaze to adjacent points in visual space. Robinson drew three important conclusions from these observations. The first was that stimulation of the colliculus did not simply cause the eye to move, rather it specified a desired eye movement and if stimulation persisted, the movement was repeated. Second, Robinson noted that stimulation produced movements of a particular amplitude and direction regardless of the starting place of the eye in the orbit. Thus, like pontine burst units, the colliculus appeared to encode saccades with regard to a rotation of the eye, a framework referred to as motor error coordinates. Finally, Robinson observed that the colliculus formed a topographic map of these eye rotations, an organization now often referred to as a **motor map** and one

which encodes movements in motor error coordinates much as visual area V1 encodes stimuli with regard to their site of activation on the retina (Chapter 27).

At this same time, Robert Wurtz and Michael Goldberg (1972) at the National Institutes of Health began to record the activity of single units in the superior colliculi of awake monkeys both while visual targets were presented and while monkeys made saccades to fixate those targets. Wurtz and Goldberg discovered many interesting types of neurons in their experiments, but perhaps most important were a group of neurons they described as collicular saccade-related burst neurons. Like pontine burst neurons, these cells fired a high-frequency burst of activity before some saccades, a burst that began about 20 ms before the saccade. What Wurtz and Goldberg discovered was that a given neuron in the colliculus fired strongly before some movements and only weakly or not at all before others. These scientists proceeded to map the strength of the presaccadic response of a cell as a function of the amplitude and direction of the movement that followed that activity. They named these plots, of unit response as a function of the horizontal and vertical amplitude of a movement, **movement fields** by analogy to the previously described receptive fields of the sensory systems. Studies of movement fields revealed three critical properties of the colliculus. First, individual cells were very broadly tuned. While a given cell was most active before a movement of a particular amplitude and direction (termed its **best movement**), it was also active for many similar movements. Second, systematic examinations of collicular burst neurons revealed that they were also organized in a topographic map; the best movements of cells varied systematically across the colliculus in a manner identical to that observed for stimulation-induced movements by David Robinson. Third, these neurons, which fired before movements of a particular amplitude and direction, did not carry information about the absolute position of the eye but rather encoded motor error.

Population Coding

These studies gave rise to an obvious hypothesis: Collicular burst neurons carry a motor error signal that is somehow used by the pontine oculomotor control circuitry to control saccadic eye movements. One problem with this hypothesis, which was noted immediately by Wurtz and Goldberg, was that the collicular burst neurons were very broadly tuned, whereas saccades were observed to be highly precise. How, these authors wondered, could the amplitude and direction of movement be coded accurately by such inaccurate elements? In 1976, David Sparks and colleagues, along with James McIlwain, suggested a solution to this problem. They proposed that the total output of the colliculus was **vector averaged**. In Sparks' proposal, each collicular burst neuron "votes" for its best direction, but the strength of its vote is described by its rate of firing. Thus, a cell with a 10° rightward best movement would vote strongly for a 10° rightward movement and more weakly for movements 10° rightward and slightly upward or downward. The vector average of these votes, Sparks proposed, could specify the amplitude and direction of the movement with tremendous precision. As shown in Chapter 30, Apostolos Georgopoulos later adopted this same proposal to describe the way in which neurons in the motor cortex may code movement direction precisely (Fig. 33.11).

In 1988, Sparks explicitly tested the hypothesis that vector averaging was used to extract, from a neural population response, the amplitude and direction of a desired movement. To do this, Sparks and his colleagues, Chungkill Lee and Bill Rohrer (Lee et al., 1988), lowered a micropipette filled with lidocaine into the superior colliculus and anesthetized a small circular portion of the structure. First, these scientists predicted that movements encoded by cells at the center of the anesthetized region would be unaffected by the anesthesia because all of the cells around the site of anesthesia would vote weakly, but equally, for movements around the correct movement. Amazingly, this is exactly what these authors observed. When the animal, however, was instructed to make a movement that placed the anesthetized region of colliculus to one side of the active population, these authors observed that movements were systematically biased away from the movements specified by the anesthetized zone. These experiments established that a vector average of a population code

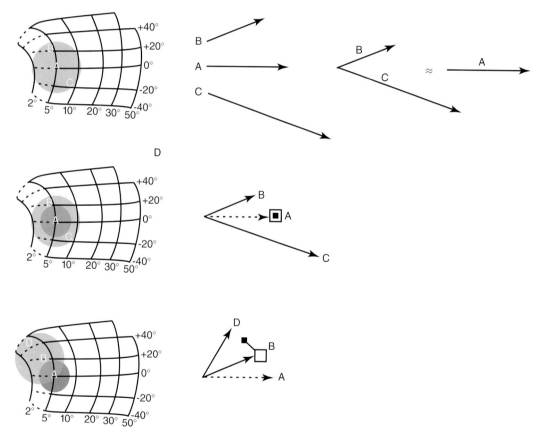

FIGURE 33.11 Population averaging scheme of Sparks and colleagues. (Top left) The stippled area represents the extent of cells within a topographically mapped superior colliculus, which would be active before a 5° rightward saccade. (Top middle) Cells at locations A, B, and C on the left fire most vigorously for movements A, B, and C plotted here. (Top right) The weighted average of activity at points B and C yields the same movement as activity at A. (Bottom). The dark stippled region plots the location of a pharmacologically deactivated collicular region. The regions of the colliculus activated during saccades A and B are plotted respectively in the left and right panels. This model predicts that saccades targeting A will be normal, whereas saccades targeting B will deviate toward D. After Lee et al. (1988).

is used to specify the desired motor error for a saccade. Perhaps more importantly, these experiments were the first to demonstrate vector averaging in a mammalian motor system.

Sensory Signals from Many Modalities Guide Saccade Planning

So far we have described how motor error is coded in the superior colliculus and what is known about how pontine circuitry uses that information to govern the actual rotations of the eye. We have not yet addressed the sources of those motor error signals. Foveate animals can shift gaze to fixate visual, auditory, and somatosensory targets. This means that if a visual stimulus is presented in the peripheral visual field, the eye can be rotated to align the fovea with that target. If a sound is presented, an eye movement can also be generated that aligns the fovea with that target. Finally, if a point on the body surface is touched, the eye can be directed so that the line of gaze intersects that point on the body surface. Each of these events involves what is known as a **sensorimotor transformation**. Information encoded by each sensory system along its own topographic maps has to be translated into motor error signals.

The simplest of these sensorimotor transformations is the use of visual information to derive motor error. This is simple because the retina, like the eye muscles, is anchored to the eye. Thus, the location on the retina activated by a visual stimulus specifies the eye rotation required to foveate a target. If a visual target activates the retina at a location 10° to the right of fixation, then a 10° rightward saccade will foveate that target. In fact, the most superficial laminae of the colliculus receive a direct retinal projection, a projection which is mapped into alignment with the collicular motor map. Similarly, most of the extrastriate visual areas learned about in Chapter 27 project directly to the collicular motor system, providing another route by which retinally sampled visual stimuli can be transformed easily into motor error signals.

The generation of saccades to auditory targets, however, presents a larger problem for sensorimotor transformation. Auditory targets are localized by comparing information received from the two ears. A sound source therefore has a location with regard to these two ears, a location with regard to the skull. Knowing that an auditory target lies straight ahead of a subject does not, however, tell what rotation of the eye will fixate it. In order to solve that problem, it is necessary to first know where the line of gaze is currently directed. If, for example, the eyes are directed leftward, then a straight-ahead target requires a rightward movement. If the eyes are directed rightward, a leftward eye movement is required. David Sparks and his colleague Martha Jay recognized this problem in the mid-1980s and conducted a series of experiments to determine how the brain solves this problem (Jay and Sparks, 1984). The first thing that they discovered was that collicular saccade-related burst neurons encoded the motor error of impending saccades to auditory targets just as they did for visual targets, irrespective of where the eyes were directed before the saccade began. Thus, the rotation required to foveate an auditory target, and not the location of the target with regard to the ears, is supplied to the pontine saccadic circuitry by the collicular burst neurons. In a second series of experiments, Jay and Sparks examined another important class of collicular neurons found in the deepest laminae of the colliculus, those that encode properties of auditory targets. These units, which had been described previously, become active when an auditory target is presented in their receptive field. What Jay and Sparks wondered was whether these "sensory" cells encoded the location of the auditory target with regard to the eye rotation required to foveate that target or with regard to the ears. If these neurons formed a coherent topographical map, aligned with the motor map of the collicular burst neurons, then to code the location of an auditory target with regard to its motor error, *they would have to shift the site of activation on the map for a single fixed target every time the eyes moved.* Jay and Sparks observed that many of the auditory-sensitive neurons that they studied were activated by a specific fixed auditory target only when the eyes were aligned so that the auditory target had a foveal motor error associated with the location of the cell on the collicular motor map. This meant that sensory stimuli received by the ears and used to compute the locations of targets relative to the ears must be transformed into motor error coordinates *before* they activate these collicular auditory units. This important discovery helped establish that *sensorimotor transformation* is a process by which stimuli from the many different sensory systems are translated into a common framework, one appropriate for activating the musculature (Fig. 33.12).

Sparks extended this principle with Jennifer Groh to a study of the way in which somatosensory targets are transformed to guide saccadic eye movements. Unlike auditory targets for which only the position of the eyes in the orbit is necessary to transform location data, somatosensory stimuli of the limbs, for example, have to be corrected both for the position of the eyes in the head and for the location of the stimulated limb with regard to the head in which the eyes are fixed. If

A

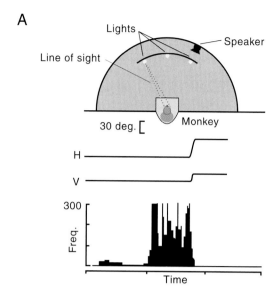

B

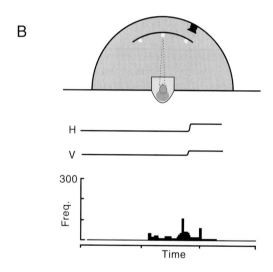

C

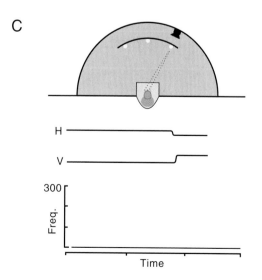

somatosensory neurons in the deeper layers of the colliculus code stimuli in motor error coordinates, then the receptive fields of these neurons on the body surface would depend both on the position of the eyes in the orbit and on the position of the body surface with regard to the eyes. Groh and Sparks found that by having a monkey shift its initial eye position, they could move the receptive field of a neuron completely off one hand of a monkey and onto the other hand! This remarkable demonstration of sensorimotor transformation makes it clear how important it is for the nervous system to take information from disparate sensory systems and to combine them in a single coordinate framework.

This work demonstrates a ubiquitous problem in motor control: the difficulty and importance of the sensorimotor transformation. Studies of skeletomuscular control must face an even more difficult version of this problem, how visual information is transformed into skeletomuscular motor error coordinates.

Coordinating the Eye and Head

Whenever we shift our line of sight more than about 10 or 15°, we accomplish this by shifting both the position of our eyes in our heads and the position of our heads on our body. Real world gaze shifts are coordinated movements of the eye and head. For technical reasons, however, most classical studies of gaze shifts have been conducted in animals mechanically prevented from making head movements. This means that most of what we know about gaze shifts is really only about shifts in the line of sight accomplished by saccadic movements of the eyes. A number of laboratories have begun to examine the activity of brain stem, superior colliculus, and frontal eye field neurons while animals make gaze shifts by moving both eyes and head. These studies are beginning to reveal that many areas thought of traditionally as eye controllers may in fact control shifts in the line of sight by simultanous effects on both eye musculature and the musculature of the neck. Studies now in progress should soon begin to explain how this eye and head coordination is accomplished.

FIGURE 33.12 Shifts in auditory response fields produced by eye movements. All three panels plot the response of a single collicular neuron to an auditory target fixed 15° to the right of the monkey. (A) When the animal is fixating a leftward target, the unit fires vigorously. (B) When the animal fixates straight ahead, the unit fires less vigorously. (C) When the animal fixates the speaker, the unit is silent to the same acoustic stimulus. After Jay and Sparks (1984).

Higher Level Saccadic Systems

Unfortunately, the sources of the collicular saccadic control signals are only vaguely understood. On anatomical and physiological grounds we do know that collicular saccade-related information is provided by the frontal eye fields, the parietal cortex, and the basal ganglia. All of these areas project directly to the colliculus and have patterns of unit activity that indicate that they play a role in activating collicular burst neurons. The most important of these areas is believed to be the frontal eye fields. Although a number of studies have shown that this structure activates neurons in the colliculus, it is also known that, unlike the parietal cortex and basal ganglia, the frontal eye fields project directly to the pontine eye movement control circuitry. It has even been shown that, after lesions of the colliculus, the frontal eye fields alone can generate saccadic eye movements (Schiller et al., 1980). (Lesions of both the superior colliculus and frontal eye fields results in a loss of the ability to make saccades.) The frontal eye fields must therefore serve a role similar to that of the colliculus. Recent studies have demonstrated that many of the collicular properties described above, like the transformation of auditory targets into saccadic motor error coordinates, are also evident in the frontal eye fields. Ongoing research seeks to understand how all of these antecedent structures give rise to the oculomotor control signals which guide collicular, pontine, and cortical eye movement control structures.

Summary

The saccadic system engages higher brainstem and cortical mechanisms to identify a target and shift gaze to it. The eye movements themselves are very fast and they minimize the time lost in visual contact while gaze is shifting to a new target.

SMOOTH PURSUIT

The optokinetic system moves the eyes at a velocity which compensates for movement of the visual field. We considered this a gaze-stabilization mechanism and pointed out that essentially all animals have this phylogenetically ancient system. Animals with foveas, can use saccades to direct the fovea to scrutinize targets throughout visual space. These animals, however, face a special challenge when they make a saccade to examine a moving target. The saccade may bring the fovea briefly into alignment with the moving visual target but unless the eye can be made to move in the same direc-

tion and velocity as the target, the shift-of-gaze cannot result in a stabilization of the target image on the retina. Matching the velocity of the eye to the velocity of the visual stimulus when the visual stimulus is the entire world is, of course, the optokinetic response. When the moving target is, however, only a tiny portion of the visual world, the optokinetic-like response needs to be driven by only a small portion of the retina. The ability to generate eye velocities which minimize the retinal slip of a small visual target, while actually producing an increased retinal slip for the rest of the visual world, is produced by the eye movement system known as *smooth pursuit*. Smooth pursuit might be viewed as a specialized form of the optokinetic response. It should be pointed out, however, that these two systems involve at least partially distinct neural architectures.

Compared to the saccadic system, little is known about the brain stem circuits that compute and represent the directions and velocities of pursuit-related motor error. In general, neurobiologists have tended to view the pursuit system as similar to the optokinetic system: Retinal slip, in this case restricted to the retinal slip of selected portions of the visual world, is minimized by adjusting eye velocity until slip is reduced or eliminated. Models of the pursuit system are thus often quite similar to models of the optokinetic system. The velocity and direction of the target's motion across the retina and knowledge about the velocity and direction of the eye's current movement are used to compute a desired velocity and direction of eye movement. This eye velocity signal is then passed, via the brain stem oculomotor nuclei, to the eye musculature to control the dynamic movement of the eye. This dynamic signal is, like the dynamic signals for other eye movements, presumed to be integrated to compute the static signal necessary to maintain the eye in its current position should the eye stop. It will come as no surprise that the site of this integrator is assumed to be the prepositus nucleus of the hypoglossal nerve nucleus. What, however, is the source of this continuous dynamic control signal? Two basic philosophies have been postulated to explain the structuring of this complex dynamic force. One proposes that the velocity and direction of retinal slip are the only visually derived inputs used by the smooth pursuit system (Robinson et al., 1986). The other hypothesis proposes that information about the position, velocity, and acceleration of the pursuit target are all combined to compute a dynamic force structure optimized for the properties of the visual stimulus (Lisberger et al., 1987). The first hypothesis can thus be thought of as muscle driven in the sense that it uses a minimum of visual information and structures its dynamic force entirely based on properties of the motor system. The second hypothesis can be thought of as sensory driven, structuring its dynamic force by a computationally exhaustive analysis of the visual target. As we examine the neural structures that generate pursuit movements, we will see that these two theories place the computational burden of pursuit at opposite ends of the neurobiological system: The sensory-driven hypothesis places this burden in the largely cortical areas which compute target motion-related information, whereas the muscle-driven hypothesis places these burdens in the oculomotor brain stem where dynamic forces are structured for other types of eye movements.

The Pursuit Brain Stem and Cerebellum

The **dorsolateral pontine nucleus** (DLPN) appears to be a critical link in the smooth pursuit system that serves as a bridge between the cortical motion processing systems shown in Chapter 27 and the oculomotor portions of the cerebellum and brain stem. The DLPN has been shown to contain neurons that encode the direction and velocity of pursuit, the direction and velocity of target motion, or both (Suzuki and Keller, 1984). Thus the DLPN could, in principle, contain both information about the sensory representations of targets and the motor error signals needed to drive the eyes. The output of the DLPN passes to the cerebellum (the flocculus, paraflocculus, and vermis) where units have been identified with firing rates that are tightly coupled to the velocity of eye rotation specifically during smooth pursuit eye movements. These units, in turn, make connections with the vestibular nuclei, presumably integrating their motor error signal into the vestibulo-pontine oculomotor systems.

Cortical Sources of Visual Target Motion Signals

The identified brain stem pursuit pathways form a portion of the complete pursuit system. Critical to their function are signals that indicate target motion. This information appears to be provided to the pursuit system by the cortical motion system composed, in part, of areas MT and MST. These areas compute the direction and velocity of moving stimuli throughout the visual field and pass this information both directly to the DLPN and to the DLPN via the posterior parietal cortex and the frontal eye fields.

How Are Visual Targets Selected for Pursuit?

In a series of experiments, Lisberger and his colleagues Vince Ferrera and Justin Gardner (Gardner and Lisberger, 2001) have begun to study how the smooth pursuit system selects a visual target for pursuit. When animal subjects are presented with two moving targets simultaneously, they almost always begin smooth pursuit in a direction that is the average of the motion of the two targets. After a brief period of this "vector average" pursuit, animals make a saccade toward one target or the other and then pursue that target exclusively. By carefully examining the relationship between these saccades and pursuit, Lisberger and colleagues have concluded that it is the saccade toward one of the two targets that actually selects that target for pursuit. This raises the possibility that the saccadic and smooth pursuit systems are intimately connected, with the saccadic system playing a causal role in the selection of targets for pursuit.

Future Research

Future studies of the smooth pursuit system will provide us with new insights into both brain stem structures for oculomotor control and cortical structures for sensory processing and target selection. Sensorimotor transforms like those employed in the saccadic system must also play a role in this system. Future experiments, such as the study of pursuit eye movements directed toward auditory targets, may well disambiguate what role different signals play in pursuit and what forms are taken by the pursuit sensorimotor transforms.

Summary

The smooth pursuit system provides insights into both brain stem structures for oculomotor control and cortical structures for sensory processing. Pursuit thus may be unique: it employs high-level visual motion signals and pontine oculomotor circuits.

VERGENCE

The function of the vergence system is to converge or diverge the lines of gaze projecting from both eyes so that they meet at the target of foveal vision. Of course, animals without binocular foveal vision do not need to align a single retinal region on both eyes with a single visual target. Thus, only a limited number of species generate vergence movements. Primates, including humans, are one group of animals that typically show this class of eye movements. Up until now we have considered eye movements that produce shifts in gaze as if a single line of sight were being redirected. In fact, current evidence indicates

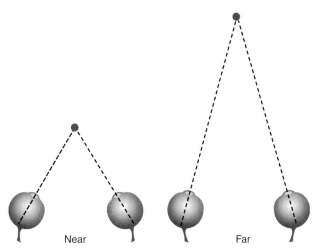

FIGURE 33.13 The convergence angle depends on target distance.

that this is exactly how the saccadic and smooth pursuit systems compute gaze shifts. How then are movements of the two eyes coordinated so that both eyes, despite the fact that they are separated by several centimeters, fixate a single target? As we learned earlier in this chapter, the German physiologist Ewald Hering proposed that an entirely separate system computes the appropriate vergence "correction" for each eye during gaze shifts and adds or subtracts that movement to the binocular saccadic or smooth pursuit motor error command. First we will examine the sources of the vergence motor error signal and then will describe physiological mechanisms that appear to compute the dynamic and static muscle forces necessary to produce these vergence eye movements (Fig. 33.13).

There Are Four Sources of Vergence Motor Error Signals

The brain generates four experimentally separable classes of vergence motor error commands. The first, and most obvious, is related to **binocular disparity**. When a visual stimulus is presented to both eyes but appears at different locations on each retina, this serves as an adequate stimulus for a vergence movement. The second class deals with **accommodation**. Apparently, the accommodative state of both lenses is monitored and this information is used to compute the distance to the target currently in focus. Based on a knowledge of this distance to target, vergence motor error can be computed and it appears that the nervous system uses this information to generate vergence motor error signals. The third class is usually referred to as **tonic**. This is the default state of convergence for the animal in

total darkness. In humans, this is about 3° of convergence. The final source of vergence motor error signals is the use of monocular (or cognitive) depth cues, such as linear perspective, to infer the distance to targets and thus compute vergence motor error. This cognitive source of vergence motor error is usually referred to as **proximal vergence**.

The Vergence Brain Stem Is Similar to the Saccadic Brain Stem

Physiological studies of the oculomotor brain stem by Mays and colleagues (Mays *et al.*, 1986; Mays and Gamlin, 1995) have revealed that a small group of neurons lying in the mesencephalic reticular formation appear to form a vergence control center much like the horizontal gaze control center of the saccadic system, which has been discussed previously. In this area, neurons of two important types have been identified: **vergence burst neurons** and **vergence burst-tonic neurons**. Vergence burst neurons are cells that fire a high-frequency burst of activity that precedes the onset of a vergence movement and whose frequency of firing is related to the velocity of the vergence movement (both convergence-specific and divergence-specific burst neurons have been identified). Further, the mathematical integral of these bursts is related to the total amplitude of the vergence movement. Vergence burst-tonic cells are neurons that appear to combine the dynamic and static responses of the vergence system. By analogy with the saccadic system, it seems likely that during a vergence eye movement, the output of the vergence burst neurons is integrated and reflected in the activity of the vergence burst-tonic neurons.

Most Gaze Shifts Involve Both Versional and Vergence Movements

As shown in Fig. 33.14, most gaze shifts for binocular foveal animals involve both a coordinated movement of the two eyes together (version) and a separate movement of each eye to adjust for differences in the depths of the targets (vergence). Thus, the point of gaze (the location at which the lines of gaze from each eye meet) must move both across and in or out. If we were to plot the location of the point of gaze during a saccade at successive points in time, it would follow the trajectory plotted in Fig. 33.14. The observed eye movement has three phases. First, notice that the eyes begin to converge quite slowly before the saccade begins. This is the vergence movement beginning. After a delay, the high-velocity saccade begins and not only does the point of gaze begin to shift from left

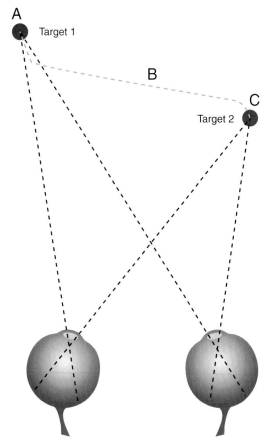

FIGURE 33.14   Trajectory of a saccade, viewed from above, that shifts the point of gaze laterally and in depth. Vergence mechanisms begin to converge the eyes prior to the saccade. The saccade then begins and the rate of vergence accelerates. After the saccade, vergence mechanisms continue to alter the convergence angle unit until both foveas are aligned with the target.

to right, but it also shifts in depth much faster. Finally, the high-velocity saccade is complete and the terminal slow portion of the vergence movement is completed. Mays and his colleague Paul Gamlin have suggested, based on simultaneous studies of the vergence and saccadic systems, that vergence bursters are normally inhibited by the saccadic omnipause neurons and this acts to limit the the firing rate of the vergence burster and hence the velocity of the vergence movement. During saccades, omnipause neurons, which act as the saccade trigger, are silent, disinhibiting the vergence bursters and hence accelerating vergence movement velocity while the saccade is in progress. After the saccade is complete, the omnipause neurons become active again, reinhibiting the vergence bursters and reducing the velocity of the remaining portion of the vergence movement. Mays' work is seminal because it reveals how the separate oculomotor systems interact during movements made by animals in the real world.

CONCLUSIONS

Oculomotor Systems Direct Gaze and Stabilize Vision

The effect of eye movements is twofold. First, eye movements stabilize the line of gaze while animals move in their environment. Unpredictable high-speed rotations of the head, which are produced whenever an animal moves, shift the line of gaze and, by smearing the optical image, reduce the resolution of the visual system. These high-velocity movements are compensated for by counterrotations of the eyes generated by the vestibulo-ocular system. Working in tandem with the VOR is the optokinetic system. The optokinetic system compensates for the slower movements of the head, which happen so gradually that the vestibular system cannot accurately detect them. Second, in animals with retinas that have a small region of high resolution, a specialized set of eye movements (saccades, smooth pursuit, and vergence) serves to direct that region to the examination of targets of interest. Together, these sets of movements permit the efficient gathering of visual information by the retina.

Dynamic Signals Are Computed, Used to Derive Static Signals, and Then Combined Neurally

Eye movements involve generating at least two classes of signals: those involved in moving the eye and those involved in holding the eye at each new position. The oculomotor system appears to combine these signals at or before the level of the motor neurons for all classes of movements. Further, the oculomotor systems all appear to employ a critical shortcut, they seem to compute explicitly only the first of these signals, the dynamic signals, and to derive the static signals from explicitly computed dynamic signals.

Sensorimotor Transformations Turn Sensory Signals into Motor Error Commands

Many classes of sensory signals are used to guide movements of the eyes. Vestibular signals, visual signals, auditory signals, and somatosensory signals are all used to compute the muscle forces necessary to generate eye rotations. In order for this single common output pathway to make use of this wide variety of input signals, each of these inputs must be used to compute a motor error signal. This process, the sensorimotor transform, is the mechanism by which

BOX 33.1

LISTING'S LAW

As described in the main text of this chapter, three pairs of muscles work together to control the position of each eye in three dimensions: horizontal, vertical, and torsional. While the horizontal dimension is controlled almost exclusively by lateral and medial rectus muscles, the other four muscles interact to control the vertical and torsional dimensions together. Try looking at a visual target 10° above and to the right of a point straight in front of you. While your eyes can move in three dimensions, those instructions specify a movement in only two dimensions horizontal and vertical. So what does the oculomotor system do with this extra dimension?

In 1847, the Dutch physician F. C. Donders noted that whenever a human rotates his/her eye to a particular horizontal and vertical position, the eye always comes to rest with exactly the same amount of torsion. From this observation he developed *Donders' law,* which states that for any given horizontal and vertical position of the eye there is a unique value for the torsional position of the eye. Torsion is thus not a free dimension at all, it can be derived from horizontal and vertical eye position.

Just what is the observed value of torsion for any particular horizontal and vertical eye position? J. B. Listing took Donders' law a step further in the 1860s with *Listing's law,* when he noted that the amount of torsion associated with any vertical and horizontal eye position could be computed geometrically. Imagine the eye looking straight ahead and slightly downward, from what is called the *primary position.* When the line of sight is moved from the primary position to any secondary position, the amount of torsion present at the secondary position is exactly the amount that would be produced if the eye had been rotated along as short a trajectory as possible to that secondary position. Listing characterized all of these legal levels of torsion as the positions that the eye would take if rotated away from the primary position around axes perpendicular to the line of sight at the primary position. Of course, this family of rotational axes would describe a single plane perpendicular to the line of sight, a slice through oculomotor space which is called *Listing's plane.*

Why and how do eye positions obey Listing's law? For many years, a debate raged around whether Listing's law was enforced actively by the brain or whether the muscles of the eye were constrained in some way so that only eye movements in accord with Listing's law could actually be produced by the six eye muscles.

Studies by Joseph Demer and colleagues at UCLA suggest that the answer to this question is that both neural and muscular constraints enforce Listing's law. Demer and colleagues used magnetic resonance images to measure the three-dimensional position of the eye, and of all six eye muscles, while human volunteers made a series of eye movements. They found that all six eye muscles pass through sheaths of connective tissue that serve as mechanical pulleys. These pulleys alter the angle with which each muscle pulls on the globe, as the eye moves, in a way that constrains the movements of the eye to conform to Listing's law. However, these pulleys do not seem to be entirely passive elements. Muscles innervated by the brain appear to adjust the exact positions of the pulleys in a way that greatly simplifies both the neural and the mechanical implementation of Listing's law.

While research is only just beginning on these pulleys, the biomechanical properties of the tissues around the eye muscles, and the innervation of the muscles that articulate the pulleys, seem to solve the puzzle of Listing's law. The most important implication of this finding is that it means that brain nuclei, which activate the six muscles of the eye, only need to concern themselves with the horizontal and vertical position of the eye, freeing the structures that control them from computations in the third dimension of torsion.

Paul W. Glimcher

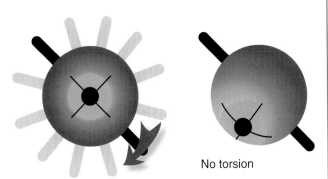

No torsion

FIGURE 33.15 When the eye comes to rest after a movement it always has exactly the amount of torsion specified by Listing's law: "When the line of fixation is brought from its primary position to any other position, the torsional rotation of the eyeball in this second position will be the same as if the eye had been turned around a fixed axis perpendicular to the initial and final directions of the line of fixation."

BOX 33.2

CLINICAL SYNDROMES OF THE MEDIAN LONGITUDINAL FASCICULUS

The median longitudinal fasciculus (MLF) carries signals that coordinate actions of the lateral rectus of one eye with the medial rectus of the other eye for lateral movement in the VOR, smooth pursuit, saccades, and maintained gaze. Thus, damage (typically a small infarct caused by occlusion of a small artery) of the right MLF (after crossing midline) will impair the coordinate adduction of the right eye that naturally accompanies abduction of the left eye on attempted left gaze. Right gaze (abduction of right eye, adduction of left) will be normal. Damage to the MLF on both sides (typically a bilateral lesion in multiple sclerosis) causes failure of adduction of both eyes, i.e., the right eye on attempted left gaze, the left eye on attempted right gaze. To be sure that it is indeed the MLF that is involved and not the third nerve itself (diabetic infarct) or the neuromuscular junction (myasthenia gravies), the clinician must show that adduction is normal in *vergence*, which does not critically involve the MLF. In contrast, damage to the midbrain convergence center (tumor of the pineal body with pressure from above) will impair adduction of both eyes in attempted convergence, but not adduction or lateral gaze.

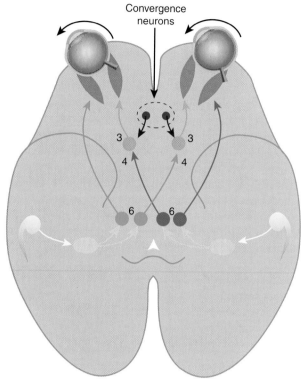

FIGURE 33.16   The 3, 4, and 6 refer to oculomotor, trochlear, and abducens nuclei and their respective cranial nerves.

retinally mapped visual signals, head-based auditory, body surface-based somatosensory, and velocity-based vestibular signals all converge on a common coordinate system, one appropriate for producing eye rotations. This property of sensory motor transformation, which has been studied so extensively in the oculomotor system, may well prove to be a general property of all or most vertebrate motor systems.

References

Baarsma, E. A., and Collewijn, H. (1974). Vestibulo-ocular and optokinetic reactions to rotation and their interaction in the rabbit. *J. Physiol.* **238**, 603–625.

Cannon, S. C., and Robinson, D. A. (1987). Loss of the neural integrator of the oculomotor system from brainstem lesions in the monkey. *J. Neurophysiol.* **57**, 1383–1409.

Dickman, J. D., and Correia, M. J. (1989). Responses of pigeon horizontal semicircular canal afferent fibers. I. Step, trapezoid and low-frequency sinusoidal mechanical and rotational stimulation. *J. Neurophysiol.* **62**, 1090–1101.

Fuchs, A. F., and Lushei, E. S. (1970). Firing patterns of abducens neurons of alert monkeys in relationship to horizontal eye movements. *J. Neurophysiol.* **33**, 382–392.

Gardner, J. L., and Lisberger, S. G. (2001). Linked target selection for saccadic and smooth pursuit eye movements. *J. Neurosci.* **21**, 2075–2084.

Groen, J. J., Lowenstein, O., and Vendrik, A. (1952). The mechanical analysis of responses from the end organs of the horizontal semicircular canal in the isolated elasmobranch labyrinth. *J. Physiol.* **117**, 329–346.

Henn, V., Young, L. R., and Finley, C. (1974). Vestibular nucleus units in alert monkeys are also influenced by moving visual fields. *Brain Res.* **71**, 144–149.

Jay, M. F., and Sparks, D. L. (1984). Auditory receptive fields in primate superior colliculus shift with changes in eye position. *Nature* **309**, 345–347.

Keller, E. L. (1974). Participation of the medial pontine reticular formation in eye movement generation in the monkey. *J. Neurophysiol.* **37**, 316–332.

Lee, C., Rohrer, W. H., and Sparks, D. L. (1988). Population coding of saccadic eye movements by neurons in the superior colliculus. *Nature* **332**, 357–360.

Lisberger, S. G. (1986). Properties of pathways subserving long-term adaptive plasticity in the vestibulo-ocular reflex in monkeys. In: "The Biology of Change in Otolaryngology" (R. W., Ruben *et al.*, eds.), pp. 171–183. Elsevier, Amsterdam.

Lisberger, S. G., Morris, E. J., and Tychsen, L. (1987). Visual motion processing and sensory-motor integration for smooth pursuit eye movements. *Annu. Rev. Neurosci.* **10**, 97–129.

Mays, L. E., and Gamlin, P. D. R. (1995). Neuronal circuitry controlling the near response. *Curr. Opin. Neurobiol.* **5**, 763–768.

Mays, L. E., Porter, J. D., Gamlin, P. D. R., and Tello, C. A. (1986). Neural control of vergence eye movements: Neurons encoding vergence velocity. *J. Neurophysiol.* **56**, 1007–1021.

Miles, F. A., and Eighmy, B. B. (1980). Long term adaptive changes in primate vestibulo-ocular reflex. I. Behavioral observations. *J. Neurophysiol.* **43**, 1406–1425.

Robinson, D. A. (1972). Eye movements evoked by collicular stimulation in the alert monkey. *Vis. Res.* **12**, 1795–1808.

Robinson, D. A. (1975). Oculomotor control signals. *In* "Basic Mechanisms of Ocular Motility and Their Clinical Implications" (P. Bach-y-Rita and G. Lennerstrand, eds.), pp. 337–374. Pergamon, Oxford .

Robinson, D. A., Gordon, J. L., and Gordon, S. E. (1986). A model of the smooth pursuit eye movement system. *Biol. Cyberne.* **55**, 43–57.

Schiller, P. H., True, S. D., and Conway, J. L. (1980). Deficits in eye movements following frontal eye field and superior colliculus ablations. *J. Neurophysiol.* **44**, 1175–1189.

Sparks, D. L., Holland, R., and Guthrie, B. L. (1976). Size and distribution of movement fields in the monkey superior colliculus. *Brain Res.* **113**, 21–34.

Strassman, A. Highstein, S. M., and McCrea, R. A. (1986). Anatomy and physiology of saccadic burst neurons in the alert squirrel monkey. II. Inhibitory burst neurons. *J. Comp. Neurol.* **249**, 358–380.

Suzuki, D A., and Keller, E. L. (1984) Visual signals in the dorsolateral pontine nucleus of the monkey: Their relationship to smooth pursuit eye movements. *Exp. Brain Res.* **53**, 473–478.

Wurtz, R. H., and Goldberg, M. E. (1972). Activity of superior colliculus in the behaving monkey. III. Cells discharging before eye movements. *J. Neurophysiol.* **35**, 575–586.

Suggested Readings

Carpenter, R. H. S. (1988). "Movements of the Eyes," 2nd Ed. Pion Limited, London.

Carpenter, R. H. S. (ed.) (1991). "Eye Movements: Vision and Visual Dysfunction," Vol. 8. CRC Press, Boston.

Collewijn, H. (1981). "The Oculomotor System of the Rabbit and its Plasticity." Springer, New York.

Fuchs, A. F., Kaneko, C. R. S., and Scudder, C. A. (1985). Brainstem control of saccadic eye movements. *Annu. Rev. Neurosci.* **8**, 307–337.

Jones G. Melvill (1991). The vestibular contribution. *In* "Eye Movements" (R. H. S. Carpenter, ed.), pp. 13–44. CRC Press, Boston.

Leigh, R. J., and Zee, D. S. (1991). "The Neurology of Eye Movements," 2nd Ed. F. A. Davis, Philadelphia.

Lisberger, S. G., Morris, E. J., and Tychsen, L. (1987). Visual motion processing and sensory-motor integration for smooth pursuit eye movements. *Annu. Rev. Neurosci.* **10**, 97–129.

Mays, L. E., and Gamlin, P. D. R. (1995). Neuronal circuitry controlling the near response. *Curr. Opin. Neurobiol.* **5**, 763–768.

Raphan, T., and Cohen, B. (1978). Brainstem mechanisms for rapid and slow eye movements. *Annu. Rev. Physiol.* **40**, 527–552.

Robinson, D. A. (1981). Control of eye movements. *In* "The Nervous System: Handbook of Physiology" (V. B. Brooks, ed.), Vol. II, pp. 1275–1320. Williams & Wilkins, Baltimore.

Sparks, D. L. (1986). Translation of sensory signal into commands for saccadic eye movements: Role of primate superior colliculus. *Physiol. Rev.* **66**, 118–71.

Paul W. Glimcher

REGULATORY SYSTEMS

34

The Hypothalamus: An Overview of Regulatory Systems

The hypothalamus is an integrative center essential for survival of an organism and reproduction of its species. Regulatory systems emerged as each organism adapted to its environment and have evolved to control the complex interactions of physiology and behavior.

The regulatory role of the hypothalamus is reflected in its structural organization and connections. Almost every major subdivision of the neuraxis, or central nervous system (CNS), communicates with the hypothalamus and is subject to its influence. In addition, the hypothalamus communicates with peripheral organ systems by converting synaptic information to blood-borne humoral signals. In turn, the hypothalamus responds to input from the peripheral systems that it regulates. The chapters in this section discuss the processes by which the hypothalamus influences physiology and behavior. This introductory chapter provides an overview of the structural and functional organization of the hypothalamus. We begin by providing a historical perspective on research that has defined the hypothalamus as an important regulatory center, continue with an overview of its structural and functional organization, and conclude with a discussion of how this region of the diencephalon functions within brain circuitry devoted to the control of motivated behavior.

HISTORICAL PERSPECTIVE

Research on the hypothalamus has a rich and storied history. Although depicted in early brain atlases, the hypothalamus was not recognized as a distinct division of the diencephalon until the work of Wilhelm His (1893). Our understanding of the structure and function of the hypothalamus developed as basic and clinical neurosciences were integrated. One important early researcher was Harvey Cushing, a neurosurgeon who studied endocrine disorders from a neuroscience perspective. He described diabetes insipidus, a neuroendocrine dysfunction of uncontrolled urinary water excretion and thirst, and identified the importance of injury to the pituitary stalk in the condition. Cushing also described the syndrome that bears his name, Cushing's syndrome, a disorder characterized by excessive secretion of adrenal corticoids. In addition, he was among the first to recognize that the hypothalamus and pituitary form a functional unit. He was a pioneer in the development of pituitary surgery and is viewed as a founder of the fields of neurosurgery and endocrinology. In 1929, summing up his work in this area shortly before his retirement, Cushing wrote of the hypothalamus, "Here in this well concealed spot, almost to be covered with a thumb nail, lies the very mainspring of primitive existence—vegetative, emotional, reproductive—on which, with more or less success, man has come to superimpose a cortex of inhibitions."

Since Cushing and others described dysfunctions associated with hypothalamic and pituitary pathology or experimental damage, technical advances have provided more and more sophisticated insights into the structural and functional organization of this region of the neuraxis. Gurdijian (1927), Kreig (1932), and Le Gros Clark et al. (1938) used histological procedures to describe the cytoarchitecture of hypothalamic nuclei. Their observations proved to be remarkably predictive of functional specialization as evidenced by the work of Ranson, Hess, and others during the same period. Work from those investigators demonstrated that lesions and localized stimulation of the hypothalamus could selectively affect appetite, weight control, water balance, autonomic control, reproductive function, and emotional behavior. This work progressed so well that in 1940 it could be summarized only in a large volume of the annual series of the "Association for Research in Nervous and Mental Disease."

In that volume, Ernst and Berta Scharrer (1940) presented evidence for "neurosecretory neurons," providing the foundation for a fundamental tenet of hypothalamic function. That is, there were neurons—in the brain—that secrete hormones directly into the bloodstream. In 1949, Wolfgang Bargmann published his studies about neurosecretory neurons with cell bodies that lay in the hypothalamus and axons that projected to the posterior lobe of the pituitary gland. Bargmann's work provided a framework for our current understanding of neuroendocrine or neurohumoral regulation, e.g., that release of peptides into the peripheral circulation allows the hypothalamus to exert a profound physiological influence on a variety of systems.

Neurohumoral regulation of the anterior lobe of the pituitary was defined by Harris and Green in the 1950s. Their identification of a neurovascular link, the portal plexus, through which the hypothalamus regulates the anterior pituitary, fundamentally altered concepts of hypothalamic function and neuroendocrine regulation. This regulatory function was further amplified in the 1970s when Guillemin and Schally independently isolated and characterized peptide hormones that act on the anterior pituitary, thereby revealing the neurochemical basis of this regulation. In subsequent years the field of neuroendocrinology built enormously on these observations, and the resulting literature documents a diverse family of hypothalamic peptides that are released into the portal plexus to stimulate or inhibit the release of other hormones from the anterior pituitary gland.

We have made great progress in improving our understanding of Cushing's "mainspring of primitive

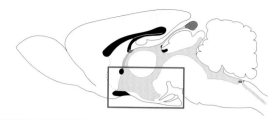

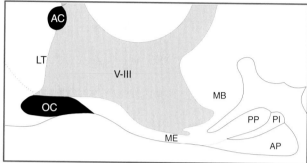

FIGURE 34.1 Boundaries of the hypothalamus of the rat (midsagittal section). The ventricular system is shaded. The boxed area shows the approximate location of the hypothalamus in the ventral quadrant of the diencephalon. The floor of the third ventricle (V-III), formed by the optic chiasm (OC), median eminence (ME), and rostral portion of the mammillary body (MB), defines a large portion of the rostrocaudal extent of the hypothalamus and is also distinguished by the infundibular stalk, which connects the pituitary to the ventral diencephalon. The rostral limit of the hypothalamus is the lamina terminalis (LT), a thin strip of tissue extending between the optic chasm and anterior commissure (AC) that also contributes to the rostral wall of the third ventricle. PP, posterior pituitary; AP, anterior pituitary, PI, pars intermedia of the pituitary.

existence." Tremendous insights into CNS function have emerged from the analysis of hypothalamic structure and function, underscoring the importance of this small, complex region of the diencephalon. Additionally, modern circuit analysis has placed the hypothalamus within a larger ensemble of neurons devoted to homeostatic and behavioral functions essential for survival.

FIGURE 34.2 Cytoarchitectural organization of the hypothalamus as viewed in six transverse Nissl-stained sections. Boundaries of the ▶ major hypothalamic nuclei and areas are designated by dotted lines. ac, anterior commissure; ADP, anterodorsal preoptic nucleus; AHA, anterior hypothalamic area; AHN, anterior hypothalamic nucleus; AMY, amygdala; ARC, arcutate nucleus; AVP, anteroventral preoptic nucleus; AVPV, anteroventral periventricular nucleus; BST, bed nucleus of the stria terminalis; CP, caudoputamen; cpd, cerebral peduncle; DMH, dorsomedial hypothalamic nucleus; FF, fields of Forel; fr, fasiculus retroflexus; fx, fornix; GP, globu pallidus; int, internal capsule; HF, hippocampal formation; LHA, lateral hypothalamic area; LM, lateral mammillary nucleus; LPO, lateral preoptic area; LS, lateral septum; MA, magnocellular preoptic nucleus; ME, median eminence; ml, medial lemniscus; mp, mammillary peduncle; MM, medial mammillary nucleus; MPN, medial preoptic nucleus; MPO, medial preoptic area; MRN, mesencephalic reticular nucleus; mtg, mammillotegmental tract; mtt, mammillothalamic tract; NDB, nucleus of the diagonal band; och, optic chiasm; opt, optic tract; PH, posterior hypothalamic nucleus; pm, principal mammillary tract; PMd, dorsal premammillary nucleus; PMv, ventral premammillary nucleus; PS, parastrial nucleus; PVH, paraventricular nucleus hypothalamus; Pvi, periventricular nucleus intermediate; PVT, paraventricular nucleus thalamus; RE, nucleus reuniens; SBPV, subparaventricular zone; SCN, suprachiasmatic nucleus; SI, substantia innoninata; SO, supraoptic nucleus; sm, stria medullaris; smd, supramammillary decussation; SN, substantia nigra; SPF, suparafascicular nucleus thalamus; STN, substalamic nucleus; SUM, supramammillary nucleus; sup, supraoptic commissure; TM, tuberomammillary nucleus; V3, third ventricle; VMH, ventromedial hypothalamic nucleus; VP, ventral posterior thalamic nucleus; VTA, ventral tegmental area; ZI, zona incerta.

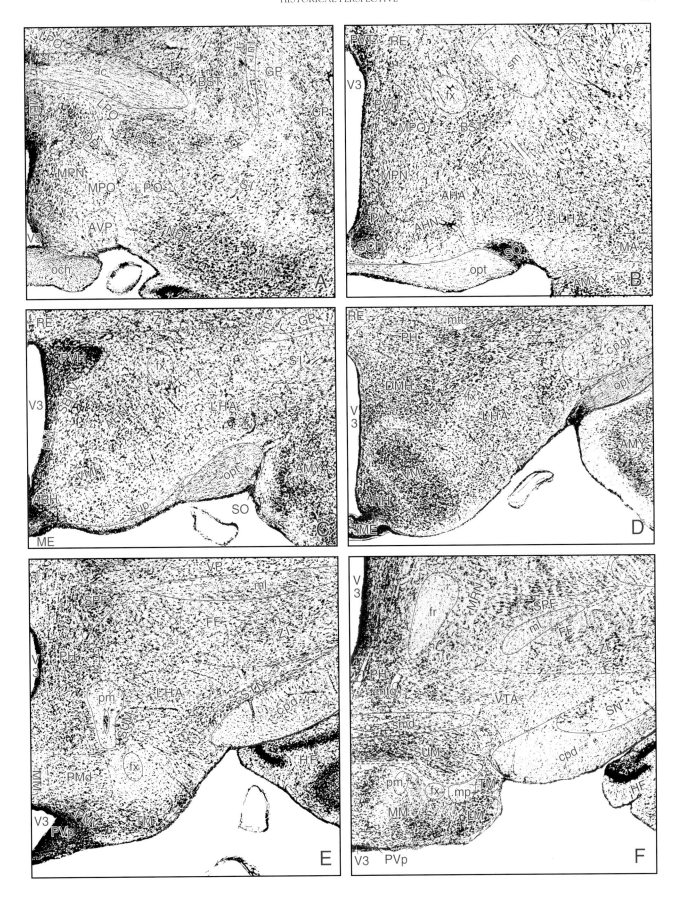

GENERAL ORGANIZATIONAL PRINCIPLES OF THE ADULT HYPOTHALAMUS

Studies of the organization and function of the hypothalamus have benefited enormously from the development of methods for defining the phenotype and connectivity of neurons. The following description provides an overview of the cellular architecture and organizational principles that underlie hypothalamic function. Because most work was done using rodents, we have based our descriptions and illustrations on data derived from the rat. Nevertheless, we have emphasized organizational principles that appear common to those found in primates, including the human.

Hypothalamic Boundaries Are Defined by Physical Landmarks

The boundaries of the hypothalamus are defined by landmarks that are apparent on the ventral surface of the brain, in medial exposures of the third ventricular wall (Fig. 34.1), and in Nissl-stained transverse sections through the diencephalon (Fig. 34.2). On the ventral surface of the brain are three prominent landmarks that define the floor of the hypothalamus. The most rostral of these is the optic chiasm, a myelinated fiber tract formed by the decussation of the optic nerves. Immediately caudal to the optic nerve is the infundibular stalk, an evagination emerging from a prominent oval protuberance, the tuber cinereum, located on the floor of the third ventricle. The infundibular stalk provides the vascular and neural connections through which the ventral hypothalamus communicates with the pituitary. The caudal limit of the hypothalamus is defined by the mammillary nuclei. In rodents, these nuclei are found caudal to the tuber cinereum but exhibit no clear external landmark. In primates, including humans, mammillary nuclei are marked externally by paired spherical protrusions located immediately caudal to the infundibular stalk. All of the structures dorsal to these landmarks and ventral to the thalamus constitute the hypothalamus.

The Hypothalamus Is Composed of Three Longitudinally Oriented Cell Columns

Historically, the hypothalamus has been divided into subdivisions that can be distinguished in both longitudinal and mediolateral axes of the diencephalon (Fig. 34.1 and Table 34.1). Current evidence favors

TABLE 34.1   Major Nuclei Contributing to Preoptic, Chiasmatic (Anterior), Tuberal, and Mammillary Subdivisions

Hypothalamic subdivision	Nucleus
Preoptic	Vascular organ of the lamina terminalis
	Median preoptic nucleus
	Preoptic periventricular nucleus
	Anteroventral periventricular nucleus
	Medial preoptic nucleus
	Lateral preoptic area
Anterior	Suprachiasmatic nucleus
	Anterior periventricular nucleus
	Anterior hypothalamic nucleus
	Paraventricular nucleus
	Subparaventricular zone
	Supraoptic nucleus
	Retrochiasmatic area
	Lateral hypothalamic area
Tuberal	Intermediate periventricular nucleus
	Arcuate nucleus
	Ventromedial nucleus
	Dorsomedial nucleus
	Lateral hypothalamic area
	Ventral premammillary nucleus
Mammillary	Posterior periventricular nucleus
	Posterior hypothalamic nucleus
	Dorsal premammillary nucleus
	Mammillary nuclei
	Supramammillary nuclei
	Tuberomammillary nuclei
	Lateral hypothalamic area

three longitudinally organized zones that can be further divided into four levels, or nuclear groups, based on position in the rostrocaudal axis of the hypothalamus.

The longitudinal subdivisions are largely consistent with the initial descriptions of Gurdjian (1927) and Krieg (1932) and consist of periventricular, medial, and lateral zones. All three zones extend through the entire rostrocaudal length of the hypothalamus. The periventricular zone, as the name implies, lies adjacent to the ependymal lining of the third ventricle. Its constituent neurons are densely packed within a narrow zone adjacent to the ependyma and occasionally expand into cytoarchitecturally distinct nuclear groups. The medial zone lies immediately adjacent to the periventricular zone and contains a series of cell groups that vary in size and cell morphology, but are organized into nuclei. This contrasts with the diffusely distributed neurons of the lateral zone. Although phenotypically and connectionally distinct, the cytoarchitecture of this zone is the least distinct of the three columns.

FUNCTIONAL ORGANIZATION OF THE HYPOTHALAMUS

To integrate a variety of physiological processes and behaviors, the hypothalamus must communicate with systems in the brain and periphery. More than any other region of the nervous system, the hypothalamus depends on conversion of synaptic information to humoral signals. In addition, the hypothalamus is subject to feedback regulation by the physiological processes that it controls. The following sections describe basic organization principles that govern hypothalamic function.

The Hypothalamus Integrates Selected Sensory and Nonsensory Information

Projections from several regions of the neuraxis terminate within the hypothalamus. In many instances, monosynaptic projections bring first-order sensory information from the periphery directly to hypothalamic nuclei. In other cases, such as limbic projections, multisynaptic cerebral pathways relay processed information to the hypothalamus. Integration of this sensory information is an essential function of the hypothalamus and has profound influence on the regulatory outputs of hypothalamic nuclei. These overlapping systems are best understood by looking at the functions that they modulate.

Olfaction

Multisynaptic pathways allow the olfactory system to influence neurons in many parts of the hypothalamus. Olfactory information passes directly to the olfactory tubercle, piriform cortex, and amygdala, which in turn relay it to the hypothalamus through the medial forebrain bundle (corticohypothalamic projections), stria terminalis, ventral amygdalofugal pathway, and fornix. In many vertebrates, olfaction is integral to behaviors involved in reproduction, defense, and feeding and this is reflected in the large amount of forebrain dedicated to the processing of olfactory stimuli. Thus, these projection systems are essential to survival and reproductive function in nocturnal animals that use olfaction as a primary sensory modality.

Visual Projections

A principal function of the hypothalamus is to impose temporal organization on hormonal and behavioral processes by virtue of the timekeeping properties of the biological clock in the rostral hypothalamus. The neurons that constitute this clock are found within the suprachiasmatic nuclei (SCN). Their endogenous circadian rhythmicity provides a timekeeping capacity that is essential to successful adaptation and, in many instances, reproduction of the organism. Importantly, the rhythmic activity of the biological clock is responsive to environmental cues, which is accomplished through central visual projections of the retina. Light transduced in the retina synchronizes the circadian activity of SCN neurons with the daily cycle of light and dark through the retinohypothalamic projection. Polysynaptic efferent influences of the clock on the functional activity of the pineal gland also provide a feedback mechanism for measuring day length and thereby controls reproduction in photoperiodic species. The responsiveness of this regulatory system to variations in photoperiod is also responsible for the "jet lag" that humans suffer when traveling across time zones.

Surprisingly, the neural projections of the SCN are relatively sparse and largely confined to the hypothalamus. Therefore, the SCN is probably part of a group of interconnected structures—the circadian timing system—that integrate a variety of sensory information important for the temporal organization of diverse functions regulated by the hypothalamus. A more detailed description of this system is presented in Chapter 41.

Visceral Sensation

Sensory information also reaches the hypothalamus through ascending projections arising in the nucleus of the solitary tract (NTS) of the caudal brain stem. The NTS is the principal visceral sensory nucleus that receives topographically organized input from the major organ systems of the body by way of cranial nerves X and IX, the vagus and glossopharyngeal nerves. As such, it is the first region in the CNS to process information about visceral, cardiovascular, and respiratory functions, as well as taste. The NTS coordinates reflex modulation of peripheral organ function and sends processed sensory information to forebrain nuclei, where it is integrated in the control of more complex physiological processes and behaviors.

A subset of hypothalamic nuclei are the principal targets of ascending NTS projections. Neurons in the paraventricular hypothalamic nucleus (PVH) and the lateral hypothalamic area (LHA) receive direct projections from the NTS and indirect projections through the ventrolateral medulla or the parabrachial nucleus in the pons. Many of these projections are bidirectional and are part of a larger system that includes the central nucleus of the amygdala, bed nuclei of the stria terminalis, and insular cortex. In addition, the NTS and parabrachial nuclei relay splanchnic visceral and nociceptive sensory information ascending from the spinal cord.

Multimodal Brainstem Afferents

The medial forebrain bundle (mfb) is a group of thin fibers that traverse the lateral zone of the hypothalamus. This bidirectional fiber tract provides extrinsic afferent projections to a number of hypothalamic nuclei and is used as a conduit for hypothalamic neurons to communicate with other regions of the neuraxis. Early nonspecific stimulation and lesion experiments incorrectly attributed certain functions to the lateral hypothalamus that are actually associated with the stimulation or loss of extrinsic axons passing through the mfb to other regions of the brain.

Several prominent cell groups contribute to the mfb. Monoamine-containing axons are an especially prominent group of ascending fibers. These axons arise from brain stem neurons, and many of them generate collaterals that terminate throughout the hypothalamus as they course rostrally to innervate other forebrain regions. Prominent among the brain stem cell groups that contribute to this projection system are noradrenergic neurons in the locus coeruleus and lateral tegmental cell groups, as well as serotoninergic neurons of the brain stem raphe nuclei. Serotonergic neurons in the midbrain raphe nuclei also generate a dense plexus of axons that enter the cerebral ventricles and arborize on the luminal surface of the ependyma. The precise function of this intraventricular plexus has not been established.

A number of systems not functionally associated with the hypothalamus also pass through the mfb. Prominent among these are dopaminergic axons arising from the substantia nigra and ventral tegmental area (VTA). The nigral component of this projection plays an important role in the regulation of movement whereas the VTA exerts a widespread influence on the cortex and also influences ventral striatal regions involved in motivated behavior and addiction. These projection systems are distinct from the dopaminergic neurons that reside within the hypothalamus (e.g., arcuate nuclei) and play an important role in neuroendocrine regulation.

Projections from Limbic Regions

The hippocampal formation with its fornix, the septum, and the amygdala with its stria terminalis maintain an intimate association with the hypo-

thalamus. In the 1930s, Papez (1937) suggested that components of this "limbic circuitry" form part of a multisynaptic pathway, classically known as Papez's circuit, responsible for the expression of emotion. Although this function has not been confirmed, modern analyses of this circuitry have established prominent functional relations among these regions that place the hypothalamus as an important functional node in the control and expression of behavior. Prominent among the observations that have forged this vision are studies demonstrating that the fornix influences the activity of the hypothalamus through direct and indirect pathways. The direct path is a prominent component of Papez's circuit and is composed of axons that arise from neurons in a distinct subdivision of hippocampal formation known as the subicular complex. This projection, known as the "postcommissural" fornix, courses behind the anterior commissure and terminates in the mammillary bodies. The indirect or precommissural fibers influence the hypothalamus via a disynaptic projection involving the septum. Risold and Swanson (1996) demonstrated that this projection arises from the hippocampus proper (Ammon's horn), is organized topographically, and terminates densely within the hypothalamus. The topography of this projection is apparent at its origin in the hippocampus and is preserved in the lateral septal nuclei, as well as the hypothalamus where second order projections innervate the three longitudinally organized columns of the hypothalamus, although not equally. Thus, different components of this projection system regulate neuroendocrine and autonomic function and ingestive behavior (periventricular zone), modulate motivated reproductive and agonistic behaviors (rostral medial zone), and also provide polysynaptic feedback projections to the hippocampus via the mammillary complex.

Limbic projections arising from the amygdala also have a prominent influence on hypothalamic function. This occurs through two projection pathways. The stria terminalis arises from neurons in the amygdala and follows a looping trajectory similar to the course of the fornix. Axons coursing through this pathway ramify within the bed nucleus and then enter the hypothalamus rostrally. Amygdala neurons also innervate the hypothalamus via the ventral amygdalofugal bundle, which passes directly over the optic tract to the hypothalamus.

Circumventricular Organs

Not all sensory information reaching the hypothalamus is of synaptic origin. Some regions of the

CNS are chemosensitive to blood-borne molecules. Such information about body fluids has a prominent influence on the maintenance of homeostasis. Circumventricular organs (CVOs) are integral to this regulation. Eight CVOs surround the ventricular system in the diencephalon, midbrain, and hindbrain. These include the subfornical organ (SFO), the vascular organ of the lamina terminalis (OVLT), the median eminence (ME), the posterior lobe of the pituitary gland (PL), the pineal gland, the subcommissural organ (SCO), and the area postrema (AP) (Fig. 37.3). Three of these regions, the OVLT, ME, and PL, are located within the hypothalamus. Two other regions, the SFO and AP, have extensive connections with

hypothalamic nuclei involved in neuroendocrine and homeostatic function. These chemosensitive regions were identified by Paul Ehrlich in the late 1800s when he noted that they selectively accumulate vital dyes injected into the peripheral vasculature. Later studies demonstrated that the accumulation of dye was due to the absence of a blood–brain barrier in the CVOs. Unlike those in the brain parenchyma, capillaries in the CVOs are fenestrated, permitting relatively large molecules to leave the vascular lumen and enter the extracellular milieu. As a result, CVO neurons are affected by blood-borne molecules that do not have access to other regions of the brain. The absence of a blood–brain barrier also allows CVOs to use neuro-

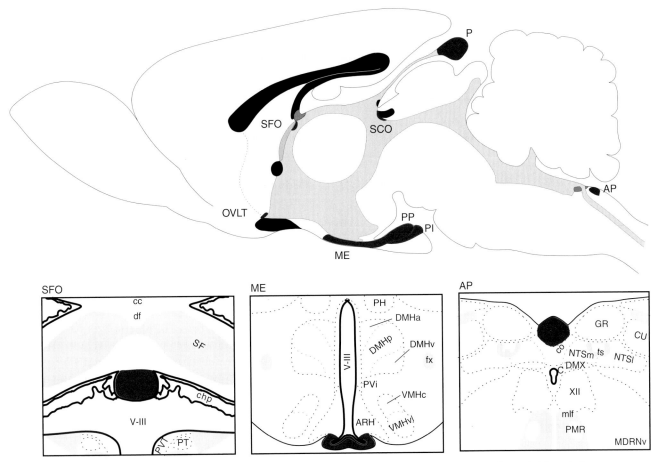

FIGURE 34.3   Location of the six circumventricular organs (shown in red) in the rat brain (midsaggital section). Three regions that have an intimate functional association with the hypothalamus are also illustrated in transverse section in the lower figures. AP, area postrema; ARH, arcuate nucleus; cc, corpus callosum; CU, cuneate nucleus; df, dorsal fornix; DMHa, anterior portion of the dorsomedial nucleus; DMHp, posterior portion of dorsomedial nucleus; DMHv, ventral portion of dorsomedial nucleus; DMX, dorsal motor vagal nucleus; GR, gracile nucleus; ME, median eminence; mlf, medial longitudinal fasiculus; co, commissural portion of the nucleus of the solitary tract; NTSl, lateral portion of the nucleus of the solitary tract; NTSm, medial portion of the nucleus of the solitary tract; OVLT, vascular organ of the lamina terminalis; PH, posterior hypothalamus; P, pineal gland; PMR, paramedian reticular nucleus; PVi, intermediate part of periventricular nucleus; SCO, subcommissural organ; SF, septofimbrial nucleus; SFO, subfornical organ; ts, tractus solitarius; V-III, third ventricle; VMHc, central part of ventromedial nucleus; VMHvl, ventrolateral part of ventromedial nucleus; XII, hypoglossal nucleus.

humoral mechanisms to influence peripheral function. Thus, CVOs represent important "windows" through which the brain can control peripheral function and, importantly, be responsive to feedback regulation by the target organs that it modulates. All of this is accomplished by humoral communication.

EFFECTOR SYSTEMS OF THE HYPOTHALAMUS ARE BOTH HUMORAL AND SYNAPTIC

The extensive influence of the hypothalamus on behavior and physiology is reflected in its effector systems. The hypothalamus has conventional synaptic connections with essentially every major subdivision of the CNS. Additionally, it has regulatory control over the pituitary gland and thereby exerts a profound influence on the function of peripheral organ systems. The basic organization of these effector systems is reviewed in the following sections.

Neuroendocrine Regulation through the Pituitary Gland

The median eminence is the gateway through which the hypothalamus exerts regulatory control over peripheral organ systems. This CVO is continu-

ous with the pituitary gland through a thin tissue bridge known as the infundibular stalk. Hypothalamic neurons exercise this regulatory control via the release of peptides and dopamine (DA) into the vasculature. The infundibular stalk is essential to this regulation. Axons of hypothalamic neurons course through the stalk to fenestrated vascular beds in the posterior division of the pituitary and it also contains blood vessels that transport hypothalamic peptides to the anterior lobe of the pituitary.

Magnocellular neurons in the supraoptic and paraventricular nuclei give rise to axons that project through the median eminence and infundibular stalk to terminate in the posterior lobe of the pituitary (Fig. 34.4). This projection system, the tuberohypophyseal tract, is the only direct neural connection between the hypothalamus and the pituitary. Normally, magnocellular neurons release either vasopressin or oxytocin into the peripheral circulation in the posterior pituitary. These peptides are well known for their influences on fluid homeostasis (vasopressin) and milk letdown in lactating females (oxytocin).

The most extensive hypothalamic control of peripheral organ systems is achieved through the release of peptides and DA in the median eminence. Fenestrated capillaries loop through the median eminence and coalesce to form long portal vessels that travel along the infundibular stalk where they are continuous with vascular sinuses in the anterior pituitary. A variety of parvicellular (small) neurosecretory neurons distinguished by peptide phenotype contribute to this regulation either by stimulating or by inhibiting the release of hormones from the anterior lobe of the pituitary (Table 34.2). The PVH and arcuate nuclei contain a large proportion of these neurons. PVH neurons are found within the parvicellular subdivisions of the nucleus and produce a diverse group of peptides, such as corticotropin-releasing hormone and thyrotropin-releasing hormone. Similarly, neurons in the arcuate

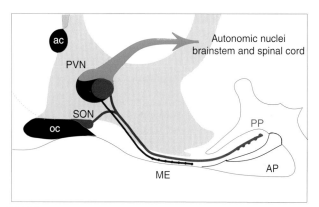

FIGURE 34.4 Functional associations of the paraventricular nucleus (PVH) and the endocrine and autonomic systems. Axons of magnocellular neurons in the PVH and supraoptic nuclei (SON) (shown in red) traverse the internal layer of the median eminence (ME) and the infundibular stalk to the posterior pituitary (PP). Parvicellular PVH neurons influence the functional activity of the anterior lobe of the pituitary (AP) through projections (shown in blue) that terminate on a fenestrated capillary plexus, the portal plexus, in the external zone of the median eminence. The terminal boutons of these axons release peptides and neurotransmitters into the portal vasculature, which carries the hormone to the anterior lobe of the pituitary. Parvicellular PVH neurons also give rise to descending projections (shown in turquoise) to autonomic nuclei in the brain stem and spinal cord. ac, anterior commissure; oc, optic chiasm.

TABLE 34.2 Hormone Systems That Project to the Median Eminence and Act on the Pituitary

Peptide or neurotransmitter	Location of perikarya
Gonadotropin hormone-releasing hormone	Diffusely within preoptic region
Somatostatin	Periventricular nucleus
Growth hormone-releasing hormone	Arcuate nucleus
Corticotropin-releasing hormone	Paraventricular nucleus
Thyrotropin-releasing hormone	Paraventricular nucleus
Dopamine	Arcuate nucleus

nucleus produce peptides, such as growth hormone-releasing hormone, and neurotransmitters, such as dopamine, that influence the secretory activity of the anterior pituitary. Thus, the synaptic activity of neurons projecting on these hypothalamic neurons is integrated, and the information is converted to a humoral signal that ultimately influences peripheral endocrine processes.

Reproductive Function

The ability of mammals to reproduce depends on the function of the hypothalamus and its ability to communicate with the pituitary gland. This is especially true for the production of gametes, whose maturation and release in both males and females require a functionally intact hypothalamic–pituitary axis. In addition, the hypothalamus plays an essential role in the organization and expression of the complex behaviors that are necessary for copulation (see Chapter 40).

Experimental studies in rodents have demonstrated that the rostral medial zone of the hypothalamus plays an important role in orchestrating reproductive behaviors. The medial preoptic region participates in the control of masculine sexual behavior, such as erection, mounting, and ejaculation, whereas ventral regions of the hypothalamus play a major role in the control of feminine sexual behaviors, such as the lordosis reflex.

A number of hypothalamic cell groups implicated in reproductive function are sexually dimorphic. For example, ultrastructural studies of a preoptic region in male and female rats demonstrated differences in the patterns of synapses that developed in response to perinatal exposure to androgens. Also, differences in the size and serotonergic innervation of the medial preoptic nuclei of male and female rats have been demonstrated. The possibility that similar dimorphisms are present in the human hypothalamus is supported by the identification of a region of the human preoptic region that is approximately twice as large in males as in females. In addition, the cytoarchitecture of the rostral hypothalamus of homosexual men appears to be different from that of heterosexual men. Although the functional significance of sexual dimorphism in the structure and connectivity of the hypothalamus remains to be established, the gender of the brain is clearly determined by the hormonal milieu present during a critical period of development.

Although abundant evidence demonstrates a role for the hypothalamus in sexual behavior, much more is known about the hypothalamic circuitry that influences the production of gametes. The production of ova and sperm is controlled by the release of gonadotropins from the anterior pituitary gland. Gonadotropin release is in turn regulated by the hypothalamus. The response of the system to gonadotropins is gender specific. For example, spermatogenesis occurs in response to constant release of gonadotropins, whereas ovulation is a cyclic event initiated by a rhythmic surge in gonadotropin release. In both cases, hypothalamic neurons produce gonadotropin-releasing hormone (GnRH) to stimulate the release of gonadotropin from the anterior lobe of the pituitary. Nevertheless, the gender-specific patterns of gonadotropin release imply that there are sexual differences in the functional organization of afferent systems that influence the activity of GnRH neurons. One postulated sexually dimorphic difference is a central pattern generator, which could be responsible for the cyclic release of GnRH in females. Dimorphism also probably exists in circuitry that integrates the sensory information underlying hormone secretion that leads to gamete production and mediates reproductive behaviors.

Central Integration of Autonomic Function

Descending projections from the hypothalamus to autonomic cell groups in the brain stem and spinal cord affect the sympathetic and parasympathetic divisions of the autonomic nervous system (ANS). Several hypothalamic cell groups also indirectly influence the ANS via projections to areas, such as the central nucleus of the amygdala, that also project to autonomic nuclei. One of the more prominent and well-described components of this projection system arises from the dorsal, medial, and lateral parvicellular parts of the PVH. These neurons project to preganglionic neurons of the sympathetic and parasympathetic divisions of the ANS. Sympathetic preganglionic neurons are found within the intermediolateral cell columns of thoracic and upper lumbar spinal cord segments. In contrast, parasympathetic neurons reside within the brain stem (e.g., dorsal motor vagal nucleus) and the sacral spinal cord. Thus, hypothalamic influences over homeostasis are achieved through both the pituitary gland and the ANS.

Immune Function

Like homeostasis, the hypothalamus exerts an influence over the immune system through neuroendocrine output and through the ANS. Szentivanyi and colleagues examined the effects of hypothalamic lesions and stimulation on anaphylactic responses and found that the diencephalon may influence immune function. Subsequent work by a number of investigators has provided compelling evidence that the nervous system exerts a direct effect on the immune system (for a review, use Ader, 1996).

Felten and colleagues (1987) demonstrated that the activity of immune cells of the spleen is influenced directly by "synaptic-like" contacts of noradrenergic neurons of the sympathetic ANS. This is but one of many examples of hypothalamic influences on immune function through sympathetic outflow. Neuroendocrine influences have also been demonstrated in work pioneered by Hugo Besedovksy. Nevertheless, the mechanisms through which regulation is achieved remain unclear, and the extent to which the nervous system controls immune function remains to be established.

Behavioral State Control

The hypothalamus plays an important role in the timing of behaviors such as sleep. A number of regions of the neuraxis, particularly components of the brain stem reticular activating system and the thalamus, are involved in sleep regulation. Substantial evidence also implicates at least three regions of the hypothalamus in this important regulatory function. For example, approximately 50 years ago Walle Nauta (1946) demonstrated that lesions of the preoptic region produce insomnia in rats. Subsequently, researchers have shown that electrical stimulation of the preoptic region, or local injection of serotonin or prostaglandin D2, induces slow wave sleep. In contrast, lesions of the caudal hypothalamus produce somnolence, suggesting that this region is involved in arousal.

Until recently, little was known regarding the specific hypothalamic cell groups involved in sleep regulation. However, recent studies have begun to provide insight into this issue. Saper and colleagues (Sherin et al., 1996) used immunohistochemical localization of the protein product of the immediate-early gene c-fos to define precisely the location of a group of hypothalamic neurons that become active at the onset of sleep in rats. These cells, located in the ventrolateral preoptic region, contain the inhibitory neurotransmitter GABA and project to the tuberomammillary nuclei in the caudal hypothalamus. The tuberomammillary nuclei, a histaminergic cell group, diffusely innervate the cerebral cortex and have been implicated in arousal. These observations reveal a circuitry whose function coincides with the opposing effects of the rostral and caudal hypothalamus in sleep regulation documented by Nauta.

Compelling evidence also supports the conclusion that the caudal hypothalamus contains another population of neurons that, like the tumberomammillary

nuclei, are diffusely projecting and implicated in the control of arousal. These neurons are found within the posterior and lateral hypothalamus and contain a recently discovered peptide known as hypocretin (or orexin). Studies of the causal mechanism underlying the sleep disorder known as narcolepsy implicate this population of neurons in the regulation of behavioral state. Narcolepsy is a disorder characterized by excessive daytime sleepiness and sudden inappropriate intrusion of sleep during waking. A defect in one of the hypocretin receptors has been demonstrated in a canine model widely employed to study the disease, and transgenic mice lacking the hypocretin gene display sleep–wake disturbances similar to narcolepsy. Additionally, cerebrospinal fluid (CSF) levels of hypocretin are reduced in humans suffering from this disorder, and postmortem analysis of the hypothalamus of narcoleptics has demonstrated substantial reductions in the number of hypocretin neurons. These findings, along with the aforementioned literature and the documented influence of the biological clock on the temporal organization of the sleep–wake cycle, are consistent with an important role for the hypothalamus in the regulation of behavioral state. However, it is important to emphasize that the hypothalamus functions within a larger ensemble of neurons devoted to behavioral state regulation. Particularly important in this regard are monoaminergic and cholinergic brain stem neurons, as well as thalamic and basal forebrain cell groups (Chapter 42). Understanding how these areas function in an integrated fashion to control behavioral state remains an important goal, but it is clear that the hypothalamus plays an important role in this regulation.

Thermoregulation

The preoptic region integrates complementary physiological and behavioral responses to thermal stress. Thermosensitive neurons identified within the preoptic region apparently provide integrative processes responsible for the control of thermoregulation and sleep. Thermosensitive neurons appear to influence arousal mechanisms integral to regulation of the sleep–wake cycle. For example, Dennis McGinty and colleagues have shown that warming the preoptic region during waking suppresses arousal-related neuronal activity in the caudal hypothalamus and in magnocellular basal telencephalon neurons that have diffuse cortical projections. The consequences of this experimental warming include decreased motor activity, reduced metabolic activity and respiratory rate, and enhanced peripheral heat loss. All these effects are similar to changes that characterize the onset of sleep. Thus, the response to thermal stress and the onset of sleep may be mediated through common circuitry. This conclusion is supported by the finding of single populations of preoptic neurons that increase their firing rate in response to warming or to onset of sleep.

To regulate temperature, the hypothalamus integrates input from the SCN and other hypothalamic nuclei. The circadian rhythm in body temperature, a well-characterized feature of mammalian physiology, and environmentally induced thermoregulation occur in large part through hypothalamic (particularly preoptic and anterior areas) control of autonomic function. The preoptic region of the hypothalamus also plays a role in producing fever. Circulating cytokines may act at or near the OVLT to elicit fever, and a "pyrogenic zone" where prostaglandin injection induces fever has been identified in the region surrounding this CVO. The precise pathways responsible for inducing fever are unknown, but a circumscribed population of neurons in central autonomic centers appears to participate. Thus, thermoregulation is complex and requires the preoptic and anterior hypothalamus to integrate information about circadian timing, homeostasis, and microbial infection.

Fluid Homeostasis and Thirst

Insight into the regions of the brain involved in fluid homeostasis has come from observing the response of neurons to dehydration and other experimental changes in milieu. The hypothalamus is a prominent component of a set of CNS nuclei in which neurons respond to dehydration (an increase in fluid osmolarity) and changes in blood volume by increasing their metabolic activity. Activated neurons have been demonstrated in the subfornical organ, the paraventricular and supraoptic nuclei, and an area of the rostral hypothalamus known as the AV3V region, which includes the median preoptic nucleus and the OVLT. These regions interact with neurons in the area postrema, the nucleus of the solitary tract, the noradrenergic cell groups of the brain stem, and the parabrachial nucleus to integrate peripheral stimuli and elicit adaptive changes in the fluid environment of the organism. CVOs appear to subserve prominent regulatory functions within this circuitry.

The SFO has dense projections to the supraoptic and paraventricular nuclei, to the region adjacent to the OVLT, and to the perifornical region of the lateral hypothalamic area. Such projections are consistent with postulated roles of the SFO in autonomic and homeostatic functions. The peptide hormone angiotensin II (AII) is integral to the way in which the SFO transduces peripheral signals and then produces compensatory neural responses. When blood pressure falls, the kidneys release renin into the bloodstream. Renin triggers a biochemical cascade that produces AII. Because of the absence of a blood–brain barrier in the SFO, circulating AII can enter the SFO and bind AII receptors on SFO neurons. Interestingly, SFO neurons appear to use AII as a neurotransmitter in projections to hypothalamic cells that are involved in the control of fluid dynamics. In this example, activation of hypothalamic systems that elicit drinking and reduce fluid excretion at the kidneys would produce the adaptive compensatory homeostatic increase in blood pressure. Further details on the components of the regulatory system are provided in Chapter 36.

Different populations of hypothalamic neurons elicit adaptive responses to changes in fluid osmolarity. Osmosensitive neurons are located primarily in the AV3V region, which includes the OVLT. The response of these neurons to alterations in fluid osmolarity elicits an adaptive compensatory thirst. The neural circuitry that modulates this response is not fully understood but is known to involve input from the OVLT, SFO, and NTS. Further, it takes advantage of the same output regulatory pathway, hypothalamic magnocellular neurons, utilized by the SFO. Chapter 39 considers the hypothalamic role in fluid homeostasis in greater detail.

Food Intake

The consumption of food is another complex behavior that involves several regions of the brain. The hypothalamus plays an essential role in this circuitry as an integrative center for a variety of sensory stimuli, both synaptic and hormonal. It also serves to modulate autonomic outflow to the viscera. This modern view of neural regulation of food intake is a substantial modification of the simple concept of opposing centers for hunger and satiety that was popular in the older literature. These centers were advanced by early studies that used hypothalamic lesions and stimulation. Chapter 38 contains a detailed discussion of more recent literature that has contributed to the modern view of the neural control of food intake. The following description summarizes the functional organization of hypothalamic nuclei that regulate food intake.

When food is consumed, hormones are released from the viscera, and sensory pathways innervating the alimentary tract are stimulated. These sensory pathways regulate neurons in the area postrema and NTS that are connected bidirectionally with hypothalamic nuclei. Hypothalamic nuclei are also subject to feedback regulation from hormonal signals arising in the gut. At least four hypothalamic nuclei are involved in the control of feeding, and a prominent part of their influence is exerted via descending projections to autonomic nuclei in the brain stem and spinal cord. Paraventricular nuclei seem to provide the primary descending hypothalamic influence. In particular, parvicellular oxytocinergic neurons in the PVH provide an important descending projection to the dorsal vagal complex (including the NTS) and the sympathetic preganglionic neurons of the thoracic spinal cord. At least some of this descending influence appears to be under the control of neuropeptide Y (NPY)-containing neurons that project from the arcuate nucleus to the PVH. In experiments, infusion of NPY into the PVH stimulates food intake. In addition, NPY-containing neurons in the arcuate nucleus are inhibited by insulin released into the peripheral circulation after a meal and by leptin, a peptide released from adipose tissue. Thus, hypothalamic nuclei regulate food intake through the autonomic nervous system, and a subset of these neurons is influenced by peripheral signals from the periphery.

Although recent work does not support the earlier conclusion that the VMH functions as a satiety center, it remains possible that neurons in this nucleus are important for caloric homeostasis and, indirectly, for food intake. As discussed in detail in Chapter 38, evidence is consistent with neurons in or near the VMH playing an important role in regulating the secretion of insulin. It is also clear that the SCN influences the temporal organization of feeding. For example, nocturnal rodents normally feed almost exclusively during the dark phase of the photoperiod, but rodents whose SCN has been ablated feed throughout the light–dark cycle.

Summary

It is clear that the hypothalamus plays a pivotal regulatory role central to the survival and propagation of vertebrate species. This regulation is achieved by output pathways that utilize both synaptic and hormonal mechanisms and is subject to feedback regulation by sensory information derived from the systems that they regulate. The integrative capacities of the hypothalamus are fundamental to its ability to orchestrate the complex and diverse adaptive behaviors that underlie homeostasis, reproduction of the species, and motivated behavior. Within this context it is important to view the hypothalamus as an integral component of ensembles of neurons devoted to specific functions rather than an individual unit. Swanson has recently advanced a conceptual frame-

work consistent with this philosophy. In this formulation, the hypothalamus is part of a "behavioral control column" that functions as a topographically organized integrative center subject to the control of cerebral hemispheres. The functional organization of this column is consistent with the distributed localization of functions classically associated with the hypothalamus. For example, the rostral portion of the column is devoted to the control of ingestive (eating and drinking) and social (defensive and reproductive) behaviors, whereas the caudal portion, which is continuous with the substantia nigra, functions in support of exploratory and foraging behaviors. Modulation of these distributed functions is under the control of the cerebral hemispheres through three descending projections involving the cortex, striatum and pallidum. The role of the hypothalamus in imparting temporal organization on the behavioral state and physiology is an important component of this organizational framework. Thus, the explosion of organizational and functional data that has accumulated over the past quarter century has expanded our understanding of hypothalamic function and established this small but complex subdivision of the diencephalon as an important integrative unit for the expression of behavior.

References

Ader, R. (1996). Historical perspectives on psychoneuroimmunology. *In* "Psychoneuroimmunology, Stress, and Infection" (H. Friedman, T. W. Klein, and A. L. Friedman, eds.), pp. 1–24. CRC Press, Boca Raton, FL.

Ehrlich, P. (1956). Uber die methylenblaureaction der lebenden Nervensubstanz. *In* "The Collected Papers of Paul Ehrlich" (F. Himmelweit, ed.), Vol. 1, pp. 500–508. Pergamon Press, London.

Felten, D. L., Felten, S. Y., Bellinger, D. L., Carlson, S. L., Akerman, K. D., Madden, K. S., Olschowka, J. A., and Livnat, S. (1987). Noradrenergic sympathetic neural interactions with the immune system: Structure and function. *Immunol. Rev.* **100**, 225–260.

Fulton, J. F., Ranson, S. W., and Frantz, A. M. (eds) (1940). "The Hypothalamus." Williams & Wilkins, Baltimore.

Gurdijian, E. S. (1927). The diencephalon of the albino rat. *J. Comp. Neurol.* **43**, 1–114.

Harris, G. W. (1948). Neural control of the pituitary gland. *Physiol. Rev.* **28**, 139–179.

Hess, W. R. (1957). "The Functional Organization of the Diencephalon." Grune & Stratton, New York.

His, W. (1893). Vorschlage zur Einteilung des Gehirns. *Arch. Anat. Entwicklungs Gesch.* (Leipzig) **17**, 157–171.

Johnson, A. K., and Gross, P. M. (1993). Sensory circumventricular organs and brain homeostatic pathways. *FASEB J.* **7**, 678–686.

Krieg, W. J. S. (1932). The hypothalamus of the albino rat. *J. Comp. Neurol.* **55**, 19–89.

Le Gros Clark, W. E., Beattie, W. E., Riddoch, W. E., and Dott, N. M. (1938). "The Hypothalamus." Oliver & Boyd, Edinburgh.

Nauta, W. J. H. (1946). Hypothalamic regulation of sleep in rats: An experimental study. *J. Neurophysiol.* **9**, 285.

Papez, J. W. (1937). A proposed mechanism of emotion. *Arch. Neurol. Psychiatry* **38**, 725–743.

Risold, P. Y., and Swanson, L. W. (1996). Structural evidence for functional domains in the rat hippocampus. *Science* **272**, 1484–1486.

Scharrer, B., and Scharrer, E. (1940). Sensory cells within the hypothalamus. *In* "The Hypothalamus" (J. F. Fulton, S. W. Ranson, and A. M. Frantz, eds.), pp. 170–194. Williams & Wilkins, Baltimore.

Sherin, J. E., Shiromani, P. J., McCarley, R. W., and Saper, C. B. (1996). Activation of ventrolateral preoptic neurons during sleep. *Science* **217**, 216–219.

Suggested Readings

Saper, C. B. (1990). Hypothalamus. *In* "The Human Nervous System" (G. Paxinos, ed.), pp. 389–414. Academic Press, San Diego.

Swanson, L. W. (2000). Cerebral hemisphere regulation of motivated behavior. *Brain Res.* **886**, 113-164.

Swanson, L. W., and Cowan, W. M. (1975). Hippocampo-hypothalamic connections—origin in subicular cortex, not Ammons Horn. *Science* **189**, 303–304.

J. Patrick Card, Larry W. Swanson,
and Robert Y. Moore

35

Central Control of Autonomic Functions: Organization of the Autonomic Nervous System

The autonomic nervous system (ANS) consists of the circuitry that controls the body's physiology. This circuitry is a morphologically, embryologically, functionally, and pharmacologically distinct division of the nervous system. Working in concert with the endocrine system, the ANS is responsible for homeostasis.

Unlike the somatic or skeletal motor system (described in Section V), which innervates striated muscles, the autonomic nervous system innervates the body's smooth muscle organs and tissues. The ANS projects to, and forms plexuses within, the hollow organs, or viscera, such as the heart and lungs in the thorax, and the gastrointestinal, genital, and urinary tracts in the abdomen. It also projects to the blood vessels, glands, and other target tissues found within trunk muscles, limb muscles, and skin.

The ANS is responsible for what Walter B. Cannon (1939) referred to as the "wisdom of the body" (see Box 35.1). In tandem with endocrine systems, the ANS orchestrates the continuous adjustments in blood chemistry, respiration, circulation, digestion, and immune responses that protect the integrity of the internal milieu and enable the coordination of skeletal muscles and exteroceptive senses into what we know as behavior. For example, Cannon (1939), in his seminal and defining physiological experiments on the ANS, found that selective surgical destruction of different autonomic pathways devastated the ability of an animal to regulate its body temperature, to respond to perturbations of its fluid and electrolyte balance, to control its blood sugar homeostasis, or to mobilize in response to threats. Autonomic adjust-

ments are often fast and phasic responses that occur with the latencies and speeds typical of neural reflexes; in contrast, endocrine responses usually occur more slowly, taking anywhere from minutes to hours to seasons for full expression.

A commonplace example illustrates autonomic operations: Occasionally, when you have been lying down resting and then jump up suddenly, you may feel dizzy, your vision may become blurred, and you may momentarily have trouble maintaining your balance—let alone doing something active and coordinated. This phenomenon is known as postural, or orthostatic, hypotension and is caused by insufficient oxygenated blood reaching your brain under the altered hemodynamic conditions produced by the rapid charge in posture. Most people experience postural hypotension only occasionally, although it can become a chronic medical problem for others. Indeed, it is a debilitating condition in people with pure autonomic failure, as well as a number of other forms of dysautonomia (Bannister, 1989). The problem in this case is that something as mundane as a change in posture requires nearly instantaneous redistribution of blood flow throughout the body to protect the privileged flow of blood, and thus oxygen and glucose, to the brain. The demands of postural adjustments require unceasing monitoring and rebalancing of the circulatory loads. The fact that these adjustments happen routinely and automatically is testimony to the efficiency of the ANS in affecting homeostatic adjustments. This example also illustrates two other characteristics of many autonomic responses: (1) The responses often are either initiated in anticipation of

BOX 35.1

DISCOVERY OF THE AUTONOMIC NERVOUS SYSTEM

The study of the autonomic nervous system has a particularly long and interesting history, and the techniques available during the different periods of research have strongly shaped descriptions of the ANS. The gross morphology of the peripheral autonomic nerves has been studied since the time of Galen, but most microscopic anatomy and embryology of the ANS have been characterized only recently. Indeed, these topics remain the subject of ongoing research. In contrast, many of the early characterizations of the autonomic nervous system were functional studies. Still other early work, such as the studies of John Langley, defined the autonomic nervous system and its separate divisions in terms of their pharmacology. Some of the more recent techniques of molecular biology and cytochemistry are now forcing revisions of our descriptions and definitions.

The terminology used in autonomic neuroscience reflects this legacy of early structural, functional, and pharmacological descriptions. The vagus, for example, takes its name from its wandering course of innervation.

Using this nerve, Loewi demonstrated acetylcholinergic (or Vagusstoff) control of smooth muscle.

Prior to the foundations laid by Langley's work, the sympathetic and parasympathetic limbs of the ANS were not consistently or clearly distinguished, and the aggregate system was often called the sympathetic system. *Sympathetic* has a history that can be traced back to Galen's concept that "sympathy," or coordination between viscera, or organs, was accomplished by the nerves. Sympathetic also connoted that the visceral nervous system might subserve the "sympathies," or emotions, described in Homeric writing.

Autonomic, which means self-governing, was introduced by John Langley. The ANS has also variously been called the automatic nervous system, the involuntary nervous system, the visceral nervous system, and the animalic nervous system. Langley is also responsible for clearly distinguishing—and naming—the parasympathetic division of the ANS.

Terry L. Powley

the perturbation or implemented so rapidly that the individual does not experience a deficit and (2) the activity of the autonomic nervous system is linked to and coordinated with activity of the somatic nervous system.

The pervasiveness and immediacy of such autonomic responses are hard to overemphasize. The range of ANS operations is illustrated by two other examples of circulatory adjustments. Differential activation of the cerebral cortex during cognitive activity, such as thinking, is associated with selective shunting of blood flow (see Chapter 13), changes achieved in part by autonomic adjustments of vascular tone. Similarly, autonomic regulation of blood flow in genitalia makes mating (tumescence, erection, etc.) possible.

The autonomous nature of ANS function is a characteristic element of autonomic control. We are rarely aware of ongoing reflex adjustments made to maintain cardiovascular and regulatory dynamics, fluid and electrolyte homeostasis, energy balance, immune system operations, and many other functions. Like the batch files of a computer, which execute without normally intruding on the screen or requiring attention, the autonomic reflex adjustments run unceas-

ingly in the "background," while other sensory events and functional decisions occupy the "foreground." In one of his delightful and trenchant essays, Lewis Thomas (1974) underscores the adaptive advantage of the autonomous operations of the ANS. Thomas speculates on how disastrous and overwhelmingly confusing it would be for his cognitive processing if he were put in charge of his liver—if he had to consider all visceral inputs and make a conscious decision for all adjustments in liver function. The ANS takes care of such hepatic, as well as all other visceral, decisions automatically, allowing the individual to focus on the behavioral and cognitive functions that typically require awareness.

The hub of the autonomic nervous system is the visceral motor outflow, which is divided into *sympathetic* (SNS) and *parasympathetic* (PSNS) divisions. Each division is organized hierarchically into pre- and postganglionic levels (see Fig. 35.1). The cell bodies of the preganglionic neurons lie within the central nervous system, specifically in the brain stem and spinal cord. Descending projections from more rostral levels of the neuraxis converge on these ANS preganglionic motor neurons in a pattern similar to that of the centrifugal projections to somatic motor

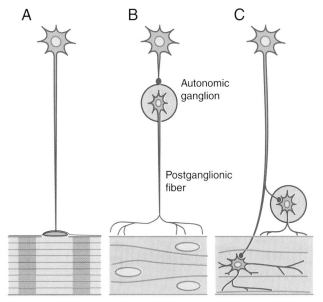

Autonomic
ganglion

Postganglionic
fiber

FIGURE 35.1 Somatic and autonomic styles of motor innervation are different. In the somatic motor pattern (A), motor neurons of the spinal cord or cranial nerve nuclei project directly to striated muscles to form neuromuscular junctions. In the autonomic or visceral pattern (B and C), in contrast, motor neurons in the central nervous system project to peripheral postganglionic neurons that in turn innervate smooth muscles. (B) The SNS has preganglionic neurons in the thoracic and lumbar spinal cord (intermediolateral cell column) that project to postganglionic motor neurons in para- and prevertebral autonomic ganglia. (C) The PSNS consists of preganglionic neurons in the brain stem cranial nerve nuclei and in the sacral spinal cord (intermediomedial cell column) that project to postganglionic motor neurons in ganglia located near or inside the viscera. From Nauta and Feirtag (1986).

TABLE 35.1 Classical Comparisons of Sympathetic and Parasympathetic Divisions of the ANS[a]

	SNS	PSNS
Location of preganglionic somata	Thoracolumbar cord	Cranial neuroaxis; sacral cord
Location of ganglia (and postganglionic somata)	Distant from target organ	Near or in target organ
Postganglionic transmitter*	Norepinephrine	Acetylcholine
Length of preganglionic axon	Relatively short	Relatively long
Length of postganglionic axon	Relatively long	Relatively short
Divergence of preganglionic axonal projection*	One to many	One to few
Functions	Catabolic	Anabolic
Innervates trunk and limbs in addition to viscera	Yes	No

[a] Langley (1921) stressed the contrasting and distinguishing traits of the two divisions of the ANS. Since his time, most texts have included several contrasting features. Most of these distinctions apply generally but not universally. Research since the time of Langley has suggested that those designated with an asterisk may be incorrect. Although many of these distinctions have blurred (e.g., transmitter) or may be completely unfounded (e.g., divergence), they are often discussed.

SYMPATHETIC DIVISION: ORGANIZED TO MOBILIZE THE BODY FOR ACTIVITY

Sympathetic Responses Predominately Produce Selective Energy Expenditure, Catabolic Functions, and Cardiopulmonary Adjustments for Intense Activity

Fight or flight, the prototypical example used extensively by Walter B. Cannon, epitomizes the operation of the sympathetic division of the ANS: You are walking alone at night in an unfamiliar part of town. Although the area is somewhat unsafe, the night is quiet, and you manage to relax. After several minutes of walking, however, you hear a sudden, loud, and unfamiliar noise close by and behind you. In literally the time of a heart beat or two, your physiology moves into high gear. Your heart races; your blood pressure rises. Blood vessels in muscles dilate, increasing the flow of oxygen and energy. At the same time, blood vessels in the gastrointestinal tract and skin constrict, reducing flow through these organs and making more blood available to be shunted to skeletal muscle. Pupils dilate, improving vision.

neurons of the brain stem and spinal cord. However, unlike the outflow pattern of the skeletal motor system, in which motor neurons of the ventral horn or the cranial nerve nuclei project directly to the effector or muscle target, autonomic preganglionic neurons project to ganglia located between the central nervous system (CNS) and the target tissues. Compared with the one-neuron final common paths of the skeletal motor system, this extra synapse interrupting the autonomic outflows at peripheral ganglia allows for more divergence, as well as the possibility of more local integrative circuitry to impinge on the outflow. These peripheral ganglia of the ANS contain the postganglionic motor neurons that project to the effector tissues. Different locations both of the preganglionic motor neurons in the CNS and of the ganglia containing the somata of the postganglionic motor neurons in the periphery are distinguishing features of the two principal divisions of the autonomic nervous system (Langley, 1921; see Table 35.1).

Digestion in the gastrointestinal tract is inhibited; release of glucose from the liver is facilitated. You begin to sweat, a response serving several functions, including reducing friction between limbs and trunk, improving traction, and perhaps promoting additional dissipation of heat so muscles can work efficiently if needed for defense or running. Multiple other smooth and cardiac muscle adjustments occur automatically to increase your readiness to fight or to flee, and almost all of them are effected by the sympathetic division of the ANS.

This fight-or-flight example illustrates important features of the autonomic nervous system, particularly its sympathetic division. First, the situation points out the need for the housekeeping functions of the ANS: If the alarming noise turns out to be a threat and it is necessary to fight or flee, skeletal muscles must be optimally tuned and provisioned. Extra quantities of oxygen and energy are essential. Second, the synergy of adjustments indicates a coordinated and adaptive program of responses, which in this case happen immediately and without cognitive evaluation. Third, the short latency of the response is characteristic (and in such a case possibly critical). Some of the physiological adjustments could be accomplished by hormonal mechanisms, but such adjustments would be too slow to be of much immediate help if the noise should signal a bona fide threat.

Not all sympathetic (or parasympathetic) responses happen on such short time scales. Operations of the ANS also involve continuous, ongoing adjustments. Textbook accounts of the emergency functions of the ANS and of single, isolated reflex adjustments sometimes leave the incorrect impression that in the absence of a threat or specific stimulus, the ANS is quiescent. Instead, the autonomic nervous system, like the somatic nervous system, always maintains an operating tone. Even during periods of inactivity, the system maintains appropriate homeostatic balances and autonomic programs. The tonic control of heart rate and cardiac output maintained by both divisions of the ANS is prototypical of such maintenance (see Chapter 36). In the case of sleep, for example, slow-wave sleep and rapid eye movement sleep have characteristic autonomic profiles (see Chapter 42). SNS innervation of brown adipose tissue is important in controlling nonshivering thermogenesis, or heat production, over extended periods of time. Similarly, after a meal, even in a resting animal, the autonomic choreography of digestion and assimilation—anabolic functions—plays out (see Chapter 38).

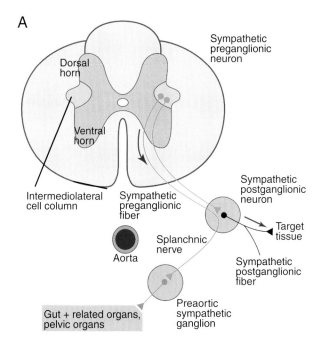

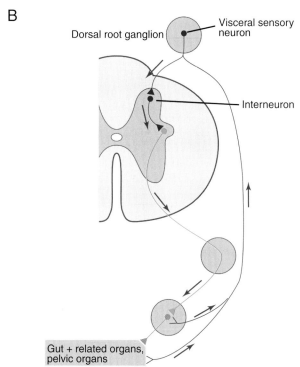

FIGURE 35.2 Details of the organization of the SNS and its sensory inputs. In thoracic and lumbar levels of the spinal cord, preganglionic cell bodies located in the intermediolateral cell column project through ventral roots to either paravertebral chain ganglia or prevertebral ganglia, as illustrated for the splanchnic nerve (A). Visceral sensory neurons located in the dorsal root ganglia transmit information from innervated visceral organs to interneurons in the spinal cord to complete autonomic reflex arcs at the spinal level (B). From Loewy and Spyer (1990).

Preganglionic Neurons of the Sympathetic Nervous System Lie in the Thoracic and Lumbar Spinal Cord

Sympathetic preganglionic neurons occupy the *intermediolateral nucleus*, a nearly continuous columnar grouping of cells running longitudinally through much of the spinal cord in the lateral horn of the spinal gray. In humans, these cells are found between the first thoracic spinal segment (T1) and the third lumbar segment (L3) (see Fig. 35.2A). The location of these preganglionic neurons and their axonal outflow gives the SNS another of its names, the *thoracolumbar division*. Cells within the intermediolateral column show a tendency to segmental aggregation. There is a rostral-to-caudal viscerotopic organization to the distribution: Preganglionic neurons controlling the smooth muscle of the eye are most rostral (e.g., T1–2); cells controlling the heart and lungs are somewhat more caudal; and neurons controlling the gastrointestinal tract, bladder, and genitalia are most caudal. The column is found bilaterally, and preganglionics on one side send their axons out the ipsilateral ventral root. The axon of a preganglionic neuron typically exits from the segment in which its soma is located. Many of the preganglionic axons are lightly myelinated, and, as they separate from the ventral root to project to the appropriate peripheral ganglion, they form a *white ramus*, a connective that takes its descriptive name from myelinated fibers.

Sympathetic postganglionic neurons are found in two distinct types of ganglia: paravertebral and prevertebral. *Paravertebral ganglia*, as the name implies, are adjacent to the spinal cord bilaterally, in a position slightly ventral and lateral to the vertebral column (see Figs. 35.3 and Fig. 35.4). Each ganglion receives a white ramus from the appropriate ventral root. These ganglia are also interconnected longitudinally into a sympathetic chain composed of axons from the preganglionic neurons that run rostrally or caudally to neighboring ganglia of the chain. Axons of the postganglionic neurons of the paravertebral ganglia course centrifugally out of the ganglion to join the peripheral nerves that will carry the individual fibers to their targets. Because most postganglionic axons in the sympathetic nervous system are unmyelinated,

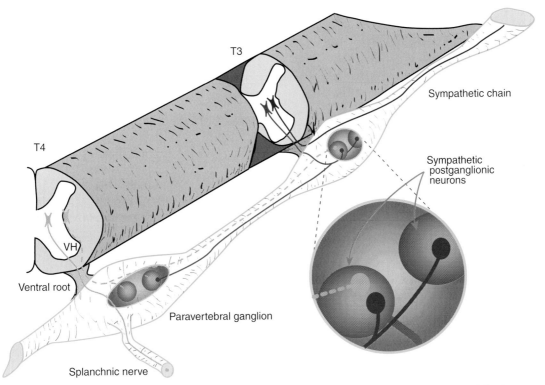

FIGURE 35.3 The SNS is organized segmentally. As illustrated here for segments T3 and T4 of the thoracic spinal cord, preganglionic axons exit through the ventral root of the segment in which the preganglionic cell body is located. These preganglionic axons can be myelinated (solid red lines) or unmyelinated (dashed red lines) and can project to the paravertebral ganglion associated with the segment, to neighboring paravertebral ganglia through the sympathetic chain, to postganglionic neurons located distally in the prevertebral ganglia, or through one of the autonomic nerves (splanchnic nerve is illustrated). T3 and T4, segments of the thoracic spinal cord; VH, ventral horn of spinal cord. From Loewy and Spyer (1990).

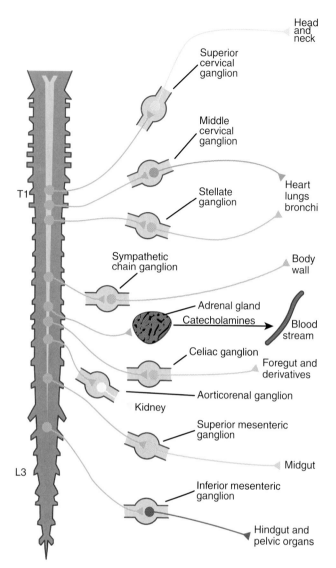

FIGURE 35.4 Summary of the major SNS ganglia and their target organs or tissues. Spinal cord is illustrated on the left. From Loewy and Spyer (1990).

these connectives joining the ventral roots are called *gray rami*.

Paravertebral ganglia of the sympathetic chain supply the postganglionic innervation of the head, thorax, trunk, and limbs. For the trunk and limbs, postganglionic axons course both alongside and within the somatic peripheral nerve innervating the region. These autonomic fibers innervate the blood vessels in the muscles (vasoconstrictor fibers), as well as different targets within the skin, including the sweat glands (sudomotor fibers) and erector pili muscles of erectile hairs (pilomotor fibers).

At the rostral end of the sympathetic chain, individual segmental ganglia are fused into aggregate

ganglionic groupings. Thus, the sympathetic chain innervates the head and the thoracic viscera in a modification of the paravertebral chain pattern (Figs. 35.4 and 35.6). The most rostral group, the superior cervical ganglion (supplied from the first and second thoracic segments), supplies the head and neck. The targets of its projections are extensive, including the eyes, salivary glands, lacrimal glands, blood vessels of the cranial muscles, and even the blood vessels of the brain. The paravertebral ganglia just caudal to the superior cervical ganglion form the middle cervical ganglion and, moving caudally, the stellate ganglion. These latter ganglia supply the postganglionic sympathetic outflows that innervate the heart, lungs, and bronchi.

Unlike the trunk, limbs, head, heart, and lungs, organs of the abdominal cavity are innervated by postganglionic neurons in ganglia situated distal to both the spinal cord and the paravertebral sympathetic chain in locations closer to the target tissue. These sites give the ganglia their distinguishing name, *prevertebral ganglia*. The preganglionic neurons innervating these sets of postganglionic neurons are located in the intermediolateral column of the spinal cord, like those innervating the paravertebral chain, but their axons pass through the white rami, the chain ganglia, and the gray rami without synapsing. They then make contact with the peripherally situated prevertebral ganglion cells (see Fig. 35.3).

There are four major prevertebral postganglionic stations. The more rostral three are located at points where major abdominal arteries separate from the descending aorta, and the ganglia take their names from their associated arteries (see Fig. 35.5). Moving from more rostral to caudal, the celiac, superior mesenteric, and inferior mesenteric ganglia innervate the gastrointestinal tract. The celiac ganglion (also commonly called the solar plexus because connectives radiate around or from it) projects predominantly to the stomach and rostralmost parts of the foregut and its embryological derivatives, such as the liver and pancreas. Consistent with their progressively more caudal locations, the middle and inferior mesenteric ganglia innervate the mid- and hindgut tissues, respectively. The inferior mesenteric ganglion also supplies the postganglionic innervation to the pelvic organs. The fourth, and most caudal, prevertebral ganglion is the pelvic–hypogastric plexus, which innervates urinary and genital tissues.

Although the paravertebral ganglia comprising the sympathetic chain are apparently structured largely as relay nuclei, prevertebral ganglia have more complex organizations. The prevertebral ganglia contain afferent neurons as well as the postganglionic

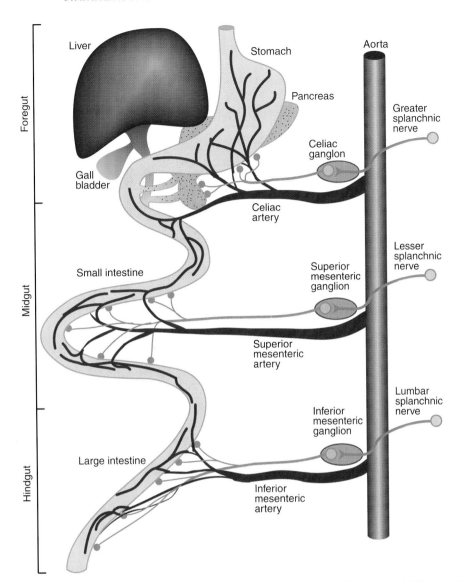

FIGURE 35.5 SNS innervation of the gastrointestinal tract. This more detailed schematic illustrates how separate segmental levels of the spinal cord and the associated prevertebral ganglia innervate targets in a topographic, specifically viscerotopic, pattern. A commonly observed association of autonomic pathways and vasculature is also shown. From Loewy and Spyer (1990).

somata. These ganglia also receive afferent inputs from neurons located in the walls of the target organs. These ganglia may have more complex neural organization than paravertebral ganglia because prevertebral ganglia are located farther from the spinal cord and closer to the target organs, and they coordinate responses of visceral organs containing separate nerve networks (the enteric nervous system is described later).

Another specialization is found among the prevertebral ganglia: The adrenal medulla is a unique variant of the sympathetic postganglionic pattern. By several standard criteria, the adrenal medulla is a sympathetic prevertebral ganglion containing post-

ganglionics. However, neurons of this medullary ganglion, rather than issuing axons to innervate target organs, function as an endocrine organ. The adrenal medulla secretes the classical postganglionic sympathetic transmitter norepinephrine, as well as epinephrine, directly into the bloodstream. These catecholamines then circulate as hormones, providing a humoral supplement to neural activation. Release of catecholamines from the adrenals during sympathetic activation provides powerful reinforcement and modulation of the more focal release of catecholamines at traditional—and local—effector sites. Although adrenal catecholamines provide dramatic amplification and divergence of sympathetic signals,

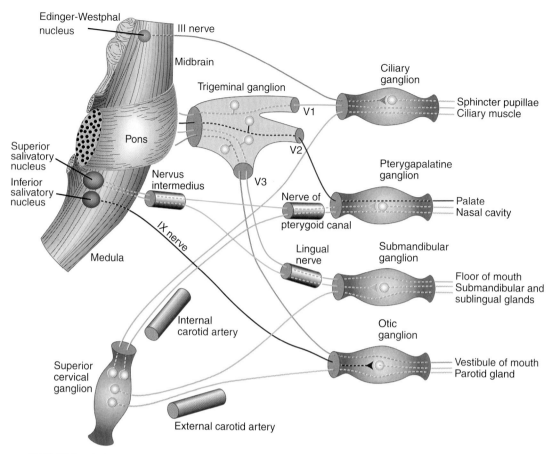

FIGURE 35.6 Autonomic innervation of the head by sympathetic (superior cervical ganglion) and parasympathetic (cranial nerve nuclei in the medulla and midbrain projecting to the several prevertebral ganglia) pathways. Visceral afferents associated with the autonomic nervous system are found in the trigeminal nerve (cranial nerve V) ganglion. From Loewy and Spyer (1990).

these secretions from the adrenal medulla, like most hormones, are slower to arrive at their targets and are slower to dissipate. In addition, they lack the point-to-point specificity of other sympathetic projections.

Summary

Overall, the two major motor outflows, or divisions, of the ANS are responsible for the maintenance of homeostasis, but the sympathetic nervous system is the branch specialized for the mobilization of energy. The SNS provides the vascular, glandular, metabolic, and other physiological adjustments that optimize behavioral responses, particularly in emergency situations and conditions requiring activity. The SNS efferent outflow consists of preganglionic neurons, which are located in the intermediolateral column of the thoracic and lumbar spinal cord; their axons, which course to paravertebral and prevertebral ganglia containing the postganglionic neurons; and

the axons of these postganglionic neurons, which project to the target tissues.

PARASYMPATHETIC DIVISION: ORGANIZED FOR ENERGY CONSERVATION

Parasympathetic Nervous System Functions Reduce Energy Expenditure and Increase Energy Stores

Functionally, the parasympathetic nervous system usually mobilizes homeostatic adjustments that are opposite and reciprocal to those activated by the SNS (see Table 35.1). In particular, PSNS adjustments are often considered "rest and digest" responses, in contrast to the "fight or flight" sympathetic activation. The parasympathetic nervous system promotes anabolic processing, whereas the sympathetic nervous system augments catabolic activity. The PSNS promotes the gastrointestinal processes required to digest and absorb nutrients effectively. This branch of the ANS also augments the efficient use of energy and the storage of extra calories as fat and glycogen. The PSNS, particularly the vagus nerve, plays a central role in controlling the dynamic flow of body reserves or energy between storage depots and the tissues that use the energy. The body's energy reserves are fat in adipose tissue and glycogen in liver and muscle. After a meal, the gastrointestinal tract serves as an additional reservoir of potential energy for the body. By mobilizing triglycerides from adipose tissue or glycogen from liver and muscle, the ANS can make reserves available for metabolism; similarly, by moving nutrient stores (e.g., from the stomach) and promoting their digestion and absorption from the intestines into the bloodstream, the ANS can supply energy to fuel metabolism or to restock triglyceride and glycogen stores, as needed. (See Chapter 38 for a more detailed discussion of autonomic influences on calorie storage.)

Preganglionic Neurons of the Parasympathetic Nervous System Lie in the Brain Stem Cranial Nerve Nuclei and the Sacral Spinal Cord

One of the features distinguishing the PSNS from the SNS is the location of preganglionic neurons. PSNS preganglionic neurons are located in two longi-

tudinal columns of neurons: one found in the brain stem and the other in the sacral spinal cord. These locations of the preganglionic neurons are responsible for the alternative name of this division of the ANS, the *craniosacral division* (or "bulbosacral" is also sometimes used). The longitudinal column of motor neurons in the brain stem is the general visceral cell column, which condenses into a number of more or less discrete nuclei just ventrolateral to the cerebral aqueduct system within the brain. These brain stem nuclei then project through their respective cranial nerves to targets in the head (cranial nerves III, VII, and IX) or thorax and abdomen (cranial nerve X) (see Fig. 35.6). Cranial nerve III, the oculomotor nerve, carries the axons of the accessory, or autonomic, nucleus of the Edinger–Westphal complex, which participate in the control of the pupillary sphincter and ciliary muscles. Cranial nerve VII, the facial nerve, carries preganglionic axons of the superior salivatory nucleus and controls the submaxillary and sublingual salivary glands, as well as the lacrimal glands. Cranial nerve IX, the glossopharyngeal nerve, carries axons of the inferior salivatory nucleus, which control the parotid salivary glands and mucus secretion.

Preganglionic motor neurons of the Xth cranial nerve, the vagus nerve, control smooth muscles and glands throughout the entire digestive tract, from the pharynx to the distal colon, including viscera such as the liver and pancreas. These Xth nerve neurons occupy a long fusiform nucleus in the medulla oblongata, the dorsal motor nucleus of the vagus (Fig. 35.7). They control numerous motor and secretomotor responses that participate in the ingestion and digestion of food, as well as in the assimilation of energy by the body. The vagus nerve also carries motor fibers

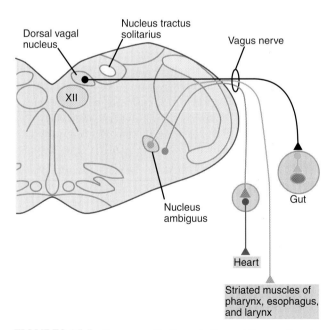

FIGURES 35.7 Parasympathetic projections of the vagal motor pathways, the most extensive of the PSNS circuits, to the viscera of the thorax and abdomen. From Loewy and Spyer (1990).

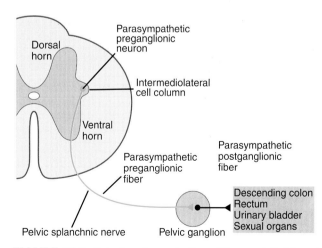

FIGURE 35.8 Spinal cord organization of the sacral division of the craniosacral, or parasympathetic, nervous system. From Loewy and Spyer(1990).

of a special visceral nucleus, the nucleus ambiguus or ventral vagal nucleus, which controls the striated muscles of the pharynx, larynx, and esophagus and the cardiac muscle of the heart. Much like the case described for sympathetic neurons, motor neurons of the dorsal motor nucleus of the vagus and the nucleus ambiguus are organized into viscerotopic subnuclei (e.g., Bieger and Hopkins, 1987; Fox and Powley, 1992).

The central representation of the much more caudal remainder of the PSNS is found in the sacral spinal cord, in humans the second (S2) through fourth (S4) sacral segments (Fig. 35.8). The parasympathetic preganglionic somata occupy two longitudinal groupings: one column immediately dorsolateral to the central canal and the other in roughly the same transverse location as that of the intermediolateral column of cells, which sympathetic preganglionics occupy in the thoracic and lumbar cord. Axons of the sacral preganglionics exit the cord in the ventral roots, run in a sacral plexus, and project to the target organs. The sacral preganglionic cell columns control parasympathetic motor, vasomotor, and secretomotor functions of the kidneys, bladder, transverse and distal colon, and reproductive organs.

The locations of their respective postganglionic neurons constitute another feature that distinguishes the PSNS from the SNS. Ganglia containing the PSNS postganglionic neurons are juxtaposed to, on the surface of, or even in, the target organ, in contrast to

---

BOX 35.2

AUTONOMIC POSTGANGLIONIC NEURONS CAN CHANGE THEIR TRANSMITTER PHENOTYPES

Generally, transmitter phenotypes of autonomic neurons seem fixed, dictated by both intrinsic and extrinsic developmental cues (see Chapter 7). One provocative observation made with tissue culture techniques and immunocytochemistry, however, is that ANS neurons can alter their phenotypes under appropriate environmental conditions. This conclusion was first reached when populations of postmitotic adrenergic and cholinergic neurons were cocultured *in vitro* in different media or in the presence of different tissues. Without changes in overall cell number, the percentages of adrenergic and cholinergic neurons in a given culture changed over time. Even more definitively, when single postganglionic cells were grown in microculture wells, the presence of a medium conditioned by heart cells caused some of these mature neurons to change from an adrenergic to a cholinergic phenotype (Potter *et al.*, 1980).

This phenotypic switching does not appear to be an artifact of cell culture situations; the change appears to occur normally *in vivo* in development to generate the specialized minority of sympathetic postganglionic neurons that are cholinergic (e.g., for innervation of sweat glands). Landis and Keefe (1983) have verified this hypothesis by using rat foot pad sweat gland innervation *in vivo* and characterizing the transmitter phenotype of the autonomic projections at different stages of development. The developing sympathetic postganglionic innervation of the sweat glands initially expresses a typical adrenergic phenotype as the axon grows toward its target. Once the sweat gland target is innervated, however, the tissue induces the change in neurotransmitter phenotype to a cholinergic one.

Such changes in transmitter are not unique to these examples. Perhaps reflecting pluripotential patterns seen earlier in phylogeny, at least some cholinergic neurons (e.g., avian ciliary ganglion cells) appear to remodel into an adrenergic phenotype, whereas other cells (e.g., maturing neural crest cells in the developing gut wall) exhibit a transient catecholaminergic stage that is lost during the ingrowth of extramural innervation.

Finally, in addition to such switching, autonomic postganglionic neurons have also been shown to exhibit plasticity in altering their levels of transmitters and cotransmitters as a function of the activity of their preganglionic inputs. For example, after preganglionic inputs are blocked or transected pharmacologically, postganglionic neurons of the superior cervical ganglion decrease their levels of tyrosine hydroxylase while increasing their level of substance P.

Terry L. Powley

References

Landis, S. C., and Keefe, D. (1983). Evidence for transmitter plasticity *in vivo*: Developmental changes in properties of cholinergic sympathetic neurons. *Dev. Biol.* **98**, 349–372.

Potter, D. D., Landis, S. C. and Funshpan, E. J. (1980). Dual function during development of not sympathetic neurones in culture. *J. Exp. Biol.* **89**, 57–71.

the para- and prevertebral locations of the SNS (see Fig. 35.1c). These juxta- and intramural stations are often called *plexuses*, rather than ganglia. Like SNS prevertebral ganglia, the PSNS postganglionic plexuses are complex integrative sites that typically receive inputs not only from preganglionic neurons, but also from afferents within the plexuses or target tissues. Because the PSNS postganglionic neurons are situated so near their targets, the parasympathetic division of the ANS has, perforce, longer preganglionic axons and shorter postganglionic fibers than the sympathetic division. The relative lengths of the postganglionic fibers in the two divisions have been taken as evidence that individual axons of the SNS may diverge more extensively and innervate larger projection fields, whereas the PSNS may exhibit less divergence and more localized projections (Box 35.2). [For counterarguments, see Wang *et al.* (1995).]

Summary

The parasympathetic nervous system or craniosacral division, i.e., the second major outflow of the ANS, is organized to digest, assimilate, and conserve energy. Its anabolic functions include not only those associated with the metabolism of nutrients, but also numerous protective reflexes, such as those that limit heat loss, reduce energy expenditure, and slow the heart. The PSNS outflow consists of preganglionic neurons located in brain stem cranial nerve nuclei or the autonomic columns of the sacral spinal cord. Their axons project to the postganglionic neurons located in ganglia situated near or in the target organs. Postganglionic neurons, in turn, project to the smooth muscle of the target viscera.

THE ENTERIC DIVISION OF THE ANS: THE NERVE NET FOUND IN THE WALLS OF VISCERAL ORGANS

When Langley articulated the classic definition of the ANS, he identified a third division of the ANS, the *enteric nervous system* (ENS). The alimentary canal, or "entrum," and the tissues derived from it, such as the pancreas and liver, contain extensive and well-formed neural networks. In particular, the gastrointestinal tract contains two well-organized major plexuses that have been estimated to contain as many neurons as the entire spinal cord (Fig. 35.9). Each plexus consists of an extensive sheet of small nodes of cells linked by connectives. One plexus, the myenteric plexus, is situated between outer longitudinal and inner circular muscle layers of the viscus. The other plexus, the sub-

mucosal or submucous plexus, is located between the circular muscle layer and the lumenal mucosal layer of the viscera. As illustrated in Fig. 35.9, there are additional, less extensive, enteric networks as well. The number of neurons in the enteric plexuses, their extensive interconnections, and their capacity to support motility have led to proposals that the enteric nervous system serves as a more or less independent "brain" in the gut.

Early descriptions emphasized the autonomy of the enteric nervous system by observing that the gastrointestinal tract could exhibit movement, peristalsis, even after all extrinsic connections to it were cut. However, more recent observations suggest that the many fully integrated or coordinated responses of the gastrointestinal tract, including motor responses other than peristalsis, as well as absorptive and secretory responses, involve extrinsic projections from the central nervous system to the enteric nervous system.

Because the preganglionic neurons of the vagus nerve project to the enteric ganglia rather than to independent postganglionic stations, the enteric nervous system serves as an extensive postganglionic station for the vagus.

Summary

The ENS or enteric nervous system, the third division of the ANS, consists of the intrinsic neurons that form ganglia and plexuses in the walls of the viscera such as with the gastrointestinal tract. This nerve network contains intrinsic afferents, interneurons, and efferents that control local functions; it also receives extrinsic inputs from autonomic preganglionic efferents, particularly those PSNS projections coursing in the vagus nerve.

ANS PHARMACOLOGY: TRANSMITTER AND RECEPTOR CODING

Early in the 20th century, pharmacological studies performed with naturally occurring agonists and antagonists provided the basis for the original chemical differentiation of the autonomic nervous system into its two major divisions—the SNS and PSNS. Dale, the contributor of "Dale's law" of neurotransmitters, Langley, and a number of other early investigators applied natural extracts such as muscarine, nicotine, *d*-tubocurarine, and others to autonomic ganglia while measuring responses in order to infer the chemical taxonomy of the ANS. Subsequent experiments have replicated the basic distinctions made by these investigators, but this newer work,

A

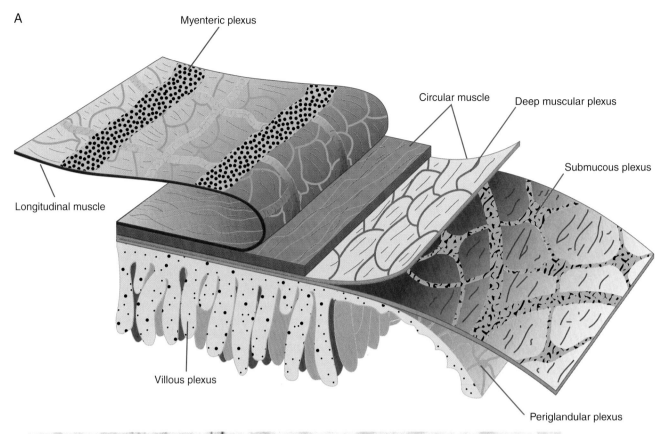

Myenteric plexus

Circular muscle

Deep muscular plexus

Submucous plexus

Longitudinal muscle

Villous plexus

Periglandular plexus

B

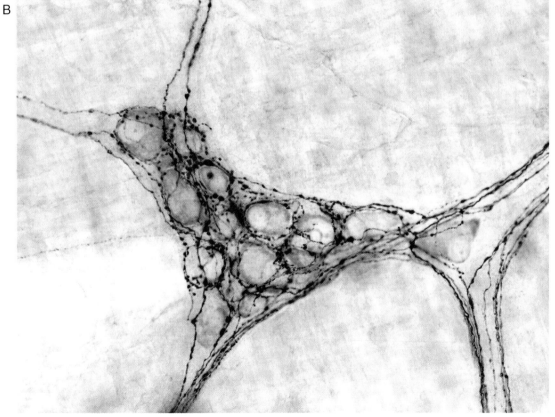

with access to an extensive pharmacopoeia of synthetic agonists and antagonists, as well as to immunocytochemistry for the characterization of transmitter substances, has described a much richer and more complicated multiplicity of neurotransmitters, neuromodulators, and receptor subtypes in autonomic nerves (Lundberg, 1996).

Preganglionic Neurons Use Acetylcholine as a Transmitter

Most preganglionic neurons of both branches of the ANS have a cholinergic transmitter phenotype. Only relatively small subpopulations of preganglionic neurons express other, e.g., dopaminergic or adrenergic, phenotypes. In the peripheral ganglia of both branches of the ANS, most postganglionic neurons, which receive inputs from the preganglionics, express a predominance of the nicotinic form of the cholinergic receptor on their somata. Specificity and response selectivity at the ganglionic level are normally maintained by the segregation of sympathetic and parasympathetic postganglionic neurons in separate ganglia, by point-to-point axonal projections, and by the spatial separation of synapses within ganglia. As discovered by the early autonomic pharmacologists, nicotine can serve as a general "ganglionic blocker" to thwart transmission at these synapses.

Sympathetic and Parasympathetic Postganglionic Neurons Use Different Transmitters

One of the cardinal defining differences between the SNS and the PSNS is the transmitter phenotype of the postganglionic neurons. The majority of sympathetic postganglionic neurons release the transmitter norepinephrine, whereas parasympathetic postganglionic neurons release primarily acetylcholine to control their targets. Such a two-transmitter chemical code makes it possible to have push–pull or positive bidirectional control of individual targets. The functional significance of this chemical code relates to the type of muscle, smooth or striated, the ANS controls. The biomechanics of smooth muscle are quite different from the biomechanics of striated muscle

(Chapters 28 and 29). Consequently, important differences exist between the two motor systems.

In contrast to skeletal muscle, smooth muscle is not always organized into antagonistic pairs, with each member of the pair being innervated by a different motor neuron. Also, the smooth muscles forming the walls of the viscera are not differentially attached to a hard frame to provide mechanical leverage through opposal activity. Reciprocal motor programs of the viscera, for the most part, involve active, phased excitation and inhibition of the same muscle to achieve coordination. To produce these patterns of excitation and inhibition, the target organs and tissues express both adrenergic and cholinergic receptors and have different, often antagonistic or complementary, responses to selective activation of the different receptors.

Response patterns of smooth muscle are further differentiated by specializations of the receptors. Adrenergic receptors, influenced by the catecholaminergic transmitter released by sympathetic fibers, are differentiated into at least four different subtypes linked to different intracellular pathways (see discussion of metabotropic receptors in Chapter 9). Similarly, the muscarinic acetylcholine receptor, influenced by the cholinergic transmitter released by parasympathetic postganglionic neurons, is differentiated into at least three subtypes with differential influences on intracellular transduction (see discussion of ionotropic receptors in Chapter 9). These heterogeneities of transmitter species and receptor types make it practical to mobilize multiple, different, and potentially highly differentiated responses from one effector tissue (see Box 35.2).

Response selection may also be facilitated by neuropeptides that the postganglionic neurons synthesize and corelease during activity. Somatostatin, neuropeptide Y, or both are found in many sympathetic neurons; vasoactive intestinal polypeptide and calcitonin gene-related peptide are often coexpressed in parasympathetic neurons. These peptides may serve as neuromodulators that vary postsynaptic responses to the conventional autonomic neurotransmitters. The release of different neuropeptides and cotransmitters can vary with different rates or patterns of firing and is not invariantly proportional to transmitter release. Thus, a heterogeneity of different cotransmitter and

FIGURE 35.9 (A) The enteric nervous system plexuses in the wall of the intestine. Enteric neurons form two conspicuous and extensive networks, or plexuses, of ganglia and connectives located between the longitudinal and circular muscle layers of the wall (the myenteric plexus) and the circular muscle layer and the inner mucosal layer (the submucous plexus). The deep muscular plexus, periglandular plexus, and villous plexus are additional networks of enteric neurons and their processes. From Costa *et al.* (1987). (B) Autonomic preganglionic terminals innervating postganglionic neurons. This example of vagal preganglionic projections (labeled with the tracer *Phaseolus vulgaris*) innervating myenteric ganglion neurons (stained with Cuprolinic blue) in the stomach wall illustrates that autonomic preganglionic axons can diverge widely to form extensive networks controlling postganglionics. From Holst *et al.* (1997).

transmitter release patterns can be produced by a single fiber or fiber type, depending on firing pattern and other local factors at the synapse (e.g., Lundberg, 1996).

Although dual innervation in an oppositional or push–pull pattern is presumed to yield faster, more responsive adjustments and to provide a mechanism that can adjust response gain, some tissues are innervated by only one arm of the ANS. The SNS has a wider distribution than the PSNS. In particular, white and brown adipose tissue, peripheral blood vessels, and sweat glands are innervated by the SNS without complementary PSNS projections. One possible explanation for this arrangement is that the functions of these particular effectors do not require the speed associated with push–pull projection patterns, particularly in terminating responses once activated. Furthermore, in the evolution of the autonomic nervous system, the SNS is thought to be the older, and correspondingly more extensive, network, whereas the PSNS occurred more recently in phylogeny and therefore has less widespread projections.

Finally, the enteric nervous system also has an extensively varied set of transmitters, cotransmitters, and neuromodulators, providing highly differentiated chemical coding of local functions (Lundberg, 1996).

Summary

Both the SNS and the PSNS use acetylcholine as a preganglionic transmitter, but they are distinguished by different postganglionic phenotypes: most SNS postganglionic neurons are catecholaminergic, whereas most PSNS postganglionics are cholinergic. The different neurotransmitter and cotransmitter elements expressed in the postganglionic neurons, as well as numerous postsynaptic receptor subtypes, provide the chemical coding for responses of the PSNS and SNS. This functional organization ensures a varied, powerful, and dynamic push–pull operation of homeostatic systems.

AUTONOMIC CONTROLS OF HOMEOSTASIS

The "self-governing" or autonomic characteristic that gives its name to the ANS is based largely on reflexes. These reflexes involve afferent inputs and efferent outputs. Two major inflows of visceral, or autonomic, afferents (see Box 35.3) establish the basic reflex arcs. These visceral afferents provide critical

---

BOX 35.3

AUTONOMIC REFLEXES: ACTIVATED BY VISCERAL AFFERENTS, AUTONOMIC AFFERENTS, OR JUST AFFERENTS?

A long-standing dispute about terminology still influences discussions of autonomic reflexes. Some authors (and textbooks) adhere to the original autonomic classification of Langley, who considered the ANS a motor system without a corresponding sensory inflow. This classic view acknowledges that autonomic effectors are influenced by afferents but considers visceral afferents, as well as somatic afferents, as independent of the ANS. Conversely, other scientists (and textbooks) consider afferents arising in and associated with the viscera as the necessary counterpart to autonomic efferents and label them autonomic afferents.

The controversy goes back to Langley's concentration on a pharmacological definition of the ANS. In his initial studies, Langley speculated about the existence of autonomic afferents, but was unable to find a neurochemical marker to distinguish visceral from somatic afferents. He sidelined the issue pending more information, focused his studies on efferents, and never returned to the search for an afferent marker. Adherents to his original motor-only classification stress that somatic and visceral afferents can elicit autonomic responses and that both classes of afferents elicit somatic responses, as well.

However, advocates for including visceral afferents within the autonomic schema argue that these afferents innervate the target tissues of the ANS efferents, share similar embryological histories with autonomic efferents, course in the same peripheral nerves as the autonomic efferents (e.g., the vagus), and form mono- and oligosynaptic reflex arcs influencing autonomic preganglionic neurons. These proponents for revision of the autonomic terminology also point out that more recent analyses have identified neuropeptide markers shared by visceral afferents (but not somatic afferents) and autonomic motor neurons. This more inclusive view of the autonomic nervous system seems to be gaining ground. It works more naturally for the discussion of reflexes, and we have adopted it in this text.

Terry L. Powley

cross-links between the sympathetic and the parasympathetic outflows, keeping them in balance. For example, sympathetic activity can increase heart rate (tachycardia) and produce constriction of vascular beds, thus leading to an increase in blood pressure. This increase in blood pressure, in turn, is detected by vagus nerve baroreceptors in the aortic arch and other sites. Visceral afferents in the vagus can then reflexively stimulate vagal parasympathetic efferents that slow heart rate (bradycardia) [see Chapter 36]. The visceral afferents monitoring the effects of autonomic activity produce positive, reciprocal, and dynamic regulation of physiological responses. When a more sustained adjust-

ment in blood pressure is required (e.g., in the general arousal of the fight-or-flight response discussed earlier), these outflows are adjusted centrally in a process akin to the α–γ linkage so that sympathetic activation is not nullified by parasympathetic responses damping the needed activation.

Visceral Afferents Connect Target Tissues and the CNS

Motor neurons of the sympathetic nervous system receive direct afferent input from most of the autonomic targets. The cell bodies of these primary

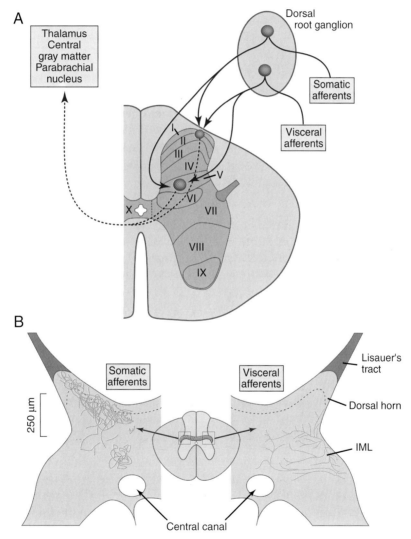

FIGURE 35.10 Visceral and somatic afferents follow parallel but distinct paths in the central nervous system. Visceral and somatic afferents consist of different populations of dorsal root ganglion neurons which project to laminae I and V of the dorsal horn of the spinal cord. These relay sites provide local spinal reflexes and also project to higher autonomic and somatic sites, respectively, in the brain (A). Although visceral and somatic afferents follow similar trajectories, more detailed tracer studies indicate the two types of afferents end in distinctly different distributions and densities within the spinal cord (B). IML, intermediolateral cell column. From Cervero and Foreman (1990).

afferents are located in the dorsal root ganglia of the spinal cord segment(s) in which the corresponding preganglionic neurons are located (see Fig. 35.2B and Fig. 35.10). Afferent somata are similar to other dorsal root ganglion cells, although they frequently are distinguishable as small, dark neurons or B afferents. From endings in the innervated viscera or tissue, the centripetally directed peripheral processes of the afferents typically course in mixed nerves that also contain the motor outflow. These processes then reach the dorsal roots through the major peripheral nerves. The central processes of these visceral afferents enter the spinal cord in association with Lissauer's tract, ending in laminae I and V of the dorsal horn (Cervero and Foreman, 1990).

Visceral afferent nerves relay sensory information about visceral volume, pressure, contents, or nocioceptive stimuli to spinal centers, where automatic responses are interpreted and functional responses are generated.

For many of these visceral afferents, their endings in the periphery and in the spinal cord (particularly in lamina V, which neighbors the intermediolateral column containing the preganglionic motor neurons) contain substance P (SP) and other neuropeptides of the tachykinin family, such as neurokinin A (NKA) and neurokinin B (NKB) [see Chapters 7 and 8; also Lundberg (1996)].

In the parasympathetic limb of the ANS are two major afferent inflows with different organization. In the cranial division, visceral afferents are most often found in the same cranial nerve as their corresponding motor counterparts. These mixed cranial nerves have sensory ganglia located outside the cranium, and the cell bodies of the afferents are found in these ganglia. Like other visceral afferents, these neurons are typically pseudounipolar neurons with a peripheral process extending to the target tissue and a central process projecting to the CNS. The central terminals of these afferents end in a cranial nerve sensory nucleus. Visceral afferents associated with the outflow of cranial nerve III are complex and enter through different channels (e.g., cranial nerve V, the trigeminal nerve). Most of the visceral afferents associated with cranial nerve autonomic reflexes terminate in the extensive nucleus of the solitary tract, which is located immediately dorsal to the general visceral column of the brain stem. Afferents of VII, IX, and X all end in the nucleus of the solitary tract. These inputs form a viscerotopy in the nucleus, with facial gustatory information projecting most rostrally and medially, the glossopharyngeal information somewhat more caudally, and the afferents of the different branches of the vagus nerve terminating most cau-

dally in different subnuclei of the nucleus of the solitary tract. As the largest and most complex of the visceral afferent relays in the brain, the nucleus of the solitary tract also receives afferent inputs from the spinal division of the trigeminal nerve and second-order inputs from the dorsal column nuclei.

Like visceral afferents associated with the SNS, visceral afferents associated with the PSNS contain SP and other tachykinins. In addition, several neuropeptides found in the gut are also found in some of these afferents. For example, the gut hormone and neuropeptide cholecystokinin (CCK) is found in vagal afferents relaying information from the gastrointestinal tract to the brain. CCK is also found in higher order ascending relays of vagal projections in the neuraxis, leading some to argue that CCK provides chemical coding for visceral afferents associated with the gastrointestinal tract (see Chapter 38).

The second major inflow of afferents to the parasympathetic limb of the ANS is associated with the sacral division. Visceral afferents in this division are organized much like the spinal afferents associated with the thoracolumbar or sympathetic division of the ANS (e.g., Morgan et al., 1991).

At the central relays of autonomic reflex arcs, the thoracolumbar circuitry of sympathetic reflexes and the craniosacral circuitry of parasympathetic responses have similar morphological elements. Their organization has been delineated with intracellular staining and axonal tracer techniques. Dembowsky and co-workers (1985) injected horseradish peroxidase intracellularly to define the morphology of the sympathetic preganglionics (Fig. 35.11). The motor neurons preferentially distribute their dendrites within the long longitudinally oriented column that constitutes the intermediolateral nucleus of the spinal cord. The neurons also distribute a subset of their dendrites dorsolaterally in an arch that brings the dendrites into contact with the incoming visceral afferents. This characteristic dendroarchitecture is consistent with the ideas that local mono- or oligosynaptic reflexes are organized segmentally within the nucleus and that preganglionic neurons are influenced heavily by activity in the intermediolateral column immediately rostral and caudal to the location of the cell. Parasympathetic preganglionics exhibit similar dendroarchitecture (e.g., Fox and Powley, 1992).

Visceral Afferents Also Organize Axon Reflexes and Signal Visceral Pain

In addition to forming conventional reflex circuits throughout the ANS, at least some visceral afferents

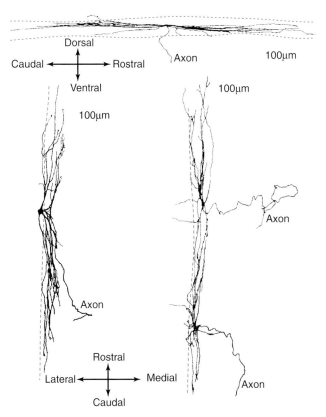

FIGURE 35.11 Examples of intracellularly labeled sympathetic neurons in the spinal cord. The preganglionics have extensive dendritic fields confined to the columnar pattern of the SNS intermediolateral cell column within the cord. From Loewy and Spyer (1990).

support responses known as an *axon reflexes*. Unlike a conventional reflex, which typically involves an afferent neuron, at least one central nervous system synapse, and an efferent neuron, axon reflexes involve only the afferent neuron and they occur in the target tissue—without a CNS relay. The phenomenon can be seen clearly in the type of experiment that was instrumental in establishing the existence of axon reflexes: If all motor axons projecting to a target tissue are eliminated by surgery or other appropriate means while sparing the afferent innervation of the site, the afferent axons can be stimulated selectively. When the afferent axons are stimulated such that their peripheral processes innervating the target are invaded antidromically, one can measure an effector response or assay the release of a neuropeptide from the peripheral afferent neurite. Such experiments performed on a variety of different visceral (and cutaneous) afferent systems have demonstrated that axon reflexes produce a number of inflammatory and vascular effector responses (Lundberg, 1996).

Presumably, when afferents are stimulated physiologically, or appropriately, axon reflexes are normally produced in peripheral collaterals contained in many and perhaps all visceral afferents (Fig. 35.12; also see the discussion of dendritic release of peptide transmitters in Chapter 12). When a peripheral ending of a visceral afferent transduces a stimulus, the resulting action potential can release extracellularly the neuropeptide contained in vesicles in that ending. The released compound then acts as a neuromodulator or neurotransmitter to affect local changes on smooth muscle—a local, or peripheral, axon reflex. The response is also relayed to neighboring tissues. When an action potential is transmitted centrally in an afferent axon, it can also be transmitted centrifugally by collaterals of the same fiber, and release of the neuromodulator from these collateral endings can propagate the reflex in the immediate area. The inflammatory responses and extravasation associated with the classic "wheal and flare" reaction to skin damage were the first axon reflexes analyzed and are a classic illustration of the phenomenon. Such local

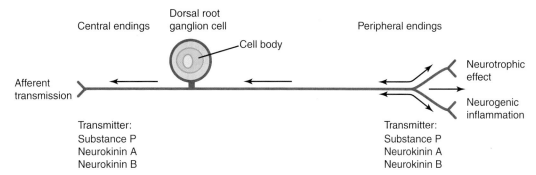

FIGURE 35.12 The architecture of visceral afferents that produce axon reflexes. Visceral and cutaneous afferents release transmitters from the tachykinin family. When action potentials (indicated by arrows) are generated peripherally, they are propagated centrally. Peripherally generated action potentials also produce a local release of tachykinins in the affected terminals and in terminals of the peripheral collaterals. From Cervero and Foreman (1990).

responses have been widely documented not only in the skin, but also in the viscera such as the lungs.

Finally, visceral afferents, particularly those associated with SNS pathways, are responsible for visceral pain (Jänig, 1996).

Summary

Visceral afferents innervate the target tissues of the ANS, and their axons frequently course in the same peripheral nerves as autonomic efferents. Also commonly called autonomic afferents, these sensory elements associated with the ANS constitute the afferent limbs of autonomic reflexes and carry the inputs recognized as visceral pain. Visceral afferents also mediate axon reflexes and are cross-linked with somatic, as well as autonomic, nervous system activity.

HIERARCHICALLY ORGANIZED CNS CIRCUITS

Homeostasis no more occurs through isolated autonomic reflexes than posture is maintained, or movement is affected, through isolated somatic reflexes. Nevertheless, methodological and historical considerations have yielded a tendency to focus on individual autonomic reflexes. Methodologically, the need for experimental control typically dictates that experiments isolate a reflex (or small set of reflexes) for examination. In addition, historically, the ANS was conceptualized primarily as a motor branch of the peripheral nervous system. One important source of the emphasis on the motor outflow of the ANS was Langley's concentration on the pre- and postganglionic leg of the circuitry in his seminal pharmacological and physiological studies. Many texts still reflect this early peripheral and motor emphasis.

The separate-reflex perspective shapes a view of the autonomic nervous system as a collection of individual motor responses, but autonomic activity typically involves finely coordinated, fully integrated adjustments of multiple outflows. Just as somatic posture and movement are coordinated by supraspinal CNS controls, autonomic integration is achieved by supraspinal controls. The preganglionic motor pools of the craniosacral and thoracolumbar outflows are final common paths for descending projections from the CNS. Similarly, the first- and second-order visceral afferent relays (e.g., the nucleus of the solitary tract and the spinal lamina V), which form short, mono- or oligosynaptic reflex arcs with these preganglionic motor pools, are targets of rostral CNS stations that coordinate and modulate the autonomic outflows.

The CNS coordination of autonomic activity provides a number of integrative functions: (1) Much like the suprasegmental organization of skeletal motor responses, central ANS stations provide coordination and sequencing of different local autonomic reflexes. These stations provide, for example, the efferent choreography necessary to coordinate the autonomic responses in the mouth, stomach, intestines, and pancreas during and after a meal. Such programs coordinate brain stem and spinal cord efferents, as well as reflexes within the SNS and PSNS divisions of the autonomic outflow. (2) Central ANS circuitry also links autonomic activity and somatic motor activity. The example used earlier of cardiovascular adjustments occurring in concert with postural adjustments illustrates such linkage between autonomic and somatic nervous system outflows. (3) The CNS stations of the autonomic nervous system also provide the information, as well as the organization and planning, that enables an organism to mobilize autonomic adjustments or responses in anticipation of environmental events. For example, both fluid and energy homeostasis involve physiological adjustments in anticipation of major imbalances or deficits, responses that cannot be explained solely by reactive reflexes (see Chapters 38 and 39).

The autonomic controls of the cardiovascular system provide prototypic examples of these principles. For example, the brain stem integrates the sympathetic and parasympathetic feedback loops controlling vasomotor tone, baroreceptor reflexes, and cardiac rate. In addition to linking these separate homeostatic reflexes into an overall adaptive program, the brain stem also cross-couples the autonomic adjustments with complementary endocrine controls involving the hypothalamo–pituitary–adrenal axis. Furthermore, CNS neural circuitry also provides the linkages by which these cardiovascular adjustments are coordinated and integrated with other homeostatic loads and challenges that must be handled simultaneously (see, for example, the role of baroreceptor reflexes in volume regulation of fluid levels in Chapter 36).

The importance and the nature of central autonomic controls are underscored by clinical disorders that result from interruptions in the connections between the central autonomic circuitry and the preganglionic motor neurons (see Box 35.4). Quadriplegia and paraplegia, which result from injuries that divide the spinal cord and separate thoracic and lumbar sympathetic loops and sacral parasympathetic pathways from higher central regions, illustrate how essential these longitudinal connections are. Interruption of the longitudinal connections causes loss of

BOX 35.4

HEALTH AND DISEASE: THE WISDOM OF THE BODY

The importance of the autonomic nervous system to health often goes unnoticed. When ANS functions operate normally, they typically occur automatically, without the individual being aware of any adjustments. Nevertheless, the loss of an autonomic response can be disruptive, and autonomic disorders can be debilitating (e.g., Bannister, 1989). In the classic example of adulthood ANS degeneration known as multiple system atrophy and autonomic failure, or the Shy–Drager syndrome, individuals may exhibit postural hypotension, urinary and fecal incontinence, sexual impotence, cranial nerve palsies, loss of sweating, and a movement disorder similar to Parkinson's disease. Disconnection of the suprasegmental autonomic stations from the spinal cord can occur in neurological disorders, such as multiple sclerosis, and traumatic spinal cord injury. As a result, bowel and bladder control are lost, and impotence is caused by a loss of autonomic genital reflexes.

Such deficits are clearly disabling, but some autonomic disorders are less conspicuous. In part, the apparently more subtle deficits may be ones that are less important in the carefully controlled environments found in industrialized and modern societies. For example, impaired thermoregulatory responses may be tolerated well by a person living in a climate-controlled environment. Also, metabolic emergencies are unlikely to occur and need autonomic compensation if a person regularly eats enough food. Nevertheless, autonomic disorders occa-

sion a number of serious, even life-threatening, health problems.

Excess activation of the ANS is implicated in various stress-related disorders, including ulcers, colitis, high blood pressure, and heart attacks.

Chronic failure of autonomic cardiovascular hemeostasis can cause debilitating postural hypotension.

Developmental autonomic disorders, such as immature or anomalous medullary respiratory circuitry, are thought to contribute to sudden infant death syndrome. Some sleep disorders, such as sleep apnea, are also thought to have autonomic components.

Furthermore, widespread autonomic dysfunction resulting from autonomic neuropathies of diabetes, alcoholism, and Parkinson's disease complicates the primary diseases.

Autonomic disturbances can also underlie metabolic disorders, such as stress-induced diabetes and reactive hypoglycemia (see Chapter 38). Autonomic disturbances have also been hypothesized to be a cause of obesity in some people.

Terry L. Powley

Reference

Bannister, R. (1989). "Autonomic Failing: A Textbook of Clinical Disorders of the Autonomic Nervous System," 2nd Ed. Oxford Medical Publications, Oxford, UK.

voluntary bladder and bowel control. Disruption of the spinal cord also causes men to become impotent because penile tumescence is a predominantly parasympathetic response and ejaculation is a sympathetic response. Although erections can occasionally be elicited as local reflexes caused by direct mechanical stimulation, ejaculations, which require suprasegmental coordination, almost universally disappear. In addition, numerous vascular and glandular reflexes are also disordered by the interruption of long autonomic pathways connecting the brain and spinal cord (see Bannister, 1989).

Early Physiological Experiments Suggested a Central Component of the ANS

Like the concept of the ANS itself, the corollary that the ANS includes a hierarchy of central mechanisms was first demonstrated by physiological

experiments. Nineteenth- and early 20th-century experiments manipulating the brain caused autonomic disturbances. In one classical experiment, for example, Claude Bernard demonstrated that localized mechanical lesions, or stab wounds, in the floor of the fourth ventricle near the dorsal vagal complex produced a "piqure glycosurique," a disturbance of blood glucose homeostasis characterized by a diabetes-like condition in which glucose spills into the urine. Making similar observations, Flourens suggested the existence of respiratory "noeud vital" in the brain stem, and Schiff pointed to a "vasoconstrictor center" in the medulla. More modern lesion and stimulation studies have identified a number of "centers" for micturation, respiration, and other autonomic functions in the medulla oblongata and pons.

Other work has implicated the hypothalamus in even more extensively coordinated and cross-linked autonomic patterns. This work led to the concept of the hypothalamus (see Chapter 34) as the "head ganglion" of the autonomic nervous system. Following an earlier application of electrical stimulation to the hypothalamus by Karplus and Kreidl, Walter Hess found that focal electrical stimulation of regions of the hypothalamus elicited coordinated patterns of sympathetic and parasympathetic adjustments (e.g., changes in pupil size, piloerection, and respiration) and affective responses that were appropriate to behavioral responses elicited from the same loci. In fact, central manipulations that affect autonomic function seem invariably to produce adjustments of both SNS and PSNS outputs, an observation that underscores the integrative role the brain plays in ANS function.

Brain lesions in virtually all limbic system regions, and notably in the septal area, amygdala, hippocampus, frontal cortex, cingulate cortex, and insular cortex, have been shown to exaggerate, dissociate,

blunt, or in other ways distort autonomic responses to environmental situations.

Tracing Experiments and Anatomical Mapping Have Revealed Multiple Hierarchically Organized, Reciprocally Interconnected Stations of the Neuraxis That Control Autonomic Activity

As neuroscience tracing tools have become more powerful, they have revealed the extensive hierarchical autonomic circuitry linking visceral afferent inputs with autonomic efferent outflows, linking the SNS and PSNS divisions of the ANS, and interconnecting the central autonomic stations with somatic and endocrine pathways in the brain (see Box 35.5). This central autonomic circuitry has been considered a "central visceromotor system" (Nauta, 1972) or a "central autonomic network" (Loewy, 1981). These

---

BOX 35.5

CENTRAL ANS CIRCUITS MAY INTEGRATE AUTONOMIC REFLEXES WITH AFFECTIVE OR EMOTIONAL RESPONSES, AS WELL AS WITH SOMATIC RESPONSES

In addition to its many other functions, the autonomic nervous system participates in emotion and motivation. Even the name of the first ANS division to be distinguished, i.e., the sympathetic, connotes an empathetic operation. More important, the central role that the limbic system plays in both the hierarchical control of both autonomic activity and the affective response repertoire supports the hypothesis that the ANS plays a pivotal role in emotional functions.

In one of the seminal early neurobiological explanations of emotion, the ANS was proposed to be the substrate. Consider the fight-or-flight example that Cannon used in his characterizations of autonomic adjustments and that was discussed earlier in this chapter: The somatic and autonomic adjustments in this emergency situation contain elements we associate with anger or fear. The central relays, including the limbic circuitry just discussed, organize the autonomic components of these responses to external environmental stimuli and coordinate them with the appropriate somatic responses. Thus, the central ANS circuitry may be involved in the expression of emotional reactions.

Some have hypothesized that in addition to being involved in the expression of emotions, the ANS might be involved in the experience of emotions. The classic

theory of this type was suggested independently by James and Lange, who speculated that afferent experience resulting from autonomic adjustments might be the basis of emotional experiences. For the fight-or-flight example, the James–Lange idea could be considered the proposition that "you do not run because you are afraid; you are afraid because you run." Cannon offered an influential refutation of the James–Lange theory, but most of his argument was based on now outmoded ideas about the ANS and a lack of distinction between expression and experience.

In an experiment designed to examine the James–Lange idea, Hohmann (1962) surveyed army veterans who had sustained spinal cord injuries at different levels. Consistent with a prediction of the theory, for self-reported experiences of both fear and anger, Hohmann found that the higher the spinal cord lesions (and thus the more of the visceral afferent inflow disconnected from the brain), the greater the reduction in affective experiences.

Terry L. Powley

Reference

Hohmann, G. W. (1962). Some effects of spinal cord lesions on experienced emotional feelings. *Psychophysiology* 3, 143–156.

studies revealed a network of multisynaptic relays descending from the hypothalamus and midbrain to preganglionic neurons in the brain stem and spinal cord. Similar projections, both direct and relayed through the hypothalamus, were also found for a number of limbic system nuclei, including most prominently the amygdala (Nauta, 1972). Neural tracers, immunocytochemical techniques, and electron microscopy have subsequently increased the resolution of the maps of this circuitry and its transmitters (e.g., Loewy, 1981).

Such experiments have established that the paraventricular nucleus of the hypothalamus (see Chapter 34) is a prototype of extensive and profound central autonomic coordination. Parvocellular neurons in the paraventricular nucleus project monosynaptically to vagal preganglionic neurons in the dorsal motor nucleus of the vagus and sympathetic preganglionics in the intermediolateral column of the spinal cord. The paraventricular nucleus also projects to the visceral afferent relay nuclei associated with each of these efferent outflows (the nucleus of the solitary tract and spinal lamina V, respectively). These descending projections influence several cardiovascular and gastrointestinal responses. Illustrating the extent of the central integration of responses, additional neurons of the paraventricular nucleus control corticotropin-releasing factor and oxytocin neuron responses, which are often activated or modulated in association with autonomic functions.

Most mesencephalic, diencephalic, and telencephalic nuclei considered part of the limbic system affect visceral motor outflows and can be included in the concept of the central visceromotor system. In addition to the central gray and paramedian regions of the mesencephalon and the entire hypothalamus, including the preoptic hypothalamus, these limbic sites include the amygdala, bed nucleus of the stria terminalis, septal region, hippocampus, cingulate cortex, orbital frontal cortex, and insular and rhinal cortexes.

Summary

Multiple central structures of the subcortical and diencephalic hierarchies can impose special controls over the ANS when required. In addition to sending descending projections, the CNS sites constituting the hierarchy of autonomic circuitry receive, reciprocally, ascending visceral afferent inputs from the medullary (nucleus of the solitary tract) and spinal (lamina V) relays. For example, second- and higher order neurons of the nucleus of the solitary tract project, by way of a relay in the pontine parabrachial nucleus (and in some cases monosynaptically), to the mid-

brain central gray, the lateral hypothalamus, the hypothalamic paraventricular nucleus, the amygdala, and the bed nucleus of the stria terminalis. Ascending connections from the spinal visceral afferents converge on many of these same stations.

A network of hierarchically organized central stations, many of them part of the limbic system, forms a central visceral neuroaxis that receives inputs from visceral afferents and issues descending projections to the ANS preganglionic neurons in the brain stem and spinal cord. This central autonomic circuitry organizes and sequences sets of separate autonomic reflexes, coordinates SNS and PSNS responses so that they are synergistic, cross-links autonomic and skeletal responses, and integrates autonomic activity with ongoing and anticipated behavior of the individual.

PERSPECTIVE: FUTURE OF THE AUTONOMIC NERVOUS SYSTEM

Our understanding of the autonomic nervous system is still incomplete and evolving, driven by the technological improvements in neuroscience. Modern techniques (e.g., molecular biology, immunocytochemistry, electron microscopy) are changing the autonomic nervous system definition that was initially derived with the techniques available to Langley and contemporaries at the beginning of the 20th century (see Box 35.1). The distinction that sympathetic postganglionic neurons are noradrenergic whereas parasympathetic postganglionics are cholinergic has been blurred by the recognition of nonadrenergic noncholinergic (NANC) neurons, nitric oxide synthetase (NOS)-containing neurons, a large number of colocalized and coreleased neuropeptides, postganglionic neurons changing their neurotransmitter phenotypes, and other exceptions that broaden the view developed by Langley's pharmacological studies. The canon that the ANS is strictly a motor system without an afferent counterpart is challenged by many who argue on functional and molecular biological grounds that "visceral afferents" belong to the ANS (see Box 35.3).

The proposal that functional differences between the two limbs of the ANS can be attributed to their contrasting patterns of projection (the sympathetic system preganglionics projecting to postganglionics in a one-to-many pattern; the parasympathetic system projecting in a one-to-few pattern) has not been substantiated by modern analyses of divergence (cf. Wang et al., 1995). Continued application of modern technologies and the prospect of continuing developments promise to define an autonomic nervous system quite different from that envisioned by Langley.

SUMMARY AND GENERAL CONCLUSIONS

The autonomic nervous system is the neural circuitry that maintains homeostasis and health. It is responsible for the neural components of Cannon's "wisdom of the body." With its sophisticated motor repertoire and complexes of reflexes, including local axon reflexes, segmental or oligosynaptic reflexes, and polysynaptic suprasegmental cascades, the ANS works continuously to adjust and defend the body's physiology. The importance of these processes was summarized succinctly by Nauta and Feirtag (1986), who wrote: "Life depends on the innervation of the viscera; in a way all the rest is biological luxury." The processes go on, for the most part, without awareness or cognitive representations. This automaticity is presumably crucial to the successful operation of the ANS and certainly frees the individual from bodily housekeeping tasks, thereby making it practical to focus on other activities and inputs from the environment.

The hub of the ANS consists of two separate motor outflows, each a hierarchical organization with preganglionic neurons stationed in the CNS and postganglionic neurons located in peripheral ganglia. The sympathetic, or thoracolumbar, division facilitates the mobilization of energy, increases catabolism, and promotes physiological responses that support activity, including emergency responses such as "fight" or "flight." The parasympathetic, or craniosacral, division facilitates conservation of energy, increases anabolism, and supports physiological responses that typically promote rest, digestion, and restoration of body reserves. The adrenergic phenotype of sympathetic postganglionic neurons, the cholinergic phenotype of parasympathetic neurons, and distinguishing complements of neuropeptides and receptor specializations provide neurochemical coding for the two divisions of the ANS.

The motor outflows of the ANS are efferent limbs of reflexes triggered by visceral and, in some cases, somatic afferents. These reflex circuits have second-order visceral afferent nuclei located adjacent to spinal and medullary nuclei of preganglionic motor neurons (laminae I and V and the nucleus of the solitary tract, respectively).

Higher order CNS circuitry, including the hypothalamus, limbic system, and a variety of cortical sites, provides hierarchical control and integration of autonomic reflexes. This hierarchy is responsible for coordinating different autonomic reflexes, integrating autonomic function with somatic activity, and executing response programs that anticipate needs and regulate physiology over more extended time scales than those represented by isolated reflexes.

References

Bannister, R. (1989). "Autonomic Failure: A Textbook of Clinical Disorders of the Autonomic Nervous System," 2nd Ed. Oxford Medical Publications, Oxford, UK.

Bieger, D., and Hopkins, D. A. (1987). Viscerotopic representation of the upper alimentary tract in the medulla oblongata in the rat: Nucleus ambiguus. *J. Comp. Neurol.* **262**, 546–562.

Cannon, W. B. (1939). "The Wisdom of the Body," 2nd Ed. Norton, New York.

Cervero, F., and Foreman, R. D. (1990). Sensory innervation of the viscera. *In* "Central Regulation of Autonomic Functions" (A. D. Loewy and K. M. Spyer, eds.), pp. 104–125. Oxford Univ. Press, New York.

Costa, M., Furness, J. B., and Llewellyn-Smith, I. J. (1987). Histochemistry of the enteric nervous system. *In* "Physiology of the Gastrointestinal tract" (L. R. Johnson, ed.), Vol. 1. Raven Press, New York.

Dembowsky, K., Czachurski, J., and Seller, H. (1985). Morphology of sympathetic preganglionic neurons in the thoracic spinal cord of the cat: An intracellular horseradish peroxidase study. *J. Comp. Neurol.* **238**, 453–465.

Fox, E. A., and Powley, T. L. (1992). Morphology of identified preganglionic neurons in the dorsal motor nucleus of the vagus. *J. Comp. Neurol.* **322**, 79–98.

Hohmann, G. W. (1962). Some affects of spinal cord lesions on experienced emotional feelings. *Psychophysiology* **3**, 143–156.

Holst, M.-C., Kelly, J. B., and Powley, T. L. (1997). Vagal preganglionic projections to the enteric nervous system characterized with PHA-L. *J. Comp. Neurol.* **381**, 81–100.

Jänig, W. (1996). Neurobiology of visceral afferent neurons: Neuroanatomy, functions, organ regulations and sensations. *Biol. Psychol.* **42**, 29–51.

Landis, S. C., and Keefe, D. (1983). Evidence for transmitter plasticity *in vivo*: Developmental changes in properties of cholinergic sympathetic neurons. *Dev. Biol.* **98**, 349–372.

Langley, J. N. (1921). "The Autonomic Nervous System," Part I. Heffer, Cambridge, UK.

Loewy, A. D. (1981). Descending pathways to sympathetic and parasympathetic preganglionic neurons. *J. Auton. Nerv. Syst.* **3**, 265–275.

Lundberg, J. (1996). Pharmacology of cotransmission in the autonomic nervous system: Integrative aspects on amines, neuropeptides, adenosine triphosphate, amino acids and nitric oxide. *Pharmacol. Rev.* **48**, 113–178.

Morgan, C., Nadelhaft, I., and de Groat, W. C. (1981). The distribution of visceral primary afferents from the pelvic nerve within Lissaure's tract and the spinal gray matter and its relationship to the sacral parasympathetic nucleus. *J. Comp. Neurol.* **201**, 415–440.

Nauta, W. J. H. (1972). The central visceromotor system: A general survey. *In* "Limbic System Mechanisms and Autonomic Function" (C. H. Hockman, ed.), pp. 21–40. Thomas, Springfield, IL.

Nauta, W. J. H., and Feirtag, M. (1986). "Fundamental Neuroanatomy." Freeman, New York.

Potter, D. D., Landis, S. C., and Furshpan, E. J. (1980). Dual function during development of rat sympathetic neurones in culture. *J. Exp. Biol.* **89**, 57–71.

Strack, A. M., Sawyer, W. B., Marubio, L. M., and Loewy, A. D. (1988). Spinal origin of sympathetic preganglionic neurons in the rat. *Brain Res.* **455**, 187–191.

Thomas, L. (1974). "Autonomy: The Lives of a Cell," pp. 64–68. Viking Press, New York.

Wang, F. B., Holst, M.-C., and Powley, T. L. (1995). The ratio of pre- to postganglionic neurons and related issues in the autonomic nervous system. *Brain Res. Rev.* **21**, 93–115.

Wood, J. D. (1987). Physiology of the enteric nervous system. *In* "Physiology of the Gastrointestinal Tract" (L. R. Johnson, J. Christensen, M. J. Jackson, E. D. Jacobson, and J. H. Walsh, eds.), 2nd Ed., Vol. 1, pp. 67–110. Raven Press, New York.

Suggested Readings

Barraco, I. R. A. (ed.) (1994). "Nucleus of the Solitary Tract." CRC Press, Boca Raton, FL.

Björklund, A., Hökfelt, T., and Owman, C. (eds.) (1988). "Handbook of Chemical Neuroanatomy," Vol. 6. Elsevier Science, Amsterdam.

Burnstock, G. (1992–2000). "The Autonomic Nervous System," Vols. 1–12. Harwood Academic, Chur, Switzerland.

Cannon, W. B. (1939). "The Wisdom of the Body," 2nd Ed. Norton, New York.

Gabella, G. (1976). "Structure of the Autonomic Nervous System." Chapman & Hall, London.

Hockman, C. H. (ed.) (1972). "Limbic System Mechanisms and Autonomic Function." Thomas, Springfield, IL.

Kuntz, A. (1953). "The Autonomic Nervous System," 4th Ed. Lea & Febiger, Philadelphia.

Loewy, A. D., and Spyer, K. M. (eds.) (1990). "Central Regulation of Autonomic Functions." Oxford Univ. Press, New York.

Pick, J. (1970). "The Autonomic Nervous System." Lippincott, Philadelphia.

Ritter, S., Ritter, R. C., and Barnes, C. D. (eds.) (1992). "Neuroanatomy and Physiology of Abdominal Vagal Afferents." CRC Press, Boca Raton, FL.

Terry L. Powley

36

Neural Regulation of the Cardiovascular System

The circulatory system includes two important major elements: the heart, which functions as a pump, and a system of vessels, the circulatory system, that exchanges gases and nutrients essential for normal cellular and organ function and, in the case of disease processes, for repair and sometimes survival. Blood circulates from the lungs, where oxygen is taken up and carbon dioxide eliminated, to all organ systems in the body. In addition, circulation of blood provides transport and distribution of nutrients from gastrointestinal and other absorptive and storage regions of the body and elimination of waste products to and from metabolically active cells in each of these organs. The heart functions as a synchronized muscular pump by providing kinetic energy that propels blood through the circulatory system so that it can be distributed in an optimal fashion, depending on the particular needs of each organ under the existing conditions. Regulation of regional distribution of blood flow allows conservation of energy and efficiency of gas and nutrient delivery. Distribution of blood flow is critically dependent on driving pressure (blood pressure) and regional vascular resistance. The nervous system regulates vascular resistance, cardiac output, and hence arterial blood pressure.

The body is exposed to conditions that require both immediate and sometimes long-term adaptation of the cardiovascular system. These situations can vary, for instance, from bed rest to maximal exercise, cold to hot environments, ocean depths to sea level to high altitude, including space flight, and fear to arousal. Pathologic conditions can be associated with hypotension or hypertension, myocardial infarction and congestive heart failure, acute asthma (bronchoconstriction), and chronic renal failure. These examples represent only a few of the many and varied conditions

to which the cardiovascular system must respond to provide optimal organ function or restoration of function of the organ(s) to as close to normal as possible.

Fortunately, a set of short-term and long-term regulatory mechanisms are in place that allow the cardiovascular system to meet these challenges. Two mechanisms, in particular, are critically important for short-term adjustments of the cardiovascular system. These include cardiovascular neural reflexes, which consist of a set of neural inputs activated by neural afferent systems that sense the internal and external environment and rapidly alter function of the heart and vascular system. Second, the organism can institute behavioral changes to profoundly influence function of the cardiovascular system so that it can cope with the environment. Examples of the latter activity include, among others, changes in body position, activity level, and voluntary changes in environmental exposure, including avoidance. Some behavioral changes are involuntary and likely constitute primitive survival mechanisms that have developed to assist reflex events. An example of one such involuntary mechanism is the feed forward or central command response that works in concert with the muscle reflex to adjust the cardiovascular and respiratory systems in preparation for and during exercise. The main focus of this chapter is on neural regulation of the cardiovascular system, rather than behavioral modifications.

DESCRIPTION OF THE SYSTEM: AN ANATOMICAL FRAMEWORK

Neural regulation of the cardiovascular system consists of two sets of interactive functional elements. One important set of regulatory elements consists of regions in the central nervous system (CNS) that maintain a basal or tonic output that, through the autonomic nervous system, continuously influences effector organ function, in this case the heart and vascular system. The second system provides phasic regulation of the cardiovascular system and consists of a large number of neural reflexes, each of which is composed of an afferent or sensory arm, regions in the CNS that integrate sensory input, and an efferent or autonomic arm. *Cardiovascular reflexes* are differentiated by unique features of their sensory component. Furthermore, the concept that the sympathetic nervous system responds in a global fashion has been replaced with the recent understanding that different reflexes (e.g., baroreceptor, chemoreceptor, and cardiopulmonary receptor) evoke individualized patterns of sympathetic activity to the heart and regional vascular systems. These patterns of reflex activation are organized in the CNS, mainly at the supraspinal level. A number of common CNS regions are involved in the integrative aspect of the reflexes, as well as in the autonomic component of the responses. It is recognized, however, that substantial differences in central processing occur, as cardiovascular responses to stimulation of two sets of afferents from even the

same organ, e.g., the heart, frequently are manifested quite differently. Work in this latter area is in its infancy.

Investigation of CNS regions involved in the regulation of blood pressure began in 1870 when Carl Ludwig performed a series of increasingly caudal transections of the brain stem and observed that blood pressure was maintained by specific regions in the medulla. Subsequent studies identified regions termed *pressor* or *depressor areas* depending on the blood pressure response when they were ablated or stimulated (Fig. 36.1) (Alexander, 1946). Since these early studies, investigations by several laboratories have recognized the existence of a system of pacemaker cells or central network generators that tonically maintain blood pressure (see later).

Since these early studies, it is now recognized that an equally important function of the nervous system is to sense changes in the environment and provide immediate short-term as well as long-term regulation of the cardiovascular system. This is accomplished through a set of neural reflexes. Short and long loop reflexes are initiated by sensory nerves positioned in organs, including blood vessels, in locations that provide them with an opportunity to sense the local

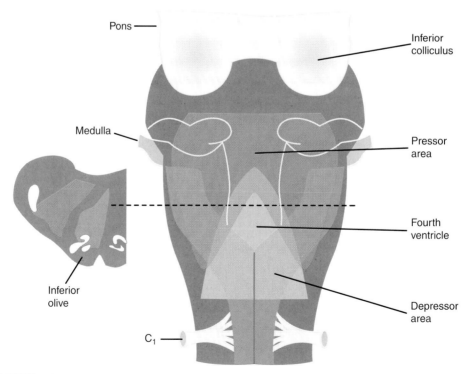

FIGURE 36.1 Pressor and depressor regions in the cat brain stem. The dorsolateral pressor region projected onto the dorsal surface (right) and in a frontal section (left at level of dashed line) is shown as a red-shaded area, whereas the ventromedial depressor region is shown as a yellow-shaded area (Alexander, 1946; Jordan, 1995).

environment. Endings of these afferent nerves are sensitive to chemical, mechanical, or thermal stimuli or to a combination of events (i.e., bimodal or polymodal in function). Their impulse activity is transmitted through pathways that are either finely myelinated or unmyelinated, termed group III or Aδ and group IV or C fibers, designating somatic and visceral afferents, respectively.

Anatomy of Somatic and Sympathetic Afferent Reflexes

One important group of sensory pathways are the sympathetic or spinal afferent systems that support somatic and visceral reflexes, including both *nociceptive* and *nonnociceptive signals* transmitted to the CNS. Cell bodies of somatic and visceral spinal afferents exist in dorsal root ganglia. Nociceptive signals from primary afferents enter the spinal cord through Lissauer's tract and terminate in laminae I and V of the dorsal horn gray matter. Many fine afferents contain substance P. Other neuropeptides present in dorsal root ganglion cells include calcitonin gene-related peptide, somatostatin, and vasoactive intestinal polypeptide. Spinal pathways ascend one or two segments before crossing to the contralateral side. Through *spinothalamic* (including a lateral and medial division), *spinoreticular, spinomesencephalic,* and *spinosolitary tracts,* these systems transmit information to the brain stem and thalamus, ultimately influencing autonomic outflow to the cardiovascular system, in addition to providing other sensory perceptions. Many cells in these tracts respond principally to noxious stimuli. They are classified as low-threshold, wide dynamic range (most common) and high-threshold (nociceptive) cells. Neurons in the lateral spinothalamic tract ascend to the ventral and ventral posterior lateral thalamus where they mediate discriminative or localization of pain. In contrast, cells in the medial spinothalamic tract, which project to the medial and intralaminar nuclear complex of the thalamus, transmit information leading to affective responses, including autonomic adjustments. Cells in the spinoreticular tract respond to chemical (bradykinin) and mechanical (premature beats) stimulation of cardiac ventricular afferents. They project to the gigantocellular tegmental field (paramedian reticular formation) and, to a lesser extent, to the caudal raphe nuclei and magnocellular tegmental field (ventromedial reticular formation), which, in turn, project to the intralaminar region of the thalamus. The medial reticular formation may mediate motor responses to visceral (including cardiac) pain and altered sympathetic function through collaterals to intermediolateral column (IML) or interneurons projecting to other

regions, such as the nucleus tractus solitarii (NTS) and rostral ventral lateral medulla (rVLM), concerned with the integration of sensory signals that drive autonomic outflow. The spinomesencephalic tract sends information to the central periaqueductal gray (PAG, also called the central gray matter) and parabrachial nucleus (PBN) in the rostral pons, and possibly the ventral lateral nucleus of the thalamus. The spinosolitary tract projects to the caudal NTS. Little information is available on the role of either the spinomesencephalic or the spinosolitary tract (Cervero and Foreman, 1990).

Central Neuroanatomy and Pharmacology of Baro- and Chemoreflex Pathways

A second set of equally important afferent pathways includes the IX (glossopharyngeal) and X (vagus) cranial nerves, which transmit signals originating from the arterial baroreceptors and chemoreceptors, as well as cardiac receptors, including both atrial and ventricular receptors.

Information from these systems is transmitted to the CNS where important temporal and spatial integration of information from the primary afferent pathway occurs, in addition to modification resulting from convergent input from other afferent pathways. A number of important CNS regions have been identified and include, among others, the NTS, caudal ventral lateral medulla (cVLM), rVLM, PBN, and lateral tegmental field (LTF). Still other areas in the medulla, hypothalamus, and midbrain identified as important sites of integration include the area postrema, PAG, and vestibular region. Each region receives input either directly from afferents or, more commonly, through interconnections (interneurons) from other nuclei. Each participates in signal conditioning to an extent dictated by the overall input and underlying conditions.

Thus, central autonomic pathways that form the anatomical substrate for many reflexes involved in regulation of the cardiovascular system have been defined. As outlined earlier, these can be separated broadly into CNS regions subserving spinal, e.g, somatosympathetic, vs CNS pathways and regions that integrate vagal and glossopharyngeal visceral afferent input. Much more information is available on the nuclei and pathways involved in the regulation of vagal afferent and other nonspinal visceral cardiovascular reflexes.

NTS

The NTS is the most important initial site receiving input from sensory nerves originating in the heart and large arteries (mechano- or barosensitive and chemosensitive regions). The NTS lies just ventral to the dorsal columns and is divided into the rostral, intermediate, and caudal NTS, relative to the obex. At the intermediate level, a central fiber bundle, the *solitary tract*, is formed from sensory input from VII, IX,

and X cranial nerves. Visceral afferents from the heart, lungs, and gastrointestinal regions project to neurons in the commissural medial NTS. Cardiovascular afferents from the heart and great vessels specifically project to the dorsolateral, medial, and commissural regions of the NTS. Surprisingly, few solitary tract

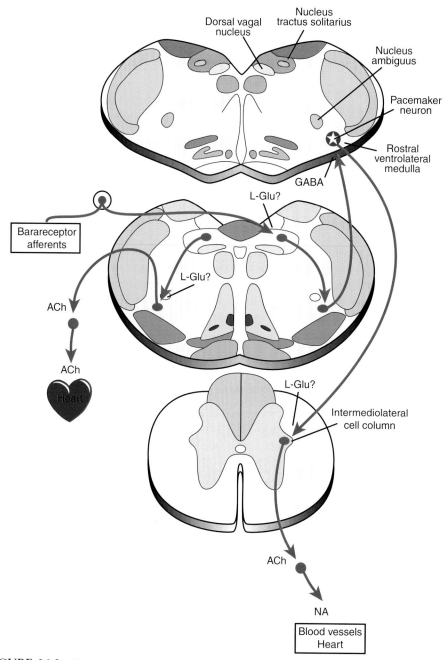

FIGURE 36.2   Neural pathways for the arterial baroreflex. Primary afferents in the IX and X cranial nerves project to the nucleus tractus solitarii (NTS). As shown on the right, interneurons forming sympathetic pathways project from the NTS to the caudal ventrolateral medulla, which in turn project to the rostral ventral lateral medulla, the source of reticulospinal projections to the intermediolateral columns in the spinal cord. Pathways from the NTS to the nucleus ambiguus form the major parasympathetic arm of the reflex, GABA, γ-aminobutyric; L-glu, L-glutamate; ACH, acetylcholine; NA, norepinephrine. (Guyenet, 1990).

neurons have pulse synchronous activity, possibly due to convergent input from multiple baroreceptor and nonbaroreceptor inputs. Non-NMDA glutamate receptors mediate fast synaptic transmission, whereas NMDA receptors function in a modulatory role. Although the excitatory amino acid glutamate appears to be the most important neurotransmitter for reflex transmission through the NTS, other neurotransmitters, neuropeptides, or neuromodulators, such as catecholamines, acetylcholine, γ-aminobutyric acid (GABA), substance P, angiotensin, nitric oxide, and opioids, also regulate the activity of these interneurons. There are important interactions between the NTS and other nearby nuclei such as the area postrema, which functions as a circumventricular organ. In turn, the NTS projects to a number of other regions, including forebrain nuclei such as the limbic system central nucleus of the amygdala, paraventricular, and median hypothalamic preoptic nuclei. There also are reciprocal connections between the NTS and the A5 cell group, caudal raphe nuclei, rVLM, PAG (or central gray matter), paraventricular, and lateral hypothalamic regions. Reciprocal connections are a major feature of this central autonomic network. The network probably functions as a microprocessor that integrates signals from receptive regions important in cardiovascular control, leading to changes in autonomic and neuroendocrine outflow (and likely behavior) to regulate function of the heart and blood vessels (Loewy, 1990).

cVLM

Second-order neurons from the NTS project to the cVLM where they provide tonic excitation mediated by an excitatory amino acid (NMDA) mechanism. Excitatory action from angiotensin II and inhibition from GABA, glycine (or a glycine-like compound), and opioids also tonically regulate activity of cVLM neurons. Third-order neurons from the cVLM, through a GABA mechanism, influence the activity of sympathetic premotor neurons in the rVLM and A5 cell group (Fig. 36.2). The cVLM contains both noradrenergic (A1) and nonadrenergic (retro or caudal periambigual area) neurons. Lesions of the cVLM increase arterial blood pressure, whereas microinjections of glutamate into this region cause depressor responses resulting from sympathoinhibition and, to a lesser extent, activation of vagal motoneurons in the nearby nucleus ambiguus (see later). Precise mapping studies suggest that depressor sites in the cVLM are primarily outside the A1 noradrenergic cell group.

rVLM

The rVLM is considered to be one of the most important sites of central integration. The rVLM, also called the *retrofacial nucleus*, is rostral to the lateral reticular nucleus and caudal to the facial nucleus. The medial region of this nucleus is the most important source of reticulospinal sympathetic premotor cells that project to the IML columns of the spinal cord. The rVLM has been subdivided into a lateral retrofacial nucleus and a medial nucleus paragigantocellularis (PGL). Both areas have been termed pressor regions because chemical lesions cause hypotension. Some studies suggest that the rostral extension of the PGL is concerned with pain control rather than cardiovascular regulation. In addition to reciprocal connections between the rVLM and the medial NTS, the rVLM receives inputs from the area postrema, cVLM, and is reciprocally connected to the parabrachial complex, PAG, lateral hypothalamic area, zona incerta, and paraventricular hypothalamus. Despite the fact that many rVLM neurons are phenotypically adrenergic (C1 group), glutamate is thought to be the principal excitatory neurotransmitter. Blockade of excitatory

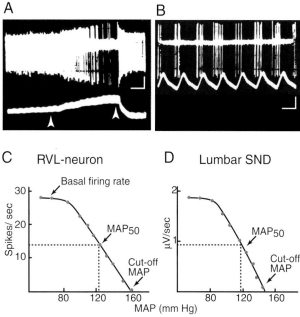

FIGURE 36.3 Bulbospinal vasomotor neurons in the rVLM identified through antidromic stimulation of the IML in the thoracic spinal cord. (A) Baroreflex inhibition of unit activity. (B) Pulse synchronous discharge activity when viewed on an expanded time scale. (C and D) The relationship between mean arterial pressure (MAP) and discharge activity of the neuron and the similar response of sympathetic discharge (SND) recorded from the lumbar chain. The unit demonstrates maximal activity at baseline followed by a linear decrease in firing rate as blood pressure is raised until the unit and sympathetic activity become silent (Sun and Guyenet, 1986).

amino acids does not alter resting blood pressure, indicating that tonic excitatory input does not exist. Conversely, blockade of GABA, which serves as the inhibitory neurotransmitter in barosensitive premotor sympathetic neurons projecting from cVLM to rVLM, increases their discharge activity and blood pressure. Other important neurotransmitters in the rVLM include acetylcholine and angiotensin, which also may be tonically active. A number of peptides such as opioids (e.g., enkephalins, endorphins), serotonin, neuropeptide Y, substance P, somatostatin, and/or thyrotropin-releasing hormone are not tonically active and may serve as neuromodulators. The network of vasomotor cells in the rVLM discharge with a cardiovascular rhythm (Fig. 36.3), which can be measured directly or with spike triggered averaging, a tech-

nique that relates intermittent unit activity to the cardiovascular cycle. In addition, many nonadrenergic cells in the rVLM display intrinsic pacemaker activity with spontaneous depolarization (see later for more detail). Approximately 50% of rVLM neurons that project to the IML are in the C1 adrenergic cell group, as they contain immunoreactive phenylethanolamine-N-methyltransferase or tyrosine hydroxylase; C1 cells do not show pacemaker activity. The rVLM contains clusters of neurons that provide selective input to regional vascular beds such as skin and muscle (Fig. 36.4) (Guyenet, 1990).

A5 Cell Group

The A5 noradrenergic cell group is located in the rostral-most portion of the ventrolateral medulla but is distinct from the rVLM. This cell group receives input from a number of regions, including the paraventricular hypothalamic nucleus, parafornical hypothalamic area, PBN, NTS, raphe obscurus, and cVLM. It projects to the NTS, dorsal vagal nucleus, PBN, lateral hypothalamic area, paraventricular thalamic nucleus, PAG, the central nucleus of the amygdala, and the IML. The function of this cell group is unclear, although it probably is not important in the tonic regulation of blood pressure (Guyenet, 1990). Stimulation of nonadrenergic neurons in this region decreases blood pressure and redistributes blood flow. However, A5 cells likely are sympathoexcitatory, as they are inhibited by baroreceptor input (Dampney, 1994).

iVLM

Between the cVLM and the rVLM is the intermediate ventrolateral medulla (iVLM), which forms an essential component of the baroreflex in rabbits and possibly in rats. Like the cVLM, the iVLM projects to the rVLM. Most neurons are not immunoreactive for tyrosine hydroxylase and therefore are distinguished from A1 cells located in this region (Dampney, 1994).

A1 Cell Group

The noradrenergic A1 cell group in the cVLM forms an important central component of the baroreflex. It projects directly to supraoptic and paraventricular regions in the hypothalamus and constitutes one of the pathways that mediates the release of vasopressin during baroreflex unloading. Cells in the A1 region are under tonic GABA inhibition from the NTS.

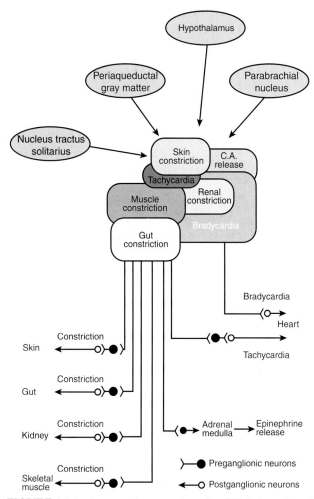

FIGURE 36.4 Inputs and outputs from the rVLM. A number of regions in the hypothalamus, midbrain and medulla project either directly or indirectly to presympathetic neurons in the rVLM. Distinct but overlapping pools of neurons are present in this region that provide separate sympathetic inputs to different regional vascular beds, the heart, and the adrenal medulla. C.A., catecholomine, (Lovick, 1987).

Other Regions Involved in Cardiovascular Control

Several other regions in the midbrain and the hypothalamus coordinate behavioral and autonomic responses.

PAG

The PAG, surrounding the cerebral aqueduct in the midbrain, receives inputs from the NTS, hypothalamus, and PBN and projects to the medullary reticular formation. Activation of the dorsolateral PAG leads to a defense reaction (see Box 36.1). Stimulation of the lateral PAG increases blood pressure. The ventrolateral PAG receives input from the somatosensory system and regulates sympathetic outflow to muscle and kidney in a viscerotopic manner by influencing activity in the medullary vasomotor centers (Jordan, 1990).

Hypothalamus

A number of specialized groups of neurons in the hypothalamus are important in cardiovascular regulation. The hypothalamus is divided into the anterior, posterior, and middle regions. The anterior region, overlying the optic chiasm, includes the circadian pacemaker (suprachiasmatic nucleus) as part of the preoptic nucleus, which controls blood pressure, cycles in body activity, body temperature, and a number of hormones. The middle portion of the hypothalamus, overlying the pituitary stalk, is composed of dorsomedial, ventromedial, paraventricular, supraoptic, and arcuate nuclei. The paraventricular nucleus projects to both sympathetic and parasympathetic premotor neurons in the medulla and spinal cord. The arcuate nucleus is an important source of opioid peptides, which function as important modulators of neuronal function in regions such as the PAG. The arcuate nucleus, along with the PAG, nucleus raphe obscurus, and rVLM, may function as a network that can be activated during somatic nerve stimulation (e.g., during acupuncture) to regulate sympathetic outflow.

The hypothalamus controls endocrine function both directly and indirectly. Large (magnocellular) neurons in paraventricular and supraoptic nuclei

---

BOX 36.1

DEFENSE REACTION

The central and autonomic nervous systems play crucial roles in providing a pattern of cardiovascular activity that allows appropriate responses to aversive stimuli. The behaviors studied have included the *flight or fight* response, frequently referred to as the defense reaction, and the *"playing dead"* response (Jordan, 1990). A number of stimuli, including visual or auditory threats, cause the defense response in several species in the awake condition. This response can also be conditioned to occur. It consists of stereotypical behaviors and cardiovascular responses, including posturing in the crouched position, retraction of the head and ears, vocalization, piloerection, pupillary dilation, heightened alertness, increased blood pressure, heart rate, myocardial contractility, and differential activation of sympathetic output to regional circulatory beds, including constriction of the mesenteric, renal, and cutaneous circulations and, at least in the naive condition, vasodilation of vessels in skeletal muscle and widespread venoconstriction. It is a preparatory reflex that sets the stage for maximal action. It can be evoked by stimulating a number of regions in the brain, including the dorsolateral PAG and other hypothalamic and midbrain regions stretching from the limbic system amygdala to the medulla. The PAG likely plays a central role in organizing and integrating this response (Fig. 36.9). Outflow from the PAG projects to neurons in the NTS (inhibiting neurons that receive baroreceptor input) and to the rVLM. Lesions in substantia nigra dorsal to the cerebral peduncles abolish vasodilation in skeletal muscle. Teleologically, this reaction conserves cardiac output by redirecting it to those regions that promote escape and ensure survival. In fewer species, such as the rabbit and opossum, the fear response of playing dead is characterized by pronounced bradycardia and hypotension (along with increased muscle blood flow), locomotor paralysis, pupillary dilation, and rapid shallow breathing. Stimulation of the central nucleus of the amygdala largely replicates the response observed in the awake animal.

John C. Longhurst

Reference

Jordan, D. (1990). Autonomic changes in affective behavior. *In* "Central Regulation of Autonomic Function" (A. D. Loewy and K. M. Spyer, eds.), pp. 349–366. Oxford Univ. Press, New York.

release vasopressin (while others release oxytocin) into the circulation from the posterior pituitary. *Vasopressin* neurons of magnocellular nuclei, as well as vasopressin-containing neurons in the paraventricular nucleus, are identified by their characteristic phasic pacemaker pattern of discharge activity.

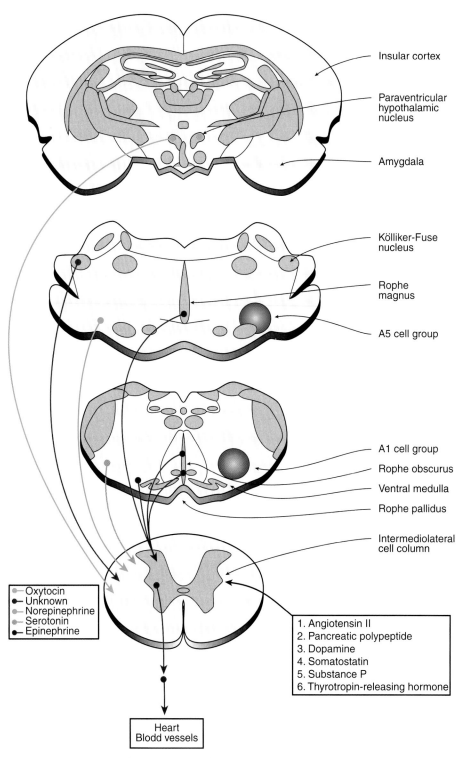

FIGURE 36.5 Direct preganglionic sympathetic inputs into the IML of the spinal cord. Projections from the raphe pallidus, obscurus, magnus, and the ventral medulla contain serotonin, whereas catecholaminergic A1 and A5 contain epinephrine and norepinephrine, respectively. The neurotransmitter for many of these neurons is glutamate or another excitatory amino acid (Loewy and Neil, 1981).

Vasopressin is produced as a prohormone in the cell bodies. Prohormones are cleaved as they are transported down axons in vesicles to the posterior pituitary where they are released as the active hormone. As suggested by its name, vasopressin causes vasoconstriction in many regional circulations, particularly in skin and muscle. However, another term for this peptide, antidiuretic hormone (ADH), signifies its action on the kidney to promote water reabsorption in collecting tubules and expansion of plasma volume; both actions of this hormone augment blood pressure. Input to the hypothalamus, leading to release of vasopressin, comes from atrial afferents, baroreceptors, chemoreceptors, and somatic (muscle) receptors.

ANATOMY AND CHEMICAL PROPERTIES OF EFFERENT AUTONOMIC PATHWAYS

Sympathetic

Outputs from the CNS to effector organs involved in cardiovascular reflex regulation course through sympathetic and parasympathetic branches of the autonomic nervous system. *Cardiovascular sympathetic premotor neurons* project from the brain stem and the diencephalon, including regions in the medulla, pons, and hypothalamus. Studies employing retrograde transneuronal viral labeling of cell bodies have defined five principal areas in the brain that innervate all levels of sympathetic outflow. These include the paraventricular hypothalamic nucleus, A5 noradrenergic cell group, caudal raphe region, rVLM, and ventromedial medulla (Fig. 36.5). Hindbrain pontine projections to the IML originate from the Kölliker–Fuse and A5 cell groups. Paraventricular and lateral hypothalamic nuclei also provide input to the IML. These cardiovascular sympathetic premotor neurons mainly project to *sympathetic preganglionic neurons* in the IML, located in the lateral horns of the spinal gray matter. To a lesser extent they also innervate the lateral funicular area (lateral and dorsal to the IML in the white matter of the lateral funiculus), intercalated cell group (medial to the IML), and central autonomic nucleus (also referred to as the nucleus intercalatus pars paraependymalis, located dorsal to the spinal central canal). There is *viscerotopographic clustering* of spinal sympathetic preganglionic neurons in restricted regions of the spinal cord, including C8, entire thoracic, and upper lumbar (thoracolumbar) and caudal lumbar regions (L_3–L_5). Sympathetic neurons exit the spinal cord through the ventral roots

and synapse with postganglionic neurons in either para- or prevertebral ganglia. Phenotypically, many terminals surrounding sympathetic preganglionic cells are catecholaminergic (e.g., from rVLM) or serotinergic (e.g., from caudal raphe, including raphe pallidus and obscurus, and ventral medial medulla). However, the principal neurotransmitter in terminals synapsing with sympathetic preganglionic cells is likely to be a fast-acting excitatory amino acid, such as glutamate (two-thirds of synaptic boutons) or an inhibitory neurotransmitter, GABA (one-third of axons). Other neurotransmitters, including serotonin, acetylcholine, enkephalins, substance P, neurotensin, leuteinizing hormone-releasing hormone, and somatostatin, are colocated in many cells and presumably function as pre- or postsynaptic neuromodulators. Ultrastructural studies have demonstrated more than 20 other transmitter-specific synapses on sympathetic preganglionic neurons.

Parasympathetic

The *nucleus ambiguus* in the ventrolateral region of the medullary reticular formation and the *dorsal motor nucleus of the vagus* in the dorsomedial region of the caudal medulla near the fourth ventricle are the sources of cardiac premotor parasympathetic fibers (Fig. 36.6). Thus, roles have been established for myelinated B fiber neurons from the nucleus ambiguus and unmyelinated C fibers from the dorsal vagal nucleus controlling heart rate and contractility and coronary flow to a lesser extent. Many premotor neurons discharge in synchrony with the cardiac cycle because they receive input from arterial baroreceptors. They also are excited by input from periph-

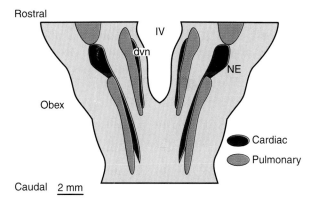

FIGURE 36.6 Horizontal view of preganglionic parasympathetic cardiac and pulmonary motoneurons in the nucleus ambiguus (nA) and dorsal motor nucleus of the vagus (dvn). The fourth (IV) ventricle and the obex are shown for reference (Jordan, 1995).

eral chemoreceptors, cardiac receptors, and trigeminal receptors (in the diving reflex). The ventral lateral portion of the nucleus ambiguus is the principal site of origin of cardioinhibitory neurons. Projections from the NTS form the major afferent input into this region. A smaller number of afferents originate from the medial and lateral PBN, paraventricular hypothalamic nucleus, Kölliker–Fuse cell group, ventrolateral nucleus of the solitary tract, caudal portion of the nucleus ambiguus, and contralateral rostral nucleus ambiguus. Although neurons in the dorsal motor nucleus and the nucleus ambiguus are phenotypically cholinergic, excitation from second order projections in the baroreflex from the NTS to the nucleus ambiguus is mediated by an excitatory amino acid. Some cardioinhibitory neurons in the nucleus ambiguus are under tonic GABA inhibitory control. Other immunoreactive substances, such as calcitonin gene-related peptide and galanin, are colocalized in some cholinergic neurons and likely function as neuromodulators. Many afferents innervating the nucleus ambiguus also contain serotonin and opioid peptides (Loewy and Spyer, 1990; Izzo and Spyer, 1997; Dampney, 1994). Laterality of cardiac motor neurons exists in the nucleus ambiguus. Electrical stimulation on the right inhibits the sinoatrial node, whereas stimulation of the left side inhibits conduction through the atrioventricular node.

Summary

Substantial information is available about the principal components of the anatomical system responsible for neural reflex control of the cardiovascular system, particularly with respect to some of the better studied visceral cardiovascular reflexes. Concepts of central integration especially have undergone substantial refinement over the last several decades. However, despite the substantial new knowledge that has been gained, it is just the beginning of an understanding of the interactive nature of the various central nuclei and pathways that are responsible for controlling the cardiovascular system under a variety of conditions.

A SYSTEM OF GENERATORS

Insurance companies have known for decades that individuals live longest with the lowest tolerated blood pressure. This pressure is the lowest basal blood pressure that allows adequate perfusion of all organs, especially the essential organs of the body, the heart and brain. Blood pressure is governed by two

major factors: the circulating volume of blood and plasma and the caliber of the lumen of blood vessels. Although blood and plasma volume depend on renal function, which, in turn, is dependent on neural and humoral input, this discussion focuses mainly on neural mechanisms regulating the caliber of blood vessels, especially on the tonic sympathetic activity that actively regulates the degree of basal constriction (i.e., *vascular smooth muscle tone*) of the small or resistance vessels. Resistance vessels are arterioles (~250 μm diameter) that are heavily innervated by a surrounding sympathetic neural meshwork. Changes in the lumen diameter of these arterioles, in response to alterations in neural input, occur to a greater or lesser extent in most regional circulatory systems and hence are important in the regulation of arterial blood pressure. Tonic sympathetic efferent neural activity, termed *sympathetic tone*, originates from higher brain centers and exists in the absence of input into these regions from external sensors. The importance of tonic sympathetic activity in maintaining blood pressure is demonstrated easily by interrupting it either physically or pharmacologically. Such studies began in the early 1850s when Claude Bernard and Brown Séquard discovered that transection of a sympathetic nerve led to vasodilation. In 1863, Claude Bernard showed that transection at the medullary-spinal level lowered blood pressure to a similar degree as pharmacological inhibition, thereby establishing the importance of supraspinal centers in generating basal sympathetic activity. When this procedure is performed, blood pressure generally decreases by 20–40 mmHg. Sherrington (1906) reinforced Bernard's conclusions during his observations on the recovery of blood pressure after spinal transection and spinal shock. Experiments by Carl Ludwig and his student, Oswjannikow, in the 1870s demonstrated that blood pressure is relatively well preserved until transection through the pons at the caudal border of the inferior colliculus. Although Dittmar (1873), working in Ludwig's laboratory and later, Schlaefke and Loeschcke, Feldberg, and Guertzenstein each identified the ventral medulla caudal to the facial nucleus as a necessary region for maintenance of resting blood pressure, their experiments did not determine specific nuclei that contribute resting sympathetic tone. More recent studies in anesthetized animals suggest that the medial diencephalon in the forebrain contributes to resting sympathetic activity (Dampney, 1994).

Chemosensitivity and pacemaker activity may contribute to the tonic activity of premotor sympathetic neurons that generate basal sympathetic tone (Dampney, 1994). Additionally, recent work by a

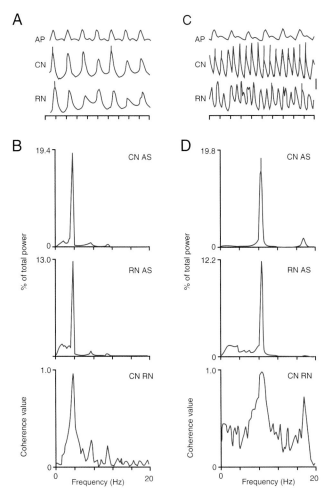

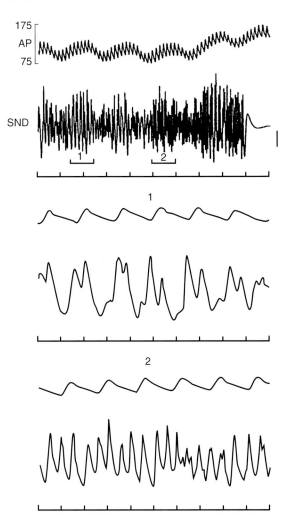

FIGURE 36.7 Spontaneous arterial pulse pressure (AP) and activity in the inferior cardiac (CN) and renal (RN) sympathetic nerves in an anesthetized baroreceptor-intact cat. Wide band-pass recordings of the time domain demonstrate activity that is phase locked with the cardiac rhythm (A) when mean blood pressure was 149 mm Hg or with a peak at 10 Hz when blood pressure was 103 mm Hg. Frequency domain autospectra (AS) of the cardiac and renal nerves and coherence between the two nerves (CN-RN) are shown in B (2–6 Hz) and D (10 Hz). Coherence analysis allows linear correlation of two signals, as a function of frequency, with 1.0 representing perfect correlation and 0 the absence of any relationship. Calibration in C is 50 μV (Barman and Gebber, 2000).

FIGURE 36.8 Unanesthetized decerebrate cat demonstrating a spontaneous change in pattern of discharge activity of inferior cardiac sympathetic nerve (SND) followed by an increase in arterial pressure (AP) that led to baroreflex inhibition of activity, recorded on a time scale of 2 s/div. The two expanded time scales (200 ms/div) at the bottom demonstrate that the animal changed from a cardiac-related (trace 1) to a 10-Hz rhythm (trace 2) (Barman and Gebber, 2000).

number of investigators, including Gebber, Barman, and Guyenet, among others, has identified a network of cells in the rVLM, caudal raphe (CMR), caudal ventrolateral (cVLP) and dorsolateral pons (rDLP), LTF, and possibly the cVLM that functions as a *network oscillator* to maintain tonic sympathetic activity (Barman and Gebber, 2000). Using the techniques of time and frequency domain analysis, including coherence analysis and spike-triggered averaging, each region has been found to demonstrate either cardiovascular or 10-Hz rhythms that are believed to underlie this tonic sympathetic activity (Fig. 36.7). The

cardiovascular rhythm of 2–6 Hz largely originates from the LTF, rVLM, cVLM, cVLP, and rDLP. These rhythms are coupled to and therefore modified by baroreceptor input, but are apparent in its absence. The *10-Hz rhythm* originating mainly in the cVLM, cVLP, and rDLP and, to a lesser extent, the rVLM and the CMR is less well understood. The change from a cardiovascular to a 10-Hz rhythm is associated with an increase in blood pressure (Fig. 36.8), whereas elimination of this rhythm leads to a fall in blood pressure. Furthermore, evidence suggests that this rhythm may underlie the differential regional vascular responses during certain alerting responses, such as the defense response (see Box 36.1) (Jordan, 1990).

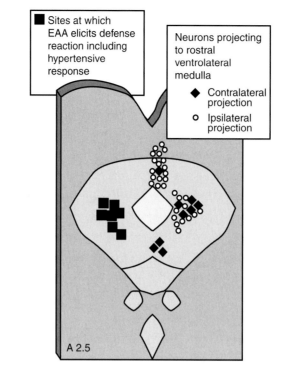

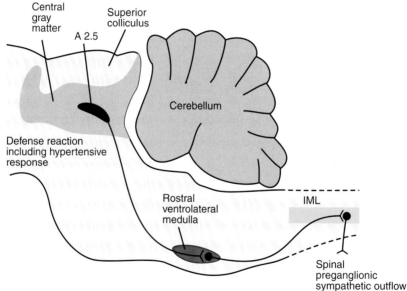

FIGURE 36.9 Coronal section displaying sites in the PAG (also called the central gray matter) that elicited a defense reaction after microinjection of excitatory amino acid (EAA) (top). Sagittal section of the area in the PAG that causes the hypertensive response, overlapping with the area projecting to sympathoexcitatory cells in the rVLM that, in turn, project to the IML (bottom). See text for abbreviations (Carrive *et al.*, 1988).

Summary

The cardiovascular system is controlled by a network of oscillators that provide for the maintenance of blood pressure, as well as the response of the cardiovascular system to a complex environment. Central generators responsible for cardiovascular and 10-Hz rhythms are distributed over a wide region in the brain stem. Additional investigation is required to understand how the rhythms are created and how the mechanisms by which this group of functionally heterogenous neurons contribute to sympathetic outflow in diverse states requiring either immediate or long-term cardiovascular responses.

BOX 36.2

EXERCISE

Voluntary exercise leads to a number of hemodynamic changes, including increases in blood pressure, heart rate, myocardial contractility, stroke volume, cardiac output, and vasoconstriction of inactive regional circulations. Vasoconstrictor responses also compete with the vasodilation caused by increased metabolic activity and flow-mediated vasodilation in active regions of the body. These changes are the result of increased neurohumoral activity. In particular, changes in autonomic neural tone include increased sympathetic and withdrawal of parasympathetic activity to the heart and vasculature. Alteration in efferent autonomic tone, particularly decreased activity in vagal motor nerves to the heart, begins immediately or soon after the start of exercise. Two processes drive these autonomic changes, including the *feed forward activity* or *central command* and the *exercise pressor reflex*. Central command or "cortical irradiation" originates in a number of supraspinal regions in the CNS, including the motor cortex, premotor cortex and supplementary motor cortex, subthalamic (hypothalamic) locomotor region or the H1 and H2 fields of Forel in the diencephalon, midbrain mesencephalic locomotor region, and the pontomedullary locomotor strip. The hypothalamic locomotor region likely is part of the defense area (see Box 36.1). Ultimately, one or more of these sites acts through medullary centers to regulate autonomic neural tone. Stimulation of the mesencephalic locomotor region in paralyzed animals either electrically or with a GABA antagonist evokes locomotion, hemodynamic, and respiratory changes quite similar to those observed during voluntary exercise. Interestingly, stimulation of the sub-

thalamic locomotor region also inhibits the baroreceptor reflex, consistent with observed suppression of this reflex during high-intensity exercise (see Box 36.4). In humans, central command is responsible for early cardiorespiratory changes that occur during dynamic and static exercise. In addition to central command, stimulation of both mechano- and chemosensitive receptors in active muscle, mediated largely (but not exclusively) by group III and IV afferents, also controls cardiovascular and respiratory changes associated with static and dynamic exercise in animal models and in humans. Changes in muscle tension and/or stretch activate predominately finely myelinated afferents to elicit early and possibly later changes in heart rate and respiration. Production of a number of chemical metabolic factors produced after a few seconds or minutes leads to slightly later activation of mainly unmyelinated muscle afferents and helps maintain the cardiorespiratory responses. The nature of the metabolic products that stimulate muscle afferents during exercise is controversial but likely is linked to an imbalance between oxygen supply and demand, i.e., a mismatch or error signal. Potential candidates include lactic acid, changes in pH, potassium, and perhaps kinins. Prostaglandins sensitize these sensory endings to the action of other metabolic products. Other metabolites, including adenosine, vasopressin, nicotine, angiotensin, catecholamines, and angiotensin, either do not cause cardiovascular responses when injected into muscle or are associated with pain rather than nonpainful reflex responses.

John C. Longhurst

SHORT-TERM CONTROL MECHANISMS

In response to internal and external changes in the environment, the cardiovascular system must respond quickly to cope with the demands placed upon it. Rapid changes in autonomic tone occur principally by one of two mechanisms, alterations in activity originating from the brain or through a reflex event. Alterations in autonomic activity originating as the result of voluntary or involuntary actions, such as exercise (see Box 36.2) or the defense reaction, in part, originate from the brain and are termed feed forward mechanisms, to be distinguished from the feedback component involving true reflexes. These feed-

forward events lack an afferent limb characteristic of reflex events, although visual or auditory input could be considered to form the necessary input that lead to their initiation. Reflex events, however, generally involve both afferent and efferent limbs, as well as a central neural integrative component.

REFLEX CONTROL OF THE CARDIOVASCULAR SYSTEM

As mentioned earlier, a primary function of the various reflex mechanisms concerned with cardiovascular control is to maintain homeostasis. Blood pressure and the metabolic environment, especially blood pH and oxygen tension, are two of the most important variables controlled. To accomplish these objectives, a number of sensory nerve ending sensors function as mechano- and chemoreceptors. This section describes several of the more important reflex pathways, including the sensory transduction mechanism, the afferent limb, central neural integration, autonomic outflow, and effector organ responses.

ARTERIAL BARORECEPTORS

Anatomy

The heart and blood vessels distribute oxygen and nutrients from the lungs, digestive, and storage regions to every cell in the body and, in turn, eliminate waste products from oxidative and nonoxidative metabolism through the lungs and kidneys. These functions are accomplished by appropriate function of the heart, which pumps blood, and optimal distribution of cardiac output to organs that need a variable supply of blood, depending on the underlying conditions. Maintenance of a constant and adequate blood pressure as the driving force for blood flow allows appropriate perfusion of organs. Mechanosensitive nerve endings are present predominately in two regions: one at the bifurcation of the common and internal carotid sinus and one in the aortic arch. Although the walls of these vessels are elastic in nature, they also contain smooth muscle, which can be stimulated to contract and unload baroreceptors. Baroreceptor nerve endings branch to form loops and rings existing as either large compact endings or terminal fibrillar expansions in adventitia or at the border of adventitia and media between muscle cells, elastic, and collagen fibers in the vessel walls; a few endings terminate in the media. The actual end organ anatomy of baroreceptors is speculative, as there are no recordings of intracellular activity in stretch sensitive endings whose anatomy has been described. Impulse activity in both A and C fiber afferent pathways is generated by changes in pressure or, more correctly, the resulting stretch and tension in vessel walls. Unmyelinated baroreceptor afferents greatly outnumber myelinated fibers. Carotid baroreceptor afferents course in the carotid sinus nerve to the glossopharyngeal or IX cranial nerve in most species; their cell bodies are in the *petrosal ganglion*. Afferents from the aortic arch are located in either a separate aortic depressor pathway or as part of the common vagus (cranial nerve X) bundle of nerves; cell bodies of aortic baroreceptor afferents are in the *nodose ganglion*.

Primary baroreceptor afferent fibers terminate mainly in the ipsilateral NTS and, to a lesser extent, in the paramedian reticular nucleus and area postrema. As noted earlier, there are secondary projections to the pontoreticular region (cVLM and rVLM), nucleus ambiguus, and dorsal motor nucleus of the vagus (Spyer, 1990).

Reflex Cardiovascular Responses

Experimental studies in animals have shown that electrical stimulation or the more physiological maneuver of stretching the vessel wall containing these endings, most commonly resulting from an increase in blood pressure, leads to negative chronotropic and inotropic events, systemic arteriolar and venular vasodilation, as well as changes in the rate of secretion of vasopressin. In the intact animal, the resulting decrease in blood pressure opposes the original change in transmural pressure and reduces baroreceptor stimulation, hence leading to the term *closed loop negative feedback reflex* (Fig. 36.10) (Sagawa, 1983).

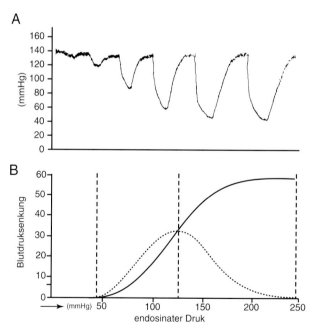

FIGURE 36.10 Reflex decreases in blood pressure in response to graded increases in carotid sinus pressure in an open loop anesthetized rabbit preparation following transection of contralateral sinus nerve and both vagi (A). The stimulus–response curve or *Blutdruckcharakteristik* shows the threshold, optimal, and saturation pressures (vertical lines from left to right) and its slope or baroreflex gain as carotid sinus pressure is increased (B). Note that gain of this negative feedback reflex is maximal at the midportion of the curve (Koch, 1931).

Chronotropic Responses

Decreased heart rate, in response to increased blood pressure, is a function of an immediate increase in vagal motor tone and a slower decrease in sympathetic activity, depending on the initial heart rate. At low basal or resting heart rates, with significant parasympathetic and little sympathetic tone, the decrease in heart rate is chiefly a function of a further increase in vagal activity. At high heart rates, both increased parasympathetic activity and withdrawal of sympathetic activity contribute to the decrease in heart rate. Conversely, arterial hypotension with underlying low heart rates leads to reflex increases in heart rate, largely from an immediate decrease in vagal efferent activity and more slowly from enhanced sympathetic activity; at high heart rates the baroreceptor-mediated positive chronotropic response is predominately a function of increased sympathetic activity.

Baroreflex sensitivity in human subjects (see Box 36.3) is increased at slow heart rates and during expiration, providing a partial explanation for sinus arrhythmia (Mark and Mancia, 1983). The influence of respiration on baroreflex sensitivity continuously oscillates throughout the respiratory cycle, either from interaction of the central respiratory generators with the reflex or from the influence of changes in arterial P_{CO_2} on the reflex–heart rate response. Changes in vagal activity in humans mediate heart rate responses to increased carotid simus pressure (after 200–600 ms latency), whereas changes in vagal and sympathetic efferent activity cause chronotropic changes during carotid sinus hypotension. Slowing of the heart rate depends on the timing of carotid sinus stimulation relative to the cardiac cycle and the duration of stimulation, with maximal changes occurring 750 ms before the P wave and with stimuli lasting 1.25 s. Such phasic enhancement and rapid adaptation provide a substantial advantage of the reflex to regulate beat-to-beat changes in the heart rate. Temporal summation occurs during maintained stimulation of the reflex and provides prolonged control of the heart rate. However, even a single brief stimulation can cause a chronotropic response that outlasts the stimulus as a result of central or effector organ prolongation of the reflex.

Dromotropic Responses

Arterial baroreceptors, through a vagal mechanism, provide tonic input to the A-V region of the cardiac conduction system, thereby influencing conduction through the His bundle in response to increases or decreases in pressure. This mechanism coordinates conduction between the upper and the lower chambers of the heart as heart rate varies, presumably to optimize preload and stroke volume. The influence of baroreceptors on atrial and ventricular conduction (both bundle branches and the Purkinje system), however, is much more modest or nonexistent.

Inotropic Responses

Baroreceptor-mediated changes in sympathetic tone lead directly to correspondingly large changes in myocardial ventricular contractility, whereas small reciprocal changes in myocardial function occur during changes in vagal motor activity. The contrasting influences of sympathetic and vagal efferent activity on inotropic performance are largely a function of differences in the degree of innervation of the ventricles by the two systems. In conscious animals, baroreflexes control myocardial contractility to a

---

BOX 36.3

METHODS OF STUDYING BAROREFLEXES IN HUMANS

The role of carotid sinus baroreceptors has been defined in humans largely through use of a neck suction/pressure device, which selectively loads or unloads this region. This technique generally has been confirmed by studies employing pharmacologic vasodilation or vasoconstriction. However, the latter methods simultaneously influence carotid and aortic regions, in addition to cardiopulmonary baroreceptors. Furthermore, this method is limited to studies of heart rate, as blood pressure is the independently manipulated variable. In contrast to the carefully controlled studies of the carotid sinus region, the role of aortic arch baroreceptors in humans is less well defined, mainly because no good methods are available to selectively stimulate these sensory nerve endings.

John C. Longhurst

small degree, if at all, presumably because there is correspondingly greater vagal tone in this condition compared to anesthetized preparations.

Regional Vascular Responses

Studies in animals and humans have examined the influence of high-pressure baroreceptors on regional vascular resistance (Sagawa, 1983). Baroreceptors in animals strongly regulate arterial vascular resistance in skeletal muscle and splanchnic regions. Similarly, carotid baroreceptors regulate skeletal muscle circulation, particularly during dynamic changes in transmural sinus pressure (Mark and Mancia, 1983). There is greater baroreflex-mediated regulation of leg vascular resistance in anesthetized compared to unanesthetized humans. Arterial baroreceptors control splanchnic vascular resistance in conscious but not in anesthetized human subjects. These studies indicate that anesthesia, presumably through its action on central vasomotor centers, variably enhances or blunts the influence of baroreceptors on regional vascular resistance. Arterial baroreceptors do not regulate either cutaneous sympathetic activity or arterial resistance, although more studies in this area are warranted. Such studies are difficult because multiunit recordings of cutaneous sympathetic activity monitor sudomotor and thermoregulatory as well as vasomotor fibers.

Integrated Cardiovascular Responses

The combination of decreased heart rate and myocardial contractility in response to arterial hypertension reduces cardiac output. Along with these changes in cardiac pump function, increased baroreceptor activity leads to the withdrawal of sympathetic tone to arteries and veins, causing corresponding increases in caliber of both resistance and capacitance vessels. Thus, increased arterial baroreceptor afferent activity in response to hypertension leads to reflex arterial vasodilation, which, along with the decreased cardiac output, returns blood pressure back to normal. Concurrent venodilation, in most animal species studied, reduces venous return and cardiac preload. In contrast to observations in animal preparations, human studies of baroreflex function have not documented significant changes in central venous pressure nor sustained changes in cutaneous venomotor tone (Mark and Mancia, 1983). Reduced stimulation of carotid baroreceptors, through decreases in sinus transmural pressure, leads to reflex arterial vasoconstriction, thereby demonstrating tonic regulation of vascular resistance by these receptors. In this

manner, high-pressure baroreceptors help maintain systemic arterial pressure around a set point. In humans, the influence of carotid baroreflex deactivation on arterial blood pressure is almost 50% greater than baroreflex activation. Conversely, the reflex influence of carotid baroreceptors on heart rate has been found to be greater with stimulation compared to inhibition of the reflex. In contrast with the immediate influence on heart rate, the latency of response of blood pressure to baroreceptor stimulation is long (3 s) and the response is prolonged (10–30 s), reflecting the slower onset and offset of sympathetic and effector organ responses vs vagal system, i.e., vascular smooth muscle vs cardiac sinoatrial node. Finally, the adrenal medulla does not play an important role in reflex vascular responses to carotid baroreceptor stimulation or inactivation in humans.

Baroreflex Interactions

Significant interactions exist between the right and left baroreceptor regions and between carotid and aortic regions (Sagawa, 1983). For example, summation of reflex responses occurs between bilateral carotid sinus inputs. This summation is nonlinear and becomes inhibitory at high intrasinus pressures as a result of central neural occlusion. At low intrasinus pressures, the interaction is facilitatory. Likewise, there is interaction between inputs from the carotid sinus and aortic arch baroreceptors. Contingent on the underlying experimental conditions, mild inhibitory, additive or even facilitatory responses have been observed.

Effective Stimuli

Carotid sinus and aortic arch baroreceptors respond to changes in mean pressure, pulse pressure, and the rate of rise of blood pressure (Fig. 36.11). Hence, they demonstrate dynamic sensitivity with greater responsiveness on the rising phase and decreased frequency on the falling phase of the sinusoidal pressure–response curve (Sagawa, 1983). Discharge activity adapts rapidly to maintained arterial pressure due to viscoelastic properties of the vascular wall but remains constant above 70 mm Hg. Aortic arch stretch receptors have a higher threshold, but once activated, they exhibit similar sensitivity as mechanosensitive receptors in the carotid sinus region.

Much more information currently is available on mechanisms of activation of myelinated compared to unmyelinated baroreceptor sensory nerve fibers and most comments mentioned earlier refer to the former

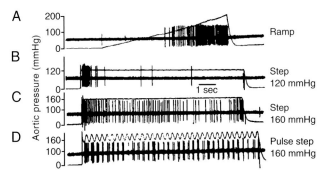

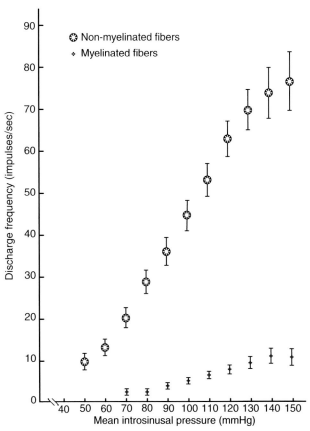

FIGURE 36.11 Responses of an unmyelinated aortic baroreceptor afferent fiber to ramp (A) and step changes in mean arterial pressure (B and C) and to phasic changes in blood pressure (D). The fiber demonstrated sparse activity at low pressures and irregular discharge activity as pressure was increased that became more constant as higher pressures were achieved. Pulse changes in pressure caused synchronous activity (Thoren and Jones, 1977).

group. However, fundamental differences between these two sets of afferents include a higher threshold, relatively reduced responsiveness, i.e., sensitivity to changes in intravascular pressure, more irregular discharge, and lower maximal frequency of discharge activity of C vs A fibers (Fig. 36.12). Thus, unmyelinated baroreceptor afferents are not very active under basal conditions. In contrast, the threshold for discharge of most myelinated baroreceptor afferents is near resting mean arterial blood pressure.

FIGURE 36.12 Adapted discharge frequency of myelinated and unmyelinated baroreceptor fibers from rabbit carotid sinus during changes in arterial blood pressure (Yao and Thoren, 1983).

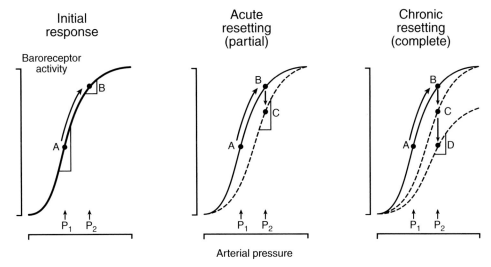

FIGURE 36.13 Acute and chronic resetting of arterial baroreceptors in response to a sustained increase in arterial blood pressure. Note that the immediate response occurring after seconds to minutes (C in middle panel) to an increase in blood pressure is to partially restore the increase in discharge frequency, whereas the complete response occurring after days to weeks (D in right panel) completely restores the activity to control (A in all panels) (Chapleau et al., 1989).

Adaptive Responses

A fundamental property of arterial baroreceptors is their ability to reset (Fig. 36.13). *Resetting*, as defined originally by McCubbin, means that myelinated (or unmyelinated) afferents respond similarly after they have been subjected to a higher (or lower) pressure for a period of time (McCubbin *et al.*, 1956; Chapleau *et al.*, 1991; Sagawa, 1983; Mark and Mancia, 1983). Alternatively, resetting can be defined as a shift in the relationship between arterial pressure and reflex hemodynamic or autonomic response. Thus, resetting translates into a shift of the pressure–discharge curve. The period required to induce this phenomenon may be as little as 15–30 min (acute resetting) and the response is promptly reversible; alternatively, it can take several hours or days (chronic resetting) and then is slowly reversible or is irreversible. Wall viscoelastic (creep/stress relaxation) and possibly changes in myogenic tone underlie acute resetting, whereas changes in wall structure are involved in chronic resetting. However, alterations in the afferents themselves, perhaps caused by changes in the biophysical properties of the sensory nerve membranes, such as ionic mechanisms or local release of substances from the endothelium and even resetting in the central nervous system, may be alter-native explanations for this phenomenon. Central resetting is defined by changes in the neural–humoral response observed during the direct stimulation of afferent nerves. Although inhibition of central processing has been observed most commonly, paradoxical central facilitation can occur and may oppose central inhibition for a period of time. With the exception of some of the localized vascular changes that lead to resetting at the receptor level, other potentially important mechanisms underlying peripheral neuronal resetting have not been defined and there is little information on the mechanisms and anatomical regions involved in central resetting.

Influence of Chemical Stimuli on Baroreflex

Although arterial baroreceptors respond primarily to changes in blood pressure, including both changes in stretch and tension, and hence function as mechanoreceptors, their function can be modified by changes in the regional chemical environment. For instance, circulating catecholamines or low concentrations of catecholamines released locally from adrenergic nerve endings constrict vascular smooth muscle and hence unload baroreceptor nerve endings (Sagawa, 1983; Chapleau *et al.*, 1991). Conversely, high concentrations

---

BOX 36.4

EFFECT OF EXERCISE ON BAROREFLEX ACTIVITY

The baroreflex accommodates normal physiological functions such as exercise when it is beneficial to maintain arterial pressure during the tremendous metabolic vasodilation in active skeletal muscle. Early studies suggested that the baroreceptor distension–response curve is shifted to the right during exercise, resulting in less discharge activity at any given blood pressure (Mark and Mancia, 1983). This observation has been challenged. Current opinion is that the sympathoadrenergic control of heart and blood vessels by baroreceptors either is not affected by exercise or that only specific components of the reflex are modified. In this regard, most studies in humans have identified no change in baroreflex sensitivity or resetting to a higher level blood pressure. Consistent with human studies, evidence in animals suggests that there is little shift in carotid sinus–blood pressure or heart rate responses during exercise. Specifically, the blood pressure portion of the cardiovascular response is similar during exercise in intact and baro-denervated animals and in humans. In contrast, a number studies have observed that the baroreflex control of heart rate is suppressed during exercise, as vagally mediated transient bradycardia is strongly inhibited by exercise. In this regard, the heart rate response during baroreceptor stimulation in humans is reset during static but not during dynamic exercise. Thus, the baroreflex–heart rate relationship either is unchanged or is reduced depending on the species studied and the type of exercise imposed. Modification of the arterial baroreflex does not appear to be essential for the hemodynamic response to mild or moderate exercise. The one exception may be attenuation of baroreflex inhibition of the chronotropic response during static exercise in humans.

John C. Longhurst

Reference

Mark, A. L., and Mancia, G. (1983), Cardiopulmonary baroreflexes in humans. *In* "Handbook of Physiology" (J. T. Shepherd, F. M. Abboud, and S. R. Geiger, eds.), Vol. III, pp. 795–813. American Physiological Society, Bethesda.

of catecholamines directly excite myelinated and particularly unmyelinated baroreceptor afferents. A number of other substances, such as atrial natriuretic factor, substance P, and vasopressin, influence baroreceptor activity largely through their action on vascular smooth muscle. Several *paracrine factors,* including nitric oxide, prostacyclin, reactive oxygen species, and various platelet-derived substances, modulate baroreceptor sensitivity by altering the excitability of nerve endings (Chapleau, 2001). Stretch, shear stress, and chemical substances may alter the discharge activity of myelinated baroreceptor nerve endings by stimulating the release of nitric oxide or prostacyclin from the vascular endothelium. However, baroreceptors can also be sensitized by prostaglandins independent of any change in mechanical deformation. Sensitization of mechanosensitive sensory endings by endogenous chemicals is not unique to baroreceptors. Group III somatic endings that respond mainly to mechanical events in muscle during contraction can also be sensitized by paracrine factors (see Boxes 36.2 and 36.4).

Several hormonal systems, including *angiotensin, arginine vasopressin,* and *atrial natriuretic factor* (ANF), strongly influence the vascular system and end organ function, such as the contribution of the kidney to body fluid balance. These hormones also influence blood pressure by regulating sympathetic tone, in part, through their effects on the baroreflex. Both angiotensin and vasopressin are potent vasoconstrictors. Angiotensin also has many actions in the peripheral and central nervous system. Angiotensin facilitates the activation of sympathetic ganglia and stimulates the adrenal medulla to increase the release of norepinephrine and epinephrine. Angiotensin also decreases baroreflex sensitivity (thereby facilitating its ability to increase blood pressure) through a central action on several *circumventricular organs* devoid of tight endothelial junctions that form the blood–brain barrier. These include the area postrema in the hindbrain, subfornical organ (SFO), anteroventral third ventricle (AV3V), and especially the organum vasculosum of the lamina terminalis and median preoptic nucleus (MNO) in the forebrain. Vasopressin acts on V_1 receptors in the area postrema to inhibit sympathetic outflow during baroreflex activation. In this manner, vasopressin facilitates the baroreceptor reflex. ANF also reduces sympathetic activity. Although controversial, ANF appears to stimulate cardiopulmonary afferents (see later) to suppress baroreflex function and promote sodium excretion by the kidney. The AV3V region is critical for fluid and electrolyte balance and likely participates as part of a long loop supramedullary pathway in the baroreflex (Dampney, 1994).

Baroreflexes in Health and Disease

The primary function of the arterial baroreflex system is to oppose changes in blood pressure (Longhurst, 1982). This system is particularly important during changes in orthostatic stress, for instance, upon assumption of the upright from the supine position. Under normal circumstances, baroreceptor endings sense changes in arterial blood pressure upon standing and prevent syncope by increasing heart rate, cardiac output, and peripheral vascular resistance. Individuals who have a defect in the baroreflex arc, e.g., in multiple systems atrophy, have a great deal of difficulty in withstanding *orthostatic challenges.* Under extreme changes in blood pressure, such as during shock resulting from a number of different disorders, e.g., 20% *hemorrhage,* baroreceptors can restore total peripheral resistance by 50–70% and can increase heart rate sufficiently to increase cardiac output by 20–25%. In these circumstances, carotid baroreceptors may be quantatively more important than aortic baroreceptors, as the threshold for reflex activation, with respect to the regulation of regional vascular resistance, is higher for mechanoreceptors in the arch region than in the sinus (100 mm Hg vs 60 mm Hg). As hemorrhage progresses, other stretch receptors in the cardiopulmonary region and both central and peripheral chemoreceptors (see later) responding to changes in central filling pressures and blood gases or pH, respectively, contribute to increased sympathetic activity. Ultimately, in profound shock when blood pressure and acid–base balance are disordered profoundly, baroreflexes fail and can even contribute to the terminal bradycardia and demise.

Abnormal baroreceptor function can also occur in both humans and animal models of disease and may contribute to the pathogenesis of certain disorders such as *hypertension* (Mark and Mancia, 1983; Oparil et al., 1991). Reduced baroreflex function does not initiate hypertension, as denervation of both carotid and aortic afferent pathways does not lead to sustained hypertension. However, baroreceptors adapt in chronic hypertension because the blood pressure–afferent nerve activity relationship is reset downward and to the right. Resetting to a higher set point prevents baroreceptor opposition of a higher blood pressure. Decreased elastin and increased collagen in the media of the walls of vessels reduce vascular compliance. Increased vascular stiffness in hypertensive animals reduces stretch of mechanosensitive nerve endings in response to increased arterial pressure. Similarly, as stiffening of vessels occurs in advancing age, baroreflex function is reduced in both humans and animals (Mark and Mancia, 1983).

Baroreflex activity has been studied in a number of experimental models of hypertension. Spontaneously hypertensive rats (SHR) display abnormal central integration leading to central resetting. Renal hypertension caused by stenosis of the renal artery in rabbits leads to an early impairment of aortic baroreflex–heart rate and sympathetic nerve reflex responses that originate from the dysfunction of baroreceptor endings. After a longer period (>6 weeks), central neural impairment contributes to the baroreflex abnormality in the renal hypertension model. Dahl-S, salt-sensitive hypertensive rats demonstrate centrally impaired baroreflex function manifested even before the onset of hypertension. This observation has led to the suggestion that there is a genetic defect. Deoxycorticosterone acetate (DOCA) salt-sensitive rats also demonstrate abnormalities in aortic baroreflex function before the onset of hypertension. Studies in both humans and rats suggest that the aortic baroreflex is more impaired than the carotid baroreflex. Studies in humans suggest that the heart rate component is affected more profoundly by hypertension than the blood pressure response, indicating that the baroreflex control of parasympathetic activity is more influenced than sympathetic activity. In addition to abnormalities in transducer function and afferent discharge in hypertension, central resetting also occurs in humans. The mechanisms underlying central neural resetting are unknown at present.

Patients with *congestive heart failure* (CHF) also experience reduced baroreflex function (Zucker, 1991). One potential mechanism for depressed baroreceptor afferent activity is retained salt and water that decreases the compliance (increases stiffness) of vessel walls. Because there is an interaction between arterial and cardiopulmonary baroreflexes, physiological and pathological alterations of the heart, particularly in the atria, may influence reflex response to changes in arterial pressure.

The syndrome of *carotid sinus hypersensitivity* is thought to be related to local and systemic diseases in the region of the carotid bifurcation (Longhurst, 1982). Thus, tumors, extensive atherosclerosis, digitalis intoxication, and Takayasu's arteritis, among other conditions, can lead to profound bradycardia, arteriolar vasodilation, or a combination of the two, and recurrent syncope or presyncope can develop.

PERIPHERAL ARTERIAL CHEMORECEPTORS

Anatomy

Arterial chemoreceptors are located primarily in two regions along the great vessels: in the *carotid bodies* at the bifurcation of the common carotid arteries and in the *aortic bodies* in the wall of the aortic arch (Biscoe, 1971; Gonzalez *et al.*, 1994). These receptors are present as clumps of *glomus* tissue that are perfused with a high blood flow by branches of the carotid artery or aorta. Chemoreceptors are known as glomera because they contain extensive capillary networks. In addition to their high flow, a characteristic feature of carotid (and presumably aortic) bodies is their very high oxygen consumption, which is four times higher than brain. Glomus tissue is composed of two cell types: type I (glomus or chemoreceptor) and type II (sustentacular, satellite, or supporting) cells. Type I cells, which account for >75% of all cells in glomus tissue, are secretory, contain various catecholamines, and are heavily innervated by sensory nerves. Although type II cells are closely associated with type I cells, they are not innervated directly; rather, they encircle unmyelinated nerve fibers. Sympathetic and parasympathetic efferent fibers innervate blood vessels as well as type I and II cells. Carotid body parenchymal cells are essential for chemotransduction, although afferent nerve endings themselves may have chemosensitive properties.

Afferents from the carotid body course in the carotid sinus (*Hering's*) *nerve*, a branch of the glossopharyngeal (IX cranial) nerve; cell bodies of carotid body sensory afferents are located in the petrosal (Andersch's) and, to a smaller extent, superior cervical (Erenritter's) ganglia (Eyzaguirre *et al.*, 1983). Sensory innervation of the aortic bodies travels in the aortic depressor (*Cyon's*) *nerve*, a branch of the vagus (X cranial) nerve, whose perikarya are located in the nodose ganglion. Both A and C fiber chemoreceptor afferents exist. Unmyelinated afferents project to the lateral NTS at levels rostral to the obex or to the medial and commissural NTS, caudal to the obex. Most chemoreceptor afferents terminate caudal to the obex, whereas baroreceptor afferents terminate mainly rostral to the obex. Chemoreceptor input in NTS excites inspiratory neurons in the ventrolateral subnucleus and converges with baroreceptor inputs on nonrespiratory neurons in both the ventrolateral subnucleus and the neighboring reticular formation. Direct chemoreceptor inputs from the NTS project to rVLM where, along with cVLM-routed signals from baroreceptors, they converge on common sympathoexcitatory premotor neurons (Spyer, 1990, 1994; Dampney, 1994).

Effective Stimuli

Carotid and aortic body chemoreceptors are stimulated by isolated decreases in the partial pressure of oxygen (PaO$_2$), with a threshold beginning ~85 mm Hg, and increases in the partial pressure of carbon

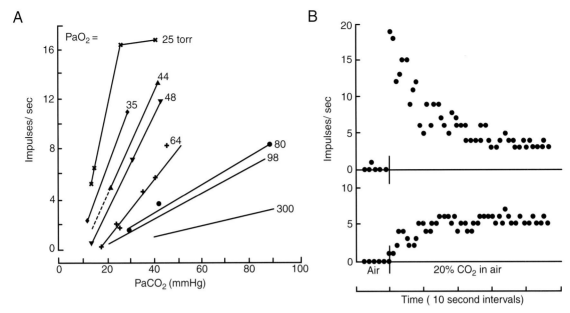

FIGURE 36.14 Response of single carotid body chemoreceptor fibers to increases in arterial P_{CO_2} (A). Note that the response is diminished as P_{O_2} is increased. Inhibition of carbonic anhydrase, which prevents the production of H^+, reduces the immediate but not the more delayed response to a step increase in P_{CO_2} (B) (McCloskey, 1968).

dioxide (Pa_{CO_2}) (Gonzalez *et al.*, 1994; Eyzaguirre *et al.*, 1983). Although stimulation of chemosensitive nerve endings by changes in Pa_{CO_2} occurs largely through carbonic anhydrase-mediated changes in H^+, CO_2 can also exert a direct effect on these sensory endings. Weak responses of aortic chemoreceptors to Pa_{CO_2}, are in sharp contrast with robust carotid body responses. However, at low Pa_{O_2} levels, aortic body afferents respond more vigorously to CO_2 (Fig. 36.14). Aortic chemoreceptors are stimulated less than carotid body chemoreceptors by changes in Pa_{O_2} (Fig. 36.15). Maneuvers that influence local Pa_{O_2}, e.g., changes in arterial O_2 content in response to carboxy-hemoglobinemia (aortic chemoreceptors), arterial hypotension (aortic chemoreceptors), or sympathetic vasoconstriction, which reduces local blood flow, increase afferent discharge activity. Conversely, stimulation of parasympathetic nerves to the carotid body reduces afferent discharge activity, either through an increase in blood flow or release of a local neurotransmitter like dopamine from type I cells. The circumstances in which autonomic input to carotid and aortic bodies modifies chemoreceptor stimulation have not been defined.

Peripheral chemoreceptors respond not only to changes in Pa_{O_2}, Pa_{CO_2}, and pH, but also are strongly stimulated by other chemicals, such as lobeline, nicotine, and cyanide (Eyzaguirre *et al.*, 1983). The latter three stimuli have been used extensively in experimental studies of chemoreceptor function. Both sets

of chemoreceptors also respond to changes in blood temperature and plasma osmolality. Their *thermosensitivity* may be explained by their high Q_{10} (75) and a high mean energy of activation (81.5 kcal/mol), which have been measured *in vitro* under basal conditions (50% O_2 in N_2). The high Q_{10} value may represent multiplication of a series of reactions, each with a low individual Q_{10}. With respect to their function as *osmoreceptors*, vasopressin (antidiuretic hormone, ADH) is released in response to either electrical stimulation of the carotid sinus nerve or hypoxic stimulation of the carotid body. For example, chemoreflex increases in blood temperature and plasma osmolality during prolonged exercise increase plasma ADH, which assists in reducing renal blood flow.

Receptor Mechanisms

A number of hypotheses of chemoreception of the carotid body have been advanced (Eyzaguirre *et al.*, 1983). These include stimulation by neurotransmitters or neuromodulators such as acetylcholine, dopamine, epinephrine, and norepinephrine, mechanosensation of sensory endings, perhaps related to sustentacular-induced changes in tension, pH sensitivity of chemoreceptor nerve endings, an O_2-binding protein or chromophore in glomus cells, or an intracellular metabolic influence on generator potentials in the nerve endings.

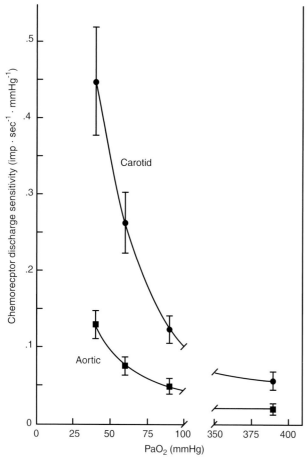

FIGURE 36.15 Sensitivity of aortic and carotid body chemoreceptors to arterial hypoxia. Compared to the discharge activity of the carotid chemoreceptors, there is a smaller response of the aortic chemoreceptors at all levels of arterial P_{O_2} (Lahiri *et al.*, 1981).

Reflex Cardiovascular Responses

Although the best known effect of these receptors is on respiration, stimulation of peripheral chemoreceptors both directly and indirectly influences the cardiovascular system (Biscoe, 1971; Marshall, 1994; Eyzaguirre *et al.*, 1983). Ventilation is increased by the stimulation of aortic or carotid body chemoreceptors, although more profound responses result from the stimulation of carotid bodies. In the intact animal, stimulation of carotid body evokes reflex hyperventilation, tachycardia, increased myocardial contractility and cardiac output, and decreased systemic vascular resistance (Fig. 36.16). When ventilation is controlled, the stimulation of carotid bodies consistently causes reflex bradycardia, decreased cardiac output, and increased total peripheral resistance. In contrast to the reflex response from carotid bodies, stimulation of aortic bodies with cyanide or nicotine while respiration is controlled causes tachycardia and hyper-

tension, resulting from increases in cardiac contractility and vasoconstriction of both veins and arteries (Fig. 36.17). Thus, the direct influence of chemoreceptor stimulation on the cardiovascular system is affected profoundly by their influence on respiration. The secondary reflex, caused by the stimulation of pulmonary stretch receptors, reverses the direct influence of the carotid chemoreceptors on the cardiovascular system. In addition, increased ventilation during chemoreceptor stimulation, e.g., with hypoxia, reduces arterial P_{CO_2}, which serves to further increase cardiac output and possibly modulate the reduced systemic vascular resistance.

Peripheral chemoreceptors are responsible for arterial hypertension and venoconstriction present in hypoxemia, although there may also be a direct effect of hypoxia on CNS chemoreceptors to facilitate reflex vasoconstriction. The vasoconstrictor response to systemic hypoxia is modified to some extent by the direct effect of low P_{O_2} in relaxing vascular smooth muscle. Despite some species variation, carotid and aortic chemoreceptors generally cause vasoconstriction in skeletal muscle, kidney, and intestine and vasodilation in skin, although this latter observation is controversial (Eyzaguirre *et al.*, 1983; Marshall, 1994). Chemoreceptor stimulation has been suggested to cause coronary vasodilation by increasing coronary parasympathetic efferent activity, although again there is controversy, as sinoaortic denervation does not alter the increase in coronary blood flow. In concert with the systemic responses noted earlier, regional vasoconstriction observed in most circulations is reduced or reversed during arterial chemoreceptor stimulation when ventilation is allowed to increase. Peripheral chemoreceptors do not regulate brain blood flow. Most neurophysiological studies involving physiological and pharmacological stimuli of peripheral chemoreceptors have been conducted in cats and rabbits, whereas investigation of the reflex circulatory adjustments to chemoreceptor stimulation has been conducted in dogs and, to a lesser extent, in rabbits. Species differences in cardiovascular responses to chemoreceptor stimulation have been noted; extrapolation of cardiovascular responses to chemoreceptor stimulation across species should thus be made with caution.

CARDIAC RECEPTORS

In 1866, Cyon and Ludwig first demonstrated a cardiovascular depressor reflex originating from pressure-sensitive nerve endings in the heart. One year later, von Bezold and Hirt documented a fall in heart rate and blood pressure following intravenous injec-

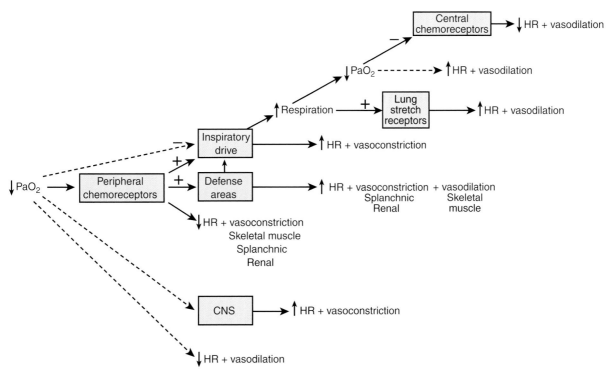

FIGURE 36.16 Cardiovascular and respiratory responses induced by systemic hypoxia. The responses are a composite of influence of low arterial P_{O_2} on the peripheral chemoreceptors and their influence on both respiratory and cardiovascular centers in the brain stem (solid arrows), as well as direct effects of low P_{O_2} on the CNS and effector organs, including the heart and blood vessels (dotted arrows) (Marshall, 1994).

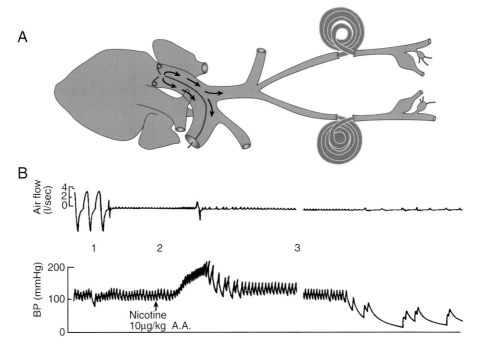

FIGURE 36.17 Influence of nicotine injected into the root of the aorta (A) on aortic bodies and carotid bodies after a delay (using interposed coils of tubing) on arterial blood pressure (B). Apnea was produced at 1 with a neuromuscular antagonist (succinylcholine) to eliminate the confounding influence of ventilatory changes caused by stimulation of the chemoreceptors. The aortic body response included tachycardia and hypertension, whereas the carotid body response consisted of bradycardia and hypotension (Comroe and Mortimer, 1964).

tion of veratridine, a response that was abolished by vagotomy. The hypotensive response to veratridine was confirmed to be of cardiac origin by Jarisch and Richter in 1939. Over time, this cardiac chemoreflex has been named the von *Bezold–Jarisch reflex*. In 1933, Adrian was the first to record discharge activity of mechanosensitive cardiac afferents in the vagus nerve. In 1948, Whitteridge observed that many vagal afferent fibers innervating atria and pulmonary veins were unmyelinated C fibers. Dawes and Comroe, in 1954, implicated the left ventricle as an additional source for cardiac depressor reflexes. Although the chemoreflex is the main stimulus for the reflex response to coronary injection of veratridine, Paintal in 1955 provided evidence that the response originates partly from cardiac mechanosensitive receptors with vagal afferent pathways. Presently, cardiac receptors are designated anatomically as either atrial or ventricular receptors. The term *cardiopulmonary baroreceptors* is used frequently to describe reflex events that arise from the four cardiac chambers as well as great veins and possibly other vessels in the lungs. Cardiac vagal afferents first synapse in the medial subnucleus of the NTS. Like arterial baroreceptors, second-order cardiac reflex pathways project from the NTS to the cVLM (via glutaminergic synapses), which in turn sends GABAergic projections to sympathetic premotor neurons in the rVLM.

Atrial Receptors and Reflexes

Receptive fields of myelinated afferents are located in the venoatrial junctions with afferent connections to the CNS principally coursing through the vagus nerve (Hainsworth, 1991; Linden and Kappagoda, 1982). These sensory endings are stimulated by stretch and often fire either in late systole just after the upstroke of the aortic pressure wave (type B recep-

tors) or just before the start of the atrial *a* wave (type A receptors). Discharge activity of the type B receptors tends to reflect atrial volume, whereas type A receptors are influenced more by heart rate. Thus, while the rate of firing of type A receptors generally is maximal for each cardiac cycle, type B receptors operate over a range of discharge frequencies (Fig. 36.18). Still other myelinated atrial afferents display both type A and B patterns of discharge activity.

In 1915, Bainbridge described a reflex increase in the heart rate in dogs in response to an infusion of saline, which is most prominent at low basal heart rates. Interestingly, despite the positive chronotropic response that originates from the activation of myelinated afferents, arterial pressure, systemic vascular resistance, and myocardial contractility do not change consistently upon stimulation of veno–atrial junctions by distending small intravascular balloons in this species. Despite the absence of change in vascular resistance during localized veno–atrial distension, obstruction of the mitral valve causes hindlimb vasoconstriction. Furthermore, distension of the entire left atrium with a balloon leads to bradycardia and a depressor response followed by tachycardia and a pressor response. The latter two maneuvers likely stimulate all types of atrial and pulmonary mechanosensitive receptors. Unmyelinated atrial vagal and sympathetic afferents also innervate atria, but their physiologic function is uncertain. Several studies have failed to document the Bainbridge reflex in humans.

Atrial Reflexes in Humans

Mild lower-body negative pressure (LBNP; see Box 36.5) reduces blood flow in both skin and muscle but has a smaller effect on splanchnic resistance vessels (Fig. 36.19) (Mark and Mancia, 1983). This latter observation contrasts with the strong influence that carotid baroreceptors have on splanchnic circulation. LBNP does not reliably influence veins in the extremities, although moderate hemorrhage reflexly decreases splanchnic capacitance. Despite the absence of a chronotropic response to volume loading, activation of cardiac chemoreceptors (i.e., the Bezold–Jarisch reflex) causes profound reflex bradycardia in humans. This latter response has implications for patients undergoing cardiac catheterization for coronary angiography. In addition, there is evidence for interaction between cardiopulmonary and other reflexes. For example, arterial depressor baroreflex function is facilitated by unloading volume receptors in the heart and lungs of humans with low-level

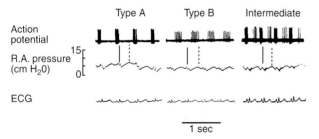

FIGURE 36.18　Type A, B, and intermediate atrial myelinated afferent patterns of discharge activity. Activity of type A receptors corresponded to the atrial *a* wave, whereas type B receptor activity occurred during the atrial *v* wave. Receptors with an intermediate response coincided with both *a* and *v* waves (Kappagoda *et al.*, 1976).

BOX 36.5

METHODS OF STUDY OF ATRIAL REFLEXES IN HUMANS

Studies in humans have relied upon a number of methods to study cardiopulmonary receptors, some of which are selective whereas others are nonselective (Mark and Mancia, 1983). *Lower body negative pressure* (LBNP) simulates gravitational pooling of blood in the lower abdomen and extremities and unloads these low-pressure receptors. Several lines of evidence suggest that mild LBNP unloads receptors primarily in the left ventricle. However, at high LBNP, above -20 mm Hg, there is sufficient pooling to lower arterial blood pressure and hence influence arterial baroreceptors. Alternatives to LBNP include inflating cuffs around extremities, hemorrhage, head-up tilt, and the Valsalva maneuver.

Unfortunately, unlike mild LBNP, these latter techniques are associated with stimulation of a number of afferent systems, in addition to those in the cardiac region. Leg elevation and lower body positive pressure increase venous return and activate cardiopulmonary receptors.

John C. Longhurst

Reference

Mark, A. L., and Mancia, G. (1983). Cardiopulmonary baroreflexes in humans. *In* "Handbook of Physiology" (J. T. Shepherd, F. M. Abboud, and S. R. Geiger, eds.), Vol. III, pp. 795–813, American Physiological Society, Bethesda.

LBNP to remove their tonic inhibitory influence. Cardiopulmonary afferents also oppose the somatic pressor reflex during exercise.

Cardiopulmonary Regulation of the Kidney

Renin release and plasma vasopressin levels are decreased more during the stimulation of cardiopulmonary receptors than during the activation of arterial baroreceptors (Fig. 36.20) (Mark and Mancia, 1983). Atrial distension in experimental preparations increases urine flow largely through a vagal reflex that causes renal vasodilation and reduces the concentration of circulating ADH and, to a lesser extent, through the release of ANF. As noted previously, in addition to a direct effect on kidney, ANF also modulates sympathetic activity, perhaps through an influence on cardiopulmonary receptors or indirectly on the arterial baroreflex. In contrast to neurohumoral responses to atrial distension, hemorrhage in dogs increases plasma ADH through an influence of cardiac ventricular receptors. Currently there is no clear consensus on the relative importance of vagal cardiopulmonary vs ventricular receptors in the regulation of vasopressin, as there is substantial variability between species. For example, studies in subhuman primates have not clearly documented an atrial stretch reflex that controls renal excretion. Studies in humans are conflicting, although both renin and ADH are regulated to varying degrees by arterial and cardiopulmonary baroreceptors depending on the stimulus (LBNP vs head-up tilt). In addition, recumbent humans have nocturnal suppression of hypervolemia-induced renal excretion. Studies of cardiac transplant recipients, although complicated by the underlying disorder, which frequently includes renal dysfunction, tend to confirm an important role of cardiac reflexes in regulating renal function.

Cardiopulmonary receptors tonically inhibit cardiovascular sympathetic activity and release of renin from the kidney, effects that originate in part from the ventricles (Goetz *et al.*, 1991). Thus, cooling or transection of the vagus nerve increases heart rate, blood pressure, renal sympathetic activity, and vascular resistances in kidney, muscle, and intestine. Animal studies suggest that inactivation of the reflex influence of low-pressure receptors during hemorrhage influences renal more than hindlimb resistance; the converse is true during unloading high-pressure (carotid) baroreceptors. Ventricular receptors in humans primarily control muscle resistance vessels, whereas arterial baroreceptors exert more control of the splanchnic circulation (see later). Thus, although it is clear that cardiopulmonary receptors tonically regulate peripheral resistance vessels, there are both regional circulatory and species differences.

Ventricular Receptors and Reflexes

Ventricular sensory receptors generally exist as bare nerve endings situated in the interstitium. Finely myelinated ($A\delta$) or unmyelinated cardiac afferent fibers (C) project to the CNS through vagus or sympathetic (spinal) pathways (Longhurst, 1984). There is little difference in sensitivity between myelinated and unmyelinated cardiac afferents. Nerve endings can be

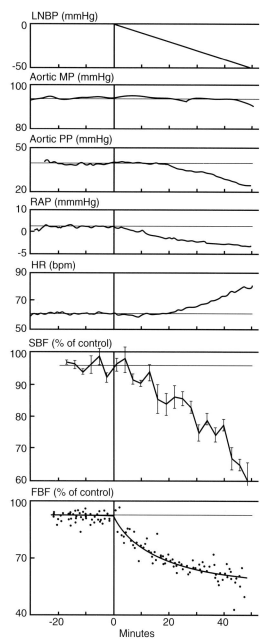

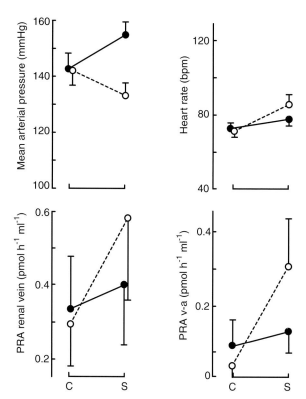

FIGURE 36.20 Contrasting responses of mean arterial pressure, heart rate, renal vein, and renal venous–arterial (v-a) plasma renin activity (PRA) to 5 min of head-up tilt to unload cardiopulmonary stretch receptors (open circles, dashed lines) or positive neck pressure to unload carotid sinus baroreceptors (closed circles, solid lines). Compared to the control state (C), unloading low-pressure cardiopulmonary receptors (S) decreased arterial pressure and reflexly increased heart rate and PRA. Conversely, reduced stimulation of high-pressure arterial baroreceptors reflexly increased blood pressure and heart rate but did not significantly influence PRA (Mancia *et al.*, 1978).

FIGURE 36.19 Effects of lower body negative pressure (LBNP) on aortic mean pressure (MP), aortic pulse pressure (PP), right atrial pressure (RAP), heart rate (HR), splanchnic blood flow (SBF), and forearm blood flow (FBF). Low-level LBNP (0–20 mm Hg) lowered venous return and RAP and, by unloading cardiopulmonary receptors, significantly decreased skin and muscle FBF and only a slight reduction in SBF. High-level LBNP (20–50 mm Hg), which reduced aortic PP and eventually aortic MP (and therefore also unloaded high-pressure arterial baroreceptors), increased HR and decreased both FBF and SBF (Johnson *et al.*, 1974).

mechanosensitive, chemosensitive, or bimodal in their sensitivity, with the latter two groups being most common. Within the physiologic pressure range, mechanosensitive cardiac C fibers respond mainly to

changes in ventricular diastolic pressure, suggesting that they may be more responsive to stretch than to compression. Convincing evidence in dogs, however, suggests that much of the reflex depressor response to changes in arterial pressure actually originates from coronary rather than from ventricular mechano-receptors. Ventricular chemosensitive C fibers respond not only to exogenous stimuli such as veratridine or contrast dye injected during angiographic procedures, but also to a number of endogenous chemical stimuli, many of which are produced during pathologic conditions such as ischemia and reperfusion (see Box 36.6). Of note, cardiac transplantation and myocardial infarction globally or regionally can interrupt ventricular afferent activity.

Reflex cardiovascular responses to stimulation of either mechano- or chemosensitive vagal endings are primarily inhibitory, resulting in reduced sympathetic nerve activity, depressor responses, and bradycardia.

BOX 36.6

FUNCTION AND RESPONSE OF CARDIAC RECEPTORS DURING MYOCARDIAL ISCHEMIA

Myocardial ischemia is associated with a number of mechanical and chemical changes in myocardium. The function of chemosensitive receptors in the heart has been studied more thoroughly. For instance, bradykinin is released, particularly during conditions of high sympathetic activity, reactive oxygen species are formed during ischemia and more so during reperfusion, and platelet activation during plaque rupture increases the regional concentration of 5-hydroxytryptamine (Longhurst et al., 2001). Prostaglandins also are released during ischemia. These cyclooxygenase products can either directly stimulate cardiac vagal afferents to induce a depressor response or, more likely, sensitize vagal and sympathetic cardiac afferents to the action of other metabolic factors such as bradykinin. Each of these chemical mediators leads to profound stimulation of both vagal and sympathetic cardiac afferents. Receptive fields of vagal afferents are located transmurally and in the inferior–posterior ventricle, whereas sympathetic afferents are located closer to the epicardial surface and more in the anterior left ventricle. Thus, ischemia and reperfusion involving the inferior surface of the heart are associated more commonly with vasodepressor reflex responses, bradyarrhythmias, nausea, and vomiting, whereas excitatory pressor responses, including pain (angina), peripheral vasoconstriction, and tachyarrhythmias, are associated more frequently with anterior ischemia and reperfusion. Depressor reflexes may reduce myocardial oxygen demand and thus lessen the

imbalance between supply and demand during ischemia. Conversely, in addition to the warning signs of angina, activation of sympathetic afferents improves coronary perfusion pressure and hence maintains myocardial blood flow. It is confusing to imagine, however, that two diametrically opposed reflexes are engendered by myocardial ischemia. Clearly, overactivity of either reflex could also result in untoward cardiac events by exaggerating ischemia, either through marked decreases in perfusion or through exaggerated increases in oxygen demand. It has been observed that simultaneous activation of both afferent pathways from the heart lessens the influence of either pathway alone due to neural occlusion that occurs in interneurons for the reflex pathways in the NTS and perhaps elsewhere (Fig. 36.21). While stimulation of ventricular sensory endings by endogenous chemical mediators almost certainly leads to complex but frequently observed clinical responses, the role of cardiac mechanoreceptor stimulation by changes in regional or global wall motion abnormalities is much less clear and deserves further study.

John C. Longhurst

Reference

Longhurst, J. C., Tjen-A-Looi, S., and Fu, L-W. (2001). Cardiac sympathetic afferent activation provoked by myocardial ischemia and reperfusion: Mechanisms and reflexes. *N.Y. Acad. Sci.*

Conversely, activation of sympathetic cardiac ventricular afferents reflexly excites the cardiovascular system, leading to an increase in blood pressure and heart rate (Fig. 36.21). Although stimulation of ventricular C fibers with vagal afferents causes bradycardia in anesthetized animals, heart rate is minimally altered in conscious animals and humans. Despite the absence of a direct effect of ventricular (or cardiopulmonary) receptors on chronotropic function, activation of ventricular vagal afferents attenuates baroreflex sensitivity and baroreflex control of heart rate.

Cardiac Reflexes in Disease

Cardiovascular reflexes originating from the atria and ventricles are associated with several clinical con-

ditions (Longhurst, 1984; Minisi and Thames, 1991). For example, high left ventricular pressures generated during stress in patients with *aortic stenosis* stimulates left ventricular mechanoreceptors with vagal afferents (and possibly chemosensitive receptors because of the subendocardial ischemia), thereby leading to peripheral vasodilation and occasionally syncope.

Another clinical condition attributed to the activation of cardiac afferents is the inappropriate diuresis associated with certain supraventricular tachyarrhythmias. In this regard, atrial fibrillation and other *paroxysmal supraventricular arrhythmias* lasting for 20 min or longer and associated with rates above 110 beats/min can be associated with substantial volume loss and orthostatic intolerance, likely because atrial type B receptors are activated by the asynchronous contraction and high atrial pressures

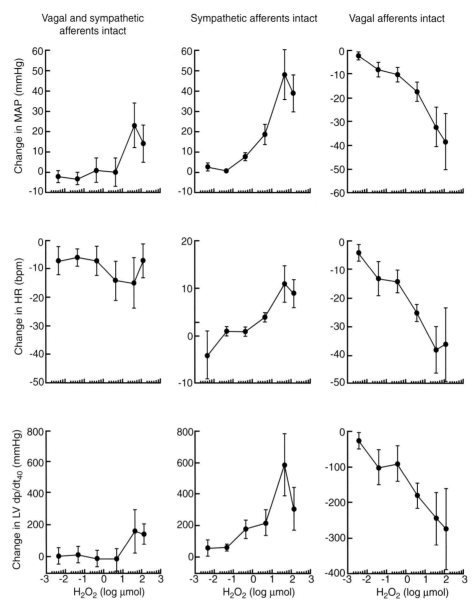

FIGURE 36.21 Changes in mean arterial pressure (MAP), heart rate (HR), and left ventricular dP/dt at 40 mm Hg developed pressure, as an index of myocardial contractile function, during stimulation of the epicardial surface of the heart with increasing concentrations of the reactive oxygen species, hydrogen peroxide (H_2O_2). Transection of both vagi to interrupt the afferents coursing in this pathway, leaving the sympathetic afferent system intact (middle panels), caused a concentration-dependent reflex pressor response in association with increases in heart rate, and myocardial contractility. Denervation of the sympathetic (spinal) afferent pathways from the heart, leaving the vagal afferent system intact (right panels), converted the response to reflex cardiovascular inhibition, consisting of graded reductions in blood pressure, heart rate, and myocardial contractility. Stimulation of the ventricle when both afferent pathways were intact (left panels) caused a small pressor response with little change in heart rate or contractility as a result of occlusive interaction in the NTS (Huang *et al.*, 1995).

associated with these conditions. The role of ANF in promoting diuresis during these arrhythmias also must be considered (Longhurst, 1984).

Although some pathological conditions such as myocardial ischemia and atrial tachyarrhythmias stimulate cardiac afferent nerve endings to engender

potentially deleterious cardiovascular reflex responses, other pathologic conditions modulate activity of these endings, much in the same way that arterial baroreceptor activity is altered (see earlier discussion). For example, patients with hypertension demonstrate less reflex forearm vasoconstriction during LBNP ranging from -5 to -40 mm Hg, suggesting that both cardiopulmonary and arterial baroreflexes are impaired in this clinical condition. Also, CHF reduces the compliance of atria, resulting in diminished responses of stretch sensitive atrial myelinated endings to elevated atrial pressure. These pathological changes impair the reflex response to increased plasma volume and promote higher levels of circulating ADH leading to additional volume retention. Thus, reduced cardiac afferent information in response to high atrial pressures contributes to peripheral edema and ascites. Interestingly, digitalis glycosides can reverse the reduced cardiac sensory receptor responsiveness associated with CHF.

VISCERAL ABDOMINAL REFLEXES

Two other visceral reflexes have been studied extensively and have yielded substantial information on the mechanisms by which visceral sensory nerve endings are activated and provide central neural input. These include the reflex cardiovascular responses manifested during the stimulation of abdominal and renal visceral afferent endings.

Reflexes from Visceral Ischemia

Occlusion of celiac or superior mesenteric arteries leads to a strong reflex increase in blood pressure that

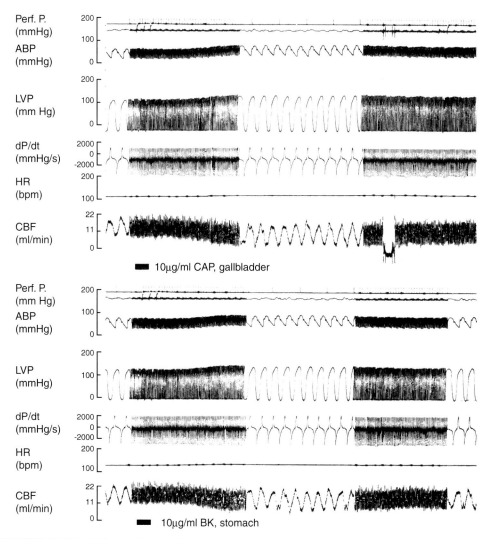

FIGURE 36.22 Reflex cardiovascular responses to application of bradykinin (BK) to serosal surfaces of the gallbladder (top) and stomach (bottom). Increases were observed in arterial blood pressure (ABP) and left ventricular pressure (LVP), whereas there were decreases in coronary blood flow (CBF) reflecting coronary vasoconstriction. Left ventricular dP/dt (contractile function) and heart rate (HR) were unchanged (Martin *et al.*, 1989).

is directly dependent on the mass of tissue involved and the temporal and spatial summation of input to cardiovascular centers in the brain stem. The increase in blood pressure in anesthetized animals is accompanied by small increases in heart rate, increased myocardial contractility, maintenance of cardiac output, and vasoconstriction of splanchnic, hindlimb, and occasionally coronary arterial circulation (Fig. 36.22). The afferent pathway follows the greater or major splanchnic nerves and spinal cord, whereas the efferent pathway includes sympathetic adrenergic and adrenal medullary systems. A number of chemical mediators formed during *mesenteric ischemia*, including bradykinin, prostaglandin E_2, hydroxyl radicals (Fig. 36.23), lactic acid, 8*R*,15*S*-dihydroxy-eicosan tetraenoic acid (diHETE), serotonin, and histamine, stimulate or sensitize predominantly unmyelinated afferent endings. Rather than directly

stimulating afferent endings, some metabolic events such as hypoxia (low Po_2) trigger sensory nerve discharge through the production of other chemical mediators. Conversely, hypercapnia, prostacyclin, thromboxane A_2, lactate, and mechanical stimulation are not involved in this ischemic reflex. Interestingly, leukotriene B_4 modulates this response. The afferent endings that respond to mesenteric ischemia are mechanically insensitive and comprise a set of high threshold nociceptors. The reflex likely is manifested during regional ischemia, e.g., in patients with splanchnic vascular atherosclerosis. Although mechanoreceptors are not activated during abdominal ischemia in the cat, graded distension or contraction of hollow viscus organs around a fixed diameter can cause reflex sympathoexcitation of the cardiovascular system. This response is mediated by unmyelinated afferents with mechanosensitive endings that project

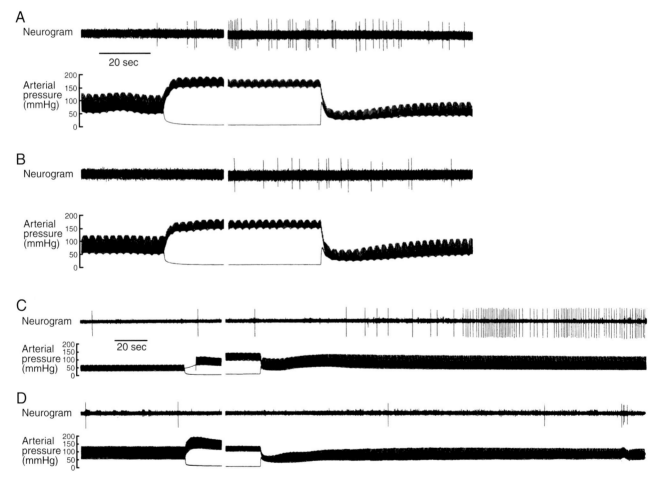

FIGURE 36.23 Single unit discharge activity of unmyelinated afferents innervating the gallbladder (top, A and B) or portal vein (bottom, C and D) during mesenteric ischemia and reperfusion before and after treatment with dimethylthiourea, a nonspecific scavenger of reactive oxygen species (ROS, A and B), or deferoxamine (B and C), an inhibitor of the Haber Weiss reaction, to prevent the formation of hydroxyl radicals. Both treatments significantly reduced the responses of the afferent fibers, indicating that ROS and particularly hydroxyl radicals stimulate the endings during ischemia and reperfusion. The increases and decreases in blood pressure reflect the proximal and distal arterial pressures during vascular occlusion (Stahl *et al.*, 1993).

to the CNS through spinal pathways. The physiologic importance of mechanoreceptor activation in the abdomen requires further investigation.

Renal Reflexes

The kidney contains myelinated mechanosensitive and chemosensitive afferents (Dietz and Gilmore, 1991; Kopp and DiBona, 1991). Mechanoreceptors may be pulse synchronous. They respond to increased ureteral pressure and distension of renal pelvis in most species, except nonhuman primates, where these receptors are very sparse. In the latter species, mechanoreceptors respond to changes in arterial pressure (pulse synchronous) or venous pressure (both pulse synchronous and asynchronous receptors), as well as to injection of a number of chemical mediators, including bradykinin, prostaglandins, histamine, adenosine, acetylcholine, and nicotine. The role of these mediators in stimulating these endings during conditions such as ischemia has not been determined. Two types of renal chemoreceptors have been described, including the CR_1 receptor that responds to renal hypoxia, ischemia or cyanide infusion, and the CR_2 receptor that responds to ion movement, including back infusion of urine, NaCl, and KCl, but not urea or mannitol. Renal spinal afferents eventually project to the NTS (to neurons that receive convergent baroreceptor input) and medulla.

Stimulation of renal afferents, either electrically or through stimulus-specific sensory nerve endings, leads to reflex cardiovascular responses, the nature of which varies depending on the species and the stimulus (Kopp and DiBona, 1991). However, reflex activation of the cardiovascular system that is quite commonly observed seems most consistent with the general observation that the stimulation of spinal afferents, such as those from the kidney, mainly (except in rabbits) leads to sympathoexcitatory pressor responses. Blood pressure is not regulated by tonic afferent activity from the kidney. Renorenal reflexes in the rat, cat, and possibly the rabbit have been observed during the stimulation of renal mechanoreceptors or chemoreceptors; they lead to diuresis and natriuresis in association with decreased contralateral efferent nerve activity.

Increased activity of renal afferents likely is a major factor in the *hypertension* consequent to renal artery stenosis (Goldblatt kidney model) or coarctation involving the renal circulation (Oparil *et al.*, 1991). Renal nerves are also partially responsible for the development of hypertension in a number of experimental models and denervation of kidneys delays or prevents the onset of hypertension in each case.

Although there are blunted responses of renal afferents to several stimuli, altered renal sympathetic efferent tone appears to be the main culprit in these conditions, as dorsal rhizotomy, to eliminate sensory output from the kidney, does not alter the hypertensive response. Similarly in humans, increased renal sympathetic activity may be important in the development of renovascular hypertension, largely through stimulation of the renin–angiotensin–aldosterone system.

Summary

Reflex control of the cardiovascular system provides a unique advantage to mammalian species by allowing them to cope with the environment. The ability to respond rapidly to changes in blood pressure, regional blood flow, the chemical composition of the blood and interstitial fluid, and adverse events such as pain or stress is managed by a set of sensory afferent systems that provide input into cardiovascular centers in the hypothalamus, midbrain, and brain stem with the end result of inducing both immediate and long-term changes in the autonomic and hormonal neuroeffector systems. Over the last century, an in-depth understanding of many neural mechanisms underlying these reflex events has been achieved. It is now known, for example, that even though these systems are largely responsible for beneficial short-term adaptations, they can play a role in a number of diseases that contribute to substantial morbidity and mortality. Future challenges are to further define the mechanisms underlying activation of the sensory endings and central neural integrative functions, including interactions of multiple systems that add complexity to the behavior of interneurons in multiple regions concerned with conditioning reflex responses. Of particular interest are some of the new opportunities for investigation that are now present as a result of recently developed molecular and genetic approaches.

References

Alexander, R. S. (1946). Tonic and reflex functions of medullary sympathetic cardiovascular centers. *J. Neurophysiol.* **9**, 205–217.

Barman, S. M., and Gebber, G. L. (2000). "Rapid" rhythmic discharges of sympathetic nerves: Sources, mechanisms of generation, and physiological relevance. *J. Biol. Rhythms* **15**, 365–379.

Biscoe, T. J. (1971). Carotid body: Structure and function. *Physiol. Rev.* **51**, 437–495.

Carrive, P., Bandler, R., and Campney, R. A. L. (1988). Anatomical evidence that hypertension associated with the defence reaction in the cat is mediated by a direct projection from a restricted portion of the midbrain periaqueductal gray to the subretrofacial nucleus of the medulla. *Brain Res.* **460**, 339–347.

Cervero, F., and Foreman, R. D. (1990). Sensory innervation of the viscera. *In* "Central Regulation of Autonomic Functions" (A. D. Loewy and K. M. Spyer, eds.), pp. 104–125. Oxford Univ. Press, New York.

Chapleau, M. W., Hajduczok, G., and Abboud, F. M. (1989). Peripheral and central mechanisms of baroreflex resetting. *Clin. Exp. Pharmacol. Physiol.* **15** (Suppl.), 31.

Chapleau, M. W. (2001). Neuro-cardiovascular regulation: From molecules to man. *N. Y. Acad. Sci.*

Chapleau, M. W., Hajduczok, G., and Abboud, F. M. (1991). Resetting of the arterial baroreflex: Peripheral and central mechanisms. *In* "Reflex Control of the Circulation" (I. H. Zucker and J. P. Gilmore, eds.), pp. 165–194. CRC Press, Boston.

Comroe, J. H., Jr. , and Mortimer, L. (1964). The respiratory and cardiovascular responses of temporally separated aortic and carotid bodies to cyanide, nicotine, phenyldiguanide and serotonin. *J. Pharmacol. Exp. Ther.* **146**, 33–41.

Dampney, R. A. L. (1994). Functional organization of central pathways regulating the cardiovascular system. *Am. Physiol. Soc.* **74**, 323–364.

Dietz, J. R., and Gilmore, J. P. (1991). The role of renal afferent nerves in circulatory control. *In* "Reflex Control of the Circulation", (I. H. Zucker and J. P. Gilmore, eds.), pp. 435–449. CRC Press, Boston.

Eyzaguirre, C., Fitzgerald, R. S., Lahiri, S., and Zapata, P. (1983). Arterial chemoreceptors. *In* "Handbook of Physiology". (J. T. Shepherd, F. M. Abboud and Geiger, S. R., eds.), Vol. III, pp. 557–621. American Physiological Society, Bethesda.

Goetz, K. L., Madwed, J. B., and Leadley Jr., R. J. (1991). "Atrial Receptors:Reflex Effects in Quadrupeds," pp. 291–311. CRC Press, Boston.

Gonzalez, C., Almaraz, L., Obeso, A., and Rigual, R. (1994). Carotid body chemoreceptors: From natural stimuli to sensory discharges. *Physiol. Rev.* **74**, 829–898.

Guyenet, P. G. (1990). Role of ventral medulla oblongata in blood pressure regulation. *In* "Central Regulation of Autonomic Functions, (A. D. Loewy and K. M. Spyer, eds. pp. 145–167. Oxford Univ. Press, New York.

Hainsworth, R. (1991). Atrial receptors. *In* "Reflex Control of the Circulation. (I. H. Zucker and J. P. Gilmore, eds.), pp. 273–289. CRC Press, Boston.

Huang, H. -S., Stahl, G. L., and Longhurst, J. C. (1995). Cardiac-cardiovascular reflexes induced by hydrogen peroxide in cats. *Am. J. Physiol.* **268**, H2114–H2124.

Izzo, P. N., and Spyer, K. M. (1997). The parasympathetic innervation of the heart. *In* "Central Nervous Control of Autonomic Function," (D. Jordan, ed.), pp. 109–127. Harwood Academic, Amsterdam.

Johnson, J. M., Rowell, L. B., Niederberger, M., and Eisman, M. M. (1974). Human splanchnic and forearm vasoconstrictor responses to reductions of right atrial and aortic pressures. *Circ. Res.* **34**, 515–524.

Jordan, D. (1990). Autonomic changes in affective behavior. *In* "Central Regulation of Autonomic Functions", (A. D. Loewy and K. M. Spyer, eds.), pp. 349–366. Oxford Univ. Press, New York.

Jordan, D. (1995). CNS integration of cardiovascular regulation. *In* "Cardiovascular Regulation", (D. Jordan and J. J. Marshall, eds.), pp. 1–14. Portland Press, London.

Koch, E. (1931). "Die reflektorische Selbststeuerung des Kreislaufes", pp. 1–234. Steinkopf, Dresden, East Germany.

Kappagoda, C. T., Linden, R. J., and Mary, D. A. S. G. (1976). Atrial receptors in the cat. *J. Physiol. (London)* **262**, 431.

Lahiri, S., Mokashi, A., Mulligan, E., and Nishino, T. (1981). Comparison of aortic and carotid chemoreceptor responses to hypercapnia and hypoxia. *Exercise Physiol.* **51**, 55–61.

Kopp, U. C., and DiBona, G. F. (1991). Neural control of renal function. *In* "Reflex Control of the Circulation", (I. H. Zucker and J. P. Gilmore, eds.), pp. 493–528. CRC Press, Boston.

Linden, R. J., and Kappagoda, C. T. (1982). "Atrial Receptors," pp. 1–363. Cambridge Univ. Press, Cambridge.

Loewy, A. D. (1990). Central autonomic pathways. *In* "Central Regulation of Autonomic Functions", (A. D. Loew and K. M. Spyer, eds.), pp. 88–103. Oxford Univ. Press, New York.

Loewy, A. D., and Neil, J. J. (1981). The role of descending monoaminergic systems in cntral control of blood pressure. *Fed. Proc.* **40**, 2778–2785.

Loewy, A. D., and Spyer, K. M. (1990). Vagal preganglionic neurons. *In* "Central Regulation of Autonomic Functions", (A. D. Loewy and K. M. Spyer, eds.), pp. 68–87. Oxford Univ. Press, New York.

Longhurst, J. C. (1982). Arterial baroreceptors in health and disease. *Cardiovasc. Rev. Rep.* **3**, 271–298.

Longhurst, J. C. (1984). Cardiac receptors: Their function in health and disease. *Prog. Cardiovasc. Dis.* XXVII, 201–222.

Longhurst, J. C., Tjen-A-Looi, S., and Fu, L-W. (2001). Cardiac sympathetic afferent activation provoked by myocardial ischemia and reperfusion: Mechanisms and reflexes. *N. Y. Acad. Sci.*

Lovick, T. A. (1987). Cardiovascular control from neurones in the ventrolateral medulla. *In* "Neurobiology of the Cardiorespiratory System" (E. W., Taylor, ed.), pp. 197–208. Manchester University Press, Manchester.

Mancia, G., Leonetti, G., Terzoli, L., and Zanchetti, A. (1978). Reflex control of renin release in essential hypertension. *Clin. Sci. Mol. Med.* **54**, 217–222.

Mark, A. L., and Mancia, G. (1983). Cardiopulmonary baroreflexes in humans. *In* "Handbook of Physiology", (J. T. Shepherd, F. M. Abboud, and S. R. Geiger, eds.), Vol. III, pp. 795–813. American Physiological Society, Bethesda.

Marshall, J. M. (1994). Peripheral chemoreceptors and cardiovascular regulation. *Physiol. Rev.* **74**, 543–594.

Martin, S. E., Pilkington, D. M., and Longhurst, J. C. (1989). Coronary vascular responses to chemical stimulation of abdominal visceral organs. *Am. J. Physiol.* **256**, H735–H744.

McCloskey, D. I. (1968). Carbon dioxide and the carotid body. *In* "Arterial Chemoreceptors" (R. W., Torrance, ed.), pp. 279–295. Blackwell, Oxford, UK.

McCubbin, J. W., Green, J. H., and Page, I. H. (1956). Baroceptor function in chronic renal hypertension. *Circ. Res.* **4**, 205.

Minisi, A. J., and Thames, M. D. (1991). Reflexes from ventricular receptors with vagal afferents. *In* "Reflex Control of the Circulation", (I. H. Zucker and J. P. Gilmore, eds.), pp. 359–405. CRC Press, Boston.

Oparil, S., Wyss, M. J., and Sripairojthikoon, W. (1991). The role of the renal nerves in the pathogenesis of hypertension. *In* "Reflex Control of the Circulation," (I. H. Zucker and J. P. Gilmore, eds.) pp. 451–491. CRC Press, Boston.

Sagawa, K. (1983). Baroreflex control of systemic arterial pressure and vascular bed. *In* "Handbook of Physiology", (J. T. Shepherd, F. M. Abboud and S. R. Geiger, eds.), pp. 453–496. American Physiological Society, Bethesda.

Spyer, K. M. (1990). The central nervous organization of reflex circulatory control. *In* "Central Regulation of Autonomic Functions", (A. D. Loewy and K. M. Spyer, eds.), pp. 168–188. Oxford Univ. Press, New York.

John C. Longhurst

37

Neural Control of Breathing

Organisms must constantly exchange various substances with the environment to maintain homeostasis. A variety of physiological systems have evolved to handle solid, liquid, and gaseous metabolic precursors and by-products. For example, aerobic metabolism consumes O_2 and produces CO_2, the so-called blood gases. Organisms with large surface-to-volume ratios, such as bacteria, yeast, plants, and insects, rely on passive diffusion for exchange of these gases with the environment. However, more complex organisms, with low external surface-to-volume ratios and high metabolic rates, such as birds and mammals, actively pump gas using a reciprocating pump (respiratory muscles) to exchange air between the environment and the lungs and a circular pump (heart) to move blood through the pulmonary to systemic circulations. The brain controls breathing by generating the motor outflow driving the rhythmic contraction and relaxation of respiratory pump muscles and by modulating the tone of skeletal and smooth muscles in the upper airways and bronchi to control resistance to air flow.

Humans breathe continuously because a constant supply of O_2 is needed to support a high metabolic rate. The central nervous system (CNS) drives respiratory muscles to produce ventilation appropriate for the regulation of blood O_2 and CO_2 adaptable over an order of magnitude range in metabolic demand (in humans from 0.25 liter $\times$ min^{-1} O_2 consumed at rest to ~3–6 liter $\times$ min^{-1} O_2 consumed during extreme exercise). In controlling breathing, the brain must also compensate for wide ranges of body posture and movement, which affect lung and musculoskeletal mechanics and compromise muscle or cardiopulmonary function. This control of ventilation must continue from birth until death without lapses of more than a few minutes. Respiratory muscles account for less than 5% of the body's metabolism at rest, but they need to be used efficiently because the metabolic cost adds up over time. Moreover, serious respiratory muscle fatigue must be avoided. During exercise, energy costs of breathing must be kept low when possible (the respiratory pump moves up to 200 liters $\times$ min^{-1} of air in world-class athletes) to maximize the amount of metabolic substrates available to other working muscles.

The drive for continuous ventilation in humans is strong. Typically, breathing is the last consequential movement to disappear following generalized depression of higher function, such as during surgical anesthesia or following insults to the brain (e.g., hypoglycemic coma). Automatic, homeostatic breathing can remain in people who have lost cortical function, resulting in ethical and emotional dilemmas over people who are "brain dead."

In experimental animals, one can take advantage of this robustness of breathing to study synaptic, neural, and network mechanisms in anesthetized or decerebrate animals that continue to breathe. The neural mechanisms underlying breathing are so robust and sufficiently self-contained that an *in vitro* tissue slice at an appropriate level in neonatal or late fetal rodent brain stem continues to generate respiratory-related patterns of motor nerve activity.

EARLY NEUROSCIENCE AND THE BRAIN STEM

The persistent absence of breathing is the surest sign of death. Many ancient cultures associated life with breathing itself. Animation, to bring to life, and animal are derived from the Latin *anima*, which

37. NEURAL CONTROL OF BREATHING

means to breathe (and also soul). Taoism holds breathing sacred and proper breathing a key to enlightenment: immortality to the man who holds his breath for the time of 1000 respirations. Buddhists believe that special states of enlightenment can be attained through effective modulation of breathing.

Although the purpose of breathing—to move air into and out of the lungs—was not established until the end of the 18th century, the sites responsible for breathing movements have been a constant source of speculation in Western culture. Perhaps the earliest suggestion that the brain was involved came from Galen (ca. 131–201 A.D.), who observed that gladiators and animals injured below the neck continued to breathe, but those injured in the neck stopped. Lorry (1760), who showed that cerebellectomized rabbits continued to breathe, concluded that the critical circuits lay within the brain stem and upper cervical

spinal cord, essentially representing the contemporary view. Legallois (1813) "extracted" brain tissue to determine what was necessary for breathing; he localized the critical sites to the rostral ventrolateral medulla, near the exit of the vagus nerve, close to the currently hypothesized site, the pre-Bötzinger complex. Later lesion-based work was consistent with a critical role of various pontine and medullary sites. These lesion studies were at variance with studies that used electrical stimulation; this latter work is mostly of historical interest, given its rather high, and therefore nonphysiologic, stimulus parameters (1- to 30-V pulses delivered via low-resistance electrodes).

Ramon y Cajal (1909), among his many brilliant contributions to neuroscience, provided an anatomic rationale for the central role of medullary structures in the control of breathing. Examining the afferent and efferent projections of respiration-related nerves, he suggested that three brain stem nuclei are important: the nucleus of the solitary tract and commissural nuclei, primary targets of pulmonary afferents, and the nucleus ambiguus, which contains cranial motor neurons that innervate the upper airway muscles. His network model for breathing is prescient (Fig. 37.1): afferent signals, containing information about the status of the lungs and components of blood, combined with intrinsic properties of brain stem neurons to produce a rhythmic outflow to spinal and cranial respiratory motor neurons. Adrian and Buytendijk (1931) recorded slow, rhythmic potentials in isolated *in vitro* goldfish brain stems. The periodicity of the potentials was similar to that of gill movements in intact goldfish (Fig. 37.2) and thus provided physiological evidence that the brain stem contained the critical circuits. Gesell and co-workers (1936) subsequently recorded individual medullary neurons discharging bursts of activity in phase with the breathing rhythm. This finding initiated a concerted effort to identify neurons that generate respiratory rhythm.

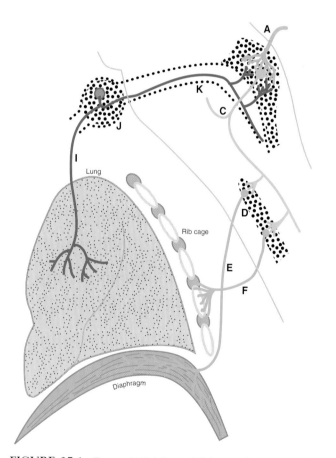

FIGURE 37.1 Ramon Y Cajal's model for respiratory control. Respiratory neurons in solitary tract (C) process signals from pulmonary afferents [K; cell bodies in nodose ganglion (J)] and some blood factor present in local capillaries (A). Descending control signals go to spinal motor neurons (D), innervating the diaphragm (E) or intercostal muscles (F). From Ramon y Cajal (1909).

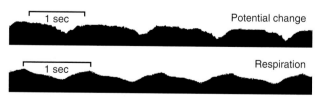

FIGURE 37.2 Oscillograph recordings of the gross electrical potential of an *in vitro* goldfish brain stem (top) compared to gill movement of an intact goldfish (bottom). From Adrian and Buytendijk (1931).

CENTRAL NERVOUS SYSTEM AND BREATHING RESPIRATORY RHYTHM GENERATION

Breathing, chewing, and locomotion are important behaviors that require rhythmic movements with periods of less than one to several seconds. The neural networks for these rhythms are programmed genetically and develop *in utero* so that newborn mammals breathe, chew, and, in some cases, locomote. The following section examines how the brain generates the rhythms underlying breathing.

Although conceptually simple and straightforward (air in, air out), breathing, from the brain's point of view, is much more than sine wave generation. Ventilation requires a patterned motor output with appropriate timing and magnitude of muscle contraction and relaxation and coordination of this activity among synergists and antagonists; it is controlled by a complex and mutable regulatory system composed of many distinct components (Fig. 37.3). The ability to adjust breathing appropriately during a full range of voluntary and reflex motor behaviors requires forebrain, brain stem, and spinal cord circuitry.

Appropriate adjustment of breathing to meet the changing metabolic needs of the animal requires sensory information on the chemical state of the blood and brain and the mechanical state of the lung, airways, and respiratory muscles. Nevertheless, even if deprived of sensory information, the central nervous system can generate a basic respiratory rhythm, and a long-standing problem has been to identify the sites and mechanisms underlying rhythmogenesis. Evidence suggests that a small cluster of neurons within the rostral ventrolateral medulla appears to contain the minimal circuitry (the kernel) necessary for the generation of respiratory rhythm.

WHERE ARE THE NEURONS THAT GENERATE THE BREATHING RHYTHM?

Breathing is a regulatory behavior, the most compelling aspect of which is its rhythmicity. In the past decade, neuroscientists have made remarkable progress toward identifying the sites of rhythm generation, but have struggled with understanding how the rhythm gets transformed into the exquisitely complex and extraordinarily efficient movements that actually generate the forces for moving air and how these movements are modulated during various states of activity (sleep to marathon running). From the

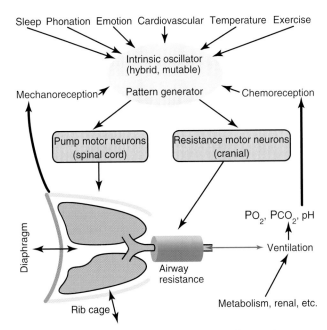

FIGURE 37.3 Functional organization of central nervous system control of breathing (see text for details).

point of view of scientific investigation into brain mechanisms, breathing is an unusually accessible behavior. Breathing is easy to measure and it is preserved in anesthetized or decerebrate mammals, even in highly reduced preparations, including tissue slices from neonatal rodent medulla. This section focuses on advances in understanding rhythm generation and discusses contemporary ideas about how this rhythm is transformed into ventilation itself.

An essential step toward an understanding of the cellular and synaptic mechanisms controlling breathing is identification of the neurons generating the basic respiratory rhythm. While it has been known since the early 19th century that the brain stem is responsible for respiratory rhythm generation, precise localization of neurons involved in this process required the development of novel *in vitro* preparations (see Box 37.1). In the 1980s, Suzue and colleagues (Ballanyi *et al.*, 1999) noted that the brain stem and spinal cord from a neonatal rat, termed the "en bloc" preparation, generated a respiratory rhythm present in the ventral roots of thoracic and cervical spinal cord in nerves that innervate respiratory muscles, which comprise a respiratory pump, as well as in cranial nerves innervating the airways, which control airway resistance. (Airways are normally constricted during expiration and dilated during inspiration, thereby adjusting the resistance to the flow of air into and out of the lungs.) The presence of rhythmic respiratory activity in cranial nerves in this

BOX 37.1

EXPERIMENTAL ANALYSIS OF VENTILATION

Neuroscientists are constrained by what they can measure. Noninvasive experiments in humans reveal the phenomenology of breathing, e.g., the relationship between ventilation and blood CO_2 levels. Brain imaging may reveal which regions are involved, but at present, spatiotemporal resolution is too coarse to show networks, much less neurons or synapses. Respiration lends itself to study because mammals suitable for experimental studies breathe much like humans. Breathing continues following anesthesia or decerebration, and the neural patterns remain following paralysis (and mechanical ventilation), making possible experimental procedures requiring highly invasive techniques, such as single neuron recording. Compared to studies of neurons in culture or in tissue slices, experiments in whole mammals have serious limitations. For example, movements of the heart and lungs make certain types of single neuron recording difficult in the brain stem and spinal cord. Moreover, in live animals, the blood–brain barrier is intact, making precise control of brain extracellular fluid impossible. Finally, the experiments are expensive and often last 36 h or more, requiring the dedicated and concurrent efforts of several investigators. Fortunately, the robust features of breathing that allow it to persist when other behaviors are suppressed by anesthesia or decerebration permit further reduction in the experimental preparation that removes these limitations. For example, a respiratory-related rhythm persists in the brain stem and spinal cord that has been removed from a neonatal rat or mouse and transplanted to an *in vitro* chamber. In addition, the rhythm persists in a particular slice of brain stem isolated from this preparation (Fig. 37.4). Using such slices, one can correlate exquisite measures of a neuron's intrinsic and synaptic properties and projections with measures of endogenous behavior, such as its firing pattern. With some common and otherwise useful *in vitro* preparations, such as the hippocampal slice, such correlations cannot be made because no endogenous behavior *in vitro* relates to known behavior *in vivo*. In general, en bloc *in vitro*, or slice, preparations play an important role in the study of basic cellular, synaptic, and integrative mechanisms underlying motor behavior.

Another model of interest lacks a direct tie to mammalian behavior but has other considerable advantages. Three neurons in the pulmonate mollusk *Lymnaea stagnalis* were identified that are essential for generating muscle movements required for oxygen gas exchange. They have isolated and cocultured these neurons to produce a three-neuron *in vitro* circuit that reproduces the repertoire of ventilatory behavior. With three large neurons *in vitro* that together have behaviorally relevant activity, the potential for analysis is virtually unlimited.

Jack L. Feldman and
Donald R. McCrimmon

in vitro preparation permitted a refinement of the "blunt spatula" brain stem transection approach used almost 200 years earlier by Legallois (1813) to identify structures critical for respiratory rhythm generation. In the contemporary case, removing thin (50–75 μm) sections from either rostral or caudal ends of the "en bloc" preparation while recording respiratory activity from spinal or cranial nerves resulted in the isolation of a small, ventral medullary region as an essential component in the rhythm generating circuitry (Smith *et al.*, 1991). This region was named the pre-Bötzinger complex. Confirmation that neurons within this region provide a minimum essential circuitry for respiratory rhythm generation, at least *in vitro*, follows from the observations that a thin transverse slice that contains this region, or even a pre-Bötzinger complex-containing "island" dissected from such a slice, can generate a respiratory-related rhythm (Johnson *et al.*, 2001). In addition, the necessary role of neurons within this region for rhythm generation blockade is suggested by the observation that the blockade of excitatory, glutamatergic neurotransmission within the pre-Bötzinger region *in vitro* abolishes respiratory rhythm (Rekling and Feldman, 1998).

The fundamental role of the pre-Bötzinger complex suggested by these *in vitro* studies is supported by numerous *in vivo* studies. For example, injection of muscimol (a $GABA_A$ agonist that inhibits spontaneous neuronal activity) into the pre-Bötzinger complex of adult rats *in vivo* eliminates respiratory activity (Rekling and Feldman, 1998). Similarly, blockade of synaptic transmission by unilateral injection of a calcium channel blocker, Ω-conotoxin GVIA, into the adult cat pre-Bötzinger complex induces central apnea (a cessation of breathing efforts). Targeted destruction of a key subset of pre-Bötzinger complex neurons in awake rats results in a pathological pattern of breathing (see later).

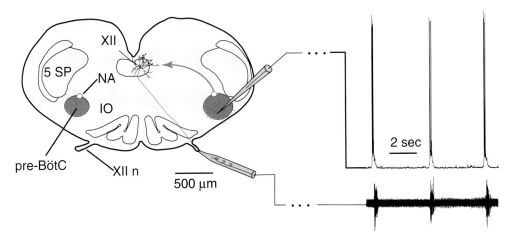

FIGURE 37.4 An "oscillating" slice preparation from a rodent brain stem exhibits endogenous respiratory rhythm in cranial nerve XII with patch-clamp recordings from a pre-BötC neuron. Diagram of a transverse slice. Patch-clamp recordings can be made from XII or pre-BötC cells while drugs (or different solutions) are supplied in a bath or applied locally. The rhythm is generated in pre-BötC and transmitted to the XII nucleus so it appears in motor axons of the XII nerve. (Right) A recording from a pre-BötC inspiratory neuron that shows periodic, inspiration-modulated depolarizations and associated action potentials (current-clamp) (upper tracing). Lower tracing is a XII nerve recording; bursts of activity correspond to inspiration.

WHICH NEURONS IN THE PREBÖTZINGER COMPLEX ARE REQUIRED FOR RESPIRATORY RHYTHM GENERATION?

While the abovementioned studies suggest that a relatively small region in the ventral medulla is critical for respiratory rhythm generation, they do not, however, provide information on which neurons are essential. A partial resolution to this problem arose when investigators took advantage of the observation that the activation of receptors for the peptide substance P and for μ opioids changes respiratory frequency. This effect could arise if the relevant peptide receptors were directly on neurons generating rhythm. Examination of the distribution of the peptide receptors, i.e., neurokinin-1 and μ-opioid receptors, revealed a restricted subset of labeled neurons within the pre-Bötzinger complex. Neurons with these receptors have respiratory activity and hence could participate in rhythm generation; if true, destruction of these neurons should disrupt breathing. A straightforward test of this possibility was undertaken using a toxin (saporin, a ribosomal toxin that interferes with the synthesis of new proteins) conjugated to substance P injected bilaterally into the pre-Bötzinger complex of anesthetized adult rats (Gray *et al.*, 2001). By itself, saporin is not taken up appreciably by neurons. However, when substance P

binds to the NK1 receptor, the ligand–receptor is internalized, and when substance P is conjugated to saporin, the toxin is dragged along into the neuron. The result is that neurons expressing the NK1 receptor in the region of the injection die after several days. This delayed effect permits injected rats to fully recover from surgery prior to determining the impact of the toxin on breathing. During this period, injected rats breathe normally. However, after several days, rats with substantial bilateral destruction of the NK1 pre-Bötzinger complex neurons develop an ataxic, i.e., highly abnormal, breathing pattern, are unable to maintain normal levels of blood O_2 and CO_2, and have pathological responses to hypoxia and hyperoxia. Nevertheless, the rats maintain sufficient ventilation to survive. These results suggest that pre-Bötzinger complex neurons are required for normal breathing, but in their absence, other neurons can generate an ataxic breathing pattern sufficient to maintain life. The identity of the neurons generating this remaining rhythm is unknown but could include neurons without NK1 receptors within the pre-Bötzinger complex or even neurons that normally generate volitional breathing movements.

Taken together, the abovementioned experiments underlie the working *hypothesis* that respiratory rhythm is generated in the pre-Bötzinger complex. They also provide a conceptual basis for experiments examining the cellular mechanisms of how the rhythm is generated.

Potential Contribution of Pacemaker Neurons to Rhythm Generation

Almost every successful explanation of brain processes underlying complex behavior is based on a combination of cellular, synaptic, and network properties. It is easy to build computational models of simple oscillatory behavior using only network, e.g., reciprocal inhibition, or only cellular, e.g., pacemaker, properties, but a true mechanistic explanation for breathing may require both. For several decades neuroscientists speculated that respiratory rhythm was driven by the same kinds of cellular properties that drive another vital rhythm, that of the heart, which is generated by the pacemaker activity of specialized cells within the sinoatrial node of the heart. With identification of the pre-Bötzinger complex, it became possible to test whether the rhythm it generates is due to pacemaker neurons. Such tests are based on the following premise: A common feature of respiratory rhythm generating network models that do *not* incorporate pacemaker neurons is the requirement for inhibitory synaptic interactions to produce phase transitions between inspiration and expiration. Thus, each phase ends when the neurons responsible for that phase are suddenly and powerfully inhibited, allowing neurons generating the complementary phase to be excited. In contrast, inhibition is not required in circuits incorporating pacemaker neurons where intrinsic membrane properties terminate each burst. This key difference suggests a straightforward experiment: block inhibition in the central respiratory networks and see if rhythm remains; if so, then a compelling case is made for a pacemaker-generated rhythm. In such experiments, neither antagonists of the known major inhibitory transmitter systems, GABA and glycine, nor ion substitution to interfere with inhibitory Cl⁻ or K⁺ currents blocks rhythm (Rekling and Feldman, 1998).

Combined calcium imaging and electrophysiological recording studies have reinforced the likelihood of a contribution of pacemaker neurons to

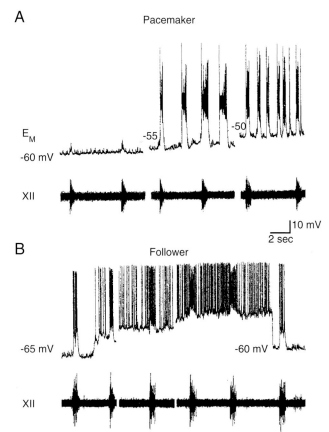

FIGURE 37.5   In an *in vitro* slice, pacemaker neurons in the pre-Bötzinger complex (A) receive a rhythmic inspiratory synaptic drive. As the membrane is depolarized by current injection, additional distinct bursts of activity appear. This response is different from that of other follower cells (B). Periodic inspiratory activity is shown in recordings from cranial nerve XII (hypoglossal nerve). Depolarization of a follower neuron, for example, a XII motor neuron, elicits tonic activity but does not produce additional bursts.

rhythm generation. A Ca²⁺-sensitive dye to labeled a population of pre-Bötzinger complex neurons, that exhibited a phasic rise in Ca²⁺ concentration and possessed underlying pacemaker properties. This suggests that pacemaker neurons constitute a subset of neurons within the respiratory rhythm generating

FIGURE 37.6   Respiratory neuroanatomy of the rat brain stem. The three major brain stem clusters of neurons controlling respiration are depicted. On the left are medium- and low-magnification views of labeled neurons in representative transverse sections of the pons and medulla after a retrograde tracer injection (not shown) within the rostral part of the contralateral VRG . The sections were photographed using reflected light so that myelinated axons appear white, retrogradely labeled neurons (immunostained with diaminobenzidine) appear gold, while the remaining cellular areas appear gray. On the right, these retrogradely labeled cells are diagrammed (red dots) within outlines of the adjacent low-magnification photomicrographs. On the right side of the diagram, the columns of respiratory neurons are identified: cVRG, pink; rVRG, green; preBötC, yellow; BötC, blue, PRG, orange; DRG, purple. Not all the (red) retrogradely labeled neurons in the medulla are included within the respiratory regions; some of these presumably represent extrinsic neuronal relays that can modulate respiration in relation to other behavioral or metabolic demands. 4V, fourth ventricle; 12, hypoglossal nucleus; AP, area postrema; BötC, Bötzinger Complex; cVRG, caudal VRG; DRG, dorsal respiratory group; IO, inferior olive; KF, Kölliker–Fuse nucleus; LPB, lateral parabrachial nucleus; MPB, medial parabrachial nucleus; NAc, ambiguus nucleus, compact division; NTS, nucleus of the solitary tract; preBötC, pre-Bötzinger complex; PRG, pontine respiratory group; rVRG, rostral VRG Sp5, spinal trigeminal nucleus; VRG, ventral respiratory group. Courtesy of George F. Alheid.

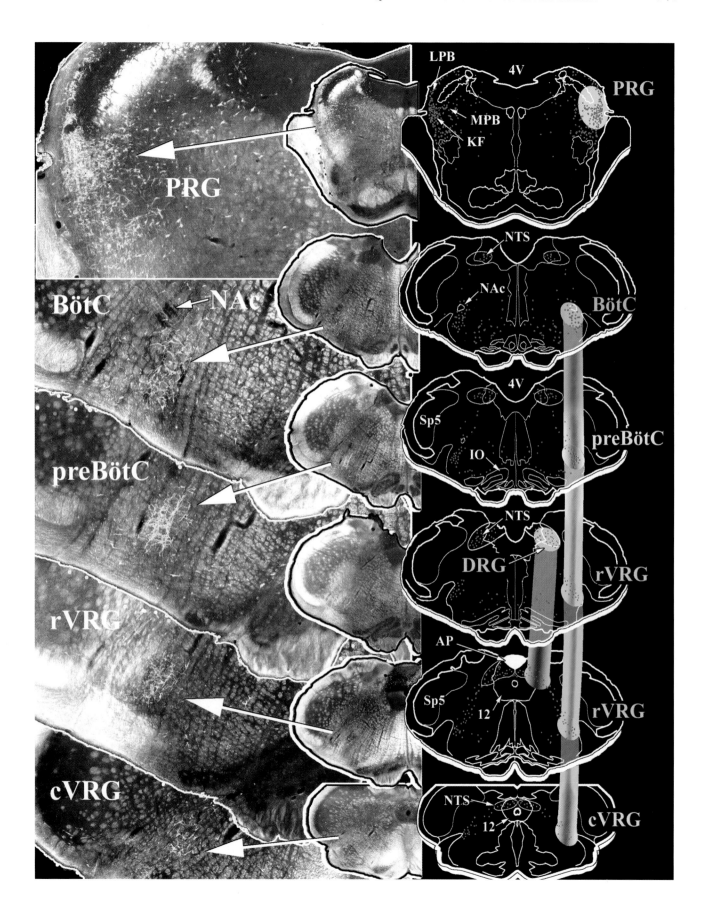

circuitry (Koshiya and Smith, 1999). Differences in the behavior of pacemaker versus nonpacemaker (follower) cells are illustrated in Fig. 37.5. Tonic injection of depolarizing current produces bursts of action potentials during the normally silent (expiratory) period of these cells. The interval between bursts is sensitive to depolarization level and hence the amount of injected current. After abolition of respiratory rhythm in a medullary slice, injection of a depolarizing current into a pacemaker neuron produces bursts of action potentials. Follower cells, in response to a similar current injection, simply increase their tonic discharge rate.

Taken together, the evidence just presented provides strong arguments that, at least *in vitro*, the pre-Bötzinger complex (1) is necessary and sufficient for the generation of respiratory rhythm and (2) pacemaker neurons (or, alternatively, groups of neurons that collectively act like a "group pacemaker"; Rekling and Feldman, 1998) within this region provide the minimal substrate (kernel) for respiratory rhythm generation. Several important questions remain: Are pre-Bötzinger complex neurons also responsible for rhythm generation *in vivo*? Do pacemaker neurons contribute to rhythm generation *in vivo*? How is the basic respiratory rhythm transformed into the diverse, but coordinated motor pattern that is distributed to the large of number of respiratory motoneurons? In addition to the pre-Bötzinger complex, where are the neurons that participate in this transformation?

WHERE ARE THE RESPIRATORY NEURONS?

Respiratory neurons are concentrated within, but not restricted to, three bilaterally symmetrical regions within the pons and medulla (Fig. 37.6; Bianchi *et al.*, 1995; Rekling and Feldman, 1998). Pre-Bötzinger complex neurons contributing to respiratory rhythm generation form a small cluster in the ventrolateral medulla, constituting a limited part of a longer column of respiratory neurons centered ventral to the nucleus ambiguus and extending from the caudal end of the facial nucleus to the rostral cervical spinal cord. This ventrolateral respiratory column is typically divided into three compartments. The most rostral of these is the Bötzinger complex, which largely contains expiratory neurons, some of which are bulbospinal but others are propriobulbar. Immediately caudal is the pre-Bötzinger complex, and then caudal to that, extending down to the spinal cord, is the ventral respiratory group (VRG). The VRG contains most of the

premotor neurons innervating inspiratory and expiratory motoneurons in the spinal cord. The VRG is subdivided into a rostral VRG (rVRG) that contains primarily inspiratory premotor neurons innervating spinal inspiratory motor neurons, including phrenic motoneurons innervating the diaphragm, the principal inspiratory muscle, and external intercostal motor neurons. The caudal VRG (cVRG) contains primarily expiratory neurons and innervates expiratory motor neurons with axons principally in the internal intercostal nerves.

A second group of medullary respiratory neurons, termed the dorsal respiratory group (DRG), is centered within the ventrolateral region of the nucleus of the tractus solitarius. DRG respiratory neurons are in close association with primary afferent fibers arising in the lungs and airways and coursing in the 9th (glossopharyngeal) and 10th (vagus) cranial nerves. The reticular formation, extending in a band dorsomedial to the nucleus ambiguus, also contains scattered respiratory neurons. The scattered nature of these cells has made them more difficult to study and less is known about their function.

Within the pons, respiratory neurons are concentrated in the rostral dorsolateral portion. These neurons are associated with the medial and lateral parabrachial and Kölliker–Fuse nuclei in a grouping referred to as the pontine respiratory group (PRG).

DISCHARGE PATTERNS OF RESPIRATORY NEURONS

The business end of breathing, which is the periodic contraction of skeletal muscles of the respiratory pump and of both skeletal and smooth muscles controlling airway resistance, requires that brain stem and spinal cord respiratory neurons generate both a rhythm and then sculpt it into a precisely coordinated, efficient pattern of muscle contraction and relaxation (Fig. 37.7). Each muscle (or muscle group) must contract with the appropriate timing and burst pattern to produce the forces on the lung appropriate to move the right amount of air. This requires precise patterns of motor neuron bursting and silence. How do individual respiratory neurons interact to produce this rhythm and pattern of respiratory motor outputs? In attempting to answer this question, much has been learned from analysis of the discharge patterns of individual neurons and the patterns of synaptic connectivity among respiratory neurons. Because breathing is cyclic, it is perhaps not surprising that the discharge of many neurons controlling breathing occurs in bursts of action

A

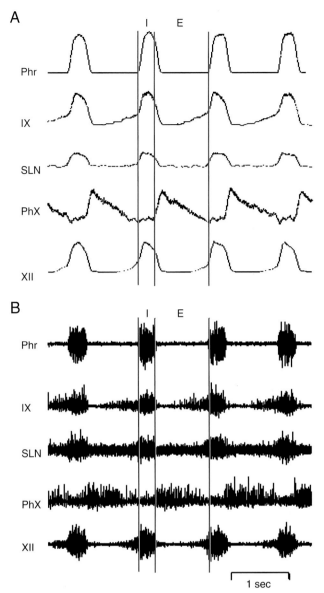

that constitute the respiratory cycle. Even among investigators in the field, there is some disagreement about the number of phases. Inspiration and expiration constitute two obvious phases. However, a close examination of the discharge patterns of inspiratory (e.g., diaphragm) and expiratory (e.g., internal intercostal) muscle activity has suggested to several investigators that there are three (or more) phases (Richter *et al.*, 1996). In this analysis, expiration consists of two phases. The onset of exhalation marks the onset of the first expiratory (E1), or postinspiratory, phase. During this phase, the diaphragm often exhibits a low level of activity (termed postinspiratory activity) that brakes diaphragmatic relaxation and slows exhalation (Fig. 37.7). Postinspiratory activity declines rapidly, frequently ending by midexpiration. At this point, an augmenting pattern of expiratory muscle activity begins, marking the onset of the second (E2) phase, characterized by active expiratory muscle contraction. The concept of two expiratory phases is contested, with the alternative explanation that during expiration there are multiple patterns of motor output within a single phase of the rhythm. The rationale that the bursts reflect motor output patterns rather than rhythm is that the transition between the two expiratory phases is often ambiguous. For example, in Fig. 37.7, a declining postinspiratory output of the pharyngeal branch of the vagus nerve, which controls the diameter of the upper airway, overlaps with the E2 pattern of activity in other nerves that affect the diameter of the upper airway, such as the glossopharyngeal and hypoglossal nerves. This overlap in activity on motor nerves raises the possibility that these neuronal activities are controlled by decrementing and incrementing aspects of a single expiratory phase.

The naming of respiratory neurons follows from the phase or phases in which their activity occurs. Thus, neurons are designated inspiratory (I), postinspiratory (P-I), or expiratory (E). Neurons that have activity in more than one phase are termed phasespanning neurons. In addition, even among neurons that discharge only during inspiration or only during expiration, neurons can have distinctly different patterns of discharge. Investigators have interpreted these diverse patterns as evidence of different roles for each group of neurons in respiratory control and have used the discharge patterns to define subgroups of inspiratory and expiratory neurons. While the total number of subgroups is relatively small, different investigators have measured neuronal activities under slightly different experimental conditions, e.g., different species, different anesthesia, or decerebration, and have used slightly different criteria to name them. The

FIGURE 37.7 A diverse pattern of respiratory motor activity is exhibited on spinal (phrenic, Phr) and cranial nerves innervating the diaphragm and airways in an anesthetized rat. (A) Low-pass filtered trace of activity showing overall pattern of discharge; (B) corresponding raw nerve recording. Red vertical lines indicate phase transitions between inspiration (I) and expiration (E). Note that the onset of inspiratory activity on cranial nerves precedes the onset of activity on the phrenic nerve. IX, glossopharyngeal nerve; PhX, pharyngeal branch of vagus nerve; SLN, superior laryngeal nerve XII, hypoglossal nerve. Adapted from Hayashi and McCrimmon (1996).

potentials that are restricted to only a portion of each breath (respiratory cycle). This distinguishing characteristic of phasic discharge permits straightforward identification of respiratory neurons.

One consideration that has impacted the classification of respiratory neurons is the number of phases

Respiratory cycle

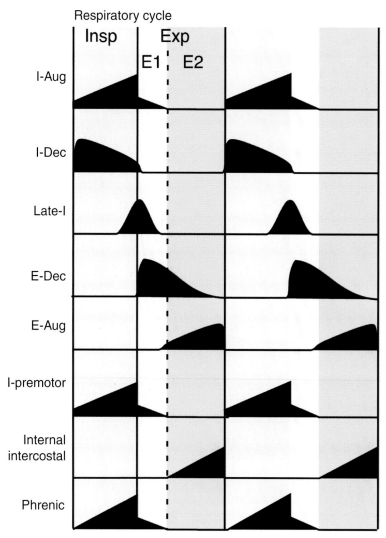

FIGURE 37.8 Discharge patterns of neuronal components of two- and three-phase models of respiratory rhythm generation. Two-phase models consist of an inspiratory phase (Insp) and an expiratory phase (Exp). In three-phase models, E is divided into E1, early expiration (or postinspiration), and E2 or late expiration. The transition from inspiration to expiration is marked by a rapid decline in phrenic nerve activity illustrated in the bottom trace. Residual, declining phrenic nerve activity (when present) marks the E1 phase. Augmenting (Aug) activity occurs on the internal intercostal nerve (second trace from bottom) and Aug- E neurons largely during the E2 phase. The ordinate for each trace is discharge frequency with higher levels representing higher frequencies. Aug, augmenting neurons; Dec, decrementing neurons; E, expiratory; I, inspiratory.

result is a confusing array of populations, even to experts in the field.

Representative changes in membrane potential and patterns of discharge are shown in Fig. 37.8 with the most common names of the predominant neuronal subgroups. Three basic discharge patterns are identified. These are augmenting (Aug), in which discharge frequency increases progressively throughout a respiratory phase, reaching a peak frequency just before the end of the phase; decrementing (Dec), in which neurons begin discharging at a high frequency and then decrease their discharge rate throughout a

phase; and constant (Con), in which a clear augmenting or decrementing pattern is not observed. Thus, inspiratory augmenting (I-Aug) neurons begin discharging near the onset of I, then depolarize progressively and increase their discharge rate during I. Inspiratory-constant (I-Con) neurons begin to discharge near the onset of inspiration and then maintain a relatively constant level of depolarization and rate of firing. Inspiratory-decrementing (I-Dec) cells depolarize abruptly at the onset of inspiration and fire at a high rate. As inspiration progresses, these neurons repolarize slowly and decrease their rate of discharge.

Two additional subgroups of I neurons have been identified. The discharge pattern of both groups resembles that of I-Aug neurons but differs in the timing of discharge onset. One of these subgroups, preinspiratory (Pre-I) neurons, has a phase-spanning discharge pattern. They begin to depolarize and fire prior to the onset of I and continue to depolarize throughout I. The other, late inspiratory (Late-I) neurons do not begin to depolarize until late in inspi-

ration and then fire a brief burst of action potentials just before the end of inspiration.

Expiratory neurons are divided into two groups. At the onset of expiration, expiratory-decrementing (E-Dec or Post-I) neurons begin to discharge at a high frequency. Throughout expiration, these cells repolarize progressively and decrease their discharge rate. Some investigators distinguish between E-Dec neurons, which discharge at a declining rate throughout

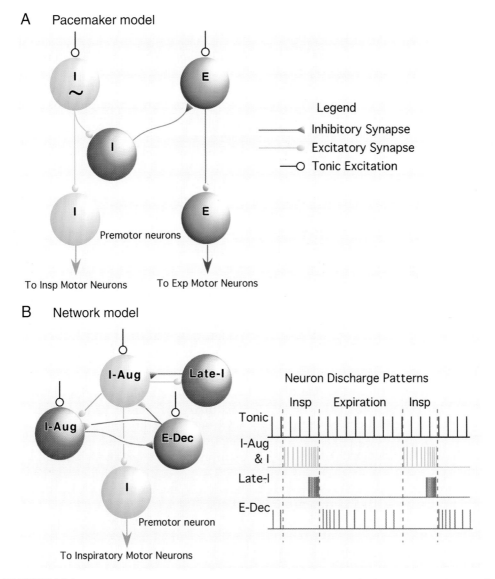

FIGURE 37.9 Simplified pacemaker and network models of respiratory rhythm generation (see text for details). For simplicity, several types of neurons have been omitted, especially several types of expiratory neurons. In addition, single neurons are used to represent populations of neurons. Neurons are identified by their discharge patterns. Patterns of discharge for individual neuron types are shown in B: E, expiratory neuron; E-Dec, inhibitory expiratory neurons that begin to fire with a high discharge rate that declines throughout expiration; I, inspiratory neurons; I-Aug, excitatory neuron that fires with progressively increasing frequency throughout inspiration; I~, pacemaker neuron; Late-I, neuron that fires a burst of action potentials at the end of I and contributes to the transition from inspiration to expiration.

expiration, and Post-I neurons, which discharge only during the early portion of expiration. Expiratory-augmenting (E-Aug) neurons typically begin discharging midway through expiration. Like I-Aug neurons, E-Aug neurons depolarize progressively, resulting in a steady increase in the firing rate. For all neurons receiving rhythmic drive, the patterns of synaptic output are constrained by the patterns of firing of their input neurons.

Given this array of neuron types, the quandary is how they form a network. In particular, how do pre-Bötzinger complex neurons interact with the rest of the network, including premotor and motor neurons, to produce the appropriate motor pattern? While investigators have produced working models that begin to address plausible mechanisms, considerably more information on intrinsic membrane properties and synaptic interactions is required before this goal can be fully realized.

Models of Respiratory Rhythm Generation Fall into Three Basic Categories

Presentations of realistic models of respiratory rhythm generation are beyond the scope of this chapter. Some of the basic elements that must be considered in generating respiratory rhythm are presented here. Those interested in reading further are encouraged to consult any of several very thoughtful and sophisticated papers on modeling (Del Negro et al., 2001; Rybak et al., 1997).

Models for the generation of respiratory rhythm can be divided into three categories: network, pacemaker, and hybrid networks. As suggested by the name, the latter combines network and pacemaker properties. In a simple model such as the one diagramed in Fig 37.9, the kernel of the rhythm generating network consists of two populations of neurons, one of which will be active during inspiration and the other during expiration. To induce activity in this circuit, both populations receive a tonic excitatory input, such as that arising from peripheral and central chemoreceptors. Reciprocal inhibition between the two populations ensures that only one fires at a time. Phase transition between inspiration and expiration can be achieved in several ways. One simple mechanism would follow if the two populations have pacemaker activity, i.e., they form a network of coupled oscillators. Intrinsic membrane properties of pacemaker neurons cause rhythmic oscillations in membrane potential. Activity of these neurons within each population is synchronized by excitatory synaptic interconnections, and their termination is due to their intrinsic properties, e.g., activation of Ca^{2+}-activated

K^+ currents during a burst terminates ongoing burst activity. As the activity of one group of neurons wanes, the other, freed from inhibition, begins to burst. As this latter burst self-terminates, the cycle repeats. Phase transitions are also triggered by active properties of the neurons,

In networks of nonpacemaker neurons, a simple mechanism for phase transition arises if the two populations have decrementing patterns of activity, e.g., inspiratory (I-Dec) and (E-Dec or Post-I) neurons. Phase switching occurs when activity in one population decreases sufficiently (due to the decrementing pattern of discharge) to reduce inhibition of the other group and allows its tonic excitatory input to bring it to threshold. Once these neurons start firing, they inhibit the first group.

An alternative network mechanism for phase termination utilizes a brief burst of action potentials in an inhibitory population. Thus, inspiration is terminated when the declining inhibition from I-Dec neurons permits a population of inhibitory Late-I neurons to burst and terminate ongoing activity in other populations of inspiratory neurons. E-Dec neurons, now no longer inhibited, begin to discharge. In network models, rhythm is generated purely by inhibitory and excitatory synaptic interactions among neurons. Pattern-forming elements then shape and time the activity of various motor neuron pools. Hybrid models incorporate pacemaker properties and synaptic interactions.

Synaptic Excitation and Inhibition Shape the Respiratory Motor Pattern

Two factors determine the firing patterns of motor neurons: rhythmic synaptic drive derived from medullary premotor neurons (see Box 37.2) and intrinsic excitability. In turn, the membrane potentials and firing patterns (see Fig. 37.8) of the premotor neurons and their predecessors leading back to rhythm-generating neurons are also determined by rhythmic and tonic synaptic drive and intrinsic excitability.

Typically, respiratory neurons other than pacemaker neurons fire when they receive phasic excitatory drive, and they are silent when they no longer receive phasic excitatory drive and typically receive phasic inhibitory drive. The excitatory drive is periodic and underlies the rhythmic discharge of all neurons, with the possible exception of pacemaker neurons (discussed later). The inhibitory drive is a bit more complex than the excitatory drive: Three types of synaptically mediated inhibition must be considered (Fig. 37.10; Rekling and Feldman, 1998).

BOX 37.2

SPINAL CORD INJURY CAN DIMINISH VENTILATION

Spinal injuries that affect the long axons of bulbospinal premotor neurons, which transmit respiratory drive to spinal motor neurons, can be life-threatening. With respect to the control of breathing, the severity of the injury depends on the spinal cord level at which the injury occurs. Damage between T1 and S1, in addition to causing sensory and motor deficits in the legs (Chapter XX), can produce loss of control of intercostal muscles below the level of the injury, leading to a diminished ability to generate inspiratory or expiratory movements. The higher the level of functional spinal cord transection, the greater the respiratory impairment. Injury between C4 and C8 can cause quadriplegia and loss of control of all intercostal musculature. Although innervation of the diaphragm may remain (with low cervical damage), the lack of control of the chest wall means the diaphragm must do more work; these patients frequently experience an alarming sense of difficulty breathing (dyspnea). Injuries between the lower brain stem and C4 result in pentaplegia, in which there are motor and sensory losses to the legs, arms, diaphragm, and neck. Such injuries require immediate artificial support of ventilation to maintain life. This type of cervical injury is common following dives into shallow pools.

Jack L. Feldman and
Donald R. McCrimmon

Reciprocal Inhibition

Between phases of excitatory inputs, e.g., during expiration in inspiratory neurons, most respiratory motor neurons and premotor neurons are actively inhibited. Because these neurons are not spontaneously active, why is it necessary to inhibit them when they are not receiving excitatory input? Most likely, reciprocal inhibition prevents their spurious activation (leading to inappropriate muscle contraction) after unexpected afferent inputs. Except for motor neurons that signal opening of the jaws, which must be activated rapidly when a hard object is unexpectedly bitten during chewing, all motor and premotor neurons involved in periodic movements appear subject to reciprocal inhibition.

Recurrent Inhibition

There is a push–pull control of neuronal firing during a burst, i.e., excitation and inhibition are concurrent, with the net balance determining the firing pattern. Reduction of inhibition, e.g., by the administration of inhibitory receptor blockers to motor neurons, results in increased amplitudes of periodic bursts.

Phase-Transition Inhibition

Inhibition has been postulated in network models for breathing to arrest the activity of neurons producing one phase, thereby allowing transition into the next phase, as the neurons of the next phase become active.

Excitatory and Inhibitory Amino Acids

The principal excitatory and inhibitory synaptic potentials that modulate membrane potentials of neurons occur on a millisecond time scale. As in the rest of the central nervous system, in the respiratory network, amino acids are the dominant transmitters and are functionally linked to ion pores. Glutamate is the primary excitatory agent, and GABA and glycine provide inhibition.

Pharmacology of Fast Excitatory Transmission

Fast excitatory drive is probably similar throughout the respiratory control system of the brain. Application of antagonists of excitatory amino acid receptors

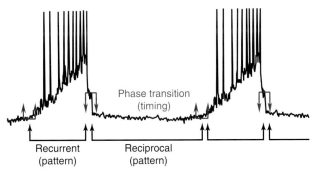

FIGURE 37.10 Membrane potential and discharge pattern of an augmenting inspiratory (or expiratory) neuron. The timing of three distinct types of inhibition is indicated.

reduces the activity of brain stem respiratory neurons, including those in the pre-Bötzinger complex and in the VRG (q.v., McCrimmon *et al.*, 1995; Rekling and Feldman, 1998). This and similar observations confirm that almost all brain stem respiratory neurons receive most of their excitatory synaptic input via glutamatergic neurotransmission. Therefore, transmission at the synapse between bulbospinal premotor neurons and phrenic motor neurons can be treated as typical excitatory communication. The relatively long distance between the somata of premotor neurons in the medulla and their synapses onto phrenic motor neurons in the cervical spinal cord makes these synapses particularly amenable to pharmacologic manipulation. In particular, drugs can be applied to the synapse onto phrenic motoneurons without the complication of drugs affecting the somata of the brain stem premotor neurons.

An amino acid, almost certainly glutamate, appears to be the primary excitatory transmitter at this synapse. In phrenic, as well as hypoglossal, motor neurons, rhythmic inspiratory drive potentials and currents are reduced by local application of drugs that block α-amino-3-hydroxy-5-methyl-4-isoxazole propionic acid (AMPA), kainate, and metabotropic receptors. Synaptically isolated motor neurons respond to exogenous glutamate, unless blocked by the appropriate receptor-selective antagonists. As further evidence, the concentration of glutamate, but not aspartate, in extracellular dialysates from the region of the phrenic nucleus is related to respiratory drive; e,g., when respiratory drive decreases, glutamate in the dialysate also decreases. In addition, bulbospinal respiratory premotor neurons are immunoreactive for glutamate. Finally, unitary postsynaptic potentials (PSPs) underlying inspiratory drive are mediated by glutamate.

Pharmacology of Fast Inhibitory Transmission

Fast synaptic inhibition in brain stem respiratory networks is associated with an increase in permeability to Cl⁻. The principal mediators of this inhibition are the amino acids GABA and glycine (McCrimmon *et al.*, 1995). In the network controlling breathing, the dominant inhibitory mechanism appears to be the result of GABA acting on postsynaptic GABA$_A$ receptors, which affects the excitability of all respiratory neurons. Blocking GABA$_A$ receptors increases the discharge of all VRG neurons. GABA appears to participate in reciprocal and phase-transition inhibitions to help maintain appropriate timing of discharges in premotor networks. In inspiratory neurons, glycinergic transmission appears to mediate the rapid inhibition at the beginning of expiration. Despite the clear

role of synaptic inhibition in maintaining appropriate patterns of activity within the premotor circuitry, respiratory rhythms can be generated in the absence of phasic synaptic inhibition, at least in *in vitro* slices.

Summary

At the heart of breathing is central rhythm generation. The site for automatic generation of this rhythm is within the brain stem. The consensus hypothesis is that the critical circuits lie within (but not necessarily restricted to) a small region of the rostral ventrolateral medulla, the pre-Bötzinger complex. Neural mechanisms undoubtedly require interactions among specialized classes of neurons and may include neurons with the burst properties of pacemaker neurons.

SENSORY INPUTS AND ALTERED BREATHING

O_2 and CO_2 Are Measured by Chemoreceptors

The discussion has focused on the central neural pathways and mechanisms for generating respiratory motor output. The principal goal of this behavior is the maintenance, within narrow limits, of levels of O_2 and CO_2 in the arterial blood (i.e., arterial P_{O_2} = 80–100 mm Hg and P_{CO_2} = 35–45 mm Hg). Changes in P_{O_2}, P_{CO_2}, and pH alter the activity in chemoreceptors, thereby causing reflex changes in breathing that restore them toward regulated levels. Decreases in either P_{O_2} or pH or an increase in P_{CO_2} stimulates breathing, whereas increases in P_{O_2} or pH or a decrease in P_{CO_2} decreases breathing.

The consequences of acute shortfalls in O_2 are catastrophic, but the effects of modestly depressed or elevated P_{O_2} are benign. In contrast, cellular metabolism is strongly sensitive to small changes in P_{CO_2} (due in large part to the effects of such changes on pH). Thus, on a breath-by-breath basis at rest and in health, ventilation is controlled mostly to regulate CO_2 rather than O_2; however, in the event of a marked drop in O_2, everything else is ignored. For example, the exceptionally low ambient pressures at the top of Mount Everest (P_{O_2} ~40 mm Hg) result in such a strong ventilatory drive that blood P_{CO_2} in climbers without supplemental O_2 is exceptionally low (~7 mm Hg compared with normal ~40 mm Hg; see Box 37.3).

O_2

The mammalian brain is extremely sensitive to O_2 deprivation. Several minutes of anoxia can initiate a cascade leading to neuronal (and, if sufficiently wide-

BOX 37.3

DISORDERS OF THE CHEMICAL CONTROL OF BREATHING ARE WIDESPREAD AND SERIOUS

Breathing is normally tightly controlled to maintain arterial P_{CO_2} within a narrow range close to 40 mm Hg. However, cardiopulmonary pathology can increase P_{CO_2} markedly. When P_{CO_2} exceeds 90–120 mm Hg, respiratory depression ensues. With further increases in P_{CO_2}, central nervous system function can be impaired severely; a life-threatening positive feedback loop can develop in which depression of breathing elevates P_{CO_2}, which further depresses breathing. In some patients with advanced chronic lung disease, and consequently elevated P_{CO_2}, any acute lung disease, such as bronchitis or pneumonia, can cause a further increase in P_{CO_2} and exacerbate respiratory depression. In these patients, the drive to breathe comes from hypoxemia (low blood Po_2) sensed by peripheral chemoreceptors. If these patients breathe O_2 without medical monitoring, the hypoxemia may disappear, and without this stimulus these patients' breathing may stop.

Drug abuse is another cause of respiratory depression sufficient to elevate P_{CO_2} to produce further respiratory depression. Narcotics, barbiturates, and most general anesthetics depress breathing and reduce the sensitivity of the chemoreceptors to elevations in P_{CO_2} or reductions in Po_2. Therefore, at high doses these drugs can cause death by respiratory failure.

Sleep apnea. Sleep is associated with a modest decrease in ventilation and a reduced responsiveness to deviations in P_{CO_2} and Po_2. As a result, during sleep, arterial P_{CO_2} increases a few mm Hg and Po_2 decreases. This change in respiratory control is associated with the loss of a wakefulness-related excitatory drive. The source of this wakefulness stimulus is not known, but it may derive from corollary activity originating in the brain stem reticular-activating system.

With the onset of sleep, the breathing pattern can become unstable, and apnea (defined as at least 10 s without breathing) can occur. Two major types of apnea have been defined (White, 1990). The most common, *obstructive sleep apnea*, occurs when inspiratory airflow reduces airway pressure (via the Bernoulli effect), pulling in on the walls of the upper airway and causing airway obstruction. During wakefulness, the activity of airway muscles counteracts this collapsing force. However, during sleep the reduction of airway muscle tone can result in vibration of the walls of the oropharynx (i.e., snoring). In more severe cases, the loss of activity in the glosso-pharyngeal nerve, which innervates the tongue, can cause the airway to become obstructed. Obstruction reduces or

abolishes ventilation, raising CO_2 and lowering O_2. This in turn can cause arousal, or waking, and restoration of airway muscle tone and airway patency. In serious cases, the cycle of sleep, airway obstruction, and hypoxia-induced waking repeats hundreds of times every night. The marked disruption of sleep can cause debilitating hypersomnolence, and severe obstructive sleep apnea can also have other sequelae, such as hypertension.

In *central sleep apnea*, a less common form of sleep apnea, pauses in breathing result from the failure of the central pattern generator for breathing to generate a rhythmic motor command. Mechanisms underlying central apneas are not understood, but the problem has been associated with a variety of neurologic disorders, including brain stem lesions, autonomic dysfunction, and encephalitis, which could impair brain stem function.

Sudden infant death syndrome (SIDS; Martin, 1990). SIDS is defined as the unexpected sudden death of an infant or young child that cannot be explained by a postmortem examination. SIDS is the leading cause of death of infants between 1 month and 1 year of age in the United States. Although a number of etiologies are likely to contribute to SIDS, current hypotheses tend to focus on abnormalities of cardiorespiratory control. The apnea hypothesis of SIDS attributes apnea to disorders of both the chemical control of breathing and the arousal response to insufficient ventilation. Infants who later succumb to SIDS have been described as exhibiting irregular breathing patterns, including periods of apnea, and depressed arousal responses to hypoxia or hypercapnia. Epidemiologically, SIDS has been associated with infants sleeping face down, where pillows, blankets, and mattress can limit the diffusion of expired air, resulting in elevated CO_2 and lower O_2 in inspired air and, consequently, in arterial blood. This in turn could depress breathing sufficiently to cause respiratory arrest and death.

Jack L. Feldman and
Donald R. McCrimmon

References

Martin, R. J. (ed.) (1990). Respiratory disorders during sleep in pediatrics. *In* "Cardiorespiratory Disorders during Sleep," pp. 283–322. Futura, Mount Kisco, NY.

White, D. P. (1990). Ventilation and the control of respiration during sleep: Normal mechanisms, pathologic nocturnal hypoventilation, and central sleep apnea. *In* "Cardiorespiratory Disorders during Sleep" (R. J. Martin, ed.), pp. 53–108. Futura, Mount Kisco, NY.

spread, brain) death. Brain hypoxia can cause loss of consciousness. Perhaps for these reasons, the principal O_2 sensors for the entire body are in the portal through which most of the O_2 enters the brain, in the *carotid bodies* at the bifurcation of the common carotid artery. The mechanisms by which O_2 levels are transduced by these *peripheral chemoreceptors* into afferent signals have been studied intensely since Corneille Heyman's discovery of the physiological function of the carotid bodies, for which he was awarded the Nobel Prize in Physiology or Medicine in 1938. Carotid chemoreceptors do not exhibit a threshold for activation, which is different from most other sensory receptors, and have a low-frequency, irregular discharge pattern at rest (Bisgard and Neubauer, 1995). O_2-related signals enter the brain via the glossopharyngeal nerve and synapse in the dorsomedial medulla in the nucleus of the solitary tract.

Under normal conditions, O_2 sensors account for only a small part of the chemical drive to breathe. Breathing 100% O_2 reduces spontaneous chemoreceptor discharge to near zero but only decreases ventilation by about 15% in awake mammals. Decreasing P_{O2} has relatively little influence on chemoreceptor activity and ventilation until the P_{O2} falls below about 60 mm Hg. With further reductions in P_{O2}, chemoreceptor discharge and ventilation increase exponentially.

CO_2

Ventilation is very sensitive to small changes in P_{CO2}, which is normally about 40 mm Hg in arterial blood. A 1 mm Hg increase in P_{CO2} leads to a 2 liter $\times$ min^{-1} increase in ventilation from a baseline value of about 5 liter x min^{-1} in an adult human. In other words, a 2.5% increase in P_{CO2} at rest leads to a 40% increase in ventilation!

The sites and mechanisms of CO_2 chemoreception remain obscure. While the carotid bodies are sensitive to changes in P_{CO2}, a robust CO_2 response is still seen in peripherally chemodenervated, decerebrate mammals, suggesting that CO_2 or related variables (pH, HCO_3^-) have additional intracranial sensors. Most attention has focused on the ventral medulla. Researchers have demonstrated that significant alterations in pH at the ventral medullary surface alter breathing in anesthetized animals. At pH 7.0, ventilation increases, and at pH 7.8, ventilation decreases (normal brain extracellular fluid pH is 7.3). These changes are in the appropriate directions, but relative to physiologically expected shifts in pH associated with significant changes in ventilation (e.g., a decrease of 0.05 unit in cerebrospinal fluid pH produces a three- to fivefold increase in ventilation) the experimental perturbations

are extreme. More recently, specific structures that appear to play a role in intracranial chemotransduction have been delineated. The most convincing experiments have utilized small injections of the carbonic anhydrase inhibitor acetazolamide (AZ); carbonic anhydrase catalyzes the reaction $CO_2 + H_2O <-> H^+ + HCO_3^-$. Injections of 1 nl of an AZ solution, which produce highly localized tissue acidosis, into various regions in cat or rat brain stem caused an increase in ventilation (Nattie, 2000). These injections were centered in three distinct regions, including the retrotrapezoid nucleus, the nucleus of the solitary tract, and the raphe nuclei. Within the raphe nuclei, serotonergic neurons have cellular properties expected of the central respiratory chemoreceptors, including a three- fold increase in the firing rate in response to a decrease in pH from 7.4 to 7.2, and projections to respiratory nuclei (Wang *et al.*, 2001). The relative role that neurons in the raphe play in the normal response to hypercapnia, compared to other brain stem regions, remains to be elucidated.

MECHANORECEPTORS IN THE LUNGS ADJUST BREATHING PATTERN AND INITIATE PROTECTIVE REFLEXES

Many patterns of muscle activity can produce alveolar ventilation appropriate for a given metabolic load; however, the chosen pattern must minimize energy expenditure. The efficiency of a pattern of respiratory muscle activity in turn depends on such factors as posture and lung and chest wall mechanics (e.g., a fibrotic, i.e., stiff, lung is harder to inflate to a given tidal volume than a normal lung, and thus for this condition, rapid, shallow breathing is more efficient). Feedback about the mechanical status of the lungs and chest wall is provided by mechanoreceptors.

Because the airways must be patent for airflow, airway receptors produce two of the most powerful and compelling reflexes: coughing and gagging. Another powerful reflex occurs at birth, when the transition from the liquid uterine environment to an air environment requires a powerful inspiratory effort (sigh) to overcome surface forces resisting the initial inflation of the lung. The obligatory sigh is stimulated by pulmonary receptors. Additional nonspecific reflex stimuli, typically mechanical or thermal, further facilitate the first inspiratory sighs. Special respiratory reflexes, such as sneezing and yawning, are also generated by pulmonary receptors.

Mechanosensory signals are critical in adapting, adjusting, and integrating breathing with other acts of brain and body. Many movements impact directly on breathing, either by using the same muscles used for breathing (e.g., phonation, posture, defecation, and emesis) or through mechanical disturbances, such as locomotion.

Lung Afferents

Sensory receptors in the lungs and airways have important roles in the control of breathing and in pulmonary defense reflexes, such as cough. There are three distinct groups of afferents, all with fibers coursing in the vagus nerve and terminating in the nucleus of the solitary tract (see Table 37.1; Kubin and Davies, 1995). Two groups consist of large, myelinated A fibers, with receptors in the airways, and include slowly adapting and rapidly adapting pulmonary stretch receptors. The third group gives rise to small, unmyelinated C fibers and responds to inhaled irritants such as smoke. The relative inaccessibility for experimentation of these stretch and irritant receptors has made it difficult to selectively activate a single type of receptor and precisely define the natural stimuli and reflex responses of each. Most natural stimuli (e.g., pulmonary edema or alveolar collapse) probably activate more than one category of receptor, and the CNS likely integrates these inputs to determine the nature of the appropriate response.

Slowly Adapting Pulmonary Stretch Receptors (SARs)

Located in airway smooth muscle, SARs are activated when the airways stretch during lung inflation (Kubin and Davies, 1995). Their activation leads to reflexes in which lung inflation shortens inspiration and prolongs expiration. This change in breathing pattern is called the Breuer–Hering reflex, which is an important determinant of inspiratory duration during normal breathing in most mammalian species, with the notable exception of humans. The activation of these receptors with each normal inspiration overrides the baseline rhythm of the respiratory pattern generator, shortening the inspiratory period and increasing the overall breathing frequency. In humans, normal breaths apparently do not activate the SAR receptors sufficiently to affect inspiratory timing. Activation of these receptors also relaxes airway smooth muscle, resulting in dilation of the airways, reducing airflow resistance to make breathing easier.

Higher Order Neurons in the Breuer–Hering Reflex

The Breuer–Hering reflex has been one of the more intensely studied vagal reflexes. Because its activation changes the respiratory rhythm, an understanding of the underlying mechanisms will illuminate aspects of the central pattern generator for breathing. SAR afferents monosynaptically activate a group of neurons within the nucleus of solitary tract termed pump (P) cells (Fig. 37.11). These neurons derive their name from the observation that in paralyzed, artificially ventilated mammals, SAR afferent input causes P cells to discharge in phase with ventilator (pump)-induced lung inflations; if the ventilator is turned off briefly, they are silent. Pump cells oligosynaptically activate several types of respiratory neurons in the ventral medulla. Among these are E-Dec neurons, which, by virtue of their hypothesized inhibitory connections, prevent firing in inspiratory neurons, thereby terminating inspiration and prolonging expiration (Hayashi et al., 1996).

TABLE 37.1 Pulmonary Vagal Afferents and Their Associated Reflexes

Receptor (fiber type)	Location	Stimulus	Reflex Response
Slowly adapting pulmonary stretch receptors (myelinated, A)	Airway smooth muscle	Lung inflation (distension of airways)	Breuer–Hering (a) inspiratory termination (b) expiratory prolongation, airway dilation
Rapidly adapting pulmonary stretch receptors (myelinated, A)	Airway epithelium and subepithelial layers of mucosa	Rapid lung inflation or deflation, edema in walls of large airways, chemical irritants	Cough, augmented inspiration (sigh), shortened expiration, airway constriction
Broncho-pulmonary C fibers (unmyelinated, C)	Throughout airways and alveolar wall	Chemical irritants, edema	Apnea (cessation of breathing), rapid shallow breathing, airway constriction, mucus secretion

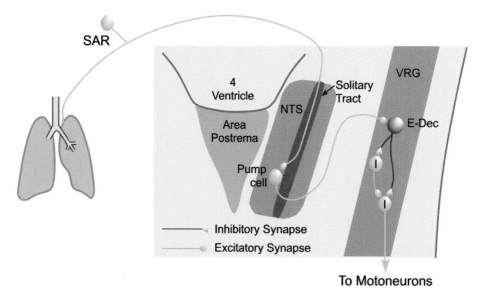

FIGURE 37.11 Dorsal view of rat brain stem showing hypothesized central pathway for producing reflex termination of inspiration and prolongation of expiration (the Breuer–Hering reflex). Slowly adapting pulmonary stretch receptor afferents (SAR) arise from receptors located in airway smooth muscle and activate second-order pump cells in the nucleus of the solitary tract (NTS). These neurons are believed to activate E-Dec neurons in the ventral respiratory group (VRG) that inhibit inspiratory neurons, thereby prolonging expiration.

Rapidly Adapting Pulmonary Stretch Receptors (RARs)

Located in airway epithelial and subepithelial layers, RARs initiate protective reflexes in response to a variety of stimuli, including large or rapid lung inflation or deflation, inhaled irritants, and, possibly, airway edema (see Table 37.1; Kubin and Davies, 1995). Inhalation of irritants such as smoke activates RARs in the large airways and elicits a cough to rid the airway of the offending material. Activation of these receptors can also result in rapid, shallow breathing. In addition, these afferents may elicit sighs in response to collapse of alveoli. As alveoli collapse, the lungs become stiffer. This change in pulmonary mechanics is sensed by RARs, and a larger than normal breath (a sigh) is elicited, inflating the lung and popping open the alveoli.

Bronchopulmonary C fibers

C fiber afferents elicit apnea followed by rapid shallow breathing. Like RARs, C fibers are poly-modal, activated by chemical and mechanical stimuli. Activation of these receptors enhances mucus secretion in the airways. Inhaled particles are trapped in the mucus and removed from the airways by the action of cilia, which continuously (in the nonsmoker) move the mucus and trapped particles toward the mouth to be swallowed or expectorated.

Summary

Chemoreceptors in the arterial system and in the brain provide sensory input to the central circuits controlling breathing to tightly regulate P_{CO_2} and P_{O_2} within narrow limits over a wide range of metabolic demand. Peripheral receptors in the carotid and aortic bodies are especially sensitive to decreases in arterial P_{O_2}, and they also sense increases in arterial P_{CO_2} and decreases in arterial pH. Central chemoreceptors in the brain stem are exquisitely sensitive to increases in tissue P_{CO_2} and decreases in pH, but central chemo-receptors respond little to changes in P_{O_2}. Mechano-receptors, especially those in the lungs, are essential for the precise regulation of the timing and amplitude of breathing and participate in reflexes, such as coughing, that protect the airways and lungs from compromises in airflow.

MODULATION AND PLASTICITY OF RESPIRATORY MOTOR OUTPUT

The generation of an appropriate motor output is not simply sine wave generation. A precise spatio-temporal pattern of motor outputs must be generated for a broad spectrum of activated muscles. For example, reflex adjustments in pattern are made as body position changes. Other adjustments produce efficient breathing patterns during physical exercise and adapt to changes in lung and chest wall mechanics that accompany postnatal development, normal aging, and pulmonary disease.

How are these challenges to the control of breathing met? Although the full answer is not yet apparent, it is clear that the activation of sensory receptors often triggers changes in breathing that outlast the stimulus by seconds to days or even weeks. For example, activation of carotid chemoafferent neurons by hypoxia increases ventilatory activity by multiple mechanisms acting in different time domains lasting seconds, minutes, and hours to days (Mitchell *et al.*, 2001). In an anesthetized and artificially ventilated rat, a single episode of hypoxia lasting 10–20 min increases ventilatory activity (assessed in neural activity to the diaphragm). When hypoxia is reversed, ventilatory activity slowly returns to the original level over a period of several minutes. This slow decrease back to the prehypoxia level of activity is referred to as *short-term potentiation*. Although ventilatory activity returns to normal after short-term potentiation has ended following a single episode of hypoxia, a unique, longer-lasting mechanism is revealed following repetitive brief episodes of hypoxia (three episodes of 5 min duration). As illustrated in Fig 37.12, immediately following the third hypoxic episode, ventilatory activity transiently returns toward prestimulation levels, but is followed by a slow, progressive augmentation of ventilatory activity, even though arterial oxygen and carbon dioxide levels are normal. This slow augmentation lasts for several hours and is known as *respiratory long-term facilitation*.

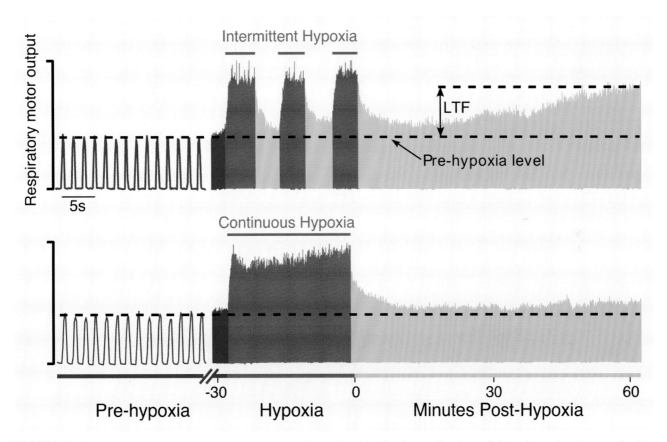

FIGURE 37.12 Respiration-related neural activity in an anesthetized and artificially ventilated rat exhibits a form of respiratory plasticity known as *respiratory long-term facilitation*. On the left in each trace, electrical activity in the phrenic nerve (the main nerve innervating the diaphragm) is integrated such that each peak represents a "fictive breath" that the artificially ventilated rat had intended to make. Under normal conditions of arterial oxygen and carbon dioxide (baseline), the phrenic bursts are rhythmic and consistent. When the rats are exposed to different patterns of decreased arterial oxygen (intermittent, upper trace; continuous, lower trace), phrenic bursts increase in amplitude, reflecting the drive to take deeper breaths when hypoxia-sensitive chemoreceptors are activated. In both types of low oxygen exposure, phrenic nerve activity returns nearly to baseline levels several minutes after the hypoxia has ended. However, in the case of intermittent but not continuous hypoxia, phrenic burst amplitude increases slowly and progressively over an hour, even though arterial oxygen and carbon dioxide are at baseline levels. This slow increase reflects a sort of "respiratory memory" that is elicited by intermittent hypoxia, or respiratory long-term facilitation. Respiratory long-term facilitation appears to result from serotonin-dependent plasticity (see text and Fig. 37.12). Courtesy of T. L. Baker and G. S. Mitchell.

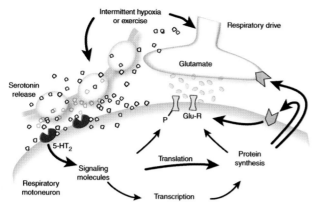

FIGURE 37.13 Schematic representation of hypothetical cellular/synaptic mechanism underlying serotonin-dependent respiratory plasticity (after Mitchell *et al.*, 2001). In this mechanism, conditions known to increase raphe serotonergic neuron activity in an intermittent pattern (e.g., intermittent hypoxia and intermittent exercise) release serotonin in the vicinity of respiratory neurons, and the glutamatergic synaptic input associated with descending respiratory drive from medullary premotor neurons. The episodic release of serotonin initiates a signaling cascade within respiratory motoneurons, leading to increased protein synthesis. These new proteins either directly or indirectly via autoreceptors modify the postsynaptic glutamate receptors, increasing respiration-related synaptic currents. Presynaptic effects are also possible. The persistence of these modifications to the respiratory synapse results in respiratory plasticity, either as respiratory long-term facilitation (Mitchell *et al.*, 2001) or as plasticity in the exercise ventilatory response (Turner *et al.*, 1997). The identity of the new proteins synthesized in this mechanism remains unknown, as do the relative contributions of presynaptic versus postsynaptic mechanisms. Courtesy of G. S. Mitchell.

The short-term potentiation of ventilation likely involves mechanisms distributed at several stages between afferent input and motor output. NMDA receptors are probably activated in the region of afferent processing in the nucleus of the solitary tract and within the phrenic nucleus. Short-term potentiation of breathing may be important in producing smoothly changing respiratory responses during rapid or large changes in afferent input. If breathing responded immediately and fully to changes in afferent signals, large swings in arterial blood gases would result, thereby causing further reflex changes in breathing, ultimately resulting in an unstable control system (e.g., Cheyne–Stokes respiration, Fig. 37.14).

The mechanism of respiratory long-term facilitation has been investigated extensively in recent years (Mitchell *et al.*, 2001). As illustrated in Fig. 37.12, this form of plasticity requires repetitive application of a short duration chemoreceptor stimulus (i.e., episodic hypoxia) rather than a single longer lasting stimulus (i.e., continuous hypoxia). Hypoxia activates peripheral chemoreceptors and initiates the release of serotonin (5-hydroxytryptamine, 5-HT) in the vicinity of respiratory motoneurons (Fig 37.13). It appears to be the episodic and repetitive nature of serotonin receptor activation that is necessary for the initiation but not the maintenance of respiratory long-term facilitation. Because respiratory long-term facilitation also requires the synthesis of new proteins, it was

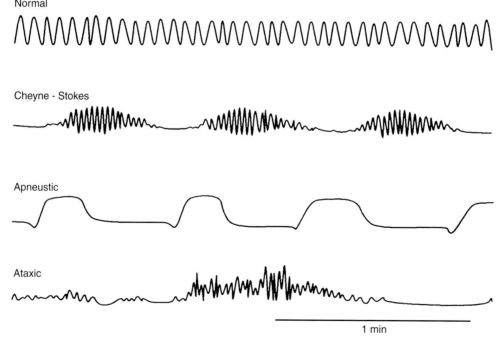

FIGURE 37.14 Abnormal breathing patterns resulting from CNS disorders. The ordinate is lung volume. Adapted from Plum and Posner (1980).

BOX 37.4

CNS LESIONS PRODUCE ABNORMAL BREATHING PATTERNS

Many brain injuries and diseases produce abnormal breathing patterns (Plum and Posner, 1980). Because many brain regions provide afferent input to the neurons generating the breathing rhythm, pathology in regions not normally associated with the generation of breathing can produce abnormal breathing patterns. Despite the diffuse nature of many pathologies that give rise to abnormal breathing patterns, Fred Plum and colleagues have systematically characterized several breathing disorders (Fig. 37.14) arising from specific CNS pathologies.

Apneustic breathing is marked by prolonged inspiratory periods. In humans, the most frequent pattern is inspirations lasting 2–3 s alternating with prolonged expiratory pauses. In cats, the prolonged inspiratory periods are associated with plateaus in inspiratory drive that can last minutes (leading to death in the absence of mechanical ventilation). Apneusis is observed in people with lesions of the pons, including, or just ventral to, the pontine respiratory group. In experimental animals, apneusis requires not only lesions of the pontine respiratory group, but also interruption of vagal afferent input.

Lesions of the corticobulbar or corticospinal tracts can lead to *Cheyne–Stokes respiration*, a rhythmic waxing and waning of the depth of breathing. Periods of no breathing (apnea) follow each period of waning inspiratory depth. Lesions of the corticobulbar and corticospinal tracts can also result in loss of voluntary control of

breathing. In pseudobulbar palsy, for example, voluntary control of breathing and of cranial motor neuron function is lost secondary to a lesion often located dorsomedially in the base of the pons.

Extensive bilateral damage to the medullary respiratory groups can severely disrupt or abolish respiratory rhythm, resulting in death unless artificial ventilation is initiated immediately. Fortunately, unilateral damage does not appear to be sufficient to cause severe disruption of respiratory rhythm- and pattern-generating mechanisms. Because two vertebral arteries supply blood to the medulla, bilateral damage from an infarct or embolism is unlikely.

Less extensive damage to medullary respiratory structures can produce *ataxic breathing*, an irregular pattern of breathing with apparent randomly occurring large and small breaths and periods of apnea. Breathing frequency tends to be low.

Jack L. Feldman and
Donald R. McCrimmon

Reference

Plum, F., and Posner, J. B. (1980). "The Diagnosis of Stupor and Coma," 3rd Ed., Contemp. Neurol. Sci. Vol. 19. Davis, Philadelphia.

hypothesized that serotonin receptor activation on respiratory motoneurons initiates a signaling cascade, resulting in the synthesis of new proteins that amplify the synaptic currents associated with descending, glutamatergic synaptic inputs from respiratory premotor neurons (Fig 37.13). Thus, in many respects, respiratory long-term facilitation has similarities with other forms of synaptic plasticity in its stimulus pattern sensitivity and requirement for protein synthesis. The requirement for episodic serotonin receptor activation is similar to serotonin-dependent plasticity at the sensorimotor synapse of *Aplysia*.

Long-term facilitation could underlie some of the adaptive changes to pathophysiological conditions that cause repeated peripheral chemoreceptor activation. For example, long-term facilitation may help restore stable respiration during sleep-disordered breathing in which repeated periods of sleep apnea result in episodic hypoxia. During sleep, the activity of serotonergic raphe neurons is reduced dramati-

cally. Repeated activation of these neurons secondary to apnea-induced chemoreceptor activation could increase ventilatory drive and reduce the probability of future apneas. Marked derangements of breathing can also occur in response to pathology within a variety of other brain regions that contain projections to respiratory neurons (see Box 37.4).

An example of unstable breathing is seen in a subset of patients in whom the central network controlling breathing responds to a change in activity of the chemoreceptors by causing too large or too rapid a change in breathing. The central circuitry controlling breathing is capable of rapidly (<200 ms) changing ventilation in response to changes in chemoreceptor activity, but the delay is much longer (several seconds) between the time ventilation changes and the detection of the resultant, corrective changes in blood gases by peripheral and central chemoreceptors. This difference between the rapid response time and the much slower detection of the resultant change in blood gases is a potential source of instability; such instability can cause Cheyne–Stokes respiration (Fig. 37.14).

Neurotransmitters Contribute to the Modulation of Breathing

The waxing and waning membrane potential underlying the periodic bursting of motor neurons can be ascribed simply to the alternating release of glutamate, GABA, and glycine at their respective postsynaptic receptors. Given the straightforward task of these motor neurons, especially for muscle as specialized as the diaphragm, one might presume that little more is required to control their excitability. Yet the picture is much richer and provides some insight into possible roles for the diversity of transmitters.

Regardless of the type of neuron considered, neurotransmitters transmit synaptic signals that shape its discharge pattern (Bianchi *et al.*, 1995; McCrimmon *et al.*, 1995). Chief among the rapidly acting neurotransmitters that sculpt the phasic discharge patterns of these neurons are the excitatory amino acids, of which glutamate is the primary member, and the inhibitory amino acids, principally GABA and glycine. GABA also appears to play a key role in regulating the baseline discharge frequency of VRG respiratory neurons. Antagonism of GABA$_A$ receptors with bicuculline results in a discharge frequency pattern that is an amplified replica of the control pattern. The magnitude of this effect is such that the discharge rate of the neurons is only about 35–50% of the rate following blockade of the GABAergic input. This phenomenon suggests that a tonic GABAergic input constrains the control and reflexly induced activities of these neurons to about 35–50% of the discharge rate without this inhibitory input. This form of gain control could provide a robust mechanism for the central respiratory controller to optimize the breathing pattern in response to changes in conditions or state.

A limited survey of other possible neurotransmitters and modulators that alter respiratory rhythm and pattern include the amine serotonin, catecholamines (norepinephrine, epinephrine, and dopamine), acetylcholine, adenosine, and numerous peptides (typically colocalized with the amines), including substance P, neuropeptide Y, galanin, Metenkephalin, cholecystokinin, and thyrotropin-releasing hormone (Fig. 37.15). Although one could look at each of these transmitters separately, little detailed information about the roles of specific transmitters in respiratory rhythm generation is available, and this reductionist approach does not address why

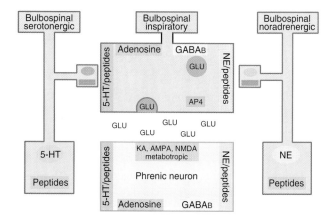

FIGURE 37.15 The diversity of synaptic control of phrenic motor neurons is essential for their proper function. The challenge is to understand how these mechanisms act in an integrated manner. Isolating and studying them one by one or out of context, e.g., in culture, may fail to reveal key properties. AMPA (see text), GLU, glutamate; 5-HT, serotonin; KA, kainate; NE, norepinephrine.

nature employs such a variety of neurotransmitters. Many of these transmitters have been identified in the phrenic nucleus, and researchers have asked why so many neurotransmitters are present at such a simple relay to a muscle with a limited repertoire of functions. Multiple transmitters and receptors may be necessary to control neuronal excitability over the broad time scales important in breathing, from the millisecond scale of synaptic currents of cycle-by-cycle respiratory drive, to the seconds required to alter ventilation in response to changes in blood gases, to the hours or days for acclimatization to altitude or adjustment to disease, development, and aging. Alternatively, multiple transmitters may allow coarse and fine control of P_{O_2}, P_{CO_2}, and pH. Multiple transmitters may also ensure that breathing is not compromised by changes in state, especially during sleep when global changes in amine levels can affect motor neuronal excitability. During rapid eye movement (REM) sleep, motor neuronal excitability produces a widespread muscle atonia, yet respiratory motor neurons must continue to drive respiratory muscles. The key to maintaining respiratory motor neuronal excitability may be related to 5-HT, which is reduced drastically during REM. Finally, multiple neurotransmitters may be needed to prevent respiratory muscle fatigue. A strong inspiratory drive will sufficiently elevate glutamate in the synaptic cleft to act via a presynaptic metabotropic receptor to reduce further release. This governor of maximal phrenic motor neuronal activity would limit the likelihood of diaphragmatic fatigue during periods of sustained high ventilatory demand (e.g., fleeing a predator).

Summary

As metabolism, posture, and sleep–wake state change, the breathing pattern must adjust rapidly to ensure appropriate and efficient ventilation. Development and disease, as well as adaptation to changes in altitude, are processes that require slower adaptations in breathing. Amino acids, amines, peptides, and other neurotransmitters coordinate circuits generating and modulating respiratory pattern to ensure that adaptations proceed smoothly and precisely by mechanisms that remain to be determined.

SUPRAPONTINE STRUCTURES AND BREATHING

The discussion has focused on the roles of the pons, medulla, and spinal cord in the control of breathing. These regions contain the minimum circuitry for generating respiratory rhythm, producing the motor output and modifying its pattern in response to afferent input from the lungs, airways, and chest. Higher brain regions have fundamental roles in producing integrated responses in which the behaviors of multiple organ systems are coordinated to produce an appropriate output. Speech, for example, requires the coordination of jaw and facial muscles, precise tongue, upper airway, and laryngeal control, and coordinated activity of breathing muscles to produce controlled subglottal pressure. The anterior limbic cortex (including the rostral anterior cingulate gyrus, the subcallosal gyrus, and gyrus rectus), midbrain periaqueductal gray, brain stem respiratory nuclei, and cranial and spinal motor neurons contribute to speech.

Sustained or repetitive movement of large muscles involved in such basic behaviors as fleeing predators, chasing prey, and exercising also involves higher CNS functions. During exercise the metabolic production of CO_2 increases as a result of increased consumption of O_2. However, arterial P_{CO_2} and P_{O_2} change little during moderate exercise because of an increase in breathing proportional to the demand for gas exchange. This increase may be produced by a feed-forward descending command from higher brain systems and sensory input from joint and muscle receptors. The latter inputs provide feedback about limb and muscle mechanics, but can be considered feed-forward with respect to the control of arterial blood gases because they may provide cues for adjusting the magnitude of the descending command. Any inadequacy in the feed-forward mechanisms to produce appropriate ventilation is immediately met by chemoreceptor feedback (mostly relevant to P_{CO_2}). Thus arterial blood gases are tightly regulated during moderate exercise.

The volitional initiation of exercise, signaled by suprapontine structures, likely involves parallel activation of spinal locomotor pathways and brain stem mechanisms controlling breathing and cardiovascular function so that pulmonary ventilation and gas transport change appropriately. It can be assumed that the commands for the activation of pulmonary and locomotor muscles arise in similar ways in the motor cortex, thalamus, and basal ganglia. Once the motor command has been initiated, respiratory and locomotor activities are believed to be coordinated at subcortical levels, including the hypothalamus. Electrical or chemical activation of the hypothalamus of an anesthetized, paralyzed cat elicits fictive locomotion paired with proportional increases in respiratory motor output (suggestive of exercise-related increases in ventilation or exercise hyperpnea) and redistribution of blood flow consistent with the induction of locomotion (Waldrop et al., 1996). Because the animals are paralyzed, muscle activation does not occur, and thus the changes in breathing are the result of feed-forward control rather than sensory feedback from joint or muscle receptors.

The exercise ventilatory response demonstrates the plasticity of the respiratory control system. An example of this modulation is evident in experiments in which goats were trained to stand or run on a treadmill (Turner et al., 1997). Normally, ventilation increases in proportion to the exercise-induced increase in metabolic rate, and arterial blood gases remain close to resting values. When the goats breathed through a tube, increasing respiratory dead space, the response was enhanced markedly and enhancement occurred within one exercise trial. A normal response was restored when the dead space was removed. Application of serotonin receptor antagonists to the spinal cord attenuated or blocked this effect. When goats were exercised repeatedly with an increased dead space, additional mechanisms came into play to further alter the ventilatory response. For example, after 2 days of exercise with increased dead space, the response without the extra dead space was augmented for up to 6 h, resulting in hyperventilation and respiratory alkalosis (i.e., decreased blood P_{CO_2} and increased pH). This longer lasting effect, in which prior experience alters ventilatory response, is a form of learning. These findings illustrate that ventilatory control is not a static, hard-wired reflex response but a complex integrative process capable of long-term adaptations to changing pathophysiological or environmental conditions, such as onset of lung disease, acclimatization to high altitude, or scuba or firefighting equipment that increase dead space.

Summary

Breathing is a basic physiologic function that must be controlled vigilantly by the brain. This chapter has explored basic mechanisms underlying rhythm generation, sensory processing, and motor output. Given the broad range of experimental systems available to study these mechanisms, from *in vitro* rodent brain stem slices to intact awake and sleeping humans, all levels of neurobiological analysis have considerable potential to unravel integrative mechanisms of brain function that may be of general importance.

References

Adrian, E. D., and Buytendijk, F. J. J. (1931). Potential changes in the isolated brainstem of goldfish. *J. Physiol. (Lond.)* **71**, 121–135.

Ballanyi, K., Onimaru, H., and Homma, K. (1999). Respiratory network function in the isolated brainstem-spinal cord of newborn rats. *Prog. Neurobiol.* **59**, 583–634.

Bianchi, A. L., Denavit-Saubié, M., and Champagnat, J. (1995). Central control of breathing in mammals: Neuronal circuitry, membrane properties, and neurotransmitters. *Physiol. Rev.* **75**, 1–45.

Bisgard, G. E., and Neubauer, J. A. (1995). Peripheral and central effects of hypoxia. *In* "Lung Biology in Health and Disease: Regulation of Breathing" (J. A. Dempsey and A. Pack, Eds.), pp. 617–668. Dekker, New York.

Del Negro, C. A., Johnson, S. M., Butera, R. J., and Smith, J. C. (2001). Models of respiratory rhythm generation in the pre-Bötzinger complex. III. Experimental tests of model predictions. *J. Neurophysiol.* **86**, 59–74.

Galen. (1968). "Usefulness of the Parts of the Body" (M. T. May, ed.). Cornell Univ. Press, Ithaca, NY.

Gesell, R., Bricker, J., and Magee, C. (1936). Structural and functional organization of the central mechanism controlling breathing. *Am. J. Physiol.* **117**, 423–452.

Gray, P. A., Janczewski, W. A., Mellen, N., McCrimmon, D. R., and Feldman, J. L. (2001). Normal breathing requires preBötzinger complex neurokinin-1 receptor-expressing neurons. *Nature Neurosci.* **4**, 927–930.

Hayashi, F., Coles, S. K., and McCrimmon, D. R. (1996). Respiratory neurons mediating the Breuer-Hering reflex prolongation of expiration in rat. *J. Neurosci.* **16**, 6526–6536.

Hayashi, F., and McCrimmon, D. R. (1996). Respiratory motor responses to cranial afferent stimulation in rats. *Am. J. Physiol.* **271**, R1054–R1062.

Johnson, S. M., Koshiya, N., and Smith, J. C. (2001). Isolation of The kernel for respiratory rhythm generation in a novel preparation: The pre-Bötzinger complex "island." *J. Neurophysiol.* **85**, 1772–1776.

Koshiya, N., and Smith, J. C. (1999). Neuronal pacemaker for breathing visualized *in vitro. Nature* **400**, 360–363.

Kubin, L., and Davies, R. O. (1995). Central pathways of pulmonary and airway vagal afferents. *In* "Lung Biology in Health and Disease: Regulation of Breathing" (J. A. Dempsey and A. Pack, eds.), pp. 219–284. Dekker, New York.

Legallois, M. (1813). "Experiments on the Principle of Life." Thomas, Philadelphia.

Lorry, M. (1760). Les mouvements du cerveau. *Mem. Math. Phys. Pres. Acad. Roy. Sci. Div. Sav. Paris* **3**, 344–377.

Lumsden, T. (1923). Observations on the respiratory centres in the cat. *J. Physiol. (Lond.)* **57**, 153–160.

Martin, R. J. (ed.) (1990). Respiratory disorders during sleep in pediatrics. *In* "Cardiorespiratory Disorders during Sleep," pp. 283–322. Futura, Mount Kisco, NY.

McCrimmon, D. R., Mitchell, G. S., and Dekin, M. (1995). Glutamate, GABA and serotonin in ventilatory control. *In* "Lung Biology in Health and Disease: Regulation of Breathing" (J. A. Dempsey and A. Pack, eds.), pp. 151–218. Dekker, New York.

Mitchell, G. S., Baker, T. L., Nanda, S. A., Fuller, D. D., Zabka, A. G., Hodgeman, B. A., Bavis, R. W., Mack, K. J., and Olson, E. B., Jr. (2001). Intermittent hypoxia and respiratory plasticity. *J. Appl. Physiol.* **90**, 2466–2475.

Nattie, E. (2000). Multiple sites for central chemoreception: Their roles in response sensitivity and in sleep and wakefulness. *Respir. Physiol.* **122**, 223–235.

Plum, F., and Posner, J. B. (1980). "The Diagnosis of Stupor and Coma," 3rd Ed., Contemp. Neurol. Ser. Vol. 19. Davis, Philadelphia.

Ramon y Cajal, S. (1909). "Histologie du Systeme Nerveux de l'homme et des Vertebres." Maloine, Paris.

Rekling, J. C., and Feldman, J. L. (1998). PreBötzinger complex and pacemaker neurons: Hypothesized site and kernel for respiratory rhythm generation. *Annu. Rev. Physiol.* **60**, 385–405.

Richter, D., Ballanyi, K., and Ramirez, J. (1996). Respiratory rhythm generation. *In* "Neural Control of Respiratory Muscles" (A. Miller, A. Bianchi, and B. Bishop, eds.), pp. 119–131. CRC Press, Boca Raton, FL.

Rybak, I. A., Paton, J. F., and Schwaber, J. S. (1997). Modeling neural mechanisms for genesis of respiratory rhythm and pattern. III. Comparison of model performances during afferent nerve stimulation. *J. Neurophysiol.* **77**, 2027–2039.

Smith J. C., Ellenberger H. H., Ballanyi K., Richter D., and Feldman J. L. (1991). Pre-Bötzinger complex: A brainstem region that may generate respiratory rhythm in mammals. *Science* **254**, 726–729.

Turner, D. L., Bach, K. B., Martin, P. A., Olson, E. B., Brownfield, M., Foley, K. T., and Mitchell, G. S. (1997). Modulation of ventilatory control during exercise. *Respir. Physiol.* **110**, 277–285.

Waldrop, T .G., Eldridge, F. L., Iwamoto, G. A., and Mitchell, J. H. (1996). Central neural control of respiration and circulation during exercise. *In* "Handbook of Physiology" (L. B. Rowell, and J. T. Shepherd, eds.), pp. 333–380. Oxford Univ. Press, New York.

Wang, W., Zaykin, A. V., Tiwari, J. K., Risso Bradley S., and Richerson, G. B. (2001). Acidosis-stimulated neurons of the medullary raphe are serotonergic. *J. Neurophysiol.* **85**, 2224–2235.

White, D. P. (1990). Ventilation and the control of respiration during sleep: Normal mechanisms, pathologic nocturnal hypoventilation, and central sleep apnea. *In* "Cardiorespiratory Disorders during Sleep" (R. J. Martin, ed.), pp. 53–108. Futura, Mount Kisco, NY.

Jack L. Feldman and Donald R. McCrimmon

38

Food Intake and Metabolism

Eating is a familiar behavior. In humans, it is strongly influenced by cultural, social, and experiential factors. Consequently, eating has been a subject of considerable interest to social and behavioral scientists. In mammals, including humans, food intake is also a regulatory behavior with the primary function of supporting the continuous energy demands of body tissues. When considered from this biological perspective, food intake is influenced by hunger, satiety, and the physiological mechanisms that couple eating with internal caloric supplies and a stable body weight. This chapter discusses the signals important for the central nervous system to control food intake and also describes mechanisms thought to integrate those signals.

Despite decades of investigation, considerable differences of opinion still exist about how food intake is controlled. The multiple views follow one of two principles. The first considers eating to be a consequence of depleted energy stores in adipose tissue, reduced use of energy-rich *metabolic fuel* (glucose or lipid) in some critical tissue, or both. In this schema, the purpose of eating is to restore energy reserves in adipose tissue or to increase fuel utilization to some desired level, thereby eliminating the signal to eat. This traditional "depletion–repletion" model is not the approach taken in this chapter. Rather, we subscribe to a second principle—one that considers animals primed to eat unless influenced by inhibitory signals that have been generated by meals. According to this view, the onset of eating does not result from acute needs, nor does the end of a meal result from a decrease in such needs. Instead, *caloric homeostasis* influences meals, albeit indirectly, and eating contributes to caloric homeostasis by providing nutrients. The storage and use of those nutrients are regulated independently by physiological

mechanisms described later. We describe the properties of caloric homeostasis before we consider the control of food intake.

CALORIC HOMEOSTASIS

Homeostatic Mechanisms Provide a Continuous Supply of Metabolic Fuels to Cells

The purpose of caloric homeostasis is to preserve cellular metabolism. Cells oxidize metabolic fuels to drive all cellular processes; thus, the higher the cellular activity, the greater the demand for energy. Because most cells have limited amounts of stored energy, they rely on a steady supply of calories and oxygen from the blood stream. Oxygen is dependably and instantaneously available via the respiratory system and is not stored in the body. In contrast, food calories can be scarce and require time after ingestion to become available to cells in significant quantities. One consequence of this functional organization is the capacity of animals to store sufficient energy to bridge long intervals during which no food is eaten.

Three categories of macronutrients—carbohydrates, lipids, and proteins—provide usable energy, but the use of specific macronutrients by the body varies depending on the tissue. Most tissues can oxidize carbohydrates in the form of *glucose* or lipids in the form of *free fatty acids*, depending on the availability of these nutrients and the levels of certain hormones in the blood. Notable exceptions are the liver, which requires lipids for proper functioning, and the brain, which has a large, continuous need for glucose despite the ability to oxidize lipids in the form of *ketone bodies*. When the supply of glucose to the brain is compromised, neurons cease to function, and in a few minutes consciousness is lost. Death will ensue unless glucose delivery to the brain is restored. Therefore, maintenance of circulating glucose in sufficient amounts to support normal brain function is a critical goal of caloric homeostasis.

Two distinct metabolic states are defined by the availability of recently consumed food to cells. The *prandial*, or fed, state is characterized by an abundance of newly ingested and absorbed nutrients in the blood. These molecules are sequestered rapidly in tissues to prevent them from being excreted wastefully in urine. The *postabsorptive*, or fasted, state is characterized by the absence of calories entering the circulation from the gastrointestinal tract and a consequent reliance on energy from metabolic fuels less recently consumed and stored. These stores are released gradually into the blood during a fast. In both states, tissues take nutrients from the blood as needed for cellular metabolism.

Many tissues store carbohydrates in the form of *glycogen*, a polymer of glucose; the liver and skeletal muscles have the largest depots. Energy is stored

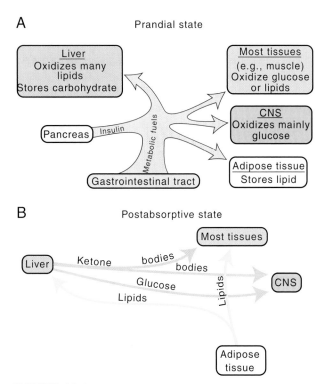

A Prandial state

B Postabsorptive state

FIGURE 38.1 Schematic diagram of the fluxes of metabolic fuels in the (A) prandial and (B) postabsorptive states. Note the absence of insulin in the postabsorptive state, which greatly facilitates the mobilization of energy stores from the liver and adipose tissue. The adult human liver stores sufficient fuel to support metabolism during fasting for about 7 h, whereas the adipose mass has a far greater capacity.

more efficiently, mainly in adipose tissue, as *triglyceride*, each molecule of which consists of glycerol with three attached fatty acids. During the prandial period, newly ingested food is used immediately by the body or is stored as glycogen or triglyceride. Excess carbohydrate is largely converted to lipid (*lipogenesis*) because glycogen storage capacity is limited, and triglyceride is a more efficient form of stored energy. During the fasting period, liver glycogen is converted back to glucose (*glycogenolysis*), which enters the blood and is available to all tissues. Similarly, stored triglycerides are mobilized from adipose tissue (*lipolysis*) and enter the circulation as fatty acids and glycerol. The fatty acids are used by tissues as needed or are converted to ketone bodies (*ketogenesis*), whereas glycerol is converted to glucose (*gluconeogenesis*) (Fig. 38.1).

The liver is the key organ in the traffic of energy. Lipogenesis (which also occurs in adipose tissue) and glycogen formation occur in the liver during the prandial period, and glycogenolysis, ketogenesis, and gluconeogenesis occur during the fasting period. These processes are regulated (discussed later), as are delivery of metabolic fuels (from the intestines into the circulation), storage of excess fuels, and mobilization of stored energy. The control system involves interplay among several hormones and the sympathetic and parasympathetic divisions of the autonomic nervous system.

Insulin Is the Key Hormone Affecting Caloric Homeostasis

Secretion of the peptide hormone *insulin* from B cells of the pancreatic islets is influenced by several factors, among which interstitial glucose is critical. Insulin secretion increases in direct proportion to the concentration of glucose in the blood and does not occur in the absence of glucose. Other substrates, such as amino acids and ketone bodies, also stimulate insulin secretion. In addition, autonomic nerves innervate the pancreatic islets: Cholinergic parasympathetic activity stimulates secretion of insulin, and α-adrenergic sympathetic activity inhibits it.

When a hungry person anticipates a meal, the aroma and, subsequently, the taste of food initiate insulin secretion via neural activity. Neural signals descend from the forebrain (where the smell and taste of food are recognized) through the hypothalamus to the dorsal motor nucleus of the vagus in the caudal brain stem and then to the pancreas by way of cholinergic fibers of the vagus nerve. This *cephalic phase* of insulin secretion helps reverse the mobilization of fuels that occurs during fasting and to prepare the

BOX 38.1

CLINICAL DISORDERS OF INSULIN SECRETION

Diabetes mellitus is a disorder characterized by abnormally high concentrations of blood glucose (*hyperglycemia*). Glucose concentrations may be so high that the kidneys cannot completely reabsorb the filtered glucose, resulting in measurable amounts of glucose in the urine. A chronically elevated concentration of glucose in the bloodstream suggests a lack of insulin, and, in fact, many diabetics have a confirmed deficiency of pancreatic B cells and of insulin (type 1 or *insulin-dependent diabetes*). A severe deficiency of insulin precludes fuel storage and the normal modulation of fuel mobilization. Therefore, in the postprandial period, metabolites of food accumulate in the circulation and are excreted, and individuals remain lean despite elevated food intake. Among humans with diabetes, however, 85 to 90% actually have substantial levels of circulating insulin but tend to be obese and resistant to the effects of insulin in promoting fuel storage (type 2 or *noninsulin-dependent diabetes*). Their impaired ability to secrete insulin rapidly during a meal results in a pronounced hyperglycemia during and following meals.

In people whose insulin production is compromised, inhibition of insulin secretion by the autonomic nervous system can mimic the symptoms of diabetes. During circumstances such as environmental stress, physical trauma, or pregnancy, an increase of sympathetic nervous activity inhibits insulin secretion sufficiently to allow the emergence of frank symptoms of diabetes, thereby revealing limited B-cell function. The symptoms disappear when the stressor is removed but reappear when stress returns or as pancreatic disease progresses.

Just as salivary secretion can be conditioned to arbitrary stimuli that herald the onset of a meal, classical conditioning similarly influences secretion of insulin at mealtimes. A parallel increase in stomach motility results in the familiar "growling" stomach. This learned reflex response provides a means for adapting the magnitude of insulin secretion to the food that is customarily eaten (Woods, 1995). Patients with *reactive hypoglycemia* have an exaggerated cephalic phase of insulin secretion and consequent hypoglycemia, which in turn triggers a compensatory secretion of epinephrine from the adrenal medulla and feelings of faintness (due to hypoglycemia) and of anxiety and arousal (due to epinephrine). The most commonly prescribed treatment is a change in daily eating habits to numerous, small, protein-rich meals because such meals elicit relatively little secretion of insulin.

Stephen C. Woods and
Edward M. Stricker

body for the entry of fuels from the gut (see Box 38.1). As ingested food enters the stomach and duodenum, several gastrointestinal hormones, which also are important in digestion, stimulate B cells to secrete more insulin. This *gastrointestinal phase* of insulin secretion ensures that the level of insulin in the circulation is high by the time digested nutrients first appear in the bloodstream. Finally, nutrients absorbed from the intestine cause even greater stimulation of insulin secretion by their direct effect on the pancreas. This *substrate phase* of insulin secretion increases insulin levels further, and this effect lasts well beyond the cessation of eating. As a result of these coordinated meal-related events, prandial insulin secretion is rapid and appropriate to the caloric load, and ingested fuels are efficiently used and stored (Fig. 38.2).

Neural and endocrine factors control the ebb and flow of metabolic fuels from body stores. Circulating insulin is the most important factor that promotes storage. Insulin enables most tissues to take up glucose from the blood for immediate oxidation or for storage during the prandial period. Conversely, the most important factor for fuel mobilization is the near disappearance of insulin from the circulation during the postprandial, postabsorptive period, when fuel delivery from the intestines has ended and parasympathetic activity to the pancreas is no longer elevated. Insulin secretion at this time is reduced greatly but is not inhibited, and therefore can be stimulated immediately if necessary. For example, when more than the needed amount of stored fuels is mobilized, substrates directly stimulate the pancreas to secrete insulin, thereby slowing substrate mobilization to a rate appropriate to need. Thus, insulin is pivotal for storing calories in the fed state and for allowing stored calories to be mobilized in measured amounts during the postabsorptive state.

Superimposed on other factors that influence insulin secretion is the amount of body fat (*adiposity*). People with low adiposity have a relatively large number of active insulin receptors on adipose tissue and skeletal muscle. Obese individuals have fewer

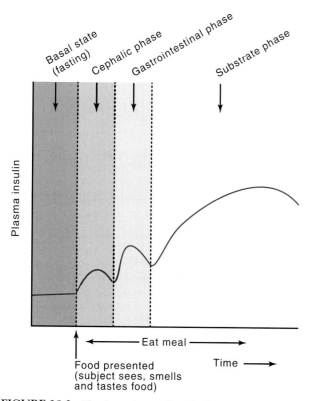

FIGURE 38.2 The three phases of meal-related insulin secretion. The cephalic phase, during which parasympathetic vagal activity stimulates the pancreas, is initiated when food is seen, smelled, and tasted. The gastrointestinal phase is mediated by the direct action of digestive hormones on the insulin-secreting B cells. The prolonged substrate phase is caused by metabolic fuels (mainly glucose) directly stimulating pancreatic B cells. When meals are prolonged, the three stimuli operate simultaneously and have additive effects.

active insulin receptors. Consequently, in response to a given stimulus, secretion of insulin is lower in people who are lean than in those who are obese, but its net effects on adipose tissue are comparable. In healthy, nondiabetic people, this reciprocal relationship between the secretion of insulin and the sensitivity of most tissues to insulin ensures efficient storage and use of fuels independent of body weight. In these individuals, plasma insulin levels in the prandial and the postprandial periods are reliable correlates of adiposity.

Summary

All cells require continuous supplies of metabolic fuels to support ongoing activity. The fuels enter the circulation from the intestines during the prandial period and from storage depots during fasting. The availability of fuels to tissues is controlled primarily by the liver and by the hormone insulin. Hepatic function and insulin secretion are in turn controlled in large part by the autonomic nervous system.

ROLE OF CALORIC HOMEOSTASIS IN CONTROL OF FOOD INTAKE

Meals Generate Biological Satiety Signals

The traditional view of caloric homeostasis is that animals eat when they need calories. However, as discussed earlier, the delivery of metabolic fuels to cells is continuous, and only infrequently do animals experience urgent needs for calories to support cellular metabolism. Instead, caloric homeostasis can be related to the control of food intake in ways that are unrelated to acute cellular needs.

Animals consume food in distinct bouts (i.e., meals); therefore, daily food intake reflects the cumulative intake of multiple meals. Control factors influence the time when each meal is initiated and the amount of food consumed before the meal is terminated. The first comprehensive study of meals was reported in 1966 by Le Magnen and Tallon. They maintained laboratory rats in cages and allowed them to eat *ad libitum* for weeks, during which time photosensors and electronic relays recorded intake. They obtained a full record of when meals were initiated, how much was eaten during each meal, how much time passed before the next meal, and so on. No relationship was found between how much a rat ate in a meal and how much time had passed since it had last eaten; in other words, meal sizes were unpredictable. However, the larger the meal, the longer the interval before the next meal, and the relationship was strongest during the night, when rats ate the largest meals. Thus, eating appeared to be inhibited by a satiety signal generated in proportion to the size of a

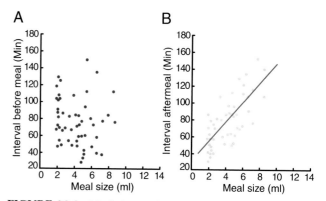

FIGURE 38.3 Meal sizes and intermeal intervals of a representative rat eating liquid food *ad libitum*. The sizes of 50 consecutive meals eaten by a neurologically normal control rat are shown. Meal size is plotted against the intervals of time that separated each meal from the one preceding it (A) and the one following it (B). Note that the premeal intervals did not predict meal sizes, whereas meal sizes did predict postmeal intervals. From Thomas and Mayer (1968).

meal, and eating resumed when that signal disappeared. Similar observations have since been made in many laboratories (Fig. 38.3).

Gastric Distension and Cholecystokinin Provide Satiety Signals

Several meal-related factors might plausibly provide satiety signals. These include factors based on the smell, taste, and texture of food. Factors arising from the stomach could also play a role, as could intestinal and postabsorptive factors that arise after ingested food has left the stomach. In studies of rats, pregastric factors have been ruled out because little satiety is achieved when ingested food is immediately drained out through an esophageal or gastric fistula; these animals eat continuously, as if they had no satiety despite the passage of very large amounts of food through the oropharynx (Fig. 38.4). Because meals end long before significant digestion and absorption occur, gastric factors have been considered a likely source of satiety signals. Gastric volume is an obvious possibility, and, in fact, meals are known to end when substantial *gastric distension* occurs. The stomach wall is richly endowed with stretch receptors whose activity increases in proportion to the volume of the stomach. Those signals are communicated by way of the vagus nerve to the *nucleus of the solitary tract* (NST) and adjacent *area postrema* in the brain stem. The signals travel to the hypothalamus and, ultimately, to the cortex, where gastric distension is perceived.

Gastric stretch that accompanies meals presumably interacts with other signals to produce satiety. For example, aside from directly affecting digestion, the intestinal peptide *cholecystokinin* (CCK), which is secreted during meals, acts on receptors located on vagal afferent fibers that carry gastric stretch signals from the pyloric region of the stomach to the brain stem. Thus, relatively small amounts of CCK can inhibit feeding in rats by acting synergistically with gastric distension. When given in larger doses, CCK can inhibit food intake even when the stomach is empty (Gibbs *et al.*, 1973). As might be expected, total or selective gastric *vagotomy* (or ablation of brain stem areas to which the gastric vagus projects) decreases the ability of gastric volume and peripherally administered CCK to reduce meal size. Conversely, systemic administration of CCK receptor antagonists increases the size of meals (see Box 38.2).

Gastric distension is one of the factors that control suckling in neonatal rats. The dam controls the timing of meals, and at each meal pups consume as much milk as their stomachs allow; gastric volume, not

caloric content, provides the signal to stop. Consistent with the importance of gastric distension to suckling, pups are particularly sensitive to the inhibitory effects of CCK on food intake, suggesting that a combination of gastric distension and CCK may be the principal signals that inhibit the initiation of spontaneous meals in suckling rats.

As rat pups mature, signals related to the caloric content of food begin to participate in the control of

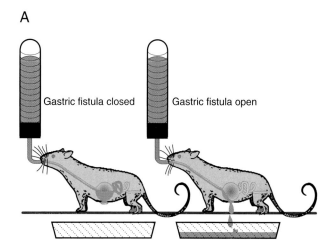

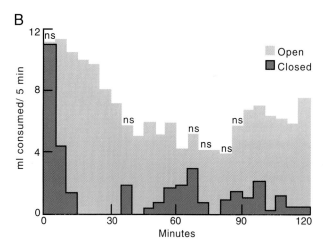

FIGURE 38.4 (A) Rats consuming liquid diet, with gastric fistula closed (real eating) or open ("sham eating"). When the gastric fistula is closed, food passes through the stomach and into the small intestine normally. When the gastric fistula is open, ingested food drains out the open fistula instead of accumulating in the stomach to distend it, and no food enters the small intestine. (B) Mean consumption of liquid diet (ml/5 min) by rats with a gastric fistula after 17 h of food deprivation. The rats consumed food in discrete meals when the fistula was closed. When the fistula was open, they ate continuously throughout the test period and never displayed satiety. Thus, rats consumed significantly more food during the 2-h test period when their fistulas were open than when they were closed. ns, intervals in which the amount of food consumed did not differ significantly between open and closed fistulas. From Smith *et al.* (1974).

BOX 38.2

SATIETY FACTORS

Several metabolically important peptides, including CCK, insulin, *glucagon*, and *bombesin*, reduce food intake when administered systemically to laboratory animals. By themselves, these findings do not prove that the peptides normally function as endogenous satiety agents; blood levels of an administered agent must be within the physiological range. In addition, the behavioral effects of the agent must be specific to the inhibition of food intake and cannot merely reflect a secondary consequence of illness, behavioral depression, or motor incapacitation. Because investigators cannot be certain what animals sense, they must infer whether animals experience satiety in association with an observed reduction in food intake.

One common approach is to determine whether the agent can cause a *learned flavor aversion* in animals. People learn readily to avoid food or drink that, when ingested, produces nausea due to the unsuspected presence of some toxic contaminant. Rats and other animals seem to respond in the same way; moreover, when a toxin is administered systemically soon after consumption of an uncontaminated, novelly flavored drink, the animals subsequently avoid fluids of that flavor and behave as if the drink had contained the toxic agent that made them sick. In addition, electrophysiological recording from the first gustatory relay nucleus in the brain stem, the nucleus of the solitary tract, shows that the response elicited by a taste that has been associated with a toxin is similar to the pattern of activity typical of naturally aversive flavor. Nausea is critical to the process; damage to the "emetic center" in the area postrema eliminates the sensation of nausea and prevents the formation of the learned taste aversion.

Another approach to distinguishing nausea from satiety is to monitor biological variables that occur in association with nausea but not satiety, or vice versa. One such variable is neurohypophyseal hormone secretion. For example, administration of lithium chloride causes nausea in humans and vomiting in monkeys and stimulates vasopressin secretion in both species. In this example, because elevated plasma vasopressin does not itself cause nausea or vomiting, it can be considered a biological marker of nausea. Curiously, rats secrete the other neurohypophyseal peptide, oxytocin (and not vasopressin), in response to large doses of lithium chloride and other nauseants. Control experiments have shown that following an ordinary meal, vasopressin is not secreted in primates nor is oxytocin secreted in rats. Thus, when rats are administered a chemical agent that stimulates pituitary oxytocin secretion, nausea, rather than satiety, is the suspected basis of the reduction in food intake.

Such experiments are helpful for interpreting the anorexia that occurs when a hormone or neurotransmitter is administered exogenously, but insight into the normal effects of endogenously secreted chemical signals requires an alternative experimental approach. For example, a drug that blocks the effect of an endogenous hormone or neurotransmitter on its receptors could be administered. If the hormone normally functions to reduce food intake, then the blocking agent should increase the size of meals. Such drugs are not yet available for all hormones suspected of being satiety factors, but experiments using drugs to reduce the activity of CCK, insulin, bombesin-like peptides, and glucagon at their respective receptors showed increases in meal size. These observations strongly suggest that these four peptide hormones normally function as endogenous satiety factors.

Stephen C. Woods and
Edward M. Stricker

meal size and become integrated with CCK, gastric distension, and other factors as satiety signals. This developmental change allows adults to ingest, assess, and respond to foods whose caloric density is not as constant as that of milk. For example, when liquid food is diluted with water, adult rats compensate by increasing the volume consumed in each meal, allowing daily caloric intake to remain stable. This observation reveals that gastric distension is but one of several possible satiety signals in adult rats and that

greater distension can be accommodated in circumstances in which the calorie-related satiety signals have diminished.

The mechanism by which caloric signals are monitored remains unknown. Although early reports suggested that the stomach monitored caloric nutrients, more recent findings have not supported this hypothesis. For example, when hungry rats were equipped with closed pyloric cuffs to prevent ingested food from entering their small intestines, the rats decreased their food intake in proportion to the volume, and not the caloric content, of intragastric infusions (Phillips and Powley, 1996). In contrast, when the cuff was open so that gastric contents could empty into the duodenum, caloric nutrients were much more effective in reducing food intake than calorie-free loads of equal volume. These observations suggest that the stomach does not detect caloric nutrients but instead contributes primarily inhibitory signals related to gastric distension.

Postgastric Effects of Meals Provide Additional Satiety Signals

Normally, some ingested food enters the intestine and is absorbed during the course of a meal, thus allowing postgastric signals to contribute to satiety. In this regard, small amounts of specific nutrients infused directly into the duodenum produce a robust suppression of eating that cannot be attributed to gastric factors. It is not clear whether the upper small intes-

---

BOX 38.3

THE GLUCOSTATIC HYPOTHESIS

Almost half a century ago, Mayer (1955) proposed that the onset and termination of meals are determined by changes in the amounts of glucose used by certain areas of the brain. Critical to Mayer's hypothesis was the observation that food intake was reliably increased by systemic injections of insulin, which reduced delivery of glucose to the brain. Another cornerstone of his theory was the observation that direct administration of the drug *gold thioglucose* (GTG) into the ventral hypothalamus destroyed local cells, after which the animals overate and became obese. Circulating insulin appeared necessary for this action because insulin-deficient (diabetic) animals were insensitive to the neurotoxic effects of GTG. Thus, Mayer hypothesized that food intake was controlled by a region of the ventral hypothalamus whose glucose utilization, unlike the rest of the brain, was sensitive to insulin. In diabetic rats, the presence of hyperphagia despite elevated blood glucose emphasized the point that diminished glucose utilization in these insulin-dependent cells (as opposed to a reduction of blood glucose levels per se) was the critical factor in removing satiety and stimulating food intake.

At first widely accepted, the glucostatic theory fell into disfavor for several reasons. For one, although eating can be induced by low availability of glucose to the brain, no evidence supports suppression of eating by high glucose availability. In addition, concentrations of blood glucose after administration of large doses of insulin are now known to be far lower than what occurs during a fast or at the normal onset of a meal. Thus, eating in response to insulin-induced hypoglycemia is now considered an "emergency" response that is not relevant to normal feeding. (A similar emergency response occurs after a systemic injection of 2-deoxyglucose induces an acute

decrease in cellular glycolysis.) Finally, the prevailing view of the ventromedial hypothalamus as a satiety center has changed considerably since the original formulation of the glucostatic hypothesis. This region of the brain is better regarded as a regulatory control center that influences many aspects of hormonal and autonomic function. Diabetic hyperphagia may therefore represent the loss of satiety promoted by insulin or leptin that activates neural systems to inhibit food intake. In contrast, the earlier glucostatic hypothesis would have explained diabetic hyperphagia in terms of a special sensitivity to insulin of hypothalamic neurons that mediate satiety.

The glucostatic theory continues to evolve. In rats allowed to eat freely, Campfield and Smith (1986) measured a decline in blood glucose that always began 15 to 20 min before an animal started to eat (Fig. 38.5). These investigators suggested that this small, transient episode of hypoglycemia causes initiation of a meal. Alternatively, this effect may result from a spurt of insulin secretion that reflects the animal's intention to begin a meal. Whether the transient decline of blood glucose is the cause or consequence of an inclination to eat remains unknown.

Stephen C. Woods and
Edward M. Stricker

References

Campfield, L. A., and Smith, F. J. (1986). Functional coupling between transient declines in blood glucose and feeding behaviour: Temporal relationships. *Brain Res. Bull.* **17**, 427–433.

Mayer, J. (1955). Regulation of energy intake and body weight: The glucostatic theory and the lipostatic hypothesis. *Ann. N.Y. Acad. Sci.* **411**, 221–235.

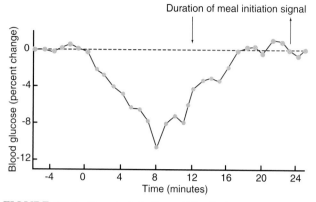

FIGURE 38.5 Transient decline of blood glucose in rats just prior to meal onset. Changes in the concentration of glucose are plotted as a percentage change from baseline against time. Values are from several experiments and are normalized to the time of onset of the decline (0 min). On average, meals began at about 12 min (↓) and ended at about 23 min (↑). From Campfield and Smith (1986).

tine or a postabsorptive site, or both, is responsible for detecting the administered calories and generating the signals that limit meal size. As discussed earlier, the liver plays a critical role in caloric homeostasis, and the delivery of nutrients absorbed from the intestine to the liver may be monitored to provide an important postgastric signal for the inhibition of food intake. Consistent with this hypothesis are findings that infusion of glucose or lipids into the hepatic portal vein reduces food intake. Furthermore, such infusions have been found to increase the activity in hepatic vagal afferent fibers, whereas infusion of fructose into the general circulation no longer reduces food intake in rats after hepatic vagotomy. Collectively, these findings suggest that the liver provides a satiety signal. That signal would disappear as absorption slows, which is when satiety diminishes as well.

Intravenously administered glucose reduces food intake but not by as much as the caloric content of the glucose. In contrast, when glucose solution is fed through a tube directly into the stomach, the compensatory reduction in food (calorie) intake is equivalent to the caloric load. In this case, gastric or intestinal signals might contribute to the increased satiety. Note that more insulin is secreted in response to infusion of glucose into the stomach than into a vein, which might contribute to the observed reduction in appetite. In fact, intravenously infused glucose reduces food intake by an equivalent caloric amount when insulin is added to the infusate. Together, these observations suggest that insulin contributes to the satiety effect of glucose whether given by gavage or ingested during a meal. Consistent with this possibility, rats made diabetic by destruction of their

pancreatic B cells eat discrete meals more frequently, as if they experienced less postprandial satiety (see Box 38.3).

In addition to providing useful nutrients, consumption of food increases *plasma osmolality*, yet another factor influencing the size of a meal. Increased plasma osmolality stimulates thirst, and for this reason water intake usually accompanies eating. The important point, however, is that food intake is lower during meals when drinking water is not available, a phenomenon known as "dehydration anorexia." Similarly, increased plasma osmolality caused by a systemic injection of hypertonic saline reduces food intake in proportion to the administered osmotic load. The well-described osmoreceptors that cause thirst and influence vasopressin secretion (see Chapter 39) apparently do not mediate this inhibitory effect on food intake, which persists after those forebrain osmoreceptors have been destroyed surgically. Instead, because the osmolality of blood in the hepatic portal vein affects the activity of visceral afferent fibers from the liver, hepatic osmoreceptors might mediate the inhibitory effect of increased plasma osmolality on food intake.

Body Weight Influences Food Intake

The control of food intake is also associated with the maintenance of body weight. For example, after a period of food deprivation and forced loss of body weight, animals (including humans) eat larger meals than normal until adiposity returns to pretreatment levels. Conversely, after a period of force feeding, during which the increased daily intake of calories causes weight gain, animals eat smaller meals than normal (or no meals at all) until normal adiposity is restored. Long-term stability of adiposity in adult animals is attributed in part to these compensatory responses to weight fluctuations that are caused by acute changes in food intake or energy expenditure.

Adiposity may indirectly influence food intake by modulating how quickly food passes through the gastrointestinal tract, how long nutrients remain in the circulation, or how nutrients interact with the liver. For example, after fasting, less prolonged gastric distension or more rapid absorption and storage of ingested calories would diminish the duration of satiety signals, thereby increasing the frequency of meals. These effects would promote the *hyperphagia* (overeating) associated with the restoration of body weight in animals that have fasted. Similarly, the satiating properties of ingested food would be reduced by diversions of ingested food calories to the fetus during pregnancy, to milk during lactation, or to skeletal muscle during exposure to cold temperatures, thereby contributing to the hyperphagia associated with each of these conditions.

Alternatively, adipose tissue may directly signal the brain to modulate food intake. Because afferent nerves from adipose tissue to brain have not been described, such communication was hypothesized to be mediated by a humoral (circulating) factor. *Parabionts*, created by surgically joining two animals at the flank muscles and skin, were used to test the hypothesis. Vascular interconnection within a parabiont is demonstrated when a dye injected into one animal appears in the blood of its partner. Because the nervous systems of the two animals remain independent, any physiologic communication between the animals must occur through the vascular system. When two lean rats were joined para-

biotically, each consumed its normal amount of food and maintained its usual body weight. Similar results were obtained when two obese rats with lesions in the *ventromedial hypothalamus* (see later) were joined together. However, when a lean animal was joined to an obese animal, the result was striking: The lean animal reduced its food intake markedly and consequently lost a considerable amount of weight. These experiments have been interpreted to mean that a circulating factor, secreted in large amounts (proportional to adiposity) by the obese animal, enters the blood of the lean animal and reduces food intake, as if the lean animal was receiving a signal that it was too fat (Coleman and Hummel, 1969).

Investigations have identified *leptin*, the hormone synthesized by adipose tissue, as a key circulating adi-

---

BOX 38.4

VARIATIONS OF STRUCTURE AND FUNCTION AMONG LEPTIN RECEPTORS

Leptin, the peptide hormone secreted by adipose cells, enters the brain through a receptor-mediated transport system in the brain capillary endothelium. Within the brain, it binds to specific leptin receptors that are expressed in discrete populations of neurons. The leptin receptor, termed Ob-R, is a member of the class I cytokine receptor family, a group of structurally similar receptors that act through JAK and STAT intracellular signaling proteins. There is only a single gene for Ob-R, and it is processed differentially by different cells such that many isoforms of the receptor are known. As depicted in Fig. 38.6, Ob-R can be considered to have three active sections. The extracellular segment, which is over 800 amino acids long in rodents, binds selectively to leptin. This segment is identical in most known isoforms of the Ob-R. The cell membrane-spanning segment has 23 amino acids and is also consistent among the isoforms. Variations in function of the different isoforms are conferred by the length of the intracellular segment, with longer intracellular segments having more sites where intracellular signaling molecules can interact. Hence, longer isoforms have a greater potential to interact with the greatest number of such signaling molecules. The longest isoform, termed Ob-Rb, has over 300 amino acids (depending on the species) and is the only form capable of initiating the full complement of JAK and STAT proteins and of stimulating transcription at the nucleus of the cell. For these reasons, Ob-Rb is known as the signal-transducing form of the leptin receptor.

Within the brain, Ob-Rb is synthesized in high quantities in various nuclei in the ventral hypothalamus, including the arcuate, ventromedial, and paraventricular nuclei. Ob-Rb is recognized as the receptor that stimulates the synthesis and secretion of α-MSH and inhibits the synthesis and secretion of neuropeptide Y and agouti-related peptide in the arcuate nucleus. Other isoforms, with shorter intracellular segments, are localized in other brain areas and in the choroid plexus. They are thought to mediate activities locally at the cell membrane such as the movement of molecules through the membrane.

Many spontaneously occurring mutations of the leptin receptor have been identified (see Fig. 38.6), and all result in an animal that is obese and hyperphagic. In the mouse, where the leptin receptor gene is called DB, at least four mutations are known. All have shortened intracellular segments and all are called db/db mice. All are also extremely obese. The fatty Zucker rat (fa/fa) has a mutation resulting in a single amino acid substitution in the extracellular segment. As its name implies, this animal is also extremely obese. The Koletsky rat has a truncated extracellular segment and lacks all leptin signaling. It is also obese. A small number of humans have been identified with mutations of the leptin receptor, and they are also hyperphagic and obese.

Stephen C. Woods and
Edward M. Stricker

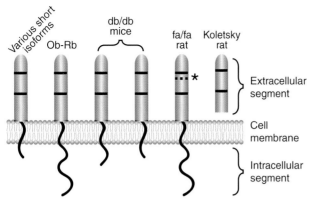

FIGURE 38.6 There are many isoforms of the leptin receptor (Ob-R). All have the same extracellular segment that binds with leptin, such that variations are in the length of the intracellular segment. Most tissues synthesize one or another "short" isoform that binds leptin and initiates cellular events locally near the cell membrane. Only the long form (Ob-Rb) is capable of triggering intracellular signaling cascades that can alter nuclear transcription. Several mutations that shorten the Ob-R occur in mice. These mice, called db/db, are all hyperphagic and obese. Two mutations of the Ob-R have also been identified in rats, and both also result in obesity. Fatty Zucker (fa/fa) rats have single amino acid substitution in the extracellular segment of Ob-R, whereas Koletsky rats have a truncated receptor.

posity signal that regulates food intake and body weight. Leptin concentration in plasma is directly proportional to adiposity, and a receptor-mediated transport process passes it into the brain. Animals that lack the gene for synthesizing leptin (ob/ob mice) are hyperphagic and obese, and administering leptin to ob/ob mice, or to normal animals, causes them to eat less and lose weight. Because lower doses of leptin have this action when administered into the ventricles of the brain than when administered systemically, leptin is believed to reduce food intake and body weight via a central site of action. Consistent with this hypothesis, the receptor for leptin has been identified and found to be located within the hypothalamus. Like ob/ob mice, animals with mutated leptin receptors (db/db mice and fatty Zucker rats) are obese (see Box 38.4), but unlike ob/ob mice, they do not respond to exogenous leptin. Hence, leptin appears to function as a negative feedback signal to the brain. When fat stores increase in adipose tissue, more leptin is secreted and enters the brain, causing a greater inhibition of food intake and loss of body fat. When circulating leptin levels are low, feeding and other anabolic responses are disinhibited. In this way, leptin acts to promote the maintenance of a relatively stable body weight over long intervals. The neural circuitry through which leptin inhibits food intake and influences caloric homeostasis is discussed later.

Insulin provides a second circulating signal that informs the brain of body fat levels. Plasma levels of insulin are directly correlated with adiposity, and, like leptin, insulin is transported through the blood–brain barrier where it can act on insulin receptors in the hypothalamus and other sites. Insulin administered into the brain reduces food intake and body weight, whereas animals that do not secrete insulin are hyperphagic. Of course, severe diabetics do not become obese because their adipocytes cannot store fat in the absence of insulin. Mice lacking insulin receptors on brain cells are both hyperphagic and obese. In short, both leptin and insulin provide blood-borne signals that enter the brain and act on their respective receptors to reduce food intake and body fat.

Summary

Three effects of eating limit the size of an ongoing meal: gastric distension (potentiated by CCK), post-gastric detection of calories (via satiety signals such as CCK, perhaps potentiated in the liver by insulin), and increased plasma osmolality. These signals reach the brain through visceral afferent fibers (especially those traveling in the vagus nerve) and the circulatory system. Meal size invariably increases after the inhibitory effects are experimentally removed by blocking the detection of gastric stretch or of CCK, diluting the food with noncaloric material, or rehydrating the animal. Inhibition appears to be integrated so that as one effect diminishes (e.g., the signal associated with gastric distension), another increases (e.g., the signal associated with the postabsorptive delivery of calories and insulin to the liver), thereby maintaining satiety and prolonging the interval between meals. When the satiety signals disappear, hunger emerges and stimulates initiation of another meal.

Food intake is also normally linked closely with body weight. In experimental animals, periods of starvation or forced feeding are followed by self-regulated compensatory changes in eating patterns until prior body size is regained. Links between body weight and food intake can be mediated indirectly by altered gastrointestinal motility and absorption as well as by the blood-borne, centrally active hormones, leptin and insulin.

CENTRAL CONTROL OF FOOD INTAKE

Early theories of the control of food intake focused on signals derived from stomach and blood. Peripheral factors, such as the concentration of glucose in

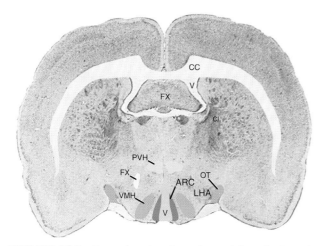

FIGURE 38.7 Coronal section through an adult rat brain at the level where the optic tract enters the two hemispheres. The lateral ventricle and third cerebral ventricle (V) are shaded, and selected fiber tracts are outlined for reference (OT, optic tract; CC, corpus callosum; FX, fornix). Key hypothalamic sites important in caloric homeostasis, present in each hemisphere, are paraventricular nuclei (PVN), ventromedial nuclei (VMN), arcuate nuclei (ARC), and the lateral hypothalamic area (LHA).

Food Intake Is Not Controlled by Hypothalamic Hunger and Satiety Centers

The strength of the traditional dual center model, in which one center mediates hunger and the other satiety, was that it provided a simple answer to the question of how the brain controls intake of food. The principal limitation of the model, however, was that it

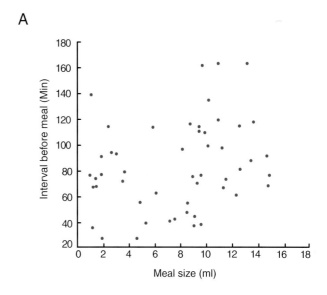

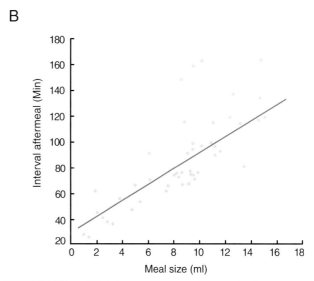

FIGURE 38.8 Meal sizes and intermeal intervals of a representative rat eating liquid food *ad libitum*. The sizes of 50 consecutive meals eaten by a rat that became hyperphagic after electrolytic lesions of the ventromedial hypothalamus are shown. The volume of each meal is plotted against the intervals of time separating it from the preceding (A) and following (B) meals. As with control animals (see Fig. 38.3), premeal intervals did not predict meal sizes, whereas meal sizes did predict postmeal intervals. Note that after a meal of any given size, hyperphagic rats returned to eat sooner than neurologically normal control rats did. From Thomas and Mayer (1968).

the blood, were plausibly associated with food intake and were accessible to experimentation. Theories involving the brain emerged after development of a stereotaxic instrument that enabled discrete lesions of the cerebrum to be made in laboratory animals, permitting evaluation of ideas about brain function (Fig. 38.7). The first findings from such experiments were striking: Bilateral electrolytic lesions of the ventromedial hypothalamus (VMH) caused marked hyperphagia and obesity in rats. This observation was interpreted to mean that the animals had become less sensitive to incoming signals of satiety and that they therefore overate and became fat. Bilateral lesions in the adjacent *ventrolateral hypothalamus* (VLH) were later found to cause *aphagia* (absence of eating), which led to death by starvation. This finding was interpreted to mean that these rats no longer detected hunger signals, and thus they starved to death while unaware of their internal state. Collectively, these results provided the foundation of a *dual center hypothesis*, in which a satiety center in the VMH was thought to suppress activity in a hunger center in the VLH. Both the syndrome of hyperphagia and obesity and the syndrome of aphagia and weight loss that result from focal hypothalamic lesions have been reproduced in multiple laboratories and in multiple species. However, additional observations have caused reinterpretation of these familiar and reliable findings, and they now have a very different meaning.

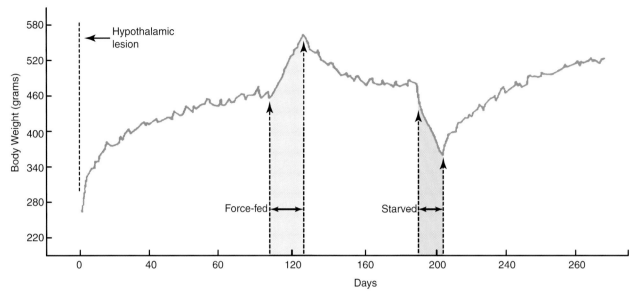

FIGURE 38.9 Changes in the body weight of rats with bilateral lesions of the ventromedial hypothalamus. After lesions are made on day 0, rats gain weight rapidly and then defend that elevated body weight when challenged with periods of weight gain due to force feeding and weight loss due to food restriction. Not shown are the associated food intakes, which increase subsequent to the lesion, decrease after the period of force feeding, and increase after the period of food restriction. From Hoebel and Teitelbaum (1966).

could not answer the next level of questions: What signals control individual meals? How are these signals integrated with physiological aspects of caloric homeostasis, including long-term maintenance of body weight? What is the influence of other neural sites and systems in the brain? How are excitatory and inhibitory influences on eating integrated? How are behaviors, such as motivation and reinforcement, explained? Investigators are addressing these and related questions, but they now usually take a perspective that does not presume the existence of brain centers mediating hunger and satiety.

In addition to causing hyperphagia, VMH lesions profoundly reduce sympathetic tone and increase parasympathetic tone and vagal reflexes. For example, the high concentration of insulin in animals with VMH lesions is not simply a secondary consequence of hyperphagia but occurs even when food intake is limited. Because of the change in autonomic tone, caloric equilibrium in adipose tissue shifts away from lipolysis and toward lipogenesis, thereby allowing more rapid storage of ingested calories after a meal. Increased parasympathetic activity also allows faster gastric emptying. Importantly, VMH lesions do not cause loss of satiety. Meal sizes continue to correlate with postmeal intervals, but the interval after a meal of any size is shorter in animals with VMH lesions than in control animals (Fig. 38.8).

Because the duration of their postprandial satiety signals is shorter than normal, rats with VMH lesions eat more frequent meals. They remain hyperphagic

until the equilibrium between lipogenesis and lipolysis is reestablished in adipocytes. For this to happen, triglyceride stores must accumulate in the cells to levels sufficient to create insulin resistance, whereupon lipogenesis subsides. Meals are eaten less frequently, and daily food intake is reduced. The animal maintains its obese state as if it had a new "set point" for body weight (Fig. 38.9). Thus, after obese rats with VMH lesions have been deprived of food and forced to lose weight, hyperphagia reoccurs until high adiposity is reattained. Similarly, when neurologically normal rats are overfed and become obese prior to receiving a lesion of the VMH, they are not hyperphagic after the lesion but rather eat to maintain their elevated weight. (Hoebel and Teitelbaum, 1966).

In sum, rats gain body fat after VMH lesions, and as fat accumulates the duration of satiety after meals increases. This explanation contrasts with early hypotheses that body weight increased after VMH lesions because animals became obligatorily hyperphagic. The primary phenomenon is now recognized as a change in autonomic tone to promote vagal reflexes and fat storage. Because the change in autonomic tone is observed even when increased food intake is prevented, hyperphagia cannot be the primary phenomenon. The key element appears to be the chronic, neurally stimulated increase in insulin secretion. When the increased insulin secretion is prevented by denervating the pancreas, obesity does not develop and hyperphagia is attenuated greatly.

In contrast to VMH lesions, rats with large VLH lesions do not eat (to the point of starvation). However, they also do not drink water when dehydrated, move about in their cages, or respond to diverse stimulation. In other words, the most prominent abnormalities in these rats are akinesia and sensory neglect. In this respect, rats with VLH lesions resemble human patients with Parkinson's disease, a neurological disorder that has been attributed to the degeneration of dopamine-containing neurons of the nigrostriatal bundle (see Chapters 30 and 31). Dopaminergic fibers course through the internal capsule just lateral to the VLH as they ascend from the ventral mesencephalon to the striatum along the medial forebrain bundle (Chapter 44). Large electrolytic lesions of the VLH area interrupt these dopaminergic fibers. More selective damage to the dopaminergic neurons by intracerebral administration of the neurotoxin

6-hydroxydopamine also produces akinesia and sensory neglect in association with loss of food intake, and it does so without disturbing parasympathetic reflexes. Thus, the aphagia induced by large VLH lesions does not result from damage to a putative hunger center in the brain but instead reflects a more general disruption of movement and sensorimotor integration (Ungerstedt, 1971), at least in part (see later).

Summary

The ability of brain circuitry to control food intake was initially based on the consequences of stereotaxic lesions of ventromedial and ventrolateral hypothalamic nuclei leading to hyperphagia or aphagia, respectively. Subsequent studies revealed that each lesion also induces changes in gastrointestinal function and in the equilibrium between lipolysis and

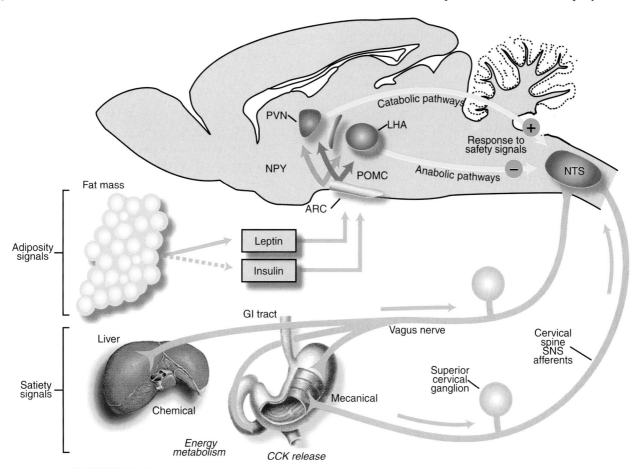

FIGURE 38.10 Schematic diagram of the signals that control caloric homeostasis. Satiety signals arising in the periphery such as gastric distension and CCK are relayed to the nucleus of the solitary tract (NTS) in the brain stem. Leptin and insulin, the two circulating adiposity signals, enter the brain and interact with receptors in the arcuate nucleus (ARC) and other brain areas. These adiposity signals inhibit ARC neurons that synthesize NPY and AgRP (NPY cells in the diagram) and stimulate neurons that synthesize proopiomelanocoritin (POMC), the precursor of α-MSH, and CART. These ARC neurons in turn project other hypothalamic areas, including paraventricular nuclei (PVN) and the lateral hypothalamic area (LHA). Catabolic signals from the PVN and anabolic signals from the LHA are thought to interact with the satiety signals in the brain stem to determine when meals will end. From Schwartz *et al.* (2000).

lipogenesis in adipocytes. In addition, these nuclei help regulate body weight through influences on spontaneous mobility and sensory responsivity to food-derived stimuli. The nucleus of the solitary tract also relays important visceral sensory cues on gastrointestinal fill that can further influence food intake.

NEUROPEPTIDES AND THE CONTROL OF FOOD INTAKE

Although the details of the central control of food intake are incompletely understood, many neuropeptides have been implicated. To simplify the discussion, we focus on two broad categories of neuropeptides: those that are mainly anabolic and those that are mainly catabolic. Both of these subgroups in turn are modified by multiple influences, including satiety signals, adiposity signals, experience, habit, emotional state, the social situation, and so on. Anabolic peptides cause increased eating, decreased energy expenditure, and, when chronically elevated, increased body fat accumulation. Catabolic peptides reduce food intake, increase energy expenditure, and lead to loss of body fat. Figure 38.10 presents a simplified model of some of the better-known components of this control system. An interesting feature of the model is that major efferent outputs from the hypothalamus to autonomic nuclei and to motor nuclei controlling ingestion per se emanate from the VMH and VLH, the central neural sites that were the main focus of attention over a half-century ago.

The Hypothalamic Arcuate Nucleus Mediates the Effect of Adiposity on Food Intake and Body Weight

The amount of body fat is signaled to the brain by leptin and insulin. Receptors for both peptides are located (among other sites) in the hypothalamic arcuate nucleus on two distinct groups of neurons. The first group of arcuate neurons synthesizes the neuropeptides, *α-melanocyte-stimulating hormone* (α-MSH) and *cocaine–amphetamine-related* transcript (CART); these neurons are activated by leptin and insulin. α-MSH and CART are potent catabolic peptides, and when either is administered locally into the third cerebral ventricle, animals eat less food, have increased energy expenditure, and lose weight (Cone, 1999). α-MSH is in the *melanocortin* family of peptides, a group that also includes *adrenocorticotrophic hormone* (ACTH). These peptides act on melanocortin (MC)

receptors, and two of these receptors, termed MC3 and MC4, are expressed in several nuclei of the hypothalamus, including the *paraventricular nucleus* (PVN), VMH, and VLH, where α-MSH-containing axons project from the arcuate nucleus and where α-MSH acts as an agonist. Animals that lack either MC3 or MC4 receptors become obese; animals with no MC3 receptors gain weight gradually over their lifetime without overeating, whereas animals without MC4 receptors are hyperphagic and become much fatter. The administration of selective MC4 antagonists causes normal animals to overeat and, if prolonged, to become obese. Hence, hypothalamic melanocortins, exemplified by α-MSH, exert a tonic catabolic effect to keep body weight from increasing (Cone, 1999). Importantly, the ability of exogenous leptin to reduce food intake and body weight is completely attenuated in the presence of an antagonist to MC3 and MC4 receptors, suggesting that the "downstream" pathway by which adiposity influences caloric homeostasis is via melanocortin signaling (Seeley *et al.*, 1997).

The other type of arcuate neuron influenced by adiposity signals synthesizes the neuropeptides, *neuropeptide Y* (NPY) and *agouti-related protein* (AgRP). Both peptides are potent anabolic compounds in that the administration of either into the third ventricle results in hyperphagia, reduced energy expenditure, and weight gain. Although NPY is synthesized in many areas of the brain, AgRP synthesis is limited to the arcuate nucleus. Neurons containing NPY and AgRP express both leptin and insulin receptors, and the local administration of either insulin or leptin near the arcuate nucleus reduces the synthesis of both NPY and AgRP. Hence, adiposity signals exert net catabolic effects through the joint mechanisms of stimulating α-MSH/CART neurons and simultaneously inhibiting NPY/AgRP neurons. For all of these reasons, the arcuate nucleus can be considered to be the brain's sense organ that detects body adiposity by monitoring the levels of leptin and insulin. In turn, axons from these two groups of arcuate neurons innervate many other hypothalamic nuclei as they modulate aspects of caloric homeostasis.

A particularly important tract includes NPY-containing axons that project from the arcuate nucleus to the PVN. The PVN expresses receptors for NPY, and careful mapping studies have identified the PVN as the most sensitive site to the orexigenic effect of exogenously administered NPY. Consistent with this finding, when antisense oligonucleotides to NPY receptors are given locally within the PVN, rats that have been deprived of food eat less than they usually would. Among the numerous sites that synthesize NPY within the brain, only those in the arcuate nucleus are sensitive to changes of food intake as signaled by leptin and insulin (Schwartz *et al.*, 2000). NPY mRNA is increased in the arcuate nucleus when animals are fasted and returns to baseline upon refeeding. Fasting also increases the levels of NPY in axon terminals in the PVN and increases secretion of NPY within the PVN. Hence, the fasted animal is primed to eat more food due in part to the action of elevated NPY in the area of the PVN. Circulating insulin and leptin are decreased during fasting, and local administration of either into the brain of a fasted rat lowers the elevation of NPY mRNA in the arcuate nucleus and lowers the amount of food eaten by food-deprived rats (Schwartz *et al.*, 2000). Hence, the metabolic state, as reflected by leptin and insulin, has a marked influence on arcuate NPY-containing neurons and consequently on neural pathways that influence energy intake and expenditure. Endogenous levels of NPY in the arcuate

–PVN system normally peak when daylight ends and nocturnal activity begins (Leibowitz, 1990), which is also the time when rats typically eat their largest meal of the day. Hence, NPY activity in the PVN appears to be a key mediator of anabolic activity.

The other neuropeptide synthesized in NPY neurons in the arcuate nucleus, AgRP, is an endogenous antagonist of MC3 and MC4 receptors (Cone, 1999). AgRP therefore promotes food intake by acting at MC receptors in the PVN and other areas to block the action of α-MSH. When exogenous AgRP is administered into the third cerebral ventricle, the resultant hyperphagia lasts for up to 6 days (Hagan *et al.*, 2000). In contrast, the hyperphagia elicited by NPY lasts only a few hours. Hence, activation of the arcuate NPY/AgRP neurons results in an acute but robust increase of food intake caused by the actions of NPY and a steady and more prolonged increase caused by the actions of AgRP.

BOX 38.5

FEEDING IN INVERTEBRATES: THE BLOWFLY AS A MODEL SYSTEM

The neural control of food intake in invertebrates is particularly well understood in the blowfly (*Phormia regina*). The central integration of excitatory and inhibitory signals is surprisingly similar to key elements of the control of food intake in rats and other well-studied mammals (Dethier, 1976).

Briefly, adult flies require merely sugar and water for their sustenance. The excitatory signal to eat is provided solely by sweet taste, which is detected by sensory receptors located on hairs on the legs of blowflics. This chemical signal causes the proboscis to extend into the sweet solution. Sucking commences and the liquid is drawn into the foregut and crop. Inhibitory signals are triggered by certain tastes (sodium chloride or acid solutions) and by distension of the crop and foregut during the meal. The flies ingest sugar until inhibition counterbalances excitation (from sweet taste), at which point consumption stops. Thus, more concentrated (i.e., sweeter) sugar solutions are consumed in larger meals. However, dilute (i.e., less sweet) sugar solutions require less gastric distension for inhibition to terminate ingestion. Inhibitory signals from the crop and foregut project to the brain via identified nerves from the abdomen. When those nerves are severed, ingestion of the sugar solution cannot be inhibited, and the flies continue their intake until they literally burst.

The crop and foregut empty as absorption occurs, and the flies then become ready to feed again. Because concentrated solutions are absorbed relatively slowly, inhibitory signals generated by such fluids last longer than those generated by dilute solutions. Thus, flies ingest concentrated solutions in large meals taken infrequently, whereas dilute solutions are consumed in smaller but more frequent meals. In either case, the flies ingest the same amount of sugar over time. Remarkably, they do so despite their inability to detect calories. The fly is unable to monitor the metabolic consequences of feeding, but because sweet taste, sugar concentration, and caloric density correlate with one another, when the fly responds to sweet taste, it effectively tracks calories.

In sum, adult blowflies attend to signals of taste and gastric distension to find food and to eat enough to survive. The blowfly appears to eat reflexively, showing no evidence of experiencing hunger or of altering its eating on the basis of learning from past experience. In these respects, the flies are reminiscent of decerebrate rats. Thus, much of the control of eating in intact rats may be found in the brain stem, but forebrain function is required to mediate the separate but interrelated phenomena of motivation, sensation (e.g., hunger and satiety), caloric homeostasis, and cognitive functions (e.g., learning and memory).

Stephen C. Woods and
Edward M. Stricker

Furthermore, the two peptides act in different ways. NPY acts through its receptors to stimulate anabolic pathways directly, whereas AgRP acts through a different receptor by antagonizing tonically active catabolic peptides. It is not known whether NPY and AgRP from the arcuate neurons act on the same or different target cells in the PVN, VLH, and elsewhere.

In sum, the arcuate nucleus appears to be a chemosensor in the brain that detects body adiposity by means of insulin and leptin receptors. One type of arcuate neuron synthesizes peptide transmitters (α-MSH and CART) having a net catabolic effect, and another type synthesizes peptide transmitters (NPY and AgRP) with a net anabolic effect. Both types of neuron project to other hypothalamic areas where they influence specific aspects of caloric homeostasis. [Another example of the role of dual excitatory and inhibitory influences on feeding can be found in an invertebrate model (see Box 38.5).]

Other Hypothalamic Peptides Also Influence Food Intake

Several newly discovered neuropeptides important in the control of caloric homeostasis are synthesized in the VLH, including *orexin A* and *melanin-concentrating hormone* (MCH) (Shimada *et al.*, 1998). Administration of either of these peptides into the brain stimulates food intake, whereas mice that lack the gene for MCH are lean and obesity resistant. It appears likely that the aphagia exhibited by animals with VLH lesions is due in part to reduced levels of these peptides and that the hyperphagia caused by electrical stimulation of the VLH is due in part to release of these peptides.

Oxytocin is a peptide synthesized in the PVN and supraoptic nuclei of the hypothalamus and is secreted from the posterior lobe of the pituitary. In the systemic circulation of female mammals, this hormone is well known for stimulating uterine contractions for parturition and stimulating milk let down in mammary glands during lactation. However, the hypothalamus and pituitary of males contain as much oxytocin as those of females; therefore, the peptide has long been suspected of being secreted in other circumstances and having additional functions. In fact, research has revealed that gastric distension, CCK administration, and plasma hyperosmolality, treatments that decrease food intake in rats, elicit pituitary oxytocin secretion in male and female rats. In addition, increases in plasma concentrations of oxytocin correlate highly with observed decreases in food intake (Fig. 38.11).

Although observations were consistent with oxytocin being an appetite suppressant, later experiments

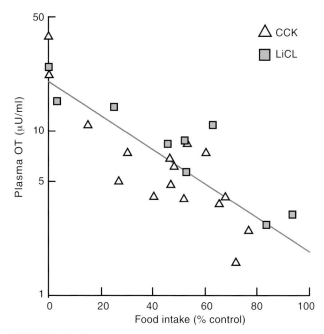

FIGURE 38.11   Relationship between plasma levels of oxytocin (OT) and inhibition of food intake by hungry rats pretreated with various doses of cholecystokinin (CCK) or lithium chloride (LiCl). Symbols represent individual rats. Food intake is expressed as a percentage of baseline for each rat. The same pattern was observed when hungry rats were pretreated with a hypertonic sodium chloride solution to induce hyperosmolality. Adapted from McCann *et al.* (1989).

showed that this was not the case: Systemic administration of oxytocin does not affect food intake. Instead, the reduced food intake seen after treatment with CCK or hypertonic saline appears to be mediated by oxytocin secreted from neurons whose cell bodies are located in the hypothalamic PVN but whose axons project within the central nervous system rather than to the pituitary gland. Consistent with this hypothesis, central injection of oxytocin into the cerebral ventricles (icv) decreases food intake in rats, an effect that is blocked by icv pretreatment of the animals with an oxytocin receptor antagonist. More to the point, the effects of exogenous CCK and hypertonic saline on food intake are blunted by icv pretreatment with an oxytocin receptor antagonist. A summary of some of the hypothalamic peptides that modulate food intake is depicted in Figure 38.12.

Stress is also well known to decrease food intake in animals, and various stressors activate the hypothalamic–pituitary–adrenal axis. A key mediator of this effect is *corticotropin-releasing hormone* (CRH), which is synthesized and secreted from the PVN. CRH stimulates the secretion of ACTH from the anterior pituitary, and ACTH in turn elicits steroid hormone secretion from the adrenal cortex (see

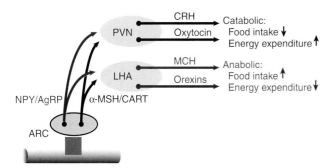

FIGURE 38.12 Hypothalamic neuropeptides that influence caloric homeostasis. The adiposity hormones, leptin and insulin, are transported through the blood–brain barrier and influence neurons in the arcuate nucleus (ARC). ARC neurons that synthesize and release NPY and AgRP are inhibited by adiposity signals, whereas ARC neurons that synthesize and release α-MSH and CART are stimulated by adiposity signals. NPY/AgRP neurons are inhibitory to the PVN and stimulatory to the LHA, whereas α-MSH/CART neurons are stimulatory of the PVN and inhibitory of the LHA. The PVN in turn has a net catabolic action, whereas the LHA has a net anabolic action.

Chapter 40). In rats, icv injection of CRH decreases food intake in the absence of stress and in association with oxytocin secretion from the posterior pituitary. In addition, icv pretreatment with an oxytocin receptor antagonist eliminates CRH-induced inhibition of food intake. These findings are consistent with central oxytocinergic neurons mediating the inhibition of food intake that occurs during stress. Such inhibitory effects on eating would complement the known inhibitory effects of central oxytocin on gastric motility and emptying.

Two additional features of these findings deserve note. First, despite prominent pituitary oxytocin secretion, central oxytocinergic pathways are not stimulated by suckling. Therefore, nursing does not inevitably reduce food intake in dams; in fact, lactating rats are hyperphagic in association with the substantial loss of calories through milk. Second, because the various stimuli for oxytocin release are not related to caloric homeostasis, oxytocin is not a factor in the termination of normal meals; in fact, oxytocin is not secreted by rats during meals taken *ad libitum*.

The Brain Stem Plays an Important Role in the Control of Food Intake

The NST and the adjacent area postrema in the brain stem receive sensory fibers from gustatory receptors in the mouth and throat (see Chapter 24), as well as afferent information from the stomach, intestines, pancreas, and liver. In the central control of food intake, these linked brain stem sites likely are

where sensory input from the viscera is first integrated with input from taste buds. This sensory information is relayed along prominent neural projections from the brain stem to the hypothalamus, amygdala, and other portions of the limbic system, as well as to the thalamus and gustatory cortex. Reciprocal neural connections to the brain stem from these rostral sites allow emotion and cognitive function to influence the control of eating. Complementary and linked efferent elements participate in the central control of the gastrointestinal tract, the liver, and autonomic function generally.

Evidence of the control of the brain stem over food intake comes from investigations of the chronic decerebrate rat in which all axonal connections between the caudal brain stem and the forebrain are severed at the midcollicular level of the midbrain (Grigson *et al.*, 1997). This animal does not seek food or initiate spontaneous meals, but, like an intact animal, will reflexively swallow liquid food put directly into its mouth via an oral fistula. The decerebrate rat will swallow a sucrose solution when its stomach is empty, such as after a period of food deprivation; however, it will not swallow water or saline when food deprived, nor will it swallow sucrose solution when its stomach is full or when it has received a systemic injection of CCK or hypertonic saline (but instead lets the administered fluid passively drip from its mouth). These experiments suggest that considerable control of food intake exists entirely within the caudal brain stem, which receives signals that arise when ingested food contacts peripheral sensory organs (i.e., taste buds, gastric stretch receptors, intestinal CCK-secreting cells). Nonetheless, decerebrate animals are incapable of receiving input from forebrain sites that could modify intake based on learning or other experience, on body adiposity, or on time of day.

Other observations provide additional support for an important role of the brain stem in the control of meal size. When the area postrema is ablated, rats eat larger meals than normal, although total daily food intake is normal; that is, they compensate for their large meals by eating less frequently, indicating that long-term controls of food intake are not impaired. A similar effect is seen in rats pretreated with capsaicin, a neurotoxin that destroys most gastric afferent vagal axons, eliminating the food intake-reducing effects of CCK and presumably damaging the signal of gastric distension.

Summary

To provide a biological context within which to consider the purpose of eating and the fate of ingested food, we began this chapter with a description of the physiology of caloric homeostasis. Two principles were emphasized. First, meal size is determined by the integrated effects of several acute stimuli. Delivery of calories to the stomach and intestines upon food consumption and postabsorptive delivery of nutrients to the liver elicit sensory neural signals from the stomach and the liver, respectively, to the brain stem. Second, food intake is also influenced by chronic signals associated with body adiposity. Adiposity indirectly affects gastric and hepatic signals of satiety. In addition, humoral signals proportional to adiposity enter the brain and affect food intake. One signal emanates from adipose tissue itself (i.e., leptin), and the other comes from the pancreas (i.e., insulin). These two peptides appear to be important in the central control of food intake; they modulate the response of the brain to the acute neural signals that affect food intake.

These neural and humoral signals are related to caloric homeostasis and are inhibitory in nature. During meals, they combine to stop ongoing ingestion; later, when these signals disappear in the postabsorptive state, new meals begin. Other inhibitory signals are unrelated to caloric homeostasis yet can have a pronounced effect on the cessation of eating. These signals include gastric distension, toxins (in the food or body), and dehydration.

The central nervous system exerts control over eating at many levels: The spinal cord and brain stem influence all aspects of caloric homeostasis via the autonomic nervous system. The hypothalamus and limbic forebrain receive signals about ingested food and body adiposity and integrate them with information about the taste of the food, the memory of that food, the experience of previous meals, the competition of other desires, and aspects of the environment. Thus, the central control of eating involves many areas of the central nervous system in the collective maintenance of caloric homeostasis. In short, food intake is a simple behavior influenced by a complex array of stimuli and situational variables, the details of which remain to be fully understood.

References

Campfield, L. A., and Smith, F. J. (1986). Functional coupling between transient declines in blood glucose and feeding behavior: Temporal relationships. *Brain Res. Bull.* **17**, 427–433.

Coleman, D. L., and Hummel, K. P. (1969). Effects of parabiosis of normal with genetically diabetic mice. *Am. J. Physiol.* **217**, 1298–1304.

Cone, R. D. (1999). The central melanocortin system and energy homeostasis. *Trends Endocrinol. Metab.* **10**, 211–216.

Dethier, V. G. (1976). "The Hungry Fly." Harvard Univ. Press, Cambridge, MA.

Gibbs, J., Young, R. C., and Smith, G. P. (1973). Cholecystokinin decreases food intake in rats. *J. Comp. Physiol. Psychol.* **84**, 488–495.

Grigson, P. S., Kaplan, J. M., Roitman, M. F., Norgen, R. and Grill, H. J. (1997). Reward comparison in chronic decerebrate rats. *Am. J. Physiol.* **273**, R479–R486.

Hagan, M. M., Rushing, P. A., Pritchard, L. M., Schwartz, M. W., Strack, A. M., Van Der Ploeg, L. H., Woods, S. C., and Seeley, R. J. (2000). Long-term orexigenic effects of AgRP-(83–132) involve mechanisms other than melanocortin receptor blockade. *Am. J. Physiol.* **279**, R47–R52.

Hoebel, B. G., and Teitelbaum, P. (1966). Weight regulation in normal and hypothalamic hyperphagic rats. *J. Comp. Physiol. Psychol.* **61**, 189–193.

Le Magnen, J., and Tallon, S. (1966). La periodicite spontanee de la prise d'aliments ad libitum du rat blanc. *J. Physiol. (Paris)* **58**, 323–349.

Leibowitz, S. F. (1990). Hypothalamic neuropeptide Y, galanin, and amines: Concepts of coexistence in relation to feeding behavior. *Ann. N.Y. Acad. Sci.* **611**, 221–235.

Mayer, J. (1955). Regulation of energy intake and the body weight: The glucostatic theory and the lipostatic hypothesis. *Ann. N.Y. Acad. Sci.* **63**, 15–43.

McCann, M. J., Verbalis, J. G., and Stricker, E. M. (1989). LiCl and CCK inhibit gastric emptying and feeding and stimulate OT secretion in rats. *Am. J. Physiol.* **256**, R463–R468.

Phillips, R. J., and Powley, T. L. (1996). Gastric volume rather than nutrient content inhibits food intake. *Am. J. Physiol.* **271**, R766–R779.

Schwartz, M. W., Woods, S. C., Porte, D., Jr., Seeley, R. J., and Baskin, D. G. (2000). Central nervous system control of food intake. *Nature* **404**, 661–671.

Seeley, R. J., Yagaloff, K. A., Fisher, S. L., Burn, P., Thiele, T. E., van Dijk, G., Baskin, D. G., and Schwartz, M. W. (1997). Melanocortin receptors in leptin effects. *Nature* **390**, 349.

Shimada, M., Tritos, N. A., Lowell, B. B., Flier, J. S., and Maratos-Flier, E. (1998). Mice lacking melanin-concentrating hormone are hypophagic and lean. *Nature* **396**, 670–674.

Smith, G. P., Gibbs, J., and Young, R. C. (1974). Cholecystokinin and intestinal satiety in the rat. *Fed. Proc.* **33**, 1146–1150.

Thomas, D. W., and Mayer, J. (1968). Meal taking and regulation of food intake by normal and hypothalamic hyperphagic rats. *J. Comp. Physiol. Psychol.* **66**, 642–653.

Ungerstedt, U. (1971). Adipsia and aphagia after 6-hydroxydopamine induced degeneration of the nigro-striatal dopamine system. *Acta Physiol. Scandin. Suppl.* **367**, 95–122.

Woods, S. C. (1995). Insulin and the brain: A mutual dependency. *Prog. Psychobiol. Physiol. Psychol.* **16**, 53–81.

Suggested Readings

Barsh, G. S., Farooqi, I. S., and O'Rahilly, S. (2000). Genetics of body-weight regulation. *Nature* **404**, 644–651.

Elmquist, J. K., Elias, C. F., and Saper, C. B. (1999). From lesions to leptin: Hypothalamic control of food intake and body weight. *Neuron* **22**, 221–232.

Friedman, M. I., and Stricker, E. M. (1976). The physiological psychology of hunger: A physiological perspective. *Psychol. Rev.* **83**, 409–431.

Langhans, W. (1996). Metabolic and glucostatic control of feeding. *Proc. Nutr. Soc.* **55**, 497–515.

Le Magnen, J. (1985). Hunger. Cambridge Univ. Press, London.

Newsholme, E. A., and Start, C. (1973). "Regulation in Metabolism." Wiley, London.

Schwartz, M. W., Figlewicz, D. P., Baskin, D. G., Woods, S. C., and Porte, D., Jr. (1992). Insulin in the brain: A hormonal regulator of energy balance. *Endocr. Rev.* **13**, 387–414.

Smith, G. P., and Gibbs, J. (1992). The development and proof of the CCK hypothesis of satiety. *In* "Multiple Cholecystokinin Receptors in the CNS" (C. T. Dourish, S. J. Cooper, S. D. Iversen, and L. L. Iversen, eds.), pp. 166–182. Oxford Univ. Press, London.

Stricker, E. M. (ed.) (1990). "Handbook of Behavioral Neurobiology," Vol. 10. Plenum, New York.

Woods, S. C., Schwartz, M. W., Baskin, D. G., and Seeley, R. S. (2000). Food intake and the regulation of body weight. *Ann. Rev. Psychol.* **51**, 255–277.

Stephen C. Woods and Edward M. Stricker

39

Water Intake and Body Fluids

Body fluids are the watery matrix in which the biochemical reactions of cellular metabolism occur. The concentration of substrates in cellular fluid is a key factor in determining the rate at which those reactions take place. All tissues depend on circulating blood to deliver the nutrients needed to support cellular metabolism and to carry away unwanted metabolites for excretion. Thus, the maintenance of solute concentrations or osmolalities—*osmotic homeostasis*—and the regulation of plasma volume—*volume homeostasis*—are essential functions in the physiology of animals.

When normal body fluid osmolality or plasma volume is threatened, various physiological and behavioral responses are stimulated to maintain or restore the basal state adaptively. For example, during water deprivation, animals decrease water lost in urine to prevent dehydration from worsening and consume water to replace the fluid they have lost. Similarly, hemorrhage stimulates the urinary conservation of water and sodium, as well as the ingestion of water and NaCl. Water retention and sodium retention are accomplished through actions of the antidiuretic hormone *arginine vasopressin* (AVP) and the antinatriuretic hormone *aldosterone*, whereas water ingestion and NaCl ingestion are motivated by *thirst* and *salt appetite*. These complementary responses are mediated and coordinated by the brain.

This chapter describes the various mechanisms by which the signals for fluid homeostasis are detected and integrated by the central nervous system. However, we first present a brief overview of body fluid physiology to provide a context in which to consider the regulated functions.

BODY FLUID PHYSIOLOGY

Water is the largest constituent of the body. It contributes 55–65% of the body weight of animals, including humans, varying mostly in relation to the amount of body fat. Total body water is distributed between *intracellular fluid* (ICF) and *extracellular fluid* (ECF) *compartments*, with approximately two-thirds in the former and one-third in the latter. The ECF can be further subdivided into the *interstitial fluid* surrounding the cells and the *intravascular fluid* within blood vessels. The intravascular fluid, the plasma (or serum) of blood, averages 7–8% of total body water, or 20–25% of the ECF.

Fluid compartments differ not only in their volumes, but also in the solutes they contain. Specifically, membrane-bound Na^+-K^+ pumps move Na^+ outside the cells and K^+ inside. Despite the differences in solute composition, the *osmotic pressure*, which reflects the concentrations of all solutes in a fluid compartment, is equivalent between ECF and ICF compartments. This equilibrium occurs because water flows freely across cellular membranes by osmosis from a relatively dilute compartment into one with a higher solute concentration until the osmotic pressures are the same on both sides of the cell membrane.

Multiple Mechanisms Help Maintain Blood Volume and Pressure

The distribution of fluid between intravascular and interstitial fluid compartments is determined by a balance between the *hydrostatic pressure* of the blood, which is maintained by cardiac output and arteriolar

1011

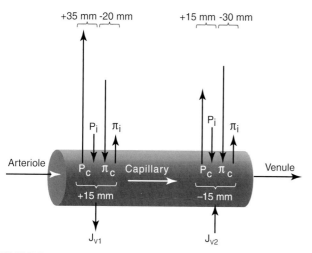

FIGURE 39.1 Starling forces governing transcapillary fluid transfer. At the arteriolar end of the capillary, the difference between the intravascular hydrostatic pressure (P_c) and the interstitial hydrostatic pressure (P_i) exceeds the oppositely oriented difference between the intravascular oncotic pressure (π_c) and the interstitial oncotic pressure (π_i); the resultant pressure gradient drives capillary fluid into the interstitial space (J_{v1}). As fluid leaves the capillary, P_c decreases due to fluid loss and p_c increases due to hemoconcentration. Consequently, at the venous end of the capillary, interstitial fluid is pulled back into the vascular space (J_{v2}). Numerical values indicate approximate net pressure differences (in mm Hg) between intravascular and interstitial spaces. Relative sizes of P and π are indicated by arrow length. Note that fluid accumulating in the interstitial space ultimately returns to the blood via the lymphatic system (not shown).

vasoconstriction, and the opposing osmotic pressure contributed by plasma proteins. Although those proteins contribute only 1–2% to overall plasma osmolality, the permeability of capillary membranes to such large molecules is low; therefore, proteins exert a pressure differential (of approximately 15–20 mm Hg), called the *colloid osmotic (oncotic) pressure*, that tends to pull interstitial fluid into the circulation. Figure 39.1 summarizes the forces governing transcapillary fluid transfer between the two extracellular compartments, a phenomenon first described by the English physiologist Starling (1896). Note that according to this arrangement, interstitial fluid acts as a reservoir for plasma. The Starling equilibrium is such that when blood pressure falls, as after hemorrhage, interstitial fluid moves into the circulation, thereby helping restore plasma volume. The reverse occurs when saline is added to the blood because plasma proteins are then diluted and the oncotic pressure they provide diminishes, allowing fluid to flow into the interstitial space.

Blood pressure is also maintained by two other mechanisms intrinsic to the cardiovascular system. First, although the arteries that receive the cardiac

output of blood have thick walls to preserve blood pressure, the veins are thin-walled, distensible vessels. After a moderate hemorrhage, veins collapse, redistributing blood to arteries, which cannot collapse and thus remain full. Consequently, arterial blood pressure is not compromised, and the blood deficit occurs primarily on the venous side of the circulation. Conversely, fluid accumulates in the veins when blood volume is expanded, again without much effect on arterial blood pressure. This property is called the *capacitance* or *compliance* of the vascular system. Second, the filtration of blood in the glomeruli of the kidneys is determined in large part by blood pressure in the renal arteries. A drop in blood pressure reduces the *glomerular filtration rate* (GFR) and decreases urine formation, whereas a rise in blood pressure elevates GFR and promotes urinary fluid loss. This normal function of the kidneys is so efficient that the development of hypertension always implicates renal dysfunction as a contributing factor because the kidneys failed to adjust to the elevated blood pressure by increasing fluid excretion in urine.

Summary

Body fluid homeostasis is directed at achieving stability in the osmolality of body fluids and the volume of plasma. Such homeostatic regulation is promoted by several mechanisms intrinsic to the physiology of body fluids and the cardiovascular system. For example, the osmotic movement of water across cellular membranes rapidly buffers changes in the osmolality of ECF. Similarly, the movement of fluid across capillary membranes buffers acute changes in plasma volume (according to the Starling equilibrium), as does venous compliance and compensatory alterations in GFR. Nevertheless, changes in body fluid osmolality and plasma volume may be so large that additional mechanisms must be recruited to maintain homeostasis. These other responses involve the central control of water and sodium excretion in urine through the actions of specific hormones, and the central control of water and NaCl consumption motivated by thirst and salt appetite.

OSMOTIC HOMEOSTASIS

Osmolality is an expression of concentration—that is, a ratio of the total amount of solute dissolved in a given weight of water:

$$\frac{\text{solute (osmoles)}}{\text{water (kilograms)}}.$$

Dehydration and the consequent need for water occur whenever this ratio is elevated, whether by a decrease in its denominator or by an increase in its numerator. In fact, both changes occur naturally and often: Body water decreases as a result of water deprivation or the loss of dilute fluids to accomplish evaporative cooling (e.g., sweating) and increases as a result of solute load (e.g., the consumption of sodium as NaCl in foods).

The water loss associated with dehydration is borne by the ECF and the ICF in proportion to their sizes because the osmolality of fluid in the two compartments remains in equilibrium. In contrast, the increase in plasma osmolality that results from a solute load results only in cellular dehydration because the water leaving cells by osmosis expands ECF volume. Thus, a solute load is a more abrupt, less complex treatment than water deprivation for stimulating AVP secretion and thirst, the two main osmoregulatory responses of the brain.

Arginine Vasopressin Is the Antidiuretic Hormone

AVP is a nine amino acid peptide that is synthesized in the magnocellular neurons in the supraoptic nucleus (SON) and the paraventricular nucleus (PVN) of the hypothalamus. The peptide is cleaved enzymatically from its prohormone (Fig. 39.2) and transported along axons projecting from the hypothalamus to the nearby posterior lobe of the pituitary gland (*neurohypophysis*). There, AVP is stored within neurosecretory granules until specific stimuli, such as an increase in the effective osmolality of body fluids,

cause its secretion into the bloodstream. The importance of AVP in maintaining water balance is underscored by the fact that its stores in the pituitary contain sufficient hormone to enable maximal antidiuresis when dehydration is sustained for more than a week.

The circulating hormone acts on a subset of AVP receptors (termed V_2) in the kidney to increase water permeability of the distal convoluted tubules of nephrons through insertion of water channels into the apical membranes of tubular epithelial cells. Permeability of the collecting duct is also increased. Antidiuresis occurs when water moves out of the distal convoluted tubule and collecting duct by osmosis. As secondary responses to the increased net water reabsorption, urine flow decreases and urine osmolality increases. See Box 39.1 for more on renal water channels (Knepper, 1997).

With refinement of radioimmunoassays for AVP, the unique sensitivity of the hormone to small changes in osmolality has become apparent, as has the remarkable sensitivity of the kidney to small changes in plasma AVP levels. Circulating AVP is linearly related to plasma osmolality above a threshold of 1–2% pg ml^{-1} (Fig. 39.3). Urine osmolality, in turn, is related linearly to AVP levels from 0.5 to 5–6 pg ml^{-1}, in association with increases in plasma osmolality to only 4% above the threshold for AVP secretion. However, because urine volume is related inversely to urine osmolality, small increases in plasma AVP concentration (e.g., from 0.5 to 2 pg ml^{-1}) have the effect of decreasing urine flow much more than subsequent larger increases (e.g., from 2 to 5 pg ml^{-1}; Fig. 39.4). This relationship emphasizes the

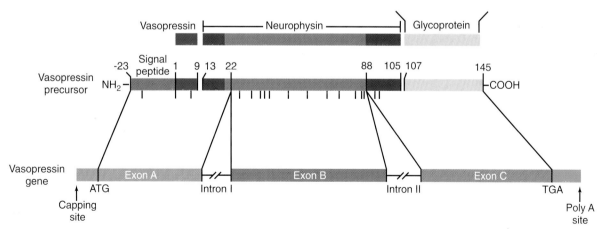

FIGURE 39.2 The vasopressin gene and its protein products. The three exons encode a 145 amino acid prohormone with an amino-terminal signal peptide. The prohormone is packaged into neurosecretory granules of magnocellular neurons. During axonal transport of the granules from the hypothalamus to the posterior pituitary, enzymatic cleavage of the prohormone generates the final products: vasopressin, neurophysin, and a carboxy-terminal glycoprotein. When afferent stimulation depolarizes the vasopressin-containing neurons, the three products are released into capillaries of the posterior pituitary. Modified with permission from Richter and Schmale (1983).

BOX 39.1

WATER CHANNELS

Water conservation by the kidney is dependent on its ability to concentrate the urine. Urine is concentrated through the combined actions of the loop of Henle and the collecting duct of the kidney. The loop of Henle generates a high osmolality in the renal medulla via a mechanism known as the countercurrent multiplier system. AVP acts in the collecting duct to increase water permeability, thereby allowing osmotic equilibration between the urine and the hypertonic interstitium of the renal medulla. The net effect of this process is to extract water from the urine into the medullary interstitial blood vessels, resulting in increased urine concentration and decreased urine volume.

AVP produces antidiuresis by virtue of its effects on the epithelial principal cells of the collecting tubule in the kidney, which are endowed with AVP receptors of the V_2 type. It has long been known that binding of AVP to G-protein-coupled V_2 receptors causes cAMP generation via activation of adenylate cyclase. However, the intracellular mechanisms responsible for the subsequent increased water reabsorption across the collecting duct cells have been elucidated only recently following the discovery of *aquaporins*, which are a widely expressed family of water channels that mediate rapid water transport across cell membranes.

Many different aquaporin water channels are expressed in various body tissues, including the brain. At the present time, four of these channels have been localized in the kidney. Aquaporin-1 is expressed constitutively in the proximal tubule and thin descending limb of the loop of Henle and is believed to be responsible for reabsorption of a large fraction of the water filtered by the glomerulus. The other three water channels, aquaporin-2, -3, and -4, are expressed in collecting duct principal cells, target cells for the action of AVP to regulate collecting duct water permeability. Aquaporin-2 is the only water channel known to be expressed in the apical membrane (i.e., the side bordering the tubular lumen, through which urine flows) of collecting duct principal cells and is also abundant in intracellular vesicles located below the apical membrane. Aquaporin-2 is the only known AVP-regulated water channel and mediates water transport across the apical plasma membrane of the principal cells of the collecting ducts. In contrast, aquaporins-3 and -4 are expressed at high levels in the basolateral plasma membranes (i.e., the side bordering the blood) of principal cells and are responsible for the constitutively high water permeability of the basolateral plasma membrane.

There are at least two ways by which AVP regulates osmotic water permeability in the collecting duct: short-term and long-term regulation (Knepper, 1997). Short-term regulation is associated with increases in water permeability within a few minutes of AVP exposure, an effect that is rapidly reversible. AVP triggers this response by binding to the V_2 receptor and increasing intracellular cyclic AMP levels by activating adenylate cyclase. Studies have demonstrated that the increase in collecting duct water permeability is a consequence of fusion of aquaporin-2-containing intracytoplasmic vesicles with the apical plasma membranes of the principal cells, a process that increases apical water permeability by markedly increasing the number of water-conducting pores in the apical plasma membrane. Dissociation of AVP from the V_2 receptor allows intracellular cAMP levels to decrease, and the water channels are reinternalized into the intracytoplasmic vesicles, thereby terminating the increased water permeability. By virtue of the subapical membrane localization of the aquaporin-containing vesicles, they can be quickly shuttled into and out of the membrane in response to changes in intracellular cAMP levels. This mechanism therefore allows minute-to-minute regulation of renal water excretion through changes in ambient plasma AVP levels. Long-term regulation of collecting duct water permeability represents a sustained increase in collecting duct water permeability in response to prolonged high levels of circulating AVP. This response requires at least 24 h to elicit and is not as rapidly reversible. Studies have demonstrated that this conditioning effect is due largely to the ability of AVP to induce large increases in the abundance of aquaporin-2 and -3 water channels in the collecting duct principal cells. Greater total expression of the number of aquaporin-2 and -3 water channels, when combined with the short-term effect of AVP to shift aquaporin-2 into the apical plasma membrane, allows the collecting ducts to achieve extremely high water permeabilities during conditions of prolonged dehydration, thereby further enhancing the urine concentrating capacity in response to elevated levels of circulating AVP.

The discovery of AVP-regulated apical water channels and the rapid growth of knowledge of their regulation and function have opened new possibilities for understanding pathological processes involving abnormalities of renal water handling. Many polyuric states have been associated with decreases in kidney aquaporin-2 expression, including animal models of Li^+ administration and physiological effects of small initial changes in plasma AVP levels. The net result of these relations among plasma osmolality, AVP secretion, urine volume, and urine osmolality is a finely tuned regulatory system that adjusts the rate of free water excretion according to plasma osmolality via changes in pituitary hormone secretion.

Thirst Is Another Effective Osmoregulatory Response to Dehydration

Accompanying the excretion of concentrated urine is reabsorption of conserved water, which can considerably dilute remaining body fluids. Thirst, and the

water intake it provokes, is a much more rapid and less limited response to dehydration than antidiuresis. Thirst may be defined as a strong motivation to seek, to obtain, and to consume water in response to deficits in body fluids. Like AVP secretion, thirst can be stimulated by cellular dehydration caused by increases in the effective osmolality of ECF (Gilman

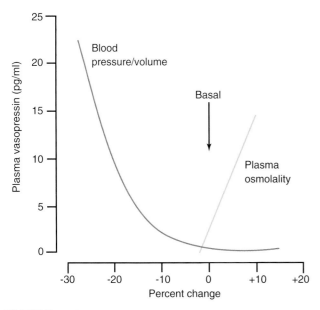

FIGURE 39.3   Plasma concentrations of AVP as a function of changes in plasma osmolality, blood volume, or blood pressure in humans. The arrow indicates the plasma AVP concentration at basal plasma osmolality, volume, and blood pressure. Modified with permission from Robertson (1986).

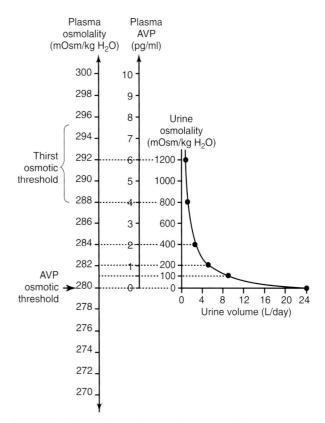

FIGURE 39.4   Relationship of plasma osmolality, plasma AVP concentrations, urine osmolality, and urine volume in humans. Note that small changes in plasma AVP concentrations have larger effects on urine volume at low plasma AVP concentrations than at high plasma AVP concentrations. Modified with permission from Robinson (1985).

BOX 39.2

DIABETES INSIPIDUS

The disease *diabetes insipidus* (DI), in which the secretion of AVP is impaired or absent, illustrates the crucial role of AVP in controlling the volume of water in the body. Early Greeks named the disease diabetes insipidus, or insipid urine, to distinguish it from *diabetes mellitus*, or sweet urine, in which abnormally high concentrations of glucose in the blood result in glucose appearing in the urine.

AVP is the only known antidiuretic substance in the body. In its absence, the kidney is unable to concentrate urine maximally to conserve water. The result is a continued excretion of copious amounts of a very dilute urine. Patients with severe cases of DI, in whom the ability to excrete AVP is completely lost, can excrete up to 25 liters of urine each day. Such patients urinate almost hourly, which renders the completion of even simple tasks and activities of daily living, including sleeping, exceedingly difficult.

Patients with DI can quickly become dehydrated if their urinary fluid losses are not replaced by drinking water. Fortunately, thirst remains intact in most patients with DI because lesions that destroy the magnocellular neurons in the SON and PVN that synthesize AVP generally leave intact the osmoreceptors in the anterior hypothalamus as well as the higher brain centers that control thirst. Consequently, extreme thirst is one of the hallmarks of this disease, leading to the characteristic symptoms of *polydipsia* (excessive drinking) and *polyuria* (excessive urination). If drinking water is unavailable, or if a person with DI is unable to drink, then the unreplaced urinary water loss leads to dehydration and death in the absence of medical intervention.

DI can be caused when tumors and infiltrative diseases of the hypothalamus destroy the magnocellular neurons that produce AVP. Because four nuclei contain magnocellular neurons, and 10–20% of AVP-producing neurons are sufficient for normal urine concentration, brain lesions that cause DI are generally large. Less commonly, DI is idiopathic (of unknown cause), perhaps with an autoimmune basis. DI can also be genetic, transmitted as an autosomal-dominant trait. In families with congenital DI, point mutations have been found in the signal peptide region and the neurophysin part of the AVP prohormone (see Fig. 39.3). Interestingly, none of these mutations is similar to the frameshift mutation responsible for the well-studied animal model of DI, the Brattleboro rat (Richter and Schmale, 1983). Some patients with DI do not have any defect in AVP secretion but rather have defects in the V_2 AVP receptors in the kidney that respond to circulating AVP. These cases are called *nephrogenic* (of kidney origin) DI.

The treatment for DI, like that of other endocrine deficiency disorders, is replacement of the deficient hormone, in this case AVP. The short half-life of AVP in the circulation allows mammals to have minute-to-minute control of their urine output. However, longer acting synthetic analogs of AVP are more convenient for treatment because they need not be taken as frequently as short-acting drugs (Robinson, 1985). These agents can restore urinary concentration and allow a person with DI to lead a more normal life.

Edward M. Stricker and
Joseph G. Verbalis

1937). Studies in animals consistently indicate that drinking behavior is elicited by 1–3% increases in plasma osmolality above basal levels, and analogous research in humans has revealed that similar thresholds must be reached to produce thirst (Robertson, 1986). This arrangement, in which the threshold for drinking is slightly higher than that for secretion of AVP (Fig. 39.4), ensures that ongoing behavior is not disrupted by thirst unless the buffering effects of osmosis and antidiuresis are insufficient to accomplish osmoregulation. It also ensures that dehydration does not become severe before thirst is stimulated. See Box 39.2 for more on how the neurohypophysis controls the volume of water in the body.

Also like AVP secretion, water intake increases linearly in proportion to increases in the effective osmolality of ECF. The dilution of body fluids by ingested water complements the retention of water that occurs during antidiuresis, and both responses occur when drinking water is available. However, there may be marked individual differences in whether dehydrated subjects respond to their need for water promptly by drinking or more slowly by increasing renal water conservation (Kanter, 1953). AVP secretion and urine osmolality are more elevated when an induced increase in plasma osmolality is not compensated for by water intake (e.g., because drinking water is not available). Conversely, water intake

BOX 39.3

RAPID INHIBITORY FEEDBACK CONTROL OF DRINKING

Water deprivation and systemic administration of hypertonic saline each increase the effective osmolality of circulating plasma and thereby activate forebrain osmoreceptor cells. Animals drink water, but 10–20 min elapse before ingested water is absorbed into the circulation and affects plasma osmolality. However, many species (e.g., dogs, humans) drink water very quickly, stopping long before the ingested water actually rehydrates them. What are the biological mechanisms that mediate this anticipatory satiety?

One possibility is that a neural message is communicated from the oropharynx to the brain in association with the act of swallowing. Thus, the more animals drink and swallow, the greater the inhibition of thirst, even before the water is absorbed. In fact, evidence is consistent with metered fluid consumption providing a preliminary signal of satiety. The main experiments were done in dogs with implanted gastric fistulas (Thrasher *et al.*, 1981). When the fistula was closed, ingested water flowed normally from the stomach into the intestine and was absorbed; water-deprived dogs drank rapidly, stopped 15 min before their plasma osmolalities began to decrease, and did not resume drinking as their stomach emptied. In contrast, when the fistula was left open, ingested water drained out from the stomach, never entering the intestine and thus never being absorbed; the dogs drank normal amounts, stopped drinking, and after 10–20 min resumed drinking. When the dogs were not allowed to drink but water was introduced into the stomach through the fistula, thus bypassing the oropharynx, the gastric load did not affect water intake until it had been absorbed.

These observations are consistent with a temporary satiety being produced by the act of water consumption, with a more long-lasting satiety occurring only after absorption of the ingested water and rehydration of the dog. AVP secretion is affected in parallel, showing that physiological and behavioral components of osmoregulation are influenced similarly. Ingestion of a concentrated NaCl solution instead of water produces the same temporary satiety and inhibition of AVP secretion, but after the saline is absorbed, the increase in plasma osmolality stimulates more drinking and AVP secretion than occurred at first. In similar experiments, people respond the same way.

Animals drink appropriate amounts perhaps because they have learned from previous experiences how much to drink to relieve their thirst. After all, when we are thirsty, we fill a glass to a volume that, based on previous experience, we think will be sufficient for satiety. No doubt animals behave equivalently. Alternatively, this drinking response may not be learned, and instead appropriate neural circuits linking the act of swallowing with satiety may be present at birth. Consistent with this possibility is the finding that the first drinking experience of newly hatched chickens is rapid and provides the correct amount of water needed for osmoregulation.

Research indicates that rats also obtain early feedback from drinking but do so by a different mechanism. In one study, rats were infused intravenously with a hypertonic NaCl solution to stimulate AVP secretion (Huang *et al.*, 2000). Water intake for 5 min was found to cause a rapid decrease in plasma levels of AVP without noticeable changes in plasma osmolality. These effects were not associated simply with the act of drinking because intake of the same volume of isotonic saline had no effect on plasma AVP levels. Thus, the animals appeared to be responding to the composition of the ingested fluid, not its volume. These and other observations suggest the existence of osmo- or Na^+-receptor cells that detect ingested water, located somewhere after the fluid leaves the stomach and before it enters the general circulation. The small intestines, hepatic portal vein, and liver all are potential sites for such receptors. Moreover, after the destruction of vagal afferent neurons from these visceral loci, or the neural projection sites in the nucleus of the solitary tract and area postrema in the caudal brain stem (Curtis *et al.*, 1996), rats drank excessive amounts of water in response to thirst stimuli, especially in the early portion of the drinking test. These thirsty animals behaved as if they did not receive inhibitory feedback until the ingested water was absorbed and had reduced plasma osmolality. Thus, whether inhibitory signals arise from the oropharynx, the hepatic portal vein, or other peripheral sites, early messages modulate drinking and AVP secretion.

Edward M. Stricker and
Joseph G. Verbalis

in response to a solute load increases in animals after their kidneys are removed or their capability to secrete AVP is compromised, thereby precluding rapid excretion of the load in urine. See Box 39.3 on the rapid inhibitory feedback control of drinking.

Osmoreceptor Cells Stimulate AVP Secretion and Thirst

All body cells lose water by osmosis when the effective osmolality of ECF is increased. Thus, cells that provoke AVP secretion and thirst do not have unique

osmosensitive properties (unlike retinal photoreceptor cells, e.g., which are specially responsive to light). Instead, the unique feature of osmoreceptor cells is thought to be their neural circuitry, which activates the central systems for AVP secretion and thirst when the cells are dehydrated.

Destruction of osmoreceptor neurons should eliminate detection of increased plasma osmolality and thus the AVP secretion and thirst responses that are elicited by dehydration. In fact, ample research has confirmed that certain brain lesions eliminate AVP secretion and thirst responses. Such studies also have

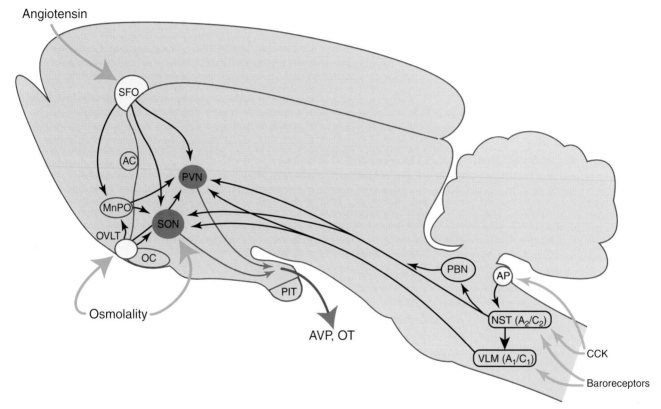

FIGURE 39.5 Summary of the main anterior hypothalamic pathways that mediate secretion of arginine vasopressin (AVP) and oxytocin (OT). The vascular organ of the lamina terminalis (OVLT) is especially sensitive to hyperosmolality. Hyperosmolality also activates other neurons in the anterior hypothalamus, such as those in the subfornical organ (SFO) and median preoptic nucleus (MnPO), and magnocellular neurons, which are intrinsically osmosensitive. Circulating angiotensin II (AII) activates neurons of the SFO, an essential site of AII action, as well as cells throughout the lamina terminalis and MnPO. In response to hyperosmolality or AII, projections from the SFO and OVLT to the MnPO activate excitatory and inhibitory interneurons that project to the supraoptic nucleus (SON) and paraventricular nucleus (PVN) to modulate direct inputs to these areas from the circumventricular organs. Cholecystokinin (CCK) acts primarily on gastric vagal afferents that terminate in the nucleus of the solitary tract (NST), but at higher doses it can also act at the area postrema (AP). Although neurons apparently are activated in the ventrolateral medulla (VLM) and NST, most oxytocin secretion appears to be stimulated by monosynaptic projections from A2/C2 cells, and possibly also noncatecholaminergic somatostatin/inhibin b cells, of the NST. Baroreceptor-mediated stimuli, such as hypovolemia and hypotension, are more complex. The major projection to magnocellular AVP neurons appears to arise from A1 cells of the VLM that are activated by excitatory interneurons from the NST. Other areas, such as the parabrachial nucleus (PBN), may contribute multisynaptic projections. Cranial nerves IX and X, which terminate in the NST, also contribute input to magnocellular AVP neurons. It is unclear whether baroreceptor-mediated secretion of oxytocin results from projections from VLM neurons or from NST neurons. AC, anterior commissure; OC, optic chiasm; PIT, anterior pituitary.

revealed that osmoreceptor cells (Johnson and Buggy, 1978; Thrasher *et al.*, 1982) appear to be located in the vascular organ of the lamina terminalis (OVLT) and areas of the adjacent anterior hypothalamus, near the anterior wall of the third cerebral ventricle (Fig. 39.5). Surgical destruction of that area of the brain in animals abolishes the AVP secretion and thirst responses to hyperosmolality but not their responses to other stimuli. The same conclusion was drawn after a study of people who were unable to osmoregulate when water deprived or when given a NaCl load; these patients were found to have focal brain tumors that destroyed the region around the OVLT.

The location of osmoreceptor cells in the OVLT is consistent with the results of pioneering investigations in which hyperosmotic solutions injected into blood vessels perfusing the anterior hypothalamus stimulated AVP secretion in dogs (Verney, 1947). The OVLT and

surrounding areas of the anterior hypothalamus have also been implicated by studies in rats. After systemic injections of hypertonic NaCl solution, modern immunocytochemical techniques were used to detect early gene products in cells associated with the production of new protein. Dense staining in the OVLT (and in AVP-secreting cells in the hypothalamus) indicated that it had been strongly stimulated by the experimentally induced dehydration. See Box 39.4 on the use of cFos immunocytochemistry in studies of brain function.

The neural pathways connecting the OVLT with magnocellular AVP-secreting cells in the hypothalamic SON and PVN have been identified, whereas the neural circuits in the forebrain that control thirst are still unknown. Early reports identified the lateral hypothalamus as a "thirst center" because its destruction in rats eliminated the drinking response, but not the associated AVP secretion, to increased osmolality

---

BOX 39.4

USE OF cFOS IMMUNOCYTOCHEMISTRY IN STUDIES OF BRAIN FUNCTION

cFos was named for its homology to an **FBR o**steogenic **s**arcoma virus protein, v-fos. The cFos protein is the product of the c-*fos* gene, which belongs to a family of genes whose products are involved in the regulation of gene transcription. The protein has a "leucine zipper" motif that promotes dimerization (pairing) with other regulatory proteins, most commonly with members of the Jun family. Genes encoding Jun and Fos are *immediate-early genes* (IEGs), the first genes expressed in response to activation of cells. Jun and Fos protein dimers bind specific DNA sequences (e.g., APS sites) to modulate the expression of genes expressed later.

The precise relationship between cFos expression and transcription of later gene products remains uncertain for most neural systems. However, many neurons are known to express cFos only on synaptic activation; therefore, the mRNA or protein product (cFos) of the c-*fos* gene can be used as a marker of neuronal activation in the brain. The protein product is especially useful because it is detected easily by antibodies directed against cFos. This immunohistochemical staining allows investigators to determine which neurons are activated in the brain in response to specific stimuli given to experimental animals (Hoffman *et al.*, 1993).

Many of the initial studies simply localized the IEG expression to magnocellular neurons in the SON and PVN, but later studies used antibodies against proteins located in cytoplasm, along with the antibody against

IEG products, and showed that the IEG products were located in the nucleus (Hoffman *et al.*, 1993). Such studies have now confirmed that in response to these treatments, IEG expression in AVP- and oxytocin-secreting neurons closely parallels pituitary AVP and oxytocin secretion. Thus, in rats, hyperosmolality, hypovolemia, and administration of AII stimulate secretion of AVP and oxytocin and activate cFos expression in AVP and OT neurons; CCK, which stimulates secretion of oxytocin but not AVP, causes expression of cFos only in neurons that secrete oxytocin. Similarly, although severe hemorrhage stimulates secretion of AVP and oxytocin and activates cFos expression in both types of neurons, lower intensity stimuli predominantly cause peptide secretion and cFos expression only in AVP neurons. During CCK administration and during hemorrhage, plasma AVP and oxytocin correlate well with cFos expression. Consequently, IEG expression is now considered a specific and sensitive marker of magnocellular secretory activity in response to most acute stimuli.

Immunocytochemical detection of cFos expression, phenotypic characterization of activated cells, and standard techniques of tract tracing together enable investigators to map brain circuits activated by specific stimuli (Hoffman *et al.*, 1993).

Edward M. Stricker and
Joseph G. Verbalis

---

of body fluids. However, later investigations showed that the critical damage was not to hypothalamic cells but to dopamine-containing fibers that coursed through the area. The induced disruption of behavior was not specific to drinking but instead reflected a general inability of the brain-damaged animals to initiate movement (Stricker, 1976). Indeed, the syndrome of behavioral dysfunctions seen in these animals generally resembled that of Parkinson's disease, which has also been attributed to the loss of dopaminergic fibers in the brain. (See Chapter 38 for the same reinterpretation of the inability of rats to eat nor-mally after dopamine-depleting lesions of the lateral hypothalamus.)

Natriuresis and Inhibition of Solute Intake Also Promote Osmotic Homeostasis during Dehydration

When body fluid is hyperosmolal, adaptive behavior includes not only drinking and conserving water (thereby increasing the denominator in the ratio that represents body fluid osmolality), but also excreting NaCl and avoiding the consumption of additional osmoles (thereby decreasing the numerator of that ratio). Endogenous natriuretic agents promote urinary sodium loss after an administered NaCl load or a period of imposed water deprivation. One such agent is the hormone *atrial natriuretic peptide* (ANP), which is synthesized in the atria of the heart and released when increased intravascular volume distends the atria. Another is the hormone *oxytocin*. Like AVP, oxytocin is synthesized in magnocellular neurons in the PVN and SON and secreted from the posterior pituitary in proportion to induced hyperosmolality (Stricker and Verbalis, 1986). In rats, oxytocin is as potent in stimulating natriuresis as AVP is in stimulating antidiuresis (Verbalis *et al.*, 1991).

Salt loads are also known to decrease the intake of osmoles, whether in the form of NaCl solution or food, complementing the stimulation of thirst and the secretion of AVP and oxytocin. However, because destruction of the OVLT eliminates the two latter effects but not the dehydration-induced reduction in NaCl intake, osmo- or Na$^+$ receptors located outside the basal forebrain must mediate the inhibition of NaCl and food intake. Possible sites for such cells include the *hepatic portal vein* and the *area postrema*, both of which have been suspected of having Na$^+$ receptor functions. In addition, cells in the hepatic portal vein are well situated to detect the sodium content of ingested food and to modulate its intake accordingly.

Diuresis and Inhibition of Water Intake Promote Osmotic Homeostasis during Overhydration

Osmoregulation is required not only under conditions of dehydration, but also during periods of acute overhydration and hypoosmolality, as may result when beverages are consumed in excess of water needs. Such consumption occurs not because of thirst but, for example, because of the palatability of or chemical substances in the beverages (e.g., caffeine, alcohol). Unlike excess food, which is stored as triglycerides in adipose tissue, excess water is not stored for later use but instead is excreted in urine. When plasma osmolality is below normal, circulating levels of AVP are reduced, and in consequence, the kidneys void dilute urine and thereby raise plasma osmolality. The major behavioral contribution of osmotic dilution to osmoregulation is inhibition of free water intake; the ingestion of osmoles in food and NaCl is not stimulated by osmotic dilution. See Box 39.5 for regulation of cell volume in brain during chronic hypoosmolality.

Summary

Osmoregulation in animals and humans is accomplished by a combination of physiological responses to dehydration, resulting in antidiuresis and natriuresis, and the behavioral response of increased water intake. Osmoreceptor cells critical for mediating these functions have been identified in the basal forebrain. These neurons respond to very small increases in plasma osmolality, and the effector systems they control correct any increase in plasma osmolality. In addition, an early stimulus must exist, generated by peripheral osmo- or Na$^+$ receptor cells, that signals the brain in anticipation of subsequent rehydration. Other osmo- or Na$^+$ receptor cells appear to mediate the inhibition of NaCl and food intake, which also contributes to osmoregulation during dehydration. Conversely, diuresis and inhibition of water intake promote osmoregulation during overhydration, whereas excitation of NaCl or food intake does not.

VOLUME HOMEOSTASIS

Like osmotic dehydration, loss of blood volume (*hypovolemia*) stimulates several adaptive compensatory responses appropriate for restoring circulatory volume. The physiological contributions to volume regulation have been studied extensively in laboratory animals subjected to a controlled loss of blood. Because behavior is compromised by the anemia and

BOX 39.5

BRAIN VOLUME REGULATION

Many different clinical disorders are associated with dehydration, either secondary to excessive loss of body fluids [e.g., gastrointestinal losses from diarrhea, kidney losses due to inability to concentrate urine properly (see Box 39.2 on diabetes insipidus), cutaneous losses from increased sweating during fever], or from inadequate fluid intake (e.g., following a stroke). Conversely, there is also a large group of disorders associated with overhydration due to an inappropriate retention of water; these are classified as the *syndrome of inappropriate antidiuretic hormone secretion*, and also can be caused by a variety of different disorders (e.g., tumors that synthesize AVP, inflammatory brain disorders that alter the balance of excitatory and inhibitory inputs to the neurohypophysis, drugs that mimic AVP or cause pituitary secretion of AVP). Whatever the causes, dehydration results in hyperosmolality of the extracellular fluid with subsequent shrinkage of cells as water moves along osmotic gradients from inside cells to the more osmotically concentrated extracellular fluid space. Conversely, overhydration causes hypoosmolality of the extracellular fluid with subsequent swelling of cells as water moves along osmotic gradients from the less osmotically concentrated extracellular fluid into cells. Such shrinkage or swelling of cells, if unchecked, would eventually lead to disruption of the normal functions of the cells and the organs that contain them. Consequently, it is not surprising that organisms have evolved effective defense mechanisms to protect against these effects of sustained perturbations of the extracellular fluid osmolality.

Most cells have the ability to regulate their volume to substantial degrees. When individual cells are placed in a hyperosmolar bath solution, they initially shrink as the osmotic gradient pulls water from the cells by osmosis. However, within minutes the cells then return toward their original volume. Conversely, when cells are placed in a hypoosmolar bath, they swell initially as the osmotic gradient pulls water into the cells, but again, within minutes this effect is reversed and the cells return toward their original volume. These rapid readjustments in cell size are, for the most part, the result of electrolyte shifts into and out of the cells; thus the cells actually alter their intracellular solute content in order to prevent changes in cell volume that might be deleterious to normal intracellular metabolic processes.

Changes in the volume of individual cells have obvious implications for the organs in which they reside. The brain must be particularly well equipped to maintain its volume in view of its fixed location inside a rigid and unyielding skull. If no cellular volume regulation occurred, then mammals would die whenever their plasma osmolality decreased by more than 10%, as the cerebrospinal fluid space available in the brain to accommodate tissue swelling would be exceeded and herniation of the brain through the foramen magnum would occur with subsequent compression of vital brain stem respiratory centers. Just as in cultured cells, brain volume regulation during hypoosmolality occurs, in part, via losses of intracellular electrolytes, particularly K^+, the major intracellular electrolyte in mammals. Although early studies of brain volume during induced hypoosmolality found that only 60–70% of the observed volume regulation was accounted for by the measured electrolyte losses, the remaining 30–40% can be explained nearly completely by losses of other solutes from brain cells, without speculating that some fraction of the intracellular solutes is somehow inactivated or compartmentalized.

Multiple studies have shown that brain cells lose many *osmolytes* (small organic molecules) in addition to inorganic solutes such as electrolytes during the process of volume regulation to chronic hypoosmolar conditions in mice and rats, and similar results have been demonstrated in humans as well. Conversely, the brain is able to accumulate larger amounts of these same compounds in response to chronic hyperosmolality. These organic osmolytes include many amino acids (glutamate, glutamine, taurine), polyhydric alcohols (*myo*-inositol), methylamines (betaine, glycerolphosphorylcholine), and urea. By adjusting the cellular content of organic osmolytes in response to chronic changes in ambient extracellular osmolality, cells are able to maintain their volume without requiring large electrolyte shifts, which might also have more detrimental effects on intracellular metabolism. In effect, during sustained periods of osmotic disequilibrium, these osmotically active compounds replace part of the initial shifts of inorganic solutes that are responsible for the acute phases of brain cell volume regulation.

Mechanisms that allow the achievement of brain volume regulation are vital for survival during hypoosmolar conditions, but such compensatory changes must eventually be reversed to allow a full recovery to normal conditions once the hypoosmolality is corrected. In some cases the reversal of the adaptive processes may be more problematical than the initial adaptation itself. Rapid correction of chronic hypoosmolality has been

---

BOX 39.5   *(cont'd)*

---

shown to cause dehydration of brain tissue and, in some cases, demyelination of white matter in various parts of the brain, producing a debilitating and sometimes fatal disorder called pontine and extrapontine myelinolysis. Moreover, the induced dehydration occurs to a greater degree in chronically hypoosmolar rats than in normal rats following equivalent increases in osmolality, suggesting that this phenomenon reflects a loss of osmotic buffering capacity by brain tissue as a consequence of the very solute losses that allowed survival in the face of hypoosmolar conditions. Thus, the compensatory mechanisms that allow successful adaptation of cells to chronic hypoosmolality become maladaptive, and potentially harmful, when the osmolality is subsequently corrected.

Studies have suggested that disruption of the *blood–brain barrier* (BBB) may be correlated with this pathophysiological process. Rapid increases in plasma osmolality have long been known to disrupt the tight endothelial junctions that constitute the BBB, but the osmotic threshold required to produce this disruption in normal rats is fairly high, approximately 370 mOsm/kg H_2O. Studies utilizing imaging techniques in rats have shown a striking decrease (50–70 mOsm/kg H_2O) in the osmotic threshold for BBB disruption, indicating that adaptation to hypoosmolality entails volume regulation of the endothelial cells of the BBB as well. This observation implies that rapidly correcting the plasma osmolality to normal ranges in chronically hypoosmolar rats can be sufficient to disrupt the BBB, and subsequent studies have shown that there is indeed a significant positive correlation between BBB disruption and the development of brain demyelination in rapidly corrected hypoosmolar rats.

Edward M. Stricker and
Joseph G. Verbalis

---

hypotension that result from extensive hemorrhage, researchers studying thirst in rats may instead produce hypovolemia by subcutaneous injection of a colloidal solution. Such treatment disrupts the Starling equilibrium in capillaries near the injection site because the extravascular colloid opposes the oncotic effect of plasma proteins. Consequently, fluid leaches out of capillaries and remains in the interstitial space. Ingested fluid is also drawn into the interstitial space by the colloid so the total fluid volume required to correct the plasma volume deficit may be substantial. Water does not move from the cells by osmosis, however, because the osmolality of the injected colloidal solutions actually is similar to that of cells.

After colloid injections, rats conserve water and Na^+ in urine and increase their consumption of water and saline solution (Stricker, 1981). When given an isotonic NaCl solution to drink, these rats ingest volumes appropriate to their needs. When given separate bottles of water and concentrated NaCl solution, remarkably the rats drink appropriate amounts of each to create an isotonic fluid mixture. These observations raise several questions: How do the hypovolemic rats detect their plasma volume depletion? How are their thirst and salt appetite coordinated so that they consume the desired isotonic mixture of fluid? How are these two behavioral responses integrated with the complementary physiological responses of water and Na^+ conservation in urine, as well as with the vasoconstrictor responses needed to support blood pressure? Research has provided answers to these and related questions, which are discussed in the following sections.

Neural and Endocrine Signals of Hypovolemia Stimulate AVP Secretion

An appropriate physiological response to volume depletion should include water conservation and urine concentration. In fact, like plasma hyperosmolality, hypovolemia is an effective stimulus for AVP secretion (Robertson, 1986; Stricker and Verbalis, 1986). However, AVP secretion does not occur until blood loss exceeds 10% of total blood volume, meaning AVP secretion is much less sensitive to hypovolemia than to increases in ECF osmolality (Fig. 39.3). The effects of hypovolemia and osmotic dehydration are additive; that is, a given increase in osmolality causes greater secretion of AVP when animals are hypovolemic than when they are euvolemic (Fig. 39.6).

Loss of blood volume is first detected by stretch receptors in the great veins entering the right atrium of the heart. These stretch receptors provide an afferent vagal signal to the *nucleus of the solitary tract* (NST) in the brain stem (see Chapter 31). Still larger decreases in blood volume may also lower arterial blood pressure and reduce the stretch of receptors in the walls of the carotid sinus and aortic arch. That information is integrated in the NST with neural mes-

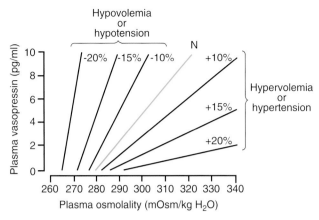

FIGURE 39.6 The relationship between the osmolality of plasma and the concentration of vasopressin (AVP) in plasma depends on blood volume and pressure. The line labeled N shows plasma vasopressin concentration across a range of plasma osmolality in an adult with normal intravascular volume (euvolemic) and normal blood pressure (normotensive). Lines to the left of N show the relationship between plasma vasopressin concentration and plasma osmolality in adults whose low intravascular volume (hypovolemia) or blood pressure (hypotension) is 10, 15, and 20% below normal. Lines to the right of N are for volumes and blood pressures 10, 15, and 20% above normal. Modified with permission from Robertson (1986).

sages from the low-pressure, venous side of the circulation. Note that these sensory neurons are not actually baroreceptors (literally, pressure receptors), although they are commonly referred to as such.

The ascending pathway between the NST in the brain stem and the SON and PVN in the hypothalamus includes noradrenergic fibers arising from A1 cells in the ventrolateral medulla. Volume depletion stimulates AVP secretion via other pathways as well. In addition, the kidneys secrete *renin* during hypovolemia, a response mediated in part by sympathetic neural input to ß-adrenergic receptors on cells that secrete renin. Renin is an enzyme that initiates a cascade of biochemical steps that result in the formation of *angiotensin II* (AII) (Fig. 39.7), an extremely potent vasoconstrictor. AII stimulates AVP secretion by acting in the brain at the *subfornical organ* (SFO) (Ferguson and Renaud, 1986), which is located in the dorsal portion of the third cerebral ventricle. Because this circumventricular organ lacks a blood–brain barrier, the AII receptors can detect very small increases in the blood levels of AII. Neural pathways from the SFO to the SON and PVN in the hypothalamus mediate AVP secretion and appear to use AII as a neurotransmitter. A branch of this pathway goes first to the OVLT, perhaps providing an opportunity for the integration of information about volume states and osmotic concentration.

Neural and Endocrine Signals of Hypovolemia Also Stimulate Thirst

In addition to the antidiuresis and vasoconstriction produced by the secretion of AVP and activation of the renin–angiotensin system, colloid treatment increases water intake in rats (Fitzsimons, 1961). Once 5–10% of the normal plasma volume has been lost, the water intake elicited by hypovolemia increases linearly in relation to further deficits in plasma volume. This stimulus for water intake and the effect of a NaCl load on thirst are additive. The stimulus of thirst during hypovolemia appears to be the same as the signal for AVP secretion,–i.e., a combination of neural afferents from cardiovascular baroreceptors and endocrine stimulation by AII (Fitzsimons, 1969). Each signal can stimulate water intake in the absence of the other. Thus, for example, water intake by hypovolemic rats is not diminished by destruction of the NST and loss of neural input from baroreceptors, nor is it eliminated by the loss of AII resulting from bilateral removal of the kidneys (Fitzsimons, 1961). Presumably, colloid treatment would not elicit thirst in rats subjected concurrently to bilateral nephrectomy and NST lesions.

Intravenous infusion of AII strongly stimulates thirst in rats and most other animals studied in the laboratory (including humans). AII adds to the thirst stimulated by an osmotic load when the two treatments are combined. There had been considerable controversy about whether AII functions as a normal physiological stimulus of thirst because the doses of AII required to stimulate significant water intake produce blood levels of AII well above the physiological range. However, such doses also increase arterial blood pressure, and it has been shown that this hypertension inhibits thirst and limits the induced water intake. For example, drinking was enhanced considerably when the hypertensive effects of AII were blunted by a simultaneous administration of vasodilating agents (Robinson and Evered, 1987). In addition, water drinking in response to intravenous AII was augmented greatly in rats with lesions of the NST, which could not receive the neural signal of hypertension from arterial baroreceptors. Note that the inhibitory effect of increased arterial blood pressure has also been seen when rats are made thirsty either by infusion of hypertonic saline or by hypovolemia.

Osmotic Dilution Inhibits Thirst and AVP Secretion during Hypovolemia

Hypovolemic rats need isotonic saline, not water alone, to repair their plasma volume deficits. When

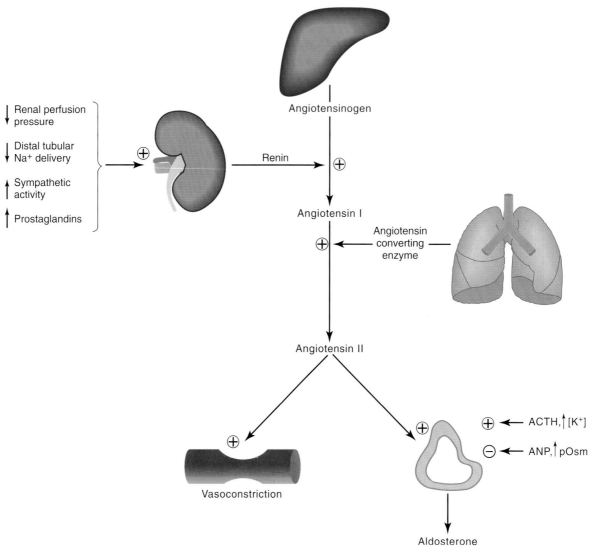

FIGURE 39.7 The renin–angiotensin cascade. Baroreceptors in the aortic arch, carotid sinus, and renal afferent arterioles sense hypovolemia and then cause the kidneys to secrete the enzyme renin. Renin cleaves angiotensinogen, which is synthesized by the liver, to produce angiotensin I. The angiotensin-converting enzyme, primarily in the lungs, cleaves angiotensin I to produce angiotensin II (AII), a peptide made of eight amino acid residues. AII is a potent vasoconstrictor and one of several stimulants of aldosterone secretion. Stimulation of aldosterone secretion from the adrenal cortex, along with possible direct intrarenal effects of AII, promotes renal conservation of sodium ions, complementing the pressor effect of AII in stabilizing arterial pressure and volume. ACTH, adrenocorticotropic hormone; ANP, atrial natriuretic peptide; pOsm, plasma osmolality. Modified with permission from Stricker and Verbalis (1992).

the rats drink only water, about two-thirds of the ingested volume moves into cells by osmosis, and much of what remains extracellular is captured by the colloid. Thus, most of the water that is consumed does not remain in the vascular compartment, and the volume deficit within the vascular compartment persists. This situation may be contrasted with the negative feedback control of osmoregulatory thirst in which the dehydration of osmoreceptor cells causes thirst and ingested water repairs dehydration, eliminating the stimulus for thirst.

Rather than repairing the volume deficit, the water consumed by hypovolemic rats causes a second serious challenge to body fluid homeostasis:-osmotic dilution. The animals cannot readily eliminate this self-administered water load because hypovolemia reduces GFR and thereby diminishes urinary excretion independent of AVP. Therefore, when water is the only drinking fluid available (and sodium is not provided in food), an appropriate response of colloid-treated rats would be to stop drinking and thereby limit the secondary problem of osmotic dilution. In experiments, colloid-treated rats actually do stop drinking water despite persistent hypovolemia, and the stimulus for the inhibition of thirst has been found to be osmotic dilution of body fluids (Stricker, 1969). A mere 4–7% decrease in osmolality is sufficient to stop drinking that has been motivated by a 30–40% loss of plasma volume. Thus, the osmoregulatory system appears dominant in the control of thirst. Comparable data demonstrate the same to be true of AVP secretion in colloid-treated rats: Osmotic dilution inhibits AVP secretion even in severely hypovolemic rats (Stricker and Verbalis, 1986).

Osmotic dilution brings to seven the number of stimuli identified in the control of thirst. Figure 39.8 summarizes these acute signals. Briefly, increases in plasma osmolality, detected by osmoreceptors in the OVLT, provide a common excitatory stimulus for thirst. Gastric NaCl loads, whether administered by the investigator or consumed by the experimental subject, increase plasma osmolality and additionally stimulate thirst more rapidly via putative Na^+ receptors in the hepatic portal vein. Similarly, the induced water intake inhibits drinking by acting rapidly in the oropharynx (in dogs, humans, and most experimental subjects) or on the visceral Na^+ receptors (in rats), and slowly when sufficient water has been absorbed to lower circulating plasma osmolality and affect the OVLT osmoreceptors. Hypovolemia provides two

signals for thirst: one neural (presumably from cardiac baroreceptors) and one humoral (when AII acts on receptors in the SFO) (Simpson et al., 1978). Decreases in arterial blood pressure also stimulate thirst when renin is secreted and AII acts on receptors in the SFO. Finally, increases in arterial blood pressure, detected by arterial baroreceptors, inhibit water intake regardless of which signal stimulates thirst. Thus, the sensation of thirst is controlled according to the integrated effects of these separate excitatory and inhibitory signals.

Hypovolemia Also Stimulates Aldosterone Secretion and Salt Appetite

As mentioned earlier, hypovolemic animals need to consume and retain water and NaCl, not just water. Appropriately, colloid-treated rats drink NaCl solution and conserve Na^+ in urine. Renal Na^+ retention is mediated largely by aldosterone secreted from the adrenal cortex, although Na^+ conservation also occurs in association with the decrease in GFR. The central nervous system does not innervate the adrenal cortex, as it does the adrenal medulla. However, a neural influence on aldosterone secretion is provided indirectly because AII is a very potent stimulus of aldosterone secretion, and renin secretion from the kidneys during hypovolemia is stimulated in part by the sym-

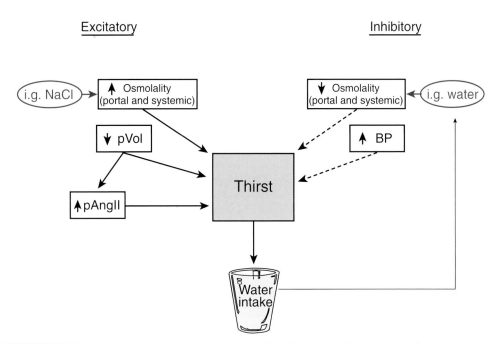

FIGURE 39.8 Schematic summary of the seven variables that control thirst in rats. Solid arrows, excitatory signals; dashed arrows, inhibitory signals. pVol, plasma volume; BP, arterial blood pressure; pAngII, plasma levels of angiotensin II; i.g. NaCl (or water), intragastric loads. See text for description.

BOX 39.6

SALT APPETITE AFTER ADRENOCORTICAL DYSFUNCTION

Fifty years ago, a 4-year-old boy was brought to the Johns Hopkins University Hospital in Baltimore with the peculiar behavior of eating large amounts of table salt. The child heavily salted all his food, even juice, and often consumed salt directly from its container. His parents tried unsuccessfully to keep him from consuming salt and brought him to the hospital in the hope that his strange behavior could be understood and stopped. The physicians were able to prevent the boy from having access to NaCl, but they were shocked when he died a few days later. An autopsy revealed that the child had bilateral tumors in his adrenal glands. In retrospect, it seems clear that he could not secrete aldosterone and therefore lost Na^+ in urine uncontrollably. Like patients with diabetes insipidus, who excrete a copious dilute urine and drink comparable volumes of water in compensation (see Box 39.2 on diabetes insipidus), this boy evidently was ingesting salt as an adaptive compensation to his recurrent need for sodium (Wilkins and Richter, 1940). He died when that response was prevented.

After surgical removal of their adrenal glands, rats increase their consumption of NaCl by amounts proportional to the sodium loss in urine (Richter, 1936). The stimulus for this salt appetite appears to be a combination of elevated circulating levels of AII and reduced activity in a central oxytocinergic inhibitory system. In humans, however, a comparable salt appetite is not common in patients with Addison disease, whose adrenocortical dysfunction causes them to lose Na^+ in urine. Nor is salt appetite stimulated in people who lose excessive amounts of Na^+ in perspiration. No explanation is available for why an adaptive salt appetite appears readily in laboratory animals but not in humans.

Edward M. Stricker and Joseph G. Verbalis

pathetic nervous system (Fig. 39.7). The secretion of aldosterone is also stimulated by another peptide hormone, *adrenocorticotrophic hormone* (ACTH), which is secreted from the anterior lobe of the pituitary gland in response to *corticotrophic-releasing hormone* (CRH). The release of CRH from the PVN is triggered by activated cardiovascular baroreceptors. Yet another stimulus of aldosterone secretion is increased plasma levels of K^+, which can develop as a consequence of reduced GFR and an associated decrease in urinary K^+ excretion. The effects of these three independent stimuli of aldosterone secretion are additive. Note that aldosterone can eliminate Na^+ from urine, whereas AVP merely diminishes urinary water loss even during maximal antidiuresis. See Box 39.6 on salt appetite after adrenocortical dysfunction.

The onset of salt appetite induced in rats by colloid treatment is curiously delayed relative to the appearance of thirst. That is, water intake increases within 1–2 h after colloid treatment, whereas the intake of NaCl solution does not increase until at least 5 h later (Stricker, 1981). Investigations showed that the delay is caused both by the gradual appearance of an excitatory stimulus of salt appetite (i.e., AII) and by the gradual disappearance of an inhibitory stimulus for NaCl intake. With regard to the latter, recall that during the delay, hypovolemic rats drank water and thereby caused an osmotic dilution of body fluids, which inhibits secretion of pituitary AVP and oxytocin. Either of these neurohypophyseal hormones might have provided an inhibitory stimulus for salt appetite that disappeared as the animals drank water. In other studies, however, rats showed a strong inverse relationship between intake of NaCl and plasma levels of oxytocin (but not AVP), suggesting that circulating oxytocin was an inhibitory stimulus of salt appetite.

Central Oxytocin Inhibits Salt Appetite

However, in tests of the hypothesis that circulating oxytocin inhibits salt appetite, an intravenous infusion of physiological doses of oxytocin did not decrease NaCl intake in hypovolemic rats, nor did infusion of an oxytocin receptor blocker increase NaCl intake. These unexpected findings were clarified by the observation that, coincident with the secretion of oxytocin from magnocellular neurons, oxytocin was released from parvicellular neurons projecting centrally from the PVN. Thus, plasma oxytocin may have been a peripheral marker of the centrally acting oxytocin that mediated the inhibition of salt appetite in rats (Blackburn *et al.*, 1992). This revised hypothesis has been strongly supported by the results of a series of investigations. For example, in colloid-treated rats, infusion of oxytocin into the cerebrospinal fluid

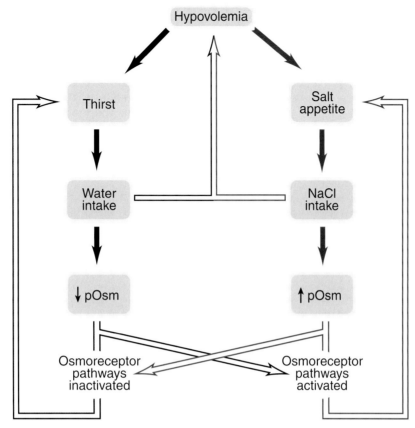

FIGURE 39.9 Schematic diagram of the mechanisms controlling thirst and salt appetite in hypovolemic rats. Solid arrows indicate stimulation, and unfilled arrows indicate inhibition. The combination of the effects of blood-borne AII on the brain and neural baroreceptor signals to the brain stem stimulates hypovolemic animals to drink water and a concentrated saline solution. The rats alternately drink the two fluids in amounts that ultimately add up to a volume of isotonic saline sufficient to repair the volume deficit. When the animals have access to only one fluid, water and salt intakes are limited by activation of the appropriate inhibitory osmoregulatory pathways. When rats drink isotonic saline (instead of water and concentrated saline), neither inhibitory pathway is activated, and consequently intake is continuous. Modified with permission from Stricker and Verbalis (1988).

inhibited NaCl intake but did not affect water intake. Similarly, salt appetite in hypovolemic rats was eliminated by a systemic injection of naloxone, an opioid receptor antagonist that disinhibits oxytocin secretion, and this effect was blocked by the prior injection of an oxytocin receptor antagonist directly into the cerebrospinal fluid. Conversely, NaCl ingestion in response to hypovolemia or AII was potentiated by diverse treatments that inhibit the secretion of oxytocin. In addition to osmotic dilution, these treatments included systemic injection of ethanol, maintenance on a sodium-deficient diet (instead of the standard laboratory diet rich in Na⁺), and peripheral administration of mineralocorticoid hormones such as aldosterone. Thus, excitatory and inhibitory components together regulate NaCl intake in a dual-control system in the brain.

Two aspects of the preceding findings deserve emphasis. First, hypovolemia stimulates two endocrine effects in the central control of NaCl intake:-acute stimulation of NaCl appetite by a peptide hormone (AII) and chronic disinhibition of NaCl intake by a steroid hormone (aldosterone). Second, hypovolemia and AII each provide conflicting stimuli for salt appetite, as each stimulates salt appetite directly but also stimulates central oxytocin secretion, which is an inhibitory signal. The coordination of thirst and salt appetite stimulated by colloid treatment in rats can be conceptualized as follows (Fig. 39.9): The combination of hypovolemia and AII stimulates thirst but provides a mixed stimulus of salt appetite. Thus, the animals at first drink water; however, by doing so, they dilute their body fluids. The osmotic dilution eventually becomes large enough to inhibit thirst. Dilution has the additional effect of reducing central oxytocin secretion, which in turn disinhibits salt appetite, and the rats begin to drink the concentrated NaCl solution. The NaCl raises plasma osmolality and thereby removes the dilution-induced inhibition of thirst and oxytocin secretion. Consequently, the rats stop drinking saline and resume drinking water. Osmotic dilution again develops, thirst is again inhibited, and salt appetite is again disinhibited. Thus, hypovolemic animals, stimulated by neural and endocrine signals of hypovolemia, alternate their intakes of the two fluids while maintaining body fluid near isotonic. Water and Na^+ are conserved in urine until the deficit in plasma volume is repaired. At that point the stimuli for adaptive physiological and behavioral responses disappear, and normal body fluid volume and tonicity are restored. Because the same neural and endocrine signals of hypovolemia stimulate thirst, salt appetite, and AVP and oxytocin secretion, these responses are integrated.

Central oxytocinergic neurons can inhibit salt intake and food intake (see Chapter 38). Thus, when osmotic dehydration activates oxytocinergic neurons, the intake of food and salt is inhibited and hyperosmolality is thereby prevented. From this perspective, food is a source of osmoles (not just of calories) and NaCl solution provides osmoles without calories. Inhibition of intake of osmoles complements the natriuretic effect of pituitary oxytocin in supporting osmoregulation.

Salt Appetite Is Also Inhibited by Atrial Natriuretic Peptide

The role of oxytocin in osmoregulation has become apparent only during the last decade, and the identification of other peptide hormones as important factors in the homeostasis of body fluids may be anticipated. One likely candidate is atrial natriuretic peptide. Like oxytocin, ANP promotes Na^+ loss in urine; in fact, ANP may mediate the natriuretric effects of OT. Also, like oxytocin, ANP is secreted by neurons within the brain, and when administered directly into the cerebrospinal fluid, it inhibits an experimentally induced salt appetite in rats. Moreover, destruction of ANP receptors in the brain eliminates the inhibition of salt appetite caused by a NaCl load (Blackburn *et al.*, 1995). Further work will be needed to understand the role of ANP-containing neurons in the central control of salt intake and the relationship of the neurons with other systems that participate in the regulation of water and NaCl intake.

Summary

Regulation of blood volume, like osmoregulation, is accomplished by a combination of physiological responses to hypovolemia, resulting in antidiuresis and antinatriuresis, and the complementary behavioral responses of increased water and NaCl intake. Cardiovascular baroreceptor cells detect hypovolemia and send neural signals to the brain stem, which communicates to the hypothalamus and forebrain structures mediating neurohypophyseal AVP and oxytocin secretion, as well as thirst and salt appetite. AII also appears to stimulate these responses while additionally supporting blood pressure as a potent vasoconstrictor. However, AII and hypovolemia both increase central oxytocin secretion, which mediates inhibition of NaCl intake, so for salt appetite to emerge this effect must be inhibited (as by osmotic dilution of body fluids, resulting from the renal retention of ingested water). The integration of these stimuli ensures that behavioral and physiological responses occur simultaneously, and their redundancy allows these vital regulatory processes to occur even when one stimulus is lost due to injury or disease. More generally, studies of water and NaCl ingestion provide insights into how the brain controls motivation and how peptide and steroid hormones interact with neural signals in the control of behavior.

References

Blackburn, R. E., Samson, W. K., Fulton, R. J., Stricker, E. M., and Verbalis, J. G. (1995). Central oxytocin and atrial natriuretic peptide receptors mediate osmotic inhibition of salt appetite in rats. *Am. J. Physiol.* **269**, R245–R251.

Blackburn, R. E., Verbalis, J. G., and Stricker, E. M. (1992). Central oxytocin mediates inhibition of sodium appetite by naloxone in hypovolemic rats. *Neuroendocrinology* **56**, 255–263.

Curtis, K. S., Verbalis, J. G., and Stricker, E. M. (1996). Area postrema lesions in rats appear to disrupt rapid feedback inhibition of fluid intake. *Brain Res.* **726**, 31–38.

Ferguson, A. V., and Renaud, L. P. (1986). Systemic angiotensin acts at subfornical organ to facilitate activity of neurohypophysial neurons. *Am. J. Physiol.* **251**, R712–R717.

Fitzsimons, J. T. (1961). Drinking by rats depleted of body fluid without increase in osmotic pressure. *J. Physiol. (Lond.)* **159**, 297–309.

Fitzsimons, J. T. (1969). The role of a renal thirst factor in drinking induced by extracellular stimuli. *J. Physiol. (Lond.)* **155**, 563–579.

Gilman, A. (1937). The relation between blood osmotic pressure, fluid distribution and voluntary water intake. *Am. J. Physiol.* **120**, 323–328.

Hoffman, G. E., Smith, M. S., and Verbalis, J. G. (1993). c-Fos and related immediate early gene products as markers of activity in neuroendocrine systems. *Front. Neuroendocrinol.* **14**, 173–213.

Huang, W., Sved, A. F., and Stricker, E. M. (2000). Water ingestion provides an early signal inhibiting osmotically stimulated vasopressin secretion in rats. *Am. J. Physiol.* **279**, R756–R760.

Johnson, A. K., and Buggy, J. (1978). Periventricular preoptic-hypothalamus is vital for thirst and normal water economy. *Am. J. Physiol.* **234**, R122–R125.

Kanter, G. S. (1953). Excretion and drinking after salt loading in dogs. *Am. J. Physiol.* **174**, 87–94.

Knepper, M. A. (1997). Molecular physiology of urinary concentrating mechanism: Regulation of aquaporin water channels by vasopressin. *Am. J. Physiol.* **272**, F3–F12.

Richter, C. P. (1936). Increased salt appetite in adrenalectomized rats. *Am. J. Physiol.* **115**, 155–161.

Richter, D., and Schmale, H. (1983). The structure of the precursor to arginine-vasopressin, A model preprohormone. *Prog. Brain Res.* **60**, 227–233.

Robertson, G. L. (1986). Posterior pituitary. *In* "Endocrinology and Metabolism" (P. Felig, J. Baxter, and L. A. Frohman, eds.), pp. 338–385. McGraw-Hill, New York.

Robinson, A. G. (1985). Disorders of antidiuretic hormone secretion. *Clin. Endocrinol. Metab.* 14, 55–88.

Robinson, M. M., and Evered, M. D. (1987). Pressor action of intravenous angiotensin II reduces drinking response in rats. *Am. J. Physiol.* **252**, R754–R759.

Simpson, J. B., Epstein, A. N., and Camardo, J. S., Jr. (1978). Localization of receptors for the dipsogenic action of angiotensin II in the subfornical organ of rat. *J. Comp. Physiol. Psychol.* **92**, 581–601.

Starling, E. H. (1896). On the absorption of fluids from the connective tissue spaces. *J. Physiol. (Lond.)* **19**, 312–326.

Stricker, E. M. (1969). Osmoregulation and volume regulation in rats, Inhibition of hypovolemic thirst by water. *Am. J. Physiol.* **217**, 98–105.

Stricker, E. M. (1976). Drinking by rats after lateral hypothalamic lesions: A new look at the lateral hypothalamic syndrome. *J. Comp. Physiol. Psychol.* **90**, 127–143.

Stricker, E. M. (1981). Thirst and sodium appetite after colloid treatment in rats. *J. Comp. Physiol. Psychol.* **95**, 1–25.

Stricker, E. M., and Verbalis, J. G. (1986). Interaction of osmotic and volume stimuli in regulation of neurohypophyseal secretion in rats. *Am. J. Physiol.* **250**, R267–R275.

Stricker, E. M., and Verbalis, J. G. (1988). Hormones and behavior, The biology of thirst and sodium appetite. *Am. Sci.* **76**, 261–267.

Stricker, E. M., and Verbalis, J. G. (1992). Ingestive behaviors. *In* "Behavioral Endocrinology" (J. B. Becker, S. M. Breedlove, and D. Crews, eds.), pp. 451–472. MIT Press, Cambridge, MA.

Thrasher, T. N., Keil, L. C., and Ramsay, D. J. (1982). Lesions of the laminar terminalis (OVLT) attenuate osmotically-induced drinking and vasopressin secretion in the dog. *Endocrinology (Baltimore)* **110**, 1837–1839.

Thrasher, T. N., Nistal-Herrera, J. F., Keil, L. C., and Ramsay, D. J. (1981). Satiety and inhibition of vasopressin secretion in dogs. *Am. J. Physiol.* **240**, E394–E401.

Verbalis, J. G., Mangione, M. P., and Stricker, E. M. (1991). Oxytocin produces natriuresis in rats at physiological plasma concentrations. *Endocrinology (Baltimore)* **128**, 1317–1322.

Verney, E. B. (1947). The antidiuretic hormone and the factors which determine its release. *Proc. Soc. (Lond.)* **B135**, 25–105.

Wilkins, L., and Richter, C. P. (1940). A great craving for salt by a child with cortico-adrenal insufficiency. *J. Am. Med. Assoc.* **114**, 866–868.

Suggested Readings

Denton, D. (1982). "The Hunger for Salt: An Anthropological, Physiological and Medical Analysis." Springer-Verlag, Berlin.

Fitzsimons, J. T. (1979). "The Physiology of Thirst and Sodium Appetite." Cambridge Univ. Press, Cambridge.

Gauer, O. H., and Henry, J. P. (1963). Circulatory basis of fluid volume control. *Physiol. Rev.* **43**, 423–81.

Gullans, S. R., and Verbalis, J. G. (1993). Control of brain volume during hyperosmolar and hypoosmolar conditions. *Annu. Rev. Med.* **44**, 289–301.

Guyton, A. C., Hall, J. E., Lohmeier, T. E., Jackson, T. E., and Manning, R. D., Jr. (1981). The many roles of the kidney in arterial pressure control and hypertension. *Can. J. Physiol. Pharmacol.* **59**, 513–9.

Ramsay, D. J., and Thrasher, T. N. (1990). Thirst and water balance. *In* "Handbook of Behavioral Neurobiology" (E. M. Stricker, ed.), Vol. 10, pp. 353–86. Plenum, New York.

Stricker, E. M., and Sved, A. F. (2000). Thirst. *Nutrition* **16**, 821–26.

Stricker, E. M., and Verbalis, J. G. (1990). Sodium appetite. *In* "Handbook of Behavioral Neurobiology" (E. M. Stricker, ed.), Vol. 10. pp. 387–419. Plenum, New York.

Verbalis, J. G. (1990). Clinical aspects of body fluid homeostasis in humans. *In* "Handbook of Behavioral Neurobiology" (E. M. Stricker, ed.), Vol. 10, pp. 421–62. Plenum, New York.

Wolf, A. V. (1958). "Thirst: Physiology of the Urge to Drink and Problems of Water Lack." Thomas, Springfield, IL.

Edward M. Stricker and Joseph G. Verbalis

40

Neuroendocrine Systems

THE HYPOTHALAMUS IS A NEUROENDOCRINE ORGAN

The hypothalamus, located at the most rostral region of the brain stem in the diencephalon, is a key center regulating numerous and diverse physiological functions, including growth, metabolism, stress responses, reproduction, osmoregulation, and circadian rhythms (also see Chapter 34). All of these functions are critically involved in maintaining the homeostasis of the animal and in coordinating the timing of physiological functions with the appropriate environmental conditions. In order to accomplish this, the hypothalamus acts as an integrator, receiving converging inputs from virtually every sensory and autonomic system related to the internal and external environment of the organism. The hypothalamus responds rapidly to this convergent information by changing its output, namely the release of its neurotransmitters and neuropeptides to its targets within the central nervous system (CNS) and to the pituitary gland.

The hypothalamus contains several groups of cells that are defined as neuroendocrine, meaning that they have both neuronal and endocrine features. Neuroendocrine cells are located in the central nervous system, have a neuronal phenotype, and release a peptide or neurotransmitter in response to a depolarizing stimulus, similar to other non-neuroendocrine neurons in the brain. However, neuroendocrine cells differ from other "traditional" neurons in their targets. Instead of releasing their neuropeptide or neurotransmitter at another neuron, e.g., via synaptic connections, these hypothalamic neuroendocrine cells release their neurotransmitter into a portal capillary plexus located in the infundibular stalk of the anterior

pituitary gland. The release of a neuroactive substance or hormone directly into the circulatory system defines the cell producing this substance as endocrine, and therefore the hypothalamic cells releasing their neurotransmitters in this way are truly endocrine cells as well as neurons. Moreover, while the substances released by most neuroendocrine cells are peptides and neurotransmitters, they can also be called hormones in that they are released into blood vessels to act remotely at a target organ. Thus, the molecules released by these hypothalamic neuroendocrine cells are often referred to as neurohormones.

The concept of a link between the hypothalamus and the anterior pituitary gland was first suggested and later demonstrated by Geoffrey Harris, who proved the existence of a tiny series of blood vessels leading from the median eminence at the base of the hypothalamus to the anterior pituitary gland (Harris, 1971). Harris proposed that the hypothalamus controls the release of anterior pituitary hormones via this vascular connection. Subsequent studies have shown that the hypothalamic–pituitary connection is critical for maintaining numerous physiological functions involved in metabolism, growth, reproduction, stress responses, and osmoregulation. The isolation and purification of the hypothalamic hormones in the late 1960s by the laboratories of Roger Guillemin, Andrew Schally, and others led to an enormous increase in knowledge of these molecules; Guillemin and Schally were awarded the Nobel prize in Physiology and Medicine in 1977 for these fundamental discoveries in neuroendocrinology.

The hypothalamic neuroendocrine cells have certain features in common (Fig. 40.1). These cells have

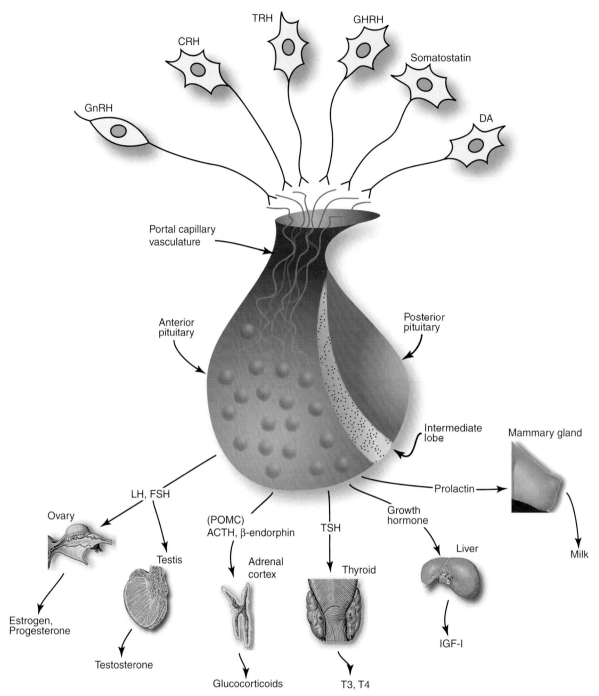

FIGURE 40.1 General features of brain–pituitary–target organ systems. Each neuroendocrine system has a hypothalamic neurosecretory cell, a corresponding pituitary hormone, and a target organ. GnRH, gonadotropin-releasing hormone; CRH, corticotropin-releasing hormone; TRH, thyrotropin-releasing hormone; GHRH, growth hormone-releasing hormone; DA, dopamine; LH, luteinizing hormone; FSH, follicle-stimulating hormone; POMC, proopiomelanocortin; ACTH, adrenocorticotrophic hormone; TSH, thyroid-stimulating hormone; T$_3$, triiodothyronine; T$_4$, thyroxine; IGF-I, insulin-like growth factor I.

perikarya in the hypothalamus and preoptic area, where the hormones are synthesized in precursor form. Each hormone is processed to a final peptide hormone, which is transported to neuroterminals located in the external zone of the median eminence. There, the hormone is released in a pulsatile manner into the portal capillary system. The hormones bind to receptors located on specific cells in the anterior pituitary gland, stimulating or inhibiting the synthesis and secretion of a corresponding pituitary hormone.

HYPOTHALAMIC RELEASING/INHIBITING HORMONES AND THEIR TARGETS

Overview of General Hypothalamic–Pituitary– Target Organ Axis Systems

Each neuroendocrine system has three levels: (1) the hypothalamic hormone that either stimulates ("releasing" hormone) or inhibits ("inhibiting" hormone) its corresponding anterior pituitary hormone; (2) the anterior pituitary hormone that is released into the general circulatory system; and (3) the target organ in the body that is regulated by the appropriate anterior pituitary hormone (Fig. 40.1). At the hypothalamic level, neuronal perikarya are localized in various hypothalamic or preoptic nuclei, depending on the neuroendocrine system. These neuroendocrine cells project neuroterminals to the median eminence, located at the floor of the hypothalamus just above the anterior pituitary gland (Fig. 40.2). The external zone of the median eminence contains the portal blood vessels that lead to the anterior pituitary gland, into which the hypothalamic hormone is released.

The anterior pituitary contains a heterogeneous group of cells that respond to a specific releasing or inhibiting hormone. The anterior pituitary cells are specialized, and each has the specific receptors that bind a specific hypothalamic hormone. The binding of the hypothalamic hormone to its receptor triggers a

cascade of biosynthetic and secretory events, triggering (or inhibiting) the synthesis and release of the pituitary hormone into the general circulatory system. The anterior pituitary gland, like the hypothalamus, is an endocrine gland, as it releases its hormones into the circulatory system, where they act remotely at receptors on organs in the body. These hormones can also feedback onto receptors in the brain and/or pituitary gland to regulate the neuroendocrine axes in a predominantly negative feedback manner, as is discussed later.

Target organs of the neuroendocrine axes have specific receptors that bind the corresponding pituitary hormone. These target organs respond to the binding of these hormones to their receptors by increasing (or decreasing) synthesis and secretion of another hormone, such as a sex steroid hormone (from the gonads), thyroxine and triiodothyronine (from the thyroid), insulin-like growth factor-I (from the liver), and glucocorticoids (from the adrenal cortex). It is the actions of these hormones at somatic targets that cause the ultimate physiological effect on the body such as growth, metabolism, lactation, mediation of stress, and reproductive function. In addition, each of these hormones feeds back at the level of the brain, hypothalamus, and/or pituitary gland or to regulate its neuroendocrine axis. In this way, the delicate hormonal balance is maintained for each system.

The hypothalamic–pituitary target organ axes are not an independent series of parallel regulatory systems. These axes have considerable crosstalk with one another and can interact at multiple levels. For example, reproductive and stress axes regulate each other at specific hypothalamic neurons, both through direct actions at the CNS, as well as through feedback from the target steroid hormones. During stressful

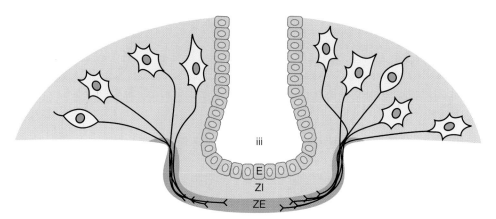

FIGURE 40.2 Depiction of a coronal section through the median eminence cell showing its three major zones and the typical projections of neuroendocrine cells to the external zone containing the portal capillaries leading to the anterior pituitary gland. iii, third ventricle; E, ependymal zone; ZI, internal zone; ZE, external zone.

situations, elevated adrenal glucocorticoids will feed-back to the brain and have actions not only at the CRH neurons, but at the GnRH neurons as well, thereby suppressing reproduction at a time when it is not optimal. Therefore these hypothalamic neurons serve as integrators of multiple, complex pieces of information about the homeostasis and environment of the organism.

The Hypothalamus Is Regulated by Inputs from the Central Nervous System and Feedback of Hormones from the Body

Previously, neuroendocrine axes have been referred to as hypothalamic–pituitary–target axes (the targets being the gonad, adrenal gland, thyroid gland, liver, mammary gland, and other somatic organs). However, while this description is accurate in that hypothalamic hormones are the primary regulators of each of these axes, the central nervous system plays a more complex role in the regulation of neuroendocrine function than simply the release of a hypothalamic hormone. For example, each hypothalamic-releasing or -inhibiting hormone neuron receives afferent inputs from other elements of the brain, such as neurons or glia, that regulate their function. Additionally, feedback of hormones released by target organs may not occur directly or exclusively at the respective hypothalamic cells, and therefore feedback regulation of hypothalamic hormones may be mediated by other cells in the brain.

A good example is provided by the hypothalamic–pituitary–gonadal system. Hypothalamic gonadotropin-releasing hormone (GnRH) neurons are the primary activators of this axis. These cells stimulate the release of the gonadotropins, LH and FSH from the anterior pituitary, and these molecules in turn target the gonads to stimulate the synthesis and release of sex steroid hormones, particularly estrogen, progesterone, and testosterone. However, GnRH neurons are not believed to possess sex steroid hormone receptors, and therefore the feedback regulation of GnRH cells by these steroid hormones is probably mediated indirectly by other central nervous system afferents to GnRH neurons. Some of these afferents may be localized in the hypothalamus, whereas others may lie in extrahypothalamic regions, as sex steroid hormone receptors are expressed throughout the brain. Thus, many researchers have begun to refer to the hypothalamic–pituitary–gonadal axis as the *brain–pituitary–gonadal axis*. This concept can be extended to the other neuroendocrine axes as well, as each is regulated by extrahypothalamic inputs, and steroid hormone feedback may occur directly on the hypo-

thalamic cells, but may also be mediated by indirect inputs to these cells. Thus, the neuroendocrine axes will subsequently be referred to as brain–pituitary–target organ axes.

Characteristics of Neurohormone Release: Ultradian, Circadian/Diurnal, and Seasonal Rhythms

The release of hypothalamic hormones occurs in a pulsatile manner. Thus, brief pulses of these hormones generally occur at intervals of 1–2 h and this rhythmic pattern is referred to as ultradian (i.e., shorter than daily rhythms) or circhoral (approximately hourly intervals of release). The corresponding anterior pituitary cells respond to each pulse of a hypothalamic hormone with a corresponding pulse of its pituitary hormone shortly thereafter (Fig. 40.3). It has been speculated that the pulsatile release of hypothalamic hormones is necessary to prevent the desensitization of their receptors in the anterior pituitary gland. Indeed, infusion of exogenous hypothalamic hormone analogs in a continuous manner results in an initial activation of pituitary hormone release, but subsequent refractoriness of the pituitary cell and overall decreases in release. In contrast, infusion of exogenous hypothalamic hormones in a pulsatile manner maintains the pituitary sensitivity to its corresponding hypothalamic hormone.

Along with these ultradian pulses of hypothalamic pulses are the circadian or diurnal rhythms of hor-

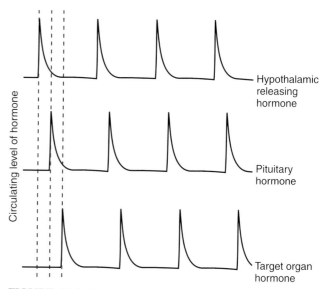

FIGURE 40.3 Representation of pulsatile hormone release in a neuroendocrine system. A representative hypothalamic-releasing hormone is released in discrete pulses at 1 to 2-h intervals. This causes pulses of the corresponding anterior pituitary hormone to occur shortly thereafter. The release of the pituitary hormone stimulates the target organ to release its hormones.

monal release that are characteristic of the neuroendocrine system (see Chapter 41). These 24-h rhythms of hormone release, which can occur independently of the light/dark cycle (circadian) or are entrained to the light/dark cycle (diurnal), have been reported for all of the neuroendocrine systems (Gore,

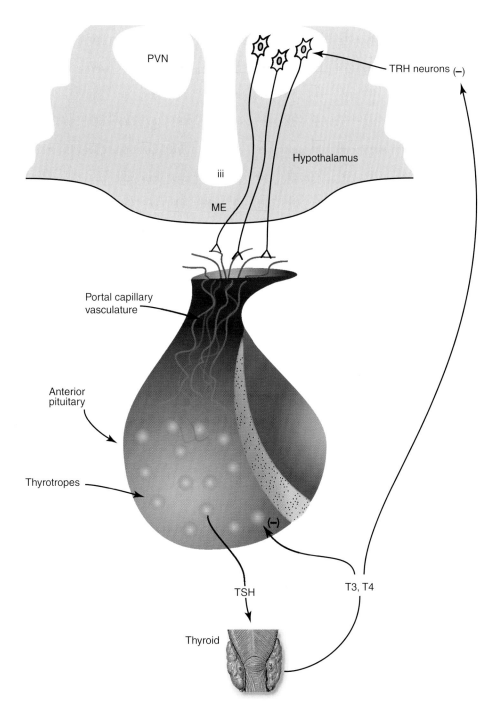

FIGURE 40.4 Schematic representation of the brain–pituitary–thyroid axis showing TRH neurons in the paraventricular nucleus projecting their neuroterminals to the external zone of the median eminence. This occurs bilaterally, although only a unilateral projection is shown. TRH travels through the portal vasculature to cause the synthesis and release of TSH from thyrotropes. This molecule acts at the thyroid gland to cause the biosynthesis and release of the thyroid hormones, T_3 and T_4. These are released into the general circulation to affect metabolism and feedback in a negative manner at the thyrotropes of the pituitary and the TRH neurons of the PVN. PVN, paraventricular nucleus; TRH, thyrotropin-releasing hormone; ME, median eminence; iii, third ventricle; TSH, thyroid-stimulating hormone; T_3, triiodothyronine; T_4, thyroxine.

1998). Circadian rhythms are driven by a part of the hypothalamus called the suprachiasmatic nucleus (SCN), and the SCN makes projections within the hypothalamus to regulate neuroendocrine release in a 24-h cycle.

Even longer cycles of hormonal release can be observed, which is most apparent for the reproductive axis. This is discussed in more detail later, but in brief, many species are seasonal breeders and are only sexually active during certain periods of the year. This enables the species to coordinate the energetically demanding process of pregnancy, lactation, and rearing of the offspring with the appropriate environmental conditions. Thus, lambs are born in the spring when food supplies are abundant, and sheep are only reproductively functional during the fall and winter so that the lambs are born during the spring. During the rest of the year, the reproductive axis is quiescent, and therefore this system is regulated and coordinated by extremely long, yearly cycles, along with the shorter circadian/diurnal and ultradian patterns of hormone release.

CHARACTERISTICS OF EACH NEUROENDOCRINE SYSTEM

Five neuroendocrine axes are involved in the control of metabolism, growth, reproduction, lactation, and stress. Each system has its own specialized neuroendocrine cells in the hypothalamus that coordinate the appropriate responses to environmental or internal homeostatic stimuli. The target cells of hypothalamic hormones in the pituitary gland, and the target organs that respond to the pituitary hormones, each have the appropriate receptors to respond to its specific hormonal activator. These systems are summarized in Fig. 40.1 and are discussed in detail later.

Metabolism: The Brain–Pituitary–Thyroid Axis

Overview and Characteristics

The proper regulation of metabolism is critical for the development and survival of the organism. The brain–pituitary–thyroid axis plays a critical role in the control of metabolic activity, stimulating an increase in metabolism in target cells. The hypothalamic hormone involved in this function is thyrotropin-releasing hormone (TRH), produced by a group of cells in a specific nucleus in the hypothalamus, the paraventricular nucleus (Fig. 40.4). As is the case for all releasing hormones, TRH is released from neuroterminals in the

external zone of the median eminence into the portal capillary system. At the anterior pituitary gland, TRH targets receptors on thyrotropes, which are stimulated to produce the thyroid-stimulating hormone (TSH). Thyrotropes constitute approximately 10% of the cells in the anterior pituitary gland. TSH is released from the anterior pituitary gland into the general circulation and acts at receptors in the thyroid gland, causing these cells to produce the thyroid hormones, thyroxine (T_4) and triiodothyronine (T_3), the latter being the more potent thyroid hormone, which are also released into the general circulation (Fig. 40.4). Thyroid hormones act at target organs throughout the body to regulate cellular metabolism and also feedback at the brain and anterior pituitary gland to regulate levels of TRH and TSH, respectively. The thyroid hormone axis is a classical negative feedback loop, as thyroid hormone feedback inhibits the secretion of these hypothalamic and pituitary hormones, thereby maintaining constant levels of free thyroid hormone in the bloodstream. The negative feedback regulation of TRH and TSH by the thyroid hormone maintains levels of free thyroid hormone in a constant level. Such precise regulation of thyroid hormone levels is critically important because elevated or depressed levels of this hormone can have substantial adverse consequences on the body, particularly during sensitive periods of development.

When the thyroid hormone is released into the circulation, it binds to binding globulins, and the free thyroid hormone constitutes only <1% of all thyroid hormone circulating in the bloodstream. The free (not protein-bound) thyroid hormone is responsible for the negative feedback regulation of TRH neurons and thyrotropes, as well as for actions at target tissues.

Physiological Functions

Thyroid hormone is critical for cellular metabolism The brain–pituitary–thyroid axis is involved in metabolism, protein synthesis, and development of the brain. Thyroid hormone receptors are located throughout the brain, highlighting their importance in central nervous system development and function. They are also found in peripheral and autonomic nervous systems, pituitary gland, bone, muscle, liver, heart, testis, lung, placenta, and other tissues. The major function of the thyroid hormone is the regulation of basal metabolic rate and calorigenic responses. In the cells, the thyroid hormone regulates ATP levels produced by mitochondria and alters protein synthesis. The maintenance of thyroid hormone levels is extremely important for adult metabolic activity, and thyroid hormone abnormalities in the developing organism can have catastrophic consequences. Thyroid hormone deprivation in the fetus causes permanent nervous system abnormalities and substantial effects on growth and bone development that may be reversed or mitigated if the thyroid hormone is replaced.

Pulsatile and circadian release of TRH and TSH TSH, and presumably TRH, is released in a pulsatile manner, with pulses occurring at approximately 90- to 180-min intervals in humans (Gore, 1998). Studies on the pulsatile release of TSH in humans demonstrate that it changes across the 24-h period, peaking from the evening through 0400 h, decreasing through noon, and remaining low until the beginning of the next cycle in the evening. The increase in TSH release during the evening is referred to as the nocturnal TSH surge. This appears to be a true circadian rhythm, driven by the suprachiasmatic nucleus of the hypothalamus.

Structures and Properties of TRH, TSH, Thyroid Hormone, and Their Receptors

TRH and the TRH receptor TRH is a tripeptide with the sequence pGlu-His-Pro-NH2 (Fig. 40.5). This tiny peptide stimulates the pulsatile release of TSH from pituitary thyrotropes rapidly and potently. As is true for other neurohormones, TRH is cleaved from a prohormone, the sequence of which was determined from the cloned TRH gene (Yamada *et al.*, 1990). The sequence for the TRH tripeptide is expressed in multiple copies in this prohormone, cleaved and processed from the prohormone as with other neuropeptides (see Chapter 8).

The TRH receptor, localized in the anterior pituitary on thyrotropes, is a G-protein-coupled membrane receptor (Gershengorn, 1993). Binding of TRH to its receptor causes the activation of membrane-bound phospholipase C and the hydrolysis of phosphatidylinositol 4,5-biphosphate (PIP_2) to inositol 1,4,5-triphosphate (IP_3) and diacylglycerol (DAG). This results in calcium mobilization and the phosphorylation or changes in the concentrations of nuclear proteins that interact with the genes involved in the synthesis of TSH and causes an increase in TSH gene transcription.

TSH and the TSH receptor TSH is a ~30-kDa glycoprotein hormone, comprising an α and β subunit, that are synthesized from two different genes. The α subunit of TSH is identical to that of the gonadotropins, LH and FSH. The β subunit confers the unique identity to TSH, LH, and FSH. The α subunit is ~92 amino acids in humans and is approximately 14 kDa. The TSH β subunit gene is ~2 kb and encodes a 105 amino acid glycoprotein in humans (Szkudlinski *et al.*, 2000).

A PyroGlu - His - ProNH2 (TRH)

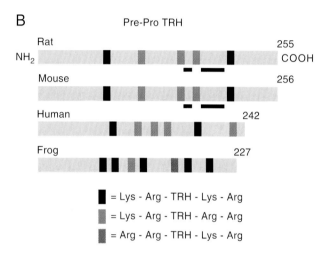

B Pre-Pro TRH

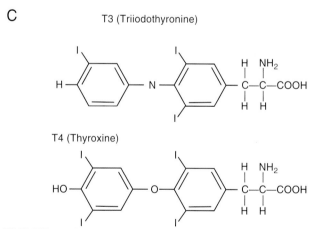

C T3 (Triiodothyronine)

FIGURE 40.5 (A) Structure of thyrotropin-releasing hormone (TRH.) (B) Structures of PreProTRH from several mammalian species. Note the multiple copies of TRH present in each precursor flanked by pairs of basic amino acids. (C) Structures of the thyroid hormones—triiodothyronine and thyroxine.

The TSH receptor is a seven transmembrane domain G-protein coupled receptor located predominately in the thyroid gland (Graves and Davies, 2000).

Binding of TSH to its receptor activates cAMP generation and stimulates the production and release of the thyroid hormone in the thyroid gland.

Thyroid hormone The two major thyroid hormones are T_4 and T_3, of which T_3 has greater biological activity (Fig. 40.5). Although thyroid hormones are structurally quite different from other steroid hormones, such as sex steroids, they are considered members of the steroid hormone family due to the presence of the two phenolic rings, which confer steroidogenic function, and their target organ receptors are members of the steroid hormone receptor superfamily. The thyroid hormones contain three (T_3) or four (T_4) iodide molecules, and in an iodine-deficient diet, thyroid hormone metabolism is impaired, leading to developmental abnormalities mentioned earlier. With respect to function of the thyroid hormone axis, T_3 binds to the thyroid hormone receptors in target tissues and also mediates negative feedback effects on TRH cells in the hypothalamus and pituitary. Although more T_4 than T_3 is released from the thyroid gland, it is likely that most T_4 is converted to T_3, as catalyzed by two enzymes, type I and type II deiodinases. Type I deiodinase is found mostly in peripheral tissues and the pituitary gland, and type II deiodinase is found in the brain, pituitary gland, and brown fat.

With respect to the negative feedback regulation by thyroid hormone, thyroid hormone receptors have been localized within TRH neurons in the paraventricular nucleus (Segerson *et al.*, 1987). Thus, these actions can be mediated directly on TRH neurons in the brain. In addition, the expression of the thyroid hormone receptor is abundant in the anterior pituitary gland, particularly thyrotrope cells, indicating direct feedback action of the thyroid hormone on this organ as well.

Along with its regulation by TSH, the thyroid gland also receives direct neuronal inputs from the autonomic nervous system. Fibers from the sympathetic and parasympathetic nervous systems penetrate the thyroid gland and terminate around arterioles, capillaries, and, less frequently, venules and near follicular cells.

The thyroid hormone receptor family The thyroid hormone receptor is a member of the steroid hormone superfamily. These are nuclear transcription factors that bind to a regulatory element on the DNA to activate or inhibit gene transcription. Several thyroid hormone receptor isoforms have been identified. These are termed thyroid hormone receptors (TR) α and β, which are derived from different genes and can be alternatively spliced. Thus, each TR subtype has a

splice variant, termed $\alpha 1$, $\alpha 2$, $\beta 1$, and $\beta 2$. $\alpha 1$ and $\beta 2$ are most abundant in the hypothalamus and are found in more than 80% of TRH neurons in the PVN (Lechan *et al.*, 1994). As is the case for most steroid hormone receptors, binding of the thyroid hormone to its receptor causes the dimerization of the receptors and facilitates the binding of the receptor–ligand complex to the promoter of the target gene, thereby modulating gene transcription.

Neuroanatomy of the TRH System

TRH neurons are concentrated in the paraventricular nucleus (PVN) of the hypothalamus (Fig. 40.4). This hypothalamic nucleus is localized at the dorsal region of the third ventricle and can be divided into a magnocellular division (large neurons) and a parvicellular division (small- to medium-sized neurons). TRH neurons exist exclusively in the parvicellular region of the PVN and are particularly concentrated along the medial and periventricular parts of the parvicellular PVN. Other non-TRH neurons are also localized in this region, including corticotropin-releasing hormone, neurotensin, galanin, enkephalin, and vasoactive intestinal peptide. It has been reported that there are also nonneuroendocrine TRH cells localized outside the PVN that do not project to the median eminence, but rather play other nonneuroendocrine roles in nervous system function.

Disruptions in the Thyrotropic Axis

Thyroid hormone excess or insufficiency can have profound effects on the central nervous system, particularly during development. Excessive thyroid hormone can result in symptoms such as tremor, nervousness, tremulousness, insomnia and sleep disorders, and impairments in memory and concentration. More profound effects include neuropsychiatric syndromes, seizure, chorea, and even coma. Deficiencies of the thyroid hormone can cause problems such as sleep apnea, hypothermia, hypoventilation, neuropsychiatric syndromes, peripheral neuropathy, cerebellar ataxia, and coma. During chronic thyroid hormone deficiency, fluids can accumulate and result in puffiness of the hands, feet, face, and tongue and cause speech impairment. This is called myxedema and is generally associated with the loss of thyroid hormone negative feedback effects.

When an organism is exposed to insufficient thyroid hormone during fetal or early neonatal development, it can develop cretinism, characterized by severe deficits in mental, neurological, and physical development (Box 40.1). The deficiencies in growth and the skeletal system can be reversed by thyroid hormone replacement, but the central nervous system

BOX 40.1

CRETINISM

Cretinism, characterized by deficits in mental, neurological, and physical development, can occur if the thyroid hormone is not available during fetal and early neonatal development. In this syndrome, severe hypothyroidism gives rise to numerous structural and functional abnormalities in the brain, including poor neurite outgrowth, less synapse formation, decreased myelination, reduced microtubule formation, and delayed axonal transport, particularly in the cerebral cortex and cerebellum. If the thyroid hormone is not replaced within the critical 1–3 months (in humans) following birth, most of these abnormalities become permanent. Even transient hypothyroidism in preterm infants is associated with an increased risk of cerebral palsy and impaired mental development. In the mature brain, thyroid hormone insufficiency and excess can also have functional, neurological, and psychological manifestations, summarized in the accompanying table.

Potential Clinical Manifestations of Thyroid Hormone Excess or Insufficiency on the Central and Peripheral Nervous Systems

Excess thyroid hormone	Insufficient thyroid hormone
Tremor	Cretinism
Nervousness	Mental deficiency, defects in hearing and speech, spastic or ataxic gait,
Tremulousness	impaired voluntary motor activity, clonus
Hyperkinesis, agitation, irritability	Sleep apnea
Insomnia	Dysarthria
Vivid dreams and nightmares	Hypothermia
Decreased memory	Hypoventilation
Impaired concentration	Cerebellar ataxia
Seizures	Coma
Chorea	Neuropsychiatric syndromes
Coma	Myxedema madness (psychosis), dementia
Neuropsychiatric syndromes	Peripheral neuropathy
Depression, anxiety, mania, dysphoria, emotional	Carpal tunnel syndrome, facial weakness
lability, attention deficit, delirium, paranoia	

Roberto Toni and Ronald M. Lechan

effects can never be corrected, and brain damage is permanent. Another thyroid hormone disease is Graves' disease, which is characterized by a diffuse goiter and exopthalmia (bulging eyes) associated with hyperthyroidism.

Growth: The Somatotropic Axis

Overview and Characteristics

Somatic growth is an obvious characteristic of the development of vertebrate organisms. This process is under the control of the somatotropic axis, comprising hypothalamic cells in the brain, corresponding pituitary cells that produce growth hormone, and target cells in the body, particularly the liver. The major somatic targets of growth hormone are the bones and muscles. In addition, the tertiary hormone produced by this axis, insulin-like growth factor I (IGF-I), which is synthesized in the liver, acts both independently and synergistically with the growth hormone to affect somatic growth.

Unlike most other neuroendocrine systems, the somatotropic axis has two hypothalamic hormones playing important but opposite roles (Fig. 40.6). One hormone, growth hormone-releasing hormone (GHRH), is stimulatory to the release of the pituitary growth hormone. The other hypothalamic hormone, somatostatin (also called somatotrope release-inhibiting hormone, SRIH), inhibits growth hormone release. These hormones are released into the portal capillary vasculature to affect the synthesis and release of growth hormone, also called somatotropin, from specialized cells in the anterior pituitary gland called somatotropes, constituting ~30% of pituitary cells.

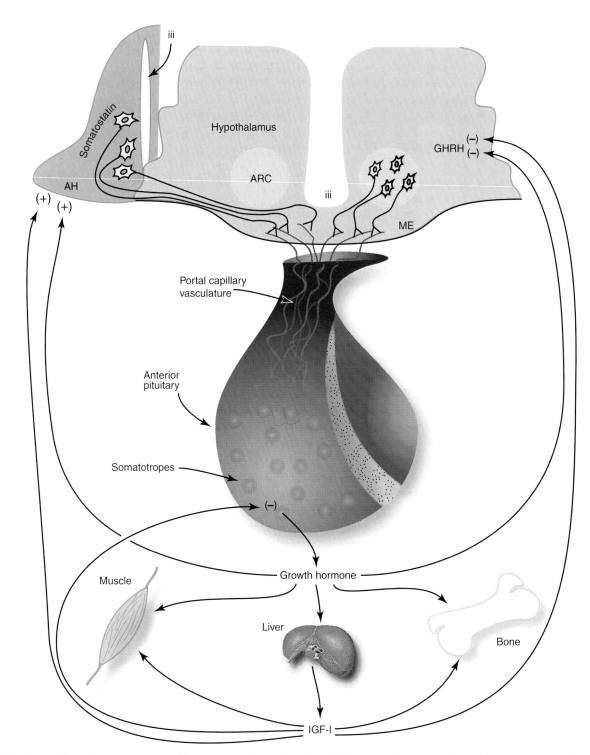

FIGURE 40.6 Schematic representation of the somatotropic axis showing GHRH neurons in the arcuate nucleus and somatostatin neurons in the periventricular region of the anterior hypothalamus projecting their neuroterminals to the external zone of the median eminence. This occurs bilaterally for both hypothalamic hormones, although only a unilateral projection is shown. GHRH and somatostatin travel through the portal vasculature to stimulate or inhibit, respectively, the synthesis and release of growth hormone from somatotropes. This molecule acts at the liver to cause the biosynthesis and release of IGF-I. Both growth hormone and IGF-I are released into the general circulation to affect somatic growth and feedback in a negative manner at the somatotropes of the pituitary and the GHRH neurons of the arcuate nucleus. IGF-I and growth hormone also feedback to stimulate somatostatin, which also causes negative feedback on the somatotropic axis. ARC, arcuate nucleus; AH, anterior hypothalamus; GHRH, growth hormone-releasing hormone; ME, median eminence; iii, third ventricle; IGF-I, insulin-like growth factor I.

The release of growth hormone into the general circulation affects a number of target organs and tissues undergoing growth, regeneration, or metabolic homeostasis, such as bone and muscle. In addition, the growth hormone binds to its receptors in the liver to stimulate the release of another hormone, IGF-I. IGF-I can travel through the general circulation and have somatotropic actions itself.

Both growth hormone and IGF-I appear to be involved in the feedback regulation of the somatotropic axis. In the case of GHRH, the growth hormone acts as a classical negative feedback molecule, downregulating the synthesis and secretion of GHRH (Fig. 40.6). For somatostatin, the growth hormone increases its gene expression, and in the absence of growth hormone, somatostatin mRNA levels are downregulated. IGF-I also acts as a feedback regulator of the somatotropic axis, negatively regulating GHRH levels and stimulating somatostatin gene expression. As shown in Fig. 40.6, this is a highly complicated and tightly regulated feedback loop.

Physiological Functions

The somatotropic axis controls somatic growth and development The growth hormone plays its major role in neonatal and postnatal growth and is particularly important in the pubertal growth spurt. Its anabolic activities are critical for metabolic homeostasis. The growth hormone stimulates protein synthesis, increases lipolysis, influences carbohydrate metabolism, enhances glucose uptake and utilization, and has lipolytic effects. At the systems level, it stimulates the growth of organs, such as the heart and kidney, and plays a role in hormone production, skeletal growth and maturation, and immune function. Many of its effects are sexually dimorphic, as are the distribution of its receptors and other proteins involved in this axis.

Pulsatile and diurnal release of GHRH and somatostatin Both GHRH and somatostatin are released into the portal circulation in a pulsatile manner, similar to other neurohormones. While it might be predicted that these neurohormones might be released out of phase, in fact, their release is often coordinated. Pulses of GHRH appear to drive pulses of growth hormone, which occur at intervals of ~1–3 h.

The growth hormone is released in a diurnal pattern. The 24-h cycle of growth hormone release is strongly associated with sleep, with highest levels occurring shortly after the onset of slow-wave sleep, and most growth hormone secretion occurring at night in humans. Thus, this is not a true circadian rhythm but rather a diurnal pattern of release.

A GHRH

H-Tyr-Ala-Asp-Ala-Ile-Phe-Thr-Asn-Ser-Tyr-Arg-
Lys-Val-Leu-Gly-Gln-Leu-Ser-Ala-Arg-Lys-Leu-
Leu-Gln-Asp-Ile-Met-Ser-Arg-Gln-Gln-Gly-Glu-
Ser-Asn-Gln-Glu-Arg-Gly-Ala-Arg-Ala-Arg-Leu-NH$_2$

B Somatostatin-14 and-28

Ser-Ala-Asn-Ser-Asn-Pro-Ala-Met-Ala-Pro-Arg-Glu-Arg-Lys-
(Ala-Gly-Cys-Lys-Asn-Phe-Phe-Trp-Lys-Thr-Phe-Thr-Ser-Cys)$_{SS14}$

FIGURE 40.7 Amino acid sequences of (A) growth hormone-releasing hormone (GHRH) and (B) somatostatin-14 and –28 (the latter is an N-terminal extension of somatostatin-14).

Structures and Properties of GHRH, Somatostatin, Growth Hormone, IGF-I, and Their Receptors

Growth hormone-releasing hormone and somatostatin GHRH is derived from a 108 amino acid precursor protein, called preproGHRH. Following a multistep processing procedure involving cleavage by endopeptidases, mature GHRH molecules are produced (Fig. 40.7). In some species, there are two GHRHs with similar biological activity; other species have a single GHRH peptide. The active GHRH peptide ranges from 42 to 44 amino acids, depending on the species (Mayo et al., 1995).

GHRH binds to its receptor on somatotropes to affect the release of growth hormone. The GHRH receptor is a member of the G-protein-coupled receptor family (Mayo et al., 1995). Binding of GHRH to its receptor triggers the G protein, in this case G$_s$, to trigger a cascade of intracellular events involving cyclic AMP (cAMP) as the second messenger. This causes calcium mobilization, the phosphorylation of proteins that are involved in the synthesis of growth hormone, and the release of growth hormone via secretory granules. The synthesis of the growth hormone that is triggered by GHRH probably involves the cAMP-induced phosphorylation of the cAMP response element-binding protein (CREB), which binds to an enhancer element in the promoter of the somatotropin gene to stimulate its transcription.

The somatostatin gene contains two exons that are transcribed into a 0.85-kb mRNA. This mRNA is translated into a 116 amino acid precursor protein, preprosomatostatin. This precursor is cleaved by endopeptidases and is a tissue-specific process. In the hypothalamus, somatostatin is cleaved into two biologically active forms, somatostatin-14 and somatostatin-28, the latter having an N-terminal extension of the somatostatin-14 molecule (Fig. 40.7).

The binding of somatostatin to its receptor causes a cascade of events involved in the inhibition of growth hormone release. To date, there are five known somatostatin receptors (SS-Rs), with different properties and affinities. All of these receptors involve an inhibitory G protein (G_i), which reduces cAMP and causes cell hyperpolarization and a diminution of Ca^{2+} influx into cells.

Growth hormone Growth hormone, or somatotropin, is a 191 amino acid peptide that contains two disulfide bonds that give it a three-dimensional conformation that is necessary for its biological activity. Release of the growth hormone is triggered by GHRH and is inhibited by somatostatin. The growth hormone plays a negative feedback role in the somatotropic axis, feeding back at the level of the GHRH neuron in the hypothalamus to inhibit GHRH mRNA levels and synthesis and stimulating somatostatin gene expression and release. Not only does the regulation of growth hormone involve the balance between GHRH and somatostatin, but it also involves other neurotransmitters and neuroactive substances, such as dopamine vasoactive intestinal peptide, pituitary adenylate cyclase-activating peptide, TRH, galanin, neuropeptide Y, motilin, and interleukins. In addition, other hormones, such as the thyroid hormone, glucocorticoids, sex steroid hormones, and metabolic fuels, can influence the release of growth hormone, highlighting the interwoven nature of the different neuroendocrine systems.

The growth hormone is released into the general circulation, where ~50% of this molecule is transported in association with a growth hormone-binding protein that is the same as the extracellular domain of the growth hormone receptor. This molecule and the growth hormone receptor (GH-R) are alternative splice products of the same precursor RNA into two distinct mRNAs: one for the growth hormone-binding protein and one for the GH-R.

The GH-R is a member of the cytokine receptor family (Behncken and Waters, 1999). Binding of growth hormone to its plasma membrane receptor causes receptor dimerization and triggers a cascade of protein phosphorylations mediated by the JAK-STAT system, the activation of nuclear transcription factors, and the stimulation of somatotropin-regulated genes.

IGF-I A major target for the growth hormone is the IGF-I system. IGF-I is a growth factor that exerts effects on neurite outgrowth and nervous system development. In addition, it is an important mediator of the somatotropic axis and, in fact, was originally referred to as somatomedin. Both growth hormone and IGF-I individually have similar effects on somatic growth and development; however, the two hormones act much more efficiently in combination. In addition, it appears that the growth-promoting effects of IGF-I are particularly important in the central nervous system. This is consistent with the observation that along with its production by the liver, IGF-I is also produced in the brain, and it is probably this central IGF-I that is responsible for many of its neurotrophic effects.

Like the growth hormone, IGF-I plays a feedback role in the inhibition of GHRH biosynthesis (Fig. 40.6). This may involve central and not peripheral IGF-I, as most animal studies have demonstrated that only centrally but not peripherally administered IGF-I has this effect. At the level of the pituitary, IGF-I appears to be the major regulator of negative feedback of growth hormone synthesis and release. Somatotropes contain IGF-I receptors, and IGF-I inhibits growth hormone gene expression and release under basal and GHRH-stimulated conditions. IGF-I can also act as a negative feedback regulator of GHRH neurons, as it can cross the blood–brain barrier to a limited extent. Moreover, IGF-I is synthesized in the central nervous system, including the hypothalamus, and therefore local IGF-I can exert an influence on GHRH neurons. It has also been shown that IGF-I can stimulate somatostatin release, albeit at higher doses than those necessary to inhibit GHRH release, suggesting that IGF-I may be more involved in the suppression of GHRH than the enhancement of somatostatin levels.

The IGF-I gene has been cloned in a number of species and encodes a polypeptide precursor molecule of 105 amino acids that is cleaved into the mature IGF-I of 70 amino acids. IGF-I in the circulation binds to several binding proteins, the major one being IGF-I binding protein 3 (IGFBP-3). Free IGF-I is more biologically active than bound IGF-I, and therefore IGFBP-3 levels are an important regulator of the actions of IGF-I. At its target tissues, IGF-I binds to its receptor, a member of the receptor tyrosine kinase family, which utilizes the MAP kinase system as its second messenger system.

Neuroanatomy of GHRH/Somatostatin Systems

Most GHRH-containing neurons are located in the basomedial hypothalamus in the arcuate nucleus, lateral to the floor of the third ventricle. These neurons project axons to the external zone of the median eminence, from which GHRH is released into the portal capillary system. GHRH neurons can also send axons to other hypothalamic regions, and this may be involved in the regulation of feeding behavior by GHRH. GHRH neurons receive inputs from other neuronal systems in the central nervous system, including α-adrenergic, dopaminergic, serotonergic, and enkephalinergic neurons.

Somatostatin neurons have a very different localization from the GHRH system. Unlike GHRH neurons, which are concentrated in a discrete nucleus, somatostatin is more dispersed throughout the central nervous system. Perikarya of the somatostatin neurons involved in the regulation of growth hormone release are found primarily in the periventricular region of the anterior hypothalamus. As is the case for other hypothalamic hormones, their axon terminals project to the external zone of the median eminence. Somatostatin neurons also make projections to GHRH neurons, and it is believed that this is the mechanism for the inhibition of GHRH neurons by somatostatin cells.

Inputs from metabolically active substances affect the somatostatin system. Amino acids are thought to stimulate and fatty acids and glucose to inhibit somatostatin secretion. There are also a number of neurotransmitters involved in the regulation of somatostatin levels. Catecholamines such as dopamine and norepinephrine are implicated in this process, as are acetylcholine and GABA. Neuropeptides, including substance P, neurotensin, and bombesin, can alter somatostatin levels, and factors involved in glucoregulation, such as glucose and glucoregulatory enzymes and hormones, modify activity of the somatostatin system.

Disruptions of the Somatotropic Axis

Somatic growth and development are affected by disruptions of the somatotropic axis, and the consequences are dependent on when during development the system is affected. In early development, growth hormone deficiency can result in an extremely short stature, with adults sometimes reaching a maximal height of less than 1 m. Growth hormone deficiency is generally treated with growth hormone replacement using recombinant growth hormone. In some cases, GHRH, rather than growth hormone, is replaced in a pulsatile manner.

If the growth hormone is oversecreted or dysregulated, the consequence can be gigantism, resulting in an extremely large stature. When growth hormone stimulation occurs after adulthood, this results in acromegaly. In adulthood, only certain tissues remain responsive to growth hormone stimulation, including the jaws, nose, orbital ridges, fingers, elbows, and knees, and these tissues are stimulated to grow while other tissues are not, causing deformations in proportions and appearance.

Stress: The Brain–Pituitary–Adrenal Axis

Overview and Characteristics

In order to survive, an animal must be able to adapt to stress, which can be manifested in a variety of forms. These stressors can include the acute stress of hunting or escaping predation or the chronic stress of a disease or the social situation or status. Thus, a stress is an internal or external cue that disrupts the homeostatic status of the animal.

The neuroendocrine system involved in mediating the stress response is the brain–pituitary–adrenal axis. The hypothalamic hormone controlling this axis is corticotropin-releasing hormone (CRH), produced in highest levels in the medial parvicellular part of the paraventricular nucleus (mpPVN; Fig. 40.8). CRH somata send projections to the external layer of the median eminence, typical of all hypothalamic neuroendocrine cells, where CRH is released. The targets of CRH in the anterior pituitary gland are the corticotropes, which have receptors for CRH. In addition, another hypothalamic hormone, arginine vasopressin (AVP), produced in the magnocellular elements of the PVN, also acts at pituitary corticotropes to exert synergistic effects on these cells. The corticotropes respond to CRH and AVP with the synthesis and release of adrenocorticotropic hormone (ACTH). ACTH is released from the pituitary gland into the general circulation, where it acts at receptors on the adrenal cortex to stimulate the production and release of glucocorticoids. The feedback of glucocorticoids onto the brain and pituitary negatively regulates the synthesis of CRH and ACTH: therefore, this neuroendocrine system is a classical negative feedback loop.

Physiological Functions

Glucocorticoids mediate stress responses and affect cellular metabolism Corticosteroids are necessary for normal fetal development. Enzymes in the liver, gastrointestinal system, lungs, and adrenal medulla are stimulated by glucocorticoids. There, glucocorticoids play important roles in the regulation of glycogen utilization and storage, with glucocorticoids promoting the production of glycogen synthase. The stress axis is subject to developmental and age-related regulation due to changes in afferent connections to the hypothalamus, glucocorticoid, and mineralocorticoid receptor-binding changes and alterations in the negative feedback of glucocorticoids on CRH neurons.

Glucocorticoids exert effects on the cardiovascular system, causing elevations in heart rate and

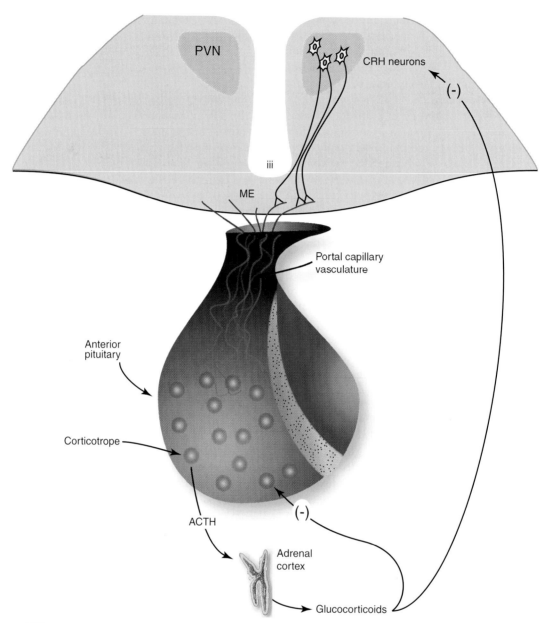

FIGURE 40.8 Schematic representation of the brain–pituitary–adrenal axis showing CRH neurons in the paraventricular nucleus projecting their neuroterminals to the external zone of the median eminence. This occurs bilaterally, although only a unilateral projection is shown. CRH travels through the portal vasculature to cause the synthesis and release of ACTH from corticotropes. This molecule acts at the adrenal cortex to cause the biosynthesis and release of glucocorticoids. These are released into general circulation to mediate the stress response and feedback in a negative manner at the corticotropes of the pituitary and the CRH neurons of the PVN. PVN, paraventricular nucleus; CRH, corticotropin-releasing hormone; ME, median eminence; iii, third ventricle; ACTH, adrenocorticotropic hormone.

blood pressure and alterations in blood flow. They act in close coordination with the autonomic nervous system to exert their effects. In general, their role is to mobilize energy stores and to improve cardio-vascular tone. Glucocorticoids may also modulate immune responses and inhibit cytokine production, thereby playing a role in the inhibition of the inflam-matory response. Glucocorticoids can interact with hormones produced by other neuroendocrine axes, such as those involved in thyroid function, repro-ductive function, and growth. Chronic stress can suppress the growth axis and reproductive func-tion and cause hyperthyroidism (O'Connor *et al.*, 2000).

Pulsatile and circadian release of CRH and ACTH
The release of stress hormones exhibits a circadian rhythmicity (Gore, 1998). That it is a true circadian rhythm and not a diurnal rhythm (attuned to the sleep/wake cycle or the light cycle) is demonstrated by studies in which the suprachiasmatic nucleus of the hypothalamus was lesioned. The SCN is the primary circadian clock of the central nervous system; when lesioned, circadian rhythms are abolished or altered, including those of the CRH rhythm. Moreover, rhythms of the brain–pituitary–adrenal axis persist in the absence of external night/day cues. The circadian rhythmicity of this axis has been best studied for glucocorticoids, the release of which peak during the early morning (~0700 h) and reach a nadir during the afternoon in humans. A similar pattern of release is seen in rats, with highest levels when the animals are awakening (in the case of rats, which are a nocturnal species, this is the evening) and lowest levels in the morning. The adrenal hormone synthesized is species dependent; in humans, the major glucocorticoid is cortisol, and in rats, it is corticosterone. However, these glucocorticoids serve similar functions as the final hormones produced by the stress axis.

Circadian rhythms in hypothalamic CRH and pituitary ACTH have also been reported. For the stress axis, the primary level at which the circadian pattern of glucocorticoid release is generated is the hypothalamus, as hypothalamic CRH mRNA levels in the mpPVN fluctuate across the 24-h cycle in the rat, and the increase in CRH mRNA levels precedes the increase in glucocorticoid release by several hours. It should also be noted that the rhythm of the brain–pituitary–adrenal axis is altered by the timing of food intake. This is relevant to the observation that glucocorticoids alter glucose metabolism and energy use, and thus, it is not surprising that levels of glucocorticoids may fluctuate depending on energy and food demands of the organism.

Structures and Properties of CRH, ACTH, Glucocorticoids, and Their Receptors

CRH Corticotropin-releasing hormone is a 41 amino acid peptide expressed in the parvicellular region of the PVN in the hypothalamus (Fig. 40.9). It is also found in other CNS regions and outside of the brain in adrenal gland, placenta, ovary, immune tissues, and at inflammatory sites. CRH is released in a pulsatile manner from neuroterminals in the external zone of the median eminence. At the anterior pituitary target cell, the corticotrope, CRH acts together with arginine vasopressin (AVP), also produced in the PVN (magnocellular region), to cause the synthesis and release of ACTH (Fig. 40.8).

Binding of CRH to its receptor in the pituitary corticotrope activates ACTH synthesis and secretion. The receptor is linked to the activation of adenylate cyclase. The CRH receptor is also found in the central nervous system, with highest concentrations in the olfactory bulb, cerebellum, cerebral cortex, and striatum and lower concentrations in the spinal cord, hypothalamus, medulla, midbrain, thalamus, pons, and hippocampus (DeSouza, 1987).

ACTH ACTH derives from the cleavage of a precursor protein, proopiomelanocortin (POMC), in the corticotropes (Fig. 40.9). POMC is cleaved to a number of smaller peptides, including β-endorphin, β-MSH, and γ-MSH. ACTH is the primary effector of the stress axis, and its release into the general circulation from the pituitary corticotrope has effects on the target organ, the adrenal cortex, to affect the production of glucocorticoids.

The ACTH receptor is a member of the melanocortin family of receptors (Naville *et al.*, 1999). It is a seven transmembrane domain G-protein-coupled receptor expressed primarily in adrenal cortex. The binding of ACTH to its receptor activates adenylate cyclase and cAMP production.

Glucocorticoids Glucocorticoids are members of the steroid hormone family (Fig. 40.9). As is the case for sex steroid hormones, they derive from a cholesterol precursor. Following a series of enzymatic reactions, the major corticosteroids, such as cortisol (in humans) or corticosterone (in rats), are synthesized.

The glucocorticoid receptor (GR) is widely distributed in the central nervous system, including the hypothalamus and, more specifically, the CRH cells of the PVN. Thus, glucocorticoid negative feedback can occur directly on the hypothalamic cells driving the stress axis. GRs are also abundant in the hippocampus, in pyramidal cells, and in dentate granule cells. The hippocampus appears to play a role in mediating the stress response, and there are multiple redundant pathways between the hippocampus and the PVN. GRs are found in many other brain regions such as the olfactory cortex, cerebral cortex, amygdala, septum, thalamus, midbrain raphe nuclei, cerebellum, and brain stem (Morimoto *et al.*, 1996). The widespread distribution of this receptor suggests important and diverse effects of glucocorticoids in the central nervous system.

Glucocorticoids can also bind to the mineralocorticoid receptor (MR), the primary ligand of which is aldosterone. Moreover, the brain MR has a higher (~10-fold higher) affinity for glucocorticoids than the GR. Both of these receptors are members of the steroid

A   SEEPPISLDLTFHLLREVLEMARAEQLAQQAHSNRKLME I I

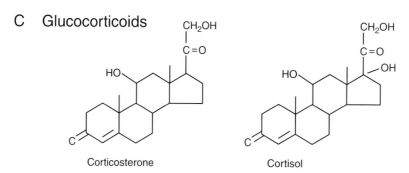

FIGURE 40.9 (A) Amino acid sequence of CRH in human and rat. (B) Structure of the proopiome-lanocortin (POMC) precursor protein that is cleaved to α- and γ-MSH, β-endorphin, adrenocorticotropic hormone (ACTH), or β-lipotropin (β-LPH). (C) Structures of the major corticosteroids— corticosterone and cortisol.

hormone superfamily. They are thought to reside in the cytoplasm of target cells in the unliganded state. When bound to their ligands, GRs or MRs translocate into the nucleus, where they bind to specific sites on the promoter of the responsive gene. Thus, GR and MR are transcription factors. Their efficacy in stimulating or inhibiting gene transcription is modulated by their binding to other molecules, such as heat shock proteins, which can alter the translocation of the receptor–ligand complex to the nucleus, or transcriptional coactivators, which modulate the histones associated with the gene (see Chapter 10).

Chronic exposure to glucocorticoids can cause damage to the brain, which is particularly apparent in the hippocampus, which is abundant in GRs. It has been observed that chronic corticosteroids changes the morphology of CA3 dendritic fields and may lead to neurodegeneration and eventually cell death. Nevertheless, whereas chronic high levels of glucocorticoids may be toxic, a lack of glucocorticoids can also be detrimental. In the dentate gyrus, maintenance of the dentate granule cell number appears to require glucocorticoids, and adrenalectomy results in the loss of granule cells. Moreover, neurogenesis in the adult dentate gyrus also appears to be glucocorticoid dependent. There are functional correlates to the effects of glucocorticoids on the hippocampus, with these hormones playing roles in learning and memory. Acute

stress can interfere with the ability of an organism to learn, and chronic stress is correlated with deficits in spatial learning.

Neuroanatomy of the CRH System

CRH neuronal perikarya are localized primarily in the medial parvicellular part of the paraventricular nucleus (mpPVN) and project neuroterminals to the external zone of the median eminence. The PVN is an important integrative region of the hypothalamus; it sums and integrates inputs from other regions throughout the brain. The primary origins of these inputs are the brain stem, the midbrain/pons groups, the limbic system, the circumventricular organs, and the hypothalamus. Inputs from the brain stem are catecholaminergic pathways involved in the transmission of visceral information. The catecholamine system plays an important role as a stress mediator, possibly as an autonomic nervous system neurotransmitter. Noradrenergic projections to the PVN arise from the nucleus of the solitary tract (A2 cell group), the A1 cell group of the ventrolateral medulla, and the locus coeruleus. Inputs from the midbrain may involve the midbrain raphe cell groups, which are serotonergic in nature. The midbrain periaqueductal gray and pontine central gray regions relay sensory information to the PVN, as do caudal thalamus, cholinergic brain stem regions (laterodorsal tegmental nucleus and the pedunculopontine nucleus).

These inputs appear to play a role in relaying somatic and special sensory information. Inputs to the PVN from the limbic system arise from the prefrontal cortex, septum, amygdala, and hippocampus, and a notable projection to the PVN is from the bed nucleus of the stria terminalis to the PVN. These inputs relay information on cognition and emotion. The circumventricular organs (subfornical organ, OVLT) convey information to the PVN from blood-borne chemosensory signals. The major neurotransmitters involved in this function are GABA and angiotensin II. Finally, the hypothalamus itself signals to the PVN, and these connections may provide signals about the motivational state of the animal or relay other stress-specific signals. However, the functions of these interhypothalamic projections are not well understood.

Disruptions in the Stress Axis

The negative feedback loop of CRH–ACTH–glucocorticoids is kept in a delicate balance. In response to stress, there is a large increase in the activity of the stress axis, but the system is downregulated rapidly by negative feedback from the glucocorticoids to the brain and pituitary gland, causing it to return the output of the stress axis to basal low levels. However, the stress axis can be disrupted by psychological stressors such as mood disorders that can chronically dysregulate the brain–pituitary–adrenal axis. For example, posttraumatic stress syndrome can cause dysfunctions of the stress axis that can last for years (Box 40.2).

Overactivity of the stress axis can increase susceptibility to infection and tumors and reduce inflammatory and autoimmune disease (O'Connor et al., 2000). For example, Cushing's disease is characterized by hypercortisolemia and abnormal secretion and/or bioactivity of ACTH. The high levels of cortisol suppress CRH release and cause alterations in immune function. People with Cushing's disease have an increase in appetite and can experience changes in fat distribution. However, the brain–pituitary–adrenal axis can adapt to overactivity, and thus the immune system suppression that occurs in Cushing's disease is milder than that which would be predicted by the high levels of circulating cortisol. Elevations in activity of the stress axis can also impair memory, probably through actions of glucocorticoids on the hippocampus.

Underactivity of the stress axis can cause the opposite effects of hyperactivity, namely resistance to infection and tumors but increased susceptibility to inflammatory and autoimmune disease. In the case of adrenocortical insufficiency, there is generally a failure of the adrenal cortex to respond to ACTH. Addison's disease is characterized by an insufficient release of glucocorticoid secretion, and its symptoms include muscle weakness and fatigue, psychological symptoms, gastrointestinal symptoms, and changes in skin

---

BOX 40.2

POST TRAUMATIC STRESS DISORDER (PTSD)

This anxiety disorder is among the few psychiatric illnesses that are caused by external traumatic events. Forty-four percent of a nationally representative sample of adults reported at least one significant stress symptom since the September 11, 2001 terrorist attack, and the prevalence of PTSD in the United States may be currently higher than the previously reported 8%. There are currently no neuroimaging, blood, or cerebrospinal fluid (CSF) tests that can definitively confirm a psychiatric diagnosis, and great reliance is placed on the patient event report of distressing symptoms.

A diagnosis of PTSD requires exposure to a trauma that involves actual or threatened death, serious injury, or a threat to the physical integrity of self or others. Rape, physical assault, witnessing or living through a terrorist attack, or natural or man-made disasters qualify for stressors that could result in PTSD, in contrast to other setbacks such as divorce or disappointments, which are within the range of usual human experience. Prominent fear, helplessness, or horror accompanying the exposure to the traumatic event is another hallmark of PTSD. A combination of reexperiencing symptoms (e.g., intrusive recollections of the event, nightmares, flashbacks, physical and psychological distress on exposure to reminders of the trauma), avoidance symptoms (e.g., avoiding thoughts and feelings or conversations about the trauma, amnesia, decreased interest, feeling detached from loved ones), and symptoms of increased arousal (e.g., insomnia, anger, difficulty concentrating, increased vigilance and startle reactions) together constitute the syndrome of PTSD, when it results in impairments in social or occupational functioning.

BOX 40.2 (*cont'd*)

The limbic hypothalamic pituitary adrenal (HPA) axis and the sympathetic adrenal medullary arms of the stress system have been investigated extensively in subjects with PTSD. Although, increased levels of corticotropin releasing hormone (CRH) are reported in patients with combat-related PTSD, plasma cortisol levels can be paradoxically low, particularly in the late evening and early morning. Cortisol levels in 24-h collections of urine are decreased, increased, or not significantly different compared to control subjects. Patients with PTSD respond to low doses of dexamethasone with a greater reduction of plasma cortisol compared to control subjects, suggesting that PTSD is associated with an increased number and sensitivity of glucocorticoid receptors. Various challenge tests of the HPA axis, e.g., CRH stimulation test, ACTH stimulation test, and metyrapone stimulation test, yielded mixed results. Preclinical data suggest that stress-induced elevations of CSF CRH result in an upregulation of mineralocorticoid receptors, which in turn lower cortisol levels. Abnormalities in mineralocorticoid receptors in patients with PTSD could explain the paradoxical observation of normal to low cortisol levels in the presence of increased CSF CRH. However this possibility has not been investigated in PTSD.

Persistent abnormalities in the sympathetic nervous system in patients are indicated by significant and consistent increases in CSF and plasma norepinephrine and plasma epinephrine in response to exposure to traumatic reminders and during the administration of drugs that stimulate the sympathetic nervous system, such as an α_2-antagonist, yohimbine.

HPA axis abnormalities in the immediate aftermath of trauma have been investigated with an aim to predict PTSD in the future. A majority of studies evaluating cortisol immediately after trauma do not show significant elevations in those who later develop PTSD. However, subjects who had elevated norepinephrine levels at 1 and 6 months after a motor vehicle accident were more likely to develop PTSD. Elevated heart rate immediately after the trauma reliably identified those who would develop PTSD after an acutely traumatic event. It is possible that abnormalities in, or an imbalance between, the HPA and sympathetic arm of the stress response system may be an important biological basis for susceptibility to developing PTSD in the future.

Preclinical studies in animal models have supported the possibility that psychosocial stress and elevated levels of cortisol result in impaired neurogenesis, decreased dendritic branching, and neuronal cell death in the hippocampus. Several studies in humans with combat and childhood sexual and/or physical abuse related PTSD found a smaller hippocampal volume; however, a twin study in Vietnam veterans with PTSD suggests that a smaller hippocampal volume could be a risk factor for developing PTSD, rather than a consequence of severe stress.

Studies using positron emission tomography and functional MRI during exposure to stimuli reminiscent of the trauma reveal a failure of activation of the medial prefrontal cortex (particularly the anterior cingulate cortex). In keeping with the hypothesis that a dysfunctional anterior cingulate cortex inadequately inhibits the amygdala, increased activation of the amygdala has been demonstrated in response to trauma-related stimuli. These and other findings support the possibility that neural processes mediating extinction to trauma-related stimuli may be impaired in patients with PTSD. Psychophysiological data confirm that patients with PTSD acquire conditioned responses more readily and take a longer time to extinguish the responses, despite the absence of the primary stimulus.

Inconsistencies in neuroendocrine and neuroimaging data may be attributed to the heterogeneity of the patients, with differences in the kind of trauma (sexual and/or physical abuse, combat, motor vehicle accidents, witnessing violence, etc.), duration of exposure to trauma (single episode versus prolonged exposure), timing of exposure (prepubertal versus postpubertal), gender, phase in the menstrual cycle, medications, and comorbid alcohol and substance use.

Medications and psychotherapy are the cornerstones for PTSD treatment. Currently, two drugs belonging to the class of selective serotonin reuptake inhibitors, sertraline and paroxetine, are FDA approved for the treatment of PTSD. Cognitive behavioral techniques, such as exposure therapy, anxiety management programs, and cognitive therapy, are effective in the treatment of PTSD. However, individual patient factors, such as high motivation and compliance, and tolerance of anxiety (in the case of exposure therapy) contribute to improved outcome. The efficacy of a combination of medications and psychotherapy has not been evaluated in PTSD.

Meena Vythilingam and Dennis S. Charney

pigmentation. Fortunately, glucocorticoid replacement can help mitigate these symptoms.

Reproduction: The Brain–Pituitary–Gonadal Axis

Overview and Characteristics

Reproduction is critical to the survival of the species. In vertebrate organisms, the reproductive axis comprises the gonadotropin-releasing hormone (also called luteinizing hormone-releasing hormone) synthesizing neurons of the hypothalamus and preoptic area; the gonadotropes of the anterior pituitary gland; and the gonads (ovary in females and testis in males). GnRH neurons of the hypothalamus and preoptic area project their neuroterminals to the median eminence, where the GnRH peptide is released in a pulsatile manner (Gore, 2002). GnRH acts at the gonadotropes to cause the production of two hormones called the gonadotropins: luteinizing hormone and follicle-stimulating hormone. These hormones in turn are released in a pulsatile manner into the general circulation and bind to receptors on specialized cells in the ovaries or testes to stimulate steroidogenesis, spermatogenesis in males, and oogenesis in females. The gonads respond to this activation by synthesizing and secreting the sex steroid hormones, predominantly estrogen and progesterone in the ovary and testosterone in the male. The sex steroid hormones, released into the circulatory system, act at receptors that are located throughout the body to exert their classical effects on secondary sex characteristic development. In addition, sex steroid hormones act on receptors in the brain, including the hypothalamus, to exert diverse effects on the CNS. One of the major effects of sex steroid hormones is as a feedback modulator of the hypothalamic GnRH neurons, probably indirectly through afferents to the GnRH cell. However, while much sex steroid hormone feedback is the usual negative feedback typical of neuroendocrine systems, in females, ovulation is controlled by *positive* feedback from estrogen. This concept of negative/positive feedback regulation is discussed later.

Physiological Functions

Activity of the reproductive axis varies during the life cycle Not surprisingly, functions of the reproductive axis change during the life cycle of the organism, as reproductive function varies with developmental stage (Plant, 1988). During the late embryonic/early postnatal period, as the GnRH system finishes its neuroanatomical development, there is increased activity of the brain–pituitary–testicular axis in males and, to a lesser extent, the brain–pituitary–ovarian axis in females. Shortly after birth, the reproductive system becomes quiescent, possibly due to the development of inhibitory inputs to GnRH neurons or the lack of stimulatory inputs to this system. This quiescent period, often called the "prepubertal hiatus," is characterized by low GnRH, gonadotropin, and steroid hormone release. At the onset of puberty, the GnRH system becomes activated, probably due to the removal of inhibitory afferents to GnRH neurons, dominated by GABAergic neurons, and the ability of stimulatory afferents to GnRH neurons to exert a stimulatory tone on GnRH regulation. To date, numerous substances have been implicated in the activation of GnRH neurons at the onset of puberty, including glutamate (through the NMDA receptor), norepinephrine, neuropeptide Y, and growth factors (transforming growth factor-α and insulin-like growth factor I). Once reproductive function has been attained (ovulation in females, viable sperm in ejaculates of males), the pulsatile release of GnRH and its regulation of the reproductive axis in males continues for much of the life cycle, whereas in most spontaneously ovulating females, reproductive cycles (estrous cycles, menstrual cycles) occur.

In human females but not most other species, menopause, the cessation of menstrual cycles and lack of ovulation, signals the end of the reproductive life cycle. The most obvious characteristic of menopause is a loss of ovarian follicles, called follicular atresia. While many other mammals undergo reproductive senescence, characterized by a lack of spontaneous reproductive cycles, this is not due to follicular atresia. Rather, in most species, reproductive senescence is probably due to the loss of drive from hypothalamic GnRH neurons and/or changes in pituitary gonadotropin responses to GnRH rather than overt ovarian changes. In humans, it is likely that there are also hypothalamic and pituitary changes that may play a role in the menopausal process that are only just beginning to be studied.

Pulsatile, diurnal, and seasonal release of GnRH and LH/FSH GnRH is released in a pulsatile manner from neuroterminals in the external zone of the median eminence. Virtually every pulse of GnRH causes a pulse of LH and, to a slightly lesser extent, FSH, although some "silent" pulses of GnRH (that occur in the absence of the corresponding release of the gonadotropins) can be observed. Although the pulsatile release of LH appears to be driven entirely by pulses of GnRH, as is evidenced by the concordance of these pulses, the regulation of pulsatile FSH also involves the gonadal peptide inhibin. Inhibin is a glycoprotein produced in the gonad that selectively acts at the pituitary gland to suppress FSH release.

The mechanism by which GnRH pulses are generated is under considerable debate, as these neurons are widely dispersed through the hypothalamus and preoptic area; although contacts between GnRH cells have been observed, these are not abundant. It is possible that GnRH neurons coordinate their pulses via some signals at the level of the median eminence where the GnRH neuroterminals converge. Alternatively, other afferent systems contacting GnRH neurons may release their neurotransmitters in a pulsatile manner, and this may be a way of coordinating the widely scattered GnRH perikarya to release pulses of GnRH in a coordinated manner.

A pulsatile manner of GnRH release is necessary for the maintenance of pituitary gonadotropin function. When GnRH is infused continuously, the GnRH receptor in the pituitary is downregulated and gonadotropin secretion is inhibited. If exogenous GnRH is infused in a pulsatile manner, the GnRH receptor is upregulated on the gonadotropes.

The pulsatile release of GnRH is more or less constant in males, with pulses occurring approximately every 1–2 h. However, in females, the nature of GnRH pulses varies across the reproductive cycle. In primates, which have a 28-day menstrual cycle, LH pulses (measured as an indicator of GnRH pulses) occur approximately once per hour during the early follicular phase, but slow to a frequency of once every 90 min later in the follicular phase as estrogen negative feedback increases. Just prior to ovulation, a large increase in GnRH release can be measured, although it is still controversial whether discrete pulses continue to be superimposed on this "GnRH surge." Nevertheless, it is likely that there is a change in the mode of GnRH release during the preovulatory period.

The pulsatile release of GnRH, LH, and FSH is superimposed upon a diurnal pattern of the release of these hormones (Gore, 1998). Thus, the timing of the preovulatory LH surge in rodents is coordinated with the 24-h light/dark cycle (i.e., it is a diurnal but not a circadian rhythm). Although in women these diurnal rhythms are not as obvious as those in rats, it appears that the release of gonadotropins has a weak diurnal rhythm in humans. Men have also been reported to have nocturnal increases in reproductive hormone release. Interestingly, the diurnal rhythm of reproductive hormone release is regulated developmentally. Prior to the onset of puberty, there is little day/night difference in GnRH, LH, or FSH release. At the onset of puberty, a diurnal rhythm develops, characterized by nocturnal increases in the release of these hormones. This nocturnal increase is most pronounced late in puberty, and once adult reproductive function is attained, the rhythm diminishes. The mechanism for, and the function of, the pubertal diurnal rhythm of GnRH and gonadotropins is currently not understood but is one of the most robust diurnal rhythms observed in all the neuroendocrine systems.

The reproductive axis can exhibit rhythms even longer than those entrained to the 24-h clock. Many species are seasonal breeders, in which reproductive processes are coordinated to a time of the year when the likelihood of the survival of the offspring is highest. Seasonal breeding animals such as sheep have an almost completely inactive reproductive axis during the nonbreeding season, with very low GnRH release, low basal and GnRH-stimulated gonadotropin release, and a lack of ovulation. In many of these species, day length is what drives the seasonal breeding cycles, although this varies among the species. For hamsters, short nights stimulate the reproductive system, whereas short nights inhibit the reproductive axes of sheep.

Structures and Properties of GnRH, Gonadotropins, Sex Steroid Hormones, and Their Receptors

GnRH   GnRH is a 10 amino acid peptide that is synthesized from a 92 amino acid precursor molecule (Fig. 40.10). During cleavage of the prohormone, GnRH is produced together with a 56 amino acid peptide referred to as GnRH-associated peptide (GAP). Both GnRH and GAP are released from neuroterminals of these cells into the portal vasculature; however, while GnRH is a strong stimulator of LH and FSH release from pituitary gonadotropes, GAP has only a weak ability in this regard. GAP is also able to inhibit prolactin secretion; nevertheless, a physiological role for GAP is still unknown.

The GnRH peptide is extremely evolutionarily conserved. All mammals studied to date, with the exception of the guinea pig, have an identical GnRH decapeptide in the hypothalamus-preoptic area. Nonmammalian vertebrates have decapeptides similar to the mammalian GnRH molecule, and the conservation is maintained all the way across the evolutionary spectrum to the jawless fish, which have a GnRH molecule that is 60–70% structurally homologous with the mammalian GnRH decapeptide.

Unlike other neuroendocrine cells, GnRH neurons have an unusual embryonic origin, deriving from cells that are first detected in the olfactory placode. During embryonic development, GnRH neurons migrate into the brain, reaching their final destinations in the preoptic area and hypothalamic regions during mid- to late embryogenesis. Also, unlike most other neuroendocrine peptide systems, GnRH neurons are relatively scattered through these regions and are not tightly concentrated in a single discrete nucleus.

GnRH binds to its receptor in pituitary gonadotropes to activate the synthesis and release of the gonadotropins. The GnRH receptor is a member of the G-protein coupled receptor family, containing seven transmembrane domains. The G protein involved in this function is probably G_q and/or G_{11}. The binding of GnRH to its receptor appears to activate several second messenger systems, including the protein kinase A and protein kinase C pathways, as well as the phospholipase C pathway (Sealfon *et al.*, 1997).

Gonadotropins The gonadotropins, LH and FSH, were originally named after their functions in the female ovary, namely their ability to cause luteinization of the follicle (hence LH) and to promote follicular development (hence FSH). However, these same gonadotropins are synthesized and released from the anterior pituitary gland of males and play a critical role in the regulation of testicular function. Thus, in the testis, LH is responsible for steroidogenesis, and FSH for spermatogenesis.

LH and FSH are glycoprotein hormones and are in the same family as TSH. These three molecules have a common α-subunit, but vary in the β-subunit. They are glycosylated polypeptides, and the α and

A GnRH pGlu - His - Trp - Ser - Tyr - Gly - Leu - Arg - Pro - Gly - NH_3

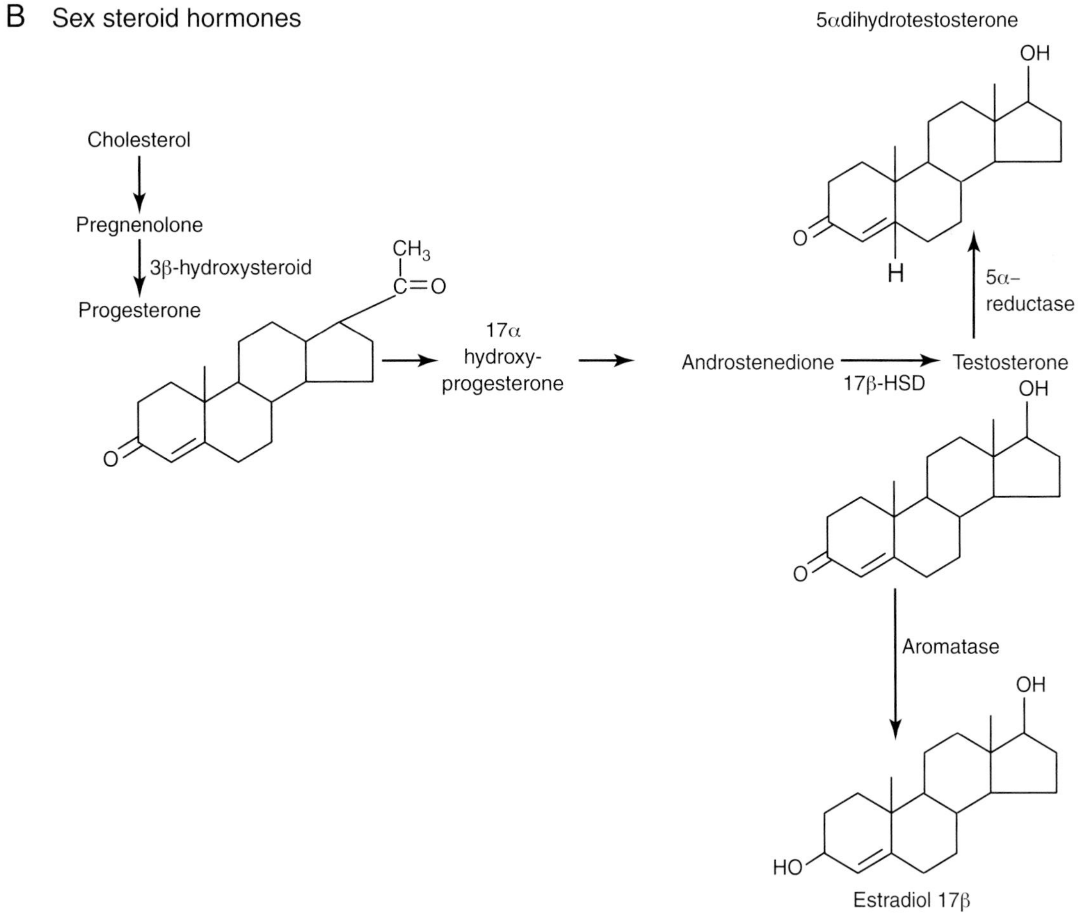

FIGURE 40.10 (A) Amino acid sequence of the GnRH decapeptide in mammals. (B) Synthesis and structures of sex steroid hormones. 17β-HSD, 17β-hydroxysteroid dehydrogenase.

β-subunits are linked covalently. Both LH and FSH are approximately 28 kDa. The common α-subunit is a 92 amino acid molecule, the LH-β molecule is 121 amino acids, and the FSH-β molecule is 111 amino acids. These hormones bind to their respective LH or FSH receptors, which are G-protein-coupled receptors found in target tissues of the ovary or testis.

Sex steroid hormones   Sex steroid hormones are synthesized from the precursor cholesterol in a multistep process (Fig. 40.10). Cholesterol is first converted to pregnenolone, which is converted to progesterone. This hormone is a major end point for biosynthesis in gonadal tissues and exerts potent effects on the body and brain. Progesterone serves as a precursor for the synthesis of testosterone (following conversion first to 17α-hydroxyprogesterone and then androstenedione). Testosterone is the major steroid hormone in males and serves as a precursor for 5α-dihydrotestosterone, which is responsible for many of the masculinizing effects of steroids in males, and for 17β-estradiol, which is the primary estrogen responsible for sexual behavior and physiology in females. The sex steroid hormones bind to their receptors, members of the steroid hormone superfamily, which are localized intracellularly in the cytoplasm and/or nucleus. The binding of a steroid hormone to its receptor, and subsequent receptor dimerization in the nucleus, allows these transcription factors to bind to specific sites on the promoter of the target gene. This enables the receptor–ligand complexes to induce or repress gene transcription in their target tissues.

Sex steroid hormones are synthesized and secreted from the ovaries or testes to regulate the expression of secondary sex characteristics. In the Leydig cells of the testis, LH released from the pituitary gland is responsible for testosterone biosynthesis. Together with FSH, testosterone acts to coordinate and stimulate spermatogenesis in testicular seminiferous tubules. The testosterone that is released from the testis acts at secondary sex targets such as the internal and external genitalia (prostate, seminal vesicles, penis) to cause their development and maintain their functions. In addition, testosterone acts at muscle to increase muscle mass, causes the growth of facial and body hair, and enlarges the epiglottis, which is responsible for the deepening of the voice. In the ovary, FSH stimulates follicular development during each ovarian cycle, and FSH together with LH stimulates ovulation. Production of the sex steroid hormones estrogen and progesterone is also stimulated by FSH and LH. These ovarian hormones are responsible for the development of female secondary sex characteristics such as the genitalia and mammary tissue.

Sex steroid hormone feedback in the male is accomplished by the usual neuroendocrine negative feedback mechanism. Pulses of GnRH cause pulses of the gonadotropins, which in turn are responsible for pulses of testosterone. Feedback of testosterone onto the brain causes an inhibition of hypothalamic GnRH neurons, and testosterone also feeds back onto the pituitary gonadotropes. At the pituitary gland, sex steroid hormones act primarily to decrease the sensitivity of pituitary gonadotropes to GnRH, resulting in a decrease in LH pulse amplitude.

In the female, the major feedback regulator of the reproductive axis is the ovarian steroid hormone estrogen. In addition, progesterone can act at the hypothalamus to provide negative feedback. During most of the reproductive cycle, estrogen feeds back at the brain and the pituitary gland to suppress the release of GnRH and the gonadotropins, respectively. However, during the mid- to late follicular stage in primates, or on the day of proestrus in rats with a 4- to 5-day estrous cycle, feedback effects of estrogen on GnRH release become positive. The stimulatory effects of estrogen on the pituitary result in the occurrence of the "preovulatory LH surge," which triggers the final maturation of the ovum in the follicle and results in ovulation and the subsequent development of the corpus luteum. Studies measuring GnRH itself, and not LH as an indicator of GnRH release, suggest that there is a large increase in GnRH release that causes the preovulatory LH surge, the former therefore called the "preovulatory GnRH surge."

Unlike the other neuroendocrine systems, the feedback site of testosterone and estrogen does not appear to be the GnRH neurons. Although this field is still somewhat controversial, in general it is thought that GnRH neurons do not express estrogen receptors or androgen receptors. However, many afferent inputs to GnRH neurons express these receptors, and therefore the regulation of the GnRH system by steroid hormone feedback appears to be mediated transsynaptically. In addition, it is possible that the "switch" between estrogen negative and positive feedback onto the GnRH neurons in females may be mediated by different neurotransmitters that inhibit or stimulate, respectively, the GnRH cells depending on their exposure to various levels of estrogen.

Neuroanatomy of the GnRH System

As mentioned earlier, GnRH neurons are not localized in a discrete hypothalamic nucleus, but are relatively widely dispersed across a continuum of the hypothalamus and preoptic area (Fig. 40.11). While the rostral–caudal extent of the localization of GnRH perikarya can vary among species, in general, most

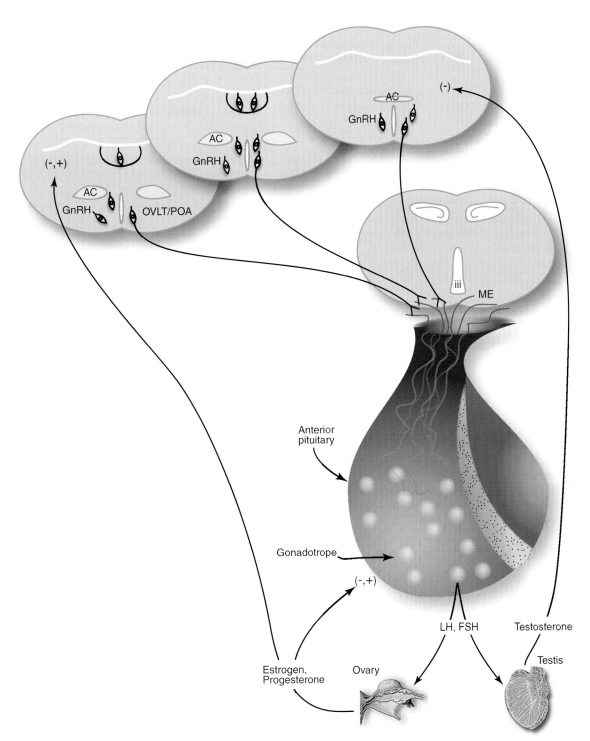

FIGURE 40.11 Schematic representation of the brain–pituitary–gonadal axis showing GnRH neurons in the preoptic area/anterior hypothalamus projecting their neuroterminals to the external zone of the median eminence. This occurs bilaterally, although only a unilateral projection is shown. GnRH travels through the portal vasculature to cause the synthesis and release of the gonadotropins, LH and FSH, from gonadotropes. These molecules act at the gonads (ovary and testis) to cause the biosynthesis and release of sex steroid hormones. These are released into general circulation to affect secondary sex characteristics and act at other somatic tissues and feedback at the brain and pituitary to regulate biosynthesis of GnRH and the gonadotropins. AC, anterior commissure; OVLT/POA, organum vasculosum of the lamina terminalis/preoptic area; LH, luteinizing hormone; FSH, follicle-stimulating hormone; GnRH, gonadotropin-releasing hormone; ME, median eminence; iii, third ventricle.

GnRH cells are found in the preoptic area, septal nuclei, diagonal band of Broca, and anterior hypothalamus (particularly basal regions). All of the neuroendocrine GnRH neurons project a process to the median eminence, where the GnRH decapeptide is released in a pulsatile manner.

The morphology of GnRH neurons is somewhat different from other neuroendocrine neurons, possibly due to differences in the cells' embryonic origin. GnRH neurons are oval or fusiform in shape and are usually unipolar or bipolar. They also receive relatively little synaptic input on their perikarya. Nevertheless, GnRH neurons are regulated by numerous neurotransmitters and neurotrophic factors, which is probably related to the integrative nature of the GnRH neuron. In order for reproduction to be successful, the organism must be able to assess the conditions of internal and external environment to determine that conditions are optimal. The numerous inputs to GnRH neurons from other sensory and neuroendocrine cells enables these key reproductive neurons to evaluate the organism's health and fitness and the external conditions (e.g., season, food availability, the presence of predators or a conspecific mate) and to coordinate the timing of reproduction, which is quite costly, with the optimal external and internal circumstances. Thus, GnRH cells are regulated by inputs from neurotransmitters such as glutamate, GABA, catecholamines and monoamines, neuropeptides such as CRH, β-endorphin, vasopressin, neurotensin, neurotrophic factors, and many other substances. In this way, GnRH neurons receive cues regarding nutritional status, thermogenesis and exercise, stress, and social cues and can integrate these inputs to coordinate the timing of reproduction with the appropriate stimuli.

Disruptions in the Reproductive Axis

There are two natural genetic mutations lacking normal GnRH systems. In humans, Kallmann's syndrome is characterized by the failure of GnRH neurons to migrate properly during embryonic development. While these patients develop essentially normally in most other ways (except that they are anosmic due to abnormalities of the olfactory placode from which both GnRH neurons and olfactory cells derive), they never enter puberty and are infertile. Replacement of pulsatile GnRH to these individuals can stimulate the onset of puberty and maturation of the secondary sex characteristics and fertility. The hypogonadal (hpg) mouse has a defect in the GnRH gene. Similar to their human Kallmann's syndrome counterparts, these animals never undergo reproductive development and can be "rescued" by GnRH replacement.

Other defects of the reproductive system involve the timing of the onset of puberty. In idiopathic central precocious puberty, GnRH is released far earlier than is normal, e.g., in patients as young as 1 year of age (Box 40.3). Although the mechanism by which the GnRH release is stimulated precocially is unknown, this results in activation of the release of pituitary gonadotropins, stimulation of the gonads, and the early development of secondary sexual characteristics. Treatment with long-lasting GnRH agonists, which initially stimulate but rapidly downregulate pituitary GnRH receptors, cause a downregulation of the reproductive axis and can halt pubertal development until the normal timing of puberty occurs. In the case of delayed puberty, the normal pubertal release of GnRH does not occur, and exogenous GnRH can be infused in a pulsatile manner to cause the stimulation of puberty in these individuals.

BOX 40.3

IDIOPATHIC CENTRAL PRECOCIOUS PUBERTY

If GnRH stimulates the pituitary in a continuous, rather than pulsatile, pattern, the pituitary rapidly downregulates its GnRH receptors. As a result, secretion of pituitary gonadotropins ceases. This finding is applied clinically to reverse pubertal development in children with idiopathic central precocious puberty, which results from an increase, of unknown origin, in GnRH drive to the pituitary prior to the normal onset time of puberty. Oral treatment with long-acting GnRH agonists, which provide a continuous GnRH stimulus to the pituitary, leads to GnRH receptor downregulation and effectively reverses pubertal development. These children are maintained on GnRH agonists until the time of normal puberty; this widely accepted method for treating precocious puberty has few side effects. When continuous exposure to GnRH is terminated, endogenous pulsatile GnRH stimulation of the pituitary occurs and onset of puberty and then normal adult reproductive function ensue.

Judy L. Cameron

Lactation and Maternal Behavior

Overview and Characteristics of the Lactotrophic Axis

The pituitary hormone prolactin is a major regulator of lactation in mammals. However, unlike the other pituitary hormones, a unique releasing hormone for prolactin has not been identified in the hypothalamus, although there is a prolactin-inhibiting factor, dopamine. Prolactin is found in pituitary cells called lactotropes. Its release into the circulatory system causes milk synthesis and secretion into the alveoli of the mammary glands in response to the suckling stimulus. Prolactin, together with oxytocin, which is involved in milk ejection, is responsible for the maintenance of lactation.

It is generally accepted that hypothalamic dopamine plays a major role in the inhibition of prolactin

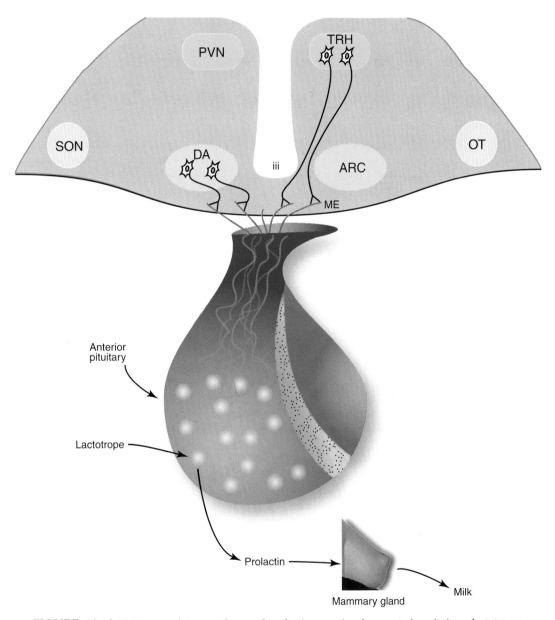

FIGURE 40.12 Major regulatory pathway of prolactin secretion from anterior pituitary lactotropes. Prolactin release is inhibited by tuberinfundibular dopaminergic neurons in the arcuate nucleus. The release of prolactin from the pituitary stimulates the mammary gland to produce and release milk. Other hypothalamic factors thought to regulate the prolactin system are also shown, although their roles are less well defined than that of dopamine. DA, dopamine; ARC, arcuate nucleus; iii, third ventricle; ME, median eminence; TRH, thyrotropin-releasing hormone; PVN, paraventricular nucleus; OT, oxytocin; SON, supraoptic nucleus.

release, and dopamine is probably the prolactin-inhibiting factor (Leong *et al.*, 1983; Fig. 40.12). Dopamine is abundant in the hypothalamus and is found in high concentrations in the median eminence, where it can be released to influence the function of the anterior pituitary gland via the portal capillary system. Evidence for a negative influence of the hypothalamus on prolactin secretion was provided by studies demonstrating that experimental isolation of the pituitary gland from the hypothalamus resulted in a large increase in basal prolactin secretion. Moreover, drugs that decrease dopamine levels in the pituitary portal circulation increase prolactin secretion, and application of exogenous dopamine can inhibit endogenous prolactin release. It was also reported that dopamine receptors are present on pituitary lactotropes, and finally, that changes in dopamine concentrations in the portal capillary system correlate with changes in prolactin release under physiological conditions.

Regarding the stimulation of prolactin release by a hypothalamic factor(s), while many molecules have been proposed, none appears to be a unique prolactin-releasing hormone, analogous to the other hypothalamic-releasing factors. TRH can stimulate prolactin release, as can GnRH-associated peptide (cleaved from the GnRH precursor peptide), but both are weak prolactin secretagogues. However, the fact that each of the other pituitary hormones has a releasing hormone, particularly the growth hormone, which is closely related to prolactin, suggests that, by analogy, prolactin should have a releasing factor as well, which has yet to be identified.

Physiological Functions of the Lactotrophic Axis

Role of prolactin in reproductive physiology and lactation   The release of prolactin varies by age, sex, and reproductive status. Levels of prolactin are higher in females than males probably due to the higher estrogen levels in females, which stimulate prolactin release. During reproductive cycles in females, prolactin levels vary, with levels being higher during the luteal than the follicular phase in humans. In rats, prolactin levels peak shortly before the preovulatory LH surge that causes ovulation, a time when estrogen levels are high. Prolactin levels also increase during pregnancy, decrease just before birth, and increase again as a response to suckling.

The role of prolactin in lactation is its best-studied and probably most important function. In all mammals, prolactin acts on the mammary gland to prepare and maintain its secretory activity. It causes the growth of ductal and lobuloalveolar tissues and causes increases in mRNA levels and translation of the milk protein, casein. Prolactin release is directly stimulated by suckling and results in the synthesis of milk. In addition, there is a relationship between suckling and the inhibition of reproductive function, as suckling can delay implantation of fetuses conceived during a postpartum estrus or cause long periods of anovulation. Prolactin may also play a role in maternal behavior, although this is not well understood.

Prolactin can influence the reproductive axis through its actions on the ovary. There, prolactin causes increases in LH receptors in the corpus luteum, progesterone synthesis by the corpus luteum, and high- and low-density lipoprotein binding in membranes of the corpus luteum. These functions may be related to uterine endometrial development and implantation of the blastocyst in rats, although it is not clear if this is the case in humans.

Other functions of prolactin include osmoregulation, primarily in fish and amphibians. The expression of prolactin receptors in kidney, gut, skin, and urinary bladder is consistent with this role. Prolactin receptors have a widespread distribution throughout the body of many species. Predictably, they are abundant in mammary gland, but they are also found in other tissues involved in reproduction, as well as the liver, kidney, gastrointestinal tract, and brain. Thus, it is likely that prolactin may play roles in these tissues that are independent of lactation or reproductive function.

Pulsatile and circadian release of prolactin   Like the other pituitary hormones, prolactin is released from the anterior pituitary in a pulsatile manner. Its release is entrained to the 24-h clock, similar to other hormones, but this appears to be a diurnal rhythm, as it is driven by sleep cues rather than the circadian clock, similar to its related hormone, growth hormone (Gore, 1998).

Structures and Properties of Prolactin and Its Receptors

Prolactin is a member of the somatotropin (growth hormone) family of molecules. Its gene shares considerable homology with the growth hormone gene. The prolactin protein is a 23- to 24-kDa protein containing three disulfide bridges, giving it a unique structure. There are multiple forms of the prolactin receptor, and its expression is widespread throughout the body. Isoforms of the prolactin receptor range in size from 329 to 591 amino acids and they have structural overlap with cytokine receptor family members. Prolactin receptors are found in the mammary gland, liver, kidney, adrenals, gonads, uterus, placenta, prostate, seminal vesicles, lymphoid tissues, intestine, choroid plexus, hypothalamus, and other tissues.

BOX 40.4

INAPPROPRIATE PROLACTIN SECRETION

Hyperprolactinemia, the elevated secretion of prolactin (more than 20 ng ml⁻¹) over a prolonged period of time, is the most common human hypothalamopituitary disorder. It has multiple causes. For example, hypothalamic hyperprolactinemia can be caused by the interruption of dopamine delivery due to stalk transection or tumors that block the connection between the basal hypothalamus and the pituitary stalk. Prolactin-secreting adenomas are a cause of pituitary hyperprolactinemia. (Most of these tumors contain DA receptors and can be treated with dopamine agonists, such as bromoergocryptine.) Many drugs that interfere with DA synthesis, reuptake, or binding lead to hypersecretion of prolactin. Thus, hyperprolactinemia and inappropriate lactation are common complications of treatment with neuroleptics, dopamine receptor blockers, antidepressants, antihypertensives, or oral contraceptives, which in various ways reduce dopaminergic suppression of prolactin secretion. The syndrome hyperprolactinemia-amenorrhea illustrates the importance of interactions between regulated prolactin secretion and the brain–pituitary–gonad axis.

In men and women, hyperprolactinemia can cause gonadal dysfunction, headaches, and visual field disturbances. Several routes of therapy have been used to restore normal prolactin levels, reduce tumor mass, reinstate normal vision, and allow normal reproductive function. Surgical resection, pituitary radiation, and dopamine agonists have been used with considerable success.

Phyllis M. Wise

Neuroanatomy of the Hypothalamic Dopamine System

The major hypothalamic population of dopamine neurons believed to regulate prolactin release are called tuberoinfundibular dopaminergic neurons, also referred to as the A12 cell group. Their perikarya lie in arcuate nuclei, and their neuroterminals project to the median eminence in the external zone, the latter projection being similar to that of other hypothalamic-releasing and -inhibiting hormones.

At the anterior pituitary gland, dopamine binds to the D2 subtype of receptor on lactotropes to cause its inhibitory effects on the synthesis and release of prolactin. The binding of dopamine to the D2 receptor causes a decrease in cAMP concentrations in lactotropes and causes an inhibition of prolactin gene transcription. Another second messenger system, the Ca^{2+}/phosphokinase C system, may also play a role in this process, although this latter mechanism is not well understood.

Prolactin release is regulated by neurotransmitters other than dopamine. The hypothalamic hormone thyrotropin-releasing hormone (TRH), the primary function of which is the regulation of the thyroid hormone axis, has also been shown to stimulate prolactin release. Another neuropeptide, vasoactive intestinal peptide (VIP), can stimulate prolactin release, and blockade of the VIP system with antisera inhibits basal prolactin secretion. GnRH-associated peptide (GAP) can inhibit prolactin release. In addition, hormones released by the posterior pituitary, such as oxytocin, are thought to regulate the prolactin system.

Disruptions in the Prolactin System

Hyperprolactinemia is the elevated secretion of prolactin (Box 40.4). This is a common human pituitary disorder and can be a result of disrupted dopamine transmission, which would normally suppress prolactin release. Hyperprolactinemia can result from pituitary adenomas that secrete prolactin. As a result of hyperprolactinemia, inappropriate lactation can occur, as can be the case with drugs that affect the dopamine system (neuroleptics, dopamine receptor blockers, antidepressants, antihypertensives, oral contraceptives).

HYPOTHALAMIC CONTROL OF SEXUAL BEHAVIOR

The control of adult sexual behavior is established very early in life, during the embryonic and early postnatal periods of development. Genetic, hormonal, and environmental factors all contribute to the development of gender-appropriate sexual behavior. For mammals, the presence of the Y chromosome plays a critical sex-determining role in the early development of the gonads (ovary or testis). Exposure to hormones produced in the fetal testis, or lack of exposure to hormones from the ovary, subsequently influences the development of the reproductive tract, as well as the central nervous system. This section reviews sexual differentiation of the reproductive system and the brain, particularly the hypothalamus, and discusses how early exposures and experiences have long-term consequences for adult behavior.

Sexual Determination of the Reproductive System

The gonad of an early embryo is *indifferent*, meaning that it has the potential to develop into a testis or ovary in response to the appropriate stimuli. Sex determination of the gonads is driven by a gene located on the Y chromosome called SRY (sex-determining region of the Y chromosome; Schafer and Goodfellow, 1996). In the presence of SRY, the bipotential gonad develops into a testis, and in the absence of SRY, an ovary develops. SRY is expressed in mammalian males, which possess a Y chromosome, or in females in which the SRY region of the Y chromosome has been translocated onto the X chromosome. Males lacking the SRY region on the Y chromosome develop ovaries and appear to be phenotypically female. Thus, SRY is necessary and sufficient for the determination of the male testis during embryonic development (Fig. 40.13; Box 40.6).

SRY is a transcription factor that binds to DNA to induce gene transcription. The downstream targets of SRY include P450 aromatase, anti-Müllerian hormone (AMH), and fra-1, a component of AP-1, another transcription factor (see Chapter 10). These first two targets are relevant to reproductive physiology and sexual development: P450 aromatase is an enzyme in the steroidogenic pathway converting testosterone to estradiol and AMH induces regression of the Müllerian ducts during male development. A role for fra-1 in sex determination is unknown, but the AP-1 site is an important one for DNA binding in many systems and mediates many pathways involved in gene activation.

The internal genitalia are not bipotential organs like the gonads, but rather the embryonic organism possesses two unipotential sets of ducts that develop into male or female organs, depending on the exposure to hormones. Thus, all mammals begin with a set of Wolffian ducts that can develop into male internal genitalia (epididymis, vas deferens, prostate) and a set of Müllerian ducts that can develop into the female internal genitalia (oviduct, uterus, upper vagina; Fig. 40.13). The sex determination of the internal genitalia is determined by two hormones: testosterone, which maintains and promotes the growth of the Wolffian ducts, and AMH, which causes the regression of the Müllerian ducts. The fetal male testis synthesizes these two hormones. Leydig cells of the immature testis produce the sex steroid hormone testosterone, which is responsible for the development of the internal genitalia. Immature Sertoli cells of the testis produce the AMH that causes Müllerian duct regression. In females, the absence of testosterone prevents maintenance of the Wolffian ducts, which regress, and the absence of AMH allows the Müllerian ducts to remain and develop into the female internal genitalia.

Finally, the external genitalia in males (penis, scrotum) and females (clitoris, lower vagina, and labia), like the gonads, are bipotential (Fig. 40.13). Instead of a genetic mechanism for sex determination as in the gonads (SRY), however, it is exposure to testosterone and its metabolite, 5α-dihydrotestosterone (DHT), produced in the testis, that causes the development of male genitalia. In the absence of testosterone, female genitalia develop.

Sexual Differentiation of the Brain

Although the most obvious targets of sex hormones during development are the reproductive tract, sex steroid hormones are released into the general circulation and can act at other targets through the body and the brain to exert potent effects. One of the major targets of sex steroid hormones during fetal development is the brain, particularly the hypothalamus (reviewed in Breedlove, 1992; Box 40.5). The brain has a widespread expression of steroid hormone receptors, including those for androgens, estrogens, and progestins, and these are particularly concentrated in the hypothalamus.

Early exposure to sex steroid hormones has permanent effects on the neuroanatomy of the brain and on subsequent sexual behaviors. Several brain regions have been shown to be particularly sensitive to sex steroid exposure, including several discrete nuclei in the preoptic area, called the sexually dimorphic nuclei, other hypothalamic regions, as well as the spinal nucleus of the bulbocavernosus (SNB), which innervates the base of the penis or clitoris. Perinatal sex steroid hormones act to alter the size of these brain regions; in general, because the fetal testis is much more active than the ovary, testicular hormones are responsible for these neuroanatomical changes. Although it might be predicted that testosterone is responsible for these effects, it is in fact estradiol that is much more potent in many of these actions in mammalian species. The mechanism is believed to involve the conversion of

BOX 40.5

SEXUAL DIFFERENTIATION OF MATING, PAIR BONDING, AND SONG IN BIRDS

In mammals the female is the homogametic (XX) sex. Most aspects of female genital and CNS development are generally thought to occur perinatally without an active endocrine stimulus, although a minority view holds that estradiol contributes actively to the differentiation of aspects of neural development in females. In avian species the male is the homogametic sex (ZZ), and, as in the case of female mammals, evidence suggests that many aspects of psychosexual differentiation occur without an endocrine stimulus. In female quail the capacity to display mounting behavior with a receptive female conspecific is normally eliminated (feminized) by the prehatching action of estradiol, presumably of ovarian origin (Adkins, 1975). When given estradiol as adults, male quail mount receptive females readily and display receptive responses to mounts by other males. Administration of estradiol to quail prior to hatching or to zebra finches after hatching feminizes mounting capacity in males, whereas administration of an aromatase inhibitor to female quail prior to hatching enhances their later mounting behavior. These results are predicted by analogy to the mammalian situation in which psychosexual differentiation occurs in the homogametic sex (i.e., females) without an active perinatal steroid signal.

An additional body of literature suggests that in male birds (which are homogametic), as in male mammals (which are heterogametic), estradiol acts shortly before or after hatching to organize male-typical patterns of mate choice (including pair bonding) and courtship song. Thus, in zebra finches, administration of estradiol (but not testosterone or DHT) to females in the weeks after hatching permanently enhances their potential to learn and perform courtship song (Gurney and Konishi, 1980). Females treated with estradiol early in life are also much more likely than normal females to form long-lasting pair bonds with other (stimulus) females. The effects of early estradiol treatment on singing behavior in female zebra finches correlated with an increase in the number of neurons in several parts of the telencephalic circuit that controls song learning and production.

Several puzzling questions remain, however, about the normal role of estradiol in the development of neural mechanisms controlling singing and pair bonding in male song birds. In the case of the song-control system, it has been difficult to duplicate the male phenotype (e.g., number of neurons in song-control nuclei) by administering estradiol to females after they have hatched. Even more puzzling is the inability of blockers of estrogen or aromatase to interfere with song-system development in male zebra finches. Likewise, such drugs failed to disrupt development of female-oriented pair bonding in male finches. Considerable uncertainty exists about the perinatal role of sex steroids in the sexual differentiation of brain mechanisms controlling song and pair bonding in male birds.

Michael J. Baum

References

Adkins, E. K. (1955). Hormonal basis of sexual differentiation in the Japanese quail. *J. Comp. Physiol. Psychol.* **89**, 61–71.

Gurney, M. E., and Konishi, M. (1980). Hormone-induced sexual differentiation of brain and behavior in zebra finches. *Science* **208**, 1380–83.

testosterone into estradiol through the P450 aromatase enzyme. This enzyme is found in the hypothalamus, as well as many other brain regions. Evidence for this was provided by studies in which the aromatization of testosterone to estradiol was blocked, which resulted in a "feminized" brain. That it is estradiol and not testosterone that is the active metabolite is also demonstrated by experiments showing that estradiol can exert similar effects of testosterone in masculinizing the brain. However, the testosterone metabolite, DHT, does not cause masculinization of several regions the central nervous system, indicating that it is not the reduction of testosterone to DHT that has masculinizing effects.

In mammals, the region of the brain that has probably been best studied for its sexual dimorphisms is the sexually dimorphic nucleus of the preoptic area (SDN-POA). This region, just rostral to the hypothalamus, is important in the regulation of male-typical sexual behavior (see later). It was reported that the SDN-POA of male rats is five to six times larger than its counterpart in females (Jacobson *et al.*, 1980). The size difference in this region between the genders relates to the prenatal/neonatal exposure to steroid hormones. Treatment of neonatal females with testosterone or its estradiol metabolite results in females with a significantly larger SDN-POA. Neonatal castra-

BOX 40.6

PSYCHOSEXUAL DIFFERENTIATION (GENDER IDENTITY AND SEXUAL ORIENTATION) IN HUMANS

Nature sometimes varies the exposure of human fetuses to sex hormones. The resultant clinical syndromes suggest that in humans, as in animals, psychosexual differentiation is organized by perinatal exposure to sex steroids. Two clinical syndromes provide parallels with animal studies showing that perinatal exposure to testosterone, which acts in part through neural conversion to estradiol, contributes to the development of male-typical patterns of sex partner preference and coital behavior.

Congenital adrenal hyperplasia is usually caused by a mutation in the gene encoding 21-hydroxylase, the enzyme that catalyzes the conversion of progesterone to cortisol in the fetal adrenal cortex. Lack of glucocorticoid and mineralocorticoid secretion leads to diagnosis soon after birth. These symptoms are treated with continuous administration of adrenal steroids. In addition to under-production of glucocorticoids and mineralocorticoids, congenital adrenal hyperplasia involves overproduction of androgens, including testosterone, which in females causes varying degrees of genital virilization. In early childhood, many of these girls have surgical reconstruction of their external genitals and are assigned a female gender role. As adults, most of these women express satisfaction with their core sexual identity and report exclusively heterosexual choices of romantic partners. Still, when compared with women matched for age and experience, women with congenital adrenal hyperplasia more often reported homosexual or bisexual romantic experience or interest (Dittman *et al.*, 1992).

Another clinical syndrome suggests that estrogenic metabolites of androgens may mediate some effects of fetal exposure to testosterone on sexual orientation. The synthetic estrogen diethylstilbestrol (DES) was prescribed to thousands of pregnant American women between 1947 and 1971 in the mistaken belief that it would reduce the incidence of spontaneous abortion. The psychosexual profile of young women exposed prenatally to DES is remarkably similar to that of women with congenital adrenal hyperplasia: Core sexual identity is typically female, and although the majority report exclusively heterosexual orientation, significantly more of these women report homosexual or bisexual orientation than matched controls.

Testicular feminizing syndrome, caused by androgen insensitivity in genetic males, is another relevant clinical syndrome. The SRY gene is normally expressed in these individuals during fetal life, leading to the differentiation of testes. In this syndrome, the Tfm gene, which encodes the androgen receptor, is mutated. Thus, testosterone and DHT cause less or none of their usual somatic and CNS effects. As a result, despite normal fetal expression of SRY and subsequent differentiation of testes, boys with Tfm mutations have female-typical external genitalia and are assigned a female gender role at birth. Breasts develop at puberty in response to estrogens formed through the peripheral aromatization of testosterone secreted by testes (which typically remain undescended in the body cavity). Typically, the core sexual identity is female, and, as adults, genetic males with Tfm mutations are attracted sexually to men. Presumably, estradiol is synthesized normally from circulating testosterone in the developing nervous system of fetuses with Tfm mutations, and estrogen receptors are present in their brains. However, male psychosexual differentiation does not occur. Nevertheless, estradiol may play a role in male psychosexual differentiation. Perhaps humans require testosterone to act through androgen receptors in the nervous system shortly after birth to complete male psychosexual differentiation begun prenatally by the action of estrogens. Absence of functional androgen receptors in individuals with Tfm gene mutations would preclude this event, leaving the Tfm male able to assume a female core identity. Also, in the absence of functional androgen receptors, female external genitalia cannot be masculinized by exogenous testosterone. This female body image is incompatible with psychosexual functioning as a male and thus may contribute to the female core identity and sexual orientation that characterizes Tfm individuals. More study of nonhuman primate models is needed to assess contributions of androgen and estrogen to psychosexual differentiation and CNS development.

Michael J. Baum

Reference

Dittmann, R. W., Kappes, M. E., and Kappes, M. H. (1992). Sexual behavior in adolescent and adult females with congenital adrenal hyperplasia. *Psychoneuroendocrinology* **17**, 153–70.

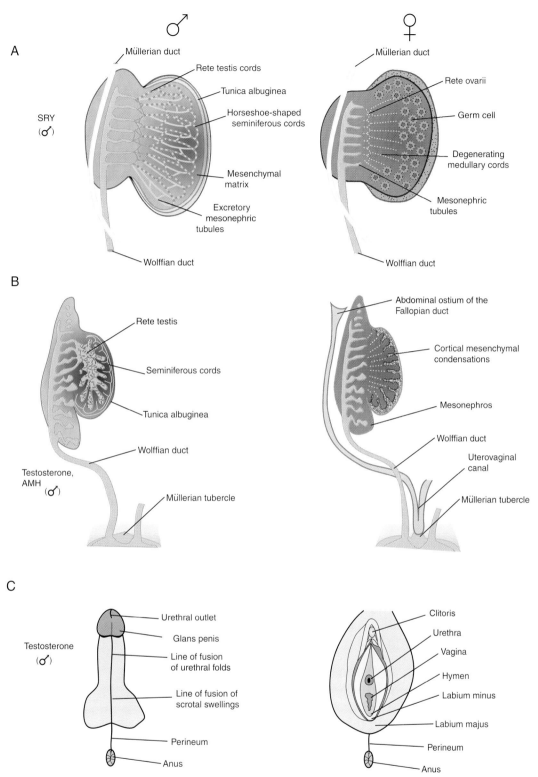

FIGURE 40.13 Sex determination of (A) gonads, (B) internal genitalia; and (C) external genitalia of males and females. (A) The presence of SRY on the Y chromosomes causes the development of the male testis, and the absence of SRY results in the development of the female ovary. (B) Testosterone and anti-Müllerian hormone (AMH) produced by the fetal testis are responsible for the development of male internal genitalia through the Wolffian duct-promoting effects of testosterone and the Müllerian duct-regressing effects of AMH. In the female, the absence of testosterone and AMH results in maintenance of the Müllerian duct and regression of the Wolffian duct. (C) Testosterone produced by the testis masculinizes male external genitalia. The lack of testosterone produced by the ovary results in female external genitalia. Modified from Johnson and Everitt (2000).

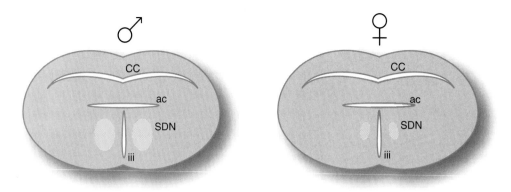

FIGURE 40.14 Schematic representation of the sexually dimorphic nucleus of the preoptic area (SDN-POA) of male (left) and female (right) rat brain, as shown in coronal sections. The SDN-POA can be five to six times larger in the brain of a male than a female. iii, third ventricle; ac, anterior commissure; cc, corpus callosum. Modified from Jacobson *et al.* (1980).

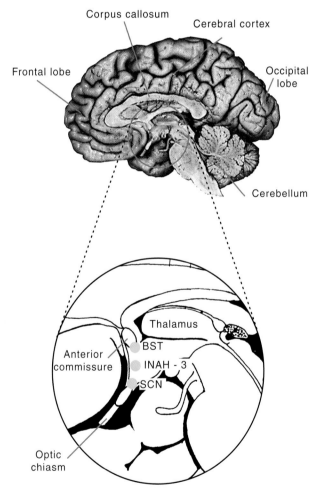

tion of males causes a decrease in the size of the SDN-POA (Fig. 40.14).

Another brain region that has been studied for its sexual dimorphism is the SNB. This region innervates the muscles of the bulbocavernosus and levator ani, which are attached to the base of the penis or the clitoris. At birth, these muscles are innervated approximately equally in males and females, but shortly thereafter, this innervation atrophies in females. Again, this is dependent on exposure to neonatal testosterone, as treatment with testosterone maintains this projection in females, and castration reduces this pathway in males (Breedlove, 1992).

The issue of sexual dimorphism in the human brain is quite controversial. Differences in the size and/or shape of the corpus callosum between men and women have been reported. Homologues to the sexually dimorphic nuclei of rats also appear to be dimorphic in humans. For example, Onuf's nucleus, which is homologous to the rat SNB, has more motor neurons in men than in women. In the human anterior hypothalamus, roughly equivalent to the rat SDN-POA, there are sex differences in the size of some of the interstitial nuclei, called INAH (for interstitial nuclei of the anterior hypothalamus), with men having larger volumes than women of some of these nuclei. This issue is particularly controversial, as it has been reported that the INAH-3 of homosexual men is intermediate in size between that of heterosexual men (having the largest INAH-3) and that of women (having the smallest INAH-3). However, further research is needed to confirm these results and to determine the implications of different sized INAHs on sexual behavior and identity (Fig. 40.15; Box 40.7).

FIGURE 40.15 Brain structures for which published data suggest that volume is sexually allomorphic [e.g., anterior commissure, central region of bed nuclei of the stria terminalis (BST), and third interstitial nucleus of the anterior hypothalamus (INAH-3)], differs in heterosexual men versus homosexual men [anterior commissure, INAH-3, suprachiasmatic nucleus (SCN)], or differs in men with male versus female gender identities (BST).

BOX 40.7

SEXUAL ALLOMORPHISMS IN HUMAN BRAIN STRUCTURE: CORRELATIONS BETWEEN SEXUAL ORIENTATION AND GENDER IDENTITY

Animal studies linking male psychosexual function to the integrity of medial preoptic neurons and neuronal inputs to them led several researchers to examine whether the human preoptic region also contains sexual allomorphisms. Despite considerable controversy about the number and nature of sex differences in the human brain, there is some agreement about the existence of a series of nuclei (interstitial nuclei 1–4 of the anterior hypothalamus; INAH) in the human hypothalamus. One of these nuclei (INAH-3) appears to be larger in heterosexual men than in women. LeVay (1991) also reported that INAH-3 was significantly smaller (similar to that of heterosexual women) in homosexual men than in heterosexual men (Fig. 40.15).

This report generated considerable controversy because many of the homosexual subjects included in the study had died of AIDS; thus, their neuronal morphology might have been affected by HIV infection. Controversy also arose regarding the openly political agenda of the author, who seeks legal sanctioning of same-sex relationships. Another report (Zhou *et al.*, 1995) links core gender identity with the volume of a central region of bed nuclei of the stria terminalis. In this study of bed nuclei, the volume shown with immunohistological staining for vasoactive intestinal polypeptide (VIP) was significantly greater in heterosexual men than in women. Furthermore, bed nuclei volume was significantly smaller (similar to women) in male to female transsexuals. These men had assumed female gender identity, usually with the aid of genital reconstructive surgery and estrogen therapy, at some point well prior to death and autopsy. Interestingly, bed nuclei volume was similar in hetero- and homosexual men whose gender identity was male.

Replication is critical to all scientific endeavors; however, replication is particularly difficult when postmortem human tissue is involved. Even if these studies were replicated, they could only correlate psychosexual orientation and sexually allomorphic morphology of the human hypothalamus. Imaging methods with high anatomic resolution will make it easier to rigorously address the question of how brain morphology and function differ between sexes and among people with different gender identities and sexual partner preferences.

Michael J. Baum

References

LeVay, S. (1991). A Difference in hypothalamic structure between heterosexual and homosexual men. *Science* **253**, 1034–37.

Zhou, J.-N., Hofman, M. A., Gooren, L. J. G., and Swaab, D. F. (1995). A sex difference in the human brain and its relation to transsexuality. *Nature* (*Lond.*) **378**, 68–70.

Hormones and Sexual Behavior

The exposure of neonatal animals to hormones has permanent effects on the development of sexual behavior at the attainment of adult reproductive function. Often, the permanent effects of neonatal hormones on the brain are referred to as "organizational." These effects are not observed until after puberty, when subsequent exposure to gonadal hormones causes the gender-appropriate behavior. The manifestation of these sex behaviors in adulthood by gonadal steroids is called the "activational" effects of hormones.

There are clearly differences in the sexual behavior of males and females. For example, copulatory behavior in male rodents comprises mounts of the female, intromissions, and ejaculations. A receptive female rodent will respond to male copulatory behaviors with a lordosis response, characterized by a rigid stance and an arched back. These behaviors are driven in large part by the responses of hypothalamic nuclei to hormones, and the nature of the adult behavior is determined by the prenatal/neonatal exposure to hormones. Thus, the hypothalamus of adult males, which has been masculinized neonatally by testicular testosterone (aromatized to estradiol), will respond to the testosterone produced by the adult gonad (reduced to DHT) by causing the typical male pattern of sexual behavior. In contrast, the female hypothalamus, which is not exposed neonatally to sufficient levels of ovarian hormones to cause masculinization of her brain, responds to estrogen produced by her adult ovary with the appropriate female lordotic response. Moreover, a normal adult male will not express lordosis behavior in response to exogenous estrogen, nor will a normal adult female exhibit male-typical sexual behaviors in response to exogenous testosterone, as their brains have not been organized in such as way as to produce a gender-inappropriate response in adulthood. However, a neonatally castrated male can respond to estradiol in adulthood with the expression of lordosis behavior, as his brain was not masculinized neonatally. Similarly, a female who was exposed to exogenous testosterone or estradiol neonatally can exhibit male-typical sexual behaviors as an adult if she is treated with testosterone.

It is necessary to distinguish between masculinizing and defeminizing effects of hormones in females, and the feminizing and demasculinizing effects of hormones in males. As mentioned earlier, female sexual behavior is characterized most overtly by lordosis. The prevention of this behavior by exposure to sex steroid hormones neonatally would be an example of a defeminizing effect. In contrast, a female whose brain has been exposed to steroid hormones at birth, and in adulthood is injected with testosterone, may exhibit male-typical sexual behavior such as mounting another female. This is an example of the masculinizing effects of hormones. For males, the feminizing effects of hormones could be seen in a neonatally castrated male who, as an adult, is exposed to female sex steroids and responds with lordosis behavior in response to the mounting by another male. Demasculinization would occur in this male if, as an adult, he fails to perform normal male-typical sexual behavior (mounts, intromissions, ejaculations) in response to a female. Thus, hormones can cause both of these effects in males or females, depending on the time and duration of exposure.

The regions of the brain responsible for sex behavior differ between males and females. Sexual behavior in males is largely driven by the preoptic area (POA) of the brain, just rostral to the hypothalamus. Lesions of the POA in males cause the loss of sexual behavior, and testosterone implanted into the POA can induce sex behavior. In females, the primary hypothalamic site regulating receptive sexual behavior is the ventromedial nucleus of the hypothalamus (VMH). Estrogen, followed by progesterone, facilitates the expression of the lordosis reflex and coordinates the timing of female receptivity with the preovulatory GnRH/LH surge that causes ovulation. Thus, the timing of mating behavior and ovulation is coordinated by the release of ovarian steroid hormones. During the reproductive cycle, circulating estrogen levels increase, and estrogen binds to its receptor in the VMH to cause the transcription of several genes, including that of the progesterone receptor. Then, progesterone levels rise and can bind to its

newly induced receptor in the VMH. This causes proceptive behaviors in females and facilitates the lordosis response. Females that have been androgenized neonatally have a large reduction in the lordosis response to exogenous estrogen and progesterone replacement.

Pheromones, the Vomeronasal Organ, and Sexual Behavior

Reproductive behavior in many species involves signals from pheromones, which are chemical signals used for communication between animals (Meredith, 1998). Pheromones are chemical messengers that are typically produced by specialized glands, such as the sebaceous glands in the flanks of animals, or released in urine or vaginal fluid. They are released not into the body but rather into the external environment to convey information about the physiological status of the animal to other individuals.

The ability to detect pheromones involves the vomeronasal organ and its projections to the accessory olfactory bulbs. Cells in these latter regions contact a number of brain regions, including the medial amygdala, cortical regions, and the bed nucleus of the stria terminalis, all of which are implicated in sex behavior. These regions in turn project to the hypothalamus and preoptic area. Thus, information from pheromones about mating status can be conveyed to parts of the brain coordinating reproductive physiology and behavior.

In most species, information about reproductive status, dominance status, or other social cues can be conveyed by pheromones, although it is still controversial whether humans have a vomeronasal organ and/or can sense pheromones. Those organisms using pheromones as chemosensory cues have developed mechanisms for depositing or releasing pheromones to "advertise" sexual competency or receptivity in order to attract a mate or to mark territory to protect food supplies, mates, or offspring. Pheromones and the systems that mediate their effects play broader roles than those involved in reproductive physiology and behavior. Pheromones can dramatically influence the timing of sexual development and function. In female mice, exposure to male urinary pheromones accelerates the timing of pubertal development. Males respond to female urinary pheromones with sharp increases in luteinizing hormone release. It has also been reported that pheromones can coordinate the timing of reproductive cycles, even in humans, although the mechanisms and functions of these pheromones are still controversial and poorly understood. Nevertheless, it is clear that pheromones play important roles in coordinating physiology and behavior.

References

Behncken, S. N., and Waters, M. J. (1999). Molecular recognition events involved in the activation of the growth hormone receptor by growth hormone. *J. Mol. Recogn.* **12**, 355–362.

Breedlove, S. M. (1992). Sexual dimorphism in the vertebrate nervous system. *J. Neurosci.* **12**, 4133–4142.

DeSouza, E. B. (1987). Corticotropin-releasing factor receptors in the rat central nervous system: Characterization and regional distribution. *J. Neurosci.* **7**, 88–100.

Gershengorn, M. C. (1993). Thyrotropin-releasing hormone receptor: Cloning and regulation of its expression. *Recent Progr. Horm. Res.* **48**, 341–363.

Gore, A. C. (1998). Circadian rhythms during aging. *In* "Functional Endocrinology of Aging" (C. V. Mobbs and P. R. Hof, eds.), pp. 127–165. Karger, Basel.

Gore, A. C. (2002). "GnRH: The Master Molecule of Reproduction." Kluwer Academic Publishers.

Graves, P. N., and Davies, T. F. (2000). New insights into the thyroid-stimulating hormone receptor: The major antigen of Graves' disease. *Endocrinol. Metabol. Clin. North Am.* **29**, 267–286.

Harris, G. W. (1971). Humours and hormones. *J. Endocrinol.* **53**, ii–xxiii.

Jacobson, C. D., Shryne, J. E., Shapiro, F., and Gorski, R. A. (1980). Ontogeny of the sexually dimorphic nucleus of the preoptic area. *J. Comp. Neurol.* **193**, 541–548.

Johnson, M. H., and Everitt, B. J. (2000). "Essential Reproduction." Blackwell Science.

Lechan, R. M., Qi, Y., Jackson, I. M. D., and Mahdavi, V. (1994). Identification of thyroid hormone receptor isoforms in thyrotropin-releasing hormone neurons of the hypothalamic paraventricular nucleus. *Endocrinology* **135**, 92–100.

Leong, D. A., Frawley, L. S., and Neill, J. D. (1983). Neuroendocrine control of prolactin secretion. *Annu. Rev. Physiol.* **45**, 109–127.

Mayo, K. E., Godfrey, P. A., Suhr, S. T., Kulik, D. J., and Rahal, J. O. (1995). Growth hormone-releasing hormone: Synthesis and signaling. *Recent Progr. Horm. Res.* **50**, 35–73.

Meredith, M. (1998). Vomeronasal, olfactory, hormonal convergence in the brain: Cooperation or coincidence? *Ann. N. Y. Acad. Sci.* **855**, 349–361.

Morimoto, M., Morita, N., Ozawa, H., Yokoyama, K., and Kawata, M. (1996). Distribution of glucocorticoid receptor immunoreactivity and mRNA in the rat brain: an immunohistochemical and in situ hybridization study. *Neurosci. Res.* **26**, 235–269.

Naville, D., Penhoat, A., Durant, P., and Begeot, M. (1999). Three steroidogenic factor-1 binding elements are required for constitutive and cAMP-regulated expression of the human adrenocorticotropin receptor gene. *Biochem. Biophys. Res. Commun.* **255**, 28–33.

O'Connor, T. M., O'Halloran, D. J., and Shanahan, F. (2000). The stress response and the hypothalamic-pituitary-adrenal axis: From molecule to melancholia. *Q. J. Med.* **93**, 323–333.

Plant, T. M. (1988). Puberty in primates. *In* "The Physiology of Reproduction" (E. Knobil and J. Neill, eds.), pp. 1763–1788. Raven Press, New York.

Schafer, A. J., and Goodfellow, P. N. (1996). Sex determination in humans. *BioEssays* **18**, 955–963.

Sealfon, S. C., Weinstein, H., and Millar, R. P. (1997). Molecular mechanisms of ligand interaction with the gonadotropin-releasing hormone receptor. *Endocr. Rev.* **18**, 180–205.

Segerson, T. P., Kauer, J., Wolfe, H., Mobitker, H., Wu, P., Jackson, I. M. D., and Lechan, R. M. (1987). Thyroid hormone regulates TRH biosynthesis in the paraventricular nucleus of the rat hypothalamus. *Science* **238**, 78–80.

Szkudlinski, M. W., Grossmann, M., Leitolf, H., and Weintraub, B. D. (2000). Human thyroid-stimulating hormone: Structure-function analysis. *Methods* **21**, 67–81.

Yamada, M., Radovick, S., Wondisford, F. E., Nakayama, Y., Weintraub, B. D., and Wilber, J. F. (1990). Cloning and structure of human genomic DNA and hypothalamic cDNA encoding human preprothyrotropin-releasing hormone. *Mol. Endocrinol.* **4**, 551–556.

Andrea C. Gore and James L. Roberts

41

Circadian Timing

In its elliptic course around the sun, the earth revolves on its axis and, at any given moment, half the earth is in light and half is in darkness. This inexorable progression of light and dark, day and night, is the most pervasive recurring stimulus in our environment and is the basis for a fundamental adaptation of living organisms—circadian rhythms (circadian is derived from circa,-about,-and diem,-day). These rhythms are expressed in nearly all living organisms, from bacteria to humans, and there are references to daily rhythms in the earliest descriptions of life. Although they were assumed to represent a passive response to the solar light–dark cycle, we now know that circadian rhythms are genetically determined, endogenously generated adaptations. In the 1729, French geologist deMairan provided the first clear description of a fundamental property of circadian rhythms, their persistence under constant conditions. Observing plants kept in a dark room, he recorded rhythmic leaf movements that continued with a daily periodicity in the absence of a light–dark cycle. Progress in understanding circadian rhythms progressed slowly until the last century, and major advances in the analysis of circadian biology have occurred since the mid-1950s.

CIRCADIAN RHYTHMS ARE A FUNDAMENTAL ADAPTATION OF LIVING ORGANISMS

Circadian rhythms probably are the most common behavioral adaptation of living organisms. With the evolution of nervous systems to coordinate the adaptation of animals, rest–activity cycles were placed under neural control. In mammals, many behavioral

and physiological functions exhibit circadian rhythms (Fig. 41.1) (Pittendrigh, 1993; Aschoff, 1965), including the sleep–wake cycle and attendant rhythms in psychomotor performance, memory and sensory perception, and a variety of physiological functions, including autonomic regulation, secretion of hormones, and regulation of core body temperature.

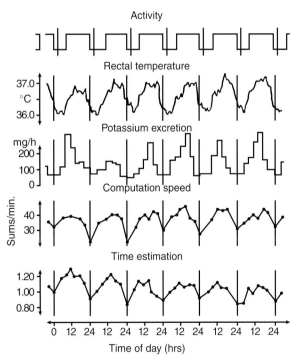

FIGURE 41.1 Daily rhythms in rest–activity, body temperature, potassium excretion, computation speed (number of computations performed per minute), and time estimation (accuracy with which short intervals of time are assessed). From Wever (1974) with permission.

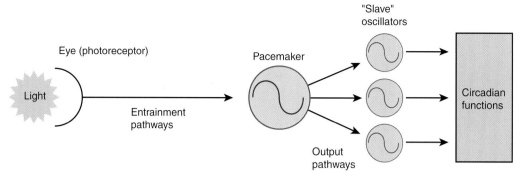

FIGURE 41.2 Overview of the basic organization of the circadian timing system (CTS). The control feature of the CTS is the circadian pacemaker. Information from photoreceptors is conveyed by entrainment pathways to the pacemaker. The pacemaker has a rhythmic output that drives "slave" oscillators, which control functions that exhibit circadian regulation.

Circadian rhythms have three principal properties. They are normally entrained to the light–dark cycle with a period of 24 h and a stable phase relationship to the timing of the solar cycle. In addition, as noted earlier, circadian rhythms persist in the absence of a light–dark cycle with a free-running period that differs slightly from 24 h. These properties require that circadian rhythms be generated and regulated by a system that is made up of three components: (1) pacemakers, (2) photoreceptors and photoreceptor input to the pacemakers, and (3) output from the pacemakers to organismal functions under circadian control (Fig. 41.2). These components may all be represented in one cell, as in prokaryotes, or they may be specialized system functions (see later). Circadian rhythms are also temperature compensated; i. e., they show minor changes in period length in response to changes in external, or internal, temperature, a property quite important to poikilothermic animals.

Circadian timing presents a particularly interesting challenge to the neuroscientist. Circadian function is inherited and, hence, established by gene expression. This allows circadian rhythms to be studied at a molecular level. Data demonstrate that the molecular basis of circadian function in virtually all organisms is an autoregulatory feedback loop of gene transcription and translation with feedback by the gene products to control transcription. The output of this process in neuronal circadian oscillators is the regulation of clock-controlled genes, which appear to regulate membrane potential and, hence, firing rate in neurons. An assembly of neuronal oscillators is coupled by synaptic interaction to become a pacemaker, and the pacemaker controls effector systems through efferent connections as part of a neural system that functions to provide circadian timing. The principal output of the circadian system in mammals is the sleep–wake cycle. In this sense, the major func-

tion of the circadian system is the control of behavioral state. Specifically, the circadian system provides a temporal organization of behavioral state to maximize the effectiveness of adaptive waking behavior. Thus, circadian timing provides a nearly unique situation in which a specialized function of the nervous system can be studied at the molecular, cellular, neural system, and behavioral levels of organization. This chapter begins with a description of the molecular basis of circadian function, outlines the organization of a mammalian circadian timing system, describes some variations in the system among vertebrates, and introduces the subject of disorders of circadian timing.

CIRCADIAN TIMING IS INHERITED

Circadian timing in plants and animals is an inherited adaptation and, as such, is determined genetically. The discovery of clock mutants in *Drosophila* (fruit fly) by Ronald Konopka and in *Neurospora* (bread mold) by Jerry Feldman provided the foundation for most of our understanding of the molecular mechanisms of circadian function. In *Drosophila* and *Neurospora*, the principal mutants have altered free-running periods. For example, in *Drosophila*, the affected flies are called *per* mutants (*per* for period). *Neurospora* mutants are designated *frq* mutants (*frq* for frequency) and express a variety of free-run phenotypes. The extensive knowledge of *Drosophila* and *Neurospora* genetics, coupled with the technology of modern molecular biology, has enabled rapid progress to be made in unraveling the molecular mechanisms of circadian function and, although some differences exist between the organisms, the fundamental molecular mechanisms appear similar (Loros and Dunlap, 2001; Williams and Sehgal, 2001; Allada *et al.*, 2001; Reppert and Weaver, 2001). A number of recent studies on mammals indicate that the basic molecular mechanism, an autoregulatory feedback loop, is conserved. Five proteins, FRQ in *Neurospora* and PER, TIM, CLK (clock), and CYC (cycle) in *Drosophila*, have been identified as candidate clock components and tested against the criteria for clock components: (1) the amount, or activity, of the component should cycle with an appropriate period; (2) the phase of the rhythm of the component must be reset by the light–dark cycle, and experimentally induced changes in the amount of the component should reset overt rhythms; (3) loss or prevention of the rhythm of the component should result in loss of overt rhythms; and (4) mutations affecting the component should affect canonical clock properties, free-running period (*Tau*), and temperature compensation, and a null mutation should abolish rhythmicity. FRQ, PER, TIM, CLK, and CYC appear to meet these criteria, although there is not agreement that each meets all criteria. We describe the current understanding of molecular mechanisms of clock function in *Drosophila* as an example.

The *Drosophila* Clock Controlling the Rest–Activity Rhythm Is Neural

The *per* gene was the first potential clock component to be identified and cloned. PER protein and *per* mRNA both show a circadian oscillation (Figs. 41.3A and 3B). The peak in *per* mRNA precedes that in PER protein. The *per* gene normally is expressed in a number of tissues, the eye, brain (in neurons and glia), gut, and reproductive system. However, the rest–activity rhythm (flies are active during the day and inactive at night) is dependent on lateral neurons of the head. Restricted expression of *per* in these neurons drives the behavioral rhythm, the *per* gene restores rhythmic behavior to *per0* flies when the gene is expressed rhythmically only in the head, flies that lack the lateral neurons (a mutant called "*disco*") are arrhythmic, ablation of lateral neurons with targeted cell death genes produces significant loss of rhythmicity, and loss of peptide-produced lateral neurons results in loss of the rhythm. Thus, rhythmic behavior in *Drosophila* appears to depend on rhythmic expression of the *per* gene in neurons of the fly brain. Another mutant, timeless, is critical to molecular clock mechanisms. Like *per0* flies, *tim0* flies are behaviorally arrhythmic and have no rhythmic *per* gene expression. In *tim0* flies, the PER protein fails to localize to the nucleus, suggesting that the *tim* mutation blocks the entry of the PER protein into the nucleus and thus blocks the feedback regulation of *per*.

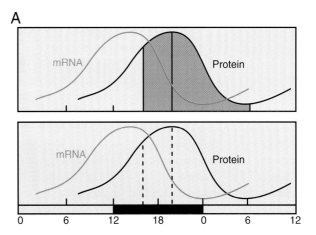

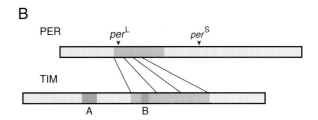

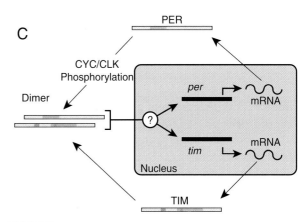

FIGURE 41.3 Features of *per–tim* interactions. (A) Profiles of PER and TIM mRNA and protein levels across a light (open bar) – dark (filled bar) cycle. The shaded area shows when PER–TIM heterodimers are present in the nucleus. (B) Structures of PER and TIM proteins. The connecting lines indicate areas of each protein thought to be involved in PER–TIM dimerization. A, acidic region; B, basic region. (C) Interdependent negative feedback control loops of per and tim. See text for description. From Reppert and Sauman (1995).

PER and TIM Interact to Provide Feedback Regulation of Clock Function

The *tim* gene encodes a protein that has no homology to *per*. Both *per* and *tim* lack a recognizable DNA-binding motif. However, PER contains a PAS dimerization domain through which PER interacts with TIM. Transcription of both genes begins in the early part of the day, and peak levels of both mRNAs are expressed from the end of the day to the beginning of the night. The two proteins accumulate in the cytoplasm and form a heterodimer that enters the nucleus to bind to the transcription factors, CYC and CLK (Fig. 41.3C). This interaction prevents CYC/CLK from binding to E-box sequences in the *per* and *tim* promoters. PER and TIM are degraded in the late night and early morning, a process in which phosphorylation plays an important role, and transcription of *per* and *tim* is initiated again. The molecular basis of entrainment appears to depend on light effects on the concentration of clock proteins (Klein *et al.*, 1991). One example is the degradation of TIM caused by light. When flies are kept in a constant environment, a light pulse between hours 2 and 10 of the circadian day (CT2 and CT10) has no effect on rhythmicity because TIM is absent during these hours. Because *per* and *tim* are transcribed during this time, PER and TIM normally are produced late in subjective day. Light, however, degrades TIM rapidly, and the protein must reaccumulate after translation from abundant tim RNA. Consequently, production of the PER–TIM heterodimer is delayed. Thus, no heterodimer enters the nucleus to suppress *per* and *tim* transcription, and a phase delay results. Later in the circadian day, CT18-CT0, a pulse of light will decrease peak TIM levels, resulting in an advance of transcription of per and tim and, hence, a phase advance. Thus, light causes a unidirectional biochemical effect beginning with degradation of TIM that results in phase delay, phase advance, or no phase change in response to light as occurs in the dead zone of the phase response curve during subjective day.

One of the important issues in understanding the molecular regulation of circadian function that has not been explored extensively is identifying genes under clock control and the mechanisms through which they are controlled.

Mammalian Clocks Are Similar but More Complex

Since the mid-1990s there has been a rapid extension of understanding of the molecular basis of circadian function to mammals. The fundamental basis of clock function in mammals is very similar to that in other species, an autoregulatory feedback loop with clock proteins regulating their own production. The situation is more complex in that there are more clock proteins, including three separate Per proteins [mPER1-3, two cryptochrome proteins (mCRY1, 2)], CLK interacts with another protein, Bmal, and a functional mammalian homologue of TIM has not been

found. The way in which the molecular components of the mammalian clock function remains to be established.

Summary

Circadian function is inherited. It is based on a highly conserved mechanism made up of an autoregulatory feedback loop of clock gene transcription, protein formation, and translocation of the proteins to the nucleus to regulate gene expression.

CIRCADIAN TIMING IN ANIMALS IS A FUNCTION OF THE NERVOUS SYSTEM

Generation of circadian rhythms is a regulatory function of the nervous system. It is mediated by the circadian timing system (CTS), a specific set of neural structures that establish a temporal organization of physiological processes and behaviors into precise 24-h patterns. As noted earlier, the fundamental properties of circadian rhythms, endogenous generation and entrainment, require that the CTS have at least three components: (1) photoreceptors and visual pathways that transduce photic entraining information, (2) pacemakers that generate a circadian signal, and (3) output pathways that couple the pacemaker to effector systems (Fig. 41.2).

Animals have evolved two different patterns of circadian timing for organizing behavior into cycles of rest and activity. In animals in which vision has evolved as the primary sense, activity typically occurs during the day, when vision best serves adaptation, and rest occurs at night. Such animals are called diurnal. In animals in which audition and olfaction dominate perception of the environment, activity typically occurs at night and rest occurs during the day, a pattern called nocturnal. In each case, the temporal order of behavior has evolved so that activity and rest occur when the dominant senses can best aid feeding and reproducing, as well as avoidance of predators. These patterns of behavior are integrated with a number of temporally organized physiological processes that further promote successful adaptive behavior. In addition, circadian timing provides the basis for successful reproduction in many mammals.

Circadian Timing Is Predominantly a Nervous System Function

The systematic study of circadian rhythms began in the first half of this century with observations of a wide variety of rhythms in diverse organisms. Studies in the 1950s and 1960s describing fundamental features of animal rhythms firmly established that the rhythms are generated by endogenous pacemakers, or clocks. This work led to the discovery of neural clocks and to the elucidation and analysis of a circadian timing system, a set of central nervous system (CNS) structures dedicated to circadian regulation. Many individuals contributed to these advances in our understanding of circadian rhythms. For example, the work of Colin

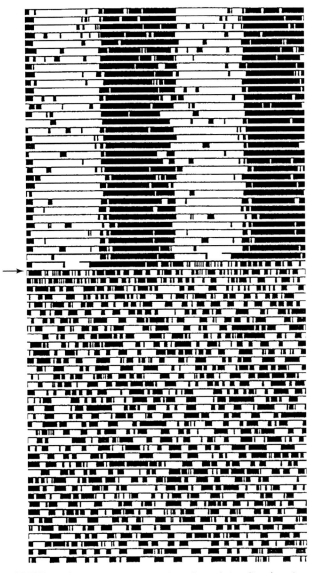

FIGURE 41.4 SCN ablation results in loss of circadian function. This is a record of activity of an albino rat maintained in a light–dark cycle. From the top of the record to the arrow, the animal exhibits a normal rhythm of activity, indicated by dark areas. The record is double plotted, which means that each line shows the preceding day and the new day to ease evaluation of the record. At the arrow, a bilateral SCN lesion was performed. Activity is distributed randomly thereafter, meaning circadian organization of rest–activity has been lost.

Pittendrigh (1993) and Jurgen Aschoff (1965) provided fundamental insights in both animals and humans. After circadian regulation was identified as a CNS function in mammals, Curt Richter, another early investigator of circadian rhythms, concluded that a circadian pacemaker controlling rest–activity cycles was likely to be located in the anterior hypothalamus.

Another important line of investigation in this era was initiated by the identification and characterization of the pineal hormone melatonin by Aaron Lerner and the demonstration of the synthetic pathways for melatonin by Julius Axelrod. Melatonin is synthesized and secreted in a circadian pattern. To identify the visual pathways that controlled the synthesis of pineal melatonin and the fluctuating pineal content of the melatonin precursor serotonin, Robert Moore and collaborators selectively ablated visual pathways until all known pathways leaving the optic chiasm had been transected. Surprisingly, the animals were blind and had no reflex responses to light but retained normal circadian entrainment. This failure to identify an entrainment pathway among the known visual pathways led to experiments that demonstrated a direct projection from the retina to the suprachiasmatic nucleus (SCN) of the hypothalamus. Transection of the retinohypothalamic tract (RHT) at its entry into the SCN abolishes entrainment without affecting other visual functions, indicating that the RHT is necessary for entrainment. Identification of the SCN as the site of RHT termination led directly to an initial test of the hypothesis that the SCN is the circadian pacemaker. Ablation of the SCN results in a loss of circadian rhythms (Fig. 41.4), indicating that the SCN plays an important role in circadian function (Klein *et al.*, 1991; Takahashi *et al.*, 2001; van Esseveldt *et al.*, 2000; Moore, 1996).

The demonstration of the RHT and the dramatic effects of SCN ablation were the introductory events to a remarkable period of intense investigation of the mammalian circadian timing system. There have also been striking advances in our understanding of the organization of the circadian timing system in invertebrates and nonmammalian vertebrates. In the sections that follow we consider the neural mechanisms of pacemaker organization, function, entrainment, and coupling to effector systems.

Summary

The circadian timing system is composed of central neural elements that function to provide a precise temporal organization of physiological and endocrine processes and behavior. Critical components include photoreceptors and visual pathways (e.g., retinohypothalamic tract), circadian "clocks" or pacemakers (such as the suprachiasmatic nucleus), and output pathways, which couple pacemakers to effectors.

THE SUPRACHIASMATIC NUCLEUS IS THE DOMINANT CIRCADIAN PACEMAKER

In mammals, the SCN is a paired nucleus of small neurons lying above the optic chiasm on each side of the third ventricle (Fig. 41.5). Four lines of evidence

support the view that the SCN is the dominant mammalian circadian pacemaker. First, as noted earlier, the SCN is the site of termination of an entraining pathway—the RHT—and SCN ablation abolishes circadian rhythms. Second, lesions of the SCN typically alter only the temporal organization of a function; the function itself is not changed. Third, isolation of the SCN, either *in vivo* or *in vitro*, does not alter its ability to generate a circadian signal. Finally, transplantation of a fetal SCN into the third ventricle of arrhythmic hosts with SCN lesions restores circadian rhythm with a period that reflects donor, not host, rhythm (Klein *et al.*, 1991; Takahashi *et al.*, 2001; van Esseveldt *et al.*, 2000).

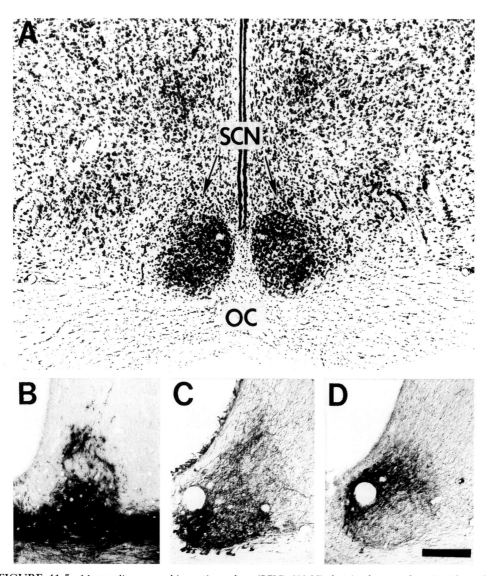

FIGURE 41.5   Mammalian suprachiasmatic nucleus (SCN). (A) Nissl-stained, coronal section through the anterior hypothalamus and optic chiasm (OC) of the rat. The SCN is two compact cell groups lying above the optic chiasm and lateral to the third ventricle, the slit-like structure in the center of the figure. (B) Photomicrograph through the same level of the SCN showing the distribution of the retinohypothalamic tract, the darkly stained material. (C) Photomicrograph showing vasoactive intestinal polypeptide-containing neurons in the ventrolateral SCN. (D) Vasopressin-containing neurons in the dorsomedial SCN.

The SCN Has Two Distinct Divisions

The SCN is made up of two distinct subdivisions, which differ in neuronal morphology, peptide phenotype, and connections. The central region of the SCN lying immediately above the optic chiasm is designated the "core" and it is surrounded by the second subdivision, the "shell." In Golgi material, neurons in the shell are quite small and have sparse dendritic arbors, whereas neurons in the core are larger and have more extensive dendritic arbors, which often extend beyond the apparent boundary of the SCN. The majority of shell neurons contain arginine vasopressin (AVP) colocalized with the inhibitory transmitter, GABA. Afferents to the SCN shell arise predominantly from the brain stem, hypothalamus, basal forebrain, and limbic cortex. Core neurons, however, typically contain vasoactive intestinal polypeptide (VIP) or gastrin-releasing peptide (GRP) colocalized with GABA. Visual afferents, the primary retinal input from the RHT and secondary visual projections from the intergeniculate leaflet (IGL) of the lateral geniculate complex, terminate in the core. Another important input to the core is from the serotoninergic neurons of the midbrain raphe nuclei (Fig. 41.6). These SCN subdivisions are found in all mammals and there is evidence that they can function as independent pacemakers (Shinohara *et al.*, 1995).

SCN Neurons Are Circadian Oscillators

There are two ways SCN neurons might be organized to form a pacemaker: (1) individual neurons are born as circadian oscillators and are subsequently coupled by neural connections to form a pacemaker and (2) pacemaker function emerges from the interaction of neurons that are rhythmic with periods of less than 24 h (ultradian rhythm). Current data strongly support the view that individual SCN neurons are born as circadian oscillators and are coupled to make a pacemaker. Individual SCN neurons maintained in cell culture each have a rhythmic firing rate that approximates 24 h. Variations in the period of SCN neurons in culture are greater than would be expected from the variations in free-running rhythms. Periods close to 24 h are observed most commonly. The coupling of individual oscillators is critical to the function of the SCN as a pacemaker. Recent work indicates that GABA is important to the process of synchronization of SCN neurons. Evidence also suggests that gap junctions and neural cell adhesion molecules participate in the coupling of SCN neurons that underlie

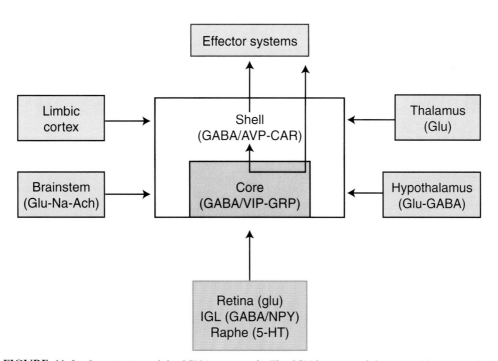

FIGURE 41.6 Organization of the SCN in mammals. The SCN has two subdivisions: (1) a core, which contains neurons in which the vasoactive intestinal polypeptide (VIP) or gastrin-releasing peptide (GRP) is colocalized with GABA; and (2) a shell in which arginine vasopressin (AVP) or calretinin (CAR) is colocalized with GABA. The sides and bottom of the figure show the pattern of distribution of entrainment pathways, Transmitters are shown for each pathway. Glu, glutamate; 5HT, serotonin; ACH, acetylcholine; NA, noradrenaline; NPY, neuropeptide Y. SCN output is shown at the top of the figure.

pacemaker function and that these factors all interact to provide the neuronal coupling that produces an SCN pacemaker that has a reliable and uniform output that can be entrained to the solar cycle (Reppert and Weaver, 2001).

In Fetal Life the SCN Pacemaker Is Entrained to Maternal Rhythms

Overt circadian rhythms are typically expressed in mammals after birth. The SCN in the rat is formed in late gestation, between embryonic days 14 and 17 (E14–E17; gestation in the rat is 21 days). Circadian function in the SCN is first expressed at E19 as an intrinsic rhythm in glucose utilization, which is entrained to maternal rhythms. Maternal rhythmicity is not necessary, however, for the development of SCN function. When the SCN of pregnant females is ablated early in gestation, before the formation of SCN neurons in the fetus, development of the fetal SCN progresses normally. In this situation, however, individual pups develop rhythms independent of one another and of their environment. The signal for entrainment to maternal rhythms is not known with certainty, but melatonin appears to play an important role.

Circadian Oscillators Occur Widely in Neural and Nonneural Tissues

As discussed in a later section, the avian circadian system is more complex than that of mammals, and in some birds, the SCN, pineal gland and eye, or combinations of these structures may be primary pacemakers controlling circadian function. The evidence for non-SCN pacemakers in mammals, however, was quite limited until a study showing a circadian rhythm in melatonin production by cultured hamster neural retina. This study provided definitive evidence that the mammalian eye contains a circadian pacemaker. This pacemaker is probably important in maintaining the circadian rhythm of visual sensitivity. With the development of understanding of the molecular basis of clock function, additional non-SCN oscillators have been described in many tissues, including brain areas outside the SCN. Most of these do not maintain circadian function in the absence of the SCN so that the CTS can be viewed as a hierarchically organized, multioscillator system (Buijs and Kalsbeek, 2001). In this respect, vertebrates are much like invertebrates (see description of the *Drosophila* circadian system, described earlier).

Summary

The suprachiasmatic nucleus is the dominant mammalian pacemaker. It is composed of two subdivisions made up of neurons that are born as individual circadian oscillators coupled to form a pacemaker. One subdivision, the shell, contains AVP/GABA neurons and receives nonvisual input. The shell surrounds the core, which contains VIP/GABA and GRP/GABA neurons that receive visual input from the retina and from the intergeniculate leaflet of the lateral geniculate.

LIGHT IS THE DOMINANT ENTRAINING STIMULUS

Light establishes both the phase and the period of the pacemaker and, thus, is the dominant entraining stimulus, or Zeitgeber (time giver), of the circadian system. The pacemaker can be viewed as a somewhat inaccurate clock, which must be reset repeatedly. It free runs with a period that is slightly off 24 h in the absence of a light–dark cycle. The light–dark cycle sets the exact timing of the pacemaker and is best understood by looking at the phase response curve (PRC) of the pacemaker to light (Fig. 41.7). The PRC shows that the pacemaker responds differently to light at different times of day. The process of entrainment can be envisioned in the following way. The SCN clock is an imperfect timepiece that is unable to maintain a period of exactly 24 h and, for that reason, requires resetting on a regular basis. It is typically reset each day in the morning and the evening at the transitions between light and dark. The PRC is a description of that process.

Entrainment Is Mediated by a Specific Photoreceptive System

The circadian system is not responsive to specialized aspects of visual stimuli. It responds to changes in luminance, the total amount of light, but not to color, shape, movement, or other visual parameters. The responsiveness of the circadian system is not altered in mutant mice lacking both rod and cone photoreceptors, which suggests that other retinal photoreceptors are used for this function. Recent data indicate that the cortical photopigment is melanopsin located in retinal ganglion cells projecting to the SCN (Hattar *et al.*, 2002; Berson *et al.*, 2002).

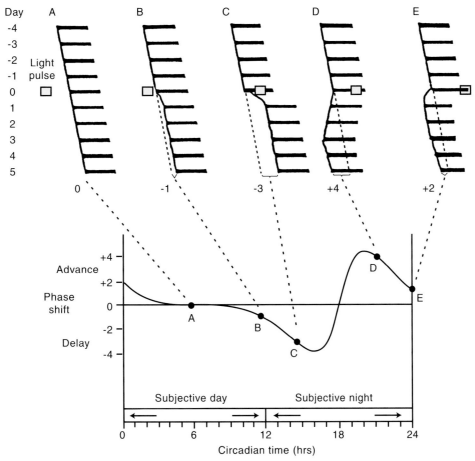

FIGURE 41.7 The phase response curve (PRC). With animals maintained in constant dark, activity is recorded (horizontal bars) and light pulses are given as indicated. The effects of light are determined and then the PRC is constructed as shown.

The Circadian Retina and Retinohypothalamic Tract Are Critical to Entrainment

The SCN is a brain structure that appears exclusively to be involved in circadian function. Similarly, entrainment is mediated by specific photoreceptors and we would expect the remaining visual structures to be unique components of the CTS. Entrainment in mammals requires the lateral eyes. As noted earlier, transection of visual pathways distal to the optic chiasm does not affect entrainment but results in blindness and loss of visual reflexes. In contrast, selective sectioning of the RHT abolishes entrainment but does not affect other visual functions. These data indicate that the RHT terminating in the SCN is the principal entrainment pathway and that it mediates only one function, circadian entrainment. This suggests that the RHT arises from a set of retinal ganglion cells separate from those projecting to other visual areas, but there was no evident way to test this hypothesis until neurotropic viruses became available as tools to

trace neural connections across synapses. To identify the ganglion cells that give rise to the RHT, a mutant swine herpesvirus lacking some components of its glycoprotein envelope protein is injected into one eye where it is taken up, replicated, and transported by ganglion cell axons to terminal sites in the SCN. The optic tracts beyond the SCN are transected so that virus does not go to other visual centers. The virus is released and taken up by SCN neurons, which replicate it and release it at sites of synaptic contact of RHT axons from the noninjected eye. Virus is then transported retrogradely to that eye where it is replicated solely in the retinal ganglion cell projecting in the RHT. The infected ganglion cells are shown with an antiserum against virus. This method allows identification of a specific subset of retinal ganglion cells that gives rise to the RHT, a homogeneous population of small retinal ganglion cells with sparse, but widely spread, dendrites that are found throughout the retina and belong to the W, or type III, ganglion cell class. No other retinal elements have been demonstrated with this method and it now appears that ganglion cells contain the photoreceptive mechanism for entrainment.

Glutamate Is the RHT Transmitter

Glutamate has long been recognized as a neurotransmitter produced by most retinal ganglion cells, and glutamate is now known to mediate the entraining effects of the RHT projecting to the SCN and IGL. Stimulation of the RHT produces a PRC essentially identical to that obtained with light, as does *in vitro* administration of glutamate to the SCN in slices, and blocking glutamate receptors block light-induced phase shifts. Glutamate is colocalized with either substance P or the pituitary adenylate cyclase-activating peptide in subsets of ganglion cells that project to the SCN.

The Intergeniculate Leaflet Carries Photic and Nonphotic Inputs to the SCN

The flow diagram shown in Fig. 41.2 implies that visual input should suffice for entrainment of the circadian system. Although this is probably correct, regulation of the SCN pacemaker is quite complex in the intact mammal and nonphotic stimuli can modulate pacemaker function. As mentioned earlier, the SCN has multiple inputs in addition to the RHT, including ones from the lateral geniculate complex and the midbrain raphe. The IGL is a distinct subdivision of the lateral geniculate complex in all mammals (Moore and Card, 1994). This small, ventral thalamic derivative contains a population of NPY- and GABA-containing neurons that project to the SCN core. Perfusion of NPY into the SCN region produces a PRC with phase advances during subjective day and phase delays during subjective night. A similar PRC is obtained by stimulating the IGL or by applying NPY to slices of SCN *in vitro*. However, the physiological significance of the phase shifts was unknown until stimuli that produce vigorous locomotor activity were shown to cause phase advances during subject day. The phase shifts are a function of activity; when activity is prevented, no phase change occurs. Furthermore, lesions that ablate the IGL eliminate activity-induced phase changes, indicating that the effects of activity on phase are mediated by the IGL–SCN projection. Thus, the IGL modulates entrainment by transmitting information about nonphotic events to the SCN. As described earlier, the IGL receives dense retinal input from retinal ganglion cells that give rise to the RHT, so it seems likely that the IGL integrates photic and nonphotic information for the CTS to affect pacemaker function (Fig. 41.8).

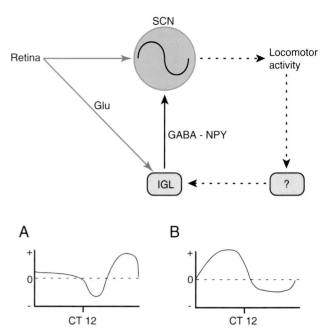

FIGURE 41.8 Actions of two entrainment pathways. The RHT projects to the SCN and IGL. The SCN controls the rest–activity cycle, and locomotor activity feeds back through the IGL projection to the SCN to affect SCN pacemaker function. The effect of RHT activation is shown by the light phase response curve (PRC) (A), and the effect of IGL–RHT activation is shown by the nonphotic PRC (B).

Raphe Modulates Photic Entrainment through Serotonergic Innervation of the SCN

Serotonergic neurons of the midbrain raphe densely innervate the core of the SCN to modulate its responses to light. Raphe neurons are usually state dependent; they fire regularly during waking, slowly during slow-wave sleep, and not at all during rapid eye move-ment sleep. During waking, visual stimulation acutely increases the activity of the neurons. Serotonin inhibits the responses of the SCN to light and optic nerve stimulation *in vivo* and *in vitro*. Data suggest that serotonin acts between the RHT and pacemaker mechanisms on the entrainment mechanisms within SCN neurons.

Summary

Entrainment is mediated by a specific photopigment, melanopsin, located in retinal ganglion cells projecting through the RHT to the SCN and the IGL independent of classical retinal efferent circuits to geniculate colliculus and accessory optic systems. The ganglion cell–SCN circuit uses Glu as a neurotransmitter, while the IGL–SCN projection provides both photic and nonphotic input through a geniculohypothalamic pathway whose cotransmitters are GABA and NPY. A serotonin-mediated projection from the raphe nuclei can modulate SCN responses to the direct retinohypothalamic input.

PACEMAKER OUTPUT IS LIMITED

Efferent projections of the SCN are largely to the hypothalamus, with the densest projections intrinsic to the SCN itself and to a region intercalated between the dorsal border of the SCN and the ventral border of the paraventricular nucleus, the subparaventricular zone (SPVZ) (Watts, 1991; LeSauter and Silver, 1998). This zone has projections that largely overlap projections of the SCN, leading to the view that its function is to reinforce the SCN control of effector systems. The SCN also projects to other hypothalamic areas: the medial preoptic area, lateral hypothalamic area, retrochiasmatic area, paraventricular nucleus, dorsomedial nucleus, and posterior hypothalamic area. Outside the hypothalamus, the SCN projects to the basal forebrain (bed nucleus of the stria terminalis and lateral septal nucleus), midline thalamus (nucleus reuniens and paraventricular nucleus), and IGL. Figure 41.9 provides a framework for how the SCN might control a myriad of functions using only these restricted projections. Circadian control of the behavioral state is a particularly important function of the CTS. Studies have provided new insights into the interactions between the CTS and areas involved in maintenance of the waking and sleep states.

What is the signal that SCN projections deliver to the innervated areas? SCN neurons have a circadian rhythm in the firing rate with peak firing rates in daytime that are about twice the trough rates at night. The rhythm has a simple, nearly sinusoidal waveform; the output of the SCN is expressed as a gradually changing frequency of neuronal firing. Firing occurs at high frequency during subjective day and low frequency during subjective night. This pattern appears to be the same in diurnal and nocturnal animals. However, simple neuronal firing with transmitter release may not be the only means by which the SCN communicates with the areas it controls. In animals in which SCN transplants restore rhythmicity that was lost due to SCN lesions, direct connections into the host brain from the -transplant, typically in the third ventricle, appear unnecessary for functional recovery. This suggests that a humoral mechanism may play a role in rhythm regulation (LeSauter and Silver, 1998). Recent studies indicate that a specific peptide, prokineticin, is important in transmitting circadian information.

Summary

The SCN projects densely to the subparaventricular zone and other hypothalamic areas and to several other nonhypothalamic structures of the diencephalon and basal forebrain. These efferent circuits

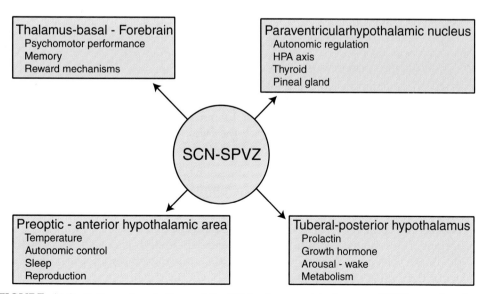

FIGURE 41.9 Pattern of projections of the SCN–subparaventricular zone (SPVZ) complex shown diagrammatically with the functions likely to be controlled by each of these pathways.

control the expression of circadian rhythmicity in the areas innervated.

THE AVIAN CIRCADIAN TIMING SYSTEM IS MORE COMPLEX THAN THAT OF MAMMALS

Studies of birds have provided remarkable insight into the organization of the vertebrate CTS. Birds typically have a highly developed visual system and a diurnal pattern of their circadian rest–activity. The circadian system of birds has been studied for many years in the common house sparrow, *Passer domesticus*. The locomotor activity of these small birds is recorded readily, and they exhibit a robust circadian rhythm with high levels of activity during the day and low levels at night. The rhythm free runs under constant lighting conditions. The pineal appears to be a primary pacemaker in these birds. Early work showed that pinealectomy leads to a loss of the circadian activity rhythm in constant darkness. The rhythm persists in a light–dark cycle, but it is driven by the light–dark cycle through action on extraretinal photoreceptors and, hence, is not a true circadian rhythm. (This response is quite different from that in mammals, in which no functional extraretinal photoreceptors are known.) The conclusive demonstration that the pineal is a circadian pacemaker in the sparrow was provided in experiments performed by Michael Menaker and colleagues in which pineals from intact animals were transplanted into the anterior chamber of the eyes of animals that were arrhythmic due to pinealectomy. The rest–activity rhythm was immediately restored in the transplant recipients, with the phase of the restored rhythms identical to that of the sparrows from which the pineals were obtained.

Communication between the pineal and brain appears to be mediated by melatonin. Continuous infusion of melatonin abolishes the activity rhythm in intact animals, whereas administration of melatonin for 12 h each day to arrhythmic, pinealectomized sparrows restores rhythmicity. If melatonin is the signal for rhythmicity, where does it act? An avian homologue of the mammalian SCN receives direct retinal input. Ablation of the SCN in the sparrow abolishes the rhythm of locomotor activity in constant illumination even when the pineal is intact. In animals with SCN lesions, rhythmicity continues in the presence of a light–dark cycle, as in animals with pinealectomy. The loss of rhythmicity in SCN-ablated animals indicates that melatonin acts through the SCN, which is known to have melatonin receptors.

Investigators initially thought that the control of circadian rhythmicity in all birds would be like that of the sparrow, but four patterns of pacemaker organization are now recognized in birds. One pattern is expressed by passerine birds, such as sparrows. A second pattern was demonstrated in the Japanese quail in which ablation of the pineal has no effect on the rhythm of locomotor activity, but removal of the eyes results in a complete loss of rhythmicity under conditions of constant lighting, indicating that the eye contains the circadian pacemaker that organizes the rest–activity cycle in these birds. The eye pacemaker requires direct neural connections to the brain to generate locomotor activity rhythm; transection of the optic nerves is as effective as removal of the eyes in abolishing the rhythm.

A third pattern of pineal and ocular pacemakers is seen in the pigeon. When these birds are kept in constant, dim light, neither pinealectomy nor enucleation alters their activity rhythm, but together the lesions result in an altered rhythm that degrades over days to arrhythmicity. This observation indicates that both the pineal and the eye contribute to generation of the rest–activity rhythm. The final variant in avian generation of circadian rhythmicity is exhibited by the domestic chicken. Singly or together, pinealectomy and enucleation do not abolish circadian function in the chicken; however, SCN ablation does. Thus, the chicken is an avian species that appears similar to mammals with respect to organization of the circadian system.

In sum, the avian and mammalian circadian systems share many characteristics, such as localization of function, but they also differ in significant ways, such as the presence of extraretinal photoreceptors in birds (Fig. 41.10). In addition, the avian system shows much more variation than the mammalian system. In mammals, the SCN is the primary pacemaker and the eye a secondary one. Although this is true in some birds, the eye and the pineal gland are the dominant pacemakers in most avian species. Mammals and birds express melatonin receptors in the SCN, but the receptors are also expressed in other areas of the avian brain, such as the visual centers.

Summary

The avian circadian timing system is more complex than that of mammals. Extraretinal photic information occurs in some but not all birds in the pineal gland and is transmitted through melatonin secretion to the SCN via the cerebrospinal fluid. In other birds, ocular pacemakers have been detected without pineal participation, and combined ocular–pineal pacemakers

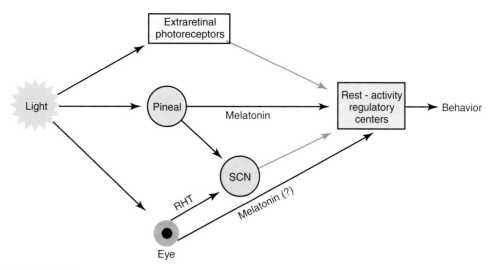

FIGURE 41.10 Organization of avian circadian systems. Depending on the type of bird, the pineal, eye, or SCN may be a circadian pacemaker driving the rest–activity rhythm. The interactions of these structures are shown diagrammatically.

have been observed in pigeons. In the chicken, the system more strongly resembles the mammalian timing system, with the SCN taking on the primary pacemaker role.

Differences between avian and mammalian CTSs are probably not as great as the aforementioned discussion might suggest. Recent observations indicate that the mammalian CTS contains circadian oscillators in areas of the brain outside the SCN and in tissues and organs outside of the brain. The SCN plays a predominant role because of the importance of rest–activity cycles to adaptation and, in those species in which reproductive function is under circadian regulation, to perpetuation of the species. The SCN in mammals has a predominant role because it is the site of termination of a crucial entrainment pathway and because its efferents are distributed in a manner crucial to sleep–wake regulation and the coordination of physiological, endocrine, and neural system function.

CIRCADIAN TIMING IS CRITICAL FOR REPRODUCTION IN SOME MAMMALS

The CTS Controls Estrus

In many female mammals, reproductive events occur in cycles called estrous cycles. The estrous cycle in the rat is 4 days long and culminates on the day of proestrus in a midafternoon surge of release of luteinizing hormone (LH). The timing of the LH surge is precise and results in ovulation followed by receptivity to males the subsequent night. The surge in LH

production and release results from release of the gonadotropin-releasing hormone (GnRH) from the median eminence into the portal circulation. [GnRH neurons are located in the preoptic anterior hypothalamic area and have axons projecting to the median eminence (see Chapter 40).] The precise timing of the release of GnRH to produce the LH surge is a function of a series of endocrine and neural events that lead to proestrus, with the SCN providing the crucial temporal signal. SCN ablation results in loss of estrous cycles and reproductive capacity. This is a further example of the CTS providing precise temporal organization to physiological processes and behavior, in this case reproductive physiology and behavior.

The CTS Also Regulates Seasonal Reproduction

In habitats with marked seasonal variation of temperature and food supply, the survival of species requires seasonal regulation of reproduction. The CTS of these animals uses production of the pineal hormone melatonin to measure day length as a means of predicting seasonal changes.

The pineal gland is a neural structure derived from the caudal portion of the dorsal diencephalic germinal epithelium. It begins as an evagination from the third ventricle and develops into a solid structure connected with the caudal thalamus by the pineal stalk (Fig. 41.11). The pineal contains two types of cells: pinealocytes, a modified neuronal element, and glia. In primates and most carnivores, the pineal stalk is short, and the pineal body lies immediately caudal to

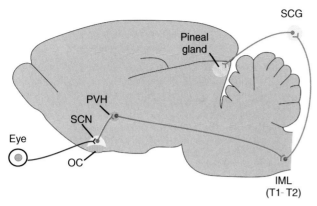

FIGURE 41.11 Diagram of a sagittal view of the rat brain showing pathways controlling pineal melatonin production. The RHT runs from the retina to the SCN, which in turn projects to the paraventricular nucleus of the hypothalamus (PVH). The PVH projects to the intermediolateral cell column of the upper thoracic cord (IML, T1–T2), which provides preganglionic input to sympathetic neurons in the superior cervical ganglion (SCG) innervating the pineal gland.

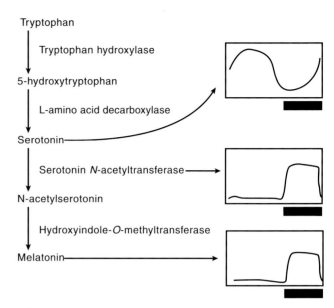

FIGURE 41.12 Metabolic pathway for the production of melatonin from tryptophan in the pineal gland. The circadian rhythms of serotonin, serotonin N-acetyltransferase, and melatonin are shown on the right.

the diencephalon above the tectum. In many rodents, however, the pineal stalk is quite long, and the pineal body lies at the top of the interhemispheric fissure, below the confluence of venous sinuses. The pineal typically has two types of innervation: a sympathetic input from the superior cervical ganglion and a direct central innervation from diencephalic nuclei. Only the sympathetic innervation is known to function in regulating melatonin production. In all mammals, the activity of superior cervical sympathetic neurons innervating the pineal increases at night. The release of norepinephrine from axon terminals acts through β-adrenergic receptors to stimulate melatonin synthesis and release. At night, exposure to light acts through the RHT to inhibit cervical sympathetic activity and thereby quickly stop the production of melatonin.

Melatonin is synthesized from the amino acid tryptophan in a series of steps, one of which involves the enzyme serotonin N-acetyltransferase. The synthesis of serotonin N-acetyltransferase, in turn, follows a circadian rhythm. Thus, regulation of melatonin production depends on sympathetic input to the pineal to affect the synthesis of serotonin N-acetyltransferase in a rhythm dependent on the SCN (Fig. 41.12). The RHT entrains the SCN and, in addition, mediates the effect of bright light in suppressing melatonin production at night. The pathway for pineal control is from the SCN to the autonomic subdivision of the paraventricular nucleus, which projects directly to the intermediolateral cell column of the upper thoracic cord. These preganglionic neurons innervate the superior cervical

ganglion, which then innervates the pineal.(Shinohara et al., 1995).

The pineal was tied to seasonal reproduction in a remarkable series of experiments in which male hamsters were shown to change their reproductive function in response to changes in day length (photoperiod). Hamsters are long-day breeders; they breed and bear young in spring and summer. The gestation period is short, as is the period required for young to develop to independence. As days shorten in the fall to a photoperiod less than about 12.5 h, the male hamsters' testes shrink and spermatogenesis stops. Thus, male hamsters are incapable of reproducing at a time of year when the survival of young would be jeopardized by cold weather and limited food. In the spring, as days lengthen, the testes recover to full function in time for the normal mating season. Pinealectomy blocks the response to short days; even in constant darkness, gonadal size and function remain unaffected in animals from which the pineal has been removed. The response to short photoperiods can be mimicked in these animals by the administration of melatonin. The response is dependent on the timing and duration of melatonin administration. It is now clear that the SCN controls this photoperiodic response by controlling the duration of melatonin secretion by the pineal. In short days, melatonin is secreted over a long portion of the night and produces a decrease in gonadal function, whereas in long days, gonadal function is maintained because the

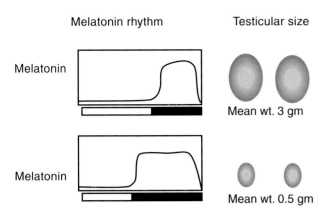

FIGURE 41.13 Melatonin rhythm and testicular size in male hamsters in different day lengths. In 14 h of light alternating with 10 h of dark (LD 14:10), the duration of melatonin secretion is short, and testes are large. In contrast, with 10 h of light and 14 h of dark (LD 10:14), the duration of melatonin secretion is long, and testes are small.

duration of the nocturnal period of melatonin secretion is short (Fig. 41.13). In essence, the duration of nocturnal melatonin production is a measure of day length.

The mechanism by which melatonin alters reproductive function is unclear. The situation is quite complex, however, as demonstrated by the pattern of reproductive function in short-day breeders, such as sheep. In contrast to hamsters, sheep predominantly exhibit estrous cycles and mate in the fall and early winter. Lambs are born in the spring, which gives them a long period of warm weather and plentiful food to grow and become independent. The reproductive cycle in sheep is also generated by endogenous mechanisms that are regulated by melatonin. The photoperiodic control of melatonin secretion synchronizes the endogenous year-long cycle, but in this case, the effect of melatonin is the reverse of that in the hamster. Long photoperiods inhibit the endogenous promotion of reproductive function, whereas short photoperiods promote it. Every day, the SCN–pineal axis provides a pulse of melatonin secretion that faithfully mirrors the lengths of day and night. Thus, the duration of the melatonin signal allows the animals to track time on an annual basis.

The Action of Melatonin Is Mediated by a Specific G-Protein-Coupled Receptor

Melatonin receptors were identified through the use of a radioactive iodine analog of melatonin, iodomelatonin, as a ligand in experiments. In the mammalian brain, melatonin receptors have a very limited distribution; they are consistently present only in the SCN and midline thalamic nuclei and in the

pars tuberalis of the anterior pituitary. The gene for the melatonin receptor has been cloned, and the receptor is a member of the family of receptors coupled to G proteins. SCN melatonin receptors are thought to mediate the feedback of melatonin on the CTS, and melatonin receptors in the pars tuberalis are thought to mediate reproductive effects (for a review, see Arendt 1995).

Substantial evidence indicates that melatonin can affect pacemaker function. For example, melatonin can lessen the symptoms of jet lag and, in elderly people, the disruptions of sleep that occur as a consequence of alterations of pacemaker function (see Box 41.1). Thus, melatonin is important not only for seasonal reproduction, but for feedback regulation of pacemaker function.

Summary

The circadian timing system can control reproduction in male mammals by controlling testicular function and in females by regulating estrus through a circuit from the SCN to the sympathetic nerves controlling pineal melatonin production. This same pathway is also used by mammals that reproduce in a seasonal pattern to regulate the timing of reproduction.

THE PRIMATE CIRCADIAN TIMING SYSTEM FUNCTIONS PRINCIPALLY TO PROMOTE BEHAVIORAL ADAPTATION

Reproduction is not under circadian control in human and nonhuman primates. The function of the CTS is to coordinate a large series of humoral, physiological, and behavioral mechanisms to promote maximally effective sleep and adaptive waking behavior. As described in detail in the next chapter, sleep and waking are controlled by two opposing factors, a homeostatic drive for sleep and a circadian arousal stimulus. Homeostatic sleep drive accumulates as a function of the time that an individual has been awake. Sleep dissipates the drive and, after a full night's sleep, homeostatic drive is absent. The nature of circadian control of the sleep–wake cycle was not understood until the early 1990s when Dale Edgar and associates showed that SCN lesions in monkeys not only alter the circadian control of sleep and wake, but also change sleep. Before the lesions, monkeys, like humans, sleep approximately 8 h a day and are awake for 16 h. After the lesions, however, the monkeys sleep 12 h a day. This indicates that one function of the SCN is to promote arousal. This works as follows. In the morning after awakening, there is

BOX 41.1

DISORDERS OF CIRCADIAN TIMING

The passenger of an aircraft flying across several time zones will experience the most common of circadian disorders, jet lag, or rapid time-zone change syndrome. Like most other disorders of circadian timing, jet lag manifests primarily as a sleep disorder. Afflicted individuals typically report nighttime insomnia and daytime sleepiness. Jet lag reflects the delay in readjustment of the circadian pacemaker to the new time zone and is a disorder of entrainment. It is self-limited, rarely lasting more than a few days and occurs typically with travel over more than three time zones. Travel from west to east is usually more troublesome than travel from east to west. Recent data show a change in cognitive function with structural changes in the brain in individuals exposed to chronic jet lag. Treatment of jet lag with melatonin is reported to be effective.

Non-24-h sleep–wake disorder occurs most frequently in blind people whose circadian rhythms, lacking visual input, typically free run with a period slightly greater than 24 h. For many years the human circadian system was erroneously believed to be insensitive to light and largely entrained to social cues. It is now clear that even dim light can reset the human clock, and some blind individuals show quite clearly that social cues may be insufficient for entrainment. These individuals fail to entrain to social cues and free run, suffering symptoms very similar to jet lag when they attempt to maintain a regular schedule temporally synchronized with the environment. In contrast, other blind individuals are entrained to social cues and yet another group is entrained to the light–dark cycle despite being totally blind. In the latter group, the RHT can be shown to be intact because their nocturnal rise in pineal melatonin secretion is blocked by light. There are also people with normal sight who exhibit a free-running sleep–wake cycle, indicating an absence of RHT function despite a normal function of other central retinal projections. Delayed sleep phase syndrome is another disorder of

entrainment, common in adolescence and sometimes continuing into adult life. Affected individuals shift their sleep–wake cycle toward going to bed late and getting up late. Such a change in the phase of the rest–activity cycle typically begins around the time of puberty. Apparently a change in the sensitivity of the pacemaker to phase-advancing stimuli disrupts the normal balance between phase advances and phase delays. This balance is disrupted differently in the advanced sleep phase syndrome, in which people (typically elderly) go to sleep early in the evening and awaken early in the morning. This sleep– wake cycle appears to represent a change in sensitivity in the phase delay portion of the PRC. There are familial cases of both phase advance and phase delay sleep disorder, and recent work indicates that these may result from mutations of one of the *mper* genes.

Disorders of pacemaker function and output appear to be less common than disorders of entrainment. Occasionally, tumors disrupt the pacemaker and result in loss of rhythm, similar to that seen in animals with SCN lesions. Also, elderly people frequently show a decrease in the amplitude of circadian rhythms, but it is unclear whether this represents an abnormality in pacemaker function or in the capacity of effector systems to respond to pacemaker output is unclear. Without a method for measuring pacemaker output in humans, these alternatives are not distinguished easily.

Seasonal affective disorder (SAD) may also fall into this category of circadian rhythm disorders. The symptoms of SAD typically begin in autumn and remit in spring. Affected individuals experience changes in mood, sleep pattern, appetite, libido, memory, and cognition. Treatment with bright light, which extends the length of the day, has been successful in treating this disorder. At the simplest level, SAD reflects a disturbance in the measurement of the length of photoperiod.

Robert Y. Moore

virtually no homeostatic drive for sleep and SCN output is low as shown by the neuronal firing rate. As the day progresses, homeostatic drive increases and is countered by an increasing SCN output. At the end of the day, SCN output decreases and, as it becomes low, homeostatic drive results in the onset of sleep. In the morning, homeostatic drive is diminished and cir-

cadian arousal influences result in awakening (Dijk *et al.*, 2000).

General Summary

Circadian rhythms are fundamental adaptations of living organisms to their environment. Circadian

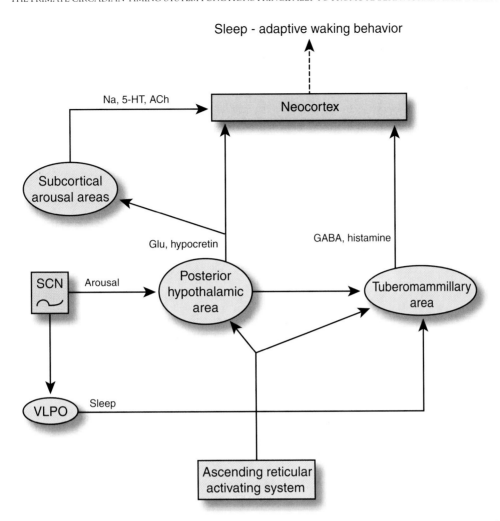

FIGURE 41.14 The SCN and behavioral state control. The SCN projects to the ventrolateral preoptic area (VLPO), an area mediating sleep. VLPO inhibits the arousal activity of the tuberomammillary nucleus during sleep. The SCN provides an arousal-promoting input to the posterior hypothalamic area, particularly to hypocretin neurons, which project upon the neocortex and subcortical arousal areas. See text and Chapter 46 for further description.

function is controlled genetically through a molecular mechanism maintained by the expression of clock genes that code for specific proteins that feed back on the nucleus to control their own production. In animals, a neural circadian timing system (CTS) establishes the temporal organization of behavior into cycles of rest and activity (sleep and wake in mammals), maximizing the adaptive success of both rest and waking behaviors. The mammalian CTS has three components: (1) photoreceptors and entrainment pathways, which determine the precise period and phase of the circadian pacemakers; (2) circadian pacemakers, which generate a circadian signal; and (3) pacemaker output to effector systems that are regulated by the CTS. Light is the dominant entraining stimulus for the CTS, and the major photic entrainment pathway is the retinolypothalamic

tract. The RHT terminates densely in the principal circadian pacemaker, the suprachiasmatic nucleus. The SCN produces a simple circadian signal, which is conveyed to hypothalamic, thalamic, and basal forebrain areas that are regulated by the CTS. Circadian control of sleep–wake cycles is accomplished by generating arousal during the wake period that counters homeostatic drive for sleep. The CTS not only provides temporal organization for behavior, but also regulates aspects of reproductive function, particularly in animals that reproduce seasonally. Finally, disorders of circadian function are common, and research on the neurobiology of circadian timing has facilitated our understanding of the disorders and led to further insights into pathophysiology and the development of new therapies.

References

Allada, R., Emery, P., Takahashi, J. S., and Rosbash, M. (2001). Stopping time: The genetics of fly and mouse circadian clocks. *Annu. Rev. Neurosci.* **24**, 1091–1119.

Arendt, J. (1995). "Melatonin and the Mammalian Pineal Gland." Chapman & Hall, London.

Aschoff, J. (1965). Circadian rhythms in man. *Science* **148**, 1427–1432.

Berson, D. M., Dienn, F. A., and Takao, M. (2002). Phototransduction by retinal ganglion cells that set the circadian clock. *Science* **295**, 1070–1073.

Buijs, R. M., and Kalsbeek, A. (2001). Hypothalamic integration of central and peripheral clocks. *Nature Neurosci. Rev.* **2**, 521–526.

Cheng, M. Y., Bullock, C. M., Li, C., Lee, A. G., Belluri, J., Weaver, D. R., Leslie, F. M., and Zhou, Q.-Y. (2002). Prokineticin 2 transmits the behavioral circadian rhythm of the suprachiasmatic nucleus. *Nature* **417**, 405–410.

Dijk, D. J., Duffy, J. F., and Czeisler, C. A. (2000). Contribution of circadian physiology and sleep homeostasis to age-related changes in human sleep. *Chronobiol. Int.* **17**, 285–311.

Edgar, D. M., Dement, W. C., and Fuller, C. A. (1993). Effect of SCN lesions on sleep in squirrel monkeys: Evidence for opponent processes in sleep-wake regulation. *J. Neurosci.* **13**, 1065–1079.

Hattar, S., Liao, H.-W., Takao, M., Berson, D. M., and Yau, K.-W. (2002). Melanopsin-containing retinal ganglion cells: Architecture, projections and intrinsic rhythmicity. *Science* **295**, 1065–1070.

Klein, D. C., Moore. R. Y., and Reppert, S. M. (eds.) (1991). "Suprachiasmatic Nucleus: The Mind's Clock." Oxford Univ. Press, New York.

LeSauter, J., and Silver, R. (1998). Output signals of the SCN. *Chronobiol. Int.* **15**, 535–550.

Loros, J. E., and Dunlap, J. C. (2001). Genetic and molecular analysis of circadian rhythms in Neurospora. *Annu. Rev. Physiol.* **63**, 757–794.

Moore, R. Y. (1996). Entrainment pathways and the functional organization of the circadian timing system. *Prog. Brain Res.* **111**, 103–119.

Moore, R. Y. (2001) Circadian rhythms: Basic neurobiology and clinical applications. *Annu. Rev. Med.* 48, 253–266.

Moore, R. Y., and Card, J. P. (1994). Intergeniculate leaflet: An anatomically and functionally distinct subdivision of the lateral geniculate complex. *J. Comp. Neurol.* **344**, 403–430.

Pittendrigh, C. S. (1993). Temporal organization: Reflections of a Darwinian clock-watcher. *Annu. Rev. Physiol.* **55**, 17–54.

Reppert, S. M., and Sauman, I. (1995). Period and timeless tango: A dance of two clock genes. *Neuron* **15**, 983–986.

Reppert, S. M., and Weaver, D. R. (2001). Molecular analysis of mammalian circadian rhythms. **63**, 647–676.

Shinohara, K., Honma, S., Katsuno, Y., Abe, H., and Honma, K. (1995). Two distinct oscillators in the rat suprachiasmatic nucleus *in vitro. Proc. Natl. Acad. Sci. USA* **92**, 7396–7400.

Takahashi, J. S., Turek, F., and Moore, R. Y. (eds.) (2001). "Circadian Clocks." Plenum Press, New York.

van Esseveldt, K. E., Lehman, M. N., and Boer, G. J. (2000). The suprachiasmatic nucleus and the circadian timing system revisited. *Brain Res. Rev.* **33**, 34–77.

Watts, A. G. (1991). The efferent projections of the suprachiasmatic nucleus: Anatomical insights into the control of circadian rhythms. *In* "The Suprachiasmatic Nucleus: The Mind's Clock" (D. C. Klein, R. Y. Moore, and S. M. Reppert, eds.), pp. 77–106. Oxford Univ. Press, New York.

Wever, R. A. (1974). "The Circadian System of Man," p. 26. Springer-Verlag, New York.

Williams, J. A., and Sehgal, A. (2001). Molecular components of the circadian system in Drosophila. *Annu. Rev. Physiol.* **63**, 729–755.

Robert Y. Moore

<h1>42</h1>

<h1>Sleep, Dreaming, and Wakefulness</h1>

Sleep is a behavioral state that alternates with waking. Sleep is characterized by a recumbent posture, a raised threshold to sensory stimulation, a low level of motor output, and a unique behavior—dreaming. The complex neurobiology of these behavioral features of sleep has been explored at the systemic, cellular, and molecular levels since the mid-1960s. Although these studies have provided substan-

tial insight into the physiology and pathology of sleep, we have yet to obtain definitive answers to the adaptive significance of sleep, the behavioral state that takes up one-third of our lives.

In contrast to sleep, the conscious behavior of waking is characterized by an active and deliberate sensorimotor discourse with the environment. For maintenance of waking behavior, neural gates must

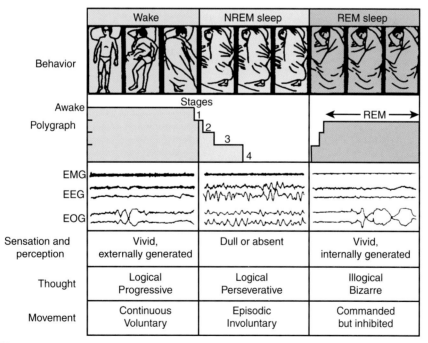

FIGURE 42.1 Behavioral states in humans. Body position changes during waking and at the time of phase changes in the sleep cycle. Removal of facilitation (during stages 1–4 of NREM sleep) and addition of inhibition (during REM sleep) account for immobility during sleep. In dreams, we imagine that we move, but no movement occurs. Tracings of electrical activity are shown in ~20-s sample records. The amplitude of the electromyogram (EMG) is highest in waking, intermediate in NREM sleep, and lowest in REM sleep. The electroencephalogram (EEG) and electrooculogram (EOG) are activated in waking and REM sleep and inactivated in NREM sleep. Reprinted with permission from Hobson and Steriade (1986).

remain open for sensory input and motor output, the brain must be tuned and activated, and the chemical microclimate must be appropriate for processing and recording of information. Wakefulness is accompanied by conscious experience that reaches its highest level of complexity in adult humans. Waking behavior includes a number of components, such as sensation, perception, attention, memory, instinct, emotion, volition, cognition, and language, that make up our awareness of the world and self and form the basis of an adaptive interaction with our environment. This chapter focuses on the mechanisms of behavioral state control that make such interactions possible, with an emphasis on sleep as a component of adaptive behavior. Because evidence so strongly favors an integration of psychological and physiological features, the substrate of conscious experience is sometimes referred to as the "brain–mind".

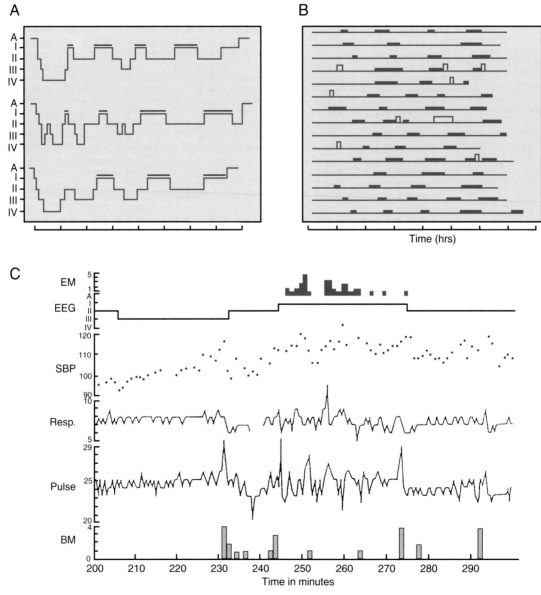

FIGURE 42.2   Periodic activation in sleep cycles. (A) The sleep stages of three people are graphed. The first two or three cycles of the night are dominated by deep stages (3 and 4) of NREM sleep, and REM sleep (indicated by red bars) is brief or nonexistent. During the last two cycles of the night, NREM sleep is lighter (stage 2), and REM episodes are longer, sometimes more than an hour. (B) Records begin at the onset of sleep. The amount of time before the first episode of REM varies, but once REM has begun, the interval between episodes is fairly constant. (C) Eye movements (EM), EEG, systolic blood pressure (SBP), respiration (Resp.), pulse, and body movement (BM) over 100 min of uninterrupted sleep. The interval from 242 to 273 min is considered the REM period, although eye movements are not continuous during that interval.

THE TWO STATES OF SLEEP: SLOW WAVE AND RAPID EYE MOVEMENT

The behavioral signs of sleep vary regularly during every period of sleep; posture, arousal, threshold, and motor output change in a stereotyped, cyclic manner. Although these changes can be observed directly, their study is facilitated by placing electrodes on the scalp to measure the electrical activity of the brain. From these electroencephalograms (EEGs) (Fig. 42.1), two distinct substates of sleep—rapid eye movement (REM) and non-REM (NREM)—can be discerned. Both show interesting contrasts with waking, and these contrasts improve our understanding of states of consciousness.

At the onset of sleep, the brain deactivates, and awareness of the outside world is lost. A well-described sequence of thalamocortical events causes the progressive slowing of brain waves, seen on EEG during this NREM phase of sleep. The threshold for arousal rises in proportion to the degree of EEG slowing, and at the greatest depth of sleep, awakenings are often difficult, incomplete, and brief. This sleep state is designated the slow wave or delta phase of NREM sleep. People have little or no recall of conscious experience in deep NREM sleep. Many autonomic and regulatory functions, such as heart rate, blood pressure, and respiration rate, diminish in NREM sleep, but neuroendocrine activity increases. The pulsatile release of growth hormone and sexual maturation hormones from the pituitary is maximal during sleep, with over 95% of the daily output occurring in NREM sleep.

At regular intervals during sleep, the brain reactivates into a state characterized by fast, low-voltage activity characterized by muscle atonia and rapid eye movements. This sleep state, termed rapid eye movement sleep because of prominent eye movements, differs from waking by an inhibition of sensory input and motor output. Postural shifts precede and follow REM sleep; eye movements, intermittent small muscle twitching, and penile erection occur during REM sleep. The presence (or absence) of REM sleep erection is used clinically to distinguish between psychological and physiological male impotence. In REM sleep, many autonomic functions change; the control of temperature and cardiopulmonary function is lost.

People aroused from NREM sleep, especially early in the night, are confused, have difficulty reporting conscious experience, and return to sleep rapidly. Subjects aroused from REM sleep, especially during periods with frequent eye movements, give detailed reports of dreams characterized by vivid hallucinations, bizarre thinking, and intense emotion. These

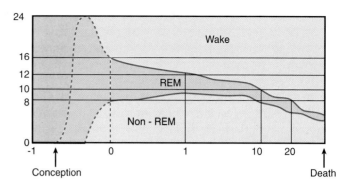

FIGURE 42.3 Portions of a 24-h day that are devoted to waking, REM sleep, and non-REM (NREM) sleep change over a lifetime. Although the timing of these changes *in utero* is not known with certainty (dotted lines), data from premature infants are consistent with REM sleep occupying most of life at a gestational age of 26 weeks. After 26 weeks, the time spent in waking increases until death.

observations indicate that dreaming is the behavior associated with activation of the brain in REM sleep.

NREM and REM Phases Alternate throughout Sleep

The two sleep states alternate at intervals of about 90 min in adult humans. NREM phases are deeper and longer early in the night (Fig. 42.2A). Together with the regularity of the periods (see Fig. 42.2B), this property has suggested that a damped oscillator is the underlying neural mechanism for NREM–REM cycles. The portion of the 24-h day devoted to NREM and REM sleep varies within and across species (Fig. 42.3 and Table 42.1).

Sleep Appears to Have Multiple Functions

As a quiescent and ecologically protected behavior, sleep fosters conservation of energy, repair of injury,

TABLE 42.1 Phylogeny of Rest and Sleep

Organism	Rest	Sleep	REM sleep
Mammals			
Adults	+	+	+
Neonates	+	+	+,–
Birds			
Adults	+	+	+
Neonates	+	+	+
Reptiles	+	+	–
Amphibians	+	–	–
Fish	+	+, –	–

Note. REM, rapid eye movement; +, present; +, –, ambiguously or inconsistently present; –, absent.

and defense from predation. The anabolic character of NREM sleep (e.g., brain and body inactivity and hormone release) suggests a rest and restoration function. In contrast, the high proportion of REM sleep in the developing brain, the high level of forebrain activity, and the stereotyped movements in REM sleep suggest a role of REM sleep in brain development and plasticity. In fact, many studies indicate a role for REM sleep in memory consolidation. The crucial role of sleep is illustrated by studies showing that sleep deprivation results in the disruption of metabolic and caloric homeostasis and, if prolonged, death.

Summary

Sleep and waking are distinct, alternate behavioral states that are mutually exclusive, but interrelated. Within sleep, two substates of behavior are readily distinguishable by electroencephalographic recordings, termed rapid eye movement and non-REM sleep. The characteristic behaviors of sleep include relaxed posture, elevated thresholds for sensory arousal, and diminished motor activity. The slow wave and REM sleep phases alternate throughout the sleep period in cycles. Although the precise function of sleep remains unknown, much scientific evid-

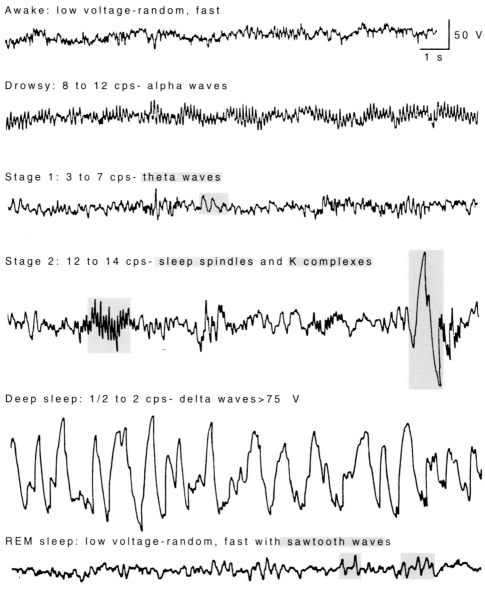

FIGURE 42.4 Electroencephalograms showing electrical activity of the human brain during different stages of sleep.

ence favors the sleep period being for rest and restoration.

SLEEP IN THE MODERN ERA OF NEUROSCIENCE

Philosophical speculation about the nature of sleep and conscious behavior is as old as recorded history, and many philosophers, including the Ionian Greeks, anticipated the physicalistic models that have only recently been articulated in modern neuroscience (for details of the following historical material, please refer to Hobson, 1988). The signal event of the modern era of neuroscience was the discovery of the electrical nature of nervous activity and, more specifically, the 1928 discovery of the human electroencephalogram (EEG) by the German psychiatrist Adolf Berger.

The state-dependent nature of the EEG helped Berger convince his skeptical critics that the rhythmic oscillations he recorded across the human scalp with his galvanometer originated in the brain and were not artifacts of movement or of scalp muscle activity. When his subjects relaxed, closed their eyes, or dozed off, the low-voltage brain waves associated with alertness gave way to higher voltage, lower frequency patterns (Fig. 42.4). These patterns stopped rapidly when the subjects were aroused.

Waking and Sleep Initially Were Viewed as Activated and Nonactivated States

Following Berger's discovery, a flurry of descriptive and experimental studies aimed at understanding the EEG itself, the full range of its state-dependent variability, and the control of that variability by the brain were performed. Loomis and Harvey were the first to describe the tendency of the EEG to show systematic changes in activity as subjects fell asleep at night (tracings 3–5 of Fig. 42.4).

Because mammals shared the same correlation between arousal level and EEG, the Belgian physiologist Frederick Bremer made experimental transections of the mammalian brain to determine the nature and source of EEG activation (the low-voltage, fast pattern of waking) and deactivation (the high-voltage, slow pattern of sleep). Thinking the activity level probably depended on sensory input, Bremer transected the brain at the level of the first cervical spinal cord segment of the cat, producing a preparation called the *encephale isole*. He was surprised to find that the isolated forebrain was activated and alert despite such

transection of a major portion of its sensory input. When he then produced the *cerveau isole* preparation, by transecting the midbrain at the intercollicular level, he observed persistent EEG slowing and unresponsiveness. Interpreting this observation, Bremer incorrectly inferred that removal of the trigeminal nerve afferents (which entered the brain stem between the level of the two cuts) accounted for the sleep-like state of the *cerveau isole*.

Sleep Can Be Induced Electrically

That sleep might be an active brain process—and not simply the absence of waking as Bremer supposed—was first experimentally suggested by the work of the Swiss Nobel laureate W. R. Hess. Hess was involved in a broad program investigating the effects of electrical stimulation of the subcortical regions mediating autonomic control (especially the hypothalamus). He discovered that by driving the thalamocortical system at the frequencies of intrinsic EEG spindles (short series of waves) and slow waves, he could induce the behavioral and electrographic signs of sleeping in unanesthetized cats. This discovery opened the door to the idea that sleep and waking might be active processes, each with its own specific cellular and metabolic mechanisms and functional consequences. This paradigm has since born abundant scientific fruit: The precise details of spindle and slow wave elaboration have been worked out (Steriade, 2000). In addition, the paradigm correctly anticipated the finding that central homologues of sympathetic neurons mediate waking, whereas central cholinergic neurons mediate REM sleep (Hobson and Steriade, 1986; Steriade and McCarley, 1990). In his concept of arousal as energy consuming and sleep as energy conserving, Hess anticipated much of our present understanding of sleep.

The intrinsic nature of brain activation was clearly demonstrated in 1949 when Giuseppe Moruzzi and Horace Magoun discovered that EEG desynchronization and behavioral arousal could be produced by high-frequency electrical stimulation of the midbrain. To explain their observation, Moruzzi and Magoun suggested that the nonspecific (i.e., nonsensory) reticular activating system operates in series and in parallel with the ascending sensory pathways. This concept allowed for the translation of afferent stimuli into central activation (Bremer's idea) and opened the door to the more radical idea that not only waking but also adaptive behavior could be autoactivated by brain stem mechanisms.

Now that we accept the idea that the spontaneous activity of neurons determines the substages of sleep,

BOX 42.1

DEAFFERENTATION VERSUS INTERNAL MODULATION: A PARADIGM SHIFT FOR SLEEP NEUROBIOLOGY

Before the discovery of the neuromodulatory systems of the brain by the Swedish team led by Kjell Fuxe in the early 1960s, scientists who studied sleep could not understand that the brain controlled its own state and that the stages of sleep were actively generated. Thus such neurobiological giants as Charles Sherrington were convinced that because sleep occurred *when* environmental stimulus levels were low (which is true), it also occurred *because* stimulus levels were low (which is false). In the light of the discovery of the reticular activating system by Giuseppe Moruzzi and Horace Magoun in 1949 and REM sleep in 1953 by Eugene Aserinsky and Nathaniel Kleitman, this theory of deafferentation was gradually replaced by the

models of active internal control of the brain by the regular variations in balance between the brain stem neuromodulators, especially NE, 5-HT, and ACh. This paradigm shift has not only led to the specification of increasingly detailed mechanisms for regulation of the brain state, but has opened the door to an appreciation of sleep as functionally significant in ways that are actively complementary to waking. The rich variety of brain activity in sleep inevitably makes the emerging panoply of sleep disorders explicable and potentially treatable via a deeper understanding of sleep neurobiology.

J. Allan Hobson and Edward F. Pace-Schott

---

it is difficult for us to appreciate the strength and persistence of its predecessor, the reflex concept of sleep. Scientific giants such as Ivan Pavlov and Charles Sherrington were so inspired by the reflex doctrine that they were convinced that brain activity simply ceased in the absence of sensory input (Box 42.1).

The Brain–Mind Is Activated during REM Sleep

In 1953, Eugene Aserinsky and Nathaniel Kleitman, working in Chicago, discovered that the brain–mind did indeed self-activate during sleep. They observed regularly timed, spontaneous desynchronization of the EEG, accompanied by clusters of rapid, saccadic eye movements and acute accelerations of heart and respiration rates. Working with Kleitman, William Dement then showed that these periods of spontaneous autoactivation of the brain–mind were associated with dreaming and that this autoactivation process was also found in another mammal, the cat (see Fig. 42.1 and tracing number 6 of Fig. 42.4).

In adult humans, the intrinsic cycle of inactivation (NREM sleep) and activation (REM sleep) recurs with a period length of 90–100 min (see Fig. 42.2). REM sleep occupies 20–25% of the recording time and NREM the remainder (75–80%) (see Hobson, 1989). The NREM phases of the first two cycles are deep and long, whereas REM phases, during which sleep lightens, occupy more of the last two or three cycles.

Input–Output Gating Occurs during Sleep

The paradoxical preservation of sleep in the face of dreaming in REM sleep began to be explained when Francois Michel and Michel Jouvet, working in Lyon in 1959, demonstrated that inhibition of muscle activity was a component of REM sleep in cats. Using transection, lesion, and stimulation techniques, the Jouvet team also discovered that the control system for REM sleep was located in the pontine brain stem. The pons is the source of EEG activation and REMs. Muscle inhibition is also mediated by pontine signals, but these are relayed via the bulbar inhibitory reticular formation to the spinal cord. Synchronous with each flurry of REMs, periodic activation signals, or ponto-geniculo-occipital (PGO) waves, are sent from the pons up to the forebrain (and down to the spinal cord). The PGO waves trigger bursts of firing by geniculate and cortical neurons and other signals originating in the brain stem damp sensory input (via presynaptic inhibition) and motor output (via postsynaptic inhibition) (Calloway *et al.*, 1987). Thus, in REM sleep the brain–mind is effectively off-line with respect to external inputs and outputs and receives internally generated signals.

The cellular and molecular bases of these dramatic changes in input–output gating have been detailed using Sherrington's reflex paradigm together with extracellular and intracellular recording techniques (see Hobson and Steriade, 1986). For example, such techniques revealed that during REM sleep, each motor neuron was subject to a 10-mV hyperpolarization, which blocked all but a few of the activation signals generated by the REM–PGO system. Furthermore, studies showed that this inhibition was mediated by glycine (Chase *et al.*, 1989). When this motor inhibition was disrupted experimentally by lesions in the pons, the cats, still in a REM-like sleep state but without the atonia, showed stereotyped behaviors (such as defense and attack postures). These behaviors reflected the activation, in REM, of the generators that produce the motor patterns for these instinctual, fixed acts (see Jouvet, 1999).

These studies indicated that in normal REM sleep, motor inhibition prevents the motor commands of the generators of instinctual behavior patterns from being acted out. As a result, during REM these patterns are unexpressed in the outside world but occur in a fictive manner within the internal world of the brain–mind. One strong significance of these findings for a theory of dream consciousness lies in their ability to explain the ubiquity of imagined movement in dreams (see Hobson *et al.*, 2000). From a sensorimotor point of view, the highly patterned (and hence nonrandom) organization of autoactivation in REM sleep may be important.

Summary

The scientific history of sleep began with the application of electroencephalography in 1928, demonstrating that the electrical activity of the brain changed but did not cease during sleep. Subsequent refinements revealed the necessary role of the reticular formation for arousal and the association of arousal with desynchronized cortical activity. In addition, emulating the oscillatory EEG spindles of thalamic projections to cortex allowed sleep to be induced by direct thalamic electrical stimulation in experimental animals. Sleep analysis in the 1950s showed REM sleep to be a "paradoxical" state in which sleep was at its deepest, yet accompanied by rapid eye movements and sympathetic signs of arousal, interpreted as dreaming, and accompanied by still further reductions of postural muscle tone. During REM sleep, pontine waves of activity arise with each flurry of eye movements, during which motor activity is deeply depressed.

ANATOMY AND PHYSIOLOGY OF BRAIN STEM REGULATORY SYSTEMS

Brain Stem Reticular Formation Contains Specific Neuronal Groups Involved in Behavioral State Regulation

Moruzzi and Magoun's original concept of a nonspecific reticular activating system has been elaborated and greatly modified by subsequent anatomical and physiological studies. Two general principles have emerged. One is that most of the classic reticular core neurons have very specific afferent inputs and highly organized outputs. The other is that the reticular formation contains small groups of neurons that send widely branching axons to distant parts of the brain, where their neurotransmitters modulate brain function.

The input–output characteristics of each of the reticular formation's multiple subsystems reflect specific sensorimotor function, modulatory function, or both. For example, many neurons of the reticular formation are involved in the integration of eye, head, and trunk positions as these change to accommodate specific behavioral challenges and tasks. These reticular neurons receive inputs from skin, muscle, bone, and joint receptors in the periphery, which they integrate and link to the vestibular and cerebellar circuits that determine posture and movement. This information must also be integrated by higher brain structures in the visual, somatosensory, and motor systems to develop the complex motor patterns of adaptive behavior.

A series of chemically specified neuronal groups also lies in the reticular formation. They have patterns of connections that differ from those of the previously discussed neurons of the reticular formation. Dahlstrom and Fuxe (1964) were the first to identify neuronal populations in the brain that produced norepinephrine (NE) and serotonin (5-hydroxytryptamine, 5-HT). (For additional discussion of these and other neurotransmitter systems discussed in this chapter, see Chapter 7 and Fig. 43.2.)

The NE neurons (designated A1–A7 by Dahlstrom and Fuxe) are located in the pons and medulla in two major groups. One group consists of scattered neurons largely located in the ventral and lateral reticular formation. The most caudal neurons (A1–A3) project rostrally to the brain stem, hypothalamus, and basal forebrain, whereas the rostral groups (A5 and A7) project caudally to the brain stem and spinal cord. These neuronal groups, together called the lateral tegmental neuron group (Moore and Card, 1984) appear to be involved in hypothalamic regulation and motor control.

The major NE cell group is the locus coeruleus (A4 and A6). This compact cell group is located in the rostral pontine reticular formation and central gray matter. The neurons of the locus coeruleus project widely but in a highly specific pattern. One group of locus coeruleus neurons appears to project largely caudally to sensory regions of the brain stem and spinal cord. Other neurons of the locus coeruleus project widely to the cerebellar cortex, dorsal thalamus, and cerebral cortex (Moore and Card, 1984). Thus, the projection patterns of the locus coeruleus appear to be primarily to sensory structures and to cortical structures involved in integration. From this we could expect the locus coeruleus to be involved in regulating sensory input and cortical activation. As we shall see, this expectation is in accord with the available information on function.

Two additional subsets of chemically identified neurons appear critically involved in behavioral state regulation. The first subset to be discovered contained the 5-HT neurons of the brain stem raphé (Dahlstrom and Fuxe, 1964) (B1–B9 in their nomenclature). These neurons extend from caudal medulla to midbrain and are located predominantly in the raphé nuclei, a set of neuronal groups located in the midline of the brain stem reticular formation. The largest numbers of 5-HT neurons are found in the midbrain nuclei, the dorsal raphé nuclei, and the median raphé nuclei (B8 and B9). These groups project rostrally, innervating nearly the entire forebrain in a pattern that also suggests a role in regulation of behavioral state.

The other important set of reticular formation nuclei involved in behavioral state control produces acetylcholine (ACh) as its neurotransmitter. ACh was well known as the transmitter of motor neurons, and early work indicated that ACh is found in nonmotor brain areas. Two sets of cholinergic neurons are involved in control of the behavioral state. The first set is two pontine nuclei: the laterodorsal tegmental nucleus and the pedunculopontine nucleus. Cholinergic neurons in these nuclei project to the brain stem reticular formation, hypothalamus, thalamus, and basal forebrain. The projection to the forebrain involves the second set of cholinergic neurons, those in the medial septum, the nucleus of the diagonal band, and the substantia innominata–nucleus basalis complex. This set projects to limbic forebrain, including the hippocampus, and to the neocortex.

In contrast to the modulatory neurons, which are characterized by their production of norepinephrine, 5-HT, and ACh, neurons in reticular formation nuclei that are involved in sensorimotor integration typically produce either the excitatory transmitter glutamate or the inhibitory transmitter GABA.

SENSORIMOTOR AND MODULATORY RETICULAR NEURONS DIFFER FUNCTIONALLY

Sensorimotor and modulatory neurons of the reticular formation differ markedly in their firing properties. Sensorimotor neurons, approximately 50 to 75 μm in diameter, can fire continuously at high rates of up to 50 Hz and can generate bursts of up to 500 Hz. Their larger axons, especially those projecting to the spinal cord, have conduction velocities in excess of 100 m/s (Hobson and Steriade, 1986), making these neurons well suited to rapid posture adjustment and motor control.

Modulatory neurons are smaller (10–25 μm in diameter) than sensorimotor neurons, and even those with long axons conduct their signals very slowly (1 m/s). They fire wider spikes (2 ms in duration) at much slower tonic frequencies (1–10 Hz) than sensorimotor neurons. In addition, they often show a very regular, metronome-like firing pattern, a reflection of the pacemaker properties they share with the Purkinje cells of the heart. As their leaky membranes spontaneously and slowly depolarize, they reach threshold, fire, and then self-inhibit, becoming refractory even to exogenous excitatory inputs. Modulatory neurons are much less likely than sensorimotor neurons to fire in clusters or bursts unless powerfully excited; even then, they adapt rapidly. Thus, modulatory neurons are well suited to detect novel input. Because of their vast postsynaptic domain, they can also help set behavioral and mental states.

The contrasting features of sensorimotor and modulatory neurons confer functionally important distinctions on their neuronal populations. The high rate of discharge of the sensorimotor neurons, acting through extensive interconnections that tie together sensorimotor neurons, causes exponential recruitment. This amplification occurs in response to novel stimuli requiring analysis and directed action (in the wake state) and in the generation of REM sleep, a state of sustained activation (when the system is off-line with respect to its inputs and outputs).

In contrast, the feedback inhibition and pacemaker potentials of modulatory neurons allow the production of highly synchronized output during waking and sleeping. These features also somehow cause an exponential decline in the firing rate of these neurons during REM sleep, until firing stops. Studies suggest that this REM sleep inhibition may involve a GABAergic action that arises in the hypothalamus at sleep onset and spreads through the brain stem as NREM sleep progresses to REM (see Fig. 42.5). These contrasting properties of sensorimotor and modulatory neurons of the reticular formation are the physical basis for the reciprocal interaction that causes NREM–REM sleep cycles.

Waking Requires Active Maintenance

Moruzzi and Magoun (1949) demonstrated that reticular formation is necessary to maintain the waking conscious state. Lesions in the midbrain reticular formation, sparing the lemniscal sensory pathways, result in a state that resembles NREM sleep. Although maintenance of the waking state often seems effortless, it requires brain mechanisms that compete with other active mechanisms that promote and mediate sleep.

Later, Dann et al. (1984) proposed that two mechanisms interact to regulate sleep–wake cycles. One of these, outlined in detail in Chapter 45, is a circadian rhythm in the propensity to fall asleep (curve C Fig. 42.6). The tendency to fall asleep is normally lowest early in the day, peaks at about late afternoon, and then declines in the evening. Thus sleepiness cycles independent of sleeping and waking. That is, if a subject is deprived of sleep, sleepiness will continue to follow a circadian rhythm. The second mechanism is a homeostatic property, designated S in Fig. 42.6. It increases as a function of the amount of time since the last sleep episode. S can be viewed as the equivalent of a sleep-promoting substance that accumulates during waking and dissipates during sleep. Although a large amount of work has been devoted to identifying a "sleep substance," whether one or more such substances is normally involved in sleep regulation remains unclear (see Strecker et al., 2000; also Krueger and Fang in Lydic and Baghdoyan, 1999). Many factors likely contribute to the homeostatic regulation of sleep.

Waking is a complex state. Its fundamental features are the maintenance of sensory input from multiple receptors, the capacity for directing attention and accessing memory, the constant readjustments of posture, the maintenance of forebrain activation, and an array of motor output. The mechanisms of many specific behaviors are discussed in Chapters 50 through 59. It is worth noting here, however, that reticular formation plays a crucial role in the initiation and maintenance of both wakefulness and sleep. We now focus on the active control of sleep.

The onset of sleep occurs when S and C factors coincide and the environmental milieu is conducive to sleep. At this point, the brain stem and cortical mechanisms of waking are relaxed: vigilance lapses, muscle tone declines, eyelids close, and the EEG slows. Because the cortex is still active, removal of ascending influences often results in sudden unresponsiveness, which may be associated with dreamlike imagery. This sleep onset mentation is usually abolished quickly by the thalamocortical oscillation of NREM sleep. As NREM sleep begins, the incomplete relaxation of the mechanisms maintaining muscle tone may result in paroxysmal twitching, a form of myoclonus often affecting the legs.

The Hypothalmus Participates in Sleep–Wake Regulation

During World War I and the following decade, an epidemic of encephalitis often resulted in a prolonged sleep-like state of unresponsiveness. The pathology of this encephalitis, called Von Economo encephalitis lethargica, included lesions in the posterior hypothalamus. Subsequent experimental animal work showed that large, posterior hypothalamic lesions produced a prolonged sleep-like state, whereas lesions in the preoptic area-anterior hypothalamus markedly suppressed sleep. These and similar observations led to the hypothesis of a sleep center in the posterior hypothalamus.

Subsequent animal studies confirmed that lesions to anterior portions of the hypothalamus (preoptic area and adjacent basal forebrain) cause insomnia, whereas stimulation of this area promotes sleep (see Hobson et al., 2000; also Shiromani et al. in Lydic and Baghdoyan, 1999). In contrast, lesions of the posterior hypothalamus cause hypersomnolence, and histaminergic tuberomammillary nucleus (TMN) neurons in this region have been shown to decrease their firing during sleep (Shiromani et al.).

We now know that during NREM sleep a small nucleus in the ventrolateral preoptic area (VLPO) activates the immediate-early gene c-fos (Sherin et al., 1996; Saper et al., 2001), indicating an increase in metabolic activity in NREM sleep. The VLPO contains GABA and galanin neurons that project to and inhibit the posterior hypothalamus, particularly the TMN whose wake-promoting, histamine-producing neurons project widely to the thalamus and cortex (Shiromani et al.). Sherin et al. thus suggest that this circuit constitutes a monosynaptic "switch" for the alternation of sleep and wakefulness. As noted earlier, orexinergic cells of the lateral hypothalamus may also play a key modulatory role in the sleep–wake cycle (Moore et al., 2001; Saper et al., 2001). See Fig. 42.5 for a schematic representation of this process.

Thus, one could conceive of a hypothalamic network in which the homeostatic and circadian regulatory processes of sleep interact at least in part at the VLPO, which in turn inhibits histaminergic activation of the thalamus and cerebral cortex by the tuberomammillary nucleus as suggested by Shiromani et al. and illustrated in Figure 42.5. Such a mechanism could link diencephalic and and brain stem mechanisms in the control of sleep onset and the REM–NREM alternation and allow the complex thalamocortical interactions of NREM sleep, as described in the next section.

NREM Sleep Requires a Thalamocortical Interaction

About 75% of sleep time is spent in the NREM phase. Detailed studies of cellular activity in thalamo-

cortical circuits have led to important, unifying concepts, such as that the forebrain, particularly the cortex, tends toward oscillation and unconsciousness unless activated by the brain stem (see Steriade, 2000; also Steriade in Lydic and Baghdoyan, 1999).

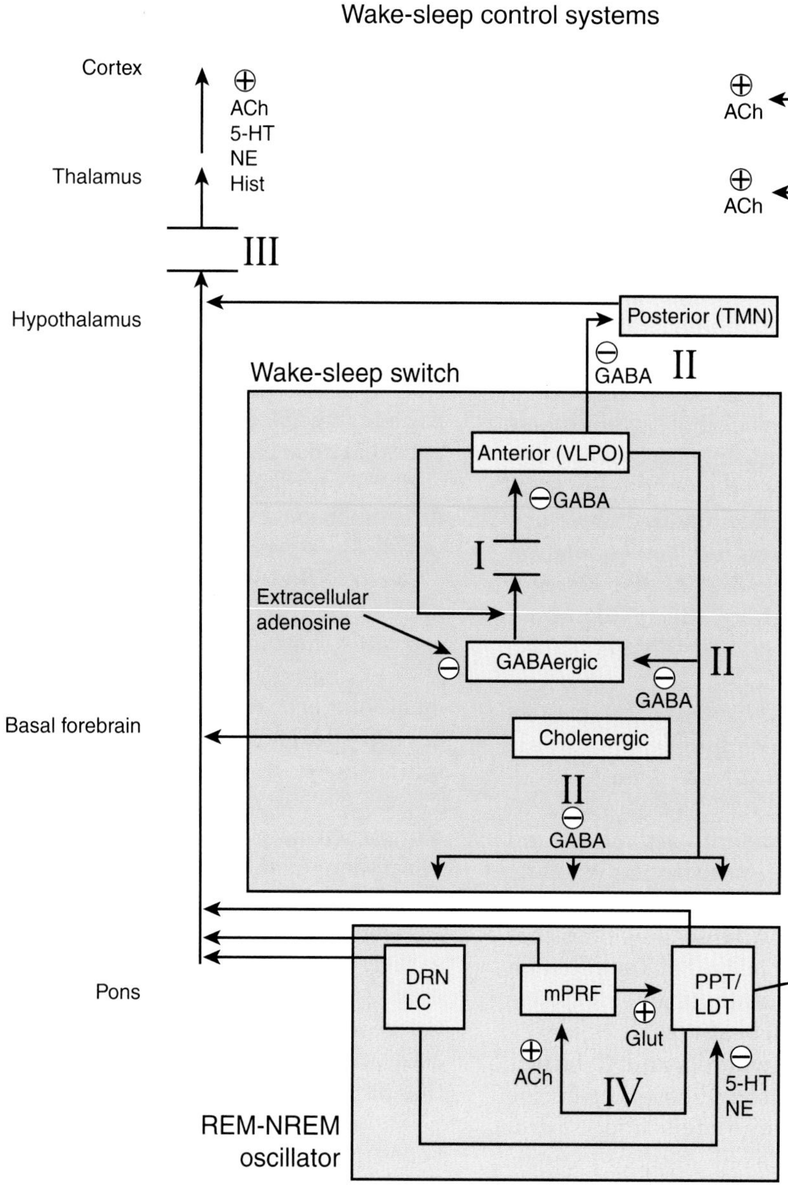

FIGURE 42.5   Integrated model of sleep onset and REM–NREM oscillation proposed by Shiromani et al. I. During prolonged wakefulness, accumulating adenosine inhibits specific GABAergic anterior hypothalamic and basal forebrain neurons, which have been inhibiting the sleep–active VLPO neurons during waking. II. Disinhibited sleep–active GABAergic neurons of the VLPO and adjacent structures then inhibit the wake–active histaminergic neurons of the TMN, as well as those of the pontine aminergic (DR and LC) and cholinergic (LDT/PPT) ascending arousal systems, thereby initiating NREM sleep. III. Forebrain activation by ascending aminergic and orexinergic arousal systems is disfacilitated. IV. Once NREM sleep is thus established, the executive networks of the pons initiate and maintain the ultradian REM/NREM cycle. ACh, acetylcholine; DRN, dorsal raphe nucleus; GABA, γ-amino butyric acid; LC, locus coeruleus; 5-HT, serotonin; LDT, laterodorsal tegmental nucleus; NE, norepinephrine; PRF, pontine reticular formation; TMN, tuberomammillary nucleus. From Pace-Schott and Hobson (2001).

The initiation of NREM sleep is gradual and is characterized by slowing of the frequency of brain waves seen on EEG (see Hobson, 1989). This initial slowing is stage 1 sleep. It is succeeded by stage 2 sleep, characterized by a further decrease in the frequency of brain waves and the presence of intermittent, high-frequency clusters of spikes of electrical activity, sleep spindles. Sleep spindles decrease in stage 3 sleep, and the amplitude of slow waves increases. Very high amplitude delta waves occur in deepest sleep, stages 3 and 4 (Fig. 42.4).

The critical circuitry (Fig. 42.7B) consists of reciprocally interconnected thalamic and cortical neurons whose dysfacilitation following sleep onset allows the emergence of underlying thalamocortical oscillatory (see Steriade, 2000; also Steriade in Lydic and Baghdoyan, 1999). The thalamocortical and thalamic reticular neurons regulating this state are shifted into this oscillatory firing mode by the deactivation and demodulation of diencephalic structures, such as the hypothalamus and basal forebrain, as well as the brain stem. In contrast, during waking, these circuits are modulated by neurons that produce ACh, NE, 5-HT, or histamine, whereas the principal modulator released during REM sleep is ACh.

After sleep onset, thalamocortical oscillations first produce the characteristic sleep spindles of stage 2 NREM. As sleep becomes deeper and spindling diminishes in NREM stages 3 and 4, GABAergic neurons of the thalamic reticular nucleus further hyperpolarize and dysfacilitate thalamic relay neurons, allowing the emergence of high-voltage delta (1–4 Hz) frequency oscillations (see Steriade, 2000; also Steriade in Lydic and Baghdoyan, 1999). The cortex may further constrain these spindle and delta wave-generating thalamocortical bursts within a newly described slow (<1 Hz) oscillation seen in cats (Steriade) and humans (Achermann and Borbely, 1997). This slow oscillation reflects a dynamic electrical oscillatory milieu among neurons within the cortex consisting of a slow (0.5 to 1 Hz) alternation of a quiescent hyperpolarization phase followed by intense spike trains during a depolarized phase (Steriade, 2000).

When high-voltage delta waves are present, people are difficult to arouse, and after waking they are confused, may confabulate, and cannot perform cognitive tests. However, the unique oscillatory physiology of NREM may underlie the transient, static but sometimes intense imagery ascribed to NREM mentation (Steriade, 2000). Thalamocortical and cortical neurons may use the oscillations in NREM sleep to balance ionic currents and intracellular regulatory mechanisms in such a way that experience from previous waking episodes is incorporated into memory

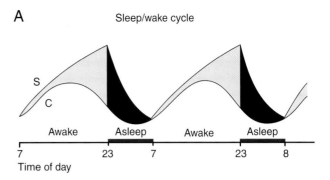

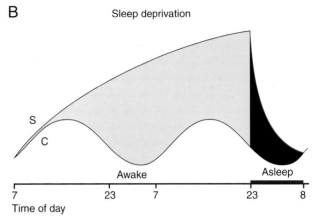

FIGURE 42.6 The Borbely and Daan model of sleep regulation. Sleep is assumed to result from the actions of process C and process S. Process C follows a circadian rhythm and is independent of sleeping and waking. Process S, on the other hand, depends on sleep–wake behavior; S declines during sleep and rises continuously during sleep deprivation. The period of recovery sleep that follows sleep deprivation is more intensive but only slightly longer than normal. If curve C represents the threshold for waking up, then at any time, "sleep pressure" is the (vertical) distance between the S and C curves. The greater the distance, the greater the pressure to fall asleep. Reprinted with permission from Daan et al. (1984).

(Steriade, 2000). Despite oscillatory activity, NREM sleep is a quiescent state for the brain relative to waking and REM, and blood flow and glucose use are decreased in slow wave NREM by more than 40% compared to waking. Positron emission tomography (PET) studies show that decreases in blood flow in NREM sleep are particularly marked in the brain stem and diencephalon (reviewed in Hobson et al., 2000).

Thus, the net brain stem and hypothalamic drive on the thalamocortical system sustains consciousness in the activated brain. In addition, the different modulatory inputs to the thalamocortical circuitry produce the different kinds of consciousness seen in waking and dreaming.

REM Sleep Is Initiated in the Brain Stem

Extracellular and intracellular recording techniques allowed detailed study of the cellular and molecular bases of the changes in input–output gating in REM sleep (Hobson, 1988). Edward Evarts used the movable microelectrode system of David Hubel to record the activity of individual brain neurons in animals sleep (reviewed in Hobson, 1988). Evarts showed that the generalized activity and the periodic PGO wave activation seen on EEG during REM sleep reflect the excitation of neurons throughout the forebrain, including the visual, motor, and association cortices and the thalamic nuclei reciprocally connected to them (see Hobson, 1988; also Hobson and Steriade, 1986) (Fig. 42.8). It may come as a surprise that we now know more about the neurophysiology of REM sleep and dreaming than we know about waking. REM sleep naturally favors neurophysiological studies because during REM sleep the normal modulation of motor and sensory systems paralyzes and partially anesthetizes animals.

REM sleep is a period of global as well as specific changes in the activation of neurons and flow of information throughout the brain. This picture of REM sleep is relevant to understanding the features that distinguish the conscious state of waking from those of NREM sleep and REM sleep, which is accompanied by dreaming (see Table 42.2). In waking, the activated brain–mind preferentially processes data from the outside world and responds by directing actions. In NREM sleep, the system is taken off-line via deactivation and therefore does not process information about the outside world. In REM sleep, in contrast to waking, the internal representations of the outside world become inputs, and the action summoned (but not executed) in response to those inputs itself becomes one of those inputs (Llinas and Pare, 1991).

The modulatory neuron system of the brain stem, particularly the noradrenergic locus ceruleus and the serotonergic pontine raphé neurons, mediates these changes in brain–mind state [for the following section, please refer to Hobson (1988), Hobson and Steriade (1986), and Hobson *et al.* (1993, 2000) for citations of original source material]. As we have seen, these aminergic populations contain pacemaker neurons that fire spontaneously throughout waking. The neurons also respond to stimuli by increasing their output. Output decreases during lulls between stimuli and at the onset of sleep. The cholinergic neurons of the pedunculopontine nucleus also respond to stimuli, but these cells are not pacemakers and tend to be otherwise quiescent in waking. Thus, the waking brain is bathed in constant levels of NE and 5-HT and receives pulsatile boosts of these two transmitters and of ACh when novel input data call for them. Because histaminergic neurons of the hypothalamus are also selectively

active in waking and inactive REM sleep, these observations suggest that the attentive, memory-forming awake state is chemically characterized as an aminergic–cholinergic collaboration.

At the onset of sleep, the activity of these subcortical modulatory neurons decreases, and the neurons contribute to the development of EEG spindles and slow waves. As NREM sleep deepens, the activity of the two pontine aminergic systems declines gradually and spontaneously, whereas the activity of the cholinergic neurons increases gradually and spontaneously. At the onset of REM sleep, the aminergic systems are completely quiet and the cholinergic system is fully active. The net effect, confirmed by measurements of transmitter release, is a shift from an aminergic microclimate in waking to a cholinergic microclimate in REM.

These physiological findings are supported by experiments showing that antiaminergic and procholinergic drugs tend to increase REM, whereas proaminergic and anticholinergic agents suppress it. In addition, these drugs have reciprocal effects on waking and NREM sleep. Among the wealth of pharmacological studies, two are particularly impressive and reveal dramatic REM sleep enhancement.

When the cholinergic agonist carbachol or the anticholinesterase (blocker of the enzyme cholinesterase, which breaks down ACh) neostig-

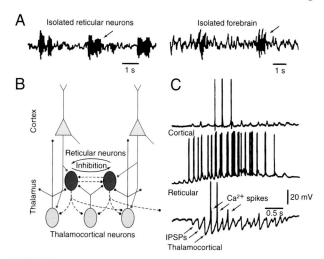

FIGURE 42.7 Thalamocortical oscillations *in vivo*. Sleep spindle oscillations are generated by synapses in the thalamus. (A, left) Potentials recorded through a microelectrode inserted in the deafferented reticular thalamic nucleus of a cat. The arrow points to one spindle sequence. (A, right) Spindle oscillations recorded from the thalamus of a cat with an upper brainstem transection that created an isolated forebrain preparation. The figure shows two spindle sequences (the second marked by an arrow) and, between them, lower frequency (delta) waves. (B) Neuronal connections involved in the generation of spindle oscillations. (C) Intracellular recordings of one spindle sequence (see A) in three types of neurons (cortical, reticular thalamic, and thalamocortical). Ca^{2+}, calcium ions; IPSP, inhibitory postsynaptic potential.

mine is injected into the paramedian pontine brain stem, an immediate, intense, and prolonged episode of REM sleep results. This effect, which disappears in about 6 h, is called short-term REM sleep enhancement. When injected into the far lateral peribrachial pons, the cholinergic agonist and acetyl- cholinesterase antagonist immediately but only unilaterally enhance PGO waves and, 24–48 h later, enhance activity in REM sleep episodes for 6–10 days; this is long-term REM sleep enhancement (Hobson *et al.*, 1993), and some of its features are illustrated in Fig. 42.9.

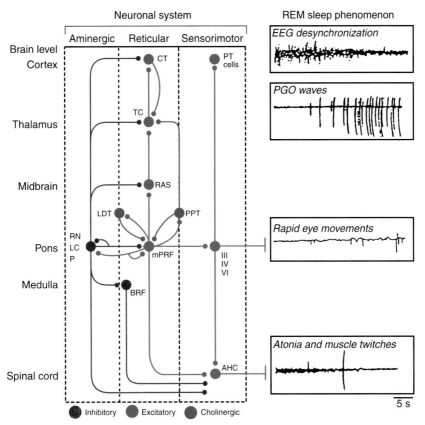

FIGURE 42.8 Schematic representation of the REM sleep generation process. A distributed network involves cells at many brain levels (left). The network is represented as comprising 3 neuronal systems (center) that mediate REM sleep electrographic phenomena (right). Postulated inhibitory connections are shown as red circles; postulated excitatory connections as green circles; and cholinergic pontine nuclei are shown as blue circles. It should be noted that the actual synaptic signs of many of the aminergic and reticular pathways remain to be demonstrated and, in many cases, the neuronal architecture is known to be far more complex than indicated here (e.g., the thalamus and cortex). During REM, additive facilitatory effects on pontine REM-on cells are postulated to occur via disinhibition (resulting from the marked reduction in firing rate by aminergic neurons at REM sleep onset) and through excitation (resulting from mutually excitatory cholinergic–noncholinergic cell interactions within the pontine tegmentum). The net result is strong tonic and phasic activation of reticular and sensorimotor neurons in REM sleep. REM sleep phenomena are postulated to be mediated as follows: EEG desynchronization results from a net tonic increase in reticular, thalamocortical, and cortical neuronal firing rates. PGO waves are the result of tonic disinhibition and phasic excitation of burst cells in the lateral pontomesencephalic tegmentum. Rapid eye movements are the consequence of phasic firing by reticular and vestibular cells; the latter (not shown) excite oculomotor neurons directly. Muscular atonia is the consequence of tonic postsynaptic inhibition of spinal anterior horn cells by the pontomedullary reticular formation. Muscle twitches occur when excitation by reticular and pyramidal tract motorneurons phasically overcomes the tonic inhibition of the anterior horn cells. RN, raphé nuclei; LC, locus coeruleus; P, peribrachial region; PPT, pedunculopontine tegmental nucleus; LDT, laterodorsal tegmental nucleus; mPRF, meso- and mediopontine tegmentum (e.g., gigantocellular tegmental field, parvocellular tegmental field); RAS, midbrain reticular activating system; BIRF, bulbospinal inhibitory reticular formation (e.g., gigantocellular tegmental field, parvocellular tegmental field, magnocellular tegmental field); TC, thalamocortical; CT, cortical; PT cell, pyramidal cell; III, oculomotor; IV, trochlear; V, trigmenial motor nuclei; AHC, anterior horn cell. From Hobson *et al.* (2000).

OTHER BRAIN STEM AND DIENCEPHALIC NEUROTRANSMITTER SYSTEMS

Despite the prominence of cholinergic and aminergic neuronal populations in the control of the sleep–wake and REM–NREM cycles, many additional neurotransmitter systems participate in the modulation of these long-period oscillators and may interact with aminergic and cholinergic control of these systems. The chemical identities and regulatory contributions of these substances have, in recent years, appeared frequently in the literature. The following section briefly summarizes these findings, referring the reader to major reviews for the original citations. Two 1999 volumes by Lydic and Baghdoyan and Mallick and Inoue (see General References) have provided exhaustive summaries of many of these systems, and we refer frequently, by chapter author, to specific sections of these volumes.

Dopamine and Histamine: Other Amines That May Be Involved in Modulating Wakefulness

The release of a third amine dopamine (DA) appears not to vary in phase with the natural sleep cycle as do the other two amines, 5-HT and NE, or as does ACh. In fact, the effects of DA on sleep may be mediated by its effects on the aminergic and cholinergic systems (Hobson et al., 2000). In animals, DA has been shown to influence both sleep–wake and REM–NREM cycles and REM deprivation has, in turn, been shown to alter dopaminergic function (Hobson et al., 2000). Human studies report REM suppression by DA reuptake inhibitors, the most well-known example being the treatment of narcolepsy with psychostimulants. However, another DA-enhancing agent, bupropion, has been shown to enhance REM, and DA may play a role in the induction or intensification of nightmares (see Hobson et al., 2000). Therefore the effects of DA on sleep are in much need of further study.

A fourth amine, histamine, is the transmitter of an arousal system originating in neurons of the posterior hypothalamus, which innervates the entire forebrain as well as brain stem (see Shiromani et al. in Lydic and Baghdoyan, 1999). Histamine is a wake-promoting substance, and lesions of histaminergic nuclei in the posterior hypothalamus result in hypersomnolence (Shiromani et al.). During sleep, these wake-active histaminergic neurons are inhibited tonically by GABAergic and galaninergic projections from the

TABLE 42.2   Physiological Basis of Changes That Occur during Dreaming

Function	Change (compared with waking)	Hypothesized cause
Sensory input	Blocked	Presynaptic inhibition
Perception (external)	Diminished	Blockade of sensory input
Perception (internal)	Enhanced	Removal of inhibition from networks that store sensory representations
Attention	Lost	Aminergic modulation decreases, causing a decrease in the ratio of signal to noise
Memory (recent)	Diminished	Because of a decrease in aminergic activity, activated representations are not stored in memory
Memory (remote)	Enhanced	Removal of inhibition from networks that store memory representations
Orientation	Unstable	Internally inconsistent signals are generated by cholinergic systems
Thought	Poor reasoning, processing hyper-associative	Loss of attention, memory, and volition leads to failure of sequencing and rule inconstancy; analogy replaces analysis
Insight	Self-reflection lost	Failures of attention, logic, and memory weaken second- (and third-) order representations
Language (internal)	Confabulatory	Aminergic demodulation frees the use of language from the restraint of logic
Emotion	Episodically strong	Cholinergic hyperstimulation of the amygdala and related structures of the temporal lobe triggers emotional storms, which are not modulated by aminergic activity
Instinct	Episodically strong	Cholinergic hyperstimulation of the hypothalamus and limbic forebrain triggers fixed motor programs, which are experienced fictively but not enacted
Volition	Weak	Cortical motor control cannot compete with disinhibited subcortical networks
Output	Blocked	Postsynaptic inhibition

anterior hypothalamus and adjacent basal forebrain (Shiromani *et al*.).

GABA And Glutamate: Amino Acids, Respectively, the Most Ubiquitous Inhibitory and Excitatory Brain Neurotransmitters

GABA is involved at many stages in the control of the sleep–wake and the REM–NREM cycle (see Jones and Muhlethaler and also Luppi *et al*. in Lydic and Baghdoyan, 1999). GABAergic inhibition plays both REM facilitory and REM inhibitory roles. For example, GABA inhibits aminergic neurons, which, in turn, suppress pontine cholinergic REM generation networks (e.g., Nitz and Siegel, 1997). It also directly inhibits mesopontine cholinergic neurons, which generate PGO waves (Datta in Mallick and Inoue, 1999). GABAergic inhibition is also important in sleep-promoting dysfacilitation of the brain stem and diencephalic arousal networks, which maintain wakefulness and prevent NREM sleep (Luppi *et al*. and Shiromani *et al*. in Lydic and Baghdoyan, 1999). During NREM sleep, GABA has been hypothesized to play key roles in the deactivation of wake-related arousal systems and in the generation of intrinsic thalamocortical oscillations (see Steriade in Lydic and Baghdoyan, 1999). Another inhibitory neurotransmitter, glycine, regulates specific physiological manifestations of REM. For example, medullary glycinergic cells are responsible for the postsynaptic inhibition of somatic motoneurons during REM atonia (Chase *et al*., 1989).

The excitatory amino acid glutamate widely interacts with cholinergic and cholinoceptive neurons to generate the exponential increase of mesopontine and pontine reticular activity associated with REM sleep activation (see Semba in Lydic and Baghdoyan, 1999). Glutamatergic cells of the pons transmit signals to inhibitory glycinergic and GABAergic cells of the medulla, which, in turn, suppress somatic motorneurons to produce REM sleep atonia (see Rye, 1997; also Lai *et al*. in Mallick and Inoue, 1999).

A Gaseous, Intercellularly Diffusable Neurotransmitter: Nitric Oxide (NO)

NO has recently been widely implicated in sleep cycle modulation and functions primarily as an intercellular messenger, which can enhance the synaptic release of neurotransmitters such as ACh and enhance capillary vasodilation (see Leonard and Lydic in Mallick and Inoue, 1999). NO is coproduced by cholinergic mesopontine neurons and may play a role in maintaining the cholinergically mediated REM

sleep state in both the pons and the thalamus (Leonard and Lydic).

Adenosine and Peptides: Endogenous Somnogens and More

Adenosine is a currently thought to be a strong candidate for the putative endogenous somnogen, which accumulates in the brain during prolonged wakefulness (Porkka-Heiskanen *et al*., 1997). Adenosine may exert inhibition over excitatory inputs to mesopontine cholinergic cells, over serotonergic raphé neurons during REM, and over basal forebrain cholinergic neurons during sleep onset (see Jones in Kryger *et al*., 2000). Certain cytokine neuropeptides have also been proposed to be endogenous somnogens (see Krueger and Fang in Lydic and Baghdoyan, 1999).

Neuropeptides are increasingly seen to play diverse roles in regulation of the sleep–wake and REM–NREM cycles. For example, the hypothalamic peptide galanin participates in the inhibition of wake-promoting centers during sleep onset (see Shiromani *et al*. in Lydic and Baghdoyan, 1999), whereas the hypothalamic peptide orexin is the agent of a newly discovered arousal system defects in which may constitute the genetic basis of narcolepsy (see Moore *et al*., 2001). Other peptides implicated in the REM–NREM and sleep–wake cycles include the vasoactive intestinal polypeptide (Steiger and Holsboer, 1997), as well as numerous hormones (see Obal and Krueger in Mallick and Inoue, 1999).

Second Messengers and Intranuclear Events

As in much of neuroscience, research on behavioral state control is now beginning to extend its inquiry beyond the neurotransmitter and its receptors to the roles of intracellular second messengers and the molecular biology of gene transcription (see Tononi and Cirelli, 2001; also Capece *et al*. in Mallick and Inoue, 1999). Behavioral state-dependent expression of immediate early genes shows that intranuclear events participate in the control of sleep–wake cycles (see Shiromani *et al*. in Lydic and Baghdoyan, 1999).

Summary

Specific neuronal groups within the hypothalamus, pons, and medulla are responsible for the regulation of behavioral states of sleep and wakefulness. Because some of these neuronal groups often lack distinct neuronal boundaries, they are a part of the so-called reticular core of the brain stem. These neuronal systems have very distinct afferent and efferent connections and very specific chemical identities, containing NE,

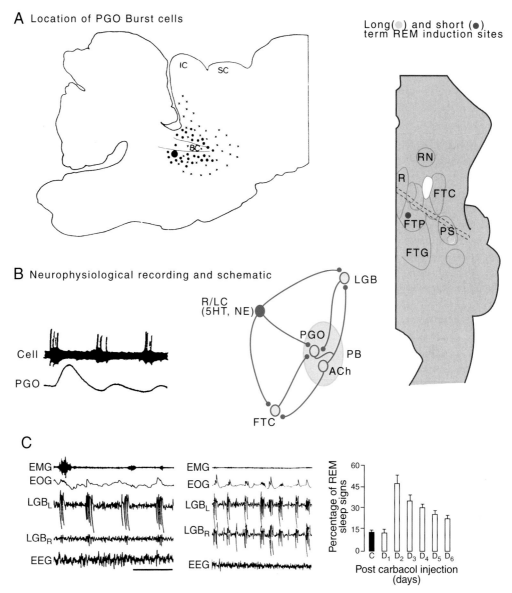

FIGURE 42.9 Sites of REM induction. (A, left) Filled circle indicates site of injection of carbachol into peribrachial pons. Small dots indicate location of cholinergic cells and crosses location of PGO burst cells. (A, right) Injection of carbachol, an acetylcholine agonist, in the perimedian pons (magenta dot) causes short-term induction of REM sleep. Injection of the peribrachial pons (yellow dot) causes long-term induction of REM sleep. After injection of a cholinergic agonist into the peribrachial pons, ponto-geniculo-occipital (PGO) burst cell activity and PGO waves can be measured immediately in the lateral geniculate body (LGB) on the same side (ipsilateral) as the injections (B, left). Hypothesized connections among the PGO trigger zone (PB), modulatory aminergic raphé (R), locus coeruleus (LC), and paramedian pontine reticular cells (FTC) are shown. (C, left) Injections of carbachol at the PB site shown in A produce immediate PGO waves in the ipsilateral LGB. After 24 h, REM sleep intensifies (C, middle) and remains so for 6 days (C, right). FTC, FTG, and FTP are reticular tegmented nuclei. ACh are cholinergic nuclei. RN, red nucleus; IC, inferior colliculus; SC, superior colliculus; BC, brachium conjunctiuum.

5HT, and ACh. These neurons are small or modest in size with extensive and elaborate axonal projections to hypothalamus, midbrain, and forebrain and include descending projections to the spinal cord. In addition, the three sets of neurons are heavily interconnected, such that NE and 5-HT neurons fire slowly in quiet waking and are reduced further as the ACh neurons activate during slow wave and REM sleep. NE neurons are actively suppressed, but with the end of REM sleep show activation by novel sensory events. 5-HT neurons fire most rapidly during continuous motor activity, such as walking or running. Both systems must be active for maintenance of the waking state. A posterior hypothalamic projection to the thalamus and cortex may serve to integrate thermal and circadian aspects of sleep and waking. Reciprocal connections between the cortex and the thalamus organized into synchronized oscillations underlie the EEG manifestations of slow-wave sleep, diminishing as sleep deepens. In REM sleep, when NE and 5-HT neurons are silent, autoactivation of the ACh neurons or pharmacological enhancement of cholinergic transmission within the reticular formation enhances REM sleep duration. Several other neurochemical systems (e.g., GABA, histamine) participate in the modulation of sleep-wake transitions and the aminergic cholinergic control of REM.

MODELING THE CONTROL OF BEHAVIORAL STATE

Two linked models—one neurobiological (McCarley and Hobson, 1975) and the other psychophysiological

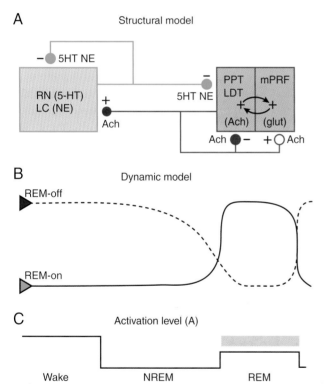

FIGURE 42.10 Structural and dynamic models of activation in REM sleep. (A) In the structural model, REM-on cells of the pontine reticular formation are excited by acetylcholine (ACh) or they produce excitatory signals using ACh in their synaptic terminals (or they do both). REM-off cells respond to or use NE or 5-HT as inhibitory neurotransmitters (or they do both). (B) In the dynamic model, during waking the pontine aminergic system (dashed line) is active continuously and inhibits the pontine cholinergic system (solid line). During NREM sleep, aminergic activity decreases, allowing cholinergic activity to rise. By the time REM sleep begins, the aminergic system is off and cholinergic excitation has peaked. (C) A result of the neuronal systems modeled in A and B.

(Hobson and McCarley, 1977; Hobson et al., 2000)—have been advanced to organize experimental findings and their implications for a theory of consciousness. According to the neurobiological model (Fig. 42.10), in waking, brain activation and open input–output gates result from a combination of continual aminergic activity and phasic (waxing and waning) aminergic and cholinergic activities. In contrast, in REM sleep the continually low level of aminergic activity and the periodic increases in cholinergic activity close input–output gates, activate the brain, and periodically stimulate the brain.

The subjective experience of waking, NREM sleep, and REM sleep can tentatively be linked to the accompanying changes in physiology (Table 42.2). Sensation and perception decline progressively during the cortical deactivation that occurs at the onset of sleep; responsiveness declines further as NREM sleep deepens. During REM sleep the brain reactivates, but presynaptic inhibition blocks sensory signals. REMs and their associated PGO waves act as internal stimuli, which take the place of stimuli from external sources. The brain stem sends information about eye movements to the thalamocortical visual system, possibly accounting for the intense visual hallucination of dreams. Furthermore, these PGO signals also drive the amygdala, perhaps accounting for such emotions as anxiety and surprise in dreams. Interestingly, PET studies of REM sleep show an increase of regional cerebral blood flow in limbic structures, including the amygdala.

In the early days of the EEG, brain waves with frequencies greater than 25 Hz were either ignored or filtered out because of the problem of interference by 50- or 60-Hz artifacts from electrical power sources. Later, researchers were able to focus on the possibility that 40-Hz EEG activity synchronizes processing in cortical areas.

Rodolfo Llinás proposed that as the cortex is scanned by the thalamus, 40-Hz waves propagate from the frontal to the occipital poles (reviewed in Kahn et al., 1997). Noting that 40-Hz activity is observed in REM sleep as well as in waking, he suggested that intrinsic neuronal oscillations are important in the genesis of both states of consciousness and that the main difference between waking and dreaming arises from differences in input–output gating (Llinas and Pare, 1991). In addition to being without temporal or spatial input, in REM sleep the brain has little background aminergic activity; this lack may contribute to the declines in attention, orientation, memory, and logic that characterize dreaming and make dreams difficult to remember (Hobson et al., 2000).

Neuroimaging and Lesion Studies of Sleep and Dreaming

Functional neuroimaging studies have revealed distinctive differences in regional brain activation between the cardinal behavioral states of waking, NREM sleep and REM sleep (for a review and original citations, see Hobson et al., 2000). In brief, widespread deactivation of the forebrain and brain stem is seen following sleep onset, and activation further decreases with the increasing depth of NREM sleep from NREM stage 1 to 2 to slow-wave sleep (SWS). Subsequently in REM, however, there is selective reactivation to waking or above-waking levels in brain stem, diencephalic, subcortical limbic, cortico-limbic, and selected cortical association areas. Notably however, during REM, significant deactivation of the dorsolateral prefrontal cortex relative to waking persists. Figure 42.11 illustrates the structures found to be

activated or deactivated in two or more of these recent neuroimaging studies.

These findings have led to an updating of the original activation synthesis hypothesis of dreaming (Hobson and McCarley, 1977), which now emphasizes that the distinctive cognitive features of dreams result from simultaneous autoactivation of the limbic brain (with consequent dream emotionality and salience) combined with the deactivation of executive structures subserving logic and working memory (with consequent dream bizarreness and disorientation) (Hobson et al., 2000).

Complementing these findings have been neuropsychological findings on brain-damaged patients by Solms (1997). In these studies, dorsolateral prefrontal damage was found to have little effect on dreaming in keeping with its relative inactivity during REM and the apparent diminution of its mnemonic, orientational, and logical functioning in dreaming. In contrast, destructive lesions of multimodal parietal areas resulted in global cessation of dreaming, whereas lesions of the visual association cortex led to nonvisual dreaming in keeping with the activation of the supramarginal gyrus and inferotemporal cortex in some PET studies and the highly visuospatial nature of dreaming. Similarly, disconnective lesions in upper brain stem-limbic-prefrontal areas led to global cessation of dreaming in keeping with their activation in REM and the highly emotional and personally salient quality of dreaming (Box 42.2).

The Brain Stem Has Three Clocks

Chapter 41 reviewed the biological basis of circadian timing. An important question is how the circadian clock(s), located in the suprachiasmatic nucleus of the hypothalamus, interacts with the NREM–REM sleep clock in the pons so that the full-amplitude oscillation of the sleep clock is confined to the rest phase of the rest–activity cycle (see Moore 1996; Fig. 42.12). The suprachiasmatic nucleus receives input from serotonergic raphé nuclei, and other connections between the two centers are beginning to be demonstrated (Saper et al., 2001). As mentioned earlier, the NREM–REM cycle free-runs when the connections between pons and hypothalamus are cut or when the hypothalamus is removed. However, we do not understand exactly how the synchronizing signals are transmitted and what their cellular and molecular basis may be (see Chapter 41).

During waking, damping of the NREM–REM oscillator is incomplete. Numerous studies have revealed a weak but significant periodicity of behavior during the activity phase of the rest–activity cycle. The period

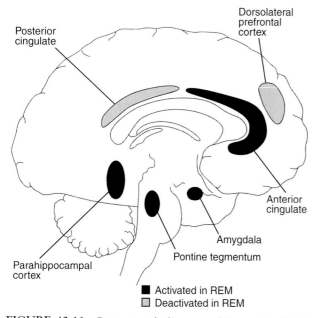

FIGURE 42.11 Convergent findings on relative regional brain activation and deactivation in REM compared to waking. A schematic sagittal view of the human brain showing those areas of relative activation and deactivation in REM sleep compared to waking and/or NREM sleep, which were reported in two or more of the three PET studies published to date (Braun et al., 1997; Maquet et al., 1996; Nofzinger et al., 1997; see Hobson et al., 2000 for citations). Only those areas that could be matched easily between two or more studies are illustrated here and a realistic morphology of the depicted areas is not implied. Note that considerably more extensive areas of activation and deactivation are reported in the individual studies; these more detailed findings are reviewed in Hobson et al. (2000). The depicted areas are thus viewed most realistically as representative portions of larger CNS areas subserving similar functions (e.g., limbic-related cortex, ascending activation pathways, and multimodal association cortex).

BOX 42.2

REGIONAL ACTIVATION AND DEACTIVATION: IMAGING THE HUMAN BRAIN AWAKE AND ASLEEP

Not only is the brain surprisingly and strongly activated during REM sleep, but its various subregions are activated and deactivated in a pattern quite different from that of waking. The mechanism of this differential activation pattern, revealed in PET, SPECT, and fMRI functional neuroimaging studies, is unknown, but it seems quite likely that the underlying shifts in regional metabolism and blood flow are orchestrated by the neuromodulators, which play this role in the rest of the body.

Compared to waking, deep NREM sleep shows a rather global deactivation pattern in keeping with the observed EEG slowing and synchronization. However, in REM, some areas are hyperactivated (among which the pontine brain stem, the limbic system, and the paralimbic cortex are most notable), whereas others are deacti-

vated (among which the posterior cingulate and the dorsolateral prefrontal cortex are most notable).

These shifts in regional blood flow, and by inference regional neuronal activity, map nicely onto the observed changes in consciousness. Thus activation of the amygdala and the parahippocampal cortex is relevant to the domination of dream consciousness by emotion, the activation of multimodal cortex is relevant to the hyperassociative quality of dreaming, whereas the inactivation of the dorsolateral prefrontal cortex seems relevant to the defects in cognition and memory. At last, the human brain and its wonderous array of conscious states is ameanable to neuobiological analysis, in real time, in real people, and in patients as well as in normals.

J. Allan Hobson and Edward F. Pace-Schott

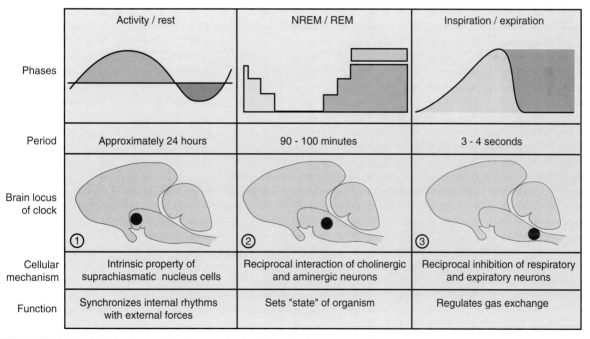

FIGURE 42.12 Biological rhythms and brain stem clocks. Three rhythms interact during sleep. Circadian rhythms have a period of about 24 h and control many cycles, including the rest–activity cycle. The circadian clock is located in the suprachiasmatic nucleus of the hypothalamus. The 90- to 100-min period of NREM–REM sleep cycles is controlled by cholinergic and aminergic neurons of the pontine reticular formation. These neurons oscillate out of phase from each other to determine behavioral state (waking, NREM sleep, or REM sleep). The circadian clock sets the threshold of the sleep cycle clock by an unknown mechanism. The respiratory oscillator is similar in neuronal design to the sleep cycle clock but has a shorter period (3 s), which is controlled by the reciprocal inhibition of expiratory and inspiratory neurons in the medulla.

is about 90–100 min, suggesting that the pontine clock may be timing at low amplitude throughout the day and thus causing the normal waxing and waning of attention and motor activity during waking. A better understanding of the interaction of this clock with the circadian clock is an important issue for research (Fig. 42.12).

Central Autonomic Control Systems Are State Dependent

Cognitive and vegetative functions are linked to changes in central modulatory systems during sleep. For example, active hypothalamic temperature control is diminished or abandoned in REM sleep (Hobson, 1989), and the sensitivity of the respiratory control system is likewise diminished. As a result, a neuron that is sensitive to temperature or pO_2 during waking loses that responsiveness during REM sleep.

Sleep, then, involves significant changes in the reflex control of autonomic function. Our understanding of changes in the control of vegetative and sensorimotor functions during waking and sleep can be applied to understand sleep-related dysfunctions such as insomnia (inability to sleep), hypersomnia (excessive sleepiness), and parasomnia (sleep with reflex responses to stimuli) (Hobson, 1989).

Sleep Disorders Result from Disrupted Control of Behavioral State

When central nervous system (CNS) aminergic activity increases, the brain is shifted in the direction of hyperarousal, and insomnia and sometimes stress result. If stress and insomnia are prolonged, the chronic sympathetic overdrive can harm cardiovascular, cognitive, and behavioral functions of an animal. Behavioral and pharmacologic interventions that

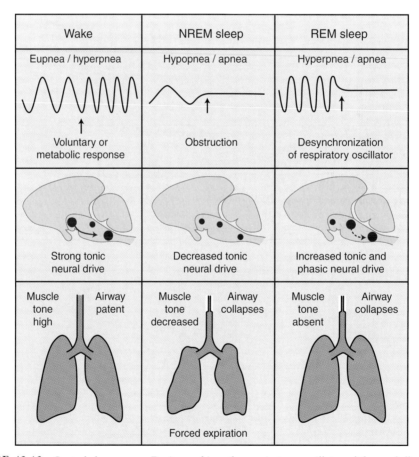

FIGURE 42.13 Central sleep apnea. During waking, the respiratory oscillator of the medulla receives tonic drive from other neural structures and can respond to voluntary and metabolic signals to change breathing pattern. Muscle tone keeps the oropharynx open to the flow of air. In NREM sleep, central drive decreases, and the rate and depth of ventilation fall. If the airway collapses, prolonged apnea (lack of breathing) may result. During REM sleep, activation of pontine generator neurons drives the respiratory oscillator, and desynchronization may lead to breathing efforts that are too frequent or strong (hyperpnea) or that stop. During REM sleep the oscillator also becomes unresponsive to metabolic signals.

decrease sympathetic output may be understood as reversals of the peripheral and central excitatory stimuli that prevent the locus coeruleus and raphé systems from gaining the periodic respite of sleep; insomnia is a form of sleep deprivation that prevents the cholinergic system from exerting its restorative effects. [For reviews of sleep disorders discussed in later, see Kryger *et al.* (2000) and Hobson (1989).]

The decrease in CNS aminergic activity (as in depression or narcolepsy) has opposite effects on cardiovascular, cognitive, and behavioral systems. With sleepiness, attention and cognition decline, and motor activity is impaired. Under these conditions, the cholinergic system is disinhibited, and the REM generator is triggered abnormally easily. The result is unwanted sleepiness or frank REM sleep attacks. These symptoms are decreased by aminergic agonists, such as blockers of amine reuptake, and anticholinergics, both of which boost sympathetic activity. Indeed, the best drugs for treating hypersomnia have both proaminergic and anticholinergic actions.

Respiratory Dysfunction Is Common in Sleep

One of the more dramatic problems associated with sleep is an exaggeration, at sleep onset, of the normal decline in respiratory drive (see Chapter 37). Also, respiratory irregularity may be provoked by the altered brain stem activity of REM sleep. This sleep-dependent disruption of respiratory function is central sleep apnea, a decrease in respiratory drive during NREM sleep (Fig. 42.13). In addition, especially in obese people, mechanical collapse or compression of the airway can result in peripheral (or obstructive) sleep apnea, in which ventilation decreases because of a mechanical problem in the oropharynx. In peripheral sleep apnea, central respiratory drive causes continued respiratory effort. Eventually, arousal results in increased muscle tone in the oropharynx, and the airway opens. As the person falls into deeper sleep again, the oropharynx relaxes and the airway becomes obstructed until arousal recurs. This cycle can repeat.

People with sleep apnea usually feel excessively sleepy during daytime because frequent arousal prevents deep, sustained sleep. They are often unaware of their sleep-dependent breathing pattern because they are never fully aroused from sleep. Instead, observant friends or family often describe seeing these signs of respiratory dysfunction. In a sleep laboratory, EEG, respiratory effort, and cardiovascular parameters (e.g., heart rate and blood pressure) are measured to quantify the problem. Sleep apnea can be treated by having the person wear a mask through which air is forced gently, helping to keep the airway open. The pressure of the air fluctuates to allow regular exhalation. People with sleep apnea are treated not only to alleviate their constant drowsiness, but to prevent long-term effects of sleep apnea, such as cardiopulmonary complications.

Motor Disturbances Occur during Sleep

Parasomnias that affect the skeletal motor system (e.g., sleep walking, sleep talking, tooth grinding, and night terrors) result from activation, in NREM sleep, of the response to central motor pattern generators. Normally, responses to these generators are disinhibited at sleep onset and later inhibited so no motor commands are enacted during REM sleep. Unlike NREM sleep phenomena, which affect mainly young people, REM sleep behavior disorder can be a sign of degenerative brain disease in the elderly. Because of a failure to inhibit the expression of motor acts in REM, people may literally enact their dream scenarios in their bedrooms.

A syndrome strikingly similar to REM sleep behavior disorder can be induced experimentally by bilateral lesions of the pontine tegmentum in cats. When in REM sleep, these animals perform stereotyped behavior sequences, such as hissing, piloerection, pouncing, and jumping. Jouvet called these "hallucinatory behaviors," and Morrison called the phenomenon "REM sleep without atonia" (see Jouvet, 1999). Because the ability of a cat to inhibit motor pattern commands during REM sleep is impaired by the lesions, they act out the commands. The instinctual aspect of these released behaviors is relevant to the psychophysiology of dreaming and has important implications for the hypothesis that REM sleep serves an active maintenance function.

Sleep Has a Function

Although it is easy to conceptualize the function of waking and to understand the adaptive value of consciousness, it has been difficult to move beyond the subjectively compelling but scientifically unsatisfactory notion of sleep as rest. Evidence strongly suggests that sleep has an anabolic and actively conservative function that is related to the complexity of the mammalian brain (see Table 42.1). In fact, Bennington and Heller (1995) propose that an important function of NREM sleep is to restore brain glycogen stores.

The most dramatic evidence of this homeostatic function comes from sleep deprivation studies in rats in which sleep deprivation was fatal when it persisted for 4 to 6 weeks. Early in the deprivation period, the rats began to eat more but could not maintain their body weight. Later, they lost their ability to maintain body temperature and developed strong heat-seeking behavior. Finally, they died of overwhelming sepsis because of immunodeficiency. The study implied that metabolic caloric balance, thermal equilibrium, and immune competence are preserved by sleep (Rechtschaffen *et al.*, 2002).

Additional evidence links immune function and sleep. Pappenheimer found that NREM sleep in rabbits was enhanced by dimuramyl peptides of bacterial cell wall origin. NREM sleep is also enhanced by the cytokines interleukin-1 and interleukin-2, both of which are released during NREM sleep (Krueger *et al.*, 1999).

Contributing to the notion that sleep has an anabolic function is the abundance of sleep in early life. REM sleep predominates *in utero*, where its stereotypic pattern of motor activation and its chemical microenvironment could promote CNS development (see Hobson, 1989). Such a function would be expected to decline in childhood, just as REM does. Also, growth and development could be enhanced by the release of growth hormone and gonadotropins in NREM sleep. Such hormone release declines, as does NREM sleep, after growth and sexual maturation are complete, around 30 years of age.

The theory of sleep as rest is supported by recognition that sleep is an energy- and heat-saving behavior that tends to occur at night, when ambient temperatures are low. In addition, sleeping with other members of the species may provide safety from predators and supply warmth.

Not only energy but also information may be conserved in sleep. Numerous studies show that animals have more REM sleep when learning a task and that REM deprivation interferes with learning (see Stickgold, 1998; Smith, 1995) Neurotransmitters needed to form recent memories (e.g., NE and 5-HT) could be conserved and their receptors could be regulated or sensitized during REM sleep if their neurons stop firing. At that time, the cholinergic environment of the brain could help consolidate memories already in the system. Finally, cognition and emotion, which most people agree benefit from sleep, could be mediated by the reversal of wake state neuromodulation in REM.

Sleep and Memory Are Interdependent

Recent findings have clearly shown an interdependence of sleep and memory (for recent reviews pertaining to the following section, see Stickgold, 1998; Stickgold *et al.*, 2001). One of the most notable examples is the discovery, in rats, by Carlyle Smith, of "REM

windows" (see Smith, 1995), which are time periods after an animal is trained on specific tasks when the animal shows enhanced quantities of REM sleep and when retention of learning could be decreased by selective REM sleep deprivation. Subsequent studies in humans have led to the theory that REM sleep is especially important for procedural learning, which can be defined as a general category of memory involving the learning of sensorimotor skills, whereas SWS has been shown to be of greater importance in the retention of explicit or declarative memory, which involves recall of specific events or knowledge. However, studies on a procedural learning visual discrimination task has shown a requirement for both REM and SWS on the night following training in order for next day improvement on the task to be observed (Stickgold *et al.*, 2000a). This finding supports an earlier theory based on animal studies in which a two-step process involving both REM and SWS was hypothesized. In humans, the requirement for sleep immediately following learning was shown when subjects who were sleep deprived the night following training but were allowed two subsequent nights of unrestricted recovery sleep showed no significant task improvement (Stickgold *et al.*, 2000b). In addition to procedural learning tasks, REM effects have been reported in humans on learning of complex logic games, foreign language acquisition, and intensive studying in general, and both REM and SWS effects have been reported for the consolidation and processing of emotional memories.

Summary

Two models attempt to explain sleep and wakefulness. In the neurobiological model, sleep and waking are the result of a hypothalamic sleep-wake switch followed by reciprocal, phasic interactions between NE and 5-HT neurons and ACh neurons. In the alternative psychophysical model, the influences of external and internal sensations are emphasized. During slow-wave sleep, thalamocortical synchronous activity diminishes responsiveness to the external world. During REM sleep, under the influence of forebrain cholinergic projections, internal representations of visual information predominate. In addition to changes in levels of sensory arousal and cognitive performance during sleeping, vegetative functions such as circadian rhythm recognition, body temperature, and autonomic activity are also regulated coordinately. Disorders of sleep influence emotional and cognitive functions adversely. Prolonged sleep deprivation is lethal, ending in a septic state of immunodeficiency, strongly suggesting that sleep serves an important but uncertainly mediated restorative function.

BOX 42.3

CONSCIOUSNESS IN WAKING, SLEEPING, AND DREAMING: A MODEL FOR MENTAL ILLNESS

Since the brain is continuously active across states of sleep, so is the mind. Every modality of conscious experience can be shown to be state dependent, and particularly strong contrasts are evident between waking and dreaming, the two conscious states associated with higher levels of brain activation.

These alterations in consciousness are particularly informative to neurologists and psychiatrists because they provide new ways of thinking about the brain basis of mental illness. When brain activation declines in NREM sleep, most aspects of waking consciousness also decline. But when the brain is activated again during REM sleep, it does not reinstate waking consciousness. Instead, consciousness changes in an almost qualitative manner: Perception, instead of being shaped by external forms, becomes hallucinatory. Cognition is similarly deranged. Instead of being oriented, the dreaming mind loses track of time place and person. Instead of thinking

actively and critically, the dreaming mind indulges in non-sequiturs, ad-hoc explanations, and other illogical whims. Memory, during dreams, instead of being declaratively faithful to recent history, is fragmented in its disconnection from current events and globally deficient in recalling them. Emotion, instead of being restrained and focused in response to percepts and thoughts, comes to dominate nd organize dreaming consciousness often in strikingly salient ways. All of these features of dream consciousness are normal and all are closely related to the changes in brain modulation. Because they are formally similar to the symptoms of the major psychoses, they suggest that mental illness may reflect genetic and environmental dysfunction of brain modulatory systems.

J. Allan Hobson and Edward F. Pace-Schott

The brain undergoes daily, complex, systematic changes that profoundly alter the nature of our consciousness, behavior, autonomic control, and physiologic homeostasis. At the root of these changes is the circadian clock. Located in the hypothalamus, this clock programs rest–activity and body temperature cycles. It also gates the NREM–REM sleep cycle control system in the pons.

Some cellular and molecular details of the brain stem diencephalic behavioral state control system are clear: For the awake state, the noradrenergic locus coeruleus and the serotonergic raphé neurons of the pons as well as the histaminergic (and possibly orex inergic) neurons of the hypothalamus must fire regularly to support alertness, attentiveness, memory, orientation, logical thought, and emotional stability. When the output of these chemical systems diminishes, drowsiness occurs. When sleep begins, the output of these systems declines further, and the brain–mind enters NREM sleep, a phase of lowered consciousness. During NREM sleep, cholinergic activity increases gradually. At the NREM–REM transition, the activity of the serotonergic and nonadrenergic systems is at its nadir, and the output of the cholinergic system increases exponentially. This chemical switch results in the cholinergic activation and autostimulation of REM sleep. Combined with the lack of aminergic stimulation, this cholinergic overdrive accounts for the charac-

teristic hallucination, delusion, disorientation, memory loss, and emotional intensity of dreaming.

Although the details of these daily changes in brain chemistry remain to be specified, consequences of their dysfunction are becoming more clearly understood through the study of insomnias, hypersomnias, and parasomnias. Integration of data from basic neurobiology, cognitive psychology, and clinical science enables the construction of specific, testable models of how waking and sleep affect our conscious experience. These models, in turn, constitute the building blocks of a scientific theory of consciousness.

References

Achermann, P., and Borbely, A A. (1997). Low frequency (<1 Hz) oscillations in the human sleep electroencephalogram. *Neuroscience* **81**, 213–222.

Aston-Jones, G., and Bloom, F. E. (1981). Activity of norepinephrine-containing locus coeruleus neurons in behaving rats anticipates fluctuations in the sleep-waking cycle. *J. Neurosci.* **1**, 876–886.

Baghdoyan, H. A., Monaco, A. P., Rodrigo-Angulo, M. L., Assens, F., McCarley, R. W., and Hobson, J. A. (1984). Microinjection of neostigmine into the pontine reticular formation of cats enhances desynchronized sleep signs. *J. Pharmacol. Exp. Ther.* **231**, 173–180.

Bennington, J. H., and Heller, H. C. (1995). Restoration of brain energy metabolism as the function of sleep. *Progress Neurobiol.* **45**, 347–360.

Callaway, C. W., Lydic, R., Baghdoyan, H. A., and Hobson, J. A. (1987). Ponto-geniculo-occipital waves: Spontaneous visual system activation occurring in REM sleep. *Cell Mol. Neurobiol.* **7**, 105–149.

Calvo, J., Datta, S., Quattrochi, J. J., and Hobson, J. A. (1992). Cholinergic microstimulation of the peribrachial nucleus in the cat. II. Delayed and prolonged increases in REM sleep. *Arch. Ital. Biol.* **130**, 285–301.

Chase, M. H., Soja, P. J., and Morales, F. R. (1989). Evidence that glycine mediates the post synaptic potentials that inhibit lumbar motorneurons during the atonia of active sleep. *J. Neurosci.* **9**, 743–751.

Daan, S., Beersma, D. G. M., and Borbely, A. A. (1984). Timing of human sleep: Recovery process gated by a circadian pacemaker. *Am. J. Physiol.* **246**, R161–R178.

Dahlstrom, A., and Fuxe, K. (1964). Evidence for the existence of monoamine neurons in the central nervous system. I. Demonstration of monoamines in the cell bodies of brain stem neurons. *Acta Physiol. Scand.* **62**(S232), 1–55.

Hobson, J. A., McCarley, R. W., and Qyzinki, P. W. (1975). Sleep cycle oscillation: Reciprocal discharge by two brainstem neuronal groups. *Science* **189**, 55–58.

Hobson, J. A., Datta, S., Calvo, J. M., and Quattrochi, J. (1993). Acetylcholine as a brain state modulator: Triggering and long-term regulation of REM sleep. *Prog. Brain Res.* **98**, 389–404.

Jacobs, B. L., and Azmitia, E. C. (1992). Structure and function of the brain serotonin system. *Physiol. Rev.* **72**, 165–229.

Kahn, D., Pace-Schott, E. F., and Hobson, J. A. (1997). Consciousness in waking and dreaming: The roles of neuronal oscillation and neuromodulation in determining similarities and differences. *Neuroscience* **78**, 13–38.

Krueger, J. M., Obal, F., and Fang, J. (1999). Humoral regulation of physiological sleep: Cytokines and GHRH. *Sleep Res.* **8** (Suppl. 1), 53–59.

Llinas, R. R., and Pare, D. (1991). Of dreaming and wakefulness. *Neuroscience* **44**, 521–535.

Lydic, R., Baghdoyan, H. A., and Lorinc, Z. (1991). Microdialysis of cat pons reveals enhanced acetylcholine release during state-dependent respiratory depression. *Am. J. Physiol.* **261**, 766–770.

Moore, R. Y., and Card, J. P. (eds.) (1984). "Noradrenaline-Containing Neuron System." Elsevier, Amsterdam.

Moore, R. Y., Abrahamson, E. A., and Van Den Pol, A. (2001). The hypocretin neuron system: An arousal system in the human brain. *Arch. Ital. Biol.* **139**, 2195–2205.

Moruzzi, G., and Magoun, H. W. (1949). Brainstem reticular formation and activation of the EEG. *Electroencephal. Clin. Neurophysiol.* **1**, 455–473.

Nitz, D., and Siegel, J. M. (1997). GABA release in the dorsal raphe nucleus: Role in the control of REM sleep. *Am. J. Physiol.* **273**, R451–R455.

Pappenheimer, J. R. (1982). Induction of sleep by moramyl peptides. *J. Physiol.* **336**, 1–11.

Rechtschaffen, A., and Beogman, B. M. (2002). Sleep deprivation in the rat: An update of the 1989 paper. *Sleep* **24**, 18–24.

Rye, D. B. (1997). Contributions of the peduculopontine region to normal and altered REM sleep. *Sleep* **20**, 757–788.

Saper, C. B., Chou, T. C., and Scammell, T. E. (2001). The sleep switch: Hypothalamic control of sleep and wakefulness. *Trends Neurosci.* **24**, 726–731.

Sherin, J. E., Shiromani, P. J., McCarley, R. W., *et al.* (1996). Activation of ventrolateral preoptic neurons during sleep. *Science* **271**, 216–219.

Smith, C. (1995). Sleep states and memory processes. *Behav. Brain res.* **69**, 137–145.

Solms, M. (1997). "The Neuropsychology of Dreams: A Clinico-anatomical Study." Lawrence Erlbaum Associates.

Steiger, A., and Holsboer, F. (1997). Neuropeptides and human sleep. *Sleep* **20**, 1038–1052.

Stickgold, R. (1998). Sleep: Off-line memory reprocessing. *Trends Cog. Sci.* **2**, 484–492.

Stickgold, R., Whidbee, D., Schirmer, B., Patel, V., and Hobson, J. A. (2000a). Visual discrimination task improvement: A multi-step process occurring during sleep. *J. Cog. Neurosci.* **12**, 246–254.

Stickgold, R., James, L., and Hobson, J. A. (2000b). Visual discrimination learning requires sleep after training. *Nature Neurosci.* **3**, 1237–1238.

Stickgold, R., Hobson, J. A., Fosse, R., and Fosse, M. (2001). Sleep, learning and dreams: Off-line memory reprocessing. *Science* **294**, 1052–1057.

Strecker, R. E., Morairty, S., Thakkar, M. M., Porkka-Heiskanen, T., Basheer, R., Dauphin, L. J., Rainnie, D. G., Portas, C. M., Greene, R. W., and McCarley, R. W. (2000). Adenosinergic modulation of basal forebrain and preoptic/anterior hypothalamic neuronal activity in the control of behavioral state. *Behav. Brain Res.* **115**, 183–204.

Tononi, G., and Cirelli, C. (2001). Modulation of brain gene expression during sleep and wakefulness: A review of recent findings. *Neuropsychopharm.* **25**, S28–S35.

Suggested Readings

Hobson, J. A. (1988). "The Dreaming Brain." Basic Books, New York.

Hobson, J. A. (1989). "Sleep." Scientific American Library.

Hobson, J. A., Pace-Schott, E. F., and Stickgold, R. (2000). Dreaming and the brain: Toward a cognitive neuroscience of conscious states. *Behav. Brain Sci.* **23**, 793–842.

Hobson, J. A., and Steriade, M. (1986). The neuronal basis of behavioral state control. *In* "Handbook of Physiology" (F. E. Bloom, ed.), Sect. 1, Vol. 4, pp. 701–823. American Physiological Society, Bethesda, MD.

Jouvet, M. (1999). "The Paradox of Sleep: The Story of Dreaming." MIT Press.

Kryger, M. H., Roth, T., and Dement, W. C. (eds.) (2000). "Principles and Practice of Sleep Medicine." Saunders, Philadelphia.

Lydic, R. and Baghdoyan, H.A. (eds.) (1999). "Handbook of Behavioral State Control: Molecular and cellular mechanisms." CRC Press.

Mallick, B. N., and Inoue, S. (eds.) (1999). "Rapid Eye Movement Sleep." Dekker.

Pace-Schott, E. F., and Hobson, J. A. (2002). Basic mechanisms of sleep: New evidence on the neuroanatomy and neuromodulation of the NREM-REM cycle. *In* (D. Charney, J. Coyle, K. Davis and C. Nemeroff, eds.), "American College of Neuropsychopharmacology, Fifth Generation of Progress." Lippincott, Williams & Wilkins, New York.

Steriade, M. (2000). Corticothalamic resonance, states of vigilance and mentation. *Neuroscience* **101**, 243–276.

Steriade, M., and McCarley, R. W. (1990). "Brainstem Control of Wakefulness and Sleep." Plenum, New York.

J. Allan Hobson and Edward F. Pace-Schott

43

Motivation and Reward

Animals adapt to change, whether external or internal, through motivated behavior. Such adjustments to change may involve the integration of endocrine, autonomic, and behavioral responses. Some adjustments are part of the regulatory process of homeostasis and act through negative feedback loops to correct an internal change. Indeed, motivation used to be explained largely in terms of reductions of needs, or "drives," such as those for sodium or water. This purely homeostatic explanation of motivation could plausibly account for ingestive and thermoregulatory behaviors. However, it fails satisfactorily to explain behavior such as aggression, mating, or exploration, for which there are obvious external triggering stimuli but no identifiable deficit state. It also fails to explain what happens when homeostatic mechanisms are apparently overridden by powerful external incentives, as occurs during drug binges and during overingestion of delicious food. Instead, such behavior often is explained by attraction to external stimuli that have appetitive or rewarding properties (incentive-motivation).

In many cases, goals such as food or a sexual partner are not available, and an animal must search or forage for them. Therefore, motivated behavior is more than simple control of consummatory responses, such as eating, drinking, and sexual mounting or lordosis, which end sequences of motivated behavior. Consummatory behavior tends to be stereotyped and reflexive and is acquired early in an animal's life. In sequences of motivated behavior, however, consummatory behavior is usually preceded by adaptive, flexible forms of appetitive behavior (e.g., foraging for food), which enables an animal to come into physical contact with its goal. This appetitive behavior may be simple locomotor approach responses to the goal or may include

exploratory behavior and complex response sequences. In addition, appetitive behavior may occur in parallel with endocrine and autonomic responses (e.g., secretion of saliva and insulin; see Chapter 38) that prepare the animal for efficient interaction with the goal.

In the absence of immediate goals, an animal usually must use past experience to predict the likelihood of an occurrence. This learning may involve classically conditioned (i.e. Pavlovian) reflexes and goal-directed instrumental (or operant) behaviors. With the latter behaviors, an outcome that increases occurrence of a preceding behavior is a positive reinforcer. This term is often used interchangeably with the more colloquial term reward, which connotes pleasure. However, accurately inferring such subjective states in animals is difficult, if not impossible. Thus, to avoid ambiguity, most behavioral neuroscientists prefer to use operational definitions of motivated behavior, such as incentive and positive reinforcement. Identification of neural structures that mediate subjective phenomena, such as pleasure, may have to depend on functional neuroimaging of humans. Incentive, however, generally refers to the attractiveness of a goal, and positive reinforcement strengthens specific responses by presenting stimuli contingent on performance. For example, rats can learn arbitrary instrumental actions, such as a lever press, to gain access to positive reinforcers, such as food or drugs—self-administration behavior (see Chapter 44)—or to stimuli associated with these primary reinforcer-conditioned reinforcers. Schedules of reinforcement vary the relationship between activity and positive reinforcement. Thus, an animal's degree of motivation can be assessed by its capacity to work for a goal. Another measure of motivation often involves the choice an animal makes, e.g., between actions that produce one stimulus associated with reward over another stimulus that is not associated. Conditioned place preference is a commonly used procedure based on this principle in which choice is made between two environments, only one of which is linked to reward. A distinctive location is associated with a reinforcer such as food or a drug (see Chapter 44). Following several learning trials, a test trial is conducted in the absence of the goal itself. In the test, the preference for that place (as measured by the time spent there) relative to another place without that association is taken as an index of the incentive properties of the goal.

The complexity of motivated behavior (see Fig. 43.1), from selection of voluntary actions based on past experience to reflexive control of consummatory behavior, involves coordination of several levels of neural control, including the neocortex, limbic system, integrative centers (e.g., hypothalamus), and the basic motor mechanisms (e.g., brain stem).

NEURAL MECHANISMS OF MOTIVATION

The Hypothalamus Plays a Role in Motivation

Guided by the concept of homeostatic centers, many investigators approached motivation as a search for specific neural or hormonal signals that could trigger a center to initiate the appropriate behavioral responses. Thus, hypothetical motivational centers were based on early concepts of brain stem centers for fundamental processes, such as respiration (see Chapter 37). Such models could explain the efficient integration of many different signals to produce coordinated sequences of behavior. The hypothalamus is an ideal structure for such integrative functions, given its rich blood supply

and exposure to cerebrospinal fluid (and thus access to a variety of chemical signals and the capacity also to deliver them), control over the pituitary, and neural connections (through brain stem and spinal centers) with visceral afferent information (e.g., taste and olfaction) and autonomic outflow. The concept of mutually inhibitory centers for the initiation (hunger) and suppression (satiety) of feeding arose from such a view (see Chapter 38).

Several Criteria can be Established for Motivational Centers

Theorists (e.g., Hoebel, 1974) defined principles for identifying motivational centers. For example, designation of the lateral hypothalamic region (LH) as a "feeding center" was based on the following: (1) Electrolytic lesions produced profound aphagia (abstention from eating). (2) Electrical stimulation of the brain (ESB) through electrodes implanted in the LH induced eating in sated rats (see Hoebel, 1974). (3) Infusions of the neurotransmitter noradrenaline into the hypothalamus also induced eating in sated rats (Leibowitz, 1980).(4) Electrophysiological recording showed that when monkeys were deprived of food, individual neurons in the LH were sensitive to the sight and taste of food (Rolls, 1975).

Hypothalamic Centers for Other Forms of Motivation

On the basis of the criteria just described, the list of hypothalamic motivational centers has been extended to include behaviors as diverse as drinking, thermoregulation, aggression, and sex (see Chapters 38–40). Thus, for example, thermoregulatory behavior,

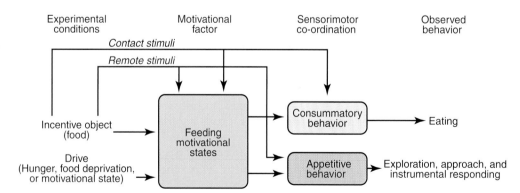

FIGURE 43.1 Theory of incentive-motivation, as applied to feeding. Note that drive (internal stimuli) and food (external stimuli) separately affect central motivation to feed. Also, incentive (i.e., food) and discriminative (i.e., sensorimotor) influences exert their effects separately to control consummatory behavior (when food is contacted) and appetitive behavior (when food remains remote). Modified after Robbins (1986), with permission.

such as reflexive shivering, panting, and grooming, is impaired by lesions of the preoptic region of the hypothalamus and is elicited by cooling or warming of this region (Satinoff, 1982). Defensive (affective) aggression and accompanying autonomic changes, such as piloerection, are produced by electrical stimulation of the ventromedial hypothalamus (VMH), whereas predatory ("quiet") aggression is produced by electrical stimulation of the lateral hypothalamus in a number of species (Flynn *et al.*, 1970).

A particularly well-studied example is that of sexual motivation. Hypothalamic nuclei contain high concentrations of steroid receptors (e.g., for estradiol and testosterone), especially in the medial preoptic region and the VMH. In rats, male copulatory behavior is abolished by medial preoptic lesions (Heimer and Larsson, 1966–1967), whereas electrical stimulation of this region elicits copulation. In female rats, lordosis is blocked (and aggression toward males increased) by lesions of the ventromedial nucleus of the hypothalamus. Lordosis is also induced by electrical stimulation of this region (see Pfaff, 1982). Most of these responses are hormone dependent. In females having had their ovaries removed, proceptive ("ear wiggling," hopping, and darting) and receptive (lordosis) behaviors can be elicited by implanting estradiol into the VMH. Similarly, the sexual behavior of castrated males can be restored by implanting testosterone into the preoptic area. This hormone dependence underlines the interaction between external (environmental) and internal (plasma steroids) states in inducing motivated responses. Also, sex hormones influence the organization of sexually dimorphic brain development (e.g., development of the sexually dimorphic nuclei in the preoptic region), as well as sexually dimorphic behavior (see Chapter 40). Maternal behavior also is dependent on hormones and is impaired by lesions of the medial preoptic area (see Chapter 40). Thus it seems clear that the hypothalamus plays a central role in the regulation of sexual behavior.

The intermingling of hypothalamic neural mechanisms controlling thermoregulation, maternal behavior, feeding, and mating suggests that these behaviors share controls in many circumstances. In summary, a wide variety of motivational states expressed as easily elicited, sometimes stereotypical and species-specific, behaviors are represented within the hypothalamus and related structures.

Critique of the Hypothalamic "Drive Center" Hypothesis

Despite this great volume of evidence, the precise importance of the hypothalasmus in motivation

remains unclear and some of the original data that were used to support the concept of hypothalamic centers have since required reinterpretation. We now know that lesions of the LH do not reduce only eating and drinking but virtually all motivated behaviors, as well as basic sensorimotor processes. Moreover, whereas residual deficits remain in the control of drinking and the response to changes in body fluids, animals can recover from many of the eating deficits caused by lateral hypothalamic lesions (see Chapters 38 and 39). Recovery probably occurs by two main processes: reorganization of the rest of the brain to compensate behaviorally and intrinsic recovery of the damaged neurotransmitter systems. The phenomenon of recovery is important because it suggests that some hypothalamic "centers" are not necessary for the control of motivation and that motivation can be affected by plastic neural systems.

The effects of experimental brain stimulation can also be misinterpreted. For example, although ESB produces behavior that resembles naturally motivated behavior, in nondeprived animals, the behaviors also differ depending on the nature of the goal–object. In addition, expression of a consummatory response often gradually evolves over a number of experiences with ESB, suggesting involvement of learning mechanisms instead of, or in addition to, local activation of a hypothetical motivational center (Valenstein, 1973). Behavior elicited by ESB could also reflect abnormal functions, such as a coping response to the stress of ESB itself. For example, sated rats will resume eating in response to sustained pinching of their tails (Antelman and Szechtman, 1975)! These results point to possible nonspecific "arousing" or "activating" effects of stimulation, which can lead to specific motivational responses based on the present context and previous experience of the animal.

Distinguishing between *Consummatory* and *Instrumental* Behavior

Many studies of the role of the hypothalamus in motivation have concentrated on measuring consummatory rather than learned instrumental behavior, a research strategy that may lead to misleading conclusions about motivational changes in general. For example, rats with preoptic lesions will not respond to thermal stress with reflex mechanisms such as shivering, adjustment of food intake, nest building, or changes in locomotion. However, they will learn to press a lever for hot or cool air and can achieve thermoregulation by this means (Carlisle, 1969). Similarly, male monkeys with preoptic lesions still show motivated behavior such as masturbation, but they are unable to copulate with females. Moreover, male rats with preoptic lesions still show displacement behaviors and locomotor excitement in the presence of a receptive female, as well as lever pressing to gain access to her, but cannot perform the consummatory behavior of copulation.

This dissociation between consummatory and instrumental behaviors is important because damage to a component of the limbic system, the amygdala, is known to produce the opposite pattern of effects—unimpaired mounting but reduced instrumental behavior (Everitt, 1990). These examples show that hypothalamic mechanisms operate mainly at the level of controlling consummatory rather than learned instrumental behavior leading to a goal. Behavioral flexibility illustrated by learning appears to require recruitment of additional neural systems, including the amygdala (see the following section).

Motivation Can Be Controlled at Other Levels of the Neuraxis

Below the Level of the Hypothalamus:

The hypothalamus is not necessary for the fundamental reflexive elements of consummatory behavior. For example, classical research showed that cats with midbrain transections (below the hypothalamus) could still perform complete responses, such as chewing, swallowing, growling, and piloerection ("sham rage"). Only when the transection was above the hypothalamus, however, did the responses look like integrated, motivated behavior. Thus, the hypothalamus appeared to coordinate and sequence motivated responses, as well as their correlated autonomic responses. The circuitry is now known to descend from the hypothalamus to the midbrain and then to integrative centers in the brain stem and spinal cord. In addition, decerebrate rats receiving transections below the hypothalamus, thus disabling its communication with the brain stem, show normal acceptance and rejection behaviors in response to pleasant and unpleasant food. They also show a normal rise in insulin secretion in anticipation of eating, as well as a decrease in response to satiety (Norgren and Grill, 1982). However, decerebrate rats cannot learn taste aversions or search for food. Thus, the hypothalamus, as well as other forebrain structures, apparently has important integrative functions, but, for the hypothalamus, this role is probably limited to the organization of simple, often consummatory, behaviors.

Above the Level of the Hypothalamus:

Structures above the level of the hypothalamus, e.g., the neocortex and limbic system, modulate motivated behavior. For instance, stimulation of the amygdala inhibits the rage elicited by stimulation of the hypothalamus. Many such descending influences are learned, including responses to novel and familiar foods, conditioned taste aversion, and control of instrumental behavior (see preceding discussion). Inhibition of motivation is not restricted to the neocortex and limbic system; e.g., inhibitory mechanisms (of food intake) apparently are located in the paraventricular nucleus and ventromedial region of the hypothalamus (see Chapter 38).

In summary, the control of motivated behavior occurs at several distinct and interactive levels of the central neurous system, probably in a hierarchical manner.

DOPAMINE AND THE LATERAL HYPOTHALAMIC SYNDROME

Electrolytic lesions of the LH cause dramatic deficits in food intake. However, not only do such lesions affect more than simply feeding behavior (see earlier discussion), they also destroy far more than the LH region itself, mainly by interrupting ascending and descending fibers in the medial forebrain bundle (Fig. 43.2). Thus, the effects of LH lesions on eating were unlikely all to be caused by damage to an LH "feeding" center. For example, the nigrostriatal dopamine (DA) pathway courses through the LH without synapsing there (see Chapter 7). Injection of a catecholamine-selective neurotoxin, 6-hydroxydopamine (6-OHDA), into the vicinity of the LH reproduced most of the classic LH syndrome (Ungerstedt, 1971a). The injected rats suffered large depletions (>90%) of DA from the striatum. They were cataleptic and had difficulty initiating head, limb, axial, and oral movements. Further experiments showed that the syndrome could be produced by injection of 6-OHDA at any of several points along the nigrostriatal DA pathway between its origin in the substantia nigra and its termination in the caudate-putamen. Thus, DA depletion at sites well away from the LH reproduced much of the LH syndrome. 6-OHDA-induced lesions of the mesolimbic, rather than the nigrostriatal, pathway minimally affected ingestion but did affect other behaviors, such as locomotion and exploration, that may accompany feeding (Koob et al., 1978). Therefore, both consummatory and appetitive behaviors are affected by DA depletion, although probably in different regions of the forebrain.

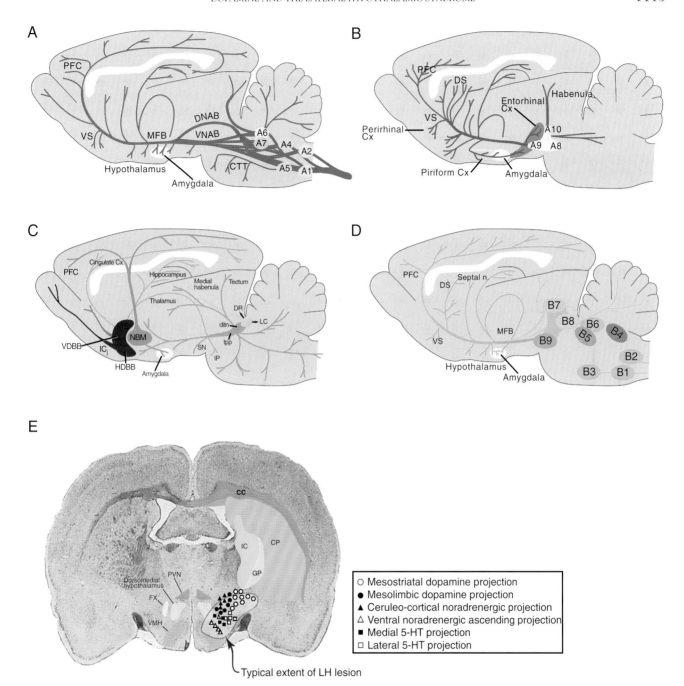

FIGURE 43.2 Ascending monoamine neurotransmitter systems. Figure shows schematic sagittal (A–D) and coronal (E) sections through the lateral hypothalamus of a rat brain. (A) Origin and distribution of central noradrenergic pathways. Note noradrenergic cell groups A1–A7, including the locus ceruleus (A6). DNAB, dorsal noradrenergic ascending bundle; VNAB, ventral noradrenergic ascending bundle. (B) Origin and distribution of central dopamine pathways. Note dopaminergic cell groups A8–A10. (C) Origin and distribution of central cholinergic pathways. Note rostral cell groups. NBM, nucleus basalis magnocellularis (Meynert in primates); MS, medial septum; VDBB, vertical limb nucleus of the diagonal band of Broca; HDBB, horizontal limb nucleus of the diagonal band of Broca. (D) Origin and distribution of central serotoninergic pathways. Note cell groups in the raphe nucleus, B4–B9. MFB, medial forebrain bundle; PFC, prefrontal cortex; VS, ventral striatum; DS, dorsal striatum. Based on T. W. Robbins and B. J. Everitt, in *The Cognitive Neurosciences*. MIT Press, Cambridge MA, 1995; reproduced with permission. (E) Schematic coronal section through the rat brain at the level of the ventromedial hypothalamus. LH lesions could disrupt various ascending monoaminergic fibers. CC, corpus callosum; CP, caudate-putamen; DMH, dorsomedial hypothalamus; IC, internal capsule; GP, globus pallidus; PVH, paraventricular hypothalamus; LH, lateral hypothalamus; FX, fornix; VMH, ventromedial hypothalamus. Modified from Robbins (1986), with permission.

LH Syndrome Is Similar but Not the Same as the Syndrome Produced by 6-Hydroxydopamine

Recovery from the LH syndrome and the syndrome produced by 6-OHDA is similar (Marshall and Teitelbaum, 1977). At first, animals show adipsia (absence of drinking), aphagia (absence of eating), sensorimotor neglect (lack of response to stimuli), and akinesia (dearth of movements). Recovery from sensorimotor neglect parallels recovery from aphagia in both syndromes. (Recovered rats do not respond normally to physiological challenges, such as hyperosmolality.) Stricker and Zigmond (1976) explained this recovery as intrinsic recovery of function in dopaminergic systems. They proposed that changes in DA turnover and reuptake, as well as increases in the number of DA receptors, combine to minimize the impact of a lesion (see Chapters 38 and 39). In fact, in animals recovered from 6-OHDA lesions, aphagia and adipsia can be reinstated by drugs that block the synthesis of catecholamines or that block DA receptors. These studies led to the hypothesis that the entire LH syndrome is caused by a deficit in behavioral activation and results from depletion of brain DA rather than damage to LH cells.

Despite these similarities, subtle differences between the two syndromes cannot be explained by this DA hypothesis. For example, 6-OHDA-lesioned rats, unlike animals with LH lesions, are not somnolent (drowsy), are less finicky about food, and have fewer deficits in thermoregulation, taste aversion, learning, and oral motor performance. However, the most compelling difference is that rats with LH lesions and the full syndrome have only 50% depletion of striatal DA, whereas 6-OHDA-lesioned rats (even with less than the full syndrome) have greater than 90% depletion of striatal DA. Therefore, damage to the LH itself or to fibers of passage, in addition to those of the ascending DA system, apparently contributes to the LH syndrome.

Cell Body Lesions in the Hypothalamus Produce a Less Severe LH Syndrome

The neurotoxins kainic, ibotenic, and quisqualic acids are structurally related to the excitatory neurotransmitter glutamate. They bind to various subtypes of glutamate receptors and essentially stimulate neurons to death (see Chapter 8). These excitotoxins can be used to produce lesions of cell bodies while sparing fibers of passage. Electrolytic and mechanical lesions, in contrast, damage soma and fibers. Despite sparing striatal DA, such cell body lesions lead to severe problems with eating, followed by long-lasting

deficits in homeostasis (Winn *et al.*, 1984) However, there are no signs of akinesia or sensorimotor neglect. Hence, at least two factors are required to explain the LH syndrome: damage to the LH disrupts homeostasis and striatal DA loss disrupts initiation and execution of feeding and related behaviors.

Animals with DA Denervation Syndrome Show Rotation and Sensorimotor Neglect

A central question for research in this area is what is the precise nature of the dopaminergic contribution to motivation? Some clues to answering this question were provided by experiments in which rats received unilateral 6-OHDA lesions of the nigrostriatal system. The rats rotated toward the side of the lesion following treatment with a DA-releasing drug, such as *d*-amphetamine (Ungerstedt, 1971b). Presumably, this rotation occurred because more DA is released on the intact side than the lesioned side of the brain and because any output pathway from the striatum influences, via crossed pathways, the opposite side of the body. Of even greater interest, the direct DA receptor agonist apomorphine caused the rat to turn away from the side of the lesion so long as the lesion was extensive. This rotation could be explained by supersensitive DA receptors on the lesioned side. These studies of drug-induced movement have been important in helping to identify mechanisms of receptor regulation that might contribute to recovery from motivational deficits following DA denervation. However, they do not by themselves help answer the central question posed earlier of the precise contribution of DA to motivation.

More relevant to this question is that unilateral lesions of the LH or nigrostriatal DA system also produce polymodal sensorimotor neglect, measured by responses to contralateral somatic, auditory, and olfactory stimuli—a syndrome initially attributed to sensory inattention (Marshall and Teitelbaum, 1977). A more detailed analysis suggests that the fundamental deficit is a failure in initiating responses rather than attending to stimuli (Box 43.1 and Fig. 43.3). This leads us to the conclusion that the nigrostriatal DA system contributes to *activation*, energizing the vigor of behavioral output (see also Chapters 42 and 49).

Mesencephalic DA Mediates Activation of Behavior

Animals with lesions of the nigrostriatal system retain the capacity for movement; they do not have an irreversible motor deficit. However, they have great difficulty in starting that movement without an intact

BOX 43.1

SEPARATION OF SENSORY AND RESPONSE FACTORS IN THE DOPAMINERGIC SYNDROME OF NEGLECT

Sensory and motor aspects of the neglect syndrome were separated in the following way (Carli *et al.*, 1985). Rats were trained to detect brief flashes of light presented to either side of the head. In one case, they were trained to respond where the light was. In the alternate case, rats were trained to respond in a location away from the side of the light (see Fig. 43.3). Rats with DA depleted from one side of the striatum could not respond properly toward the contralateral side, whether or not the stimulus was presented on that side. Measurement of reaction time showed that the problem was in initiation, rather than completion, of the movement. Consistent with these data, DA-depleted rats could detect a con-

tralateral stimulus and respond to it with an unlateralized response. Thus, their deficit was in initiation of movement in response to stimuli rather than in detection of the stimuli.

Trevor W. Robbins and
Barry J. Everitt

Reference

Carli, M., Evenden, J. L., and Robbins, T. W. (1985). Depletion of unilateral striatal dopamine impairs initiation of contralateral actions and not sensory attention. *Nature* (*Lond.*) **312**, 679–682.

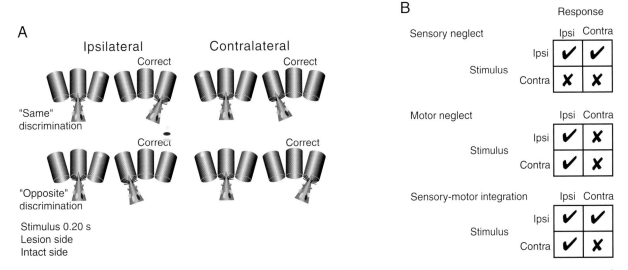

FIGURE 43.3 Distinguishing between sensory and response factors. Rats were trained to move toward the same or opposite side on which a brief (0.2 s) visual stimulus was presented. If a rat did not respond to the stimulus, it remained in a central location. After training, unilateral striatal lesions (oval) were made. Rats were then observed for their ability to respond to stimuli presented ipsilateral or contralateral to their lesions. Based on the responses of lesioned rats to stimuli, conclusions were drawn about the sensory and motor nature of the deficits caused by striatal lesions. Figure 43.3B shows the hypothetical pattern of behavioral results obtained in the different test conditions following unilateral DA depletion. Data were, in fact, consistent with a deficit in responding to contralateral space (i.e., motor neglect).

DA system. It is instructive to compare this with the problems that patients with Parkinson's disease have with movement initiation, since they too have a severe deficit in nigrostriatal DA (see Chapter 31). To identify the circumstances in which the DA system normally becomes active, *in vivo* neurochemical techniques, such as microdialysis and voltammetry (Phillips *et al.*, 1991), have been used to monitor the

release of DA in animals exhibiting particular behaviors. In addition, researchers have examined the firing of DA cells in response to particular stimuli (Schultz *et al.*, 1995). For example, DA cells have been identified in the ventral tegmental area that responds to rewards such as food. However, if the food is reliably predicted by a conditioned stimulus, then, as a consequence of learning, the firing is initiated instead

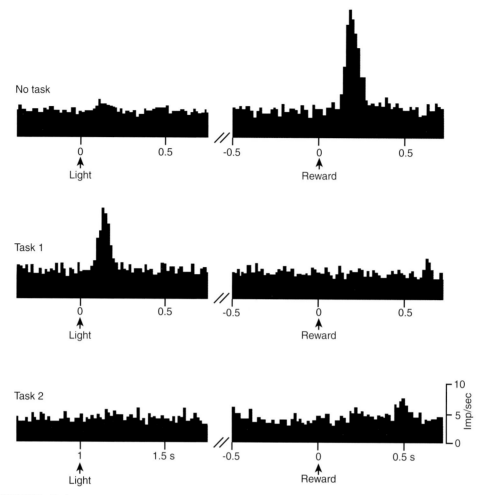

FIGURE 43.4 Responses of dopamine neurons to unpredicted primary reward (top) and the transfer of this response to progressively earlier reward-predicting conditioned stimuli with training (middle). The bottom record shows a control baseline task when the reward is predicted by an earlier stimulus and not the light. From Schultz *et al.* (1995), with permission.

in response to the previously neutral stimulus (see Fig. 43.4). This and other findings support the theory that the DA cells provide an *error correction signal* that enables reinforcement learning by networks in the striatum to influence appetitive behaviors.

Summary

Different DA systems (i.e., mesocortical, mesolimbic, and mesostriatal; see Chapter 8) probably have different roles in the activation of behavior, depending on the target structures they innervate. Two broad generalizations can be made. (1) Nigrostriatal DA projections to the caudate-putamen participate in the activation of behavior triggered by stimuli of endogenous origin (e.g., as in anticipation of movement). (2) The mesolimbic DA system is involved in

the activation of responses to external stimuli with incentive-motivational properties.

REINFORCEMENT SYSTEMS

Electrical Stimulation of the Brain Can Be a Positive Reinforcer

In 1954, Olds and Milner discovered that rats learned new responses when their learning was positively reinforced by electrical stimulation of the brain. That finding affirmed the importance of incentive factors in instrumental behavior. The best natural parallel appeared to be behavior in response to large incentives by animals in low states of drive (e.g., chocolate milk in undeprived rats). However, equating rewarding brain stimulation with subjective feel-

BOX 43.2

PSYCHOPHYSICS OF HEDONISM AS MEASURED BY BRAIN STIMULATION REWARD

Electrical stimulation of the brain can be used as positive reinforcement of learned behaviors. An apparatus is set up so that when an animal presses a lever, its brain is stimulated. An advantage of using stimulation to measure motivation is that the strength of the reward can be titrated easily by adjusting the amount of current delivered for each lever press. If the current is adjusted too low (i.e., below the threshold for reinforcement), then the animals will not press the lever. As current is increased, the relationship between the rate of lever pressing and the strength of current typically follows a sigmoidal curve called rate–intensity function. Pharmacologic manipulation of catecholamine neurotransmitter systems can shift the function to the left (e.g., treatment with amphetamine or cocaine) or to the right (e.g., treatment with α-methyl-p-tyrosine, reserpine, or the dopamine receptor antagonist pimozide) (Fig. 43.5). Such shifts mean the amount of current required to support lever presses varies while the maximal response rate is unchanged. Thus, these drugs affect reward processes, rather than motor function. The threshold of reinforcement can also be measured by allowing rats to adjust the strength of the current. In this setup, a process is employed in which rats press lever one to produce ICSS, but each lever-one press also reduces the intensity of the current. To reset current intensity, rats must press

lever two. Such "self-titration" experiments yield conclusions similar to those based on rate–intensity functions.

Trevor W. Robbins and
Barry J. Everitt

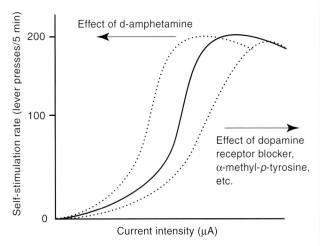

FIGURE 43.5 Rate–intensity function for electrical self-stimulation of the brain. Pharmacologic agents shift the curve left (e.g., amphetamine or cocaine) or right (e.g., catecholamine-depleting agents, such as α-methyl-p-tyrosine and reserpine, and catecholamine receptor blockers, such as chlorpromazine and pimozide).

ings of pleasure and hedonism seemed inappropriate when literature on human intracranial self-stimulation (ICSS) was considered because the subjects, often people with schizophrenia or intractable pain, frequently had difficulty verbalizing their responses. Measurement of the strength of reinforcers in microamperes (Box 43.2, Fig. 43.5) promised a pragmatic, as well as objective, new approach to the psychophysics of an operational hedonism. However, its greatest contribution was to enable the anatomical mapping of the central reward or reinforcement mechanisms of the brain (see Phillips, 1984).

Reward and Punishment Regions

Using the rate of responses that elicited rewarding brain stimulation, researchers mapped sites of ICSS in the rat and other species to the medial forebrain bundle. Response rates were high and were often accompanied by stimulus-bound behavior, such as

eating whenever food was present or locomotion despite absence of a goal object (Hoebel, 1974). At first, theorists assumed that the consummatory behavior was caused by ESB mimicking the effect of natural rewards within hypothalamic centers. This response contrasted with that seen at other, often limbic, sites (e.g., septum, amygdala, hippocampus, and prefrontal cortex). At these sites, response rates were lower and behavioral activation was less evident. When ESB occurred in negatively reinforcing regions of the brain, rats' new responses would allow them to escape from or avoid the stimulation (see section on Aversion Systems).

Catecholamine Hypothesis of Rewarding Brain Stimulation

Later work showed that animals can also learn behaviors to stimulate other sites through ICSS (e.g., the locus ceruleus, midbrain central gray, cerebellum,

BOX 43.3

MAJOR DEPRESSIVE DISORDER

A major depressive episode (MDE) is a pathological mood state in which persistent negative emotions and thoughts coexist with disturbances of motivation, sleep, energy, appetite, and libido. Such episodes may arise in the absence of clear medical or psychiatric antecedents as primary, idiopathic disorders [termed "major depressive disorder" (MDD), when only depressive episodes occur, or "bipolar disorder" (BD), when manic as well as depressive episodes occur (see Box 43.5)]. They may also arise secondarily to specific neurological, endocrinological, or psychiatric disorders or in response to pharmacological substances. The most common of these conditions, MDD, rivals hypertension as the most frequently encountered illness in primary health care. MDD is ranked fourth as a cause of disability by the World Health Organization, and by 2015 its ranking is expected to rise to second.

The emotional experience during a MDE may be dominated by anxiety, irritability, or anhedonia (inability to derive pleasure or reward from activities or appetitive stimuli) rather than by depressed mood, and patients often report that terms such as "psychic pain" describe their mood state more accurately. Emotional symptoms may be eclipsed in clinical salience by prominent fatigue, weight loss, insomnia, psychomotor retardation (decrease in the rate and amount of movement and speech), or agitation. The psychological manifestations of an MDE include preoccupation with death, suicide, and hopelessness. About 15% of patients hospitalized for a MDE eventually suicide, and about one-half of completed suicides occur within the context of a MDE. The intrusive and perseverative nature of thoughts of death, suicide, or guilt and their responsiveness to antidepressant drugs or electroconvulsive therapy suggest that abnormal brain processes may underlie and maintain such symptoms.

The usual course of MDD consists of recurrent depressive episodes separated by a (usually only partial) return toward the premorbid level of function. The average frequency of episodes is about 6 per 20-year period, although some depressives experience multiple recurrences per year and others develop chronic episodes lasting several years. Antidepressant treatment shortens the duration of depressive episodes, reduces the likelihood of chronicity, and, if continued, decreases the risk of recurrence.

Epidemiological measures of the lifetime prevalence for a MDE vary between 6 and 18% across studies. The variability in this rate partly reflects the limitations in establishing diagnosis in mild cases and the nonavailability of objective diagnostic tests. Illness onset can occur throughout the life span, although the first episode usually occurs after puberty.

The etiologies of MDD and BD are unknown. Twin, adoption, and family studies indicate that genetic factors contribute substantially to the liability for developing both disorders. Nevertheless, these data also support a role for acquired factors in disease expression. Moreover, the variability in the clinical course, illness antecedents, response to somatic or psychological treatments, and neurobiological data evident in depressed samples indicates that the MDD syndrome, in particular, encompasses an etiologically heterogenous group of disorders.

Because the symptoms of a MDE resemble those of a severe stress or bereavement response, adverse life events are expected to constitute "acquired factors" which may interact with genetic susceptibility in the development of mood disorders. A link between stressors and MDEs has been difficult to establish, however. Patients with recurrent episodes often report that their pattern of depressive symptoms is uncoupled from stressful life situations. The life events that are clearly associated with the development of MDE are pregnancy and delivery, as the postpartum period comprised the epoch of greatest risk in females.

The function of the hypothalamic–pituitary–adrenocortical (HPA) axis is abnormal in at least a substantial proportion of MDD cases. Severe depression is associated with increased CSF levels of corticotropin-releasing factor (CRF), hypersecretion of ACTH and cortisol, pituitary and adrenal gland enlargement, and reduced sensitivity to negative feedback inhibition of cortisol secretion. In addition, suicide victims studied postmortem have decreased CRF receptor density in the frontal cortex along with pituitary mRNA levels indicative of chronic HPA axis activation.

In addition, MDD has been associated with abnormalities in serotonergic, dopaminergic, noradrenergic, cholinergic, GABAergic, and peptidergic (i.e., CRF and opiate) function. The serotonin (5-HT) system has received particular interest, as selective 5-HT reuptake inhibitors exert antidepressant effects, and other antidepressant drugs also increase 5-HT transmission. This effect may compensate for reduced 5-HT function in MDD, as neuroendocrine responses to 5-HT receptor agonists are blunted, CSF concentrations of the 5-HT are metabolite 5-HIAA are reduced in MDD, and the binding of some 5-HT receptors is abnormal in MDD or depressed suicide victims. The

BOX 43.3 (cont'd)

dopaminergic, noradrenergic, and cholinergic systems are functionally interrelated with the serotonergic system, and abnormalities in these systems are hypothesized to give rise to the deficits of reward processing and cognitive function evident in severe MDD.

Functional neuroimaging studies show that cerebral blood flow (CBF) and glucose metabolism are increased in the depressed relative to the nondepressed states in parts of the posterior orbitofrontal cortex and ventral anterior cingulate cortex where CBF increases during experimentally induced emotional states in healthy humans, and where glucose utilization and Fos-like immunoreactivity increase in experimental animals subjected to stressors. During the depressed phase of recurrent, familial MDD, CBF, and metabolism are also abnormally elevated in the amygdala, medial thalamus, and ventral striatum and are reduced in the dorsal anterolateral and dorsomedial prefrontal cortices. Many of these regions have been shown to have abnormal reductions of the gray matter volume by *in vivo* MRI and *postmortem* neuropathological studies. *Postmortem* histopathological studies of the ventral anterior cingulate cortex, amygdala, subiculum of the hippocampus, and posterior orbital cortex suggest that the reduction in gray matter volume is accounted for by a reduction in neuropil, as neuron density is increased, synaptic markers and contacts are decreased, and glial cell counts and glia-to-neuron ratios are decreased.

These data converge with evidence from lesion analysis studies to implicate circuits involving parts of the frontal and temporal cortex along with related parts of the striatum, pallidum, and thalamus in the pathophysiology of depression. Lesions involving the frontal cortex and de-

generative diseases of the basal ganglia (e.g., Parkinson's and Huntington's diseases) are associated with higher rates of depression than other similarly debilitating conditions. Because the neuropathological correlates of these conditions would affect synaptic transmission through the limbic-cortical-striatal-pallidal-thalamic circuitry in diverse ways, it appears that an abnormal interaction between elements of these circuits, rather than increased or decreased activity in any single structure, may produce MDE. These circuits are generally implicated in the modulation of stress and emotional responses and in the guidance of goal-directed behavior as reinforcement contingencies change.

Wayne C. Drevets

Suggested Readings

Carroll, B. J. (1994). Brain mechanisms in manic depression. *Clin. Chem.* **40**, 303–308.
Chaput, Y. deMontigny, O. and Blier, P. (1991). Presynaptic and postsynaptic modifications of the serotonin system by long-term adminstration of antidepressant treatments: An in vitro electrophysiologic study in the rat. *Neuropsychopharmacology* **5**: 219–229.
Charney, D. S., Delgado, P. L., Southwick, *et al.* (1991). Current hypothesis of the mechanism of antidepressant treatments: implications for the treatment of refractory depression. *In*: "*Refractory Depression*" (J. D. Amsterdam, ed.), pp. 23–40. Raven Press, New York.
Drevets, W. C. (2000). Neuroimaging studies of mood disorders. *Biol. Psychiatry* **48**, 813–829.
Drevets, W. C., and Todd, R. D. (1997). Depression, mania and related disorders. *In* "*Adult Psychiatry*" (S.B. Guze, ed., vol. 8, pp. 99–141. Mosby Press, St Louis.
Manji, H., Drevets, W. C., and Charney, D. (2001) The cellular neurobiology of depression. *Nature Med.* **7**(5); 541–547.

trigeminal motor nucleus, substantia nigra, caudate nucleus, and nucleus accumbens) (Phillips, 1984). The diversity of these sites has not been fully explained. Many of them are known to lie along the trajectory of catecholamine-containing neurons. Although this includes both norepinephrine and DA projections, most pharmacologic data can be interpreted in terms of dopaminergic mechanisms (Box 43.2, Fig. 43.5). In particular, very high rates of responding for ICSS were found in the ventral tegmental area, ventral striatum (including the nucleus accumbens to which DA neurons project), and limbic system. However, of several, possibly independent neural systems that may subserve rewarding brain stimulation, only some depend on DA. The difficulty in interpreting the role

of striatal DA in ICSS lies in distinguishing motor from reward effects (see Box 43.2). The phenomenon of human drug dependence and the discovery in the early 1960s of drug self-administration in animals opened the way to an analysis of reward effects, the neurochemical basis of reinforcement (see Chapter 44).

The Mesolimbic DA System Plays a Key Role in Natural Rewards

Wise (1982) proposed that drugs and natural reinforcers are perceived as rewards because they increase activity of the mesolimbic DA system (see Chapter 44). If Wise's hypothesis is correct, the mesolimbic DA system should mediate natural

BOX 43.4

SUICIDE

Understanding the neuroscientific substrates of suicidal behavior will lead to better understanding of the reasons for suicide and may enhance predictability in at-risk individuals and the development of more effective treatment strategies. The goal is to create a road map of brain functioning and neurochemistry correlated with suicidal behavior, taking advantage of the powerful modern methods of molecular biology, quantitative morphometrics, and neurochemistry. Additional impetus for the neurobiological study of suicide comes from the implications of a genetic contribution to the risk for suicidal acts.

The two main strategies used to study the neurobiology of suicide are neuroendocrine challenges (e.g., HPA axis) and neurotransmitter (e.g., serotonin) measures. Neuroendocrine systems have not been investigated as intensively as neurotransmitter systems. Nevertheless, neuroendocrine studies are noteworthy in representing some of the initial endeavors to identify biological correlates of suicide.

The earliest report of a biological abnormality derives from the observation of metabolic abnormalities and adrenocortical dysfunction in a seriously suicidal patient with Cushing's syndrome (among whom emotional and mental disturbances are frequent). Subsequent reports in Cushing's syndrome also suggested endocrine abnormalities in suicide. The most severe depressive clinical presentations have significantly elevated ACTH levels. These data support the hypothesis that suicidal behavior, at least in a subgroup of patients with hypercortisolism, may be associated with dysregulation of the hypothalamic–pituitary–adrenal (HPA) axis.

The possibility that hyperactivity of the HPA axis might have a special relationship to suicidal behavior was initially suggested by investigators of the National Institute of Mental Health who observed elevated urinary 17-hydroxycorticosteroids, an indirect measure of daily cortisol production, in patients who later committed suicide. Subsequent studies investigating this association have yielded mixed results. In addition, investigations of relationships between suicidal behavior and plasma cortisol levels, before and after administration of dexamethasone, have also yielded contradictory results. Most studies found higher rates of nonsuppres-

sion on the desamethasone suppression test (DST) in patients who had attempted or completed suicide compared to nonsuicide attempters. There are, however, some negative studies reporting no association of recent suicidal behavior and nonsuppression of DST. More recently, suicide victims have been found to have reduced binding of corticotropin-releasing factor (CRF) in the frontal cortex. Inasmuch as it is thought that CRF hypersecretion is the basis of cortisol dysregulation in depression, this finding is consistent with the hypothesis that CRF is hypersecreted in depression with resulting receptor downregulation.

The majority of clinical neurobiological studies of suicide have concentrated on the serotonin (5-HT) system. A rationale for the intensive study of 5-HT is that it occupies a key role in other-directed aggression and impulsivity, as well as a variety of other physiologic and behavioral functions of animals. The link between other directed aggression/impulsivity and self-directed aggression (suicidal behavior) has been commented upon frequently. Serotonergic function bears a similar relationship to aggression in animal models of aggression and clinical studies of suicide and aggression. Most 5-HT studies of suicide attempters have demonstrated abnormalities in related 5-HT indices, leading to the hypothesis that lower serotonergic activity is associated with an increased suicide risk. One of the earliest studies of the relationship between 5-HT function and attempted suicide comes from a cerebrospinal fluid (CSF) study of 5-hydroxyindoleacetic acid (5-HIAA), the principal metabolite of 5-HT, in depressive illness. The finding that the CSF 5-HIAA concentration was distributed bimodally in depressed patients generated interest in discovering clinical correlates of the two modes of the CSF 5-HIAA distribution. More lethal suicide attempts are associated with lower CSF 5-HIAA concentration. Studies of 5-HT function in suicide attempters have also employed the platelet serotonin transporter, and 5-HT$_{2A}$ receptor and neuroendocrine strategies, and results suggest hypofunction. Alterations in the serotonergic system in the brain of suicide victims also support the hypothesis that lower serotonergic activity is associated with suicide. Similar to the majority of studies showing low CSF 5-HIAA in attempters, brain stem levels of 5-HT and 5-HIAA are also lower compared

BOX 43.4 (cont'd)

with controls in most studies of suicide victims. Paralleling the CSF 5-HIAA findings in attempters, low brain stem 5-HT and 5-HIAA are independent of psychiatric diagnosis, occurring in suicide in several diagnostic groups (major depression, schizophrenia, personality disorders, and alcoholism). Investigators have turned their attention to mapping changes in serotonin receptors or transporter sites in discrete brain regions of suicide victims. These postmortem studies localize changes to the ventral prefrontal cortex, an area involved in behavioral inhibition. Impaired serotonin input to that brain region may explain the greater impulsivity noted in suicide attempters, which may contribute to the probability of acting on suicidal thoughts.

J. John Mann

Adapted from Stoff and Mann, New York Academy of Sciences Annals Series, 1999

rewards, such as food and sex. In fact, depletion of DA in the nucleus accumbens does not impair consummatory behavior in rats (unlike DA depletion from the caudate-putamen), but it does reduce incentive-motivational responses. For example, proceptive behaviors (such as "ear wiggling," hopping, and darting, all of which serve to solicit the attention of the male) are reduced in female rats. Also, depletion of DA from the nucleus accumbens decreases locomotor excitement of hungry rats in the presence of food (Koob *et al.*, 1978).

Mesolimbic DA may also control behavior motivated by reward. For example, it was shown in studies of Taylor and Robbins (see Robbins *et al.*, 1989) that when a previously neutral light became a predictor of the occurrence of a primary reinforcer, water, rats learned a new behavior to turn on the light. Injection of amphetamine into the nucleus accumbens (but not the caudate) increased the frequency of the behavior. This increased frequency of response suggested that amphetamine enhanced the motivational properties of this reward-related stimulus (i.e., the light, which was related to the reward, water). Amphetamine itself was well known to suppress eating and drinking; thus, the increased frequency of behavior was not due to increased thirst, for example. Furthermore, amphetamine did not increase the frequency of response for a randomly paired stimulus. Finally, amphetamine-induced facilitation was completely blocked by the depletion of DA in the nucleus accumbens (but not by DA depletion in the caudate). These results indicated that increased activity in the mesolimbic DA system could enhance the motivational properties of stimuli predictive of natural rewards (Robbins *et al.*, 1989). Excessive activation of this and other systems may result in emotional disorders such as mania (see Box 43.5).

The Amygdala Also Has a Role in Appetitive Conditioning and Motivation

Less is known about the role of the amygdala in positive affective functions than its role in aversive functions (see Chapter 51). However, monkeys with lesions of the temporal pole, including the amygdala, poorly learn new stimulus–reward associations, suggesting an altered emotional response to reward. In rats, excitotoxic, axon-sparing lesions of the amygdala diminish the capacity of stimuli associated with reward to motivate behavior. Such lesions also impair responses that are rewarded with access to female rats. However, mating per se is unaffected, in contrast with the effect of preoptic lesions (see Everitt *et al.*, 2000). This separation of control of consummatory and learned aspects of sexual behavior indicates that motivated sequences of behavior are constructed through the coordination of neural systems that are at least partly independent. Lesions of the basolateral amygdala also impair the phenomenon of place preference in which experimental animals will consistently return to locations—generally in a well-defined environmental enclosure—where they were previously given reward. Overall, portions of the amygdala clearly function in associative processes that contribute to appetitive behavior.

Motivated Behavior Is Controlled in Part by Learning

The ventral striatum (see Chapter 31) is part of a system that receives afferents from several limbic cortical structures, including the basolateral amygdala, the hippocampal formation, and the prefrontal cortex, and projects to structures such as the lateral hypothalamus and ventral pallidum (Fig. 43.6). Output from

BOX 43.5

MANIA

Mania is a syndrome characterized by a pathologically euphoric, labile, or irritable mood along with motor restlessness, insomnia, racing thoughts, and impairment of attention, insight, and judgment. This syndrome is seen most commonly in the primary, idiopathic condition of bipolar disorder (BD; "manic-depressive illness"), although it may also arise secondarily to the effects of certain pharmacological agents or neurological conditions. In BD, both manic and depressive episodes generally alternate with the normal, or "euthymic," state. Mania and depression reflect phenomenological antitheses of one another, being characterized by increases and decreases, respectively, in mood, motivation, energy, psychomotor activity, self-esteem, libido, and hedonic perception.

The hedonic state of mania reflects an abnormal elevation of the sense of pleasure and reward derived from social, work-related, or creative activities. Patients consequently increase their engagement in such activities, often continuing them throughout the night. This "hyper-motivational" state is fueled by a sense of having boundless energy and needing less sleep. The euphoria often interrelates with grandiose ideas of having special talents, prowess, or religious significance and, in some cases, with delusions of having supernatural powers, possessing great wealth, or being a famous political or religious figure. While productivity may increase in the initial stages, as mania worsens the work performance deteriorates and thought processes become disorganized. The increased engagement in pleasurable activities and the impairment of judgment may further lead to ruinous buying sprees, sexual indiscretions, or alcohol abuse. Moreover, the coincident agitation and irritability associated with mania increase the risk for violent behavior.

The age of onset for BD is usually in adolescence or young adulthood, and the lifetime prevalence is about 1%. Once the bipolar course is established, manic episodes are typically followed by depressive episodes. Untreated episodes typically last several months. Treatment with lithium, valproate, or antipsychotic drugs decreases episode length and severity, and maintenance treatment with these agents can reduce episode frequency. Despite treatment, a sizable minority of bipolar patients have multiple episodes per year or continue to manifest mood instability and occupational impairment between episodes.

Adult twin and adoption studies indicate that the transmission of bipolar disorder is largely due to genetic factors. While there have been several claims of linkage of particular genetic loci to bipolar disorder, at present none of the putative linkage locations or associations are widely accepted and few positive studies have been replicated.

The pathophysiology of mania is poorly understood. Because the dopaminergic projections from the ventral tegmental area into the ventral striatum and medial prefrontal cortex (PFC) appear to play a role in mediating hedonia, motivation, behavioral reinforcement, and psychomotor activity, this system has been implicated as a neural substrate where dysfunction may result in the emotional and behavioral features of BD. Pharmacological data are compatible with this hypothesis, as manic symptoms are reduced by DA receptor antagonists or DA synthesis inhibitors and can be precipitated in euthymic or depressed bipolar patients by DA receptor agonist or precursor administration. Nevertheless, the observations that psychotic symptoms in either mania or depression respond to DA receptor antagonists and the existence of mixed episodes characterized by both manic and depressive features suggest that if DA dysfunction exists in BD, it likely involves complex interactions with other neurotransmitter systems.

Moreover, assessments of cerebrospinal fluid chemistry, neuroendocrine responses to pharmacological challenge, and neuroreceptor and transporter binding have demonstrated abnormalities involving serotonergic, noradrenergic, cholinergic, and peptidergic systems and in the functioning of the hypothalamic–pituitary–adrenal (HPA) axis in BD. While dysfunction within these neurotransmitter and neuroendocrine systems is likely to play roles in the pathophysiology of BD, there is a growing expectation that they represent downstream effects of other, more primary abnormalities in signal transduction pathways, which would be capable of affecting the functional balance between multiple neurotransmitter systems. Elucidation of the biochemical effects of lithium has supported such hypotheses, as lithium has been shown to inhibit adenylate cyclase, alter certain types of protein phosphorylation, affect expression of some G-protein and adenylate cyclase subtypes, and influence the coupling between neurotransmitter receptors and G proteins.

Analyses of the lesions that can result in secondary mania implicate the ventral PFC, basotemporal cortex,

BOX 43.5 (cont'd)

and striatum in the pathogenesis of BD. Within these regions, neuroimaging and *postmortem* neuropathological studies have shown abnormal reductions of gray matter volume, glial cell counts, and/or synaptic contacts or proteins in the ventral anterior cingulate cortex, ventral striatum, and subiculum of the hippocampus in primary BD. These regions have shown to play major roles in reward-directed behavior and emotional processing by studies in both humans and experimental animals.

Wayne C. Drevets

Suggested Readings

Drevets, W. C., and Todd, R. D. (1997). Depression, mania and related disorders. *In* "Adult Psychiatry" (S. B. Guze, ed.), Vol. 8, pp. 99–141. Mosby, St. Louis, MO.

Goodwin, F. K., and Jamison, K. R. (1990). "Manic-Depressive Illness" Oxford, New York.

Manji, H., Drevets, W. C., and Charney, D. (2001). The cellular neurobiology of depression. *Nature Med.* **7**(5), 541–547.

Willner, P. (1995). Dopaminergic mechanisms in depression and mania. *In* "Psychopharmacology: The Fourth Generation of Progress" (F. E. Bloom and D. J. Kupfer, eds.), Chapter 80, pp. 921–932. Raven Press, New York.

the pallidum is routed in several different ways, including to brain stem motor regions and looping back to the prefrontal cortex through the mediodorsal thalamus. This circuit (limbic cortex-ventral striatum-pallidum) could, in principle, provide "a neural mechanism by which motivation gets translated into action" (Mogenson *et al.*, 1980). To understand the function of this circuit, Mogenson and colleagues used electrophysiological experiments to demonstrate interactions among its components, e.g., between the amygdala and the nucleus accumbens.

As described earlier, the basal and lateral amygdala convey associative information about stimuli that predict the occurrence of reinforcers. The recipients of this information are systems that select responses. A link between the amygdala and the ventral striatum is important in the translation of emotion (and motivational effects of stimuli) to behavioral output, or action (Everitt *et al.*, 2000). In some circumstances, therefore, reinforcement involves glutamatergic inputs from these limbic afferents to the striatum. These inputs interact with the ascending DA system and together they determine the output of the ventral striatal GABAergic medium spiny neurons that project to the globus pallidus (ventral pallidum) (see Chapter 31). The nucleus accumbens has turned out to be a heterogeneous structure. Its medial "shell" and lateral "core" can be distinguished anatomically, neurochemically, and functionally. The shell region is considered by some to be part of an extended amygdala encompassing the central nucleus of the amyg-

dala and the bed nucleus of the stria terminalis (Heimer *et al.*, 1995, see Chapter 44).

Summary

Appetitive motivational systems organize responses to regulatory and incentive (external sensory) influences and integrate these responses with higher order controls dictated by learning. These controls probably require coordination of several levels of the central nervous system, including limbic, hypothalamic, and brain stem structures. Integration of the activity of these structures appears to be modulated by ascending monoaminergic neurotransmitter systems, such as the mesencephalic DA neurons. This modulation probably optimizes the vigor of behavioral responses and enables the reward process to contribute to the learning of behavioral sequences (through associative functions of the limbic system).

BRAIN AVERSION SYSTEMS

The system that mediates aversion was identified by a combination of anatomical and behavioral experiments. For example, mapping studies identified sites eliciting escape from brain stimulation, sites at which ESB elicits defensive responses, and sites at which fear or pain naturally evokes aggressive responses. Many of these pathways are like central reflex path-

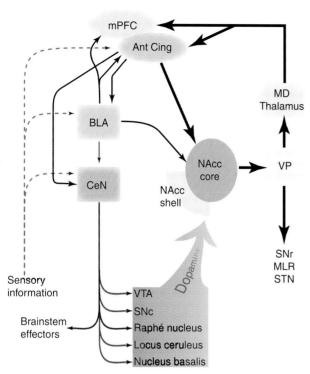

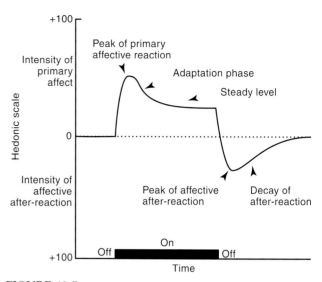

FIGURE 43.7 Opponent motivational system. The graph shows the standard time course of the dynamic control of affect. Five distinctive features of affect result from a typical, square-wave input (black bar). The B process becomes apparent after the A process ends. Modified with permission from Solomon and Corbit (1974).

FIGURE 43.6 Schematic of cortico-limbic-striatal-pallidal-brain stem circuitry. Processing of motivational and emotional information occurs in limbic and cortical regions of the brain such as the medial prefrontal cortex (mPFC), anterior cingulate cortex (Ant Cing), hippocampus (not shown), and basolateral amygdala (BLA). This interacts with dopamine-dependent functions of the nucleus accumbens (NAcc). The cortico-striatal-cortical "loop" is completed via a relay in the mediodorsal (MD) thalamic nucleus. Dopamine pathways originate in the ventral tegmental area (VTA) and substantia nigra, pars compacta (SNc). The shell and core of this structure act as interfaces with motor (behavioral), endocrine, and autonomic outputs to the hypothalamus (not shown) and brain stem, e.g., midbrain locomotor region (MLR) via the ventral pallidum (VP) and substantia nigra, pars reticulata (SNr). Outflow from the central nucleus, in contrast to the BLA, is also routed to brain stem behavioral and physiological effector mechanisms, as well as to origins of the ascending neuromodulatory influences, of the noradrenergic system (from the locus coeruleus), the basal forebrain cholinergic system (nucleus basalis), and the midbrain serotoninergic system (raphe nucleus), as well as to the dopamine cells of the VTA and SNc.

ways, with both ascending and descending components modulated by influences from the central nucleus of the amygdala.

Some ESB sites (e.g., VMH) produced markedly ambivalent reinforcing effects, which were interpreted as an interaction between positive reinforcement and aversion systems. ESB itself has been suggested to have both appetitive and aversive properties, as have drugs of abuse and, in some situations, electric shock. In fact, animal learning theory has led to the concept of opponent motivational processes (one appetitive, one aversive) (see Chapter 44).

Aversion May Be Mediated by Opponent Motivational Processes

It has been suggested that many reinforcers produce affective and hedonic effects (A processes) that are opposed by B processes of opposite affective sign in a simple, dynamic control system for affect (Fig. 43.7) (Solomon and Corbit, 1974). The A process follows the reinforcing event with short latency and then decays. Its size decreases with repeated presentation of the reinforcer. The B process has a longer latency of onset, reaches its maximum only after repeated trials, and decays very slowly. These components of emotional responses are exhibited in response to many reinforcers, including not only drugs such as heroin (see Chapter 44), but also natural rewards that may also lead to different forms of "dependence," such as attachment of offspring to a mother. So, for example, either heroin or the mother elicits a hedonic A process, which is followed by a rebound negative or aversive B process when the heroin wears off (or the mother leaves). These effects may get stronger with repeated experiences of heroin (or the mother at a critical period of development), leading to a form of dependence in each case. The opponent process can also work in reverse. For example, if tolerance develops for an initially aversive experience, a rebound hedonic response can occur when this experience stops. Indeed, this may partly explain the "pleasure" of jogging.

How might these opponent processes be represented in the brain? Evidence of functional antagonism between systems using different neurotransmitters, such as norepinephrine and serotonin, led researchers to postulate a noradrenergic reinforcing system balanced by a serotoninergic punishment system. Although this particular interaction is now in doubt, the general idea of opposed chemical systems remains plausible. For example, opposing interactions may occur between central dopaminergic and serotoninergic systems. (See Chapter 44 for hypotheses based on studies of drug withdrawal.) Another consideration for research is that the same limbic–striatal interactions that mediate the conditioning of appetitive behavior may also affect the conditioning of aversive responses. For example, the amygdala is involved in aversive conditioning as well as the appetitive learning described earlier (see Chapter 51).

Summary

Neural systems controlling aversive motivation are probably distinct from those controlling appetitive motivation. However, opponent relationships involving mutual inhibition have been theorized to exist between the two systems. These interactions are hypothetically subserved by brain regions where appetitive and aversive systems overlap and may underline complex forms of motivation, such as dependence.

Motivation is thus a complex behavioral process that depends on controls provided both by internal stimuli (homeostasis) and by external incentives, the latter often dependent on learning. These stimuli together enable state-dependent selection and coordination of different sequences of behavior that have flexible anticipatory elements and more stereotyped terminal elements. Neural control of these processes is distributed throughout the brain and is powerfully modulated by the activity of neurotransmitter systems such as DA.

References

Antelman, S. M., and Szechtman, H. (1975). Tail-pinch induces eating in hungry rats which appears to depend on nigrostriatal dopamine. *Science* **189**, 731–733

Carli, M., Evenden, J. L., and Robbins, T. W. (1985). Depletion of unilateral striatal dopamine impairs initiation of contralateral actions and not sensory attention. *Nature (Lond.)* **313**, 679–682.

Carlisle, H. J. (1969). The effects of preoptic and anterior hypothalamic lesions on behavioral thermoregulation in the cold. *J. Comp. Physiol. Psychol.* **69**, 391–402.

Everitt, B. J. (1990). Sexual motivation: A neural and behavioral analysis of the mechanisms underlying appetitive copulatory responses of male rats. *Neurosci. Biobehav. Rev.* **14**, 217–232.

Flynn, J. P., Vanegas, H., Foote, W., and Edwards, S. (1970). Neural mechanisms involved in a cat's attack on a rat. *In* "The Neural Control of Behaviour" (R. Whalen, R. F. Thompson, M. Verzeano, and N. M. Weinberger, eds.), pp. 135–173. Academic Press, New York

Heimer, L., and Larsson, K. (1966–1967). Impairment of mating behaviour in male rats following lesions in the preoptic-anterior hypothalamic continuum. *Brain Res.* **3**, 248–263

Heimer, L., Zahm, D. S., and Alheid, G. F. (1995). Basal ganglia. *In* "The Rat Nervous System" (G. Paxinos, ed.), 2nd Ed., pp. 579–614. Academic Press, Sydney.

Koob, G. F., Riley, S., Smith, S. C., and Robbins, T. W. (1978). Effects of 6-hydroxydopamine lesions to nucleus accumbens septi and olfactory tubercle on food intake, locomotor activity and amphetamine anorexia in the rat. *J. Comp. Physiol. Psychol.* **92**, 917–927

Leibowitz, S. F. (1980). Neurochemical systems of the hypothalamus: Control of feeding and drinking behaviour and water-electrolyte excretion. *In* "Handbook of the Hypothalamus" (P. J. Morgan and J. Panksepp, eds.), Vol. 3, Part A, pp. 299–437. Raven Press, New York.

Norgren, R., and Grill, H. (1982). Brain-stem control of ingestive behavior. *In* "The Physiological Mechanisms of Motivation" (D. W. Pfaff, ed.), Vol. 4, pp. 99–131. Springer-Verlag, New York.

Phillips, A. G. (1984). Brain reward circuitry: A case for separate systems. *Brain Res. Bull.* **12**, 195–201.

Phillips, A. G., Pfaus, J. G., and Blaha, D. C. (1991). Dopamine and motivated behavior. *In* "The Mesolimbic Dopamine System: From Motivation to Action" (P. Willner and J. Scheel-Kruger, eds.), pp. 199–224. Wiley, Chichester.

Robbins, T. W. (1986). Hunger. *In* "Neuroendocrinology" (S. L. Lightman and B. J. Everitt, eds.), pp. 252–303. Blackwell, Oxford.

Rolls, E. T. (1985). The neurophysiology of feeding. *In* "Psychopharmacology and Food" (M. Sandler and T. Silverstone, eds.), pp. 1–16. Oxford Univ. Press, Oxford.

Satinoff, E. (1982). Are there similarities between thermoregulation and sexual behaviour? *In* "The Physiological Mechanisms of Motivation" (D. W. Pfaff, ed.), pp. 217–251. Springer-Verlag, New York.

Schultz, W., Romo, R., Ljungberg, T., Mirenowicz, J., Hollerman, J. R., and Dickinson, A. (1995). Reward-related signals carried by dopamine neurons. *In* "Models of Information Processing in the Basal Ganglia" (J. R. Houk, J. L. Davis, and D. Beiser, eds.), pp. 233–248. MIT Press, Cambridge, MA.

Solomon, R. L., and Corbit, J. D. (1974). An opponent-process theory of motivation: I. Temporal dynamics of affect. *Psychol. Rev.* **81**, 119–145.

Stricker, E. M., and Zigmond, M. J. (1976). Recovery of function after damage to central catecholamine-containing neurons: A neurochemical model for the lateral hypothalamic syndrome. *Prog. Psychol. Physiol. Psychol.* **6**, 121–188.

Ungerstedt, U. (1971a). Adipsia and aphagia after 6-hydroxydopamine induced degeneration of the nigrostriatal dopamine system. *Acta Physiol. Scand. Suppl.* **367**, 95–122.

Ungerstedt, U. (1971b). Striatal dopamine release after amphetamine or nerve degeneration revealed by rotational behavior. *Acta Physiol. Scand. Suppl.* **367**, 49–68.

Winn, P., Tarbuck, A., and Dunnett, S. B. (1984). Ibotenic acid lesions of the lateral hypothalamus: Comparison with the electrolytic lesion syndrome. *Neuroscience* **12**, 225–240.

Wise, R. (1982). Neuroleptics and operant behavior: The anhedonia hypothesis. *Behav. Brain Sci.* **5**, 39–87.

Suggested Readings

Blackburn, J. R., Pfaus, J. G., and Phillips, A. G. (1992). Dopamine functions in appetitive and defensive behaviors. *Prog. Neurobiol.* **39**, 247–279.

Dickinson, A., and Balleine, B. (1994). Motivational control of goal-directed action. *Anim. Learn. Behav.* **22**, 1–18.

Everitt, B. J., Cardinal, R. N., Hall, J., Parkinson, J. A., and Robbins, T. W. (2000). Differential involvement of amygdala sub-systems in appetitive conditioning and drug addiction. *In* "The Amygdala: A Functional Analysis." (Aggleton, J. P. ed), pp. 353–390. Oxford Univ. Press, Oxford.

Hoebel, B. G. (1974). Brain reward and aversion systems in the control of feeding and sexual behavior. *In* "Nebraska Symposium on Motivation" (J. Cole and T. Sonderegger, eds.), pp. 49–112. University of Nebraska Press, Lincoln.

Marshall, J. F., and Teitelbaum, P. (1977). New considerations in the neuropsychology of motivated behaviors. *In* "Handbook of Psychopharmacology" (L. L. Iversen, S. D. Iversen, and S. H. Snyder, eds.), Vol. 7, pp. 201–229. Plenum, New York.

Mogenson, G. J., Jones, D. L., and Yim, C. Y. (1980). From motivation to action: Functional interface between the limbic system and the motor system. *Prog. Neurobiol.* **14**, 69–97.

Pfaff, D. W. (ed.) (1982). "The Physiological Mechanisms of Motivation," pp. 217–251. Springer-Verlag, New York.

Robbins, T. W., Taylor, J. R., Cador, M., and Everitt, B. J. (1989). Limbic-striatal interactions and reward-related processes. *Neurosci. Biobehav. Rev.* **13**, 155–162.

Sachs, B. D., and Meisel, R. L. (1988). The physiology of male sexual behavior. *In* "The Physiology of Reproduction" (E. Knobil and J. Neill, eds.), pp. 1393–1485. Raven Press, New York.

Stellar, E. (1954). The psychology of motivation. *Psychol. Rev.* **61**, 5–22.

Toates, F. (1980). "Animal Behaviour: A Systems Approach." Wiley, Chichester.

Valenstein, E. T. (1973). "Brain Control." Wiley, New York.

Trevor W. Robbins and Barry J. Everitt

Drug Reward and Addiction

Drug abuse is one of the world's major public health problems. For example, statistics from the 1999 *National Household Survey on Drug Abuse* of the National Institute on Drug Abuse of the United States reveal that approximately 14.8 million Americans were current users of illicit drugs and 3.5 million were dependent on illicit drugs. In addition, 8.3 million individuals were listed as dependent on alcohol and 47 million were current smokers. The cost of drug abuse to society is staggering. Total economic costs of alcohol abuse per year in the United State is listed as 166.5 billion dollars, smoking 138 billion dollars, and that of illicit drugs 109.9 billion dollars. This totals over 400 billion dollars in lost productivity due to illness or death, health care expenditures, motor vehicle crashes, social welfare, and so on (Robert Wood Johnson Foundation, Princeton, New Jersey, 2001).

A common characteristic of most definitions of drug dependence and addiction is a *compulsion to take a drug* with a loss of control in limiting intake (American Psychiatric Association, 1994). The criteria used by the "Diagnostic and Statistical Manual of Mental Disorders IV" to diagnose drug dependence incorporate changes in behavior that, when presented in a person's daily repertoire, are likely to reflect a compulsion to take drugs and loss of control over drug intake (Table 44.1). In this chapter, drug *addiction* is equated with *substance dependence* as defined by the American Psychiatric Association (1994). Drug *abuse*, in contrast, is defined as the harmful use of a drug. It is important to distinguish among drug use, abuse, and dependence because they represent a continuum of increased drug ingestion that conveys different effects on the brain and body. Many individuals learn to drink limited amounts of alcohol in a social

TABLE 44.1 Diagnostic Criteria for Substance Abuse and Substance Dependence (DSM-IV, the American Psychiatric Association)

Substance abuse	Substance dependence
A maladaptive pattern of substance use leading to clinically significant impairment or distress, as manifested by one or more of the following occurring over the same 12-month period.	1. Tolerance 2. Withdrawal. 3. The substance is often taken in larger amounts over a longer period than was intended.
1. Recurrent substance use resulting in a failure to fulfil major role obligations at work, school, or home. 2. Recurrent substance use in situations in which it is physically hazardous.	4. Any unsuccessful effort or a persistent desire to cut down or control substance use. 5. A great deal of time is spent in activities necessary to obtain the substance or recover from its effects.
3. Recurrent substance-related legal problems.	6. Important social, occupational, or recreational activities given up or reduced because of substance use.
4. Continued substance use despite having persistent or recurrent social or interpersonal problems caused by substance.	7. Continued substance despite knowledge of or having had a persistent or recurrent physical or psychological problem that is likely to be caused or exacerbated by the substance. 8. Three or more symptoms occurring during the last year.

BOX 44.1

SOURCES OF REINFORCEMENT

Addiction component	Behavioral construct
Pleasure	Positive reinforcement
Self-medication	Negative reinforcement
Habit	Conditioned positive reinforcement
Habit	Conditioned negative reinforcement

The motivating factors for the development, maintenance and persistence of drug addiction can be broken down into four major sources of reinforcement in drug dependence: positive reinforcement, negative reinforcement, conditioned positive reinforcement, and conditioned negative reinforcement. Clearly, positive reinforcing effects are critical for establishing self-administration behavior, and some have argued the hypothesis that positive reinforcement is the key to drug dependence. However, while alleviation of withdrawal symptoms (negative reinforcement) may not be a major motivating factor in the *initiation* of compulsive drug use, a compelling case can be made for compromises in hedonic processing associated with drug abstinence as a driving force of addiction. The construct of negative reinforcement plays an important role in the *maintenance* of drug use after the development of dependence. Largely unexplored has been the issue of individual differences in vulnerability to this transition to drug dependence. Thus, while initial drug use may be motivated by the positive affective state produced by the drug, continued use leads to neuroadaptation to the presence of drug and to another source of reinforcement, the negative reinforcement associated with relieving negative affective consequences of drug termination. The defining feature of drug dependence has been argued to be the establishment of a negative affective state. However, an even more compelling motivational force is the hypothesis that negative affective states, even during protracted abstinence, can contribute to the reinforcement associated with drug taking by changing the "set point" for hedonic processing. Much progress has been made in identifying the neuronal substrates for the acute positive reinforcing effects of drugs of abuse. A more recent focus has been on the neuronal substrates for negative reinforcement and the conditioned reinforcing effects that contribute to relapse.

George F. Koob

---

context, which may even have health benefits, whereas others use alcohol to the point of such abuses as driving under the influence of alcohol or drug dependence with all of its harmful sequelae. Reinforcement and motivation are crucial parts of substance dependence. *Reinforcement* can be defined operationally as the process by which stimuli increase the probability of a subject's responding, whereas *motivation* can be defined as the tendency to produce organized activity (see Chapter 43). Motivation as a construct involves many sources of reinforcement, which can combine to produce powerful tendencies of organized activity (see Box 44.1).

Most views of substance dependence also involve development of tolerance and withdrawal. *Tolerance* is the loss of an effect of a drug with repeated administration. *Withdrawal* is defined as the appearance of symptoms associated with the termination of chronic drug use. Tolerance and withdrawal are key elements supporting the idea that adaptive processes are initiated to counter acute effects of a drug, and our understanding of this subject emphasizes tolerance and withdrawal associated with affective measures, not physical signs (American Psychiatric Association,

1994). Another neuroadaptive process that has been proposed as a key element in the development of drug dependence is *sensitization*–the increased response to a drug that follows its repeated, intermittent presentation (Koob and Le Moal, 2001). These three neuroadaptive processes—tolerance, withdrawal, and sensitization—can persist long after a drug has left the brain, and they have been explored at all levels from the behavioral to the molecular (Koob and Le Moal, 2001).

ASSESSING THE REINFORCING ACTIONS OF DRUGS

A variety of behavioral tests are used in the study of drug reinforcement. This section studies three of these: drug self-administration, intracranial self-administration, and place conditioning.

Animals will self-administer drugs both orally and intravenously. In general, drugs that are self-administered correspond to those that have high abuse potential (Schuster and Thompson, 1969). This relationship

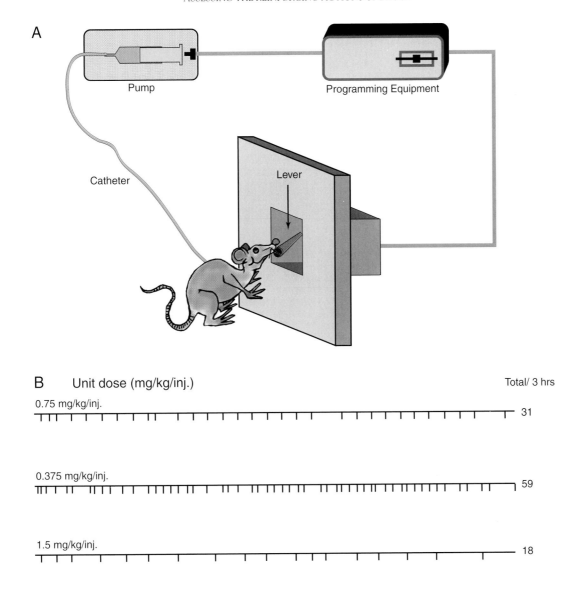

A

Pump

Programming Equipment

Catheter

Lever

B   Unit dose (mg/kg/inj.)   Total/ 3 hrs

0.75 mg/kg/inj.   31

0.375 mg/kg/inj.   59

1.5 mg/kg/inj.   18

0.75 mg/kg/inj. + pretreatment with 20µg/Kg SCH23390   67

0   60   120   180

Time (min)

FIGURE 44.1   Intravenous self-administration by rats. (A) Drawing illustrating the setup for intravenous self-administration of cocaine by rats. (B) Event records for different unit doses of cocaine show a dose–response relationship relating dose of cocaine to number of infusions. Rats implanted with intravenous catheters and trained to self-administer cocaine with limited access (3 h per day) show stable and regular drug intake over each daily session. No obvious tolerance or dependence develops. Rats generally are maintained on a fixed ratio (FR) schedule of drug infusion, such as FR-1 or FR-5. In an FR-1 schedule, one lever press is required to deliver an intravenous infusion of cocaine; in an FR-5 schedule, five lever presses are required to deliver an infusion of cocaine, and so on. With an FR schedule, rats appear to regulate the amount of drug self-administered. Lowering the dose from the training level of 0.75 mg/kg per injection increases the number of self-administered infusions; raising the unit dose decreases the number of infusions. Pretreatment with the dopamine antagonist SCH23390 also increases the number of self-administered infusions. Reprinted with permission from Caine *et al.* (1993).

is so strong that animal models of drug self-administration have predictive value for abuse potential in humans, and these models now are used for preclinical assessment of the abuse liability of new pharmaceutical agents. Animals equipped with long-term intravenous catheters readily learn to intravenously self-administer cocaine or heroin. A typical pattern of cocaine self-administration in a rat maintained on a simple fixed ratio schedule is shown in Fig. 44.1. Note the relationship between dose of the self-administered drug and number of self-administered infusions

(termed a *dose–response* or *dose–effect* function). The impact of changes in dose depends in part on the route of administration. For example, with *intravenous* self-administration of drugs within the range of doses that maintain stable responding, as the dose received per self-injection increases, animals increase the interval between injections. Said differently, animals decrease their rates of self-administration, apparently compensating for the increased dose received with each self-injection. However, for *oral* self-administration of drugs such as alcohol, the relationship

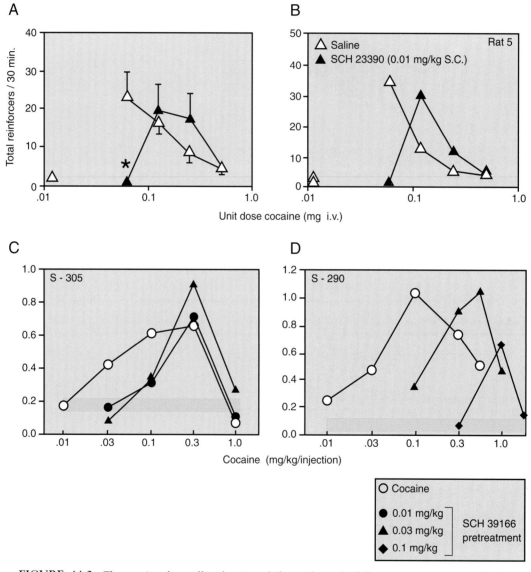

FIGURE 44.2 The cocaine dose–effect function shifts to the right following pretreatment with the dopamine (DA) D-1 receptor antagonists SCH23390 and SCH39166. (A) Effects of pretreatment with SCH23390 (0.01 mg/kg subcutaneous) on the dose–effect function of intravenously self-administered cocaine (0.06–0.05 mg) measured using the within-session dose–effect paradigm (*n*=4). (B) Same as in A but for an individual rat. Reprinted with permission from Caine and Koob (1995). (C and D) Effects of pretreatment with SCH39166 on cocaine self-administration in two squirrel monkeys. Points are means based on the last three sessions at each dose of drug. Reprinted with permission from Bergman *et al.* (1990).

between dose and number of deliveries of the liquid reinforcer is more of a monotonic function, with higher doses producing a higher intake of drug and in effect producing an inverted u-shaped dose–effect function. Competitive antagonists of drugs shift a dose–effect function to the right, as more drug is required to overcome antagonism (see Fig. 44.2). For example, with intravenous drug self-administration, pharmacologic antagonists of dopamine (DA) shift the dose–effect function to the right (representing a decrease in the reinforcing potency of cocaine) and cause increases in self-administered infusions of cocaine.

Another behavioral test that has been used extensively to measure positive reinforcing effects of drugs of abuse is *rewarding brain stimulation*, or *intracranial self-stimulation* (ICSS). Electrical self-stimulation of certain brain areas is rewarding for animals and humans, as demonstrated by subjects that will readily self-administer such stimulation (Liebman and Cooper, 1989; see also Chapter 43). The high reward value of ICSS has led to the hypothesis that ICSS directly activates neuronal "reward circuits." Because ICSS bypasses much of the input side of these neuronal circuits, it provides a unique tool in neuropharmacological research with which to study the influence of various substances on reward and reinforcement processes. ICSS differs significantly from drug self-administration in that animals work to directly stimulate presumed reinforcement circuits in the brain that are activated by conventional reinforcers (e.g., food, water, and sex). Drugs of abuse appear to make ICSS *more* rewarding, or decrease thresholds for ICSS, and there is a good correlation between the ability of drugs to decrease ICSS thresholds and their potential for abuse (Liebman and Cooper, 1989).

The third major behavioral test used to measure reinforcing actions of drugs of abuse is *place conditioning*. In effect, this is a Pavlovian conditioning procedure in which a drug state is paired with experience in a particular environment. In a simple version of the *place preference* paradigm, animals experience two distinct neutral environments that are paired spatially and temporally with distinct drug states, the unconditioned stimuli. Then, in the absence of the drug, the animal is given an opportunity to enter and explore either environment. Positive reinforcing effects of the drug are reflected in the choice of the animal to spend more time in the environment that was paired with the drug. Of course, the opposite also can occur—an aversive experience can become a negative reinforcer. One of the earlier demonstrations of place preference was the observation by Olds and Milner (1954) that

rats stimulated through an intracranial electrode would return to the location in which they received the stimulation.

Summary

Compulsive drug-seeking behaviors are the result of positive and negative reinforcement associated with chronic drug taking. These multiple sources of reinforcement serve to strengthen the power of drugs in the abuser's life and are hypothesized to result from powerful actions on brain reward systems.

NEUROBIOLOGICAL SUBSTRATES OF DRUG REWARD

Positive Reinforcing Effects of Drugs Are Mediated by Multiple Systems Converging on Common Targets in the Basal Forebrain

The midbrain and forebrain appear to be involved in motivated behavior through connections of the medial forebrain bundle, composed of ascending and descending pathways including most of the brain monoamine systems (Koob, 1992; see Chapters 8 and 43). The medial forebrain bundle is involved in brain stimulation reward and natural rewards, and work in the neurobiology of addiction has led to an understanding of the neurochemical and neuroanatomical components of this system. The principal components of this system include the ventral tegmental area (VTA), the basal forebrain (the nucleus accumbens, olfactory tubercle, frontal cortex, and amygdala), and the DA connection between the VTA and the basal forebrain, called the mesolimbic DA system. Additional components are the opioid peptide systems, γ-aminobutyric acid (GABA) systems, and serotonin (5-hydroxytryptamine; 5-HT) systems that interact with the VTA and the basal forebrain (Koob, 1992) (see Fig. 44.3; see also Fig. 43.2). The functional role of each component of this mesolimbic system is discussed in the following sections, and a concept called the *extended amygdala* is introduced to provide important insight into the relationship between drug reward and natural reward systems. This chapter also explores the actions of several groups of drugs with respect to this system, including general stimulants (cocaine and amphetamine), opiates (heroin), nicotine, general depressants and anxiolytics (alcohol, barbiturates, and benzodiazepines), and tetrahydrocannabinol (THC).

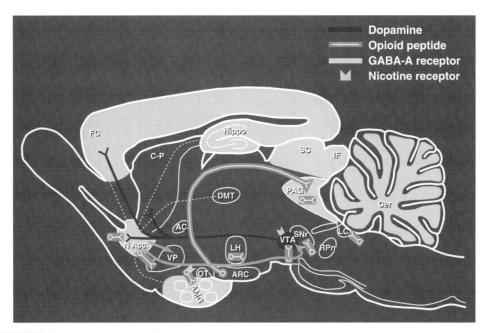

FIGURE 44.3 Sagittal section through the brain of a rat depicting the neurochemical systems implicated in the reinforcing effects of drugs of abuse. Yellow indicates limbic afferents to the nucleus accumbens (N. Acc.). Orange represents efferents from the nucleus accumbens thought to be involved in psychomotor stimulant reward. Red indicates a projection of the mesocorticolimbic DA system thought to be a critical substrate for psychomotor stimulant reward. This system originates in the A10 cell group of the ventral tegmental area (VTA) and projects to the nucleus accumbens, olfactory tubercle, and ventral striatal domains of the caudate-putamen (C-P). Green indicates opioid peptide-containing neurons that may be involved in opiate and alcohol reward. These opioid peptide systems include the local enkephalin circuits (short segments) and the hypothalamic midbrain ß-endorphin circuit (long segment). Blue shows the approximate distribution of GABA$_A$ receptor complexes, some of which may mediate sedative–hypnotic (alcohol) reward, determined by binding of tritiated (e.g., radioactively labeled) flumazenil to GABA receptors and by expression of the α, ß, and γ subunits of the GABA$_A$ receptor. VP, ventral pallidum; LH, lateral hypothalamus; SNr, substantia nigra pars reticulata; DMT, dorsomedial thalamus; PAG, periaqueductal gray; OT, olfactory tract; AC, anterior commissure; LC, locus coeruleus; AMG, amygdala; Hippo, hippocampus; Cer, cerebellum, FC, frontal cortex. Modified with permission from Koob (1992).

The Positive Reinforcing Effects of Cocaine and Other Indirect Sympathomimetics Depend Critically on the Mesolimbic DA System

Amphetamine and cocaine are psychomotor stimulants that, in humans, have behavioral effects such as suppressing hunger and fatigue and inducing euphoria in humans. In animals, these drugs increase motor activity, decrease food intake, stimulate operant behavior, enhance conditioned responding, and produce place preferences (Koob, 1992). Psychomotor stimulants also decrease thresholds for reinforcing brain stimulation and act as reinforcers for drug self-administration (Koob, 1992; see Figs. 44.1 and 44.4).

Psychomotor stimulants with a high potential for abuse have effects that lead to increases in the availability of monoamine neurotransmitters at synapses. By blocking reuptake or enhancing release, cocaine and amphetamine increase the synaptic availability of DA, norepinephrine (NE), and 5-HT. However, the acute reinforcing effects of these drugs depend critically on DA (Koob, 1992). Studies of intravenous self-administration have provided the most direct evidence implicating DA, and more specifically the mesolimbic DA system, in the reinforcing actions of cocaine and amphetamine drugs. Low doses of DA receptor antagonists injected either systemically or centrally into the nucleus accumbens, amygdala, or bed nucleus of the stria terminalis block cocaine and amphetamine self-administration in rats (Koob, 1992). A specific role for the mesolimbic DA system in the reinforcing properties of cocaine and amphetamine was deduced from the observation that, over days, neurotoxin-induced lesions of the terminal regions of the mesolimbic DA system in the nucleus accumbens produce a significant and long-lasting decrease in self-administration of cocaine and amphetamine (Koob, 1992). The neurotoxin, 6-hydroxydopamine (6-OHDA), is an analog of DA that, when injected into the brain, is taken up by presynaptic DA nerve termi-

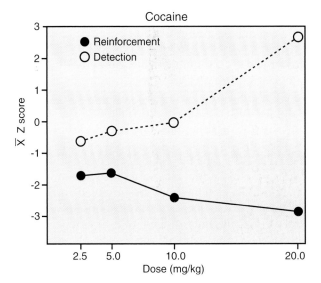

Cocaine

FIGURE 44.4 Effects of cocaine on thresholds of brain stimulation reward and brain stimulation detection. For measurement of detection threshold, the initial, noncontingent stimulus varied in intensity (at subreward levels), whereas the second, or response-contingent, stimulus was held constant at a rewarding intensity to maintain responding. Each point is the mean z $score$ $\pm$ SEM, the difference between the means of the thresholds after administration of vehicle and drug, divided by the standard deviation of all thresholds after vehicle administration. A z $score$ of 2 indicates significant difference from vehicle treatment sessions. These results show that an acute administration of cocaine can lower thresholds of brain stimulation (i.e., facilitate central reward). The cocaine treatment does not affect the ability of the rat to discriminate because detection of a nonrewarding stimulus is not altered (detection threshold). Error bars not shown indicate SEM less than the diameter of the symbols in this illustration. Reprinted with permission from Kornetsky and Bain (1982).

nals, converted to reactive oxygen species, and destroys the terminals. 6-OHDA-induced lesions of the DA terminals in the nucleus accumbens even decrease the amount of work an animal will perform for

cocaine without affecting many other reinforcers, such as food. The specific sites within the mesolimbic DA system that appear particularly important for the reinforcing actions of cocaine correspond with specific subregions of the limbic region, such as the shell (medial part) of the nucleus accumbens and the central nucleus of the amygdala.

Neurobiological Substrates for the Acute Reinforcing Effects of Opiates Involve Opioid Peptide Systems

Much like psychostimulants, opiate drugs such as heroin are readily self-administered intravenously by animals. When provided an opiate for a few hours per day, rats and primates maintain stable daily opiate intake without major signs of physical dependence when not taking the drug (Schuster and Thompson, 1968). Advances in opiate pharmacology, such as identification of high specific binding for opiates in the brain and discovery of endogenous opioid peptides, provided insight into the brain systems responsible for the reinforcing effects of these drugs (Koob, 1992; see Box 44.2). Both systemic administration and central administration of competitive opiate antagonists into the nucleus accumbens and ventral tegmental area decrease intravenous opiate self-administration. The reinforcing actions of heroin and morphine appear to be mediated largely by the μ-opiate receptor subtype (see Chapter 9). μ-Opioid antagonists produce dose-dependent decreases in heroin reinforcement, and μ-knockout mice show loss of morphine-induced reward and loss of morphine-induced analgesia. Intracerebral opioid antagonists block heroin self-administration in nondependent rats when these drugs are injected into the VTA or the

BOX 44.2

OPIATE RECEPTORS

In 1978, Professors Solomon H. Snyder, John Hughes, and Hans W. Kosterlitz were awarded the Lasker award for their combined discovery of opiate receptors in the brain and for the even more amazing discovery of the existence of endogenous ligands for opiate receptors. The endogenous brain compounds were peptides, called enkephalins and endorphins, which shared all the physiologic properties of opiates. These observations opened a rich field of inquiry into the mechanism of action of opiate drugs, and these findings began a new outlook on

neuropeptide neurotransmitters, an area of intense research. First, many new neuropeptides have been discovered with brain receptors potentially amenable to nonpeptidergic agonists and antagonists. Second, because neuropeptides are contained within neurons that are also more conventional amino acid or amine transmitters, the possibility of multiple mediators for any specific synapse had to be considered (see Chapter 7).

George F. Koob

region of the nucleus accumbens. Microinjections of opioids into the VTA also lower thresholds for ICSS and produce robust place preferences and these effects appear to be dependent on mesolimbic DA function (Di Chiara and North, 1992). Rats will self-administer opioid peptides in the region of the nucleus accumbens. However, heroin self-administration is not blocked by DA antagonists given in doses that block cocaine self-administration (Koob, 1992) nor by large neurotoxin-induced lesions of the mesolimbic DA system. These results demonstrate that neural elements in the regions of the VTA *and* the nucleus accumbens are responsible for the reinforcing properties of opiates, suggesting both DA-dependent and DA-independent opiate action (Di Chiara and North, 1992; Koob, 1992).

Nicotine Activates Mesolimbic DA and Opioid Peptide Systems

Nicotine has antifatigue, stimulant-like, and antianxiety effects and appears to improve cognitive performance in animals and humans. It has direct reinforcing actions, as measured by intravenous self-administration in animals and humans. Smoking one to two packs of cigarettes per day leads to nicotine dependence (addiction), characterized by tolerance, withdrawal, craving, and continued use despite repeated efforts to stop use.

Nicotine is a direct agonist at nicotinic acetylcholine receptors of the brain (see Chapter 9) and the drug also appears to activate both the mesolimbic DA system and endogenous opioid peptide systems. Antagonism of dopaminergic systems can block nicotine self-administration, whereas administration of nicotinic acetylcholine antagonists and the opiate antagonist naloxone can precipitate nicotine withdrawal in rodents (Watkins *et al.*, 2001). The relative importance of opioid, cholinergic, and dopaminergic neurotransmitter systems in the motivational aspects of nicotine dependence remains to be determined

Alcohol Has Multiple Neurochemical Substrates within Brain Reinforcement Systems

Alcohol (i.e., ethanol), barbiturates, and benzodiazepines all have measurable sedative–hypnotic actions, including euphoria, disinhibition, anxiety reduction, sedation, and hypnosis. All of these drugs also have anxiolytic (or antianxiety) effects, reflected in conflict situations as a reduction of behavior suppressed by punishment. The neurobiological basis of the anxiolytic properties of these sedative–hypnotic

drugs has provided clues to their reinforcing properties and their abuse potential. For example, GABAergic antagonists reverse many of the behavioral effects of alcohol, an observation that has led to the hypothesis that GABA has a role in the intoxicating effects of alcohol. Further support for a role of brain GABA in alcohol reinforcement is the observation that potent antagonists of GABA receptor function decrease alcohol reinforcement; one particularly affected brain site is the central nucleus of the amygdala (Koob, 1992). Several studies also have suggested that brain DA systems may be involved in the reinforcing properties of alcohol. DA receptor antagonists reduce lever pressing for alcohol in nondeprived rats (Koob, 1992), and extracellular DA levels increase in nondependent rats orally self-administering low doses of alcohol (Koob and Le Moal, 2001). However, virtually complete destruction of DA terminals in the nucleus accumbens by 6-OHDA failed to alter voluntary responding for alcohol (Tabakoff and Hoffman, 1992). Combined with pharmacologic data discussed earlier, these results suggest that although mesolimbic DA transmission may be associated with important aspects of alcohol reinforcement, it is not critical for the reinforcing properties of alcohol and that multiple neurotransmitters combine to orchestrate the reward profile of this drug (Tabakoff and Hoffman, 1992). For example, alcohol in a physiologic dose range may antagonize the actions of glutamate (Tabakoff and Hoffman, 1992). Also, increases in synaptic availability of 5-HT (e.g., via blockade of 5-HT reuptake or via the central injection of 5-HT) reduce the voluntary intake of alcohol (Tabakoff and Hoffman, 1992). Activation of opioid peptide systems also has been implicated in alcohol reinforcement by numerous reports that the opiate antagonists naloxone and naltrexone reduce alcohol self-administration in several animal models (Tabakoff and Hoffman, 1992). Thus, interactions of alcohol with opioid neurotransmission may contribute to alcohol reinforcement as well.

Tetrahydrocannabinol Has Effects Similar to Other Drugs of Abuse

Tetrahydrocannabinol shares effects in animal models of drug reinforcement similar to those of other drugs of abuse. Upon acute administration, THC decreases ICSS reward thresholds and produces a place preference in rats. It maintains self-administration behavior in squirrel monkeys, and a synthetic THC analog is self-administered intravenously in mice. THC binds to the cannabinoid-1 receptor that is distributed widely throughout the brain, particularly in the basal ganglia, and is thought to mediate the actions of the endogenous ligand anandamide (see Chapter 8). THC activates the mesocorticolimbic DA system, and data suggest that THC can selectively increase the release of DA in the shell of the nucleus accumbens similar to other drugs of abuse (Gardner and Vorel, 1998).

The Extended Amygdala May Be a Common Substrate for Drug Reward and Natural Rewards

Neuroanatomic and functional data have provided the basis for the hypothesis that neuroanatomical substrates for the reinforcing actions of drugs may involve neural circuitry that forms a separate entity within the basal forebrain, termed the *extended amygdala* (Heimer and Alheid, 1991) (Fig. 44.5). The concept of an extended amygdala implies a macrostructure and was originally described by Johnston (1923) as composed of several basal forebrain structures: the bed nucleus of the stria terminalis, the centromedial amygdala, the medial portion (or shell) of the nucleus accumbens, and continuous cell columns in the sublenticular substantia innominata. The func-

tional entity called the extended amygdala is based on similarities in morphology, immunohistochemistry, and connectivity among these structures (Heimer and Alheid, 1991). Afferent connections to this complex include frontal, entorhinal, and olfactory cortices, the hippocampal formation, basolateral amygdala, thalamic nuclei, VTA, ventral pallidum, lateral hypothalamus, and lateral septum. Efferent connections from this complex project to the posterior medial (sublenticular) ventral pallidum, medial VTA, reticular formation, and central gray area. Also included are a small projection to the raphé nuclei and, perhaps most intriguing from a functional point of view, the lateral hypothalamus (see Chapter 43). There are also numerous connections among the components of the extended amygdala, particularly between the central nucleus of the amygdala and the bed nucleus of the stria terminalis (Heimer and Alheid, 1991).

The concept of the extended amygdala links extensive developments in the neurobiology of drug reward with knowledge of the substrates for natural rewards, bridging what have been largely independent research pursuits. For many years in the search for neurochemical components that are the basis of brain reward circuits, the neuroanatomical focus has

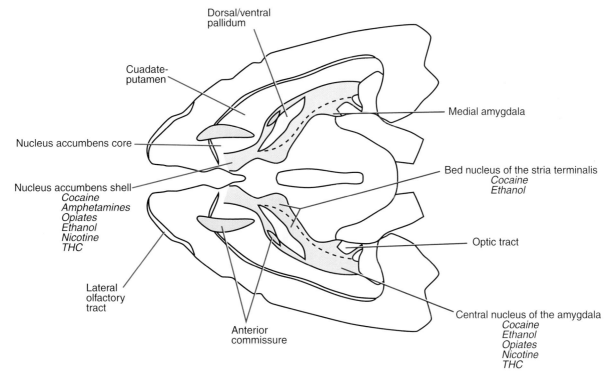

FIGURE 44.5 Effects of drugs of abuse on subregions of the extended amygdala. Horizontal section of a rat brain depicting the principal structures of the extended amygdala, including the central nucleus of the amygdala, the shell part of the nucleus accumbens, and the bed nucleus of the stria terminalis. The drugs listed below each structure refer to potential sites of action of drug reinforcement during the addiction cycle, either positive or negative. Reprinted with permission from Koob *et al.* (1998).

been the medial forebrain bundle (see earlier discussion and Chapter 43). Neurobiological studies show important neurochemical links to drug reward within the extended amygdala and important neuroanatomical connections from the extended amygdala to the hypothalamus. These studies may provide the substrates of drug reward and the neurochemical key to natural reward mechanisms.

Summary

The positive reinforcing effects of drugs are mediated by multiple systems converging on common targets in the basal forebrain. The positive reinforcing effects of cocaine and other psychostimulants depend on the mesolimbic DA circuits, which may prove to be true for THC. Within these forebrain reward systems, the acute reinforcing effects of opiates involve opioid peptide-mediated circuits. Nicotine activates both ascending DA and, possibly, intrinsic opioid peptide-mediated circuits. Alcohol-induced effects rely on DA, opioid, and probably other transmitter systems. The outer boundaries of the drug-sensitive forebrain roughly resemble the extended boundaries of the amygdala complex.

NEUROBIOLOGICAL SUBSTRATES FOR MOTIVATIONAL EFFECTS OF DRUG DEPENDENCE

Negative Affect Is a Common Result of Withdrawal from Chronic Administration of Drugs of Abuse

Withdrawal signs associated with cessation of chronic drug administration usually are characterized by responses that are opposite to the initial effects of the drug. Thus, all drugs of abuse produce rewarding effects, and withdrawal commonly is associated with subjective symptoms of dysphoria, negative affect, and anxiety (Koob and Le Moal, 2001). However, details of the withdrawal experience can vary depending on the nature of the effects of the drug itself. For example, whereas few physical signs of withdrawal usually are observed during cocaine withdrawal in humans, cessation of cocaine use often is characterized by severe depressive symptoms combined with irritability, anxiety, and anhedonia lasting several hours to several days (i.e., the "crash") and may be a motivating factor in the maintenance of the cocaine dependence cycle (Koob and Le Moal, 2001). However, in the case of opiate withdrawal, subjective symptoms such as dysphoria, anxiety, craving for drugs, and malaise are

accompanied by both physical symptoms of extreme discomfort, including pupillary dilation, hot and cold flashes, goose bumps, and a flu-like state. In the case of alcohol withdrawal, humans show tremor and increases in heartbeat rate, blood pressure, and body temperature, as well as subjective signs, including dysphoria, anxiety, insomnia, and malaise. Withdrawal from nicotine is characterized by anxiety, negative affect, fatigue, irritability, sleep disturbances, and an intense craving for cigarettes. Withdrawal from THC resembles a mild sedative–hypnotic or opiate withdrawal with irritability, restlessness, hot flashes, sweating, disturbances in appetite and sleep, and low-level dysphoria. Withdrawal from benzodiazepines resembles that of alcohol withdrawal but generally is more prolonged in onset and less intense.

Chronic Drug Administration Compromises the Brain Reward Systems

In animal studies, withdrawal from chronic administration of stimulants has been studied using ICSS after repeated administration of cocaine or amphetamine over several weeks or 12–48 of cocaine self-administration. Withdrawal from prolonged self-administration of cocaine in rats increases ICSS reward thresholds. The increase in threshold dose is time dependent and is an effect opposite to that of acute cocaine (Koob and Le Moal, 2001) (Table 44.2). Similar effects have been observed in withdrawal from chronic amphetamine administration. Opiate withdrawal induced by the administration of low doses of the opiate antagonist naloxone also elevates brain stimulation thresholds, as does spontaneous withdrawal from alcohol (Koob and Le Moal, 2001). Withdrawal from chronic nicotine and THC also produces profound increases in ICSS reward thresholds, suggesting that brain reward dysregulation is a common element of acute withdrawal from drugs of abuse.

TABLE 44.2 Drug Effects on Thresholds of Rewarding Brain Stimulation

Drug class	Acute administration	Withdrawal from chronic treatment
Psychostimulants (cocaine amphetamines)	↓	↑
Opiates (morphine, heroin)	↓	↑
Nicotine	↓	↑
Sedative–hypnotics (ethanol)	↓	↑

Summary

Negative affect is a common consequence of acute withdrawal from the continuous use of abusable drugs. This chronic use of drugs of abuse compromises the effectiveness of the brain reward systems on which drugs of abuse impose their effects.

NEUROCHEMICAL ADAPTATION IN REWARD NEUROTRANSMITTERS

DA and 5-HT Systems Show Neuroadaptive Changes with Substance Dependence

Monoamines, including the DA and 5-HT systems, have been implicated in the reinforcing actions of each of the drugs discussed: stimulants, opiates, nicotine, alcohol, and THC. One way of assessing the prolonged effects of drug self-administration is to measure extracellular levels of a neurotransmitter during ongoing behaviors, such as intravenous self-administration of a drug or withdrawal from the drug after a period of chronic self-administration. Such measurements can be made by using the technique of *in vivo* microdialysis, which involves implanting into a specific site in the brain a guide tube through which a probe with a semipermeable membrane at the tip perfuses and collects the neurotransmitter in extracellular fluid. Several studies using this technique have shown that extracellular DA and 5-HT levels in the nucleus accumbens decrease during acute withdrawal from cocaine, opiates, and alcohol (Koob and Le Moal, 2001), an effect opposite to that of acute drug administration (Fig. 44.6).

Signal Transduction Mechanisms Show Neuroadaptative Changes with Substance Dependence

Not only can the functional activity of neurotransmitters increase due to the increased presynaptic

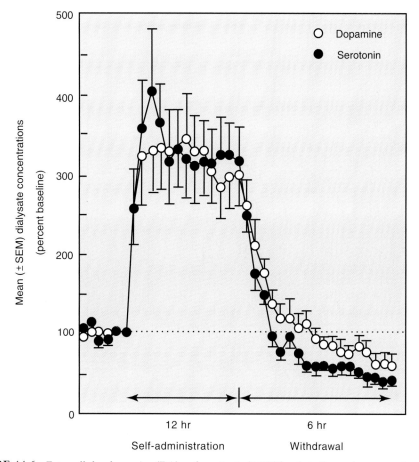

FIGURE 44.6 Extracellular dopamine (DA) and serotonin (5-HT) levels in the nucleus accumbens during and following a 12-h binge of cocaine self-administration in rats. For 12 h, rats had unlimited access to cocaine self-administration. The mean (± SEM) presession baseline dialysate concentrations of DA and 5-HT were 5.3 ± 0.5 and 1.0 ± 0.1 nM, respectively (n=7). Reprinted with permission from Parsons *et al.* (1995).

activity of chronic drug use, but these increases can also be translated to postsynaptic signal transduction. The changes in signal transduction can be long lasting and may result in long-term changes in receptor function. These changes take place at the level of receptor binding or in the impact that the association of a drug with its receptor has on a postsynaptic cell. For example, whereas chronic opiate use has minimal effects on the binding of opiate receptors by opioid peptides, it dramatically changes signal transduction in the terminal regions of the mesolimbic DA system, such as the nucleus accumbens (Nestler, 2001). This occurs at least in part by increasing adenylate cyclase activity and intermediate-early gene expression. Many of these effects presumably occur postsynaptic to DA release, but some of the same effects may be observed on DA neurons themselves. These changes can result in the expression of novel proteins and, consequently, changes in neuronal function that could explain clinical phenomena, such as protracted abstinence and vulnerability to relapse, in people formerly addicted to drugs.

The persistence of changes in drug reinforcement mechanisms that characterize drug addiction suggests that the underlying molecular mechanisms are long lasting, and considerable attention has been given to the drug regulation of gene expression. Current research focuses on several types of transcription factors, including cAMP response element binding protein (CREB) and novel Fos-like proteins termed chronic Fos-related antigens (FRAs). More recently, FosB, a member of the Fos family of transcription factors that dimerizes with a member of the Jun family to form activator protein-1 (AP-1) transcription factor complexes (see Chapter 10), has been implicated in the adaptation to chronic exposure to drugs of abuse. AP-1 complexes bind to sites in the regulatory regions of many genes. Acute administration of several drugs of abuse activates c-fos and FRAs, but chronic administration of drugs of abuse eliminates these activations and produces a gradual accumulation of FosB. This highly stable protein is hypothesized to function as a sustained molecular switch contributing to vulnerability to relapse after prolonged periods of abstinence (Nestler, 2001). These transcription factors may be possible mediators of chronic drug action. However, it has not yet been possible to relate regulation of a specific transcription factor to specific features of drug reinforcement or addiction.

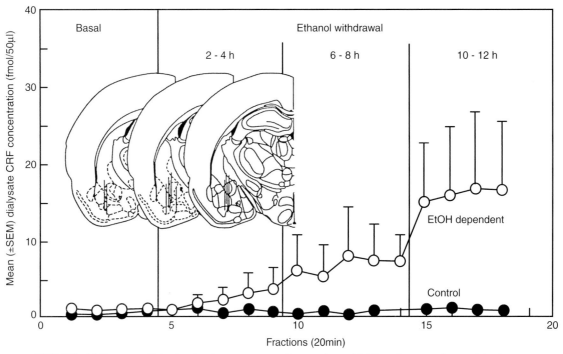

FIGURE 44.7 Extracellular levels of corticotropin-releasing factor (CRF) in the central amygdala during withdrawal from chronic alcohol administration. Dialysate was collected over four 2-h periods, which alternated with nonsampling 2-h periods. The four sampling periods correspond to the basal collection (before removal of alcohol) and 1–4 h, 6–8 h, and 10–12 h after withdrawal of alcohol. Fractions were collected every 20 minutes. Data are represented as means ± SEM ($n=5$ per group). ANOVA confirmed significant differences between the two groups over time ($p<0.05$). (Inset) An anatomical analysis identifying these locations (vertical lines) as sites where changes in CRF concentration were detected in the alcohol experiment ($n=10$) and as being within the amygdaloid complex. Reprinted with permission from Merlo Pich et al. (1995).

Brain Corticotropin-Releasing Factor and NE Systems Show Neuroadaptive Changes with Substance Dependence

Anxiety and stress are common elements of substance dependence and acute withdrawal from drugs of abuse in humans and produce stress-like behavior in animals (Sarnyai *et al.*, 2001). Stress can be defined simply as *any challenge to or alteration in psychological homeostatic processes*. Animal studies exploring the role of corticotropin-releasing factor (CRF) in the actions of alcohol, opiates, and cocaine have provided evidence of a neurochemical basis for the stress associated with abstinence following chronic drug administration. Not only is CRF a major hypothalamic releasing factor controlling the classic stress response, but also appears to have a neurotrophic role in the central nervous system, modulating behavioral responses to stress. CRF itself produces stress-related behaviors, and CRF antagonists reverse a number of behavioral responses to stress. Rats treated repeatedly with drugs such as alcohol, opiates, and cocaine show significant stress-like responses in behavioral tests that follow cessation of drug administration, and these responses are reversed by administration of a CRF antagonist directly into the brain. For example, injection of a CRF antagonist into the central nucleus of the amygdala reverses the stress-like effects of alcohol withdrawal in rats. Withdrawal from alcohol is associated with an increase in the release of CRF into the amygdala, suggesting that alcohol withdrawal can activate CRF systems previously implicated in behavioral responses to stress (Fig. 44.7). Also, stress-induced reinstatement of drug self-administration following extinction can be reversed by CRF antagonists (Sarnyai *et al.*, 2001). NE in the limbic forebrain also has been associated with the physical and motivational signs of opiate withdrawal. More recent evidence suggests that projections to the bed nucleus of the stria terminalis—a critical part of the extended amygdala—may have a role in the motivational effects of opiate withdrawal (Delfs *et al.*, 2000). In addition, the bed nucleus of the stria terminalis is rich in CRF neurons and has been implicated in a feed-forward NE-CRF-NE system that may be involved in stress and drug dependence. In this hypothesized feed-forward system, CRF activates brain stem noradrenergic activity, which in turn activates forebrain CRF activity, effectively closing the loop. This mechanism could explain the potentiation of stress responses with repeated exposure that could lead to psychopathology. However, note that behavioral and autonomic responses may be activated in both the brain stem and the forebrain as partial exits from the loop (Koob, 1999).

NEUROADAPTATION, PROLONGED ABSTINENCE, AND RELAPSE

Adaptation to Chronic Exposure to Drugs of Abuse Can Be Modeled as an Opponent Process

Drug tolerance and withdrawal appear to involve neuroadaptation, and changes in reward threshold in the medial forebrain bundle reflect such adaptations, as do accompanying neurochemical changes (Koob and Le Moal, 2001). A number of conceptual frameworks for adaptation to chronic drug use have been proposed. One hypothesis, termed the *opponent process model* and discussed briefly in Chapter 43, was developed specifically to explain changes in the hedonic state (Solomon, 1977). According to this model, the initial hedonic response to a drug (*A process*) is followed by a negative affective state (*B process*). Theoretically, the *A process* becomes smaller and smaller with repeated drug administration (tolerance), and the *B process* becomes larger and larger (affective withdrawal). The neurochemical changes in DA, 5-HT, and CRF described earlier represent system level changes that contribute to the *B process* — decreased function of reward neurotransmitters and increased brain stress neurotransmitters (Table 44.3).

Neural Substrates of Sensitization Involve Changes in the Mesolimbic DA System and Activation of Brain Stress Systems

Under certain circumstances, repeated administration of stimulants and opiates results in increasingly larger motor activating effects, and these effects have been hypothesized to contribute to the development of the neuroadaptations associated with addiction. This sensitization to the activating effects of stimulants and opiates appears to involve activation of the mesolimbic DA system (Robinson and Berridge, 1993). For example, injections of opiates directly into the VTA produce sensitization. Also, repeated

TABLE 44.3   Neurotransmitters Implicated in the Motivational Effects of Withdrawal from Drugs of Abuse

Change in neurotransmitter	Effect
↓ Dopamine	Dysphoria
↓ Opioid peptides	Pain, dysphoria
↓ Serotonin	Pain, dysphoria, depression
↓ GABA	Anxiety, panic attacks
↑ Corticotropin-releasing factor	Stress

microinjections of amphetamine into the somatodendritic region of the VTA DA cells, at doses that do not cause behavioral activation, are sufficient to sensitize the DA cells to later systemic injections of amphetamine or morphine. Thus, changes in the activity of these DA cells are sufficient to produce sensitization.

Multiple mechanisms for sensitization have been proposed, and a common theme is a time-dependent chain of adaptations that ultimately leads to long-lasting changes in the function of the mesolimbic DA system (Robinson and Berridge, 1993). For example, repeated administration of cocaine produces a decrease in the sensitivity of impulse-regulating somatodendritic D2 receptors on DA neurons (termed *autoreceptors* because the neuron is itself responding to the transmitter it releases). Because these autoreceptors normally exert an inhibitory influence on the activity of dopaminergic neurons, this change in sensitivity could translate into enhanced DA availability with subsequent injections of cocaine (Robinson and Berridge, 1993). However, the decrease in dopaminergic sensitivity lasts only 4–8 days, and behavioral sensitization can last for weeks; thus, other mechanisms must also be involved. The hypothalamic–pituitary–adrenal stress axis (see Chapter 40) may also have an important role in sensitization. Stressors can cause sensitization to stimulant drugs, and both the stress axis and the extrahypothalamic CRF system appear to be important in stress-induced sensitization. Finally, N-methyl-D-aspartate (NMDA) glutamate receptor antagonists selectively block the development of sensitization to psychomotor stimulants, suggesting a role for brain glutamate systems and specific glutamate receptors in sensitization (Koob and Le Moal, 2001).

Neuroadaptive Processes Underlie Substance Dependence

Substance dependence is defined as compulsive, uncontrollable drug use; however, the etiology of that compulsive use is controversial. One position is that positive reinforcing effects of a drug are critical for addiction. Partially as a result of this concept, another position—substance dependence as the alleviation of withdrawal symptoms—fell out of favor as an explanation for compulsive drug use. However, although simple positive reinforcement clearly is necessary for the development of drug use, it falls short in explaining the development of compulsive use. For example, tolerance or apparent tolerance develops to drug reward during chronic use with positive reinforcement either being absent or subsumed by negative reinforcement. Indeed, this issue raises the question of what factors distinguish drug *use* from *abuse* and *dependence* or addiction. Sensitization theory addresses this issue by invoking a shift to a state of *incentive salience*, defined as a hypersensitive neural state that produces the experience of craving. It has been hypothesized that this state of incentive salience is produced by drug-induced sensitization of the mesolimbic DA system (Robinson and Berridge, 1993). According to this model, the pathologically strong craving or yearning encountered during protracted abstinence would be due in large part to an overactive mesolimbic DA system.

In contrast, to the sensitization theory, neuroadaptation theories such as the opponent process theory postulate that the processes of tolerance to the positive affective state (hedonic tolerance) and subsequent

---

BOX 44.3

ALLOSTASIS

Counteradaptive processes, such as opponent process, that are part of normal homeostatic limitation of reward function can fail to return within the normal range and are hypothesized to contribute to the allostatic state of addiction. Allostasis from the addiction perspective is defined as the process of maintaining apparent reward function stability by changes in brain reward mechanisms. The allostatic state is fueled not only by dysregulation of reward circuits per se, but also by the activation of brain and hormonal stress systems (Koob and Le Moal,

2001). The following definitions apply: (1) *allostasis*, the process of achieving stability through change; (2) *allostatic state*, a state of chronic deviation of the regulatory system from its normal, or homeostatic, operating level; and (3) *allostatic load*, the cost to the brain and body of the deviation, accumulating over time, and reflecting in many cases pathological states and accumulation of damage.

George F. Koob

development of the negative affective state (affective withdrawal) play important roles in the transition from drug use to drug dependence (Solomon, 1977). Whereas initial drug use may be motivated by the positive affective state produced by a drug, continued drug use leads to neuroadaptation to the presence of the drug, to development of a negative affective state, and ultimately to self-medication of that affective state. Some theorists have gone so far as to argue that the presence of a negative affective state is the defining feature of addiction and that dysregulation of the residual reward system represents a state of allostasis, the process of obtaining stability through change. The *allostasis* hypothesis suggests that *both* sensitization and opponent process mechanisms contribute to increases in hedonic set points that convey the vulnerability to relapse for drug addiction (see Box 44.3).

Conditioning Has an Important Role in Sustaining Substance Dependence

Another explanation for the chronic relapsing nature of drug addiction is that reinforcement can be derived from secondary sources that motivate continued drug use. Both positive and negative affective states can become associated with stimuli in the drug-taking environment through classical conditioning processes. When the drug taker is reexposed to these conditioned stimuli, compulsive drug use is reestablished.

Conditioning to the positive affective states induced by drugs has been demonstrated in animals. Stimuli associated with drugs of abuse can maintain responding in rats and monkeys when presented without the drug. It is also possible to demonstrate conditioned withdrawal. For example, when previously neutral stimuli are paired with naloxone-induced withdrawal, the neutral stimuli themselves elicit signs of opiate withdrawal. Conditioned withdrawal has been observed in opiate-dependent animals and humans.

Neurobiological substrates for conditioned drug effects have only begun to be explored. The enhancement of conditioned reinforcement produced by psychomotor stimulants appears to involve activation of the mesolimbic DA system (Koob and Le Moal, 2001) and the basolateral amygdala, a main projection to the extended amygdala. The neurobiological substrates for conditioned withdrawal may also depend on the basolateral amygdala. It is possible that NE is involved in some of these processes. Thus, conditioned opiate withdrawal can be reversed by the administration of clonidine, a NE α-2 receptor agonist that decreases firing of the locus coeruleus NE system and has been used clinically for opiate detoxification (Koob and Le Moal, 2001).

Summary

Much is known about the neurobiological substrates for the acute reinforcing actions of drugs of

---

BOX 44.4

NONDRUG ADDICTIONS

Many substances that humans consume to produce chemical dependency act to achieve common end events; namely activation of neuronal circuits at key sites in the extended amygdala. As described in the text, each class of drugs does so in a unique way (Fig. 44.8). In fact, life events that may be reinforcing to a given individual's behaviors may have the same end result. Specific recurrent behaviors that escaped from the individual's ability to control have been termed *impulse control disorders* and share common clusters of symptoms with the chemical dependencies: (a) anticipation and obsession with performing the act, (b) repeated performance of the act

leading to binges of action and "intoxication," and (c) the withdrawal phase accompanied by severe unpleasant feelings (dysphoria). Behaviors that can be qualified as impulse control disorders when no longer under control include, but are not limited to, gambling, shopping, eating, exercise, and sex. Very few data exist regarding the neurobiological bases for mediating these nondrug impulse control disorders. One exception is pathological gambling where there is evidence of activation of some of the same neurotransmitters (e.g., DA) and some of the same neurocircuits involved in mediating drug reward.

George F. Koob

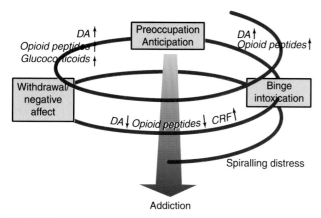

FIGURE 44.8 Diagram describing the hypothetical spiraling distress-addiction cycle from a neurobiological perspective. Small arrows refer to increased or decreased functional activity. The addiction cycle is conceptualized as a spiral that increases in amplitude with repeated experience, ultimately resulting in the pathological state of addiction. DA, dopamine; CRF, corticotropin-releasing factor. Reprinted with permission from Koob and Le Moal (1997).

abuse. The mesolimbic DA system is critical for the reinforcing actions of psychomotor stimulants and has a role in opiate, nicotine, and alcohol reinforcement. Opioid peptide systems have important roles in opiate, nicotine, and alcohol reinforcement. Other neurotransmitter systems, including GABA, 5-HT, and glutamate, localized within the extended amygdala area of the basal forebrain appear to have an important role in alcohol reinforcement. However, much less is known about the neurobiological substrates for the reinforcement associated with *chronic* drug use. Compulsive use that characterizes substance dependence produces neuroadaptive, opponent process-like changes in these neurotransmitter systems, resulting in a compromised reward system. Acute abstinence is characterized by functional decreases within motivational systems mediating acute drug reinforcement (e.g., the DA, 5-HT, and opioid peptide systems) and increases in stress systems recruited during development of dependence (e.g., CRF and locus coeruleus). Protracted abstinence and the propensity for relapse are probably the keys to maintenance of addiction, but only a little is known about the neurobiology of protracted abstinence. Sensitization probably involves development of a hypersensitive DA system and activation of brain stress mechanisms. Conditioned drug effects are only beginning to be explored but may involve limbic elements that project to the extended amygdala. Study of the changes in the central nervous system that are associated with such allostatic dysregulation may provide the key to drug addiction and the etiology of psychopathologies associated with mood and anxiety disorders (see Boxes 44.3 and 44.4).

References

American Psychiatric Association (1994). "Diagnostic and Statistical Manual of Mental Disorders," 4th Ed. American Psychiatric Press, Washington, DC.

Bergman, J., Kamien, J. B., and Spealman, R. D. (1990). Antagonism of cocaine self-adminstration by selective DA D1 and D2 antagonists. *Behav. Pharmacol.* **1**, 355–363.

Caine, S. B., Lintz, R., and Koob, G. F. (1993). Intravenous drug self-administration techniques in animals. *In* "Behavioral Neuroscience: A Practical Approach" (A. Sahgal, ed.), Vol. 2, pp. 117–143. Oxford Univ. Press, New York.

Caine, S. B., and Koob, G. F. (1995). Pretreatment with the DA agonist 7-OH-DPAT shifts the cocaine self-administration dose-effect function to the left under different schedules in the rat. *Behav. Pharmacol.* **6**, 333–347.

Delfs, J. M., Zhu, Y., Druhan, J. P., and Aston-Jones, G. (2000). Noradrenaline in the ventral forebrain is critical for opiate withdrawal-induced aversion. *Nature* **403**, 430–434.

Di Chiara, G., and North, R. A. (1992). Neurobiology of opiate abuse. *Trends Pharmacol. Sci.* 13, 185–193.

Gardner, E. L., and Vorel, S. R. (1998). Cannabinoid transmission and reward-related events. *Neurobiol. Dis.* **5**, 139–148.

Heimer, L., and Alheid, G. (1991). Piecing together the puzzle of basal forebrain anatomy. *In* "Advances in Experimental Medicine and Biology" (T. C. Napier, P. Kalivas, and I. Hanin, eds.), Vol. 295, pp. 1–42. Plenum, New York.

Johnston, J. B. (1923). Further contributions to the study of the evolution of the forebrain. *J. Comp. Neurol.* **35**, 337–481.

Koob, G. F. (1992). Drugs of abuse: Anatomy, pharmacology, and function of reward pathways. *Trends Pharmacol. Sci.* **13**, 177–184.

Koob, G. F., and Le Moal, M. (1997). Drug abuse: Hedonic homeostatic dysregulation. *Science* **278**, 52–58.

Koob, G. F., and Le Moal, M. (2001). Drug addiction, dysregulation of reward, and allostasis. *Neuropsychopharmacology* **24**, 97–129.

Koob, G. F., Sanna, P. P., and Bloom, F. E. (1998). Neuroscience of addiction. *Neuron* **21**, 467–476.

Kornetsky, C., and Bain, G. (1982). Biobehavioral bases of the reinforcing properties of opiate drugs. *Ann. N.Y. Acad. Sci.* **398**, 240–259.

Liebman, J. M., and Cooper, S. J. (1989). "The Neuropharmacological Basis of Reward." Clarendon Press, Oxford.

Merlo Pich, E., Lorang, M., Yeganeh, M., Rodriguez de Fonseca, F., Koob, G. F., and Weiss, F. (1995). Increase of extracellular corticotropin-releasing factor-like immunoreactivity levels in the amygdala of awake rats during restraint stress and alcohol withdrawal as measured by microdialysis. *J. Neurosci.* **15**, 5439–5447.

Nestler, E. J. (2001). Molecular basis of long-term plasticity underlying addiction. *Nature Rev. Neurosci.* **2**, 119–128.

Olds, J., and Milner, P. (1954). Positive reinforcement produced by electrical stimulation of septal area and other regions of rat brain. *J. Comp. Physiol. Psychol.* **47**, 419–427.

Parsons, L. H., Koob, G. F., and Weiss, F. (1995). Serotonin dysfunction in the nucleus accumbens of rats during withdrawal after unlimited access to intravenous cocaine. *J. Pharmacol. Exp. Ther.* **274**, 1182–1191.

Robinson, T. E., and Berridge, K. C. (1993). The neural basis of drug craving: An incentive-sensitization theory of addiction. *Brain Res. Rev.* **18**, 247–291.

Sarnyai, Z., Shaham, Y., and Heinrichs, S. C. (2001). The role of corticotropin-releasing factor in drug addiction. *Pharmacol. Rev.* **53**, 209–243.

Schuster, C. R., and Thompson, T. (1969). Self administration and behavioral dependence on drugs. *Annu. Rev. Pharmacol. Toxicol.* **9**, 483–502.

Solomon, R. L. (1977). The opponent-process theory of acquired motivation: The affective dynamics of addiction. *In* "Psychopathology: Experimental Models" (J. D. Maser and M. E. P. Seligman, eds.), pp. 124–145. Freeman, San Francisco.

Tabakoff, B., and Hoffman, P. L. (1992). Alcohol: Neurobiology. *In* "Substance Abuse: A Comprehensive Textbook" (J. H. Lowenstein, P. Ruiz, and R. B. Millman, eds.), 2nd Ed., pp. 152–185. Williams & Wilkins, Baltimore MD.

Watkins, S. S., Koob, G. F., and Markou, A. (2001). Neural mechanisms underlying nicotine addiction: Acute positive reinforcement and withdrawal. *Nicotine Tobacco Res.* **2**, 19–37.

Suggested Readings

Cador, M., Robbins, T. W., and Everitt, B. J. (1989). Involvement of the amygdala in stimulus-reward associations: Interaction with the ventral striatum. *Neuroscience* **30**, 77–86.

Engel, J. A., Enerback, C., Fahlke, C., Hulthe, P., Hard, E., Johannessen, K., Svensson, L., and Soderpalm, B. (1992). Serotonergic and dopaminergic involvement in ethanol intake. *In* "Novel Pharmacological Interventions for Alcoholism" (C. A. Naranjo and E. M. Sellers, eds.), pp. 68–82. Springer, New York.

Hardman, J. G., and Limbird, L. E., (eds.), (2001). "Goodman and Gilman's The Pharmacological Basis of Therapeutics," 10th Ed. McGraw Hill, New York.

Koob, G. F., and Bloom, F. E. (1988). Cellular and molecular mechanisms of drug dependence. *Science* **242**, 715–723.

Koob, G. F., Heinrichs, S. C., Menzaghi, F., Pich, E. M., and Britton, K. T. (1994). Corticotropin-releasing factor, stress and behavior. *Semin. Neurosci.* **7**, 221–229.

Kornetsky, C., and Esposito, R. U. (1979). Euphorigenic drugs: Effects on reward pathways of the brain. *Fed. Proc.* **38**, 2473–2476.

Mucha, R. F., van der Kooy, D., O'Shaughnessy, M., and Bucenieks, P. (1982). Drug reinforcement studied by the use of place conditioning in rat. *Brain Res.* **243**, 91–105.

Nestler, E. J. (1992). Molecular mechanisms of drug addiction. *J. Neurosci.* **12**, 2439–2450.

Russell, M. A. H. (1976). What is dependence? *In* "Drugs and Drug Dependence" (G. Edwards, M. A. H. Russell, D. Hawks, and M. MacCafferty, eds.), pp. 182–187. Saxon House/Lexington Books, Westmead.

Wikler, A. (1973). Dynamics of drug dependence: Implications of a conditioning theory of research and treatment. *Arch. Gen. Psychiatry* **28**, 611–616.

George F. Koob

BEHAVIORIAL AND COGNITIVE NEUROSCIENCE

Human Brain Evolution

Much of the allure of the neurosciences stems from the common conviction that there is something unusual about the human brain and its behavioral capacities. Nevertheless, modern neuroscientists have paid rather little attention to the study of brain evolution, and so our understanding of how the human brain differs from that of other animals is very rudimentary. In part, this neglect is due to a widely held belief that mammalian brains are all essentially similar in their internal structure and that species differ mainly in the size of the brain. This chapter reviews the modern evidence concerning brain evolution and shows that brain structure, far from being uniform across species, exhibits some remarkable variations. Because the subject is vast, the discussion is necessarily selective. Thus, after a brief review of evolutionary principles, this chapter describes the evolutionary history of three groups of vertebrates that are of special interest to people: mammals, primates, and humans themselves. The major steps are outlined in the evolution of our large, complex, and extremely useful brains from the smaller, simpler brains of the first mammals, focusing on the neocortex, as this part of the brain has been studied most extensively. The neocortex is disproportionately large in humans and is critically involved in mental activities and processes that are considered to be distinctly human.

EVOLUTIONARY AND COMPARATIVE PRINCIPLES

How Do We Learn about Brain Evolution?

There are three main ways to learn about how different brains have evolved. First, the fossil record can be studied. Much of what we have learned about the evolution of vertebrates in general has come from studying fossils. However, because bones frequently fossilize, whereas soft tissues seldom do, we know a lot about the bones of our ancestors, but much less about everything else. Of course, one can infer much about some soft tissues, such as muscles, from their effects on bones, and this is true for brains as well. The brains of mammals fill the skull tightly, and thus the skull cavity of fossils rather closely reflects the size and shape of the brain, and even the locations of major fissures. Much has been learned and written about the changes in brain size from the fossil record (Jerison, 1973), and we could learn more by considering changes in the proportions of brain parts and even the proportions of parts of neocortex. For example, early primates already differed from most early mammals by having more neocortex in proportion to the rest of the brain, and more neocortex devoted to the temporal lobe where visual processing occurs. This implies a greater emphasis on functions mediated by neocortex and a greater emphasis especially on the processing of visual information. We can even learn something about the functional organization of the neocortex from fossils. For instance, subdivisions of the body representation in the primary somatosensory cortex are often marked by fissures in the brain, and fissure patterns revealed by endocasts (internal casts of the brain case) from fossil skulls have been used to suggest specializations of the somatosensory cortex in extinct mammals. More recently, David Van Essen (1997) has proposed that an important factor in the development of brain fissures is the pattern of connections within the developing brain. According to this theory, densely interconnected regions tend to resist separation during brain growth and form bulges (gyri) that limit the separation distance, whereas poorly interconnected regions are free to fold and form fissures (sulci) that would increase the separation distance. Thus, it is because the hand and face regions of the somatosensory cortex are poorly interconnected that a fissure may develop between the two. If this explanation of fissures is correct, then the locations of brain fissures seen in fossil endocasts can potentially tell us something about anatomical connections in the brains of extinct mammals.

Unfortunately, little of the brain's great internal complexity is revealed by its size, shape, and fissures. Thus, to learn more about brain evolution, it is neces-

sary to study the brains of extant (living) species and use comparative methods to deduce the organization of ancestral brains. There has been great progress since the early 1980s in understanding how to use comparative approaches to study evolution, and even studies of the fossil record involve a comparative approach. It is never or seldom known, for example, that any given fossil was an actual ancestor of another fossil, but only that the comparative evidence, together with suitable times of existence, suggested that they could be.

As Darwin (1859) recognized, each living species represents the living tip of a largely dead branch of an

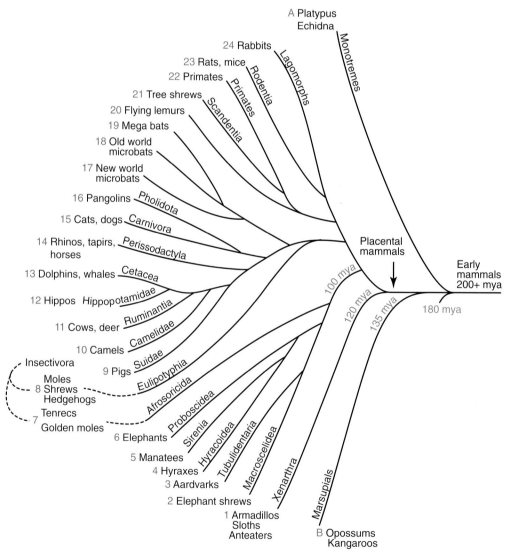

FIGURE 45.1 The probable course of the major branches of mammalian evolution (e.g., mammalian orders). Proposed clades of placental mammals are numbered, whereas monotremes (A) and marsupials (B) are lettered. Each branch of the tree also has branched many times given the great numbers of present-day species. Note how this branching pattern differs from long-standing notions of a scale of nature from simple to complex. Based on Springer and deJong (2001).

extremely bushy tree of life. By examining other living tips of the tree, we can infer much about the organizations of the brains (and other body parts) of ancestors that occupied the branch points of this tree. Theories of brain evolution, including those of the evolution of the human brain, depend on reconstructing the probable features of the brains of ever more distant relatives.

The comparative method depends on (1) examining the brains of suitable ranges of extant species and (2) determining what features they share and whether these features are shared because they were inherited from a common ancestor or because they evolved separately. The 50-year-old field of cladistics provides guidelines for making such judgments. The choice of species for comparison depends on the question being asked. For example, to deduce what the brains of early mammals were like, one should examine brains from each of the major branches of the mammalian evolutionary tree (Fig. 45.1), and thus consider members of the monotreme, marsupial, and placental mammal branches. To know about early primates, members of the major branches of primate evolution should be considered. In principle, the more branches considered, the better, because a broad comparative approach is required to accurately reconstruct ancestral brain organization.

Because brain studies can be difficult, time-consuming, and labor intensive, it is not always possible to study a large number of species, and one must concentrate on the most informative species. While the brains of all living mammals contain mixtures of ancestral and derived features, and comparative studies are needed to distinguish the two, one might first consider the brains of those mammals that are likely to have changed the least since the time of their divergence. Because we know from the fossil record that early mammals had small brains with little neocortex, mammals with large brains and much neocortex have obviously changed quite a bit, and it is likely to be more informative for reconstructing the brain organization of early mammals to concentrate on present-day mammals with brain proportions similar to those of early mammals. While the very large brains of humans and whales undoubtedly share features inherited from a small-brained common ancestor, it may be difficult to detect the common features in the multitude of changes. As early primates more closely resembled many of the living prosimian primates in brain size and proportions than monkeys, apes, and humans, studies of the brains of prosimians are likely to be especially relevant for theories of early primate brain organization. Also, it is useful to consider the probable impact of obvious specializations

on the brain organizations of living mammals. While monotremes represent a very early major branch of the mammalian tree, the living monotremes, consisting of the duck-billed platypus with a "bill" and a capacity for electroreception and the spiny echidna with spines and a long sticky tongue for eating ants, are quite specialized, as are their somatosensory systems.

Nevertheless, while the brains of some mammals may have retained more primitive characteristics than others, it is dangerous to assume that the brain of any living mammal fully represents an ancestral condition. Brain features need to be evaluated trait by trait in a comparative context, as any particular feature could be primitive or derived. To reconstruct the course of brain evolution, we need to distinguish ancestral and derived characters rather than ancestral and derived species. The existence of a mixture of ancestral and derived features in members of a single species is referred to as *mosaic evolution.*

A third source of information about brain evolution is based on understandings of the mechanisms and modes of brain development and the constraints they impose on evolution. For example, Finlay and Darlington (1995) have presented evidence that there is an orderly pattern of brain change as brains get bigger. In general, larger brains have proportionately more neocortex and less brain stem. Finlay and Darlington suggest this is the case because the late-maturing neocortex of large brains grows proportionately longer and larger. Another difference between large and small brains is that large brains have more neurons and longer connections. The increase in neurons makes it difficult for each neuron in a large brain to maintain the same proportion of connections with other neurons as do neurons in a small brain, and to maintain the same transmission times over longer axons. Thus, as larger brains evolve, changes in organization are needed to reduce the commitment to connections, especially connections requiring long, thick axons. Further understandings of the genetic, developmental, and structural constraints on brain design could allow us to better postulate how brains are likely to change in organization with changes in brain size.

Cladistics and Phylogenetic Trees

To understand brain evolution, we must first understand the evolutionary relationships among mammals, which are summarized in biological classifications (taxonomies). The science of classification (known as "systematics") has a long history, but the early classification that divided the world into "things that belong to the Emperor and things that don't" is clearly outmoded. Our modern understanding of plant and animal relationships emerged from the efforts of the Swedish naturalist Linnaeus (1707–1778), who grouped species into larger and larger categories (species, genus, family, order, class, phylum) according to degrees of resemblance and dissimilarity. We now understand why life forms exhibit the particular pattern of similarities and differences they do, and we have a logic for extending and refining the Linnaean system. In brief, complex life on Earth appears to have evolved only once. It is based on a molecular template that is passed on from generation to generation and yet is modifiable. Because this molecular material usually is not exchanged between individuals from different species (horizontal transfer), a phylogenetic classification can be derived that reflects times of divergence from common ancestors. Similarities retained over time reflect the preservation of parts of the code, whereas differences reflect alterations in the code. The many different modifications of the genome in the many diverging lines of descent over billions of years have led to the great diversity of life that we see today. Our current classification scheme is based on our understanding of phylogenetic (ancestral) relationships. Because this understanding continues to grow, parts of the classification scheme are occasionally modified with new advances in knowledge.

Phylogenetic relationships are deduced from comparative evidence. The entomologist Willi Hennig helped reinvigorate this field of study when he formulated a rigorous comparative method of reconstructing phylogenetic relationships, sometimes known as "cladistics." The term reflects Hennig's emphasis on the correct identification of "clades," i.e., groups of organisms that share a common ancestor. A clade is simply a branch of the evolutionary tree, which is connected through a set of ancestors (which are the branching points of the tree) to all the other branches in the tree. In Hennig's method, evolutionary relationships are reconstructed by a process of "character analysis." A character is any observable feature or attribute of an organism. A character could be a feature of the brain, such as the corpus collosum between the two cerebral hemispheres, or a feature of any other part of the body, or (as is often the case today) a molecule or a DNA sequence. By considering the states of as many characters as possible, e.g., whether a corpus collosum is present (as it is in placental mammals) or absent (as in other vertebrates), and by adopting the assumption that closely related species will share more character states than distantly

related species, one can arrive at a hypothesis about the relationships of the groups being examined. Because a given character state can evolve independently in different lineages (e.g., forelimbs that function as wings evolved independently in birds and bats), not every character will yield an accurate picture of evolutionary relationships. It is therefore important to base reconstructions of evolutionary relationships on as many characters as possible. Typically, a very large number of possible trees can be generated from a given character analysis; the tree that requires the smallest number of changes to account for the observed pattern of character states (the maximum-parsimony solution) is usually considered to be the best estimate of the correct tree. The growth of molecular biology has provided a new source of comparative information to supplement character analyses based on anatomical characteristics, helping to improve the resolution of modern mammalian trees (Fig. 45.1). These trees guide our interpretation of the evolutionary history of brain organization.

To communicate precisely, comparative biologists have developed a specialized nomenclature. The concepts of *homology* and *analogy* are central to comparative biology (see Box 45.1). A group of species that all share a common evolutionary history is a *natural taxon* or a *monophyletic group*, which is the same thing as a *clade*. Unnatural taxa are groups that either exclude one or more of an ancestor's descendants (*paraphyletic groups*) or combine descendants of multiple ancestors (*polyphyletic groups*). The great ape family Pongidae (consisting of orangutans, gorillas, chimpanzees) is now known to be paraphyletic because it excludes humans, which share a recent common ancestor with chimpanzees and gorillas. If a character state is found throughout a monophyletic group, it likely was present in the common ancestor of the group or even earlier. Thus, comparisons are necessary with members of a *sister group*, which is the monophyletic taxon thought to be related most closely to the group under study. To determine whether a character is derived (new) or ancestral, one examines members of one or more *outgroup*, the more distant relatives of the group under examination. The direction of change is called its *polarity*. For example, mammals include forms that lay eggs, the monotremes, whereas the sister group of monotremes, the marsupial–placental group, gives birth to live offspring. We can determine the polarity of these character states (egg laying, live birth) by examining out groups, i.e., by examining other vertebrates like reptiles and amphibians. Because most nonmammalian vertebrates lay eggs, we conclude that egg laying is ancestral for mammals, and live birth derived.

BOX 45.1

HOMOLOGY AND ANALOGY

Homology and analogy are two of the most important concepts in evolutionary biology. Both terms refer to similarity, but to similarity arising from different sources. The terms can be applied to any biological characteristic or feature, including brain structures and even behavior. In our efforts to understand brain evolution, features of brains are compared across species, and it is important to deduce if these features have been inherited from a common ancestor or emerged independently. The two terms reflect conclusions based on the available evidence, and uncertainty is common.

Homology

When different species possess similar characteristics because they inherited them from a common ancestor, the characteristics are said to be homologous. This does not mean they are identical in structure or function. For example, all mammals appear to have a primary somatosensory area, S1, as a subdivision of neocortex. This structure appears to be involved in electroreception in the duck-billed platypus, a monotreme, but not in other mammals. Humans and monotremes have inherited an S1 from a distant ancestor (at least 150 million years ago), but subsequently, ancestors have specialized S1 in quite different ways.

Analogy and Homoplasy

Characteristics that have evolved independently are referred to as analogous or homoplaseous. Some authors prefer to refer to similarities in function as analogous and similarities in appearance as homoplaseous, whereas others use the terms interchangeably or prefer analogous as the more common term. As an example, most primates and some carnivores such as cats divide the primary visual cortex, V1, into alternating bands of tissue activated mostly by one eye or the other, the so-called ocular dominance columns or bands. Because carnivores and primates almost certainly diverged from a common ancestor that did not have ocular dominance columns, we conclude that this way of subdividing visual cortex evolved independently at least two times. When analogous similarities evolve, the process is called *convergent* or *parallel* evolution (parallel if the sequences of changes were similar).

Both homology and analogy can be applied to structures or to specific features of structures. The forelimbs of bats and birds are homologous as forelimbs because both bats and birds inherited forelimbs from their common ancestors. The common ancestor of bats and birds did not fly, however, and the modifications that have transformed the forelimbs of bats and birds into wings evolved independently; these wing-like characteristics are therefore analogous. Correctly identifying homologies is a very important step in deducing the course of evolution of the human brain. Features such as S1, which are homologous in most or nearly all mammals, must have evolved early with the first mammals or before, whereas features common to only primates, such as the middle temporal visual area (MT), would have emerged much later in only the line leading to the first primates. Some brain features related to language production may have arisen quite recently with the emergence of archaic or modern humans. Identifying homologies and their distributions across groups of related mammals (clades) allows us to reconstruct the details of brain evolution in the different lines of descent, including the one leading to modern humans. The problem of distinguishing homologies from analogies is that both are identified by similarities. However, analogous structures have similarities based on common adaptations for functional roles, and thus they should also vary greatly in details unrelated to function. In contrast, homologous structures likely have retained many details from a common ancestor that may not be functionally necessary. Thus, aspects of structures that appear to be unessential may count more in judging homologies. Much can also be deduced from studying brain development and the development of similarities. Of course, knowledge about the phyletic (cladistic) distribution of similarities is critical, as is accounting for differences in structures by finding species with intermediate types. Ultimately, one hopes to have evidence for so many similarities that the independent evolution of them all seems extremely improbable, or sufficient evidence from differences to indicate that the similarities in structures were acquired independently. Often the evidence is far from compelling, and opinions may change with new evidence.

Jon H. Kaas and Todd M. Preuss

Misconceptions about Brain Evolution

Probably the most serious misconception about brain evolution is that theories of evolutionary change are necessarily highly speculative (see Striedter, 1998). As in other historical sciences, direct observation of the process of brain evolution is usually not possible, but objective criteria for evaluating theories and reconstructions of ancestral brains do exist (e.g., character analysis). It is not the case that one opinion is as good as the next, although such a view has allowed poorly founded theories to persist. A similar problem exists for those interested in objective approaches to the study of consciousness. While nearly everyone seems to have a theory, not all theories are equally well informed.

Another serious misconception is that evolution has a single goal or direction. This stems from the persistent belief in a "phylogenetic scale" that starts with lowly forms such as sponges, proceeds with insects, fish, amphibians, reptiles, and various mammals at successively higher levels and reaches its pinnacle with humans (Hodos and Campbell, 1969). This view that the history of life is like a scale or ladder reflects the popular idea that evolution is primarily a process of progressive improvement, a philosophical and religious viewpoint that reassuringly identifies us as the most perfect. However, evolutionary biologists have long recognized the great diversity of life and have adopted from Darwin the branching tree as a metaphor for the process whereby parent species divide to form daughter species, with each branch becoming adapted to its particular environment through natural selection. This perspective still leaves a place for progress in evolution, if progress means to become better adapted, but there are so many different ways organisms can become better adapted—most of which do not involve becoming bigger brained or smarter—that there can be no single dimension of progress, as the phylogenetic scale implies. Progress, for example, might mean reducing the size of the visual system to reduce metabolic costs in mammals living underground. Thus, there is also no universal trend toward increased complexity, as evolving brains sometimes simplify by reducing or losing parts. Overall, the brains of many mammalian groups evolved to get bigger (Jerison, 1973), but this change partly reflects the fact that they started off small, and it was more often adaptive to get bigger than smaller. However, mammals with very small brains, near the theoretical limit of smallness in mammalian brain size, persist today and there is reason to think that small brain size is not the primitive condition in all these groups, but resulted from relatively recent reductions in brain size. Interestingly, domestic mammals, with our efforts to improve a wild stock, have generally reduced brain size. Evolutionary biologists make a distinction between traits that are ancestral (also termed primitive or *plesiomorphic*) from those that are recently acquired (also known as derived or *apomorphic*), but this distinction does not imply that primitive is simple and that derived is complex.

A third misconception is that ontogeny recapitulates phylogeny. At one time, evolution was thought to proceed by sequentially adding new parts (*terminal addition*), and that in the development of complex forms, the newest parts were those added last. Thus, the evolutionary history of any organism would be revealed in its sequence of development. While this is not the case in general, the study of brain development remains relevant to the study of brain evolution because evolution occurs through alterations in the course of development. It is also the case that many changes in the course of development that have led to new adaptations have occurred in the later stages of development, primarily because alterations in early stages often are lethal or produce profoundly different and maladaptive adult forms. Nevertheless, it is important to recognize that the course of development can be altered in many ways and at many stages. Studies of brain development are useful because they can indicate how homologous structures that appear dissimilar in adults arose from forms that were more similar early in development.

The concepts of progress and terminal addition have led some investigators to consider certain features of the brains of such mammals as humans, monkeys, and cats as either relatively old or new on the basis of their histological appearance. Poorly differentiated areas of neocortex, i.e., areas with indistinct lamination, were considered to be ancient, and well-differentiated areas were thought to be new. For example, because the primary visual cortex (V1) has very highly differentiated layers in many primates, including humans, V1 was considered by some to be a recently acquired area of the cortex. However, a comparative analysis indicates that the primary visual cortex (V1) is as old as the first mammals, perhaps much older. The laminar organization of V1 happens to have been poorly differentiated in early mammals, and it remains poorly differentiated in many living species. Moreover, humans are not the species with the most highly laminated V1: this distinction belongs to the tarsier, a tiny, nocturnal primate with enormous eyes. As another example, the superior colliculus or optic tectum, an ancient visual structure, is well differentiated in many birds and reptiles, poorly or moderately differentiated in many mammals (including humans), and yet is well differentiated in still other mammals, such as squirrels and tree shrews.

Summary

Our understandings of brain evolution come from measurements of brain size and shape from the casts of the fossil skulls of extinct mammals, inferences made from comparative studies of the brains of present-day mammals, and from deductions stemming from understanding how brains are likely to have changed in internal structure as they enlarged in some lines of evolution. Interpretations of comparative data depend on an understanding of the evolutionary relationships or taxonomy of mammals. The premise that closely related species are likely to share more biological features or characters than distantly related species allows hypotheses about relationships between groups to be evaluated through the process of "character analysis." Characters in different species may resemble each other because they are homologous (inherited from a common ancestor) or because they are analogous and independently came to resemble each other. Comparative biologists have developed objective criteria for evaluating theories about the course of evolution and evolutionary change. Evolution results from many different types of adaptive changes in characters, and thus there has not been a single direction of change from lower to higher or from simple to complex as often supposed. Parts or features of brains that emerged early in evolution are not necessarily simpler or less differentiated than more recently evolved parts.

EARLY STAGES OF BRAIN EVOLUTION

Did Vertebrates Turn Their Brain Upside Down?

All multicellular animals are thought to be monophyletic, i.e., to stem from a common ancestor. Thus, modern insects and other arthropods are our distant relatives, with the chordate line leading to vertebrates and the arthropod line having diverged from a primitive bilateral animal some 600 million years ago. Yet arthropods and vertebrates have quite different body plans. In all vertebrates, the brain and spinal cord are dorsal to the mouth and gut, whereas in arthropods, the central nervous system is located below the gut. How did these two apparently different nervous systems evolve? An early theory, long considered discredited, was that the ancestors of vertebrates inverted

their bodies so that the nervous system shifted from ventral to dorsal. As strange as this theory seems, recent results from molecular biology on the dorsoventral patterning of organizing proteins support the inversion theory. Furthermore, the results of other molecular studies suggest that a primitive common ancestor had photoreceptive cells from which the eyes of insects and vertebrates evolved. Thus, it now seems possible to trace aspects of the evolution of human

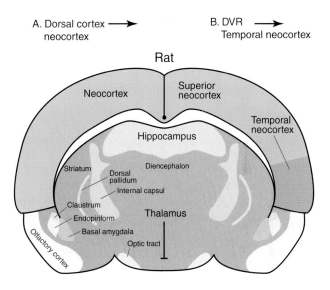

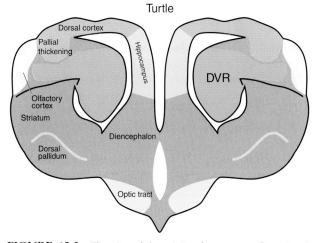

FIGURE 45.2 Theories of the origin of neocortex. One view is that (A) only the dorsal cortex of ancestral reptiles gave rise to the neocortex. Another current view is that (B) the dorsal cortex gave rise to the superior part of the neocortex, whereas the dorsal ventricular ridge (DVR) gave rise to the temporal neocortex of extant mammals such as rats (top) and reptiles such as turtles (bottom). The neocortex and dorsal cortex are much different in size, as well as in cellular organization (see text). Modified from Kaas and Reiner (1999).

brains back to the simpler nervous system of an ancestor some 600 million years ago.

Origin of the Neocortex

The hallmark of the evolution of mammalian brains from reptilian ancestors was emergence of the neocortex. The cerebral cortex (or pallium) covers the deeper parts of the forebrain (telencephalon). In mammals, the cortex is generally divided into three parts: the lateral *paleocortex* or olfactory piriform cortex, the medial *archicortex* or hippocampus and subiculum, and the *neocortex* or *isocortex* lying in between (Fig. 45.2). The archicortex and paleocortex can be recognized in reptiles, and their names reflect the early conclusion that they are phylogenetically old parts of the forebrain. While all extant mammals have an obvious neocortex, and the presence of a neocortex in early mammals is clearly indicated in the endocasts, nothing quite like the neocortex exists in reptiles. Hence, the term *neo*cortex was used to refer to this seemingly new part of the brain. Nevertheless, the neocortex as a structure is not really new, as it is homologous with the dorsal cortex of reptiles and possibly also with a subcortical region in reptiles called the dorsal ventricular ridge (opinions still vary on this possibility). However, the dorsal cortex of reptiles is a rather small and thin sheet of tissue with hardly more than a single row of neurons. In contrast, all living mammals have a thick cortex that is divided into layers having different cell types and packing densities. An imaginary line drawn through the thickness of the neocortex would likely encounter over 100 neurons. Thus, the neocortex is much different in structure than the dorsal cortex. Unfortunately, no mammal-like reptiles exist today to show us what intermediate states were like in the evolution of the mammalian neocortex. Because the neocortex as a structure did not really originate with mammals and because it is not "new," some investigators refer to the neocortex as the *isocortex*, using a term that refers to the relatively uniform appearance of the neocortex throughout all regions. However, the changes in the dorsal cortex that produced the neocortex are impressive, and no other vertebrates have a structure that clearly resembles the neocortex. Thus, mammals are characterized as much by their neocortex as a modified structure as they are by their mammary glands.

While the neocortex has a somewhat uniform histological appearance, its considerable variability in size and organization is what allows mammals to differ so much in behavior and abilities. To understand how variations in the neocortex make this possible, it is necessary to identify ancestral features of the neocortex, i.e., features that were present in the last common ancestor of living mammals, and then determine how this organization was modified in different lineages of living mammals, such as primates.

The laminar organization of the neocortex appears to be similar in most mammals, suggesting that the ancestral design was so useful that many features have been retained in modern groups. For example, in most mammals and over most of the neocortex, six layers can be recognized (Brodmann, 1909). Of the six layers of neurons, layer 4 receives activating inputs from the thalamus or from other parts of the cortex. Layer 3 communicates with other regions of the cortex, layer 5 projects to subcortical structures, and the deepest layer 6 sends feedback to the thalamic nuclei or cortical area providing activating inputs. This ancestral framework for cortical neural circuits has been modified and elaborated in various lines of descent to give us the great variability in brain function we see today. The neocortex has changed by diversifying its neuron types, differentiating its laminar structure in various ways, altering connections, changing in overall size and in the sizes of individual cortical areas, adding cortical areas, and dividing areas into specialized modular processing units or cortical "columns." What was achieved through these changes ranges from echolocation to language. Of course, changes in the neocortex have been accompanied by modifications occurring in other parts of the brain because cortical and subcortical structures often have integrated functions. For example, the superior colliculus of the midbrain has been variously modified in function, largely by changing and expanding the direct inputs from neocortex, but also through other alterations. To understand how cortical organization has changed to produce the remarkable human brain, the next section focuses on the neocortex of early mammals.

Brains of Early Mammals

Early mammals had small brains with little neocortex. By comparing the histological appearance of the neocortex in extant mammals of differing lines of descent, we can conclude that the neocortex of early mammals was not as highly differentiated in terms of distinct layers and neuron types as is the cortex of many modern mammals. However, the cortex likely was not homogeneous in appearance either. In present-day mammals, the primary sensory areas typically have a noticeably different layer 4 (the receiving layer) with somewhat smaller and more densely packed neurons than in other areas. From such slight regional differences in appearance, early investigators such as Brodmann (1909) surmised that all mammals had functionally significant subdivisions of the cortex, called *areas*, that some areas were shared by many species (homologous areas), and that mammals differed in numbers of areas. What was difficult for Brodmann and other early investigators was to reliably identify areas by their histological appearance, especially in the poorly differentiated cortex of many small-brained mammals, but sometimes even in the large expanses of the rather homogeneous cortex in large-brained mammals. As a result, areas were often incorrectly delimited, and the sometimes radical changes in the appearance of certain areas that took place across species resulted in mistaken interpretations of homology. To Brodmann's credit, he correctly identified the primary visual cortex in species as different from each other as humans, where the task is easy because of the area's histological distinctiveness, and hedgehogs, insectivores with poor cortical differentiation. However, many of Brodmann's proposed areas and proposed homologies have little validity, although his subdivisions for human and other brains are commonly portrayed in textbooks today. Fortunately, modern methods allow us to compare many features of cortical biology in great detail, including connection patterns, neuron response properties, and cortical histochemistry, which allows us to identify cortical areas and evaluate homologies with a high degree of assurance. From these methods, we can conclude that the neocortex of early mammals was subdivided into a small number of functionally distinct areas, on the order of 10–20, and these areas have been retained in most lines of descent.

The neocortex of small-brained North American opossums (Fig. 45.3) reflects many of the features of other small-brained mammals. Much of the limited expanse of the neocortex is dominated by sensory inputs relayed from the thalamus. Caudally, the neocortex includes a large primary visual area, V1, bordered laterally by a strip-like second visual area, V2. More laterally, an additional strip of cortex responds to visual stimuli, but the organization of this cortex is not known. Nearly all existing mammals have a V1, V2, and a more lateral zone of visual cortex, and this pattern likely emerged with (or before) the first mammals. More rostrally, opossums have a primary somatosensory area, S1, bordered laterally by two additional representations of tactile receptors, the second somatosensory areas, S2, and the parietal ventral area, PV. Connection patterns indicate that narrow bands of the cortex rostral and caudal to S1 are also involved in processing somatosensory inputs. This collection of five somatosensory fields is seen

Opossum cortical areas

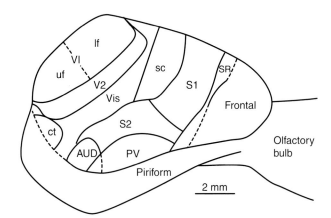

FIGURE 45.3 Some of the proposed neocortical areas in North American opossums. Somatosensory areas include the primary area, S1, a secondary area, S2, a parietal ventral area, PV, and caudal (sc) and rostral (SR) somatosensory belts. The auditory cortex (AUD) is limited and likely contains a primary field A1 and possibly another area or two. The visual cortex includes primary (V1) and secondary (V2) areas and a visual (Vis) belt. The caudotemporal (ct) field is probably visual. In V1, the upper visual field (uf) is represented caudal to the lower visual field (lf). Modified from Beck *et al.* (1996).

repeatedly in small-brained mammals, although S2 and PV are not always distinct from each other. A region of cortex caudal to S2 and PV responds to auditory stimuli, and much of this region is occupied by the primary auditory area, A1, which is present in all or nearly all living mammals. However, the auditory cortex contains a number of additional areas in most mammals, including many of the studied small-brained mammals, although homologies are presently uncertain. Thus, early mammals probably had several auditory fields. More rostrally, the frontal cortex of opossums is very small and does not contain any obvious motor areas. Instead, motor-related information from the cerebellum is relayed to S1. However, opossums are marsupials (Fig. 45.1), and most or all placental mammals have a primary motor area, M1, just rostral to S1 (and the narrow somatosensory band bordering S1), and possibly a second motor area, M2, also known as the supplementary motor area, SMA. The frontal cortex also includes an orbitofrontal region, which mediates autonomic responses to exteroceptive stimuli. On the medial wall of the cerebral hemisphere, opossums and other mammals share several divisions of the limbic cortex with inputs from the anterior and lateral dorsal nuclei of the thalamus. In addition, narrow strips of the entorhinal cortex are present that connect the neocortex with the hippocampus.

From this ancestral pattern, a great variety of brain organizations have evolved through alterations in the number of parts and connections. Consider, for example, the variations of the primary somatosensory cortex. The duck-billed platypus devotes most of S1 to representing receptors present in its highly sensitive bill, and it has added inputs from electroreceptors (Krubitzer, 1995). The star-nosed mole devotes most of S1 to its long, fleshy nose appendages, rats mostly activate S1 with their facial whiskers, and human S2 has a large representation of the hand, lips, and mouth. In addition to variations in the way particular areas are organized, mammals differ in the complement of areas they possess. The amount of neocortex varies greatly across species of mammals (Jerison, 1973), and some of this variation may be due to differences in numbers of cortical areas present in different groups of mammals (Kaas, 1995). The number of sensory areas increased independently in several lines of evolution, which has important implications. Both cats and monkeys have a large number of visual areas, but the carnivore and primate lines appear to have acquired most of these areas independently rather than from a common ancestor. Thus, many of the visual areas in cats have no homologies in monkeys or humans. A similar situation holds for other regions of the brain. New areas were added most commonly to unimodal sensory regions rather than to multimodal "association" cortex as once thought. Humans, monkeys, and cats do have bimodal and multimodal areas, but these areas occupy relatively little neocortex. Thus, mammals in various lines of descent developed new cortical areas, as well as other unique brain specializations. As a long-known example of the emergence of a new brain feature, the corpus callosum, the major pathway interconnecting the neocortex of the two cerebral hemispheres, is a derived character of placental mammals, having emerged in the ancestors of placentals after they diverged from marsupials. Whereas connections between the two hemispheres are mediated by the anterior commissure in marsupials and monotremes, most of these connections are carried in the shorter, more direct callosal pathway in placental mammals.

Much of our further understanding of how the human brain evolved will depend on comparisons of the brains of various primates. Primates have specializations of the visual system such as a unique type of retinotopic organization of the superior colliculus, a characteristic lamination pattern in the lateral geniculate nucleus, and areas of visual cortex not found in other mammals.

Summary

Some features of the human brain may have originated in the early nervous systems of multicellular animals before the first vertebrates evolved. The hallmark of the emergence of mammalian brains was a distinctive thick, six-layered neocortex which was considerably modified from the thin dorsal cortex of reptiles. Early mammals had small brains with little neocortex that was dominated by a few sensory and motor representations of areas. These areas have been commonly retained in present-day mammals, some of which still have small brains and little neocortex. A great variety of brain organizations have evolved through alterations, especially in the neocortex. In several lines of evolution, the number of cortical areas has increased by the addition of new areas. Patterns of connections between areas and the internal organizations of areas have also changed.

EVOLUTION OF PRIMATE BRAINS

Evolution of Primates

Early primates emerged from small-brained, nocturnal, insect-eating mammals some 60–70 million years ago and soon branched into three main lines leading to present-day prosimians, tarsiers, and anthropoids (Fig. 45.4). The prosimian suborder of primates includes lorises, lemurs, and bushbabies; the anthropoid suborder consists of New World monkeys, Old World monkeys, and the ape–human group. Tarsiers are small, prosimian-like animals. Two main schemes of classification of primates have been in use, mainly because it has not been obvious where to place tarsiers. Many authors use a traditional classification and distinguish prosimian from anthropoid primates and include tarsiers with prosimians. However, this is now thought to be an unnatural paraphyletic grouping because tarsiers, despite their generally prosimian-like appearance, are generally considered to be more closely related to anthropoids than to lemurs, lorises and galagos. This conclusion is reflected in the cladistic classification preferred by other authors, in which lemurs, lorises, and galagos are placed in the suborder, Strepsirhini, a group that has retained ancestral features, including a naked, moist rhinarum (wet nose). Tarsiers and anthropoids, which have a reduced olfactory system (and thus a dry nose), are placed in the suborder Haplorhini, and tarsiers are placed into their own infraorder. The remaining anthropoid primates are divided into the

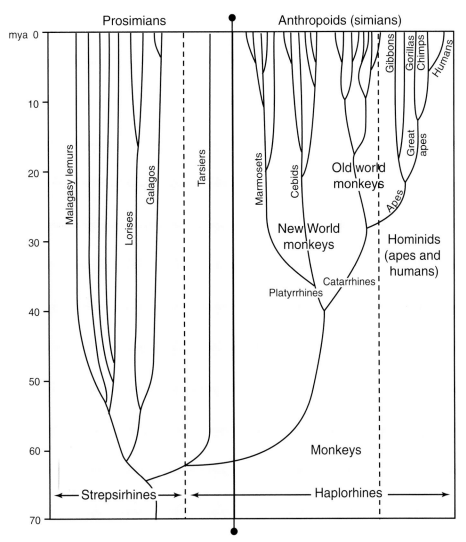

FIGURE 45.4 The evolution and classification of primates. Tarsiers are generally considered to be prosimians, but they are related more closely to anthropoids, so they are recognized as haplorhine primates. Despite the ancient split of prosimian and anthropoid primates, they share many brain features that are unique to primates. Tree shrews, bats, and flying lemurs are thought to be close relatives of primates, forming the superorder Archonta, but the composition of Archonta is in doubt. mya, millions of years ago. Based largely on Kay *et al.* (1997) and Purvis (1995).

infraorders Platyrrhini (New World monkeys) and Catarrhini (Old World monkeys, apes, and humans).

The earliest primates are thought to have been small-bodied, nocturnal visual predators living on insects and small vertebrates, as well as fruit. They adapted to the tropical rainforests by emphasizing vision and visually-guided reaching and grasping. This involved having larger, forward-facing eyes, opposable big toes and thumbs, and digits tipped with nails. These primates produced the largely nocturnal strepsirhine radiation with its varied forms, including some species now living in Madagascar that have become diurnal. The haplorine primates emerged about 60 million years ago in association

with a shift from nocturnal to diurnal life, together with an increased emphasis on fruit eating (Ross, 1996). With the shift to diurnality came reduced dependence on olfaction, enhancement of the visual system, enlarged body size, and sometimes a more gregarious mode of life. Specifically, the olfactory apparatus was reduced in size and the eyes enlarged, with the result that the eyes were brought close together. The reflecting surface at the back of the eye (tapetum lucidum), an adaptation to nocturnal vision present in prosimians and many other nocturnal mammals, was lost. The ratio of cones to rods in the retina increased greatly, and a morphological specialization—the fovea—evolved, which was packed with small cones, enhancing central visual acuity. The cone system itself was modified: many anthropoid primates are apparently unique in having trichromatic vision, which is made possible by having cones sensitive to three different wavelengths, rather than two as in most mammals. All catarrhine primates have trichromatic color vision, whereas platyrrhine species display a variety of dichromatic and trichromatic phenotypes. The enhancement of color discrimination with trichromatic vision is plausibly regarded as an adaptation for identifying ripe, edible fruits. The shift to diurnality was also marked by larger social groupings, which may offer enhanced protection from predation. These changes were accompanied by an increased brain size, including increases in the temporal lobe visual region, and in regions of the parietal and frontal cortex mediating motor control and social interactions.

The ancestors of present-day tarsiers evidently abandoned the diurnal niche to become nocturnal visual predators again. Tarsiers retain a fovea and two types of cones, but have evolved a rod-dominated retina and have enormous eyes to create sensitivity at low light levels without the aid of a reflecting tapetum. The primary visual cortex has become very large relative to the rest of the brain and is extremely well differentiated, with a multiplicity of layers and sublayers. Tarsiers have become such extremely specialized visual predators that they eat no plant food. Other haplorhines (anthropoids) remained diurnal and spread to many niches, including those outside the rainforest and niches based more on eating leaves a well as fruits. Some increased considerably in body size. Later anthropoids were able to process hard, husked fruits with their hands and teeth. Some early anthropoids managed to reach South America from Africa, apparently by rafting, to form the New World monkey radiation. All modern anthropoids are diurnal with the exception of owl monkeys, a New World monkey group, that has (like tarsiers) become secondarily nocturnal.

In Africa, early anthropoids diverged some 25–30 million years ago into lines leading to modern Old World monkeys and to apes. At first, apes were the most successful radiation, coming to occupy a range of rainforest and open woodland environments, while monkeys were quite rare. Perhaps as many as 30 different types of apes existed at one time. This condition changed radically some 10 million years ago when monkeys became abundant and apes rare. This change may have resulted from the advent of a more seasonally variable and drier climate. Ancestral Old World monkeys acquired specialized teeth suited to a leaf and fruit diet in drier climates. Also, the more

rapid reproduction of monkeys may have made them more resistant to extinction than apes.

Some 5–6 million years ago, a line of apes diverged into two branches: one that gave rise to modern common chimpanzees and bonobos (pygmy chimpanzees) and a second branch that led to hominids, the group of bipedal apes that includes modern humans (Fig. 45.5). The oldest known hominids, the so-called australopithecines, date back at least 4 million years. These early hominids were bipedal, but skeletal traits suggest they retained considerable ability for climbing trees. Body size was rather small and males were bigger than females. The brain was only slightly larger than for apes of similar body size. Hominid traits may have emerged as adaptations to a drier environment with grassland and savanna. Early australopithecines soon gave rise to a number of species differing in body size and limb proportions, as well as in characteristics of the jaws and teeth and brain size. Primitive members of our own genus began to emerge some 2 million years ago with *Homo habilis* (or "handy man," due to its use of stone tools). *Homo habilis* had a slightly increased cranial capacity compared to australopithecines, reduced face and teeth, and pelvic modifications for improved bipedal locomotion and the birth of neonates with larger heads. About 1.7 million years ago, *H. habilis* appears to have been replaced by *H. erectus*, a larger hominid with a further reduction in face and teeth and a larger brain. Shortly thereafter, *Homo erectus* spread out of Africa to central Asia. Early *Homo sapiens* emerged from an African population of *H. erectus* some 250,000 to 300,000 years ago, and archaic forms of *H. sapiens* persisted until about 35,000 years ago. Modern human forms and behaviors appeared in Africa before that time. One line of archaic *H. sapiens* became Neanderthals (*H. sapiens neanderthalensis*), who adapted to a colder Europe and southwest Asia over 130,000 years ago. They disappeared and were replaced by modern *H. sapiens* some 35,000 years ago, apparently without contributing genetically to present-day humans. Thus, modern *H. sapiens* replaced Neanderthals without effective interbreeding. Neanderthals were shorter and more heavily built than modern humans, but they had a comparable or slightly larger cranial capacity. Over the last 15,000 years, some populations of humans have become smaller and have reduced their brain size, apparently as a result of a poorer diet as agriculture replaced hunting and gathering.

Chimpanzees appear to be our closest surviving relatives. The major phenotypic differences between chimps and humans are based on an estimated 1.5% difference in genes, and we have surprisingly few

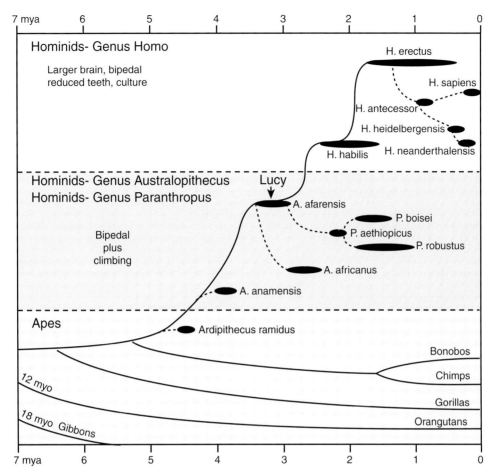

FIGURE 45.5 The evolution of apes and humans. Apes include living apes and a late fossil judged to not be bipedal (*Ardipithecus ramidus*). *Australopithecus* and *Paranthropus* appear to have been bipedal. The age of the famous fossil, Lucy, is indicated. Relationships are somewhat uncertain, and more branches on the tree exist.

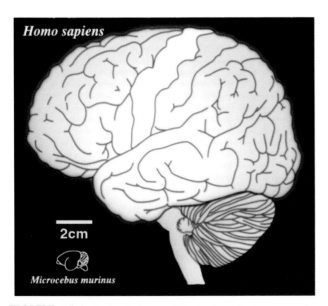

FIGURE 45.6 Lateral views of the brains of a human and a small prosimian primate, the mouse lemur, to illustrate the great range of sizes for present-day primates.

genes (~35,000). Greater differences in genes occur between sister species of some genera. The reasons for our great phenotypic differences, including those in brain size and presumably brain organization, are not well understood, but factors affecting gene expression, including differences in gene position on chromosomes that affect the timing of gene expression, are likely to be important. Gene expression in the neocortex may actually be more different between chimps and humans than between chimps and macaques.

Brains of Early Primates

The brains of primates vary greatly in size and fissure patterns. Humans have the largest of primate brains, whereas mouse lemurs have the smallest (Fig. 45.6). Judging from fossil endocasts and other parts of the skeleton, early primates were lemur-like in body form, and their brains were shaped like those of present-day lemurs, although smaller. The modern mouse lemur has moderately expanded temporal and occipital lobes, indicating an emphasis on vision, a calcarine fissure or fold in the primary visual cortex, and a lateral (Sylvian) fissure separating somatosensory areas of the parietal lobe from auditory areas of the temporal lobe. Nearly all primates share these two fissures. Many early as well as present-day primates also have an additional prominent fissure in the temporal lobe (the superior temporal sulcus). Other fissures are more variable.

Among living prosimians, evidence about brain organization comes mostly from studies of galagos, nocturnal animals from Africa that are cat-sized or smaller and eat mainly fruit, tree gums, and insects. Their brains have only a few fissures (Fig. 45.7). Their visual system contains several features that are common to all primates that have been examined, including a distinctive type of lamination in the lateral geniculate nucleus of the visual thalamus (with magnocellular and parvocellular layers) and a pulvinar complex with the distinct inferior and lateral

pulvinar divisions. As in other primates, the superior colliculus of the midbrain represents only the contralateral half of the visual field, whereas other mammals have a more extensive representation that includes the complete visual field of the contralateral eye. The visual cortex includes areas V1 and V2, both retained from nonprimate ancestors but with primate modifications including "blobs," which are cytochrome oxidase-rich modules in V1, and band-like modules that span the width of V2. Other visual areas apparently shared with all other primates include V3, a dorsomedial area (DM), and a middle temporal visual area (MT), all with inputs from V1. Other areas, such as the dorsolateral area (DL or V4), are also shared, but not enough is known about visual cortex organization in various primates to be certain of how many of the more than 30 proposed visual areas (Felleman and Van Essen, 1991) are shared. Some or most of these areas, such as MT, are not found in nonprimates, or at least not in a primate-like form, and these areas are distinctive features of primate brains.

Organization of the auditory system of galagos and other prosimians is not well understood, but they appear to share two primary or primary-like areas, A1 and R ("rostral"), with other primates, and they likely share several nonprimary areas as well. A1 and possibly R are likely to have been retained from nonprimate ancestors. The somatosensory cortex appears to be relatively unchanged from nonprimate ancestors (Kaas, 1983), as an S1, S2, and PV have been identified in galagos, and there are additional, narrow belts of somatosensory cortex along the rostral and caudal borders of S1. S2 and PV retain the primitive feature of being activated directly by inputs from the ventro-

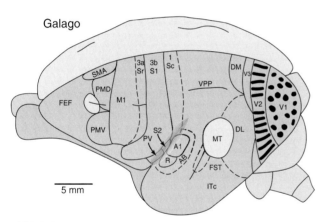

FIGURE 45.7 A lateral view of the brain of a prosimian primate, *Galago garnetti*, showing some of the proposed visual, somatosensory, auditory, and motor areas. Visual areas include the primary (V1) and secondary (V2) areas, common to most mammals, but with the modular subdivisions (blobs in V1; bands in V2) characteristic of primates. As in other primates, galagos have a third visual area (V3), a dorsomedial area (DM), a middle temporal area (MT), a dorsolateral area (DL), a fundal-sucal-temporal area (FST), an inferior temporal caudal area (IT$_c$), and a visually related ventral posterior parietal cortex (VPP). The auditory cortex includes a primary field (A1), a rostral area (R), and an auditory belt (AB), which includes several areas and regions of the parabelt auditory cortex. The somatosensory cortex includes a primary area (S1 or 3b), a parietal ventral area (PV), a secondary area (S2), a somatosensory rostral belt (SR or 3a), and a somatosensory caudal belt (SC or possibly area 1 or areas 1 plus 2). Motor areas include a primary area (M1), ventral (PMV) and dorsal (PMD) premotor areas, a supplementary motor area (SMA), a frontal eye field (FEF), and other motor areas on the medial wall of the cerebral hemisphere. See Wu *et al.* (2000) for details.

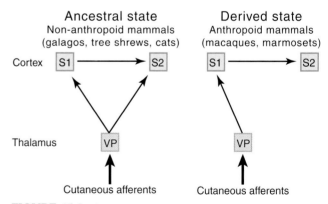

FIGURE 45.8 Somatosensory processing in prosimian primates and anthropoid primates. The processing in anthropoids is serial, rather than parallel and serial. Because the prosimian type is also found in a number of nonprimate mammals, we infer that this is the ancestral state. The ventroposterior nucleus (VP) of the somatosensory thalamus and the first (S1) and second (S2) somatosensory areas of the cortex are shown.

posterior nucleus of the thalamus (Fig. 45.8). Motor cortex organization is surprisingly advanced, with the five or more premotor areas also found in anthropoid primates (Wu *et al.*, 2000).

Although the brains of prosimians are not especially large, they appear to share a number of primate-specific areas with anthropoids over and above the complement inherited from their mammalian ancestors. The further study of prosimians is critical for understanding the emergence of features of brain organization that are distinctive of primates.

Brains of Early Anthropoids

As noted earlier, the anatomy of early anthropoids suggests that an emphasis on high-acuity, diurnal vision and reduced emphasis on smell were important in their evolution. The endocasts of early anthropoids reveal a greater expansion of the temporal lobe than is evident in prosimians.

Collectively, New World and Old World monkeys cover a wide range of body and brain sizes. The extent to which fissures develop on the brain surface depends on absolute brain size. All primates, no matter how small, have a deep calcarine fissure in the occipital lobe. Most also have a deep lateral sulcus (Sylvian fissure). These are the only well-developed sulci in marmosets, the smallest of the New World monkeys. Slightly larger New World monkeys, such as owl monkeys and squirrel monkeys, also have a shallow central sulcus and a shallow superior temporal sulcus. The largest New World monkeys, including spider monkeys and cebus monkeys (capuchins), have even more sulci and resemble (at least superficially) the well-fissured brains of Old World monkeys, such as macaques and baboons.

Both Old World and New World monkeys have all of the areas of the neocortex described for prosimians, as well as some additional areas. Most notably, the somatosensory cortex has been altered so that areas 3a, 3b, 1, and 2 are well differentiated from each other, with each area corresponding to a separate representation of receptors of the contralateral body surface (Kaas, 1983). Within S1 (area 3b), the proportional representation of body parts varies somewhat across species, so that in some monkeys as much as half of the area is devoted to the face and oral cavity. The hand is also prominently represented, especially in monkeys such as macaques. Some New World monkeys, such as spider monkeys, have a large representation of their highly tactile, prehensile tail. Marmosets appear to have a relatively poorly differentiated somatosensory region, which lacks a definite area 2, a field that is responsive to tactile stimuli and

muscle movements in other monkeys. This may be a consequence of brain size reduction in marmosets, which have evolved smaller brains and bodies from larger ancestors. In all anthropoids, S2 and PV appear to have lost activating inputs from the ventroposterior nucleus of the somatosensory thalamus, and they depend on inputs from areas 3a, 3b, 1, and 2 (Fig. 45.8). S2 and PV receive modulatory inputs from the ventroposterior inferior nucleus. Thus, processing in the somatosensory system became more serial than parallel with the advent of monkeys. Other differences likely exist between anthropoids and prosimians in the somatosensory portions of the lateral sulcus and posterior parietal cortex, but more research is needed. Both of these regions of somatosensory processing have expanded greatly in anthropoids compared to prosimians, and several areas involved in visually guided reaching have been described in macaque monkeys.

There is currently much interest in how the visual system of monkeys is subdivided into cortical areas and how these visual areas function in behavior. Elaborate proposals have been presented, but considerable uncertainty remains. In Old World monkeys, over 30 visual areas have been proposed (Felleman and Van Essen, 1991), and it seems likely that anthropoids in general have more visual areas than prosimians, although the full extent of this difference is not yet clear. In the auditory cortex, a core of three primary-like areas, a belt of seven to eight additional fields, and a "parabelt" of several additional areas have been proposed (Kaas and Hackett, 2000), but not enough is known about prosimians to know what differences exist. The proposed subdivisions of the motor cortex in prosimians and simians are quite similar (Wu *et al.*, 2000). Finally, a comparison of cortical connections and architectonics in galagos and macaque monkeys led to the conclusion that macaques have several areas of dorsolateral prefrontal cortex in addition to those found in galagos (Preuss and Goldman-Rakic, 1991). Brodmann (1909) also thought that anthropoids have more prefrontal subdivisions than prosimians.

Evolution of Hominid Brains

In trying to determine the recent course of the evolution of the human brain, we depend more on the fossil record than on a comparative approach, as we are the only hominid that is surviving. Human brains are much bigger than those of our closest living relatives, the African apes. From the fossil record (Fig. 45.9), we can see that early australopithecines had brains that were only 10–25% larger than the

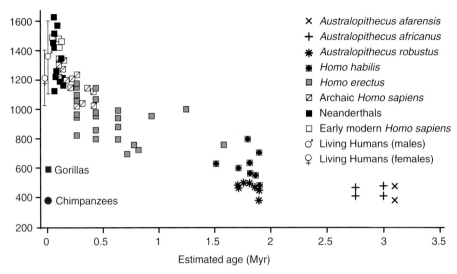

Brain size (in cm³) plotted against time (Myr) for specimens attributed to Hominidae

FIGURE 45.9 Evidence for the rapid growth of brains of hominids over the last 2 million years. The brain sizes of modern chimpanzees and gorillas have been added for comparison. Modified from McHenry (1994).

brains of present day African apes when body size is taken into account. However, brains increased rapidly in size as the various species of *Homo* evolved over the last 2 million years. Early hominids had brains in the 600- to 800-cc range; *H. erectus*, about 500,000 years ago, had brain volumes close to 1000 cc; and soon thereafter brains reached the volumes within the range of modern *H. sapiens* (1400 cc).

In deducing the changes in internal organization that likely occurred over this remarkable increase in brain size, it would be useful to know more about the organization of the brains of the living apes. However, only limited information is available from early motor and somatosensory mapping experiments on apes, and further noninvasive studies, as in humans, are needed. Fortunately, much can be learned by studying the histology of tissue from brains of apes that have died natural deaths using modern histochemical techniques (see Preuss, 2001). For now, however, we have only a limited understanding of how the brains of apes differ from those of monkeys. Nevertheless, even studies of brain proportions have been useful. For example, a surprising outcome of a recent comparative study was that apes devote proportionately nearly as much of their forebrain to the frontal lobe as do humans. This result argues against the long-held premise that a major feature of hominid brain evolution was the great relative expansion of the frontal lobe. Of course, with our much larger brains, our frontal lobes are also much

bigger, but they are not disproportionately so. However, parts of the frontal lobe of humans might be disproportionately large, if, for example, we exclude the motor areas and only consider the prefrontal cortex. If we assume that "theory of mind" is a human psychological specialization (Povinelli and Preuss, 1995) and that this specialization depends on the prefrontal cortex, then we have good reason to suppose that the frontal lobe underwent extensive modification in human evolution. However, there presently is no clear anatomical evidence that humans have a different frontal lobe organization than apes, and even monkeys.

We also assume that brain specializations evolved to support the ability for language, such as Wernicke's area in the temporoparietal cortex and Broca's area in the frontal lobe. Human brains are not symmetrical in shape, so that the planum temporale, the sheet of cortex on the lower surface of the lateral sulcus (the upper face of the temporal lobe), is usually larger in the left cerebral hemisphere than on the right. As the left hemisphere usually becomes dominant for language, the larger size of the left planum temporale has long been assumed to be related to language. Interestingly, there is some evidence for a temporal lobe asymmetry from the length and shape of the lateral fissure in the brain casts of fossil hominids, and to some extent even in the great apes, which do not normally develop language (although they may have some limited capacity to do so). However, it is not known when language emerged in hominids, which remains an issue of much speculation. What seems likely is that previously existing brain regions not originally used for language, such as the ventral premotor area and dorsal-stream auditory areas of monkeys, became specialized for language in the ancestors of humans, especially in the left cerebral hemisphere. Broca's area may include cortex homologous to the ventral premotor area.

Summary

Early primates were small, nocturnal, insect-eating mammals that evolved into lines leading to present-day prosimians, tarsiers, and anthropoids (monkeys, apes, and humans). The early primates resembled present-day prosimian lemurs in body form and brain size. Comparative studies suggest that these primates had many of the brain features shared by galagos and other primates today. In the visual system, these include a lateral geniculate nucleus with magnocellular and parvocellular layers, a superior colliculus with only a contralateral hemifield representation, and areas V1, V2, V3, DM, MT, and DL (V4) of the visual cortex. Early anthropoids had larger brains, and the anterior parietal cortex was differentiated into four strip-like fields, somatosensory areas 3a, 3b, 1, and 2. The visual cortex was expanded and apparently contained more areas. Early hominids (bipedal primates) had brains that were similar in size to those of present-day African apes, but brains of hominids rapidly increased three times in size over the last 2 million years leading to modern humans. Over this time, more cortical areas were added, hemispheric specialization for language and other functions emerged, and changes in the prefrontal cortex allowed for new cognitive functions.

WHY BRAIN SIZE IS IMPORTANT

A general assumption is that larger brains are better because they can do more. This does not imply that brains of the same size (or same size in proportion to the body) do the same things because brain organization is modified for different functions. Nevertheless, larger brains do have obvious design problems that are likely to have been solved in similar ways in the different lines of evolution. All organs and systems of the body confront design problems and limits as they become larger or smaller, and the smallest mammals seem to be close to their minimal possible size. To some extent, neurons enlarge as brains get bigger, but dendrites and axons cannot enlarge much without

compromising their functions. To maintain passive cable conduction in dendrites, Bekkers and Stevens (1970) calculated that dendrites increase four times in diameter when they are doubled in length. Similarly, when axons are doubled in length, axon diameter must also be doubled to maintain conduction times. As brain size increases, some dendrites and axons do become lengthened and enlarged disproportionately. However, given the problems associated with scaling up neuron size, the major way of increasing brain size is to increase the number of neurons. This introduces a related problem. It becomes increasingly difficult to maintain the connections of each neuron with the same percentage of other neurons, as the number of connections needed grows much faster than the number of neurons. Larger brains do devote much more of their mass to connections. As a result, cell body densities decrease and cortical thickness increases, but the increase in connections is not nearly enough to maintain ratios of connectivity or to fully compensate for longer connection distances (Ringo et al., 1994; Kaas, 2000).

There are two major ways in which larger brains can be modified to reduce the design problems produced by larger distances and more neurons. First, the brain can become more modular so that most connections of individual neurons are with neighboring, rather than distant, neurons. This can be done by (1) increasing the number of processing areas so that areas are smaller and (2) confining most connections within an area. In addition, areas can be subdivided into smaller functional divisions (columns or modules) that limit long connections in a similar manner. Thus, large brains are likely to have larger numbers of cortical areas, and large areas are likely to contain several types of modules. Second, connections that require long, thick axons should be reduced as much as possible. Functionally related areas can be grouped so that necessary connections between areas are shorter. Another way of reducing the need for long connections is to increase the degree of specialization of each cerebral hemisphere. As brains get bigger, it becomes more and more inefficient to send information from one hemisphere to the other. Thus, the total proportion of callosal axons is less than expected in larger brains, and proportionately fewer of the axons are of the larger diameters needed to preserve conduction times (Ringo et al., 1994). Regions and areas of each hemisphere become differently specialized so that major interconnections can remain within the same hemisphere. Large brains should, therefore, be less symmetrical than small brains, and the large human brain appears to be extreme in this respect.

Another issue is that large cortical areas are unlikely to function in the same manner as small cortical areas. Unless neurons compensate with larger dendrites and intrinsic connections as areas get larger, the computational window or scope of neurons will decrease. For example, as a visual area gets bigger, individual neurons would evaluate information from less and less of the total visual field (Fig. 45.10). This implies that as areas get bigger, their neurons become less capable of global center-surround comparisons and more devoted to local center-surround comparisons, and some of their more integrative functions

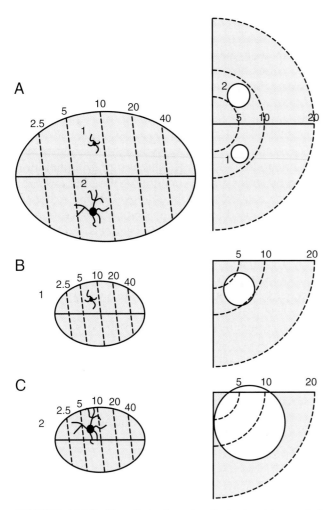

FIGURE 45.10 The effects of varying the horizontal spread of dendritic arbors of neurons in large (A) and small (B and C) visual areas. An increase in arbor size (1 to 2) in a large area (A) produces little change in receptive field size (circles 1 to 2 in the central 20° of the visual hemifield on the right), whereas such a change (B to C) in a small area changes the scope of the receptive field greatly . Thus, the functions of small areas are changed more dramatically by small morphological adjustments. Surface view schematics of retinotopically organized visual areas are on the left, whereas schematics of receptive fields in the visual hemifield and the lower visual quadrant are on the right. From Kaas (2000); see Elston *et al.* (1999).

are displaced to smaller areas. It is also apparent that changes in the sizes of dendritic arbors and the lengths of intrinsic axons in smaller areas would have more impact on the sizes of computational windows of neurons. Comparable changes in dendrites and axons would enlarge or reduce receptive field sizes more in a small than a large visual area (Fig. 45.10). Because their functions are more modifiable by small structural modifications, smaller areas may be specialized more easily for different functions. Recent measurements suggest that neurons in large areas do not have longer dendritic arbors and larger intrinsic connections, and indeed they may have smaller dendritic arbors (e.g., Elston *et al.*, 1999). In addition, primary sensory areas are typically larger in larger brains, but they are not proportionately larger (Fig. 45.11). Thus, the primary visual cortex is less than three times larger in human brains than in the brains of macaque monkeys, whereas the neocortex as a whole is over 10 times larger (Fig. 45.10). We suggest that lack of proportional growth reduces the impact of changing functions with size and reflects the addition of other smaller cortical areas.

Other size-related constraints relate to mechanisms of development. We often assume that natural selection can act independently on each brain trait, but this is unlikely to be the case. Instead, selection may operate on a few developmental mechanisms, such as those that control the number of neurons or the extent that correlated activity is used to maintain functional connections. Along this line of reasoning, Finlay and Darlington (1995) have provided evidence that late-developing brain structures enlarge disproportionately in larger brains ("late makes large"). As we learn more about the genetics and mechanisms of development and how development is modified in evolution, we should be able to form more accurate models of brain evolution and understand more fully how the human brain emerged from those of our ancestors. We might also benefit from considerations of other possible constraints on brain size. A larger brain creates more heat, and thus needs a better cooling system (Falk, 1990), and the higher metabolic costs of a larger brain may require a better diet or the reduction in size of other metabolically expensive tissue (gut).

CONCLUSIONS

Based on comparative studies and the fossil records, we conclude that early mammals had small brains with little neocortex and few functional subdivisions (areas or fields) of cortex. Vision was empha-

A

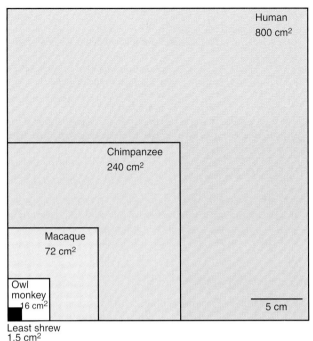

B

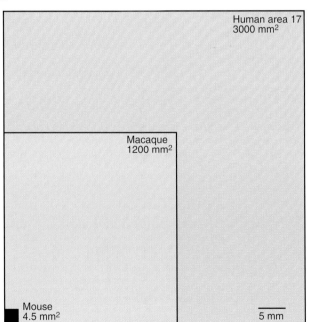

FIGURE 45.11 Species differences in (B) the surface area of the neocortex and (A) of the primary visual cortex in one cerebral hemisphere. The neocortex of humans is over 500 times larger in surface area and over twice as thick as the neocortex in the smallest mammals that resembled those leading to the first primates and over three times the surface area of our closest living relatives, the chimpanzees. Some of the areas of the brain are also larger in humans, but not to the extent expected from the great enlargement of the neocortex. From Kaas (2000).

sized in the early primates, and the visual cortex in the temporal and occipital lobes enlarged. These primates also had several unique features of the visual system, including new visual areas such as MT, distinctive kinds of modules in V1 (blobs) and V2 (bands), separate magnocellular and parvocellular layers in the lateral geniculate nucleus, and a representation in the superior colliculus restricted to the contralateral visual hemifield. Several premotor areas were present, whereas the somatosensory system was relatively primitive. Later anthropoid primates had larger brains, more neocortex, and more areas of neocortex. The somatosensory cortex had expanded and included the four striplike areas on the anterior parietal lobe, areas 3a, 3b, 1, and 2. It remains uncertain how new cortical areas evolve, but they may result from a gradual process of differentiation and consolidation of module classes or by duplication of existing areas and subsequent specialization. We know little about possible specializations of the brains of early apes. However, over the last 6 million years of evolution from early apes to modern humans, brains increased three to four times in size. This expansion was probably accompanied by a further increase in the number of cortical areas, modifications leading to functional and anatomical asymmetries in the two cerebral hemispheres, specializations for language and cognition, more prefrontal cortex, and larger expanses of occipitoparietal and inferotemporal cortex. The larger brains had many more neurons with a greater proportion of tissue devoted to connections relative to cell bodies, and presumably had a higher ratio of local connections to long-distance connections.

Further progress in understanding the course of the evolution of the human brain can be achieved with current methods of investigation. We have the opportunity to learn much about the similarities and differences among the brains of various primates. Neuroscientists have generally concentrated on studies of brain features that are widely shared, but differences in brain structure and function are what make us distinctively human. One goal of future research should be to understand these brain differences.

References

Beck, P. D., Pospichal, M. W., and Kaas, J. H. (1996). Topography, architecture, and connections of somatosensory cortex in opossums: Evidence for five somatosensory areas. *J. Comp. Neurol.* **366**, 109–133.

Bekkers, J. M., and Stevens, C. F. (1970). Two different ways evolution makes neurons larger. *Prog. Brain Res.* **83**, 37–45.

Brodmann, K. (1909). "Vergleichende Lokalisationslehre der Grosshirnrhinde." Barth, Leipzig. [Reprinted as Brodmann's "Localisation in the Cerebral cortex," translated and edited by L. J. Garey, Smith-Gordon, London, 1994.]

Darwin, C. (1859). "On the Origin of Species." John Murray, London. [Facsimile of the first edition: Harvard Univ. Press, Cambridge, MA, 1984].

Elston, G. N. Tweedale, R., and Rosa, M. G. P. (1999). Cortical integration in the visual system of the macaque monkey: Large-scale morphological differences in the pyramidal neurons in the occipital parietal and temporal lobes. *Proc. R. Soc. Lond. B* **266**, 1367–1374.

Falk, D. (1990). Brain evolution in Homo: The "radiator" theory. *Behav. Brain Sci.* **13**, 339–381.

Felleman, D. J., and Van Essen, D.C. (1991). Distributed hierarchical processing in the primate cerebral cortex. *Cereb. Cortex* **1**, 1–47.

Finlay, B. L., and Darlington, R. B. (1995). Linked regularities in the development and evolution of mammalian brains. *Science* **268**, 1578–1584.

Hodos, W., and Campbell, C. B. A. (1969). *Scala naturae*: Why there is no theory in comparative psychology. *Psych. Rev.* **4**, 337–350.

Jerison, H. J. (1973). "Evolution of the Brain and Intelligence." Academic Press, New York.

Kaas, J. H. (1983). What, if anything, is S1? Organization of the first somatosensory area of cortex. *Physiology* **62**, 206–231.

Kaas, J. H. (1995). The evolution of isocortex. *Brain Behav. Evol.* **46**, 187–196.

Kaas, J. H., and Reiner, A. (1999). The neocortex comes together. *Nature* **399**, 418–419.

Kaas, J. H. (2000). Why is brain size so important: Design problems and solutions as neocortex gets bigger or smaller. *Brain Mind* **1**, 7–23.

Kaas, J. H., and Hackett, T. A. (2000). Subdivisions of auditory cortex and processing streams in primates. *Proc. Natl. Acad. Sci. USA* **97**, 11793–11799.

Krubitzer, L. (1995). The organization of neocortex in mammals: Are species differences really so different? *Trends Neurosci.* **18**, 408–417.

McHenry, H. M. (1994). Tempo and mode in human evolution. *Proc. Natl. Acad. Sci. USA* **91**, 6780–6786.

Povinelli, D. J., and Preuss, T.M. (1995). Theory of mind: Evolutionary history of a cognitive specialization. *Trends Neurosci.* **18**, 418–424.

Preuss, T. M. (2001). The discovery of cerebral diversity: An unwelcome scientific revolution. *In* "Evolutionary Anatomy of the Primate Cerebral Cortex" (D. Falk and K. R. Gibson, eds.), pp. 138–164.

Preuss, T. M., and Goldman-Rakic, P. S. (1991). Ipsilateral cortical connections of granular frontal cortex and surrounding regions in the stepsirhine primate, galago and the anthropoid primate, macaca. *J. Comp. Neurol.* **310**, 429–474.

Purvis, A. (1995). A composite estimate of primate phylogeny. *Phil. Trans. R. Soc. Lond. B.* **348**, 405–421.

Ringo, J. L., Doty, R. W., Demeter, S., and Simard, P. Y. (1994). Time is of the essence: A conjecture that hemispheric specialization arises from interhemispheric conduction delay. *Cereb. Cortex* **4**, 331–343.

Ross, C. (1996). Adaptive explanation for the origins of the Anthropoidea (Primates). *Am. J. Primatol.* **40**, 205–230.

Springer, M. S., and deJong, W. W. (2001). Which mammalian supertree to bark up? *Science* **291**, 1709–1711.

Striedter, G. F. (1998). Progress in the study of brain evolution: From speculative theories to testable hypotheses. *Anat. Rec. (New Anat.)* **253**, 105–112.

Van Essen, D. C. (1997). A tension-based theory of morphogenesis and compact wiring in the central nervous system. *Nature* **385**, 313–318.

Wu, C. W. H., Bichot, N. P., and Kaas, J. H. (2000). Converging evidence from microstimulation, architecture, and connections for multiple motor areas in the frontal and cingulate cortex of prosimian primates. *J. Comp. Neurol.* **423**, 140–177.

Suggested Readings

Allman, J. M. (1999). "Evolving Brains." Freeman, New York.

Butler, A. B., and Hodos, W. (1996). "Comparative Vertebrate Neuroanatomy." Wiley-Liss, New York.

Deacon, T. W. (1997). "The Symbolic Species: The Co-Evolution of Language and the Brain." Norton, New York.

Falk D., and Gibson, K. R (2001). "Evolutionary Anatomy of the Primate Cerebral Cortex." Cambridge Uni. Press, Cambridge.

Fleagle, J. G. (1999). "Primate Adaptation and Evolution," 2nd Ed. Academic Press, San Diego.

Futuyma, D. J. (1998). "Evolutionary Biology," 3rd Ed. Sinauer, Sunderland, MA.

Hennig, W. (1966). "Phylogenetic Systematics." University of Illinois Press, Urbana.

Jones, E. G. and Peters, A (1990). "Cerebral Cortex," Vol. 8B. Plenum Press, New York.

Northcutt, R. G., and Kaas, J. H. (1995). The emergence and evolution of mammalian neocortex. *Trends Neurosci.* **18**, 373–379.

Preuss, T. M. (2000). "The Diversity of Cerebral Cortex." *Brain Behav. Evol.* **55**, 283–347.

Jon H. Kaas and Todd M. Preuss

Cognitive Development and Aging

The human brain has evolved over a very extensive period (Chapter 45), but an individual human brain develops rapidly over the first few years of life, allowing the nearly helpless human infant to gain control of locomotion, language, and thought. The story of brain development in the early years of infancy through adolescence occupies the first part of this chapter. This is followed by consideration of the cognitive changes that occur during this period of the life span and how these capacities are altered over the course of normal aging. The final parts of the chapter discuss pathological processes that (1) affect cognitive development in childhood and adolescence and (2) can cause devastating cognitive impairment in the elderly.

BRAIN DEVELOPMENT

Basic Concepts of Brain Development

Brain Maturation Progresses Well into Adolescence

Brain development is an organized, predetermined, and highly dynamic multistep process that continues beyond birth into the postnatal period, well into adolescence in humans. This complex process remains rapid through the first several years after birth and then slows sharply toward the end of the first decade of life.

Most of our knowledge about human brain development has been obtained through analyses of postmortem specimens and, more recently, powerful neuroimaging techniques. These approaches have provided extensive information on how the size and shape of different brain regions change from conception through adulthood (Fig. 46.1). Total brain weight more than doubles during the first 9 months after

birth to reach over 90% of average adult weight by the 6th year. The development of the cerebral cortical surface proceeds gradually from the flat (lissencephalic) brain of the fetus to the adult gyral pattern at birth. Primary sulci (Sylvian fissure, and rolandic, parietal, and superior temporal sulci) and gyri (pre- and postcentral gyri, superior temporal and middle temporal gyri, superior and middle frontal gyri, and superior and inferior occipital gyri) become well defined between 26 and 28 weeks of gestation. Development of secondary and tertiary gyri occurs later in gestation, and in the last trimester the sulci become deeply enfolded.

Cortical Development Can Be Divided in Two Phases

Cortical development in most mammals can be broadly divided into two phases. The first is a genetically determined sequence of events occurring *in utero* that can be modified by manipulations of either the local environment within the fetal nervous system or the maternal environment. The second phase is one that occurs in the perinatal period where the connectivity of the cortex becomes sensitive to patterns of neural activity. Cortical development is first driven by spontaneous activity in the sense organs and subsequent activation of afferents to the cortex, plus spontaneous activity in the cortical neurons themselves *in utero*. After birth, sensory information driven by external events starts to modulate the synaptic connections that are being built. This lability of cortical connectivity wanes as sexual maturation occurs and cortical synaptic connectivity is pruned to a final stable adult pattern (Chapter 20). The second developmental phase is characterized by a variety of events, including the proper alignment, orientation, and layering of cortical neurons, dendritic and axonal

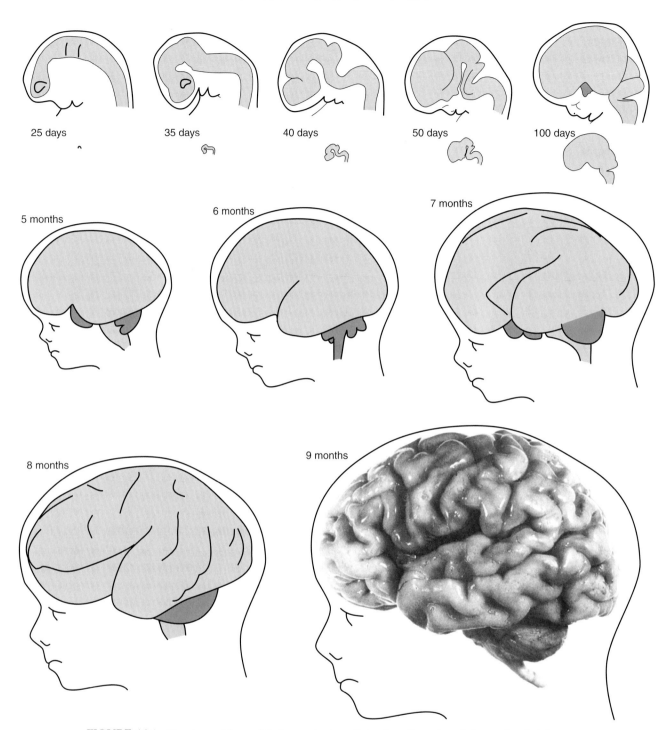

FIGURE 46.1   The size and form of the human brain as it develops through gestation and early infancy.

differentiation, synaptic development, synaptic pruning, cell death and/or the selective elimination of neuronal processes. Glial processes also critically participate in normal development, supporting cell proliferation, differentiation and guidance, and the formation of myelin sheets around axons.

The Cortex Thickens during Development

Development of the cortical mantle in the human brain was documented extensively in the classic studies of Conel (1939–1963). The primary visual cortex increases in thickness until around the 6th postnatal month, when it attains values observed in adults. Cell densities and overall structure are also mature by this time. In contrast, other cortical areas, including visual association areas, display a long and variable increase in cortical thickness that approaches maturity around 10 years after birth. Longitudinal neuroimaging studies in large samples of children (Giedd *et al.*, 1999) have shown changes in volume of cortical gray matter that are nonlinear and regionally specific. Volume of gray matter in the frontal and parietal lobes increases during preadolescence with a maximum occurring around 11–12 years of age, followed by a decline in post-adolescence. Temporal lobe gray matter also follows a nonlinear developmental course, but maximum volume is not reached until 16 years, with a slight decline thereafter. Although neuroimaging techniques lack the resolution necessary to identify the specific structural modifications that underlie changes in cortical volume during development (i.e., cell number, synapse density, myelination), they do indicate that development of the human cerebral cortex is highly dynamic over time and varies across different cortical areas.

Dendritic Spine Number Increases during Development

The formation of dendritic spines and the time course of changes in the length and branching patterns of dendrites have been described for visual and frontal cortical areas in humans. Within the visual cortex, peak spine density is achieved around 5 months of age; this number then decreases until adult values are obtained around 21 months of age. Progressive elongation of dendrites occurs up to 24 months. Thus, during the period from 5 to 24 months, the major event may be a decrease in spine density rather than an actual decline in total spine number. Dendritic development in the visual system reaches mature levels in deep cortical layers earlier than in superficial layers, displaying the "inside-out" pattern of development that is characteristic of neurogenesis and migration (Chapter 15).

Development and maturation of the frontal cortex proceed more slowly. Whereas neuronal density in the primary visual cortex (V1) reaches adult levels by 4–5 months, neuronal density in the frontal cortex has still not reached adult levels by 7 years of age. Additionally, by 2 years of age, the dendritic length in frontal cortex (which is mature by 18–24 months in V1) is only half that found in adults. Left–right asymmetries exist in the dendritic branching patterns of pyramidal neurons within layer V of the inferior frontal and anterior precentral cortex. During the first year, growth is more advanced on the right side, but by 6–8 years of age, the maturation of distal dendrites on the left exceeds that of the right.

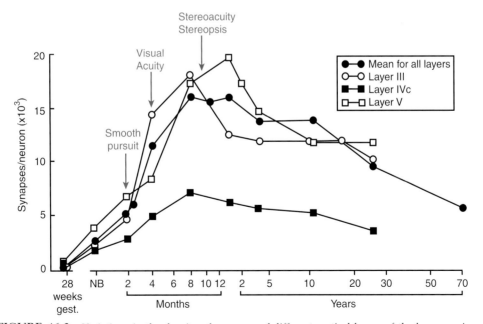

FIGURE 46.2 Variations in the density of synapses of different cortical layers of the human primary visual cortex during development. Arrows point to the emergence of various visual functions in relation to the increase in synapses in the visual cortex. NB, newborn. Adapted with permission from Huttenlocher and De Courten (1987).

Synapses First Increase and Then Decrease in Number

As in the brains of other animals (Chapter 20), the immature human brain contains many more synapses than the mature brain (Huttenlocher, 1990). Within the primary visual cortex, synaptic density increases gradually during late gestation and early postnatal life; it then displays a steep increase from 2 to 4 months of age, during which period the density doubles. After 1 year of age, however, there is a decline in synaptic density until adult values (50–60% of the maximum) are attained at about 11 years of age. The time course of the decrease in synaptic density varies within different cortical layers (see Fig. 46.2). The decrease does not display the "inside-out" pattern of development; rather, there is a considerable decrease, over time, in the number of synapses in every layer.

The other cortical area for which data on synaptogenesis are available in humans is the middle frontal gyrus (layer III). This area also shows a postnatal increase in synaptic density followed by a decrease, but these changes take place over a longer time course in the frontal cortex than in the primary visual cortex (see Fig. 46.3). The maximum density of synapses occurs around 1 year of age (compared to 4 months in the visual cortex). Adult values are not obtained until around 16 years of age (compared to 7–11 years for the visual cortex). Overall synaptic density in mature humans is greater in the frontal and motor cortex than in the visual cortex.

In summary, these quantitative anatomical results suggest that, in contrast to other animals (Chapter 19), programmed cell death plays only a limited role in human brain development. Synapse elimination in humans and other primates exceeds that observed in many species, however, suggesting that modifications in synaptic connectivity may be particularly important for the development of complex nervous systems. Current findings are consistent with a role for incoming afferent input in selectively stabilizing functional synapses and in eliminating or suppressing inactive contacts. The exuberant connectivity observed during development may also support compensatory processes in cases of early brain trauma, allowing surviving synapses to assume functions normally subserved by damaged inputs.

Postnatal Refinement of Synaptic Contacts Occurs in the Neostriatum and Hippocampus as Well

Although the morphological development of certain subcortical structures, such as the thalamus and cerebellum, is nearly complete at birth, other structures continue to mature into early postnatal life.

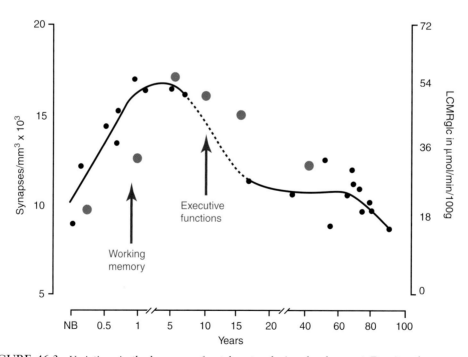

FIGURE 46.3 Variations in the human prefrontal cortex during development: Density of synapses in layer III of the medial frontal gyrus (black circles) and resting glucose uptake (LCMRglc) in the frontal cortex (blue circles). Arrows point to the approximate periods of emergence of various prefrontal cortex functions. NB, newborn. Adapted with permission from Huttenlocker (1990) and Chugani et al. (1993).

In the neostriatum, synaptic density continues to increase until the end of the first postnatal month, and changes in neuronal and neuropil morphology are observed until 2–4 months postnatally. Refinement of synaptic contacts proceeds until the end of the first postnatal year when the striatal neurochemical mosaic attains adult characteristics. In the hippocampus, neurons have reached their destination at birth, although the development of dendrites and the formation of synapses continue for several postnatal years. Indeed continued dendritic remodeling in the hippocampus has been observed as late as the 5th postnatal year in humans (Seress, 2001).

Axons Myelinate during Development

Myelination involves the formation of a sheath of myelin membranes around the axons. Growth of the cerebral white matter lags behind that of the cortical cell layers during fetal development and continues postnatally long after the gray matter has reached its definitive volume (Yakovlev and Lecours, 1967). Both morphological and neuroimaging studies show that myelination proceeds rapidly within the brain up to 2 years of age. The process slows markedly after 2 years, although fibers to the association areas of the brain continue to myelinate well into the 3rd or 4th decade of life. In general, myelination progresses from caudal to cephalic. Thus, the brain stem myelinates prior to the cerebellum and basal ganglia. Similarly, the cerebellum and basal ganglia myelinate prior to the cerebral hemispheres. Sensory and motor systems display mature myelination within the first 2 years of life. However, nonspecific thalamic radiations do not reach mature levels until 5–7 years of age, and intracortical fibers continue their myelination processes well into the 3rd decade of life. Numerous morphological studies have demonstrated that the corpus callosum is uniformly thin in the first month postnatally. The genu and then the splenium undergo rapid growth spurts during the next 5 months, resulting in their characteristic "bulbous" appearance.

Cerebral Metabolic Rate Increases and Then Decreases after Birth

Increases in neuronal activity have been linked to increases in cerebral metabolism, as measured by neuroimaging techniques. Data show substantial subcortical activation in newborns, notably in the thalamus and phylogenetically old portions of the cerebellum, but little activation of the cerebral cortex. However, over the first 3–4 years of life, the cortical metabolic rate increases until it reaches levels twice those observed in adults. After 4 years of age, metabolic

activity decreases gradually until adult levels are reached, around age 15. The time course of the rise and decline of activity, as revealed by positron emission tomography (PET), varies from one cortical region to the other but parallels the rise and decline in the number of synapses in these cortical regions, sug-

A

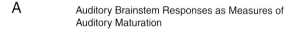

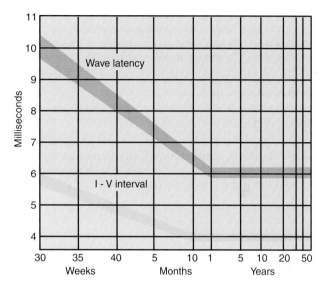

B

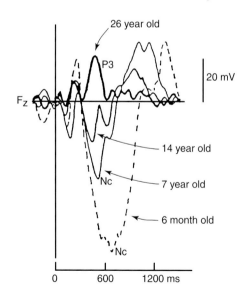

FIGURE 46.4 Changes in electrophysiological activity of the brain (Holcombe *et al.*, 1992). (A) Declines over the first year of life in the latency of components of the auditory ERP that are generated by subcortical structures. (B) Changes in the ERP waveform at varying ages. The later components generated by cortical structures change dramatically as development progresses (for a discussion of the ERP method, see Chapter 49, Box 49.1).

gesting that the exuberant cortical synapses observed during development are metabolically active. As these synapses are eliminated, metabolic activity decreases.

Electrophysiological Activity also Undergoes Postnatal Change

Averaged scalp recordings [event-related potentials (ERPs)] largely reflect postsynaptic potentials of apical dendrites. These recordings show a highly variable and protracted course of brain development in their response to sensory and cognitive processing (Courchesne, 1990). Measures of brain stem and thalamic electrical activity (e.g., auditory brain stem responses) reveal rapid decreases in latency from 30 weeks of gestation onward that attain adult values by 2 years of age. In contrast, the early cortical sensory responses (the N100-P200 vertex potential or N1-P2) do not appear mature until around 13–15 years of age (Fig. 46.4). In addition, several of the later ERP events (P300 and N400) linked to cognitive functions, such as attention and language, do not display a mature pattern until even later, at 15–20 years of age.

Dorsolateral Prefrontal Cortex Is One of the Last Brain Regions to Develop

In the dorsolateral prefrontal cortex, there is a spurt of growth and differentiation of pyramidal neurons and inhibitory interneurons, which involves morphological changes in the dendrites. Synaptic density reaches adult values shortly after birth, but there is a further postnatal increase that plateaus between 1 and 2 years at 150% of levels observed in adult. The number of synapses per neuron also increases during this period. These changes are accompanied by a spurt of increasing glucose uptake in the dorsolateral prefrontal cortex during the same period (Fig. 46.3). The expression of neurotransmitter receptors in the monkey dorsolateral prefrontal cortex, as measured by quantitative receptor autoradiography, also appears to undergo a distinctive pattern of postnatal development. Whereas the density of dopaminergic receptors in this region is low at birth, it increases to reach a peak around 2 months of age and then declines progressively to adult levels around the age of 3 years.

Refinement in the circuit organization of the dorsolateral prefrontal cortex, like that of the hippocampal formation (see earlier discussion), continues until quite late in development. In the case of the dorsolateral prefrontal cortex, a gradual decline in synaptic density continues well into late adolescence and suggests that connectivity in this cortical region undergoes substantial change until 15–20 years of age. It is believed that changes in the neuromodulatory effects

of dopamine may influence the adolescent refinement of excitatory and inhibitory inputs to layer III pyramidal neurons and that dopamine may have a particularly strong influence on cortical information processing around the time of puberty (for the relevance of this late prefrontal cortex development in the emergence of psychopathologic states, such as schizophrenia, see the section on pathological processes).

Brain Development Differs in Boys and Girls

Structural neuroimaging investigations in normal children and adolescents demonstrate that the brains of boys and girls develop differently (Giedd et al., 1996). When adjusted for total cerebral volume, basal ganglia show sex differences in mean volume such that the caudate is relatively larger in females and the globus pallidus is larger in males. The volume of the amygdala and hippocampus increases for both sexes, with the amygdala volume increasing significantly more in males than females and hippocampal volume increasing more in females. Many sex differences in brain structure and function result from the differential exposure of males and females to the sex steroid hormones (testosterone in males, estradiol and progesterone in females). These hormones play an important role in regulating plastic changes in neuronal structure and function throughout development and adulthood.

Summary

Structural, metabolic, and physiological indices of human brain development all point to a long postnatal time course that displays considerable variability from region to region and from system to system. Thus, while postnatal development in the hippocampus proceeds until approximately 4–5 years of age, it continues until 7–11 years for the visual cortex and until around 16 years of age for the frontal cortical areas. The dorsolateral portion of the prefrontal cortex appears to be one of the last regions of the brain to develop. Interestingly, the development of myelin has been observed as late as the 3rd to 4th decade of life for fibers within the association areas of the neocortex.

COGNITIVE DEVELOPMENT AND AGING: A LIFE SPAN PERSPECTIVE

Investigators are now attempting to link the types of neural changes described in the preceding section to the maturation of sensory, behavioral, and cognitive capacities in infants and children. At present, such studies are limited in number. Until recently, the predominant view was that postnatal development of the cortex is largely intrinsically determined. However, new studies of both animals and humans have revealed a central role for extrinsic factors in shaping the organization of neural systems and in permitting recovery from brain damage. Indeed, calculations showing that information in the genome is not sufficient to specify the connectivity of the brain, together with evidence for the long-lasting existence of transient, redundant connections in primates, suggest that neural changes under the influence of environmental input play a significant and persistent role in the development of the functional specificity of the human brain.

Cognitive Development in the First Years of Life

Early Subcortical Behavioral Responses Are Inhibited by Cortical Development

The increasing metabolic rate observed in basal ganglia and many cortical regions during the second and third postnatal months is correlated with several organizational changes that occur in the infant brain during this period. During this period, the frequency of several subcortical reflexes (e.g., the tonic neck reflex, the grasp reflex, as well as the frequency of endogeneous smiles and spontaneous crying) decreases, presumably as a consequence of increased cortical drive on the brain stem centers that control these reflexes. A similar mechanism may underlie the observation that the risk of sudden infant death syndrome peaks during this postnatal interval. Specifically, this syndrome is thought to be associated with a developmentally regulated increase in cortical inhibition of the brain stem centers that control normal respiration.

Anatomical Development of the Visual System in Infants Is Linked to Functional Development

Several parallels have been noted between anatomical changes and the emergence of function in human visual systems. Looking preferences are used to examine visual functions in infancy. To study acuity, for example, infants are given a choice between two displays that differ in some way such as spatial frequency by varying the thickness of stripes. Preference for one of the two patterns, measured by the time spent looking at each of the stimuli, reflects the infant's capacity for discriminating between the items.

The visual abilities of the newborn have been linked to subcortical structures that show mature anatomy and high metabolic rates during this period.

The limited visual abilities of the newborn are augmented by the appearance of smooth pursuit tracking around 6–8 weeks. The emergence of this capacity may be related to the maturation of cortical layers IV, V, and VI in V1 (see Fig. 46.2). These layers connect magnocellular afferents from the lateral geniculate nucleus and the middle temporal (MT) region, a pathway important for visual movement. Visual acuity and visual alertness increase dramatically around 4 months of age, when the volume of visual cortex reaches adult levels and the highest density of synapses is present. Shortly thereafter, cortically mediated binocular interactions become apparent. These interactions, which include stereoacuity, binocular summation of the light reflex, and stereopsis (binocular depth perception), appear in the same time frame as maturation of the middle cortical layers and rapid synaptogenesis in V1. This period of rapid growth appears to be a time of increased vulnerability to altered afferent input. Strabismic amblyopia and amblyopia due to the absence of patterned input (i.e., centrally mediated visual impairments) are reported to occur at this age unless corrected early. The time period during which visual impairments can be corrected is different for different visual functions. For example, correction for an absent lens (aphakia) due to cataracts may be completely effective only when performed prior to 2 months of age, i.e., just prior to the onset of exuberant synaptogenesis in V1. However, very high synaptic density persists to at least the age of 4 years in V1. The presence of this extensive connectivity may account for the ability to recover from amblyopia (with forced use of the strabismic eye) during this time. If the disruption of binocular convergence by strabismus is not corrected within the first year of life, the ability to see stereoscopically may not develop even though the development of acuity and contrast sensitivity is normal. Thus, there may be separate critical periods for the development of resolution acuity and stereopsis. Because the parvocellular system is thought to underlie acuity, whereas disparity detection is mediated by the magnocellular system, the magnocellular system may be more modifiable by environmental input than the parvocellular system. This differential sensitivity may be due to the slower maturation of the magnocellular system and/or to differences in the number of exuberant synapses within these systems.

Studies of individuals born deaf and blind suggest that in humans, as in other animals, there is a time period when cortical areas that normally process information from the deprived modality can be reorganized to process information from intact modalities. From the alteration of visual functions seen in indi-

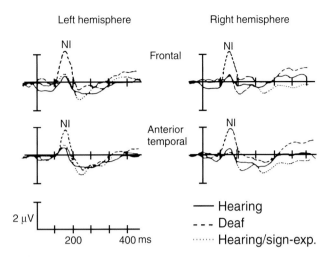

Left hemisphere   Right hemisphere

NI   Frontal   NI

NI   Anterior temporal   NI

2 μV

200   400 ms

—— Hearing
- - - Deaf
······ Hearing/sign-exp.

FIGURE 46.5 Visual-evoked potentials to peripheral stimuli recorded from congenitally deaf subjects and from hearing subjects who had early exposure to sign language (hearing/sign-exposed) and those who did not. Only deaf subjects showed enhanced ERPs over temporal areas (Neville *et al.*, 1983).

viduals born deaf, it appears that areas of the auditory cortex have been recruited for visual function (see Fig. 46.5). Deaf subjects, by comparison, show abnormally strong electrical responses to peripheral visual stimuli. These responses are not found in normally hearing individuals, even those exposed to sign language by deaf parents. The prolonged persistence of exuberant cortico-cortico connections may provide the substrate for such cortical reorganization.

Development of the Ventral Visual Stream and Object Representation

A multitude of visual cortical areas located in the striate and extrastriate cortex contribute to different aspects of visual processing (Chapter 47). These visual areas have been divided into two visual processing systems, one coursing ventrally from the striate and extrastriate areas to the ventrolateral temporal cortex and the other coursing dorsally from the striate and extrastriate cortex to the parietal cortex. The dorsal stream mediates spatial processing associated with attention to movement and location, whereas the ventral stream is involved primarily in processing information about patterns and objects. Both streams project rostrally, each reaching common and adjacent areas of the prefrontal cortex.

Major functions of the ventral stream include the ability both to segment a pattern into a set of constituent parts (local level of processing) and to integrate those parts into a coherent whole (global level of processing). In adults, systematic differences exist in the distribution of global and local levels of processing within the brain, such that global levels of pro-

cessing are associated with the right posterior temporal region and local levels of processing with the left posterior temporal regions. Around 4 months of age, infants show hemispheric differences for global and local processing that are similar to the hemispheric differences observed in the adults. Thus, at this age, children segment out well-formed units and use simple associations to organize these units into a configuration. With further maturation, children show changes in the way they decompose objects into parts and in the relations that they use to organize the parts. These changes may reflect the protracted development of the posterior temporal cortical areas, a finding consistent with ERP studies in human infants indicating functional activation within the temporal cortical areas around 6 months of age. The latter observation parallels the emergence, around the same age, of object representation and visual rule learning (Alvarado and Bachevalier, 2000).

Development of the Dorsal Visual Stream and Spatial Attention

A variety of spatial processes have been associated with activation of the dorsal visual pathway, such as the processing of information about spatial attention and spatial location (Chapter 48). Considerable clinical and experimental evidence show that the posterior parietal lobes play a crucial role in the ability to shift attention to different spatial locations. By at least 6 months of age, infants, like adults, show facilitated stimulus detection as a function of prior cueing, i.e., they take less time to detect an object if it is presented in a box that has been cued previously. They also demonstrate, as do adults, that the detection of the target is quicker when the interval between the cue and the target is short than when this interval is long. While this basic attentional response may be robust as early as 4 months of age, the timing parameters that elicit the responses may change with development, suggesting that further maturational processes occur in the parietal cortex.

Early Development of Recognition Memory as a Precursor of Declarative Memory

Looking preference has been used to study the emergence of recognition memory abilities in both human infants and infant monkeys (Alvarado and Bachevalier, 2000). In both species, the most common procedure is to first present the infant with an attractive stimulus for a period of time (generally 20 to 30 s). After an intervening delay that can vary from a few seconds to many hours, the familiar stimulus is shown together with a new item. Human infants as young as 1 day old display a strong preference for looking at the novel object with delays as long as 24 h, demonstrating that they recognize the previously presented item as familiar. This early emergence of recognition memory has also been observed in infant monkeys, and, in this species, surgical removal of the hippocampal formation and adjacent tissue before the age of 3 weeks abolishes this memory ability. These findings point to the importance of these limbic structures for recognition memory early in development.

The early emergence of recognition memory is consistent with what is currently known about maturation of the hippocampal formation in both humans and monkeys (see earlier discussion). In both species, the hippocampal formation is almost adult-like at birth, although there are a number of postnatal morphological refinements that continue until the end of the first year in monkeys and until about 4–5 years of age in humans. These protracted modifications in hippocampal circuitry, together with the further maturation of cortical areas in the temporal and prefrontal lobes, may in turn support the emergence of spatial and relational memory abilities (Chapters 51 and 53) around 1 year of age in monkeys and 4–5 years of age in humans.

Orientation to Faces, Recognition of Mother's Face, and Imitation of Facial Expressions Are Present at Birth

The human face is a powerful visual source of social information, and the development of face-processing abilities appears to follow a delayed postnatal development. Newborns preferentially orient to faces, recognize the mother and other familiar faces, and imitate facial expressions. These precocious tendencies appear to be mediated by a subcortical retinotectal pathway. For example, newborns display preferences selectively for moving stimuli presented in the peripheral visual field (i.e., under conditions that engage the subcortical systems), but not when they are displayed in the central visual field.

The fact that newborns just hours to days after birth look longer at the mother's face than a stranger's face (even when cues from her smell and voice are eliminated) indicates that, from very early on, there is a mechanism capable of learning about individual faces based on experience. This early learning system may be mediated by the hippocampal formation, as this area is known to be involved in memory and it matures early relative to memory-related neocortical areas (see earlier discussion). Nevertheless, the face-processing abilities of the newborn are qualitatively different than the sophisticated capacities present in the adult, and none of these tendencies are necessarily the direct precursors of the cortically mediated, adult face-processing system (Chapter 47). Instead, these responses might serve the purpose of providing input to developing cortical circuits that will at some later time functionally emerge to mediate face processing.

At 3 Months of Age Infants Are Able to Form Categories of Visual Stimuli

A marked change in infants' visual attention to faces occurs at approximately 8 weeks of age. At this time, infants' preferential following of peripheral moving faces declines, and a preference emerges for fixating faces compared to other patterns presented in the central visual field. This behavioral change is thought to be due to the functional development of visual cortical pathways that inhibit the preferential following response and mediate the new preferential fixation response. At 2 months of age, infants become more sensitive to the internal facial features of static faces. In addition, within the face, the eyes are a more salient feature of the face than the nose or mouth, but where the eyes are located is immaterial to the babies' preference for face-like drawings. Furthermore, during this age, infants begin to relate information between individual faces and to form categories; i.e., they perceive visual stimuli with comparable features as being more similar than visual stimuli with different features. They also exhibit inversion effects (i.e., recognition of upright faces is easier than recognition of inverted faces). The change between 1 and 3 months has been associated with the functional development of temporal cortical areas and their connections with the hippocampus and adjacent structures. However, at this early age, the change may not be specific to faces, as 3-month-old infants can form perceptual categories of a variety of other complex categories, such as tables and trees.

Hemispheric Differences in Face Processing Emerge Around 4 Months of Age

By 4–9 months, hemispheric differences in face processing emerge, as babies at this age move their eyes more quickly to the mother's face than a stranger's face when the stimuli are presented in the left visual field, but not when they are presented in the right visual field. In contrast, simple geometric shapes are discriminated equally well in either visual field. These results suggest that by this age the right hemisphere may be more proficient than the left in recognizing faces. Finally, during childhood, the child's prototype of the face becomes more tuned to the types of faces that the child sees most often, and with this may emerge race effects and other species effects seen in adult face processing. Other race effects refer to the ability to distinguish among faces of one's own race more quickly than faces of other races. Other species effects refer to the ability to distinguish between human faces more quickly than faces of other species. These last changes may be based on experience due to increased exposure to faces, the number and type of features children attend to and encode, and the maturation of a posterior temporal cortical area (the fusiform area) that is known to be involved in face processing in adults.

Fear of Unfamiliar Faces Emerges between 7 and 9 Months

Although infants are able to discriminate among some facial expressions of emotion by 3 months of age, they do have difficulty discriminating between sadness and surprise. It is only by 7 months of age that infants, like adults, show categorical perception of facial expressions. For example, with pictures of faces in which emotional expressions are progressively degraded from happy to fear, human infants and adults exhibit more accurate discrimination for pictures of faces that cross emotional categories (happy versus fear) than for pictures of faces within the same emotional category, despite equal physical differences in the pictures. With this increased ability to categorize faces, and the increased exposure to familiar faces, two remarkable events occur between 7–9 months of age: the emergence of fear for unfamiliar people and anxiety during temporary separation from the caretaker. Distress under both conditions must involve more than the ability to discriminate strangers from parents because 3 month-olds can make this discrimination, but do not show fear reactions.

One speculation concerning the phenomena of stranger and separation fear is that improvements in working memory, and an enhanced ability to retrieve memories of a past event, are required for the appearance of fear reactions. This change appears to be associated with the maturation of the orbital frontal cortex (Schore, 1996), a region of the prefrontal cortex intimately interconnected with limbic areas in the temporal lobe (temporal pole cortex and amygdala), with subcortical drive centers in the hypothalamus, and with dopamine neurons in reward centers in the ventral tegmental area. By the end of the first year, the initial phase of orbital frontal maturation is achieved and allows for developmental advances that enable the individual to react to situations on the basis of stored representations, rather than on information immediately present in the environment. In the case of the orbital frontal cortex, this capacity applies specifically to socioemotional information. Indeed, by

10 months, infants are first able to construct and store abstract prototypes of human visual facial patterns, and can use these prototypes to evaluate novel information.

For example, a preferential looking paradigm was used to habituate 10-month-old infants to pictures of faces. One condition presented faces of different females, and in the other condition, the same female face was presented in various poses. After infants habituated to the stimuli (i.e., decreased their looking), they were given two test trials: one with a face of a familiar female and another with a face of a novel female. When infants were previously habituated using different female faces, they spent equivalent amounts of time gazing at familiar and novel faces on the test trials. However, when infants were habituated to the same face with different poses, they generalized their looking response to the familiar face but dishabituated (or looked longer) at the novel face. This pattern of results suggests that infants can abstract relevant categorical information by 10 month of age.

Changes in Visual Search Are Related to Development of the Prefrontal Cortex

Infants younger than 7 or 8 months of age will not uncover a hidden object. If a cloth is thrown over a toy while an infant of 5 or 6 months is reaching for it, the infant will withdraw his or her hand and stop reaching. By 7 or 8 months, most infants who watch an object being hidden can retrieve it. However, if the infant then watches as the object is hidden at a second location, most infants of 7–8 months search for the object at its first hiding location, which is now empty. Jean Piaget called this the A-not-B error because the infant is correct at the first hiding place (A) but not at the second (B). It is rare to see this error when there is no delay between when the object is hidden and when the infant is allowed to reach. However, a delay as brief as 1, 2, or 3 s is sufficient to produce the error in infants 7–8 months of age. As they grow older, the error is still seen, but only if the delay between hiding and retrieval is increased. The A-not-B error suggests that during the second half of the first year the brain has matured sufficiently to enable the infant to hold a representation of the object's location in mind (working memory) for a few seconds (Chapter 54) or to understand the relationship of (a) their previous action of retrieving the object, (b) the subsequent hiding of the object in a different location (even though they observed the hiding), and (c) the object's present whereabouts (Diamond, 1990). The enhanced working memory observed in the 7- to 10-month-old infant parallels the protracted maturation and refinement of dorsolateral prefrontal cortex circuitry (see Fig. 46.3). After 12 months of age, it is difficult to elicit the A-not-B error.

Language Undergoes Rapid but Prolonged Development

In humans, the prolonged structural, metabolic, and neurophysiological maturation of "association" cortical areas, which continues well into adolescence, provides the substrate for the panoply of higher cognitive functions that continue to develop during this time. Attempts have been made to link the very rapid development of speech and language skills over the first 3 years of life to these general changes. This goal has remained elusive, probably because so many aspects of the brain and behavior are changing together. Moreover, key elements of language appear to be processed at cellular and synaptic levels of organization that are difficult to investigate in humans with even the most sophisticated techniques available.

There is wide agreement that language is strongly dependent on structures within the left perisylvian region (Chapter 52). Very early on (by 28 weeks of gestation), structural asymmetries appear between the temporal lobes; these may provide the substrate for the functional asymmetries that appear later. The rapid and early acquisition of phonological information and speech production and comprehension, and the subsequent burst in size of the vocabulary, may be linked to the rapid rise in the number of synapses and the marked increases in cortical metabolism that occur during the second year of life. Also, the persistence of large numbers of exuberant synapses through adolescence may provide the anatomical substrate for prolonged neural plasticity and recovery of language skills following cortical damage in the first decade of life. It is well established that language skills can display considerable recovery following large lesions to the left hemisphere during the first 7–10 years of life. The impressive recovery of language skills in children in whom the left hemisphere has been removed is even more striking in light of the enduring language impairment of specifically language-impaired children or reading difficulties encountered by dyslexics, in whom macroscopic aspects of brain structure are basically normal. These findings underscore the importance of characterizing microscopic structural aspects of the brain and the functional organization of the brain in relation to processing.

The prolonged time course of development that may confer plasticity on the immature brain appears to be characterized by optimal or critical periods (Chapter 21) for language acquisition. Several studies report that both first and second language acquisi-

tions are impaired and cerebral organization is altered when language is acquired after the first decade of life. Moreover, as has been observed for vision (see Fig. 46.2), different aspects of language appear to display different critical periods. Vocabulary items can be acquired long past the first decade of life, but the grammatical rules of a language appear to be acquired most readily before the age of 10. Along with other evidence, this pattern suggests that different neural systems, with differing developmental time courses, mediate these various aspects of language.

Summary

Cognitive development parallels some of the most important changes in brain development. Thus, the visual abilities of the newborn are limited and mediated by subcortical functions. With the maturation of visual cortical areas in the first few postnatal months, visual acuity, visual alertness, and stereopsis develop. With further development of visual cortical areas within the temporal lobe, an infant's ability to recognize faces using internal facial features, mostly the eye region, emerges around 3 months of age. However, it is only by 7–9 months of age that infants develop fear for unfamiliar people. It is believed that this behavior is associated with the development, around this age, of the orbital frontal cortex, a cortical area that enables the infant to react to situations on the basis of stored representations (working memory). The enhanced spatial working memory abilities observed by the middle of the first year parallel the protracted maturation and refinement of the dorsolateral prefrontal circuitry. Finally, the maturation of association areas of the cortex, which continues well into adolescence, provides the substrate for the development of higher cognitive functions, such as language. In the future, it will be possible to analyze the neural basis of cognition in increasing detail by using high-resolution methods for imaging brain structure and function in normally developing children and children with specific structural or functional deficits.

Cognitive Aging

Average Human Life Expectancy Has Increased Dramatically

The world's population is growing older. Whereas life expectancy in the United States was approximately 50 years in 1900, infant mortality rates decreased dramatically during the last century, and combined with advances in disease treatment and prevention, current life expectancy is approaching 80 years in most industrialized countries. A significant consequence of these and other demographic trends is that the percentage of the population over 65 years of age is projected to double over the next several decades, with the most rapid growth occurring among those over 85. Neurodegenerative disorders such as Alzheimer's disease are among the most devastating and feared consequences of advanced age (see section on Dementia, this chapter). There is increasing recognition, however, that many otherwise healthy aged individuals experience deficits in memory and other aspects of cognitive function that, although relatively modest in severity, significantly compromise the quality of life. The following sections outline key concepts that have emerged from the study of normal cognitive aging in the absence of frank disease.

Effects of Normal Aging on Memory in Humans Are Variable

A theme developed throughout Section VII of this volume is that cognition encompasses a variety of dissociable capacities, such as perception, attention, executive function, and memory. Long viewed as primarily psychological constructs, it is now accepted that different domains of cognitive function are dissociable at a neurobiological level of analysis and are mediated by partially distinct neural circuitry. This organization yields a valuable framework for the study of cognitive aging. In particular, through careful analyses aimed at documenting the specific types and severity of cognitive deficits that accompany aging, neuropsychological research has provided important clues about the brain systems that are likely to mediate dysfunction. This strategy has been most widely exploited to examine the effects of normal aging on learning and memory, where a rich background of information is available concerning the characteristics of impairment that follows damage to selective brain regions in young adults.

An important concept to emerge from studies in humans and animal models is that the effect of aging on the type of memory mediated by the hippocampal formation and related medial temporal lobe structures is highly variable among older individuals. As detailed in Chapter 51, the integrity of this system is critical for establishing a consciously accessible record of ongoing experience; a domain of function termed explicit, episodic, or declarative memory. Figure 46.6 illustrates the results of a study documenting the effect of aging on this form of memory in healthy individuals ranging from roughly 35 to 90 years of age using a test of delayed recall as an assessment instrument. A central feature of this investigation is that, prior to neuropsychological testing, subjects

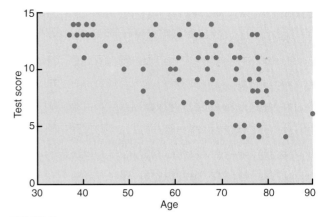

FIGURE 46.6 Scores for young adults and optimally healthy aged human subjects on a test of delayed recall that requires the integrity of the medial temporal lobe memory system. Note that although there is a significant overall decline with age, performance is highly variable across aged individuals. Data courtesy of M.S. Albert, Massachusett General Hospital, Harvard University.

were screened carefully to exclude individuals with a history of neurological impairment, major depression, cardiovascular disease, or other conditions that can influence memory function. In this way, the aim was to document the effects of normal aging on declarative memory in optimally healthy elderly individuals in the absence of disease. The findings illustrate two key points. On average, memory declines significantly as a function of age. This decline is shown in Fig. 46.6 by the increase in lower recall scores for many individuals over 60 years of age relative to younger adults. Equally noteworthy, there is marked variability among aged individuals such that, even at 80 years of age, some people retain levels of memory function comparable to much younger subjects. These findings suggest the important conclusion that marked deterioration in memory is not an inescapable consequence of aging and that in a substantial proportion of aged individuals, the functional integrity of the medial temporal lobe system is preserved. The next section considers related research conducted in animal models, where it is feasible to ask what neurobiological alterations might account for individual differences in normal cognitive aging.

Animal Models of Cognitive and Neurobiological Aging

Research on aging in animal models has taken advantage of testing procedures that have been useful for understanding the neurobiology of learning and memory in young adult subjects. In the widely used spatial, or "place," version of the Morris water maze, for example, rats learn across a series of trials the location of an escape platform hidden in a pool of clouded water. As described in Chapter 51, normal adult rats solve this procedure by learning and remembering the escape location in relation to the configuration of cues surrounding the testing apparatus, and this capacity requires the functional integrity of the hippocampal formation. Guided by this background, many laboratories have used the Morris water maze and other tests of spatial information processing to examine the effects of aging on learning and memory that are mediated by the hippocampal system (see Gallagher *et al.*, 1993).

In gerontological research, rats are generally considered "aged" at approximately 24–28 months of age, roughly equivalent to humans in their 70s. Numerous behavioral investigations have demonstrated that, relative to young adults, aged rats are significantly slower to learn the hidden platform location in the place version of the water maze. Although these findings are consistent with a possible hippocampal contribution to cognitive aging, an important alternative to consider is that impaired visual acuity, motor function, or other factors could account for the water maze deficits observed in older subjects. One means of addressing this possibility involves the use of control testing procedures that make many of the same sensory, motor, and motivational demands as the hidden platform task, but that lack a spatial learning component. In a common variant of the water maze, for example, rats are tested for their ability to swim to a platform that protrudes above the surface of the water and provides a salient visual goal that animals can navigate toward in order to escape. Because the position of the cued platform is varied randomly across trials, learning and memory for spatial information are not required. Many aged rats acquire this task normally, demonstrating that they can swim as rapidly as young adults and are motivated to escape (Gallagher *et al.*, 1993). Thus, although certain aspects of motor and visual function are indeed susceptible to age-related decline, these impairments fail to explain the deficits that aged rats exhibit in the spatial version of the water maze. Rather, the overall profile that emerges during aging—impaired learning and memory for spatial information against a background of intact goal-approach learning—is qualitatively similar to the effects of damage to the hippocampal system in young subjects. Research using other testing procedures confirms that learning and memory mediated by the hippocampus and related brain structures are susceptible to an age-related decline (Gallagher and Rapp, 1997).

Earlier in this chapter it was emphasized that memory decline during normal human aging is variable and that a substantial proportion of individuals

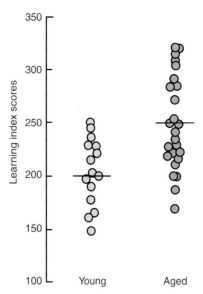

FIGURE 46.7 Learning scores for young adult and aged rats on a water maze test of spatial learning that requires the hippocampus. This measure of performance reflects the average distance of an animal from the goal location over the course of testing, and lower scores reflect better learning. Note that although the performance of the aged group is worse than for the younger cohort (compare group means represented by the horizontal bars), there is substantial variability among the aged rats and about half learn as well as young adults. Data courtesy of M. Gallagher, Johns Hopkins University.

retain levels of functioning on a par with younger adults. The same appears to be true in vertebrate animal models. Figure 46.7 illustrates learning scores obtained in the spatial version of the water maze for 15 adult rats and a sample of 25 aged animals. The specific measure of performance displayed in Fig. 46.7 reflects each rat's average cumulative distance from the escape platform, assessed over multiple trials during the course of learning. Therefore, low scores represent more accurate searching focused on the escape location. Similar to the results for humans presented in Fig. 46.6, spatial learning scores for aged rats are distributed continuously across a broad range such that some perform as well as even the most proficient young subjects. By comparison, approximately half of the older animals exhibit marked deficits, scoring outside the range of the young adult group.

Variability in the cognitive effects of aging has been documented in other animal models as well. The neuropsychology of aging in nonhuman primates has been examined using testing procedures adopted from studies on the effects of medial temporal lobe damage in young adult monkeys (Chapter 51). In the delayed nonmatching to sample task, subjects are tested for their ability to recognize a visual stimulus across delay intervals ranging from seconds to many minutes or more. Young adult monkeys with sufficiently extensive damage to any component of the medial temporal lobe memory system display significant deficits on this task, particularly when the memory demands are increased by lengthening the retention interval. Recognition memory also declines during aging in the monkey, and as in humans and rats, the degree of impairment varies substantially across individual subjects. Variability in the cognitive effect of aging has sometimes been considered a complicating or nuisance factor in gerontological research that makes it difficult to draw firm conclusions about the consequences of growing older. As discussed in the next section, however, the current perspective is that this variability makes it possible to ask what neurobiological alterations distinguish the brains of individuals with age-related memory impairment from other age-matched subjects with preserved function. By this approach the aim is to identify those changes in the structure and physiology of the aged brain that are specifically coupled to individual differences in the cognitive outcome of normal aging.

Neurobiology of Age-Related Memory Decline

Age-Related Learning and Memory Impairment Is Associated with Compromised Hippocampal Physiology

Behavioral studies suggest that the functional integrity of the hippocampal system declines during aging. Electrophysiological investigations extend these observations by directly assessing the functional and computational properties of the aged hippocampus. Models of learning-related cellular plasticity, such as long-term potentiation (LTP; Chapter 50), have been particularly well-characterized in the hippocampus. These normative findings establish a useful background against which to explore the effects of aging. A prominent theme is that aging influences hippocampal physiology in a highly selective manner and that many properties of hippocampal function are spared (reviewed in Barnes, 2001). Significant parameters that exhibit little or no change in older subjects include the resting potential, the input resistance, and the amplitude and duration of evoked action potentials of principal hippocampal neurons. By comparison, other aspects of cellular physiology are reliably compromised. For example, although the peak magnitude of LTP is comparable in the young adult and aged hippocampus, the intensity and frequency of stimulation necessary to achieve that response increase with advanced age. Once established, LTP also decays to prepotentiated baseline levels more rapidly in aged subjects than in young

animals. This enhanced rate of decay is correlated with the rapid forgetting that aged rats exhibit on tests of spatial memory, consistent with the conclusion that a reduced capacity for synaptic enhancement in the hippocampus contributes to this behavioral deficit.

Electrophysiological studies of ongoing hippocampal neuronal activity in awake-behaving rats shed additional light on how information processing in this structure is affected during normal aging. As described in Chapter 51, a particularly well-characterized phenomenon is that the firing rate of individual hippocampal neurons increases dramatically as animals navigate through a restricted area within a testing environment. This so-called "place field" activity is largely independent of specific behaviors exhibited during exploration, and instead seems to be controlled by geometric relations between the multiple sensory cues that define a particular spatial location. Recapitulating a theme from studies of LTP, many aspects of place field firing remain relatively normal in the aged hippocampus, including the percentage of neurons that exhibit location-specific firing, and the spatial selectivity of place fields. The informational content encoded by the aged hippocampus, however, is reliably altered (Barnes *et al.*, 1997; Tanila *et al.*, 1997a,b). For example, hippocampal pyramidal cells in old rats are abnormally prone to confuse familiar environments that share some of the same stimulus elements, unpredictably engaging the wrong distribution, or "map," of place fields during successive bouts of exploration in a given setting. Related findings demonstrate that hippocampal encoding also becomes increasingly rigid with age such that a relatively narrow subset of available spatial cues comes to control place field activity. Taken together, the significant implication is that aging is accompanied by a reduction in the overall scope of information encoded by the hippocampus. Supporting this interpretation, the severity of abnormalities in place field activity predicts the degree of spatial learning impairment among individual aged rats. Research on the structural integrity of the hippocampus, discussed in the following sections, points to a potential link between the behavioral and electrophysiological consequences of aging.

Early Findings Suggested Neuron Loss Is Distributed Diffusely throughout the Aged Brain

Traditionally, one of the most widely held notions about brain aging is that a substantial number of neurons inevitably die as we grow older. Early studies provided support for this view, suggesting that neuron death occurs throughout life, with the cumulative loss exceeding 50% in many neocortical areas by age 95 (for a history review, see Brody, 1970). While not all regions of the brain seemed to be affected to the same degree, significant age-related neuron loss was reported in every region examined, including both primary sensory and association areas of the cortex. On the basis of these early observations, it seemed reasonable to suppose that widely distributed neuron death might account for many of the cognitive deficits associated with normal aging. A direct experimental test of this proposal has become feasible only recently. One significant concern had been that the finding of widespread neuronal loss might reflect undiagnosed, preclinical dementing disease in an unknown proportion of the aged individuals who were examined. This confound is overcome effectively in studies using animal models of cognitive aging because rats and monkeys do not develop dementia spontaneously. In addition, as described next, robust quantitative methods are now widely available for examining neuron loss in the aged brain.

Memory Impairment during Normal Aging Does Not Require Substantial Hippocampal Neuron Loss

Improved methods for quantifying cell number have led to a significant revision of traditional views on age-related neuron loss (for a detailed discussion, see West, 1993). Until recently, most investigators had focused on cell density, defined as the number of neurons present in a fixed area or volume of tissue. This parameter is measured experimentally by counting the number of neurons in multiple small samples within a brain region of interest. Typically, this is accomplished using standard histological staining procedures to visualize cells microscopically. One then counts stained profiles of cell bodies, nuclei, or nucleoli, either manually or with automated image detection routines. A significant limitation of this approach, however, is that density can vary widely in the absence of any actual difference in cell number. Assume, for example, that total neuron number is identical in a region of interest in two brains, but that the overall size of the brains differs due to normal biological variability among individuals, gliosis, white matter abnormalities, or other neuropil alterations. Under these conditions, average neuron density is likely to be lower in the larger brain, simply as a consequence of the cells being distributed in a larger total volume. In this way, volumetric differences between young and aged brains (whether real or artifacts of differential shrinkage during histological processing) could substantially influence

cell density in the absence of any actual age-related difference in the number of resident neurons. Other limitations of traditional cell counting methods for research on aging have also been recognized (West, 1993).

The field of stereology has provided standardized tools for directly estimating the total number of neurons in any defined brain region, yielding an unequivocal measure for examining potential neuron loss during normal aging (see Box 46.1). This approach has been used most widely in studies of the aged hippocampus. Early studies measuring cell density had suggested that the hippocampus is especially susceptible to age-related cell death and that the magnitude of this neuron loss is greatest among aged individuals with the most pronounced deficits in learning and memory. The surprising conclusion from investigations using modern stereological methods, however, is that the total number of principal neurons (i.e., the granule cells of the dentate gyrus and pyramidal neurons in the CA3 and CA1 fields) is generally preserved in the aged hippocampus. Similar results have been observed in all species examined, including rats, monkeys, and humans. Data from animal models of cognitive aging are particularly compelling, demonstrating that neuron number in the hippocampus remains stable even among aged individuals with pronounced learning and memory deficits indicative of dysfunction in this system. In one study, for example, young and aged rats were behaviorally characterized prior to morphometric analysis using the hippocampus-dependent spatial version of the Morris water maze (Rapp and Gallagher, 1996). As illustrated in Fig. 46.8, subsequent stereological analysis revealed that the total number of principal hippocampal neurons was comparable in young adult subjects and aged rats, regardless of their capacity for spatial learning and memory. Although there is evidence for modest neuron death in other subfields of the hippocampal formation (i.e., the hilar region of the dentate gyrus and the subiculum) in humans, results from lesion studies in young animals provide little basis for supposing that this regionally selective, numerically limited loss could be sufficient to account for the effects of normal aging on memory. Overall, findings indicate that widespread hippocampal neuron loss is not inevitable, as was assumed traditionally, and that age-related impairment in learning and memory can occur in the absence of significant neuron death in the hippocampus. Prompted by these observations, researchers have looked toward changes in synaptic connectivity and other markers of functional deterioration as a more likely basis for normal cognitive aging.

BOX 46.1

THE OPTICAL FRACTIONATOR STEREOLOGICAL METHOD

The figure shows the key features of a new stereological technique designed to provide accurate and efficient estimates of total neuron number in a brain region of interest. The hippocampal formation of the rhesus monkey brain is used as an example. The method consists of counting the number of neurons in a known and representative fraction of a neuroanatomically defined structure in such a way that each cell has an equal probability of being counted. The sum of the neurons counted, multiplied by the reciprocal of the fraction of the structure that was sampled, provides an estimate of total neuron number.

Serial histological sections are prepared through the entire rostrocaudal extent of the hippocampus and are stained by routine methods for visualizing neurons microscopically. An evenly spaced series of the sections is then chosen for analysis (represented schematically by dotted

lines at top left). This first level of sampling, the "section fraction," is therefore defined as the fraction of the total number of sections examined. For example, if every 10th section through the hippocampus is analyzed, the section fraction equals 1/10. The appropriate sections are then surveyed according to a systematic sampling scheme, typically carried out on a microscope with a motorized, computer-controlled stage. The lower right part of the figure illustrates this design in which the microscope stage is moved in even X and Y intervals, and neurons are counted within the areas defined by the small red squares. The second level of the fractionator sampling scheme is therefore the "area fraction," or the fraction of the XY step (XYarea) from which the cell counts are derived ("a" in the inset).

The last level of sampling is counting cells only within a known fraction of the total section thickness, avoiding a

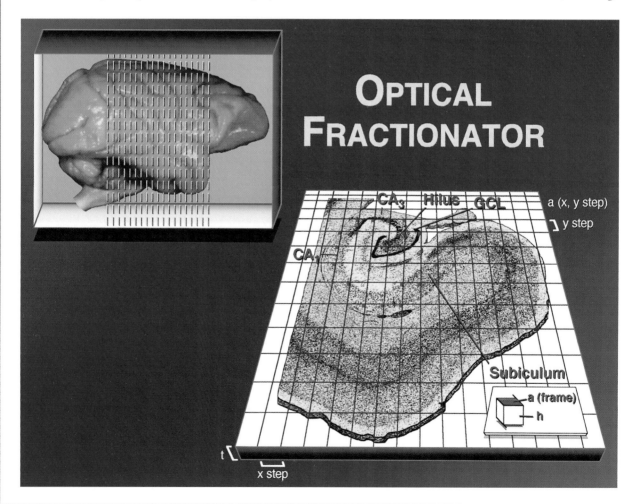

BOX 46.1 *(cont'd)*

variety of known errors introduced by including the cut surfaces of the histological preparations in the analysis. This is accomplished using a high-magnification microscope objective (usually 100×) with a shallow focal depth. In the illustration provided, the "thickness fraction" is defined as h/t. Neurons are counted as they first come into focus, according to an unbiased counting rule, called the "optical disector," that eliminates the possibility of counting a given cell more than once.

Finally, total neuron number in the region of interest (N) is estimated as the sum of the neurons counted

(sumQ-), multiplied by the reciprocal of the three sampling fractions; the "section fraction," "area fraction," and the "thickness fraction." For the present example, the total estimated neuron number is given by

$$N = (\text{sumQ--}) \times (10/1) \times (\text{XYarea}/a) \times (t/h).$$

Original illustration design by J. P. Stanisic and P. R. Rapp.

Peter R. Rapp and Jocelyne Bachevalier

Hippocampal Connectivity Is Compromised during Normal Aging

The entorhinal cortex originates the major source of cortical input to the hippocampus, giving rise to the so-called perforant path, which synapses on the distal dendrites of dentate gyrus granule cells in the outer portions of the molecular layer. More proximal portions of these same dendrites receive a prominent intrinsic input arising from neurons in the hilar region of the dentate gyrus. Cells in the entorhinal cortex that originate the perforant path projection to the dentate gyrus also innervate other fields of the hippocampus, including the most distal aspects of CA3 pyramidal cell dendrites. Multiple lines of investigation suggest that the integrity of these entorhinal cortex inputs is compromised with age. Ultrastructural quantification using modern stereological methods, for example, has documented that aging is associated with significant loss among a morphologically distinct subset of synapses in the outer molecular layer (i.e., the zone innervated by the entorhinal cortex) (Geinisman *et al.*, 1992). Alternative experimental approaches that have been used to examine connectivity throughout the hippocampus also reveal age-related changes in other targets of the perforant path projection. Together, these results have prompted speculation that, among the principal relays of hippocampal circuitry (i.e., the major connections within and between the subfields of the hippocampal formation), input originating in the entorhinal cortex may be especially vulnerable to aging. Because this circuitry conveys much of the cortically derived information that the hippocampus uses to support normal learning and memory, it seems reasonable to suppose that the disruption

of entorhinal–hippocampal connectivity might contribute to the cognitive outcome of aging. Consistent with this proposal, the magnitude of the morphological alterations observed in the hippocampal termination zones of the entorhinal cortex is greatest among aged animals with documented deficits on tasks that require the hippocampus and among older rats that exhibit abnormalities in various physiological measures of hippocampal plasticity.

Executive Function Mediated by the Prefrontal Cortex Declines during Normal Aging

Normal aging is sometimes thought of as a generalized process of nonspecific deterioration in which the function of many neural systems declines gradually. By this view, age-related cognitive decline might be best understood as the cumulative effect of subtle alterations distributed diffusely throughout the brain. There is actually little empirical support for this notion, however, and as we have seen in the case of hippocampal circuitry, the current perspective is that the neurobiological consequences of aging are remarkably selective. At the same time, it is important to recognize that the effects of aging on memory do not occur in isolation and that cognitive capacities mediated by other neural systems are also susceptible to decline.

As discussed in Chapter 53, the functionally and neuroanatomically heterogenous areas comprising the prefrontal cortex of the mammalian brain support a constellation of capacities referred to as "executive function." Whereas damage to these regions typically does not produce the frank amnesia that follows medial temporal lobe lesions, significant deficits are observed in a variety of information processing

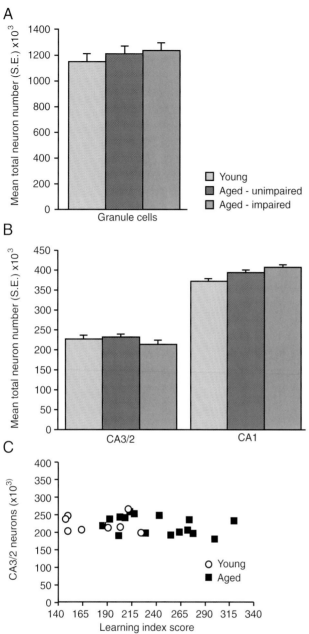

FIGURE 46.8 Estimated total neuron number in principal cell layers of the hippocampus for behaviorally characterized young and aged rats. Values are for one hippocampus from each brain. Half of the aged rats exhibited substantial spatial learning deficits in the Morris water maze (aged impaired); the other half performed within the range of learning scores for the young group (aged unimpaired). (A) Mean estimated total neuron number (+standard error) in the granule cell layer for young, aged-unimpaired, and aged-impaired rats. Average granule cell number is comparable across the groups. (B) Mean estimated total neuron number (+SE) in CA3/2 (left) and CA1 (right) pyramidal cell fields of the hippocampus for behaviorally characterized young and aged rats. Neuron number does not differ with age or cognitive status. (C) Scatter plot of total neuron number in the CA3/2 hippocampal field for individual rats plotted as a function of spatial learning scores (lower values indicate better learning). Neuron number is stable with age and across a broad range of learning capacities. Adapted with permission from Rapp and Gallagher (1996).

domains that influence memory performance, including the strategic use and manipulation of remembered information and the ability to identify the source and order in which information was acquired. It is therefore of interest that a qualitatively similar profile of deficits emerges during the course of normal aging (reviewed in Gallagher and Rapp, 1997). Elderly humans, for example, frequently experience difficulty recalling the original source of remembered information, even under conditions in which recollection of a target item is successful. These failures in "source memory" also predict performance on other tests of frontal lobe function, suggesting that a common neurobiological basis might underlie these deficits. Another parallel with the consequences of direct frontal lobe damage is that memory for temporal order (the ability to reproduce the sequence of items on a remembered list, for example) is reliably impaired in elderly humans relative to younger adults.

Neuropsychological studies in animal models reinforce the conclusion that dysfunction localized to the prefrontal cortex contributes to certain features of cognitive aging. One of the best-documented deficits associated with aging in the monkey, for example, is poor performance under testing conditions that emphasize the spatial and temporal, or the "where and when," components of memory (reviewed in Gallagher and Rapp, 1997). In the classic delayed response task, subjects observe while a food treat is hidden in one of two locations that are then covered with identical plaques (see Fig. 53.7). Because each of the reward locations are baited frequently across trials within a single test session, there is substantial opportunity for interference, and accurate performance depends on the ability to keep in mind the location that was baited most recently. The task also involves an explicit demand on short-term spatial memory, a capacity known to require the integrity of the dorsolateral prefrontal cortex. Damage involving this area of the prefrontal cortex in young monkeys produces impairment at retention intervals of just a few seconds or more in the delayed response procedure. This pattern is different than that seen following lesions of the hippocampal system, where impairment is selectively observed at longer delays. Numerous studies since the late 1970s have documented that aged monkeys exhibit a profile of delayed response deficits qualitatively similar to the effects of prefrontal cortex lesions in young animals. Consistent with the interpretation that this effect reflects age-related prefrontal dysfunction, the severity of impairment observed with other testing procedures increases when demands on the spatial and temporal attributes of memory are emphasized. Additional signs of prefrontal decline have also been documented in the aged monkey, including marked perseveration and behavioral rigidity when older subjects are confronted with shifting task contingencies. For example, whereas young adult monkeys quickly cease responding to a previously positive stimulus when it is no longer rewarded, aged subjects are slower to make this behavioral adjustment.

Are the effects of normal aging on capacities mediated by the prefrontal cortex coupled to other signatures of cognitive decline, consistent with the view of aging as a generalized process of nonspecific deterioration? Available evidence suggests that this is not the case. For example, age-related deficits on tests of prefrontal cortex function tend to emerge earlier during the course of aging than alterations in declarative memory supported by the medial temporal lobe system. In addition, when impairments indicative of both frontal and medial temporal lobe dysfunction cooccur in the same subject, these effects are statistically unrelated to each other (reviewed in Gallagher and Rapp, 1997). This issue has been examined by testing healthy elderly human subjects on a battery of neuropsychological assessments that includes measures of both frontal lobe function and declarative memory. Statistical analysis of results from this type of experiment indicates that whereas measures of information processing within each domain are correlated with each other (e.g., the severity of impairment on different tests of hippocampal memory are correlated), there is no apparent relationship in performance across tests of frontal and medial temporal lobe function. The implication of these observations is twofold: different aspects of cognitive function can decline independently during aging and these effects are not the consequence of generalized deterioration distributed widely throughout the frontal lobe and hippocampal system.

Neurobiology of Aging in the Prefrontal Cortex

Although the basis of age-related decline in executive function supported by the prefrontal cortex remains to be established, an outline of neurobiological aging in the frontal lobe has begun to emerge. Similar to the hippocampal system, neuron death is not a prominent feature of normal aging in areas of the frontal lobe, such as the dorsolateral prefrontal cortex, that mediate information processing functions known to decline with age. Other structural alterations have been documented in this region, however, including a substantial decline in the density of synapses, marked changes in dendritic architecture, and a variety of abnormalities in the myelination of

axons (Peters *et al.*, 1998). These parameters have been correlated with measures of cognitive aging in monkeys, raising the possibility that, like the hippocampal system, changes in the organization of critical prefrontal circuitry may play a significant role. A growing body of evidence from *in vivo* imaging studies in humans also supports this interpretation. One finding to emerge from this approach is that cognitive processing efforts sufficient to produce prefrontal cortical activation in young subjects fail to do so in older individuals. In addition, age-related deficits observed in memory for temporal order (see earlier discussion) have been linked specifically to changes in frontal lobe activation during aging revealed by PET. Medial temporal lobe activation, by comparison, appears less affected (reviewed in Gallagher and Rapp, 1997). These results point to the likely involvement of the prefrontal cortex and underscore the more general theme that the neurobiological effects of normal aging are regionally specific, resulting in independent influences on the information processing capacities mediated by different neural systems.

Neurochemically Specific Subcortical Systems Are Susceptible to Aging and Positioned to Broadly Influence Behavior

The preceding discussion challenges the view that normal aging is associated with generalized deterioration distributed diffusely throughout the brain. It is important to note, however, that aging does affect the integrity of neurochemically specific classes of cells whose long-ascending projections influence widespread areas of the brain. Cholinergic cell groups in the basal forebrain have been studied particularly intensively because this system is the site of pronounced degeneration in pathological disorders of aging, including Alzheimer's disease. Less severe effects are also observed during normal aging, involving acetylcholine-containing neurons that project to the hippocampus, amygdala, and neocortex. A significant implication is that cholinergic cell loss might disrupt the information processing functions of these target regions, and consistent with this possibility, reliable correlations between the magnitude of cholinergic cell loss and behavioral impairment have been reported in aged individuals. At the same time, cholinergic abnormalities alone are not likely to account for the full profile of cognitive deficits observed during aging because neurotoxin lesions that selectively destroy these neurons fail to reproduce certain key features of the behavioral decline observed in older individuals. Nonetheless, age-related cholinergic impairment might comprise an important component of a broader constellation of alterations that leads to cognitive dysfunction. Other neurochemical systems whose function is compromised during aging include dopamine-containing circuitry that originates in mid-brain cell groups and noradrenergic inputs that arise from the locus coeruleus. These systems innervate a variety of more anterior brain regions, and consistent with this broad distribution, neurochemical alterations have been linked to a diverse array of behavioral deficits ranging from age-related cognitive impairment to disturbances in motor function. These findings encourage the view that appropriately designed pharmacological interventions might have beneficial effects on a similarly broad profile of outcome measures of aging.

Summary

This section considered the cognitive and neurobiological effects of normal aging in humans and animal models. Key themes include the observation that the impact of aging on memory can vary widely from one individual to the next. Whereas neuron death was previously presumed to be the proximal cause of many cognitive deficits associated with aging, including impairments in learning and memory, it is now clear that age-related cognitive decline does not require marked neuron loss in the hippocampus and related cortical areas. Instead, it now appears that subtle alterations in connectivity, and downstream changes in cellular function, are more likely the causative factors. Building on emerging data concerning the neural circuitry that is most vulnerable to aging, it should be possible to achieve substantial advances toward a cell biological account of normal cognitive aging.

PATHOLOGICAL PROCESSES IN COGNITIVE DEVELOPMENT AND AGING

Developmental Psychopathologies

Developmental disabilities are typically defined by performance on specific psychological tests and are frequently classified as mental disorders, distinct from other physically characterized disorders of childhood, such as cerebral palsy, muscular dystrophy, spina bifida, and congenital malformations. This classification suggests that developmental or childhood disorders can be neatly divided into categories of physical and mental disability. However, this is not necessarily the case. Developmental disabilities such

as mental retardation can, for example, co-occur with physical disorders such as neural tube defect. Moreover, an increasing body of research demonstrates that there are physical (e.g., neural, genetic, and biochemical) anomalies associated with specific developmental (mental) disabilities, such as attention-deficit and hyperactivity disorders, schizophrenia, and autism.

Research in this field employs behavioral data to make the evaluation or clinical diagnosis. The brains of behaviorally identified subjects are then studied for differences from normal controls. In other words, developmental problems, as expressed by behavior, bring a child to clinical attention, and then researchers work to understand the underlying neural bases of the disorder. Recent advances in neuroimaging and gene linkage technology have vastly expanded research possibilities for noninvasive clinical studies. Even with a new arsenal of research technologies, however, it has not been possible to isolate and define characteristics of each developmental disability. Such efforts are limited by several factors.

1. Disagreement regarding the criteria for diagnosis. Because different researchers often use differing behavioral criteria, cross-study comparisons frequently show inconsistencies in results.
2. Heterogeneity of disorders. Even when consistent behavioral criteria are carefully applied, different underlying etiologies can result in the same behavioral profile.
3. Difficulties inherent in the study of children. Although modern brain imaging techniques such as magnetic resorance imaging are considered noninvasive, they are stressful and time-consuming, and parents will not always allow their affected children to participate in such studies. Although studies can be conducted using adults who have been affected since childhood, data obtained from such studies may not accurately reflect anomalies that characterize the early disruption of brain development because brains change over time. Moreover, retrospective diagnoses of childhood disorders frequently rely on memory (e.g., a patient is asked "Did you have difficulty reading as a young child?") and hence can be unreliable.

Despite these challenges, ongoing research has uncovered important neurological and genetic features that seem to be associated with specific developmental disorders. The following sections outline what is known about how specific injuries or anomalies in development of the brain may result in specific patterns of cognitive and behavioral impairment. Two examples of developmental psycho-

BOX 46.2

DYSLEXIA

Reading is a complex process that depends upon the prior establishment of a variety of supporting cognitive skills. Rapid mastery of reading skills is becoming increasingly important in early education, and failure to acquire reading competency can adversely affect acquisition of a fundamental knowledge base. Therefore, reading skill stands in a uniquely important position in overall cognitive development, strongly dependent on antecedent skill acquisition and critically supportive of further educational success.

After accounting for the effects of inadequate instruction, the most common cause of severe reading problems in childhood is **developmental dyslexia**, a disorder whose behavioral manifestations are extremely complex. In developmental dyslexia poor reading is typically characterized by the inability to apply the sound–correspondence rules necessary to decode print (see Chapter 52), resulting in inaccurate and slow reading. In contrast to spoken language, which is acquired with great ease by children, reading involves skills that have to be explicitly, and sometimes painstakingly, taught. Although reading impairment is common, with an incidence of 5–10% among school-age children, our understanding of its biological roots is relatively recent.

Neurobiological studies of dyslexia are challenging, as the behavioral manifestations of this disorder are complex. Although defined by poor reading performance, dyslexia is characterized by additional deficits, including poor phonological processing, poor verbal working memory, and slow naming ability. Recent research has demonstrated that dyslexics frequently show subtle deficits in motor control and early sensory processing, most notably in the visual system. With structural and functional brain imaging, investigators may now explore the neural mechanisms underlying reading and explore how these representations change as reading skills are acquired during early schooling. With these methods it is now possible to localize brain activity in children from their first attempts at letter recognition until reading has become an automatic and effortless process.

Dyslexic brain structure differs from that seen in individuals with normal reading skills. In dyslexia,

micro and macroscopic structural abnormalities have been detected in perisylvian language regions (temporal and parietal banks of the sylvian fissure as well as the insula), visual system structures, the thalamus, and the corpus callosum. The planum temporale is an expanse of neocortex on the temporal bank of the sylvian fissure, its anterior border defined by Heschl's gyrus. From the time of birth the left planum temporale is larger than the homologous region in the right hemisphere in 70–80% of individuals. Reductions or reversal of this leftward asymmetry has been documented in individuals with developmental dyslexia. The functional concomitants of these anatomical variations have been explored in functional imaging studies that have revealed differences in patterns of task-related activity between dyslexics and controls during the performance of reading and phonological decoding tasks. Interestingly, the cortical areas identified are similar in English, French, and Italian dyslexics, supporting a biological origin for this reading abnormality, independent of cultural upbringing. Similarly, candidate genes for dyslexia have been identified and replicated in different countries, suggesting the multigenetic contribution to reading disability.

Besides the problems related to reading, dyslexics also exhibit subtle abnormalities in visual processing. Evidence for selective involvement of magnocellular pathways of the visual system (see Chapter 27) has accumulated, beginning with the demonstration that cell bodies in the magnocellular layers of the lateral geniculate nucleus are smaller in dyslexics compared to a control group. The fact that both contrast sensitivity and visual persistence are abnormal in reading disabled children is consistent with the notion that these children have disturbances in the magnocellular system, which is specialized for temporally demanding visual processing. These behavioral results are supported by functional imaging studies demonstrating less task-related activity in extrastriate and parietal cortex during visual motion detection by dyslexics.

Future studies will determine the nature of the neural mechanisms that link deficits in early visual processing

---

BOX 46.2   (cont'd)

with more cognitive skills such as phonological awareness. Also remaining to be clarified are issues concerning which of these deficits is a primary cause of dyslexia as opposed to a consequence of having partially compensated for a reading disorder. Such information will aid in identifying better avenues for reading remediation. To date, the best methods for improving the reading abilities of dyslexics

focus on structured teaching of the code that allows individuals to sound out words (phonological awareness) in the context of fluency and comprehension exercises.

Guinevere F. Eden

---

pathology are described: autism and schizophrenia. Both disorders appear to involve an early brain dysfunction that results in the development of behavioral and cognitive symptoms, very early in infancy in the case of autism, but only in adolescence and early adulthood in the case of schizophrenia.

Autism

Autism is a rare neurodevelopmental syndrome affecting about 1 child in 2500. The main characteristics include deficits in social reciprocity and communication and unusual repetitive behaviors that begin in infancy or by the end of the third year of life at the latest. Parents often first become concerned because their child fails to use words to communicate, even though he/she recites passages from videotapes or says the alphabet. Like other kinds of abnormal behavior, autism is a heterogeneous condition that can range widely in severity.

Characteristics of Autism

A multitude of symptoms occur in autism, including social isolation (the autistic child largely ignores other people, shows little attachment to parents or other relatives, and retreats into a world of his or her own), stereotyped behaviors (the autistic child rocks back and forth, stares at neutral stimuli, rotates an object, or engages in other repetitive behaviors for long, uninterrupted time periods), resistance to change in routine, abnormal responses to sensory stimuli (the autistic child may ignore visual stimuli and sounds, especially speech sounds, sometimes to such an extent that it might be thought the child is deaf), inappropriate emotional expressions (the autistic child has sudden bouts of fear and crying for no obvious reason; at other times the child displays utter fearlessness and

unprovoked laughter), and poor use of speech. Individuals with autism can also exhibit symptoms that fall along a continuum of disorders. For example, many have mental retardation and show delays in the development of language. Others display neither language delay nor mental retardation, although they are clearly socially inept. For a long time, autism was thought to be the result of poor parenting. However, a growing number of studies over the last two decades provide mounting evidence that autism results from an early onset brain dysfunction.

Neuropathological Alterations in Autism

Several studies of autistic individuals provide evidence for megalencephaly (whole brain enlargement) and for increased head circumference. The nature of this enlargement has yet to be studied carefully, but it is specifically observed in the occipital, parietal, and temporal lobes. Postmortem analyses of the brains of autistic individuals have revealed increased cortical thickness and abnormalities in cortical morphology. Furthermore, abnormalities in the size and density of neurons in the medial temporal lobe and limbic system, including the amygdala, hippocampus, and entorhinal cortex, septal nuclei, and cingulate cortex, have also been documented. These neuropathological abnormalities make sense with respect to certain major symptoms of autism because the limbic system is known to play a central role in coordinating social–emotional functioning. Other evidence implicating this neural system in autism includes (a) case studies of patients with temporal lobe lesions and autistic-like behaviors, (b) a significant and specific association between temporal lobe lesions from tuberous sclerosis and autism, (c) a volumetric decrease in the amygdala in autism, (d) reduced functional activity on SPECT scans in the temporal lobe in autism,

BOX 46.3

TRIPLET REPEAT DISORDERS

Not all neurogenetic diseases follow simple inheritance patterns; not all developmental disorders reveal themselves immediately; and diseases with similar genetic etiologies can have widely different manifestations. **Trinucleotide repeat mutations**, or **dynamic mutations**, were discovered only in the early 1990s but are responsible for a number of important neurodegenerative disorders, such as Huntington Disease (see Box 31.5), Fragile X mental retardation, and myotonic dystrophy. To date, 14 neurological disorders have been found to result from such a mutational mechanism, and the list will probably continue to grow.

Triplet repeat mutations are unstable and prone to expand as alleles are passed from one generation to the next, although contractions can occur. Repeats at different loci differ markedly in their rates and extents of expansion, and the instability of repeats at each locus often depends upon the sex of the transmitting parent.

Fragile X syndrome, an X-linked dominant mental retardation syndrome, was the first disease shown to result from a triplet repeat mutation. There is a CGG repeat expansion at a locus (Xq27.3) giving rise to a folate-sensitive fragile site (FRAXA). The CGG repeat ranges in length in the general population from 5 to 50 triplets. Affected individuals carry more than 230 repeats, up to several thousand triplets. CGG tracts between 45 and 200 repeats in length are termed "premutations"; they are not long enough to result in mental retardation, yet are prerequisite for further expansion to the full mutation. Escalating risk of affected offspring is associated with increasing size of premutations in female carriers. Curiously, offspring of male carriers of premuations are not at risk for fragile X syndrome, as these alleles have not been observed to expand to full mutations upon male transmission. The normal function of the affected protein FMR1 remains to be fully determined, but it appears to play a role in RNA metabolism, likely in the areas of transport, stability and/or translation.

Myotonic dystrophy (DM) remains a particularly enigmatic triplet repeat disorder affecting multiple systems, causing myotonia, muscle weakness, cardiac conduction defects, diabetes, cataracts, premature balding, and sometimes dysmorphyic features and mild mental retardation. There is a tendency for these features to appear in more severe form in subsequent generations of a family. In DM there is a CTG repeat in the 3' untranslated region of the myotonin protein kinase gene (DMPK). This CTG tract is small in the general population (5–37 triplets)

but can expand dramatically to thousands of repeats. Slightly increased lengths (70–100) can result in mild effects, such as late-onset cataracts, and the classic symptoms of early adulthood myotonia are found in individuals with hundreds of repeats. Very large expansions can cause severe disease in newborns.

The mechanism(s) by which the mutation leads to the various clinical symptoms remains uncertain. A variety of effects have been described and the repeat expansions clearly affect both the DMPK gene and nearby genes. It is also likely that the expanded CTG repeat carrying mRNAs can act to diminish the levels of nuclear proteins that bind at these sequences, resulting in mis-regulation of genes not linked to DMPK. Mutations in equivalent mouse genes have not provided a complete model of the human disease. The phenotype in DM results from multiple effects of the repeat expansion, rather than a simple loss or gain of function mechanism.

Friedreich's ataxia (FA) causes both limb and gait ataxia, loss of position and vibration sense, decreased tendon reflexes, cardiomyopathy, diabetes, and, in some patients, optic atrophy and deafness. FA is a recessive disorder and the only triplet repeat disorder known to involve a GAA sequence. Carriers of FA are rather common (1/85), and, consequently, so is the GAA expansion. Members of the general population carry between 7 and 34 repeats, while pathogenic alleles can number in the hundreds. The affected frataxin gene product appears to be involved in mitochondrial iron homeostasis, and its absence affects postmitotic cells rich in mitochondria. The mechanism by which the GAA repeat affects gene function appears to be inhibition of primary RNA transcripts.

A second class of triplet repeat disorders includes those caused by expansion of translated CAG repeats which encode a polyglutamine tract in each of the respective proteins. These "polyglutamine" disorders share many features, suggesting that a common pathogenetic mechanism is at play in spite of the fact that the mutated genes share no homology outside of the CAG repeats. They are progressive neurologic diseases with onset of symptoms in young to mid-adulthood with only a specific group of neurons vulnerable in each disease. Symptoms develop when the number of uninterrupted repeats exceed ~ 35 glutamines. The phenotype is caused not by loss of function of the relevant protein but rather by a gain of function conferred by the expanded polyglutamine tract.

The **spinocerebellar ataxias (SCA)** are genetically distinct but overlap a great deal in their clinical presentation

BOX 46.3 *(cont'd)*

—between subtypes and even within families affected by the same disease. It is nearly impossible to distinguish one subtype from another on the basis of clinical signs alone. **Spinocerebellar Ataxia Type 1 (SCA1)** was the first of the inherited ataxias to be mapped. Patients with SCA1 suffer from progressive ataxia (loss of balance and coordination), dysarthria and eventual respiratory failure. SCA1 is characterized pathologically by cerebellar atrophy with severe loss of Purkinje cells and brain stem neurons. Patients with SCA1 have an expanded "perfect" CAG repeat tract encoding ataxin-1 the function of which is largely unknown.

Studies of human patients with deletions of, for example, the HD, or SCA1 genes (and of mice lacking these genes) confirm that disease is not due to loss of function of the respective proteins. More importantly, studies of mouse and fruit fly models that over-express full-length or truncated forms of either ataxin-1, ataxin-3, huntingtin, AR, atrophin-1, or ataxin-7 demonstrate progressive neuronal dysfunction consistent with a gain of function mechanism. Several illuminating findings have emerged from the study of human patients, cell culture systems, and the various animal models. In transgenic mice, expression of truncated polypeptides containing expanded glutamine tracts caused widespread dysfunction that extends beyond the specific groups of neurons affected by the full-length protein. The expanded polyglutamine tracts may cause the respective proteins to misfold or resist degradation. Aberrant protein-protein interactions or alterations in levels of proteins essential for the normal functioning of neurons (such as proteins that regulate Ca^{+2} levels and neurotransmitters) could, in turn, exacerbate neuronal dysfunction and lead to neuronal death.

The finding that chaperone overexpression mitigates the phenotype in one vertebrate and several invertebrate models of polyglutamine disorders, and the identification of several additional modifiers of the neuronal phenotype, provide a platform for identifying key pathways of pathogenesis and potential therapeutic targets.

Adapted by Graham V. Lees with permission from Nelson, D., and Zoghbi, H. (2003). Disorders of Trinucleotide repeat expansions. *In* "Encyclopedia of the Human Genome." Nature Macmillan, London.

Suggested Readings

Wells, R. D., and Warren, S. T. (eds.) (1998). "Genetic Instabilities and Hereditary Neurological Diseases." Academic Press, San Diego.
Cummings, C. J., and Zoghbi, H. Y. (2000), Trinucleotide repeats: Mechanisms and pathophysiology. *Ann. Rev. Genom. Hum. Gen.* **1**, 281–328.

and (e) animal models of autism based on early lesions to medial temporal lobe structures.

A fMRI study of autism has documented dysfunction localized to the ventral temporal lobe using a face recognition task (Baron-Cohen *et al.*, 1999). In this study (see top of Fig. 46.9), high-functioning individuals with autism and matched controls were presented with a series of photographs of eyes while their brains were being scanned to assess brain regions activated by two different tasks. In the first task (experimental condition), each photograph was presented simultaneously with words (either unconcerned or concerned, or sympathetic or unsympathetic). Participants were asked to indicate by pressing a button which word best describes what the person in the photograph is feeling or thinking. In the second task (control condition), each photograph was presented with the words "male" or "female" and the subjects were asked to make a gender recognition by pressing a button. In both tasks, the performance of autistic individuals and controls was above chance. However, the controls were more accurate in the two tasks than the autistic individuals. To investigate the brain regions activated by the experimental task, brain maps obtained during the control task were subtracted from brain maps obtained during the experimental task. For each brain slice shown at the bottom of Fig. 46.9, the activation maps were computed separately from control and autistic group data and superimposed. In the control group (shown in yellow and blue), the experimental task activated two main regions of the brain: the fronto-temporal neocortical areas, including the left dorsolateral prefrontal cortex and supplementary motor areas, bilateral temporo-parietal regions, and

A

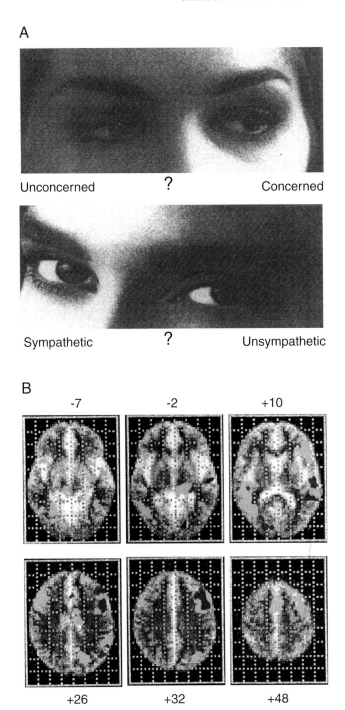

FIGURE 46.9 Examples of stimuli used in a fMRI study of facial expression recognition in autism. Subjects were presented with a choice of mental state words to select from and were also requested to identify the gender of the person in the photograph. For the example shown at the top, the correct answer is concerned and female. For the example shown below, the correct answer is sympathetic and female. The brain activation maps were computed separately from the control and autistic groups and are superimposed on standard brain space. Yellow corresponds to activation found in control subjects only. Red corresponds to activation found in autistic subjects only. Blue corresponds to activation found in both groups. Numbers refer to 2 coordinates (mm) relative to intercommissural line in the standard space. Adapted with permission from Baron-Cohen *et al.* (1999).

subcortical structures, including the left amygdala and parahippocampal gyrus. The autism group (shown in red and blue) activated the frontal components but did not activate the amygdala. The significance of these data is that one critical role of the amygdala is to identify the mental states or emotions of other individuals and that this structure appears to be dysfunctional in persons with autism.

Significant atrophy of the vermal lobules in the cerebellum has also been reported in autistic individuals, although this effect does not appear specific to autism and is found widely in neurodevelopmental disorders. By comparison, there is now extensive evidence for the involvement of higher association areas in the pathophysiology of autism, particularly the frontal and parietal cortices.

Autism Is a Complex Genetic Disorder

The most compelling evidence for a genetic contribution to autism comes from studies of monozygotic (identical) and dizygotic (fraternal) twins. When one member of a pair of monozygotic twins is autistic, the other twin has more than a 50% probability of being autistic. However, if one member of a pair of dizygotic twins is autistic, the other twin has only a 3% probability of developing autism. Using conventional nomenclature, we say that monozygotic twins have a 50% or higher concordance for autism and that dizygotic twins have a 3% concordance. The relative risk factor for siblings is one of the highest for a complex genetic disorder.

The most significant genetic finding relevant to autism is the recent identification of genes responsible for Rett's syndrome and fragile X syndrome, two conditions associated with autistic features. Rett's syndrome is caused by mutations in the methyl-CpG binding protein 2 (MECP2) gene. Decreased expression of this gene leads to a failure to suppress expression of genes regulated by methylation. Fragile X syndrome is a disorder caused by mutation of the gene FMR1 (see Box 46.3). A better understanding of how reduced expression of the MECP2 and FMR1 genes leads to mental retardation as well as social and language disorders will likely provide a better understanding of the autistic disorder.

Schizophrenia

Schizophrenia is a catastrophic illness with an onset typically in adolescence or early adulthood (see also Box 54.1). It was identified and defined in the early 20th century as "dementia praecox" (Latin for deterioration of the mind at an early age). In 1911, Eugen Bleuler introduced the term schizophrenia. This term can be confusing because its translation from the Greek means "split mind," which is sometimes interpreted as multiple personality, a condition in which a person alternates between one personality and another. A schizophrenic person has only one personality and the split in the schizophrenic mind is between emotional and intellectual realms. The combination of significant incapacity, onset early in life, and chronicity of illness makes schizophrenia a particularly tragic disorder, occurring in 0.5 to 1% of the population.

Characteristics of Schizophrenia

The clinical symptoms of schizophrenia are often divided into two broad categories: positive and negative. Positive symptoms include delusions, hallucinations, disorganized speech, and disorganized or bizarre behavior. These symptoms are referred to as positive because they represent distortions or exaggerations of normal cognitive or emotional functions. The negative symptoms of schizophrenia reflect a loss or diminution of functions that are normally present. Negative symptoms include alogia (marked poverty of speech or speech that is empty of coherent content), affective flattening (diminution in the ability to express emotion), anhedonia (inability to experience pleasure or loss of interest in social interactions); avolition (inability to initiate or persist in goal-directed behavior), and attentional impairment. Although the positive symptoms of schizophrenia are often colorful and draw attention to the patient's illness, the negative symptoms are an important feature of the disease that impair the person's ability to function normally in daily life.

The profound and pervasive cognitive and emotional disturbances that characterize schizophrenia suggest that it is a serious brain disease affecting multiple functions and systems. The various symptoms suggest possible involvement of a variety of cortical and subcortical brain regions. Auditory hallucinations and disruptions in linguistic expression suggest involvement of the auditory cortex and perisylvian language regions. Other positive symptoms, such as delusions or disorganized behavior, are more difficult to localize to specific regions and suggest dysfunction distributed across multiple neural systems and circuits. Negative symptoms may be related to the prefrontal cortex, which mediates goal-directed behavior and fluency of thought and speech. The affective flattening and asociality suggest involvement of the limbic areas within the temporal lobe.

The Dopamine Hypothesis of Schizophrenia

A great deal of research since the 1950s has made it clear that schizophrenia is associated with abnormalities in the dopaminergic synapses of the brain. Still, the exact nature of this perturbation remains elusive. The strongest link between dopamine synapses and schizophrenia comes from studies of drugs that alleviate the symptoms of schizophrenia. A large number of antischizophrenic, or neuroleptic, drugs have been found, most of which belong to two chemical families, the phenothiazines, which include chlorpromazine, and the butyropherones, which include haloperidol. All of these drugs have two properties in common: they block postsynaptic dopamine receptors and they inhibit the release of dopamine from the presynaptic neuron. One interpretation of these results is that schizophrenia is due to excess activity at dopamine synapses. Establishing cause-and-effect relationships in human psychiatric disorders, however, is challenging. For example, although a substantial increase in the number of dopaminergic receptors is observed in the schizophrenic brain, because virtually all patients receive neuroleptic medication, it is not known if increased receptor density is a consequence of the disease itself or a response to an extended use of antidopaminergic drugs. An additional complication for the dopamine receptor hypothesis of schizophrenia concerns the time course for the effects of neuroleptic drugs. Although these treatments block dopamine receptors almost at once and reach their full pharmacological effectiveness within a few days, effects on behavior emerge more slowly, over 2 or 3 weeks. Clearly the symptomatic relief achieved with neuroleptic intervention involves mechanisms in addition to the blockade of dopamine receptors.

One possibility is that the prolonged use of neuroleptic drugs decreases the number of spontaneously active dopamine neurons in what is known as the mesolimbic system, a set of neurons that project from the midbrain tegmentum to the limbic system. Another possibility is that the underlying problem in schizophrenia is not an excess of dopamine activity at all, but a deficit of glutamate activity. Glutamate is the predominant excitatory amino acid released by neurons in the cerebral cortex that project widely throughout the limbic system, and dopamine synapses are known to inhibit glutamate release in these target regions. If glutamate release is reduced in the schizophrenic brain, one way to correct this deficiency would be to block activity at dopaminergic receptors, relieving glutamate synapses from inhibition

Neuropathological Alterations in Schizophrenia

The most consistently described structural alterations in schizophrenia are ventricular enlargement and decreases in the volume of temporal lobe structures, including the hippocampus, amygdala, and entorhinal cortex. Cytoarchitecture and cell densities are also reportedly altered in limbic structures: reduced cell number and size have been observed in the hippocampus, parahippocampal gyrus, and entorhinal cortex, along with disturbed cytoarchitecture involving a cellular disarray in hippocampus, and the entorhinal and cingulate cortices. This distribution of structural abnormalities may help account for the symptoms of schizophrenia in that these limbic structures link neocortical association areas with the septum–hypothalamic complex and are therefore key in sensory information processing and sensory gating. Defects in this neural circuit could lead to a dissociation between neocortically mediated cognitive processing and limbic–hypothalamic emotional reactions and to a disturbed emotional experience of external sensory perceptions. Some studies have also described morphometric and anatomical alterations in other brain regions, namely enlargement of the basal ganglia, a decrease in the density of certain classes of neurons in the thalamus, and reductions of cortical volume and central gray matter.

The structural alterations reported in schizophrenia are often subtle and certainly heterogeneous, contributing minimally to the elucidation of the disease if symptoms are to be attributed to defects in single brain regions. Alternatively, it is currently hypothesized that the variety and severity of symptoms observed in schizophrenia can be explained by defects in several brain regions affecting the neural circuits that mediate higher cognitive functions. Such neural circuitry would include neocortical association areas, the limbic system and midline thalamic structures, with possible involvement of the basal ganglia.

The Neurodevelopmental Hypothesis of Schizophrenia

Several clinical observations point to neurodevelopmental abnormalities in schizophrenia: onset in adolescence in most patients and earlier onset among males, pronounced premorbid neurodevelopmental abnormalities, such as asociality and "soft" neurological signs, impaired cognitive and neuromotor functioning, minor physical anomalies, presence of structural abnormalities at the onset of the illness, which may predate the illness, and the absence of neurodegenerative processes.

Post mortem morphological observations in the brains of schizophrenic patients suggest that multiple aspects of neural development may be disrupted. The spatial disorganization of neurons found in the hippocampus and the inappropriate laminar location of cells in the entorhinal cortex, for example, suggest a potential defect in neuronal migration. Other evidence indicates that the organization of synaptic connectivity is affected. The functional circuitry of the frontal cortex undergoes significant remodeling until adolescence, mediated by an NMDA receptor-dependent mechanism. The number of these receptors is reduced in the brain of schizophrenics. Still other abnormalities involve biochemical alterations of membrane phospholipids in the dorsolateral prefrontal region. These changes include a decrease in phosphomonoesters and an increase in phosphodiesters. Such biochemical changes in membrane phospholipids are known to occur during normal synaptic pruning in adolescence, but appear to be exaggerated in the dorsolateral prefrontal cortex of schizophrenics. These enhanced biochemical changes may lead to greater synaptic pruning in schizophrenics than in normal individuals and contribute to the reduction in prefrontal neuropil volume that accompanies the disease.

The precise timing of neurodevelopmental abnormalities in schizophrenia remains controversial. Some implicate a fixed neural lesion from early life interacting with normal neurodevelopmental events that take place much later. Others posit that schizophrenia is caused by a deviation from normal brain maturational processes during late adolescence, involving large-scale synaptic elimination or pruning in brain regions critical for cognitive development. Still others propose that early brain pathology acts as a risk factor rather than a sufficient cause so that its effects can only be understood in the light of the individual's later exposure to other risk and protective factors.

Genetics Play a Role in Schizophrenia

As for autism, a substantial body of evidence indicates that schizophrenia is associated with both genetic and environmental factors. Findings pointing to a significant genetic contribution come from family, twin, and adoption studies. Evidence for environmental factors derives from studies of prenatal intrauterine environment, neonatal obstetric complications, and postnatal brain insults. Currently, it remains an open question whether these environmental factors play a necessary role in the neurodevelopmental abnormalities responsible for psychotic brain disorders or whether their role is additive or interactive with genetic contributions.

People with schizophrenia are more likely than others to have schizophrenic relatives. The most compelling evidence is the 50% concordance rate for monozygotic twins relative to 15% concordance for dizygotic twins. Several neuroimaging studies have been performed on discordant monozygotic twins, which consistently indicate more prominent structural brain abnormalities in the ill twin. More importantly, a neuroimaging study demonstrated that schizophrenia is associated with dysfunction of a prefrontal-limbic network (Weinberger *et al.*, 1992). In this study, monozygotic twins discordant for schizophrenia underwent PET blood flow scans while they performed a task known to activate the dorsolateral prefrontal cortex in normal subjects. This task, known as the Wisconsin Card Sorting Task (WCST), is depicted at the top of Fig. 46.10, and measures abstract problem solving requiring attention and working memory. The participant sees four cards bearing designs that differ in color, form, and number of elements. The subject's task is to sort the stack of cards into piles in front of one or another of the stimulus cards. The subject is told whether the sorting choice is correct or incorrect. The test follows this principle: the correct solution is first color; once the subject has figured out this solution, without warning the correct solution then becomes form. Thus, the

subject must now inhibit classifying cards on the basis of color and shift to classifying on the basis of form. Once the subject has succeeded at selecting form, the correct solution again changes unexpectedly, now to the number of elements. Shifting response strategies is difficult for patients with frontal lobe dysfunction. As shown on the graphs (Fig. 46.10), in the affected schizophrenic twin, prefrontal activation correlated strongly with both left and right hippocampal volumes; a relationship that was not found in the unaffected twins. These data suggest that schizophrenia could result from a dysfunction of a distributed neural network involving the prefrontal cortical areas and the limbic structures.

Molecular studies have also demonstrated schizophrenia to be a complex genetic disorder and have implicated several possible susceptibility loci, including regions on chromosomes 1q, 6p, 8p, 13q, and 22q. Of genes mapped, the 22q11 gene [a common functional polymorphism of catechol-*O*-methyltransferase (COMT), which is a methylation enzyme that metabo-

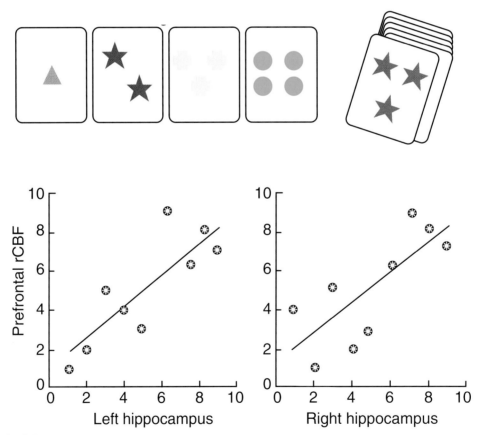

FIGURE 46.10 The Wisconsin Card-Sorting Task showing test materials as presented to the subject. For the twins affected with schizophrenia, there was a positive correlation between prefrontal regional cerebral blood flow measured by PET while the subjects performed the tasks and volume of left and right hippocampi estimated from magnetic resonance imaging scans. Such a correlation was not found in the unaffected twins. Values represent rank ordering for each variable. Adapted with permission from Weinberger *et al.* (1992).

lizes released dopamine] has been a popular candidate because of the long-hypothesized role of dopamine in schizophrenia.

Sex Hormones May Influence Neurodevelopmental Disorders

There are gender differences in the occurrence of neurodevelopmental disorders. The gender ratio of incidence is skewed toward boys for a variety of developmental disabilities, including severe mental retardation (1.3 boys/1 girl), speech and language disorders (2.6/1), learning difficulties (2.2/1), dyslexia (4.3/1), schizophrenia (1.9/1), and autism (4/1). Why? Although the existence of sex differences in the area of language and learning disorders has been contested on the grounds that it is a result of teacher and clinician bias in identifying these disorders, studies have supported the existence of a significant gender difference in the incidence of these disorders (Flannery et al., 2000). Moreover, gender differences are also seen in clear-cut phenomena such as complications of pregnancy and birth, which are more common in male infants, and these differences cannot be explained as a reflection of investigator or clinician bias. Several theories have attempted to explain these gender differences.

One theory posits that male but not female fetuses invoke a form of "antigenic" response from the mother during pregnancy, being recognized by the immune system as "foreign." The hostile environment thus created for the male fetus in utero would explain not only a higher incidence of developmental disorders among boys, but also the finding that later-born sons are increasingly likely to be affected adversely (consistent with increased immune responsiveness on repeated exposure).

Another theory (the Geschwind theory, as it came to be known, after the neurologist Norman Geschwind) proposed that the uneven gender ratios in developmental disorders are associated with exposure to some "male factor" (possibly androgen) during the last trimester of fetal development. This factor acts to slow cortical maturation in male fetuses, particularly in the left hemisphere, rendering them more susceptible to perturbation during the normal course of development. This exposure to a male hormone would explain the higher incidence of developmental disorders among boys. Conversely, faster central neurons system development in female fetuses would enable them to better withstand insult during late pregnancy and birth. This idea is supported by evidence that female infants appear to show better cognitive recovery than male infants from intracranial hemorrhage associated with prematurity.

Summary

This section examined two forms of developmental abnormalities: autism and schizophrenia. In both cases it is possible to link the behavioral manifestations of the disorder to anomalies in neurobiological systems and to identify a genetic component. In both disorders, too, affected individuals do not show localized damage in circumscribed brain regions, but show evidence of cellular disturbance early in brain development (i.e., during neuromigration), which gives rise to pervasive and dysfunctional reorganization of critical neural systems underlying complex behaviors. Emerging evidence suggests that similar mechanisms may characterize other developmental disabilities, including dyslexia, mental retardation, and attention deficit disorders. Current findings also support the existence of sex differences in brain development and organization, which may in turn differentially affect the response of the brain to early injury.

Pathological Manifestations of Cognitive Aging: Dementia

Dementia is a generic term that refers to debilitating deterioration in more than one domain of cognitive function. The involvement of multiple capacities distinguishes dementia from other disorders, such as amnesia and aphasia, that affect a single functional domain (memory and language, respectively). Approximately 50 disorders are known to cause dementia. Most of these are progressive in nature, increasing in severity over time. The age at onset and the rate of progression of symptoms differ dramatically among the major dementing disorders. Most have an insidious onset and develop slowly, sometimes over a period of many years. These include Alzheimer's disease, Huntington's disease, frontotemporal dementia, and the dementia observed in a subpopulation of patients with Parkinson's disease. The rare neurodegenerative disorder Creutzfeldt–Jakob disease also develops insidiously, but is distinguished by a very rapid rate of progression, often spanning a year or less from the onset of dementia to death. Vascular dementia (or multi-infarct dementia) follows still another pattern of decline. Initial cognitive symptoms develop acutely, but in this case the clinical course typically proceeds in a step wise fashion over many years, with periods of relative stability punctuated by abrupt deterioration. Age is a major risk factor for dementing illnesses, and the following sections focus on the most well-studied and common example of age-related dementia; Alzheimer's disease.

Alzheimer's Disease Is the Most Common Cause of Dementia

In 1906, the German scientist Alois Alzheimer reported a case study of a woman in her late 40s who developed memory impairment and deficits in other mental faculties that progressively worsened in severity until her death in her early 50s. Subsequent neuropathological examination of this patient's brain revealed grossly apparent and widespread neocortical atrophy that Alzheimer concluded was inconsistent with any previously described disease. Although the disorder that would come to bear Alzheimer's name was originally thought to be quite rare, it is now recognized as the most common form of dementia, accounting for an estimated 50% of all cases. Approximately 4 million people in the United States, and 12 million people worldwide, are currently diagnosed with Alzheimer's disease. The prevalence of the disease is tightly coupled to age and increases after the fourth decade of life. The disease affects about 10% of persons over the age of 65, and by 85, at least one in four individuals is afflicted. Demographic trends indicate that the elderly comprise the fastest growing segment of the population, and as a consequence, the number of people suffering the devastating impact of Alzheimer's disease is projected to more than triple during the first half of the 21st century. Not surprisingly, efforts to understand the basis of this and related disorders are among the most active research areas in modern neuroscience.

Memory Impairment Is a Central Feature of Alzheimer's Disease

Alzheimer's original case study provided an accurate description of the clinical course for many patients with this disease. Impairment in establishing and maintaining memories for recent events is frequently the initial sign that brings the patient to the attention of health care professionals. At this early stage, memory for the remote past is relatively preserved, as are other forms of memory that do not require the hippocampal formation and related medial temporal lobe structures. By comparison, patients with Huntington's disease display a different profile in which declarative memory is relatively spared against a background of substantial impairment in procedural, or habit-like, memory that is thought to rely on cortico-striatal circuitry. Thus, the neuropsychological profile of the Alzheimer's patient provides important clues about the neuropathological progression of this disorder, suggesting that the systems responsible for declarative memory are especially vulnerable. Neuroanatomical studies of the diagnostic hallmarks

of Alzheimer's disease confirm this proposal (described in the next section). Progression of the disorder is marked by inexorable decline across multiple cognitive capacities. Although generally alert and responsive in early and middle phases of the disorder, Alzheimer's patients often experience difficulty identifying the meaning of simple words, uses for common household objects, or the meaning of numbers. Other accompanying disturbances can include general confusion, agitation, delusions, social disinhibition, and paranoia. Language abilities can deteriorate progressively, and at the end stage of disease, patients are often mute and densely amnesic for both recent and more remote events. As might be predicted on the basis of this broad profile of impairment, the distribution of neuropathology in individuals dying with late-stage Alzheimer's disease is extensive, involving widespread areas of the limbic system and association cortices, along with many subcortical brain regions, including the basal forebrain cholinergic system, striatum, thalamus, and cerebellum.

Amyloid-Containing Plaques and Neurofibrillary Tangles Are Diagnostic Hallmarks of Alzheimer's Disease That Preferentially Target Memory-Related Brain Regions

There are two types of neuropathological lesions that, when present in sufficiently high numbers, are the diagnostic hallmarks of Alzheimer's disease. Plaques comprise extracellular deposits of amyloid β-protein (Aβ) that, in their mature form, are typically surrounded by a shell of dystrophic neurites. Because of this arrangement, plaques often assume a star-like appearance in standard microscopic preparations (see Fig. 46.11B). The neuritic component of plaques consists of morphologically abnormal dendrites and axons of multiple neuronal types, typically associated with substantial numbers of glial cells. The amyloid core of plaques can contain multiple species of Aβ, including a form ending at amino acid 42 that is prone to aggregation ($A\beta_{42}$), and a slightly shorter species ($A\beta_{40}$) that is normally produced more abundantly in neurons. Plaques vary substantially in size, and although the time it takes for mature neuritic plaques to form is not known precisely, they are likely to evolve slowly, over many years.

In contrast to extracellular plaques, the second neuropathological hallmark of Alzheimer's disease is localized intracellularly. Generally referred to as neurofibrillary tangles, these are composed of densely packed, abnormal fibers that occupy much of the cytoplasm and proximal neuronal processes of affected cells (Fig. 46.11A). Indeed the density of these fibers in many tangle-bearing neurons is sufficiently

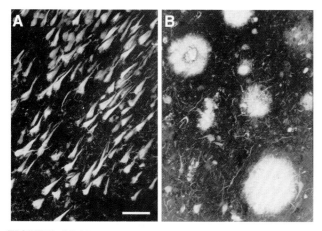

FIGURE 46.11 Photomicrographs of neurofibrillary tangles (A) and amyloid-containing plaques (B) in the hippocampal formation of a patient that died with late-stage Alzheimer's disease. Note that the size and morphological characteristics of plaques in B vary widely. Scale bar: 50 μm. Courtesy of P. Hof, Mount Sinai School of Medicine.

high that the cell body appears swollen and the nucleus displaced. The term paired helical filaments (PHF), sometimes used to describe this type of pathology, derives from electron microscopic evidence that tangles consist of pairs of twisted filaments with a highly regular periodicity. Studies using biochemical and immunocytochemical methods have demonstrated that PHF are composed of a cytoskeletal protein found in normal, healthy neurons; the microtuble-associated protein tau. Cytoskeletal abnormalities can disrupt intracellular trafficking of materials that are critical for cell viability, culminating in neuron death. Defining the mechanisms that initiate the hyperphosphorylation of tau and its aggregation into mature neurofibrillary pathology is a prominent avenue of research on Alzheimer's disease.

Investigations aimed at mapping the neuroanatomical distribution of pathology during early and later stages of Alzheimer's disease help account for the progression of clinical symptoms in patients with this disorder. Early in the course of the disease, when memory impairment is often the predominant complaint, plaques and tangles are particularly abundant in the entorhinal cortex and associated projection targets in the hippocampus. Indeed, in many cases virtually all of the neurons in layer II of the entorhinal cortex (i.e., cells that originate the perforant path projection to the hippocampus) exhibit neurofibrillary tangles. Thus, the neuropathology of Alzheimer's disease appears to initially target circuitry critical for normal declarative memory, disrupting a major source of neocortical input that the medial temporal lobe system uses to establish memory for ongoing events.

Consistent with this proposal, evidence from imaging studies indicates that abnormalities localized to the entorhinal cortex are correlated with memory impairment early in the course of Alzheimer's disease and can be used to increase the accuracy of clinical diagnosis. As the severity of cognitive impairment progresses, the distribution of neuropathology becomes more widespread, affecting cortical and subcortical systems that support language, semantic knowledge, abstract reasoning, and other capacities. Defining the mechanisms that confer the differential vulnerability of different brain regions to Alzheimer pathology is an active area of investigation .

Genetic Contributions to Alzheimer's Disease

Important clues about the basis of Alzheimer's disease have come from the study of people afflicted with an "early onset" form of the disorder that emerges before the age of 65. This relatively rare and aggressive condition exhibits an increased prevalence in certain families and is therefore thought to have a significant genetic component. To date, three gene mutations linked to early onset Alzheimer's have been identified: one involving the amyloid precursor protein gene on chromosome 21, another in the presenilin 1 gene on chromosome 14, and the third in the presenilin 2 gene on chromosome 1. Each of these mutations is expressed in an autosomal-dominant fashion such that half the offspring of an affected parent will develop the disease. Importantly, the common thread among gene mutations associated with early onset Alzheimer's disease is that each of them influences processing of the amyloid precursor protein (reviewed in Selkoe, 2001).

Several additional lines of evidence support the suggestion that the deposition of amyloid is central to the pathogensis of Alzheimer's disease. By far the most common form of the disorder (accounting for an estimated 98% of cases) has a relatively late onset, after age 65. Among a number of recently identified candidate genes, one risk factor for late-onset Alzheimer's disease is the allelic composition of the apolipoprotein E gene on chromosome 19 (ApoE); i.e., a gene that codes for a glycoprotein involved in cholesterol transport and metabolism. The ApoE gene has three alleles (designated ApoE2, ApoE3 and ApoE4), and patients with Alzheimer's disease carry the ApoE4 allele with a frequency greatly exceeding individuals without the disease. Moreover, the risk of disease is coupled to the number of copies of this specific allele: individuals with no copies of ApoE4 are less likely than the general population to develop Alzheimer's disease, the presence of one ApoE4 allele increases the disease risk four times, and people with two copies of ApoE4 are eight times more likely than the population at large to develop Alzheimer's. Although the precise mechanism by which ApoE4 mediates disease susceptibility is the subject of intensive investigation, one hypothesis is that it involves the disruption of processes responsible for scavenging and clearing amyloid peptide from the extracelluar space in brain.

Additional findings relevant to the role of amyloid in Alzheimer's disease come from research on Down's syndrome. The most common cause of mental retardation, Down's syndrome results from the presence of an extra copy of the same chromosome that carries the gene for the amyloid precursor protein; chromosome 21. Thus, it is of considerable interest that people with Down's syndrome who survive until the fourth decade of life almost invariably develop a distribution of amyloid plaques in the brain similar to that observed in Alzheimer's patients. To the degree that aberrant processing or clearance of amyloid comprises the single common pathogenic mechanism of Alzheimer's disease, current findings encourage the view that interventions targeting this pathway might be developed to prevent or reverse this defect, realizing an effective treatment for the most common cause of age-related dementia.

Prospects for the Treatment of Alzheimer's Disease

Although Alzheimer's disease is presently incurable, several pharmacological treatments have been approved for the clinical management of cognitive impairment associated with the disorder. These interventions all target the function of the neurotransmitter acetylcholine. The rationale for this approach was based on the observation that pharmacological disruption of cholinergic function in young subjects leads to a pattern of cognitive deficits resembling the effects of aging and dementia and that Alzheimer's disease is accompanied by substantial degeneration among cholinergic neurons in the basal forebrain that project to the hippocampal formation and widespread regions of the cortical mantle. Two drugs currently in use for the symptomatic treatment of cognitive deficits in Alzheimer's disease (tacrine and donepezil) augment the function of surviving cholinergic neurons by inhibiting the activity of acetylcholinesterase, thereby increasing the availability of released acetylcholine at the synapse. The therapeutic benefit achieved with such intervention is limited, however, and results in a modest slowing in the rate of cognitive decline, rather than reversal of impairment. In addition, only some patients respond to treatment. Alternative approaches targeting this transmitter system are under active development, including the use of exogenous cells grafts engineered to secrete neurotrophic factors that are known to promote the survival of cholinergic neurons. Other strategies for intervention include treatment with compounds that protect against the oxidative damage observed in the Alzheimer's brain, the use of hormone replacement therapies that appear to reduce the risk and delay the age at onset of Alzheimer's disease in postmenopausal women, and the development of drugs that might block the formation of plaques.

While currently available treatments offer modest, transient benefit for certain Alzheimer's patients, they fall far short of an effective cure or prevention. Encouraging preliminary progress toward the latter goal is based on the proposal that aberrant amyloid deposition represents the central pathogenic event responsible for the disorder. Whereas laboratory animals fail to develop Alzheimer's disease spontaneously, one can take advantage of a transgenic mouse model that accumulates amyloid-containing plaques in an age-dependent manner. These mice also develop spatial learning deficits relatively early in life, in temporal correspondence with the emergence of amyloid deposits. When transgenic animals were vaccinated at multiple time points during the first 4 months of life with Aß, and subsequently examined for the effects of immunization on behavior and neuropathology, treatment attenuated the spatial learning deficits substantially (Janus et al., 2000). Nevertheless, performance remained mildly impaired relative to nontransgenic controls. This partial protection from cognitive decline was also accompanied by roughly a 50% reduction in the number and size of mature, Aß-containing plaques, relative to nonimmunized, age-matched transgenic controls. Related findings using a similar experimental approach also demonstrate that immunization with Aß is even effective in reducing the degree and progression of amyloid deposition when provided to older animals at a point in the life span when this pathology is already well established (reviewed in Selkoe, 2001). The development of similar approaches for clinical use faces a number of significant challenges, including the possibility that humans will fail to mount an effective immune response to Aß. Nonetheless, these recent findings encourage the view that vaccine therapies might ultimately yield an effective route for the treatment and prevention of Alzheimer's disease.

Summary

This chapter has considered the neurobiological basis of cognitive development and aging. Early cognitive development is marked by the emergence of a remarkably complex set of adaptive capacities, includ-

BOX 46.4

EPILEPSY

Epilepsy is among the most prevalent of the serious neurological disorders, affecting from 0.5–1% of the world's population. Epilepsy is the condition of spontaneously recurrent seizures. A seizure is a stereotyped episode, with a defined start and finish, involving altered sensory, motor, autonomic function, consciousness, and due to abnormal electrical discharge in the brain. Some seizures result from an acute insult, such as head trauma. Others result from metabolic derangements or structural abnormalities such as tumors. Unfortunately, the majority of seizures have no known cause.

Epilepsy is not a disease, but a family of disorders. The location of the seizure in the brain, and its pattern of spread, determines how a seizure presents itself. For example, a seizure in the motor cortex will cause uncontrolled movements in the part of the body controlled by that region of motor cortex. In adults, the most common type of seizure originates in medial temporal lobe structures, including hippocampus, amygdala, and adjacent cortex. These seizures, called complex partial seizures, usually present as confusion, memory loss, and automatic behavior, sometimes with auras (warnings) of distorted emotions or perceptions.

The "International Classification of Seizures" divides seizures into "partial" seizures that start focally, and "generalized" seizures that begin in widespread regions of brain. Partial seizures are subclassified as simple partial seizures, which involve no alteration in cognitive state, and complex partial seizures, which are associated with loss of consciousness or memory. Generalized seizures are further divided into absence ("petit mal"), tonic-clonic ("grand mal"), atonic (drop seizures), myoclonic (brief jerks), and a few less common types.

Most recurrent seizures are treated with medications. Medications adequately control seizures in about two-thirds to three-fourths of patients. Some of the remainder can be cured by surgical procedures to interrupt the seizure focus. About two-dozen antiseizure medications are available, some better for particular seizure types, and each with a slightly different profile of side effects. Seizure medicines typically enhance function of GABA, partially block excitatory neurotransmission, or alter sodium channels to prevent rapid firing of neurons. Common side effects include sleepiness, dizziness, blurry vision, cognitive impairment, and gastrointestinal upset.

People with epilepsy often consider the psychosocial consequences of epilepsy to be a greater problem than the seizures. Epilepsy is unreasonably stigmatized, and people with epilepsy face hurdles in the workplace and can have problems in school. Yet, most people with epilepsy do succeed. Mechanisms of epilepsy are linked intimately to mechanisms of brain function. Continuing advances in neuroscience and molecular biology should lead to better treatment and ultimately a real cure.

Robert S. Fisher and Maslah Saul

ing language skills, reasoning abilities, attention, declarative memory, and executive functions. The vast majority of neurons—the essential building blocks of the central nervous system—are present at birth in humans, and rather than depending on the recruitment of new neurons, cognitive development appears to involve the fine tuning and establishment of appropriate circuitry among existing cells. Given this complex orchestration of processes, it is not surprising that many major disorders affecting cognitive function appear to result from a disruption of normal neurodevelopmental events. Higher order cognitive capacities are also vulnerable to deterioration during normal aging. Whereas widely distributed neuron death was previously presumed to underlie these deficits, it now appears that regionally selective changes in connectivity and cell biological function in critical circuits are the causative factors. Aging is also associated with some of the most devastating pathological conditions affecting cognitive function, including Alzheimer's disease. The dramatic

progress realized in recent years has, for the first time, established a basis for the rationale development of strategies for disease prevention and treatment. Continued advances in basic research will fuel these efforts and, in the process, establish a comprehensive neurobiology of cognitive development and aging.

References

Alvarado, C. M., and Bachevalier, J. (2000). Revisiting the development of medial temporal lobe memory functions in primates. *Learn. Memory* **7**, 244–256.

Barnes, C. A. (2001). Plasticity in the aging central nervous system. *Int. Rev. Neurobiol.* **45**, 339–354.

Barnes, C. A., Suster, M. S., Shen, J., and McNaughton, B. L. (1997). Multistability of cognitive maps in the hippocampus of old rats. *Nature* **388**, 272–275.

Baron-Cohen, S., Ring, H. A., Wheelwright, S., Bullmore, E. T., Brammer, M. J., Simmons, A., and Williams, S. C. R. (1999). Social intelligence in the normal and autistic brain: An fMRI study. *Eur. J. Neurosc.* **11**, 1891–1898.

Brody, H. (1970). Structural changes in the aging nervous system. *Interdisc. Top. Gerontol.* **7**, 9–21.

Chugani, H. T., Phelps, M. E., and Mazziotta, J. C. (1993). Positron emission tomography study of human brain functional development. *In* "Brain Development and Cognition: A Reader", (M. H. Johnson, ed.), Chap. 8, pp. 125–143. Blackwell, Cambridge, MA.

Conel, J. L. (1939–1963). "The Postnatal Development of the Human Cerebral Cortex," Vols. I–VI. Harvard Univ. Press, Cambridge, MA.

Courchesne, E. (1990). Chronology of postnatal human brain development: Event-related potential, positron emission tomography, myelinogenesis, and synaptogenesis studies. *In* "Event-Related Brain Potentials," (J. Rohrbaugh, R. Parasuraman, and R. Johnson, eds.), Chap. 14, pp. 210–214. Oxford Univ. Press, New York.

Diamond, A. (1990). The development and neural bases of memory functions as indexed by the AB and delayed response tasks in human infants and infant monkeys. *Ann. N. Y. Acad. Sci.* **608**, 637–676.

Flannery, K. A., Liederman, J., Daly, L., and Schultz, J. (2000). Male prevalence for reading disability is found in a large sample of black and white children free from ascertainment bias. *J. Int. Neuropsychol. Soc.* **6**, 433–442.

Gallagher, M., Burwell, R., and Burchinal, M. (1993). Severity of spatial learning impairment in aging: Development of a learning index for performance in the Morris water maze. *Behav. Neurosci.* **107**, 618–626.

Gallagher, M., and Rapp, P. R. (1997). The use of animal models to study the effects of aging on cognition. *Annu. Rev. Psychol.* **48**, 339–370.

Geinisman, Y., de Toledo-Morrell, L., Morrell, F., Persina, I. S., and Rossi, M. (1992). Age-related loss of axospinous synapses formed by two afferent systems in the rat dentate gyrus as revealed by the unbiased stereological disector technique. *Hippocampus* **2**, 347–444.

Giedd, J. N., Blumenthal, J., Jeffries, N. O., Castellanos, F. X., Liu, H., Zijdenbos, A., Paus, T., Evans, A. C., and Rapoport, J. L. (1999). Brain development during childhood and adolescence: A longitudinal MRI study. *Nature Neurosci.* **2**, 861–863.

Giedd, J. N., Vaituzis, A. C., Hamburger, S. D., Lange, N., Rajapakse, J. C., Kaysen, D., Vauss, Y. C., and Rapoport, J. L. (1996) Quantitative MRI of the temporal lobe, amygdala, and hippocampus in normal human development: Ages 4–18 years. *J. Comp. Neurol.* **366**, 223–230.

Holcombe, P. J., Coffey, S. A., and Neville, H. J. (1992). Visual and auditory sentence processing: A development analysis using event-related brain potentials. *Dev. Neuropsychol.* **8**, 203–241.

Huttenlocher, P. R. (1990). Morphometric study of human cerebral cortex development. *Neuropsychologia* **28**, 517–527.

Huttenlocher, P. R., and De Courten, C. (1987). The development of synapses in striate cortex of man. *Hum. Neurobiol.* **6**, 1–9.

Janus, C., Pearson, J., McLaurin, J., Mathews, P. M., Jiang, Y., Schmidt, S. D., Chishti, M. A., Horne, P., Heslin, D., French, J., Mount H. T., Nixon, R. A., Mercken, M., Bergeron, C., Fraser, P. E., St. George-Hyslop, P., and Westaway, D. (2000). Aß peptide immunization reduces behavioral impairment and plaques in a model of Alzheimer's disease. *Nature* **408**, 915–916.

Neville, H. J., Schmidt, A., and Kutas, M. (1983). Altered visual evoked potentials in congenitally deaf adults. *Brain Res.* **266**, 127–132.

Peters, A., Morrison, J. H., Rosene, D. L., and Hyman, B. T. (1998). Are neurons lost from the primate cerebral cortex during normal aging? *Cerebr. Cort.* **8**, 295–300.

Rapp, P. R., and Gallagher, M. (1996). Preserved neuron number in the hippocampus of aged rats with spatial learning deficits. *Proc. Natl. Acad. Sci. USA* **93**, 9926–9930.

Schore, A.N. (1996). The experience-dependent maturation of a regulatory system in the orbital prefrontal cortex and the origin of developmental psychopathology. *Dev. Psychopathol.* **8**, 59–87.

Selkoe, D. J. (2001). Alzheimer's disease: Genes, proteins, and therapy. *Physiol. Rev.* **81**, 741–766.

Seress, L. (2001). Morphological changes of the human hippocampal formation from midgestation to early childhood. *In* "Handbook of Developmental Cognitive Neuroscience," (C. A. Nelson and M. Luciana, eds), Chap. 4, pp. 45–58. MIT Press, Cambridge, MA.

Tanila, H., Shapiro, M., Gallagher, M., and Eichenbaum, H. (1997a). Brain aging: Changes in the nature of information coding by the hippocampus. *J. Neurosci.* **17**, 5155–5166.

Tanila, H., Sipila, P., Shapiro, M., and Eichenbaum, H. (1997b). Brain aging: Impaired coding of novel environmental cues. *J. Neurosci.* **17**, 5167–5174.

Weinberger, D. R., Berman, K. F., Suddath, R., and Torrey, E.F. (1992) Evidence of dysfunction of a prefrontal-limbic network in schizophrenia: A magnetic resonance imaging and regional cerebral blood flow study of discordant monozygotic twins. *Am. J. Psychiat.* **149**, 890–897.

West, M. J. (1993). New stereological methods for counting neurons. *Neurobiol. Aging* **14**, 275–285.

Yakovlev, P. I., and Lecours, A. R. (1967). The myelogenetic cycles of regional maturation of the brain. *In* "Regional Development of the Brain in Early Life" (A. Minkowski, ed.), pp. 3–70. Blackwell, Oxford.

Suggested Readings

Bauman, M. L., and Kemper, T. L. (1994). "The Neurobiology of Autism," Johns Hopkins Univ. Press, Baltimore, MD.

Grady, C. L. (2000). Functional brain imaging and age-related changes in cognition. *Biol. Psychol.* **54**, 259–281.

Dean, R. L., and Bartus, R. T. (1988). Behavioral models of aging in nonhuman primates. *In* "Handbook of Psychopharmacology" (L. L. Iversen, S. D. Iversen, and S. H. Snyder, eds.), Vol. 20, pp. 352–392. Plenum, New York.

Deboysson-Bardies, B., de Schonen, S., Jusczyk, P., McNeilage, P., and Morton, J. (1993). "Developmental Neurocognition: Speech and Face Processing in the First Year of Life." Kluwer Academic, Boston.

Foster, T. C. (1999). Involvement of hippocampal synaptic plasticity in age-related memory decline. *Brain Res. Rev.* **30**, 236–249.

Keshavan, M. S., and Murray, R. M. (1997). "Neurodevelopment and Adult Psychopathology." Cambridge Univ. Press, Cambridge.

Morrison, J. H., and Hof, P. R. (1997). Life and death of neurons in the aging brain. *Science* **278**, 412–419.

Nelson, C. A., and Luciana, M. (2001). "Handbook of Developmental Cognitive Neuroscience." MIT Press, Cambridge, MA.

Stromswold, K. (1995). The cognitive and neural bases of language acquisition. *In* "The Cognitive Neurosciences" (M. Gazzaniga, ed.), pp. 855–870. MIT Press, Cambridge, MA.

Winkler, J., Thal, L. J., Gage, F. H., and Fisher, L. J. (1998). Cholinergic strategies for Alzheimer's disease. *J. Mol. Med.* **76**, 555–567.

Peter R. Rapp and Jocelyne Bachevalier

Visual Perception of Objects

THE PROBLEM OF OBJECT RECOGNITION

Accurate perception and recognition of objects is a crucial ability for visually dependent organisms such as humans, but it is also a complex one. As object and viewer move with respect to one another, the images cast by the object on the retinas of the observer can change radically. Not only will image position and size change, but surfaces may be foreshortened, occluded, or newly revealed. Similarly, changes in ambient illumination can reveal new surfaces, hide others in shadow, or introduce spurious edges where light ends and shadow begins. However, the viewer is quite accurate in object recognition. This means that the visual system is able to extract a reasonably constant "representation" for the shapes and identities of meaningful objects despite such transformations. Image processing by the retina, visual thalamus, and primary visual cortex begins this process by extracting features and representing them over increasingly large receptive fields. However, in order to understand how the brain represents the identity of an object—its defining, invariant features of shape, relations among parts, and its significance—one must examine how circuits beyond the primary visual cortex encode and retain crucial information of a more global or "high-level" nature.

In general, vision can be thought of as having low-level, intermediate-level, and high-level components. The initial, low-level stages are those by which the brain extracts information about the physical properties of the stimulus, such as the edges, brightness, color, and motion of objects present in scenes (Chapter 27). This processing is often described as *bottom up* because it can proceed from low or input levels on up through the visual system largely without feedback from cognitive processes such as memory. Intermediate-level vision involves putting information about these physical properties together in order to detect global properties of an object, such as object shape and the orientation of the object in depth. High-level processes include those that endow the stimulus with meaning, leading to object recognition and classification. Recognition and classification, in particular, depend on object knowledge and context and can therefore be thought of as *top down* in that the neural processing involved is influenced directly and profoundly by cognitive factors. However, some top-down mechanisms, such as selective attention, can operate at even early stages of visual processing (see Chapter 49).

This chapter is concerned primarily with the neural basis of the high-level components of object vision. First, historical evidence is reviewed that helped localize the crucial circuitry involved to the ventral parts of the temporal lobes. Next, the main pathways are described for object perception and recognition as they have been studied in nonhuman primates, as well as some of the kinds of neural codes that precede and lead up to object vision. Then, neuroimaging and electrophysiological studies are reviewed to show that very similar processing pathways and mechanisms exist in humans. In addition, human studies are reviewed to consider ways in which specialized classes of visual objects may be treated differently by the brain and to discuss ways in which experience with objects tunes their neural representations. Finally, visual object perception is considered in the broader context of general object knowledge and memory.

1201

SUBSTRATES FOR OBJECT PERCEPTION AND RECOGNITION: EARLY EVIDENCE FROM BRAIN DAMAGE

Early Studies of Human Patients Pointed to the Inferior Temporal Cortex as a Site for Object Agnosia

The earliest clues about the neural bases of object perception and recognition came from the study of brain-damaged humans with *visual agnosia*. Visual agnosia is a term for a set of disorders affecting object recognition, in which elementary visual capacities such as acuity and visual fields are preserved or grossly intact (for review, see Farah, 1990). Early attempts to generalize about the lesions in such cases appeared mainly in the German neurological literature of the early 1900s. Writers as early as Potzl in 1928 noted the importance of inferior regions of the temporal lobes, along with adjacent ventral occipital cortex, in the etiology of most cases of visual agnosia.

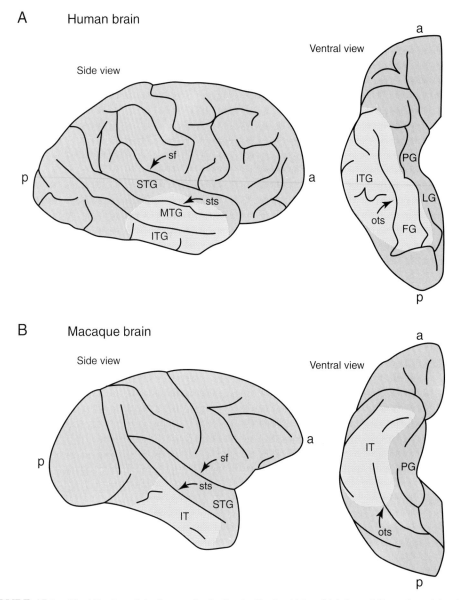

FIGURE 47.1 (Top) Region of the human brain (in shading) within which large bilateral or right-sided lesions cause associative visual agnosia. FG, fusiform gyrus; ITG, inferior temporal gyrus; LG, lingual gyrus; MTG, middle temporal gyrus; PG, parahippocampal gyrus; STG, superior temporal gyrus; ots, occipito-temporal sulcus; sf, Sylvian or lateral fissure, sts, superior temporal sulcus. (Bottom) Region in the macaque monkey (in shading) referred to as the inferior temporal cortex, within which bilateral lesions cause visual discrimination and recognition deficits analogous to agnosic syndromes in humans. a, anterior; p, posterior.

Subsequent studies upheld these general findings and confirmed the central role of the lingual and fusiform gyri (Fig. 47.1). Patients with visual agnosia typically have bilateral or, less commonly, right-sided damage to these regions.

Two Types of Visual Agnosia Have Been Distinguished Historically

Lissauer, who is credited with the first detailed discussion of visual agnosia in 1890, drew a functional distinction between two types, which he termed *apperceptive* and *associative*; these terms are still used commonly today. Agnosic patients whose elementary perception of shape is impaired, despite intact or roughly normal visual acuity, are classified as apperceptive agnosics because their impairment is presumed to be at an early stage of the perceptual processing needed for object recognition. Patients with such deficits are relatively rare and usually have suffered diffuse brain damage, often from carbon monoxide poisoning, as opposed to the more localized damage to posterior cortex and inferior temporal regions seen in the majority of agnosics. Agnosics whose elementary shape perception is grossly intact are classified as associative agnosics following Lissauer's contention that they suffer from an inability to associate a percept with its meaning, i.e., its visual representation stored in memory.

Although the notion that these latter patients show a deficit in association *per se* has been called into question, the impairments they show reveal critical features of how the object recognition system tends to break down. To be considered an associative visual agnosic, the patient is tested to determine the presence of the following features. First, the patient must show difficulty recognizing visually presented objects, as measured by both naming and nonverbal tests of recognition, such as sorting objects by category (e.g., grouping kitchen utensils together, separate from sports equipment) or pantomiming the uses of the object. Second, the patient must show knowledge of the objects through sensory modalities other than vision, i.e., be able to recognize items by sound or touch or through verbal questioning ("What is an egg beater?"). Third, the patient must have sensory and perceptual capacity sufficient to allow him or her to describe the appearance of an unrecognized object, to draw it, or identify whether it is the same as or different from a second item. An illustrative case of associative visual agnosia is summarized in Box 47.1. Figure 47.2 shows some copies drawn by this patient, who nevertheless did not recognize the pictures he copied.

Associative Visual Agnosia Involves Deficits in Invariant Object Representations

Closer examination of the manner in which agnosics copy and match pictures they cannot identify shows that they are often abnormally attentive to the small details of the image rather than being guided by the overall shape or "gestalt" of the object itself; the copying is done in a slow, line-by-line fashion, and patients may classify two pictures as different because of a small flaw in the printing. These observations suggest that the associative agnosic patients are not able to match what is in front of them to a unified, stored visual representation of the object. Such stored representations likely include knowledge about the *invariant*, distinguishing visual attributes (such as the general body shape and relative placement of features of the pig in Fig. 47.2) and/or stored semantic knowledge (the identity of the object as a pig). The underlying problem in visual agnosia could thus result from an inability to generate a high-level representation of the object (a perceptual deficit), a permanent loss of previously stored representations (a memory deficit), or an inability to link the two. In fact, there is some evidence that different agnosic patients are impaired differentially in these different stages. At the same time, recent work suggests that, at the neural level, "perceptual" and "memory" processes for objects may use the same circuitry and could be in principle largely inseparable, as discussed in later sections of this chapter.

Object Recognition in Monkeys Depends on the Inferior Temporal Cortex

Ablation studies in monkeys have both confirmed the crucial role of the temporal lobes in visual object perception and recognition and shed light on the nature of the visual representations used in the object recognition process. One of the earliest experimental studies on the role of the temporal cortex in visual recognition was that of Kluver and Bucy, who described in the 1930s what is now known as the Kluver–Bucy syndrome. When these researchers removed the temporal lobes of monkeys bilaterally, the monkeys demonstrated complex changes in visual, social, sexual, and eating behavior. These changes appeared to result from a combination of perceptual, memory, and motivational impairments. Subsequent researchers eventually specified the region now known as inferior temporal (IT) cortex as the critical area for producing the visual deficits. Monkeys with bilateral IT lesions are impaired both in learning to distinguish between different visual

BOX 47.1

CASE STUDY OF ASSOCIATIVE VISUAL AGNOSIA

The subject was a 47-year-old man who had suffered an acute loss of blood pressure with resulting brain damage. His mental status and language abilities were normal, and his visual acuity was 20/30, with a right homonymous hemianopia (blindness in the right visual hemifield). His one severe impairment was an inability to recognize most visual stimuli. For the first 3 weeks in the hospital, the patient could not identify common objects presented visually and did not know what was on his plate until he tasted it. He identified objects immediately on touching them.

When shown a stethoscope, he described it as "a long cord with a round thing at the end" and asked if it could be a watch. He identified a can opener as a key. Asked to name a cigarette lighter, he said, "I don't know" but named it after the examiner lit it. He said he was "not sure" when shown a toothbrush. He was never able to describe or demonstrate the use of an object if he could not name it. If he misnamed an object, his demonstration of use would correspond to the mistaken identification. Identification improved very slightly when given the category of the object (e.g., something to eat) or when asked to point to a named object instead of being required to give the name. When told the correct name of an object, he usually responded with a quick nod and often said, "Yes, I see it now." Then, often he could point out various parts of the previously unrecognized item as readily as a normal subject (e.g., the stem and bowl of a pipe and the laces, sole, and heel of a shoe). However, if asked by the examiner, "Suppose I told you that the last object was not really a pipe, what would you say?" He would reply, "I would take your word for it. Perhaps it's not a pipe." Similar vacillation never occurred with tactilely or aurally identified objects.

After he had spent 3 weeks on the ward, his object-naming ability improved so that he could name many common objects, but this was variable; he might correctly name an object at one time and misname it later. Performance deteriorated severely when any part of the object was covered by the examiner. He could match identical objects but could not group objects by categories (clothing, food). He could draw the outlines of objects (key, spoon, etc.) that he could not identify.

He was unable to recognize members of his family, the hospital staff, or even his own face in the mirror. Sometimes he had difficulty distinguishing a line drawing of an animal face from a man's face but always recognized it as a face. The ability to recognize pictures of objects was impaired greatly, and after repeated testing he could name only 1 or 2 of 10 line drawings. He was always able to name geometrical forms (circle, square, triangle, cube). Remarkably, he could make excellent copies of line drawings and still fail to name the subject. He easily matched drawings of objects that he could not identify and had no difficulty discriminating between complex nonrepresentational patterns, differing from each other only subtly. He occasionally failed in discriminating because he included imperfections in the paper or in the printer's ink. He could never group drawings of objects by class unless he could first name the subject. Reading, both aloud and for comprehension, was limited greatly. He could read, hesitantly, most printed letters but often misread "K" as "R," and "L" as "T" and vice versa. He was able to read words slowly by spelling them aloud.

Hillary R. Rodman, Luiz Pessoa,
and Leslie G. Ungerleider

Excerpted from Rubens, A. B., and Benson, D. F. (1971). Associative visual agnosia. *Arch. Neurol.* **24**, 305–316.

patterns or objects and in retaining previously acquired visual discriminations. Figure 47.1 shows the location of this area in the macaque brain, relative to the areas implicated in agnosia in humans.

What type of stimulus representation is impaired after IT lesions? Much research has been aimed at answering this question. The general approach has been to infer which stimulus properties are normally encoded (or not encoded) in IT representations by showing which stimulus properties monkeys with IT lesions are impaired at using (or not impaired at using) when attempting to tell objects apart. On the basis of our current knowledge, a reasonable short answer might be that the IT cortex represents aspects of the intrinsic shape of the stimulus that are useful for recognition (e.g., the salient features in a face and their relative positions) and omits most aspects of stimulus appearance that depend on viewing conditions, as described later.

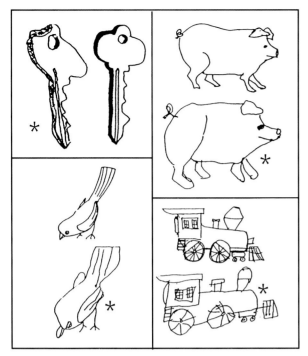

FIGURE 47.2 Pictures that a patient with associative visual agnosia did not recognize but was able to copy. Asterisks indicate the patient's copies. From Rubens and Benson (1971).

Position in the visual field is one visual property that is clearly not necessary for object recognition, and normal monkeys will easily generalize a visual discrimination learned in one hemifield to the other. In other words, if monkeys learn to tell apart stimuli in one half of visual space, they will easily be able to perform the discrimination when the same stimuli are presented to the other half of visual space. The fact that monkeys with IT lesions are impaired at this generalization implies that they have lost representations that are invariant across visual field locations. Retinal image size of a stimulus is another visual property that depends on viewing conditions and not just intrinsic object geometry, and this is another property that gives monkeys with IT lesions trouble. For example, monkeys trained to discriminate between two disks of different absolute sizes are unable to perform the discrimination when those disks are presented at variable distances (and hence with variable retinal image sizes). Instead, they respond on the basis of retinal size or distance. This result implies that representations within the IT cortex normally encode the absolute size of an object, an intrinsic object property useful for recognition, rather than its distance *per se* or its retinal image size. Finally, variations in illumination prevent monkeys with IT lesions from seeing the equivalence of objects, implying that

representations in the IT cortex are unaffected by patterns of shadow and light falling on object surfaces.

Summary

Studies of brain damage in humans and experimental lesions in monkeys both point to the crucial role of tissue in the inferior parts of temporal cortex for object perception and recognition. In both species, moreover, analysis of the ensuing deficits suggests that this tissue participates in creating and storing neural representations of the defining features and invariant aspects that identify a visual object or class of objects.

VISUAL PATHWAYS FOR OBJECT PROCESSING IN NONHUMAN PRIMATES

The Visual Cortex of Monkeys Can Be Divided into Occipitotemporal and Occipitoparietal Pathways

Much of our detailed knowledge of visual cortical organization derives from studies of Old World monkeys of the genus *Macaca*. Similar regions and processing stages are now known to exist in both New World species (Chapter 45) and in humans, as described later in this chapter. The original evidence that the visual cortex is divided into separate processing streams was based on the contrasting effects of inferior temporal and posterior parietal cortex lesions in monkeys. Whereas, as described earlier, inferior temporal lesions cause severe deficits in visual discrimination tasks, they do not affect animals' performance on visuospatial tasks (e.g., visually guided reaching and judging which of two objects lies closer to a visual landmark). In contrast, parietal lesions do not affect visual discrimination ability but instead cause severe deficits on visuospatial performance. On the basis of behavioral results such as these, Ungerleider and Mishkin (1982) proposed the existence of two processing streams: an occipitotemporal or ventral processing stream for mediating the visual recognition of objects ("what" an object is) and an occipitoparietal or dorsal processing stream for mediating the appreciation of the spatial relationships among objects and the visual guidance toward them ("where" an object is). The dorsal processing stream and its importance for spatial cognition is the topic of Chapter 48. As described in Chapter 27, physiological studies of cell properties also support the functional distinction between ventral and dorsal pathways. Neurons in areas (or modules of areas) within the ventral stream (areas V1, V2, V4, and inferior temporal areas TEO and TE) respond selectively to visual features relevant for object identification, such as color, shape and texture, whereas neurons in areas (or modules of areas) within the dorsal stream (areas V1, V2, V3, middle temporal area MT, medial superior temporal area MST, and further areas in inferior parietal and superior temporal sulcal cortex) instead respond selectively to spatial aspects of stimuli, such as the direction and speed of stimulus motion, and also respond when the animal visually tracks a moving target. The remainder of this section specifies details of the anatomical arrangement of components of the *occipitotemporal pathway* for object recognition.

The Object Recognition Pathway in Monkeys Consists of an Interconnected Set of Cortical Areas

Cortical regions that make up the object recognition pathway in monkeys lie directly anterior to the primary visual cortex (V1) in the occipital lobe and in progressively more anterior and ventral portions of the temporal lobe. Figure 47.3 illustrates the location of these areas and diagrams the forward flow of information within this occipitotemporal pathway in the context of the overall organization of the visual cortex of the macaque. The cortical analysis of objects begins in V1, where information about contour orientation, color composition and brightness is represented in subsets of neurons responsible for each point in the visual field (Chapter 27). Information from V1 is then sent forward to subdivisions or modules—interdigitating thin, thick, and interstripe regions—within V2 (Chapters 27 and 45). From the thin and interstripe regions in V2, representing color and form information, respectively, neural signals proceed forward to area V4 on the lateral and ventromedial surfaces of the hemisphere and to a posterior inferior temporal area just in front of V4, area TEO. From both V4 and TEO, signals related to object form, color, and texture proceed forward to area TE, the last exclusively visual area within the ventral stream for object recognition. Together, areas TEO and TE make up the IT cortex.

Progressing forward along the occipitotemporal pathway from V1 to TE, there is a gradual shift in the nature of connectivity, which is significant for the eventual extraction of invariant object features. At successive stages, patterns of cortical projections become successively less topographic or "point to point." While connections from V1 to V2 maintain topographic order, they are looser between V2 and V4, and inputs to area TE from V4 and TEO retain no obvious retinotopic organization. Moreover, pathways interconnecting areas of the ventral stream on the two sides of the brain via the corpus callosum and/or the anterior commissure tend to be restricted to the representation of the midline of visual space early in the pathway, but their representation becomes more widespread at higher levels in the pathway. This loss of retinotopy within area TE means that single neurons respond to objects anywhere in the visual field. Thus, explicit information about the spatial location of an object is not retained at the highest levels of the ventral stream.

Neural processing in the object recognition pathway is not, however, a simple matter of successive elaboration of information from lower order to higher order areas. At all stages connections are reciprocal, such that an area receiving feed-forward projections from an area earlier in the ventral stream also provides feedback projections to that area. Long-range nonreciprocal connections, such as from area TE back to V1, also exist. Whereas feed-forward projections provide bottom-up, sensory-driven inputs to subsequent visual areas, and severing these projections disconnects subsequent areas from their visual input, the precise functions of reciprocal, feedback projections are still unknown. However, these feedback projections are thought to play a top-down role in vision, such as in selective attention, by modulating activity in earlier areas of the ventral pathway (Chapter 49). In addition to feed-forward and feedback projections, there appear to be "intermediate-type" projections that link areas at the same level of the visual hierarchy. These are seen most notably between areas of the dorsal and ventral streams. For example, area V4 is interconnected with motion-

FIGURE 47.3 (A) Schematic diagram of the macaque monkey brain illustrating the two cortical visual system model of Ungerleider and Mishkin (1982). According to this model, there are two major processing pathways, or "streams," in the visual cortex, both originating in the primary visual cortex: a ventral stream, directed into the temporal lobe and crucial for the identification of objects, and a dorsal stream, directed into the parietal lobe and crucial for spatial perception and visuomotor performance. The shaded region indicates the extent of the visual cortex in the monkey, and the labels (OC, OB, OA, TEO, TE, PG) indicate cytoarchitectonic areas according to the nomenclature of von Bonin amd Bailey. Adapted from Mishkin *et al.* (1983). (B) A lateral view of the monkey brain illustrating the multiplicity of functional areas within both processing streams. (C) Some of the pertinent connections of the inferior temporal cortex with other cortical areas and medial temporal lobe structures. Red lines indicate the main afferent pathway to area TE, which includes areas V1, V2, V4, and TEO. For simplicity, only projections from lower order to higher order areas are shown, but each of these feed-forward projections is reciprocated by a feedback projection. Faces indicate areas in which neurons selectively responsive to faces have been found. Adapted from Gross *et al.* (1993).

A

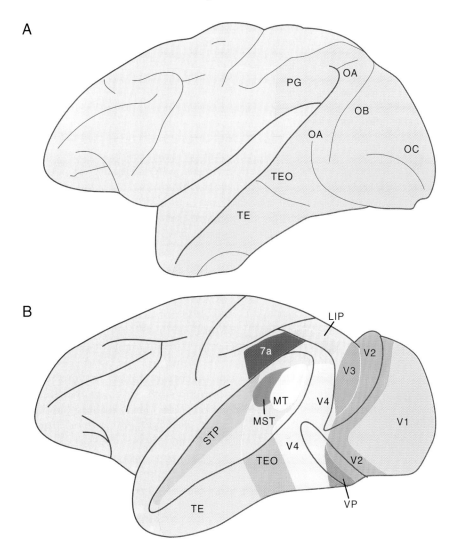

B

C

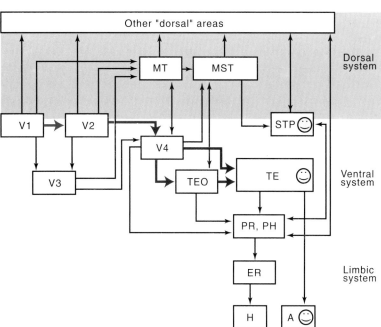

A	amygdala
ER	entorhinal cortex
H	hippocampus
LIP	lateral intraparietal area
MST	medial superior temporal area
MT	middle temporal area
PH	parahippocampal cortex
PR	perirhinal cortex
STP	superior temporal polysensory area
TE	ant. inferior temporal cortex
TEO	post. inferior temporal cortex
V1	first visual area
V2	second visual area
V3	third visual area
V4	fourth visual area
VP	ventral posterior area

sensitive areas MT and MST. Thus, an anatomical substrate exists for interactions between the two processing streams, and these might serve to integrate what an object is with where an object is.

All areas within the ventral stream also have heavy interconnections with subcortical structures, most notably the pulvinar, claustrum, and basal ganglia. In addition, each receives subcortical modulatory inputs from ascending cholinergic projections from the basal forebrain and ascending noradrenergic projections from the locus coeruleus. These projections are thought to play a role in the storage of information in the cortex and the influence of arousal on information processing, respectively. Finally, visual information is sent *from* the IT cortex to the most ventral and anterior reaches of the temporal lobe, notably the perirhinal cortex and parahippocampal areas TF and TH. These regions in turn project, via the entorhinal cortex, to medial temporal lobe structures, such as the hippocampus, which contribute to forming long-term memories of visual objects and their contexts (Chapter 51). Information is also sent from the IT to the prefrontal cortex, which plays an important role in working memory, holding an object briefly in mind when it is no longer visible (Chapters 53 and 54). Finally, there are direct projections from the IT cortex to the amygdala, which is important for attaching emotional valence to a stimulus (Chapter 51).

Summary

Areas along the occipitotemporal pathway of the monkey are organized hierarchically proceeding from V1 to V2 through V4 and TEO to TE. At progressive stages of this hierarchy there is a progressive loss of retinotopic information, such that information about the spatial location of the object is gradually lost. In addition to bottom-up information being supplied by feed-forward projections from lower order to higher order visual areas within this pathway, there are also reciprocal, feedback projections from higher order to lower order visual areas. These projections are thought to play a top-down role in vision.

NEURONAL PROPERTIES WITHIN THE OBJECT RECOGNITION PATHWAY

Cells along the Occipitotemporal Pathway Are Sensitive to Increasingly More Complex Physical Features of Objects

The different cortical areas in the occipitotemporal pathway share a number of physiological characteristics. Consistent with a role in object recognition, all areas in the pathway contain populations of cells sensitive to the shape, color, or texture of visual stimuli or some combination of these features. Despite the fact that visual areas within the ventral stream are selective for a variety of stimulus attributes, progressing forward along the pathway reveals a general trend toward selectivity for increasingly complex stimulus features or combinations of features. For example, whereas many V1 neurons function as local spatial filters (e.g., signaling the presence of contours at particular positions in the visual field), some V2 cells respond to so-called illusory contours of whole figures; a V2 cell selective for the horizontal orientation of an edge placed in its receptive field (RF) may respond similarly to an edge that is not physically present but implicitly suggested by stimulation of surrounding regions. Other cells in V2 are jointly selective for wavelength and small dimensions of stimuli; such cells represent an early stage of integration of stimulus features. Moving forward to V4, the trend continues in that a greater proportion of cells are conjointly tuned for multiple dimensions of a stimulus (such as length, width, and/or wavelength of a bar of light). In addition, about a third of neurons in V4 show selectivity to contour features such as curves and angles with particular properties, suggesting an intermediate stage of processing.

Another important property of V4 neurons is the existence of large silent suppressive zones surrounding the excitatory receptive fields of cells. These zones are termed "silent" because stimulation of the zones does not normally cause any change from the baseline activity of the cell but can have a powerful effect on the response to a stimulus placed in the receptive field (what is now called by many the "classical" receptive field). The stimulus-selective properties of the excitatory receptive field and the suppressive surround are often matched. As a consequence, many V4 cells respond maximally to a stimulus only if it stands out from its background on the basis of a difference in form. This sensitivity to receptive field/surround differences is thought to be useful for figure/ground segregation—the parcellation of scenes into a collection of objects within them.

Moving forward successively into area TEO and then into posterior and anterior portions of area TE, there is a further increase in the complexity of the critical features needed to activate many neurons and an increase as well in the proportion of cells that are selectively driven by some kind of complex pattern or object (Gross *et al.*, 1972). Although some percentage of cells selectively responsive to simple parameters of length, width, orientation, spatial frequency, and wavelength (or little selectivity at all) can be found in each of these regions, at the level of TE many cells require moderately complex features for their activation. Importantly, the critical features that drive single cells are typically not complex enough to specify a particular object. To represent individual objects would instead require activation of a few to several tens of cells with different critical features.

The work of Tanaka (1993) has shown that a key property of TE is that it is composed of columns, in many ways similar to those in V1, in which cells with related but slightly different selectivity cluster together (Fig. 47.4). For example, some cells in a column responsive to faces might respond optimally to different face components, others might be sensitive to the overall configuration of a face regardless of viewpoint, and still others might respond well to faces specifically in profile. Thus, a given object feature is apparently not represented by the activity of a single cell, but by the activity of many cells within a column. Representation by multiple cells in a column in which the selectivity

varies, but overlaps, from cell to cell satisfies two apparently conflicting requirements in visual recognition: robustness to subtle changes in input and precision of representation. Given this clustering of cells responsive to related features, an object in its entirety would then be represented by a pattern of activity distributed across multiple columns, each of which may participate in representing multiple objects. Whereas the image of an object projected on the retina changes in response to variations in illumination and viewing angle, the pattern of activity in TE should be largely maintained, insofar as the clustering of cells with overlapping but slightly different selectivity should serve as a buffer to absorb such changes.

Some Cells in the Occipitotemporal Pathway Are Face Selective

One of the more striking characteristics of monkey temporal cortex is the presence of neurons with responses selective for face stimuli, first described by

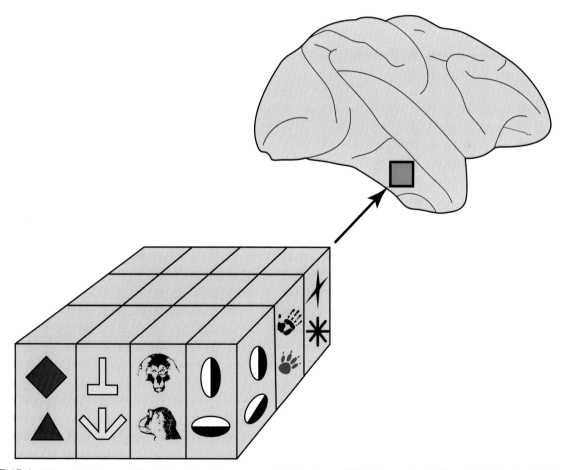

FIGURE 47.4 Schematic diagram illustrating the columnar organization in area TE of the monkey. Cells with similar but slightly different selectivity tend to cluster in elongated vertical columns perpendicular to the cortical surface. Stimuli shown are examples of the critical features for the activation of single cells in TE. Most cells, as shown, require moderately complex features for their activation, although some can be driven by simpler stimuli, such as color, orientation, and texture. Adapted from Tanaka (1993).

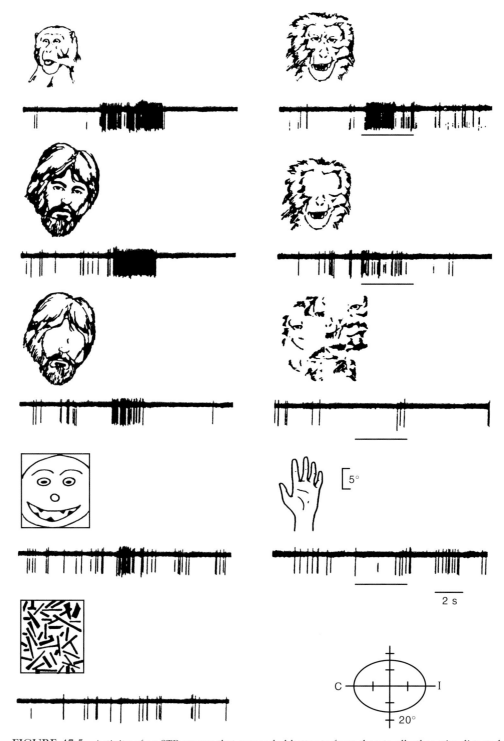

FIGURE 47.5 Activity of an STP neuron that responded better to faces than to all other stimuli tested. Removing eyes on a picture or representing the face as a caricature reduced the response. Cutting the picture into 16 pieces and rearranging the pieces eliminated the response. All the unit records are representative ones chosen from a larger number of trials. The receptive field of the neuron is illustrated on the lower right. C, contralateral; I, ipsilateral visual field. From Bruce *et al*. (1981).

Bruce *et al*. (1981) and Perrett *et al*., (1982). Although the overall numbers of these *face-selective cells* are small (1–5% of all neurons recorded in these regions), their concentration is much higher in the cortex of the lower and upper banks of the superior temporal sulcus, where they are found together in clumps and where they may make up as much as 10–20% of all cells studied. The lower bank of the superior temporal sulcus is part of area TE, whereas the upper bank is part of the superior temporal polysensory area (STP), which responds to auditory and somatic as well as visual stimuli.

Face-selective cells vary in the degree and nature of their preference for face stimuli. Many respond well to both real faces or face pictures, but give nearly no response to any other stimuli tested, including other complex objects, texture patterns, and images in which the features making up the face are rearranged or scrambled (Fig. 47.5). Thus, at least some face-selective neurons appear to be sensitive to very general or global aspects of a face, such as the proto-typical arrangement of the eyes, nose, and mouth into a face-like configuration. Other neurons in TE and STP respond to specific face components, such as the presence of eyes per se, the distance between the eyes, or the extent of the forehead. While such neurons may merely be sensitive to facial features, they are nonetheless likely to participate in circuits responsi-ble for recognizing a particular individual. One subset of face cells that responds to whole faces is particu-larly sensitive to the direction of gaze of the eyes (looking back directly or turned to the side), which is an important social signal for both monkeys and humans.

Finally, some neurons in area STP respond selec-tively to *biological motion*, i.e., motion patterns consis-tent with what one sees when one observes the gait of another animal. For example, these cells respond when viewing a monkey or human walking, or to equivalent motion patterns generated by so-called Johanssen point-light stimuli (i.e., stimuli generated by attaching lights to the joints of a moving animal, which is otherwise in the dark). Together, all these observations have led to the proposal that the primate temporal lobe has evolved specialized mechanisms for the encoding and recognition of biologically significant stimuli. Consistent with this idea is the finding that face-selective neurons are present very early in life in monkeys. Later in the chapter, addi-tional lines of evidence for specialized neural machin-ery for face recognition are considered. Alternative interpretations of such *category-specific* phenomena are also discussed, which take into account the learning history of the subject.

The Occipitotemporal Pathway Extracts Some Invariant Aspects of Objects

As suggested at the start of the chapter, visual information impinging on the retina is a two-dimensional projection of a three-dimensional world, a projection that varies dramatically as a function of changes in the position, distance, illumination, and orientation of an object relative to the viewer. Thus, the function of the occipitotemporal pathway can be defined in large measure as determining and encod-ing those *invariant* features of objects that are useful for recognition across myriad cirumstances. On the one hand, exactly how this might be best done is not clear even at a theoretical level. On the other hand, there have been a number of findings regarding the occipitotemporal pathway that provide useful hints as to how this process begins.

As described earlier, as one progresses forward from V1 to TE, RFs become larger and the retinotopic maps less precise. By area TE, RFs are large and bilat-eral, typically encompassing the central 20° or more, and in far anterior TE can include the entire visual field. As we have seen, the large RFs of TE neurons signal the presence of a given feature, collection of features, or object, regardless of where in the visual field they fall. In other words, they exhibit invariance of stimulus coding across changes in retinal position.

In addition to invariance over position, many neurons in TE show maintained selectivity for their "preferred" stimuli over more complex kinds of trans-formations, such as size, distance from the subject in depth, or degree of ambient illumination, so that they show invariance over a number of the changes that normally take place as a moving object is viewed under naturalistic conditions. Also, many TE neurons show *form-cue invarance*: for example, a neuron selec-tive for a particular shape defined by luminance borders (e.g., white star on a black background) will be selective for the same form defined by relative texture and motion cues instead (e.g., a star-shaped region of speckles of the same average luminance as the background moving in a different direction from the background). These various types of response invariance or *generalization*, taken together, make it possible to understand the types of deficits seen in experimental monkeys when the IT cortex is removed, as discussed earlier.

Finally, as discussed in Box 47.2, one central ques-tion in object recognition has been the degree to which neural representations of objects are object-centered (view independent) or viewer-centered (view dependent). The question of *view dependence* has been addressed by a number of single-unit studies of neurons in TE. For example, in one study, monkeys were trained to recognize specific novel three-dimen-sional objects from any viewpoint after experience with a few prototypical views in a discrimination task (Logothetis *et al.*, 1995). After months of such training,

BOX 47.2

THE ISSUE OF VIEWPOINT DEPENDENCE IN OBJECT RECOGNITION

Although we know something of the underlying anatomy and physiology, the mechanisms by which object recognition is actually accomplished by the brain have been a matter of heated debate. The pioneering theoretical work of Marr in the late 1970s set the stage for current theories, which can be divided into two main groups: object-centered (view independent), and viewer-centered (view dependent) theories.

According to *object-centered* accounts, objects are represented in the brain as hierarchies of parts that are, to a large degree, independent of any particular viewpoint. One of the best known examples is Biederman's (1990) recognition by components (RBC), which postulates that objects can be defined as a set of 30 or so primitive shapes, so-called *geons*. In this theory, geons are three-dimensional component building blocks, which, when combined, form the objects that we know (Fig. 47.6). Thus, any arbitrary object may be described as a collection of elementary geons. For example, the telephone in Fig. 47.6 can be constructed from geons 1, 3, and 5. One compelling feature of geons for object recognition is that particular ones can be inferred from the presence of *nonaccidental relations* between image contours or parts. Nonaccidental relations are those unlikely to occur by chance, such as parallel or colinear edges, closure, and symmetry. Also, because the same nonaccidental features can be derived across a wide range of image variations, detection of geons and their spatial relations would be preserved over changes in position, distance, illumination, and orientation; the telephone, for example, looks pretty much the same (in terms of its constituent geons and how they sit relative to one another) from a variety of angles. Therefore, according to RBC, recognizing an object amounts to determining the set of geons that compose the object and determining the spatial relations between them.

Viewer-centered theories, however, suggest that recognition is linked to the appearance of objects as originally seen. In other words, the brain is not thought of as storing a central, invariant representation of an object, but instead as storing information from multiple independent views (e.g., a view of the telephone as in the figure, but also an end-on or side view, a view from above, etc.). A potential problem with this idea is that it might seem that for reliable object recognition, stored representations for *all* views of objects would need to

exist. The solution is to suggest that a small set of characteristic or *prototypical* views would suffice. Proponents of this approach have offered a variety of different theoretical normalization mechanisms for generalizing from unfamiliar views to the familiar, protoypical stored views (Bulthoff *et al.*, 1995). For example, the visual system might mentally rotate the object as currently seen to bring it into line with a prototypical view or do an interpolation or comparison of the current view with multiple stored views. Therefore, according to viewer-centered theories, recognizing an object amounts to explaining the appearance of an incoming stimulus in terms of transformations or combinations of previously stored representative views.

At first glance, object-centered theories appear more compelling, as they attempt at the outset to solve the central problem associated with object recognition, namely reliable recognition despite variation in the precise retinal image. However, one serious challenge is how the brain chooses the correct structural interpretation among the possible ones, as a given set of geons may be compatible with several different objects. Psychophysical testing also indicates that object-centered encoding is not the whole story; studies have shown substantial and robust viewpoint effects even for extremely simple three-dimensional volumes resembling proposed geon primitives.

However, viewer-centered approaches also face challenges. Viewer-centered theories have been most successful in accounting for *exemplar-level* recognition, i.e., discriminating between individual visually similar objects within a relatively homogeneous class of objects such as faces, cars, or birds. While recognition at the exemplar level is often important, there is little question that so-called *class-level* recognition actually constitutes much of the job of recognition. For example, for objects such as chairs, telephones, and toasters, we rarely need to discriminate two instances of the class and instead we learn to recognize such objects at a basic category or class level. Viewer-centered models suggest that the brain represents the appearance of a specific individual example of an object from specific viewpoints, and thus seem unsuitable or unnecessary for class-level recognition. Moreover, even for a single exemplar, it is uncertain how many prototypical views are enough for robust recognition. One solution would be to store as many views of an object as possible so that new views would always be similar

BOX 47.2 (cont'd)

enough to some previously stored view. However, it is unclear that there can ever be sufficient memory to do so for all the objects that the observer becomes proficient at recognizing under varied conditions.

Hillary R. Rodman, Luiz Pessoa, and Leslie G. Ungerleider

References

Biederman, I. (1990) Higher-level vision. *In* "Visual Cognition and Action" (D. H. Osherson, S. M. Kozzlyn, and Z. M. Hollerbach, eds.), Vol. 2, pp. 41–72. MIT Press, Cambridge, MA.

Bulthoff, H. H., Edelman, S. Y., and Tan, M. J. (1995). How are 3-dimensional objects represented in the brain. *Cereb. Cortex* **5**, 247–260.

the monkeys were found to have neurons in TE that exhibited strong selectivity for precisely those views on which the animal had been trained. These results support the view dependent account of object recognition. Studies of face-selective neurons in area TE also initially provided strong support for view dependence by finding separate populations of cells tuned for front and profile views in both adult and infant monkeys. However, other studies have shown that at least small subsets of TE neurons respond to faces or objects independent of view, providing evidence for view-independent representations as well. Overall, the issue of view dependence remains an open question, with some evidence for both accounts to be found in the neurophysiological literature as well as in psychophysical studies (Fig 47.6)

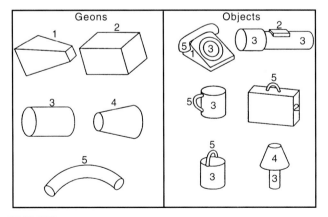

FIGURE 47.6 Illustration of geons and how they are arranged to form objects. (Left) A given view of an object can be represented by an arrangement of simple primitive volumes, or geons, five of which are shown here. (Right) Only two or three geons are required to uniquely specify an object. The relations among the geons matter, as illustrated with the pail and cup. From Biederman (1990).

Response Properties of Cells in the Object Recognition Pathway Are Affected by Experience

The previous sections illustrated how the object recognition pathway, especially area TE, represents features that are useful for recognition. For example, some neurons respond selectively to the salient features in a face, or their relative positions, while ignoring aspects of stimulus appearance that depend on viewing conditions, such as absolute size and luminance. However, in ecological terms, what is useful and salient within the image of an object or scene changes with experience and context, and these changes are reflected in the way the brain represents stimuli over time. Neurons in the IT cortex and the adjacent perirhinal cortex show effects of both recent viewing history and long-term experience with stimuli.

Experiments by Miller and Desimone (1994) have shown how short-term changes in response properties of temporal neurons encode aspects of both stimulus recency and short-term stimulus significance. For example, for many of these cells, responses to an object that is presented repeatedly decrease in a systematic fashion, potentially signaling that the object has been seen recently. Such reduced signals may be useful for redirecting attention to novel objects. This kind of response decrement, termed *repetition suppression*, has been found both under anesthesia and for stimuli which an awake animal is trained to ignore. This habituation-like response is therefore a passive, automatic mechanism by which the visual system edits out recently seen objects. In contrast, if a monkey is trained to do a matching task in which it must hold a particular visual pattern in memory over

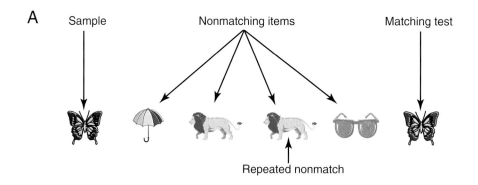

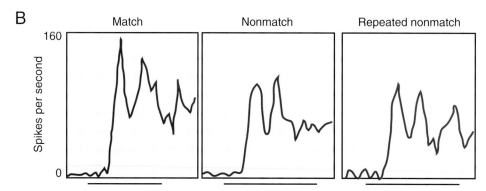

FIGURE 47.7 Experiment demonstrating mnemonic enhancement. (A) On each trial, the monkey was shown a sample stimulus, and then between zero and four intervening nonmatching items appeared before the matching stimulus was presented. Repeated nonmatches appeared after zero (as shown) or one intervening stimulus between them. The task of the monkey was to respond to the matching test stimulus and ignore repeated nonmatches. (B) Responses of a neuron to a single stimulus appearing as a match, non-match, and repeated nonmatch. Horizontal bars under the histograms indicated when the stimuli were on, which was 500 ms for nonmatch and repeated nonmatch stimuli. The match stimulus was terminated when the animal made its response. Results show mnemonic enhancement to the match stimulus but not to a stimulus that repeats but is not held in mind (i.e., repeated nonmatch). Adapted from Miller and Desimone (1994).

a short delay, some temporal neurons increase their firing rates specifically when the to-be-remembered stimulus is recognized. This phenomenon, termed *mnemonic enhancement*, can be thought of as a mechanism in which bottom-up processing of the stimulus is affected by top-down, cognitive factors, namely, expectation of the relevant stimulus (Fig. 47.7). Stimuli that are repeated but are not behaviorally relevant in the context of the task do not show this enhancement effect.

Experiments such as these demonstrate that the magnitude of responses of neurons can be affected by the experience of the subject with the stimulus and by its significance, at least in the short term. Other studies suggest that the kind of familiarity gained over longer periods of time—akin to the development of "expertise" as discussed later in the chapter—can also be reflected in the responses of TE cells. For example, in monkeys that have been trained for as long as a year to discriminate between objects, more

than 30% of the cells show selectivity for those objects compared to untrained monkeys in which roughly 10% of the cells show such selectivity (Kobatake *et al.*, 1998).

Even more fascinating perhaps is the finding that some TE and perirhinal cells come to represent the *history of association between objects* in the activity patterns they exhibit in response to members of a set of stimuli. Some research groups have examined mechanisms of visual memory by using *paired-associate* tasks in which monkeys are trained to associate arbitrary patterns with one another for reward. In experiments conducted by Sakai and Miyashita (1991), for example, monkeys were first shown one member of a learned pair and then were required to choose the associated "match" from a display of two stimuli while single-unit activity in the anterior IT cortex was recorded. Across the population of cells as a whole, they found neurons that responded best to stimuli that had been paired together during training. In other words, some cells in temporal cortex developed conjoint selectivity (*pair coding*) for the members of associated pairs. It was shown that pair coding by TE cells was decreased by surgically interrupting the feedback projections to them from the perirhinal and entorhinal cortices. Thus, return projections appear to play a specific role in associating objects because the pair-coding property depends on them.

Furthermore, although associative learning effects have typically been seen in studies after weeks or months of training, there is evidence that small but detectable shifts in neuronal population selectivity occur even after only a day or so of experience, suggesting that TE cells tend to develop pair-coding properties more rapidly than previously thought (Ericksen et al., 2000; Messinger et al., 2001). Thus, the pattern of selectivity shown by TE cells at any given moment in time may partly reflect a record of their exposure to stimuli seen together. Overall, TE circuits as a whole appear to represent not only complex visual features, but also the history of their meanings and relationships in a behavioral context.

Summary

At successive levels of processing along the occipitotemporal pathway more complex kinds of information about objects are extracted. At the highest levels of the pathway, within area TE and neighboring STP, some neurons are preferentially responsive to faces and other biologically significant stimuli. In addition, TE neurons extract some invariant aspects of objects. For example, TE neurons show similar selectivity for objects regardless of large changes in their retinal position, size, distance in depth, and degree of ambient illumination. Finally, as the result of experience, some TE neurons come to represent novel objects and/or the associative relations between objects.

FUNCTIONAL IMAGING AND ELECTROPHYSIOLOGY OF OBJECT RECOGNITION IN HUMANS

The Human Brain Also Has Ventral and Dorsal Processing Streams

The differential visual impairments produced by focal lesions in clinical cases suggest that the human visual cortex, like that of the monkey, contains two anatomically distinct and functionally specialized pathways: the ventral and dorsal streams. In one study, for example, a double dissociation of visual recognition (face perception camouflaged by sha-

dows) and visuospatial performance (stylus maze learning) was demonstrated in two men with lesions of the occipitotemporal and occipitoparietal cortex, respectively, confirmed by postmortem examination (Newcombe *et al.*, 1987). The specific clinical syndromes produced by occipitotemporal lesions include visual object agnosia, as noted earlier, as well as prosopagnosia, an inability to recognize familiar faces, and achromatopsia, or cortical color blindness. In contrast, syndromes produced by occipitoparietal lesions include optic ataxia (misreaching), visuospatial neglect, constructional apraxia, gaze apraxia, akinetopsia (an inability to perceive movement), and disorders of spatial cognition. Interestingly, imagery disorders involving descriptions of either objects (especially faces, animals, and colors of objects) or spatial relations (e.g., geographic directions) are also dissociable following temporal and parietal lesions.

The advent of functional brain imaging, both *positron emission tomography* (*PET*) and *functional magnetic resonance imaging* (*fMRI*), has made it possible to map the organization of the human visual cortex with far greater precision than is possible with human lesion studies, and without the confounding influence of compensatory responses to brain injury (Chapter 13, Box 13.1). In experiments by Haxby and colleagues (1994) designed to investigate the possible existence of separate object vision and spatial vision pathways in humans, changes in regional cerebral blood flow were measured using PET while subjects performed object identity and spatial location matching-to-sample tasks (Fig. 47.8). In the object identity task, the subjects indicated on each trial which of two choice faces matched the sample face, whereas in the spatial location task, the subjects indicated which of two choice stimuli contained a small square in the same location, relative to a double line, as the small square in the sample stimulus. Faces for the object identity task were contained within the small squares so that identical stimuli were used for face and location matching, with only the task requirements changing. The results identified occipitotemporal and occipitoparietal regions associated with face and location matching, respectively, and posterior occipital regions associated with both visual functions. In addition, regions in the ventral and dorsal frontal cortex were selectively activated by face and location matching, respectively. These findings thus indicate the existence in humans, as in monkeys, of two functionally specialized and anatomically segregated visual processing pathways, both of which receive their inputs from early visual areas. The findings further suggest the extensions of each into the frontal lobe, which plays a role in working memory for objects and their spatial locations (Chapter 53).

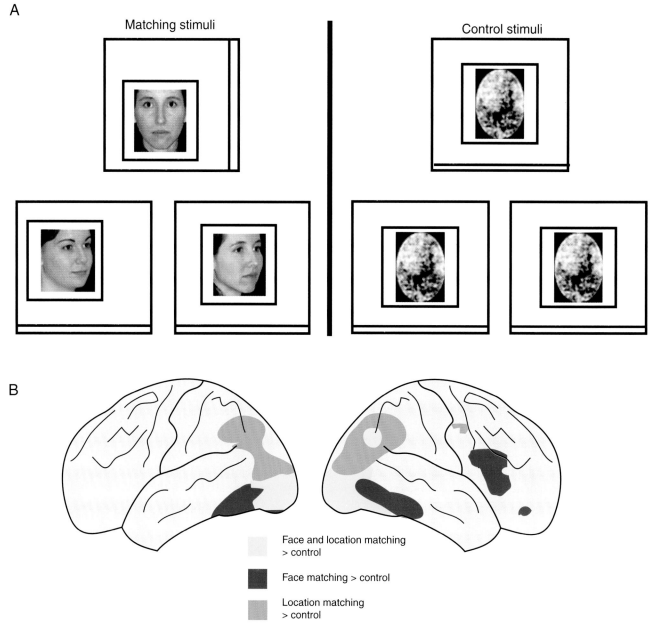

FIGURE 47.8 Ventral and dorsal processing streams in the human cortex, as demonstrated in a PET imaging study of face and location perception. (A) Sample stimuli used during the experiment. (Left) Stimuli for both face and location matching tasks. During face matching trials, subjects had to indicate with a button press which of the two faces at the bottom was the same person shown at the top. In this example, the correct choice is the stimulus on the right. During location matching trials, subjects had to indicate with a button press which of the two small squares at the bottom was in the same location relative to the double line as the small square shown at the top. In this example, the correct choice is the stimulus on the left. (Right) Control stimuli. During control trials, subjects saw an array of three stimuli in which the small squares contained a complex visual image. In these trials, which controlled for both visual stimulation and finger movements, they alternated left and right button presses. (B) Areas shown in red had significantly increased activity during the face matching but not during the location matching task, as compared with activity during the control task. Areas shown in green had significantly increased activity during the location matching but not during the face matching task, as compared with activity during the control task. Areas shown in yellow had significantly increased activity during both face and location matching tasks. Adapted from Haxby *et al*. (1994).

The Building Blocks of Object Recognition in Human Cortex Include Early Visual Areas and the Lateral Occipital Complex (LO)

Functional imaging studies have also revealed a number of distinct visual areas within the ventral and dorsal streams in humans. Many of these areas appear to be equivalent (and perhaps homologous) to specific monkey visual areas, including V1, V2, V3, V4, and the middle temporal area (MT). Some of these areas have been defined on the basis of retinotopic mapping strategies, as in the monkey, whereas others have been defined on the basis of their functional properties. For example, studies that measure activation in tasks requiring perception of, or attention to, color, shape, and faces, tend to find foci in the vicinity of

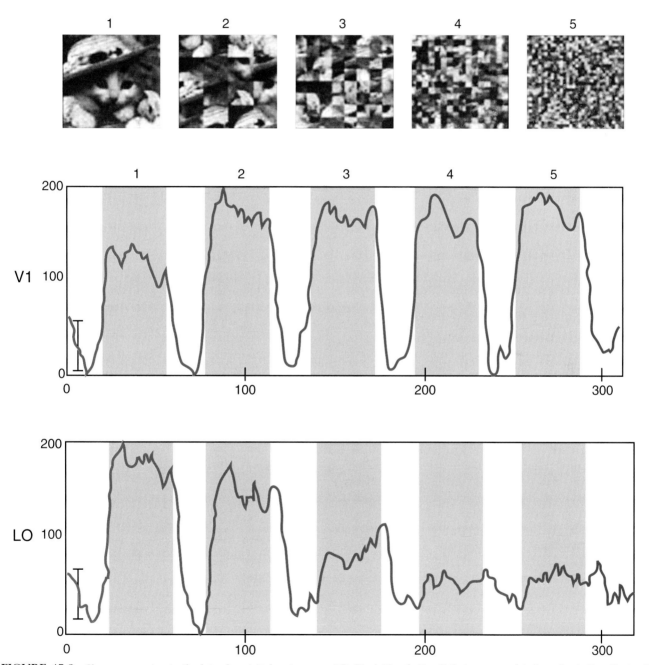

FIGURE 47.9 Shape processing in the lateral occipital cortex, area LO. (Top) Visual stimuli that were used to investigate the effects of image scrambling on activity in LO, as measured by fMRI. Subjects viewed the stimuli and were instructed to covertly name them, even the scrambled images. Stimulus 1 is the original image, and stimuli 2–5 are increasingly scrambled. (Bottom) fMRI time series illustrating the averaged activations in V1 and LO to each of the images shown at the top. Note that LO is very sensitive to image scrambling, whereas V1 is not. Adapted from Grill-Spector *et al.* (1998).

areas termed V2 and V4 on the basis of retinotopy, as well as in more anterior ventral stream areas in the temporal lobe (see later), all of which contain cells selective for these features in the monkey. In contrast, studies that measure activation during perception of, or attention to, motion often find foci in areas associated with the dorsal stream, particularly in a region that seems homologous to MT, an area in the monkey that contains a high proportion of cells selective for visual motion.

Within the ventral stream of humans, it is generally thought that because areas V1–V4 are organized retinotopically, they represent low-level stages in object processing. How can one separate the low-level processing performed by these areas from higher level processes associated with object recognition *per se*? The approach adopted by Grill-Spector and colleagues (1998) has been to compare the cortical activation evoked by pictures of a variety of objects to the activation evoked by pictures of various texture patterns, which match the object pictures in their low-level properties, such as contrast and spatial frequency (Fig. 47.9). Areas responding more to objects than to textures are interpreted as being involved in object-related processing. A major focus of activation in these studies was found to be located at the lateral-posterior aspect of the occipital lobe, just abutting the posterior aspect of the motion-sensitive area MT, in a region termed the *lateral occipital complex* (LO).

A number of properties of the fMRI responses obtained by Grill-Spector and colleagues strengthen the interpretation that LO is an important stage in human object processing. First, a four-fold change in visual size does not affect LO activation, although it changes some stimulus properties greatly (e.g., local contrast). Second, LO exhibits a high sensitivity to image scrambling. In contrast, early visual areas V1–V3 respond similarly to intact, recognizable stimuli and highly scrambled, unrecognizable pictures (in fact, scrambled pictures tend to elicit stronger responses). Third, LO is an area of convergence of visual cues. For example, the shape of an object can be defined by luminance, by texture, or by motion cues alone; objects defined by any one or more of these cues reliably evoke LO responses. Fourth, responses in LO exhibit some invariance to changes in image position. Fifth, and most importantly, objects that vary widely in their recognizability, such as famous faces and unfamiliar three-dimensional abstract sculptures, produce similar activations in LO. Taken together, these findings indicate that LO is an intermediate link in the processing of objects, i.e., a stage following low-level processing and preceding object processing stages that involve memory. It may be that LO in humans is equivalent to area TEO in the posterior IT cortex of monkeys in that

both LO and TEO exhibit a crude central-to-peripheral retinotopic organization.

While the processing of general object shape observed in LO is very important for object perception and recognition, LO probably is not responsible for object recognition *per se*. Whereas LO responds to essentially any three-dimensional shape, areas in the ventral stream anterior to LO, most notably on the fusiform gyrus in the ventral temporal cortex, respond preferentially to recognizable objects. It is therefore thought that object recognition is critically dependent on the ventral temporal cortex. Indeed, as later sections describe, it is likely that the storage of object representations takes place in the ventral temporal cortex as well. The next section considers the processing of specific categories of objects and the functional architecture of the ventral temporal cortex.

Summary

Evidence from both lesion studies and neuroimaging indicates the existence in humans, as in monkeys, of two visual processing pathways: a ventral stream for object vision and a dorsal stream for spatial vision. Within the ventral stream, early visual areas, including V1–V4, are organized retinotopically and appear to be homologous to areas studied in monkeys. In humans, LO appears to play an important role at the next stage of processing, where general object shape is processed. Activation of LO is highly sensitive to image scrambling, but insensitive to image size or the visual cues that define the shape of an object. Activation in LO, however, is not sensitive to object recognizability, suggesting that it precedes processing stages that involve memory.

PERCEPTION AND RECOGNITION OF SPECIFIC CLASSES OF OBJECTS

Prosopagnosia Is a Specific Deficit of Face Recognition

Evidence from neuropsychology and neurophysiology suggests that certain kinds of objects may have special significance to primates. *Prosopagnosia*, a selective deficit in recognizing familiar faces, has been known since at least the end of the 19th century. Although patients with this syndrome are aware that faces are faces, i.e., they know the basic stimulus category, they fail to reliably identify or even achieve a sense of familiarity from the faces of co-workers, family members, famous persons, and other individuals previously well known to them. Typically, they also have trouble forming memories of new faces, even if other new objects can be learned. Because the voice of a visually unrecognized person usually enables the patient to identify and feel familiar with that person, prosopagnosia (or face agnosia) appears to be a specifically visual impairment.

A number of explanations for the apparent selectivity of the prosopagnosic deficit have been offered. One explanation is that face perception and recognition are indeed unique behavioral capacities and reflect unique, dedicated neural circuits that can be selectively damaged. Such dedicated neural circuits may have developed through evolution due to the biological significance of faces and facial expressions for social communication. A second explanation suggests that face processing reflects subtle and difficult discriminations between highly similar exemplars within a category and that it is this general capacity, not the processing of the facial configuration *per se*, that is disrupted in prosopagnosia. This view is consistent with the observation that prosopagnosia is often accompanied by varying levels of object agnosia of other types. A third and intriguing suggestion, discussed in more detail shortly, is that face processing represents the acquisition of a type of expertise derived from very protracted experience with a category of complex visual stimuli. Reports of persons with prosopagnosia who have associated deficits in types of object recognition in which they had previously acquired expertise over long periods of time (e.g., a show dog expert who lost the ability to differentiate breeds) are consistent with this idea. These cases are also consistent with the idea, described earlier, that prosopagnosia stems from a problem in making subtle, difficult discriminations between exemplars within a category.

Since the 1980s, a number of cases with prosopagnosia have come to autopsy. The damage common to these lay within the *lingual and fusiform gyri* (Fig. 47.1), very ventrally and medially within the cortex at the occipitotemporal junction. However, in all such cases, this area (or at least the underlying white matter) was damaged bilaterally, and consequently bilateral damage has been thought by many to be a necessary precondition for prosopagnosia. Several cases with prosopagnosia and right cortical damage alone, along with the results of imaging studies, have reopened the debate over the locus of the critical lesion in prosopagnosia.

Imaging and Electrophysiological Studies Also Suggest Specialized Processing Modules

The existence of prosopagnosia suggests that certain regions of the ventral stream should be very responsive to faces. This is exactly what has been observed in imaging studies. For example, a number of early imaging studies revealed that a region on the fusiform gyrus is significantly more active when subjects view faces than when they view common objects. In addition, the fusiform gyrus is more active during face matching than location matching and during the viewing of faces than during the viewing of scrambled faces, letter strings, or textures. Face-selective regions are not confined, however, to the fusiform gyrus; face-selective regions also include ventral occipital regions (see later), LO, and portions of the superior temporal sulcus.

The strong responses to faces in ventral visual cortex, especially the fusiform gyrus, are not surprising given the effects of lesions of this region in patients and the nature of single-cell responses to faces in monkey TE. Similar to face-selective neurons, the fusiform gyrus of humans responds significantly more strongly to passive viewing of intact versus scrambled faces. The fusiform gyrus also responds more vigorously to photos of faces than photos of human hands, indicating that the responses are not to animate objects in general. Furthermore, the face selectivity of this region has been linked to face perception. In one imaging study the differential sensitivity of the ventral cortex to different visual stimuli was explored in a *binocular rivalry* paradigm in which different stimuli were presented to the right and left eye (Tong *et al.*, 1998; Fig. 47.10). (The resulting percept, however, is not a combination of the two stimuli. Instead, under appropriate conditions, subjects report perceiving an alternation between the two stimuli. Thus, while the retinal stimulation is kept constant, the percept alternates between the two stimuli every few seconds.) This study was based on the fact that faces are effective in driving the fusiform cortex. Other research had shown that a neighboring region, the parahippocampal gyrus, responds strongly to outdoor scenes of stimuli such as houses. In the binocular rivalry study (Fig. 47.9), a face and a house stimulus were presented to different eyes. As expected, subjects' perceptions fluctuated between houses and faces. Critically, however, a change from a house to a face percept was accompanied by increasing activation in the fusiform gyrus and decreasing activation in the parahippocampal gyrus. Perceived changes from a face to a house led to the opposite pattern of responses. Collectively, these findings suggest that the fusiform gyrus plays an important and specialized role in face perception.

Evidence from electrophysiological recordings in patients with implanted electrodes (as part of the preparation for neurosurgery to treat epilepsy) also

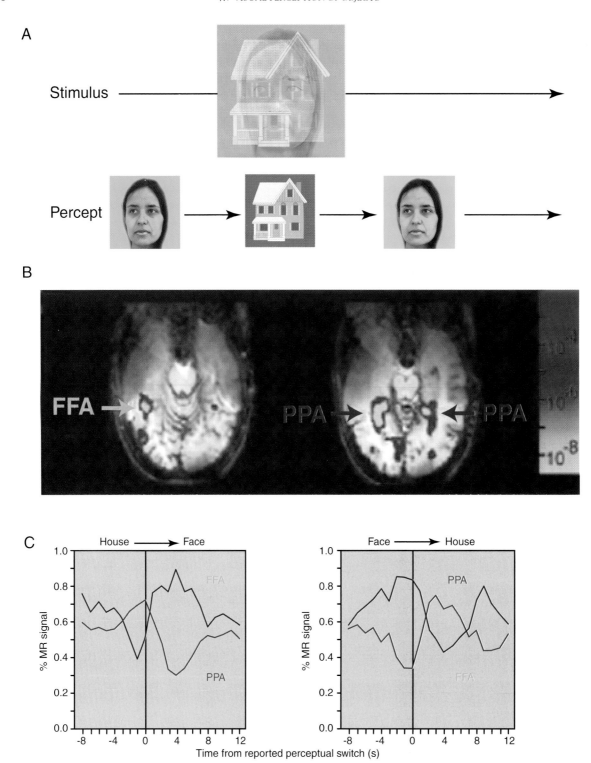

FIGURE 47.10 Design and results from an fMRI experiment on binocular rivalry. (A) The top illustration shows the ambiguous face/house stimulus used to produce rivalry. When viewed through red and green filter glasses, only the face could be seen through one eye and only the house through the other eye. This arrangement led to binocular rivalry, with a face percept alternating with a house percept every few seconds. (B) Two adjacent axial slices through the brain of a single subject showing, in the left slice, the area on the fusiform gyrus that responded more to faces than houses (FFA) and, in the right slice, the area on the parahippocampal gyrus that responded more to houses than to faces (PPA). In the slices shown, left is the right hemisphere and right is the left hemisphere. (C) fMRI time series showing FFA and PPA activity for a single subject illustrating that the activity in these two regions correlated with the subject's visual percept. Adapted from Tong *et al.* (1998). PPA, parahippocampal place area.

reveals face-selective processing in the ventral stream (Allison *et al.*, 1999). A large evoked potential, called the *N200* because it occurs roughly 200 ms after stimulus onset, is generated in small regions (i.e., typically at only one electrode within an electrode array) in the ventral occipitotemporal cortex. The selectivity of the N200 has been studied most thoroughly for face stimuli. In this case, it has been found that the N200 amplitude does not vary substantially whether evoked by colored or gray-scale faces, by normal, blurred, or line-drawing faces, or by faces of different sizes. The N200 amplitude is largest to full faces and decreases progressively to eyes, face contours, lips, and noses viewed in isolation. Interestingly, a region just lateral to face-selective N200 sites is more responsive to internal face parts than to faces, and some sites in ventral occipitotemporal cortex are face-part specific.

Electrophysiological studies can provide information about the time course of the response at the millisecond time scale, unlike imaging studies that have a time scale on the order of seconds. Thus, while the N200 is a response occurring roughly 200 ms after stimulus onset, longer latency response components are also observed (Fig. 47.11). This allows researchers to compare how the different components are modulated by experimental conditions and make inferences

about the types of computations taking place at specific moments in time. For instance, the face-selective N200 response is not affected by the familiarity or unfamiliarity of faces or by face-name learning (Puce *et al.*, 1999). These results have been interpreted as evidence for computations associated with face perception *per se*, i.e., not involving explicit recognition and memory processes. At the same time, at face-selective N200 sites, other response components such as P290 and N700 (occurring 290 ms and 700 ms after stimulus onset, respectively) are affected by face-name learning, suggesting that these components reflect processes associated with recognition and memory and that they are potentially subject to top-down influences. Thus, it appears that the face-selective N200 component reflects the automatic processing of faces, whereas the later components reflect processes associated with face recognition and memory.

In other small, circumscribed locations in the ventral occipitotemporal cortex, N200 potentials are selectively elicited by visual stimuli other than faces, such as letter strings (including words and non-words), numbers, complex objects, and gratings. Importantly, the responses are not elicited by control stimuli, such as scrambled versions of the pictures. The small regions, which vary in their exact location

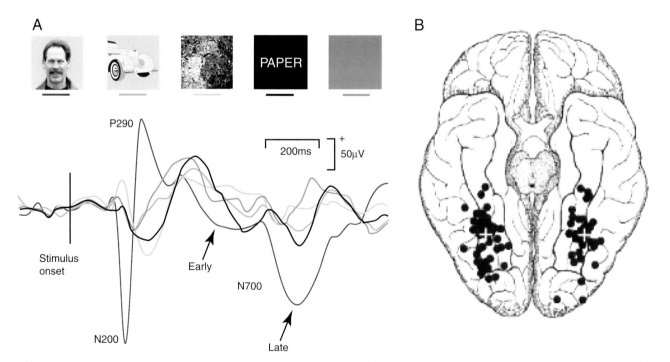

FIGURE 47.11 (A) Event-related potential specific to faces (red line) elicited from the occipitotemporal cortex of humans. Potentials elicited by other stimuli are also shown. (B) Summary of locations (black dots) on the ventral surface of the human brain from which a surface-negative potential (N200) was recorded when patients were shown faces but not when other categories of objects were tested. Locations are primarily along the fusiform gyrus. Adapted from Allison *et al.* (1999).

among individuals, are reminiscent of clumps of object-selective neurons found in area TE of monkeys.

The Role of Expertise Provides an Alternative Explanation of Selectivity

Data from imaging, single-cell recording, and lesion studies have been interpreted by some to indicate the existence of a special face-perception module in the fusiform gyrus of the ventral temporal cortex. One alternative proposal is that the fusiform gyrus is involved in a mode of processing not limited to faces. In particular, it has been suggested that expertise in handling certain types of objects is a key determinant of the function of the fusiform gyrus.

The idea that expertise underlies responses in ventral temporal cortex raises an important distinction between two interpretations. One interpretation suggests that activation is based on visual features (e.g., the visual features composing a face, such as eyes, nose, and mouth). Another interpretation emphasizes the *processes* associated with perceiving or recognizing objects. In this latter view, the ventral stream contains areas that are best suited for different computations. This might involve encoding subtle differences between visually similar objects or, conversely, finding underlying similarities between visually dissimilar objects. Another important process may involve encoding objects in terms of spatial layout. Accordingly, different recognition goals would be associated through experience with different categories of objects, which would lead to automatic processing biases. For example, we learn to recognize faces at the individual level while very young, and this ability is crucial to most of our social interactions. In contrast, for many objects, such as chairs, telephones, and toasters, we are rarely placed in a situation where we need to discriminate two instances of the class. Instead we learn to recognize such objects at a higher class level.

Support for this expertise view has been obtained for the part of the fusiform gyrus shown to be selective for faces. For example, pictures of nonface objects produce more activation in the fusiform gyrus when subjects match them with very specific labels rather than with more categorical ones (e.g., pelican versus bird). This observation demonstrates that the fusiform gyrus may be involved in processing exemplar-based information (such as discriminating different species of birds) to a greater extent than class-level information (such as identifying a pelican as belonging to the class "birds"). The activation seen in the fusiform gyrus has also been found to increase with intensive training with objects from a novel category that sub-

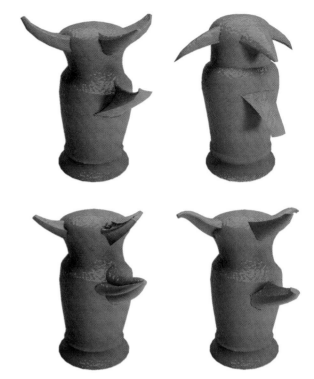

FIGURE 47.12   Four examples of "greebles." Adapted from Gauthier *et al.* (1998).

jects are unfamiliar with. For example, acquisition of expertise with so-called "greebles", computer-generated novel objects with distinctive features (Fig. 47.12), leads to increased activation in the same region of the fusiform gyrus that is ordinarily activated by faces (Gauthier *et al.*, 1999). Interestingly, the fusiform gyrus is also more activated by greebles in "experts" than in novices, even when the experts passively look at them. This finding supports the idea that experience may lead to automatic processing biases. The effect of expertise on fusiform gyrus activation has also been extended to other categories. In another study, bird and car "experts" were tested with fMRI during tasks with faces, familiar objects, cars, and birds. Within-category exemplars (i.e., cars and birds) activated the fusiform gyrus more than between-category familiar objects, with the right hemisphere showing significant expertise effects. Taken together, these results suggest that the level of categorization and expertise are important determinants of fusiform gyrus activation. This may help explain why some patients with prosopagnosia may also have associated deficits in areas of acquired expertise, such as a farmer who lost the ability to tell his cows apart or the show dog expert mentioned earlier who lost the ability to differentiate breeds.

Alexia Is a Specific Deficit in the Recognition of Written Words

In addition to faces, other visually complex and behaviorally important classes of stimuli may also have specialized substrates in the ventral stream. For example, studies of brain lesions in patients suggest that there is a specialized region for the processing of *written words* in the inferior temporal lobe. Patients with *alexia* cannot read normally despite intact visual capabilities, and despite their ability to understand spoken language and to write. Accordingly, alexia has been conceptualized as essentially a visual agnosia for verbal material. Studies investigating the neural substrates of the processing of words and letter strings have compared activations elicited by face and texture stimuli with activations elicited by (unpronounceable, non-word) letter strings. Regions responding more strongly to letter strings primarily involved the left occipitotemporal and inferior occipital sulci. The suggestion is that these regions comprise a prelexical, presemantic stage of word-form processing in the reading system.

Because learning to read is a very recent event in evolution, regions of the cortex specialized for words and letter strings are presumably not present at birth. Thus, the existence of these specialized regions must develop through protracted experience with written words, demonstrating that the environment helps shape the architecture of the visual system. One manner in which this may happen is that neural "learning" extracts correlations from the environment. Stimuli within a category, such as letters, tend to occur together and would therefore be encoded in close temporal proximity. Thus, many years of repeated experience with letters could lead to regions in the ventral temporal cortex specialized to process letters, similar to the development of conjoint selectivity by monkey TE cells for visual images that are shown together. Consistent with this proposal, brain-damaged patients can be selectively impaired at letter recognition compared to, for example, number recognition and vice versa.

Studies in Humans Support "Distributed" Rather Than Highly Localized Representations of Objects in the Ventral Visual Stream

Brain imaging and electrophysiological recording studies in humans have reported discrete cortical regions in the posterior ventral temporal cortex that respond preferentially to faces, other types of objects, and even written letter strings. These findings have suggested to some a *category-specific*, anatomically segregated *modular organization* of the object recognition pathway. A strong version of this view would imply that face-selective regions in the ventral temporal cortex would respond little, or not at all, to other classes of stimuli. A test of this idea would be then to determine the types of responses elicited to several types of stimuli. In an fMRI study employing several categories of stimuli, such as faces, houses, and chairs, it was found that three distinct regions of the ventral temporal cortex respond preferentially to these categories of objects (Ishai *et al.*, 1999). However, each category also evokes significant responses in the regions that respond maximally to other stimuli. For example, a region that responds maximally to faces (such as the fusiform gyrus) also elicits significant responses to both chairs and houses. Moreover, each category is associated with its own pattern of response across the ventral temporal cortex with a highly consistent spatial arrangement across subjects. These findings led to the suggestion that the representation of an object is not restricted to a region that responds maximally to that object, but rather is distributed across a broader expanse of cortex. The distributed patterns of response to object categories have been found to be similar across tasks (passive viewing, delayed matching) and presentation formats (photographs, line drawings), strengthening the interpretation that they provide the neural substrate of object representation.

Thus, in this alternative framework, the functional architecture of the ventral stream is not viewed as composed of category-specific modules but instead as a distributed representation of information about object form that has a highly consistent and orderly spatial arrangement (Haxby *et al.*, 2001). Within this distributed system, however, the representation of faces appears to be less extensive as compared to the representation of nonface objects. This finding may help explain why it is possible for lesions to produce prosopagnosia while leaving the recognition of nonface objects intact.

Summary

Prosopagnosia, a selective deficit in recognizing faces, is associated with damage to the occipitotemporal cortex, including the fusiform gyrus. Consistent with this impairment, imaging and electrophysiological studies have demonstrated that the fusiform gyrus responds selectively to faces and that this activation is linked to face perception. Although these findings suggest the existence of a specialized module for processing faces, another equally plausible interpretation is that the fusiform gyrus performs specialized computations associated with perceiving certain objects, including but not limited to faces. Such computations would presumably apply to many objects with which one has expertise. Moreover, the existence of a region in the occipitotemporal cortex selectively activated by letter strings and words demonstrates the role of experience in shaping the functional architecture of the object recognition pathway. With the possible exception of faces, whose cortical representation appears to be relatively circumscribed, objects appear to be represented by a distributed pattern of activity across a broad expanse of ventral temporal cortex.

OBJECT KNOWLEDGE IS STORED IN A DISTRIBUTED NETWORK OF CORTICAL AREAS

Although the distinction between perception and memory might at first seem sharp, in reality these two processes are intimately connected. Indeed, each time one identifies an object one automatically retrieves stored knowledge about that object. In other words, identifying an object necessarily implies knowing what that object is. Further, it is generally believed that the same neural tissue devoted to object processing also serves to store the long-term representations of objects. For example, when a subject mentally imagines houses or faces (requiring the retrieval of stored object representations from long-term memory), the same patterns of activation across ventral temporal cortex are seen as those observed when actually viewing houses or faces.

Object knowledge implies not only familiarity with the shape of an object, but also other attributes, such as its typical color and function. For example, how does one know that bulldozers are usually yellow and are used for digging? One imaging study that examined this question asked subjects to name either the associated color or the associated action in response to the presentation of black and white line drawings of objects (Martin *et al.*, 2000). By associated action the investigators meant the typical motion associated with an object, such as the motion produced by the arm of the bulldozer digging. Results showed that the generation of color names associated with objects selectively activated a region in the ventral occipital cortex just in front of the area involved in the perception of color, whereas the generation of action names activated a region dorsally in the middle temporal gyrus just in front of the area involved in the perception of motion. These findings suggest that information about the different attributes of an object is not stored in a unified fashion in any single area of the cortex. Rather, object knowledge seems to be stored in

a distributed fashion such that information about specific attributes is stored close to the specific regions of the cortex that mediate the perception of those attributes. How these stored attributes may be linked to create complete object representations, such as the concept of "pencil", is considered in Box 47.3.

For some objects, stored knowledge involves not only perceptual attributes, but also associated movements that are used when one manipulates the objects (e.g., the movements of our fingers when we use a scissors). This issue was investigated in an imaging study that examined brain activity in response to viewing and naming both animals and tools (Martin *et al.*, 2000). Results of this study revealed that a widely distributed network of both sensory and motor areas stores information about object attributes. In this study, viewing and naming both animals and tools produced strong activity in the posterior portion of the fusiform gyrus of the temporal lobe, as would be expected given the role of the fusiform gyrus in object perception. However, other brain regions were differentially activated by animals and tools. First, viewing and naming tools were associated with activity dorsally in the middle temporal gyrus, in precisely the same region found by Martin *et al.* (2000) to be active when subjects generated action words in response to line drawings of objects (i.e., just in front of the area involved in the perception of motion). Second, viewing and naming tools were also associated with activity in the premotor cortex, in the same region found to be active when subjects imagine grasping objects with their hands. Thus, identifying individual tools was dependent on accessing information about object-associated patterns of visual motion (stored in the posterior region of the middle temporal gyrus) and about object-associated patterns of motor movements (stored in premotor cortex). In contrast, viewing and naming animals were associated with the activation of early visual areas within the medial occipital cortex, which may be related to the fine visual details used when differentiating animals.

These imaging results provide a basis for understanding category-specific disorders of knowledge resulting from patterns of focal brain damage (Fig. 47.13). This type of deficit, seen most commonly for animals and tools, involves a selective difficulty in naming and retrieving information about objects from a single category. If the distinction between different categories of objects, such as animals and tools, is dependent on access to information about different types of attributes, and if such attributes (e.g., form, color, motion and object-use associated motor movements) are stored in separate regions of the brain,

BOX 47.3

HOW ARE THE ATTRIBUTES OF AN OBJECT BOUND TOGETHER?

On your desk is a collection of pens and pencils of diverse colors and shapes. Scanning it, you search around and finally retrieve the yellow highlighter pen you wanted to use. This seemingly trivial activity poses a potentially serious challenge. How is it that the color of another pen does not get misattributed to the pen you wish to retrieve? In other words, how does the visual system correctly link up all the different features of complex objects? This so-called *binding problem* has been considered extensively by visual neuroscientists.

In an experimental setting, when subjects identify items in briefly presented arrays, they sometimes report seeing a stimulus made up of the color from one element and the shape from another. For example, subjects may report seeing a red, vertical bar when the display contains only red horizontal bars and orange vertical and horizontal bars. These so-called *illusory conjunctions* involve features such as color, shape, and size and occur not only when stimuli are presented very briefly, but also when subjects are required to split attention between two tasks (a so-called divided attention task), such that the amount of attention paid to the stimuli is reduced. Thus, perceptual features can be recombined to form new object representations, suggesting that they may be unbound initially and only later grouped or bound.

The idea that object attributes are analyzed separately and later combined also has support from physiology. As discussed in Chapter 27, different features are processed to some extent by different areas within the visual cortex. For example, some cells in V2 and V4 respond selectively to the orientation of an object, independent of color, whereas others respond selectively to color, independent of orientation. For accurate object perception, the visual system must somehow combine their activity. If all cells were highly selective for spatial location, binding might be accomplished by associating features in a given small region of the visual field as belonging to the same object, e.g., by integrating orientation and color for neurons sharing the same receptive field. However, progressing through the ventral stream, receptive field size increases dramatically. Indeed, receptive fields in area TE can include the entire visual field, which would appear to preclude successful binding when multiple objects appear together in the visual field.

Various ideas have been offered to help conceptualize the binding problem. One is that attention works as a "glue" to associate features of objects in the part of the visual field focused upon; this would explain why illusory conjunctions are seen most commonly in divided attention tasks. The idea that attention functions as a glue does not, however, specify how it is actually instantiated in the brain

(see Chapter 49). A possible mechanism that has attracted considerable attention is *binding by synchrony* (Gray *et al.*, 1989), which proposes that cells coding attributes belonging to the same object are distinguished from others by firing in unison. Oscillations of firing in the 30- to 60-Hz range have been reported and are thought to maintain the synchronization, especially for widely separated populations of cells. In this view, while the synchrony lasts, the cells sharing it represent the same object. Thus, binding is solved by a temporal code that links distinct features of a stimulus.

The main alternative to a temporal code is a place code, as originally suggested by Barlow in the early 1970s. In this proposal, cells from lower levels representing a given region of space converge onto cells in higher cortical areas (e.g., TE) so that these latter cells become sensitive to conjunctions of more elementary features. Objects are thus represented by feature combinations, such as coding a face through a set of detectors for combinations of face parts, e.g., eye, nose, eyebrow, and hairline. Finally, another proposal is that feature binding involves interactions between ventral and dorsal pathways. If so, elimination of such interactions via dorsal stream damage should lead to illusory conjunctions even with the ventral stream object recognition pathway intact. This prediction was confirmed in a patient with bilateral parietal damage that led to *simultanagnosia*, the inability to perceive more than one object at a time (Friedman-Hill *et al.*, 1995). This patient had an exaggerated tendency to perceive illusory conjunctions, suggesting that spatial information from the dorsal stream is normally combined with object information from the ventral stream in order to correctly link them into a unified percept.

The binding problem is a matter of current heated debate. Some researchers even question whether there is a binding problem to solve in the first place! Instead, they suggest that the complex, emergent pattern of activity in different regions *is* the representation of the object, and no linking—temporal or otherwise—is required for perception.

Hillary R. Rodman, Luiz Pessoa,
and Leslie G. Ungerleider

References

Friedman-Hill, S. R., Robertson, L. C., and Treisman, A. (1995). Parietal contributions to visual feature binding: Evidence from a patient with bilateral lesions. *Science* **269**, 853–855.

Gray, C. M., Konig, P., Engel, A. K., and Singer, W. (1989), Oscillatory responses in cat visual cortex exhibit intercolumnar synchronization which reflects global stimulus properties. *Nature* **338**, 334–337.

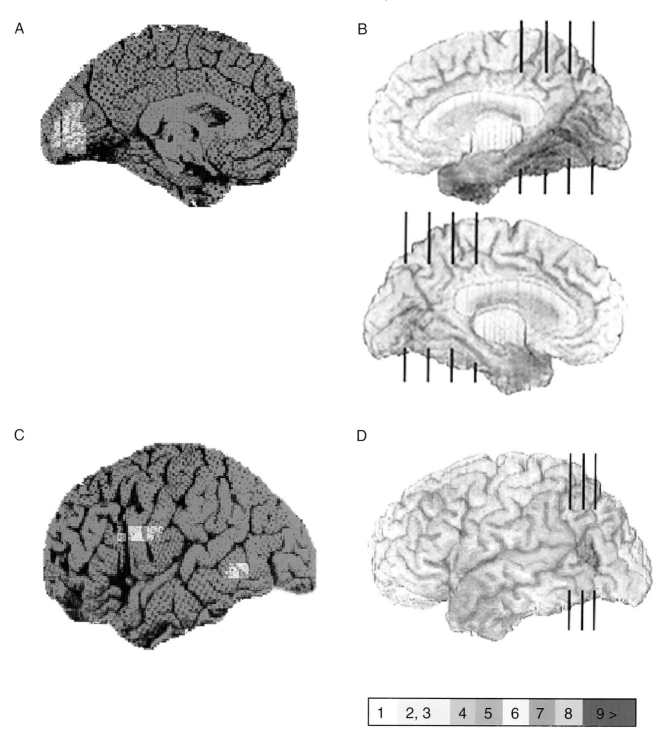

FIGURE 47.13 Comparison of results from an fMRI study comparing activations when subjects named drawings of animals and tools (A and C, respectively) to lesion sites in subjects with impaired recognition and naming of drawings of animals and tools (B and D, respectively). (A) View of the medial surface of the left hemisphere showing the region of activation in the medial occipital cortex when subjects named drawings of animals relative to drawings of tools. (B) View of the medial surface of the right and left hemispheres showing the location of lesions in 28 subjects with impaired recognition and naming of drawings of animals. (C) View of the lateral surface of the left hemisphere showing activated regions in the premotor cortex and middle temporal gyrus when subjects named drawings of tools relative to drawings of animals. (D) View of the lateral surface of the left hemisphere showing the location of lesions in 8 subjects with impaired recognition and naming of drawings of tools. Color bar indicates the number of subjects with a lesion at that site for B and D. Vertical lines in brains of B and D indicate planes of coronal sections not shown. Adapted from Martin *et al.* (2000).

then one may find a category-specific deficit depending on the site of the lesion. Indeed, consistent with the imaging data, it has been found that the locations of lesions in patients with impaired recognition and impaired naming of drawings of animals included the medial aspects of the occipital lobe, nearly the same region active during animal naming. In contrast, the locations of lesions in patients with impaired recognition and impaired naming of drawings of tools all included the middle temporal gyrus, nearly the same region active during tool naming (Tranel *et al.*, 1997). It is important to note that the impairment in patients with category-specific deficits is not limited to visual recognition. These deficits occur when knowledge is probed visually or verbally, and therefore they reflect disorders of stored knowledge and not simply disorders of perception.

Overall Summary

Early studies of brain damage in humans and lesions in monkeys pointed to the crucial role of tissue in the ventral parts of the temporal cortex for object perception and recognition. After many decades of intensive research, one can now say that the ventral portions of the temporal cortex form the last stations of an occipitotemporal ventral pathway, beginning in the primary visual cortex and progressing through multiple visual areas beyond it. In macaque monkeys, important regions for object perception and recognition include areas TEO and TE of the inferior temporal cortex. In humans, homologous circuits appear to exist in both occipital and temporal regions, including the lateral occipital complex, the fusiform gyrus, and nearby regions in the ventral temporal cortex and the superior temporal sulcus.

Single-neuron recording studies in monkeys show a progressive increase in the complexity of object features needed to "trigger" cells at progressively more anterior stations in the occipitotemporal pathway. Many TE neurons show preservation of their selectivity over transformations that change the physical stimulus, such as retinal position, size, distance in depth, and degree of ambient illumination. At the highest levels of the pathway, within area TE and neighboring STP, some neurons are preferentially responsive to faces and other biologically significant stimuli.

More recently, neuroimaging and evoked potential studies in humans with implanted electrodes have also shed light on the mechanisms by which the primate brain represents objects. Descriptions of prosopagnosia, a selective deficit of face recognition following damage to ventral occipitotemporal cortex, foreshadowed discoveries of cortical zones that are activated preferentially by face stimuli. At the same time, selectivity for letter strings and even for learned arbitrary stimuli (such as greebles) has suggested that expertise also markedly influences activity in the ventral pathway. With the possible exception of faces, whose representation appears to be relatively circumscribed, objects are likely to be represented by a distributed pattern of activity across the ventral temporal cortex. Finally, more general knowledge about objects (what they are used for and how to manipulate them) appears to be stored in an even more distributed network of sensory and motor cortical areas.

References

Allison, T., Puce, A., Spencer, D. D., and McCarthy, G. (1999). Electrophysiological studies of human face perception. I: Potential generated in occipitotemporal cortex by face and non-face stimuli. *Cerebr. Cortex* **9**, 415–430.

Biederman, I. (1990). Higher-level vision. *In* "Visual Cognition and Action" (D. H. Osherson, S. M. Kosslyn, and J. M. Hollerbach, eds.), Vol. 2, pp. 41–72. MIT Press, Cambridge, MA.

Bruce, C., Desimone, R., and Gross, C. G. (1981). Visual properties of neurons in a polysensory area in superior temporal sulcus of the macaque. *J. Neurophysiol.* **46**, 369–384.

Bulthoff, H. H., Edelman, S. Y., and Tarr, M. J. (1995). How are 3-dimensional objects represented in the brain? *Cereb. Cortex* **5**, 247–260.

Erickson, C. A., Jagadeesh, B., and Desimone, R. (2000). Clustering of perirhinal neurons with similar properties following visual experience in adult monkeys. *Nature Neurosci.* **3**,1143–1148.

Farah, M. J. (1990). "Visual Agnosia: Disorders of Object Recognition and What They Tell Us About Normal Vision." MIT Press, Cambridge, MA.

Friedman-Hill, S. R., Robertson, L. C., and Treisman, A. (1995). Parietal contributions to visual feature binding: evidence from a patient with bilateral lesions. *Science* **269**, 853–855.

Gauthier, I., Tarr, M. J., Anderson A. W., Skudlarski P., and Gore, J. C. (1999). Activation of the middle fusiform "face area" increases with expertise in recognizing novel objects. *Nature Neurosci.* **2**, 568–573.

Gauthier, I., Williams, P., Tarr, M. J., and Tanaka, J. (1998) Training "greeble" experts: A framework for studying expert object recognition processes. *Vis. Res.* **38**, 2401–2428.

Gray, C. M., Konig, P., Engel, A. K., and Singer, W. (1989). Oscillatory responses in cat visual cortex exhibit inter-columnar synchronization which reflects global stimulus properties. *Nature* **338**, 334–337.

Grill-Spector, K., Kushnir, T., Hendler, T., Edelman, S., Itzchank, Y., and Malach, R. (1998). A sequence of early object processing stages revealed by fMRI in human occipital lobe. *Hum. Brain Mapp.* **6**, 316–328.

Gross, C. G., Rocha-Miranda, C. E., and Bender, D. B. (1972). Visual properties of neurons in inferotemporal cortex of the Macaque. *J. Neurophysiol.* **35**, 96–111.

Gross, C. G., Rodman, H. R., Gochin, P. M., and Colombo, M. W. (1993). Inferior temporal cortex as a pattern recognition device. *In* "Computational Learning and Cognition" (E. Baum, ed.), pp. 44–73. Society for Industrial and Applied Mathematics, Philadelphia.

Haxby, J. V., Horwitz, B., Ungerleider, L. G., Maisog, J. M., Pietrini, P., and Grady, C. L. (1994). The functional organization of human extrastriate cortex: A PET-rCBF study of selective attention to faces and locations. *J. Neurosci.* **14**, 6336–6353.

Haxby, J. V., Gobbini, M. I., Furey, M. L., Ishai, A., Schouten, J. L., and Pietrini, P. (2001). Distributed and overlapping representations of faces and objects in ventral temporal cortex. *Science* **293**, 2425–2430.

Ishai, A., Ungerleider, L. G., Martin, A., Schouten, J. L., and Haxby, J. V. (1999). Distributed representation of objects in the human ventral visual pathway. *Proc. Natl. Acad. Sci. USA* **3**, 9379–9384.

Kobatake, E., Wang, G., and Tanaka, K. (1998). Effects of shape-discrimination training on the selectivity of inferotemporal cells in adult monkeys. *J. Neurophysiol.* **80**, 324–330.

Logothetis, N. K., Pauls, J., and Poggio, T. (1995). Shape representation in the inferior temporal cortex of monkeys. *Curr. Biol.* **5**, 552–563.

Martin, A. J., Haxby, J. V., Lalonde, F. M., Wiggs, C. L., and Ungerleider, L. G. (1995). Discrete cortical regions associated with knowledge of color and knowledge of action. *Science* **270**, 102–105.

Martin, A., Ungerleider, L. G., and Haxby, J. V. (2000). Category specificity and the brain: The sensory/motor model of semantic representations of objects. *In* "The New Cognitive Neurosciences" (M. S. Gazzaniga, ed.), pp. 1023–1036. MIT Press, Cambridge, MA.

Messinger, A., Squire, L. R., Zola, S. M., and Albright, T. O. (2001). Neuronal representatives of visual stimulus associations develop in the temporal lobe during learning. *Proc. Nat. Acad. Sci. USA* **98**, 12239–12244.

Miller, E. K. and Desimone, R. (1994). Parallel neuronal mechanisms for short-term memory. *Science* **263**, 520–522.

Mishkin, M., Ungerleider, L. G., and Macko, K. A. (1983). Object vision and spatial vision: Two cortical pathways. *Trends Neurosci.* **6**, 415–417.

Newcombe, F., Ratcliff, G., and Damasio, H. (1987). Dissociable visual and spatial impairments following right posterior cerebral lesions: Clinical, neuropsychological and anatomical evidence. *Neuropsychologia* **25**, 149–161.

Perrett, D. I., Rolls, E. T., and Caan, W. (1982). Visual neurones responsive to faces in the monkey temporal cortex. *Exp. Brain Res.* **47**, 329–342.

Puce, A., Allison, T., and McCarthy, G. (1999). Electrophysiological studies of human face perception. III Effects of top-down processing on face-specific potentials. *Cereb. Cortex* **9**, 445–458.

Rubens, A. B., and Benson, D. F. (1971). Associative visual agnosia. *Arch. Neurol.* **24**, 305–316.

Sakai, K., and Miyashita, Y. (1991). Neural organization for the long-term memory of paired associates. *Nature* **354**, 152–155.

Tanaka, K. (1993). Neuronal mechanisms of object recognition. *Science* **262**, 685–488.

Tong, F., Nakayama, K., Vaughan, J. T., and Kanwisher, N. (1998). Binocular rivalry and visual awareness in human extrastriate cortex. *Neuron* **21**, 753–759.

Tranel, D., Damasio, H., and Damasio, A. R. (1997). A neural basis for the retrieval of conceptual knowledge. *Neuropsychologia* **35**, 1319–1327.

Ungerleider, L. G. and Mishkin, M. (1982). Two cortical visual systems. *In* "Analysis of Visual Behavior" (D. J. Ingle, M. A. Goodale, and R. J. W. Mansfield, eds.), pp. 549–586. MIT Press: Cambridge, MA.

Suggested Readings

Barlow, H. B. (1972) Single units and sensation: A neuron doctrine for perceptual psychology? *Perception* **1**, 371–394.

Damasio, A. R. (1990). Category-related recognition deficits as a clue to the neural substrates of knowledge. *Trends Neurosci.* **13**, 95–98.

Desimone, R. (1991). Face-selective cells in the temporal cortex of monkeys. *J. Cogn. Neurosci.* **3**, 1–8.

Desimone, R., and Ungerleider, L. G. (1989). Neural mechanisms of visual perception in monkeys. *In* "Handbook of Neuropsychology" (F. Boller and J. Grafman, eds.), Vol. 2, pp. 267–299. Elsevier; Amsterdam, The Netherlands.

Forde, E. M. E., and Humphreys, G. W. (1999). Category-specific recognition impairments: A review of important case studies and influential theories. *Aphasiology* **13**, 169–193.

Logothetis, N. K., and Sheinberg, D. L. (1996). Visual object recognition. *Annu. Rev. Neurosci.* **19**, 577–621.

Marr, D. (1982). "Vision: A Computational Investigation into the Human Representation and Processing of Visual Information" Freeman, San Francisco, CA.

Tanaka, K. (1996). Inferotemporal cortex and object vision. *Annu. Rev. Neurosci.* **19**, 109–139.

Ullman S. (1996). "High-Level Vision." MIT Press, Cambridge, MA.

Ungerleider, L. G., and Haxby, J. V. (1994). "What" and "where" in the human brain. *Curr. Opin. Neurobiol.* **4**, 157–165.

Hillary R. Rodman, Luiz Pessoa, and Leslie G. Ungerleider

Spatial Cognition

As we move through the world, new visual, auditory, vestibular, and somatosensory inputs are continuously presented to the brain. Given such constantly changing input, it is remarkable how easily we are able to keep track of where things are. We can reach for an object, look at it, or even kick it without making a conscious effort to assess its location in space, but how do we construct a representation of space that allows us to act so effortlessly? This chapter outlines the contributions of several brain areas in the parietal, frontal, and hippocampal cortices to spatial representation, spatial memory, and the generation of actions in space.

NEUROANATOMY OF SPATIAL COGNITION

Dorsal Stream Areas Process Visuospatial Information

Within the cerebral hemispheres, visual information is processed serially by a succession of areas progressively more distant from the primary visual cortex of the occipital lobe. Within this hierarchical system, there are two parallel chains, or streams, of areas: the ventral stream, leading downward into the temporal lobe, and the dorsal stream, leading forward into the parietal lobe (Ungerlieder and Mishkin, 1982)(see Chapter 47). Although the two streams are interconnected to some degree, it is a fair first approximation to describe them as separate parallel systems. Areas of the ventral stream play a critical role in the recognition of visual patterns, including faces, whereas areas of the dorsal stream contribute selectively to conscious spatial awareness and to the

spatial guidance of actions, such as reaching and grasping. Dorsal stream areas have at least two distinctive functional characteristics: (1) they contain a comparatively extensive representation of the peripheral visual field and (2) they appear to be specialized for the detection and analysis of moving visual images. Both traits would be expected in any system processing visual information for use in spatial awareness and in the visual guidance of behavior.

Although visual input is important for spatial operations, awareness of space is more than just a visual function. It is possible to apprehend the shape of an object and know where it is, regardless of whether it is seen or sensed through touch. Accordingly, spatial awareness, considered as a general phenomenon, depends not on visual areas of the dorsal stream but rather on higher order cortical areas to which they send their output. The transition from areas serving purely visual functions to those mediating generalized spatial awareness is gradual, but has been accomplished by the time the dorsal stream reaches its termination in the association cortex of the posterior parietal lobe.

Association Areas Responsible for Spatial Cognition Form a Tightly Interconnected System

The posterior parietal cortex is thought to be preeminent among cortical areas responsible for spatial awareness because lesions of the posterior parietal cortex lead to the most devastating and specific impairments of spatial cognition. However, numerous other association areas in the cerebral hemisphere mediate cognitive functions that depend in some way on the use of spatial information. These areas occupy a continuous region of the cerebral hemisphere, encompassing large parts of the frontal, cingulate, temporal, parahippocampal, and insular cortices. They are connected to each other anatomically and to the parietal cortex by a parallel distributed pathway through which signals shuttle back and forth (Goldman-Rakic, 1988). The functions of some parts of this system are especially well understood. For example, the frontal cortex is involved in the generation of voluntary behavior, and the medial temporal lobe, including the hippocampus, is important for memory. In most individuals, the association areas of the right hemisphere are particularly important for spatial cognition. In nonhuman species, lateralization is much less pronounced. In general, spatial functions are represented in the same cortical areas in humans, monkeys, and rats. The following sections describe the spatial functions of the parietal cortex; how frontal areas program voluntary movements in spatial terms; and, finally, how the hippocampus and parahippocampal areas mediate the formation of memories with a spatial component.

PARIETAL CORTEX

The Parietal Cortex Contributes to Spatial Perception and Attention

The parietal lobe is divided into superior and inferior parietal lobules. Within each lobule, several subdivisions are distinguished by anatomical and functional properties (Colby and Duhamel, 1991). In

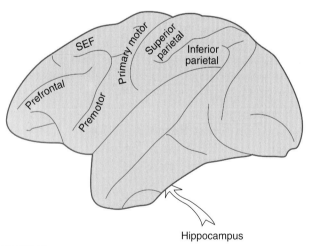

FIGURE 48.1 Lateral view of the left cerebral hemisphere of a rhesus monkey. Areas in the parietal and frontal cortex responsible for motor and cognitive processes of a spatial nature. SEF, supplementary eye field. Brain drawing, courtesy of Laboratory of Neuropsychology, NIMH.

both humans and monkeys, the superior parietal lobule serves functions related primarily to somesthesis, or tactile perception, whereas the inferior parietal lobule serves functions related primarily to visuospatial cognition (Fig. 48.1). The intraparietal sulcus runs in between the superior and the inferior lobules. Within the sulcus there are several functionally distinct areas with independent representations of space. In monkeys, these include the lateral intraparietal area (LIP), which is important for spatial attention, and the ventral intraparietal area (VIP), where visual and somatosensory representations of space are brought together. Recent functional imaging studies suggest that there are corresponding cortical areas in humans.

Injury to the Human Posterior Parietal Cortex Causes Impairments of Spatial Function

A group of behavioral impairments specifically associated with damage to the parietal lobes was first described by the neurologist Balint in 1909. Balint's syndrome includes difficulty in executing eye movements to engage visual targets, inaccuracy in reaching for visual targets, and a tendency not to see things in the peripheral visual field. This collection of symptoms reflects an impairment in the visual guidance of movement and, more generally, in spatial cognition. The following sections describe three of the specific impairments of spatial behavior known to arise from injury to the parietal lobe.

Simultanagnosia: An Inability to See Multiple Objects Simultaneously

After injury to the posterior parietal cortex, some patients experience difficulty in the visual perception of spatial relations. They can see objects, but cannot judge whether two objects are the same size or which of two objects is closer. When asked to copy simple line drawings, they may omit or transpose parts, as if unable to judge accurately the spatial arrangement of the object's components. In some patients, failure on visuospatial tests arises from a specific inability to see more than one object at a time (Coslett and Saffran, 1991). This condition, called simultanagnosia, is commonly observed after bilateral damage to the parietal cortex. When looking at the flame of a match, a patient with simultanagnosia may be unable to see the hand holding it. When tested in controlled situations, simultanagnosic patients demonstrate a profound inability to perceive more than one object simultaneously (see Box 48.1).

A particularly illuminating test carried out on simultanagnosic patients is shown in Figure 48.2

SIMULTANAGNOSIA

Disorders of spatial awareness arising from parietal lobe injury are not merely a laboratory phenomenon, but can have a profound impact on the patient's daily life, as described in the following case study of simultanagnosia (from Coslett and Saffran, 1991).

When first examined by the authors 4 months after a right hemisphere infarction, the patient's major complaint was that her environment appeared fragmented; although she saw individual items clearly, they appeared to be isolated and she could not discern any meaningful relationship among them. She stated, for example, that she could find her way in her home (in which she had lived for 25 years) with her eyes closed, but she became confused with her eyes open. On one occasion, for example, she attempted to find her way to her bedroom by using a large lamp as a landmark; while walking toward the lamp, she fell over her dining room table. Although she enjoyed listening to the radio, television programs bewildered her because she could only "see" one person or object at a time and therefore could not determine who was speaking or being spoken to; she reported watching a movie in which, after hearing a heated argument, she noted to her surprise and consternation that the character she had been watching was suddenly sent reeling across the room, apparently as a consequence of a punch thrown by a character she had never seen. Although she was able to read single words effortlessly, she stopped reading because the "competing words" confused her. She was unable to write, as she claimed to be able to see only a single letter; thus when creating a letter, she saw only the tip of the pencil and the letter under construction and "lost" the previously constructed letters.

Carol L. Colby and
Carl R. Olson

Reference

Coslett, H. B., and Saffran, E. (1991). Simultanagnosia: To see but not to see. *Brian* **114**, 1523–1545.

(Humphreys and Riddoch, 1993). When patients were presented with a set of randomly intermingled red and green circles (random condition), they were unable to say whether the circles were of different colors. Presumably this was because they could see only one circle at a time. When the circles were joined by line segments into red or green barbells (single color condition), these patients still could not say that more than one color was present. Only when pairs of circles of different colors were joined by line segments, unifying them into a single object, were patients able to report that there were different colors present (mixed condition). Note that the average distance between circles of different colors was the same in all three conditions. This indicates that the inability of patients to see and compare pairs of circles in the

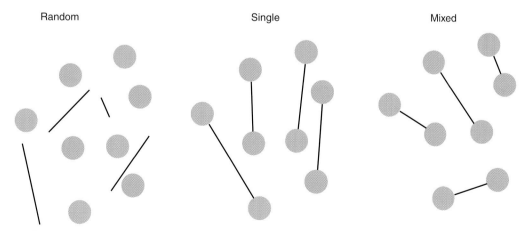

FIGURE 48.2 Three stimuli used for assessing simultanagnosia in human patients. Patients were consistently able to report that circles of different colors were present only in the mixed condition, in which red and green circles were unified into a single object by connecting line segments. From Humphreys and Riddoch (1993).

random and single conditions was the result of the circles belonging to separate objects and not simply a result of their being separated by a certain distance. Simultanagnosia, by preventing simultaneous vision of two objects, gives rise to poor performance on tests requiring a comparison between objects. However, when tests are confined to a single object, this condition appears to leave spatial perception intact. Simultanagnosic patients are able to make accurate judgments of spatial relations so long as the judgments pertain to a single object.

Optic Ataxia: An Impairment of Visually Guided Reaching

After damage to the parietal cortex, some patients experience difficulty in making visually guided arm movements. This condition is referred to as misreaching, or optic ataxia (Perenin and Vighetto, 1988). Patients with optic ataxia experience difficulty in real-life situations requiring them to reach accurately under visual guidance. For example, a patient cutting food with a knife and fork may miss the plate altogether and hit the table when attempting to move the knife toward the food. Neuropsychologists have been able to characterize the reaching deficits of such patients in considerable detail by testing them in controlled situations.

In the test illustrated in Figure 48.3, patients were required to reach out and insert one hand into a slot in the center of a disk held by the experimenter. The disk could be held in either the right or the left visual hemifield, and the patient could be asked to reach with either the right or the left hand. To perform the task, the patient had to both direct the hand toward the center of the slot and orient the hand correctly so that it would pass into it. Pictures in the top row of Fig. 48.3 show one patient with right parietal lobe damage reaching with the left hand. When the disk was positioned in the right (ipsilesional) visual field, the patient was able to reach accurately (Fig. 48.3A). However, when the disk was in the left (contralesional) visual field, the patient committed errors of hand orientation (Fig. 48.3B) and of reaching direction (Fig. 48.3C). The lower row of Fig. 48.3 shows reaching by a patient with damage to the left parietal lobe. When using the left hand in the left (ipsilesional) visual field, this patient was also able to reach accurately (Fig. 48.3D). However, when using the right hand in the right (contralesional) visual field, the patient committed errors of hand orientation (Fig. 48.3E) and of reaching direction (Fig. 48.3F).

These results demonstrate that optic ataxia may be lateralized, occurring only when the patient is required to point to targets in one visual hemifield or only when one hand is used for pointing. Generally,

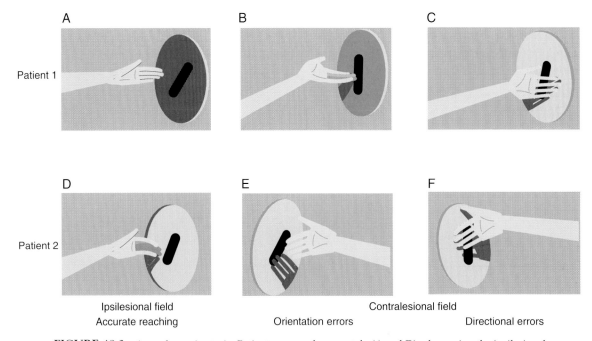

FIGURE 48.3 A test for optic ataxia. Patients can reach accurately (A and D) when using the ipsilesional hand in the ipsilesional visual field, but they make errors of hand orientation (B and E) and of direction (C and F) when reaching into the contralesional visual field. The top and bottom rows show the performance of two different patients. From Perenin and Vighetto (1988).

in cases where the deficit is restricted to a single hemifield or a single arm, the affected hemifield or arm is opposite the injured parietal lobe. This is what would be expected if the parietal lobe of each hemisphere mediates communication between more posterior visual areas (which represent the contralateral half of visual space) and more anterior motor areas (which represent the contralateral arm). There are, however, cases in which the problem is bilateral or occurs for specific combinations of arm and hemifield. Optic ataxia is not simply a problem with visuospatial perception, as indicated by the fact that performance with one arm may be perfectly normal. Nor is it simply a motor problem, as indicated by the fact that patients unable to reach accurately for visual targets can commonly touch points on their own bodies accurately under proprioceptive guidance. Optic ataxia is best characterized as an inability to use visuospatial information to guide arm movements.

Hemispatial Neglect: Unawareness of the Contralesional Half of Space

Hemispatial neglect is a classic symptom of injury to the posterior parietal cortex. It is a condition in which a lateralized failure of spatial awareness is present. Patients fail to notice things in the contralesional half of space (the half of space opposite the injured hemisphere). The most common form of neglect arises from damage to the right parietal lobe and is manifested as a failure to detect objects in the left half of space. Patients with neglect experience problems in daily life, such as colliding with obstacles on the contralesional side of the body or mistakenly identifying letters on the contralesional side of a written word. When asked to copy pictures or to draw simple objects from memory, they leave out details on the affected side. When asked to say whether two objects are the same or different, they tend to indicate that two dissimilar objects are the same if the differentiating details are on the contralesional side. Whether the problem underlying neglect is a failure of attention to one half of space or a failure of the ability to form a mental representation of that half of space is not clear.

Neglect involves more than just a defect of attention to contralesional sensory events. For example, patients fail to report detail on the left half of an object even when they are asked to form a mental representation of the object by viewing it one part at a time as it passes slowly behind a vertical slit. In a famous set of experiments, patients were asked to imagine themselves in a familiar public setting and then to report what they would be able to see around them (Bisiach

and Luzzatti, 1978). When they imagined standing at one end of the town square, patients described the buildings on the right side and failed to report buildings on the left. However, when instructed to imagine themselves standing at the other end of the square, facing the opposite direction, they now failed to mention buildings on the left that they had described just moments before and were able to describe buildings on the right that they had previously omitted.

Given that neglect affects the half of space opposite an injured parietal lobe, each parietal lobe must represent the opposite half of space. On the face of it, this proposition does not sound particularly surprising. Most visual areas in each hemisphere represent the opposite half of the visual field, most somatosensory areas represent the opposite half of the skin surface, and most motor areas represent muscles on the opposite half of the body. Injury to these areas leads to a sensory loss or motor impairment that affects the opposite half of a functional space defined with respect to some anatomical reference frame (the retina, the skin surface, or the muscles). In striking contrast, injury to the posterior parietal cortex gives rise to a neglect that may be defined with respect to any of several spatial reference frames. These fall into two broad classes: egocentric reference frames, in which objects and locations are represented relative to the observer; and allocentric reference frames, in which locations are represented in coordinates extrinsic to the observer. Examples of egocentric reference frames include those centered on the hand or the body. Allocentric reference frames include those in environmental coordinates (e.g., room centered) and those centered on an object of interest. The full range of reference frames used by the brain is just beginning to be explored. Patients with neglect often show deficits with respect to more than one reference frame. The following sections describe evidence for impairments of multiple spatial reference frames in neglect.

A patient with left hemispatial neglect, looking straight ahead at the center of some object, will tend not to see detail on its left side. This observation is open to several interpretations. The simplest interpretation is that stimuli presented in the left visual field tend not to be registered. However, the fundamental problem might actually be with registering stimuli that are to the left of the head, of the torso, or of the object itself. These possibilities cannot be distinguished without disentangling the various reference frames. Experiments aimed at identifying the spatial reference frame in neglect have indicated that the patient's failure to detect a stimulus is affected not only by its location relative to the retina but also by its location relative to the object or array within which it is contained, by its location relative to the body, and even by its location relative to a gravitationally defined reference frame. Patients span a continuum from exhibiting predominantly egocentric forms of neglect to predominantly allocentric neglect.

In many patients, a component of neglect is object centered. If these patients are presented with an image anywhere in the visual field, they tend to ignore its left side. In one experiment, patients with left hemispatial neglect were required to maintain fixation on a small spot while chimeric faces (images formed by joining at the midline half-images representing the faces of two people) were presented at various visual field locations. Their reports of what they saw were based predominantly on the right halves of the chimeric images. This was true even when the entire composite face was presented within the right visual hemifield. In a second experiment, patients with left hemifield neglect were required to maintain fixation on a small spot while four stimuli in a horizontal row were presented. One of the stimuli was a letter that was to be named aloud. When the letter was in the leftmost location, patients were slower to name it, even when the entire array was in the right visual field.

A particularly dramatic way of demonstrating the object-centered nature of neglect is to ask patients to make copies of simple line drawings (Marshall and Halligan, 1993). When asked to copy a picture of two flowers, a patient with right parietal lobe damage saw and copied each flower but omitted the petals on the left half of each, thus showing evidence of left object-centered neglect (Fig. 48.4, top). When the same two flowers were joined by a common stem, the patient saw and copied the plant, but omitted details on its left side, including all of the leftmost flower, thus showing neglect for the left half of the larger composite object (Fig. 48.4, bottom).

Patients with parietal lobe damage can exhibit deficits with respect to other allocentric reference frames in addition to the object-centered neglect described earlier. The role of a gravitational reference frame in neglect has emerged from studies in which patients face a display screen either while sitting upright or while lying on their side (Ladavas, 1987). When the patient sits upright, the right and left halves of the screen coincide with the right and left retinal visual fields. However, when the patient lies on one side while facing the screen, the situation is changed. Reclining on the right side, the patient

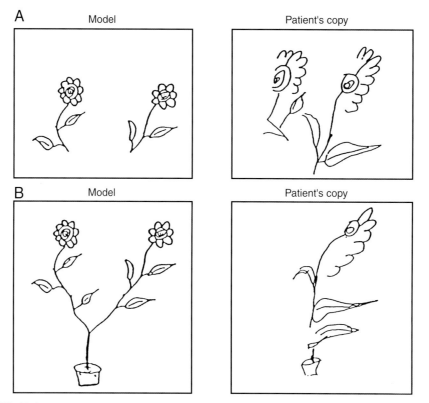

FIGURE 48.4 A test for object-centered neglect. When asked to copy the two drawings on the left, a patient made the two copies on the right. Detail is omitted from the left half of each object rather than from the left half of the drawing as a whole. From Marshall and Halligan (1993).

sees the right and left halves of the screen as being in the upper and lower visual fields, respectively. Applying this procedure to patients with left hemispatial neglect enables the investigator to pose the question: Is the neglect specific for the left retinal visual field or is it specific for the left half of the screen? Neglect turns out to depend in part on each of these factors.

Further evidence that the parietal cortex represents the locations of objects relative to an external framework has come from the observation that neglect, in some patients, is restricted to stimuli within a certain range of distances from the body. The form of neglect termed peripersonal or proximal is specific for stimuli in the immediate vicinity of the body. Another form of neglect, termed extrapersonal, is specific for more distant stimuli. The implication of these findings is that there is a localization of function within the parietal cortex and that neurons in discrete areas process sensory input from objects at different distances. Discrete areas of the parietal cortex are known to be specialized for relaying sensory information to different motor systems. Sensory input from peripersonal space is uniquely significant for guiding reaching movements. In contrast, sensory input from greater distances (extrapersonal space) is linked primarily to the control of eye movements.

Lesions of the Parietal Cortex in Monkeys Produce Spatial and Attentional Problems

The original distinction between dorsal and ventral processing streams in the primate visual system was based in part on differences in the effects of lesions of the posterior parietal cortex and the inferior temporal cortex (Ungerleider and Mishkin, 1982). Monkeys with posterior parietal lesions are selectively impaired in visuospatial performance, such as judging which of two identical objects is located closer to a visual landmark. In contrast, inferior temporal cortex lesions produce deficits in visual discrimination (e.g., shape or pattern recognition; see Chapter 47).

In addition to spatial perceptual deficits, parietal lesions also produce spatial motor deficits. After parietal lesions, monkeys have difficulty directing eye movements toward targets in the hemispace opposite the side of the lesion (Lynch and McLaren, 1989). Further, when two targets are presented simultaneously in the ipsilesional and contralesional fields, lesioned monkeys tend to ignore the contralesional stimulus, an effect termed visual extinction. Parietal lesions also have profound effects on the ability of a monkey to reach toward an object. Lesions confined to the inferior parietal cortex impair reaching with the

contralesional limb toward a target in contralesional space. Lesions extending across the intraparietal sulcus to include the superior parietal cortex produce impairments in reaching with the contralateral arm into either half of space. In sum, monkeys with parietal lesions are unable to assess spatial relations between objects or to judge locations of objects relative to themselves.

Parietal Neurons Have Response Properties Related to Spatial Information Processing

To understand more precisely how the parietal cortex contributes to spatial cognition, several groups of investigators have measured the electrical activity of single neurons during the performance of spatial tasks. These studies were done in alert monkeys trained to make eye movements to visual targets. Because brain tissue itself has no sensory receptors, microelectrodes can be introduced into the brain without disturbing the performance of a animal on a task. By recording single neuron activity during specially designed tasks, neural activity can be related directly to the sensory, cognitive, and motor processes that underlie spatial behavior. The next three sections describe how neurons in different areas within the parietal cortex are selectively activated during spatial tasks and how they contribute to spatial representation.

Area LIP

Neurons in the lateral intraparietal area (area LIP) exhibit several different kinds of task-related activities (Colby et.al., 1996). First, LIP neurons, like neurons elsewhere in the striate and extrastriate visual cortex (Chapter 27), respond to the onset of a visual stimulus in the receptive field of the neuron. Second, these visual responses are enhanced when the monkey attends to the stimulus: the amplitude of the visual response is increased when the stimulus or stimulus location becomes the focus of attention. This enhancement occurs no matter what kind of movement the animal will use to respond to the stimulus. Regardless of whether the task requires a hand movement or an eye movement or requires that the monkey refrain from moving toward the stimulus, the visual response of an LIP neuron becomes larger when the stimulus is made behaviorally relevant. This means that the same physical stimulus arriving at the retina can evoke very different responses in cortex as a result of spatial attention.

A third interesting feature of LIP neuron activity is the sustained responses observed when the monkey must remember the location at which the stimulus appeared. In this task, a stimulus is flashed only briefly but the neuron continues to fire for several seconds after the stimulus is gone, as though it were holding a memory trace of the target location. A particularly intriguing question in understanding spatial representation concerns the fate of this memory-related activity in area LIP following an eye movement, as will be described later. A fourth kind of activation commonly observed in LIP neurons is specifically related to performance of a saccade—a rapid eye movement—toward the receptive field. LIP neurons fire just before the monkey initiates a saccade that will move the fovea onto a target presented in the receptive field. LIP neurons have overlapping sensory and motor fields, just like neurons in the superior colliculus (see Chapter 33). Finally, LIP neuron activity can be modulated by the position of the eye in the orbit (Andersen *et al.*, 1990). For instance, the visual response of a given cell may become larger when the monkey is looking toward the left part of the screen than when it is looking toward the right. This property is striking because it suggests that neurons in

area LIP may contribute to spatial representations that go beyond a simple replication of the retinal map. This idea is discussed in more detail in the next section.

In sum, individual LIP neurons have receptive fields at particular retinal locations and carry visual, memory, and saccade-related signals that can be modulated by attention and by eye position. Activity in area LIP cannot be characterized as a simple visual or motor signal. Rather, the level of activation in a given LIP neuron reflects the degree to which attention has been allocated to a location within the receptive field.

Spatial Representation in Area LIP

Every time we move our eyes, each object in our surroundings activates a new set of retinal neurons. Despite this constantly changing input, we experience a stable visual world. How is this possible? More than a century ago, Helmholtz proposed that the reason the world appears to stay still when we move our eyes is that the "effort of will" involved in making a saccade simultaneously adjusts our perception to take

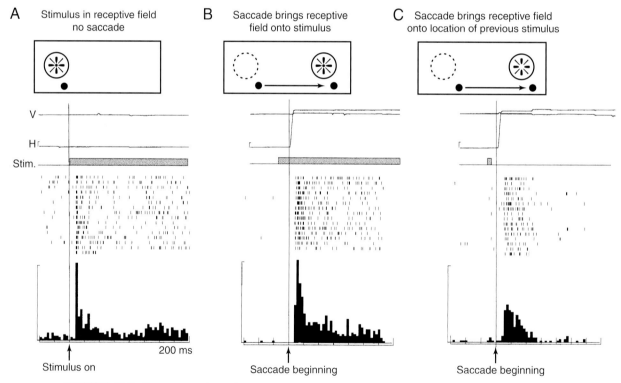

FIGURE 48.5 Remapping of visual memory trace activity in area LIP. The activity of a single neuron was recorded under three different conditions. (A) Simple visual response to a constant stimulus in the receptive field, presented while the monkey is fixating. The rasters and histogram are aligned on the time of stimulus onset. (B) Response following a saccade that brings the receptive field onto the location of a constant visual stimulus. (C) Response following a saccade that brings the receptive field onto the location where a stimulus was presented previously. The stimulus is extinguished before the saccade begins so it is never physically present in the receptive field. The neuron responds to the updated memory trace of the stimulus. V, vertical eye position; H, horizontal eye position. From Duhamel *et al.* (1992).

that specific eye movement into account. He suggested that when a motor command to move the eyes is issued, a copy of that command, or corollary discharge, is sent to brain areas responsible for generating our internal image of the world. This image is then updated so as to be aligned with the new visual information that will arrive in the cortex after the eye movement. A simple experiment shows that Helmholtz's account must be essentially true. When the retina is displaced by pressing on the eye, the world does seem to move, presumably because there is no corollary discharge. Without that internal knowledge of the intended eye movement, there is no way to update the spatial representation of the world around us.

Experiments indicate that neurons in area LIP contribute to this updating of the internal image (Duhamel *et.al.*, 1992). The experiment illustrated in Fig. 48.5 shows that the memory trace of a stimulus is updated when the eyes move. The activity of a single LIP neuron was recorded under three different conditions. In the first set of trials, the monkey looked at a fixed point on the screen while a stimulus was presented in the receptive field (Fig. 48.5A). In the diagram at the top of Fig. 48.5A, the dot is the fixation point, the dashed circle shows the location of the receptive field, and the asterisk represents the visual stimulus. The time lines just below the diagram show that the vertical and horizontal eye positions remained steady throughout the trial, demonstrating that the monkey maintained fixation. The stimulus time line shows that the stimulus appeared 400 ms after the beginning of the trial and continued for the entire trial. The raster display shows the electrical activity of a single LIP neuron in 16 successive trials. In these rasters, each dot indicates the time at which an action potential occurred, and each horizontal line of dots represents activity in a single trial. The rasters show that in each trial there was a brief initial burst of action potentials shortly after the stimulus appeared, followed by continuing neural activity at a lower rate. The histogram at the bottom of Fig. 48.5 shows the average firing rate as a function of time. The visual response shown in Fig. 48.5A is typical of that observed in neurons in many visual areas: the neuron fired when a stimulus appeared in the receptive field of the neuron.

In the second set of trials (Fig. 48.5B), a visual response occurred when the monkey made an eye movement that brought a stimulus into the receptive field. At the beginning of the trial, the monkey looked at the fixation point on the left, and the rest of the screen was blank. Then, simultaneously, a new fixation point appeared on the right and a visual stim-

ulus appeared above it. The monkey made a saccade from the old fixation point to the new one, indicated by the arrow. The eye movement was straight to the right so only the horizontal eye position trace shows a change. At the end of this saccade, the receptive field had been moved to the screen location containing the visual stimulus. The rasters and histogram in Fig. 48.5B are aligned on the time that the saccade began. In each trial, the neuron began to respond after the receptive field had landed on the stimulus. This result is just what would be expected for neurons in any visual area with retinotopic receptive fields.

The surprising finding is shown in Fig. 48.5C. In this third set of trials, the monkey made a saccade that would bring a stimulus into the receptive field, just as in the second set of trials. The only difference was the duration of the stimulus, which lasted for a mere 50 ms instead of staying on for the entire trial. As can be seen on the stimulus time line, the stimulus actually disappeared before the saccade began. This means that the stimulus was never physically present in the receptive field. Nevertheless, the neuron fired as though there were a stimulus in its receptive field. This result shows that LIP neurons respond to the memory trace of a previous stimulus. Moreover, the representation of the memory trace is updated at the time of a saccade. The general idea of how a memory trace can be updated is as follows. At the beginning of the trial, while the monkey is looking at the initial fixation point, the onset of the stimulus activates those neurons whose receptive fields encompass the stimulated location. Some of these neurons will continue to respond after stimulus offset, encoding a memory of the location at which the stimulus occurred. When the monkey moves its eyes toward the new fixation point, a copy of the eye movement command is sent to parietal cortex. This corollary discharge causes the active LIP neurons to transmit their activity to the new set of neurons whose receptive fields will encompass the stimulated screen location after the saccade. By this means, LIP neurons encode the spatially updated memory trace of a previous stimulus.

The significance of this finding lies in what it illustrates about spatial representation in area LIP. It indicates that the internal image is dynamic rather than static. Tonic, memory-related activity in area LIP not only allows neurons to encode a salient spatial location after the stimulus is gone but also allows for dynamic remapping of visual information in conjunction with eye movements. This updating of the internal visual image has specific consequences for spatial representation in the parietal cortex. Instead of spatial information being encoded in purely retinotopic coordinates, tied to the specific neurons initially activated by the stimulus, the information is encoded in eye-centered coordinates. This is a subtle distinction but a very important one in generating accurate spatial behavior. Maintaining visual information in eye-centered coordinates tells the monkey not just where the stimulus was on the retina when it first appeared, but where it would be on the retina following an intervening eye movement. The result is that the monkey always has accurate information with which to program an eye movement toward a real or a remembered target. Further results from this series of experiments indicate that humans also depend on this kind of remapping for accurate spatial representation.

Area VIP

In contrast to the eye-centered spatial representation found in area LIP, some neurons in the adjacent ventral intraparietal area (area VIP) encode locations with respect to a head-centered reference frame. These neurons have several interesting properties. They respond strongly to moving stimuli and are selective for both the speed and the direction of the stimulus (Colby, et al. 1993). In this respect, VIP neurons are similar to those in other dorsal stream visual areas that process stimulus motion, especially areas MT and MST (see Chapter 27). An unexpected finding in area VIP is that most of these visually responsive neurons also respond to somatosensory stimuli (Duhamel, et al,, 1991). These neurons are truly bimodal in the sense that they can be driven equally well by either a visual or a somatosensory stimulus. Most of these bimodal neurons have somatosensory receptive fields on the head and face that match their visual receptive fields. This correspondence is illustrated in Fig. 48.6, which shows visual and somatosensory receptive fields for 14 individual VIP neurons.

Three kinds of correspondence are shown. First, for each neuron, receptive fields in each modality match in location. For example, a neuron that responds to a visual stimulus in the upper left visual field also responds when the left brow is touched (Fig. 48.6, top right). Second, receptive fields match in size. A neuron with a restricted visual receptive field also has a small somatosensory receptive field. The smallest visual receptive fields are those located at the fovea. It

is striking that the corresponding somatosensory receptive fields for these neurons are not centered around the eye but are found around the mouth. In terms of sensitivity, the mouth can be thought of as the fovea of the facial somatosensory system. Hence it is logical that the two regions of highest spatial acuity should be linked. The third type of correspondence is in the preferred directions of movement. For example, a neuron responsive to a visual stimulus moving toward the right also responds when a small probe is brushed lightly to the right across the face of the monkey (Fig. 48.6, lower left). In sum, visual and somatosensory receptive fields for individual VIP neurons match in location, size, and directional preference.

This observation of correspondence in receptive field location immediately raises a question: What happens to the relative locations of the visual and somatosensory receptive fields when the eyes move? If the visual receptive field were simply retinotopic, it would move when the eyes do; if the somatosensory receptive field were purely somatotopic, it would be unchanged by eye movements. There could not be a consistent correspondence in location if visual receptive fields were defined only with respect to the retina while somatosensory receptive fields were defined only with respect to the skin surface.

The answer is that visual receptive fields are linked to the skin surface and not to the retina. A neuron that responds best to a visual stimulus approaching the forehead and has a somatosensory receptive field on the brow will continue to respond best to a visual stimulus moving toward the brow regardless of where the monkey is fixating. Thus, both visual and somatosensory receptive fields are defined with respect to the skin surface. In this sense, the receptive fields are head centered: a given VIP neuron responds to stimulation of a certain portion of the skin surface and to the visual stimulus aligned with it no matter which part of the retina is activated.

In sum, neurons in area VIP encode bimodal sensory information in a head-centered representation of space. This kind of representation would be most useful for guiding head movements. Anatomical studies indicate that area VIP sends information to the specific region of the premotor cortex that is involved in generating head movements. In contrast, neurons in area LIP encode sensory information in an eye-cen-

FIGURE 48.6   Matching visual and somatosensory receptive fields of 14 neurons from area VIP. On each outline of the head of the monkey, the patch of color corresponds to the somatosensory receptive field of one neuron. On the square above the head, the patch of texture corresponds to the visual receptive field of the same neuron. The square can be thought of as a screen placed in front of the monkey so that its center is directly ahead of the monkey's eyes. From Duhamel et al. (1991) with permission of Oxford University Press.

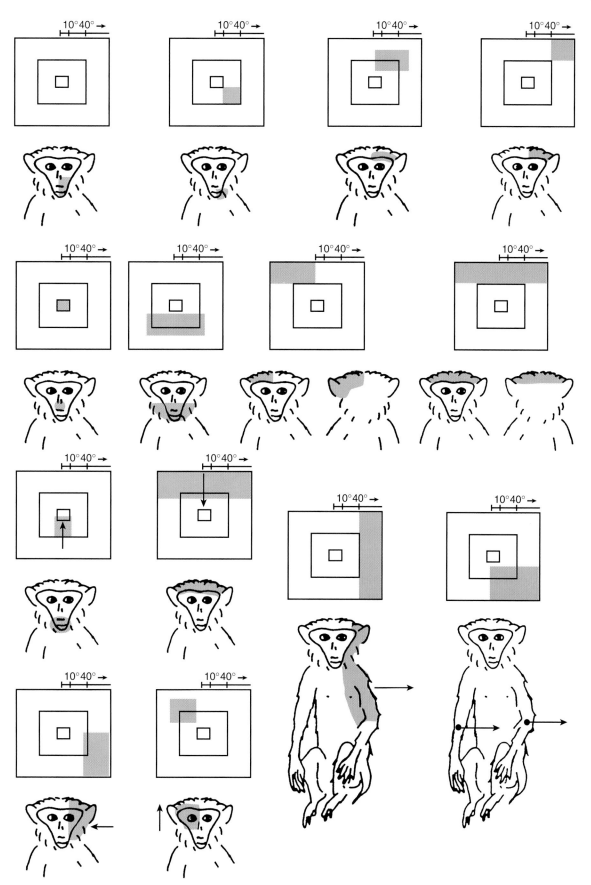

tered representation of space in a form most useful for guiding eye movements. Area LIP sends projections to both the superior colliculus and the frontal eye fields, regions that are involved in generating eye movements. The parietal cortex contains a number of other areas, especially within the intraparietal sulcus, each of which may be specialized for particular types of stimuli and particular regions of space. The general point is that the problem of spatial representation may be solved in several ways, and each solution may contribute to the generation of a different kind of action.

Summary

The posterior parietal cortex plays a critical role in spatial awareness. Injury to the parietal cortex in humans and monkeys leads to deficits in spatial perception and action. Physiological studies in monkeys have shown that parietal neurons construct a representation of space by combining signals from multiple sensory modalities with motor signals. An intriguing physiological finding is that parietal neurons represent spatial locations relative to multiple reference frames, including ones centered on the eye and the head. In accord with this physiology, human neuropsychological studies have shown that neglect resulting from parietal lobe injury can be expressed with respect to several different reference frames.

FRONTAL CORTEX

The Frontal Cortex Contributes to Voluntary Movement and the Control of Behavior

The frontal lobe is involved in spatial functions as a natural result of its being involved in behavioral control. The three main divisions of the frontal lobe are the primary motor cortex; located on the precentral gyrus, the premotor cortex, including the supplementary eye field, located in front of the primary motor cortex, and the prefrontal cortex (see Fig. 48.1). The motor, premotor, and prefrontal areas all contribute to behavioral control, but they differ with respect to the quality of their contribution. This difference is seen in the effects of brain injury. Injury to the primary motor cortex leads to weakness and paralysis of the contralateral muscles. In contrast, injury to the premotor cortex leads to difficulty in producing movements in certain circumstances, e.g., when the patient is asked to mime the use of a tool or to learn arbitrary associations between stimuli and

responses. Finally, injury to the prefrontal cortex results in a classic syndrome characterized by a lack of drive and an impaired ability to execute plans (see Chapter 53). These effects indicate that progressively more anterior parts of the frontal cortex contribute to progressively more abstract aspects of behavioral control. Each of these divisions participates in spatial processes insofar as the kind of behavioral control to which it is dedicated has a spatial component. The next four sections describe aspects of spatial representation and function in the primary motor cortex, in the premotor cortex, in the supplementary eye field, and in the prefrontal cortex.

Neurons in the Primary Motor Cortex Represent Movement Direction Relative to a Spatial Frame

The primary motor cortex contains a map of the muscles of the body in which the leg is represented medially, the head laterally, and other body parts at intermediate locations. Within this map are patches of neurons that represent different muscles. Neurons within a given patch receive proprioceptive input from a muscle or small group of synergistic muscles and send their output back to that muscle or group of synergists by way of a multisynaptic pathway through the brain stem and spinal cord. There have been many studies in which the electrical activity of neurons in the primary motor cortex is monitored while animals move. The general conclusion of these studies is that neurons in the primary motor cortex are active when the corresponding muscles are undergoing active contraction. It is important to note, however, that neurons in the primary motor cortex probably do more than simply encode the levels of activation of individual muscles. One proposal is that they encode movement trajectories. Every voluntary movement can be described in two quite different, but perfectly complementary, ways: in terms of the lengths of the muscles or in terms of the position of the part of the body being moved. For example, during an arm movement, changes take place both in the lengths of muscles acting on the arm and in the position of the hand. Could it be that neurons in the primary motor cortex encode a spatial variable, such as the direction of movement of the hand, rather than a muscle variable?

Evidence supporting the idea that neurons of the primary motor cortex encode movement direction has come from studies in which monkeys make reaching movements in various directions. Individual neurons are selective for a specific direction of movement: a given neuron may fire most strongly during movements up and to the right and progressively less strongly for movements that deviate from the preferred direction (Schwartz, *et al.*, 1988). The patterns of selectivity are well defined and the preferred directions of different neurons cover the range of possible movements fairly evenly. By recording the activity of the entire population of neurons one could, in principle, quite accurately describe the movement. The question remains whether these neurons are selective for the direction of movement in space or for the specific patterns of muscle activation associated with particular movements. In an elegant series of studies, Kakei, *et al.*, (1999) recorded from neurons in the primary motor cortex while the monkey moved its arm in a constant direction using different combinations of muscles. They discovered that the primary motor cortex contains both neurons selective for movement direction and neurons selective for patterns of muscle activation.

Neurons in the Premotor Cortex Have Head and Hand-Centered Visual Receptive Fields

One of the functions of premotor cortical areas is to act as a conduit through which sensory signals are relayed to the motor system. The sensory information that reaches these areas has been highly processed already in the posterior cerebral hemispheres. Thus it is not surprising that the sensory receptive fields of some neurons in the premotor cortex are defined with respect to an external spatial framework in a form suitable for use by the motor system.

Both head and hand-centered visual receptive fields have been described in the premotor cortex. First, in portions of the premotor cortex representing orofacial movements, neurons respond to visual stimuli at a certain location relative to the head (Fogassi *et al.*, 1992). These neurons have been characterized by recording from them while objects approach the head of the monkey along various trajectories. A typical experiment is illustrated in Fig. 48.7. In the first phase of the experiment, shown in the left column, the monkey looked straight ahead at a fixation target (F) while an object approached the face and then receded. The stimulus moved along a trajectory that brought it either to the right side of the head (trajectory 1) or to the left side (trajectory 2). Records of neuronal activity showed that the neuron fired when the object approached along trajectory 1 but not when it approached along trajectory 2. Accordingly, it appears that the neuron had a visual receptive field located in the right visual field (shaded area in Fig. 48.7A).

To determine whether the receptive field was head or retina-centered required a second phase of testing (right column). In this phase, the monkey looked far to the left at a fixation point (F). While he maintained a leftward gaze, objects again approached the face, following trajectories 1 and 2. If the receptive field of this neuron were head centered, one would predict that it should continue to respond as the object approached along trajectory 1. However, if the receptive field were fixed to the retina, then the neuron should respond as the object approached along trajectory 2. Records of the activity of the neuron clearly indicate that the neuron had a head-centered visual receptive field. It was responsive to stimuli presented to the right of the midline of the head, but not to stimuli presented to the right of the midline of the retina. This head-centered spatial selectivity of premotor cortex neurons in the premotor cortex is similar to that found in area VIP. That neurons in these two areas should exhibit consistent patterns of spatial selectivity is not surprising because the parietal and premotor cortices are strongly interconnected.

A second type of body-centered spatial representation in the premotor cortex has been observed in areas representing arm movements. Here, neurons respond to visual stimuli if they are presented in the vicinity of the hand (Graziano, *et al.*, 1994). When the hand moves to a new location, the visual receptive field moves with it. The visual receptive field remains fixed to the position of the hand regardless of where the monkey is looking and, thus, regardless of the part of the retina on which the image is cast. The two distinct forms of body-centered visual responsiveness seen in the premotor cortex presumably reflect the involvement of these neurons in the visual guidance of orofacial and arm movements.

Neurons in the Supplementary Eye Field Encode the Object-Centered Direction of Eye Movements

A particularly striking form of allocentric spatial representation is found in the supplementary eye field (SEF). The SEF is a division of the premotor cortex with attentional and oculomotor functions. Neurons here fire before and during the execution of saccadic eye movements. Two characteristics of the SEF set it apart from subcortical oculomotor centers and suggest that its contribution to eye movement control occurs at a comparatively abstract level. First, neurons here fire while the monkey is waiting to make an eye movement in the preferred direction, as well as during the eye movement itself. Second, some SEF neurons become especially active when the monkey is

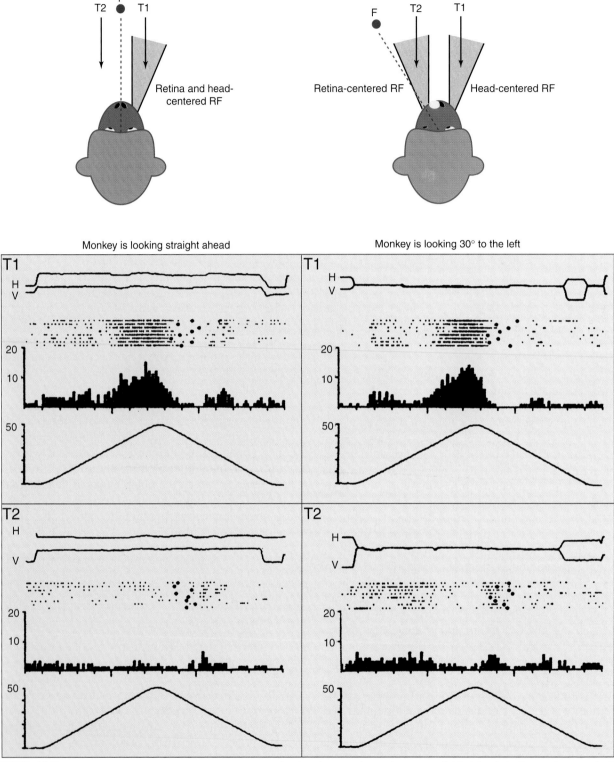

FIGURE 48.7 Data from a neuron in the premotor cortex with a head-centered visual receptive field. (A) While the monkey was looking straight ahead at a fixation point (F), an object approached and receded, traveling either along trajectory 1 (T1, to the right of the head) or along trajectory 2 (T2, to the left of the head). The neuron fired strongly only when the object approached along trajectory 1. (B) When the monkey looked at a new fixation point on the far left, the neuron still responded only when the object approached along trajectory 1, indicating that the receptive field is tied to the location of the head and not to the location of the retina. The time lines above each raster and histogram show the horizontal (H) and vertical (V) eye position during one trial. The time line below shows the position of the visual object as it comes toward and then moves away from the monkey. From Fogassi *et al.* (1992).

learning to associate arbitrary visual cues with particular directions of eye movements.

SEF neurons exhibit a unique form of spatial selectivity in monkeys trained to make eye movements to particular locations on an object. In this context, SEF neurons encode the direction of the impending eye movement as defined relative to an object-centered reference frame (Olson and Gettner, 1995). Regardless of where in space an object appears, these neurons respond when the animal is planning to make an eye movement to a specific location on that object. An experiment demonstrating this point is shown in Fig. 48.8. This figure shows the activity of a single SEF neuron while the monkey performed an eye movement task. At the beginning of each trial, the monkey fixated a dot at the center of a screen. While the monkey fixated, a sample and cue were presented in the right visual field. The cue flashed on either the right or the left end of the short horizontal sample bar. Following extinction of the sample–cue display, the monkey maintained fixation for a brief time. Then, simultaneously, the central spot was extinguished and a target bar appeared at an unpredictable location in the upper

visual field of the monkey. The monkey had to make an eye movement to the end of the target bar corresponding to the cued end of the sample bar. Across the set of eight conditions, the object-centered direction of the eye movement was completely independent of its physical direction.

This situation made it possible to ask whether the activity of the neuron was related to the object-centered direction of the movement or to its physical direction. To the right of each panel in Fig. 48.8 is shown the average firing rate as a function of time during the trial. Regardless of the direction of the physical movement of the eye, firing was clearly stronger on trials in which the monkey made an eye movement to the left end of the target bar than on trials in which the target was the right end of the bar. For example, in panels 1 and 2, the physical direction of the eye movement was exactly the same, and yet firing was much stronger when the left end of the bar was the target (panel 1) than when the right end of the bar was the target (panel 2). This neuron exhibited object-centered direction selectivity in the sense that it fired most strongly before and during movements to a certain location on an object.

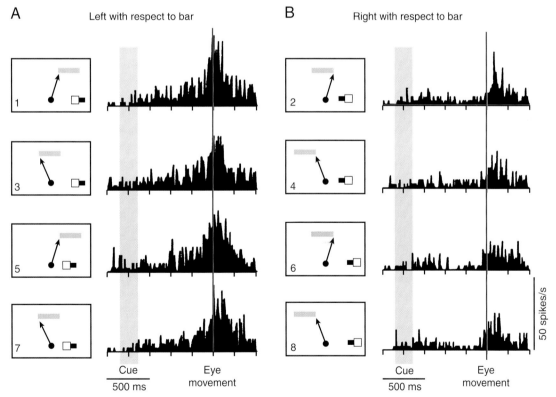

FIGURE 48.8 Data from a neuron in the SEF selective for the object-centered direction of eye movements. The monkey was trained to make eye movements to the right or left end of a horizontal bar. A cue appeared on the small sample bar shown in the lower right of each panel (1–8) to tell the monkey which end of the target bar (top in each panel) was relevant on a given trial. The arrow in the panel next to each histogram indicates the direction of the eye movement. The neuron fired strongly when the eye movement was directed to the left end of the target bar (left column) regardless of whether the physical movement of the eye was up and to the right (panels 1 and 5) or up and to the left (panels 3 and 7). From Olson and Gettner (1995).

Object-centered direction selectivity serves an important function in natural settings. In scanning the environment, we sometimes look toward locations where things are expected to appear, but which, at the time, contain no detail, e.g., the center of a blank screen or the center of an empty doorway. Our eyes are guided to these featureless locations by surrounding features that define them indirectly. It is specifically in these cases that the SEF may contribute to the selection of the target for an eye movement.

The Prefrontal Cortex Mediates Working Memory for Spatial Information

Working memory is required to hold a plan in mind and carry it out step by step (see Chapters 53 and 54). The fact that this ability is severely impaired in some patients following prefrontal injury indicates that this region plays a crucial role in working memory. Insofar as plans and working memory have a spatial component, operations carried out by the prefrontal cortex should also be spatial in nature. Single neuron-recording experiments in monkeys performing delayed-response tasks have demonstrated the importance of the dorsolateral prefrontal cortex for both spatial and nonspatial forms of working memory (Funahashi et al., 1991). A delayed-response task consists of several trials, each several seconds long. At the beginning of each trial, a cue is presented briefly, instructing the monkey which response to make, but the reponse must be withheld until the end of the trial. Delayed-response tasks can be designed so that both cues (e.g., spots flashed to the right or left of fixation) and responses (e.g., eye movements to the right or left) may be spatial. In the context of these spatial tasks, prefrontal neurons are active during the period between the cue and the signal to respond, when the monkey is holding spatial information in working memory. Just as for visual responses, some neurons are selective for the direction of the motor response. The simple interpretation of this pattern of activity is that it is a neural correlate of the monkey actively remembering the cue and holding in mind the intended response. This interpretation is also supported by recent experiments based on the imaging of brain activation in humans.

The idea that the prefrontal cortex mediates spatial working memory has received further support from lesion experiments in monkeys. After injury to or inactivation of specific locations in the prefrontal cortex, monkeys are impaired at remembering locations in the opposite half of space. Their delayed responses are spatially inaccurate and the inaccuracy is exacerbated by longer delays. An experiment

demonstrating the importance of the prefrontal cortex for spatial working memory is illustrated in Fig. 48.9, which shows behavioral data from a monkey trained to perform an oculomotor delayed-response task (Sawaguchi and Goldman-Rakic, 1994). At the beginning of each trial, the monkey fixated a spot at the center of the screen. While the monkey maintained fixation, a cue was flashed at one of six possible locations at positions. Following presentation of the cue, a delay of 1.5–6 s ensued before the monkey was permitted to make an eye movement to the cued location.

Data from a normal monkey are shown in the left column of Fig. 48.9. In each panel, the six bundles of radiating rays represent the eye trajectories on trials when the cue was at the six different locations. Even when required to remember the cue for 6 s, the monkey made accurate eye movements. Data in the right column are from the same monkey after a

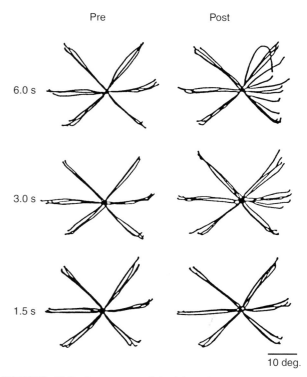

FIGURE 48.9 Inactivation of the left prefrontal cortex disrupts spatial working memory in the right half of space. A monkey was trained to fixate a central spot while a peripheral cue was presented briefly at one of six locations. After an interval of 6, 3, or 1.5 s, the fixation spot was extinguished and the monkey made an eye movement to the remembered location. Each set of diverging rays shows the trajectories of eye movements executed under a certain set of conditions. The left column shows eye movement performance before inactivation by a dopamine antagonist. The right column shows performance after inactivation. When the cue was in the right hemifield and the monkey was required to remember its location over long delays, the movements became highly inaccurate. From Sawaguchi and Goldman-Rakic (1994).

dopamine antagonist was injected into the left prefrontal cortex. The ability of the monkey to remember the location of the cue remained intact when the cue was in the left (ipsilesional) visual field, as shown by the accurate eye movements. However, performance deteriorated on trials when the cue was in the right (contralesional) visual field. Especially after long delays (top panel), the direction of the eye movement began to deviate from the location of the cue, as if the working memory of the monkey were fading. The fact that this deficit was specific to long delays is noteworthy because it rules out any simple explanation based on interference with visual or motor processes as opposed to working memory itself.

Summary

Neurons in the frontal cortex represent spatial information as a natural consequence of their role in controlling behavior. Neurons in the primary motor cortex encode the directions of movements. Neurons in the premotor cortex encode locations relative to the body, even when these locations are not the immediate targets of actions. SEF neurons encode locations in an allocentric, object-centered representation. Finally, neurons in the prefrontal cortex encode the locations of objects being held in short-term memory.

HIPPOCAMPUS AND ADJACENT CORTEX

The Hippocampal System Is Associated with Memory Formation

Spatial functions of the hippocampus center on its role in memory formation (see Chapter 51). The hippocampus is an area of primitive cortex, or allocortex, hidden on the underside of the temporal lobe. It is connected to a set of immediately adjacent cortical areas, including the perirhinal, entorhinal, and parahippocampal cortices (Zola-Morgan and Squire, 1993).

Amnesia Resulting from Hippocampal Injury in Humans Includes a Spatial Component

Extensive evidence implicates the hippocampus and related medial temporal structures in the formation of declarative memories in humans. Memories dependent on the hippocampus include, although they are by no means restricted to, memories for spatial material. In addition to many other impairments, the amnesia of the noted patient H.M. was manifested by his inability to learn to find his way through new neighborhoods. Patients with damage to the hippocampus, especially the right hippocampus, are impaired on tests requiring them to inspect a scene with many objects and then to recall the locations of individual objects.

Neurons of the Hippocampal System Have Place Fields and Are Sensitive to Directional Orientation of the Head

Recordings from hippocampal neurons in rats running mazes or exploring open areas have revealed a remarkable degree of spatial selectivity. Many neurons throughout the hippocampus have place fields; i.e., a given neuron will fire most strongly when the rat is within a certain sector of the workspace (see Chapter 51). Different neurons have different place fields so that, collectively, they cover the workspace. Place fields are defined relative to prominent environmental landmarks. If a radially symmetric eight-arm maze is rotated relative to a surrounding room containing salient landmarks, then the place fields remain fixed with respect to the room. Even in darkness, however, neurons continue to fire when the rat is in their place field, indicating that these responses are not simply visual. If the rat is placed in a new environment, hippocampal neurons develop new place fields rapidly. The location of the place field of a neuron relative to the new environment is not predictable from its location relative to the old environment. This is true even in cases where the workspace is changed without any change in the surrounding room, e.g., through replacement of an eight-arm radial maze by an open field.

Some hippocampal system neurons are sensitive not only to the location of the rat, but also to the direction in which the head is pointing. Sensitivity to heading, although not the most distinctive feature of hippocampal neurons, is dominant in the postsubiculum, a cortical area adjacent to and closely linked to the hippocampus. Each postsubicular neuron fires most strongly when the head of the rat is pointing in its preferred direction and fires progressively less strongly as the orientation of the head of the rat deviates farther from that direction. In a room that is suddenly darkened, postsubicular neurons remain sensitive to the heading of the rat so long as the rat retains a sense of spatial orientation, as reflected by error-free performance on spatial tests. When the sense of spatial orientation drifts away from veridicality during prolonged darkness, as evidenced by the occurrence of systematic errors on spatial tests, then the preferred headings of postsubicular neurons exhibit a commensurate drift. These observations establish that neurons of the hippocampal system are sensitive to the spatial orientation of the rat. How the hippocampus uses spatial information, along with nonspatial information, to form new memories is taken up in Chapter 51.

Summary

The hippocampal system mediates the formation of memories, including memories with spatial content. Injury to the hippocampal system, both in humans and in other animals, leads to profound deficits of memory, including navigational memory. In accord with these findings, single neuron recording in rats has revealed that neurons of the hippocampal system can exhibit place fields, encoding the location of the rat in its environment, and directional sensitivity, encoding head direction relative to the environment.

SPATIAL COGNITION AND SPATIAL ACTION

The preceding sections described how spatial information is processed by numerous cortical areas that serve distinct functions, such as motor control, attention, and working memory. Even within the motor system, there appears to be a fractionation of spatial functions in that neurons controlling movements of the eyes, head, and arm represent the locations of visible targets relative to eye, head, and hand-centered reference frames, respectively. In addition to these distinctions, there may be another fundamental distinction within brain systems mediating spatial functions. Areas mediating conscious awareness of spatial information may be partially separate from those mediating the spatial guidance of motor behavior. These functions may seem inseparable insofar as one must be aware of the location of a thing in order to look at it or reach for it. However, this is not necessarily the case. An indication that spatial awareness and spatially programmed behavior are distinguishable has come from studies of patients with "blindsight" (Weiskrantz, 1996). This condition arises as a result of injury to the primary visual cortex. Patients experience a scotoma, an area of blindness, in the part of the visual field represented by the injured cortex. The blindness is total in the sense that patients do not report seeing visual stimuli when stimuli are presented within the confines of the scotoma. Nevertheless, if patients are asked to look toward or to reach for an unseen stimulus, choosing the target by guesswork, their responses are directed to the correct location. Similar findings have been reported in patients with diffuse pathology affecting widespread areas, including the prestriate visual cortex (Goodale et al., 1994). When asked to express spatial judgments (e.g., to indicate the size of a visible object by spreading the thumb and forefinger), these patients perform poorly. Nevertheless, when asked to make visually guided movements (e.g., to reach for an object), they accurately adjust their grip size and hand orientation under visual control to grasp the object efficiently. The fact that intact visuomotor performance coexists with profoundly impaired visuospatial perception in these patients seems to argue for the existence of distinct brain systems specialized for conscious spatial awareness and motor guidance, respectively.

Summary

Spatial cognition is a function of several different brain areas. No one area is uniquely responsible for the ability to carry out spatial tasks. Nevertheless, some generalizations can be made about the part of the problem that is solved in each brain region. The parietal lobe plays a crucial role in many aspects of spatial awareness, including spatially focused attention. The representation of space in the parietal cortex takes several forms. Each subdivision within the parietal cortex contributes to different kinds of representations, designed to help guide different kinds of actions.

In contrast to the parietal cortex, the frontal lobe transforms spatial awareness into actions. The motor cortex uses a spatial framework to encode intended actions. The premotor cortex contains a set of different spatial representations to generate eye, hand and arm movements. The SEF contains neurons with very high-order, abstract spatial representations, whereas the prefrontal cortex mediates spatial working memory. Finally, the hippocampus mediates spatial declarative memories, including those that underlie spatial navigation.

Beneath the unity of our spatial perception lies a diversity of specific representations. The distributed nature of spatial cognition and the many purposes it serves means that we construct internal representations of space not once but many times in parallel. A challenge for the future is to understand how these many representations function together so seamlessly.

References

Andersen, R. A., Bracewell, R. M., Barash, S., Gnadt, J. W., and Fogassi, L. (1990). Eye position effects on visual, memory, and saccade-related activity in areas LIP and 7a of macaque. *J. Neurosci.* **10**, 1176–1196.

Bisiach, E., and Luzzatti, C. (1978). Unilateral neglect of representational space. *Cortex* **14**, 129–133.

Colby, C. L., and Duhamel, J.-R. (1991). Heterogeneity of extrastriate visual areas and multiple parietal areas in the macaque monkey. *Neuropsychologia* **29**, 517–537.

Colby, C. L., Duhamel, J.-R., and Goldberg, M. E. (1993). Ventral intraparietal area of the macaque: Anatomic location and visual response properties. *J. Neurophysiol.* **69**, 902–914.

Colby, C. L., Duhamel, J.-R., and Goldberg, M. E. (1996). Visual, presaccadic and cognitive activation of single neurons in monkey lateral intraparietal area. *J. Neurophysiol.* **76**, 2841–2852.

Coslett, H. B., and Saffran, E. (1991). Simultanagnosia: To see but not two see. *Brain* **114**, 1523–1545.

Duhamel, J.-R., Colby, C. L., and Goldberg, M. E. (1991). Congruent representations of visual and somatosensory space in single neurons of monkey ventral intraparietal cortex (area VIP). *In* "Brain and Space" (J. Paillard, ed.), pp. 223–236. Oxford Press, Oxford.

Duhamel, J.-R., Colby, C. L., and Goldberg, M. E. (1992). The updating of the representation of visual space in parietal cortex by intended eye movements. *Science* **255**, 90–92.

Fogassi, L., Gallese, V., di Pellegrino, G., Fadiga, L., Gentilucci, M., Luppino, G., Matelli, M., Pedotti, A., and Rizzolatti, G. (1992). Space coding by premotor cortex. *Exp. Brain Res.* **89**, 686–690.

Funahashi, S., Bruce, C. J., and Goldman-Rakic, P. S. (1991). Neuronal activity related to saccadic eye movements in the monkey's dorsolateral prefrontal cortex. *J. Neurophysiol.* **65**, 1464–1483.

Goldman-Rakic, P. S. (1988). Topography of cognition: Parallel distributed networks in primate association cortex. *Annu. Rev. Neurosci.* **11**, 137–156.

Goodale, M. A., Meenan, J. P., Bulthoff, H. H., Nicolle, D. A., Murphy, K. J., and Racicot, C. I. (1994). Separate neural pathways for the visual analysis of object shape in perception and prehension. *Curr. Biol.* **4**, 604–610.

Graziano, M. S., Yap, G. S., and Gross, C. G. (1994). Coding of visual space by premotor neurons. *Science* **266**, 1054–1057.

Humphreys, G. W., and Riddoch, M. J. (1993). Interactions between object and space systems revealed through neuropsychology. *In* "Attention and Performance" (D. E. Meyer and S. Kornblum, eds.), Vol. XIV, pp. 143–162. MIT Press, Cambridge, MA.

Kakei, S., Hoffman, D. S., and Strick, P. L. (1999). Muscle and movement representations in the primary motor cortex. *Science* **285**, 2136–2139.

Ladavas, E. (1987). Is the hemispatial deficit produced by right parietal lobe damage associated with retinal or gravitational coordinates? *Brain* **110**, 167–180.

Lynch, J. C., and McLaren, J. W. (1989). Deficits of visual attention and saccadic eye movements after lesions of parietooccipital cortex in monkeys. *J. Neurophysiol.* **61**, 74–90.

Marshall, J. C., and Halligan, P. W. (1993). Visuo-spatial neglect: A new copying text to assess perceptual parsing. *J. Neurol.* **240**, 37–40.

Olson, C. R., and Gettner, S. N. (1995). Object-centered direction selectivity in the macaque supplementary eye field. *Science* **269**, 985–988.

Perenin, M.-T., and Vighetto, A. (1988). Optic ataxia: A specific disruption in visuomotor mechanisms. I. Different aspects of the deficit in reaching for objects. *Brain* **111**, 643–674.

Sawaguchi, T., and Goldman-Rakic, P. S. (1994). The role of D1-dopamine receptor in working memory: Local injections of dopamine antagonists into the prefrontal cortex of rhesus monkeys performing an oculomotor delayed-response task. *J. Neurophysiol.* **71**, 515–528.

Schwartz, A. B., Kettner, R. E., and Georgopoulos, A. P. (1988). Primate motor cortex and free arm movements to visual targets in three-dimensional space. I. Relations between single cell discharge and direction of movement. *J. Neurosci.* **8**, 2913–2927.

Ungerleider, L. G., and Mishkin, M. (1982). Two cortical visual systems. *In* "Analysis of Visual Behavior" (D. J. Ingle, M. A. Goodale, and R. J. W. Mansfield, eds.), pp. 549–586. MIT Press, Cambridge, MA.

Weiskrantz, L. (1996). Blindsight revisited. *Curr. Opin. Neurobiol.* **6**, 215–220.

Zola-Morgan, S., and Squire, L. R. (1993). Neuroanatomy of memory. *Annu. Rev. Neurosci.* **16**, 547–563.

Suggested Readings

Bisiach, E., Luzzatti, C., and Perani, D. (1979). Unilateral neglect, representational schema and consciousness. *Brain* **102**, 609–618.

DeRenzi, E. (1985). Disorders of spatial orientation. *In* "Handbook of Clinical Neurology" (J. A. M. Frederiks, ed.), Vol. 1, pp. 405–422. Elsevier, Amsterdam.

Driver, J., and Halligan, P. W. (1991). Can visual neglect operate in object-centered coordinates? An affirmative single-case study. *Cognit. Neuropsych.* **8**, 475–496.

Hyvarinen J. (1982). Posterior parietal lobe of the primate brain. *Physiol. Rev.* **62**, 1060–129.

Kakei, S., Hoffman, D. S., and Strick, P. L. (2001). Direction of action is represented in the ventral premotor cortex. *Nature Neurosci.* **4**, 1020–1025.

O'Keefe, J., and Nadel, L. (1978). "The Hippocampus as a Cognitive Map." Oxford Univ. Press, Oxford.

Olson, C. R., and Gettner, S. N. (1996). Brain representation of object-centered space. *Curr. Opin. Neurobiol.* **6**, 165–170.

Rizzolatti, G., Fogassi, L., and Gallese, V. (1997). Parietal cortex: from sight to action. *Curr. Opin. Neurobiol.* **7**, 562–567.

Stein, J. F. (1991). Space and parietal association areas. *In* "Brain and Space" (J. Paillard, ed.), pp. 185–222. Oxford Univ. Press, Oxford.

Carol L. Colby and Carl R. Olson

49

Attention

INTRODUCTION

Intuition, together with cognitive and psychophysical experiments, shows that the brain is limited in the amount of neural processing it can carry out at any moment in time. For instance, when people are asked to identify the objects of a briefly presented scene, they become less accurate as the number of objects increases. Similarly, when people concentrate on one demanding task (e.g., mental arithmetic) they invariably do so at the expense of performance on other simultaneous activities (e.g., recalling a familiar tune). The inability to carry out more than one cognitive or perceptual task at a time reflects the limited capacity of some stage or stages of sensory processing, decision-making, or behavioral control. As a result of such computational bottlenecks, it is necessary to have neural mechanisms in place to ensure the selection of stimuli, or tasks, that are immediately relevant to behavior. "Attention" is a broad term denoting the mechanisms that mediate this selection.

Over the past several decades, research has concentrated on the relation between attention and sensory perception. Clearly, it is possible to focus on selected stimuli in any sensory modality—sights, sounds, smells and touch. Most studies, however, have examined vision, the dominant sensory modality for humans and nonhuman primates. Experiments have investigated the neural mechanisms of visual attention at the level of the neuron and cortical circuit and related operation of these mechanisms to behavior and perception. This chapter outlines the main findings of these studies.

A key observation is that attending to an object greatly enhances the ability to perceive and report the object's visual attributes; conversely, withdraw-

ing attention, either by force of the behavioral context or following certain brain lesions, can render observers practically blind to certain visual events. A second key point is that the attentional processes that underlie perceptual selection may also guide the voluntary eye movements with which foveate animals, such as monkeys and humans, scan the environment. In terms of neural organization, while some neural centers have been closely linked with the control of attention, attention appears to affect the activity of neurons at almost all levels of the visual system. Finally, the chapter considers the activity of neuromodulatory systems that originate in the brain stem, which are important in regulation of the overall level of alertness.

VARIETIES OF ATTENTION

In natural behavior, individuals have great flexibility as to how and when they attend and what they attend to. Attending to an object is often accompanied by overt orienting toward that object using the eyes and possibly also the head and body. When a person enters a room, it is natural to turn in that person's direction. However, one can also attend covertly to objects that are not in the center of gaze, without looking directly at them. When driving, one can monitor a passing car while continuing to look straight ahead. Covert attention can improve peripheral visual acuity, thereby extending the functional field of view. Although one can direct attention without moving the eyes, the converse does not appear to be true: experiments show that covert attention must be deployed to an object before that object can be targeted with an eye movement. Indeed, saccades—rapid eye movements used most commonly for scanning the environment—may be considered a motor manifestation of visual attention, a relationship that is discussed in more detail later.

Certain external stimuli can summon attention in and of themselves. These can be physically salient objects, such as especially large, bright or loud objects, or stimuli with special learned significance, such as one's own name or a mother's face. This mode of attentional engagement, known as *exogenous* or *stimulus driven*, ensures that salient and potentially important external events do not pass unnoticed even if they are not being actively sought out. However, purposeful behavior often requires that attention is directed voluntarily, or *endogenously*, based on internally defined goals and against potential external distractions. When reading, one purposefully directs one's attention from one word to the next, tuning out noise and other distractions. In natural behavior, endogenous and exogenous factors interact continuously to control attentional resources (Egeth and Yantis, 1997).

Another important issue is *what* is attended. One can attend to a location in space, regardless of what happens to be at that location. This ability is known as spatial attention. One can also attend to specific objects regardless of their location. Early psychophysical studies showed that observers can attend to one stimulus while suppressing attention to another stimulus, even when the two stimuli are superimposed and cannot be selected by spatial attention alone (Neisser and Becklen, 1975; Rock and Guttman, 1981).

Attentional processes, therefore, are highly flexible. Attention can be deployed in a manner that best serves the organism's behavioral goals: either to locations or to objects, based on internal goals or the external environment, with or without accompanying orienting movements. It is important to keep in mind that although these phenomena can be demonstrated in laboratory experiments, all varieties of attention are closely related and they operate seamlessly during natural behavior.

COVERT SPATIAL ATTENTION HAS BEEN STUDIED INTENSIVELY WITH THE CUING PARADIGM

As mentioned earlier, it is possible to attend selectively to particular spatial locations. Spatial attention is often conceived of as a mental spotlight, which improves perception of any and all objects within the attended ("illuminated") region. No prior visual processing, such as scene segmentation or object identification, is needed for spatial attention. All that is required is an intact ability for spatial orientation.

Spatial attention has been studied in the laboratory using a paradigm known as spatial cuing (Posner and Petersen, 1990). In a typical cuing task, subjects look at a fixation point at the center of a computer screen and are shown a brief cue that instructs them to attend to a peripheral spatial location (e.g., to the right or left of the display) where a visual stimulus is expected to appear. Subjects have to direct attention covertly, while continuing to maintain gaze on the central fixation point (Fig. 49.1). At variable delays following this cue, a visual stimulus (the target) is flashed very briefly (for a few hundreds of milliseconds), and subjects are asked to make some judgment about that target as quickly and accurately as they can. On the majority of trials (typically, 80%) the target appears at the cued, presumably attended, location. These are known as valid trials. On other trials the target appears at an uncued and presumably unattended location. These are termed invalid trials. The difference in performance on the judgment task between valid and invalid trials reflects the effect of attention on the perception of the target.

Attending to a location dramatically improves the accuracy and speed of report for targets at that location. Attention has been shown to increase perceptual sensitivity for target discrimination, to reduce the interference caused by nearby distractors, and to improve the ability to discriminate high spatial frequencies at the cued locations. In the plane of fixation, the perceptual benefits conferred by attention decline with distance from the cued location. Less is known about the way attention is deployed in depth, which is likely of major importance in natural behavior.

Cuing tasks can be distinguished according to the type of cues that are used to direct the subjects' attention (Fig. 49.1). Symbolic cues indicate the most likely target location abstractly without themselves appearing at the target location. Such cues can be verbal instructions or central arrows that point toward the expected target location. In contrast, peripheral cues are visual stimuli that are flashed directly at the expected location of the target. Peripheral cues produce fast orienting of attention to the target location, usually within 100 ms. In contrast, attentional benefits following symbolic cues can take 300–400 ms to reach their peak, most likely because it takes longer to decode the meaning of a symbolic than of a peripheral cue.

A

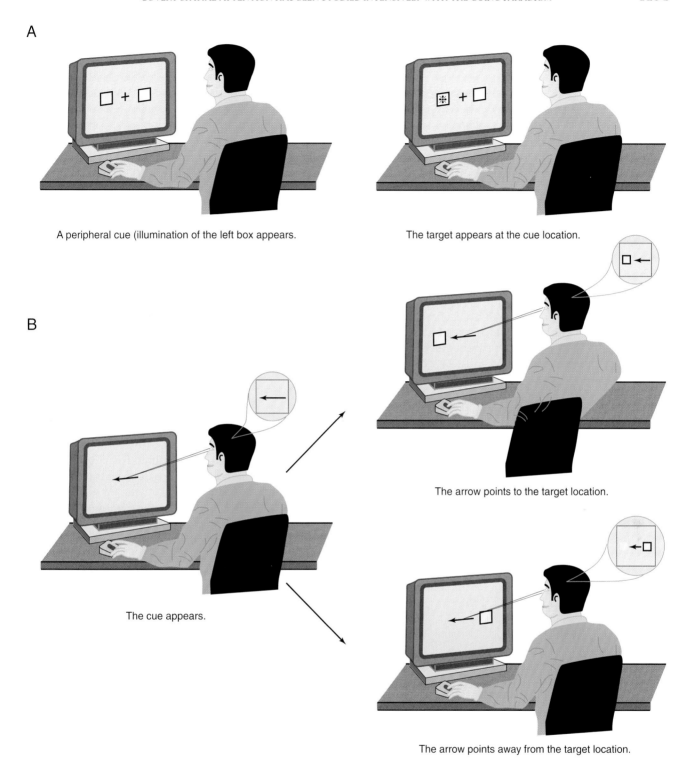

A peripheral cue (illumination of the left box appears.

The target appears at the cue location.

B

The cue appears.

The arrow points to the target location.

The arrow points away from the target location.

FIGURE 49.1 Cuing task (see text).

It is important to note that flashed stimuli used as peripheral cues are powerful attentional attractors in and of themselves, regardless of the information they convey about the likely target location. Indeed, suddenly appearing objects, rare in the natural world, can capture attention even if they are uninformative or detrimental to the task at hand (Yantis and Jonides, 1984). Following the initial fast orienting toward a peripheral cue, a *decrement* in performance may be seen at the location of that cue. This phenomenon is known as inhibition of return because it is thought to reflect the tendency of attention to be allocated away from, or to avoid revisiting a recently inspected, irrelevant location. Inhibition of return may be useful in counteracting the ineluctable pull of an abrupt onset when that onset proves of little value to the organism.

NEGLECT SYNDROME: A DEFICIT OF SPATIAL ATTENTION

Studies of patients with brain lesions have identified regions of the brain that are involved in attention. Unilateral brain lesions in humans may cause a profound inability to attend to certain spatial regions, a syndrome known as spatial neglect. In severe cases, patients with neglect behave as if the world contralateral to their lesioned hemisphere (the contralesional world) has ceased to exist. For example, a patient with neglect following a right hemisphere lesion may fail to read from the left side of a book, may ignore the food on the left side of the plate, or may remain unaware of the numerals on the left side of a clock (Fig. 49.2). Neglect patients may also be reluctant to initiate movement in contralesional space, with or without external sensory stimulation. Because the critical feature causing an object to be ignored is its location, this type of neglect is thought of as primarily a disorder of spatial attention.

The behavioral impairments in neglect cannot be explained by simple sensory or motor deficits (Mesulam, 1999). Neglect patients have normal vision in the contralesional visual field once their attention has been directed there, and they have no hemiparesis that could account for their reluctance to move. In addition, the extent of their difficulty is not immutable, as a sensory or motor deficit would be, but is strongly affected by the goals, expectations, and motivational state of the patient. Thus, neglect represents a failure to select, in some circumstances, the appropriate portions of a sensory representation. Neglect operates on high-level representations that differ considerably from the raw sensory input. For example, visual neglect is not confined only to retinal visual coordinates (affecting only objects in the contralesional visual field), but can affect objects in the contralesional space relative to the patient's body, relative to the patient's gaze, or relative to an external object or scene. Thus, neglect affects a visual representation that incorporates information about the position of the body with high-level visual information. Neglects affects not only the perception of present sensory environment, but also the processing of memorized or imagined scenes.

A related but milder attentional deficit, known as extinction, can follow more limited brain lesions or can occur during recovery from the acute phase of neglect. In visual extinction, patients are able to orient toward a contralesional stimulus presented in isolation, but fail to notice it if the same stimulus is presented simultaneously with an ipsilateral distractor. Extinction-like deficits are demonstrated readily with the spatial cuing task (Posner et al., 1984). In these tasks, neglect patients are slowed only mildly in their ability to detect targets in the contralesional visual field following valid symbolic or peripheral cues in the same field. However, they have enormously prolonged latencies for detecting contralateral targets if their attention had been misdirected

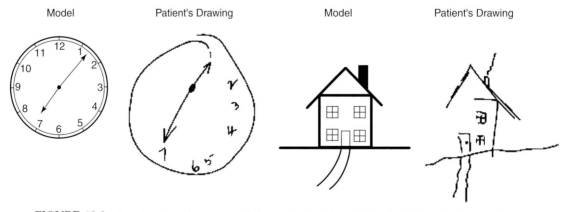

FIGURE 49.2 Two drawings that were made by a patient with spatial neglect. The patient was asked to copy the two models (clock, house). In each case, the copies exclude important elements that appeared on the left side of the model, indicating that the patient was unable to process information about the left side of the model.

to the ipsilesional field by means of an invalid cue. No impairment is seen when patients are cued to the contralesional field but asked to detect an ipsilesional target. Extinction-like phenomena have also been demonstrated in search tasks in which patients are asked to find a target object located at various locations in a complex scene. The time needed to find a target in contralesional space increases in proportion with the number and salience of ipsilesional distractors.

THE NETWORK MEDIATING SPATIAL ATTENTION IN HUMANS CENTERS AROUND FRONTAL AND PARIETAL CORTICAL AREAS

Spatial neglect in humans can result from unilateral lesions at several cortical sites, most notably the parietal lobe, the frontal lobe, and the anterior cingulate cortex (Heilman, 1979; Vallar, 1993). These observations suggest that a highly interconnected fronto-cingulo-parietal network is crucial for the control of spatial attention (Mesulam, 1999) (Fig. 49.3). The parietal, frontal, and cingulate cortices are sites of heavy sensory and motor convergence. Each area receives visual, somatosensory, auditory, and proprioceptive information and contains representations of several kinds of movement, including eye and head

movements, locomotion, reaching, and grasping. Further, the network has access to limbic system information regarding motivational value or behavioral significance of various objects. This network is thus well positioned to gate behaviorally relevant information from across sensory modalities toward the appropriate motor output channels and conscious perception. At the subcortical level, lesions of the basal ganglia or of the pulvinar thalamic nucleus, which is heavily connected with the parietal cortex, can also cause neglect.

In the human cortex, the anatomy and physiology of the human spatial attention network has been studied noninvasively by measuring event-related potentials (ERPs) and by acquiring functional images of the brain. With ERPs, voltage fluctuations from scalp electrodes are averaged over many trials (see Box 49.1). With functional brain imaging techniques, such as positron emission tomography (PET) or functional magnetic resonance imaging (fMRI), hemodynamic changes are measured—blood flow in the case of PET and blood oxygenation in the case of fMRI—and these are used as indirect measures of neural activity (see Box 13.1).

Functional brain imaging studies agree with neuropsychological studies in identifying areas in the parietal, frontal, and cingulate cortices as being especially active in relation to spatially directed attention (Fig. 49.4). However, there are two notable differences

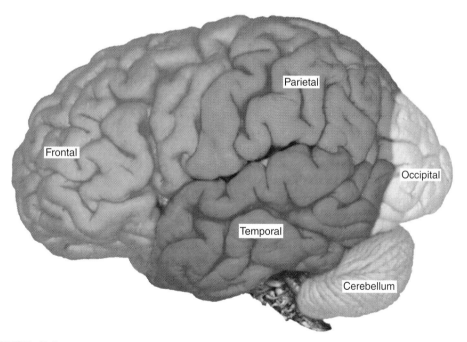

FIGURE 49.3   Lateral view of a human brain. Frontal (purple), parietal (orange), temporal (blue) and occipital (yellow) lobes are outlined.

between the results from neurological patients and functional brain imaging studies. First, studies of neglect patients suggest that the right parietal lobe is much more specialized for visuospatial attention than the left. Spatial neglect is much more severe and occurs more often following right than following left cortical lesions (Vallar, 1993). This specialization, which has not been found in monkeys or other animals, may be related to the complementary specialization of the human left hemisphere for language. A right hemispheric specialization for attention, however, has not been supported unequivocally by functional brain imaging studies. Some investigators have found stronger or even exclusive activation of areas in the right parietal lobe whether attention is directed to the right or to the left hemifield, suggesting that whereas the right hemisphere controls direction of attention to both the right and the left, the left hemisphere has a more limited role in directing attention to the right hemispace. However, other imaging studies have found largely symmetrical activations in the right and left parietal lobes, which appear to be independent of which visual hemifield is attended (for review, see Kastner and Ungerleider, 2000).

A second difference between results from patients and functional brain imaging studies concerns which portion of the parietal lobe plays the key role in attention. The patient literature has consistently identified the inferior parietal lobe, including the temporo-parietal junction, as the critical lesion site causing neglect. This classical view has been challenged recently by the finding that the lesion site of patients with visuospatial hemineglect may be the superior temporal lobe rather than the inferior parietal lobe (Karnath *et al.*, 2001). In contrast, most functional brain imaging studies point to the superior parietal lobe as the area most active in visuospatial attention tasks. The extent of lateralization of function in visual attention and the precise demarcation of parietal areas involved in attention are currently under investigation in many laboratories.

HUMAN FRONTAL AND PARIETAL CORTICAL AREAS PROVIDE TOP-DOWN SIGNALS CONTROLLING SPATIAL ATTENTION

Functional brain imaging studies have shown that areas in the superior parietal lobule (SPL), the frontal eye field (FEF), and the supplementary eye field (SEF) extending into the anterior cingulate cortex are activated in a variety of visuospatial tasks requiring spatially directed attention (Fig. 49.4; for review, see Kastner and Ungerleider, 2000). These areas were acti-

vated in tasks in which subjects were asked to maintain fixation at a central point and to direct attention covertly to peripheral target locations in order to detect a stimulus, to discriminate it or to track its movement (see meta-analysis in Fig. 49.4D).

One functional brain imaging study distinguished between activity associated with spatially directed attention and activity associated with visual sensory input (Kastner *et al.*, 1999). Subjects were asked to direct attention to a blank peripheral location and to anticipate the onset of visual stimuli at that location (expectation period). After stimulus onset, the task was to count the occurrences of a target stimulus in the peripheral location (attended visual stimuli). On different trials, the same visual stimuli were also presented when the subjects attended to a different location of the visual field (unattended visual stimuli). The same distributed network, consisting of the FEF, the SEF, and the SPL, was activated when subjects waited attentively for a target as when the target itself later appeared (Figs. 49.4B and 49.C). That is, there was an increase in activity in these frontal and parietal areas due to directed attention in the absence of visual input. During presentation of the visual stimuli at the attended location, this activity did not further increase. Thus, in FEF, SEF, and the SPL there was sustained activity throughout the expectation period and the attended presentations (Fig. 49.5B). In these areas, the sustained activity did not appear to reflect the visual processing of the stimuli but rather the attentional operations themselves. An increase in activity in the absence of visual input was also seen in several areas in the visual cortex. However, this increase in baseline activity was followed by a further increase after the onset of the visual stimuli (see later and Fig. 49.5A), indicating that these areas were driven by both attentional feedback signals and by the stimulus itself. The sustained pattern of activity and the larger increase of activity in SPL, FEF, and SEF taken together suggest that the parietal and frontal areas are the sources of the top-down biasing signals seen in the visual cortex. Hence, studies of patients with brain lesions and functional brain imaging studies in healthy subjects suggest that a distributed fronto-parietal network of areas is involved in attentional control.

VISUAL SALIENCE MAPS IN MONKEY PARIETAL AND FRONTAL CORTICES GUIDE THE DEPLOYMENT OF SPATIAL ATTENTION

In monkeys, neurophysiologists have recorded the electrical activity of individual neurons and correlated this activity with cognitive and sensory aspects of

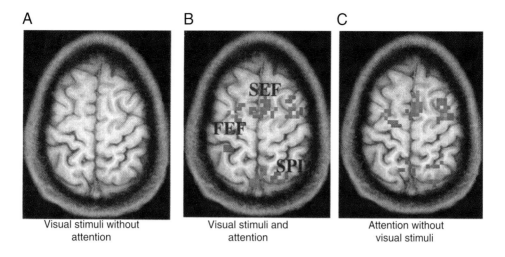

A
Visual stimuli without
attention

B
Visual stimuli and
attention

C
Attention without
visual stimuli

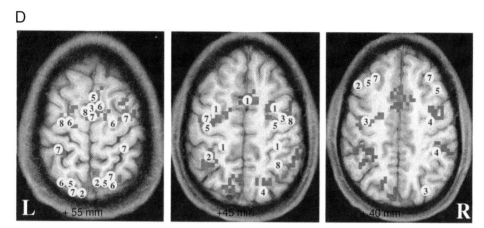

D

FIGURE 49.4 Regions in human brain activated by attention and regions associated with neglect. (A) Visual stimulation did not activate the frontal or parietal cortex reliably when attention was directed elsewhere in the visual field. (B) When the subject directed attention to a peripheral target location and performed an object discrimination task, a distributed fronto-parietal network was activated, including the SEF, the FEF, and the SPL. (C) The same network of frontal and parietal areas was activated when the subject directed attention to the peripheral target location in the expectation of the stimulus onset, i.e., in the absence of any visual input whatsoever. This activity therefore may not reflect attentional modulation of visually evoked responses, but rather attentional control operations themselves. (D) Meta-analysis of studies investigating the spatial attention network. Axial slices at different Talairach planes are indicated. Talairach (peak) coordinates of activated areas in the parietal and frontal cortex from several studies are indicated (for references, see Kastner and Ungerleider, 2000). R, right hemisphere; L, left hemisphere.

behavioral tasks that monkeys are performing concurrently. The first evidence of a correlation between selective visual attention and neural activity in the monkey came from a now classic study of posterior parietal cortex neurons (Bushnell *et al.* ,1981). Neurons were first recorded during a standard "passive visual task" in which monkeys were rewarded simply for maintaining gaze on a small spot of light located straight ahead (the fixation spot). While the monkey fixated, a second spot of light—the visual stimulus— was flashed briefly at a peripheral location in the

monkey's field of view, but the monkey was not required to respond to this stimulus in any way. Many parietal neurons, like many neurons throughout the visual system, had strong bursts of action potentials whenever the peripheral stimulus appeared within a specific spatial region called the receptive field (e.g., Fig. 49.6A). Because the monkey did not respond overtly to the peripheral stimulus, the neurons were assumed to encode the presence and location of a visual stimulus, regardless of the behavioral significance of that object.

In a second, "peripheral attention" task, the monkey maintained fixation of the central point as before but, in addition, also monitored the peripheral stimulus and released a lever upon detecting its dimming. Thus, the only difference between this task and the passive visual condition was in the behavioral relevance of the peripheral stimulus. More than half of posterior parietal neurons had stronger visually evoked responses in the peripheral attention task than in the passive viewing condition. Other experiments showed that the enhancement of neural activity was specific for the task-relevant stimulus and did not occur in response to other, irrelevant stimuli that were presented simultaneously in the field of view. Furthermore, enhancement generalized to other conditions requiring attention, e.g., when the monkey had to make a saccade or a hand reach toward the peripheral stimulus. Therefore, enhanced neural activity appears to be a suitable signal for spatially directed attention: it strengthens the representation only of stimuli that were attended and generalizes across several behavioral tasks.

A later study demonstrated that the attentional modulation in the parietal the cortex area is even greater than originally thought (Gottlieb et al., 1998). In this study, investigators asked whether the responses usually labeled as "passive visual" might in fact have been due to the unusual salience of the flashed stimuli used to elicit them. As noted earlier, suddenly appearing objects are among the most powerful exogenous attentional attractors. Is it possible then that flashed stimuli used in the passive visual task captured the monkey's attention automatically, even though they were nominally "irrelevant" to the task, and that this attentional capture, rather than the mere presence of a stimulus, accounted for the robust neural responses?

To see if this were true, a "stable-array task" was devised in which a circular array of eight stimuli appeared once and remained stably lit for several minutes without moving or flashing on or off. Monkeys were rewarded for making saccades (rapid eye movements) that brought one of the stable stimuli from the outside to the inside of the receptive field of the neuron being studied. Figure 49.6A shows a neuron in the lateral intraparietal area (LIP, a subdivision of posterior parietal cortex) that responded strongly on the standard visual task when a stimulus was flashed within its receptive field. In a separate block of stable-array trials (Fig. 49.6, middle), the monkey made saccades that brought a stable stimulus (physically identical to that used before) into the receptive field of the neuron. However, in this case the neuron had almost no response.

To see if this difference in response was indeed due to the stability of the stimulus in the stable-array task,

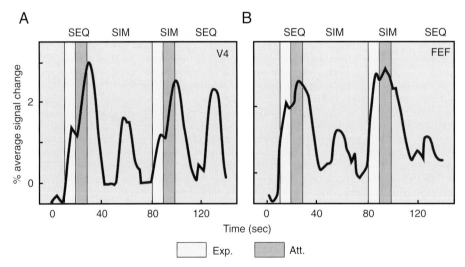

FIGURE 49.5 Directed attention in humans with and without visual stimulation. (A) Time series of fMRI signals in V4. Directing attention to a peripheral target location in the absence of visual stimulation led to an increase of baseline activity (textured blocks), which was followed by a further increase after the onset of stimuli (gray-shaded blocks). Baseline increases were found in both the striate and the extrastriate visual cortex. (B) Time series of fMRI signals in FEF. Directing attention to the peripheral target location in the absence of visual stimulation led to a stronger increase in baseline activity than in the visual cortex; the further increase of activity after the onset of stimuli was not significant. Sustained activity was seen in a distributed network of areas outside the visual cortex, including SPL, FEF, and SEF, suggesting that these areas may provide the source for the attentional top-down signals seen in visual cortex. Adapted from Kastner et al. (1999).

the investigators used a recent-onset version of the stable array task. In this version, the stable array contained only seven stimuli, and the eighth stimulus—the one that was brought into the receptive field by the saccade—was turned on and off on each trial (Fig. 49.6B, right). The stimulus was turned on outside the receptive field of the neuron (while the monkey fixated peripherally) and was turned off again at the end of the trial so that the visual stimulation around the time of the saccade was identical to that in the standard condition. Most LIP neurons responded strongly to stimuli that were rendered salient by repeatedly appearing and disappearing (Fig. 49.6, right). Note that the difference in response between the recent-onset and the stable condition cannot be explained by simple habituation of the responses to a continuously visible object (such as

may be encountered in retinal ganglion cells, for example), as LIP neurons tracked the location of the recently appeared object across a change of retinal position.

These experiments show that LIP neurons do not respond automatically to most stable, inconspicuous objects of the kind monkeys encounter in everyday viewing. Instead, LIP neurons are extremely selective for stimuli that are especially salient, even if these stimuli do not require an overt response. Area LIP thus appears to contain a selective "salience map," highlighting objects or locations of special exogenous salience.

To ask if these neurons also signal the behavioral relevance of a nonsalient object, a cued-saccade version of the stable array task was used (Fig. 49.7). In this version, all eight stimuli were stable on the

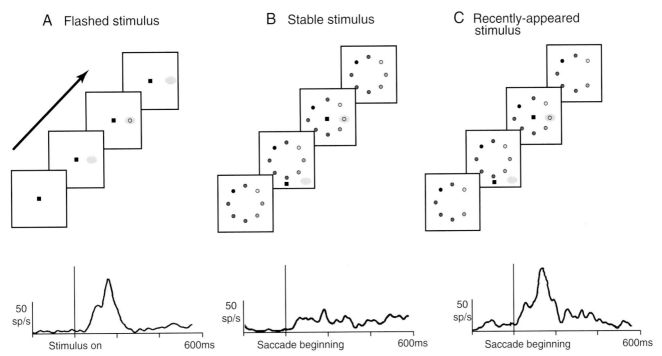

FIGURE 49.6 Monkey posterior parietal cortex neurons respond selectively to flashed or recently-appeared stimuli. (A) Neuron in the lateral intraparietal area responds strongly in a passive visual task to a stimulus flashed in its receptive field (shaded area). The wavy bottom line shows the firing rate averaged across repeated stimulus presentations. The time of stimulus onset is indicated by the vertical bar. The schematic at the top shows the task. A fixation point (square) is visible throughout the trial. After the monkey looks at this point (second panel), a stimulus is flashed for 200 ms at 15° right in the receptive field of the neuron (RF; third panel). The monkey continues to maintain fixation after the stimulus is extinguished (fourth panel) in order to obtain a reward. (B) The responses of the same neuron on the stable array task. The stimulus array, with a 15° radius and centered directly in front of the monkey, appears and remains on for the duration of the experiment (first panel). The monkey fixates the fixation spot that appears outside the array, thereby bringing the RF of the neuron to a blank location on the screen (second panel). The fixation point then jumps to the center of the array and, when the monkey follows it with a saccade, the RF of the neuron falls on one of the array elements (third panel). The array remains unchanged even as the monkey looks away at the end of the trial (fourth panel). Neural responses in the bottom part are aligned to the beginning of the saccade that brought the stable array stimulus into its RF. (C) Same as B but now the stable array has only seven stimuli (first and last panels). The stimulus entering the RF after the saccade appears while the animal fixates in the periphery. The neuron responds strongly to the entrance of this recently-appeared stimulus into its RF.

screen, and the monkey first made a saccade to the center of the array, thereby bringing one of the stable stimuli into the receptive field of the neuron. A cue was then flashed briefly near the center of gaze, outside the receptive field of the neuron. The cue matched one of the stable array objects, chosen at random on each trial, and the cue instructed the monkey to make a saccade to that object after a delay of a few hundred milliseconds. LIP neurons remained quiescent if the stable stimulus in their receptive field did not match the cue, i.e., if it was not relevant to the monkey on that trial. However, they began responding during the delay period only on those trials in which the cue matched the stimulus in the receptive field. Other experiments showed that this response did not reflect preparation for the saccade to the receptive field, but rather the selection of the stable stimulus as the saccade target. Thus, endogenous and exogenous salience—both drawing on the same pool of attentional resources—appears to be encoded in the same representation by the same, or closely overlapping, sets of neurons. A map of visual salience may also exist in another parietal area adjacent to area LIP—area 7a—although in this case it remains unclear whether the enhanced responses reflect exogenous salience, task relevance, or both.

A number of observations suggest that the parietal cortex might be important for shifting attention after it is already engaged at some location. In one task (Constantinidis and Steinmetz, 2001), monkeys were shown displays consisting of mostly like-colored stimuli, with one stimulus being of a contrasting color (red among other green stimuli or green among red stimuli). After the array disappeared, a sequence of individual stimuli appeared at some of the locations that had been occupied by the array objects. Monkeys were required to release a lever whenever a stimulus appeared at the location where the odd stimulus had been. During the initial array presentation, most 7a neurons encoded the location of the salient, task-relevant stimulus and had little or no response to the uniformly colored distractors. However, during presentation of the subsequent stimulus sequence, neurons had the opposite selectivity: they were suppressed when a stimulus appeared at the cued location (even though the monkey responded to it). It is likely that this suppression was due to the fact that the monkey was already attending to the cued location and that area 7a neurons responded preferentially when attention had to be shifted to a new location. A similar suggestion had been made earlier for neurons in area LIP. In that case, a spatial cuing task was used similar to that used in humans (see earlier disccussion).

Although monkeys were faster to detect validly cued than invalidly cued targets, a small group of LIP neurons had the opposite preference: they responded less for validly cued than for invalidly cued targets. Other tasks suggested that this relative suppression was due to the fact that the monkey was already attending at the validly cued location. The suggestion that the parietal cortex is most active when attention is already engaged but must now be moved elsewhere is consistent with the pattern of deficits found in neglect patients. Their greatest difficulties arise if attention has to be moved following invalid cuing to the ipsilateral hemifield. An alternative formulation of this idea is that the parietal cortex is most important for redirecting attention in the face of multiple competing attentional demands.

Area LIP is strongly interconnected with the frontal eye field (FEF), a prefrontal area lying along the anterior bank of the arcuate sulcus. The FEF was first defined on functional grounds according to its participation in the control of saccades—rapid eye movements used for visual exploration. Many FEF neurons respond strongly before saccades of specific directions and amplitudes, which define their movement fields. Furthermore, saccades can be evoked with very low intensity microstimulation from many FEF sites. However, experiments suggest that the FEF also participates in the control of attention, and not only in saccade production. FEF neurons can discriminate between targets and non-targets in visual search tasks. Selectivity for the target in easy search tasks is found whether or not monkeys make saccades to the target stimulus. Furthermore, evolution of target-related activity on easy and more difficult searches varies with the similarity between target and distractors and correlates with the behavioral latency for finding the target. These observations suggest that FEF activity reflects the search process itself and is not a stereotyped saccade-planning signal (Bichot et al., 2001). Finally, electrical microstimulation of FEF sites below the intensity level that triggers an eye movement increases the ability of monkeys to detect a faint stimulus, provided that the stimulus appears at the spatial location represented by neurons at the stimulation site. These findings strongly suggest that the FEF is involved both in saccade planning and in covert attentional selection. The complex relationship between covert attention and saccades is discussed further in a separate section later.

In monkeys, as in humans, lesions of the parietal cortex or of the frontal lobe can cause contralateral neglect or extinction. Neglect following experimental lesions of these structures in the monkey, however, is often much milder than that found in humans. It is not known whether this observation reflects differ-

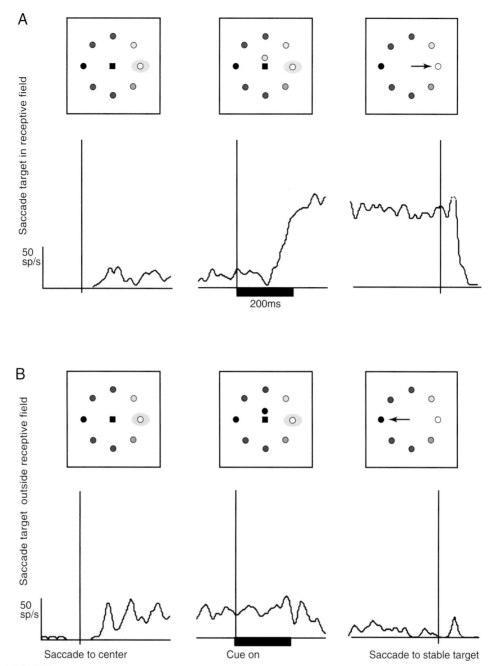

FIGURE 49.7 Neurons in the lateral intraparietal area respond to nonsalient objects if, and only if, these become task relevant. A stable array remains on the screen at all times as in Fig. 49.6. The monkey begins by making a saccade to the center of the array at the time indicated by the vertical bar in the left panels (both top and bottom). There is only a minimal response, even though this saccade brings one of the array stimuli into the receptive field (RF) of the neuron under study, which is indicated by the oval. A cue is shown briefly outside the RF, which matches one of the array elements (middle column, top and bottom). In the top row the cue matches the element inside the RF, whereas in the bottom row it matches the element opposite the RF. After a brief delay the monkey makes a saccade to the element matching the cue (third column). The neuron responds during the delay period between cue presentation and saccade only if the saccade is directed to the stimulus inside the RF (top row). If the saccade is directed to the stable stimulus opposite the RF (bottom row), the neuron is slightly inhibited, even though the visual stimulus in its RF is identical to that in the trials shown in the top row. Thus, neurons respond to stable stimuli only if these become relevant to the current behavior of the monkey.

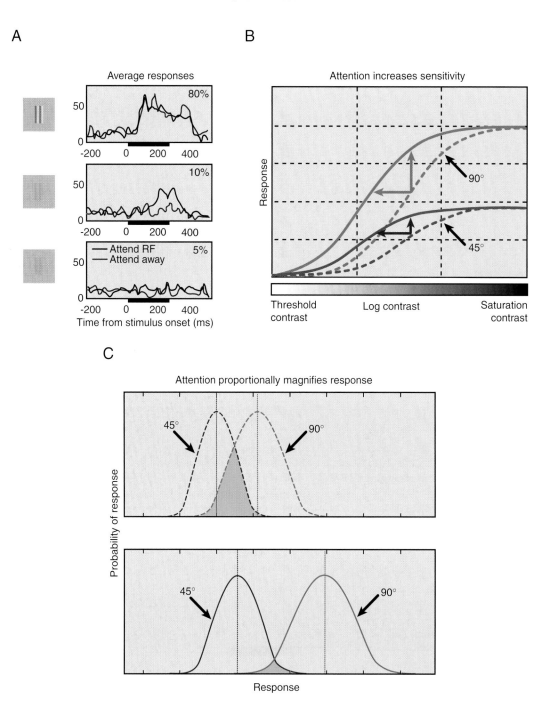

FIGURE 49.8 Attention to a single stimulus in the receptive field increases neuronal sensitivity and separates responses elicited by different stimuli, enabling the neuron to better discriminate between them. (A) Each of the three panels shows responses that were elicited by a vertically oriented grating when it was presented at different levels of contrast, indicated by the gratings on the left of each panel. Contrast increases from 5% in the bottom panel to 10% in the middle panel up to 80% in the top panel. The two lines in each panel show the mean response of a V4 neuron when attention was directed either away from the receptive field (pink line) or toward the receptive field (black line). The stimulus elicited a robust response when it was presented at 80% contrast, whether or not it was attended. The faintest stimulus (5% contrast) was too faint to be detected by the neuron, even when the monkey was attending to its loca-tion. However, attention enabled the cell to detect a 10% contrast stimulus, which it did not detect when attention was directed elsewhere. That is, attention shifted the response threshold of the neuron, making it more sensitive to stimuli appearing at the attended location (Reynolds *et al.*, 2000). (B) Contrast response functions of a hypothetical neuron that illustrate responses observed in area V4 of the macaque extrastriate visual cortex. Dashed lines show average responses to a

ences in the organization of the spatial attentional system in the monkey and human.

ATTENTION INCREASES SENSITIVITY AND BOOSTS THE CLARITY OF SIGNALS GENERATED BY NEURONS IN PARTS OF THE VISUAL SYSTEM DEVOTED TO PROCESSING INFORMATION ABOUT OBJECTS

While frontal and parietal areas have been associated with the control of spatial attention, they are not usually considered crucial for visual processing or object recognition. How does attention affect information processing in areas of the brain that encode stimulus features such as color, motion, texture, and shape?

One important finding is that when attention is directed to a single stimulus in the receptive field, there is often an increase in the firing rates of neurons that respond to the attended stimulus. Fig. 49.8A shows the effect of attention on the responses of a neuron in macaque area V4, a stage of visual processing in the extrastriate cortex that helps process information about the form and identity of visual stimuli. The neuron did not respond to a very faint stimulus, regardless of whether it was attended or not. A slightly higher contrast stimulus also did not elicit a response when it was ignored, but elicited a clear response when it was attended. A very high-contrast stimulus elicited a strong response whether or not it was attended. Thus, attention increased the sensitivity of the neuron to stimuli, enabling it to detect a stimulus that was too weak to elicit a response when it was unattended. Thus, the effect of attention is to cause a leftward shift in the contrast response function of a neuron, as illustrated in Fig. 49.8B (Reynolds *et al.*, 2000).

How could such a change in sensitivity improve an observer's ability to identify properties of stimuli that appear at an attended location? A likely answer is that by increasing neuronal responses, attention enables neurons to send signals that better differentiate between stimuli with different physical characteristics (McAdams and Maunsell, 1999). Consider what happens when attention shifts the contrast response functions illustrated in Fig. 49.8B. At a given level of contrast, a leftward shift in the contrast response func-

tion for the preferred stimulus of the neuron (90° orientation, indicated by blue lines) results in an increase in response. An identical shift in the contrast response function for a poor stimulus (45° orientation, indicated by red lines) results in a smaller increase in response. As a result, mean responses to the two stimuli are better separated by attention.

Why would this enable the neuron to more reliably signal the identity of the attended stimulus? The reason is that neuronal signals are noisy. Some presentations of the poorer 45° orientation stimulus will therefore elicit responses that are higher than responses observed on some presentations of the 90° orientation stimulus. This is illustrated in Fig. 49.8C, which shows the distribution of responses elicited by each of the two stimuli. The two curves in the upper part of Fig. 49.8C indicate the distributions of responses elicited by the two stimuli, without attention. Although the distributions are not identical, they overlap a great deal. Responses within this area of overlap cannot be uniquely associated with either stimulus. The lower part of Fig. 49.8C illustrates the effect of attention: to shift response distributions of both stimuli to the right. This shift is larger for the 90^0 orientation stimulus, and so with attention, the two distributions overlap less. As a result, the neuron can more reliably signal which of the two stimuli is present.

ATTENTION AFFECTS NEURAL ACTIVITY IN THE HUMAN VISUAL CORTEX IN THE PRESENCE AND ABSENCE OF VISUAL STIMULATION

There is converging evidence from event-related potential (ERP) and functional imaging studies that selective attention can affect the neural processing of visual information in the human visual cortex. In a typical experiment, identical visual stimuli are presented simultaneously to corresponding peripheral field locations to the right and to the left of a central fixation point. Subjects are instructed to direct attention covertly to the right or the left by a symbolic cue presented at the fixation point and to detect the occurrence of a visual stimulus, all while ERPs are measured or functional brain images are acquired. In functional imaging studies, directing attention to the left hemifield

◀ preferred (blue dashed line) and a poor stimulus (red dashed line) across a range of luminance contrasts, when the monkey attends away from the stimulus in the receptive field of the neuron. Attention shifts these contrast response functions to the left (solid lines), causing the neuron to lower its contrast response threshold. The largest increases in response are observed for stimuli at intermediate contrasts. The increase in response is proportionally larger for the preferred stimulus than for the poor stimulus. (C) Response distributions of the neuron illustrated in B to a 45 and 90^0 grating at fixed contrast. With attention directed away from the receptive field (top), there is substantial overlap between the distributions; consequently, the response on a given trial does not reliably indicate which stimulus is present. Attention boosts responses elicited by the preferred stimulus by more than it boosts responses to the poor stimulus, reducing the ambiguity in the signal.

BOX 49.1

MEASURING BRAIN WAVES

Scientists have been measuring brain waves for more than 50 years, ever since Hans Berger showed that electrical activity from the brain could be measured by placing conducting material on the scalp and amplifying the resultant electrical signal so that it could be written out by a pen recorder. His instrument, the electroencephalograph (EEG), has been a standard tool for diagnosing brain damage in the years since.

The EEG did not become suitable for cognitive studies, however, until G. D. Dawson developed a method of averaging the EEG signal following a stimulus. The concept is simple. The stimulus is presented many times to the same subject. At each electrode, the electrical activity is recorded at fixed intervals following the stimulus—say, every 4 ms. The electrical values at each interval are taken from many trials and averaged together so that electrical activity not caused by the stimulus averages to zero and the resultant signal shows only the activity produced by the stimulus. Usually 10 to 100 presentations of the stimulus suffice to produce a reliable potential that reflects characteristics of both the individual brain and the particular stimulus. The waveform can be described by giving the direction (positive or negative) and the delay to the appearance of each of the bumps in the wave.

To improve the chances of finding an electrical signal from the areas where brain activity has been found with

PET or other neuroimaging methods is a complex task. First, a large number of electrodes are used to achieve as thorough a sample of electrical activity from the surface as possible. Second, the activity of each electrode is compared to the average activity of all other electrodes. Finally, a subtractive strategy similar to that used in PET studies helps isolate the effects of a particular mental operation.

For example, one study (Fig. 49.9) measured event-related potentials in tasks similar to those used in PET. One task involves the presentation of visual words. Each trial starts with a fixation cross that serves as a warning signal. During the entire procedure, the subject's eye position is monitored through a TV camera to make sure that the eyes have not wandered from the fixation point. After half a second a word replaces the cross and remains present for another half to one second. Half a second after it is taken away, a prompt tells the subject to press a key to give his or her response. Brain waves are recorded just before the warning signal and continue to be recorded throughout the trial. Later the event-related potentials for a given condition (e.g., words or nonsense strings) are averaged for each subject, and grand averages over all subjects are computed.

G. S. Aston-Jones, R. Desimone, J. Driver,
S. J. Luck, and M. I. Posner

increased stimulus-evoked activity in the extrastriate visual cortex of the right hemisphere, whereas directing attention to the right hemifield increased activity in the extrastriate visual cortex of the left hemisphere (Heinze *et al.*, 1994). Thus, responses to stimuli were enhanced on the side of the extrastriate cortex that contained representations of the attended hemifield. These and other studies suggest that spatial attention effects are topographically organized and retinotopically specific; i.e., only the activity of neurons coding the attended location is modulated by spatial attention. ERP studies with similar experimental paradigms have found that early components of the sensory ERP, which begins about 80 ms after stimulus onset, can be modulated by covert spatial attention toward or away from the stimulus (Hillyard and Vento, 1998). Indeed, spatially directed attention to a stimulus in the cuing paradigm described earlier may affect the sensory ERP recorded over the extrastriate visual cortex as early as 100 ms after stimulus onset (Fig. 49.9). Taken together, these findings

suggest that spatial attention modulates visual processing by amplifying the neural signals for stimuli at an attended location. At the same time, signals evoked by stimuli at unattended locations can be attenuated relative to the signals evoked by attended stimuli. Thus, attention affects not only the activity of neurons that code an attended location, but also the activity of neurons that code an attended stimulus attribute.

In functional brain imaging studies, activity evoked within different visual cortical areas has been compared while subjects perform a task requiring selective attention to particular features of identical visual stimuli. One such study found that selective attention to shape, color, or speed enhanced activity in the regions of the extrastriate visual cortex that selectively process these same attributes. Attention to shape and color led to response enhancement in regions of the posterior portion of the fusiform gyrus, including area V4. Attention to speed led to response enhancement in areas MT/MST (Corbetta *et al.*, 1991). In other studies,

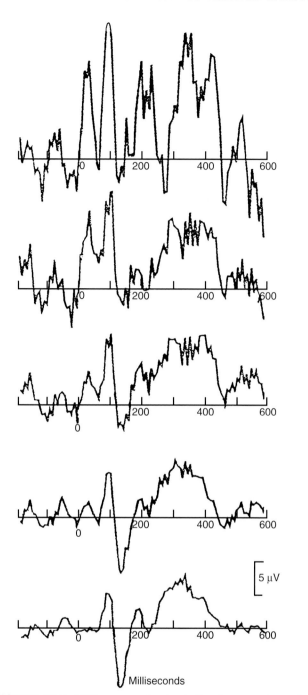

FIGURE 49.9 ERP responses to visual stimuli, summed over 1 (top panel) to 32 (bottom panel) trials. The horizontal axis indicates time from stimulus onset. Electrical activity prior to that is clearly noise.

attention to faces or houses led to response enhancement in areas of the midanterior portion of the fusiform gyrus, areas responsive to the processing of faces and objects. Taken together, these results support the idea that selective attention to a particular stimulus attribute modulates neural activity in those extrastriate areas that preferentially process the selected attribute.

Attentional response modulation has been found at all stages of visual processing, including V1. However, attentional effects are stronger in more anterior extrastriate areas, such as V4 and MT/MST (Kastner *et al.*, 1998), suggesting that these latter areas are the primary targets of attentional top-down effects. One interpretation of these findings is that attentional effects in V1 may be caused by feedback effects from higher order extrastriate areas. This idea is supported by single cell recording studies, which have shown that attentional effects in area TE of the inferior temporal cortex have a latency of about 150 ms, whereas attentional effects in V1 have a longer latency of about 235 ms.

Functional brain imaging and ERP studies suggest that attentional top-down signals can occur not only in response to visually driven activity, but also in the absence of any visual stimulation whatsoever. In one such study (Kastner *et al.*, 1999), subjects were cued to direct attention covertly to a target location in the periphery of the visual field and to anticipate the onset of visual stimuli. Visual stimuli occurred with a delay of several seconds. Neural activity associated with spatially directed attention in the absence and in the presence of visual stimulation could therefore be distinguished. It was found that fMRI signals increased when attention was directed to the target location and before any visual stimulus was present on the screen. As illustrated in Fig. 49.5A for area V4, this increase in baseline activity was followed by a further increase of activity that was evoked by the onset of the stimulus presentations. Increases in baseline activity due to spatially directed attention in the absence of visual input were found only in visual areas with a representation of the attended location, indicating the topographic specificity of the effect.

This increased baseline activity likely reflects attentional top-down feedback, which biases neurons that represent an attended location. The result is to favor stimuli that will appear at that location at the expense of those appearing at unattended locations. At the same time, the activity of neurons representing unattended regions of the visual field appears to be reduced. As discussed earlier, these biasing signals appear to be generated from a distributed fronto-parietal network of areas involved with attentional control.

Like the attentional modulation of stimulus-evoked responses described earlier, attention-induced increases in baseline activity during anticipation of a visual stimulus have both a spatial and a nonspatial, feature-based component. For example, the anticipation of a motion stimulus leads to greater increases of activity in motion-selective areas than in other visual areas. Similarly, anticipation of a color stimulus leads to greater increases in baseline activity in visual areas that preferentially process color information. These attentional signals can also be modulated by the difficulty of the anticipated discrimination. That is, anticipation of a low-contrast grating stimulus that is difficult to discriminate leads to greater increases in baseline activity across the visual cortex than anticipation of a high-contrast grating stimulus that is easy to discriminate.

In summary, attention affects neural activity in sensory representation areas of the human cortex both in the presence and in the absence of sensory input. Functional brain imaging and ERP studies suggest that attentional enhancement mechanisms operate in a strikingly similar way in human and monkey visual cortices.

THE VISUAL SEARCH PARADIGM HAS BEEN USED TO STUDY THE ROLE OF ATTENTION IN SELECTING RELEVANT STIMULI FROM WITHIN A CLUTTERED VISUAL ENVIRONMENT

So far this chapter has considered the situation when attention is cued to a location (or a feature) in the visual field. However, one is rarely told in advance to attend to a particular location. Normally, one needs to find a particular object in a complex visual world that is composed of a large number of stimuli. Psychologists have used a visual search paradigm to understand how attention selects behaviorally relevant stimuli out of a group of other stimuli.

In a typical task, observers are asked to search among an array of stimuli and indicate whether a particular target is present in the array. This task is easier under some conditions than others. For example, it is easy to determine whether a horizontal green bar is present in Fig. 49.10A. It takes longer to make this judgment for stimuli in Fig. 49.10B. Treisman and Gelade (1980) found that searches for a target with a unique feature, like the one illustrated in Fig. 49.10A, can be completed quickly regardless of the number of elements in the search array—the target seems to "pop out" of the search array. Such searches are often referred to as efficient. In contrast, Treisman and Gelade (1980) found that the amount of time required to find a target that is defined by conjunctions of elementary features (e.g., a horizontal green among horizontal reds and vertical greens, as in Fig. 49.10B) increases linearly with the number of elements in the array. Such searches are often referred to as inefficient. The amount of time added

per item depends on stimulus conditions, but a rule of thumb is that each additional item in the array adds about 50 ms to the amount of time taken to locate the target. The fact that it takes time to locate the target in Fig. 49.10B implies that the visual system is limited in capacity. If it were not, the target could be identified immediately by evaluating every element in the array simultaneously.

WHERE IS THE COMPUTATIONAL BOTTLENECK AS REVEALED BY SEARCH TASKS?

Considerable debate exists regarding the locus and nature of the computational bottleneck that causes the capacity limitations that are revealed by visual search tasks. One influential theory, feature integration theory (FIT, Treisman and Gelade, 1980), proposes that capacity limitations occur at very early stages of cortical processing where "elementary" features are bound into coherent objects. This theory proposes that in the "pop-out" case, where the target differs from distractors in a single elemental feature, a search can be completed efficiently because there is no need to bind together different elementary features. Thus, a green target among red distractors (Fig. 49.9A) can be found in parallel by V1 neurons that respond to green but not red stimuli, without the need for visual attention. However, in a conjunction search, where each of the elementary target features (color and orientation) is shared with distracters, the observer must bind elementary features into coherent object representations before search can occur. Capacity limitations are revealed in this condition because attention is needed for this binding operation. Accordingly, one cannot process multiple objects simultaneously because in order to avoid misconjoining features from different objects, attention selects features from one location at a time. Consistent with this idea, patient RM, who suffered damage to his parietal attentional control system, often misconjoins the shape and color of letters, even after viewing them for up to 10 s; i.e., he mixes up which letters are presented in which colors.

However, the idea that limited capacity occurs at early stages of processing has been challenged. For example, some studies suggest that parts of objects are integrated into wholes prior to the application of attention. Consider the task of searching for the oddly shaped object appearing at the bottom of Fig. 49.10 (adapted from Rensink and Enns, 1998). This odd shape pops out from among the squares and circles in Fig. 49.10C, but it is harder to find the same shape in

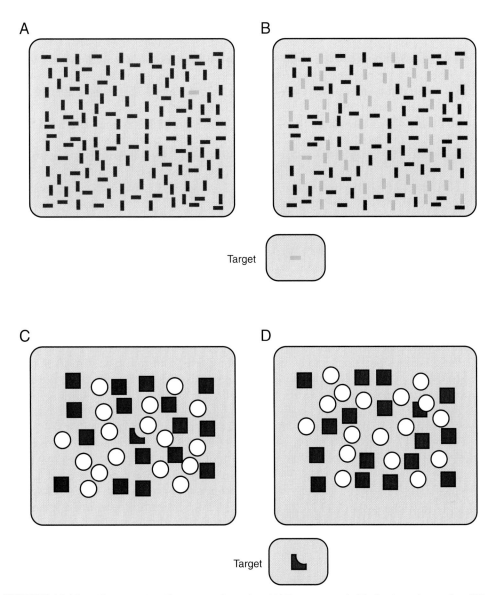

FIGURE 49.10 Efficient and inefficient visual searches. (A) Pop-out search. The horizontal green bar differs from all other array elements in a single feature, color. As a result, it pops out immediately, regardless of how many elements are in the array. (B) The same target is difficult to find when it is embedded among elements that cannot be differentiated from it on the basis of a single feature (color or orientation). (C) The dark target pops out among squares and circles. (D) When the same target is perceived to be a square occluded behind a circle, it is difficult to find among squares and circles. Because this arrangement of the array interferes with visual search, this suggests that integration of objects into wholes occurs prior to the activation of attentional mechanisms used in visual search. Thus, these mechanisms are evidently not necessary for completion. Adapted from Rensink and Enns (1998.)

Fig. 49.10D. The difference is that in Fig. 49.10D, the oddly shaped part appears to be a square that is occluded by a superimposed circle; i.e., the visual system completes the shape of the occluded square, hiding it among the other squares. Because this completion stops the square from popping out, the completion operation must occur prior to visual search.

Further evidence that features can be integrated preattentively into objects comes from the finding that when an observer attends to one feature of an object (e.g., its orientation), other features of the object are selected automatically as well. In a now classic study, Duncan (1984) found that observers could easily make simultaneous judgments about two features of the same object (e.g., its orientation and whether or not it contained a gap). Making the second judgment did not interfere with the first judgment. However, observers were severely impaired when they simultaneously judged the same two features, one on each of two different stimuli. This finding suggests that when attention is directed to one feature of an object, all of the features that make up the object can automatically be selected together because the features are already linked together into objects. These sorts of observations suggest that limited capacity results from information processing bottlenecks that occur relatively late in processing, after features are already integrated into wholes. One possibility is that the bottleneck occurs when objects enter a limited capacity working memory. Under this view, attention plays the role of selecting which objects pass through the bottleneck.

These two perspectives are not mutually exclusive. Some feature integration may occur preattentively (e.g., Rensink and Enns, 1998), but other types of stimulus integration might require spatial selection. As described earlier, attention has been found to modulate neural activity at all stages of visual processing including early stages (Motter, 1993), where neuronal responses first show signs of grouping the features and parts of objects into wholes, as well as late stages, which are likely involved in selecting stimuli for storage in working memory. Thus, both early and late stages of processing may act as limited capacity bottlenecks.

NEURONAL RECEPTIVE FIELDS ARE A POSSIBLE NEURAL CORRELATE OF LIMITED CAPACITY

Extracellular recording studies of attention in awake, behaving monkeys have revealed that the receptive fields of individual neurons might contribute to the limitation in visual capacity. As visual information traverses the successive cortical areas of the ventral stream that underlie object recognition (Ungerleider and Mishkin, 1982), the sizes of receptive fields increase from less than a degree of visual arc in primary visual cortex (area V1) to about $20°$ of visual arc in area TE, the last purely visual area in the ventral visual processing stream (see Chapter 47). Similar increases in receptive field size are observed in the dorsal visual processing stream. In a typical scene, such large receptive fields will contain many different objects. Therefore, a likely explanation for why one cannot process many different objects in a scene simultaneously is that neurons, whose signals are limited in bandwidth, cannot simultaneously send signals about all of the stimuli inside their receptive

fields. This idea implies that processing limitations exist at all levels of processing but that they become more pronounced in higher order visual areas, where receptive field sizes are larger. How then do neurons transmit signals about behaviorally relevant stimuli in their receptive fields?

One proposal is that the selective processing of behaviorally relevant stimuli is accomplished by two interacting mechanisms: competition among potentially relevant stimuli and biases that determine the outcome of this competition. For example, when an observer is asked to detect the appearance of a target at a particular location, this task is thought to activate spatially selective feedback signals in cortical areas, such as parts of the parietal cortex discussed earlier. These cortical areas provide a task-appropriate spatial reference frame and transmit signals to the extrastriate cortex, where they bias competition in favor of stimuli that appear at the attended location. Similarly, when an observer searches for an object in a cluttered scene, feature-selective feedback is thought to bias competition in favor of stimuli that share features in common with the searched-for object. When competition is resolved, the winning stimulus controls neuronal responses, and other stimuli are effectively filtered out of the visual stream.

Studies in monkeys have compared the effect of attention on neuronal responses with single and multiple stimuli in the receptive field. Consistent with the proposal just outlined, larger changes in firing rate occur when multiple stimuli appear within the receptive field (and one stimulus must be attended), as compared to when the attended stimulus appears alone and there is no competition to be resolved (Moran and Desimone, 1985). According to the biased competition model just described, neurons that respond to a stimulus should be suppressed when a second stimulus is added that activates a competing population of neurons. To test this idea, pairs of stimuli were presented that activated two nearby populations of neurons (Reynolds et al., 1999). Monkeys attended away from the receptive fields of the neurons. The first stimulus was chosen to be of a color and orientation that would strongly activate the recorded neuron. Then, a second stimulus, which elicited a response in a nearby population of neurons, was added. As predicted, the addition of this second stimulus partially suppressed the response of the neuron to its first stimulus. To test whether attentional feedback would resolve competition in favor of the neurons that responded to the attended stimulus, attention was then directed to the poor stimulus. As predicted, this magnified the suppressive influence of the poor stimulus, reducing the firing rate of the neuron to a level

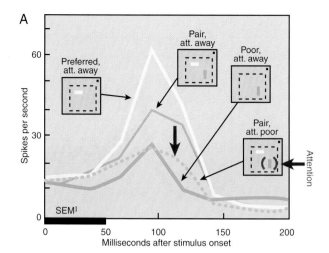

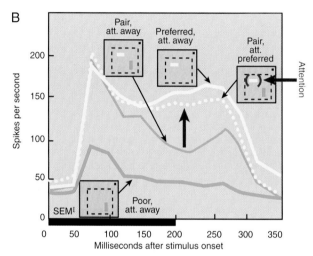

FIGURE 49.11 Attention to one stimulus of a pair filters out the effect of the ignored stimulus. (A) The x-axis shows time (in milliseconds) from stimulus onset, and the thick horizontal bar indicates stimulus duration. Small iconic figures illustrate sensory conditions. Within each icon, the dotted line indicates the receptive field, and the small dot represents the fixation point. The location of attention inside the receptive field is indicated in red. Attention was directed away from the receptive field in all but one condition. The preferred stimulus is indicated by a horizontal yellow bar and the poor stimulus by a vertical blue bar. In fact, the identity of both stimuli varied from cell to cell. The yellow line shows the response of a V2 neuron to the preferred stimulus. The solid blue line shows the response to the poor stimulus. The green line shows the response to the pair. The addition of the poor stimulus suppressed the response to the preferred stimulus. Attention to the poor stimulus (red arrow) magnified its suppressive effect and drove the response down to a level (dotted blue line) that was similar to the response elicited by the poor stimulus alone. (B) Response of a second V2 neuron. The format is the same as in A. As in the neuron above, the response to the preferred stimulus was suppressed by the addition of the poor stimulus. Attention directed to the preferred stimulus filtered out this suppression, returning the neuron to a response (dotted yellow line) similar to the response that was elicited when the preferred stimulus appeared alone inside the RF. Adapted from Reynolds *et al.* (1999).

comparable to what was observed when the poor stimulus was presented alone (see Fig. 49.11A). In a final experiment, attention was directed to the preferred stimulus. Consistent with the resolution of competition in favor of the neurons that responded to the preferred stimulus, directing attention to the preferred stimulus strongly reduced the suppressive effect of the poor stimulus (see Fig. 49.11B).

Similar results have been reported in the dorsal stream of visual processing (Recanzone and Wurtz, 2000). Thus, when multiple stimuli appear together within the receptive fields of neurons in the later stages of the ventral visual processing stream and in motion-sensitive areas MT and MST of the dorsal stream, the neuronal response is driven primarily by the attended stimulus. In this way, attention helps determine which stimuli are selected for processing in these areas.

COMPETITION CAN BE BIASED BY NONSPATIAL FEEDBACK

The findings just summarized support the proposal that competitive neural circuits can be biased by spatially selective feedback signals. As illustrated in Fig. 49.12, feature-selective feedback can also bias competition. Responses of neurons in area TE were recorded when monkeys searched for a target (Chelazzi *et al.*, 1998). On each trial, the monkey viewed a cue stimulus that appeared at the fixation point. After a delay, an array of stimuli (the search array) appeared within the receptive fields of neurons in area TE. The monkey's task was to indicate whether a target matching the cue stimulus was present in the array, by making a saccade to the target. Locations of the stimuli were selected at random so that the monkey could not know where the target would appear, if it appeared at all. During the delay period, many TE neurons had a higher baseline firing rate when the cue stimulus was a preferred stimulus for the cell than when it was a poor stimulus; i.e., neurons that were tuned to respond to the target were activated while the monkey prepared to search for the target. An interesting possibility is that this activation might bias the visual system toward detecting the target object, just as spatially specific feedback is thought to bias the system toward a particular location. Consistent with this, within 150–200 ms after the search array appeared, the response of the neuron increased or decreased, depending on whether the target was, respectively, a preferred or a poor stimulus for the cell. That is, shortly after the appearance of the search array, the activity of the cell reflected the identity of the target stimulus and was no longer influenced by the nontar-

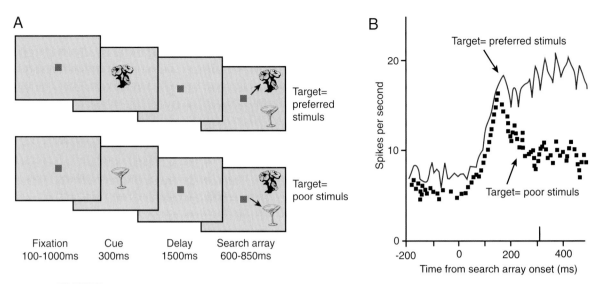

FIGURE 49.12 Responses of inferior temporal (IT) neurons during a memory-guided visual search. (A) Task. Monkeys fixated a spot on a computer screen and were shown a central cue (here, either the flower or the cup). After a delay, two (or more) stimuli appeared within the receptive field and the monkey had to saccade to the stimulus that had appeared earlier as the cue. Sometimes (top four images), the cue was a preferred stimulus for the cell (the flower) and the monkey had to saccade to the preferred stimulus. On separate trials (lower four images), the cue was a poor stimulus (the cup) and the monkey had to saccade to the poor stimulus. (B) Neuronal responses. During the delay period, IT neurons showed an elevated baseline activity that reflected the cue stored in memory. The spontaneous firing rate was higher on trials in which the cue was a preferred stimulus for the cell, relative to trials when the cue was a poor stimulus. After the search array appeared, the responses separated, increasing or decreasing depending on whether the cue was, respectively, a preferred or poor stimulus for the cell. This separation occurred well before the onset of the saccade, which is indicated by the vertical bar on the horizontal axis.

get stimulus, even though the nontarget stimulus was still present physically within its receptive field.

FILTERING OF UNWANTED INFORMATION IN HUMANS

Functional brain imaging studies suggest that in the human visual cortex, just as in the monkey cortex, mechanisms exist such that multiple stimuli compete for neural representation and unwanted information can be filtered out (Kastner *et al.*, 1998, 2001). In one fMRI study, subjects maintained fixation while they were presented with colorful visual stimuli in four nearby locations in the periphery of the visual field (Kastner *et al.*, 1998). Stimuli were presented under two different conditions. In a sequential condition, a single stimulus appeared in one of the four peripheral locations, then another appeared in a different location, and so on, until each of the four stimuli had been presented in the four different locations. In a simultaneous condition, the same four stimuli appeared in the same four locations, but they were presented at the same time. Thus, physical stimuli were identical in the two conditions except that in the second case, all four stimuli appeared simultaneously, which should

encourage competitive interactions among the stimuli. The subjects' task was to count letters at fixation, thereby ignoring the peripheral stimulus presentations. Activation of V1 and ventral stream extrastriate areas V2 to TEO was found under both presentation conditions. Although the fMRI signal was similar in the two presentation conditions in V1, activation was reduced in the simultaneous condition compared to the sequential condition in V2. This reduction in activity was especially pronounced in V4 and TEO. The most straightforward interpretation of this result is that simultaneously presented stimuli interacted in a mutually suppressive way. This sensory suppression effect may be a neural correlate of competition in the human visual cortex. Importantly, the suppression effects appeared to be scaled to the receptive field size of neurons within visual cortical areas; i.e., the effects were larger in areas with larger receptive fields. This observation suggests that, as in the monkey visual cortex, competitive interactions occur most strongly at the level of the receptive field (Kastner *et al.*, 1998).

The effects of spatially directed attention on multiple, competing visual stimuli have been studied in a variation of the same paradigm (Kastner *et al.*, 1998). In addition to the two different visual presentation conditions, sequential and simultaneous, two different attentional conditions were tested, unattended and attended. During the unattended condition, attention was directed away from the visual display by having subjects count the occurrences of letters at the fixation point. In the attended condition, subjects were instructed to attend covertly to the stimulus location that was closest to the fixation point and to count the occurrences of one of the four stimuli. The attended condition led to greater increases in fMRI signals to simultaneously presented stimuli than to sequentially presented stimuli. Thus, in this case, attention partially cancelled out the suppressive interactions among competing stimuli. The magnitude of the attentional effect was greater where the suppressive interactions among stimuli had been strongest, such that the strongest reduction of suppression occurred in areas V4 and TEO. These findings support the idea that directed attention enhances information processing of stimuli at attended locations by counteracting the suppression induced by nearby stimuli that are competing for limited processing resources. In this way, unwanted distracting information is filtered out effectively.

CLOSELY RELATED MECHANISMS GOVERN COVERT ORIENTING AND TARGET SELECTION FOR EYE MOVEMENTS

To this point, this chapter has considered the effects of covert visual attention on perception. However, attentive behavior is also closely related to overt orienting, particularly when saccadic eye movements shift gaze rapidly from one object to the next. Saccades are strongly related to the task at hand and to the composition of the scene. How does the brain select the target of the next saccade? Does covert visual attention accomplish this selection or do saccades have their own separate target selection mechanisms?

To characterize the relationship between saccades and attention, investigators have used a dual-task paradigm in which subjects are asked to identify a particular item in a multi-item display while simultaneously preparing a saccade either to the same or to a different item. In one experiment subjects were shown a circular array of letters and were instructed to make a saccade from the center of the array, where they were initially fixating, to one of the array letters (randomly selected on each trial) (Kowler *et al.*, 1995). After the eye movement, the letter array was extinguished and subjects were queried about the identity of a letter at one of the locations, again selected ran-

domly on each trial. Subjects accurately reported only the identity of the letter they had made a saccade to and performed at chance for all other nontarget letters. Clearly, the subjects' natural strategy was to attend to (and hence, identify and remember) the saccade target, while ignoring the other elements in the display.

Can subjects voluntarily split the loci of attention and saccade if asked to do so? The dual task was given under three sets of instructions: give priority to the saccade task, give priority to the perceptual identification task, or give equal priority to both tasks. The clear-cut finding was that improved performance on one task could not be achieved without a cost for the other task. Better identification accuracy was always accompanied by longer saccadic reaction times. Conversely, shorter saccadic reaction times were always achieved at the cost of lower identification accuracy. Interestingly, the planning and execution of saccades appeared to require only a small amount of attention: a relatively large increment in perceptual accuracy was achieved with only small lengthening of saccadic latencies.

These results strongly argue that the mechanisms underlying attentional selection are closely related to those that select saccade targets. In the authors words: "It is not possible to prepare to look to one location, while simultaneously, and without cost, making accurate perceptual judgments about an eccentric target located elsewhere" (Kowler *et al.*, 1995, p. 1912). Using similar methodology, a strong reliance on visual attention was also found for smooth pursuit eye movements—the slow, continuous movements used to track selected moving targets.

Consistent with these behavioral findings, electrophysiological investigations in humans show that the same brain structures are often activated by visual attention and by saccade planning. In the monkey, prominent centers associated with saccade planning are the frontal eye field in the prefrontal cortex, the lateral intraparietal area in the parietal lobe, and the superior colliculus. In all three areas, large numbers of neurons have spatially selective activity when monkeys plan saccades to visual targets at specific retinal locations. However, many of these neurons also respond selectively to salient or behaviorally relevant visual stimuli even if saccades to such stimuli are purposefully withheld. Accordingly, such cells may be part of a substrate that is common to both covert attention and saccade target selection. Alternatively, such cells may participate exclusively in attentional control, and saccade planning might be accomplished by a separate class of neurons that is intermixed with these cells within the same structures. Thus, although the control of covert attention and of saccades is shared by certain brain regions, it is not yet known whether the same neurons within these regions participate in both functions.

A relatively unexplored question regards the relation between visual attention and other kinds of movement, such as head and body rotations or arm movements. In daily behavior, one habitually coordinates movements of the eyes, arms, and body so that it is possible to look at, turn the body, and reach toward the same object. Visual attention is likely to be involved in any task when one must select a target for coordinated motor behavior.

ATTENTIONAL STATE

In order for mechanisms of selective attention to operate, an organism must maintain a certain level of alertness. The maintenance of alertness is mediated by a number of pathways that use acetylcholine (ACh), norephinephrine (NE), dopamine (DA), or 5-hydroxytryptamine (5-HT) as their transmitters. These so-called neuromodulatory systems originate in the brain stem and send widespread projections into cortical and subcortical regions. Unlike neurons using classical neurotransmitters such as γ-aminobutyric acid (GABA) or glutamate, neurons that use neuromodulators do not directly excite or inhibit their postsynaptic targets. Instead, they modulate the responses of target neurons to classical neurotransmitter inputs (Box 49.2).

MONOAMINES ACT AS NEUROMODULATORS

The best understood neuromodulatory system is the noradrenergic system, whose cells of origin lie in the locus ceruleus of the brain stem (the NE–LC system). Monoaminergic neurons in the LC project to the thalamus, the cerebral cortex, and the cerebellum. In these structures, NE potentiates responses to sensory inputs while reducing spontaneous or low-level activity, thereby improving the signal-to-noise ratio. For example, in the cerebellum, NE increases responses evoked by GABA or glutamate relative to the basal activity of the cell.

LC neurons show three types of task-related activity that are thought to influence behavior: spontaneous discharge, phasic stimulus-evoked responses, and phasic responses related to physical orienting toward a given stimulus. Spontaneous LC activity in the monkey is much faster during waking than during sleep or drowsiness (Aston-Jones and Bloom, 1981). During alert task performance, spontaneous LC activity does not vary continuously but appears to switch between two discrete levels of tonic activity: an "intermediate" level and an "elevated" level. The difference between these two levels is statistically robust, but quite small, on the order of one to two spikes per second.

Variations in the level of spontaneous activity correlate closely with task performance. In one study, monkeys were trained on a visual discrimination task in which they were required to maintain gaze on a central fixation point and depress a lever while viewing a stimulus—either a vertical or a horizontal bar—that was presented at the center of gaze (Aston-Jones et al., 1998). Monkeys had to release the lever after the presentation of one of these stimuli (e.g., the horizontal bar), but to continue holding the lever if the other stimulus appeared (e.g., the vertical bar). Good task performance was associated with trials in which spontaneous LC activity was in the intermediate range. In contrast, during periods of elevated tonic LC activity, monkeys appeared distractible and unable to focus on the task. They foveated the central fixation point less frequently, broke fixation more often, and tended to respond erroneously to nontarget stimuli (false alarms). Thus intermediate-level spontaneous LC activity appears necessary for focused task performance (Fig. 49.12).

LC neurons also respond phasically to the appearance of visual stimuli. In the visual discrimination task described earlier, these responses were not selective for stimulus orientation but were highly sensitive to the behavioral relevance of the stimuli. Specifically, neurons responded only to the target stimulus—the one that required lever release. Reversing the behavioral significance of the stimuli reversed the selectivity of the stimulus-evoked activity. The stimulus-evoked responses preceded the behavioral responses by about 200 ms, and their latencies (on the order of 100 ms) were correlated positively with the manual response latency of the monkey. Stimulus-evoked activity was highest and differentiated best between relevant and nonrelevant stimuli during periods of intermediate spontaneous activity and was weaker and less well differentiated during periods of elevated spontaneous activity.

In both rats and monkeys, the strongest phasic activation of LC neurons is associated with physical orienting toward an external stimulus. LC activity is most intense when ongoing behavior such as sleep, grooming, or feeding is suddenly disrupted and the animal orients (Aston-Jones and Blum, 1981).

BOX 49.2

PANIC DISORDER

Panic disorder (PD) is an anxiety disorder characterized by recurrent unexpected panic attacks, with at least one of the attacks being followed by one or more of the following symptoms: (a) persistent concern about having additional attacks (termed anticipatory anxiety); (b) worry about the implication of the attack or its consequences; and (c) a significant change in behavior related to the attacks. Epidemiological studies indicate that PD affects about 3.5% of the population. PD can be effectively treated by both medication and psychotherapy. Selective serotonin reuptake inhibitors (SSRI), and tricyclic antidepressants, compounds which alter monoamine function as well as benzodiazepine drugs have been demonstrated to work well for PD patients. Similar efficacy has been shown for psychotherapies developed based upon cognitive behavioral principles.

There have been substantial advances in our understanding of the brain circuits mediating the symptoms of anxiety disorders. For example, evidence suggests that the amygdala may play a crucial role in conditioned fear and anxiety. It has been shown that the amygdala exerts inhibitory effects on prefrontal neuronal activity. Children with anxiety disorders show exaggerated amygdala responses to fearful faces compared with healthy children. In adults with PD, imaging studies evaluating brain metabolism and blood flow at rest and during symptom provocation with pharmacological challenges, show metabolic alterations in the hippocampus and the adjacent areas, decreased regional cerebral blood flow in the left posterior parietal-superior temporal cortex, and blunted frontal cortex activation.

Specific neurotransmitters and neuropeptides have been found to be involved in the pathophysiology of PD. Linking together preclinical and clinical data, there is strong evidence for noradrenergic dysregulation in PD. Stress produces regional selective increases in norepinephrine turnover in the locus coeruleus, limbic regions (hypothalamus, hippocampus, and amygdala), and cerebral cortex. Extensive clinical evidence suggests abnormal central noradrenergic function in at least a subgroup of anxiety disorders patients. The α_2-adrenoreceptor antagonist yohimbine, which activates noradrenergic neurons, produces panic attacks and greater increases in anxiety, somatic symptoms, blood pressure, and norepinephrine metabolites in patients with panic disorder than in healthy controls. Thus, it is believed the panic attacks in at least some patients with PD are mediated by excessive noradrenergic neuronal activity. Effective medication and psychotherapy may work by suppressing this hyperactivity.

Substantial evidence shows that central benzodiazepine receptors are also involved in the pathogenesis of PD. The animal model of inescapable stress has been used as a model for human anxiety disorders and for the development of medications for these disorders. Animals exposed to inescapable stress during a time period between 7 days and several months developed a number of behaviors that were noted to parallel symptoms of anxiety disorders in humans. It was shown that these animals develop a 20%–30% decrease in benzodiazepine receptor binding in the frontal cortex, cerebral cortex, with some studies showing reductions in the hippocampus. The major behavioral effects of benzodiazepine agonists and antagonists are mediated through saturable high-affinity benzodiazepine receptor sites located on α subunit of the GABA$_A$ receptor. Hypotheses regarding the role of GABA$_A$/benzodiazepine receptor function in anxiety disorders have proposed either changes in the GABA$_A$/benzodiazepine macromolecular complex or alterations in the concentration of receptors. The latter hypothesis is supported by recent brain imaging findings of a decrease in the density of benzodiazepine receptors in left hippocampus and precuneus in PD patients relative to healthy controls. These data are consistent with the therapeutic effects of benzodiazepine drugs in PD.

Animal studies link together serotonin (5-HT) and GABA systems. Recent gene knockout experiments suggest that a 5-HT$_{1A}$ receptor deficit leads to an anxiety phenotype. Moreover, 5-HT$_{1A}$ receptor knockout mice show abnormalities in GABA$_A$ function consistent with reduced sensitivity to benzodiazepine drugs. Clinical research studies are now in progress studying 5-HT$_{1A}$ receptor density in vivo in patients with PD, and the interaction between 5-HT$_{1A}$ receptor systems and benzodiazepine receptor systems in PD patients.

In the coming years increased knowledge of the genetic basis of human anxiety and gene-environment interactions will improve diagnostic precision and identify new molecular targets for the development of new therapeutic drugs for PD.

Dennis S. Charney and
Alexander Neumeister

These findings suggest a way of understanding the action of the NE–LC system. Robust LC activity, such as found during waking, results in a heightened release of NE throughout the neuraxis, which enhances the signal-to-noise ratio for responses evoked by external stimuli. Conversely, very low spontaneous LC activity may facilitate internally driven vegetative programs, such as sleep, by reducing neural responsiveness to the external world. During waking, a very specific spontaneous activity level—in the intermediate range—is required to maintain the ability to respond selectively to meaningful stimuli while suppressing inappropriate behaviors. Slightly higher LC activity causes less differentiated interaction with the sensory environment and high distractibility. This state may be adaptive for promoting quick physical reactions in dangerous or unpredictable environments.

CONCLUSIONS

"Everyone knows what attention is. It is the taking possession of the mind in clear and vivid form of one out of what seem several simultaneous objects or trains of thought." Thus did William James define the elusive entity commonly known as "attention." A century later, experimental neuroscience and cognitive psychology afford a closer look at the neural mechanisms enabling this "taking possession" to occur.

The behavioral manifestations of attention are clearly not the result of operations in any one dedicated neural center. Selective attention affects neural activity at all levels of the visual system and other sensory systems, with the possible exception of neurons in the sensory periphery. A few structures located at the top of the visual system hierarchy in the parietal, frontal, and cingulate cortices are thought to be relatively more specialized for generating the signals that guide selective attention and less specialized for analyzing the physical properties of the sensory environment.

Answers are beginning to be available to the question of why attention is necessary in the first place. A possible computational bottleneck may be built into all levels of the visual system in the form of spatial receptive fields. The fact that several objects within a certain spatial region can activate the same neuron reduces the ability of such neurons to transmit accurate information about each one of these objects. Mechanisms are therefore required to shrink the functional receptive field around the object(s) that needs greater scrutiny in a particular situation. Other bottlenecks will doubtlessly be revealed in future research.

References

Aston-Jones, G., and Bloom, F. E. (1981). Activity of norepinephrine-containing locus coeruleus neurons in behaving rats anticipates fluctuations in the sleep-waking cycle. *J. Neurosci.* **1**(8), 876–886.

Aston-Jones, G., Rajkowski, J., Ivanova, S., Usher, M., and Cohen, J. (1998). Neuromodulation and cognitive performance: Recent studies of noradrenergic locus ceruleus neurons in behaving monkeys. *Adv. Pharmacol.* **42**, 755–759.

Bichot, N. P., Thompson, K. G., Chenchal Rao, S., and Schall, J. D. (2001). Reliability of macaque frontal eye field neurons signaling saccade targets during visual search. *J. Neurosci.* **21**(2), 713–725.

Bushnell, M. C., Goldberg, M. E., and Robinson, D. L. (1981). Behavioral enhancement of visual responses in monkey cerebral cortex. I. Modulation in posterior parietal cortex related to selective visual attention. *J. Neurophysiol.* **46**, 755–772.

Chelazzi, L., Duncan, J., Miller, E. K., and Desimone, R. (1998). Responses of neurons in inferior temporal cortex during memory-guided visual search. *J. Neurophysiol.* **80**(6), 2918–2940.

Constantinidis, C., and Steinmetz, M. (2001). Neuronal responses in area 7a to multiple stimulus displays: II responses are suppressed at the cued location. *Cereb. Cortex.* **11**(7), 592–597.

Corbetta, M., Miezin, F. M., Dobmeyer, S., Shulman, G. L., and Petersen, S.E. (1991). Attentional modulation of neural processing of shape, color, and velocity in humans. *Science* **248**, 1556–1559.

Duncan, J. (1984). Selective attention and the organization of visual information. *J. Exp. Psychol. Gen.* **113**(4), 501–517.

Egeth, H. E., and Yantis, S. (1997). Visual attention: Control, representation, and time course. *Annu. Rev. Psychol.* **48**, 269–297.

Gottlieb, J. M., Kusunoki, M., and Goldberg, M. E. (1998). The representation of visual salience in monkey parietal cortex. *Nature* **391**, 481–484.

Heilman, K. M. (1979). Neglect and related disorders. *In* "Clinical Neuropsychology" (E. Valenstein, ed.), pp. 268–307. Oxford Univ. Press. New York.

Heinze, H. J., Mangun, G. R., Burchert, W., Hinrichs, H., Scholz, M., *et al.* (1994). Combined spatial and temporal imaging of brain activity during visual selective attention in humans. *Nature* **372**, 543–546.

Hillyard, S. A., and Vento, L. A. (1998). Event-related brain potentials in the study of visual selective attention. *Proc. Natl. Acad. Sci. USA* **95**, 781–787.

Karnath, H. O., Ferber, S., and Himmelbach, M. (2001). Spatial awareness is a function of the temporal not the posterior parietal lobe. *Nature* **411**, 950–953.

Kastner, S., De Weerd, P., Desimone, R., and Ungerleider, L. G. (1998). Mechanisms of directed attention in the human extrastriate cortex as revealed by functional MRI. *Science* **282**, 108–111.

Kastner, S., Pinsk, M. A., De Weerd, P., Desimone, R., and Ungerleider, L. G. (1999). Increased activity in human visual cortex during directed attention in the absence of visual stimulation. *Neuron* **22**, 751–761.

Kastner and Ungerleider (2000). Mechanisms of visual attention in the human cortex. *Annu. Rev. Neurosci.* **23**, 315–342.

Kowler, E., Anderson, E., *et al.* (1995). The role of attention in the programming of saccades. *Vision Res.* **35**(13), 1897–1916.

McAdams, C. J., and Maunsell, J. H. (1999). Effects of attention on the reliability of individual neurons in monkey visual cortex. *Neuron* **23**(4), 765–773.

Mesulam, M.M. (1999). Spatial attention and neglect: Parietal, frontal and cingulate contributions to the mental representation and attentional targeting of salient extrapersonal events. *Philos. Trans. R. Soc. Lond. B Biol. Sci.* **354**(1387), 1325–1346.

Moran, J., and Desimone, R. (1985). Selective attention gates visual processing in the extrastriate cortex. *Science* **229**(4715), 782–784.

Motter, B. C. (1993). Focal attention produces spatially selective processing in visual cortical areas V1, V2, and V4 in the presence of competing stimuli.

Neisser, U., and Becklen, R. (1975). Selective looking: Attending to visually significant events. *Cog. Psychol.* **7**, 480–494.

Posner, M. I., and Petersen, S. E. (1990). The attention system of the human brain. *Annu. Rev. Neurosci.* **13**, 25–42.

Posner, M. I., Walker, J. A., Friedrich, F. J., and Rafal, R. D. (1984). Effects of parietal lobe injury on covert orienting of visual attention. *J. Neurosci.* **4**, 1863–1874.

Recanzone, G. H., and Wurtz, R. H. (2000). Effects of attention on MT and MST neuronal activity during pursuit initiation. *J. Neurophysiol.* **83**(2), 777–790.

Rensink, R.A., and Enns, J.T. (1998). Early completion of occluded objects. *Vision Res.* **38**(15–16), 2489–2505.

Reynolds, J. H., Chelazzi, L., and Desimone, R. (1999). Competitive mechanisms subserve attention in macaque areas V2 and V4. *J. Neurosci.* **19**(5), 1736–1753.

Reynolds, J. H., Pasternak, T., and Desimone, R. (2000). Attention increases sensitivity of V4 neurons. *Neuron.* **26**(3), 703–714.

Rock, I., and Gutman, D. (1981). The effect of inattention on form perception. *J. Exp. Psychol. Hum. Percep. Perform.* **7**(2), 275–285.

Treisman, A.M., and Gelade, G. (1980). A feature-integration theory of attention. *Cognit Psychol.* **12**(1), 97–136.

Ungerleider, L. G., and Mishkin, M. (1982). Two cortical visual systems. *In* "The Analysis of Visual Behavior" (D. J. Ingle, R. J. W. Mansfield, and M. A. Goodale, eds.), pp. 549–586. MIT Press, Cambridge, MA.

Vallar, G. (1993). The anatomical basis of spatial neglect in humans. *In* "Unilateral Neglect: Clinical and Experimental Studies" (I. H. Robertson and J.C. Marshall eds.), pp. 27–62. Lawrence Erlbaum, Hillsdale, NJ.

Yantis, S., and Jonides J. (1984). Abrupt visual onsets and selective attention: Evidence from visual search. *J. Exp. Psychol. Hum. Percept. Perform.* **10**(5), 601–621.

Suggested Readings

Colby, C. L., and Goldberg, M. E. (1999). Space and attention in parietal cortex. *Annu. Rev. Neurosci.* **22**, 319–349.

Connor, C. E., Preddie, D. C., Gallant, J.L., and Van Essen, D.C. (1997). Spatial attention effects in macaque area V4. *J. Neurosci.* **17**(9), 3201–3214.

Corbetta, M. (1998). Frontoparietal cortical networks for directing attention and the eye to visual locations: Identical, independent, or overlapping neural systems? *Proc. Natl. Acad. Sci. USA* **95**(3), 831–838.

Desimone, R., and Duncan, J. (1995). Neural mechanisms of selective visual attention. *Annu. Rev. Neurosci.* **18**, 193–222.

Driver, J., Davis, G., Russell, C., Turatto, M., and Freeman, E. (2001). Segmentation, attention and phenomenal visual objects. *Cognition* **80**, 61–95.

Heeger, D. J. (1999). Linking visual perception with human brain activity. *Curr. Opin. Neurobiol.* **9**(4), 474–479.

Itti, L., and Koch, C. (2001). Computational modelling of visual attention. *Nature Rev. Neurosci.* **2**(3), 194–203.

Mangun, G. R. (1995). Neural mechanisms of visual selective attention. *Psychophysiology* **32**(1), 4–18.

Posner, M. I. (1994). Attention: The mechanisms of consciousness. *Proc. Natl. Acad. Sci. USA* **91**(16), 7398–7403.

Treue, S. (2001). Neural correlates of attention in primate visual cortex. *Trends Neurosci.* **24**(5), 295–300.

John H. Reynolds, Jacqueline P. Gottlieb, and Sabine Kastner

Learning and Memory: Basic Mechanisms

Significant advances have been made since the mid-1970s in understanding how the nervous system encodes and retrieves information. Current research focuses on understanding learning and memory at the cellular level, where the information-encoding process can be traced to changes in the properties of neurons. The encoding process is known to take place through modifications in the biophysical properties of neurons and the strength of synaptic connections among neurons. One emerging and overarching neurobiological principle is that no single universal mechanism for learning and memory exists. Instead, different memory systems (see Chapter 51) can use different mechanisms, and any single memory system can use a variety of cellular mechanisms. Therefore, a comprehensive understanding of memory mechanisms requires an understanding of the general ways in which neurons are changed by learning and the ways in which those changes are maintained and expressed at the cellular level.

The forerunners of modern theories of learning and memory can be traced back more than a century. The American psychologist William James was among the first to discuss the physiological basis of the manner in which information is encoded into brain cells. In 1890 James formulated the "law of neural habit," which states that the formation of associations is driven by the coactivity of elementary brain processes. Although James did not specifically identify the locus of the physiological modifications, others were quick to do so. In 1893 the Italian anatomist Tanzi advanced the hypothesis that the connection between neurons was the locus of the change that encodes experience. Similarly, in 1911 the Spanish neuroanatomist Ramón y Cajál reasoned that if signaling between neurons takes place at the con-

nections between neurons, it follows that changes in the signal strength could alter the flow of activity within the brain and, consequently, the way an organism responds to experiences. In 1949, Donald Hebb later advanced the argument that learning involved coincident pre- and postsynaptic activity, which came to be known as the "Hebb synapse" and will be discussed later.

Research during the past several decades on several vertebrate and invertebrate model systems has led to the development of several general principles. A list of these principles (Byrne, 1987) might include the following.

1. Multiple memory systems are present in the brain (see also Chapter 51).
2. Short-term forms of learning and memory require changes in existing neural circuits.
3. These changes may involve multiple cellular mechanisms within individual neurons.
4. Second-messenger systems play a role in mediating cellular changes.
5. Changes in membrane channels are often correlated with learning and memory.
6. Long-term memory requires new protein synthesis, whereas short-term memory does not.

This chapter describes several of the types of neural and molecular mechanisms implicated in learning and memory. The chapter first considers some of the paradigms that have been used to study simple forms of nonassociative and associative learning and provides an example of mechanistic analyses that have been performed in a selected invertebrate model system. The later sections of the chapter describe the mechanisms of two phenomena, which are known as long-term potentiation (LTP) and long-term depression (LTD). Both LTP and LTD occur in forebrain structures, and LTP and LTD are thought to be mechanisms for memory storage in the central nervous system. LTD appears to be particularly important for memory storage in the cerebellum. Chapter 51 considers different types of memory systems and their anatomical loci.

PARADIGMS HAVE BEEN DEVELOPED TO STUDY ASSOCIATIVE AND NONASSOCIATIVE LEARNING

Associative Learning

Associative learning is a broad category that includes many of our daily learning activities: learn-

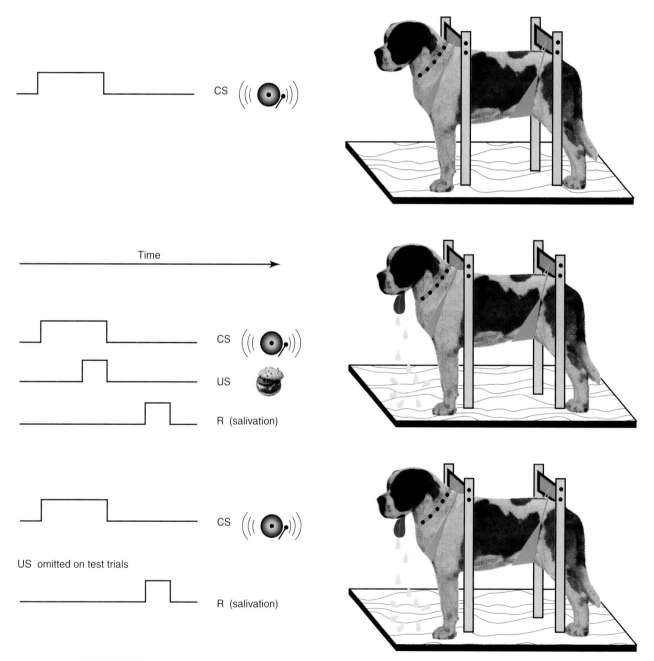

FIGURE 50.1 Classical conditioning. In the procedure introduced by Pavlov, the production of saliva is monitored continuously. Presentation of meat powder reliably leads to salivation, whereas some "neutral" stimulus such as a bell initially does not. With repeated pairings of the bell and meat powder, the animal learns that the bell predicts the food and salivates in response to the bell alone. Modified from Rachlin (1991).

ing to be afraid, learning to talk, learning a foreign language, or learning to play the piano. In essence, associative learning involves the formation of associations among stimuli and/or responses. It is usually subdivided into classical conditioning and instrumental conditioning. Classical (or Pavlovian) conditioning is induced by a procedure in which a generally neutral stimulus, termed a *conditioned stimulus* (CS), is paired with a stimulus that generally elicits a response, termed an *unconditioned stimulus* (US). Two examples of unconditioned stimuli are food, which elicits salivation, or a shock to the foot, which elicits limb withdrawal. Instrumental (or operant) conditioning is a process by which an organism learns to associate consequences with its own behavior. In an operant conditioning paradigm, the delivery of a reinforcing stimulus is contingent upon the expression of a designated behavior. The probability that this behavior will actually be expressed is then altered. This chapter focuses on classical conditioning, as it is mechanistically the best understood type of associative conditioning.

An astute observation by Ivan Pavlov, a Russian physiologist who had been studying digestion in dogs, led to his discovery of classical conditioning in a celebrated case of serendipity. He first noticed that the mere sight of the food dish caused dogs to salivate. He continued the experiments to see if dogs would also salivate in response to a bell rung at feeding time. Pavlov trained dogs to stand in a harness and, after the sound of a bell, fed them meat powder (Fig. 50.1). He then recorded the salivary responses of the dogs. At first, the bell by itself did not elicit any response, but the meat powder elicited reflex salivation, which was termed the *unconditioned response* (UR). He noted that after a few pairings of the bell and meat powder the dogs began to salivate when the bell rang, before they received the meat powder. This response is termed the *conditioned response* (CR). This type of conditioning came to be called reward or appetitive *classical conditioning*. If the bell or another stimulus was followed by an unpleasant event, such as an electric shock, then a variety of autonomic responses became conditioned. This type of conditioning is often termed aversive or fear conditioning. Skeletal muscle movements appropriate to deal with the US (e.g., leg flexion after a shock delivered to a paw) are also learned in aversive classical conditioning.

Traditionally, classical or Pavlovian conditioning is an operation that pairs one stimulus, the conditioned stimulus or CS, with a second stimulus, the unconditioned stimulus or US, as noted earlier. The US reliably elicits a response termed the unconditioned response or UR. Repeated pairings of the CS and US result in the CS eliciting a response, which is defined as the conditioned response or CR. Conditioning procedures in which the CS and US overlap in time are called *delay conditioning*, whereas in *trace conditioning* a short time interval is interposed between the CS and the US. Often, the CR is similar to the UR (e.g., in Pavlov's experiment both were salivation). Although the traditional view of Pavlovian conditioning emphasized the contiguity of the CS and US, a more general and contemporary view of Pavlovian conditioning emphasizes the informational relation between the CS and the US. In other words, the information that the CS provides about the occurrence of the US is the critical feature for learning.

Nonassociative Learning

Three examples of nonassociative learning have received the most experimental attention: habituation, dishabituation, and sensitization. *Habituation* is defined as a reduction in the response to a stimulus that is delivered repeatedly. *Dishabituation* refers to the restoration or recovery of a habituated response due to the presentation of another, typically strong, stimulus to the animal. *Sensitization* is an enhancement or augmentation of a response produced by the presentation of a strong stimulus. The following sections introduce the *Aplysia* and focus on the neural and molecular mechanisms of sensitization.

INVERTEBRATE STUDIES: KEY INSIGHTS FROM *Aplysia* INTO BASIC MECHANISMS OF LEARNING

Since the mid-1960s, the marine mollusc *Aplysia* has proven to be an extremely useful model system to gain insights into the neural and molecular mechanisms of simple forms of memory. Indeed, the pioneering discoveries of Eric Kandel using this animal were recognized by his receipt of the Nobel Prize in Physiology or Medicine in 2000. A number of characteristics make *Aplysia* well suited for the examination of the molecular, cellular, morphological, and network mechanisms underlying neuronal modifications (plasticity) and learning and memory. The animal has a relatively simple nervous system with large, individually identifiable neurons that are accessible for detailed anatomical, biophysical, biochemical and molecular studies. Neurons and neural circuits that mediate many behaviors in *Aplysia* have been identified. In several cases, these behaviors have been shown to be modifiable by learning. Moreover, specific loci within neural circuits at which modifications occur during learning have been identified, and aspects of the cellular mechanisms underlying these modifications have been analyzed and modeled (Byrne *et al.*, 1993; Byrne and Kandel, 1996; Hawkins *et al.*, 1993).

The Siphon–Gill and Tail–Siphon Withdrawal Reflexes of Aplysia

Within the mantle cavity of *Aplysia* lies the respiratory organ of the animal, the gill, and protruding from the mantle cavity is the siphon (Fig. 50.2). The siphon–gill withdrawal reflex is elicited when a tactile or electrical stimulus is delivered to the siphon; the stimulus causes withdrawal of the siphon and gill (Fig. 50.2A). A second behavior that has been examined extensively is the tail–siphon withdrawal reflex. Tactile or electrical stimulation of the tail elicits a coordinated set of defensive responses composed of a reflex withdrawal of the tail and the siphon (Fig. 50.2B).

These two defensive reflexes in *Aplysia* can exhibit three forms of nonassociative learning: habituation, dishabituation, and sensitization. A single sensitizing stimulus, such as a brief several second-duration electric shock, can produce a reflex enhancement that lasts minutes (short-term sensitization), whereas prolonged training (e.g., multiple stimuli over an hour or more) produces an enhancement that lasts from days to weeks (long-term sensitization). *Aplysia* also exhibit several forms of associative learning, including classical conditioning and operant conditioning.

A prerequisite for successful analysis of the neural and molecular basis of these different forms of learning is an understanding of the neural circuit that controls the behavior. The afferent limb of the siphon-gill withdrawal reflex consists of a population of approximately 24 sensory neurons with somata in the abdominal ganglion. The siphon sensory neurons (SN) monosynaptically excite a population of approximately 13 gill and

A   B

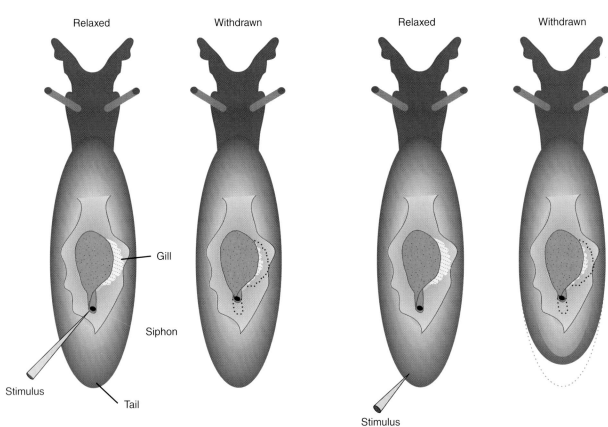

FIGURE 50.2 Siphon–gill and tail–siphon withdrawal reflexes of *Aplysia*. (A) Siphon–gill withdrawal. Dorsal view of *Aplysia*. (Left) Relaxed position. (Right) A stimulus (e.g., a water jet, brief touch, or weak electric shock) applied to the siphon causes the siphon and the gill to withdraw into the mantle cavity. (B) Tail–siphon withdrawal reflex. (Left) Relaxed position. (Right) A stimulus applied to the tail elicits a reflex withdrawal of the tail, the siphon, and the gill.

A B

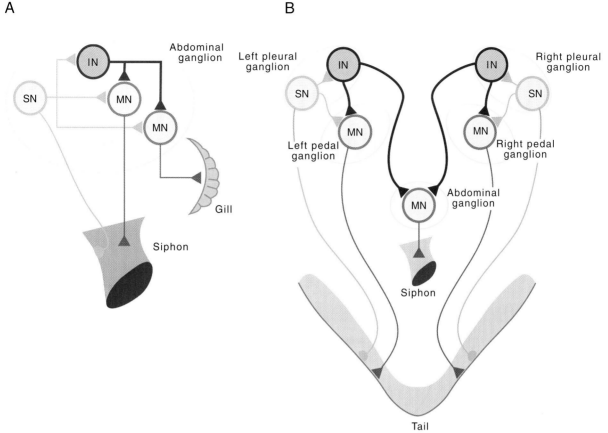

FIGURE 50.3 Simplified circuit diagrams of siphon–gill (A) and tail–siphon (B) withdrawal reflexes. Stimuli activate the afferent terminals of mechanoreceptor sensory neurons (SN) whose somata are located in central ganglia (abdominal, pedal, and pleural). The sensory neurons make excitatory synaptic connections (triangles) with interneurons (IN) and motor neurons (MN). The excitatory interneurons provide a parallel pathway for excitation of the motor neurons. Action potentials elicited in the motor neurons, triggered by the combined input from the SNs and INs, propagate out peripheral nerves to activate muscle cells and produce the subsequent reflex withdrawal of the organs. Modulatory neurons (not shown here, but see Fig. 50.6A1), such as those containing serotonin (5-HT), regulate the properties of the circuit elements and, consequently, the strength of the behavioral responses. Modfied from Cleary *et al.* (1995).

siphon motor neurons (MN) that are also located in the abdominal ganglion (Fig. 50.3A). Activation of the gill and siphon motor neurons leads to contraction of the gill and siphon. Excitatory, inhibitory, and modulatory interneurons (IN) in the withdrawal circuit have also been identified, although only excitatory interneurons are illustrated in Fig. 50.3. The afferent limb of the tail-siphon withdrawal reflex consists of a bilaterally symmetrical cluster of approximately 200 sensory neurons located in the left and right pleural ganglia. These sensory neurons make monosynaptic excitatory connections with at least three motor neurons in the adjacent pedal ganglion, which produce withdrawal of the tail (Fig. 50.3B). In addition, the tail sensory neurons form synapses with various identified excitatory and inhibitory interneurons. Some of these interneurons activate motor neurons in the abdominal ganglion, which control reflex withdrawal of the siphon. Moreover,

several additional neurons modulate the tail–siphon withdrawal reflex (Cleary *et al.*, 1995; see Fig. 50.4A1).

Sensory neurons for both siphon-gill and tail-siphon withdrawal reflexes are similar and appear to be important, although probably not exclusive (e.g., Cleary *et al.*, 1998), sites of plasticity in their respective neural circuits. Changes in their membrane properties and the strength of their synaptic connections (synaptic efficacy) are associated with sensitization.

Multiple Cellular Processes Mediate Short- and Long-Term Sensitization in Aplysia

A discussion of memory mechanisms can be divided into three parts: induction, expression, and maintenance. *Induction* refers to the initial events that trigger or initiate the modification process; *expression* concerns how the modification process is ultimately

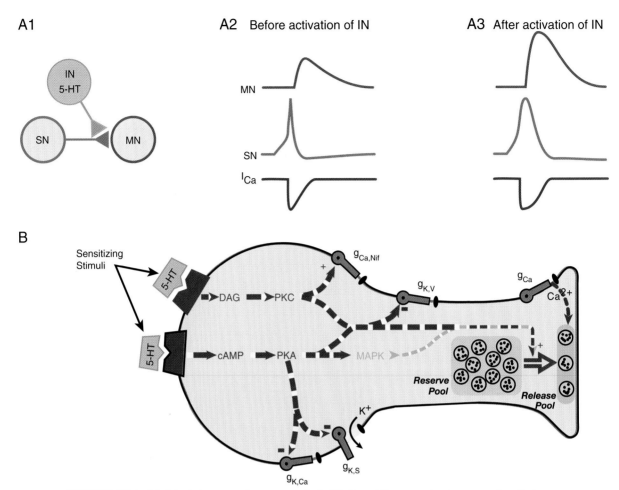

FIGURE 50.4 Model of short-term heterosynaptic facilitation of the sensorimotor connection that contributes to short- and long-term sensitization in *Aplysia*. (A1) Sensitizing stimuli activate facilitatory interneurons (IN) that release modulatory transmitters, one of which is 5-HT. The modulator leads to an alteration of the properties of the sensory neuron (SN). (A2 and A3) An action potential in SN after the sensitizing stimulus results in greater transmitter release and hence a larger postsynaptic potential in the motor neuron (MN, A3) than an action potential before the sensitizing stimulus (A2). For short-term sensitization, the enhancement of transmitter release is due, at least in part, to broadening of the action potential and an enhanced flow of Ca^{2+} (I_{Ca}) into the sensory neuron. (B) Model of a sensory neuron that depicts the multiple processes for short-term facilitation that contribute to short-term sensitization. 5-HT released from facilitatory neurons binds to at least two distinct classes of receptors on the outer surface of the membrane and leads to the transient activation of two intracellular second messengers, DAG and cAMP, and their respective kinases (PKC and PKA). 5-HT can also activate MAPK apparently via the activation of cAMP. These three kinases affect multiple cellular processes, the combined effects of which lead to enhanced transmitter release when subsequent action potentials are fired in the sensory neuron (see text for additional details). Modified from Byrne and Kandel (1996).

expressed; and *maintenance* addresses the manner in which the modification is made to endure over time.

Short-Term Sensitization

Short-term (minutes) sensitization is induced when a single brief train of shocks to the body wall results in the release of modulatory transmitters, such as serotonin (5-HT), from a separate class of interneurons referred to as facilitatory neurons (Fig. 50.4A1). These facilitatory neurons regulate the properties of the sensory neurons and the strength of their connec-

tions with postsynaptic interneurons and motor neurons through a process called *heterosynaptic facilitation* (Byrne and Kandel, 1996; Figs. 50.4A2 and 50.4A3). The molecular mechanisms contributing to short-term heterosynaptic facilitation are illustrated in Fig. 50.4B. The first step is the binding of 5-HT to one class of receptors on the outer surface of the membrane of the sensory neurons. This leads to the activation of adenylyl cyclase, which in turn leads to an elevation of the intracellular level of the second messenger cyclic adenosine 3′,5′-monophosphate [cyclic

AMP (cAMP)] in sensory neurons. When cAMP binds to the regulatory subunit of cAMP-dependent protein kinase [protein kinase A(PKA)], the catalytic subunit is released and can now add phosphate groups to specific substrate proteins and therefore alter their functional properties. One consequence of this protein phosphorylation is an alteration in the properties of membrane channels. Specifically, the increased levels of cAMP lead to a decrease in the serotonin-sensitive potassium current [S-K$^+$ current ($I_{K/S}$)], a component of the calcium-activated K$^+$ current ($I_{K,Ca}$) and the delayed K$^+$ current ($I_{K,V}$). (See Chapter 6 for more information on these channel types.) These changes in membrane currents lead to depolarization of the membrane potential, enhanced excitability, and an increase in the duration of the action potential (i.e., spike broadening). Reflections of enhanced excitability include an increase in the number of action potentials elicited in a sensory neuron by a fixed extrinsic current injected into the cell or by a fixed stimulus to the skin.

Cyclic AMP also appears to activate a facilitatory process that is independent of membrane potential and spike duration. This process is represented in Fig. 50.4B (large open arrow) as the translocation or mobilization of transmitter vesicles from a reserve pool to a releasable pool. The translocation makes more transmitter-containing vesicles available for release, with subsequent action potentials in the sensory neuron. The overall effect is a short-term, cAMP-dependent enhancement of transmitter release.

Serotonin also acts through another class of receptors to increase the level of the second messenger diacylglycerol (DAG). DAG activates protein kinase C (PKC), which, like PKA, contributes to facilitation that is independent of spike duration (e.g., mobilization of vesicles). In addition, PKC regulates a nifedipine-sensitive Ca^{2+} channel ($I_{Ca, Nif}$) and the delayed K$^+$ channel ($I_{K,V}$). Thus, the delayed K$^+$ channel ($I_{K,V}$) is dually regulated by PKC and PKA. The modulation of $I_{K,V}$ contributes importantly to the increase in duration of the action potential (Fig. 50.4A3). Due to its small magnitude, the modulation of $I_{Ca, Nif}$ appears to play a minor role in the facilitatory process.

Prolonged treatments of 5-HT (1.5 h) activate mitogen-activated protein kinase (MAPK) (Martin *et al.*, 1997). This pathway was originally suggested to be important only for the induction of long-term processes (see later). However, recent work indicates that MAPK is involved in the phosphorylation of synapsin by a brief (5 min) application of 5-HT (Angers *et al.*, 2002). Synapsin is a synaptic vesicle-associated protein that tethers synaptic vesicles to cytoskeletal elements and thus helps control the

reserve pool of vesicles in synaptic terminals (see Chapter 8). Phosphorylation of synapsin would allow vesicles in the reserve pool to migrate to the releasable pool and thus contribute to enhanced transmitter release. Of general significance is the observation that a single modulatory transmitter (i.e., 5-HT) activates at least three kinase systems. The involvement of multiple second messenger systems in synaptic plasticity also appears to be a theme emerging from mammalian studies. For example, as discussed in a later section of the chapter, the induction of LTP in the CA1 area of the hippocampus appears to involve MAPK, PKC, calcium/calmodulin-dependent protein kinase (CaM kinase II), and tyrosine kinase (reviewed in Dineley *et al.*, 2001).

The consequences of activating these multiple second-messenger systems and modulating these various cellular processes are expressed when test stimuli elicit action potentials in the sensory neuron at various times after the presentation of the sensitizing stimuli (Fig. 50.4A3). More transmitter is available for release as a result of the mobilization process and each action potential is broader, allowing a larger influx of Ca^{2+} to trigger release of the available transmitter. The combined effects of mobilization and spike broadening lead to the facilitation of transmitter release from the sensory neuron and consequently a larger postsynaptic potential in the motor neuron. Larger postsynaptic potentials lead to enhanced activation of interneurons and motor neurons and thus to an enhanced behavioral response.

The maintenance of short-term sensitization is dependent on the persistence of the PKA-, PKC-, and MAPK-induced phosphorylations of the various substrate proteins.

Long-Term Sensitization

Sensitization also exists in a long-term form, which persists for at least 24 h. Whereas short-term sensitization can be produced by a single brief stimulus, the induction of long-term sensitization requires a more extensive training period over an hour or more.

A substantial amount of data indicates that both short- and long-term sensitization share some common cellular pathways during their *induction*. For example, both forms activate the cAMP/PKA cascade (Fig. 50.5). However, in the long-term form, unlike the short-term form, activation of the cAMP/PKA cascade induces gene transcription and new protein synthesis (Byrne *et al*, 1993; Hawkins *et al.*, 1993). Repeated training leads to a translocation of PKA to the nucleus where it phosphorylates the transcriptional activator CREB1 (cAMP responsive element

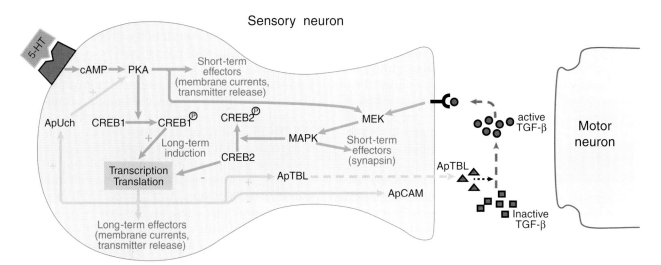

FIGURE 50.5 Simplified scheme of the mechanisms in sensory neurons that contribute to long-term sensitization and some aspects of short-term sensitization. Sensitization training leads to cAMP-dependent regulation of short-term effectors (see Fig. 50.4 for details) and phosphorylation of CREB1. cAMP also activates MAPK, which regulates the repressor CREB2. The combined effects of activation of CREB1 and derepression of CREB2 lead to regulation of the synthesis of at least 10 proteins, only 3 of which (ApTBL, ApCAM, and ApUch) are shown. Two of these proteins (ApTBL and ApUch) appear to be components of positive feedback cycles. ApTBL is believed to activate latent forms of TGF-β, which can then bind to receptors on the sensory neuron. TGF-β activates MAPK, which can have both acute and long-term actions. One of its acute effects is the regulation of transmitter release. MAPK may also act by initiating a second round of gene regulation by affecting CREB2-dependent pathways. Increased synthesis of ApUch leads to enhanced degradation of the regulatory subunit of PKA, leading to enhanced activation of the catalytic subunit and increased phosphorylation of CREB1. The third protein ApCAM is downregulated. Downregulation of ApCAM is involved in regulating growth processes associated with long-term facilitation.

binding protein). CREB1 binds to a regulatory region of genes known as CRE (cAMP responsive element). Next, this bound and phosphorylated form of CREB1 leads to increased transcription. cAMP also leads to the activation of MAPK, which phosphorylates the transcriptional repressor CREB2. Phosphorylation of CREB2 by MAPK leads to a derepression of CREB2 and therefore promotes CREB1-mediated transcriptional activation (Bartsch *et al.*, 1995). The combined effects of activation of CREB1 and derepression of CREB2 lead to changes in the synthesis of specific proteins. So far, more than 10 gene products that are regulated by sensitization training have been identified, and others are likely to be found in the future. These results indicate that there is not a single memory gene or protein, but that multiple genes are regulated, and they act in a coordinated way to alter neuronal properties and synaptic strength. The following section discusses three regulated proteins of particular significance.

The down-regulation of a homologue of a neuronal cell adhesion molecule (NCAM), ApCAM plays a key role in long-term facilitation. This down-regulation has two components. First, the synthesis of ApCAM is reduced. Second, preexisting ApCAM is internalized via increased endocytosis. The internalization and degradation of ApCAM allow for the restructuring of

the axon arbor (Bailey *et al.*, 1992). The sensory neuron can now form additional connections with the same postsynaptic target or make new connections with other cells. Another protein whose synthesis is regulated by long-term facilitation is *Aplysia* tolloid/BMP-like protein (ApTBL-1). Tolloid and the related molecule BMP-1 appear to function as secreted Zn^{2+} proteases. In some preparations, they activate members of the transforming growth factor β (TGF-β) family. Indeed, in sensory neurons, TGF-β mimics the effects of 5-HT in that it produces long-term increases in the synaptic strength of the sensory neurons (Zhang *et al.*, 1997). Interestingly, TGF-β activates MAPK in the sensory neurons and induces its translocation to the nucleus. Thus, TGF-β could be part of an *extracellular* positive feedback loop, possibly leading to another round of protein synthesis (Fig. 50.5) to further consolidate the memory (Zhang *et al*, 1997). A third important protein, *Aplysia* ubiquitin hydrolase (ApUch), appears to be involved in an *intracellular* positive feedback loop. During the induction of long-term facilitation, ApUch levels in sensory neurons are increased, possibly via CREB phosphorylation and a consequent increase in *ApUch* transcription. The increased levels of ApUch increase the rate of degradation, via the ubiquitin-proteosome pathway, of proteins including the regulatory subunit of PKA (Chain *et al.*, 1999). The catalytic subunit of PKA, when freed from the regulatory subunit, is highly active. Thus, increased ApUch will lead to an increase in PKA activity and a more protracted phosphorylation of CREB1. This phosphorylated CREB may act to further prolong *ApUch* expression, thus closing a positive feedback loop.

One simplifying hypothesis is that the mechanisms underlying the *expression* of short- and long-term sensitization are the same, but extended in time for long-term sensitization. Some evidence supports this hypothesis. For example, long-term sensitization, like short-term sensitization, is associated with an enhancement of sensorimotor connections. In addition, K$^+$ currents and excitability of sensory neurons are modified by long-term sensitization (Cleary *et al.*, 1998). Based on the model for short-term sensitization, one would expect action potential duration to be affected by long-term sensitization. Surprisingly, this hypothesis has never been examined rigorously. Although some of the expression mechanisms are common, the expression of long-term sensitization has been associated with unique mechanisms. Structural changes such as neurite outgrowth and active zone remodeling have been correlated with long-term sensitization, but not with short-term sensitization (Bailey and Kandel, 1993). Another recently identified correlate of long-term sensitization, and a correlate of procedures that mimic sensitization training, is an increase in high-affinity glutamate uptake (Levenson *et al.*, 2000). A change in glutamate uptake could potentially exert a significant effect on synaptic efficacy by regulating the amount of transmitter available for release, the rate of clearance from the cleft, and thereby the duration of the EPSP and the degree of receptor desensitization. Moreover, long-term sensitization has been correlated with changes in the postsynaptic cell (i.e., the motor neuron, Cleary *et al.*, 1998). Thus, as with other examples of memory, multiple sites of plasticity exist even within this simple reflex system.

Persistent phosphorylation also contributes to intermediate-term facilitation (see later) and may contribute to the induction and maintenance of long-term facilitation as well. For example, one way that new protein synthesis regulates synaptic strength is by reducing levels of the regulatory subunit of PKA (see earlier discussion), resulting in persistent phosphorylation of target proteins (Chain *et al.*, 1999). An interesting hypothesis is that TGF-β could also be part of the maintenance mechanism. Its late activation by ApTBL-1 could feed back through an extracellular loop to reactivate MAPK in the sensory neurons and therefore engage some acute MAPK-dependent effectors (Fig. 50.5).

Other Temporal Domains for the Memory of Sensitization

Historically, memory has been divided into two temporal domains, short term and long term. It has become increasing clear from studies of a number of memory systems that this distinction is overly simplistic. For example, in *Aplysia*, Carew and colleagues (Sutton *et al.*, 2001) and Kandel and colleagues (Ghirardi *et al.*, 1995) have discovered an intermediate phase of memory that has distinctive temporal characteristics and a unique molecular signature. The intermediate-phase memory for sensitization is expressed at times approximately 30 min to 3 h after the beginning of training. It declines completely prior to the onset of long-term memory. Like long-term sensitization, its induction requires protein synthesis, but unlike long-term memory it does not require mRNA synthesis. The expression of the intermediate-phase memory requires the persistent activation of PKA.

In addition to intermediate-phase memory, it is likely that *Aplysia* has different phases of long-term memory. For example, at 24 h after sensitization training there is increased synthesis of a number of proteins, some of which are different from those whose synthesis is increased during and immediately after training. However, blocking protein synthesis at times between 12 and 24 h after training does not block long-term facilitation at 24 h. These results suggest that the memory for sensitization that persists for times greater than 24 h may be dependent on the synthesis of proteins occurring at 24 h and may have a different molecular signature than the 24-h memory.

Mechanisms Underlying Associative Learning of Withdrawal Reflexes in *Aplysia*

The withdrawal reflexes of *Aplysia* are subject to classical conditioning (Byrne *et al.*, 1993; Hawkins *et al.*, 1993). The short-term classical conditioning observed at the behavioral level reflects, at least in part, a cellular mechanism called *activity-dependent neuromodulation*. A diagram of the general scheme is presented in Fig. 50.6. The US pathway is activated by a shock to the animal, which elicits a withdrawal response (the UR). When a CS is paired consistently with the US, the animal will develop a withdrawal response (CR) to the CS. Activity-dependent neuromodulation is proposed as the mechanism for this pairing-specific effect. The US activates both a motor neuron (UR) and a modulatory system. The modulatory system delivers the neurotransmitter serotonin to all the sensory neurons (parts of the various CS pathways), which leads to a nonspecific enhancement of transmitter release from the sensory neurons. This nonspecific enhancement con-

A. Learning

B. Memory

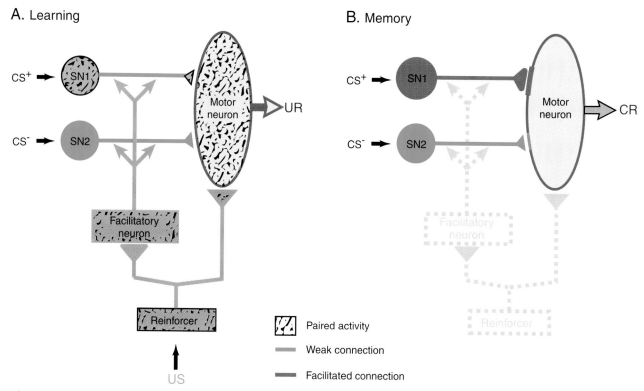

FIGURE 50.6 Model of classical conditioning of a withdrawal reflex in *Aplysia*. (A) Activity in a sensory neuron (SN1) along the CS+ (paired) pathway is coincident with activity in neurons along the reinforcement pathway (US). However, activity in the sensory neuron (SN2) along the CS– (unpaired) pathway is not coincident with activity in neurons along the US pathway. The US directly activates the motor neuron, producing the UR. The US also activates a modulatory system in the form of the facilitatory neuron, resulting in the delivery of a neuromodulatory transmitter to the two sensory neurons. The pairing of activity in SN1 with the delivery of the neuromodulator yields the associative modifications. (B) After the paired activity in A, the synapse from SN1 to the motor neuron is selectively enhanced. Thus, it is more likely to activate the motor neuron and produce the conditioned response (CR) in the absence of US input. Modified from Lechner and Byrne (1998).

tributes to short-term sensitization (see prior discussion). Sensory neurons whose activity is temporally contiguous with the US-mediated reinforcement are additionally modulated. Spiking in a sensory neuron during the presence of 5-HT leads to changes in that cell relative to other sensory neurons whose activity was not paired with the US. Thus, a subsequent CS will lead to an enhanced activation of the reflex (Fig. 50.6B). Figure 50.7 illustrates a more detailed model of the proposed cellular mechanisms responsible for this example of classical conditioning. The modulator (US) acts by increasing the activity of adenylyl cyclase (AC), which in turn increases the levels of cAMP. Spiking in the sensory neurons (CS) leads to increased levels of intracellular calcium, which greatly enhances the action of the modulator to increase the cAMP cascade. This system determines CS–US contiguity by a method of coincidence detection at the presynaptic terminal.

Now, consider the postsynaptic side of the synapse. The postsynaptic region contains NMDA-type receptors (see Chapters 9 and 11). These receptors need concurrent delivery of glutamate and depolarization in

order to allow calcium to enter. The glutamate is provided by the activated sensory neuron (CS), and the depolarization is provided by the US (for review, see Lechner and Byrne, 1998). Thus, the postsynaptic neuron provides another example of coincidence detection. The increase in intracellular calcium putatively causes a retrograde signal to be released from the postsynaptic to the presynaptic terminal, ultimately acting to further enhance the cAMP cascade in the sensory neuron. The overall amplification of the cAMP cascade acts to raise the level of PKA, which in turn leads to the modulation of transmitter release. These activity-dependent changes enhance synaptic efficacy between the specific sensory neuron of the CS pathway and the motor neuron. Thus, the sensory neuron along the CS pathway will be better able to activate the motor neuron and produce the CR.

Summary

Certain invertebrates display an enormous capacity for learning and offer particular experimental

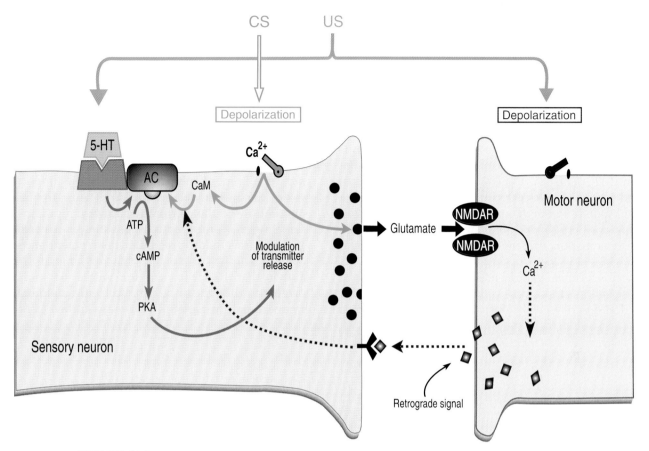

FIGURE 50.7 Model of associative facilitation at the *Aplysia* sensorimotor synapse. This model has both a presynaptic and a postsynaptic detector for the coincidence of the CS and the US. Furthermore, a putative retrograde signal allows for the integration of these two detection systems at the presynaptic level. The CS leads to activity in the sensory neuron, yielding presynaptic calcium influx, which enhances the US-induced cAMP cascade. The CS also induces glutamate release, which results in postsynaptic calcium influx through NMDA receptors if paired with the US-induced depolarization of the postsynaptic neuron. The postsynaptic calcium influx putatively induces a retrograde signal, which further enhances the presynaptic cAMP cascade. The end result of the cAMP cascade is to modulate transmitter release and enhance the strength of the synapse. Modified from Lechner and Byrne (1998).

advantages for analyzing the cellular and molecular mechanisms of learning. For example, behaviors in *Aplysia* are mediated by relatively simple neural circuits, which can be analyzed with conventional anatomical and electrophysiological approaches. Once the circuit is specified, the neural locus for the particular example of learning can be found, and biophysical, biochemical, and molecular approaches can then be used to identify mechanisms underlying the change. The relatively large size of some of these cells allows these analyses to take place at the level of individually identified neurons. Individual neurons can be removed surgically and assayed for changes in the levels of second messengers, protein phosphorylation, RNA, and protein syntheses. Moreover, peptides and nucleotides can be injected into individual neurons. This chapter

has focused exclusively on *Aplysia*, but many other invertebrates have proven to be valuable model systems for the cellular and molecular analysis of learning and memory. Each has its own unique advantages. For example, *Aplysia* is excellent for applying cell biological approaches to the analysis of learning and memory mechanisms. Other invertebrate model systems such as *Drosophila* and *Caenorhabditis elegans*, are not well suited for cell biological approaches because of their small neurons, but offer tremendous advantages for obtaining insights into mechanisms of learning and memory through the application of genetic approaches. See Byrne (1987) and Carew (2000) for a review of several selected invertebrate model systems that have contributed importantly to the understanding of memory mechanisms.

VERTEBRATE STUDIES: LONG-TERM POTENTIATION

In contrast to the studies on invertebrates like *Aplysia* described earlier, in vertebrates it has been more difficult to link synaptic plasticity with specific examples of learning. However, one exciting and extensively studied candidate memory mechanism is the synaptic phenomenon termed long-term potentiation (LTP). This phenomenon is defined as a persistent increase in synaptic strength (as measured by the amplitude of the EPSP in a follower neuron) that can be induced rapidly by a brief burst of spike activity in the presynaptic afferents. The intense experimental interest in LTP is driven by the working hypothesis that this form of synaptic plasticity may participate in information storage in several brain regions. This section describes the properties of LTP and how it is

studied, reviews its underlying mechanisms, and explores the possibility of linkages between LTP and learning and memory.

Long-Term Potentiation Occurs in a Variety of Neural Synapses

The first evidence that long-term modification of mammalian synapses could be induced by experimental means appeared in 1973, when Timothy Bliss and Terje Lomo demonstrated LTP in the hippocampus of the anesthetized rabbit. Brief, high-frequency stimulation of the perforant-pathway input to the dentate gyrus produced a long-lasting enhancement of the extracellularly recorded field potential. Subsequent studies of nonanesthetized animals have shown that LTP can last for weeks or months. Originally thought to be unique to the mammalian hippocampal formation, LTP is now known to occur

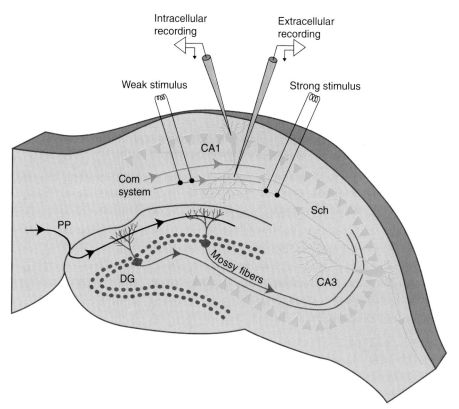

FIGURE 50.8 Schematic of a transverse hippocampal brain slice preparation from the rat. Two extracellular stimulating electrodes are used to activate two nonoverlapping inputs to pyramidal neurons of the CA1 region of the hippocampus. By suitably adjusting the current intensity delivered to the stimulating electrodes, different numbers of Schaffer collateral/commissural (Sch/com) axons can be activated. In this way, one stimulating electrode was made to produce a weak postsynaptic response and the other to produce a strong postsynaptic response. Also illustrated is an extracellular recording electrode placed in the stratum radiatum (the projection zone of the Sch/com inputs) and an intracellular recording electrode in the stratum pyramidale (the cell body layer). Also indicated is the mossy fiber projection from granule cells of the dentate gyrus (DG) to the pyramidal neurons of the CA3 region. Adapted from Barrionuevo and Brown (1983).

in the cerebellum, neocortical regions, subcortical regions such as the amygdala, mammalian peripheral nervous system, the arthropod neuromuscular junction, and the *Aplysia* sensorimotor synapse. It is important to bear in mind that no universal mechanism exists for inducing LTP. Indeed, different mechanisms may be used at the same synapse, depending on the experimental conditions. This chapter focuses primarily on the LTP at the synapse made by a pyramidal neuron in the CA3 region of the hippocampus to a pyramidal neuron in the CA1 region of the hippocampus.

Long-Term Potentiation at the CA3–CA1 Synapse

Within the hippocampus proper, by far the best studied synapse is that from the Schaffer collateral/commissural (Sch/com) fibers of the CA3 pyramidal cells to the CA1 pyramidal cells (Fig. 50.8). In fact, this is probably the most commonly studied synapse in the mammalian brain, due in part to its relatively simple circuitry and its laminar organization. These features make it possible to extract useful data from extracellular recordings, which are easier to perform than intracellular recordings and preferable for some purposes. Examples of LTP induction are illustrated in Fig. 50.9B. The lower waveforms are extracellularly recorded field EPSPs recorded in the CA1 region in response to a single weak stimulation of the Schaffer collateral pathway. Brief electric stimuli delivered to this pathway lead to the initiation of action potentials in the individual axons in the pathway. These action potentials then propagate to the synaptic terminals. The release of transmitter from the multiple afferent terminals produces a summated EPSP in the postsynaptic cell, which can be detected with an extracellular electrode. Test stimuli are delivered repeatedly at a low rate that produces stable EPSPs in the postsynaptic cell (Figs. 50.9A and B1). After a baseline period, a brief high-frequency tetanus is delivered. Subsequent test stimuli produce enhanced EPSPs (Fig. 50.9B2). The enhancement persists for many hours. Although the synaptic enhancement is stable after the tetanus,

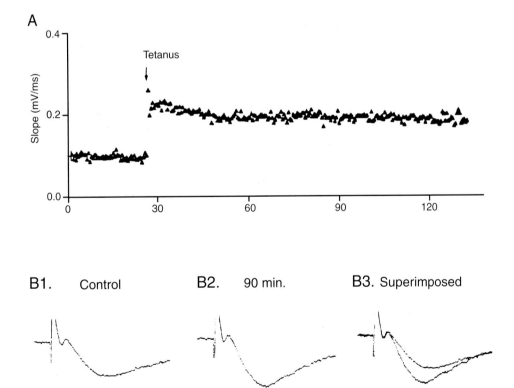

FIGURE 50.9 LTP at the CA3–CA1 synapse in the hippocampus. (A) Test stimuli are delivered repeatedly once every 10 s while the strength of the synaptic connection is monitored. Strength can be assessed by the *amplitude* of the extracellularly recorded EPSP or, as was done in this example, as the *slope* of the rising phase of the EPSP, which provides an accurate reflection of its strength. To induce LTP, two 1 s, 100 Hz tetani were delivered with a 20 interval. Subsequent test stimuli produce enhanced EPSPs. The enhancement is stable and persists for at least 2 h. Examples of extracellulary recorded field EPSPs before (B1) and 90 min after the induction of LTP (B2). In B3 the traces from B1 and B2 are superimposed. Modified from Nicoll *et al.* (1998).

LTP, like heterosynaptic facilitation of the sensori-motor synapse in *Aplysia*, has multiple temporal domains. One domain is associated with an enhancement of the EPSP that persists for about 90 min. This form of LTP is referred to as early LTP (E-LTP). A second domain referred to as late LTP (L-LTP) is associated with synaptic enhancement that persists for periods of time greater than about 90 min. As described later, different mechanisms underlie the induction and maintenance of E- and L-LTP.

Properties of Long-Term Potentiation at the CA3–CA1 Synapse Include Cooperativity, Associativity, and Input Specificity

The CA3–CA1 synapses exhibit a form of LTP characterized by "classical" properties that have been variously termed "cooperativity," "associativity," and "input specificity" (Fig. 50.10) (Brown *et al.*, 1990; Bliss and Collingridge, 1993). These "classical properties" are actually different manifestations of the same underlying mechanism that is responsible for this type of LTP. Other less commonly studied types of LTP have different signatures.

Cooperativity refers to the fact that the probability of inducing LTP, or the magnitude of the resulting change, increases with the number of stimulated afferents. Weak high-frequency stimulation, which activates fewer afferents, often fails to induce LTP (Fig. 50.10A). In contrast, strong stimulation, which activates more afferents, produces LTP more reliably (Fig. 50.10B). Thus, the additional axons recruited by higher stimulation intensities "cooperate" to trigger LTP.

Associativity was shown in preparations in which two distinct axonal inputs converged onto the same postsynaptic target. Consider the interactions between two stimulus pathways, one termed the *weak*

pathway with a small number of stimulated afferents, and the other, termed the *strong* pathway, with a large number of stimulated afferents (Fig. 50.10C). Tetanic (high-frequency) stimulation of the *weak* input by itself failed to produce LTP in that pathway unless this stimulation was paired with tetanic stimulation of the *strong* input. Thus, LTP was induced in a *weak* input only when its activity was associated with activity in the *strong* input.

Input specificity means that LTP is restricted to only the inputs that received the tetanic stimulation. The unstimulated *weak* pathway was not facilitated after the tetanus to the *strong* pathway (Fig. 50.10B).

A Hebbian Mechanism Explains the Properties of Long-Term Potentiation at the CA3-CA1 Synapse in the Hippocampus

How can these classical properties of LTP in the CA1 region of the hippocampus be explained? In the late 1940s, the Canadian psychologist Donald Hebb (1949) formulated a postulate regarding the conditions that cause synapses to change. His thinking proved to be influential and guided later experiments that probed the mechanisms behind LTP. According to Hebb's postulate:

When an axon of cell A is near enough to excite a cell B and repeatedly or persistently takes part in firing it, some growth process or metabolic change takes place in one or both cells such that A's efficiency, as one of the cells firing B, is increased. (Hebb, 1949, p. 62)

In short, coincident activity in two synaptically coupled neurons was proposed to cause increases in the synaptic strength between them. Numerous modern interpretations of Hebb's postulate exist, but most are captured by the mnemonic: "Cells that fire together, wire together."

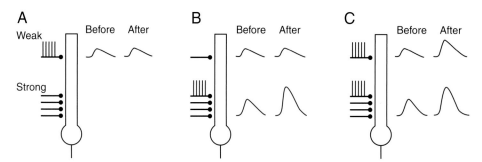

FIGURE 50.10 Features of LTP at CA3–CA1 synapses in the hippocampus. A single hippocampal pyramidal cell is shown receiving a weak and strong synaptic input. (A) Tetanic stimulation of the weak input alone does not cause LTP in that pathway (compare the EPSP before and after the tetanus). (B) Tetanic stimulus of the strong input alone causes LTP in the strong pathway, but not in the weak pathway. (C) Tetanic stimulation of both the weak and the strong pathway together causes LTP in both the weak and the strong pathway. Modified from Nicoll *et al.* (1998).

Could the classical properties of LTP all be consequences of synapses that obey a Hebbian rule? Possibly so if a critical amount of postsynaptic depolarization were a necessary condition for inducing LTP in active synapses. In this case, cooperativity would result when enough input fibers were stimulated to produce the critical amount of postsynaptic depolarization. Associativity would emerge from the fact that the strong input caused sufficient depolarization of the postsynaptic membrane during the presynaptic activity in the weak input. Input specificity would occur because LTP was induced only in those inputs to a neuron that were active at the same time that the cell was sufficiently depolarized by the strong input to that neuron. In other words, these classical phenomena could all be manifestations of a single

underlying Hebbian mechanism at the CA3–CA1 synapse.

Not all forms of LTP are Hebbian, however. Examples of non-Hebbian LTP can be found at the mossy fiber–CA3 synapse in the hippocampus and at the parallel fiber–Purkinje cell synapse in the cerebellum. These results indicate that the classical properties of cooperativity, associativity, and input specificity are not universal.

Mechanisms for Induction, Expression, and Maintenance of Long-Term Potentiation

LTP Induction

It is currently thought that there are multiple mechanisms or at least multiple second-messenger

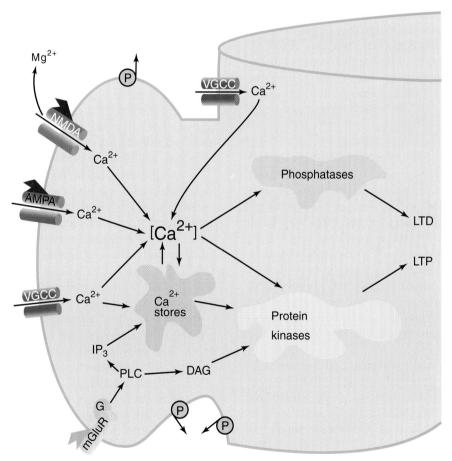

FIGURE 50.11 Events leading to LTP or LTD. The schematic depicts a postsynaptic spine with various sources of Ca²⁺. The NMDA receptor channel complex admits Ca²⁺ only after depolarization removes the Mg²⁺ block in the presence of bound glutamate. Calcium may also enter through the ligand-gated AMPA receptor channel or voltage-gated calcium channels (VGCC), which may be located on the spine head or dendritic shaft. Also, certain subtypes of metabotropic glutamate receptors (mGluRs) are coupled positively to phospholipase C (PLC), which cleaves membrane phospholipids into inositol triphosphate (IP₃) and diacylglycerol (DAG). Increased levels of IP₃ lead to the release of intracellular Ca²⁺ stores, whereas increases in DAG can activate protein kinases. Calcium pumps, located on the spine head, neck, and dendritic shaft, are hypothesized to help isolate Ca²⁺ concentration changes in the spine head from those in the dendritic shaft

pathways that can lead to persistent synaptic enhancement. Multiple mechanisms may also contribute to expression and maintenance.

Calcium ions and LTP   It is generally agreed that the induction of LTP depends on an increase in the intracellular concentration of calcium ions ($[Ca^{2+}]_i$) in some key compartment of pre- and/or postsynaptic cells (Bliss and Collingridge, 1993; Johnston *et al.*, 1992; Nicoll and Malenka, 1995). The exact role of calcium in the induction process depends on the particular form of LTP and the synaptic system. In the CA1 region of the hippocampus, LTP induction in the Sch/com synapse depends on changes in postsynaptic $[Ca^{2+}]_i$.

It is currently thought that many different pathways modulate or control $[Ca^{2+}]_i$ in the critical subcellular compartment(s) (Bliss and Collingridge, 1993; Nicoll and Malenka, 1995; Teyler *et al.*, 1994) (Fig. 50.13). Three pathways that have been studied extensively may be implicated in some aspect of LTP induction: calcium influx through ionotropic GluRs, especially the *N*-methyl-*D*-aspartate receptor (NMDAR); calcium influx through voltage-gated calcium channels (VGCCs); and calcium release from intracellular stores.

NMDAR-dependent LTP   Recall that the classical form of LTP in the CA1 region of the hippocampus has properties that can be explained in terms of a Hebbian mechanism. For this form of LTP, considerable evidence shows a role for the NMDAR (Bliss and Collingridge, 1993). Numerous pharmacological studies have shown that competitive antagonists of NMDA, such as D-2-amino-5-phosphonopentenoic acid (D-AP5, also termed AP5 or APV) or NMDA ion channel blockers, such as the noncompetitive antagonist (+)-5-methyl-10,11-dihydro-*5H*-dibenzo[*a,d*] cyclohepten-5,10-imine (MK-801), can prevent the induction of LTP.

The NMDAR has two properties that immediately suggest the nature of its role in LTP induction at Hebbian synapses (Brown *et al.*, 1990; Bliss and Collingridge, 1993). First, NMDARs are permeable to Ca^{2+} (in addition to Na^+ and K^+). This property is significant because postsynaptic $[Ca^{2+}]_i$ plays a critical role in inducing NMDAR-dependent LTP. Second, the chan-nel permeability is a function of both pre- and postsynaptic factors. Channel opening requires the neurotransmitter glutamate (or some related agonist) to bind to the NMDA site. This in turn requires presynaptic activity for glutamate release. At the usual resting membrane potential, the ionic channels of NMDARs are normally blocked by magnesium ions

(Mg^{2+}), but this channel block is relieved by sufficient depolarization of the postsynaptic membrane. Thus, the NMDAR-mediated conductance is voltage dependent, allowing Ca^{2+} entry only when presynaptic release is combined with postsynaptic depolarization.

At this point, you should recall the distinction between the properties of the NMDAR and those of the AMPAR (α-amino-3-hydroxy-5-methyl-4-isoxazole propionic acid receptor) (see Chapters 9 and 11 for details), which are also found in the postsynaptic membrane. The AMPAR does not exhibit voltage-dependent Mg^{2+} block, has relatively lower Ca^{2+} permeability, and the AMPAR-mediated conductance is essentially voltage independent. Released glutamate can potentially act on both the AMPARs and the NMDARs associated with the membrane on the dendritic spine (Fig. 50.11). With this knowledge, one can easily envision a possible role for the AMPAR and NMDAR in a Hebbian modification. Nearly concurrent presynaptic activity (producing glutamate release and binding) and postsynaptic depolarization (relieving the Mg^{2+} block) allow Ca^{2+} influx into the dendritic spine of the postsynaptic neuron. The increased $[Ca^{2+}]_i$ in some critical region of the dendritic spine, presumably very close to the NMDAR, is thought to activate Ca^{2+}-dependent enzymes, such as calmodulin-dependent kinase II (CaM kinase II), which play a key role in LTP induction (Fig. 50.11).

In qualitative terms, one can understand how these molecular events could help account for the properties of cooperativity, associativity, and spatiotemporal specificity. Active synapses release glutamate, which can bind to the NMDAR, causing Ca^{2+} influx into dendritic spines on the postsynaptic cell. This Ca^{2+} influx acts locally and results in input-specific LTP. However, the Ca^{2+} influx occurs only when the synaptic input is strong enough to depolarize the postsynaptic membrane sufficiently to relieve the Mg^{2+} block, giving rise to cooperativity (see Fig. 50.10). The depolarization itself is mediated in large part by the (voltage-independent) AMPARs, which are also colocalized on the dendritic spine (Fig. 50.11). Note that activity in a weak input by itself would not depolarize the postsynaptic cell sufficiently to relieve the Mg^{2+} block unless this activity were properly timed in relationship to activity in a strong input to the same cell. The combined depolarization of the two inputs gives rise to associativity and input specificity (Fig. 50.10).

NMDAR-independent LTP   Most of the preceding accounts of the Hebbian, NMDAR-dependent form of LTP apply only to certain synapses under some conditions, and even then it may be only one aspect of the story (Johnston *et al.*, 1992; Nicoll and Malenka, 1995). In many synapses, LTP induction does not appear to require the NMDA receptor (Johnston *et al.*, 1992; Teyler *et al.*, 1994). Even within the hippocampus, some synapses exhibit NMDAR-independent forms of LTP. For example, in the presence of the competitive antagonist APV, even the Sch/com inputs to CA1 pyramidal neurons, which are known to exhibit the classical Hebbian form of LTP that relies on the NMDAR, can exhibit an NMDAR-independent type of LTP. The onset of NMDAR-independent LTP is relatively slow (20-30 min), exhibits input specificity, and is prevented by a blocker of voltage-gated calcium channels (VGCCs). Thus, a distinction exists between "NMDA LTP" and "VGCC LTP." Other work has suggested that VGCCs are likely to be responsible for certain types of LTP in the CA3 region of the hippocampus and in the visual cortex.

The general case may be that both NMDAR-dependent and NMDAR-independent forms of LTP may coexist in the same brain region, among different classes of synaptic inputs onto the same postsynaptic neuron, and even among the same class of synaptic inputs to the same postsynaptic neuron.

LTP and mGluR   Another LTP induction mechanism involves the metabotropic glutamate receptor (mGluR) (Bashir *et al.*, 1993). Like the NMDAR, this receptor complex is found on the postsynaptic cell, but unlike the NMDAR, it is also found presynaptically. There are a variety of mGlu receptors. Class I mGluR subtypes (mGluR1 and mGluR5) are coupled to phospholipase C (PLC), which enzymatically breaks down membrane phospholipids to

form diacylglycerol and inositol 1,4,5-trisphosphate (IP$_3$) (see Fig. 50.11). DAG modulates channel activity through protein kinase C (PKC), whereas IP$_3$ mobilizes the release of Ca^{2+} from intracellular stores (Fig. 50.11), a process that does not raise intracellular Ca^{2+} concentrations as quickly as the opening of VGCCs. In contrast, class II mGluR subtypes (mGluR2 and mGluR3) are coupled to G-protein-mediated inhibition of adenylyl cyclase, an action that causes a depression of the second messenger cAMP (not shown in Fig. 50.11). The role of mGluR has been studied most extensively in the Sch/com input to hippocampal region CA1. Collingridge and co-workers reported (Bashir *et al.*, 1993) that application of the mGluR antagonist (+)-α-methyl-4-carboxyphenylglycine (MCPG) blocked LTP induction in synapses that had not previously received high-frequency stimulation (HFS), but did not prevent the induction of additional LTP at synapses that had prior exposure to HFS.

Induction of late LTP   A common requirement for the induction of both early LTP and late LTP at the CA3–CA1 synapse is the elevation of levels of intracellular calcium in the postsynaptic (i.e., CA1) neuron. Additional steps are involved in the induction of L-LTP, however. As was the case for the induction of long-term facilitation of the sensorimotor synapse in *Aplysia*, activation of PKA appears to be necessary for the induction of L-LTP (Huang *et al.*, 1996). However, in the CA1 neuron the cAMP pathway is engaged directly by the activation of a calcium-sensitive adenylyl cyclase rather than being activated by 5-HT as in *Aplysia*. (Transmitters that

---

BOX 50.1

IS MEMORY MORE THAN CHANGES IN SYNAPTIC STRENGTH?

The search for the biological basis of learning and memory has led many of the leading neuroscientists of the 20th century to direct their efforts to investigating the synapse. The focus of most recent work on LTP (and indeed the bulk of this chapter) has been to elucidate the mechanisms underlying changes in synaptic strength. Although changes in synaptic strength are certainly ubiquitous, they are not the exclusive means for the expression of neuronal plasticity associated with learning and memory. Both short-term and long-term sensitization and classical conditioning in *Aplysia* are associated with an enhancement of excitability of the sensory neurons in

addition to changes in synaptic strength. Changes in excitability of sensory neurons in the mollusc *Hermissenda* are produced by classical conditioning. In vertebrates, classical conditioning of eye-blink reflexes produces changes in the excitability of cortical neurons. Eye-blink conditioning also produces changes in the spike afterpotential of hippocampal pyramidal neurons. Finally, as described in their original report on LTP, Bliss and Lomo found that the expression of LTP was also associated with enhanced excitability.

John H. Byrne

regulate cAMP in CA1 neurons can profoundly modulate LTP, however.) Thus, at the CA1 neuron elevated levels of calcium lead to activation of adenylyl cyclase, increased synthesis of cAMP and activation of PKA. Also, like long-term facilitation in *Aplysia*, MAPK kinase is necessary for the induction of L-LTP (Dineley *et al.*, 2001). The mechanisms of activation of MAPK in CA1 neurons have not been elucidated in detail, but may involve PKA, PKC or both acting together. The final steps in the induction of L-LTP involve a PKA- and MAPK-dependent phosphorylation of CREB and induction of CREB responsive genes. These genes would encode the proteins underlying changes at the synapse (Box 50.1).

LTP Expression

Up to this point, evidence related to early events in the causal chain that triggers the induction process has been emphasized. Another question follows naturally: What biochemical and biophysical changes incorporate this modification once it has been triggered? Most of the ideas about enhanced synaptic transmission concern either increased transmitter release or increased receptivity to released transmitter. The former entails presynaptic changes, the latter, postsynaptic. Although some of the induction mechanisms discussed previously implicated a postsynaptic increase in $[Ca^{2+}]_i$, this does not necessarily imply that expression must also be postsynaptic. Ample evidence is available for ongoing two-

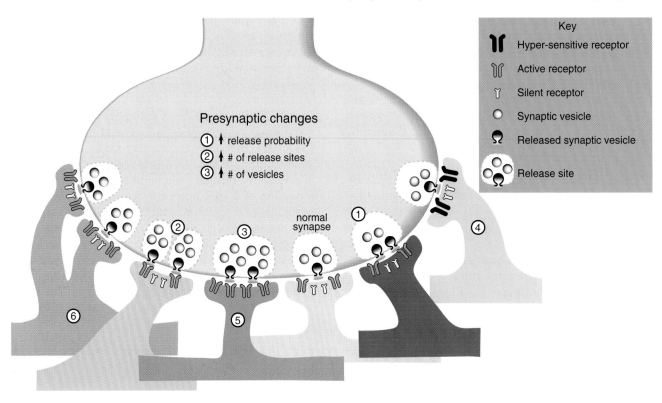

FIGURE 50.12 Schematic representation of possible loci for cellular changes involved in the enhancement of synaptic efficacy. The efficacy of a synapse can be potentiated through at least six mechanisms. First, there could be an increase in the fraction (release probability) of available presynaptic vesicles that undergo exocytosis. For example, in *mechanism 1*, two out of four available vesicles are released (i.e., 50% release probability), in contrast to the *normal synapse*, where only one out of four vesicles is released (i.e., 25% release probability). Second, there could be an increase in the number of release sites at the presynaptic neuron (*mechanism 2*). Third, the synapse could be potentiated through an increase in the number of vesicles available for release. For example, at a release site with eight vesicles, two of them will be exocytosed (instead of one) (*mechanism 3*), even if the release probability (25%) is the same as at the normal synapse. Fourth, there could be an increase in the sensitivity of the preexisting receptors to presynaptically released neurotransmitter (*mechanism 4*). Fifth, there could be an increase in the number of functional receptors (illustrated as an increase from two active receptors at the normal synapse to four at the potentiated synapse; *mechanism 5*). Finally, the synapse could also be potentiated through coordinated presynaptic and postsynaptic morphological changes, such as the growth of new synaptic contacts between the same pair of neurons (*mechanism 6*). Adapted from Wang *et al.* (1997).

way communication across the synaptic cleft, so a post-synaptic trigger could, in principle, give rise to a pre- and/or postsynaptic modification (see also Fig. 50.7). There are extensive and seemingly conflicting accounts in the literature regarding the nature of the changes responsible for the observed increase in synaptic efficacy following LTP induction. Some of the possibilities are illustrated schematically in Fig. 50.12. Regarding LTP at the CA3–CA1 synapse, evidence is growing that the expression of LTP is associated with an increase in the number of functional AMPA receptors in the post-synaptic neuron (*mechanism No. 5* in Fig. 50.12). In contrast, at the mossy fiber CA3 synapse LTP appears to involve an increase in transmitter release.

LTP Maintenance

Regardless of the ultimate nature and locus of the modification that gives rise to LTP expression, the more general problem remains of how a synaptic change can endure over long periods of time in the face of constant molecular turnover.

Maintenance of early LTP The maintenance of E-LTP is due to the persistence of phosphorylation of substrate proteins involved in expression mechanisms (see earlier discussion). This phosphorylation, in turn, is regulated by the engagement of protein kinases and phosphatases. For E-LTP, autonomously active forms of PKC and CaM kinase II appear to be particularly important.

Maintenance of late LTP The maintenance of persistent forms of LTP ultimately involves alterations in gene expression and changes in protein synthesis. High-frequency electrical stimulation in the rat hippocampus raises levels of specific mRNAs that encode transcription factors (e.g., fos, zif268), cytoskeletal proteins (e.g., arc), and signal transduction molecules such as CaM kinase II. Moreover, protein synthesis inhibitors block the late phase of LTP but not earlier phases. One interesting observation is that brain slices that received protein synthesis inhibitors just 2 h after high-frequency stimulation showed no decline in enhancement, indicating that there is a critical time window during which protein synthesis might be necessary to maintain long-term plasticity. Other work conducted *in vivo* has pointed to a still later stage of LTP that lasts for weeks and that is blocked by treatment with protein synthesis inhibitors during the tetanus (Krug *et al.*, 1984). As indicated earlier, similar multiple stages of long-term synaptic plasticity have been identified in *Aplysia*. They also are found in bees, *Drosophila*, and *Hermissenda*.

Although the involvement of new protein synthesis is consistent with the data, it immediately raises the

problem of synaptic input specificity. If neural activity ultimately affects gene expression in the nucleus, then the proteins produced in the soma could, in principle, travel to any synapse within the cell. The problem is how to modify only the appropriate synapses. One solution is for the synapse to produce a local "marker" that makes it especially susceptible to proteins sent from the nucleus (Frey and Morris, 1997; Martin *et al.*, 1997). Support of a more permanent modification might require a self-perpetuating marker and/or an enduring modification in local transport.

Links between Long-Term Potentiation and Learning

Long-term potentiation has properties that have long been considered necessary for the encoding and retrieval of information. Hebbian forms of LTP exhibit associativity, which appears to be a desirable property, and all forms of LTP appear to be well suited to rapid learning. One of the more important challenges entails linking LTP (and LTD, see later) to learning and memory (Martin *et al.*, 2000). This task has proven rather difficult to achieve, although evidence is accumulating for a causal link between LTP and memory.

Several different experimental strategies have been used to search for links between LTP and learning. These include correlating changes in synaptic efficacy with learning and blocking or saturating LTP mechanisms to show that learning has been blocked. Correlating synaptic enhancement with memory has been possible in several systems such as in amygdala circuits that mediate fear conditioning (see Chapter 51). However, there has been only limited success so far. The first obstacle to surmount is the "needle in the haystack" problem. The synaptic changes underlying learning are presumably rather specific and localized. Consequently, it is virtually impossible to place a recording electrode in the correct anatomical location. Moreover, as described later, learning may involve decreases as well as increases in synaptic strength. Coarse recording techniques might see no net change. Saturation of LTP by the massive stimulation of afferents has blocked learning, but the concern here is that the saturation may affect the basic operation of the circuit. The most widely used approach has been to block LTP with pharmacological or gene knockout techniques. This approach has generated many successes but also some striking dissociations, as blocking experiments have two problems. First, it is difficult to be sure that the agent used to block LTP does not cause some secondary effect. Thus, if memory is blocked successfully, it may be because of a block of some other process critical for memory and not the block of LTP. Second, if, for example, an agent that blocks NMDAR-*dependent* LTP fails to block learning, it may not necessarily imply that LTP does not mediate learning, but rather that the animal simply has used another non-NMDAR-*independent* memory mechanism to solve the problem.

Some of the more promising work in this area has come from studies of genetically engineered knockout mice. The first generation of knockouts prevented the expression of some factor that was thought to be necessary for LTP, such as CaM kinaseII. Although these studies were intriguing, they suffered from the fact that the consequences of a gene knockout might alter brain development and might not be confined to a specific part of the brain under study. Some of these problems have been overcome in a second generation of knockouts that have temporal as well as spatial specificity. For example, temporal and spatial control of gene expression can now be achieved using binary transgene systems such as tetracycline transactivating systems and Crc/LoxP recombination systems. The NMDAR gene in only CAI pyramidal cells of the hippocampus has been knocked out using the Crc/LoxP system (Tsien *et al.*, 1996). The results provide strong evidence in favor of the notion that NMDA receptor-dependent synaptic plasticity at CAI synapses is required for the acquisition of spatial memory. This general approach holds tremendous promise for testing hypotheses about the functional role of various forms of LTP in specific brain regions.

LONG-TERM DEPRESSION

LTD is believed by many to be the mechanism by which learning is encoded in the cerebellum (Ito, 2001), as well as a process whereby LTP could be reversed in the hippocampus and neocortex (Bear and Malenka, 1994). In the hippocampus, brief, high-frequency stimulation (e.g., four trains of 10 shocks at 100 Hz) can induce classical LTP, whereas low-frequency stimulation (LFS) over longer periods (1 Hz for 10 min) can induce LTD.

Some forms of LTD appear to be mediated by the NMDAR and seem to result from depotentiation (removal of LTP). In addition, NMDAR-independent forms of LTD exist. For example, in some brain regions, non-NMDAR-dependent LTD is due to the activation of metabotropic glutamate receptors. Another example of NMDAR-independent LTD is found in the parallel fiber input to Purkinje cells in the cerebellum. In this case, LTD is induced by the combined increase in intracellular levels of Ca^{2+} (by

activity) in postsynaptic Purkinje cells and activation of metabotropic glutamate receptors produced by the release of glutamate from parallel fibers.

It should be clear that LTD, like LTP, occurs in many forms. Furthermore, these forms may vary in different brain regions and sometimes among different inputs to the same brain region. Even within the CA1 region, the Sch/com input may exhibit both NMDAR-dependent and NMDAR-independent forms of LTD, and the latter could be mediated partly by Ca^{2+} entry through VGCCs.

Calcium levels in the dendritic spines appear to be a common locus for the induction on NMDAR-dependent LTP and LTD. For example, at the Sch/com input to CA1, both LTP and LTD can be blocked by injecting Ca^{2+} chelators into the postsynaptic cell. If both LTP and LTD are triggered by Ca^{2+} entry, then how are their induction processes different? Presumably, more Ca^{2+} influx occurs during an LTP-inducing HFS than during an LTD-inducing LFS. One formal molecular model developed by John Lisman incorporates this Ca^{2+}-dependent, bidirectional control of synaptic strength. In this model, high $[Ca^{2+}]_i$ activates a protein kinase that phosphorylates a protein causing LTP induction, whereas low $[Ca^{2+}]_i$ activates a protein phosphatase that dephosphorylates this protein and causes LTD. The synaptic strength thus depends on which of these competing processes is most active, which in turn will be a function of the pattern of activity experienced by the cell (Fig. 50.11).

Summary

The understanding of LTP and LTD is evolving rapidly (Malenka and Nicoll, 1999). For example, whereas the *N*-methyl-D-aspartate receptor was once the pivotal focus of long-term potentiation research, it is now clear that voltage-gated calcium channels and metabotropic glutamate receptors as well as other mechanisms should be considered. It has also become evident that high-frequency stimulation is but one end of a spectrum of stimulations that can induce synaptic changes. Lower stimulation frequencies can induce long-term depression, which may share some common molecular mechanisms with LTP. Finally, several stages in the maintenance of LTP have been identified, and probably more will be found. A remaining challenge is to clarify the varieties of LTP and LTD mechanisms and to demonstrate their functional significance by establishing convincing links to the encoding and retrieval of information.

HOW DOES A CHANGE IN SYNAPTIC STRENGTH STORE A COMPLEX MEMORY?

The relationship between the synaptic changes and the behavior of conditioned reflexes can be straightforward because the locus for the plastic change is part of the mediating circuit. Thus, the change in the strength of the sensorimotor synapse in *Aplysia* can be related to the memory for sensitization (e.g., Fig. 4A1). However, the idea that an increase in synaptic strength leads to an enhanced behavioral response,

and a decrease in synaptic strength leads to a decreased behavioral response, can be misleading. For example, a decrease in synaptic strength in a postsynaptic neuron that exerts an inhibitory action can be translated into an enhanced behavioral response. Indeed, in the parallel fiber-to-Purkinje cell connection in the cerebellum, such a disinhibition is precisely the mechanism that has been proposed to mediate classical conditioning of the eye-blink reflex (see Chapter 51 for a discussion of this form of conditioning). Nevertheless, for relatively simple reflex systems in which the circuit is well understood, it is possible to directly relate a change in synaptic strength to

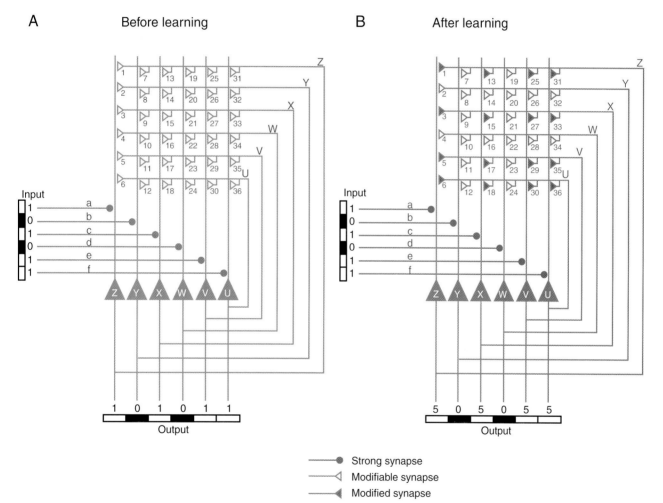

FIGURE 50.13 Autoassociation network for recognition memory. The artificial circuit consists of six input pathways that make strong connections to each of six output neurons. The output neurons have axon collaterals that make synaptic connections (numbered 1–36) with each of the output cells. (A) A pattern represented by activity in the input lines or axons (a, b, c, d, e, f) is presented to the network. A 1 represents an active axon (e.g., a spike), whereas a 0 represents an inactive axon. The input pathways make strong synapses (•) with the postsynaptic output cells. Thus, output cells (u, v, w, x, y, z) generate a pattern that is a replica of the input pattern. The collateral synapses were initially weak and do not contribute to the output. Nevertheless, the activity in the collaterals that occurred in conjunction (assume minimal delays within the circuit) with the input pattern led to a strengthening of a subset of the 36 synapses. (B) A second presentation of the input produces an output pattern that is an amplified, but an otherwise intact, replica of the input. An incomplete input pattern can be used as a cue to retrieve the complete pattern.

learning. However, in most other examples of memory, it is considerably less clear how the synaptic changes are induced and, once induced, how the information is retrieved. This is especially true in memory systems that involve the storage of information for patterns, facts, and events. Neurobiologists have turned to artificial neural circuits to gain insights into these issues.

A simple network that can store and "recognize" patterns is illustrated in Fig. 50.13. The network is artificial, but nevertheless is inspired by actual circuitry in the CA3 region of the hippocampus. In this example, six different input projections make synaptic connections with the dendrites of each of six postsynaptic neurons (Fig. 50.13A). The postsynaptic neurons serve as the output of the network. Input projections can carry multiple types of patterned information, and these patterns can be complex. In order to simplify the present discussion, consider that the particular input pathway in Fig. 50.13A carries information regarding the pattern of neural activity induced by a single brief flash of a spatial pattern of light. For example, activity in the top pathway (line a) might represent light falling on the temporal region of the retina, whereas activity in the pathway on the bottom (line f) might represent light falling on the nasal region of the retina. Thus, the spatial pattern of an image falling upon the retina could be reconstructed from the pattern of neuronal activity over the n (in this case 6) input projections to the network.

Three aspects of the circuit endow it with the ability to store and retrieve patterns. First, each of the input lines makes a sufficiently strong connection with its corresponding postsynaptic cell to activate it reliably. Second, each output cell (z to u) sends an axon collateral that makes an excitatory connection with itself as well as the other five output cells. This pattern of synaptic connectivity leads to a network of 36 synapses (a total of 42, including the 6 input synapses). Third, each of the 36 synaptic connections are modifiable through an LTP-like mechanism (see earlier discussion). Specifically, the strength of a particular synaptic connection is initially weak, but it will increase if the presynaptic *and* postsynaptic neurons are active at the same time. The circuit configuration with the embedded synaptic "learning rule" leads to an autoassociation or autocorrelation matrix. The autoassociation is derived from the fact that the output is fed back to the input where it associates with itself.

Now consider the consequences of presenting the patterned input to the network of Fig. 50.13A. The input pattern will activate the six postsynaptic cells in such a way as to produce an output pattern that will be a replica of the input pattern. In addition, the pattern will induce changes in the synaptic strength of the active synapses in the network. For example, synapse 3 will be strengthened because the postsynaptic cell, cell z, and the presynaptic cell, cell x, will be active at the same time. Note also that synapses 1, 5, and 6 will be strengthened as well. This occurs because these input pathways to cell z are also active. Thus, all synapses that are active at the same time as cell z will be strengthened. When the pattern is presented again as in Fig. 50.13B, the output of the cell will not only be governed by the input, but also by the feedback connections, a subset of which were strengthened (Fig. 50.13B, filled synapses) by the initial presentation of the stimulus. Thus, for output cell z, a component of its activity will be derived from input a, but components will also come from synapses 1, 3, 5, and 6. If each of the initially strong and newly modified synapses is assumed to contribute equally to the firing of output cell z, the activity would be five times greater than the activity produced by input a before the learning. After learning, the output is an amplified version of the input but the basic features of the pattern are preserved.

Note that the "memory" for the pattern does not reside in any one synapse or in any one cell. Rather, it is *distributed* throughout the network at multiple sites. The properties of these types of autoassociation networks have been examined by James Anderson, Teuvo Kohonen, David Marr, Edmond Rolls, David Wilshaw, and their colleagues and found to exhibit a number of phenomena that would be desirable for a biological recognition memory system. For example, such networks exhibit pattern completion. If a partial input pattern is presented, the autoassociation network can complete the pattern in the sense that it can produce an output that is approximately what is expected for the full input pattern. Thus, any part of the stored pattern can be used as a cue to retrieve the complete pattern. For the example of Fig. 50.13, the input pattern was {101011}. This pattern led to an output pattern of {505055}. If the input pattern were degraded to {101000}, the output pattern would be {303022}. Some change in the strength of firing occurs, but the basic pattern is preserved. Autoassociation networks also exhibit a phenomenon known as graceful degradation, which means that the network can still function even if some of the input connections or postsynaptic cells are lost. This property arises from the distributed representation of the memory within the circuit.

Summary

The concept of distributed representation of memory crosses multiple levels of organization of memory systems. Multiple brain systems are involved in memory, and memory is distributed among synapses in a particular memory circuit (Fig. 50.13). Also, memory at any one synapse is represented by multiple cellular changes (Figs. 50.4, 50.6, and 50.11). The reductionist approaches described in this chapter have provided key insights into cellular memory mechanisms. In the near future, a major experimental question to be answered is the extent to which the mechanisms for learning are common both within any one animal and between different species. Although many common features are emerging, there seem to be some differences. Thus, it will be important to understand the extent to which specific mechanisms are used selectively for one type of learning and not another. Irrespective of the particular example of learning and memory that is analyzed, whether it be simple or complex, it will be important to pay attention to three major details: details of the circuit interactions, details of the learning rule, and details of the intrinsic biophysical properties of the neurons within the circuit.

Acknowledgments

I thank A. Eskin, D. Fioravante, D. Johnston, M. Mauk, G. Phares, P. Smolen, and D. Sweatt for helpful comments on the chapter.

References

Bailey, C. H., Chen, M., Keller, F., and Kandel, E. R. (1992). Serotonin-mediated endocytosis of apCAM: An early step of learning-related synaptic growth in *Aplysia. Science* **256**, 645–649.

Bailey, C.H., and Kandel, E.R. (1993). Structural changes accompanying memory storage. *Annu. Rev. Physiol.* **55**, 397–426.

Barrionuevo, G., and Brown, T. H. (1983). Associative long-term potentiation in hippocampal slices. *Proc. Natl. Acad. Sci. USA* **80**, 7347–7351.

Bartsch, D., Ghirardi, M., Skehel, P. A., Karl, K. A., Herder, S. P., Chen, M., Bailey, C. H., and Kandel, E. R. (1995). Aplysia CREB2 represses long-term facilitation: Relief of repression converts transient facilitation into long-term functional and structural change. *Cell* **83**, 979–992.

Bashir, Z. I., Bortolotto, Z. A., Davies, C. H., Beretta, N., Irving, A. J., Seal, A. J., Henley, J. M., Jane, D. E., Watkins, J. C., and Collingridge, G. L. (1993). Induction of LTP in hippocampus needs synaptic activation of glutamate metabotropic receptors. *Nature (Lond.).* **363**, 69–72.

Bliss, T. V. P., and Collingridge, G. L. (1993) A synaptic model of memory: Long-term potentiation in the hippocampus. *Nature (Lond.).* **361**, 31–39.

Brown, T. H., Ganong, A. H., Kairiss, E. W., and Keenan, C. L. (1990). Hebbian synapses: Biophysical mechanisms and algorithms. *Annu. Rev. Neurosci.* **13**, 475–512.

Byrne, J. H., and Kandel, E. R. (1996). Presynaptic facilitation revisited: State- and time-dependence. *J. Neurosci.* **16**(2), 425–435.

Byrne, J. H., Zwartjes, R., Homayouni, R., Critz, S., and Eskin, A. (1993) Roles of second messenger pathways in neuronal plastic-ity and in learning and memory: Insights gained from *Aplysia. Adv. Second Messenger Phosphoprotein Res.* **27**, 47–108.

Chain, D. G., Casadio, A., Schacher, S., Hegde, A. N., Valbrun, M., Yamamoto, N., Goldberg, A. L., Bartsch, D., Kandel, E. R., and Schwartz, J. H. (1999) Mechanisms for generating the autonomous cAMP-dependent protein kinase required for long-term facilitation in *Aplysia. Neuron.* **22**, 147–156.

Cleary, L. J., Byrne, J. H., and Frost, W. N. (1995). Role of interneurons in defensive withdrawal reflexes in *Aplysia. Learn Memory* **2**, 133–151.

Cleary, L. J., Lee, W. L., and Byrne, J. H. (1998). Cellular correlates of long-term sensitization in *Aplysia. J. Neurosci.* **18**, 5988–5998.

Frey, U., and Morris, R. G. M. (1997). Synaptic tagging and long-term potentiation. *Nature (Lond.) .* **385**, 533–536.

Ghirardi, M., Montarolo, P. G., and Kandel, E. R. (1995). A novel intermediate stage in the transition between short- and long-term facilitation in the sensory to motor neuron synapse of *Aplysia. Neuron* **14**, 413–420.

Hawkins, R. D., Kandel, E. R., and Siegelbaum, S. (1993). Learning to modulate transmitter release: Themes and variations in synaptic plasticity. *Annu. Rev. Neurosci.* **16**, 625–665.

Hebb, D. O. (1949). "The Organization of Behavior." Wiley (Interscience), New York.

Huang, Y.-Y., Nguyen, P. V., Abel, T., and Kandel, E. R. (1996). Long-lasting forms of synaptic potentiation in the mammalian hippocampus. *Learn. Mem.* **3**, 74–85.

Johnston, D., Williams, D., Jaffe, D., and Gray, R. (1992). NMDA-receptor-independent long-term potentiation. *Annu. Rev. Physiol.* **54**, 489–505.

Krug, M., Loessner, B., and Ott, T. (1984) Anisomycin blocks the late phase of long-term potentiation in the dentate gyrus of freely moving rats. *Brain Res. Bull.* **13**, 39–42.

Lechner, H. A., and Byrne, J. H. (1998). New perspectives on classical conditioning: A synthesis of Hebbian and Non-Hebbian mechanisms. *Neuron* **20**, 355–385.

Levenson, J., Endo, S., Kategaya, L. S., Fernandez, R. I., Brabham, D. G., Chin, J., Byrne, J. H., and Eskin, A. (2000). Long-term regulation of neuronal high-affinity glutamate and glutamate uptake in *Aplysia. Proc. Nat. Acad. Sci.* **97**, 12858–12863.

Martin, K. C., Michael, D., Rose, J. C., Barad, M., Casadio, A., Zhu, H., and Kandel, E. R. (1997) MAP kinase translocates into the nucleus of the presynaptic cell and is required for long-term facilitation in *Aplysia. Neuron* 18, 899–912.

Martin, K. C., Casadeo, A., Zhu, H. E. Y., Rose, J. C., Chen, M., Bailey, C. H., and Kandel, E. R. (1997). Synapse-specific, long-term facilitation of *Aplysia* sensory to motor synapses: A function for local protein synthesis in memory storage. *Cell* **91**, 927–938.

Nicoll, R. A., Kauer, J. A., and Malenka, R. C. (1988). The curent excitement of long-term potentiation. *Neuron* **1**, 97–103.

Nicoll, R. A., and Malenka, R. C. (1995) Contrasting properties of two forms of long-term potentiation in the hippocampus. *Nature (Lond.)* **377**, 115–118.

Rachlin, H. (1991). "Introduction to Modern Behaviourism," 3rd Ed. Freesman, New York.

Sutton, M. A., Masters, S. E., Bagnall, M. W., Carew, T. J. (2001). Molecular mechanisms underlying a unique intermediate phase of memory in *Aplysia. Neuron* **31**, 143–154.

Teyler, T. J., Cavus, I., Coussens, C., DiScenna, P., Grover, L., Lee, Y. P., and Little, Z. (1994) Multideterminant role of calcium in hippocampal synaptic plasticity. *Hippocampus* **4**(6), 623–634.

Tsien, J. Z., Huerta, P. T., and Tonegawa, S. (1996). The essential role of hippocampal CA1 NMDA receptor-dependent synaptic plasticity in spatial memory. *Cell* **87**, 1317–1326.

Wang, J. H., Ko, G. Y., and Kelly, P. T. (1997). Cellular and molecular basis of memory: Synaptic and neuronal plasticity. *J. Chin. NeuroPhysiol.* **14**, 264–293.

Zhang, F., Endo, S., Cleary, L. J., Eskin, A., and Byrne, J. H. (1997) Role of transforming growth factor-b in long-term facilitation in *Aplysia. Science* **275**, 1318–1320.

Suggested Readings

Agners, A., Fioravante, D., Chin, J., Cleary, L. J., Bean, A. J., and Byrne, J. H. (2002). Serotonin stimulates phosphorylation of aplysia synapsin and alters its subcellular distribution in sensory neurons. *J. Neurosci.* **22**, 5412–5422.

Bear, M. F., and Malenka, R. C. (1994). Synaptic plasticity: LTP and LTD. *Curr. Opin. Neurobiol.* **4**, 389–399.

Byrne, J. H. (1987). Cellular analysis of associative learning. *Physiol. Rev.* **67**, 329–439.

Bliss, T. V. P., and Collingridge, G. L. (1993). A synaptic model of memory: Long-term potentiation in the hippocampus. *Nature (Lond.)* **361**, 31–39.

Carew, T. J. (2000). "Behavioral Neurobiology." Sinauer, Sunderland, MA.

Dineley, K. T., Weeber, E. J., Atkins, C., Adams, J. P., Anderson, A. E., and Sweatt, J. D. (2001). Leitmotifs in the biochemistry of LTP induction: Amplification, integration and coordination. *J. Neurochem.* **77**, 961–971.

Ito, M. (2001). Cerebellar long-term depression: Characterization, signal transduction, and functional roles. *Physiol. Rev.* **81**(3), 1143–1195.

Malenka, R. C., and Nicoll, R. A. (1999). Long-term potentiation: A decade of progress? *Science* **285**, 1870–1874.

Martin, S. J., Grimwood, P. D., and Morris, R. G. (2000). Synaptic plasticity and memory: An evaluation of the hypothesis. *Annu. Rev. Neurosci.* **23**, 649–711.

John H. Byrne

51

Learning and Memory: Brain Systems

Memory is a remarkable property of the brain. It allows us to accomplish numerous tasks that are essential to our everyday lives: recalling personal experiences, learning facts and gaining conceptual knowledge, recognizing objects and people, acquiring coordinated skills and habits, and forming attractions and aversions to specific stimuli. The initial scientific studies of memory were guided by the reductionistic view that memory is a unitary or monolithic entity—a single faculty of the mind and brain. In recent years, however, the assumption of a unitary memory has been overturned by converging evidence from psychology and neuroscience indicating the existence of multiple memory systems that can be dissociated from one another. These studies have led to the current view that memory should be conceived as a fundamental property of brain systems, and a natural outcome of the various processing activities of the brain. According to this view, memory is a critical element of, and is integrally tied to, the various functions of many brain systems. It is both a part and a product of the ongoing activities of each functional system.

This chapter begins with a historical introduction and with a summary of key concepts and pertinent early findings from humans and experimental animals. The chapter then presents a current conceptualization of multiple memory systems in the brain. This will be followed by a description of experimental analyses of the distinct memory systems and then by a characterization of the role of the cerebral cortex in several types of memory.

EARLY PROPOSALS ABOUT DIFFERENT FORMS OF MEMORY

The idea of multiple forms of memory has roots in the 19th century. Two early proponents of the idea were the European thinkers Franz Joseph Gall and Maine de Biran. Gall, founder of the phrenological movement, focused on the notion that each specialized faculty of the mind is concerned with particular contents (e.g., music, mathematics) and maintains its own memory. Gall believed that the differential development of these separate faculties accounted for the common observation that some people can remember certain kinds of information very well but have great difficulty remembering other kinds of information. While Gall's specific characterizations of cortical areas were entirely wrong, later 19th-century neurologists and neurophysiologists demonstrated the existence of distinct cortical zones that are specialized to process different kinds of information, including centers for auditory, visual, and motor functions. In the 20th century, studies would show that these areas are involved in modality-specific memory functions. Thus, as is described later, Gall's general notion that the cortex is composed of distinct modules that are dedicated to specific faculties of information processing and memory was essentially correct.

The philosopher Maine de Biran distinguished among three different types of memory: *representative memory*, concerned with recollection of ideas and events; *mechanical memory*, concerned with acquisition of habits and skills; and *sensitive memory*, concerned with memory for feelings. The latter two kinds of memory had in common that they could operate without conscious recall and could be the source of relatively inflexible behavior. Biran's formulation did not involve consideration of the anatomy or function of brain systems, and there is no record that his theory influenced subsequent research on memory. Yet, as it turns out, he was prescient in describing a division of memory systems that is strongly supported by modern cognitive neuroscience.

At the end of the 19th century, the philosopher and psychologist William James maintained the distinction between habits and conscious memory. He envisioned walking, writing, fencing, singing, and other routines as mediated by the concatenation of habits, organized to generate the serial production of unconscious movements and sensations. In contrast, James viewed memory as the conscious recollection of events and facts. He argued that the underlying foundation of recall was a complex, yet systematically organized set of associations. The goodness of memory, he believed, was as much dependent on the number and variety of associations in the network as on the strength of those associations. In addition, James was first to separate a *short-term memory* capacity by which one can hold new information on-line, e.g., in carrying on a conversation or repeating a telephone number, from *long-term memory*, the permanent store of information that is not maintained in consciousness and must be retrieved during subsequent recollection.

After this promising beginning, ideas about multiple forms of memory were overwhelmed in the first half of the 20th century by a drive toward reductionism in the form of rigorous behavioral analysis, which sought to account for memory in terms of simple associative mechanisms. This approach was reflected strongly both in the systematic analysis of human verbal memory, begun in the 1880s by Herman Ebbinghaus, and in the "behaviorist" school that led to behavioral investigations of animal learning. However, the reductionist approach was not universally accepted, generating spirited debate about whether the phenomena of memory could be explained satisfactorily by simple habit-like mechanisms or instead required a more complex, more cognitive explanation.

EMERGENCE OF THE MODERN CONCEPTION OF MEMORY SYSTEMS

By the middle of the 20th century, there were several proposals that offered reconciliation by returning to a distinction between habit-like and cognitive forms of memory. However, it was not until the 1960s and 1970s that experimental evidence for different types of memory appeared and the study of memory systems emerged as a central research topic in psychology and neuroscience. With the introduction of cognitive neuroscience, the issue has now been largely resolved by evidence for the existence of different types of memory supported by distinct brain systems.

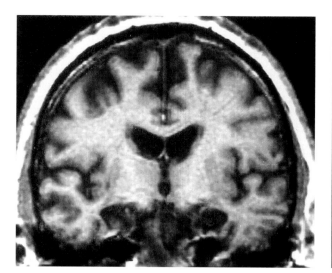
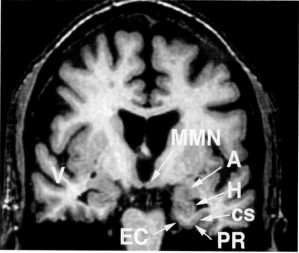

FIGURE 51.1 (Left) Magnetic resonance imaging scan showing the removal of medial temporal lobe structures in patient H.M. The lesion included all of the entorhinal cortex, most of the perirhinal cortex, and amygdala, and about one-half of the hippocampus. (Right) Scan of a normal control subject showing the structures removed in H.M. A, amygdala; cs, collateral sulcus; EC, entorhinal cortex; H, hippocampus; MMN, medial mammillary nucleus; PR, perirhinal cortex. From Corkin *et al.* (1997).

The Discovery of Selective Memory Deficits Supports Distinctions between Memory Systems

A major breakthrough came with observations of the amnesic patient H.M., who in 1953 sustained a large bilateral resection of the medial temporal lobes in an effort to relieve severe epilepsy (Scoville and Milner, 1957; Fig. 51.1; see Box 51.1). Following surgery, H.M. exhibited a profound impairment in retaining and recollecting virtually any kind of new information. He performed extremely poorly on tests of memory for short stories, word lists, pictures, and a wide range of other materials. Thus his impairment was characterized as a "global" amnesia. However, despite the severity and broad scope of his deficit in forming new lasting memories, H.M. had a normal capacity for immediate memory, confirming the distinction between short-term and long-term memory proposed by William James. Furthermore, it was observed that H.M. and other amnesic patients could learn new motor skills and could benefit in identifying objects or words following recent exposure to them (see discussion of "priming," later). Although the implications of these observations for the notion of separate memory systems were not immediately

---

This 27-year-old motor winder, a high school graduate, had had minor seizures since the age of 10 and major seizures since the age of 16. Despite heavy and varied anticonvulsant medication, the major attacks had increased in frequency and severity throughout the years until the patient was quite unable to work. The etiology of this patient's attacks is not clear. He was knocked down by a bicycle at the age of 9 and was unconscious for 5 min afterward, sustaining a laceration of the left supraorbital region. Later radiological studies, however, including two pneumoencephalograms, have been completely normal, and the physical examination has always been negative. Electroencephalographic studies have consistently failed to show any localized epileptogenic area. On September 1, 1953, bilateral medial temporal-lobe resection was carried out, extending posteriorly for a distance of 8 cm from the midpoints of the tips of the temporal lobes, with the temporal horns constituting the lateral edges of resection. (MRI images obtained by Corkin *et al.*, 1997 indicate that the rostrocaudel extent of the resection is just over 5 cm.)

After operation, the patient was drowsy for a few days, but his subsequent recovery was uneventful apart from the grave memory loss already described. There has been no neurological deficit. An electroencephalogram taken 1 year after operation showed increased spike-and-wave activity, which was maximal over the frontal areas and bilaterally synchronous. He continues to have seizures, but these are less incapacitating than before.

A psychological examination was performed on April 26, 1955. The memory defect was immediately apparent. The patient gave the date as March 1953 and his age as 27. Just before coming into the examining room, he had been talking to Dr. Karl Pribram, yet he had no recollection of this at all and denied that anyone had spoken to him. In conversation, he reverted constantly to boyhood events and seemed scarcely to realize that he had had an operation.

On formal testing, the contrast between his good general intelligence and his defective memory was most striking. On the Wechsler–Bellevue Intelligence Scale, he achieved a full-scale IQ rating of 112, which compares favorably with the preoperative rating of 104, the improvement in arithmetic being particularly striking. An extensive test battery failed to reveal any deficits in perception, abstract thinking, or reasoning ability, and his motivation remained excellent throughout. On the Wechsler Memory Scale, his immediate recall of stories and drawings fell far below the average level, and on the "associate learning" subtest of this scale he obtained zero scores for the hard word associations, low scores for the easy associations, and failed to improve with repeated practice. These findings are reflected in the low memory quotient of 67. Moreover, on all tests, we found that once he had turned to a new task, the nature of the preceding one could no longer be recalled nor the test recognized if repeated.

In summary, this patient appears to have a complete loss of memory for events subsequent to bilateral medial temporal lobe resection 19 months before, together with a partial retrograde amnesia for the years leading up to his operation, but early memories are seemingly normal and there is no impairment of personality or general intelligence.

Edited from Scoville and Milner (1957).

Howard B. Eichenbaum

apparent, the finding that amnesic patients could exhibit some kind of new learning despite poor recollection of their recent experiences proved central to later ideas about multiple memory systems.

Another major advance came when Cohen and Squire (1980) proposed that examples of spared abilities in amnesia were indicative of a large domain of preserved learning capacities mediated by different brain systems. Their conclusion was based on the observation in amnesic patients of complete preservation of the acquisition and retention of a perceptual skill (reading mirror-reversed words). These patients showed fully intact skilled performance, yet were markedly impaired both in recognizing the particular words on which they trained and in recollecting their training experiences. Thus, the patients could acquire skilled performance at a normal rate, as they participated in a series of training experiences, but they had a diminished capacity to explicitly remember or consciously recollect those training experiences or their contents. Cohen and Squire attributed the observed dissociation between spared and impaired performance to the operation of distinct forms of memory, which they called *procedural memory* and *declarative memory*, respectively. These forms of memory were viewed as functionally distinct memory systems, one dedicated to the tuning and modification of networks that support skilled performance and the other to the encoding, storage, and retrieval of memories for specific facts and events. A similar distinction was subsequently made by Daniel Schacter and colleagues between *implicit* and *explicit* expression of memory. The dissociation of these different forms of memory in patients with circumscribed brain damage permitted a link to neuroanatomy, with declarative or explicit memory critically dependent on the medial temporal lobe (hippocampus and surrounding cortical areas) and midline diencephalic structures damaged in the amnesic syndrome. Procedural or implicit memory was viewed as mediated by various brain systems that are specialized for particular types of skilled performance in different perceptual, motor, or cognitive domains. In recognition of the large number of such abilities, the kind of memory that is intact in amnesia, and independent of the medial temporal lobe and diencephalic structures, is sometimes referred to as nondeclarative.

Observations on Experimental Animals Provided Parallel Evidence for Multiple Memory Systems

Studies of experimental animals have also identified distinct domains of memory mediated by different brain structures and systems, and these are now viewed as largely congruent with the current conception of amnesia in human patients. In early studies, this line of work focused particularly on the hippocampus. In one proposal, O'Keefe and Nadel (1978) summarized a large body of literature on the effects of hippocampal damage on different behavioral tasks and concluded that animals with damage to the hippocampus are severely impaired at many forms of spatial learning. They proposed that the hippocampus is important for spatial cognition and memory. Furthermore, they characterized this kind of memory as rapidly acquired and driven by curiosity rather than by rewards and punishments, properties that are consistent with characterizations of declarative memory in humans.

Despite strong evidence of a role for the hippocampus in some kinds of spatial learning, the narrow view that hippocampal function is limited to space in rats did not match the global memory function that had been identified for the hippocampal region in humans. Also, a number of the subsequent studies using animals demonstrated deficits in many types of nonspatial learning following hippocampal damage (see examples in the section on Declarative Memory). The view of hippocampal function that has emerged as a result of these studies suggests that the hippocampus mediates the organization of related memories and the flexible expression of memory, i.e., the ability to use memories to guide behavior in situations other than a repetition of the learning event. In contrast, direct modifications in performance systems that support stimulus–response or stimulus–reward associations proceed without hippocampal involvement. Although a full consensus on how to characterize these capacities has not emerged, there is general agreement on two points: (1) some type of organized representation of multiple stimuli and experiences is dependent on hippocampal function and (2) specific stimulus–reward and stimulus–response associations are mediated by other brain systems.

Memory Systems Defined and Identified

Initially the separate lines of investigation on humans and animals were divergent, and suggested to some that the functions of the hippocampal region might differ between species. However, subsequent findings from these two areas have converged, both in their characterizations of the kind of memory that is dependent on the hippocampal region and in their identification of functional domains and anatomical pathways associated with other types of memory. Although concepts of memory systems are still evolving, evidence from psychology and neuroscience has identified specific sets of memory systems in humans and in animals, and these putative systems overlap substantially across species.

In recent years, considerable progress has been made in both humans and animals in identifying the brain system that supports declarative memory and brain systems that mediate the different forms of non-declarative memory (Eichenbaum and Cohen, 2001). The current conceptualization that encompasses much of the data from these studies incorporates both psychological and anatomical distinctions between memory systems. Within this scheme, a *memory system* is defined by both a unique set of operating characteristics and by unique brain structures and connections. Memory systems are not separated according to conventional distinctions between stimulus modalities (e.g., vision, audition) or between response modalities (e.g., manual, verbal). All the known memory systems have access to all sensory modalities and all the systems can reach multiple output routes. The critical distinctions between systems involve differences in the nature of the memory representation, its organization, and the flexibility with which memory can be expressed. Each system has at least some brain structures that are unique to that system. However, it is important to recognize that the anatomical pathways of the various memory systems are not entirely separate. For example, large areas of the cerebral cortex play a role in most systems (see later).

A sketch of some of the most prominent memory systems currently under study is provided in Fig. 51.2. One system supports *declarative memory* and involves connections from the cortical association areas to the hippocampus via the cortical areas immediately surrounding the hippocampus. The main output of hippocampal processing is back to the same cortical areas, which are thought to be the long-term repository of declarative memories. The second major memory system is specialized for *procedural memory* and is composed of two main subsystems. One subsystem involves the neostriatum as a nodal stage in the association of sensory and motor cortical information and mediates habit and skill learning. The other main subsystem involves cortical and subcortical sensory pathways through the cerebellum and mediates sensori-motor adaptations. The third major memory system is specialized for *emotional memory*. This system involves the amygdala as a nodal stage in the association of exteroceptive sensory inputs via the cortex and subcortical areas to emotional outputs effected via the hypothalamic–pituitary axis and autonomic nervous system, as well as other brain areas. In addition, the amygdala has outputs to both of the other major memory systems, and these pathways subserve the capacity for emotional arousal to modulate memory processing in those systems.

In this scheme, a major structure in each memory system is the expanse of the cerebral cortex, in particular the so-called "association" areas. Circuits within

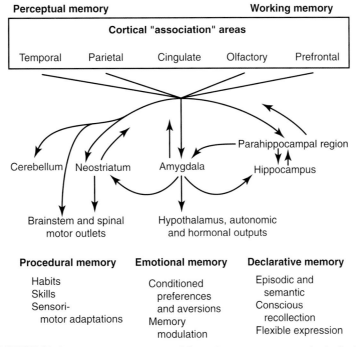

FIGURE 51.2 A current conception of the major memory systems in the brain.

the cerebral cortex mediate *perceptual memory*, the ability to tune and bias the processing of sensory stimuli, and *working memory*, the ability to hold and manipulate information in consciousness. Furthermore, the cortex provides major inputs to the systems that support distinct memory functions in declarative memory, procedural memory, and emotional memory. However, this is not to say that all memory requires cortical storage. In some cases, learning can also be supported by subcortical structures (see examples of fear conditioning and classical eyeblink conditioning later).

Summary

The notion that there are different forms of memory has a long history. Early proposals distinguished among different faculties of the mind and included ideas about fundamentally distinct types of memory based on philosophical, neuroanatomical, and psychological considerations. Most of the 20th century was dominated by reductionistic attempts to find a unitary explanation of memory based on simple associative mechanisms, although these efforts were balanced by evidence that memory is richly organized in both humans and other animals.

The modern era of research on memory systems began with the discovery that brain damage could result in severe impairment in memory without affecting other functions. In addition, the existence of multiple memory systems has now been demonstrated in both humans and animals, and there is considerable convergence in the findings from these lines of study. There is broad consensus that one system, including the hippocampus and surrounding cortex, supports declarative memory. This system mediates a capacity for the organization of memories and flexible memory expression. Several forms of nondeclarative memory are mediated by other identified brain systems. These systems include a procedural memory system that involves a cortical-neostriatal circuit and the cerebellum, and an emotional memory system that mediates attractions and aversions to specific stimuli and that modulates memory processing in the other systems. Each of these main memory systems utilizes information from the cerebral cortex. The following sections provide further details on the distinctions between these systems.

DECLARATIVE MEMORY

Studies of H.M. and other amnesic patients have revealed characteristics of memory dependent on the hippocampus and surrounding cortex. Amnesic patients suffer a pervasive disorder in memory, a deficit that is "global" with respect to stimulus modalities and verbal and nonverbal memory expression. Yet pure amnesia is a disorder that is highly selective in three important ways. First, the impairment is selective to memory. Other higher order perceptual, motor, and intellectual functions are intact. Across a broad range of neuropsychological tests, amnesic patients perform well on assessments of sensory capacities, motor coordination, intelligence, and language performance.

Second, even within memory function, the disorder is selective to temporally defined domains of learning and memory capacity. Typically, amnesic patients can remember material learned long before the accident, disease, or operation that caused the amnesia. Thus, memory for language and childhood events are intact. In contrast, memory for events for some period of months or years preceding the onset of amnesia is impaired. In addition, the capacity for short-term memory (working memory) is typically intact. Amnesic patients can immediately reproduce a list of six or seven numbers as well as control subjects. Thus the "span" of short-term memory is normal. However, the memory deficit becomes evident as soon as immediate memory span is exceeded or after a delay is interposed that includes some distraction to interrupt rehearsal.

Third, the deficit in forming long-term memories is specific to declarative memory. Typically, amnesic patients are impaired at learning specific personal events (*episodic memory*) and at learning new facts (*semantic memory*). Moreover, they are impaired whenever the memory task requires the explicit expression of memory, as in free recall or recognition. In contrast, amnesic patients demonstrate normal acquisition of a broad variety of tasks that involve implicit expression of biases, skills, or habits. Amnesic patients can demonstrate robust "priming," an increase in the speed or ability to reproduce recently perceived stimuli, even when they cannot recall or recognize the previously studied items. Amnesic patients can also perform perfectly normally in the acquisition of motor skills, such as tracing a mirror image of a line drawing, and in sequence learning, such as in the acquisition of a repetitive sequence of spatial positions tapped on a keyboard. Amnesic patients can also learn a set of "grammatical" rules for linking letter strings and show a normal facilitation in the speed of rereading a section of text. For each of these successful learning performances, amnesic subjects typically do not recall the tests or the materials that guided their successful performance. Combining all of the results across a large range of tests, amnesic patients succeed whenever they do not have to recollect a specific fact or previous experience, and instead simply have to perform a task guided by the conditions and strategies at hand. New memory is revealed in changes of task performance itself, typically either in a change in the speed of responding or in a bias for one of the response choices that is readily available.

Anatomy of the Declarative Memory System

The declarative memory system is composed of three major components: cerebral cortical areas, a collection of cortical areas surrounding the hippocampus, and the hippocampus itself (Fig. 51.3; Burwell *et al.*, 1995; Suzuki, 1996) and the major pathways of the system are very similar in rats and monkeys. The cerebral cortical areas comprise diverse and widespread "association" regions that are both the source of information to the hippocampal region and the targets of hippocampal output. They project to the cortical region adjacent to the hippocampus, including the perirhinal cortex, the parahippocampal cortex (in the monkey, it is called the postrhinal cortex in the rat), and the entorhinal cortex. This region serves as a convergence site for input from the cortical association areas and mediates the distribution of cor-

tical afferents to the hippocampus. These cortical areas are interconnected and send major efferents to multiple subdivisions of the hippocampus itself, the dentate gyrus, the CA3 and CA1 areas, and the subiculum. Within the hippocampus, there are broadly divergent and convergent connections that mediate a large network of associations (Amaral and Witter, 1989), and these connections support forms of long term potentiation that could participate in the rapid coding of novel conjunctions of information (see Chapter 50). The outcomes of hippocampal processing are directed back to the adjacent cortical areas, and the outputs of that region are directed in turn back to the same areas of the cerebral cortex that were the source of its inputs. Additional structures have been included as components of this system, including medial diencephalic structures.

A Model of Amnesia in Nonhuman Primates

Neuroscientists have used a specific, carefully selected set of behavioral tests in developing a nonhuman primate model of human amnesia to identify the particular medial temporal lobe structures that support declarative memory. The tasks involve learning about three-dimensional objects or complex pic-

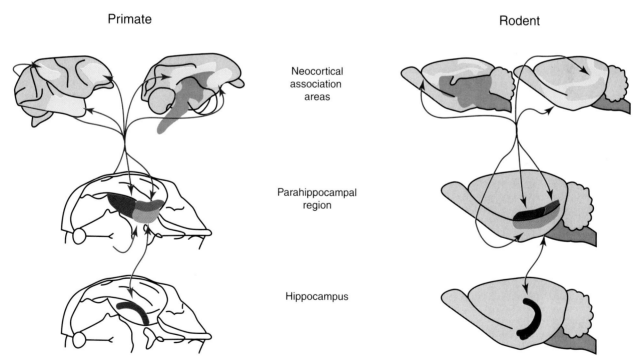

Primate   Rodent

Neocortical association areas

Parahippocampal region

Hippocampus

FIGURE 51.3 The anatomy of the hippocampal memory system in monkeys and rats. Multiple association areas in the cerebral cortex send outputs that converge on subdivisions of the cortex surrounding the hippocampus, which in turn sends its outputs to the hippocampus. The output path involves return projections from the hippocampus to the surrounding cortical region, which in turn projects back to the same cortical association areas. From Eichenbaum (2001).

A   B

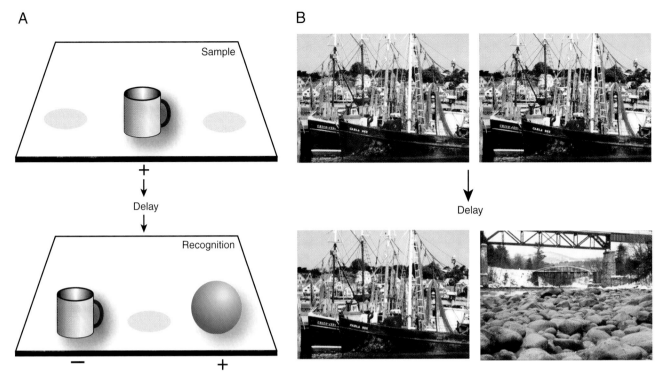

FIGURE 51.4 Recognition memory tasks used for studies of memory in nonhuman primates. (A) The delayed nonmatching-to-sample task using unique objects as stimuli. The subject is initially presented with a single novel object as the sample and must displace the object. This is followed by a variable delay during which the subject cannot see any objects. In the subsequent recognition test, two objects are presented, one of which is the same as the sample and the other of which is novel. Correct performance requires the subject to recognize and avoid the sample object and instead choose the novel one to receive a food reward. (B) Visual paired comparison task. During the sample phase the monkey looks at two identical pictures. In the test phase, one of the sample pictures is represented along with a novel picture. Memory is measured, by the disproportional time that the monkey spends looking at the novel test picture.

tures. In one task, delayed nonmatching to sample, subjects are shown an object once and then, after a delay, are shown two objects (the original object and a new one). The task of the monkeys is to select the new object (Fig. 51.4A). When the delay is only a few seconds, monkeys with experimental lesions that include the same medial temporal lobe structures damaged in H.M. (including the hippocampus, amygdala, and adjacent cortices) performed as well as normal monkeys (Mishkin, 1978). As the delay was increased, the monkeys became progressively more impaired. Thus, monkeys with medial temporal damage, like humans with amnesia, have intact short-term memory but are forgetful. Monkeys with medial temporal lobe damage also perform poorly when they must retain rapidly acquired object discriminations for a prolonged period. In contrast to these impairments in object memory, monkeys with medial temporal lobe damage have intact capacities for skill acquisition as measured in a task that involves learning to retrieve a candy by manipulating it along a bent rod. Thus, the pattern of both preserved and impaired memory in human amnesic patients is

closely modeled by the performance of monkeys with similar brain damage (Zola-Morgan and Squire, 1985).

Retrograde amnesia is another aspect of the amnesic syndrome that has been studied in monkeys. Patients with amnesia due to medial temporal lobe damage suffer not only a deficit in learning new material (anterograde amnesia), but also loss of memories that were acquired before the brain damage (retrograde amnesia). Importantly, the retrograde deficit is graded, and material acquired shortly before the damage is affected most severely, whereas items learned earlier in life are relatively spared. Parallel to these observations, studies have also shown that simple object discriminations that were learned by monkeys shortly before medial temporal lobe damage are poorly retained, but discriminations learned remotely are spared. This pattern of memory impairment, along with the other characteristics of memory impairment in monkeys that have been described, validates the nonhuman primate model of human amnesia.

Using this animal model, investigators were able to identify the structures of the medial temporal lobe critical to supporting declarative memory. In H.M. the damage included the amygdala, the hippocampus, and the surrounding cortical region. However, studies with the monkey have shown that the amygdala is not a part of the declarative memory system. In addition, the severity of memory impairment depends on the extent and locus of damage within the medial temporal lobe. Damage limited to the hippocampus, or to its major connections through the fornix, produces only a modest impairment. In contrast, damage to the adjacent cortices produces severe amnesia. Thus, the perirhinal and parahippocampal cortical regions themselves make major contributions to memory, and the hippocampus itself is a critical component of the system. For example, hippocampal damage impairs recognition memory performance on the visual paired-comparison task (Zola *et al.*, 2000; Fig. 51.4B). In this task, the monkey is initially shown a pair of duplicate pictures. Then, following a variable delay, two pictures are again shown. One picture is identical to the initial sample and the other is a novel picture. Memory for the sample picture is measured by monitoring the animal's eye movements during picture presentation. Normal monkeys (and humans) spend less time looking at the familiar picture than the novel one. On this test, damage limited to the hippocampus results in a time-dependent memory impairment, such that at a brief interval memory is intact, but after a few seconds memory is severely impaired. The overall pattern of findings supports the view that both the hippocampus and the adjacent cortical areas support performance on these and other tests of recognition memory.

Models of Hippocampal Function in Rodents

Studies with rodents have identified specific contributions of the hippocampus in this species and offer insights into the nature of memory representations in networks of hippocampal neurons. These findings have implications for hippocampal memory function in humans and nonhuman primates.

Many studies have demonstrated that damage to the hippocampus results in deficits in a variety of spatial learning and memory tasks. A particularly useful example is place learning in the Morris water maze task (Morris *et al.*, 1982; Fig. 51.5). In this task, rats are trained to find a hidden escape platform submerged just below the surface in a pool of cloudy water. Because there is no specific cue at the escape site, the rat must learn the location of the platform on the basis of spatial relationships among the cues that are visible in the room. Rats with hippocampal

damage are severely impaired at this task. However, the same rats are completely intact at a so-called "cued" version of the test in which they learn to swim toward a platform that is visible above the water surface and that can be located in any one of several places. This distinction between hippocampal-dependent "place" learning and hippocampal-independent "cued" learning has been influential in formulating views of hippocampal function in animals.

During learning

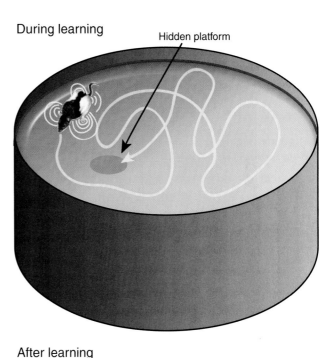

After learning

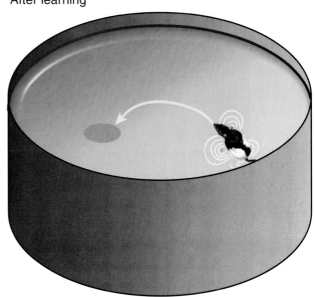

FIGURE 51.5 The Morris water maze task. Early in training, rats search for the submerged platform for extended periods. After training the rat swims directly to the platform.

Although these data suggest a selective role for the hippocampus in spatial learning, this notion does not accommodate the pattern of findings across the full range of spatial and nonspatial memory tasks. For example, rats with hippocampal damage can learn simple spatial discriminations, e.g., to turn left rather than right in a T maze. However they are impaired if they are forced initially to visit either the left or the right arm of the maze, and then asked to remember that experience and choose to visit the opposite arm. Rats with hippocampal damage can also learn to locate the escape platform in the Morris water maze when they are trained to find the platform from a single starting point. However, they cannot learn if trials from different starting points are intermixed. These studies show that rats with hippocampal

damage can use spatial stimuli to guide performance, but they cannot organize information gained from different episodes to express memory flexibly according to the demands on a particular trial.

Other experimental evidence indicates that the hippocampus is also critically involved in the organization and flexible expression of nonspatial memories. For example, in an experiment using olfactory cues that exploited the natural foraging strategies of rats, animals were trained with distinctive odors, which were added to sand (Bunsey and Eichenbaum, 1996). The rats had to dig through the sand to obtain a cereal reward (Fig. 51.6). Initially, the rats learned a set of odor "paired associates," i.e., a list of associations between pairs of odors. Then they learned a second set of associates, and each association involved one of the

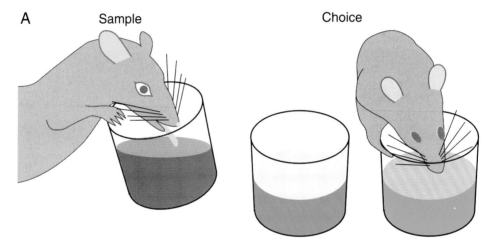

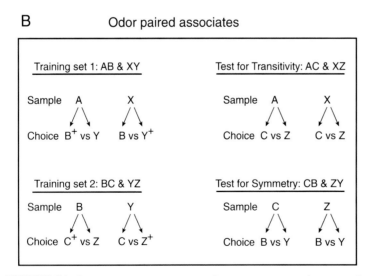

FIGURE 51. 6 Associative transitivity and symmetry in paired associate learning. (A) On each training trial, one of two odors is presented as the sample. On the subsequent choice trial the animal must select the assigned associate, indicated by a "+". (B) Outline of odor pairings used in training on two sequential sets of paired associates, plus stimuli used in tests for transitivity (C for A; Z for X) and symmetry (B for C; Y for Z). From Bunsey and Eichenbaum (1996).

odors from the first set. Subsequently, the rats were given probe tests to determine the extent to which learned representations supported two forms of flexible memory expression. One of these tests, a test for transitivity, measured the ability to infer an association between two odors that shared a common associate. For example, having learned that odor A is associated with odor B and that odor B is associated with odor C, could they infer that A is associated indirectly with C? The other test, a test for symmetry, measured the ability to recognize associated odors when they were presented in the reverse of their training order. For example, if B is associated with C, is C associated with B? Intact rats learned paired associates rapidly, and hippocampal damage did not affect the acquisition rate on either of the training sets, presumably because they engaged a nondeclarative strategy (see Procedural Memory below; note that humans with hippocampal damage have great difficulty learning paired associates). Intact rats also showed strong transitivity across the sets, and successfully inferred an association that had been learned only indirectly. In contrast, rats with selective hippocampal damage were severely impaired in that they showed no evidence of transitivity. In the symmetry test, intact rats showed their associations were indeed symmetrical. In contrast, rats with hippocampal damage again were severely impaired, showing no detectable capacity for symmetry. These findings show that the role of the hippocampus in rats extends beyond spatial memory and suggest that the hippocampus is important for declarative, flexible memory.

Complementary evidence for this framework of thinking about hippocampal function comes from recordings of the firing patterns of hippocampal neurons in behaving rats. A major early finding in studies of hippocampal cells was that many of these neurons fire when the rat is in a particular location in its environment. This activity was shown to reflect an encoding of the spatial relationships among physical stimuli in the environment, leading experimenters to call these neurons "place cells" (O'Keefe, 1976). However, numerous recording studies in rats have since shown that hippocampal cells also fire in association with the animal's behavior and in association with conjunctions or combinations of multiple visual, auditory, and olfactory stimuli. For example, in one experiment, rats performed a variant of the delayed nonmatching to sample task, which was guided by olfactory cues that were presented at several locations in an open field (Fig. 51.7 top; Wood et al., 1999).

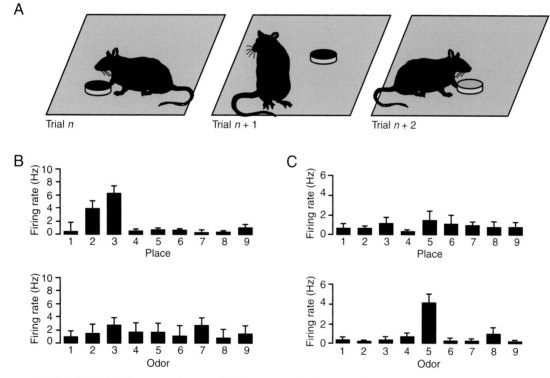

FIGURE 51.7 Hippocampal neuronal firing patterns. (A) A rat performing the delayed nonmatching to sample task with odorized cups as stimuli. The three panels indicate a sequence of trials that vary the position of the odor and whether the presented odor matches the odor used on the previous trial. (B) Example of a cell that fires when trials are performed at two adjacent places (2 and 3), regardless of the odor presented. (C) Example of a cell that does not fire differentially in association with trials at different locations, but fires selectively on trials when odor 5 is presented. From Wood et al., 1999.

Hippocampal cells fired in association with each relevant event and important place in the task. Some cells were activated only in association with an almost unique event defined by both spatial and nonspatial features. For example, some cells fired when the rat sniffed a particular odor at a particular place and when the trial was a nonmatch, i.e., when the odor presented was different from the odor presented on the previous trial. Some cells fired as the rat performed the trial at a particular location, regardless of what odor was presented, as might be expected of a "place" cell (Fig. 51.7B). However, other cells fired in association with nonspatial features of the task that were common across many trials. For example, some cells fired as the rat approached the odor stimulus or as it sniffed a particular odor, regardless of where the trial was performed (Fig. 51.7C). Thus the hippocampal network represents combinations of events and places where they occur that are unique to particular types of trials, and it represents events and places that are common across different trial types.

Observations also suggest that hippocampal neurons can represent sequences of events and places that compose episodic memories. For example, evidence of episodic-like coding was found in a study when rats performed a spatial alternation task on a T maze (Wood et al., 2000; Fig. 51.8). Each trial began when the rat traversed the stem of the "T" and then selected either the left- or the right-choice arm. To alternate successfully, the rats were required to distinguish between their left-turn and right-turn experiences and to use the memory for their most recent previous experience so they could turn in the opposite direction on the next trial. Different hippocampal

cells fired as the rats passed through the sequence of locations within the maze during each trial. These cells could be considered canonical place cells. However, in addition, the firing patterns of many of the cells depended on whether the rat was in the midst of a left- or right-turn episode, even when the rat was in the stem of the T and running similarly on both types of trials. That is, minor variations in the animal's speed, direction of movement, or position within areas on the stem did not account for the different firing patterns on left-turn and right-turn trials. While the majority of the cells strongly preferred one trial type, most of the cells fired at least to some extent when the rat was at the same point in the stem on either trial type. Thus, the hippocampus encoded the left-turn and right-turn experiences using distinct representations, and these representations included information that could link them by their common features. These results suggest that the representations of event sequences, linked by codings of their common events and places, could constitute the substrate of a network of episodic memories, consistent with the idea that the hippocampus has a broad role in declarative memory.

A Prolonged Period of Memory Consolidation

The term consolidation has been used to characterize two kinds of brain events that affect the stability of memory after learning. One event involves the fixation of plasticity within synapses over a period of minutes or hours through a sequence of protein synthesis and morphological changes at synapses (see Chapter 50). The other event involves a reorganization of memories, which occurs over weeks to years following new learning. This prolonged consolidation occurs in the declarative memory system and is thought to involve interactions between the medial temporal region and the cerebral cortex. Several experiments have now shown that damage to the hippocampus or adjacent cortex after learning can impair later retention of memories in a wide range of tasks in several species. In most cases, long-term retention is impaired if the damage occurs shortly after learning. However, if the damage is delayed by several days or weeks, subjects perform normally. These findings show that a process involving the hippocampus or the surrounding cortical region is required for postlearning processing over a period of at least several days.

Several models have been proposed to account for how the hippocampus might interact over a prolonged period in memory consolidation. These models assume that widespread areas of the neo-

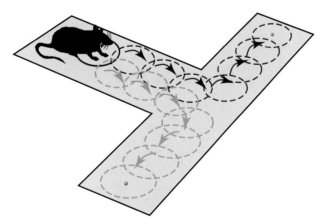

FIGURE 51.8 Selective firing during different types of memory episodes in rats performing a T maze alternation task. On left turn trials, different cells fire as the rat runs forward through a series of locations on the maze. On right turn trials, a different set of cells fire, even when the overt behavior and places are the same. From Eichenbaum (2000).

cortex contain the details of the information that is to be remembered and that medial temporal areas support the capacity to retrieve the memory during the period shortly after learning. Medial temporal areas reactivate the cortical representations repeatedly, inducing plasticity in intracortical connections that provide the permanent linkages and organization of the cortical memory. One possibility is that the same representational function the hippocampus provides in encoding and linking episodic memories at the time of learning continues for a period to support the establishment of intracortical linkages of memories within a large-scale memory network.

Summary

Amnesia associated with damage to the medial temporal region in humans is characterized by an inability to retain and consciously recollect memories of facts and events. Studies with animal models of declarative memory provide a framework for thinking about medial-temporal function in terms of memories that are organized according to relations among distinct experiences and that are accessible through a variety of routes and forms of behavioral expression. Furthermore, declarative memory supports the capacity to make generalizations and inferences from memory, which is a hallmark of declarative memory expression. Structures important for declarative memory include association areas of the neocortex, the cortical region surrounding the hippocampus, and the hippocampus, each of which likely plays a different role.

PROCEDURAL MEMORY

Among the most prevalent kinds of memory we use everyday is "procedural memory," the habits, skills, and sensori-motor adaptations that occur constantly in the background of all of our intentional and planned behavior. Because this kind of memory generally falls outside of consciousness, we take it for granted. However, without it we would be forced to "think" our way through virtually every step we take and every motion we make in our daily tasks.

Procedural Memory Is Mediated by Two Anatomically and Functionally Distinct Subsystems

Procedural memory can be separated into two general subtypes. One type involves the acquisition of habits and skills, the capacity for a broad variety of stereotyped and unconscious behavioral repertoires. These can involve simple refinements of particular, often repeated motor patterns, and can extend to the learning of long action sequences in response to highly complex stimuli. Thus, they include both the acquisition of skills (e.g., skiing, piano playing) and the unique elements of personal style and tempo reflected in the expression of these behaviors. A key structure in this subsystem is the neostriatum, a major component of the basal ganglia (Packard and Knowlton, 2002). The neostriatum receives its cortical inputs from the cerebral cortex, and these projections are capable of activity-dependent changes in responsiveness that could underlie procedural memories. The projections are organized topographically into divergent and convergent projections into modules within the neostriatum that might sort and associate somatosensory and motor representations. The neostriatum projects to other components of the basal ganglia and to the thalamus, which project back to both the premotor and motor cortex and the prefrontal association cortex. Notably, there are minimal projections from this system to the brain stem motor nuclei and none to the spinal motor apparatus, which suggests the system operates mainly to modify cortical motor representations rather than control behavior through direct motor outputs (for further details, see Chapter 31).

The other type of procedural memory involves specific sensory-to-motor adaptations and adjustments of reflexes, such as changing the force that one exerts to compensate for a new load or acquiring conditioned reflexes that involve associating novel motor responses to a new stimulus. A key structure of this subsystem is the cerebellum. The cerebellum receives cortical input from a much more restricted cortical area than the neostriatum, including only the strictly sensory and motor areas that project via brain stem nuclei into the lateral cerebellar cortex. Like the neostriatal subsystem, the cerebellum has a thalamic output route to the cerebral cortex, albeit this subsystem is limited to the motor and premotor cortex. In addition, the cerebellum receives somatic sensory inputs directly from the spinal cord and has major bidirectional connections with brain stem nuclei associated with spinal cord functions. Thus the cerebellar subsystem, in contrast to the neostriatal subsystem, may influence motor outputs directly (see Chapter 32). The functional roles of these two subsystems are discussed in turn.

The Neostriatal Subsystem

The neostriatum is critical for many forms of response or habit learning. The neostriatal habit system was introduced in studies that dissociated this system from the hippocampal and amygdala memory systems. Those experiments provided evidence indicating a role for the neostriatum in the acquisition of specific stimulus–response associations, as contrasted with declarative memory and emotional memory functions of the hippocampal and amygdala systems, respectively.

In one study the role of the neostriatum in learning specific behavioral responses was demonstrated using a simple T maze apparatus where two different strategies in solving the maze could be compared directly (Packard and McGaugh, 1996; Fig. 51.9). In this task the rat begins each trial at the base of the T maze and is rewarded with food at the end of one choice arm. Accordingly, the rats could acquire the task by learning to make a specific turning response (left or right). Alternatively, the rat could remember where the reward was located during previous encounters in the test room, independent of any particular behavioral response required to obtain it. The critical test to distinguish these two strategies is to rotate the maze by 180° so that the choice arms still end at the same two loci (albeit which arms reach those loci are now exchanged). Additionally, the start point is now at the opposite end of the room. If the rat had learned a particular turning response, it would continue to make the previously reinforced turning response at the choice point, leading it to a different goal location than the one where the food was provided during

training. In contrast, if the rat remembered the location of the reward, then it should turn in the opposite direction as it did previously in order to arrive at the same place in the room where food had been found previously.

Rats were trained for a week on the T maze task and were then given the rotated maze probe trial. Then they were trained for another week with the maze in its original orientation and were then presented with an additional probe trial. Initially, normal rats adopted a "place" strategy, as reflected in their strong preference for the location of the previous goal during the first probe trial. However, after the additional week of overtraining, normal rats switched and on the final probe test indicated that they had adopted a "response" strategy. So, under these training circumstances, initial acquisition of the task was guided by memory of the reward locus, but subsequent overtraining led to development of a habitual turning response.

Packard and McGaugh also examined whether different brain systems supported these different strategies. All animals had been implanted with indwelling cannulae that allowed injection of a local anesthetic or saline directly and locally into one of two brain structures, the hippocampus or the neostriatum, prior to the probe tests. The effects of the anesthetic were striking. On the first probe trial, when the neostriatum was inactivated, animals behaved just as controls; i.e., they were predominantly "place" learners and the

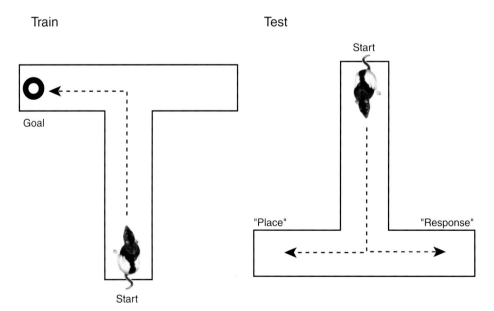

FIGURE 51.9 "Place" versus "response" learning. The rat is trained initially to turn left in order to obtain a reward at a particular location. In a subsequent test, the maze is rotated and the rat is allowed to select whether it will perform the same left turning "response" or remember the "place" of the previous reward.

place strategy did not depend on the neostriatum. In contrast, when the hippocampus was inactivated, the animals showed no preference on the first probe trial, indicating that the hippocampus was essential for the place strategy and that this was the only strategy that was normally available in the early stage of learning.

On the second probe test, a different pattern of results emerged. Whereas control subjects had by now acquired the response strategy, animals with the neostriatum inactivated lost the turning response and instead showed that they were relying on the place strategy. In contrast, animals with the hippocampus inactivated performed like controls and demonstrated a response strategy. A clear picture emerges from these data. Animals normally develop an initial place strategy that depends on the hippocampus. No turning response has developed in this initial period. With overtraining, a response habit mediated by the neostriatum is acquired, and it predominates over the hippocampal place strategy. The latter is not, however, lost. It can be "uncovered" by inactivating the neostriatum and suppressing the turning response strategy. These findings offer compelling evidence that there are distinct types of memory that guide "place" and "response" strategies. These forms of memory are distinguished by their performance char-

acteristics, as well as by the brain systems that support them.

Neostriatal Memory Function in Humans

Research indicates that the neostriatal system plays a critical role in the acquisition of arbitrary habitual responses to complex stimuli in humans, as it does in animals. For example, Knowlton and colleagues (1996) contrasted habit learning in amnesic patients with that of patients in the early stages of Parkinson's disease, which is associated with the degeneration of neurons in the substantia nigra and a resulting major loss of input to the neostriatum. Subjects were trained in a probabilistic classification learning task formatted as a weather prediction game (Fig. 51.10). The task involved predicting on each trial one of two possible outcomes (rain or shine) based on cues that were presented to the subject. On each trial, one, two, or three cards from a deck of four were presented. Each card was associated with the sunshine outcome independently and probabilistically, 75, 57, 43, or 25% of the time, and the outcome with multiple cards was determined by the conjoint probabilities. After the cards were presented on each trial, the subject was asked to choose between rain and shine and was then given

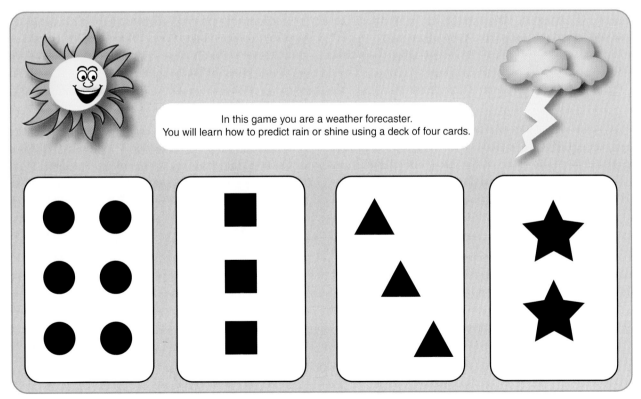

FIGURE 51.10 Weather prediction task. View of the computer screen presented to subjects showing all four stimulus cards and the "sun" or "rain" response choices. From Knowlton *et al.* (1996).

feedback (correct or incorrect). The probabilistic nature of the task made it difficult for subjects to improve by recalling specific previous trials because the same configuration of cues could lead to different outcomes. The most useful information was the probability associated with particular cues and combinations of cues, which could be acquired gradually across trials much as habits and skills are acquired. Over a block of 50 trials, normal subjects gradually improved from pure guessing (50% correct) to about 70% correct. However, patients with Parkinson's disease failed to show significant learning, and the failure was particularly evident in those patients with more severe parkinsonian symptoms. In contrast, amnesic patients were successful in learning the task, achieving levels of accuracy similar to the controls by the end of the 50-trial block.

Subsequent to training on the weather prediction task, these subjects were given a set of multiple-choice questions about the nature of the task and the kinds of stimulus materials they had encountered. Normal subjects and patients with Parkinson's disease performed very well in recalling the task events. In contrast, the amnesic patients were severely impaired. These findings demonstrate a double dissociation, with habit or skill learning disrupted by neostriatal damage and declarative memory for the learning events impaired by hippocampal or diencephalic damage. Furthermore, these findings provide additional evidence that different types of memory representations for identical learning materials are formed within parallel brain systems.

Taken together, the literature from studies of damage to the neostriatum suggests that the deficit following neostriatal damage is, or includes, an impairment in generating decisions or behavioral responses toward important environmental stimuli. The deficit extends to both approach and avoidance responses and to both spatial and nonspatial stimuli across many modalities (for a more complete characterization, see Eichenbaum and Cohen, 2001).

The Cerebellar Subsystem

The anatomy and functions of the cerebellum have long been associated with aspects of motor learning, and many studies have focused on its highly organized circuitry and emphasized its mechanisms for reflex adaptations. Considerable attention has focused on Pavlovian eye-blink conditioning as a model learning paradigm in which to study the role of the cerebellum. In this paradigm, rabbits are placed in restraining chambers where they can be presented with a well-controlled tone or light as the condition-

ing stimulus (the CS). In classic delay conditioning, this CS lasts 250–1000 ms and coterminates with an air puff or mild electrical shock to the eye (the unconditioned stimulus or US) that produces a reflexive, unconditioned eyeblink (the UR). After many pairings of CS and US, the rabbit begins to produce the eye blink after onset of the CS and prior to presentation of the US. With further training, the conditioned response (CR) occurs earlier, and its timing becomes optimized so as to be maximal at the US onset.

The role of the cerebellum and associated areas has been studied extensively by Thompson and colleagues (Fig. 51.11; Thompson and Kim, 1996). In their studies, permanent lesions or reversible inactivation of one particular cerebellar nucleus, the interpositus nucleus, resulted in impaired acquisition and retention of classically conditioned eye-blink reflexes, without affecting reflexive eye blinks (URs). Additional compelling data indicating a selective role for the interpositus in this kind of motor memory come from studies using reversible inactivations of particular brain regions during training. These studies showed that drug inactivation of motor nuclei that are essential for production of the CR and UR prevented the elicitation of behavior during training. However, in trials immediately following removal of the inactivation, CRs appeared in full form, showing that the neural circuit that supports UR production is not critical for learning *per se*. A similar pattern of results was obtained with inactivation of the axons leaving the interpositus or their target in the red nucleus, showing that the final pathway for CR production is also not required to establish the memory trace. In contrast, inactivation of the anterior interpositus nucleus and overlying cortex by drugs (muscimol, lidocaine) or temporary cooling did not affect reflexive blinking, yet resulted in failure of CR development during training and failure of retention after removal of the inactivation. These results point to a small area of the anterior interpositus nucleus and overlying cerebellar cortex as the essential locus of plasticity in this form of motor learning. As in animals, damage to the cerebellum in humans also retards the classically conditioned eye-blink reflex. Notably, this type of learning can be accomplished without involvement of the cerebral cortex.

Summary

There are at least two different brain pathways that mediate the learning of skills, habits, and sensorimotor adaptations. These involve a pathway through the cortex and neostriatum that plays an important role in the acquisition of habits and learned sequences

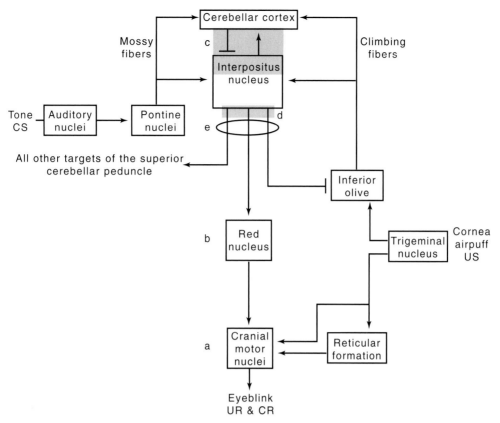

FIGURE 51.11 A schematic diagram of principal pathways involved in classical conditioning of the eyeblink reflex. The role of structures at points a–e has been studied using reversible inactivation with a local anesthetic. Inactivation at point "c" (shaded areas) prevents learning, whereas inactivation at "a," "b," "d," or "e" prevents the behavioral response during inactivation, but does not block learning. From Thompson *et al.* (1996).

and a pathway that involves the cerebellum that mediates conditioned reflexes as well as other sensorimotor adaptations (e.g., adaptation of the vestibular ocular reflex). Both of these memory subsystems are impressive in their capacity to acquire information about complex stimuli and support complicated routines in the absence of conscious recollection.

EMOTIONAL MEMORY

Emotional memory, like procedural memory, is a nondeclarative form of memory that we rely on in everyday life. This kind of memory mediates preferences and aversions that can be learned unconsciously and independent of declarative memory for the events in which the bias was acquired. Studies of emotional memory focus primarily on the amygdala, a component of the limbic system that receives a wide variety of sensory inputs from the thalamus and cortex and sends outputs to response systems that mediate different forms of emotional expression (e.g., changes in heart rate, blood pressure, sweating, and alterations in startle response), as well as hypothalamic structures that mediate hormone release. Damage to the amygdala in humans and animals impairs the perception of both emotional stimuli and emotional expression. In addition, many studies have now demonstrated a critical role for the amygdala in the acquisition of both positive and negative biases toward previously neutral stimuli. These studies indicate that the same brain system that mediates the perception and appreciation of emotional stimuli, as well as emotional expression, is also critical to the acquisition, consolidation, and expression of emotional memories.

The selective role of the amygdala—the acquisition of positive affective biases, independent of declarative and procedural memory—was demonstrated in a particularly instructive "triple dissociation" experiment by McDonald and White (1993). Rats were trained on a radial maze, i.e., a maze with a central platform with eight arms radiating outward. By carefully manipulating the task demands, McDonald and White created three different versions of the task for which experimental damage to only one of three structures prevented normal learning. The hippocampus, but not the amygdala or neostriatum, was critical when the rats were reinforced only for entering arms not visited that day, a task requiring memory for specific earlier experiences and flexible memory expression. The integrity of the neostriatum, but not the amygdala or hippocampus, was critical to learning when rats were given food reinforcement for approaching a maze arm that was illuminated, regardless of its location. The amygdala, but not the neostriatum or hippocampus, was critical when rats were confined separately to an illuminated maze arm containing food and a dark arm without food and were then tested for their preference for the illuminated or dark arm. These findings indicated that the role of the amygdala was critical when performance relied on an acquired preference for the illuminated location, independent of memory for previous experiences or the acquisition of a specific approach response.

In addition to its role in rats in developing biases toward rewarding stimuli, the amygdala plays a critical role in fear conditioning. This research has focused on the specific elements of the pathways through the amygdala that support the learning of fearful responses to a simple auditory or visual stimulus. Perhaps the best studied example of emotional memory involves a simple tone-cued fear-conditioning task (Fig. 51.12A). Rats are initially habituated to an operant chamber and are then presented with multiple pairings of a tone that terminates with a brief electric shock delivered through the floor of the cage. Subsequently, conditioned fear is assessed by measuring autonomic responses, as reflected in changes in arterial pressure in response to the tone, and motor responses, as reflected in stereotypic crouching or freezing behavior when the tone is presented. Unconditioned responses to the tone were evaluated by presenting other animals with unpaired tones and shocks.

The brain system that mediates this and other forms of Pavlovian fear conditioning has been studied extensively (Fig. 51.12B; LeDoux, 1992; Davis, 1992). The relevant amygdala pathways include sensory inputs sent via the brain stem to sensory nuclei of the thalamus, which, in turn, project directly to the lateral amygdaloid nucleus. Other sensory thalamic projections follow a route to posterior areas of cortex and then to the perirhinal cortex, both of which are additional sources of sensory input to the amygdala, particularly lateral and basolateral nuclei. Those areas of the amygdala project into the central nucleus, which is the source of outputs to subcortical areas controlling a broad range of fear-related behaviors, including autonomic and motor responses.

The role of several structures within this pathway has been identified. Animals with selective lesions in the lateral amygdala show dramatically reduced conditioned responses to the tone in measures of both autonomic and motor responses. Unconditioned responses to the foot shock (consequent to unpaired presentations of the tone and shock) are not affected. Thus the site where most sensory information enters the amygdala is a critical point in this memory system. In addition, it has been determined that critical sensory information can take one of two routes into the amygdala. While destruction of all auditory areas of the thalamus eliminated conditioned responses, selective ablation of either of the two prominent direct inputs to the lateral amygdala were individually ineffective. Thus lesions of the medial division of the medial geniculate (including all three nuclei that project directly to the lateral amygdala) or lesions of the entire auditory cortex that projects to the amygdala did not reduce either the autonomic response or freezing. However, elimination of both of these inputs produced the full effect seen after lateral amygdala lesions. Thus, for this simple type of conditioning, either the direct thalamic input, which presumably provides a crude identification of a sound, or the thalamo-cortical input pathway, which provides more detailed information about the auditory signal, is sufficient to mediate conditioning.

Another interesting observation is that when rats are placed in the conditioning chamber after learning, they begin to freeze even before the tone is presented. Thus rats appear to condition both to the tone and to the environmental context in which paired tones and shock have previously been presented. This "contextual" fear conditioning is selective to the environment in which conditioning occurs. Trained animals do not freeze prior to tone presentation in a new environment, but they do freeze when the tone is presented. Contextual fear conditioning is also different from tone-cued fear conditioning in another important way. Amygdala lesions blocked conditioned freezing to both the context and the tone. In contrast, damage to the hippocampus selectively blocked contextual fear conditioning, but spared the conditioned response to the tone. These findings provide a dissociation between amygdala-dependent acquisition of fear and hippocampal-dependent memory for the context in which the fearful experience occurred.

The Amygdala and Fear Conditioning in Humans

A similar dissociation between functions of the amygdala and hippocampus in fear conditioning has been observed in human patients with selective

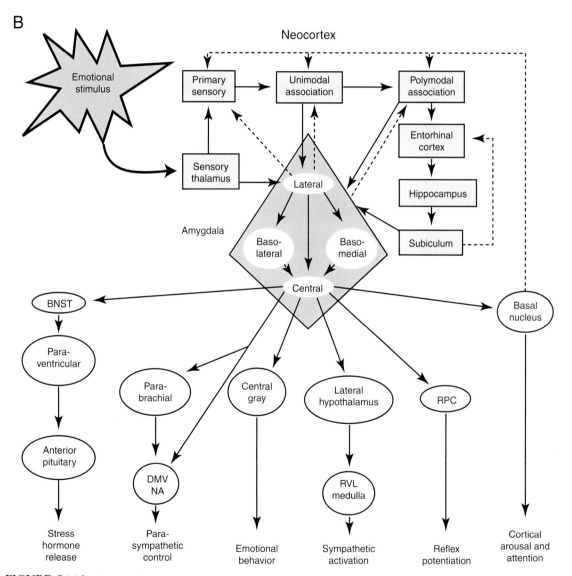

FIGURE 51.12 Fear conditioning. (A) Prior to training, the tone produces a transient orienting response. During training the tone is followed by a brief foot shock. Following training, the rat is reintroduced into the chamber and freezes when the tone is presented. (B) Anatomical pathways that mediate fear conditioning. A hierarchy of sensory inputs converges on the lateral amygdala nucleus, which projects to other amygdala nuclei and then to the central nucleus, which send outputs to several effector systems for emotional responses. BNST, bed nucleus of the stria terminalis; DMV, dorsal nucleus of the vagus; NA, nucleus ambiguus; RPC, nucleus reticularis pontis oralis; RVL, rostral ventral nucleus of the medulla. From LeDoux (1995).

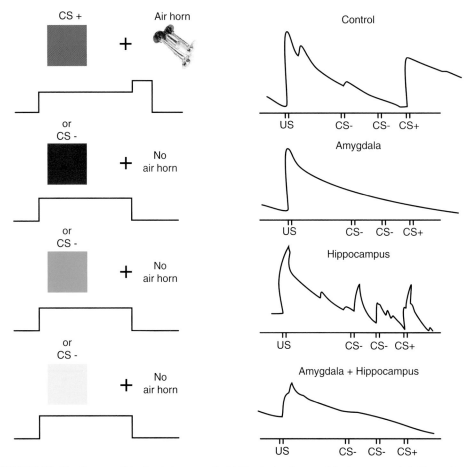

FIGURE 51.13   Fear conditioning in humans. (Left) Discriminative conditioning protocol. Subjects viewed a blue screen ending with a loud, aversive boat horn sound or screens with other colors not paired with the boat horn. (Right) Changes in skin resistance resulting from the boat horn unconditioned stimulus (US), from the paired blue conditioning stimulus (CS+), or from unpaired conditioning stimuli (CS-). From Bechara *et al.* (1995).

damage to these structures (Bechara *et al.*, 1995). Subjects were trained in a discriminative fear-conditioning protocol in which, on some trials, a monochrome color stimulus (CS+; presented on a computer screen) was presented for 2 s and was then terminated just as an unconditioned stimulus was sounded briefly (US; a loud boat horn) (Fig. 51.13). Autonomic responses to these stimuli were measured as skin conductance changes through electrodermal recordings. On other trials, different colors (CS-) were presented without the boat horn. Normal control subjects typically showed strong electrodermal responses to the US and, with training, came to show conditioned responses to the CS+ but smaller or no responses to CS- stimuli. Thus, the subjects acquired a specific fearful response to the CS+. Three patients with selective damage to the hippocampus or amygdala were also tested. One patient suffered from Urbach–Wiethe disease, a genetic developmental disorder resulting in selective bilateral calcification of the tissue of the amyg-

dala, sparing the adjacent hippocampus. This patient showed normal unconditioned responses to the US, but failed to develop conditioned responses to CS+ stimuli. In contrast, a patient with selective hippocampal damage showed robust skin conductance changes to the US and normal conditioning to CS+ stimuli and appropriately smaller responses to CS- stimuli. A subject with combined amygdala and hippocampal damage failed to condition, even though he did respond appropriately to the US. After the conditioning sessions, subjects were debriefed with several questions about the stimuli and context of contioning. Control subjects and the patient with selective amygdala damage answered most of these questions correctly, but the patients with hippocampal damage were severely impaired in recollecting the training events. These findings demonstrate a double dissociation. A form of emotional conditioning was disrupted by amygdala damage, and declarative memory for the learning situation was impaired by hippocampal damage.

Role of the Amygdala in the Modulation of Memory

Memories of emotionally arousing events are often more vivid, more accurate, and longer lasting than memories of more neutral events. Indeed, it is adaptive for organisms to remember important events better than trivial events. Thus, it also makes sense that the brain should have evolved mechanisms for storing information in accordance with how much the information is worth remembering. Research suggests that specific neural mechanisms serve to modulate the strength of newly formed memories. These memory-modulating mechanisms are thought to underlie, at least in part, the beneficial effects of emotional arousal on memory. Emotional arousal increases our attention toward particularly salient events (Gallagher and Holland, 1994) and can also improve the retention of events even when the arousal occurs within a brief period after the events (McGaugh, 2000).

Emotionally arousing events that activate the sympathetic nervous system and pituitary–adrenal adrenal axis result in the release of epinephrine and glucocorticoids by the adrenal glands. These hormones have a variety of effects associated with the "flight-or-fight" response, including increased heart rate and blood pressure, diversion of blood flow to the brain and muscles, and mobilization of energy stores. There is now a wealth of evidence that another effect of this activation is to improve memory storage for experiences that are accompanied by stress and that the amygdala is critical to this influence on memory. Thus, posttraining injections of neurohormones released during stress, such as norepinephrine or glucocorticoids, or drugs that enhance their effects, facilitate subsequent memory. Conversely, drugs that interfere with neurohormonal responses to stress responses retard memory. In addition, direct stimulation of the amygdala can modulate (enhance or impair) memory, and the effects of amygdala stimulation on memory depend on the integrity of the adrenal glands. Evidence from animal studies indicates that lesions of the amygdala or the stria terminalis, a major afferent–efferent pathway of the amygdala, block the memory-enhancing or memory-impairing effects of many drugs and hormones (Fig. 51.14) and block the memory-impairing effects of adrenalectomy. Moreover, the memory-modulatory effects of many drugs, including treatments affecting adrenergic, GABAergic, and opioid peptidergic mechanisms, are blocked by infusions of the β-adrenergic antagonist propranolol administered into the amygdala. Although infusions of naloxone into the amygdala enhance memory, this enhancement depends on an intact noradrenergic function in the amygdala. These findings indicate that systemically administered drugs and hormones influence memory storage through effects involving noradrenergic mechanisms within the amygdala.

The memory-modulatory effects of glucocorticoids depend on the integrity of the basolateral nucleus of the amygdala, whereas glucocorticoid-induced memory enhancement is not affected by lesions of the central amygdala nucleus. Similarly, the memory-impairing effects of systemic injections of diazepam (valium) are blocked by lesions of the basolateral nucleus, but not by lesions of central or lateral nuclei. Thus, the basolateral nucleus appears to play a crucial role in modulating memory storage. This view is further supported by the finding that the infusion of drugs selectively into the basolateral nucleus induces memory modulation, whereas infusions into the central nucleus are ineffective. This specificity is understandable in terms of the anatomy of the amygdala. The basolateral nucleus is reciprocally connected with brain regions involved in memory storage such as the hippocampus and neocortex.

As noted previously, one characteristic of a memory-modulatory system is that although it may

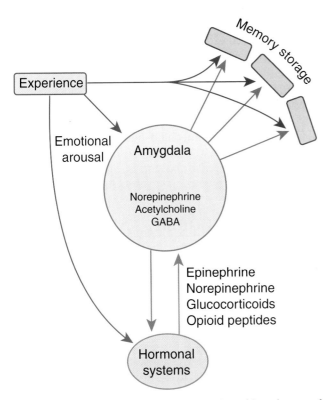

FIGURE 51.14 A schematic representation of how hormonal systems and the amygdala complex can modulate the storage of memory for emotionally arousing events through influences on other brain systems. See text for details. From McGaugh *et al.* (1992).

participate in memory storage, it is not required for normal retrieval of information once it is stored. Many experiments indicate that the amygdala exhibits this characteristic. For example, posttraining amygdala stimulation (via intraamygdala infusions of amphetamine) modulates memory for both a hippocampus-dependent and a neostriatum-dependent task. However, inactivation of the amygdala (via injection of the local anesthetic lidocaine) prior to retention testing has no effect on the enhancement of memory due to posttraining amygdala stimulation in either task. Thus, the amygdala is important in modulating storage in emotionally stressful situations, but not in the maintenance or retrieval of the memory that has been modulated.

Memory Modulation in Humans

The effects of emotional arousal in facilitating memory and the role of the amygdala in this facilitation have also been demonstrated in humans. Cahill and colleagues (1994) examined the influence of emotional content on declarative memory. Their test involved presentation of a series of slides and an accompanying narrative that told a story about a mother and son who were involved in a traumatic accident, or it told a control story with neutral emotional content. In subsequent memory testing, normal subjects recalled the emotional component of the story better than the less emotional parts of the first story and also better than the neutral story. Manipulation of hormone release associated with the stress response influenced this facilitation. For example, subjects given a β-adrenergic antagonist showed no facilitation of declarative memory for the emotional parts of the first story, even though they rated those parts of the story as strongly emotional and even though memory performance on the less emotional parts of the story was fully normal. Performance on the neutral story was not affected by the β-adrenergic antagonist. Thus, there was no general effect of the drug on story memory. Conversely, treatment with an adrenergic agonist enhanced memory for the emotional component of the story.

The amygdala has been strongly implicated in the enhancement of memory for emotional events in humans. A patient with Urbach–Wiethe disease, the genetic disorder referred to earlier, was tested in the emotional story paradigm. Compared to control subjects, this patient failed to show enhancement of memory for the emotional part of the story. However, the patient performed as well as controls on neutral story material, and all subjects rated the emotional material as affectively strong. In a complementary brain imaging study with normal human subjects, the amygdala was activated during the viewing of emotional material, and this activation was related to enhanced memory for that material, as tested later. In separate scanning sessions, subjects viewed film clips that were either strong or neutral in emotional content. The amount of activation in the amygdala was greater for the emotional than the neutral stories, and memory for this material was greater than that for the neutral stories. Furthermore, the amount of amygdala activation during presentation of the emotional material was correlated with performance in a later memory test of that material. There was no correlation between activation of the amygdala and memory performance with neutral material.

Summary

Considerable evidence indicates that pathways from the thalamus and cortex to the amygdala and then to a large number of autonomic and brain stem skeletal response mechanisms, as well as to the cerebral cortex, constitute a system for the expression of emotional memories. This system is well suited to rapidly attach positive and negative bias to a broad range of stimuli and to mediate the acquisition of such biases in the absence of conscious recollection of the circumstances of the emotional experience. In addition, components of the amygdala also mediate the modulation of memory storage during and after emotional events by regulating responses to peripheral mechanisms of the adrenomedullary and adrenocortical stress hormones and central mechanisms mediated by the amygdala. Memory-modulation mechanisms are an efficient, evolutionarily adaptive method of ensuring that the strength of a memory tends to be proportional to its importance.

CEREBRAL CORTEX AND MEMORY

The discussion of memory systems so far has focused on the different kinds of memory processing by anatomically separate structures that are components of distinct memory systems. The cerebral cortex provides some of the most detailed information to each of these systems, and so contributes substantially within each of these systems. In addition, circuits within the cerebral cortex support other aspects of memory, including perceptual memory and working memory, neither of which require other components of the memory systems discussed so far. Beginning with its more general role in the representation of information for all memory systems, this section con-

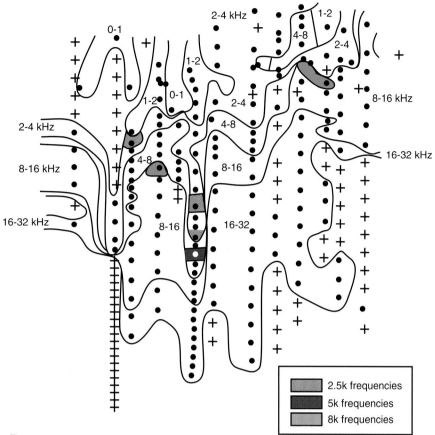

A CM2 passive stimulation at 5 kHz

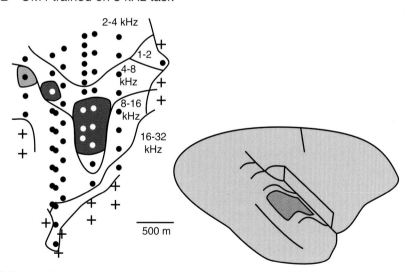

B OM4 trained on 5 kHz task

FIGURE 51.15 Plasticity of auditory cortex maps associated with training on a frequency discrimination. (A) Mapping of the auditory cortical area (see insert at bottom right) in a monkey following passive stimulation at 5 kHz. In this case the zone of auditory cortex responsive to that frequency is small. (B) In contrast, the zone responsive to 5 kHz tones is much larger in another monkey trained to discriminate that frequency. From Recanzone *et al.* (1993).

siders the organization and plasticity of cortical representations. The role of the cortex as the storehouse of semantic memory by which functionally specific zones of cortex perform both perceptual processing and serve as storage sites for particular categories of knowledge is then discussed. Then the role of the cortex in a form of perceptual memory called "priming" is outlined. Finally, the role of cortical circuits, especially the role of the prefrontal area, in working memory as well as episodic memory is discussed.

Functional Organization and Plasticity of the Cerebral Cortex

Although Gall's phrenological approach to cortical localization was discredited, the notion that the cerebral cortex is composed of multiple, functionally distinct processing regions has proven correct. Importantly, Gall was also prescient in his proposal that memory is tied integrally to these various processing systems.

As discussed in Chapter 2, the posterior half of the cerebral cortex contains many functionally distinct areas that are organized into hierarchies of serial and parallel processing for each sensory modality. Additionally, there are cortical areas where information from different modalities converges (so-called "association" areas) in the parietal and temporal lobes. The anterior cerebral cortex contains a similar hierarchy of motor areas, as well as association areas in the prefrontal cortex involved with motor planning, higher order cognition, and working memory (Fuster, 2001; see Chapters 53 and 54). Each cortical area is capable of considerable plasticity in its representations and, for each area, the modification of functional organization underlies its participation in memory.

It has been clear for some time that experience early in life can powerfully influence the functional organization of early stages of sensory processing. More recently it has also been found that there is considerable experience-driven plasticity in the adult cerebral cortex. Several studies have shown that the removal of sensory input to primary sensory areas causes a reorganization such that the zone of cortex that would normally represent the deprived information is invaded by neighboring inputs. For example, if a small part of the retina is lesioned, the area of the primary visual cortex that normally represents that part of the visual field is initially unresponsive, but later becomes responsive to neighboring parts of the visual field (Gilbert and Wiesel, 1992). Similar findings have been observed in the primary auditory,

somatosensory, and motor cortical areas in rodents as well as primates.

Specific training experiences can achieve the opposite result: experience that activates a particular cortical area results in the expansion of that part of the cortex. For example, in one study, monkeys were trained over a period of several weeks to discriminate small frequency differences in tone stimuli. In subsequent recordings, increases were observed in the size of the auditory cortex representation of the task-relevant frequencies and the sharpness of tuning to these frequencies (Recanzone et al., 1993; Fig. 51.15). Furthermore, changes in area of the cortical representation were correlated with the improvement in task performance. In other studies using classical conditioning in anesthetized guinea pigs, the tuning curves of single neurons in the auditory cortex were first characterized. Subsequently, the animal was presented with repeated pairings of a nonoptimal tone and foot shocks. This training resulted in long-lasting shifts in the tuning curves of auditory neurons toward the frequency of the training stimulus. A similar expansion of perceptual representations for training stimuli has been observed in the somatosensory cortex of monkeys following acquisition of a tactile discrimination. The reorganization of the sensory cortex following experience is thought to contribute to adaptations and tuning of perceptual representation systems and, in coordination with reorganization of cortical motor representations, may also contribute to procedural memories. In both cases, this contribution is derived specifically from alterations in the perceptual and motor processing for the relevant learning tasks.

Semantic Memory and Category-Specific Knowledge

There is general agreement among cognitive scientists that semantic knowledge is organized into categories (animals, plants, rocks, tools, furniture, rivers, stars, body parts, fruits, appliances, etc.) that are embedded in hierarchically structured frameworks. Consistent with this organization, cognitive neuropsychologists have reported numerous cases of category-specific deficits in patients with localized brain damage, suggesting that category-specific knowledge may be encoded within circumscribed regions of the brain. In their seminal work on category-specific localization, Warrington and Shallice (1984) studied four patients with bilateral damage in the temporal cortex. These patients exhibited an impairment in the ability to identify living things (i.e., animals and plants) and foods but were spared in their ability to identify nonliving things (i.e., artifacts, gems, weather terms, earth formations). This pattern of selective impairment in identifying living but not nonliving things has been replicated with several other patients, all suffering from temporal damage. Moreover, the converse pattern of selective impairment has been reported. Such patients show impaired ability to identify nonliving things and spared ability to identify living things. This dissociation between living and nonliving things is consistent with models of semantic memory, based on studies of nonclinical populations, in which knowledge is organized into distinct categories whose representations are embodied in distinct cortical areas.

These ideas have generated a number of attempts to explain selective impairments as the result of differences in the familiarity of different categories of stimulus materials, differences in the complexity of items among the categories, or as differences in the modality of information processing (e.g., visual versus auditory) rather than as a result of differences in the meanings of the items in the category. Functional brain imaging studies with normal subjects are consistent with the idea that category specific-deficits are based on differences in the meaning of the items. For example, one study imaged the cortex while subjects named tools and animals. Naming tools selectively activated two regions of the cortex. One of these regions was in the left middle temporal gyrus, identical to the region active when subjects generated action words. The other region was in the left premotor cortex, identical to an area active when subjects imagined manipulating objects with their right hand. In contrast, naming animals produced selective activation of the medial occipital cortex, a location known to be involved in the early stages of visual processing and a location that is active during detailed, object imagery. Thus, identifying and naming tools may require activation of previously acquired information about the pattern of motion and the sequence of motor acts associated with tool use, whereas naming animals may involve the activation of previously acquired visual information needed to distinguish one animal (e.g., a tiger) from another (e.g., a leopard). Within this framework, category-specific disorders arise when a lesion disrupts storage sites associated with one type of information (e.g., patterns of motion and action), but not the other (e.g., visual features; for further discussion, see Chapter 47).

Neuronal Basis of Semantic Representations in Cortical Association Areas

Cortical association areas are involved in complex aspects of perceptual processing and memory. The perceptual responses of neurons in these areas are affected profoundly during memory performance. For example, one of the association areas that has been studied extensively is the inferotemporal cortex (IT) of monkeys. IT is the highest order cortical visual processing area, whose function is the identification of objects by their visual qualities (see Chapter 47); this area is thought to be the site of long-term storage of memory about visual objects. Damage to IT in humans results in visual agnosia, a selective deficit in visual object recognition, and this area has been observed to be activated in neuroimaging studies of neurologically intact individuals performing tasks requiring visual object recognition. Damage to IT in monkeys results in deficits in visual learning and memory. Correspondingly, IT neurons respond maximally to three-dimensional objects, and their responses are typically invariant despite changes in orientation and location in the visual field, i.e., these cells seem to encode the meaning of the objects. The responses of IT neurons are sometimes highly selective and involve stimuli with which the monkey has had significant experience, such as the silhouette of a monkey's hand, a banana, a toilet brush (used to clean monkey cages), and faces.

In addition, neurons in IT change their firing patterns in accordance with their recent past history. In studies of monkeys performing short-term memory tasks, IT neurons can maintain a stimulus-evoked firing pattern during a memory delay period when the animals must hold a (working) memory for the sample stimulus. Thus visual memory is encoded in the capacity of IT cells to sustain or reactivate their normal sensory responses in the absence of the stimulus ordinarily required to evoke the representation. Also, cells in IT can respond differently to the same sample stimulus, depending on whether it matches a stimulus that is being held in memory. Different IT cells show either reduced responses ("match suppression") or increased responses ("match enhancement") to the match stimulus when it is a repetition of the sample stimulus.

Other studies have revealed that IT can also maintain long-term representations of stimulus associations. In a study designed explicitly to evaluate associative responses, complex visual patterns were paired arbitrarily, and the responses of IT neurons were recorded after learning (Sakai and Miyashita, 1991). Each trial involved presenting one stimulus of a trained association and then, after a brief empty interval, providing a choice between the other stimulus of that association and a stimulus from a different pairing. Two different findings suggested that representations of the stimulus associations had been established. "Pair-coding" neurons fired maximally upon presentation of the two cues that were paired associates, more so than for any other cues (Fig. 51.16A). "Pair-recall" neurons increased the firing rate during the delay period following presentation of the associate of the optimal cue (Fig. 51.16B). The capacity to generate these associative representations depended on the integrity of the cortical areas of the medial temporal lobe, suggesting that these codings may reflect declarative memories.

Perceptual Memory and "Priming"

Studies of humans with damage to cerebral cortex, as well as functional brain imaging investigations, have shed light on the role of the cerebral cortex in generating perceptual memories in humans. Some of these studies have focused on a phenomenon known as repetition priming, or simply "priming." Priming involves initial presentation of a list of words, pictures of objects, or nonverbal materials and then subsequent reexposure to fragments or very brief presentation of the whole item. In the reexposure phase, learning is measured by an increased ability to reproduce the whole item from a fragment or by increased speed in making a decision about the item. It appears that priming for different materials depends on distinct areas of the cerebral cortex. For example, one case study compared the performance of a patient with a large lesion in the right visual cortex with the performance of amnesic patients. Subjects initially read a list of words. In a subsequent test, they were

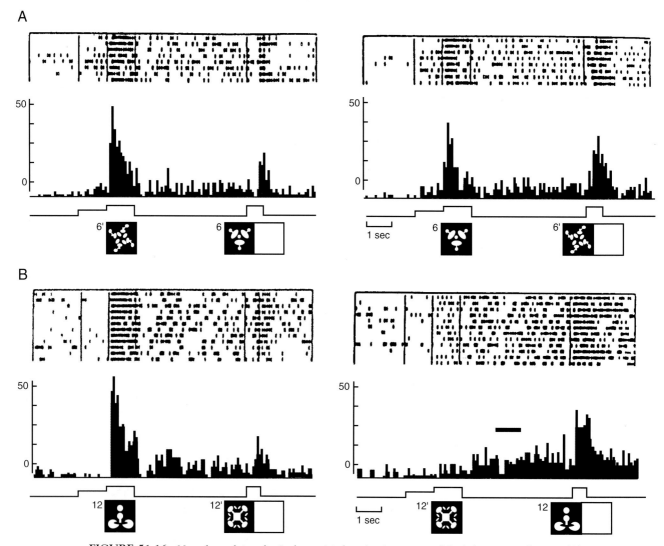

FIGURE 51.16   Neural correlates of paired associate learning in neurons of the inferotemporal cortex. (A) Responses of a "pair-coding" neuron, which fired strongly to stimulus 6' as well as to its associate, stimulus 6. (B) Responses of a "pair-recall" neuron, which fired strongly to stimulus 12 and also during the memory delay when stimulus 12' signaled the forthcoming presentation of stimulus 12. From Sakai *et al.* (1994).

asked to identify briefly presented words, including words initially read and other words not read. Normal subjects and amnesic patients performed better on the previously presented words (priming), but the patient with visual cortex damage did not. However this patient performed normally on conventional memory tests. In independent functional brain imaging studies, the visual cortex showed decreased activation to recently presented materials, suggesting that less neural activity is required to identify words recently processed. These findings suggest that the neuronal basis of priming is an increase in the efficiency and bias in the direction of cortical sensory processing associated with perceptual identification.

Working Memory and the Special Role of the Prefrontal Cortex

Working memory involves the capacity to hold information on line, i.e., in consciousness, during the manipulation of information associated with a wide range of cognitive functions. Many neuropsychological studies have shown deficits in working memory following damage to areas of the cerebral cortex. In addition, numerous functional imaging studies have examined the activation of cerebral cortical areas in humans during encoding and retrieval of memories and during working memory performance. These studies typically show activation associated with verbal and nonverbal memory performance in the left hemisphere and right hemisphere, respectively. During a large variety of tasks, large networks of cortical areas are activated. Specific perceptual processing areas in the posterior cortical zones are activated selectively during remembering specific type of materials (e.g., auditory, visual, verbal; Nyberg *et al.*, 2000; Wheeler *et al.*, 2000). In addition, the prefrontal cortex is reliably activated during effortful encoding and recall and during working memory across a broad range of materials and task protocols.

It has long been known that the prefrontal cortex is especially important to working memory. However, defining the role of the prefrontal cortex in memory is a complex issue that requires consideration of both the type of mnemonic processes and the precise regions of the frontal cortex involved (see Chapters 53 and 54). Early studies of the role of the prefrontal cortex in working memory demonstrated that monkeys with lesions of the prefrontal cortex have severe deficits on delayed-response tasks where the monkeys must remember for brief periods the location where food was placed most recently. Subsequent findings have indicated that damage to the cortex of the sulcus principalis (area 46) results in a selective

impairment in spatial working memory, whereas lesions in other parts of the lateral prefrontal cortex result in impairments on nonspatial as well as spatial memory tasks, especially in working memory tasks where the number of stimuli to be held in memory increases and when the subject must remember the precise serial order in which events have occurred (called self-ordered monitoring).

Consistent with the findings from lesion studies, data from single cell recordings indicate both regional differentiation and a considerable capacity for integration of information across prefrontal regions. Some studies have described cells in the cortex of the sulcus principalis that were specifically active during spatial working memory performance, whereas cells in other parts of the lateral prefrontal cortex seemed to be specifically active during visual object working memory performance. However, several other studies have reported that prefrontal cells with delay activity related to working memory for spatial and object information are mixed within prefrontal regions when these different types of information must be combined to solve the task. The combination of findings from lesion and recording studies suggests that while there are some indications of regional specialization within the prefrontal cortex, it is also clear that this information can be combined within prefrontal circuits such that the entire prefrontal cortex contributes to working memory (see Chapter 53).

Human patients with prefrontal damage perform normally on several standard tests of verbal and nonverbal memory. However, performance can be impaired severely in certain circumstances, e.g., on short-term memory tasks that require comparisons among a small set of recurring stimuli or judgments of the relative recency of stimuli. These tests are very similar in requirements to those of the classical delayed-response tasks, where two stimuli recur repeatedly, and the requirement is to discriminate their most recent occurrence from several earlier ones. In addition, patients with dorsolateral prefrontal lesions have severe impairments monitoring events within working memory. These impairments are illustrated in a self-ordered working memory task in which the patients are presented with a set of stimuli and are required to select a different stimulus on each trial until all the stimuli are selected. From the moment they begin responding, the patients must keep track of stimuli that have already been selected and compare them with stimuli that remain to be selected, similar to the tasks on which monkeys show impairments following damage to the middorsal part of the lateral frontal cortex (i.e., dorsal area 46 and area 9).

Prefrontal Contributions to Episodic Memory

Although patients with selective damage to prefrontal regions do not develop a profound amnesia for recent events, they have great difficulty remembering when and where recent events occurred—the defining features of episodic memory. Patients with frontal lobe lesions have great difficulty remembering the temporal order of two events. Similarly, frontal lobe damage often produces a phenomenon known as source amnesia, in which patients can acquire new facts but fail to recollect when or where they learned them. Source memory problems have also been noted in elderly adults, who often exhibit signs of frontal lobe pathology, and in young children, who have immature frontal functions (see Chapter 46). Damage to the frontal lobes can also produce striking distortions of episodic memory in which patients claim to remember events that never occurred.

Episodic memory has also been investigated using modern neuroimaging techniques. These studies have consistently revealed frontal lobe activation during episodic memory tasks. In some studies, right frontal regions show greater activation than left frontal regions during episodic retrieval, and left frontal regions show greater activation than right frontal regions during episodic encoding. In contrast, activation in the medial temporal lobe, including the hippocampus, is observed during both encoding and retrieval. Prefrontal regions show activation when subjects make extensive efforts to recall recently presented information, whereas the hippocampal formation becomes active during the actual recollection of that information. Thus, both prefrontal and medial temporal regions play important roles in episodic memory, although their contributions are distinct.

Summary

Studies in both animals and humans show that the cerebral cortex is highly plastic in that its representations can be altered after experience. All cortical information processing inherently involves adaptations to stimulus regularities and contingencies, and cortical plasticity reflects storage of the information that is processed. These observations serve to emphasize a fundamental theme, specifically that memory should be conceived as intimately intertwined with information processing in the cortex, indeed so much so that "memory" and "information processing" are difficult to distinguish.

Consistent with this view, the cortex participates in memory in several ways. Distinct cortical areas are reorganized by specific training experiences to meet demands for specific types of perceptual representation and memory. Specific cortical association areas process particular categories of knowledge and perform specific types of information processing associated with particular categories of knowledge. Also, modality-relevant cortical circuits are able to support the priming of perceptual representations. Finally, operating in conjunction with other cortical areas, the prefrontal cortex mediates executive functions, and this processing is critical to monitoring the flow of information processing during working memory and to retrieving the temporal and contextual organization of memories in episodic recall.

CONCLUSIONS

The present chapter has reviewed the evidence that there are multiple memory systems in the brain. One major system involves the cortical association areas, multiple cortical areas surrounding the hippocampus and hippocampus, and this system mediates the establishment and consolidation of declarative memories. Other brain systems mediate nondeclarative forms of memory. These include a stimulus–response or habit-learning system that is dependent on the neostriatum, a system for sensori-motor adaptations dependent on the cerebellum, a stimulus–reinforcer or emotional memory system dependent on the amygdala, and a memory modulation system that also centers on the amygdala. In addition, areas of the cerebral cortex support specific aspects of semantic memory and perceptual learning, and large networks of cortical areas, including the prefrontal cortex, mediate working memory and contribute to episodic memory. These systems support specific aspects of memory peformance independently, but operate in concert to support the various ways that behavior and mental life can be modified by experience.

References

Amaral, D. G, and Witter, M. P. (1989). The three-dimensional organization of the hippocampal formation: A review of anatomical data. *Neuroscience* **31**, 571–591.

Bechera, A., Tranel, D., Hanna, D., Adolphs, R., Rockland, C., and Damasio, A. R. (1995). Double dissociation of conditioning and declarative knowledge relative to the amygdala and hippocampus in humans. *Science* **269**, 1115–1118.

Bunsey, M., and Eichenbaum, H. (1996). Conservation of hippocampal memory function in rats and humans. *Nature* **379**, 255–257.

Burwell, R. D., Witter, M. P., and Amaral, D.G. (1995). Perirhinal and postrhinal cortices in the rat: A review of the neuroanatomical literature and comparison with findings from the monkey brain. *Hippocampus* **5**, 390–408.

Cahill, L., Prins, B., Weber, M., and McGaugh, J. L. (1994). β-adrenergic activation and memory for emotional events. *Nature* **371**, 702–704.

Cohen, N. J., and Squire, L. R. (1980). Preserved learning and retention of pattern analyzing skill in amnesics: Dissociation of knowing how and knowing that. *Science* **210**, 207–210.

Corkin, S., Amaral, D. G., Gonzalez, R. G., Johnson, K. A., and Hyman, B. T. (1997). H. M.'s medial temporal lobe lesion.' Findings from magnetic resonance imaging. *J. Neurosci.* **17**, 3964–3979.

Davis, M. (1992). The role of the amygdala in fear and anxiety. *Annu. Rev. Neurosci.* **15**, 353–1375.

Eichenbaum, H., and Cohen, N.J. (2001). "From Conditioning to Conscious Recollection: Memory Systems of the Brain." Oxford Univ. Press.

Fuster, J. M. (2001) The prefrontal cortex—An update: Time is of the essence. *Neuron* **30**, 319–333.

Gallagher, M., and Holland, P.C. (1994). The amygdala complex: Multiple roles in associative learning and attention. *Proc. Nat. Acad. Sci. USA* **91**, 1171–1776.

Gilbert, C. D., and Wiesel, T. N. (1992). Receptive field dynamics in adult primary visual cortex. *Nature* **356**, 150–152.

Knowlton, B. J., Mangels, J. A., and Squire, L. R. (1996). A neostriatal habit learning system in humans. *Science* **273**, 1399–1401.

LeDoux, J. E. (1992). Brain mechanisms of emotion and emotional learning. *Curr. Opin. Neurobiol.* **2**, 191–197.

McDonald, R. J., and White, N. M. (1993). A triple dissociation of memory systems: Hippocampus, amygdala, and dorsal striatum. *Behav. Neurosci.* **107**, 3–22.

McGaugh, J. L. (2000). Memory—a century of consolidation. *Science* **287**, 248–251.

McGaugh, J. L., Introini-Collison, I. B., Cahill, L., Kim, M., and Liang, K. C. (1992). Involvement of the amygdala in neuromodulatory influences on memory storage. *In* "The Amgydala: Neurobiological Aspects of Emotion, Memory, and Mental Dysfunction" (J. P. Aggleton, ed.), pp. 431–451. Wiley-Liss, New York.

Mishkin, M. (1978) Memory in monkeys severely impaired by combined but not separate removal of the amygdala and hippocampus. *Nature* **273**, 297–298.

Morris, R. G. M., Garrud, P., Rawlins, J. N. P., and O'Keefe, J. (1982). Place navigation impaired in rats with hippocampal lesions. *Nature* **297**, 681–683.

Nyberg, L., Habib, R., McIntosh, A. R., and Tulving, E. (2000) Reactivation of encoding related brain activity during memory retrieval. *Proc. Nat. Acad. Sci. USA* **97**, 11120–11124.

O'Keefe, J. (1976). Place units in the hippocampus of the freely moving rat. *Exp. Neurol.* **51**, 78–109.

O'Keefe, J., and Nadel, L. (1978). "The Hippocampus as a Cognitive Map." Oxford Univ. Press (Clarendon), London.

Packard, M. G., and Knowlton, B. J. (2002). Learning and memory functions of the basal ganglia. *Ann. Rev. Neurosci.* **25**, 563–593.

Packard, M. G., and McGaugh, J. L. (1996). Inactivation of hippocampus or caudate nucleus with lidocaine differentially affects expression of place and response learning. *Neurobiol. Learn. Memory* **65**, 65–72.

Recanzone, G. H., Schreiner, C. E., and Merzenich, M. M. (1993). Plasticity in the frequency representation of primary auditory cortex following discrimination training in adult owl monkeys. *J. Neurosci.* **13**, 87–103.

Sakai, K., and Miyashita, Y. (1991). Neural organization for the long-term memory of paired associates. *Nature* **354**, 152–155.

Scoville, W. B., and Milner, B. (1957). Loss of recent memory after bilateral hippocampal lesions. *J. Neurol. Neurosur. Psychiatry* **20**, 11–21.

Suzuki, W. A. (1996). Neuroanatomy of the monkey entorhinal, perirhinal, and parahioppocampal cortices: Organization of cortical inputs and interconnections with amygdala and striatum. *Semin. Neurosci.* **8**, 3–12.

Thompson, R. F., and Kim, J. J. (1996). Memory systems in the brain and localization of a memory. *Proc. Nat. Acad. Sci. USA* **93**, 13438–13444.

Tulving, E. (1972). Episodic and semantic memory. *In* "Organization of Memory" (E. Tulving and W. Donaldson, eds.), pp. 381–403. Academic Press, New York.

Warrington, E. K., and Shallice, T. (1984). Category-specific semantic impairments. *Brain* **107**, 829–854.

Wheeler, M. E., Petersen, S. E., and Buckner, R. L. (2000). Memory's echo: Vivid remembering reactivates sensory specific cortex. *Proc. Nat. Acad. Sci.* **97**, 11125–11129.

Wood, E. R., Dudchenko, P. A., and Eichenbaum, H. (1999). The global record of memory in hippocampal neuronal activity. *Nature* **397**, 613–616.

Wood, E., Dudchenko, P., Robitsek, J. R., and Eichenbaum, H. (2000). Hippocampal neurons encode information about different types of memory episodes occurring in the same location. *Neuron* **27**, 623–633.

Zola-Morgan, S., and Squire, L. R. (1985). Medial temporal lesions in monkeys impair memory on a variety of tasks sensitive to human amnesia. *Behav. Neurosci.* **99**, 22–34.

Zola, S. M., Squire, L. R., Teng, E., Stefanacci, L., Buffalo, E. A., and Clark, R. E. (2000). Impaired recognition memory in monkeys after damage limited to the hippocampal region. *J. Neurosci.* **20**, 451–463.

Suggested Readings

Cahill, L., and McGaugh, J. L. (1998). Mechanisms of emotional arousal and lasting declarative memory. *Trends Neurosc.* **21**, 273–313.

Bloedel, J. R., Ebner, T. J., and Wise, S. P. (eds.) (1996). "The Acquisition of Motor Behavior in Vertebrates." MIT Press, Cambridge, MA.

Fuster, J. M. (1995). "Memory in the Cerebral Cortex: An Empirical Approach to Neural networks in the Human and Nonhuman Primate." MIT Press, Cambridge, MA.

McClelland, J. L., McNaughton, B. L., and O'Reilly, R. C. (1995). Why there are complementary learning systems in the hippocampus and neocortex: Insights from the successes and failures of connectionist models of learning and memory. *Psychol. Rev.* **102**, 419–457.

Schacter, D. L. (1987). Implicit memory: History and current status. *J. Exp. Psychol. Learn. Memory Cogn.* **13**, 501–518.

Schacter, D. L., and Tulving, E. (eds.) (1994). "Memory Systems." MIT Press, Cambridge, MA.

Squire, L. R. (1992). Memory and the hippocampus: A synthesis from findings with rats, monkeys, and humans. *Psychol. Revi.* **99**, 195–231.

Suzuki, W., and Clayton, N.S. (2001). The hippocampus and memory: A comparative and ethological perspective. *Curr. Opin. Neurobiol.* **10**, 768–773.

Ungerleider, L. G. (1995). Functional brain imaging studies of cortical mechanisms for memory. *Science* **270**, 760–775.

Zola-Morgan, S. (1995). Localization of brain function: The legacy of Franz Joseph Gall (1758–1828). *Annu. Revi. Neurosci.* **18**, 359–383.

Howard B. Eichenbaum

Language and Communication

Language is one of the pillars of human intellect. It is the principal way we formulate thoughts and convey them to others. It plays a role in how we analyze the world, reason, solve problems, and plan actions. It lets us convey memories of the past and beliefs about the future, engage others in thinking about events that have not taken place, and express the relationships we perceive between items and events in the world.

Language is also an indispensable part of human culture. Without it, our systems of jurisprudence, commerce, science, art, and other human endeavors could not exist in the forms we know them, if at all. Language is itself an esthetic object, and many people find that linguistic renderings can capture the essence of profound emotions such as love and grief. Without language, each person's discoveries would die with him or her; language makes it possible for the achievements of one individual to be transmitted to the rest of the human species. Language skills are therefore vital to the success of societies and of individuals within societies.

The way the human brain represents and processes language has been approached in many ways. Studies of the communication systems of other species give some hints about neural mechanisms that might support language. More direct evidence comes from the effects of diseases that affect language and from observations of brain activity that occurs while individuals are performing language tasks.

This chapter discusses aspects of language and the relationship of language to the brain. It begins with a discussion of animal communication, from which human language evolved and which provides a guide to the basic neural elements and processes that underlie our own system of communication. The next

section of the chapter provides a brief summary of what human language is and how it is processed. The third section looks at how human language is related to the brain, relying on studies of patients with various types of neurological diseases and on brain imaging in normal subjects.

ANIMAL COMMUNICATION

Communication Is Important for Individual Survival

The ultimate goal of most animal communication, like that of behavior in general, is reproduction. Thus, signals that indicate the sender's species, gender, and degree of reproductive readiness account for the vast majority of natural communication. These are the messages being broadcast by chirping crickets, flashing fireflies, pheromone-releasing moths, and singing birds. Frequently, the mate-attraction call is also used to warn off potential rivals; e.g., bird and cricket songs are also used to identify the boundaries of territories or personal space. Differences in signal quality are the usual basis of mate choice in species for which some degree of discrimination is evident. This competition for the attention of members of the opposite sex has led to the development of more conspicuous signals and, in many cases, to the evolution of displays, signaling morphology (i.e., sounds vs shapes vs color vs movement vs odors), and messages that go far beyond the basic needs of species and sexual identification (Gould and Gould, 1996).

Most animals are solitary except when mating; they abandon their eggs or larvae before the offspring are born. However, a number of species engage in some degree of parental care. For them, signals between parent and offspring are often very important. Most birds, for instance, have about two dozen innate calls that communicate mundane messages such as the need to eat, defecate, take cover, and so on. In cases in which both parents tend the young—the usual circumstance in birds, for instance—additional signals are required to agree on a nest site, synchronize brooding shifts, and guard the nestlings. Most primates also come equipped with two to three dozen innate signals.

The minority of species that are highly social have the most elaborate communication systems of all. They need messages for a variety of elements of social coordination, including, in many cases, group hunting or foraging, defense, and working out of a social hierarchy.

Animal Communication Strategies and Mechanisms

Attracting a mate is vital to species survival. To ensure species specificity in mating, most organisms rely on more than one cue to identify a sexual partner. (Exceptions include some of the species that rely on pheromones.) Thus, multiple signals are sent, and a choice must be made between sending simultaneous messages and sending sequential messages (or a combination of the two). The sequential strategy has the advantage that the individual signals must be correct *and* the order must be appropriate. A female stickleback, for instance, requires the male to have a red ventral stripe, perform a zig-zag dance, poke his nose in a nest, and then vibrate her abdomen; the odds of this concatenation of signals occurring together in this order by chance are remote. However, sequential signaling is time-consuming. A faster strategy is to provide all the cues in parallel, an approach that accepts the larger chance that these cues can occur together by chance. For example, when a parent herring gull waves its bill in front of chicks to see if they need to be fed, the young simultaneously see a vertical beak, a red spot, and a horizontal motion, each of which is a discrete cue that combine in the mind of the chick to elicit pecking.

Nearly all animal communication is innate: the sender produces the appropriate signal in the correct context even without any opportunity for learning, and it can be recognized for what it is by equally naive conspecifics. The basis of innate recognition appears to lie with feature detectors in the nervous systems—the inborn circuits that automatically isolate iconic visual or acoustic elements. In the visual system the simplest elements include spots, lines, and

movement. To the extent that the issue has been studied, innate recognition can usually be correlated with such feature detectors. In the case of European toads, the signals unwittingly emitted by prey (e.g., a line moving along its long axis, which corresponds to a worm crawling) and the behavior of the predator correlate perfectly with neural responses recorded simultaneously from the nervous system (i.e., when the prey-detector neurons fire, the toad snaps at the prey). In the jargon of ethology, innately recognized features with special salience for an organism are known as "sign stimuli"; the roughly equivalent term in psychology is "unconditioned stimuli" (Gould, 1982).

The availability of many visual, auditory, tactile, and olfactory feature detectors, which can, in theory, be used in any specific combination or order, accounts for most of the diversity of animal communication, and reliance on these single feature detectors, rather than pattern detection, accounts for its limitations. For instance, female crickets initially approach male conspecifics on the basis of a calling song. The carrier frequency and time intervals within the song are important, but the actual pattern of the song, so memorable to our ears, is lost on the females: the call is equally attractive played forward and backward. This makes sense because pattern detectors are rare in the nervous system. So, too, young gull chicks find a hand-held knitting needle with several "spots" more stimulating than an adult gull; the ability to recognize a gull head and beak as a holistic unit, although it might be adaptive, is absent, reflecting the rarity of complex innate pattern recognition.

Innate Communication Mechanisms

A common misapprehension is that complex behaviors must be learned. In fact, complex behavior in relatively short-lived species is usually innate, reflecting the reality that intricate activities are very difficult to learn and may require more time and risk of errors than an animal can afford (Gould and Gould, 1999). Thus, so far as is known, all bird nests are built on the basis of innate instructions, although some improvement with experience is also evident. Therefore, looking at just how complex innate communication can be is a useful calibration for the often-made assumption that something as intricate as human speech must be largely learned.

In terms of its ability to communicate information, the most complex system of nonhuman communication known at present is the dance of honeybees (Gould and Gould, 1995). The system has some properties that are reminiscent of human language: it uses

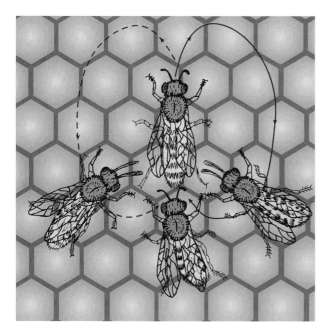

FIGURE 52.1 The waggle dance of honeybees follows a figure eight; the two intersecting straight runs are emphasized by waggling of the body and the production of sound.

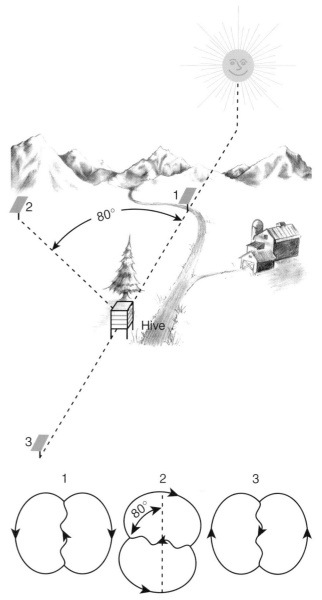

FIGURE 52.2 Direction is encoded into the dance as the angle of the waggle runs left or right of vertical on the comb, which corresponds to the angle to the food relative to the sun's azimuth in the field.

arbitrary conventions to describe objects distant in both space and time; i.e., it does not reflect a real-time emotive readout, as might be the case when a primate gives an alarm call or grunts at a banana. The dance simultaneously specifies the distance, direction, and quality of a food source, water supply, or potential nest site. The dance consists of a figure eight pattern of movement on the part of the signaling forager, with a simultaneous waggling of the body (at about 13 Hz) and buzzing (consisting of 280-Hz bursts occurring at 30 Hz) during the central parts—the waggle runs—of the dance (Fig. 52.1). The dance normally takes place on the vertical surface of the comb within the darkness of the hive cavity.

Direction is indicated by the orientation of the waggle runs: straight up is taken to be the direction of the sun, so that a dance whose average waggle-run angle is 80° to the left of vertical is indicating a site 80° to the left of the sun's current azimuth (Fig. 52.2). Because the sun moves from east to west over the course of the day, dances indicating a specific site precess counterclockwise to compensate. This compensation is evident in the extended dances of foragers that have had no opportunity to see the sun for minutes or even hours: as time passes, the dance angle shifts counterclockwise at just the rate the sun's azimuth shifts clockwise. That "up" should mean "the direction of the sun" seems arbitrary, as "down" would work equally well so long as encoder and decoder agreed on the convention; the dance direction could also be referenced to some other cue—magnetic north or the direction the hive entrance faces.

Distance is indicated by the duration of the waggle run or one of the several factors that correlate with it—duration of sound production, number of sound bursts, and so on. The conversion of meters flown to waggle duration differs among subspecies: for the Egyptian honeybee, a waggle is equivalent to less than 10 m, whereas Italian honeybees value a waggle at about 20 m, and German honeybees peg the exchange rate closer to 50 m (Fig. 52.3). These dialects are innate.

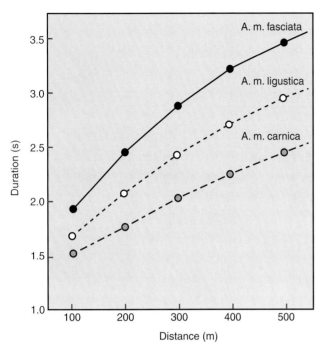

FIGURE 52.3 Distance is encoded as the duration of the waggle run. Different subspecies have different dialects.

In terms of information content, a honeybee dance is second (albeit a very distant second) only to human speech, and so far as is known is far richer than the language of any primate. However the dance language suffers from at least two limitations: It is a closed system—there seems to be no way to introduce new conventions to deal with novel needs. It is also graded; instead of discrete signals for different directions or distances, single components are varied over a range of values (angles and durations). The less complex but more flexible systems of birds and primates illustrate the likely evolutionary precursors of speech.

Innate Communication Systems Coupled with Learning

Some birds have innate songs. In these species, individuals raised in isolation produce songs that are indistinguishable from their socially reared peers and respond to calls appropriately without prior experience. Chickens, doves, gulls, and ducks are familiar examples. Most songbirds, however, illustrate a different pattern: Isolated chicks sing a schematic form of the species song, but the richness of a normal song is absent. Adult conspecifics can recognize innate songs as coming from members of their species, but in general these impoverished vocalizations produce lower levels of response. Typically, there is a sensitive period during which exposure to song must occur, if it is going to have any impact (Fig. 52.4). In most species, there is a gap

between this sensitive period and the process of overt song development; i.e., that is, practice and perfection of the adult song are based on the bird's memory of what it heard during its sensitive period (Gould and Marler, 1987).

Given a range of possible song models during isolated rearing, a chick selects an example from its own species and memorizes it. If it hears only songs of other species, the mature song is the unmodified innate song (Fig. 52.4). Thus there is an innate bias in the initial learning. Where this bias has been studied, it appears to depend on acoustic sign stimuli (i.e., species-specific "syllables"). Indeed, chicks are able to extract syllables of their species embedded in foreign songs, or scored in a way never found in their species (e.g., a syllable that is repeated at an accelerating rate presented to a species that sings syllables at a constant rate, or vice versa will be extracted and used in the species-typical manner).

Practice is essential in the normal development of birdsong, and part of this practice occurs in a babbling phase known as subsong, which begins at a species-typical age. A bird deafened after its sensitive period, but before it begins producing notes in preparation for singing (subsong), is unable to produce even an innate song (Fig. 52.4). During the earliest parts of subsong, birds try out a number of notes. These notes are typical of the species, but most are absent from the song they eventually sing. The learning process may involve producing each member of an innate repertoire of notes, listening to them, checking to see if they match any element in the memorized song, discarding the unnecessary ones, and rearranging, scoring, and modifying the others to produce a reasonable copy of the original song heard during the sensitive period.

There is some flexibility in song development. For example, when the chick has heard two very different specimens of its own species' song, it will often incorporate elements from each. Similarly, when the chick has been exposed to the sight of a singing conspecific and simultaneously the sound of a heterospecific song, it may pick out elements of the abnormal song and adapt them as best it can into its own species-specific organization.

Birdsong, therefore, depends on two processes that involve an interaction between innate capacities and learning: imprinting the song in memory and then learning to perform it. This system is flexible, but only within clear limits.

Communication Systems in Primates

Primates are the species with the closest evolutionary links to humans, and therefore the communica-

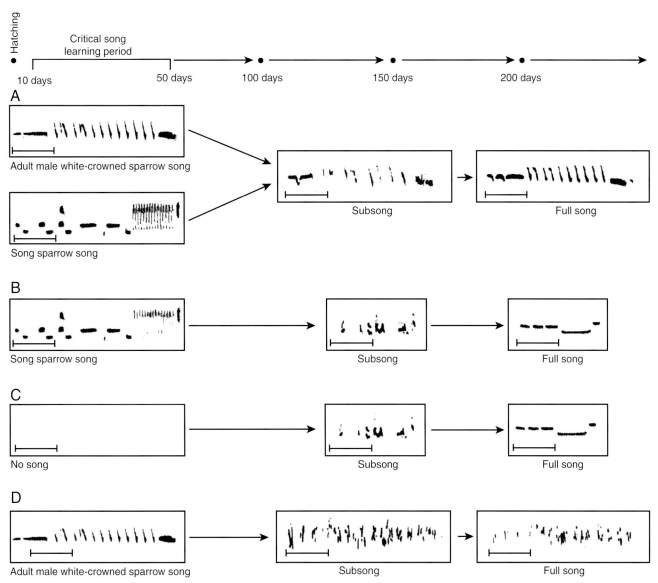

FIGURE 52.4 Birdsong development in most species is characterized by a sensitive period during which a song of the species must be heard. Later, during subsong, the bird practices making notes and assembles them into the correct order and pattern (A). Birds not allowed to hear their species' song sing a schematic version of the song (B and C); birds deafened before subsong cannot sing (D).

tion systems found in these animals are important to study for clues regarding the neural basis of human language.

Vervets, a species of monkey, provide a good case study. Vervets, like all social primates, have a large repertoire of innate calls used for social communication. Among these approximately three dozen signals are four alarm calls (Cheney and Seyfarth, 1990). In some parts of their range, one of the calls is specific for martial eagles; in another the same call is used for certain hawks. In either case, the call causes monkeys to look up; those at the tops of trees drop to the interior, whereas those on the ground move into bushes or under trees. A second call, specific to leopards in one region and to other solitary hunters elsewhere, sends the warned individuals up to the tree tops. A third, specific for snakes, induces the other members of the troop to stand up and look around in the grass. A fourth call is heard in the presence of humans or group-hunting predators.

The development of calling is revealing. Young vervets appear to understand the class of animals each call refers to, but not the particular species that are dangerous. Thus, infants will give the eagle call to harmless vultures, storks, and even falling leaves, but not to snakes or leopards. Consequently, adults generally respond to the alarm calls of infants with a casual look around, followed by their own alarm if there is a genuine danger. Juveniles make fewer mistakes, and adult errors are confined to calls produced when the potential threat is so far away that human observers require binoculars to identify the species. In short, young vervets seem to learn the details of how to apply an innate categorical vocabulary.

Neural Structures for Animal Communication Systems

The neural mechanisms that underlie animal communication may give clues as to those that allow for human language. These systems of course differ in different phyla and species. This section briefly reviews aspects of the neural basis for birdsong and primate communication. It would be of great interest to report on the neural basis for the dance of the bees, but nothing is known about this subject.

Birdsong

Birdsong appears to be produced by a small number of nuclei (collections of nerve cells). In the canary, four important nuclei are involved: HVc, RA, DM and nXIIts. Lesions in any of these nuclei destroy or seriously impair song production. These nuclei also respond when song is presented, and some neurons in some nuclei in some species (e.g., neurons in nXIIts in the zebra finch and the white-crowned sparrow) respond specifically to particular aspects of song. This indicates an overlap in the neural mechanisms involved in song perception and production, a feature that may carry over to humans as well.

Birdsong is produced by a structure between the trachea and the bronchi called the syrinx. There is one syrinx on each side of the trachea. In some species, song is entirely, or mainly, produced by one of these two structures; in other species, both syrinxes participate in song, with each producing different parts of the song. Each syrinx is controlled by structures in its corresponding side of the brain and, when one syrinx is responsible for song, these structures are larger on that side. The perceptual system is also duplicated on both sides of the brain, and, in some species, the two sides of the brain respond to different aspects of song.

In species in which only male birds sing (most species), song nuclei are much larger in males than in females ("sexual dimorphism"). This is not true in those species in which males and females perform duets. In general, there is a correlation between song nucleus size and song complexity in individual birds. Furthermore, song nuclei grow by a factor of almost 100% during the spring mating season (when birds sing) compared to the fall and winter (when they do not).

Changes in the size of song nuclei are related to testosterone production (they can be induced in females by testosterone injection in some circumstances) and by other factors usually related to daylength—part of the birds' innate calendar. They are due to many changes in nerve cells: increase in the number of dendrites, increase in cell size, and, most interestingly, increase in the number of cells. Studies using labeled thymidine, which is taken up by dividing DNA, have shown neurogenesis in neurons in the HVc nucleus in relationship to periods of increased song, indicating that new nerve cells are formed. These neurons project to the RA nucleus, strongly suggesting that they play a role in song.

Primates

The neural basis for primate vocalizations is beginning to be charted. Unlike humans, vocalizations in primates do not appear to begin in a lateral cortical region but rather in the medial portion of the brain (the cingulate), a region involved in connecting basic instinctual to more advanced cognitive functions. Actual motor planning appears to involve mainly brain stem nuclei. On the perception side, there are neurons in the auditory cortex of some species of macaque monkeys that selectively respond to conspecific calls. These regions show some degree of functional asymmetry in some species, with responses from cells in the left hemisphere and not the right.

Possible Lessons from Nonhuman Species Regarding Language and Its Neural Basis

It is dangerous to infer too much about human language, or about how the human brain may support language, from studies of species that are very distant, such as birds. However, these species provide evidence for the possibility of certain aspects of language and its neural basis that could have developed several times in evolution or that could date to a distant common ancestor

At a behavioral level, human speech and language could have developed from the repertoire of two to three dozen innate calls typical of birds and primates. In that case, we would expect to find that language contains elements that are innately recognized and that may be distinguished by the sorts of acoustic features that provide the basis for the innate discrimination of sign stimuli in other species. In fact, babies have an innate ability to discriminate a small number of sounds found in human languages, which function as acoustic sign stimuli. The evolution of human speech could also have retained the sorts of sensitive periods and innate learning biases so evident in song birds and vervet monkeys. In this case, we might expect to see a species-typical babbling phase, and perhaps a sensitive period for easy learning of new languages. If the evolution of speech and language preserves the use of preexisting (innate) forms, we might expect there to be innate aspects of human language, which would presumably be found in all languages and which might surface in situations where we see a "default grammar," not unlike the unlearned and impoverished songs of birds reared in isolation.

From the neurological perspective, several features of the neural organization for communication systems appear to be found in humans in a way that is relevant to language. These features are the fact that there are specialized neural nuclei for song production; that the neural basis for song production is often asymmetric, with one hemisphere producing most of song or the two hemispheres producing different aspects of song; that production and perception of song make use of same structures to some degree; and that there is a relationship of size to function. However, other important features of the neurobiology of birdsong, such as the neurogenesis that is important in the seasonal changes in song production, are not known to play a role in human speech and language. As for primates, the neural system responsible for call production is quite different from that in humans, being based in the cortex that is transitional from limbic to association regions (reflecting the limited semantic content and immediate biological relevance of most calls). Asymmetries in the neural basis for call perception, and the existence of neurons in the auditory association cortex that selectively respond to conspecific calls, may be quite direct evolutionary precursors of the human neural substrate for language.

HUMAN LANGUAGE

Although animal communication systems can be quite sophisticated and some of them share attributes with human language, human language is far more complex than animal communication. There are many features of human language that make it special.

One is what messages human language can convey. As we have seen, most animal communication systems serve the purposes of identifying members of a species. These systems do sometimes designate items of immediate biological significance, such as designation of *predators* by monkeys or food sources by bees. Human language differs from these systems with respect to the number of items that can be designated and the relationship of these items to present

biological necessity. Human language allows us to designate an infinitely large number of items, actions, and properties of items and actions, and to do so with respect to items that are not immediately biologically compelling.

Human language also allows us to relate items, actions, and properties to one another. This propositional level of semantic content is beyond the scope of any known animal communication system. At a yet higher level, human language allows us to express relationships between events and states of affairs in the world, such as temporal order and causation. Again, this level of meaning is far beyond anything available to other species as far as we know.

The power of language to express so many aspects of meaning is due to the fact that language has many types of representations. It consists of words, words made from other words, groupings of words into phrases and sentences, and groupings of sentences into a discourse. Each of these levels of linguistic representation consists of specific forms that are related to specific aspects of meaning. The forms at each level are intricately structured, and there are an infinite number of different structures that can be built at each level of the system. This leads to a situation in which items can be elaborated on in infinitely many ways. The result is a powerful and complex system of representation.

Human language develops naturally in the auditory-oral modality. However, humans who are deaf can develop language in the visual and gestural modalities, and the structures of these language are essentially the same as those of spoken language, once allowances are made for the fact that they are signed instead of spoken. Languages can also be represented orthographically. Orthographies range from alphabetical scripts such as English, to syllabic, consonantal, and ideographic orthographies. Orthography is not acquired in the way spoken and signed language is; reading and writing require instruction to master. This chapters deal only with spoken language. For an introduction to signed language and its neurology, see Bellugi *et al.* (1990); for a discussion of orthographic representational systems, see Henderson (1982).

Words

Simple words are defined and distinguished from each other primarily by their phonemes. A phoneme is a single distinct sound that contrasts with another (see Fig. 52.5) and makes it possible to determine the existence of a word in a language. For instance, in English /p/ and /b/ are different phonemes because they determine the separate existence of the members

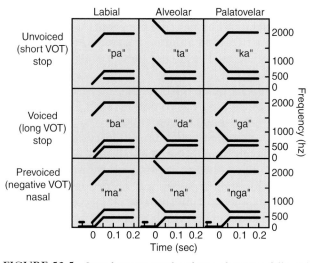

FIGURE 52.5 Sound spectrographs of nine phonemes followed by a short "a" sound. The sound bands are called "formants." The first (bottom) two formants are independent; the third is a harmonic of the second.

TABLE 52.1 Phonemes of American English[a]

Consonants		Vowels	
Symbol	Example	Symbols	Example
/w/	wet	/i/	heed
/ʍ/	whet	/I/	hid
/b/	bill	/e/ or /ei/	rain
/d/	dig	/ɛ/	head
/g/	give	/æ/	had
/p/	pick	/a/	odd
/t/	tin	/ɔ/	bought
/k/	key	/ʊ/	hood
/m/	men	/u/	too
/n/	nine	/ˆ/	ton
/η/	ring	/ə/	the
/f/	fast	/ɚ/	earth
/v/	vice	/ai/	hide
/θ/	thigh	/ɔi/	boy
/ð/	thy	/au/	out
/s/	sick	/oʊ/	boat
/z/	zip	/iu/	few
/ʃ/	shy		
/ʒ/	measure		
/l/	lie		
/r/	rock		
/j/	you		
/h/	hello		
/tʃ/	charm		
/dʒ/	joke		

[a] Phonemic symbols corresponding to the consonants are shown on the left along with an example of a typical word that includes each sound as indicated by the underlined letter or letters in each word. Right-hand columns present a similar list of vowel sounds and words that include these.

of word pairs such as pat-bat, pale-bale, pull-bull, lap-lab. A major distinction between different types of phonemes is the difference between vowels and consonants. Consonants involve some degree of constriction of the vocal tract; vowels are produced with a relatively open vocal tract. Each language "selects" its inventory of phonemes from a relatively small set of phonemes found across languages. American English phonemes have 25 consonants and 17 vowels, as listed in Tables 52.1 and 52.2.

At the semantic level, put in very simple terms, words designate concrete objects, abstract concepts,

TABLE 52.2 Articulatory Classification of English Consonant Sounds[a]

Place of articulation	Manner of articulation					
			Stop		Fricative	
	Glide	Nasal	Voiced	Unvoiced	Voiced	Unvoiced
Front						
Bilabial	w, ʍ	m	b	p		
Labiodental					v	f
Middle						
Dental					ð	θ
Alveolar	j,l	n	d	t	z	s
Palatal	r				ʒ	ʃ
Back						
Velar	w, ʍ	η	g	k		
Pharyngeal						h
Glottal		ɔ				

[a] The articulatory features of manner, place, and voicing classify the consonant sounds according to similarities and differences that exist in the way in which each sound is produced. Note that the voicing distinction is relevant only for stops and fricatives in English.

actions, properties, and logical connectives. Many philosophers and psychologists, and most neurologists who have considered the subject, have thought that the meaning of a word consists of a set of features of objects and actions that are associated with the word's sound through one's experience. However, the meaning of a word also includes unobserved properties of the item that the word designates, such as our knowledge that cats can swim even if we have never observed one swimming. This knowledge may be based on inductive generalizations, logical inferences, or innate concepts regarding the structure of items. Tulving (1972), who called the complex set of properties that make up word meaning "semantic memory," emphasized that the hallmark of this type of knowledge is the relations that items have to one another.

Words Formed from Other Words

The word-formation level of language allows words to be formed from other words. Language uses many devices to accomplish this—compounding, affixation, agglutination, and others. English affixation provides a useful illustration. There are two main types of affixes in English: inflection and derivation. Inflection is related to the syntactic structure of a sentence, as in agreement between subjects and objects (I see; he sees). English is relatively poor in overt inflectional features; languages such as Dutch and German have more complete and complex agreement systems that affect adjective–noun agreement, verb inflections, and the case markers on nouns. Derivational processes are those that create new syntactic categories of words (e.g., destroy → destruction; happy → happiness). Derivation allows the meaning associated with a simple lexical item to be used as a different syntactic category without coining a large number of new lexical forms that would have to be learned.

Affixation has semantic consequences. Agreement features convey the semantic features inherent in the agreement. For example, the third-person present tense marker s conveys the information that an action is being accomplished (or is habitually accomplished) by an individual (or a set of individuals considered as a whole) who is neither the speaker nor the listener. Derivational morphology also has effects on semantics. For instance, the thematic roles assigned by a verb (information about who is doing what to whom) are reassigned to different nouns when certain adjective-formation suffixes are added (a noun is understood as the theme of the action of hugging when it is modified by the adjective huggable, as in "The boy is huggable," as opposed to being understood as being the agent of

the action of hugging, as when it is the subject of the verb hugging, as in "The boy is hugging ...).

Sentences

The sentential level of language consists of syntactic structures (Chomsky, 1965, 1981, 1986) into which words are inserted. Individual words are marked for syntactic category [e.g., cat is a noun (N); read is a verb (V); of is a preposition (P)]. These categories combine in a hierarchy to create nonlexical nodes (or phrasal categories), such as noun phrase (NP), verb phrase (VP) and sentence (S). The way words are inserted into these higher order phrasal categories determines a number of different aspects of sentence meaning. For instance, in the sentence "The dog that scratched the cat killed the mouse," there is a sequence of words—the cat killed the mouse—that would, in isolation, mean that the cat killed the mouse. However, "The dog that scratched the cat killed the mouse" does not assert that the cat killed the mouse, but rather that the dog did. This is because the cat is not the subject of killed and does not play a thematic role around killed. The cat is the object of the verb scratched in the relative clause—that scratched the cat—and is the theme of scratched. The dog is the subject of the verb killed and is the agent of that verb. The syntactic structure of "The dog that scratched the cat killed the mouse" is shown in Fig. 52.6, which demonstrates these relationships.

At the sentence level the set of semantic values that language can express expands greatly (Pinker, 1994). Sentences convey aspects of the structure of events

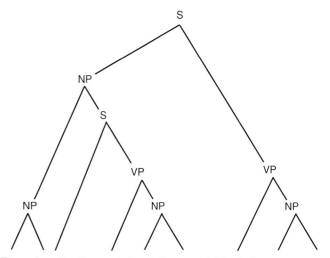

FIGURE 52.6 Syntactic structure of the sentence "The dog that scratched the cat killed the mouse" indicating the hierarchical structure responsible for its meaning.

and states in the world. These semantic values are collectively known as the propositional content of a sentence. These values include thematic roles (information about who did what to whom), attribution of modification (information about which adjectives go with which nouns, such as the fact that in the sentence "The big boy chased the little girl," the boy is big and girl is little), scope of quantification (information about what items are included in the scope of quantifiers, such as the fact that in the sentence, "None of the boys wearing hats was cold," the quantifier "none" applies to the boys wearing hats, not just to the boys), the reference of pronouns and other anaphoric elements (information about which words in a set of sentences refer to the same items or actions, such as the fact that in the sentence "The brother of the visitor shaved himself," "himself" refers to "brother" and not to "visitor"), and so on.

Sentences are a crucial level of the language code because the propositions they express make assertions about the world. These assertions can be added to an individual's knowledge of the world. Because they can be true or false (something that is not possible with words), they can be entered into logical systems. They can serve to add information to semantic memory, they can serve to plan actions, and they can serve other purposes. While the number of words that are available distinguishes human language from animal communication systems, as we have seen, the ability to refer to items is present in a rudimentary form in some nonhuman species. The combinatorial mechanism that produces an infinite number of propositions, however, is distinctly human.

Discourse

The propositional meanings conveyed by sentences are entered into higher order structures that constitute the discourse level of linguistic structure. Discourse includes information about the general topic under discussion, the focus of a speaker's attention, the novelty of the information in a given sentence, the temporal order of events, causation, and so on. Information conveyed by the discourse level of language also serves as a basis for updating an individual's knowledge of the world and for reasoning and planning action.

The structure of discourse involves relationships between propositions, and it also includes information about the syntactic role of words in sentences, intonation, and nonlinguistic items such as the intentions of a speaker and listener and their attentional foci. The discourse level of language is therefore not a purely linguistic structure but integrates several types of representations.

Universal Features of Linguistic Representations

By some counts, there are over 6500 languages in the world. These languages differ in many ways from one another: they have different vocabularies, use different sounds, and have different ways of forming words and different syntactic rules. However, beyond these surface level differences, there are features that are common to all human language. For instance, the sound systems of all human languages consist of alternations of consonants and vowels; no language forms different words by varying features of sound such as its loudness or whether a word is whispered. These "linguistic universals" form a framework within which the features of individual languages occur.

Linguistic universals can arise because of universal features of motor or sensory systems or, possibly, because of constraints on cognitive computational capacities. Linguistic research on language universals investigates those that may reflect abstract aspects of linguistic structure itself. Chomsky's work in the area of syntax is the best known and most controversial example of such analyses.

The syntactic structures of different languages appear to differ enormously. Some languages use agreement to express relationships between lexical items, others use morphology, and others use word order. Languages that use word order differ in the order of words they require (verb-medial, such as English; verb-last, such as Japanese). Despite these differences, Chomsky and his colleagues and students have argued that basic features of syntax are common to all languages. A famous example of his work in this area is the study of constraints on how items at a distance can be related to one another. For instance, in sentence 1, the boat is related to painted.

1. The boat that you believe John painted is red.

There are limitations on these long-distance relationships. For instance, sentence 2 is ungrammatical.

2. The boat that you believe the claim John painted is red.

What makes sentence 2 unacceptable? It cannot be its meaning because it means the same thing as sentence 1. It must be some aspect of its form. What seems to be the problem is that the presence of the words "the claim" makes the distance between the boat and painted too great for this relationship to be established. Chomsky's insight was that the notion of "distance" is not defined in terms of the number of words between the boat and painted. Sentence 3 is perfectly acceptable, even though it has many more words between these phrases.

3. The boat that you believe the workman told Mary John painted is red.

What makes sentence 2 unacceptable is the nature of the syntactic boundaries that occur between the boat and painted. Chomsky and other have developed theories of what kinds of syntactic boundaries can and cannot occur between nouns and the verbs they are related to. These "constraints" differ in different languages, but all languages have restrictions on the syntactic categories that can intervene between elements that are related in certain ways, and these restrictions are always expressed in quite similar terms.

The theoretical issue that makes this analysis important is that Chomsky has argued that universal features of language such as the constraints on the relationship of items are innate. They must be innate, he argues, because it is impossible that a child would ever learn such constraints on the basis of the fragmented and limited exposure he or she has to language. Not only must they be innate, he argues, but the evidence suggests that these universal features of syntax are very abstract and specific to language. Indeed, the exact constraints on the relationship of items as just reviewed are only defined over syntactic structures. Chomsky argues that the child comes to the task of learning a language with a great deal of highly abstract knowledge of what language is like; his or her task is to set a few parameters of these models (such as how many and what types of nodes constrain the connections between particular types of items) to generate the language he or she is exposed to.

Other models of language make very different claims about the nature of innate features of language and the balance between innate knowledge and learning in the development of language abilities. In the past few years, some theorists have argued that the bulk of language acquisition is the result of a massive pattern-association process, supported by mechanisms that can be simulated in "connectionist" (or "neural net") models (Seidenberg, 1997). While such models have had important successes in simulating a few isolated domains of language processing (see, e.g., Seidenberg and MacClelland's (1988) model of learning to read), they have not begun to account for the vast majority of features of language that linguists have described. However, these models tend to be more realistic from a neurological point of view, whereas the neural mechanisms that underlie the representation of the abstract categorical features of language proposed by Chomsky and many linguists remain quite mysterious.

Creoles Suggest That Language May Have a "Default" Grammar

If certain aspects of language are universal and innate, and languages preferentially contain the most elementary structures consistent with these universal features of language, perhaps these features can be seen in some situations in which a language does not become fully developed. Bickerton (1990) has proposed that this is the case for spontaneously created languages. These include the sign languages created by untutored deaf children to allow them to communicate with one another and the many creoles that have developed across the globe. Of the two, creoles are the easiest to study.

Creoles are languages with simple syntactic structures that develop when speakers of several different languages are forced to communicate with one another. This can occur through immigration and invasion or when individuals are brought together from different cultures to work. The adults in such situations develop a crude pidgin, an impoverished communication system in which a limited number of nouns, verbs, and modifiers are combined with extensive gesturing. Children of the pidgin speakers learn their parents' language, but not the pidgin; instead, in addition to using their parents' language, they also create a creole for communication with one another that is based on the pidgin. All creoles share a set of common features, which can contrast with those in fully developed languages.

1. The grammar is based on word order; in contrast, most human languages rely largely on inflection (agreement and derivation—see earlier discussion).
2. There are seven parts of speech: nouns, pronouns, adjectives, verbs, adverbs, articles, and conjunctions; many human languages omit one or more of these categories or add new ones.
3. Nouns are distinguished as singular, plural, or indefinite in number; many languages lack the latter category.
4. There are three particles used as auxiliary verbs to indicate whether an action is successful, unsuccessful, or repeated; many languages lack these distinctions.
5. There is a single verb conjugation system; most languages have a general rule for most verbs, but special-case rules for most of the commonly used (irregular) verbs.
6. Questions are based on intonation rather than word order; many languages use both.

Bickerton points out that, in many cases, these universal features of creoles are not present in the languages spoken by the parents of the children who created the creole. Therefore, creoles are very likely to be related to innately specified features of language.

However, even creoles do not illustrate such features directly. If all the features of creoles just listed were innate, it would be impossible to explain how any languages have any other features. Innate properties of language must be more abstract than the fea-

tures found in creoles and must allow all the different forms of language that are currently found to develop. Instead of thinking of creoles as demonstrating universal features of language directly, we might better think of them as showing us what features of language develop most easily. It is possible that these features characterized human languages at an early stage of their development. If they did, our

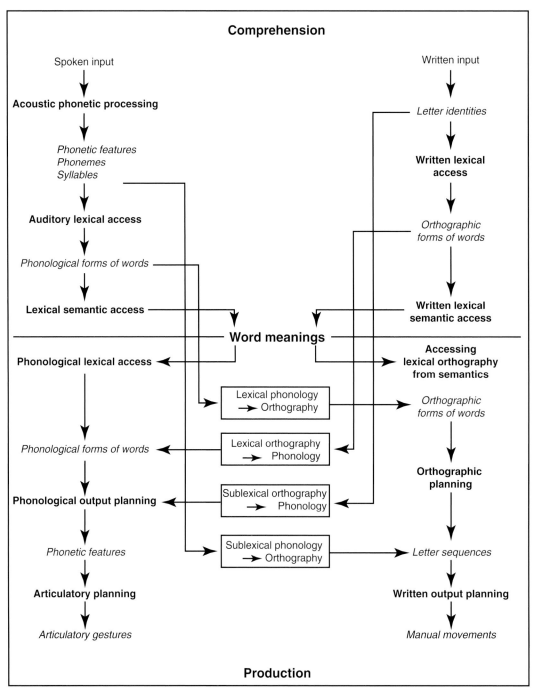

FIGURE 52.7   A model of the major psycholinguistic operations involved in processing simple words.

goal must be to understand these properties of early human languages and also the processes that drove the diversification of the original human languages into the thousands of distinct tongues that exist today.

Language Processing

Every time a speaker produces an utterance and a listener recovers the meaning of that utterance, all the complex structures of a language must be activated. How is this done?

Current models of language processing subdivide functions such as reading, speaking, auditory comprehension, and writing into many different, semi-independent components, which are sometimes called "modules" or "processors." These components can be further divided into variable numbers of highly specialized operations, such as those involved in mapping features of the acoustic signal onto phonemes or in constructing syntactic structures from words. Each operation accepts only particular types of representations as input and produces only specific types of representations as output.

Models of language processing are often expressed as flow diagrams (or "functional architectures") that indicate the sequence of operations of the different components that perform a language-related task. Fig. 52.7 presents a model indicating the sequence of activation of components of the lexical processing system. Fig. 52.7 simplifies information flow in four ways. First, it does not specify the nature of the operations in each of the major components of the system. Second, it does not fully convey the extent to which the components of the system operate in parallel. Third, it does not convey the extent of feedback among the components of the system. Lastly, not all components are represented. Despite these simplifications, the model captures enough aspects of information processing in the language system to give an idea of what functional architectures of language processing look like.

Beyond specifying the flow of information through the language processing system, researchers have begun to understand the operating characteristics of its components. Several important features of language processing operations have been demonstrated in experimental laboratories or in studies of patients.

1. They are specialized for language. For instance, recognition of phonemes is probably accomplished by mechanisms that separate very early in the processing stream from those that recognize other auditory stimuli.

2. They are obligatorily activated when their inputs are presented to them. For instance, if we attend to a sound that happens to be the word "elephant," we must hear and understand that word; we cannot hear this sound as just a noise.

3. They generally operate unconsciously. We usually have the subjective impression that we are extracting another person's meaning and producing linguistic forms without being aware of the details of the sounds of words, sentence structure, and so on.

4. They operate quickly and accurately. For instance, it has been estimated on the basis of many different psycholinguistic experimental techniques that spoken words are usually recognized less than 125 ms after their onset, i.e., while they are still being uttered. The speed of the language processing system as a whole occurs because of the speed of each of its components, but also is achieved because of the massively parallel functional architecture of the system, which leads to many components of the system being simultaneously active.

5. They require processing resources. Although we do not appreciate it consciously, language processing demands some effort. It is unclear whether there are separate pools of processing resources for each language processing component or for language processing as a whole or whether language processing can "borrow" resources from other systems if it needs to.

The operations of the language processing system are regulated by a variety of control mechanisms. These control mechanisms include both ones internal to the language processor itself and those that are involved in other aspects of cognition. The first category—language-internal control mechanisms—consists of a large number of operations that schedule psycholinguistic operations on the basis of the ongoing nature of a given psycholinguistic task. The second category of control mechanisms—those that are related to cognitive processing outside the language system—determine what combinations of processors become active in order to accomplish different tasks such as reading, repeating what one has heard and taking notes on a lecture. Functional communication involving the language code occurs when people use these processors to inform others, to ask for information, to get things done, and so on. The use of language is thus one type of intentional action. There are conventions (or rules) that regulate the use of language for these purposes. However, it is a mistake to think that language is only used, or even mainly used, for functional communication and that language is, at its core, a communication system. The heart of human language is a system of representations relating forms to meaning. In fact, as Chomsky has pointed out, far and away the most common use of language is not interpersonal communication at all, but talking to oneself.

Neural Organization for Language

Sources of Evidence Regarding Language and the Brain

This last part of this chapter reviews the functional neuroanatomy of language. The major techniques used to study the neural basis of language are listed. These techniques have also been used to study other human cognitive functions.

1. Correlating lesions with deficits. This is the approach that first gave insights into how language is organized in the brain. It originally consisted of studying a patient's language and performing an autopsy on the patient after death to determine what part of the brain was affected by a disease. By looking at many patients, a picture of what deficits occurred after damage in particular brain regions can emerge. Today, instead of autopsy data, neuroscientists can obtain images of the living brain. Areas of both structural and metabolic damage can be identified using magnetic resonance imaging (MRI) and positron emission tomography (PET), and these areas can be analyzed by computer to identify the size and location of lesions quite accurately. Although autopsies remain the "gold standard" for determining where a lesion is located and what type of disease caused it, there are advantages to the use of radiological images compared to the use of autopsy material. Many more patients can be studied radiologically than come to autopsy. Images can be obtained at the time the patient has a particular deficit, not years after the patient has been studied, so there is no chance that new diseases can affect the brain, confusing the correlation. The ability to reliably analyze these images is thus a great step forward in allowing deficit-lesion correlations to be studied.

2. Recording electrophysiological responses to language stimuli. The brain generates electrical charges and magnetic fields as it processes information. It is possible to record these charges and fields using event-related potentials (ERPs) and magnetoencephalography (MEG). By designing experiments in which participants process certain language structures while ERPs and MEG are measured, researchers can relate changes in ERPs and MEG to specific aspects of language processing. These changes in ERPs and MEG are rapid (they occur in milliseconds) and capture the time course of language processing.

ERPs can be analyzed to indicate the general regions of the brain that are active during a particular process, and MEG can give much more detailed information about where these regions are.

3. Temporarily interrupting brain activity by local stimulation. Interestingly, stimulating the brain electrically usually results in interfering with language functioning, not producing it. Neurosurgeons first used this technique during operations in an effort to locate—and spare—the neural tissue involved in language. Now this approach is also used as part of looking for the location of tissue responsible for seizures in patients. In this approach, electrodes are temporarily placed above the brain (in the subdural space) for days to weeks, allowing a greater number of observations to be made. Some researchers have stimulated the brain across the skull, with no operation involved, using magnetic fields (transcranial magnetic stimulation or TMS). This approach also interferes with function and can be used to localize a language process.

4. Recording cell responses to language stimuli intraoperatively. A few neurosurgeons have recorded responses from cells during operations and related these responses to language functions. It is also possible to record from subdural electrodes (see earlier discussion); and this technique has been used to localize language.

5. Recording vascular responses to language stimuli using PET and functional magnetic resonance imaging (fMRI) (see Box 13.1). A rapidly expanding field is the recording of changes in blood flow and other responses of circulation to cognitive processes using PET and fMRI. As with ERPs and MEG, these approaches can be used in normal subjects, where they measure normal brain responses to language processing. They therefore provide a complementary type of information to the analysis of permanent or temporary lesions. PET and fMRI records can be analyzed to identify the location of increases and decreases in activity. The time scale of PET is somewhat slow (minutes), but adequate to study many language functions; the time scale of fMRI is faster (seconds). These techniques require careful experimental design to yield information about the neural tissue involved in supporting particular language functions.

The development of all of these techniques has been extremely rapid in the past decade. Neuroscience is in a period in which an enormous amount of data regarding brain and language is being collected. One result has been that our ideas about how the brain is organized to support language have changed considerably in the past decade or so. A second is that many new questions are being posed about the way the brain is organized to process language, and we do not have the answers to all of them yet. However, a fair amount is known about language-brain relationships.

Inventory of Brain Structures Related to Language

Human language depends on the integrity of the unimodal and multimodal association cortex in the lateral portion of both cerebral hemispheres. This cortex surrounds the sylvian fissure and runs from the pars triangularis and opercularis of the inferior frontal gyrus [Brodman's areas (BA) 45, 44: Broca's area] through the angular and supramarginal gyri (BA 39 and 40) into the superior temporal gyrus (BA22: Wernicke's area) (Fig. 52.8). For the most part, the connections of these cortical areas are to one another and to the dorsolateral prefrontal cortex and lateral inferior temporal cortex. These regions have only indirect connections to limbic structures. These areas consist of many different types of association cortex, devoted not to sensation or motor function but to a more abstract type of analysis. The nature of this cortex and its patterns of connectivity are thought to combine to give language its enormous representational power and to allow its use to transcend biological immediacy.

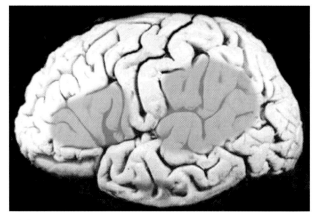

FIGURE 52.8   A depiction of the left hemisphere of the brain showing the main language areas. The area in the inferior frontal lobe is known as Broca's area, and the area in the superior temporal lobe is known as Wernicke's area, named after the 19th century physicians who first described their roles in language. Broca's area is adjacent to the motor cortex and is involved in planning speech gestures. It also serves other language functions, such as assigning syntactic structure. Wernicke's area is adjacent to the primary auditory cortex and is involved in representing and recognizing the sound patterns of words.

The evidence that language involves these cortical regions was originally derived from deficit-lesion correlations. Patients with lesions in parts of this cortex have been described who have had long-lasting impairments of language ("aphasia"). Disorders affecting language processing after perisylvian lesions

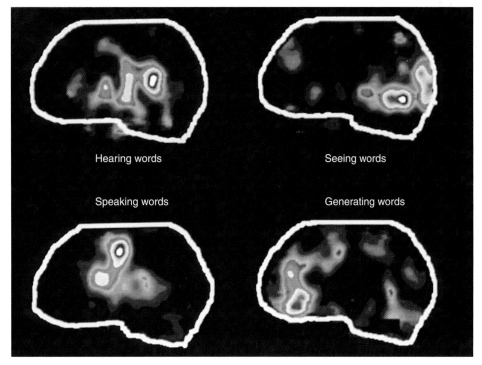

FIGURE 52.9   Activation of parts of the language area by language tasks, as demonstrated by PET scanning.

have been described in many different types of disease, in all languages that have been studied, in patients of all ages and both sexes, and in both first and subsequent tongues, indicating that this cortical region is involved in language processing independent of these factors. Functional neuroimaging studies have documented increases in regional cerebral blood flow (rCBF) using PET or blood oxygenation level-dependent (BOLD) signal using fMRI in tasks associated with language processing in this region (Fig. 52.9). Event related potentials whose sources are likely to be in this region have been described in relationship to a variety of language processing operations. Stimulation of this cortex by direct application of electrical current during neurosurgical procedures interrupts language processing. These data all converge on the conclusion that language processing is carried out in the perisylvian cortex.

Regions outside the perisylvian association cortex also appear to support language processing. Working outward from the perisylvian region, evidence shows that the modality of language use affects the location of the neural tissue that supports language, with written language involving the cortex closer to the visual areas of the brain and sign language involving brain regions closer to those involved in movements of the hands than movements of the oral cavity. Some ERP components related to processing improbable or ill-formed language are maximal over high parietal and central scalp electrodes, suggesting that these regions may be involved in language processing. Both lesion studies in stroke patients and functional neuroimaging studies suggest that the inferior and anterior temporal lobe is involved in representing the meanings of nouns. Activation studies also implicate the frontal lobe just in front of Broca's area in word meaning. Injury to the supplementary motor cortex along the medial surface of the frontal lobe can lead to speech initiation disturbances; this region may be important in activating the language processing system, at least in production tasks. Activation studies have shown increased rCBF and BOLD signal in the cingulate gyrus in association with many language tasks. This activation, however, appears to be nonspecific, as it occurs in many other, nonlinguistic, tasks as well. It has been suggested that it is due to increased arousal and deployment of attention associated with more complex tasks.

Subcortical structures may also be involved in language processing. Several studies report aphasic disturbances following strokes in deep gray matter nuclei (the caudate, putamen, and parts of the thalamus). It has been suggested that subcortical structures involved in laying down procedural memories for motor functions, in particular, the basal ganglia, are involved in "rule-based" processing in language, such as regular aspects of word formation, as opposed to the long-term maintenance of information in memory, as occurs with simple words and irregularly formed words. The thalamus may play a role in processing the meanings of words. In general, subcortical lesions cause language impairments when the overlying cortex is abnormal (often the abnormality can be seen only with metabolic scanning techniques), and the degree of language impairment is better correlated with measures of cortical than subcortical hypometabolism. It may be that subcortical structures serve to activate a cortically based language processing system but do not themselves process language.

The cerebellum has also increased its rCBF in some activation studies involving both language and other cognitive functions. This may be a result of the role of this part of the brain in processes involved in timing and temporal ordering of events, or in its being directly involved in language and other cognitive functions.

The other major component of the subcortical region of the cerebral hemispheres is the white matter. White matter tracts transmit representations from one area to another. Lesions of white matter tracts disconnect regions of the brain from others and make the operations performed in one region unavailable to others. This can cause language disorders. The best known such disturbance is pure alexia, in which a patient can write but not read—not even read his/her own writing. This can result from a lesion that destroys the primary visual cortex in the left hemisphere and extends forward in the white matter so that visual information cannot get from the right to the left hemisphere (Fig. 52.10). As discussed later, because the left hemisphere is responsible for many aspects of language (this is called "cerebral dominance" for language), this lesion disconnects visual input from language, resulting in the inability to read. Because the language hemisphere still has access to the motor system, the patient can write, however. In addition to these "disconnection" syndromes, language disturbances of all sorts occur with lesions affecting many white matter tracts, while sparing of language functions can follow lesions in the same areas in different patients. The fact that multiple language processing disturbances occur following subcortical strokes that affect white matter is consistent with the idea that a wide variety of information is carried by white matter fibers. This also implies that many of the areas of the cortex and/or subcortical nuclei that carry out sequential language processing

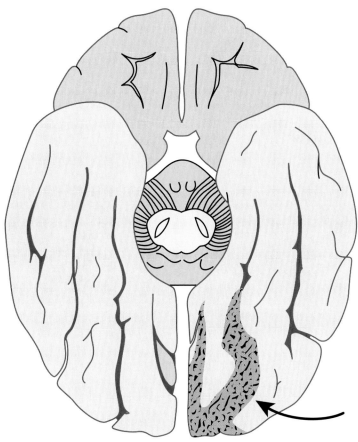

FIGURE 52.10   Diagram from Dejerine's 1892 paper showing the lesion that results in pure alexia. The lesion is shown from the inferior surface of the brain. It has destroyed the left visual cortex and interrupted fibers from the right visual cortex on their way to language centers in the left hemisphere.

operations are not contiguous. The fact that lesions in the same location can affect a particular function in one patient and spare it in another indicates that the areas in which functions are carried out are different in different individuals to some extent, or that white matter routes carry different information from one region to another in different individuals.

In summary, a large number of brain regions are involved in representing and processing language. Ultimately, they all interact with one another as well as with other brain areas involved in using the products of language processing to accomplish tasks. In this sense, all these regions are part of a "neural system," but this concept should not obscure the fact that many of these regions appear to compute specific linguistic representations in particular tasks. The most important of these regions is the dominant (usually left) perisylvian cortex. It is likely that if there are universal features of language structure that are innate, these features of language are related to features of this region of the brain. However, except for the macroscopic asymmetries between left and right

hemispheres that appear to correlate grossly with lateralization (see later), these features are not yet understood.

Lateralization

Most language processing goes on in one hemisphere, called the "dominant" hemisphere. Which hemisphere is dominant shows considerable individual differences and bears a systematic relationship to handedness. In about 98% of right-handed individuals, the left hemisphere is dominant. The extent to which left hemisphere lesions cause language disorders is influenced by the degree to which an individual is right handed and by the number of nonright handers in his/her family. About 60–65% of nonright-handed individuals are left hemisphere dominant; about 15–20% are right hemisphere dominant; and the remainder appear to use both hemispheres for language processing. The relationship of dominance for language to handedness suggests a common determination of both, probably in large part genetic.

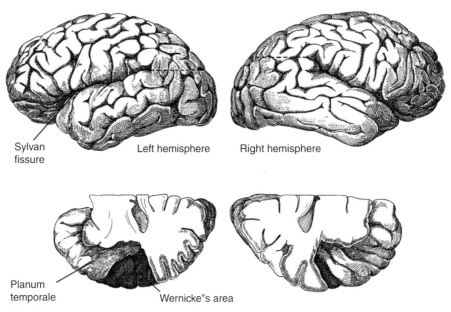

Sylvan fissure   Left hemisphere   Right hemisphere

Planum temporale   Wernicke"s area

FIGURE 52.11   Depiction of a horizontal slice through the brain showing asymmetry in the size of the planum temporale related to lateralization of language

The neural basis for lateralization was first suggested by Geschwind and Levitsky (1968), who discovered that part of the language zone (the planum temporale—a portion of the superior temporal lobe; Fig. 52.11) was larger in the left than in the right hemisphere. Subsequent studies have confirmed this finding and identified specific cytoarchitectonically defined regions in this posterior language area that show this asymmetry. Several other asymmetries that may be related to lateralization have also been identified. The exact relationship between size and function is not known, as there are instances of individuals whose dominant hemisphere is not the one with the larger planum temporale. In general, however, relative size is a good predictor of lateralization. This is another example of the "bigger is better" principle that we saw applied to song nuclei in birds.

Although language was the first function known to be lateralized, and is still the best example of a lateralized function, it is not completely lateralized. Although not as important in language functioning as the dominant hemisphere, the nondominant hemisphere is involved in many language operations. Evidence from the effects of lesions and split brain studies, experiments using presentation of stimuli to one or the other hemisphere in normal subjects, and activation studies all indicates that the nondominant hemisphere understands many words, especially concrete nouns, and suggests that it is involved in other aspects of language processing as well (see later). Some language operations may be carried out primarily in the right hemisphere. The best candidates for

these operations are ones that pertain to processing the discourse level of language, interpreting nonliteral language such as metaphors, and appreciating the tone of a discourse, e.g., the fact that it is humorous. Some scientists have developed models of the sorts of processing that the right hemisphere carries out. For instance, it has been suggested that the right hemisphere codes information in a more general way compared to the left, representing the overall structure of a stimulus as opposed to its details. This may be true for language as well as for other functions, such as visual perception. This and other suggestions provide the bases for ongoing research programs into the nature of language processing in the right hemisphere.

Organization of the Perisylvian Cortex for Language Processing

Because the perisylvian cortex is essential to the representation and processing of language, the way it is organized to support these functions has been the subject of much investigation. Two general classes of theories of the relationship of parts of the perisylvian association cortex to components of the language processing system have been developed. One is based on "holist" or distributed views of neural function and one on localizationist principles. The basic tenet of holist/distributed theories is that linguistic representations are distributed widely and that language processing components rely on broad areas of the association cortex. Localizationist theories maintain that language processing components are localized in specific parts of the cortex.

Holist Theories

Lashley (1950) identified two functional features of holist/distributed models that determine the effects of lesions upon performance: equipotentiality (every portion of a particular brain region carries out a particular function in every individual) and mass action (the larger the neuronal pool that carries out a function, the more efficiently that function is accomplished). The features of equipotentiality and mass action jointly entail that (1) lesions of similar sizes anywhere in a specified brain region have equivalent effects on function and (2) the magnitude of any functional deficit is directly proportional to the size of a lesion in this specified area. Modern work with parallel distributed processing models provides formal models of holist concepts.

There is some evidence for holist theories. Lesions throughout the language area have been found in some studies to have similar effects on language functions, consistent with the principle of equipotentiality. There is an effect of lesion size on the overall severity of functional impairments in several language spheres, consistent with the principle of mass action. These results are consistent with a distributed, or holistic, neural basis for linguistic representations and processes. However, they do not necessarily show that these models are correct because they also could result from variability in the localization of language processing components across the population.

Holist models may be better models of how individual areas of the brain work to support language. A behavioral finding supporting holist theories is the frequent observation of so-called "graceful degradation" of performance within specific language domains after brain damage. For instance, certain dyslexic patients read irregularly spelled words according to a regularization strategy (e.g., pint is read with a short i). Some of these patients are more likely to make these regularization errors in words that are less frequent. This observation implies that frequent exposure to an irregular word makes its pronunciation less susceptible to disruption; that is, the "degradation" of the connection between a whole word and its sound is related to an individual's experience with that word. Modern work with parallel distributed processing models indicates that such patterns of performance can arise following lesions in systems in which information is represented and processed in massively parallel, distributed forms. A very reasonable view is that different neural areas support differ-

ent language functions and that each of these areas works as a whole, as holist models claim. Holism may not be wrong; it just needs to be applied on the right scale. As has been said, the brain may be "globally local and locally global."

Localizationist Theories

Evidence against any holist model is the finding that multiple individual language deficits arise in patients with small perisylvian lesions, often in complementary functional spheres. For instance, some patients have trouble producing the small grammatical function words of language (such as *the, what, is, he*), whereas others have trouble producing common nouns. The existence of these two disorders indicates that the tissue involved in producing function words is not involved in producing common nouns in the first set of patients, and *vice versa* in the second set. Strong evidence against holist models also comes from activation studies that demonstrate vascular responses to particular types of language stimuli in restricted cortical areas. How language is organized at this finer-grained level in the perisylvian association cortex is an ongoing topic of research.

Classical Clinical Localizationist Models

The first localizationist theories emerged from clinical observations in the mid- and late 19th century. The pioneers of aphasiology—Paul Broca, Karl Wernicke, John Hughlings Jackson, and other neurologists—described patients with lesions in the left inferior frontal lobe whose speech was hesitant and poorly articulated and other patients with lesions more posteriorly, in the superior temporal lobe, who had disturbances of comprehension and fluent speech with sound and word substitutions. These correlations led to the theory that language comprehension went on in the unimodal auditory association cortex (Wernicke's area, Brodman area 22) adjacent to the primary auditory cortex (Heschl's gyrus, Brodman areas 41) and that motor speech planning went on in the unimodal motor association cortex in Broca's area (Brodman areas 44 and 45) adjacent to the primary motor cortex (Brodman area 4). These theories incorporated the idea that localization of a language operation depends on the way it is related to sensory and motor processes. According to this view, speech planning goes on in Broca's area because Broca's is immediately adjacent to the motor area responsible for movement of the articulators and Wernicke's area is involved in comprehension because it is immediately adjacent to primary auditory cortex.

These ideas and models were extended by Norman Geschwind and colleagues in the 1960s and 1970s.

TABLE 52.3 Classical Aphasic Syndromes

Syndrome location	Clinical manifestations	Hypothetical deficit	Classical lesion location
Broca's aphasia	Major disturbance in speech production with sparse, halting speech, often misarticulated, frequently missing function words and bound morphemes	Disturbances in the speech planning and production mechanisms (Broca's area)	Posterior aspects of the third frontal convolution
Wernicke's aphasia	Major disturbance in auditory comprehension; fluent speech with disturbances of the sounds and structures of words (phonemic, morphological, and semantic paraphasias); poor repetition and naming	Disturbances of the permanent representations of the sound structures of words	Posterior half of the first temporal gyrus and possibly adjacent cortex (Wernicke's area)
Pure motor speech disorder	Disturbance of articulation Apraxia of speech, dysarthria, anarthria, aphemia	Disturbance of articulatory mechanisms	Outflow tracts from motor cortex
Pure word deafness	Disturbance of spoken word comprehension repetition	Failure to access spoken words often impaired	Input tracts from auditory system to Wernicke's area
Transcortical motor aphasia	Disturbance of spontaneous speech similar to Broca's aphasia with relatively preserved repetition; comprehension relatively preserved	Disconnection between conceptual representations of words and sentences and the motor speech production system	White matter tracts deep to Broca's area connecting it to parietal lobe
Transcortical sensory aphasia	Disturbance in single word comprehension with relatively intact repetition	Disturbance in activation of word meanings despite normal recognition of auditorily presented words	White matter tracts connecting parietal lobe to temporal lobe or portions of inferior parietal lobe
Conduction accurate aphasia	Disturbance of repetition and spontaneous speech (phonemic paraphasias); good comprehension	Disconnection between the sound patterns of words and the speech production mechanism	Lesion in the arcuate fasciculus and/or corticocortical connections between Wernicke's and Broca's areas
Anomic aphasia	Disturbance in the production of single words, most marked for common nouns. Intact comprehension and repetition	Disturbances of concepts, and/or the sound patterns of words	Inferior parietal lobe or connections between parietal lobe and temporal lobe; can follow many lesions
Global aphasia	Major disturbance in all language functions	Disruption of all language processing components	Large portion of the perisylvian association cortex
Isolation of the language zone	Disturbance of both spontaneous speech (sparce, halting speech) and comprehension, with some preservation of repetition; echolalia common	Disconnection between concepts and both representations of word sounds and the speech production mechanism	Cortex just outside the perisylvian association cortex

Geschwind added the hypothesis that word meaning was localized in the inferior parietal lobe (Brodman areas 39 and 40) because word meanings consist of associations between sounds and properties of objects, and the inferior parietal lobe is an area of multimodal association cortex to which fibers from the unimodal association cortex related to audition, vision, and somasthesis project. Geschwind's model remains the best-known localizationist model of the functional neuroanatomy of language and is widely cited in clinical practice. The model is said to receive support from the existence of about 10 aphasic syndromes, described in Table 52.3, which serve the clinical purpose of helping to localize lesions.

However, despite its widespread use, this model has distinct limitations. It deals only with words, not with other levels of the language code. From a linguistic and psycholinguistic point of view, the syndromes are all composed of many processing deficits, which are different in different patients. The correlations between syndromes and lesions may reflect the fact that speech fluency is a critical dimension along which patients are classified, and nonfluent aphasias tend to be due to anterior lesions that affect motor structures whereas fluent aphasias tend to be due to posterior lesions that do not. The syndromes themselves do not provide a guide to the localization of more specific components of the language processing system. Ongoing work seeks to address this question.

The next sections review localizationist models in three areas: processing of phonemes, word meaning, and syntactic structures. These areas cover a spectrum with respect to abstractness of linguistic representations.

Localization of Phonemic Processing

A great deal of research on auditory perception indicates that complex auditory patterns provoke responses in cells in the auditory association cortex in the superior temporal lobe. It has long been theorized that phonemic perception, a quintessential example of complex auditory processing, takes place in this region. However, many lesion-deficit studies show that impairments in both discrimination and identification of phonemes follow strokes throughout the perisylvian cortex, with perhaps the greatest frequency following strokes in the inferior parietal lobe. Activation studies using PET, fMRI, and MEG have added to this picture. In many studies, contrasts between simply listening to speech and listening to a low-level auditory baseline (such as white noise) activate both left and right temporal lobes, whereas more complex tasks involving phonological representations, such as rehearsal, making rhyme judgments, and recognizing specific sequences of phonemes, have activated parts of a larger area that includes the left inferior parietal lobe and Broca's area.

To account for these results, it has been suggested that the superior temporal lobe of both hemispheres is involved in perceiving phonemes in an unconscious, automatic fashion as part of the process of recognizing words and that parietal and frontal areas, particularly in the left hemisphere, are involved in the conscious use of these representations (Hickok and Poeppel, 2000). Storage of these forms in short-term memory is thought to involve inferior parietal structures and rehearsal to involve Broca's area. Some researchers have gone further in localizing phonemic processing within the superior temporal lobe. Binder (2001) has argued that, contrary to a century-old belief, phoneme recognition involves the anterior, not the posterior, part of the auditory association cortex (Fig. 52.12). The area of the superior temporal sulcus, anterior to the primary auditory cortex, has been specifically identified as a possible site for this type of processing.

This recent work has made the case that phonemic processing involves several different functional operations and that each of them is localized in small parts of the language area. It retains the classical idea that phonemic recognition takes place in the auditory association cortex, but claims that this is the case only when the listener is recognizing words unconsciously

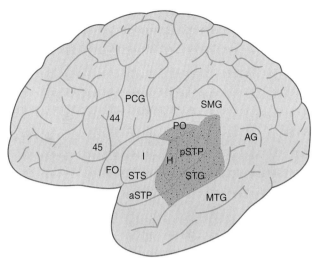

FIGURE 52.12 Depiction of the lateral surface of the brain showing areas involved in the functional neuroanatomy of phonemic processing. H is Heschl's gyrus, the primary auditory cortex. STP is the superior temporal plane, divided into posterior and anterior areas. STG is the superior temporal gyrus. Traditional theories maintain that pSTP and STG are the loci of phonemic processing. Hickok and Poeppel (2000) argue that these areas in both hemispheres are involved in automatic phonemic processing in the process of word recognition. Other research suggests that more anterior structures, aSTP and the area around the superior temporal sulcus (STS), are involved in these processes. The inferior parietal lobe (AG, angular gyrus; SMG, supramarginal gyrus) and Broca's area (areas 44 and 45) are involved in conscious controlled phonological processes such as rehearsal and storage in short-term memory.

and that this unconscious type of phonemic processing occurs bilaterally. Consciously controlled tasks that involve phonemes are thought to take place in other areas of the brain—the inferior parietal and inferior frontal cortex.

Localization of Word Meaning

As noted earlier, traditional neurological models of the neural basis for word meaning maintained that the meanings of words consist of representations of physical properties, which are associated with word sounds in the inferior parietal lobe. It is now known that most lesions in the inferior parietal lobe do not affect word meaning. Functional neuroimaging studies designed to require word meaning do not tend to activate this region. The idea that word meaning resides in this area therefore appears to be incorrect. Damasio (1989) developed a closely related model, suggesting that the meanings of words included "retroactivation" of neural patterns all the way back to the primary sensory cortex. In an extension of this model, Damasio proposed that these associations were more likely to reside in the frontal cortex for verbs and in the parietal and occipital cortex for nouns because verbs refer to actions, memories for which would involve motor planning that had taken place in the primary and unimodal association motor cortex, and nouns refer to static items, memories for which would involve sensory processing that had taken place in the primary and unimodal sensory association cortex. As noted previously, the meaning of a word includes much more than its sensory and motor associations, so activating neural tissue in which such associations are stored would not account for all of word meaning.

Word meaning is affected by lesions in the inferior temporal lobe. This may be partly due to visual agnosia, which results from the disruption of high-level visual processing involved in object recognition that occurs in this location. However, this is not likely to be the entire reason for the effects of lesions in this region on word meanings. Patients with a condition known as semantic dementia, a degenerative disease that affects the anterior inferior temporal lobe, have major problems with many aspects of semantic memory and word meaning that extend beyond visual object recognition disorders. The important lesions in these patients are in the left hemisphere, corresponding to left hemispheric specialization or lateralization of semantic memory and lexical semantic representations and processing. Patients with lesions due to herpes encephalitis, which also affects the inferior and medial temporal lobe (in many cases, somewhat more posteriorly than in lesions in semantic dementia), also exhibit semantic deficits. Activation studies have implicated the inferior temporal cortex in representing word meanings. ERP studies have documented a robust wave—the N400—that arises when subjects are presented semantically anomalous sentences, such as *I take my coffee with cream and cement*. The N400 is also found in the unrelated trials in word priming experiments in which subjects are presented with sequences of related and unrelated words. The N400 has thus been interpreted as a wave that arises when semantically unexpected material occurs and, as such, a wave that reflects some aspect of semantic processing. Although the intracerebral sources of ERPs are hard to determine with certainty, there is some evidence that this wave originates in the inferior temporal lobe.

Activation studies using PET and fMRI have also shown increases in blood flow in semantic tasks in the inferior frontal lobe, just in front of what is usually taken to be Broca's area. In the earliest PET studies on language, Petersen and colleagues (1988) found inferior frontal activation when subjects generated verbs associated with nouns compared to when they repeated the nouns. Petersen and colleagues interpreted this as evidence for involvement of this frontal cortex in processing word meaning. This interpretation has been controversial since it was first proposed, with alternative accounts being suggested, such as the possibility that the activation reflects the category-shifting aspect of the verb-generate task or the production of verbs (for the reasons outlined above). However, other studies support the interpretation that this frontal activity is due to semantic processing and is not restricted to verbs. For instance, one study found that making judgments about whether sentences contained synonyms or only closely semantically related words activated the left inferior frontal lobe, and decreased activation in the left inferior prefrontal cortex has been reported during repeated semantic processing of both words and pictures.

The picture that is currently emerging about lexical semantics is that it is represented multifocally. To explore this issue further will likely require making fine contrasts regarding the nature of the semantic representations that are being localized and the tasks that utilize these representations. In this respect, the picture that may emerge could be similar to that currently suggested in the domain of phonemic processing, where different uses of phonemic representations seem to involve different cortical regions.

Localization of Syntactic Operations

Syntactic comprehension deficits are typically established by showing that patients can understand sentences with simple syntactic structures (e.g., *The boy chased the girl*) and sentences with complex syntactic structures in which the relationships between nouns and verbs can be inferred from a knowledge of real-world events (e.g., *The apple the boy ate was red*), but not sentences with complex structures in which the relationships between nouns and verbs depend on a syntactic structure that needs to be constructed (e.g., *The boy the girl pushed was tall*). Deficits in syntactic processing in sentence comprehension occur in all aphasic syndromes and after lesions throughout the perisylvian cortex (Caplan *et al.*, 1985, 1996). Conversely, patients of all types and with all lesion locations have been described with normal syntactic comprehension (Caplan *et al.*, 1985). These data are most compatible with the idea that syntactic operations are localized, but in different locations in different individuals.

Functional neuroimaging sheds additional light on this topic. Using fMRI, Just *et al.* (1996) reported an increase in activity (BOLD signal) in both Broca's area and in Wernicke's area of the left hemisphere, as well as smaller but reliable increases in rCBF in the homologous regions of the right hemisphere when subjects

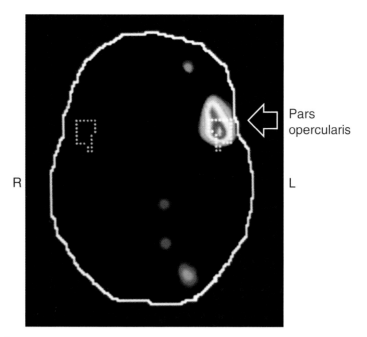

FIGURE 52.13 Horizontal section through the brain showing activation of Broca's area while subjects processed syntactically complex sentences. (The left side of the brain is shown on the right.) From Stromswold *et al.* (1996).

read and answered questions about sentences that contained syntactically complex relative clauses. In a different series of studies, PET activity associated with making plausibility judgments about syntactically simple sentences was subtracted from that associated with making judgments about sentences with the same words and propositions phrased in syntactically more complex forms. Broca's area was activated in subjects who performed the task quickly and accurately (Fig. 52.13), whereas subjects who were much slower activated other structures. This may be because different areas support the same syntactic operation in high- and low-proficient subjects. Alternatively, the reason that subjects who are less proficient in performing syntactically based comprehension tasks activate other brain regions may be that they utilize supporting cognitive mechanisms, such as short-term memory or visual imagery, to help them perform the task.

Overall, these data are consistent with localization. They appear to suggest variation in the localization of syntactic processing within the language area across the adult population. Alternatively, at least some of the data can be understood by supposing that performing sentence comprehension tasks is a complex process that engages support mechanisms to different degrees in different individuals, in part as a reflection of how proficient they are at assigning syntactic structure and determining the meaning of sentences.

CONCLUSIONS

Human language is a unique representational system that relates aspects of meaning to many types of forms (e.g., phonemes, lexical items, syntax), each with its own complex structure. Animal communication systems are neither as complex nor as powerful as human language. Nonetheless, they have some similarities to language and provide clues as to the neural basis of human language. Perhaps the most important lessons learned from animal studies are that complex communication systems can be innate, that learning can shape an innately specified range of behavioral possibilities, and that communication systems can rely on specific nuclei within the brain. Assuming that there are important universal structural features of human languages, human language may have similar neural features. Animal studies also provide evidence for lateralization and localization of the neural basis for communication systems, which are features of the functional neuroanatomy of human language. Other features of the neural basis for animal communication systems, such as seasonal variation in the size of birdsong nuclei and the mechanisms that underlie this phenomenon, are not obviously relevant to human language.

Deficit-lesion correlations and neuroimaging studies are beginning to provide data about the neural structures involved in human language. It appears that one area of the brain—the left perisyl-vian association cortex—is especially important in representing and processing language (although other regions are involved as well), and that, within this area, particular language operations are localized in specific regions. The exact details of these localizations are just beginning to be understood, as the modern tools of cognitive neuroscience are applied to this problem.

References

Bellugi, U., Poizner, H., *et al.* (1990). Mapping brain function for language: Evidence from sign language. *In* "Signal and Sense: Local and Global Order in Perceptual Maps" (G. Edelman, W. Gall, and W. Cowan, eds.), pp. 521–543. Wiley-Liss, New York.

Bickerton, D. (1990). "Language and Species." University of Chicago Press, Chicago.

Binder, J. (2000). The new neuroanatomy of speech perception. *Brain* **123**, 2371–2372.

Caplan, D., Baker, C., and Dehaut, F. (1985). Syntactic determinants of sentence comprehension in aphasia. *Cognition* **21**, 117–175.

Caplan, D., Hildebrandt, H., and Makris, N. (1996). Location of lesions in stroke patients with deficits in syntactic processing in sentence comprehension. *Brain* **119**, 993–949.

Cheney, D. L., and Seyfarth, R. M. (1990). "How Monkeys See the World." University of Chicago Press, Chicago.

Chomsky, N. (1957). "Syntactic Structures." Mouton, The Hague.

Chomsky, N. (1965). "Aspects of the Theory of Syntax." MIT Press, Cambridge, MA.

Chomsky, N. (1981). "Lectures on Government and Binding." Foris, Dordrecht, The Netherlands.

Chomsky, N. (1986). "Knowledge of Language." Praeger, New York.

Damasio, A. (1989). Time-locked multiregional retroactivation: A systems-level proposal for the neural substrates of recall and recognition. *Cognition* **33**, 25–62.

Geschwind, N. (1965). Disconnection syndromes in animals and man. *Brain* **88**, 237–294, 585–644.

Geschwind, N. and W. Levitsky (1968). Human brain: Left-right asymmetries in temporal speech region. *Science* **161**, 186–187.

Gould, J. L. (1982). "Ethology." Norton, New York.

Gould, J. L., and Gould, C. G. (1995). "The Honey Bee," 2nd Ed. Freeman, New York.

Gould, J. L., and Gould, C. G. (1996). "Sexual Selection," 2nd Ed. Freeman, New York.

Gould, J. L., and Gould, C. G. (1999). "The Animal Mind," 2nd Ed. Freeman, New York.

Gould, J. L., and Marler, P. (1987). The instinct to learn. *Sci. Am.* **256**(1), 74–85.

Grosz, B. J., Pollack, M. E., and Sidner, C. L. (1989). Discourse *In* "Foundations of Cognitive Science" (M. Posner, ed.), pp. 437–468. MIT Press, Cambridge, MA.

Henderson, L. (1982). "Orthography and Word Recognition in Reading." Academic Press, London.

Hickok, G. and Poeppel, D. (2000). Towards a functional neuroanatomy of speech perception. *Trends Cogn. Sci.* **4**, 131–138.

Just, M. A., Carpenter, P. A., Keller, T. A., Eddy, W. F., and Thulborn, K. R. (1996). Brain activation modulated by sentence comprehension. *Science* **274**, 114–116.

Lashley, K. S. (1950). In search of the engram. *Symp. Soc. Exp. Biol.* **4**, 454–482.

Petersen, S. E., Fox, P. T., *et al.* (1988). Positron emission tomographic studies of the cortical anatomy of single-word processing. *Nature* **331**, 585–589.

Pinker, S. (1994). "The Language Instinct." Harper Collins, New York.

Seidenberg, M. (1997). Language acquisition and use: Learning and applying probabilistic constraints. *Science* **275**, 1599–1603.

Seidenberg, M. S., and McClelland, J. L. (1988). A distributed, developmental model of visual word recognition and naming. *Psychol. Rev.* **96**, 523–568.

Tulving, E. (1972). Episodic and semantic memory. *In* "Organization of Memory" (E. T. A. W. Donaldson, ed.), pp. 381–403. Academic Press, New York.

Van Dijk, T. A., and Kintsch, W. (1983). "Strategies of Discourse Comprehension." Academic Press, New York.

Suggested Readings

Caplan, D. (1987). "Neurolinguistics and Linguistic Aphasiology." Cambridge University Press, Cambridge, UK.

Hauser, M. (1996). "The Evaluation of Communication." MIT Press, Cambridge, MA.

Posner, M., and Raichle, M. E. (1997). "Images of Mind." W. H. Freeman, New York.

David N. Caplan and James L. Gould

The Prefrontal Cortex and Executive Brain Functions

What controls your thoughts? How do you decide what to pay attention to? How do you act appropriately while dining in a restaurant or listening to a lecture? How do you plan and execute errands? How do you manage to pursue long-term goals, such as obtaining a college degree, in the face of the many distractions that can knock you "off task"? In short, how does the brain manage to orchestrate the activity of millions of neurons to produce behavior that is willful, coordinated, and extended over time?

This is called cognitive control, the ability we have to wrest control of our brain's processes away from reflexive reactions to the environment in order to direct them toward future goals. This ability reaches its apex in the primate brain, as does the elaboration of the brain region thought to be most central to it, the prefrontal cortex (PFC) (Fig. 53.1).

The subject of this chapter is the PFC and its role in cognition. The chapter discusses its anatomy, behavioral effects of its damage, its neural properties, and theories of its function. First, it will be helpful to elaborate on what is meant by "cognitive control."

CONTROLLED VERSUS AUTOMATIC PROCESSING

Many of our behaviors are direct reactions to our immediate environment that do not tax our attention. For example, if someone suddenly throws a baseball at your face, you might reflexively duck. You may not have willed this behavior; it seems as if your body reacts and then your mind "catches up" and realizes what has happened. Many such reflexive, automatic processes are wired into our nervous systems by evolution, but others can be acquired through a great deal of practice as learning mechanisms gradually (and thor-

oughly) stamp in highly familiar behaviors. For example, consider a walk to work. The route is highly familiar and if traffic is light, your mind can wander and before you know it you have gone a distance (and even negotiated turns) with little awareness of having done so. In these cases, your behaviors are driven in a "bottom-up" fashion: they are determined largely by the nature of sensory stimuli and their strong associations with certain behavioral responses. In neural terms, they are dependent on well-established neural pathways waiting to be fired off by the correct triggering conditions.

However, during a walk to work you may encounter a lot of traffic or something unexpected might happen. Then, you need to "take charge" of your actions. You pay attention to the people and nearby cars to anticipate and accommodate their actions, or you may decide to take an alternate route. Now, your behaviors are not governed by straightforward stimulus–response relationships; additional information is needed. You use knowledge of the current objective (arriving at work intact) and results from previous experiences to weigh the alternatives and consequences. During this controlled mode, the basic sensory, memory, and motor processes that mediated automatic behavior are also engaged. Only now, they are not simply triggered by the environment in a bottom-up fashion, they are shaped and controlled in a "top-down" fashion by the knowledge you have acquired about what goals are available and the means to achieve them.

The Characteristics of Controlled Processing

Controlled Behaviors Are Goal Directed and Learned

Automatic processes can be either innate (such as a startle reflex) or well learned (such as your route to

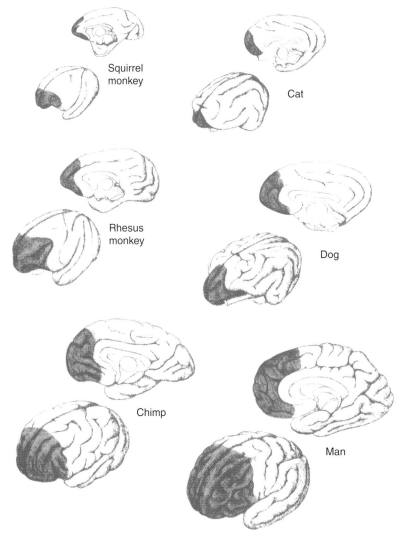

FIGURE 53.1   The relative size of the prefrontal cortex (PFC) in different animals. From Fuster (1995).

work). However, virtually all controlled behaviors are learned. Directing behavior toward unseen goals requires learning what goals are available and what types of behaviors have been successful at achieving them in similar circumstances in the past. We are not born knowing the route to work. It follows that one of the essential characteristics of a system that co-ordinates goal-related process, i.e., for cognitive control, is that it can acquire and represent this knowledge.

Cognitive Control Is Multimodal

"Divide and conquer" would seem to be the theme for sensory analyses. The external world is processed in separate systems specialized for different sensory modalities as well as subsystems within them that emphasize different stimulus attributes (albeit with some intermixing). Learning and memory has the opposite theme: synthesis. To plan and execute complex, goal-directed behaviors, one must figure out how the world works. One must learn the "rules of the game": predictive relationships between disparate sensory cues, their context, possible actions, and the consequences they produce. Insofar as primates are capable of navigating situations that involve relation-ships among diverse combinations of stimuli, internal states, and responses, a system for cognitive control must have access to and encode relationships between a similarly wide range of information from brain systems that process this information.

Controlled Processing Depends on Maintaining Relevant Information "On-Line"

Because of their prospective (forward-looking) nature, gaps in time are a fundamental problem facing controlled processing. They are not an issue for automatic reflexive reactions because those are immediate: a stimulus simply triggers an already established circuit. However, controlled behaviors often extend over time. Goal-relevant information must be brought to mind in anticipation of achieving the goal and must be kept there while we wait for new information or for a more appropriate time to act until the goal is achieved. The "in mind" maintenance of goal-relevant information is known as working memory and is critical for any system mediating cognitive control.

Controlled Processing Is Limited in Capacity

Automatic processes have a high capacity; any number of them can be triggered at a given moment as long as there is no direct conflict between them. One can answer one's cell phone while walking without fear that one's feet will stop moving. In contrast, a fundamental fact of controlled processing is a severe capacity limitation. This is apparent to anyone who has tried to talk on the phone and answer an email at the same time; you can only think about one or, at most, a few things at any given moment. The limited capacity of our high level cognitive functions was famously described by George Miller as "the magic number seven plus or minus two," the maximum number of items that an average person can hold in mind at a given moment.

Limited Capacity Requires Selection

If controlled processing is limited in capacity, then what is processed must be selected. Indeed, it has been argued that selection is central to the function of the cognitive control system. It does not analyze sensory information or program exact movements; these are handled by specialized sensory and motor systems. Instead, the cognitive control system selects among these processes by favoring some over others. In the sensory domain, this is commonly referred to as attention and, indeed, attention and cognitive control are often treated as synonymous. Thus, just as any system for cognitive control must have access to processes in a wide range of brain systems, it must also have the means to influence them.

Controlled Behaviors Are Flexible

Primates are remarkably flexible with their controlled behaviors. One may learn how to navigate a specific circumstance, but one can quickly generalize this to new situations, conjoin them with others, and rearrange them to produce novel behaviors. Take, for example, the coordinated set of goal-directed behaviors involved in dining in a restaurant. Your exact behaviors, as well as their sequence, can vary depending on the type of restaurant (e.g., casual or fine) and you can readily adapt your previous experiences to a new restaurant. Also, goal-directed behaviors can be temporarily interrupted and resumed at ease. One might temporarily divert oneself from wine shopping, for example, to pick up some cheese. In contrast, automatic behaviors are characterized by their rigidity. They are initiated by specific trigger events and are "ballistic"; once activated they tend to run off in pretty much the same way every time.

Relationship between Controlled and Automatic Processes

Most theories of cognitive function propose the type of hierarchical relationship between controlled and automatic processes that is depicted in Fig. 53.2. It is based on a model of cognition proposed by Norman and Shallice (1986).

At the lower level, there are the automatic processes that underlie sensory analysis, stored knowledge, motor acts, and well-learned skills. A doctrine of modern neuroscience is that information is stored in the patterns of connections between neurons and that learning and memory can result from modifying these connections. Thus, processing can be thought of (in a simple way, of course) as a problem of

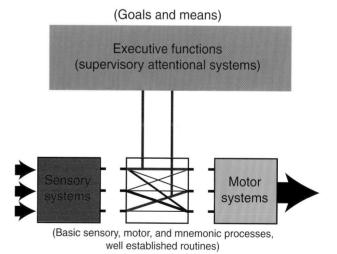

FIGURE 53.2 Two levels of cognitive processes proposed by Norman and Shallice among others. Represented here is the notion that specialized functions that acquire information about goals and means select and coordinate among innate and well-established routines. Active processing lines are indicated by red.

connecting inputs to outputs. In the architecture depicted in Fig. 53.2, automatic processing occurs when activity flows unheeded through the lower level of processing, from input to output along well-established pathways as inputs trigger basic sensory analyses, which then trigger other strongly connected functions leading to thought and actions (output).

In the primate brain, activity related to sensory experiences and voluntary behaviors flows mainly into primary sensory areas through the higher order sensory and premotor "association" cortex and, ultimately, to primary motor structures. This is oversimplified, of course—there are many interactions and connections between the cerebral cortex and subcortical structures—but it is true in a general way. Many of these connections are preprogrammed by genetics, some with help from experience during developmental periods early in life. Others are modified by experience as we learn. To aid in the modification of these pathways, the brain has evolved specialized subsystems, such as the hippocampus, to help modify connections in the cerebral cortex that underlie long-term storage.

However, if brain processing were nothing more than sculpting pathways and then triggering them with a sensory input, we would be automatons, always reacting in the same way to whatever stimuli happen to flow into our brains and whatever outputs they were

strongly connected with. To give the system intelligence, virtually all theories of cognition posit a higher level of processing, executive or supervisory functions specialized for processing information about goals and means. They send "top-down" signals that control the flow of processing in the lower level functions that deal more directly with the outside world. These signals bias their processing along goal-related lines, activating some processes and suppressing others. Because of this role, Norman and Shallice refer to executive functions as the "supervisory attention system." Another example of this two-level processing hierarchy is Baddeley's working memory model, which posits an executive controller that selects the information that is held in lower level short-term sketchpads.

Summary

There are two general modes of information processing that underlie thoughts and behaviors: automatic and controlled. Automatic processes are relatively simple, straightforward, reflexive reactions to whatever information happens to be flowing into the senses at a given moment. In contrast, controlled processes are engaged when a task has additional constraints and requires knowledge about goals and means.

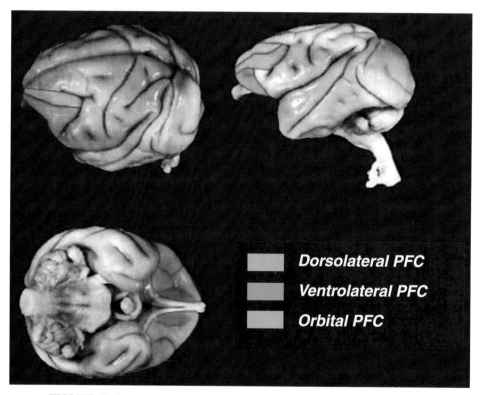

FIGURE 53.3   Brain of the macaque monkey with major subdivisions indicated.

From this brief review of some of the main characteristics of controlled processing, it is possible to make some predictions about the nature of any brain system involved in the executive control of cognitive functions.

1. It must have extensive and diverse connections to other regions of the brain in order to have access to information from, as well as be able to influence, processing in sensory systems, memory, and motor systems.

2. It needs to have information about goals and the means to achieve them, and this necessarily involves representing diverse multivariate relationships between a wide variety of sensory information, stored knowledge, actions, and consequences. It needs to be plastic and modifiable by experience in order to acquire this information.

3. There must be short-term storage mechanisms to keep goal-related information "on-line" and available until the goal is achieved.

4. It must represent goal-related information in a form that is flexible and easy to modify.

For many reasons, many investigators have argued that the neural instantiation of executive functions is, to a large degree, in the PFC. The remainder of this chapter discusses why.

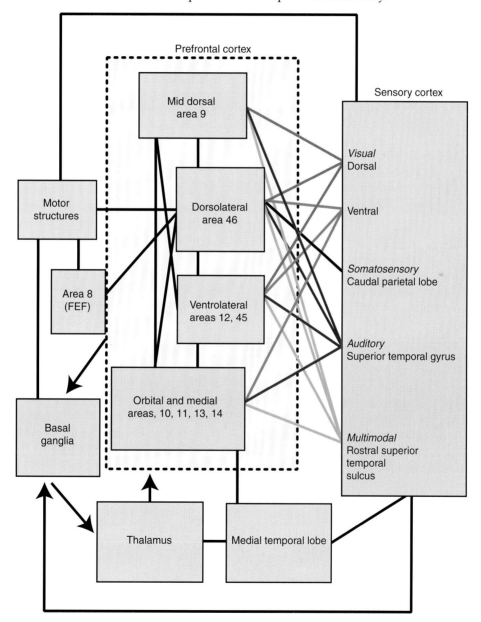

FIGURE 53.4   Schematic diagram of some of the extrinsic and intrinsic connections of the PFC. Most connections are reciprocal; exceptions are noted by arrows. From Miller and Cohen (2001).

ANATOMY AND ORGANIZATION OF THE PREFRONTAL CORTEX

The PFC consists of a collection of cortical areas that differ from one another on the basis of size, density, and distribution of their neurons. The major divisions are shown in Fig. 53.3, but these can be further subdivided into at least 18 distinct areas. The PFC is well positioned for a central role in cognitive control. Collectively, these areas have interconnections with brain areas processing external information (with all sensory systems and with cortical and subcortical motor system structures), as well as internal information (limbic and midbrain structures involved in affect, memory, and reward). The subdivisions have partly unique, but overlapping, patterns of connections with the rest of the brain, which suggests some regional differences in function (Fig. 53.4). As in much of the neocortex, however, local connections between different PFC areas can result in an intermixing and synthesis of disparate information needed for cognitive control. Indeed, the PFC has long been suggested to be the great integrator, a brain region that synthesizes information about the external and internal world for the purpose of producing goal-directed behavior.

The PFC Is Connected with Sensory Systems

The dorsolateral and ventrolateral portions of the PFC are more closely associated with the sensory neocortex than is the orbitofrontal cortex (see Fig. 53.4). They receive visual, somatosensory, and auditory information from the occipital, temporal, and parietal cortices. Many PFC areas receive converging inputs from at least two sensory modalities. For example, the dorsolateral (areas 8, 9, and 46) and ventrolateral (12 and 45) areas both receive projections from the visual, auditory, and somatosensory cortex. Further, the PFC is interconnected with other cortical regions that are themselves sites of multimodal convergence. Many PF areas (9, 12, 46, and 45) receive inputs from the rostral superior temporal sulcus, which has neurons with bimodal or trimodal (visual, auditory, and somatosensory) responses to external stimulation. The arcuate sulcus region (areas 8 and 45) and area 12 seem to be particularly multimodal. They contain zones that receive overlapping inputs from all three sensory modalities. In all of these cases, the PFC is not connected directly with primary sensory areas, but is instead interconnected with secondary or "association" sensory cortex.

The PFC Is Connected with Motor System Structures

The dorsal PFC, particularly dorsolateral area 46, has preferential connections with many motor system structures and may be the primary region by which the PFC exerts control over behavior. Dorsolateral area 46 is interconnected with motor areas in the medial frontal lobe such as the supplementary motor area (SMA), pre-SMA, and the rostral cingulate, with the premotor cortex on the lateral frontal lobe, and with cerebellum and superior colliculus. Dorsolateral area 46 also sends projections to area 8, which contains the frontal eye fields, a region important for voluntary shifts of gaze. As with the sensory cortex, there are no direct connections between the PFC and the primary motor cortex; the PFC is instead connected with premotor areas that, in turn, send projections to the primary motor cortex and the spinal cord. Also important are the dense interconnections between the PFC and basal ganglia (BG), a structure that is likely to be crucial for automating behavior (see later).

The PFC Is Connected with the Basal Ganglia

The basal ganglia are a set of subcortical structures that are closely associated with both the motor system and the PFC. The anatomy of the BG is similar to that of the PFC in that they receive converging inputs from virtually every cortical system and many subcortical structures. The region of the BG that receives inputs, the striatum (which includes the caudate and putamen), receives a heavy projection from the PFC. Information then travels through loops of subcortical nuclei, which project back to the frontal cortex via the thalamus. While the PFC projects back to the same wide range of cortical areas that give input to the BG, the BG project largely to frontal lobe motor system structures and the PFC. Thus, the BG are well positioned to influence a wide range of brain functions, albeit with an emphasis on motor output. The anatomical "loops" between the PFC and the BG have inspired theories of their close interdependency. Passingham (1993) has suggested that the BG are a major conduit by which reward signals from dopaminergic midbrain ventral tegmental areas (VTA) neurons can influence the PFC. BG anatomy, physiology, and function are discussed in Chapter 31.

The PFC Is Connected with the Limbic System

The orbitofrontal PFC is more closely associated with medial temporal limbic structures critical for long-term memory and "internal" information, such as affect and motivation, than are other PFC regions. It has direct and indirect (via the thalamus) connections with the hippocampus and associated neocortex, the amygdala, and the hypothalamus. It has strong connections with olfactory and gustatory cortices, but weaker connections than the lateral PFC to parietal and temporal cortices.

Intrinsic PFC Connections May Provide a Substrate for Diverse Information to Interact

Like most of the neocortex, many PF connections are local. Not only are there interconnections between the major subdivisions, but also interconnections between their constituent areas. The lateral PFC is particularly well connected. Ventrolateral areas 12 and 45 are interconnected with dorsolateral areas 46 and 8 and with dorsal area 9, as well as with orbitofrontal areas 11 and 13. Intrinsic PFC connections presumably allow information from a given PFC afferent or from a given process within a PFC subregion to be distributed to other parts of the PFC.

Summary

The PFC is anatomically well situated to play a role in cognitive control. It receives information from and sends projections to forebrain systems that process information about the external world, motor system structures that produce voluntary movement, systems that consolidate long-term memories, and systems that process information about affect and motivational state. This anatomy has long suggested that the PFC may be important for synthesizing external and internal information needed to produce complex behavior.

BEHAVIORAL EFFECTS OF DAMAGE TO THE PREFRONTAL CORTEX

PFC Damage in Humans Results in a "Dysexecutive Syndrome"

The PFC occupies a far greater proportion of the human cerebral cortex than in most other animals, suggesting that it might contribute to those elusive cognitive capacities that separate humans from animals. However, unlike electrical stimulation of more posterior regions that produce hallucinations or motoric responses, stimulation of the PFC produces no obvious effect. This led it to be termed the "silent cortex." Similarly, at first glance, PFC damage has

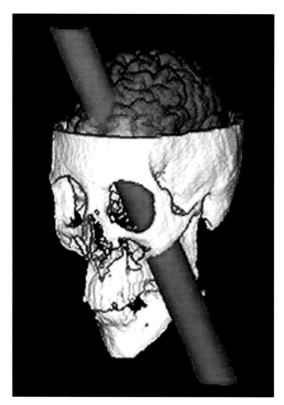

FIGURE 53.5 Reconstruction of damage to Phineas Gage's brain. From Damasio *et al.* (1994).

remarkably little overt effect; patients can perceive and move, there is little impairment in their memory, and they can appear remarkably normal in casual conversation. The most infamous case is that of Phineas Gage, a railway construction foreman. In 1848 he suffered an accident in which an iron bar exploded and was projected up through his chin and out of the top of his head, destroying much of his medial PFC in the process (Damasio *et al.*, 1994) (Fig. 53.5). However, as the *Boston Post* reported, "The most singular circumstance connected with this melancholy affair is, that he was alive at two o'clock this afternoon, and in full possession of his reason, and free from pain." However, it soon became clear that Gage had not escaped the accident wholly unscathed. While he had once been an efficient foreman, he was now irreverent and profane, rude to his co-workers, and unable to organize and plan the work that needed carrying out. He was soon fired as foreman.

Despite the superficial appearance of normality, PFC damage seems to devastate a person's life. Take the case of Elliot, a successful, happily married accountant, and by all accounts a responsible person. In his late thirties, he was diagnosed as having a prefrontal meningioma, and during the removal of the tumor his PFC was damaged. Within a few years of the operation, Elliot had divorced his wife, got married and divorced again, lost touch with his family and friends, acquired a disreputable business partner, and lost his business. All of Elliot's basic mental functions seemed to be intact, his language and memory abilities seemed normal, and on tests of

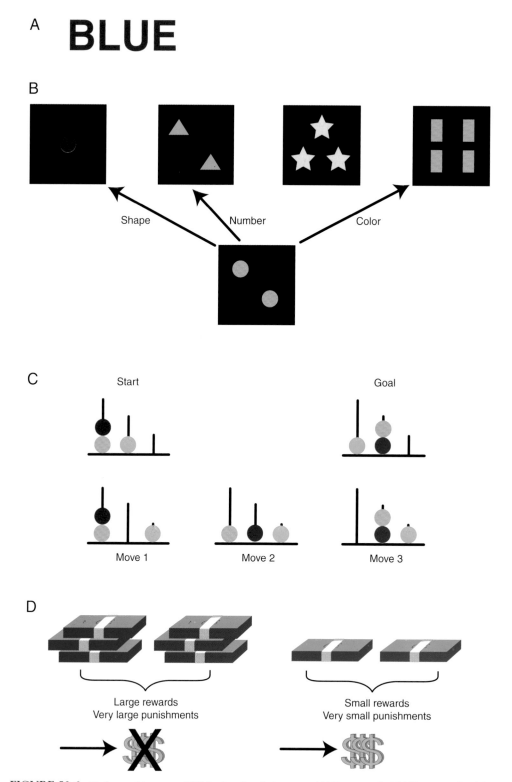

FIGURE 53.6   Tasks used to assess PFC dysfunction in humans. (A) Stroop task. (B) Wisconsin Card Sort. (C) Tower of London task. (D) Gambling task. See text for explanation of tasks.

intelligence he consistently performed in the superior range. What Elliot seemed to lack was the ability to coordinate his mental functions in a manner that took long-term concerns (unseen goals) into account. He became impulsive, lurching from one catastrophe to another based on his momentary whims.

Note that this scenario is exactly what would be expected from the two-level cognitive architecture of Norman and Shallice and others (Fig. 53.2). Damage to the higher order, executive functions leaves the components of complex behavior intact (which reside in the lower level) and able to be elicited by the appropriate external trigger. However, the individual would not be able to coordinate these behaviors with respect to goals and task-specific constraints. For example, there was a PFC patient who, when preparing coffee, first stirred and then added cream. Because of this apparent dysfunction in the top-down control over behavior, the pattern of deficits following frontal lobe damage has been thought to reflect a lack of goal directedness. The result is called the dysexecutive syndrome.

Humans with Frontal Damage Are Disinhibited

One of the most striking features of prefrontal patients is their disinhibition and lack of behavioral control. The patients are often impulsive, are quick to anger, and are prone to making rude and childish remarks. For example, one patient complained of being "much more outspoken" since her injury, while another stated, "I've become impulsive since the accident. If I have something to say I can't wait and have to say it straight away."

An example of disinhibition is utilization behavior. During a medical examination, a patient with PFC damage will pick up and use items that have been left on the doctor's desk. For example, the doctor might leave a comb on the desk, and the patient will pick the comb up and start combing their hair. In one extreme case, a patient used a urinal that the doctor had left on the desk! More formal tests of disinhibition include the Stroop test (Fig. 53.6A). It requires the patient to name aloud the color of the ink in which a word is written. The catch is that the word is the name of another color. Patients have difficulty inhibiting the saying of the word itself because the word elicits a strong, prepotent tendency to read it.

Such tests require patients to inhibit previously established specific responses, but PFC patients are also impaired at inhibiting more abstract behavioral demands like rules. Consider the Wisconsin Card Sorting Test (WCST)(Fig. 53.6B). The patient is required to sort a deck of cards on which are printed a number of symbols. The cards differ from one another in the color and shape of the symbols, and the number of symbols per card. The patient's task is to sort the cards according to a given criterion, e.g., "sort by shape." At this point the patients perform the task as well as control subjects. However, when the criterion is changed, e.g., to "sort by number," the patients are impaired; they are unable to inhibit sorting by the previous rule. This behavior, i.e., continuing to perform a previously reinforced behavior even though it is no longer rewarded, is called perseveration and is characteristic of a prefrontal patient's performance on a wide variety of tasks.

This inability to ignore irrelevant stimuli and the actions they trigger has led PFC patients to be described as stimulus bound, and disruption of the patient's ability to think and plan has been termed goal neglect (Duncan et al., 1996). Such impairments can also be understood within the framework of the architecture depicted in Fig. 53.2. Without the influence of goal-related signals from the executive functions, the systems always respond reflexively to an input with whatever output is strongly connected to it.

Humans with Frontal Lobe Damage Have Emotional Impairments

PFC damage produces a marked alteration of a patient's moods and emotions. In the case of Phineas Gage, these changes were so profound that his friends commented, "Gage is no longer Gage." Patients typically display an emotional shallowness, being indifferent and apathetic both to their own situation and to the needs of others. For example, one patient stated, "If I saw someone cry I'd just laugh—people look silly getting upset." Formal tests show that patients are less able to recognize the emotional expressions of others, although their ability to identify faces remains intact. Patients also become more irritable, aggressive, and prone to angry outbursts. Their humor, termed *Witzelsucht*, becomes compulsive, puerile, and facetious. The patients are aware of these changes even if they are indifferent to them. For example, one patient commented, "Emotion, tears, that's all gone out of the window," while another stated "I'm much more aggressive, and I feel much less fear. I go fighting for no reason: I don't get anxious."

Humans with Frontal Damage Have Difficulty in Planning

Prefrontal patients have a great deal of difficulty planning and organizing their lives. Wilder Penfield, a noted neurosurgeon of the mid-20th century, described the case of his sister, whom he operated on to remove a large frontal tumor. Prior to the surgery she had been an excellent cook, and while her basic culinary skills remained subsequent to the operation, she seemed unable to organize her behavior so that all the elements of the meal were ready simultaneously. Instead she would move haphazardly from preparing one part of the meal to another so that some parts of the meal would be burnt while others had hardly been started.

Formal tests have been developed to measure the ability of patients to organize their behavior. For example, the "tower of London test" requires the patient to think several moves in advance (Fig. 53.6C). There are three vertical posts that have three colored rings that can be placed on the posts. The three posts are of different lengths such that the first post can accommodate all three rings, the second post can accommodate two, and the third post just one. From an initial starting position the patient is asked to move the rings one at a time, from one post to another, to attain a specified goal position. This task requires the patient to plan a number of subgoal positions in order to reach the final goal. Patients with prefrontal damage are greatly impaired at this task, making many more moves than necessary to reach the final goal position. The "multiple errands test" taxes more everyday planning abilities. The test takes place in a shopping center, and the patient is required to perform various errands, such as obtaining a copy of the previous day's newspaper. The patients take much longer than control subjects. They go into inappropriate (irrelevant) shops as they pass them and repeatedly become distracted from their principal goal.

Impairments in planning might be related partly to difficulties evaluating the consequences of actions. Faced with a number of different, competing actions, patients might not choose wisely because they are less sure of the consequences of those actions. Evidence for this arises from a "gambling" task (Fig. 53.6D). The patient has to choose cards from four different decks in an effort to win play money from the experimenter. Each card wins the patient some money, but some cards also lose money and the patient has to pay the experimenter. Unbeknownst to the patient, cards from the first two decks will win large amounts of money, but are also occasionally associated with very large losses, and repeatedly choosing from these two decks will result in a net loss. In contrast, cards in the other two decks win smaller amounts of money, but the losses are also a lot smaller, and, overall, choosing from these two decks will result in a net profit. Control subjects initially choose from the two decks associated with the larger rewards, but after a few very large losses, they switch to choosing from the other decks and earn a profit. Patients with PFC damage also initially choose from the decks associated with larger rewards, but then fail to alter their behavior until they lose all their money. This task is appealing because it is closely related to the types of problems that prefrontal patients experience in real life.

Humans with Frontal Lobe Damage Have Impaired Working Memory

Patients might also have difficulties in planning due to a problem with holding information in mind for a short while. This is the kind of short-term memory that one relies on when reading a phone number and then going to dial that number. This function is called working memory because the information is forgotten as soon as it is no longer relevant. The concept of working memory is influenced by the observation that monkeys with lesions of the PFC have deficits on a spatial delayed-response task that requires them to remember the location of a stimulus or behavioral response over a brief delay of several seconds. Early studies failed to find this deficit in humans with prefrontal damage, possibly because the patients verbalized the location of the stimulus (e.g., "it's on the left"), which presumably makes the task much easier. Later studies, however, in which the prefrontal damage was more extensive and bilateral, did show a spatial delayed response deficit. Other studies used abstract patterns that could not be verbally encoded easily, and found that the patient's nonspatial working memory was also impaired.

Effects of Circumscribed PFC Damage Can Be Tested in Monkeys

We have seen that the PFC poses a complex problem. Damage to a relatively circumscribed region of the cortex in humans produces a bewildering array of symptoms. However, one caution in interpreting clinical studies concerns the size of the damage that typifies the prefrontal patient. Not only does the damage often encompass many different PFC regions, each of which may have different functions, but it also often encroaches onto neighboring regions, such as the premotor cortex, the cingulate cortex, and the insular cortex. In addition, it should be remembered that the PFC comprises many different anatomically defined areas, each possessing unique patterns of connections with the rest of the brain; it might be that each component of the dysexecutive syndrome arises from damage to different areas of the PFC. These matters are difficult to explore in humans because the damage is typically so extensive that it encompasses many brain regions both within and external to the PFC. However, focal lesions can be produced experimentally in monkeys.

In evaluating this work, it is important to bear in mind a number of points. First, in order to conclude that two different prefrontal areas are performing, or at least are important for, two different functions, it is necessary to demonstrate a double dissociation. A monkey with lesion X must be impaired at process A, but not process B, whereas a monkey with lesion Y must be impaired at process B, but not process A. A single dissociation, e.g., showing that lesion X impairs process A, but not process B, is insufficient evidence because this pattern of results could be achieved simply because the test used to assess A is more sensitive than the test used to assess process B. In many studies, monkeys were tested on just one task and any evidence for a double dissociation can only be inferred across different studies and (often) different laboratories. This complicates the interpretation because any differences in training and testing procedures and in the extent of the lesions are potential confounding factors. Second, early studies employed large lesions. These lesions often produced damage to the underlying white matter, potentially disconnecting regions of the cortex outside of the site of the lesion and often damaging underlying structures such as basal ganglia. In recent years, excitotoxins have been developed. These drugs can be injected into an area and overexcite the cells located there. The cells subsequently die, but the underlying white matter is left intact.

Monkeys with PFC Damage Are Impaired on Delayed Response Tasks

In 1935, Jacobsen published a seminal paper showing that lesions of the frontal lobe in monkeys produced deficits on a spatial delayed response task. In this task, the monkey sees a reward hidden at one of two locations and then, after a brief delay, is allowed to retrieve it (Fig. 53.7A). Monkeys with large PFC lesions behave as if they forgot where the reward was hidden, even after delays of just a few seconds. Subsequent experiments showed that lesions restricted to the dorsolateral PFC alone could produce the same deficit. In contrast, damage to the ventrolateral PFC impaired object delayed response tasks. Monkeys with such damage have difficulty with delayed matching-to-sample (DMS) tasks in which they are shown an object (the sample) and then, after

a brief delay of several seconds, must choose the same object (the match) from one or more nonmatching objects (Fig. 53.7B). The most severe deficits are observed when the same two objects are used repeatedly, requiring the monkey to remember which of the two objects it has seen most recently as the sample. Monkeys with orbital (ventral) PFC lesions tend to show the greatest deficit in tasks requiring reversal of previously successful actions. For example, they are impaired at spatial reversal tasks, in which the reward is alternated between two locations (Fig. 53.7C) and object reversal tasks, in which a reward is alternated between each of two objects (Fig. 53.7D). In both tasks the monkeys perseverate, continuing to choose the location or object under which the reward had first been hidden. Such observations led to the suggestion that the dorsal PFC might be responsible for processing spatial information, the ventral PFC for object-related information, and the orbital PFC for inhibitory control in accord with their preferential connections with the parietal, inferior temporal, and limbic system structures, respectively.

The picture, however, is not so simple and straightforward; a clear double dissociation between these impairments has not been demonstrated. Consider the hypothesized spatial versus object dissociation in the PFC. Dorsolateral PFC can impair performance on tasks that do not have a spatial component, such as object self-ordered search tasks. In this task the monkey is presented with three objects covering rewards. They must move each object in turn to obtain the reward, but after each choice a screen is lowered and the positions of the objects are shuffled (Fig. 53.7E). Thus, the monkey must remember continually which of the three objects it has already checked for a reward. Also, as noted earlier, monkeys with ventral (orbital) PFC lesions are impaired on both object and spatial reversal tasks. Neurophysiological studies paint a similar picture. While there may be some bias in the distribution of neurons that are sensitive to object identity or location in space (especially for the small population of highly specialized "face cells"), there is also a good deal of intermixing of neurons encoding these attributes, especially when the integration of these attributes is relevant to task performance.

Likewise, the notion that orbital PFC is responsible for inhibitory control is not so straightforward. It has subsequently been shown that inhibitory control is not unique to the orbital PFC. If the appropriate test is used, inhibitory control deficits can also be observed in monkeys with lesions of dorsolateral PFC. Marmosets were trained on a task similar to the WCST. They had to choose complex stimuli on the

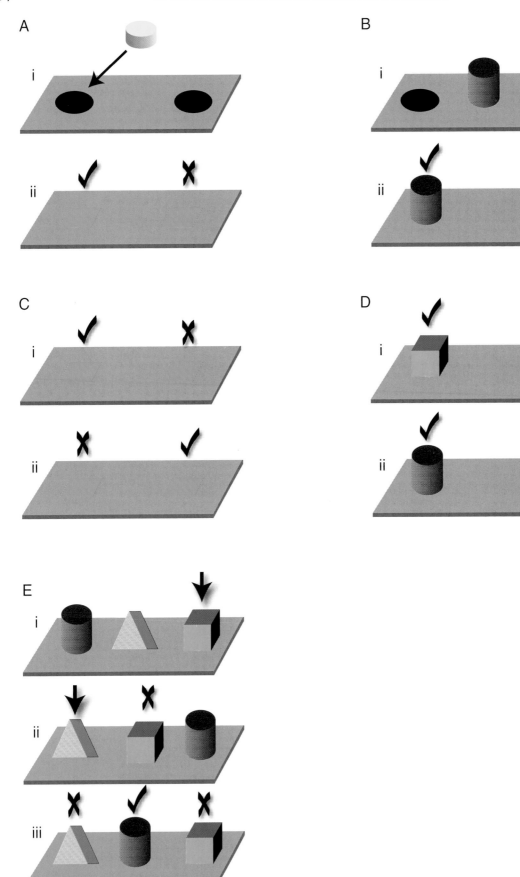

BOX 53.1

FUNCTIONAL TOPOGRAPHY

Information about topography of neural properties in the PFC can provide important insights into its function. For example, knowing that the primary visual cortex is organized into groups of neurons with similar tuning for orientation provides important clues to how it analyzes visual inputs. The anatomically complex nature of the PFC, coupled with the unique patterns of connections that each prefrontal area possesses, would certainly suggest a degree of functional fractionation. However, one immediate problem that investigators face when trying to address this issue is that it is not clear how to subdivide cognitive processing. It is far easier to specify the sensory attributes of an apple than it is to list the different processes involved in planning or reasoning.

One possibility is that PFC is organized by function, with different regions carrying out qualitatively different operations. One long-standing view is that the orbitofrontal area is associated with behavioral inhibition, whereas ventrolateral and dorsolateral regions are associated with memory or attentional functions (Goldman-Rakic, 1987; Fuster, 1989). Other suggestions include the idea that ventrolateral regions support the maintenance of information (memory), whereas dorsolateral regions are responsible for the manipulation of such information, as well as schemes based on stimulus dimensions such as segregation of information about object form and color (what) from information about its location (where). None of these schemes is mutually exclusive.

While there is undoubtedly some topographical organization of processing within the PFC, no clear global scheme has emerged. There is no overwhelming evidence for any one hypothesis and for some there are counter-vailing data. Perhaps this is not surprising. We do not yet understand the functional topography of the higher order sensory and motor cortical areas that are interconnected with the PFC. We can, however, make some general predictions. First, PFC functional topography is likely to be based on broad categories or gradients of organization with overlap and intermixing of diverse information. Complex behavior requires that we recognize and respond to relationships across diverse dimensions, and representing these relationships is a prerequisite for cognitive control. Indeed, because the majority of outputs of a given prefrontal area are to other prefrontal areas, it is not surprising that many prefrontal neurons are multimodal. Second, because learning is central to cognitive control and modulates the properties of many PFC neurons (see Neurophysiology of the Prefrontal Cortex), learning should have a large influence on PFC topography. Indeed, the flexible nature of controlled behaviors likely requires a dynamic anatomy, with neuronal properties changing to reflect the demands of the current task.

Earl K. Miller and
Jonathan D. Wallis

Reference

Fuster, J. M. (1997). "The Prefrontal Cortex," 3rd edition. Raven Press, New York.
Goldman–Rakic, P. S. (1987). Circuitry of primate prefrontal cortex and regulation of behaviour by representational memory. *In* "Handbook of Physiology: The Nervous System" (F. Plum, ed.), pp. 373–417. Am. Physiol. Sve., Bethesda.

basis of a rule, such as "choose by shape." When they were required to switch between different rules, monkeys with lesions of the dorsolateral PFC perseverated by continuing to choose on the basis of the previous rule, whereas monkeys with lesions of the orbital PFC were unimpaired. In contrast, when the same stimuli were used in an object reversal task, monkeys with lesions of the orbital PFC perseverated by continuing to choose the stimulus that had initially been rewarded, but the performance of monkeys with lesions of the dorsolateral PFC was normal. This suggests that both the dorsolateral and the orbital PFC contribute to inhibitory control. However, that the dorsolateral PFC may be more engaged by inhibitory control over rules, whereas the orbital PFC may be more engaged by inhibitory control over choices based on objects and rewards. For more discussion of the issue of PFC functional topography, see Box 53.1.

FIGURE 53.7 Some of the tasks on which monkeys with PFC damage are impaired. Check indicates correct choice, X indicates incorrect choice. Arrow in E indicates monkey's choice in self-ordered task. (A) Spatial delayed response. (B) Delayed matching to sample. (C) Spatial reversal. (D) Object reversal. (E) Object self-ordered search task.

Monkeys with PFC Damage Are Impaired on Conditional Learning Tasks

Conditional learning tasks are often used to test the ability to gain volitional control over behavior. Conditional learning refers to a class of tasks in which associative relationships must be learned that are arbitrary and extend beyond the simple one-to-one mappings that underlie reflexive reactions. Whether or not a given response is successful depends on additional, contextual, information. For example, reaching for popcorn at the cinema can be rewarding, but only if one takes other information into account; if the popcorn belongs to another patron, the result could be disastrous. The need to take into account complex relationships in order to decide among alternative actions is presumably why cognitive control has evolved.

Monkeys with PFC damage are impaired at such tasks. For example, when monkeys are trained to learn associations between, for example, three visual cues and three directional movements of a joystick, simply moving the joystick is not enough to produce reward. Rather, the specific movement direction is dependent on the specific cue. One cue means "up," another "down," and so on. Bilateral damage to the ventrolateral and orbital PFC impairs this learning severely. Depriving the PFC of its inputs from the high-order sensory cortex also results in conditional learning impairments. Humans with PFC damage are impaired on conditional learning tasks analogous to those conducted in monkeys. Conditional learning impairments seem to be dependent on which PFC region is damaged; some studies report no conditional learning deficit following dorsolateral PFC damage in monkeys.

Monkeys with PFC Damage Show Emotional Impairments

Like humans, monkeys with large PFC lesions display marked changes in social and emotional behavior. Monkey society is dictated by a dominance hierarchy, and each monkey knows its place; monkeys are submissive to monkeys higher in the hierarchy (e.g., the monkey grooms them) and are aggressive and threatening to monkeys lower in the hierarchy. Monkeys with large PFC lesions, however, disregard this hierarchy and also decrease their interactions with troop members. This typically results in their being ostracized from the troop.

Monkeys with PFC Damage are Impaired at Object Recognition

Monkeys with lesions of the ventromedial PFC show impairments in visual recognition. This ability is tested using a delayed nonmatching-to-sample task (DNMS). The monkey is presented with an object, and then after a brief delay of a few seconds, they are presented with that same object along with a novel object. New objects are used on each trial so the monkey can solve the task by recognizing which of the two objects it has previously seen in order to pick the novel object (Chapter 51). However, human patients with damage to the ventromedial PFC do not show these recognition deficits. One possibility for this discrepancy is that the deficit does not lie in recognition per se, but rather in the ability to learn the rules of the task. In particular, it has been suggested that the difficulty lies in making the association between the abstract quality of novelty and receiving a reward. This aspect of the task is not required in human patients because the patients are told the rules of the task explicitly; monkeys have to learn them by trial and error.

Summary

Humans with damage to the PFC present a wide variety of symptoms, including a lack of inhibitory control, a shallowness of emotion, difficulty planning and organizing behavior, and impaired working memory. In general, they seem to have difficulty in exerting volitional control and organizing their mental processes and actions in order to direct them toward unseen goals. As a result, their behaviors are simple, reactive, and emitted without concern for future consequences.

Just like humans, monkeys with extensive prefrontal damage can appear remarkably unimpaired to the casual observer. They have no motoric impairments, and their ability to discriminate a variety of sensory stimuli remains intact. They are also capable of simple learning, such as Pavlovian and instrumental conditioning. However, they are impaired when behavioral demands extend beyond this to include additional task-specific constraints and/or involve overcoming a previously established response. Localizing a specific deficit to any one PFC subregion has proven difficult; double dissociations between different PFC regions are rare.

The pattern of deficits observed after PFC damage in humans and monkeys makes sense in light of the cognitive architecture depicted in Fig. 53.2. The deficits seem to reflect a selective loss of higher level functions. Lower level, well-established routines are intact, but without the information about future goals and means provided by the higher level functions, processing would be at the mercy of the environment. Behavior would be ruled by whatever sensory inputs happen to flow into the system and by whatever

BOX 53.2

ATTENTION DEFICIT HYPERACTIVITY DISORDER

Do you pay attention to captivating yet irrelevant stimuli? Do you have trouble acting appropriately, fidgeting while listening to a lecture? Do you have difficulty planning and pursuing long-term goals? Do distractions knock you "off task"? When these not uncommon difficulties occur to a severe degree, they are symptoms of attention deficit hyperactivity disorder (ADHD), a disorder seen in children and adults. It is estimated that 3–5% of children have this disorder, with about half retaining problems into adulthood. The symptoms of ADHD involve dysfunction of the prefrontal cortex (PFC) and its cortical and subcortical connections.

Criteria for the diagnosis of ADHD include symptoms of "inattention" and "hyperactivity/impulsivity." Patients can have either the combined type, or predominantly "inattentive" or predominantly "hyperactive/impulsive" types. Many of the symptoms for "inattention" used to diagnose ADHD relate to attentional abilities of the PFC: e.g., difficulty sustaining attention or organizing, easily distracted, and forgetful. Similarly, many of the symptoms of "hyperactivity/impulsivity" describe PFC deficits: e.g., difficulty awaiting turn. The PFC controls attention via its projections to the parietal and temporal cortices (see Chapter 49), while it controls motor responses via its projections to the motor cortices and striatum. These circuits appear to be impaired in patients with ADHD. ADHD symptoms are especially evident in "boring" settings that require endogenous rather than exogenous regulation of behavior. For example, ADHD children can sit still and play video games for hours, but have trouble attending in school. ADHD patients have difficulty sustaining a behavior or thought over a delay. As described in this chapter, PFC cells exhibit sustained firing over a delay that regulates thought and behavioral output.

Structural and functional imaging studies show consistent alterations in PFC-striatal-cerebellar circuits in ADHD patients. Volumetric measures have detected smaller right-sided PFC regions (the right side is most associated with attention; see Chapter 49). Changes in the size of the striatum also have been reported, and functional imaging studies have shown abnormal activity of both the PFC and the striatum in ADHD patients performing tasks that require PFC inhibitory or attentional functions. Structural imaging studies have also shown consistent decreases in the size of the cerebellar vermis, a region that may exert regulatory influences on noradrenergic (NE) cells of the locus coeruleus (LC) and dopaminergic (DA) cells of the ventral tegmental area.

These NE and DA cells in turn have profound influences on PFC-striatal circuitry (see later). Thus, a smaller vermis in ADHD patients may lead to impaired catecholamine inputs to PFC and striatum. Some evidence supports this idea: a neuroreceptor imaging study suggests that there are reduced numbers of catecholamine terminals in the PFC of adults with ADHD.

NE and DA have a critical influence on PFC-striatal circuits, and thus changes in these inputs can have tremendous impact on PFC cognitive functions. This chapter describes how DA has an important effect on PFC function, and the same is true for NE. NE cells fire when a stimulus is of interest to the animal, releasing NE in the PFC. NE stimulates postsynaptic α_{2A}-adrenoceptors, enhancing delay-related firing and strengthening regulation of behavior and attention. However, very high levels of NE and DA, such as are released during stressful conditions, can impair PFC function via a_1-adrenoceptors and D1 receptors, respectively. Thus, the PFC has to have just the right neurochemical conditions to function optimally.

What causes ADHD? ADHD appears to be at least partially inherited, and one can imagine that genetic alterations that interfere with NE or DA signalling could have large effects on PFC function. Several studies indicate that two DA genes, the DA transporter and the DA D4 receptor, may be associated with susceptibility to ADHD. (The D4 receptor also has very high affinity for NE.) Environmental factors may also lead to the disruption of PFC-striatal circuits. For example, some kinds of infection may lead to autoantibodies that attack PFC-striatal circuits.

Medications for ADHD likely reduce symptoms of inattention and impulsivity by optimizing the neurochemical environment in the PFC and in the striatum. All effective treatments for ADHD interact with catecholamines: Stimulants such as Ritalin (methylphenidate) and Adderall (a mixture of amphetamines) increase NE and DA release and/or block catecholamine reuptake. Research in rats suggests that low doses of these compounds preferentially increase the release of NE. Consistent with these data, NE reuptake blockers are also used to treat ADHD (e.g., desipramine), including highly selective NE agents (atomoxetine). Drugs that mimic NE at α_{2A}-adrenoceptors (guanfacine and clonidine) are effective, especially in decreasing impulsivity. Wellbutrin (also known as Zyban or bupropion) is a DA reuptake blocker that is used to treat ADHD. How do these medications actually work to ameliorate ADHD symptoms?

BOX 53.2   (*cont'd*)

There have been several ideas proposed: (1) the etiology of ADHD involves insufficient catecholamine innervation of PFC-striatal circuits, and drugs that increase catecholamine receptor stimulation correct this; (2) ADHD involves excessive catecholamine release, and low doses of these medications correct this by promoting negative feedback, decreasing phasic catecholamine release; or (3) catecholamines are normal in ADHD patients (e.g., it is simply that their cortex is immature or inflamed), and amplification of catecholamine mechanisms enhances PFC function and reduces symptoms. Support for this latter idea arises from the fact that normal individuals are improved by small doses of these medications as well, as when college students sometimes take low doses of stimulants to focus on writing a paper.

All of us experience PFC dysfunction as part of daily life, especially when we are tired or stressed. These effects are likely due to neurochemical changes, e.g., in NE and DA, that have great impact on the functional integrity of the PFC. However, for people with ADHD, dysfunction of the PFC is much more constant and often beyond their control. Perhaps it is this prevalence of PFC dysfunction in otherwise healthy individuals, and its association with stress, that leads to the dismissal of ADHD by some as not a real disorder. It is hoped that as we come to better understand the neurobiological bases of ADHD, we will gain a fuller perspective of ADHD and its symptoms.

Amy F. T. Arnsten

Suggested Readings

The Neuropharmacology of Stimulant Drugs: Implications for AD/HD (2000). M. Solanto, A. Arnsten and F. X. Castellanos, eds. Oxford University Press, New York, NY.

---

thoughts, emotions, and actions are strongly associated with these inputs. Behavior would seem impulsive and disinhibited, and emotional reactions inappropriate, because they would be emitted reflexively without any consideration of the future. Further, without the influence of future goals to continually drive task-appropriate processes, individuals would be distractible and would easily go "off track" when there are temporal gaps between sensory inputs or between those inputs and the individual's responses (Box 53.2).

NEUROPHYSIOLOGY OF THE PREFRONTAL CORTEX

PFC anatomy suggests it has the means for executive functions, and the effects on behavior after damage to the PFC support this idea. So do neurophysiological studies; they have shown that PFC neurons have the properties one would expect from a region involved intimately in goal-directed behavior.

The PFC Is Multimodal

PFC anatomy indicates that it is interconnected with many different brain systems, a prerequisite for cognitive control. This high degree of connectivity is reflected in the neural activity observed in the PFC. Its neurons are activated by visual, auditory, tactile, and gustatory stimulation (and their memory), as well as by voluntary limb and eye movements. Further, these neurons seem capable of synthesizing this information in accord with task demands. For example, after monkeys are trained to make arm movements to visual and auditory targets appearing in different locations, many lateral PFC neurons are activated by both kinds of targets. Interestingly, few bimodal neurons were found in studies in which monkeys experienced visual and auditory stimuli passively. This finding suggests that task demands can exert a strong modulatory influence on PFC activity, which is consistent with its putative role in cognitive control.

PFC Neurons Can Sustain Their Activity

The first observations of PFC neural activity that were related to a cognitive process were made in the 1970s by Fuster, Niki, and their colleagues (Kubota and Niki, 1971; Fuster, 1973). Guided by lesion studies in monkeys, they recorded from the PFC while monkeys performed delayed response tasks. They found that, during the memory delay, many PFC neurons showed sustained activity that seemed to keep information about a spatial or object cue on-line (Fig. 53.8). In spatial delayed response tasks, cue-

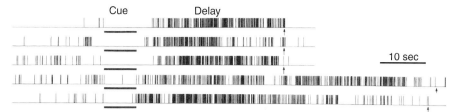

FIGURE 53.8 PFC delay activity. The activity of a single PFC neuron during five trials of a spatial delayed response task is shown. The arrow indicates the monkey's behavioral response at the end of the memory delay. Each small vertical line indicates an action potential from the neuron. Note the increased activity in the delay relative to other epochs. From Fuster (1973).

related "delay activity" could, in principle, reflect either sensory information related to the cue or movement information related to the behavioral response. Both are found in the PFC, each with different tempo-

ral characteristics. Sensory-related activity tends to be stronger nearer in time to the cue and then weakens as time passes, whereas movement-related neurons tend to increase their activity over time as the move-

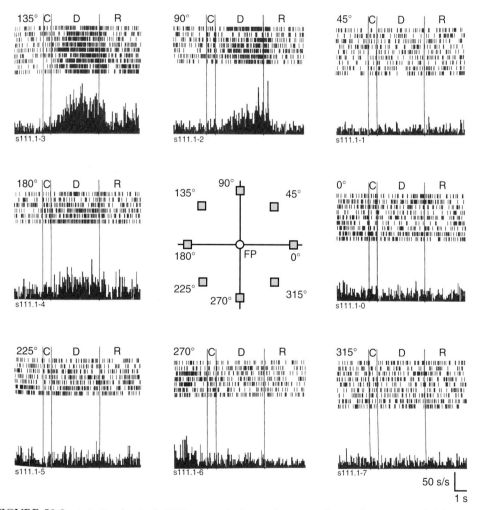

FIGURE 53.9 Activity of a single PFC neuron during performance of an oculomotor spatial delayed response task. Each trial started with the monkey fixating the central fixation point (FP) indicated in the central diagram. Then, a cue light (C) was flashed briefly on in one of the eight locations indicated in the central diagram. After a delay (D), the monkey was allowed to respond (R) by moving its eyes to the remembered location of the cue. Neural activity from cuing each location is shown by the corresponding histogram. This neuron exhibited delay period activity when the cue to be remembered was presented in the upper left quadrant of the visual field. Scale bars in the lower right indicate 1 s of time (1 S) and 50 spikes per second of neural activity (50 S/S). From Funahashi *et al.* (1989).

ment draws nearer. Goldman-Rakic and colleagues used a refined oculomotor version of the delayed response task to demonstrate that dorsolateral PFC neurons have precise tuning for memories of particular visual field locations (Funahashi *et al.*, 1989) (Fig. 53.9). They also demonstrated that PFC delay activity depends on dopamine receptors, a neurotransmitter implicated in signaling reinforcements and thus central to acquiring and sustaining goal-directed behaviors.

PFC delay activity has been shown to convey a wide range of behaviorally relevant cues: objects, colors, sounds, the frequency of a vibration to the hand, and forthcoming eye and arm movements. Similar activity is also evident in the sensory cortical areas and motor areas primarily responsible for analyzing inputs and generating behaviors, especially the higher order areas that are one or more steps removed from the primary sensory and motor cortex. This is not surprising; sustained activity is apparent in many brain structures and must play a role in many neural processes. For example, it is likely to underlie iconic memory, the very brief lingering "after image" of recent sensory events. However, what separates more "cognitive" working memory processes from such lower level processes as iconic memory is their ability to robustly sustain memories over potential distractions. PFC neurons do have this ability. For example, when monkeys are required to sustain the memory of a sample object across a delay period filled with visual distractors that require attention and processing, sustained activity within the prefrontal cortex can still maintain a memory of the sample object. In contrast, sustained activity in visual cortical areas seems more labile; activity is disrupted by the presence of distractors. Following a distracting stimulus, neural activity reflects the distractor rather than the stimulus the monkey is retaining in working memory. This particular ability is not unique to the PFC. Some neurons in the entorhinal cortex, a region critical for memory, can also maintain sample-specific delay activity across intervening stimuli.

How does the PFC "latch" onto goal-relevant information and maintain it without disruption? Several ideas have been suggested. These typically employ a form of gating signal that instructs the PFC network when to maintain a given activity state. This gating signal may come from dopaminergic (DA) neurons in the midbrain and basal ganglia. These neurons respond when monkeys are rewarded or, importantly, when monkeys can first predict that a reward is forthcoming. In many behavioral tasks, presentation of the cue at the start of the trial is a good predictor that a reward is soon coming. Such a well-timed DA burst

could strengthen current PFC representations, protecting them against interference from disruption by irrelevant, distracting information until another DA influx reinforces another representation. Local injection of DA antagonists in the PFC does block delay activity in the PFC. Anatomical loops between the PFC and basal ganglia have been suggested to play a role here. Neural activity propagating around the loops may help sustain activity, and the basal ganglia have been suggested to provide a means by which DA signals can influence PFC activity.

PFC Neural Activity Reflects Task Demands

Playing the game requires knowing the rules. To explore how these rules might be represented in the PFC, experimenters manipulate task demands: monkeys are trained on tasks in which the physical cues are held constant while their behavioral meaning changes.

In one study, monkeys learned contingencies between visual cues and directional eye movements(Asaad *et al.*, 1998). Through trial and error, they learned to saccade to the right after one object was presented and saccade to the left after another object was presented. After this was learned (in about 10–15 trials) and practiced (for about 15 more trials), the associations were reversed and monkeys modified their behavior to acquire the opposite contingencies, to saccade leftward after presentation of the object that had previously been associated with a rightward saccade and vice versa. Many PF neurons (44% of a randomly selected population) reflected the learned contingencies; they encoded specific associations between cues and saccades. For example, a given cell might be strongly activated only when object "A" instructed "saccade left" and not when object "B" instructed the same saccade or when object "A" instructed another saccade (Fig. 53.10A). Other studies have shown that many PFC neurons encode whether visual and auditory cues signal that reward will or will not be delivered and encode learned, arbitrary, associations between visual and auditory stimuli. PFC neurons can even reflect the degree to which a stimulus instructs a specific behavioral response. Over a delay, activity related to a forthcoming response increases more sharply if there is a perfect relationship between the cue and the response than if the association is less predictable.

These studies suggest that PFC neurons represent task contingencies, the associative relationships that describe the logic needed to perform a task. Further support comes from investigations that have shown that PFC activity reflects more complex task informa-

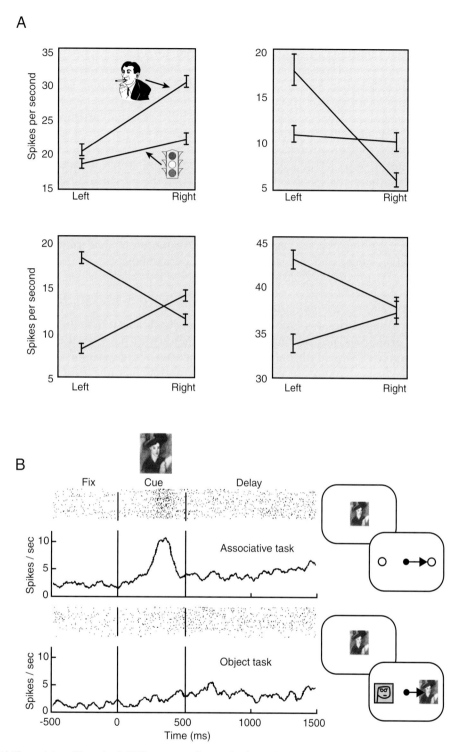

FIGURE 53.10 (A) The activity of four single PFC neurons when each of two objects, on different trials, instructed either a saccade to the right or a saccade to the left. Different objects were used for each neuron. Lines connect the average values obtained when a given object cued one or the other saccade. Error bars show the standard error of the mean. Note that in each case, the activity of the neuron depends on both the cue object and the saccade direction and that the tuning is nonlinear or conjunctive. That is, the level of activity to a given combination of object and saccade cannot be predicted from the response of the neuron to the other combinations. Adapted from Asaad *et al.* (1998). (B) A PFC neuron whose neural response to a cue object was highly dependent on the rule the monkey was currently using. The figure shows an example of the response of a single PFC neuron to the same cue object during an object task (delayed matching to sample, bottom half) and during an associative task (conditional visual motor, top half), where the object instructs either a leftward or rightward saccade. Note that the neuron is responsive to the cue during one task but not during the other, even though sensory stimulation is identical across the tasks. Adapted from Asaad *et al.* (2000).

tion such as rules. Monkeys can be taught to alternate rapidly between different rules. For example, following a given cue, they can learn to direct a response to either the location of the cue (spatial matching rule) or an alternate location associated with the cue (associative rule), depending on which rule is currently in effect. When tested in this fashion, many PFC neurons show rule-specific activity (Fig. 53.10B). For example, a PFC neuron might respond to a given visual cue when the monkey is using an associative rule but exhibit weak or no activity under identical sensory and attentional conditions that differed only in that the monkey was instead using a spatial rule. Such effects have been found in PFC for associative versus spatial rules, for object matching versus spatial matching versus associative rules, and for shape matching versus object matching rules (Asaad *et al.*, 2000).

Primate behavior is not limited to following literal associations and specific rules. Primates can also abstract general rules or principles, not tied to any particular stimulus or response. This ability allows behavior to extend beyond specific circumstances that have been experienced directly. For example, humans learn the "rules" for restaurant dining from specific experiences and can then generalize and apply them to new restaurants. Wallis and colleagues (2001) investigated this process in monkeys by recording from single neurons in the PFC. Monkeys were trained to use two abstract rules; they indicated whether two successively presented pictures were either the same ("match") or different ("nonmatch"). The monkeys could perform this task with novel pictures, thus demonstrating that they had learned two general principles that could be applied to stimuli that they had not experienced directly. The most prevalent neuronal activity observed in the dorsolateral, ventrolateral, and orbital PFC reflected the coding of the abstract "match" and "nonmatch" rules. This finding suggests that rule representation may be a cardinal PFC function.

PFC Neurons Are Flexible

Another hallmark of primates is the ability to learn new behaviors quickly. PFC neurons are capable of a correspondingly rapid modification of their properties to meet task demands. Monkeys can learn new conditional visuomotor associations in just a few trials and as they do, PFC neural activity modifies rapidly to reflect the new contingencies. Striking examples of rapid experience-dependent neural plasticity come from studies of the frontal eye fields, part of Broadmann's area 8 that is important for voluntary

shifts of gaze (Bichot and Schall, 1999). Normally, neurons in this area are activated selectively by saccade targets that appear in certain visual field locations. Monkeys were also trained to search for a target defined by a particular visual attribute (e.g., red). In this case, neurons in the frontal eye fields acquired sensitivity to that attribute. When monkeys were trained to search for a different target every day neurons discriminated not only the current target, but also discriminated distracting stimuli that had been a target on the previous day from stimuli that had been targets even earlier. Monkeys were also more likely to make errors in choosing that distracting stimulus. It was as if the previous day's experience left an impression in the brain that influenced neural activity and task performance.

PFC Neurons Encode Rewards

Feedback about the consequences of actions is key to acquiring new goal-directed behaviors. Consequently, a large proportion of PFC neurons encode information about rewards. For example, some neurons are activated by the delivery of a reward, whereas others respond when an expected reward is not delivered. PFC neurons also encode the type of reward that the monkey expects to receive, e.g., a piece of cabbage versus a raisin, as well as the quantity of reward the monkey expects. Further, the neurons appear to encode the monkey's relative preference for the rewards that are available, rather than some absolute measure of reward. Thus, a neuron might prefer reward A when the monkey's choice of reward is between A and B, but reward B when the choice is between B and C. Orbital PFC is the area of the PFC that receives gustatory and olfactory information, and indeed neurons responsive to rewards are found there. However, many neurons responsive to reward are also found in the dorsolateral PFC.

Summary

As might be expected from a brain region thought to orchestrate complex behavior, neural activity in the PFC conveys information about a wide range of external and internal information, but its activity is not limited to simple responses to sensory events or actions. Rather, the behavioral context has a pervasive influence on PFC activity. After training, many (up to half) of dorsolateral, ventrolateral, and orbital PFC neurons encode information about the formal demands of behavior: contingencies between a wide range of stimuli, actions, and reward consequences, and behavior-guiding rules. By sustaining their activity robustly, PFC neurons can keep this and other behaviorally relevant information on-line to guide behaviors that extend over time. Also consistent with its role in guiding goal-directed behavior, PFC neurons process information about the expected results of achieving goals: rewards.

THEORIES OF PREFRONTAL CORTEX FUNCTION

Working Memory

One proposal is that the cardinal function of the PFC is to hold recent sensory inputs and movement-related information in active short-term memory, or working memory (Goldman-Rakic, 1987). In this view, the PFC acts as a temporary scratch pad that sustains the inputs it receives from other cortical areas. This hypothesis has its roots in observations of deficits in the performance of delayed response tasks following PFC damage and in observations of PFC neurons that show sustained activity over a memory delay. Other deficits following PFC damage are also thought to be sequelae of a working memory deficit. For example, patients might be impaired at planning because they are unable to keep in mind all the different variables that need to be considered. This in turn might make them appear disinhibited as their behavior becomes directed toward more immediate goals, rather than toward longer term, more delayed goals.

Working memory maintenance functions are central to cognition; complex, goal-directed behaviors are typically drawn out and thus are impossible without mechanisms that extend information over time. There is ample evidence that these mechanisms are abundant in the PFC. Working memory is unlikely to be the whole story, however. Many of the tasks on which prefrontal patients and monkeys show impairment do not have an obvious working mem-ory component, such as the Wisconsin Card Sorting Test and reversal tasks.

Studies have investigated this issue explicitly, by examining the performance of monkeys with lesions of the ventrolateral PFC on a simultaneous color-matching task. In this task the monkey is presented with a sample color and two test colors simultaneously. The monkey must choose the test color that matches the sample color. PFC-lesioned monkeys were impaired at this task, despite the fact that the task involved contains no delays and therefore no working memory requirements. The task does, however, require conditional rules (e.g. "if the sample color is red, then choose the red test stimulus"), and the role of the PFC in the representation of such rules (see later) might explain this impairment.

Somatic Marker Hypothesis

It has been suggested that the orbitofrontal PFC is responsible for labeling people, objects, or situations with an "affective significance" (Damasio, 1994). This labeling is achieved by associating memories of past, affectively laden events with a representation of the somatic state which that event evoked. Thus, the memory of the past event is labeled with a "somatic marker" that helps individuals make decisions. Rather than having to evaluate all the pros and cons of prior circumstances to decide on the present, one can simply recall the associated somatic marker, providing the individual with the appropriate affective state and, in effect, a "gut feeling" of which alternative is correct. Patients with damage to this system might be unable to reach a decision, simply because they become incapacitated by contemplating irrelevant information. None of the outcomes of their actions will be obviously more emotionally preferable than alternative outcomes, and patients might make decisions randomly or impulsively, and as such appear to be disinhibited.

A deficient somatic marker system would explain the impairments that patients with damage to the orbitofrontal PFC exhibit on the "gambling task" (Fig. 53.6D). The reward contingencies associated with each deck of cards are designed to be too complex to be ascertained purely by logical reasoning. Control subjects succeed at the task because they associate a somatic marker with each deck of cards, warning the subject as to whether the choice they are about to make is risky. Further support comes from measures of skin conductance responses (SCRs) that reflect autonomic nervous system processing. Control subjects show SCRs prior to the selection of a card, and choices from risky decks are preceded by a larger SCR than choices from less risky decks. Patients with damage to the ventromedial PFC showed no anticipatory SCRs, although their SCRs when actually receiving the reward or punishment are intact.

This hypothesis is similar to one advanced by William James in the 19th century. He proposed that emotional feelings depend on feedback from the autonomic nervous system. For instance, running from a bear because we are afraid evokes a particular autonomic state (such as increased heart rate and blood pressure) that makes us feel afraid. Thus, as James stated, we do not run because we are afraid, but we are afraid because we run. A problem with simply using autonomic nervous system signals to identify emotional states, however, is that autonomic states associated with different emotions can be identical. Later studies showed that mani-pulations of the autonomic nervous system, e.g., by administering adrenaline, could alter the magnitude but not necessarily the type of emotion experienced in human subjects. These problems are avoided if the orbitofrontal cortex does not need to access the autonomic nervous system directly, but rather can use a conditioned association between the autonomic state and various cortical representations. For example, associations with the somatosensory cortex or other cortical areas responsible for representing bodily states, may be involved in emotional interpretations; patients with damage to the somatosensory cortex have difficulty recognizing facial emotions, as do patients with orbital frontal damage.

Multiple Processing Levels

It has been proposed that the PFC is organized by level of processing, much as there are primary and higher order sensory cortices (Petrides, 1996). The ventrolateral PFC is primary. It receives inputs from the sensory cortex and is responsible for their simple maintenance in working memory and for retrieval of information from long-term memory. The dorsolateral PFC then takes this information and performs more executive processes, such as monitoring multiple behaviors and manipulating information. For example, simply rehearsing a phone number is a ventrolateral PFC function while saying that same number backward is a dorsolateral PFC function. It should be noted that such an arrangement would preclude the possibility of demonstrating a functional double dissociation between these two areas, as the dorsolateral PFC is only able to perform executive processes on information after it has been received by the ventrolateral PFC. Thus, removing the dorsolateral PFC would impair higher level processes, whereas removing the ventrolateral PFC would impair both.

This hypothesis has been supported by evidence from neuroimaging in humans. Subjects were required to perform five spatial working memory tasks while they were scanned using positron emission tomography. This technique enables the visualization of areas of the brain with the increased blood flow that is related to neural activity (see Box 13.1). Two of the tasks had simple maintenance requirements; they activated the ventrolateral PFC. The three other tasks also had manipulation requirements and they activated the dorsolateral PFC.

Rule Representation

Several investigators have pointed out that because knowledge about goals, means, and consequences is vital to planning and implementing complex goal-directed behavior, the PFC is likely to play a central role in its acquisition and representation. The neural instantiation of task demands in the PFC was first proposed by Fuster (1989). Based on behavioral and neurophysiological experiments in monkeys, he hypothesized that sustained activity in the PFC was not used merely to retain recent sensory events, but also to link together behavioral relevant, but temporally separate, events and actions into a representation of task contingencies.

Other investigators have reached similar conclusions. Grafman (1994) suggested that the PFC contains managerial knowledge units (MKUs), sets of task contingencies linked under common themes that can be combined flexibly into extended routines. A MKU may describe the expected events and appropriate responses for dining in a restaurant, for example. Passingham (1993) suggested that many of the deficits following PFC damage can be explained by a loss of the ability to acquire conditional if-then rules. Wise et al. (1996) proposed complementary roles in rule learning for the PFC and basal ganglia. The PFC is thought to act when new rules are learned, whereas the basal ganglia are thought to potentiate (select) the previously learned rules that are appropriate for the current situation.

Cognitive control has also been studied by developing simulated neural network models that can perform tasks that depend on controlled processing, such as the Stroop test. These models invariably include units dedicated to representing task rules and contingencies. Analogies are often drawn between these units and the PFC.

How might the PFC acquire rule information and use it for cognitive control? Miller and Cohen (2001) proposed that reward signals from midbrain dopamine systems act on the multimodal circuitry in the PFC to strengthen connections between neurons that process the information that led to the reward. This action results in a model of the task contingencies, which in neural terms amounts to a representation of the pattern of connections among the sensory, motor, and mnemonic representations needed to solve that task. Maintenance mechanisms in the PFC sustain this representation during task performance. This produces feedback signals to the posterior cortex that bias the flow of activity along lines that match the PFC representation, i.e., along task-relevant neural pathways. In short, the PFC plots a "map" of which neural pathways in the forebrain are successful at solving a task and then holds it on-line in the PFC so that the rest of the neocortex can follow it.

Evidence for this proposal comes from the finding that PFC neurons show neural activity that reflects behaviorally relevant associations between disparate and arbitrary events and actions, behavioral context and rules. Behavioral and neurophysiological studies of focal attention also point to the operation of top-down signals on the visual cortex (presumed to come from the PFC) that enhance representations of behaviorally relevant stimuli and visual field locations at the expense of irrelevant ones. Evidence that such signals come from the PFC was supported by an observation that disconnecting the PFC from the temporal cortex prevented the activation of stored memories in the latter and caused monkeys to fail at a recall test (Tomita *et al.*, 1999).

Flexibility and Limited Capacity of Controlled Processing

Sustained activation is central in many views of PFC functions. This is not surprising considering the importance of working memory for cognitive control and that sustained activity is common in the PFC. However, as O'Reilly and Munakata (2000) have pointed out, representing information through sustained activity offers more than just the ability to bridge gaps; it has other advantages for cognitive control.

It is universally supposed that long-term storage in the brain depends on changing synaptic weights by strengthening some neural connections and weakening others. Encoding information in structural changes has obvious advantages for long-term storage, but the resulting memories are relatively inflexible. Also, changing synaptic weights has local effects; only the two neurons sharing the synapse are affected. Information contained in a set of synaptic weights is thus expressed only when the circuit is fired. In contrast, the information needed to guide goal-directed behavior must be expressed in a format that allows it to affect the ongoing processing in other brain systems. Sustained activity is such a format. It is extended over time, and information contained in a pattern of activity can be propagated across the brain. Thus, the ability of sustained activity to tonically influence other brain systems is likely important for coordinating diverse processing around a specific goal. It also affords flexibility; if cognitive control stems from a pattern of information maintained in the PFC, changing behavior is as easy as changing the pattern (O'Reilly and Munakata, 2000; Miller and Cohen, 2001).

Finally, the neuronal mechanisms by which information needed for cognitive control is expressed might explain the severely limited capacity of controlled processes. A vast amount of information can be stored by changing synaptic weights of a network that contains many neurons, each with many potential connections. At any given time, however, most of this information is latent; it is expressed only when the relevant circuit is activated. In contrast, if the information for cognitive control is expressed in a unique pattern of ongoing activity distributed across many simultaneously active neurons—a population code—then there will be a natural capacity limitation. Trying to represent more than just a few items at the same time would degrade information because the unique patterns impinging on a given set of neurons might overwrite and interfere with one another.

Summary

The ability to take charge of one's actions and direct them toward future aims is called cognitive control. Virtually all theories of cognition posit that cognition depends on functions specialized for the acquisition of information about goals and means. These functions exert a top-down influence on the lower level automatic processes that mediate sensory analysis, memory storage, and motor outputs, orchestrating and directing them toward a given goal.

The PFC, a brain structure that reaches its greatest complexity in the primate brain, seems to play a central role in cognitive control. It has the requisite anatomical infrastructure. It has access to, and the means to influence processing in, all major forebrain systems and can provide a means to synthesize the diverse information related to a given goal. Indeed, its damage in humans and monkeys results in a dysexecutive syndrome; individuals are stimulus bound and seem capable only of reacting to the immediate environment. Information about unseen goals and potential consequences of actions has little influence on behavior. PFC neurons also have properties consistent with their participation in cognitive control: they are multimodal, reflect task demands, and can sustain their activity to keep task-relevant information on-line during task performance.

Theories of PFC function suggest that the PFC makes several contributions important for cognitive control: maintenance and manipulation of information in working memory, the assignment and recall of the affective tags related to different choices, and the acquisition and representation of behavior-guiding rules that help orchestrate goal-directed behaviors. None of these theories is mutually exclusive, and indeed, different theories may be focusing on different aspects of a complex system that is involved in a wide range of brain processes.

References

Asaad, W. F., Rainer, G., and Miller, E. K. (1998). Neural activity in the primate prefrontal cortex during associative learning. *Neuron* **21**, 1399–1407.

Asaad, W. F., Rainer, G., and Miller, E. K. (2000). Task-specific activity in the primate prefrontal cortex. *J. Neurophysiol.* **84**, 451–459.

Bichot, N. P., and Schall, J. D. (1999). Effects of similarity and history on neural mechanisms of visual selection. *Nature Neurosci.* **2**, 549–554.

Damasio, A. R. (1994). "Descartes' Error: Emotion, Reason, and the Human Brain." Putman, New York.

Damasio, H., and Grabowski, T., Frank, R., Galaburda, A. M., and Damasio, A. R. (1994). The return of Phineas Gage: Clues about the brain from the skull of a famous patient. *Science* **264**, 1102–1105.

Duncan, J., Emslie, H., Williams, P., Johnson, R., and Freer, C. (1996). Intelligence and the frontal lobe: The organization of goal-directed behavior. *Cognit. Psychol.* **30**, 257–303.

Funahashi, S., Bruce, C. J., and Goldman-Rakic, P. S. (1989). Mnemonic coding of visual space in the monkey's dorsolateral prefrontal cortex. *J. Neurophysiol.* **61**, 331–349.

Fuster, J. M. (1973). Unit activity in prefrontal cortex during delayed-response performance: neuronal correlates of transient memory. *J. Neurophysiol.* **36**, 61–78.

Fuster, J. M. (1989). "The Prefrontal Cortex." Raven Press, New York.

Goldman-Rakic, P. S. (1987). Circuitry of primate prefrontal cortex and regulation of behavior by representational memory. *In* "Handbook of Physiology: The Nervous System" (F. Plum, ed.), pp. 373–417. Am. Physiol. Soc., Bethesda.

Grafman, J. (1994). Alternative frameworks for the conceptualization of prefrontal functions. *In* "Handbook of Neuropsychology" (F. Boller and J. Grafman, eds.), p. 187. Elsevier, Amsterdam.

Kubota, K., and Niki, H. (1971). Prefrontal cortical unit activity and delayed alternation performance in monkeys. *J. Neurophysiol.* **34**, 337–347.

Miller, E. K., and Cohen, J. D. (2001). An integrative theory of prefrontal function. *Annu. Rev. Neurosci.* **24**, 167–202.

Norman, D. A., and Shallice, T. (1986). Attention to action: Willed and automatic control of behavior. *In* "Consciousness and Self-Regulation: Advances in Research and Theory" (R. J. Davidson, G. E. Schwartz, and D. Shapiro, eds.), pp. 1–48. Plenum, New York.

O'Reilly, R. C., and Munakata, Y. (2000). "Computational Explorations in Cognitive Neuroscience: Understanding the Mind." MIT Press, Cambridge.

Passingham, R. (1993). "The Frontal Lobes and Voluntary Action." Oxford Univ. Press, Oxford.

Petrides, M. (1996). Specialized systems for the processing of mnemonic information within the primate frontal cortex. *Phil. Trans. Roy. Soc. Lond. B. Biol. Sci.* **351**, 1455–1461.

Tomita, H., Ohbayashi, M., Nakahara, K., Hasegawa, I., and Miyashita, Y. (1999). Top-down signal from prefrontal cortex in executive control of memory retrieval. *Nature* **401**, 699–703.

Wallis, J. D., Anderson, K. C., and Miller, E. K. (2001). Single neurons in the prefrontal cortex encode abstract rules. *Nature* **411**, 953–956.

Wise, S. P., Murray, E. A., and Gerfen, C. R. (1996). The frontal-basal ganglia system in primates. *Crit. Rev. Neurobiol.* **10**, 317–356.

Suggested Readings

Adolphs, R. (2001). The neurobiology of social cognition. *Curr. Opin. Neurobiol.* **11**, 231–239.

Braver, T. S., and Cohen, J. D. (2000). On the control of control: The role of dopamine in regulating prefrontal function and working memory. *In* "Attention and Performance 18" (S. Monsell and J. Driver, eds.), pp. 713–738. MIT Press, Cambridge.

Dehaene, S., Kerszeberg, M., and Changeux, J. P. (1998). A neuronal model of a global workspace in effortful cognitive tasks. *Proc. Natl. Acad. Sci. USA* **95**, 14529–14534.

Fuster, J. M. (1995). "Memory in the Cerebral Cortex." MIT Press, Cambridge, MA.

Fuster, J. M. (2001). The prefrontal cortex—an update: Time is of the essence. *Neuron* **30**, 319–333.

Goldman-Rakic, P. S. (1994). Working memory dysfunction in schizophrenia. *J. Neuropsychiat. Clin. Neurosci.* **6**, 348–357.

Miller, E. K. (2000). The prefrontal cortex and cognitive control. *Nature Rev. Neurosci.* **1**, 59–65.

Roberts, A. C., and Wallis, J. D. (2000). Inhibitory control and affective processing in the prefrontal cortex: Neuropsychological studies in the common marmoset. *Cereb. Cortex* **10**, 252–262.

Shimamura, A. P. (2000). The role of the prefrontal cortex in dynamic filtering. *Psychobiology* **28**, 207–218.

Earl K. Miller and Jonathan D. Wallis

54

Executive Control and Thought

INTRODUCTION

Examples of Active Thought

There are many kinds of human mental activities that we label as thought, ranging from daydreaming to solving a difficult mathematical problem. This chapter focuses on the kind of thinking that corresponds to on-line mental computations; the kind of thought that is tapped in some subtests of IQ exams and referred to as "fluid intelligence" by psychometricians. Neuroimaging research has made some progress in determining the neurological components of on-line computations. Before these are considered, the chapter first provides some examples of the kind of thought that occurs as on-line computation.

On-line computations involve keeping active a mental representation of a problem, operating on that representation, storing the altered representation, operating on that, and so forth. A good first example is mental arithmetic, such as the mental multiplication of two 2-digit numbers (e.g., 17×28). Behavioral experiments and computer simulations of this task indicate that the processing typically goes as follows. First one represents the problem in working memory—a system for the temporary storage and processing of information. Then one selectively attends to the digits in the one's column (7 and 8 in the example), mentally multiplies them, and stores the partial product in working memory. Then one selectively attends to the digit in the ten's column of the upper number and the one's column of the lower number, mentally multiplies them (adding the carry, which is also being held in working memory), again updates working memory with the partial product, and so on. From this somewhat informal analysis of

the task, it appears that the basic components of the task include storing information in working memory, updating working memory, selectively attending to some part of the information, implementing task-specific processes (the arithmetic operations), and switching attention between updating working memory and task-specific processes. The microstructure of the task involves a cycle of processing and updating the contents of working memory, modulated by shifts of attention.

The same cycle and components are apparent in other on-line thinking situations. Consider the Tower of Hanoi problem, a standard task for studying breakdowns in reasoning in frontal lobe patients (also see Tower of London problem, Chapter 53). As shown in Fig. 54.1, in its simplest version, the task involves three pegs and three disks differing in size. The disks

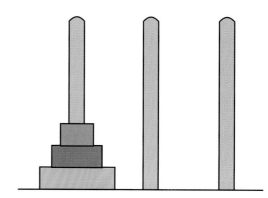

FIGURE 54.1 A schematic of the Tower of Hanoi problem. At the start of the problem, the three disks are arranged in a particular configuration on peg 1. The task is to recreate that configuration on peg 3, with the constraints that only one disk can be moved at a time, and that a larger disk can never be placed on a smaller one. Adapted from Carpenter et al. (1990).

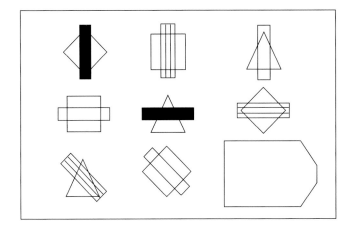

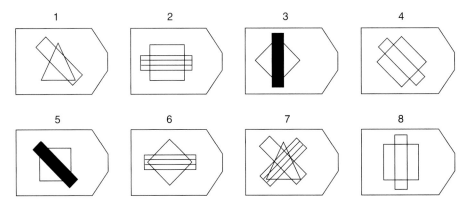

FIGURE 54.2   Example of a problem that is similar to ones on the Raven Progressive Matrices Test. The problem is not on the actual test to preserve the test's security. As described in the text, the goal is to choose one of the eight alternatives that best fits in the missing cell to complete the matrix. From Carpenter *et al.* (1990).

are arranged on peg 1 in an initial configuration, and the subject's task is to recreate that configuration on peg 3, with the constraints that only one disk can be moved at a time and that a larger disk can never be placed on a smaller one. In addition, subjects are often asked to solve the problem "in their head." Behavioral experiments plus computer simulations indicate that one of the major strategies used is this: The subject represents the whole array in working memory, selectively attends to the top disk on peg 1, mentally moves it to peg 3, updates working memory with the new array, then selectively attends to the middle sized disk on peg 1, moves it to peg 2, updates working memory with a new configuration, and so on. Again the microstructure of the task involves a cycle of task-specific processing and updating the contents of working memory, modulated by selective attention and shifts of attention between task-specific process and updating working memory.

Note that in this case the task-specific processes themselves involve a kind of thinking, one in which goals and subgoals are generated according to some plan, and then subplans are formulated for obtaining the subgoals. Theorists have argued that this too involves working memory (e. g., the subgoals and subplans must be stored and updated in working memory). Some planning may even be needed in mental multiplication, at least for young children. Planning also plays a role in the next example. However, because the neural foundations of planning are poorly understood, what follows continues to emphasize the basic working-memory cycle and its attentional modulation.

The final example is the Ravens Progressive Matrices Test. This is a standard nonverbal test of fluid intelligence, which is thought to provide an optimal measure of processes widely used in fluid reasoning. An illustrative problem is presented in

Fig. 54.2. The subject's task is to examine the incomplete 3x3 matrix of geometric forms in the box and to determine which of the eight alternative figures beneath the box fits in the bottom right of the matrix in order to properly complete it. The problem solver has to determine the rules that govern the orderliness of the rows and columns of the matrix, and then use these rules to select the correct alternative. Simulations of this task (e.g., Carpenter *et al.*, 1990) imply a process that unfolds as follows. The subject compares adjacent figures in the top row, selectively attending to each feature of the figure, notes that the geometric objects mismatch, and notes further that each figure contains a vertical bar through it that differs in shading. These comparisons give rise to tentative hypotheses about the rules that relate the figures in a row, and these hypotheses are stored in working memory; then the subject switches attention to the second row, compares adjacent figures, selectively attending to features identified as critical by the stored hypotheses. The subject then notes that some of them are again supported, but that the orientation of the bar has changed. He/she uses this to update the hypothesis in working memory, and so on. Again the processing involves storage in working memory, updating working memory, task-specific processing (including comparing features of geometric objects, and generating hypotheses about these comparisons), selective attention, and switching attention. Indeed, Carpenter *et al.* (1990) demonstrated that performance on a working memory task that contains all of these components except the task-specific processes correlates highly with performance on the Ravens Progressive Matrices Test.

Basic Components Research Strategy

This breakdown into components leads naturally to a research strategy for studying the neural bases of on-line computation. First try to determine the neural bases of each component process (e.g., selective attention) and then image cases of on-line computation like those described earlier to determine if the neural circuitry for each component is present. This componential strategy can be contrasted with a less analytic strategy, which might assume that there is a single factor for fluid intelligence and that all demanding on-line-computation tasks recruit this factor [see Duncan *et al.* (2000) for an application of this strategy using neuroimaging]. The componential strategy is the one pursued in this chapter.

Recall that the basic components of on-line computation include (1) working memory as a storage device, (2) updating working memory, (3) selective attention, (4) switching attention, and (5) task-specific processes. The last factor is not a single component, of course, but rather a placeholder for myriad different processes (e.g., arithmetic operations, mentally manipulating spatial configurations, comparing visual objects, inducing hypotheses from patterns of commonalities and differences, and on and on). Because there is an indefinite number of such processes, each in need of an analysis of its components, it makes little sense to pursue this factor. It is more useful to concentrate on components 1 through 4. Ideally, one would prefer to isolate each component and examine it separately, but because the updating and storage functions of working memory have proven to be difficult to separate, these are discussed together. A final section reviews experiments in which on-line thought corresponding to the three aforementioned examples has been the subject of neuroimaging studies.

A methodological comment is in order before turning to substance. Much of the research discussed here has used neuroimaging techniques, both positron emission tomography (PET) and functional magnetic resonance imaging (fMRI) (see Box 13.1). Typically, subjects have their brains scanned while engaging in various cognitive tasks and control tasks, and then the images for these tasks are compared to determine which neural areas are selectively activated (or deactivated) during the cognitive tasks. Such patterns of activation provide a map of brain regions that mediate task performance. However note that data are only correlational: all that is really known is that area A is activated when cognitive process P (e.g., attention) is required, not that A is necessary or sufficient for P to occur. To establish that A is necessary for P, one needs to show that if A is damaged (lesioned), then performance on any task requiring P will be compromised. Hence it is important to connect imaging data to lesion or patient data, and this connection will be made frequently in what follows.

WORKING MEMORY: STORAGE AND UPDATING

The preceding might seem to imply that there is just one working memory, as if the same storage system is used regardless of the contents that have to be maintained. This assumption is almost certainly incorrect, as shown by single cell studies of nonhuman primates and neuroimaging studies of humans (see Smith and Jonides, 1999). Recordings from the dorsolateral prefrontal cortex of adult monkeys have shown that some neurons respond only when spatial information has to be stored, whereas other neurons respond only when visual-object information has to be maintained briefly. In addition, PET studies with humans have found different patterns of activation depending on whether the material stored briefly is spatial, visual-object, or verbal in nature. Therefore, one needs to specify which working memory is under discussion. What follows focuses on verbal working memory because so many problem-solving and reasoning tasks have a verbal component. (However, note that two of the three starting examples have clear visual-spatial components as well.)

Verbal Working Memory Retains Items in a Speech-Based Code

Verbal working memory is the system involved when one must remember briefly a series of numbers, letters, words, or other verbal items. For example, after reading the following letters, look away from the text for about 5 s and then report these letters in order: E B T G V C P. Most people who do this task report that during the 5-s retention interval they implicitly spoke or "rehearsed" the names of the letters to themselves. This introspection is supported by objective behavioral data. For example, the faster one's rate of implicit speech, the better one performs the task (because it is less likely that a letter will have faded from memory before it can be rehearsed again). The upshot of this line of behavioral research is that verbal working memory represents items in a phonological code (the sounds of the items), and these phonological representations can be maintained by a rehearsal process that consists of internal speech (Baddeley, 1992).

Rehearsal and Storage Components of Working Memory Have Separate Anatomy

With regard to the neural basis of working memory, consider first some evidence from neuropsychology. Brain damage can result in an impairment known as the "short-term memory syndrome" (Shallice, 1988), in which the primary deficit is an inability to store verbal information for a period of seconds (the deficit is particularly severe for the auditory presentation of material). Consider one frequently studied patient, K.F. When K.F. is presented with a sequence of one to seven digits and is required to immediately repeat them back in order, he gets only one digit correct (normal is 7). In contrast, when K.F. is given a long-term memory task—say, learning a list of 20 words over a number of trials—he performs normally. Thus K.F.'s memory deficit is confined to verbal working memory (and to long-term memory tasks that depend directly on the phonological code of working memory, such as the task of learning a list of words in a foreign language). Importantly, part of KF's brain damage includes the parietal cortex, in the region of the supramarginal gyrus of the left hemisphere. This region is the most frequent site of damage in patients manifesting the short-term memory syndrome.

Neuroimaging studies with normal subjects provide additional support for the involvement of the left hemisphere posterior parietal cortex. In one PET study, volunteers were scanned while they performed in two working-memory conditions that required only storage of material but differed in the amount to be stored. In both conditions, on each trial a target set of four letters was presented briefly (200 ms), followed by a blank retention interval of 3000 ms, followed by presentation of a probe letter. The volunteer's task was to decide as quickly as possible whether the probe named one of the target letters (volunteers indicated their decision by pressing one of two response buttons). This is a standard test of verbal working memory referred to as the "item recognition" task. A major difference between the two conditions was that in the experimental condition, four different letters were presented, and hence four different items had to be stored and retrieved. In the control condition, all four letters presented were the same so only one item had to be stored and retrieved. A comparison of the two conditions, therefore, isolated verbal working memory (low-level perceptual processes as well as response processes had essentially been subtracted out). Data obtained from experimental and control conditions consisted of sets of images, with each image showing the relative changes in blood flow in a particular horizontal slice of cortex. Because increases in blood flow are assumed to be monotonic with increases in neural activity, each brain image revealed which regions had relative increases in neural activity during performance of the condition of interest (Fig. 54.3).

When the images of the control task were subtracted from those of the experimental task, a number of regions were significantly activated. Presumably, these regions mediate storage and rehearsal in verbal working memory. Importantly, one of these regions in the posterior cortex of the left hemisphere is the same region implicated by the neuropsychological studies of the short-term memory syndrome [Brodmann area (BA) 40]. However, other regions were activated as well. They include anterior, left hemisphere regions known to be involved in the production and planning of speech, including Broca's area (BA 44), the premotor area (BA 6), and the supplementary motor area (or SMA) (also in BA 6). Given their role in overt speech, it seems plausible that these last areas may mediate covert speech (i.e., rehearsal) as well.

Verbal WM

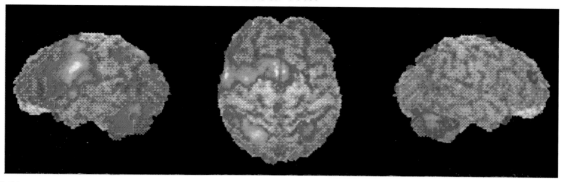

FIGURE 54.3   PET activations in an item recognition task, designed to isolate verbal working memory. Shown are left and right lateral views, as well as a superior view. PET activations are superimposed on a surface rendering of a brain created from a standard fMRI image. PET activations are shown as areas of increased brightness on the background fMRI image with the brightest possible areas corresponding to a z score of 7.0 and the lowest activations corresponding to a z of 1.65. From Reuter-Lorenz *et al.* (2000).

Neuroimaging experiments in other laboratories provide corroborative evidence for a distinction between posterior storage mechanisms and anterior rehearsal mechanisms. For example, the item recognition task was associated with activation in the left hemisphere posterior parietal cortex, as well as in anterior speech-related regions (Paulesu *et al.*, 1993). In this study, when activation in a task requiring rehearsal but not storage was subtracted from the activation associated with the item recognition task, which requires storage as well as rehearsal, significant activation remained in the posterior region but not in the anterior regions. This pattern of results gives a picture of verbal working memory that includes a storage component in posterior cortex (BA 40) and a rehearsal component in anterior cortex (BAs 44 and 6), both in the left hemisphere.

Does Updating Verbal Working Memory Lead to a Different Pattern of Activation?

The item recognition task just considered requires an updating of working memory on each trial—the old targets have to be dropped and replaced by a new set. This is quite different from the kind of updating of working memory considered in the initial three examples, in which existing representations had to be modified rather than replaced. It is possible that the kind of updating that modifies representations might recruit new brain regions. The problem in assessing this possibility is that experiments that have required updating as modification have also required processes in addition to storage. Still, it is instructive to describe one kind of working memory paradigm that clearly requires extensive updating as modification and that has been influential in the literature on working memory.

The paradigm of interest is the "*n*-back task." In one neuroimaging study using this task (Awh *et al.*, 1996), volunteers saw a continuous sequence of letters, and for each one had to decide whether it was identical to the one presented two letters earlier, or two back. This two-back task requires a storage load of two to three items (the last two letters presented plus the current one). It also requires participants to update their current working memory representation constantly so that the earliest-entered letter in that set be dropped and the current letter added. This updating involves modification of an existing representation that is more like that described in the three original examples. However, the two-back task also requires individuals to temporally code the items currently in working memory because only the letter that entered two back is a proper match.

The questions of interest are: Do brain images for this task show evidence of the working-memory neural network described earlier? Also, do new regions of activation emerge that may correspond to the updating operations needed in this task? The answer to both questions is "yes." When activations associated with a suitable control condition are subtracted from those in the two-back memory condition, the resulting images again show activation in the left hemisphere posterior parietal region that presumably mediates storage, as well as the left hemisphere anterior regions that presumably mediate inner speech (Broca's area, the premotor area, and SMA). Importantly, other regions that are not active in pure memory tasks (like item recognition) are active in this *n*-back task. Some of the additional regions are right hemisphere homologues of left hemisphere areas already described, including right hemisphere SMA. These additional regions may reflect mainly the added difficulty of this task compared to the item recognition tasks. The right hemisphere homologues are helping out in a particularly difficult version of what is normally a left hemisphere task.

Another result, however, suggests that the n-back task is qualitatively different from a pure memory task. When more sensitive statistical analyses are conducted, an area in the dorsolateral prefrontal cortex (DLPFC, BA 46) also shows evidence of activation. More generally, a number of researchers have presented summaries, or meta-analyses, of tasks requiring only working-memory storage and those that require partial updating (or some other executive process) as well and found that a major difference is that the latter tasks show more activation in the general vicinity of DLPFC (e.g., Smith and Jonides, 1999). One of these meta-analyses is presented in Fig. 54.4.

These data are consistent with the idea that updating working memory in a manner akin to real on-line computation tasks requires a special neural process. However, the added activation is also consistent with the hypothesis that the requirement to temporally code each item is the feature responsible for the activation in DLPFC. Although there is some independent evidence that the prefrontal cortex is involved in

temporal coding, neuroimaging studies suggest that such coding is more the province of the parietal cortex (e.g., Chochon *et al.*, 1999). Thus, these results are no more than suggestive of dedicated neural machinery for updating working memory.

Summary

On-line mental computation appears to involve a cycle of task-specific processing and updating the contents of working memory, modulated by selective attention and shifts of attention between task-specific processes and updating working memory. One way to study the neural basis of on-line computation then is to try to determine the neural basis of these components (save the task-specific processes). A review of recent findings indicates that verbal working memory involves two distinct mechanisms: a storage component that is mediated by left hemisphere posterior parietal regions and a rehearsal component that is mediated by left hemisphere frontal regions known to be involved in the production and planning of speech. The updating of working memory appears to bring other brain regions into play, including the DLPFC, but this idea remains speculative.

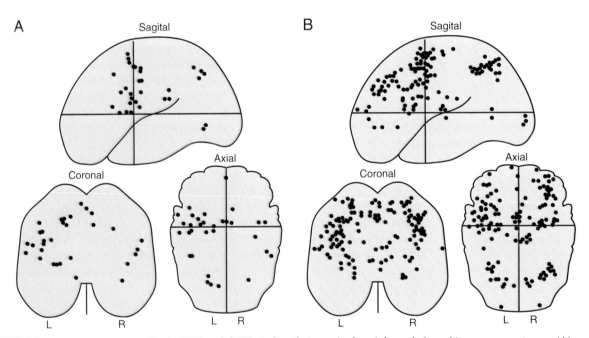

FIGURE 54.4 Neuroimaging results for PET and fMRI studies that required mainly verbal working-memory storage (A) or verbal working-memory storage *plus* partial updating (and possibly other executive processes) (B). Results are summarized by sets of three projections, with each containing points and axes conforming to a standard anatomical space (Talairach and Tourneaux, 1988). Each projection collapses one plane of view for each activation focus; i.e., the sagittal view collapses across the *x* plane as though one were looking through the brain from the side; the coronal view collapses across the *y* plane as though one were looking through the brain from the front or back; and the axial view collapses across the *z* plane as though one were looking through the brain from the top. Most of the studies represented in A are item recognition tasks (see text), whereas most of the studies represented in B are two- and three-back tasks (see text). The critical point to note is that tasks that require only working-memory storage lead to activations that typically do not extend into DLPFC, whereas tasks that require partial updating (or other executive processing), as well as storage, lead to activations that include DLPFC (after Smith and Jonides, 1999).

SELECTIVE ATTENTION

Selective attention is needed whenever there are multiple sources of information competing for processing resources (see Chapter 49). Many, if not all, cases of on-line computation have this character (e.g., selectively attending to the relevant digits in mental multiplication or to the relevant features in the Raven's test). In discussions of executive processes—those processes that comprise executive control—selective attention always looms large, and is sometimes taken to be the *only* executive process (e.g., Baddeley, 1992). Understanding the neural bases of selective attention then becomes critical for understanding on-line computation or fluid thought.

Before considering this topic in more detail, it is important to address a conceptual and terminological issue. In cases in which there are competing sources of information, one can talk about "attending" to the *relevant* source, or of "inhibiting" the *irrelevant* source. In most experiments, one cannot tell whether attention, inhibition, or both are at work, and for this reason the terms are sometimes used interchangeably. However, the two notions are conceptually distinct, and there will be times when inhibition seems the right term to use.

Studies of Selective Attention

Behavioral Studies of Attention/Inhibition

In the laboratory, the Stroop task is perhaps the best-studied paradigm in which two sources of information compete for control over responses, thus recruiting attention and inhibition processes. In this task, individuals are presented color names that are themselves printed in ink colors (see also Chapter 53). When the task is to name the color of the ink, individuals are slowed if the color name differs from the ink being named compared to a condition in which the color word is the same as the ink being named. For example, it takes longer to say "green" to the word "blue" printed in green ink (an "incompatible" condition) than to say "green" to the word "green" printed in green ink (a "compatible" condition). The most frequent account of this task is that naming words is a better learned skill than the skill of naming ink colors, with the result that the color responses from the two sources of information (lexical and hue) conflict with one another. To resolve this conflict, there must be a mechanism that allocates attention to one source of information or response (or inhibits attention from the other).

Other behavioral effects also depend on the resolution of interference. One such effect is the stimu-lus–response compatibility effect: stimuli that are naturally (compatibly) associated with responses yield faster and more accurate responses than stimuli that are associated arbitrarily with their responses (Kornblum *et al.*, 1990). For example, responding with a right key press to a stimulus presented on the right of a screen and with a left key press to a stimulus on the left yields faster and more accurate responses than if the mapping is reversed. Another relevant phenomenon is the flanker effect (e.g., Eriksen and Eriksen, 1974). When individuals are required to respond to a stimulus presented foveally, they display poorer performance if that stimulus is surrounded by irrelevant stimuli that have been associated with a different response. Beyond these examples, there are other tasks, such as the go/no-go task, which can be construed as having two sources of information, which compete against each other (Carter *et al.*, 1998). In a popular version of the go/no-go task, subjects are required to produce a response to a stimulus in one context, but to withhold that response to the same stimulus in another context.

What all these tasks share in common is that each features a competition between two or more sources of information that vie for control over responses. In the Stroop task, the two sources are the hue and lexical value of the stimulus. In the stimulus–response compatibility paradigm, the two sources are natural or well-learned stimulus–response mappings and arbitrary mappings defined by the experimenter. In the flanker task, they are the stimulus–response association of the central item and the stimulus–response association of the flankers. In the go/no-go task, they are the trained tendency to respond to a stimulus and the need to withhold that same response when the context is inappropriate. This similarity among tasks leads naturally to the question of whether there is a neural basis of conflict resolution that is common to all such tasks.

Neural Bases of Attention/Inhibition

Normal young volunteers have been imaged in all of the tasks described earlier. The Stroop task, in particular, has been imaged numerous times. Although normal individuals show substantial variation in regions of activation, two broad regions in the frontal cortex appear to be involved when one compares incompatible to compatible (or control) conditions. These frontal regions are the anterior cingulate cortex and the DLPFC (e.g., Pardo *et al.*, 1990). The anterior cingulate and DLPFC have also appeared in tasks varying stimulus–response compatibility (e.g., Taylor, *et al.*,1997), the flanker task (Hazeltine *et al.* [2000]), and the go/no-go task (Casey *et al.*, 1997).

Jonides *et al.* (2002) conducted a meta-analysis of some 15 published imaging studies involving the four tasks described earlier. The purpose of the meta-analysis was to determine whether certain common regions were activated in all these tasks of attention/inhibition. The analysis was based on Brodmann areas, and relatively few significant clusters were found, but the anterior cingulate was prominent among these. BA 24 was reliably present in the left hemisphere, and BA 32 was reliable in both hemispheres. A second significant cluster was in left hemisphere BA 6, a region that mingles with the anterior cingulate cortex at its most ventral extent medially. Finally, there was a significant cluster in right DLPFC (see Fig. 54.5). These results fit

relatively well with what may be the dominant theory of the neural bases of selective attention, as espoused by Cohen and Servan-Schreiber (1992) and Carter *et al.* (1998). According to this theory, the anterior cingulate *monitors* for conflict (at the level of partially activated responses), whereas the DLPFC *resolves* the conflict by selectively attending (activating) the task-relevant source of information.

How well do these neuroimaging findings fit with relevant results from neurological patients? Patients with damage in PFC are selectively impaired in the incompatible condition of the Stroop task (e.g., Vendrell *et al.*, 1995). This is in broad agreement with the imaging results. Indeed, so widespread is Stroop impairment in frontal patients that an abnormality in Stroop performance has been used to diagnose decreases in frontal lobe integrity in a variety of patient populations, including, schizophrenia (Box 54.1), Huntington's disease and Parkinson's disease (see, e.g., Cohen and Servan-Schreiber, 1992).

Other Kinds of Attention/Inhibition

Attention/Inhibition in Working Memory

The picture becomes more complicated for another kind of inhibition phenomena, which is based on proactive inhibition in working memory. In these cases, a previous association between a stimulus and a response intrudes on the encoding or retrieval of a new association. Neuroimaging studies have used the item recognition task that was described in the previous section. In an initial PET experiment (Jonides *et al.*, 1998), there were two critical conditions. In the "low-conflict" condition, a set of four letters was presented briefly, followed by a 3-s delay, followed by a probe letter. Participants decided as quickly as possible whether the probe was the same as one of the targets. Importantly, the negative items—probes that required a no response—had not occurred on a recent trial. No cognitive conflict was involved in the task.

A simple change in some of the negative items, however, can bring attention and inhibition into play. In the "high-conflict" condition, half of the negative probes had appeared in the previous target set of items. Because these "recent negatives" had been rehearsed just a few seconds ago, they should have been in an active state and highly familiar. This in turn should have set up a conflict between the familiarity of the probe, which points toward an incorrect yes response, and the fact that the representation of the probe does not contain a marker indicating it is a member of the current target set, which points to a correct no response. Such a conflict in processes is assumed to trigger the executive processes of atten-

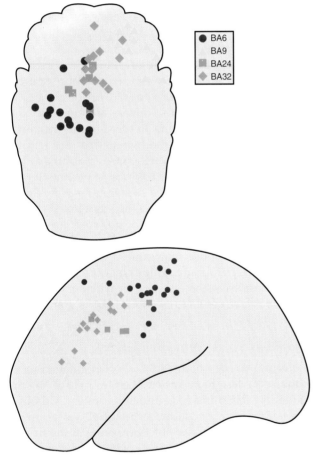

FIGURE 54.5 Neuroimaging results for PET and fMRI studies of Stroop and Stroop-like attention/inhibition tasks. Results are summarized by two projections, an axial view (top) and a sagittal view (bottom). (See legend for Fig. 54.4 for further explanation.) Plotted points represent the areas of activation that survived statistical analyses of commonality; they show the areas of common activation across the studies included in the meta-analysis (after Jonides *et al.*, 2002).

BOX 54.1

SCHIZOPHRENIA

Sometimes serious disorders of thinking can occur, and the most common disorder is schizophrenia (also see Chapter 46). The Swiss psychiatrist Eugene Bleuler coined the term in a famous book, first published in 1911. In this book Bleuler proposed that this disorder is characterized by four types of symptoms regarding (1) thinking (disordered associative processes), (2) affect (inappropriate, depressed, or manic affect), (3) will (ambivalence, i.e., indecisiveness), and (4) social behavior (autism, social withdrawal).

The following writing of a patient exemplifies the disturbed thought processes in patients with schizophrenia, driven by inappropriate, associative links between concepts rather than by logical, goal-directed thinking.

> I am writing on paper. The pen which I am using is from a factory called 'Perry & Co.' This factory is in England. I assume this. Behind the name of Perry & Co. the city of London is inscribed; but not the city. The city of London is in England. I know this from my schooldays. Then, I always liked geography. My last teacher in that subject was Professor August A. He was a man with black eyes. I also like black eyes. There are also blue and gray eyes and other sorts, too. I have heard it said that snakes have green eyes. All people have eyes. There are some, too, who are blind. These blind people are led about by a boy. It must be very terrible not to be able to see. There are people who can't see and, in addition, can't hear. I know some who hear too much. One can hear too much. There are many sick people in Burgholzli; they are called patients. One of them I like a great deal. His name is E. Sch. He taught me that in Burgholzli there are many kinds, patients, inmates, attendants. Then there are some who are not here at all. They are all peculiar people. ... (Bleuler, 1911/1950, p. 80)

Schizophrenia is also associated with the development of psychotic features, such as delusions (persistent false beliefs of being persecuted, monitored, or controlled), auditory hallucinations, and bizarre motor behaviors. The most clinically intractable manifestations of schizophrenia, however, involve deficits in the capabilities for pursuing goal-directed activities, forming appropriate emotional responses and maintaining social interaction, and cognitive impairments on tasks requiring working memory, shifts between concepts or mental sets, maintenance of attention, and utilization of abstract information.

Schizophrenia poses a major public health problem worldwide, with a lifetime prevalence of about 1% in most cultures and geographic locations studied. Its clinical manifestations usually appear in late adolescence and early adulthood. Prognosis varies widely, with some patients showing a stable illness course with minimal disability during maintenance treatment and others a more severe, deteriorating course that eventually stabilizes at a level of marked disability.

The etiology of schizophrenia is unknown. Early hypotheses regarding the neurobiological basis for schizophrenia emphasized abnormalities of the mesocorticolimbic dopaminergic system, based on observations that dopamine receptor agonists can produce psychotic symptoms in healthy humans, whereas drugs that reduce psychotic symptoms exert dopamine receptor antagonist effects. *In vivo* neuroreceptor imaging studies have demonstrated that the amount of dopamine release in the striatum in response to amphetamine is abnormally elevated in schizophrenia.

However, the observations that schizophrenia is associated with an elevated rate of environmental risk factors arising during the pre- and perinatal period (e.g., obstetric complications) and that subtle cognitive disturbances are evident premorbidly during childhood and adolescence (i.e., prior to onset of psychosis) have suggested that schizophrenia is a disorder of neural development. Family, twin, and adoption studies establish a role for genetic factors in the etiology of schizophrenia, but also suggest the involvement of acquired factors (e.g., concordance rates among monozygotic and dizygotic twins are about 50 and 20%, respectively). Schizophrenia is thus thought to result from a combination of genetic susceptibility and acquired neuropathology arising early in life.

Current neurodevelopmental models attempt to account for the relatively long latency between the developmental period and the onset of clinical symptoms in schizophrenia. One model is based on evidence that lesions placed in specific frontal cortical or hippocampal areas during the perinatal period in experimental animals result in cognitive impairment and hyperdopaminergic behaviors that are not pronounced until after puberty. Another model capitalizes on the observation that NMDA-glutamatergic receptor antagonists (e.g., phencyclidine) can produce the spectrum of psychotic, behavioral/social, and cognitive symptoms seen in schizophrenia in nonschizophrenic, postpubertal humans, whereas these agents rarely produce such reactions in children (who receive NMDA receptor antagonists as part of anesthetic regimens). The development of sensitivity to the psychotomimetic effects of NMDA hypofunction thus has an age dependency similar to that seen for the onset of psychosis in schizophrenia. Moreover, when introduced *in utero* to rats at critical developmental stages, NMDA receptor antagonists can

BOX 54.1   (cont'd)

produce neurodegenerative changes in the limbic cortex. These observations led to the hypothesis that schizophrenia is associated with NMDA receptor hypofunction, which, during cortical development, produces excitotoxic damage and consequent microscopic abnormalities, and during the postpubertal period, produces susceptibility to psychosis.

Wayne C. Drevets

References and Suggested Readings

Bleuler, E. (1911/1950). "Dementia Praecox or the Group of Scizophrenias" (J. Ziskin and N. D. Lewis, transl.). International Universities Press, New York.

Kendler, K. S., *et al.* (1993) The Roscommon family study. I. Methods, diagnosis of probands and risks of schizophrenia in relatives. *Arch. Gen. Psychiat.* **50**: 645–652.

LaRuelle, M., Abidargham, A., Vandyck, C. H., *et al.* (1996). Single photon emission computerized tomography imaging of amphetamine-induced dopamine release in drug-free schizophrenic subjects. *Proc. Nat. Acad. USA. Sci.* **93**(17), 9235–9240.

Lewis, D. A., and Lieberman, J. A. (2000). Catching up on schizophrenia: Natural history and neurobiology. *Neuron* **28**(2), 325–334.

Thompson, P. M., Vidal, C., Giedd, J. N., Gochman, P., Blumenthal, J., Nicolson, R., Toga, A. W., and Rapoport, J. L. (2001). Mapping adolescent brain change reveals dynamic wave of accelerated gray matter loss in very early-onset schizophrenia *Proc. Natl. Acad. Sci. U S A.* **98**(20), 11650–11655.

tion and inhibition, which involve inhibiting the outcome of the irrelevant familiarity process and selectively attending to the process that inspects the relevant list marker. (See Fig. 54.6 for a comparison of negative probes in low- and high-conflict conditions.)

The prediction is that only the high-conflict condition should invoke attention and inhibition. Behavioral support for this prediction is provided by the finding that participants took longer to respond correctly to recent negatives than to nonrecent negatives. Of greater interest are the neuroimaging results. The critical PET comparison is that between high- and low-conflict conditions. This comparison revealed that a portion of left hemisphere ventrolateral PFC (BA 45) was the only significant focus of activation, implying that this area is critically involved in attentional and inhibitory processing. Note that this area is not among those obtained in the meta-analysis of Stroop-like tasks (see Fig. 54.5).

This same finding was obtained in a follow-up experiment by D'Esposito and colleagues (1999), which employed fMRI and single-trial analysis. Only the high-conflict condition was tested, and now the critical comparison was between "no" trials where the

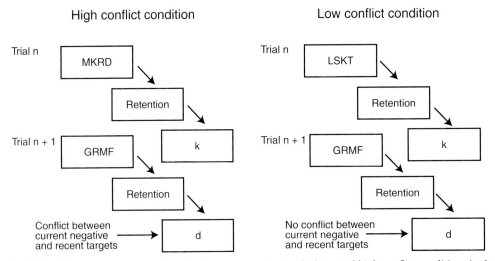

FIGURE 54.6 A comparison of the critical negative probes in the low- and high-conflict conditions in the Jonides *et al.* (1998) study.

probes had appeared recently (recent negatives) and "no" trials where the probes had appeared more remotely (nonrecent negatives). In the left hemisphere ventrolateral prefrontal region (BA 45), there was more activation for recent than nonrecent negatives. In addition, this difference between the two trial types occurred only during the interval when the probe was presented (see Fig. 54.7). These findings fit well with the hypothesis that the activation in question reflects inhi-biting familiarity information and selectively attending to information about list membership when a response is being selected.

In keeping with the need to augment neuroimaging findings with converging evidence from neuropsychology, patient performance was examined in a version of these item recognition tasks. Thompson-Schill and colleagues (1999) examined the contrast between high- and low-conflict conditions in a patient (R.C.) who had damage to middle and inferior gyri of the PFC, including the left hemisphere ventrolateral prefrontal area (BA 45) identified by the original PET study. When compared with a group of neurological controls (i.e., they had PFC lesions sparing BA 45/46), there was nothing exceptional about R.C.'s performance on the low-conflict task. However, R.C. had a marked impairment, reflected in both response time and accuracy, on trials with recent negatives in the high-conflict condition. This impairment resulted in a significantly exaggerated difference between recent negatives and nonrecent negatives, which is in line with R.C. having a deficit in attention and inhibition. It seems clear that

left hemisphere BA 45 is critically involved in the attention and inhibitory demands of this task.

Two Kinds of Attention/Inhibition?

The site of activation in this working memory task—inferior left hemisphere PFC—clearly differs from the results obtained in the meta-analysis of Stroop-like tasks (anterior cingulate cortex and the DLPFC). For one thing, the hemisphere of dominant activation differs (left for working memory, more right for Stroop-like tasks). Beyond this, the peak of the site found in the working-memory studies is inferior and posterior to the sites found in studies of the Stroop task, the stimulus–response compatibility task, and other similar tasks. In addition, working-memory studies do not elicit activation in the anterior cingulate when comparing high- and low-conflict trials, yet this is the most dominant region of activation in Stroop-like tasks. These neural differences imply that two different kinds of inhibition are in play.

How can one characterize this difference functionally? One possibility is that Stroop-like tasks involve attention/inhibition late in the processing sequence, including inhibition of partially prepared responses, whereas the working-memory task involves attention/inhibition at an earlier point in processing, e.g., when familiarity and list membership codes are compared. The idea of late inhibition seems particularly plausible for tasks such as go/no-go, where individuals can even consciously report that they are suppressing responses. This distinction between early

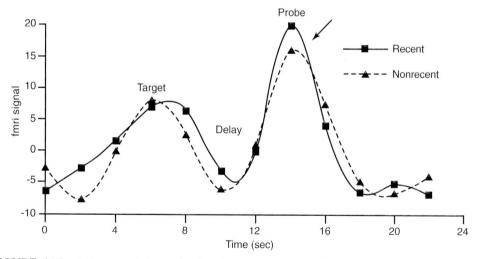

FIGURE 54.7 Trial-averaged time-series data for a representative subject in a study of item recognition. Probes were either recent negatives (■) or nonrecent negatives (▲) (see text). Data were extracted from voxels demonstrating a main effect for the probe period across both recent negative and nonrecent negative trials. Activity in these two conditions differed only during the probe portion of the task (see arrow). To determine the target, delay, and probe portions of each 24-s trial, we considered when each trial event began (target at 0 s, delay at 1.5 s, and probe at 8 s), and then added another 5–6 s since the peak of the fMRI signal is known to be delayed from its triggering neural event by about 5–6 s. After D'Esposito *et al.* (1999).

and late attention/inhibition is well known in behavioral science, and though alternatives to his distinction are considered next, it may be the most likely account of the two kinds of attention/inhibition.

Another possibility about the two kinds of attention/inhibition stems from a comparison of the sheer sizes of the interference effects in question. Reports included in the meta-analysis are of behavioral phenomena that are substantial in size. For example, the Stroop interference effect is often measured in hundreds of milliseconds. In contrast, interference effects found in the just-reviewed working-memory studies are substantially smaller, typically 50 ms or so in magnitude. Perhaps this difference in magnitude reveals a fundamental property of conflict–resolution mechanisms. It may be that conflict must be substantial in size in order to be spotted by a detection mechanism in the anterior cingulate that then turns on an attention–allocation mechanism in DLPFC. Conflict that is smaller in magnitude may be handled by other mechanisms. Possibly related to this, individuals performing tasks such as Stroop are often aware of the conflict that is present on incongruent trials, whereas individuals performing the working- memory task often have no awareness of the difference between high- and low-conflict trials. It may take awareness to trigger the detection of conflict by the anterior cingulate (which then triggers the DLPFC).

A rather different kind of possibility is that activation found in the anterior cingulate for some conflict tasks represents not so much detection of conflict as response to conflict after it has been detected. By this account, tasks in which the effect of conflict is sufficiently substantial to evoke awareness of it may trigger an affective response that is a consequence of either the conflict directly or the perceived difficulty of the task in the face of conflict. This affective response may be the source of the signal in the anterior cingulate that is found in tasks such as Stroop or other tasks in which conflict is substantial. By this account, activation in the anterior cingulate represents not a detection of conflict for later resolution by other mechanisms, but rather a response to conflict that has elicited awareness. It remains a task for future research to distinguish among these alternative accounts.

SWITCHING ATTENTION

Switching attention requires people to move their focus of attention. It involves scheduling processes in addition to attention/inhibition. By this view, there is

something in switching attention that is not in attention, namely the scheduler (also referred to as the "switcher"). Under this conceptualization, switching attention could involve neural structures in addition to those mediating selective attention, i.e., there may be a separate switching mechanism. Alternatively, although the notions of selective attention and switching seem distinct, their common reliance on the allocation of attention may mean that there will be little difference in the neural structures involved in the two kinds of tasks. Under this conceptualization, one might expect more activation in relevant regions when switching of attention is called for as opposed to just focused attention, but the relevant regions will be the same in the two kinds of tasks. The basic question then is, "Is there a separate region (regions) for the switcher?"

It is important to note at the outset that rather different kinds of tasks have been used in neuroimaging studies of switching attention and have produced somewhat different kinds of results. Thus, some relatively simple tasks require only that subjects switch their attention from one attribute of an object to another attribute of that same object, whereas other more complex tasks require that subjects switch back and forth between two entirely different tasks. In what follows, some illustrative studies of the various types of switching paradigms are considered, starting with the simpler kinds and finishing with the more complex ones.

Switching between Attributes of the Same Object

One of the best-known neuropsychological tests of frontal brain damage is the Wisconsin Card Sort Task (also see Chapter 53). In this task, individuals are presented a series of cards, each containing objects that vary on four attributes—color, shape, number, and shading. Individuals must sort each card into one of four piles depending on which attribute they think is relevant (e.g., if they think color is the relevant attribute, they would sort red objects into one pile, blue objects into a second pile, and so on). Individuals receive feedback about their choices and typically converge on the valid attribute relatively quickly. However, then the relevant attribute is switched unexpectedly, and individuals must determine what the switched attribute is, which requires switching attention from one attribute to another. Patients with frontal lobe damage are particularly impaired on this task compared to other neurological patients, and the nature of their behavioral impairment is that they persist in sorting on the no-longer relevant attribute. Here is evidence suggesting that switching attention involves more than just selectively attending (frontal patients have little problem attending to the first relevant attribute) and that the switching mechanism is located in PFC.

Neuroimaging Studies of Attribute Switching

There have been a few neuroimaging experiments of attribute-switching paradigms, and they show increased activation in PFC when attention switching is required. For the present purposes—determining whether there is a separate switching mechanism—it is useful to consider in detail a fMRI study by Pollman *et al.* (2000). The behavioral paradigm is referred to as the "pop-out" task. On each trial a volunteer sees a large array of squares and has to determine whether one of them differs from all the others on some critical attribute. Such an outlier is a "target" and the rest of the squares are "distracters." As examples, on some trials all the distracter squares might be green, while the target square is blue, or all the distracters might be moving in a leftward direction while the target has a sinusoidal direction of motion. In all cases, when the target occurs it seems to "pop out" and is readily detected. Importantly, detection of the target takes longer when the relevant dimension switches from trial to trial (color vs movement) than when it remains the same; this difference is referred to as a "switching cost."

Pollman *et al.* (2000) imaged subjects while performing this task and found that trials on which the relevant dimension changed were accompanied by increased activation in various regions of PFC, including the left hemisphere frontopolar cortex (BA 10) and inferior frontal gyrus (BA 47), and right hemisphere frontal gyrus (BA 11), as well as the anterior cingulate. Numerous nonfrontal areas were also activated, including higher level parietal and temporal areas, as well as extrastriate regions. Regarding the frontal activations, while some of them also appear in selective-attention studies (left BA 47 and the anterior cingulate—see last section), there are some new activations here, particularly the frontopolar cortex, which was the most significant frontal activation in the study. Hence the frontopolar cortex may house a separate switching mechanism. On the bases of detailed analyses, Pollman *et al.* (2000) argued that the frontopolar cortex is involved in switching attention between attributes and that higher level parietal and temporal areas mediate the consequences of the reallocation of attention.

Switching between Objects in Working Memory

Some other neuroimaging studies of attention switching have used a behavioral paradigm devel-

oped by Garavan (1998). In this task, one of two kinds of objects is presented on each trial for a series of 15–25 trials, and individuals must keep in mind cumulative counts of the two kinds of objects. For example, the objects might be small and large squares, and when individuals see a small (or large) square, they update their appropriate mental counter by one. Individuals indicate that they have completed their updating by pushing a button, which brings on the next stimulus. Individuals are tested on the cumulative counts at the end of the sequence. Presumably, the two counters are in working memory, and updating a counter requires attending to it. As a consequence, when large and small squares are presented on successive trials, attention must be switched from one counter to the other, whereas when two small (large) squares are presented in succession, no attention switch is necessary. Individuals take longer on switch trials, and switching costs are very substantial.

Garavan *et al.* (2000) used fMRI with a blocked design to image performance on this task. The blocks contained a low, medium, or high number of switches in the sequences, and Garavan and co-workers looked for regions that increased in activation as the number of switches increased. They found many regions that fit this bill, several of them in PFC, including the right hemisphere medial frontal gyrus (BA 10), the bilateral inferior prefrontal gyrus (BA 9/6), and the anterior cingulate. Note again that there is activation in an anterior frontal region (BA 10, which is anterior to DLPFC). However, Garavan *et al.* (2000) found numerous other areas of heightened activation as well and concluded that attention switching is mediated by a widely distributed neural circuit.

In a follow up to the aforementioned study (Badre *et al.*, 2002), an event-related fMRI design was used, which made it possible to separately image each trial in a sequence rather than rely on images averaged over blocks of trials. The two types of items were arrows on the left versus arrows on the right side of the screen (so individuals now needed to keep separate cumulative counts of the two kinds of arrows). But there was a further wrinkle. A left or right arrow could point either up or down. If an arrow pointed up, the appropriate counter was to be incremented by one, whereas if it pointed down it was to be decremented by one (e.g., if a left arrow pointed up, the participant had to increment their left counter by one, whereas if a left arrow pointed down the participant had to decrement their left counter by one)). Hence it was possible to determine whether successive trials require the same or a switched operation independently of whether trials require a counter switch or not. Behavioral data showed that either a switch in counter (left or right) or a switch in operation (add or subtract) took extra time. fMRI results showed that switch trials led to specific activations compared to baseline trials, particularly in anterior PFC. Both counter switching and operation switching led to activations in the frontopolar region of the right hemisphere (BA10).

Overall then, the relatively simple studies of attention switching imply that, compared to attention/inhibition, switching activates additional regions of the cortex, particularly PFC regions anterior to DLPFC. Thus there is some evidence for separate switching mechanisms.

More Complex Switching Tasks

There have been a number of neuroimaging studies in which individuals are required to perform different tasks on successive trials (unlike the studies reviewed thus far, which require a switch in attribute or mental object, but keep the task the same). A subset of the research under discussion has used paradigms in which individuals complete one task before moving onto the next, and these studies have yielded mixed results. Given the interest in connecting executive processes to fluid thinking, the paradigm to be described next is of particular interest.

In this paradigm, individuals must switch between updating working memory and some other task. An example of this general paradigm, called the "operation span," is illustrated in Fig. 54.8. On every trial a sequence of items (e.g., five) is presented, with each item consisting of a simple equation and an unrelated word. The subject has to determine whether the equation is correct and then commit the word to memory, maintaining the words in order. At the end of the trial, memory is tested by a probe that contains the words

in a particular order, and individuals must indicate whether the probe order is identical to the input order. This is a dual task that requires switching between doing specific math processes and updating working memory. It thus captures the basic cycle illustrated at the outset of this chapter in the examples of mental arithmetic, Tower of Hanoi, and the Raven's test—namely a cycle of task-specific processing and updating working memory, modulated by selective attention and switching of attention.

In a study by Smith *et al.* (2001), younger and older subjects were PET scanned while they performed either the operation span or each component task alone (math verification only or memory only). In the component tasks, no attention switching was required, whereas the operation scan required frequent attention switches per trial. Behavioral data showed that the operation scan engendered substantial switching costs on both memory and math scores (e.g., memory accuracy was lower in the operation span than in the memory-only component task). The major question of interest was whether there were PFC areas that were active in the operation scan that were not active in either component task—were there dedicated switching areas?

For older subjects, such switching areas were found in left hemisphere PFC (BA 9), which again is in anterior PFC (see bottom of Fig. 54.9). The same PFC area appeared to be a switching area for younger subjects who performed relatively poorly, but not for those who performed relatively well (see middle and top of Fig. 54.9). For the latter, the operation-span task may not have been sufficiently demanding—a trial contained only five items—or PET was too insensitive an imaging modality—it cannot "home in" on the latter part of an operation-span trial when the working-memory load is relatively high.

In sum, there is some evidence that regions anterior to the DLPFC are involved in the switching mechanism.

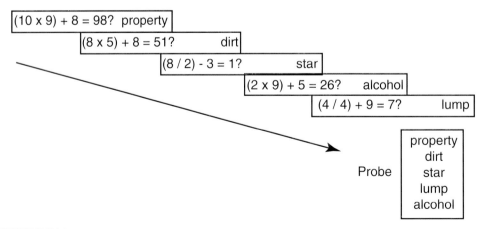

FIGURE 54.8 Illustration of the sequence of events in a five-item trial in the operations span. See text for explanation. Each equation-word pair was presented for 3 s, while the probe was presented for 4 s.

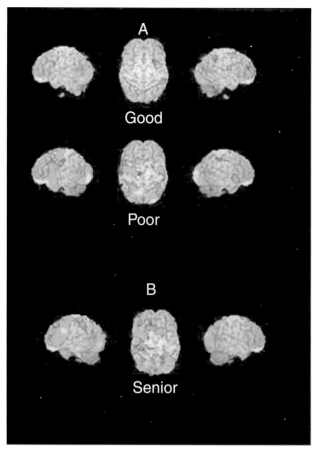

FIGURE 54.9 PET activations in the task shown in Fig. 54.8. Results are shown for young subjects, divided on the basis of their performance (A), and results for older subjects (B). Activations are for the operation span task with activations for the constituent tasks (math and memory) subtracted out. Left and right hemisphere views, as well as a superior view are shown. For the superior views, the front of the brain is at the top. PET activations are superimposed on the surface rendering of a brain created from a standard fMRI image. PET activations are shown as areas of increasing brightness on the background fMRI image (see legend for Fig. 54.3 for further details). Adapted from Smith *et al.* (2001).

Summary

The last two sections have examined the neural bases of selective attention and switching attention. There are numerous cognitive tasks that involve a competition between two or more sources of information that vie for control over responses, and attention or inhibition is required to ensure that the relevant source of information controls processing. Extensive research suggests that such an attentional mechanism is mediated by prefrontal structures, including the anterior cingulate and DLPFC. Other research indicates that when the competition is between information sources in working memory, an earlier form of attention/inhibition may occur, and this is mediated by the left hemisphere ventrolateral PFC (see, e.g., the D'Esposito *et al.* study on

p. 1387, and the ensuing discussion). The switching of attention may recruit additional prefrontal areas.

WHAT ARE THE COMPONENTS IN COMPLEX TASKS?

The chapter began with three examples of tasks involving on-line mental computation, and it was argued that each of these sample tasks involves the components of (1) working-memory storage, (2) updating working memory, (3) selective attention/ inhibition, and (4) attention switching, as well as task-specific processes that changed from task to task. This final section presents some evidence that the neural bases of these components are evident in neuroimaging studies of the three example tasks with which the chapter began.

Mental Arithmetic

In discussing mental arithmetic, it is important to distinguish between tasks that require true calculation (like the initial 17x28 example) and tasks that may involve an estimation or analog component. An impressive body of research indicates that estimation and calculation are mediated by different mechanisms, with estimation involving mostly parietal rather than frontal areas (see, e.g., Chochon *et al.*, 1999). What follows considers tasks that seem to involve mainly calculation (like the original example).

In one study of mental multiplication (Rickard *et al.*, 2000), volunteers were scanned while verifying single-digit multiplications (e.g., 4x7=35?). At least half the areas activated were "component" areas that were described earlier in this review and that are thought to support the component operations of many tasks but require online computations. These include Broca's area (BA 44), which is known to be involved in working-memory storage for alphanumeric materials and which presumably is used to hold the product of the left side of the equation. Left and right hemisphere anterior PFC areas (BAs 9 and 10) were also activated, and these had been identified in studies of attention and attention switching.

In another study that included simple multiplication and subtraction problems (Chochon *et al.*, 1999), again roughly half the significant activations were in component areas. For multiplication, these include Broca's area and the supplementary motor area (BAs 44 and 6), which are known to be involved in working-memory rehearsal; the DLPFC (BA 46), known to be involve in selective attention and possibly attention switching; and the anterior cingulate, known to be involved in selective attention.

Much the same point emerges in other studies of mental arithmetic, even when the only operations required are addition and subtraction, as long as the problem is sufficiently difficult, e.g., subtracting 17 from a number greater than 500. What is perhaps most striking is the extent to which working-memory areas are salient in, or even dominate, the activation patterns underlying mental calculation.

Tower of Hanoi

Recall the basic Tower of Hanoi problem, used frequently as a measure of planning (see Fig. 54.1). The basic task involves three pegs and three disks; the disks are arranged initially on peg 1, and the participant's task is to recreate that same configuration on peg 3, moving only one disk at a time and never placing a larger disk on a smaller one. Computerized variants of tasks similar to this one have been imaged numerous times, with the most frequent variant being the Tower of London task, in which beads of different colors are stacked on the pegs instead of disks. Because some of these variants allow the individuals to move the elements one at a time (rather than plan the whole solution in their heads), many of these studies have found extensive activation in motor areas, as well as extensive activation in visual areas when compared to simple control conditions. These visual and motor activations clearly reflect the visual and motor aspects of the task, not the planning component, which is of interest here. Can the planning component be isolated more successfully?

An experiment by Dagher *et al.* (1999) accomplishes this. These authors imaged subjects with PET while performing Tower of London problems at five different levels of complexity, where complexity may be measured objectively by the minimum number of moves needed to solve the problem. Dagher and colleagues then determined the neural areas whose activations increased with task complexity, subtracting out the role of motor movements by using a control task in which subjects simply copied a solution. The authors found a number of areas where activation increased with complexity, including the premotor cortex (BA 6), anterior cingulate, bilateral DLPFC, and right hemisphere dorsal caudate nucleus. Aside from the last mentioned area, the others are all known to be involved in the working-memory and attention components already discussed. Thus the premotor cortex figures in working memory, whereas the anterior cingulate and the DLPFC are signature areas for selective attention.

Raven's Progressive Matrices Test

Recall that in the Raven's test, the task is to examine an incomplete 3x3 matrix of geometric forms

and to determine which of several alternatives is needed to properly complete the matrix (see Fig. 54.2). There are few studies that have imaged volunteers during performance on the Raven's test, and for the present purposes it suffices to consider in detail one of these (Prabhakaran *et al.*, 1997).

Like the last study reviewed, Prabhakaran presented problems that varied in complexity. The easier problems are "figural" ones and require only visual-perceptual operations (such as continuation or superposition); the more difficult problems are "analytic" ones and require applying conceptual operations to features of the figures, operations such as generating hypotheses about the features and their relations. The distinction between figural and analytic problems has proved useful in behavioral analyses of performance on this task, and the two kinds of problems are illustrated in Fig. 54.10. The critical fMRI contrast is between analytic and perceptual problems because this contrast should eliminate low-level perceptual processes, as well as all response processes.

The contrast of interest is shown in Fig. 54.11. As usual, the important question is whether many of the significantly activated areas correspond to the component areas that have been identified in other studies. The answer seems to be "yes." The contrast revealed a number of bilateral frontal activations, all of them

A

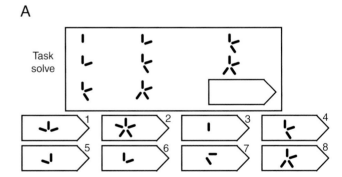

B

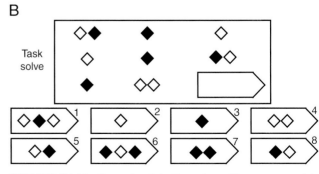

FIGURE 54.10 Example of the Raven's problem types used in the Prabhakaran *et al.* (1997) fMRI study: a figural problem (A) and an analytic problem (B).

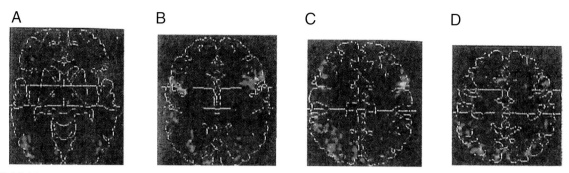

FIGURE 54.11 Neuroimaging results during performance of the Raven's test (Fig. 54.10). Images show the contrast between analytic and figural problems. An axial slice just below the plane that includes the anterior and posterior commissures (A), and parallel axial slices that are progressively higher in the brain (B–D). The analytic-figural comparison shows bilateral action in the frontal lobes (see B and C). From Prabhakaran *et al.* (1997).

having some correspondence to component areas. These include the premotor area (BA 6), Broca's area (BA 44), early selective attention area (BA 45), and late selective attention areas (BA 46 and 9). While many of these areas were left lateralized in the studies of working memory reviewed earlier, note that the review has considered only *verbal* working memory, whereas in the current Raven's study, *spatial* and *visual-object* working memory systems were likely in play, and the latter systems are known to be mediated in part by some right hemisphere regions such as the premotor area and DLPFC (see, e.g., Smith and Jonides, 1999).

In addition to frontal areas, the contrast between analytic and figural problems also reveals activations in parietal, temporal, and occipital areas. Some of these are in component areas, such as the left hemisphere supramarginal gyrus (BA 40), which is thought to be involved in storing information in working memory. Others of these areas may be involved in spatial and object working memory, such as BA 7 (superior parietal cortex) and BA 19 (extrastriate visual cortex). The authors conclude that the neural network for the Raven's test may be characterized "...as the sum of domain-dependent and domain-independent working memory systems" and that performance on the Raven's test may provide a survey of working memory abilities.

Summary

The chapter began by offering an informal analysis of the cognitive processes, or functions, involved in three representative fluid-thinking tasks that require on-line computations. Four processes seem to be involved in all of the tasks: (1) working-memory storage, (2) updating work-ing memory, (3) selective attention/inhibition, and (4) switching of attention.

The chapter then surveyed neuroimaging studies that tried to isolate each of these components and found some distinct neural substrates for the different components. Verbal working memory involved mainly left hemisphere structures, including posterior parietal (BA 40) as well as posterior frontal structures (BAs 6 and 44). Partial updating of working memory sometimes activated DLPFC, but the evidence here was relatively weak. Attention/inhibition processes that may occur relatively late in processing consistently activated bilateral DLPFC and the anterior cingulate, whereas attention/inhibition processes that may occur earlier activated left hemisphere, ventrolateral PFC (BA 45). Switching of attention studies were less consistent in their outcome, in part because rather different kinds of studies were involved, but there was some evidence for the distinctive involvement of anterior PFC, including the frontopolar region.

Finally, imaging studies of the three representative thinking tasks showed that these components were operative, particularly working memory and attention/inhibition. These results counter the hypothesis that a single undifferentiated mechanism is responsible for all cases of fluid thinking.

References

Awh, E., Jonides, J., Smith, E. E., Schumacher, E. H., Koeppe, R. A., and Katz, S. (1996). Dissociation of storage and rehearsal in verbal working memory: Evidence from PET. *Psychol. Sci.* **7**, 25–31.

Baddeley, A. D. (1992). Working memory. *Science* **255**, 556–559.

Badre, D., Jonides, J., and Smith, E. E. Hernandez, L., Noll, D. C., Bryck, R. L., Gehring, W. and Albin, R. (2002). The heterogeneous executive: Evidence of independent executive functions.

Carpenter, P. A., Just, M. A., and Shell, P. (1990). What one intelligence test measures: A theoretical account of the processing in the Raven Progressive Matrices Test. *Psychol. Rev.* **97**, 404–431.

Carter, C. S., Braver, T. S., Barch, D. M., Botvinick, M. M., Noll, D. C., and Cohen, J. D. (1998). Anterior cingulate cortex, error detection, and the online monitoring of performance. *Science* **280**, 747–749.

Casey, B. J., Trainor, R. J., Orendi, J. L., Schubert, A. B., Nystrom, L. E., Giedd, J. N., Castellanos, F. X., Haxby, J. V., Noll, D. C., Cohen, J. D., Forman, S. D., Dahl, R. E., and Rapoport, J. L. (1997). A developmental functional MRI study of prefrontal activation during performance of a go-no-go task. *J. Cogn. Neurosci.* **9**, 835–847.

Chochon, F., Cohen, L., van de Moortele, P. F., and Dehaene, S. (1999). Differential contributions of the left and right inferior parietal lobules to number processing. *J. Cogn. Neurosci* **11**(6), 617–630.

Cohen, J. D., and D. Servan-Schreiber (1992). Context, cortex, and dopamine: A connectionist approach to behavior and biology in schizophrenia. *Psychol. Rev.* **99**(1), 45–77.

Dagher, A., Owen, A. M., Boecker, H., and Brooks, D. J. (1999). Mapping the network for planning: a correlational PET activation study with the Tower of London task. *Brain* **122**(10), 1973–1987.

D'Esposito, M., Postle, B. R., Jonides, J., and Smith, E. E. (1999). The neural substrate and temporal dynamics of interference effects in working memory as revealed by event-related functional MRI. *Proc. Natl. Acad. Sci.* **96**, 7514–7519.

Duncan, J., Seitz, R. J., Kolodny, J., Bor, D., Herzog, H., Ahmed, A., Newell, F. N., and Emslie, H. (2000). A neural basis for general intelligence. *Science* **289**, 457–460.

Eriksen, B. A., and Eriksen, C. W. (1974). Effects of noise letters upon the identification of a target letter in a nonsearch task. *Percept. Psychophys.* **16**, 143–149.

Garavan, H. (1998). Serial attention within working memory. *Memory Cogn.* **26**, 263–276.

Garavan, H. Ross, T. J., Li, S.-J., and Stein, E. A. (2000). A parametric manipulation of central executive functioning. *Cerebr. Cortex* **10**(6). 585–592.

Hazeltine, E., Poldrack, R., and Gabrieli, J. D. E. (2000). Neural activation during response competition. *J. Cogn. Neurosci.* **12**(6, Suppl. 2), 118–129.

Jonides, J., Badre, D., Curtis, C., Thompson-Schill, S., Smith, E. E. (2002). Mechanisms of conflict resolution in prefrontal cortex. *In* "The Frontal Lobes" (D. T. Stuss and R. T. Knight, eds.). Oxford Univ. Press, Oxford.

Jonides, J., Smith, E. E., Marschuetz, C., Koeppe, R. A., and Reuter-Lorenz, P. A. (1998). Inhibition in verbal working memory revealed by brain activation. *Proc. Natl. Acad. Sci. USA* **95**, 8410–8413.

Kornblum, S., Hasbroucq, T., and Osman, A. (1990). Dimensional overlap: Cognitive basis for stimulus-response compatibility-a model and taxonomy. *Psychol. Rev.* **97**(2), 253–270.

Pardo, J. V., Pardo, J., Janer, W., and Raichle, M. E. (1990). *Proc. Natl. Acad. Sci. USA* **95**, 876–882.

Paulesu, E., Frith, C. D., and Frackourak, R. S. J. (1993). The neural correlates of the verbal component of working memory. *Nature* **362**, 342–344.

Pollman, S., Dove, A. Y., von Cramon, D., and Wiggins, C. J. (2000). Event-related fMRI: Comparison of conditions with varying BOLD overlap. *Hum. Brain Mapp.* **9**(1), 26–37.

Prabhakaran, V., Smith, J. A. L., Desmond, J. E., Glover, G. H., and Gabrieli, J. D. E. (1997). Neural substrates of fluid reasoning: An fMRI study of neocortical activation during performance of the Raven's progressive matrices test. *Cogn. Psychol.* **33**, 43–63.

Reuter-Lorenz, P. A., Jonides, J., Smith, E. E., Hartley, A., Miller, A., Marshuetz, C., and Koeppe, R. A. (2000). Age differences in the frontal lateralization of verbala and spatial working memory revealed by PET. *J. Cogn. Neurosci.* **12**, 174–187.

Rickard, T. C., Romero, S. G., Basso, G., Wharton, C., Flitman, S., and Grafman, J. (2000). The calculating brain: A fMRI study. *Neuropsychologia* **38**, 325–335.

Shallice, T. (1988) "From Neuropsych. to Mental Structure." Cambridge Univ. Press, Cambridge.

Smith, E. E., Geva, A., Jonides, J., Miller, A., Reuter-Lorenz, P., and Koeppe, R. A. (2001). The neural basis of task switching in working memory: Effects of performance and aging. *Proc. Natl. Acad. Sci.* **98**, 2095–2100.

Smith, E. E. and Jonides, J. (1999). Storage and executive processes in the frontal lobes. *Science* **283**, 1657–1661.

Talairach, J., and Tourneaux, P. (1988). "Co-planar Stereotaxic Atlas of the Human Brain." Thieme, Stuttgart.

Taylor, S. F., Kornblum, S., Lauber, E. J., Minoshima, S., and Koeppe, R. A. (1997). Isolation of specific interference processing in the Stroop task: PET activation studies. *Neuroimage* **6**, 81–92.

Thompson-Schill, S. L., Jonides, J., Marshuetz, C., Smith, E. E., D'Esposito, M., Kan, I. P., Knight, R. T., and Swick, D. (1999). Impairments in the executive control of working memory following prefrontal damage: A case study. *Abstr. Soc. Neurosci.* **25**, 1143.

Vendrell, P., Junque, C., Pujol, J., Jurado, M. A., Molet, J., and Grafman, J. (1995). The role of the prefrontal regions in the Stroop task. *Neuropsychologia* **33**, 341–352.

Suggested Readings

Dahaene, S. (2000). Cerebral bases of number processing and calculation. *In* "New Cognitive Neurosciences" (M. S. Gazzaniga, ed.), 2nd Ed., pp. 987–998. MIT Press, Cambridge, MA.

D'Esposito, M., Zarahn, E., and Aguirre, G. K. (1999). Event related functional fMRI: Implications for cognitive psychology. *Psychol. Bull.* **125**, 155–164.

Duncan, J. (2000). Attention, intelligence and the frontal lobes. *In* "The New Cognitive Neurosciences" (M. S. Gazzaniga, ed.), 2nd Ed., pp. 721–734. MIT Press, Cambridge, MA.

Fuster, J. M. (1995). "Memory in the Cerebral Cortex." MIT Press, Cambridge, MA.

Fuster, J. M. (1997). "The Prefrontal Cortex: Anatomy, Physiology, and Neuropsychology of the Frontal Lobes." Raven Press, New York.

Gazzaniga, M. S., Ivry, R., and Mangun, G. R. (1998). "Cognitive Neuroscience: The Biology of the Mind." Norton, New York.

Goldman-Rakic, P. S. (1987). Circuitry of primate prefrontal cortex and regulation of behavior in representational memory. *In* "Handbook of Physiology," Section 1, 5, pp. 373–417.

Pollman, S. (2001). Switching between dimension, locations, and responses: The role of the left frontopolar cortex. *Neuroimage* **14**, 5118–5124.

Shallice, T. (1988). "From Neuropsychology to Mental Structure." Cambridge Univ. Press, Cambridge.

Smith, E. E., and J. Jonides (1999). Storage and executive processes in the frontal lobes. *Science* **283**, 1657–1661.

Edward E. Smith and John Jonides

Permissions

Neuroscience is a collective endeavor that has blossomed through the activities and pursuits of researchers and scholars from a wide variety of backgrounds and interests. Their findings are reported in a great number of general and specialized scientific journals and books, published by a large number of organizations and publishers. These all play a role in developing and distributing advances in the field.

The Editors, Contributors, Elsevier Science, and Academic Press thank all the providers of original sources of text and figures that have been used throughout to enhance and illustrate this book. We have tried to identify the original source of material and the correct reference to that material in order for the volume to be as scholarly a work as possible.

The publishers who have provided permissions include: American Association for the Advancement of Science, American Medical Association, American Physiological Society, American Societies for Experimental Biology, American Society of Biochemistry & Molecular Biology, American Society for Pharmacology and Experimental Therapeutics, American Scientist, Annual Reviews, Biophysical Society, Blackwell Science Publishers, Cambridge University Press, Cell Press, The Company of Biologists, CRC Press, Elsevier Science Publishers, Gale Group, Harvard University Press, Humana Press, Indiana University Press, John Wiley & Sons, Kluwer Academic/Plenum Publishers, Lippincott Williams & Wilkins, MacMillan Publishers Ltd., McGraw–Hill, the MIT Press, the National Academy of Sciences, the New York Academy of Sciences, Nature, Oxford University Press, The Physiological Society, Rapid Science Publishers, Rockefeller University Press, the Royal Society, S. Karger, Scandinavian Physiological Society, Society for Industrial and Applied Mathematics, Sinauer Associates, Society for Neuroscience, Springer-Verlag, Stanford University Press, The New York Times, The Nobel Foundation, University of Chicago Press, W. B. Saunders, W. H. Freeman, and Yale University Press.

We thank them for their cooperation and contribution.

Contributors

Amy F. T. Arnsten   Yale University School of Medicine, New Haven, CT

Frances M. Ashcroft   University Laboratory of Physiology, Oxford, United Kingdom

G. S. Aston-Jones   University of Pennsylvania, Philadelphia, PA

Jocelyne Bachevalier   University of Texas School of Medicine, Houston, TX

James F. Baker   Northwestern University Medical School, Chicago, IL

Robert W. Baloh   UCLA Medical Center, Los Angeles, CA

Michael J. Baum   Boston University, Boston, MA

Curtis C. Bell   Oregon Health Sciences University, Beaverton, OR

Darwin Berg   University of California, San Diego, La Jolla, CA

Floyd E. Bloom   The Scripps Research Institute, La Jolla, CA

Scott Brady   University of Texas Southwestern Medical Center, Dallas, TX

Marianne Bronner-Fraser   Caltech, Pasadena, CA

Peter Brophy   University of Edinburgh, Edinburgh, Scotland

M. Christian Brown   Massachusetts Eye and Ear Infirmary, Boston, MA

Steven J. Burden   NYU Medical Center, New York, NY

John H. Byrne   University of Texas Health Science Center, Houston, TX

Judy L. Cameron   University of Pittsburgh School of Medicine, Pittsburgh, PA

David N. Caplan   Massachusetts General Hospital, Boston, MA

J. Patrick Card   University of Pittsburgh, Pittsburgh, PA

Dennis S. Charney   National Institute of Mental Health, Bethesda, MD

Luz Claudio   Mount Sinai School of Medicine, New York, NY

Carol L. Colby   University of Pittsburgh, Pittsburgh, PA

David R. Colman   Mount Sinai School of Medicine, New York, NY

Carl W. Cotman   University of California, Irvine, CA

Robert B. Darnell   Rockefeller University, New York, NY

Valina L. Dawson   Johns Hopkins University School of Medicine, Baltimore, MD

Ted M. Dawson   Johns Hopkins University School of Medicine, Baltimore, MD

R. Desimone   National Institute of Mental Health, Bethesda, MD

Ariel Y. Deutch   Vanderbilt University Medical Center, Nashville, TN

Jean de Vellis   University of California School of Medicine, Los Angeles, CA

Wayne C. Drevets   University of Pittsburgh Medical Center, Pittsburgh, PA

J. Driver   University College London, London, United Kingdom

Guinevere F. Eden   Georgetown University, Washington, DC

Howard B. Eichenbaum   Boston University, Boston, MA

Barry J. Everitt   University of Cambridge, Cambridge, United Kingdom

Jack L. Feldman UCLA Medical Center, Los Angeles, CA

Robert S. Fisher Stanford University School of Medicine, Stanford, CA

Mary Kay Floeter National Institute of Neurological Disorders and Stroke, Bethesda, MD

Alfred G. Gilman University of Texas Southwestern Medical Center, Dallas, TX

Paul W. Glimcher New York University, New York, NY

Andrea C. Gore Mount Sinai School of Medicine, New York, NY

Jacqueline P. Gottlieb Columbia University, New York, NY

James L. Gould Princton University, Princeton, NJ

Paul Greengard Rockefeller University, New York, NY

Sten Grillner Karolinska Institute, Stockholm, Sweden

William A. Harris University of Cambridge, Cambridge, United Kingdom

Volker Hartenstein University of California, Los Angeles, CA

Mary Beth Hatten The Rockefeller University, New York, NY

Stewart H. Hendry Johns Hopkins University, Baltimore, MD

Karl Herrup Case Western Reserve School of Medicine, Cleveland, OH

J. Allan Hobson Harvard Medical School, Boston, MA

Patrick R. Hof Mount Sinai School of Medicine, New York, NY

Sandra L. Hofmann University of Texas Southwestern Medical Center, Dallas, TX

James C. Houk Northwestern University Medical School, Chicago, IL

Steven S. Hsiao Johns Hopkins University, Baltimore, MD

James E. Johnson Bowman Gray School of Medicine, Winston-Salem, NC

John Jonides University of Michigan, Ann Arbor, MI

Jon H. Kaas Vanderbilt University, Nashville, TN

Michael G. Kaplitt New York Hospital–Cornell University Medical College, New York, NY

Sabine Kastner Department of Psychology, Princeton University, Princeton, NJ

Seymour Kaufman National Institutes of Health, Bethesda, MD

Sue C Kinnamon Colorado State University, Ft. Collins, CO

Chris Kintner The Salk Institute for Biological Studies, San Diego, CA

Eric I. Knudsen Stanford University, Stanford, CA

George F. Koob The Scripps Research Institute, La Jolla, CA

Gabrielle G. Leblanc National Institute of Neurological Disorders and Stroke, Bethesda, MD

Ronald M. Lechan New England Medical Center Hospital, Boston, MA

Graham V. Lees Corpus Alienum, San Diego, CA

Jeffrey W. Lichtman Washington University School of Medicine, St. Louis, MO

Arthur D. Loewy Washington University School of Medicine, St. Louis, MO

John C. Longhurst University of California, Irvine, Orange, CA

S. J. Luck University of Iowa, Iowa City, IA

Andrew Lumsden UMDS, Guy's Hospital, London, United Kingdom

Peter R. MacLeish Morehouse School of Medicine, Atlanta, GA

Pierre J. Magistretti University of Lausanne, Lausanne, Switzerland

J. John Mann New York State Psychiatric Institute, New York, NY

David A. McCormick Yale University School of Medicine, New Haven, CT

Donald R. McCrimmon Northwestern University Medical School, Chicago, IL

Robert W. Meech School of Medical Science, Bristol, United Kingdom

Earl K. Miller Massachusetts Institute of Technology, Cambridge, MA

Jonathan W. Mink University of Rochester School of Medicine and Dentistry, Rochester, NY

Aage R. Møller The University of Texas, Dallas, TX

Robert Y. Moore University of Pittsburgh School of Medicine, Pittsburgh, PA

Enrico Mugnaini Northwestern University Medical School, Chicago, IL

Alexander Neumeister National Institute of Mental Health, Bethesda, MD

Dennis D. M. O'Leary The Salk Institute, La Jolla, CA

Carl R. Olson Carnegie Mellon University, Pittsburgh, PA

Ronald W. Oppenheim Wake Forest University School of Medicine, Winston-Salem, NC

Edward F. Pace-Schott Harvard Medical School, Boston, MA

Luiz Pessoa National Institute of Mental Health, Bethesda, MD

M. I. Posner University of Oregon, Eugene, OR

Terry L. Powley Purdue University, West Lafayette, IN

Todd M. Preuss University of Louisiana at Lafayette, New Iberia, LA

Wilfrid Rall Roseland, VA

Jonathan Raper University of Pennsylvania, Philadelphia, PA

Peter R. Rapp University of Cambridge, Cambridge, United Kingdom

R. Clay Reid Harvard Medical School, Boston, MA

John H. Reynolds The Salk Institute, La Jolla, CA

Trevor W. Robbins University of Cambridge, Cambridge, United Kingdom

James L. Roberts University of Texas Health Science Center, San Antonio, TX

Hillary R. Rodman Emory University, Atlanta, GA

Christopher A. Ross Johns Hopkins University School of Medicine, Baltimore, MD

Robert H. Roth Yale University School of Medicine, New Haven, CT

Joseph Santos-Sacchi Yale University School of Medicine, New Haven, CT

Maslah Saul Stanford University School of Medicine, Stanford, CA

Marc H. Schieber University of Rochester School of Medicine and Dentistry, Rochester, NY

Jeremy D. Schmahmann Massachusetts General Hospital, Boston, MA

Howard Schulman Stanford University Medical Center, Stanford, CA

Thomas L. Schwarz Children's Hospital, Boston, MA

Gordon M. Shepherd Yale University School of Medicine, New Haven, CT

David V. Smith University of Tennessee Health Science Center, Memphis, TN

Edward E. Smith University of Michigan, Ann Arbor, MI

Solomon H. Snyder Johns Hopkins University School of Medicine, Baltimore, MD

Sara A. Solla Northwestern University Medical School, Chicago, IL

Stephen R. Sprang University of Texas Southwestern Medical Center, Dallas, TX

Edward M. Stricker University of Pittsburgh, Pittsburgh, PA

Ueli Suter Switzerland Federal Institute of Technology, Zurich, Switzerland

Larry W. Swanson University of Southern California, Los Angeles, CA

Neal R. Swendlow University of California, San Diego, School of Medicine, San Diego, CA

Marc Tessier-Lavigne Stanford University, Stanford, CA

Roberto Toni University of Bologna School of Medicine, Bologna, Italy

Bruce D. Trapp Cleveland Clinic Foundation, Cleveland, OH

Leslie G. Ungerlieder National Institute of Mental Health, Bethesda, MD

Joseph G. Verbalis Georgetown University, Washington, DC

Meena Vythilingam National Institute of Mental Health, Bethesda, MD

Jonathan D. Wallis Massachusetts Institute of Technology, Cambridge, MA

M. Neal Waxham University of Texas Health Science Center, Houston, TX

Clayton A. Wiley University of Pittsburgh, Pittsburgh, PA

Phyllis M. Wise University of Kentucky College of Medicine, Lexington, KY

Rachel O. L. Wong Washington University School of Medicine, St. Louis, MO

Stephen C. Woods University on Cincinnati Medical Center, Cincinnati, OH

Susan Wray National Institutes of Health, Bethesda, MD

Index